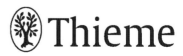

Total Otolaryngology—Head and Neck Surgery

Anthony P. Sclafani, MD, FACS
Director of Facial Plastic Surgery
Department of Otolaryngology-Head and Neck Surgery
New York Eye and Ear Infirmary of Mt. Sinai
Professor of Otolaryngology
Icahn School of Medicine at Mount Sinai
New York, New York

Robin A. Dyleski, MD
Assistant Professor of Otolaryngology
Chief of Pediatric Otolaryngology
Department of Otolaryngology–Head and Neck Surgery
Loma Linda University Medical Center
Loma Linda, California

Michael J. Pitman, MD
Associate Professor
Department of Otolaryngology–Head and Neck Surgery
New York Eye and Ear Infirmary of Mount Sinai
New York, New York

Stimson P. Schantz, MD, FACS
Professor of Otolarygology
Icahn School of Medicine of Mount Sinai
Division of Head and Neck Surgery
New York Eye and Ear Infirmary
New York, New York

Christopher J. Linstrom, MD CM, FRCSC, FRSCE
Professor of Otolaryngology
Surgeon Director of Otology and Neurotology
Department of Otolaryngology–Head and Neck Surgery
Icahn School of Medicine at Mount Sinai
New York, New York

Steven David Schaefer, MD, FACS
Director of Sinus Surgery and Academic Development
New York Head and Neck Institute
North Shore LIJ Health System
Former Professor and Chair
Department of Otolaryngology
New York Eye and Ear Infirmary of Mount Sinai
New York, New York

Edward J. Shin, MD, FACS
Chair
Department of Otolaryngology
New York Eye and Ear Infirmary of Mount Sinai
Professor of Otolaryngology
Department of Otolaryngology–Head and Neck Surgery
Icahn School of Medicine at Mount Sinai
New York, New York

Jill K. Gregory, MFA, CMI and Courtney A. McKenna, MA, CMI
Medical Illustrators

667 illustrations

Thieme
New York • Stuttgart • Delhi • Rio

Executive Editor: Timothy Hiscock
Managing Editor: J. Owen Zurhellen IV
Assistant Managing Editor: Heather Allen
Production Editor: Mason Brown
International Production Director: Andreas Schabert
Senior Vice President, Editorial and E-Product
    Development: Cornelia Schulze
International Marketing Director: Fiona Henderson
International Sales Director: Louisa Turrell
Director of Sales, North America: Mike Roseman
Senior Vice President and Chief Operating Officer: Sarah Vanderbilt
President: Brian D. Scanlan
Medical Illustrators and Cover Illustration: Jill K. Gregory, MFA, CMI
    and Courtney A. McKenna, MA, CMI; printed with permission
    from © Mount Sinai Health System

Library of Congress Cataloging-in-Publication Data

Total otolaryngology-head and neck surgery / [edited by] Anthony
P. Sclafani.
    p. ; cm.
  Includes bibliographical references.
Summary: "Otolaryngology-Head and Neck Surgery has developed
as a specialty in recognition of the highly focused attention necessary
to fully comprehend and master the intricate anatomic and physiologic relationships of the structures located between the thoracic
inlet and the foramen magnum. Our specialty originally developed
out of a need to manage the intricacies of this area of the body, but as
the depth of our knowledge grew subspecialties within the discipline
branched off, and often it may seem that we are a collection of
otologists, neurotologists, head and neck oncologists, laryngologists,
pediatric otolaryngologists, rhinologists, facial plastic surgeons, and
general otolaryngologists. This text should serve as a concise yet
practical review and reference textbook for anyone interested in the
full scope of otolaryngology-head and neck surgery"–Provided by
publisher.
  ISBN 978-1-60406-645-6 (hardback : alk. paper)
  I. Sclafani, Anthony P., editor.
  [DNLM: 1. Otorhinolaryngologic Diseases–surgery. 2. Otorhinolaryngologic Surgical Procedures–methods. WV 168]
  RF46.5
  617.5'1–dc23
                            2014017980

© 2015 Thieme Medical Publishers, Inc.
Thieme Publishers New York
333 Seventh Avenue, New York, NY 10001 USA
+1 800 782 3488, customerservice@thieme.com

Thieme Publishers Stuttgart
Rüdigerstrasse 14, 70469 Stuttgart, Germany
+49 [0]711 8931 421, customerservice@thieme.de

Thieme Publishers Delhi
A-12, Second Floor, Sector-2, Noida-201301
Uttar Pradesh, India
+91 120 45 566 00, customerservice@thieme.in

Thieme Publishers Rio, Thieme Publicações Ltda.
Argentina Building 16th floor, Ala A, 228 Praia do Botafogo
Rio de Janeiro 22250-040 Brazil
+55 21 3736-3631

Cover design: Thieme Publishing Group
Typesetting by Thomson Digital, India

Printed in China though Asia Pacific Offset   5 4 3 2 1

978-1-60406-645-6

Also available as an e-book:
978-1-60406-646-3

Of all the blessings I have received, the most important is the encouragement and love of the smartest person I know—my dear Peg—and three very impressive young men, Anthony, James, and Matthew. Without their love and support, I could never have completed this book, and it is to them that I dedicate this work.

-APS

Contents

Foreword

As a specialty, otolaryngology–head and neck surgery covers a diverse set of clinical problems, most of which can be managed by a general otolaryngologist. It seems that most practicing otolaryngologists prefer certain aspects of our field and frequently concentrate their practice in one or several of these areas. Some of the more complicated problems within otolaryngology–head and neck surgery require additional subspecialization and training, advanced equipment, and/or specialized facilities to obtain the best outcomes. For medical students, and even colleagues in other fields, it is frequently difficult to appreciate the breadth of the specialty. For residents and fellows, it can be intimidating to consider the mastery of otolaryngology-head and neck surgery.

The editors of *Total Otolaryngology–Head and Neck Surgery* have successfully created a single volume covering all aspects of our specialty, in an accessible format that is well organized and beautifully illustrated. The book is organized into sections which include Emergency Management, General Otolaryngology, Head and Neck Surgery, Facial Plastic Surgery, Pediatric Otolaryngology, Laryngology, Rhinology and Otology. The chapters are concise and efficient, containing the most relevant information. Illustrations within the text are easy to understand, while clinical pictures clearly demonstrate the underlying clinical condition. Many chapters also contain algorithms and tables to help provide quick overview of the accompanying text. Recommended reading lists are also included, which refer the reader to the most important references on a specific topic.

Total Otolaryngology–Head and Neck Surgery provides a framework for understanding the extent and depth of our field. This format provides important context for those trying to master the field and serves as a great reference, especially for practitioners who are focused on other areas of the specialty who need an update about advances in other aspects of the specialty. Congratulations to Dr. Sclafani and his coeditors on creating an up-to-date, well-illustrated, and comprehensive resource covering otolaryngology–head and neck surgery, which will aid in the training of future residents and fellows and serve as an excellent reference for practicing otolaryngologists.

Ronald B. Kuppersmith, MD, FACS
Texas ENT and Allergy
College Station, Texas

Preface

Otolaryngology-head and neck surgery has developed as a specialty in recognition of the highly focused attention necessary to fully comprehend and master the intricate anatomic and physiologic relationships of the structures located between the thoracic inlet and the foramen magnum. Our specialty originally developed out of a need to manage the intricacies of this area of the body, but as the depth of our knowledge grew, subspecialties within the discipline branched off. Often, it may seem that we are a collection of otologists, neurotologists, head and neck oncologists, laryngologists, pediatric otolaryngologists, rhinologists, facial plastic surgeons, and general otolaryngologists. There are times when, as a group, we seem to speak different dialects of a common tongue.

The true otolaryngologist–head and neck surgeon, however, is well-versed in the broad spectrum of the field and, if not an expert, can certainly understand the issues managed by other subspecialists. The facial plastic surgeon performing microtia repair should understand the issues faced by the otologist in providing aural rehabilitation to the patient; the pediatric otolaryngologist appreciates the implications of airway surgery on the development of voice and speech; the rhinologist may encounter malignant disease involving the anterior skull base and may coordinate treatment with the head and neck oncologic surgeon. Probably, most commonly and most important, the practicing general otolaryngologist is faced with the dilemma of deciding which patients and disease can be safely and appropriately handled in a general hospital and which should be referred to trusted subspecialty colleagues.

The need to pursue continuing education and to maintain board certification in the field is evident. This text is designed to provide full and comprehensive coverage of the breadth of our field in a concise, yet thorough way. The authors who have contributed to this book have distilled their topics into the most pure and concentrated forms, so that the reader is presented with practical information on these topics as concisely as possible. Illustrations have been limited to only those which illustrate key topics of the each chapter. Chapter highlights are provided in "Roundsmanship." Selected readings have been provided for more in-depth detail for the reader interested in a specific topic. This text should serve as a concise yet practical review and reference textbook for anyone interested in the full scope of otolaryngology–head and neck surgery.

–APS

Acknowledgements

Heartfelt thanks are offered to all of the colleagues who have contributed chapters to this textbook; their generosity in sharing their expertise and knowledge to create a comprehensive textbook is truly humbling. The outstanding illustrations were drawn by Jill Gregory and Courtney McKenna, who seemed to understand intuitively the important concepts to be conveyed in each illustration. Additional thanks is offered to the editorial staff of Thieme Publishers, especially Timothy Hiscock and J. Owen Zurhellen, for their assistance in the writing of this book.

I have been fortunate to have had many special mentors (including several of the authors in this book) in my personal journey through otolaryngology, including Hyun Cho, MD, Peter Schindler, MD, Richard Bellucci, MD, Robert Eberle, MD, and John Conley, MD, who in their own individual ways nurtured my development in otolaryngology.

Very special thanks and recognition are offered to Claude Douge, MD, and the late Paul Chodosh, MD, for providing me with true role models of the "total otolaryngologist." These men showed me that the practice of otolaryngology requires not only a complete fund of knowledge, but an inquisitive nature, a willingness to think "outside the box" and to challenge thoughtfully the status quo, and the dedication to serve as the patient's strongest advocate. These physicians, above all, taught me to always keep the patient foremost.

–APS

Contributors

Jihad Achkar, MD
Laryngologist
Clemenceau Medical Center in affiliation with
  Johns Hopkins International
Beirut, Lebanon

Lee M. Akst, MD
Assistant Professor, Otolaryngology-Head and Neck Surgery
Director, Division of Laryngology
Johns Hopkins University School of Medicine
Baltimore, Maryland

George Alexiades, MD, FACS
Associate Professor of Clinical Otolaryngology
Program Director
Department of Otolaryngology-Head and Neck Surgery
Icahn School of Medicine at Mount Sinai
New York, New York

Homere Al Moutran, MD
Department of Otolaryngology–Head and Neck Surgery
New York Head and Neck Institute
Staten Island University Hospital
Northshore LIJ Health System
Staten Island, New York

Sumeet M. Anand, MD
Otolaryngology–Head and Neck Surgery
Head and Neck Surgical Oncology and Reconstructive
  Surgery
Clinical Lecturer
University of Toronto
Toronto, Canada

James Azzi, MD
Department of Otolaryngology
New York Eye and Ear Infirmary of Mount Sinai
New York, New York

Jean-Paul Azzi, MD
Director
The Palm Beach Center for Facial Plastic and Laser Surgery
Jupiter, Florida

Seilesh C. Babu, MD
Physician
Michigan Ear Institute
Farmington Hills, Michigan

Rebecca L. Bagdonas, MD
Attending Physician
Department of Anesthesiology
New York Eye and Ear Infirmary of Mount Sinai
New York, New York

Joshua R. Bedwell, MD, FAAP
Division of Pediatric Otolaryngology
Children's National Medical Center
Assistant Professor of Surgery and Pediatrics
George Washington University School of Medicine
Washington, DC

Craig E. Berzofsky, MD
Assistant Professor
Department of Otolaryngology
New York Medical College
Valhalla, New York

Neel Bhatt, MD
Department of Otolaryngology-Head and Neck Surgery
Washington University
St. Louis, Missouri

Morgan R. Bliss, MD
Division of Otolaryngology–Head and Neck Surgery
University of Utah Hospital
Salt Lake City, Utah

Jonathan M. Bock, MD, FACS
Assistant Professor
Division of Laryngology and Professional Voice
Department of Otolaryngology and Communication Sciences
Medical College of Wisconsin
Milwaukee, Wisconsin

Helen Yoo Bowne, MD
Clinical Adjunct Assistant
Icahn School of Medicine at Mount Sinai
New York, New York
Assistant Professor
Otolaryngology–Head and Neck Surgery
Drexel University College of Medicine
Philadelphia, Pennsylvania

Thomas L. Carroll, MD
Assistant Professor
Department of Otolaryngology
Harvard Medical School
Brigham and Women's Hospital
Director
Brigham and Women's Hospital Voice Center
Boston, Massachusetts

John A. Carucci, MD, PhD
Chief, Mohs Micrographic and Dermatologic Surgery
Section of Dermatologic Surgery
Ronald O. Perelman Department of Dermatology
New York University Langone Medical Center
New York, New York

Edwin K. Chan, MD
Attending Physician
Department of Otolaryngology and Head and Neck Surgery
New York Eye and Ear Infirmary of Mount Sinai
New York, New York

Pat Colley, MD
Department of Otolaryngology
New York Eye and Ear Infirmary of Mount Sinai
New York, New York

Jennifer S. Collins, MD
Medical Director
Gramercy Allergy and Asthma
Attending Physician
 Department of Allergy and Immunology
Mount Sinai-Beth Israel Medical Center
New York, New York

Amy L. Cooper, MS, CCC-SLP
Director of Speech Pathology
New York Eye and Ear Infirmary of Mount Sinai
New York, New York

Maura K. Cosetti, MD
Assistant Professor of Otolaryngology and Neurosurgery
Department of Otolaryngology-Head and Neck Surgery
Louisiana State University School of Medicine
Shreveport, Louisiana

David J. Crockett, MD
Department of Pediatric Otolaryngology–Head and Neck
  Surgery
Arizona Otolaryngology Consultants
Phoenix Children's Hospital
Phoenix, Arizona

Seth H. Dailey, MD
Chief of Laryngology
Associate Professor
Division of Otolaryngology
Department of Surgery
University of Wisconsin Hospital and Clinics
Madison, Wisconsin

E. Ashlie Darr, MD
Clinical Instructor
Department of Otology and Laryngology
Harvard Medical School
Boston, Massachusetts

Clare Dean, MD
Department of Otolaryngology
New York Eye and Ear Infirmary of Mount Sinai
New York, New York

Robert Deeb, MD
Senior Staff Surgeon
Department of Otolaryngology–Head and Neck Surgery
Henry Ford Health System
Detroit, Michigan

Robin A. Dyleski, MD
Assistant Professor of Otolaryngology
Chief of Pediatric Otolaryngology
Department of Otolaryngology–Head and Neck Surgery
Loma Linda University Medical Center
Loma Linda, California

Michele M. Gandolfi, MD
Department of Otolaryngology
New York Eye and Ear Infirmary of Mount Sinai
New York, New York

Christopher R. Gilbert, DO, MS
Assistant Professor of Medicine
Bronchoscopy and Interventional Pulmonology
Department of Medicine, Division of Pulmonary, Allergy,
  and Critical Care
Penn State College of Medicine–Milton S. Hershey Medical
  Center
Hershey, Pennsylvania

Stacey L. Halum, MD, FACS
Research Professor
Department of Speech and Hearing Sciences
Purdue University
West Lafayette, Indiana

Louis B. Harrison, MD, FASTRO
Chair
Department of Radiation Oncology
Senior Member
H. Lee Moffitt Cancer Center and Research Institute
Tampa, Florida

Tina Qingxin He, MD
Attending Physician
Department of Otolaryngology
New York Eye and Ear Infirmary of Mount Sinai
New York, New York

David Henry Hiltzik, MD
Director
Department of Otolaryngology–Head and Neck Surgery
Staten Island University Hospital
New York Head and Neck Institute
Northshore LIJ Healthcare System
Staten Island, New York

Ajay Hira, MD, MBA
Radiologist
Lake Medical Imaging and Vascular Institute
Leesburg Regional Medical Center
Leesburg, Florida

Ronald A. Hoffman, MD, MHCM
Director
Ear Institute
New York Eye and Ear Infirmary of Mount Sinai
Professor of Otolaryngology–Head and Neck Surgery
Icahn School of Medicine of Mount Sinai
New York, New York

Robert Hong, MD, PhD
Attending Physician
Michigan Ear Institute
Farmington Hills, Michigan
Assistant Professor
Department of Otolaryngology
Wayne State University
Detroit, Michigan

Amanda Hu, MD, FRCSC
Assistant Professor
Department of Otolaryngology–Head and Neck Surgery
Drexel University College of Medicine
Philadelphia, Pennsylvania

Kenneth S. Hu, MD
Associate Professor of Radiation Oncology
Department of Radiation Oncology
Icahn School of Medicine at Mount Sinai
New York, New York

Bryan D. Hujsak, PT, DPT, NCS
Director, Vestibular Rehabilitation
The Ear Institute, Balance, and Hearing Center
The New York Eye and Ear Infirmary of Mount Sinai
New York, New York

Codrin E. Iacob, MD, FCAP
Associate Clinical Professor of Pathology and Ophthalmology
Icahn School of Medicine at Mount Sinai
Assistant Director of Pathology and Laboratory Medicine
New York Eye and Ear Infirmary of Mount Sinai
New York, New York

Tova Fischer Isseroff, MD
Department of Otolaryngology
New York Eye and Ear Infirmary of Mount Sinai
New York, New York

Chandra M. Ivey, MD, FACS
Assistant Professor
Department of Otolaryngology and Director,
Columbia University Medical Center
New York, New York

Adam S. Jacobson, MD
Associate Professor
New York University
Langone Medical Center
New York, New York

Nisha Jayani, MD
Los Angeles, California

Dhruve S. Jeevan, MD
Clinical Instructor
Department of Neurosurgery,
New York Medical College
Valhalla, New York

Ameet R. Kamat, MD
Rhinology and Endoscopic Skull Base Surgery
ENT Faculty Practice, LLP
Westchester, New York

Ana H. Kim, MD
Associate Professor
Department of Otolaryngology–Head and Neck Surgery
Icahn School of Medicine at Mount Sinai
New York, New York

Nancy King, MD
Department of Otolaryngology
New York Eye and Ear Infirmary of Mount Sinai
New York, New York

Matthew L. Kircher, MD
Assistant Professor
Department of Otolaryngology–Head and Neck Surgery
Loyola University Medical Center
Maywood, Illinois

Jamie A. Koufman, MD, FACS
Director, Voice Institute of New York
Professor of Clinical Otolaryngology
Adjunct Associate Surgeon
New York Eye and Ear Infirmary of Mount Sinai
New York, New York

Miguel Krishnan, DO
Assistant Professor of Otolaryngology and Pediatrics
Department of Otolaryngology–Head and Neck Surgery
Loma Linda University Medical Center
Loma Linda, California

Melda Kunduk, PhD, CCC-SLP
Associate Professor
Our Lady of the Lake Voice Center
Department of Communication Sciences and Disorders
Department of Otolaryngology–Head and Neck Surgery
Louisiana State University
Baton Rouge, Louisiana

John F. Kveton, MD, FACS
Clinical Professor
Department of Surgery/Otolaryngology and Neurosurgery
Yale University School of Medicine
New Haven, Connecticut

Jason G. Lai, MD
Anesthesiologist
Department of Anesthesiology
Danbury Hospital
Danbury, Connecticut

Laura Lei-Rivera, PT, DPT, GCS
Senior Physical Therapist
Center Coordinator of Clinical Education
Department of Vestibular Rehabilitation
The Ear Institute, Balance, and Hearing Center
New York Eye and Ear Infirmary of Mount Sinai
New York, New York

Jesse M. Lewin, MD
Procedural Dermatology
Ronald O. Perelman Department of Dermatology
New York University Langone Medical Center
New York, New York

Christopher J. Linstrom, MD CM, FRCSC, FRSCE
Professor of Otolaryngology
Surgeon Director of Otology and Neurotology
Department of Otolaryngology–Head and Neck Surgery
Icahn School of Medicine at Mount Sinai
New York, New York

Catherine Rees Lintzenich, MD
Physician
Riverside ENT Physicians and Surgeons
Williamsburg, Virginia

Andrew M. Malinow, MD
Professor of Anesthesiology Obstetrics/Gynecology and
   Reproductive Sciences
Vice-Chair for Faculty Affairs
Department of Anesthesiology
University of Maryland School of Medicine
Baltimore, Maryland

Kristin K. Marcum, MD
Director
Allergy Clinic
Center for ENT
Houston, Texas

Grigorly Mashkevich, MD
Assistant Professor
Department of Otolaryngology–Head and Neck Surgery
New York Eye and Ear Infirmary of Mount Sinai
Icahn School of Medicine at Mount Sinai
New York, New York

Ted Mau, MD, PhD
Associate Professor
Department of Otolaryngology–Head and Neck Surgery
Director, Clinical Center for Voice Care
Department of Otolaryngology–Head and Neck Surgery
University of Texas Southwestern Medical Center
Dallas, Texas

Andrew J. McWhorter, MD
Associate Professor
Director
Our Lady of the Lake Voice Center
Department of Otolaryngology–Head and Neck Surgery
Louisiana State University Health Sciences Center
New Orleans, Louisiana

Saral Mehra, MD, MBA
Assistant Professor
Department of Surgery (Otolaryngology)
Yale University School of Medicine
New Haven, Connecticutt

Hasit Mehta, MD
Assistant Professor
Department of Radiology–Neuroradiology
New York Medical College Westchester Medical Center
Valhalla, New York

Vikas Mehta, MD, FACS
Assistant Professor
Department of Otolaryngology–Head and Neck Surgery
LSU Health Sciences Center
Louisiana State University
Shreveport, Louisiana

Jeremy D. Meier, MD
Assistant Professor
Division of Otolaryngology–Head and Neck Surgery
University of Utah School of Medicine
Salt Lake City, Utah

Tanya K. Meyer, MD
Associate Professor
Department of Otolaryngology–Head and Neck Surgery
University of Washington
Seattle, Washington

Maurice Miller, PhD
Professor Emeritus
Department of Communication Sciences and Disorders–
  Audiology
New York University Steinhardt School of Culture, Education,
  and Human Development
New York, New York

Augustine L. Moscatello, MD, FACS
Professor of Clinical Otolaryngology
Vice Chair
Department of Otolaryngology–Head and Neck Surgery
New York Medical College
Valhalla, New York

Moustafa Mourad, MD
New York Eye and Ear Infirmary
New York, New York

Harlan R. Muntz, MD
Professor
Department of Surgery
Adjunct Professor
Department of Pediatrics
Otolaryngology–Head and Neck Surgery
University of Utah Health Care
Medical Director of Surgical Services
Primary Children's Hospital
Salt Lake City, Utah

Raj Murali, MD, FACS, FAANS, FRCSEd, FRCS (Eng), FRCS (C)
Professor and Chairman
Department of Neurosurgery
New York Medical College
Valhalla, New York

Jayson A. Neil, MD
Clinical Instructor
Department of Neurosurgery
New York Medical College
Valhalla, New York

Alexander Ovchinsky, MD
Department of Otolaryngology–Head and Neck Surgery
New York Eye and Ear Infirmary of Mount Sinai
Assistant Professor
Icahn School of Medicine at Mount Sinai
New York, New York

Neha A. Patel, MD
Department of Otolaryngology–Head and Neck Surgery
New York Eye and Ear Infirmary
New York, New York

James M. Pearson, MD, FACS
Private Practice
Facial Plastic and Reconstructive Surgery
Beverly Hills, California

Mark S. Persky, MD
Professor
Department of Otolaryngology–Head and Neck Surgery
New York University School of Medicine
New York, New York

Michael J. Pitman, MD
Associate Professor
Department of Otolaryngology–Head and Neck Surgery
New York Eye and Ear Infirmary of Mount Sinai
New York, New York

Ryan G. Porter, MD
Otology, Neurotology, and Skull Base Surgery
Carle Physician Group
Clinical Assistant Professor
University of Illinois College of Medicine at
  Urbana-Champaign
Urbana, Illinois

Mila Quinn, BS
Tufts University School of Medicine
Boston, Massachusetts

Miriam I. Redleaf, MD, FACS
Louis J. Mayer Professor of Otology and Neurotology
University of Illinois Hospital and Health Sciences Systems
Chicago, Illinois

William R. Reisacher, MD, FACS, FAAOA
Associate Professor
Department of Otolaryngology–Head and Neck Surgery
Weill Cornell Medical College
New York, New York

Rick M. Roark, PhD
Associate Professor of Otolaryngology
Department of Otolaryngology
New York Medical College
Valhalla, New York

Alan F. Rope, MD
Department of Medical Genetics
Northwest Kaiser Permanente
Portland, Oregon

Kenneth M. Rosenstein, MD
Physician
Becker Nose and Sinus Center, LLC
Sewell, New Jersey

Joseph J. Rousso, MD
Assistant Professor
Icahn School of Medicine at Mount Sinai
Division of Facial Plastic and Reconstructive Surgery
New York, New York

Boris Sagalovich, MD, FCCP, FAASM
Medical Director
Comprehensive Sleep Disorders Institute
Brooklyn, New York

Helen R. Salus, PhD, AuD
Graduate School University Center
City University of New York
New York, New York

Steven David Schaefer, MD, FACS
Director of Sinus Surgery and Academic Development
New York Head and Neck Institute
North Shore LIJ Health System
Former Professor and Chair
Department of Otolaryngology
New York Eye and Ear Infirmary of Mount Sinai
New York, New York

Stimson P. Schantz, MD, FACS
Professor of Otolarygology
Icahn School of Medicine of Mount Sinai
Division of Head and Neck Surgery
New York Eye and Ear Infirmary
New York, New York

Monica Dorin Schwarcz, MD
Assistant Professor
Division of Endocrinology and Metabolism
New York Medical College
Valhalla, New York

Anthony M. Sclafani
Center for Facial Plastic Surgery
Chappaqua, New York

Anthony P. Sclafani, MD, FACS
Director of Facial Plastic Surgery
Department of Otolaryngology–Head and Neck Surgery
New York Eye and Ear Infirmary of Mount Sinai
Professor of Otolaryngology
Icahn School of Medicine at Mount Sinai
New York, New York

James A. Sclafani
Center for Facial Plastic Surgery
Chappaqua, New York

Edward J. Shin, MD, FACS
Chair
Department of Otolaryngology
New York Eye and Ear Infirmary of Mount Sinai
New York, New York
Professor of Otolaryngology
Department of Otolaryngology–Head and Neck Surgery
Icahn School of Medicine at Mount Sinai
New York, New York

Shlomo Silman, PhD
Presidential Professor
Broecklundian Professor
Claire and Leonard Tow Professor
Audiology and Hearing Sciences
Brooklyn College, City University of New York
Professor
Doctor of Audiology Program and PhD Program
Speech-Language-Hearing Sciences
Graduate Center, City University of New York
New York, New York

Carol A. Silverman, PhD, MPH
Hearing Scientist and Epidemiologist
New York Eye Infirmary of Mount Sinai
New York, New York
Professor
Director of Audiology Program and PhD Program in Speech-
  Language-Hearing Sciences
Graduate Center, City University of New York
Professor
Speech-Language Pathology and Audiology
Hunter College, City University of New York
New York, New York
Adjunct Professor of Otolaryngology–Head and Neck Surgery
New York Medical College
Valhalla, New York

Phillip C. Song, MD
Associate Director of the Voice and Speech Laboratory
Massachusetts Eye and Ear Infirmary
Clinical Instructor in Laryngology and Otology
Harvard Medical School
Boston, Massachusetts

Thomas C. Spalla, MD
Assistant Professor
Cooper Medical School of Rowan University
Camden, New Jersey
Adjunct Professor
Drexel University College of Medicine
Department of Otolaryngology–Head and Neck Surgery
Philadelphia, Pennsylvania

Edward M. Stafford, MD
Washington Ear, Nose, and Throat
Washington, Pennsylvania

Katrina R. Stidham, MD
Associate Professor of Otolaryngology
Department of Otolaryngology–Head and Neck Surgery
New York Medical College
Valhalla, New York

Emily Z. Stucken, MD
Department of Otolaryngology–Head and Neck Surgery
New York Presbyterian Hospital
Columbia University and Weill–Cornell
New York, New York

Corbin D. Sullivan, MD, MA
Department of Otolaryngology and Communication Sciences
Medical College of Wisconsin
Milwaukee, Wisconsin

Melin Tan, MD
Assistant Professor
Department of Otorhinolaryngology–Head and Neck Surgery
Montefiore Medical Center
The University Hospital for Albert Einstein College of
  Medicine
Bronx, New York

Theresa N. Tran, MD, FACS
Assistant Professor
Department of Otolaryngology–Head and Neck Surgery
Icahn School of Medicine at Mount Sinai
Institute for Head and Neck and Thyroid Cancer
New York, New York

Joshua W. Trufant, MD
The Ronald O. Perelman Department of Dermatology
New York University School of Medicine
New York, New York

Gene Ukrainsky, MD, DDS
Assistant Professor
Department of Otolaryngology
The New York Eye and Ear Infirmary
New York, New York

Guy Valiquette, MD
Department of Endocrinology
Westchester Institute for Human Development
Valhalla, New York

Sunil P. Verma, MD
Director, University Voice and Swallowing Center
Medical Director
Department of Otolaryngology–Head and Neck Surgery
Assistant Professor
University of California–Irvine School of Medicine
Irvine, California

Philip A. Weissbrod, MD
Director, Center for Voice and Swallowing
Assistant Professor of Otolaryngology
UC San Diego Health System
San Diego, California

YuShan L. Wilson, MD
Department of Otolaryngology–Head and Neck Surgery
University of Massachusetts Memorial Medical Center
Worcester, Massachusetts

Sean R. Wise, MD
Assistant Professor
Department of Otolaryngology–Head and Neck Surgery
Naval Medical Center
San Diego, California

Kenneth M. Wong, MD
ENT and Sleep Specialists
Greenbelt, Maryland

Zhenqing Brett Wu, MD
Associate Adjunct Surgeon
New York Eye and Ear Infirmary of Mount Sinai
New York, New York

Mike Yao, MD
Clinical Associate Professor
Department of Otolarynology
New York Medical College
Valhalla, New York

Lonny Yarmus, DO, FCCP
Assistant Professor of Medicine
Clinical Chief
Division of Pulmonary and Critical Care
Fellowship Director
Section of Interventional Pulmonology
Johns Hopkins Medical Institutions
Baltimore, Maryland

Guo-Pei Yu, MD, MPH
Professor of Epidemiology and Vice Director
Medical Informatics Center, Peking University
Beijing, China
Associate Professor
Department of Otolaryngology
New York Medical College
Vahalla, New

Craig H. Zalvan, MD, FACS
Medical Director
The Institute for Voice and Swallowing Disorders
Phelps Memorial Hospital Center
Sleepy Hollow, New York
Associate Professor
New York Medical College
Valhalla, New York

1 Head and Neck Emergencies

Stimson P. Schantz, Jean-Paul Azzi, and James Azzi

1.1 Introduction

The head and neck contain a multitude of vital structures in proximity. It is therefore vital to identify those pathologies and insults that may require emergent treatment in order to prevent death or permanent disability. This chapter outlines some of the possible etiologies, organized by anatomical structure, and will serve to provide a framework for the management of head and neck emergencies.

1.2 Oral Cavity and Oropharynx Emergencies

- Post-tonsillectomy hemorrhage
  - Eschar sloughs off tonsillar fossa 7 to 10 days postoperatively
  - Suction clots from tonsillar fossa; bleeding may minimize or stop as bleeding vessel allowed to retract
  - If bleeding continues, start intravenous (IV) line and administer fluids
  - Obtain stat hemoglobin and hematocrit
  - Pressure packing, hemostatic agents
  - If unsuccessful, take to operating room (OR)
- Infections
  - Ludwig angina
    - Bilateral cellulitis involving fascial spaces of floor of mouth
    - Neck swelling and induration, drooling, respiratory distress
    - Upward displacement of tongue
    - Potential rapid airway compromise
    - Awake tracheotomy to protect airway
    - Drainage of submental space through external skin incision, IV antibiotics
  - Peritonsillar abscess
    - Unilateral otalgia, odynophagia, uvular deviation, trismus, drooling, "hot potato" voice; potential airway compromise
    - Intraoral incision and drainage with culture
    - Antibiotics

1.3 Neck Emergencies

- Postoperative complications
  - Hematoma
    - Neck swelling, pain, dyspnea, stridor
    - Remove bandaging, open surgical incision at bedside if airway compromise
    - Manage in OR if signs of active expansion
  - Thyroid storm
    - Tremor, nausea, altered mental status, progression to coma.
    - Tachycardia, cardiac arrhythmia, hyperthermia
    - Administer β-blockers, propylthiouracil (PTU), sodium iodide, steroids

- Administer cooled IV fluids, place cooling blanket
  - Severe symptomatic hypocalcemia
    - Circumoral paresthesias, tetany, seizures, mental status changes, laryngospasm
    - Chvostek sign (tapping on the face anterior to tragus and below zygomatic arch elicits ipsilateral facial twitching)
    - Trousseau sign (inflating blood pressure cuff for several minutes elicits wrist, metacarpophalangeal, and thumb flexion, interphalangeal hyperextension)
    - QT prolongation, cardiac arrest
    - Administer IV calcium gluconate (1 g over 10 minutes; if still symptomatic, infuse at 1 to 2 mg/kg/h until symptoms resolve)
- Deep space neck infection
  - Fascial compartments adjacent to deep musculature act as potential spaces
  - Spread from oral cavity, dentition, pharynx, salivary glands, sinuses, or temporal bone
  - Fever, chills, neck swelling, posterior pharyngeal swelling, pain, referred ear pain, dysphagia, trismus, torticollis
  - Culture throat, blood, sputum, aspirate
  - Computed tomography, anteroposterior (AP) and lateral neck radiographs
  - Manage airway
    - Oxygen saturation monitoring
    - Tracheotomy tray at bedside
  - Surgical drainage, broad-spectrum antibiotics
  - If *Actinomyces israelii* identified on histology, penicillin for 6 to 12 months
  - Complication: mediastinitis
    - Severe dyspnea, chest pain, fever
    - Chest X-ray (mediastinal widening)
    - Aggressive drainage, IV antibiotics
  - Complication: Lemierre syndrome
    - Thrombosis of internal jugular vein
  - Complication: carotid artery rupture
    - Bleeding from nose, mouth, or external auditory canal
    - Ipsilateral Horner syndrome
    - Cranial nerve IX, X, XII palsies
- Penetrating neck trauma
  - Unstable
    - Hypotensive shock, not responsive to fluid resuscitation
    - Airway, breathing, circulation (ABC)
    - Large-bore IV lines with fluids and blood running
    - Proximal and distal control of bleeding major vessels
    - Emergent exploration
  - Stable, zone I
    - Angiography
    - Consider swallow studies, direct laryngoscopy, bronchoscopy, and esophagoscopy
  - Stable, zone II
    - Symptomatic: surgical exploration
    - Asymptomatic: 48-hour observation
  - Stable, zone III
    - Angiography
    - Regular intraoral examinations

– Consider swallow studies, esophagoscopy, and direct laryngoscopy

1.4 Trachea and Esophagus Emergencies

- Tracheal foreign body
  - Persistent, nonproductive cough.
  - Transient episodes of respiratory distress
  - Inspiratory and expiratory stridor
  - Unequal breath sounds on auscultation
    - Early: obstructive emphysema, hyperinflation, distant breath sounds
    - Later: atelectasis, prominent breath sounds
  - Most often right main bronchus
  - Chest radiograph
    - Hyperaerated lung (mediastinal shift away, flattening of hemidiaphragm)
    - Atelectatic lung (mediastinal shift toward, elevation of hemidiaphragm)
  - Rigid bronchoscopy
- Esophageal foreign body
  - AP and lateral chest X-rays
  - Frequently at cricopharyngeal area
  - Potential for aspiration
  - Rigid esophagoscopy
  - Rule out esophageal injury (observe for several hours before feeding)
- Caustic ingestion
  - Lye
  - Liquefying necrosis
  - Prevent development of stricture
    - Antibiotics
    - Steroids
    - Serial dilations

2 Otologic Emergencies

Christopher J. Linstrom and Michele M. Gandolfi

2.1 Introduction

Otologic emergencies include foreign bodies in the ear, certain infections, trauma that can destroy ear structure, and idiopathic pathologies that cause hearing loss. This chapter is meant to be a guide for the initial assessment and management of major otologic emergencies.

2.2 External Auditory Canal Foreign Body

Certain foreign bodies do require emergent attention, such as a button battery. These can cause liquefaction necrosis and erosion of the ear in a short time.

▶ Evaluation
- History
  - Object known or unknown
  - Duration
  - Otalgia
  - Hearing loss
  - Vertigo
  - Otorrhea
  - Pruritus
- Physical examination
  - External auditory canal: otorrhea, edema, necrosis
  - Tenderness
  - Tympanic membrane integrity
- Testing
  - Audiogram if tympanic membrane injured and test immediately available

▶ Treatment
- Caustic foreign bodies like batteries are a true emergency and must be removed as soon as possible.
- A foreign body is best removed with a looped cerumen curet fashioned as an angled hook to get behind the foreign body and pull it forward. An alligator can also be used to grasp soft foreign bodies. Irrigation lavage should not be used for beans or seeds that can expand in the external auditory canal when exposed to water.
- Antibiotics/anti-inflammatory eardrops can be given if the external auditory canal is abraded/bleeding or if there is a visible perforation. Water precautions are also necessary in this case.
- If hearing impairment persists after removal, consider audiogram.

2.3 Malignant Otitis Externa

A potentially life-threatening osteomyelitis of the skull base that commonly affects elderly diabetic or immunocompromised patients. The most common pathogens are *Pseudomonas aeruginosa, Staphylococcus aureus*, and rarely *Aspergillus* and *Proteus*.

▶ Evaluation
- History
  - Multiple-weeks course of severe otitis externa in an immunocompromised patient that is not responsive to the typical medical therapy of steroid/antibiotic drops and oral antibiotics
  - Severe otalgia
  - Pruritus
  - Decreased hearing due to edema of the external auditory canal
  - Foul-smelling discharge
  - Fever is rare
  - Typically, a gradual progression of disease, with waxing and waning of symptoms possible
- Physical examination
  - Granulation tissue along the tympanomastoid suture line
  - Possible cranial nerve neuropathies (cranial nerves VII, IX, X, XI)
  - Exudate in the external auditory canal with edema
- Testing
  - Culture of external auditory canal debris/granulation tissue with a calcium alginate swab
  - Complete blood cell count (CBC) for white blood cells and erythrocyte sedimentation rate (ESR)
  - Computed tomography (CT) to document extent of disease
  - Initial bone scan with technetium Tc 99 m, a sensitive but nonspecific test that may stay positive for months
  - Gallium 67 scintigraphy is more specific. Used to monitor resolution of disease during treatment every 4 to 6 weeks

▶ Treatment
- Prolonged intravenous (IV) antibiotic treatment (6 to 12 weeks); often two-drug therapy is used (e.g., third-generation cephalosporin plus a quinolone)
- Follow-up cultures to make sure appropriate antibiotics are used, starting with broad-spectrum antibiotics
- Fastidious débridement of external auditory canal. Clinical examination and gallium scans to assess improvement
- Surgical intervention for intratemporal or extratemporal abscesses
- A normal external auditory canal is not a sensitive indicator of resolution. Gallium scan is more sensitive

2.4 Complications of Acute Otitis Media

2.4.1 Acute Mastoiditis/Subperiosteal Abscess

Acute mastoiditis typically occurs when there is contiguous spread of an acute otitis media to the mastoid portion of the temporal bone. *Streptococcus pyogenes* (group B β-hemolytic) is the most common cause of acute mastoiditis. Other species include *Streptococcus pneumoniae, Haemophilus influenzae, P. aeruginosa*, and anaerobes.

► Evaluation
• History
  ○ Onset of symptoms
  ○ Prior antibiotic course
  ○ Improvement of symptoms
  ○ Any other associated symptoms suggesting extracranial/intratemporal disease, such as the following:
    – Headache
    – Fever/chills
    – Retro-orbital pain
    – Diplopia
    – Cranial nerve paresis/paralysis
    – Photophobia
    – Altered mental status/drowsiness
• Physical examination
  ○ Retroauricular pain
  ○ Ear protrusion due to postauricular tenderness to palpation and edema
  ○ Bulging tympanic membrane with hyperemia and middle ear serous/purulent effusion
  ○ Weber and Rinne tests consistent with a conductive hearing loss
  ○ Neck stiffness, Kernig sign, Brudzinski sign
• Testing
  ○ CBC
  ○ CT of temporal bone to evaluate extent of disease, degree of mastoid osteitis and abscess formation (IV contrast should be used whenever an abcess is suspected)
  ○ Audiogram
  ○ Culture of middle ear effusion if tympanocentesis or myringotomy performed

► Treatment
• If no mastoid abscess formation (coalescence) seen on CT, then begin with nonsurgical treatment.
• Noncoalescent mastoiditis can be treated with myringotomy and drainage of middle ear and culture.
• Before culture results, empiric therapy is begun with a second-generation cephalosporin or an antipseudomonal aminopenicillin IV.
• Subsequent antibiotics should be culture-directed.
• After symptoms resolve, oral antibiotics should continue for 10 to 14 days.
• If no clinical improvement is noted after 24 to 48 hours of antibiotic therapy, mastoidectomy should be considered.
• Indications for surgical intervention
  ○ Coalescent mastoiditis on CT scan
  ○ Clinical nonresponsiveness after 24 to 48 hours of IV antibiotics
  ○ Significant abscess (subperiosteal, cervical, occipital, or temporal)
  ○ Suspected intracranial extension
• Surgery
  ○ Coalescent mastoiditis: simple mastoidectomy to the level or the mastoid antrum with wound drainage
  ○ Extratemporal abscess formation: incision and drainage
  ○ Additional mastoidectomy if accompanied by coalescent mastoiditis or if the abscess fails to respond to incision and drainage and antibiotics.

2.4.2 Petrous Apicitis

The internal auditory canal divides the petrous apex into anterior and posterior compartments. The anterior compartment is then divided into the peritubal and apical regions. Petrous apicitis can develop rapidly as a consequence of acute otitis media and mastoiditis. Chronic petrositis evolves as a complication of chronic serous otitis media. It can be found in asymptomatic patients on radiographic imaging. For etiology, see Acute Mastoiditis (above).

► Evaluation
• History
  ○ Deep pain
  ○ Symptoms similar to those of mastoiditis
  ○ Persistent aural discharge after mastoidectomy
  ○ Suboccipital headache and/or retro-orbital pain
• Physical examination
  ○ Pain as a result of trigeminal nerve involvement, and sixth nerve involved as it enters the Dorello canal.
  ○ Gradenigo syndrome: petrositis associated with retro-orbital pain, sixth nerve palsy, and persistent otorrhea.
• Testing
  ○ CT of the temporal bone: clouding of the petrous apex region with varying degrees of erosion.
  ○ Magnetic resonance (MR) imaging: when intracranial extension is suspected.

► Treatment
• Noncoalescent petrositis managed with culture-directed IV antibiotics obtained during myringotomy.
• Indications for surgical intervention
  ○ CT reveals coalescence; symptoms and clinical signs such as fever, leukocytosis, and otorrhea fail to respond to IV antibiotics.
  ○ A significant abscess, especially an intracranial abscess, exists. Consultation with a neurosurgeon is frequently useful to help manage the associated intracranial complications.

2.5 Auricular Trauma

Whether the patient has a simple laceration, avulsion, or blunt trauma, treatment is needed immediately. Injuries may be physical (lacerations, avulsions, or blunt trauma) and/or thermal (burns, frostbite).

► Evaluation
• History
  ○ Mechanism
  ○ Agent
  ○ Timing
• Physical examination
  ○ Presence of all structures of auricle, pieces missing
  ○ Viability of tissue
  ○ Foreign bodies in wound
  ○ Signs of infection

► Treatment
• Lacerations
  ○ Cleaning and débridement (only of devitalized tissue), irrigation with sterile saline

- Three-layer suturing of cartilage/perichondrium, skin on both sides of auricle
  - Absorbable suture to close perichondrium (5–0 or 6–0 Polyglactin 910; DemeTech, Miami Lakes, FL)
  - Nonabsorbable sutures to close skin (5–0 or 6–0 nylon)
  - Prophylactic antibiotic treatment: ciprofloxacin, amoxicllin/clavulanate
- Avulsions
  - Cleaning and débridement
  - Can require complex closure requiring staging, flap reconstruction
    - Superficial defects of the skin may be repaired with the use of vascularized skin flaps based on postauricular skin. This works well in the presence or absence of the perichondrium. Careful attention is paid to provide a flap of non–hair-bearing skin. Full-thickness skin grafts are generally not recommended for the helical rim.
    - Small helical rim defects may be amenable to chondrocutaneous advancement flaps, especially if the defect is smaller than 2 cm.
    - For defects larger than 2 cm, a staged tube flap from the postauricular skin may be necessary.
    - For large avulsions, isolate cartilage from avulsed segment. Incise temporal scalp at the superior border of the auricular remnant. Suture medial skin of auricular remnant to inferior temporal skin edge. Place avulsed cartilage in a temporal pocket dissected above the incision, and suture the avulsed cartilage to the remnant cartilage with Polyglactin 910 suture. Close the superior temporal skin edge to the lateral skin of the auricular remnant. After 6 to 8 weeks, elevate temporal skin and cartilage, skin grafting the medial side of the reattached cartilage.
  - Prophylactic antibiotic treatment as above
  - Mastoid dressing to protect ear
- Hematomas
  - Incision and drainage
    - Incision through the perichondrium under the helix just within the scaphoid fossa along the length of the hematoma. If the hematoma is located within the conchal bowl, the incision can be made on the conchal side of the antihelix. Drain the hematoma and irrigate the pocket with sterile saline.
    - Apply a pressure dressing created from soft red rubber catheters on either side of the scaphoid fossa that are sutured together through the auricle with 4–0 nylon.
  - Reevaluation every 24 to 48 hours for the next 3 to 4 days
  - Prophylactic antibiotics for 7 to 10 days
- Burns
  - Determine extent and depth of injury.
  - Fluid resuscitation for patient
  - Tetanus prophylaxis
  - Wound care and observation
    - Topical antibiotics
    - No pressure applied
- Frostbite
  - Bring patient to warm environment as soon as possible.
  - Warm auricle in water bath at 38 to 42°C slowly (pain control needed, as rewarming can be very painful).
  - Delayed surgical débridement only if necessary

2.6 Sudden Idiopathic Sensorineural Hearing Loss

Idiopathic sudden sensorineural hearing loss usually happens abruptly or rapidly and progressively over minutes, hours, or a few days. It is defined as 30 dB or more of sensorineural hearing loss over at least three contiguous audiometric frequencies occurring within 3 days or less. Possible causes include infection (measles, mumps, rubella, HIV infection, herpes, toxoplasmosis, syphilis, menigococcal infection, cryptococcal infection, Lyme disease); autoimmune disease (lupus, Wegener granulomatosis, polyarteritis nodosa, Cogan syndrome, relapsing polychondritis, ulcerative colitis); vascular disease (diabetes, vertebrobasilar insufficiency, sickle cell disease); neurologic disease (multiple sclerosis, pontine ischemia); neoplastic disease (acoustic neuroma, metastasis to internal auditory canal); trauma (perilymph fistula, barotrauma, otologic surgery); and iatrogenic causes (ototoxins).

▶ Evaluation
- History
  - Time course (treatment most successful within first 2 weeks of hearing loss)
  - Associated symptoms (tinnitus, vertigo, aural fullness, otalgia, cranial neuropathies)
- Physical examination
  - Signs of infection
  - Evaluation for trauma
  - Cranial nerve paresis/paralysis
- Testing
  - Audiogram
  - CT of temporal bone (if trauma, congenital deformity suspected)
  - MR imaging with gadolinium to evaluate internal auditory canal and cerebellopontine angle for mass
  - Electroneurography (ENG)/videonystagmography (VNG) when associated with vertigo
  - Laboratory testing
    - CBC with differential
    - ESR
    - Fluorescent treponemal antibody-absorbed (FTA-ABS) or rapid plasma reagin (RPR)
    - Thyroid function testing
    - Lipid profile
    - Antinuclear antibody (ANA)
    - HIV testing
    - Fasting glucose

▶ Treatment
- Steroids
  - Systemic: prednisone 60 to 80 mg daily for 7 days (1 mg/kg/d), then begin slow taper.
  - Intratympanic injections: superior–posterior quadrant injections 1 to 2 times a week with audiograms between injections to monitor improvement, up to 3 to 4 injections
    - Dexamethasone 0.4 to 0.7 mL of 24 mg/mL
    - Methylprednisolone 0.4 to 0.7 mL of 62.5 mg/mL
  - Antiretrovirals (acyclovir 1 g 2 times daily for 5 to 7 days)

○ Diuretics and salt restriction if Meniere disease suspected (hydrochlorothiazide/triamterene 50 mg daily)
○ Medical management of suspected underlying cause (diabetes, hypothyroidism, hyperlipidemia)

2.7 Idiopathic Facial Nerve Paralysis

Idiopathic facial paralysis (Bell palsy) is the most common cause of acute facial paralysis, with an incidence of 15 to 40 per 100,000 per year. Possible causes include infection (herpes type 1, herpes zoster [Ramsay Hunt syndrome], mononucleosis, mumps, Lyme disease, severe complicated otitis media, malignant otitis externa); autoimmune disease (Guillain-Barré syndrome, myasthenia gravis, sarcoidosis, Wegener granulomatosis); congenital syndromes (Melkersson-Rosenthal syndrome [unilateral facial palsy, facial edema, fissured tongue] and Mobius syndrome [bilateral facial and abducens palsies]); neoplasms; and trauma.

▶ **Evaluation**
• History
  ○ Time course
  ○ Associated symptoms: dysgeusia, hyperacusis, decreased lacrimation, facial hypesthesia
  ○ Exposure to pathogen/toxin
• Physical examination
  ○ Cutaneous vesicles in external auditory canal and conchal bowl with otalgia; cochlear and vestibular symptoms (Ramsay Hunt syndrome)
  ○ Complete otolaryngic examination
  ○ Cranial nerve examination (House-Brackmann classification)
• Testing
  ○ Nerve excitability test (NET) and electroneuronography (ENOG) should not be done in the first 3 days.
    – ENOG: 90% or greater degeneration of compound muscle action potentials (CMAPs) suggests poor recovery and is an indication for surgical exploration and decompression. ENOG should be performed daily until nadir is reached.
    – NET: 2.0- to 3.5-mA difference between sides suggests unfavorable prognosis.
  ○ Electromyography (EMG) measures motor unit potentials (MUPs) and may be useful in first 3 days. MUPs in 4 to 5 groups in first 3 days associated with return of function in more than 90%. EMG is good for assessing reinnervation potential of the muscle 2 to 3 weeks after onset of paralysis. Polyphasic potentials are seen in regeneration, while fibrillation potentials portend a poor prognosis.
  ○ Imaging: MR imaging is performed in cases of progression of palsy over 3 weeks, recurrent palsy, facial hyperkinesias, cranial neuropathies.

▶ **Treatment**
• Medical
  ○ Prednisone (1 mg/kg) divided into 3 daily doses for 10 days with a 10-day taper afterward
  ○ Antiretrovirals
    – Acyclovir 800 mg 5 times a day for 10 days
    – Valacyclovir more effective for Ramsay Hunt syndrome
• Surgical
  ○ Decompression from mastoid to geniculate ganglion if ENOG shows more than 90% degeneration of CMAPs

2.8 Temporal Bone Trauma

Temporal bone fracture is a frequent manifestation of head trauma. In the adult population, approximately 90% of temporal bone fractures are associated with concurrent intracranial injuries and 9% with cervical spine injuries. Motor vehicle accidents are the cause of 31% of temporal bone fractures; other causes include physical assaults, falls, motorcycle accidents, pedestrian injuries, bicycle accidents, and gunshot wounds. Two different classification systems are in use. Fractures are often mixed and oblique and do not fit into one classification.

▶ **Etiology**
• Longitudinal fractures comprise 80% of all temporal bone fractures. They are frequently caused by a lateral force over the mastoid or temporal squama, usually produced by temporal or parietal blows. Typically spare otic capsule and run anterolateral to otic capsule.
• Transverse fractures comprise 20% of all temporal bone fractures. They are usually caused by a frontal or parietal blow but may result from an occipital blow. Typically run into otic capsule, damaging cochlear and semicircular canals.

▶ **Evaluation**
• History
  ○ Etiology of trauma
  ○ Direction of impact
  ○ Time course
  ○ Associated symptoms (tinnitus, vertigo, hearing loss)
• Physical examination
  ○ Glasgow Coma Scale score
  ○ Associated injuries
  ○ Battle sign
  ○ Bloody or clear otorrhea
  ○ Cranial nerve palsy/paralysis
  ○ Tympanic membrane perforation
• Testing
  ○ High-resolution CT of temporal bone; evaluate fracture site
  ○ Eventual audiogram (when feasible)
  ○ Eventual VNG/ENG (when feasible)
  ○ NET/ENOG/EMG if facial nerve involved

▶ **Classification**
• Longitudinal (80%)
  ○ Conductive hearing loss due to ossicular chain disruption at the incudostapedial joint. Hemotympanum and external auditory canal fractures also possible. Approximately 20% of these patients have temporary/delayed facial nerve injury, usually in the horizontal segment.
  ○ Cerebrospinal fluid (CSF) otorrhea common but temporary
  ○ Tympanic membrane perforation common
  ○ Less intense vertigo
• Transverse (20%)
  ○ Severe sensorineural hearing loss

○ Vertigo common and intense
○ Facial nerve injury in 50%, which is usually permanent, severe, and early in onset
○ Occasional CSF otorrhea
○ Rare to have a tympanic membrane perforation

▶ **Treatment**
- Medical: a patient with delayed facial paralysis is managed conservatively with 10 to 14 days of systemic corticosteroids unless medically contraindicated.
- Surgical: dependent on facial nerve status

○ A patient with complete paralysis of immediate onset undergoes initial testing with the Hilger nerve stimulator between days 3 and 7. If ability to stimulate nerve is not lost, patients are observed.
○ If ability to stimulate nerve is lost within 1 week, or more than 90% degeneration on ENOG occurs within 2 to 3 weeks, then facial nerve decompression is offered to the patient.
○ Surgical exploration may also be indicated for a CSF fistula that lasts longer than 14 days and does not resolve with conservative management.

3 Pediatric ENT Emergencies

Robin A. Dyleski and Moustafa Mourad

3.1 Airway Foreign Body

Assess respiratory status, patency of airway, and ability to move air, as indicated by crying or speaking. If the patient is not exchanging air well, emergent airway control is required. Nonsurgical management includes the Heimlich maneuver or bedside direct laryngoscopy and endotracheal intubation followed by transfer to the operating room (OR) for further management/removal of the foreign body. Surgical management (rarely needed in children, especially young children) includes tracheotomy or cricothyroidotomy. For a patent airway, proceed with evaluation of the patient (Heimlich maneuver is contraindicated).

▶ **Evaluation**
- History
  - Was the aspiration witnessed?
  - Type of foreign body, if known
  - Duration of symptoms
  - Dyspnea, labored breathing
  - Dysphagia
  - Drooling
  - Cough
  - Pain
  - Ability to cry/speak
  - History of tracheoesophageal or bronchial abnormalities
  - Previous treatment for symptoms (i.e., nonresolving stridor during treatment of croup, recurrent pneumonia, recurrent bronchitis)
- Physical examination
  - Mental status
  - Presence of stridor
    - Inspiratory: glottic, subglottic, or supraglottic obstruction
    - Expiratory: subglottic or bronchial obstruction
    - Biphasic: glottic obstruction
  - Asymmetric breath sounds
  - Respiratory distress: paradoxical breathing, cyanosis, use of accessory muscles, low oxygen saturation
  - Wheezing, especially "unilateral" wheezing

▶ **Management**
- High clinical suspicion of airway foreign body
  - Witnessed aspiration episode with coughing/choking
  - Asymmetric breath sounds
  - Loss of voice or vocal changes
  - Wheezing, especially if unilateral
  - Stridor
- Nondiagnostic history and physical examination with medium to low clinical suspicion of airway foreign body
  - Chest X-ray shows indirect evidence of airway obstruction
    - Hyperinflation of one lung
    - Atelectasis
    - Bronchiectasis due to long-standing chronic bronchial obstruction
    - Soft-tissue neck X-ray (usually lateral and anteroposterior [AP])
  - Computed tomography (CT): infrequently used but may be helpful in the event that clinical suspicion remains high but plain radiography is nondiagnostic.
- Definitive treatment
  - Rigid bronchoscopy in operating room with foreign body retrieval
  - Flexible bronchoscopy is not advised when there is strong evidence for a foreign body. The flexible bronchoscope working channel is too small to permit use of appropriate forceps to grasp the object in young children. Flexible bronchoscopy is a useful diagnostic tool for the patient who arrives already intubated with a questionable history of foreign body aspiration. If a foreign body is seen, then rigid bronchoscopy for foreign body removal under general anesthesia is recommended. Only very small foreign bodies may be able to be removed with flexible bronchoscopy.

3.2 Esophageal Foreign Body

▶ **Evaluation**
- History
  - Describe object (blunt, sharp, disk battery)
  - Duration of ingestion (< 24 hours vs > 24 hours)
  - Symptoms
    - Dysphagia
    - Odynophagia
    - Drooling
    - Vomiting
    - Chest pain
  - History of gastrointestinal abnormalities such as prior tracheoesophageal fistula or esophageal stenosis
  - Intake/nutritional status (assess need for intravenous [IV] hydration)
- Physical examination
  - Respiratory status
  - Mental status
  - Complete cardiovascular, pulmonary, and abdominal examination
- Testing
  - Chest X-ray: AP and lateral
  - Avoid barium swallow because barium will interfere with subsequent endoscopy

▶ **Management**
- Blunt-edged foreign body (not a battery)
  - If foreign body located at lower esophageal sphincter, patient may be monitored for spontaneous passage with follow-up radiographs 24 hours after ingestion.
  - Thoracic inlet or midesophageal area, esophagoscopy (flexible or rigid) with general anesthesia (for airway protection)
- Sharp-edged object
  - Rigid esophagoscopy with foreign body removal. If possible, the sharp portion of the foreign body may be placed within the lumen of the esophagoscope in order to protect the esophageal mucosa.

- Alkaline disk battery
  - A chest X-ray is often able to distinguish between coins and disk batteries by the appearance of the edge of the object; disk batteries appear to have a "ring" around the edge, raising suspicion that the object is a battery.
  - Indications for immediate endoscopic retrieval
    - Any battery in esophagus
    - Battery larger than 15 mm in stomach
    - Battery smaller than 15 mm in stomach that has failed to pass within 48 hours or patient becomes symptomatic (abdominal pain, nausea, vomiting, or fevers)
- Esophagoscopy considerations
  - Esophagoscopy for foreign body should always be performed under general anesthesia for airway protection.
  - Always have pediatric bronchoscopy set up and available during esophagoscopy because of risk for loss of object into airway during retrieval.
  - After removing the foreign body, reinsert the esophagoscope to examine the site of impaction and also check for second foreign body.
  - Consider steroids and prophylactic antibiotics if significant edema noted at site of impaction.

3.3 Croup

▶ **Evaluation**
- History
  - Age: typically younger than 5 years old
  - Sudden onset
  - Barking cough
  - Hoarseness
  - Fevers variable
- Physical examination
  - Alertness of child
  - Stridor, usually high pitched and inspiratory
  - Wheezing
  - Signs of impending respiratory distress
    - Accessory muscle use
    - Cyanosis
    - Paradoxical breath
    - Chest retractions
  - Complete cardiovascular and pulmonary examination
- Testing
  - Anterolateral chest X-ray: steeple sign indicates subglottic narrowing.
  - Oxygen saturation (pulse oximetry) and in severe cases arterial blood gas

▶ **Management**
- Mildly symptomatic, with stable respiratory status and adequate hydration
  - Supportive home care
  - Humidification of air: cool mist
- Moderately symptomatic with moderately labored breathing
  - Intramuscular dexamethasone
  - Nebulized racemic epinephrine
- Severely symptomatic, acute respiratory distress
  - Emergency supportive respiratory care including treatment with dexamethasone and nebulized racemic epinephrine

- If respiratory distress continues or progresses, endotracheal intubation is necessary. Use of endotracheal tube 0.5 to 1.0 mm smaller than normal size for patient age.

3.4 Epiglottitis

Several hours, history of high fever, stridor, difficulty swallowing, drooling, muffled voice, and difficulty breathing. Patients may present in the "sniffing position" or with the neck flexed and head extended.

Typically patients have no cough, in contrast to those with croup. The diagnosis is typically based on clinical examination and history. Radiographs may be used showing an edematous epiglottis ("thumb print" sign) and obliteration of the vallecula (vallecula sign). Most cases of epiglottitis are diagnosed clinically, and ultrasound is emerging as a noninvasive and accurate method of diagnosis.

▶ **Evaluation**
- History
  - Acute onset is typical
  - Dysphagia, drooling
  - Increasing respiratory distress
  - Acute onset of high fever; up to 40°C is common
- Physical examination
  - Posture: sitting up with head thrust forward, "tripod position"
  - Drooling
  - Respiratory status
    - Accessory muscles
    - Paradoxical breathing
    - Chest retractions
    - Cyanosis
  - Mental status (obtunded patients at high risk for acute respiratory failure, requiring airway to be secured)
  - Complete cardiopulmonary examination

▶ **Management**
- Maintain a high index of suspicion
  - Avoid upsetting patient; do not separate patient from parent/caregiver, minimize situations that might induce crying.
  - Transport immediately to OR for evaluation and treatment if patient is in respiratory distress.
  - Have emergent tracheostomy tray open and available in OR.
  - Direct laryngoscopy and intubation
    - Intubate with endotracheal tube or use rigid bronchoscope
    - Consider percutaneous transtracheal jet ventilation if epiglottis is too edematous to visualize the true vocal cord.
  - Culture and sensitivity of epiglottis after airway is secured
- Treatment and monitoring
  - Intensive care unit setting for both intubated and nonintubated patients
  - Antibiotic coverage of *Streptococcus pneumoniae*, *Haemophilus influenzae*, and *Staphylococcus pyogenes*
    - Third-generation cephalosporin
    - Amoxicillin/clavulanate

○ Epiglottal edema should be monitored with flexible laryngoscopy.
○ Extubation typically possible after antibiotic treatment for 48 to 72 hours
○ Corticosteroid use controversial

3.5 Stridor with Respiratory Distress

▶ **Etiology**
- Foreign body
- Infectious
  ○ Epiglottitis/supraglottitis
  ○ Croup
  ○ Retropharyngeal abscess
- Mechanical
  ○ Subglottic stenosis
  ○ Vocal cord palsy
  ○ Airway edema
- Congenital
  ○ Airway anomalies such as laryngomalacia and tracheomalacia
  ○ Vascular malformations
- Neoplasm
  ○ Laryngeal papillomatosis

▶ **Evaluation**
- History
  ○ Age
  ○ Duration
  ○ Onset
  ○ Dysphagia
  ○ Dyspnea
  ○ Is fever present?
  ○ Birth history, especially prematurity; mechanical ventilation; intracranial, neck, or chest surgical intervention
- Physical examination
  ○ Alertness of patient
  ○ Cyanosis: presence or absence of congenital cardiac disease is important
  ○ Accessory muscle use: indicates degree of respiratory effort needed
  ○ Chest retractions, sternal retractions
  ○ Paradoxical breathing
  ○ Full head and neck examination, including flexible laryngoscopy
  ○ Full cardiopulmonary examinations, including neck auscultation for location of loudest stridor
  ○ Abdominal examination
  ○ Vital signs including continuous pulse oximetry, respiratory rate
- Testing
  ○ Laboratory data
    – Arterial or venous blood gas: unusual to require except in most severe cases or intubated cases
    – Complete blood cell count (CBC)
    – Blood electrolytes and metabolic panel
  ○ Plain radiographs
    – AP and lateral chest X-rays
    – AP and lateral neck X-rays
  ○ Barium esophagram (if suspect involvement of esophagus)
  ○ CT with contrast: may show vascular anomalies, compressions due to neoplastic masses, presence of pneumonia.
  ○ Magnetic resonance (MR) imaging, MR angiography: may allow improved delineation between neoplastic and vascular causes.

▶ **Management**
- Determine need for emergent airway management on the basis of the respiratory distress and the diagnosis.
  ○ Intubation
  ○ Tracheostomy
  ○ Cricothyroidotomy
  ○ Percutaneous transtracheal jet ventilation
- Treat underlying cause of respiratory condition.

3.6 Post-tonsillectomy Hemorrhage and Other Oropharyngeal Bleeding

3.6.1 Emergent Management

Assess the need for emergent resuscitation. Assess airway: if bleeding is severe and there is a compromised airway and hemodynamic instability, then pack oral cavity after oral endotracheal intubation, tracheotomy, or cricothyroidotomy.

Assess circulation; if hemodynamically unstable, then secure two large-bore peripheral IV lines and administer bolus fluids by weight. Type and cross match, obtain CBC, and assess for possible transfusion. Prepare the patient for emergent return to OR to control and stop bleeding.

3.6.2 Nonemergent Management

▶ **Evaluation**
- History
  ○ Vital signs: monitor oxygen saturation, heart and respiratory rates, blood pressure
  ○ Time and date of procedure, timing of postoperative bleeding
  ○ Onset/duration/quantity of bleeding
  ○ Personal or family history of bleeding or easy bruising: possible undiagnosed coagulopathy or use of medications (nonsteroidal anti-inflammatory drugs) impairing platelet function
  ○ Fever
  ○ Recent oral intake, dehydration status
- Physical examination
  ○ Signs and symptoms of acute blood loss
  ○ Complete cardiopulmonary examination
  ○ Oral cavity
    – Determine if there is localizable area of active bleeding.
    – Assess for presence of clots
    – Is the patient still bleeding?

▶ **Management**
- Notify OR for possible OR need to control post-tonsillectomy hemorrhage.

- If no gross acute/active bleed, but evidence of old clotted blood, then consider in older patients to gargle with 50:50 hydrogen peroxide and water solution, then reassess oral cavity.
- If localizable area of bleeding
  - Attempt to cauterize with silver nitrate (only in older, highly cooperative patients).
  - If bleeding does not stop or patient does not tolerate, take to OR for examination under anesthesia and electrocautery.
- Admit patient to observe for recurrence of bleeding.

3.7 Retropharyngeal Abscess

▶ Evaluation
- History
  - Precedent upper respiratory infection
  - Fever
  - Dysphagia/poor oral intake (in infants)
  - Limitation of neck range of motion, either from side to side or up and down; may mimic meningitis symptoms
  - Shortness of breath or stridor
  - Sore throat
  - Cough
  - Neck swelling
- Physical examination
  - Vital signs
  - Neck lymphadenopathy
  - Posterior pharyngeal swelling/bulge
  - Torticollis
  - Stridor
  - Drooling
  - Agitation
  - Presence of tonsillar or peritonsillar exudates
- Testing
  - Laboratory data
    - CBC
    - Blood cultures
    - Oral exudate culture
  - Imaging: lateral neck X-ray
    - Widening of the retropharyngeal soft tissues and prevertebral space
    - Gas–fluid levels in abscess cavity
    - Foreign body: while most retropharyngeal abscesses are from suppurated retropharyngeal lymph nodes, a foreign body may be the etiology.
  - Imaging: CT with IV contrast
    - Used in setting of nondiagnostic radiographs but high clinical suspicion
    - Demonstrates typical rim enhancement when abscess present
    - Allows diagnosis of extent of abscess into the lower neck/upper thoracic area (allows differentiation between retropharyngeal abscess and prevertebral space abscess)

▶ Management
- Emergent intubation or surgical airway, as indicated
- Supplemental oxygen, if needed
- IV fluids
- IV antibiotics

- Operative drainage
- Most retropharyngeal abscesses are transoral
  - Use mouth gag for exposure to the posterior pharyngeal wall
  - Injection of lidocaine with epinephrine in the proposed vertical incision site (low on the abscess for enhanced drainage after incision)
  - Incise the mucosa vertically (about a 1-cm incision), then using a tonsil clamp, bluntly enter the abscess cavity (spreading vertically between the muscle fibers).
  - Sample of abscess contents for Gram stain, culture, and sensitivity
  - No closure of incision needed
  - May begin feeding with clear liquids after operation.

3.8 Soft Palate Lacerations and Other Oropharyngeal Injuries

▶ Evaluation
- History
  - Mechanism of injury
    - Fall from seated position or while running at maximum speed
    - Grade mild, moderate, or severe size of laceration
  - Neurologic complaints: if present then need vascular surgery consultation.
  - Fever
  - Torticollis
  - Neck pain
  - Dysphagia
  - Drooling
  - Chest pain
- Physical examination
  - Primary survey: assess airway, breathing, and circulation (ABC) after trauma and possible need for emergent intubation and volume resuscitation.
  - Secondary survey in the stable patient
    - Wound assessment and characterization, including location of the laceration (midline vs lateral soft palate/lateral pharyngeal wall area)
    - Neurologic examination
    - Neck auscultation over carotid artery (e.g., carotid bruit)
    - Examination of teeth (fracture, subluxation, avulsion)
    - Examination of tongue
    - Assess for trismus and drooling (e.g., infection)
    - Assess for neck crepitus and subcutaneous air
- Testing
  - Laboratory data
    - CBC (indicated only in cases of severe bleeding)
    - Blood cultures and C-reactive protein if an infection is suspected
  - Imaging: plain radiographs of chest and neck
    - Pneumomediastinum.
    - Retropharyngeal widening
    - Foreign bodies
  - Imaging: CT angiogram of chest and neck
    - The test of choice
    - Demonstrates thrombus and/or dissection of carotid artery from a blunt or penetrating injury

- Imaging: MR angiography (limited use because of need for anesthesia in young children)
- Imaging: carotid artery angiography
  - Gold standard for internal carotid artery imaging
  - Risk for stroke with carotid artery angiography
  - Reserved for children with neurologic findings, severe mechanism of trauma, evidence of internal carotid artery (ICA) injury with other imaging

▶ **Management**
- Primary survey in severe trauma
  - Assess need for airway stabilization (endotracheal intubation vs surgical airway)
  - Assess need for volume resuscitation
  - Cervical spine immobilization
  - Do not alter or remove protruding objects
- For high-risk injury (high-force trauma, such as motor vehicle accident)
  - Angiography
  - Endoscopy
  - Surgical exploration
- For moderate-risk injury (retained oropharyngeal object)
  - Hospital admission
  - CT angiography (or less commonly MR angiography)
  - If concerning findings on CT angiography for ICA injury (ICA abnormality, subcutaneous air near ICA, or disruption of ICA sheath), proceed to carotid artery angiography. For ICA injury (e.g., intimal tear), consider vascular surgery consultation.
  - If CT angiography or MR angiography indicates non-ICA injury, then
    - Local oral cavity wound care
    - Discharge home with close monitoring for development of fevers, neurologic paresis, neck stiffness, torticollis, dysphagia, or dyspnea. Can be considered only in patients with extremely reliable parents.
    - May admit to hospital for 24 to 48 hours for serial neurologic examinations.
- For low-risk injury (superficial laceration, midline lacerations)
  - Local wound care
  - Discharge home with close follow-up
- Wound care
  - Wounds smaller than 2 cm (e.g., puncture wounds) do not require surgical wound closure.
  - Indications for operative repair
    - Palatal flaps
    - Avulsed tonsils
    - Retained or protruding foreign body
    - Gross contamination
  - Tetanus prophylaxis
  - IV/oral empiric antibiotics

4 Facial Plastic and Reconstructive Surgery Emergencies

Grigorly Mashkevich

4.1 Facial Trauma

4.1.1 General

- Initial evaluation
  - "ABC": airway, breathing, and circulation.

Vascular access with two large-bore intravenous (IV) lines.
- Protection of the cervical spine (Philadelphia collar); plain X-rays to rule out cervical spine fracture
- Stabilization of vital signs in the emergency room setting.
- Secondary survey
  - Examination of wounds
  - Head and neck radiography: computed tomography (CT) of the facial bones for suspected fractures, plain or CT angiography of the neck for penetrating trauma or suspected vascular injuries.
  - Assess potential for central nervous system, ophthalmic injury; consult other services when appropriate.

4.1.2 Facial Fractures

General

- Radiographic evaluation with thin-cut, noncontrast CT of the maxillofacial region
- Preoperative ophthalmologic evaluation when appropriate to rule out intraocular injuries before any manipulation of the frontal, orbital, or maxillary regions.
- Delayed (up to 5 to 10 days) fracture repair to allow reduction of tissue edema, improve surgical access, and diminish intraoperative bleeding.
- Open reduction with internal rigid fixation is the optimal solution for most facial fractures.

Frontal Sinus Fracture

- Radiographic evaluation with CT to assess anterior and posterior tables of the frontal sinus.
- Surgical repair depending on the degree of table displacement and comminution.
- Consider neurosurgical consultation, especially if posterior wall violated.

Nasal Fracture

- Preliminary assessment should be followed by more detailed secondary evaluation in 4 to 6 days once acute edema has partially subsided.
  - Minimal bony displacement: observation with secondary reconstruction 2 to 3 months later if necessary.
  - Clinically apparent bony displacement: closed reduction with external cast stabilization within 10 to 14 days; secondary reconstruction 2 to 3 months later if necessary.

Orbital Fracture

- Palpate orbital rims for step-off deformities.
- Assess extraocular motion.
- Assess globe position (enophthalmos/exophthalmos).
- Assess sensory function.
- Assess stability of medial canthus.
- Medial orbital fracture
  - Consider naso-orbito-ethmoid (NOE) fracture.
- Infraorbital rim fracture
  - Consider associated orbital floor fracture.
- Orbital floor fracture
  - Repair in cases of enophthalmos and radiographic evidence of orbital content displacement into the maxillary sinus.
  - Exploration of orbital floors with comminution of more than half of the total surface area.
- Lateral orbital rim fracture
  - Consider zygomaticomaxillary complex (ZMC) fracture.
  - Treat as indicated.
- Maxilla and mandible fracture
  - Soft diet
  - Empiric antibiotics
  - Cold compresses (edema reduction in preparation for surgery)
  - Restoration of proper occlusion via maxillomandibular fixation (MMF) is the most important consideration during reduction of fractures involving this region.

Temporal Bone Fracture with Facial Nerve Paralysis

- CT of temporal bone
- Electroneurography (ENOG)
- Stable patients: consider surgical exploration and nerve repair.
- Unstable patients: steroids to reduce nerve inflammation, followed by reassessment at a later date.

4.2 Lacerations of the Face

4.2.1 Skin and Soft Tissue

- Tetanus protocol
- Clean wounds
  - Within 12 hours of injury
    - Layered primary closure
  - More than 12 hours after injury
    - Antibiotics and delayed primary closure
- Grossly contaminated wounds or any evidence of pus or cellulitis
  - Wound care and packing, followed by delayed repair.

4.2.2 Bites

- Empiric antibiotics
- Uninfected wounds
  - Animal bite: rabies protocol, consider primary closure
  - Human bite: HIV and hepatitis protocols, wound care, delayed primary closure
- Grossly contaminated wounds or any evidence of pus or cellulitis: wound care and packing, followed by delayed repair

4.3 Facial Nerve Paralysis

- Operating room for exploration and repair (optimal time frame for repair is within 3 days, during which time distal nerve ends can still be stimulated).

4.4 Parotid Duct Injury

- Operating room for exploration and repair
  - Clean ductal laceration without tissue loss: direct suture repair over a stent.
  - Ductal loss: segmental replacement with an interposition vein graft sutured over a stent
  - Intraparotid ductal injury: watertight closure of parotid fascia, botulinum toxin A injection to extinguish salivary production

4.5 Penetrating Neck Wounds

- Vascular imaging (including CT angiography)
  - Surgical repair versus embolization for vascular injuries
- Evaluation of aerodigestive tract injury
  - Surgery in appropriate cases

4.6 Hematomas: Septal and Auricular

- Incision and drainage
- External splinting for apposition of separated tissues
- Insertion of small drain (short segment of a sterile rubber band)

4.7 Postoperative Emergencies

4.7.1 Rhinoplasty/Nasal Surgery

Toxic Shock Syndrome

- Early recognition is key!
  - Early: postoperative fever, facial flushing
  - Later: hypotension and cardiovascular collapse
- Remove nasal packing.

- Broad-spectrum antibiotics
- Fluids, cardiovascular support, and intensive care monitoring

4.7.2 Blepharoplasty

Bleeding/Intraorbital Hematoma

- Lateral canthotomy and cantholysis, performed urgently at bedside.
- Removal of any nasal packing, intermittent globe massage
- Stat ophthalmologic evaluation to monitor pressure and vision
- Stress dose of IV corticosteroids
- Mannitol (1 to 2 g/kg IV over 30 minutes)
- Operating room for wound exploration

4.7.3 Facelift

Hematoma

- Small: aspiration and pressure dressing, with possible drain placement
- Medium: open incision and express clots, place drain
- Large or expanding: operating room for wound exploration

Facial Nerve Paralysis

- Observe for several hours until local anesthetic wears off.
- Consider exploration depending on the index of suspicion.

4.7.4 Microvascular Reconstruction

Venous Obstruction

- Examination: engorged and bluish skin paddle, rapid capillary refill, "water hammer" Doppler signal, rapidly flowing dark blood on pricking of the skin paddle
  - Operating room for exploration of anastomosis and flap vasculature
  - Leech therapy in partially obstructed flaps

Arterial Obstruction

- Examination: pale skin paddle, absent capillary refill, absent Doppler signal, absent or significantly delayed blood flow on pricking of the skin paddle
  - Operating room for exploration of anastomosis and flap vasculature

4.7.5 Tissue Expansion

- Expander exposure
  - Early: remove the expander
  - Late: continue expansion and use expanded tissue for reconstruction.

5 Rhinologic Emergencies

Steven David Schaefer

5.1 Epistaxis

- Initial evaluation

Assess general appearance of patient.
- Obtain vital signs as warranted.
- Obtain brief history to permit focusing on the site and potential cause of hemorrhage.
- Initial control of hemorrhage
  - Manually compress the lower half of nose or use a nose clip to reduce anterior hemorrhage. If bleeding is controlled, maintain compression continuously for 15 minutes before checking for cessation of bleeding. Compressing the upper nose or nasal bones will not affect hemorrhaging.
  - Clear the nose of blood clots with suction and/or gentle nose blowing.
  - Spray the nose with a vasoconstrictive agent, such as oxymetazoline (Afrin; Merck Consumer Care, Cleveland, TN).
  - Continue manual compression of the lower nose while preparing to perform anterior rhinoscopy with a nasal speculum, or preferably with a nasal endoscope.
  - Place cotton pledgets, approximately 0.5 x 3 to cm long, along the floor of the nose and, if possible, at the site of bleeding.
  - If the site of hemorrhage is in the posterior third of the nose, consider a transpalatal injection of the sphenopalatine artery.
- Inspection of the nose
  - Perform rhinoscopy with a 0-degree nasal endoscope. If an endoscope is not available, a nasal speculum and a bright headlight will permit visualization of the anterior nose.
- Control of anterior epistaxis
  - Cauterize site of minor bleeding with silver nitrate or chromic acid.
  - Avoid chemical cauterization in patients with abnormal wound healing, such as those with lupus. In such patients, the cauterization site will become necrotic and rehemorrhage; instead, place a dissolvable agent that will facilitate clotting, such as Gelfoam (Pfizer, New York, NY), at the bleeding site.
  - Anterior nasal packing is reserved for anterior epistaxis refractory to the above measures. Place the nasal pack along the floor of the nose and against the site of hemorrhage. Vaseline gauze should be progressively layered along the floor of the nose until the site of bleeding is compressed. Commercially available packs, such as Merocel (Medtronic, Minneapolis, MN), are simpler to use but require the same careful attention to placement. Do not shove something in the nose and expect it to control hemorrhage.
  - Avoid nonbiodegradable nasal packing in patients with impaired wound healing. Biodegradable products such as Gelfoam or oxidized cellulose (Surgicel; Johnson & Johnson, New Brunswick, NJ) should be applied in the same way as other forms of nasal packing. Overall, such products are preferable because they do not require removal in 3 to 4 days, as do the nonbiodegradable nasal packs.
  - Place the patient on broad-spectrum antibiotics to avoid sinusitis.
- Control of posterior epistaxis
  - Reserve posterior nasal packing for identifiable bleeding sites or failure to control hemorrhage with anterior packing.
  - Posterior packing must tamponade the choana and sphenopalatine artery. A commercial nasal balloon or a Foley catheter is placed into the posterior nose and inflated with saline. The balloon must be pulled forward and a clamp placed over the anterior aspect of the device. Cotton gauze is placed between the clamp and the nasal ala to prevent necrosis of the nose.
  - Most patients with posterior nasal packing should be hospitalized to monitor respiratory function and oxygen saturation, and many require oxygen by face mask.
  - Place the patient on broad-spectrum antibiotics to avoid sinusitis.
  - After 2 days of nasal packing, patients with persistent hemorrhage should be considered for either endoscopically directed electrocautery, intranasal ligation of the sphenopalatine artery, or arterial embolization of the internal maxillary artery.

5.2 Iatrogenic Cerebral Spinal Fluid Rhinorrhea

- Acute, intraoperative cerebrospinal fluid (CSF) rhinorrhea
  - Immediately obtain careful hemostasis within the nose by placement of cottonoids at all bleeding sites and consider bipolar electrocautery as indicated.
  - Identify the site of CSF rhinorrhea and inspect the integrity of the bony skull base, dura, and brain. Intracranial hemorrhage requires neurosurgical consultation. Low-volume venous bleeding on the cortex can be temporarily mitigated by direct placement of neurosurgical cottonoids, and if it is available and the surgeon has the proper skills, bipolar electrocautery is useful.
  - After hemostasis has been obtained, the 1 cm or more of mucous membrane surrounding skull base defect should be removed. This will later permit adhesion of the graft to the bony skull base.
  - A watertight seal should be obtained by intrathecal grafting. Although many grafting materials are available, fat is the easiest and most reliable graft. One continuous piece of abdominal or ear lobule fat measuring several times the size of the dural defect is placed intrathecally. Approximately 25% of the fat should protrude into the nasal side of the dura to help anchor the graft.
  - After placement of the fat graft, the anesthesiologist should perform a Valsalva maneuver to raise the intracranial pressure, and the surgeon should observe the defect for persistent CSF rhinorrhea. A properly placed graft should provide a watertight seal.

○ A second graft may be placed intranasally along the bony skull base. Mucous membrane or various commercial products are excellent grafts and can be made to adhere to the skull base with tissue glues. The graft should be applied only to the exposed bone of the skull base to permit optimal adherence.

○ Biodegradable or dissolvable packing, such as Gelfoam, is applied to the underlay or intranasal graft to further secure it. As most iatrogenic fistulas occur in the roof of the ethmoid sinus, the packing should fill only part of this sinus. If possible, any packing requiring removal should be avoided because its removal may dislodge the graft.

○ Intraoperatively, an intravenous (IV) broad-spectrum antibiotic should be administered to prevent meningitis.

○ Patients should avoid straining or other activities that increase intracranial pressure, and they should be made aware of the signs of meningitis.

○ Patients should avoid flying for 6 weeks.

- Late or post-sinus surgery CSF rhinorrhea
  ○ Post-sinus surgery CSF fistulas should be repaired as soon as recognized.
  ○ Patients should be informed of the signs of meningitis and should avoid flying, nasal cleaning, nose blowing, and nasal lavage. Antibiotics should be considered with concurrent acute sinusitis.
  ○ Post-sinus surgery meningitis with or without CSF rhinorrhea should alert the physician to a communication between the subarachnoid space and the nose. Potential fistulas may cease after meningitis and later recur.
  ○ High-resolution coronal 2-mm computed tomographic (CT) images are helpful in identifying or confirming the site of the fistula. Contrast CT cisternography can be helpful if the site of the fistula is questionable, provided the patient has active rhinorrhea. In Europe, intrathecal hypodense fluorescein (10 mg/mL) is employed to endoscopically visualize fistulas.
  ○ In fistulas that are more than several weeks old, 3 days of lumbar drainage may be considered to divert the excessive CSF produced to compensate for the rhinorrhea. If lumbar drainage is employed, 1 to 2 mL of hypodense fluorescein can be placed intrathecally via the drain. The fluorescein enhances identification of the fistula site and intraoperatively ensures the detection of post-grafting rhinorrhea.
  ○ Repair of the fistula and post-hospitalization care are the same as outlined for acute injuries.

5.3 Complications of Acute Sinusitis

- Etiology of acute sinusitis complications
  ○ The proximity and venous drainage of the sinuses may result in the spread of infections to the orbit and brain.
  ○ Obstruction of the drainage pathways of the sinuses, or masses or tumors of the sinuses, may first present as eye or brain complications. Spread of infection to the orbit is more common from ethmoid sinusitis, and to the brain or epidural space from frontal and sphenoid infections. Maxillary sinusitis may be secondary to dental infections.
- Orbital complications of acute sinusitis

○ The periosteum of the orbit (periorbita) initially confines the extension of infection from the sinuses into the orbit.

○ Preseptal (anterior to the septum orbitale) infections present with swelling of the eyelids and a minimal chemosis and injection of the conjunctivae.
  – Preseptal infections are initially treated with broad-spectrum oral antibiotics, with IV antibiotics reserved for more aggressive infections or in compromised patients. Ophthalmology consultation is indicated.

○ Subperiosteal abscesses of the orbit arise from direct extension of the sinus infection into the subperiosteal space between the periorbita and the bony walls of the orbit. Such infections are not within the orbit proper and do not involve the extraocular muscles, fat, or globe. Ethmoid sinusitis is the most common etiology of such infections. Patients present with variable degrees of proptosis due to displacement of the orbital contents by the abscess.
  – Subperiosteal abscess requires surgical drainage and broad-spectrum antibiotics. Surgical drainage includes ethmoidectomy or sinusotomy (drainage) of the involved sinus. Subperiosteal abscess arising from ethmoid sinusitis can be drained into the ethmoid cavity by removal of the lamina papyracea endoscopically at the time of ethmoidectomy, or externally via a Lynch incision. Subperiosteal abscesses involving the superior orbit are approached through direct incision over the abscess or orbitotomy. Management should be in conjunction with ophthalmology.

○ Intraorbital cellulitis or abscesses result from the progression of infection from the sinuses through the periorbitae. Involvement of the extraocular muscles presents as diplopia, with proptosis resulting from the mass effect of the abscess.
  – Visual acuity and intraocular pressure must be monitored. As pressure rises, retinal perfusion is compromised, leading to potential blindness and requiring urgent care.
  – Intraorbital abscesses are treated by IV broad-spectrum antibiotics and incision and drainage of the orbit (orbitotomy). Management should be in conjunction with ophthalmology.

○ Localization of infection and/or abscess to the superior orbital fissure presents as loss of extraocular movement as the third, fourth, and sixth cranial nerves are compromised.
  – Treatment is urgent and the same as for intraorbital infections because both processes have the same etiology and simply differ in localization.
  – Management should be in conjunction with ophthalmology.

○ Loss of vision and afferent pupillary defect (Marcus Gunn pupil, or positive swinging flashlight test) implies compromise of the optic nerve between the retina and the optic chiasm.
  – In conjunction with ophthalmology, management focuses on relieving pressure or infection involving the optic nerve.

○ Cavernous sinus involvement is heralded by contralateral visual or ocular movement findings.
  – Treatment consist of IV antibiotics with prevention and/or amelioration of cavernous sinus thrombosis.

- Intracranial complications of acute sinusitis

○ The proximity of the ethmoid, frontal, and sphenoid sinuses to the intracranial cavity permits direct extension of infection and/or abscesses to the meninges, epidural space, cavernous sinus, internal carotid artery, and optic nerve.

– Treatment is urgent and is directed toward the site of infection. Symptoms vary with the site of infection. CT or magnetic resonance imaging is useful in identifying abscesses, thrombosis of the dural sinuses, and evidence of increased intracranial pressure.

– A complete neurologic examination, including assessment of the cranial nerves, deep tendon reflexes, and abnormal posturing on sensory stimulation, often helps to localize the site and severity of infection or abscess.

– Prior treatment with oral antibiotics may mask signs of meningitis (lack or minimal evidence of meningeal tenderness, papilledema, confusion, lethargy, and cranial neuropathies).

– Lumbar puncture must be wisely employed and can precipitate brainstem herniation in the setting of increased intracranial pressure. When appropriate, lumbar puncture should be performed to diagnose meningitis, and bacteria/fungus should be obtained for culture.

– Broad-spectrum antibiotics are employed and vary with the age and nature of the infection. For example, patients after neurologic or sinus procedures have a higher incidence of *Staphylococcus aureus* and pneumonia infections.

– Abscesses require drainage by neurosurgery.

○ Hematogenous spread to the subarachnoid space and brain

– Depending on the site of infection, diagnosis and management are similar to those for the site of infection.

– Timing of the drainage of brain abscess depends on the neurologic consequences of the abscess and its maturity (cerebritis vs mature abscess).

6 Laryngologic Emergencies

Philip A. Weissbrod

6.1 Introduction

Integral to breathing, swallowing, protection of the airway, and phonation, the larynx is a vital component of the upper respiratory tract. This chapter will serve to outline possible etiologies and provide a framework for the management of laryngologic emergencies.

6.2 Acute Upper Airway Obstruction

Obstruction can occur for many reasons at different levels of the upper airway, including the oral cavity, pharynx, larynx, and trachea. Often, a careful history and physical examination can point to a clear etiology and anatomical location. Management consists of establishing a safe, secure airway and reversing the underlying cause. Severe airway compromise is best managed in a controlled setting, such as the operating room, intensive care unit, or trauma bay, before patient decompensation.

▶ **Etiology**
- Anaphylaxis
- Angioedema
- Autoimmune
  - Amyloidosis
  - Sarcoidosis
  - Wegeners granulomatosis
- Foreign body
- Granulation tissue
- Granulomatosis
- Hemorrhage
  - Postsurgical
  - Traumatic (intraluminal vs extraluminal/compressive)
- Infectious
  - Deep neck space infection
  - Ludwig angina
  - Peritonsillar abscess
  - Respiratory papillomatosis
  - Retropharyngeal abscess
  - Supraglottitis/epiglottitis
- Neoplasm
- Neurologic
  - Bilateral vocal fold paralysis
- Stenosis.
- Trauma
  - External trauma.
  - Intubation-related trauma.
- Other
  - Laryngospasm.
  - Laryngomalacia/tracheomalacia
  - Paradoxical vocal fold motion

▶ **Evaluation**
- History
  - Allergy history
  - Cough
  - Duration of symptoms
  - Dysphagia
  - Dyspnea
  - Fever/chills
  - Hoarseness
  - Odynophagia
  - Pain
  - Recent intubation for airway trauma
- Physical examination
  - Vital signs
  - Stridor: noisy respiration
    - Inspiration: localizes to glottis and above
    - Biphasic: localizes to glottis or subglottis
    - Expiration: localizes to subglottis and below
  - Observed patient discomfort/anxiety
  - Mental status change
  - Examination of the head and neck with a focus on the airway column from nose to lungs to locate and grade the obstruction
  - Observe for signs of respiratory fatigue: shallow, rapid respiration; supraclavicular retractions; recruitment of accessory respiratory muscles; paradoxical breathing; intercostal retractions.
  - Chest and neck auscultation
  - Flexible laryngoscopy: while performing fiber-optic examination, it is important to avoid stimulation of the pharynx and larynx to prevent laryngospasm, which can precipitate a clinical decompensation.
- Testing
  - Arterial blood gas
  - CT scan (if there is concern for abscess, framework injury, or tumor)

▶ **Treatment**
- Determine site/level of obstruction and reverse the cause.
- Control airway distal to obstruction by either endotracheal intubation or surgical airway if warranted by the severity and location of obstruction.
- Nonsurgical airway management
  - Mask ventilation
  - Continuous positive airway pressure (CPAP)/bilevel positive airway pressure (BiPAP)
  - Laryngeal mask airway (LMA)
  - Endotracheal intubation
    - Macintosh or Miller blade
    - Rigid laryngoscope
    - Fiber-optically assisted
    - Rigid bronchoscope
  - Observation in intensive care unit or emergency department setting.
  - When appropriate, consider treatment with
    - Steroids
    - Antibiotics
    - Racemic epinephrine
    - Heliox

- Surgical airway management
  - Cricothyroidotomy.
  - Tracheotomy.
  - Cricothyroid puncture
  - During emergent surgical airways, placement of the airway below the second ring is ideal to avoid trauma to the larynx and subglottis; however, this is a lifesaving measure, and securing the airway is the priority.

6.3 Laryngeal Blunt Trauma

The management of blunt laryngeal trauma is dictated by the extent of injury to cartilaginous structures and mucosa. Care must be taken not to exacerbate a tenuous airway during the diagnostic process.

▶ Etiology
- Clothesline infury
- Motor vehicle accident
- Strangulation

▶ Evaluation
- History
  - Dyspnea
  - Hoarseness/aphonia
  - Hemoptysis
  - Mechanism of injury
  - Odynophagia
  - Pain
- Physical examination
  - Stridor
  - Dysphonia
  - Respiratory fatigue
  - Blunting of thyroid ala
  - Crepitus
  - Neck ecchymosis
  - Tenderness
- Flexible laryngoscopy (note the following if present)
  - Airway narrowing
  - Ecchymosis/hematoma
  - Edema
  - Mucosal or vocal fold laceration
  - Vocal fold immobility
  - Exposed cartilage
- Testing
  - Computed tomography: look for fracture (displaced, nondisplaced)

▶ Treatment. Treatment is dictated by the category of injury (types I, II, III, IV). Initial management should determine if the patient is in respiratory extremis or in danger of compromise. If at risk for obstruction, regardless of subtype, emergent tracheotomy or cricothyroidotomy should be considered as the first step in management without endotracheal intubation if it can be avoided. Laryngeal injury can be missed because of intubation before examination. In the presence of significant laryngeal trauma, injuries to the esophagus are frequent and can be missed. Esophagrams or rigid/flexible esophagoscopy should be performed, especially for zone I penetrating injuries.

- Type I
  - Diagnostic criteria: patients have no airway compromise, soft-tissue injury only (including mucosal abrasions, hematomas, small lacerations)
  - Management
    - Medical: close observation, no oral intake, serial fiber-optic examination
- Type II
  - Diagnostic criteria: patients with possible airway compromise, moderate soft-tissue laceration or tearing, nondisplaced or minimally displaced cartilaginous framework fracture
  - Management
    - Medical: close observation, steroids, humidified oxygen, voice rest, antireflux medication, esophagram
    - Surgical: possible tracheotomy, direct laryngoscopy, esophagoscopy
- Type III
  - Diagnostic criteria: displaced or unstable laryngeal fractures, significant mucosal or vocal fold lacerations, and/or intraluminal cartilage exposure
  - Management
    - Surgical: awake tracheotomy, direct laryngoscopy, open reduction with internal fixation, repair of mucosal lacerations, esophagoscopy
- Type IV
  - Diagnostic criteria: similar but more severe injuries than type III
  - Management
    - Surgical: same as type III but with placement of laryngeal stent for support of cartilaginous fractures, mucosal repairs, and exposed cartilage

6.4 Laryngeal Penetrating Trauma

Penetrating trauma to the neck can be life-threatening. The initial evaluation should be dictated by patient stability. If a patient is hemodynamically unstable from a neck injury, immediate exploration is indicated. As many as one-third of patients with vascular injury from penetrating trauma are asymptomatic. Otherwise, diagnostic modality and management are dictated by the location of the injury.

▶ Etiology
- Low-velocity injury (e.g., stab wounds, broken glass)
- High-velocity injury (e.g., gunshot wounds, shrapnel)

▶ Evaluation
- History
  - Dysphagia
  - Hematemesis
  - Hemoptysis
  - Hoarseness
  - Nerve weakness or paralysis
  - Odynophagia
  - Pain
- Physical examination
  - Bruits
  - Examine for both entry and exit wounds when applicable.

○ Hematoma
○ Hemorrhage
○ Impaired mental status (potential vascular injury)
○ Neurologic deficits
○ Respiratory obstruction/compromise
○ Subcutaneous emphysema
○ Stridor
○ Unequal pulses
- Surgical exploration and imaging is not indicated for injuries that do not pierce the platysma.
- Testing and treatment for zone I injury
  ○ Inferior border: sternal notch
  ○ Superior border: inferior border of cricoid
  ○ Obstacles to surgical access: sternum, clavicles
  ○ Structures at risk: brachiocephalic artery and vein, internal jugular vein, common carotid artery, subclavian artery and vein, vertebral artery, trachea, esophagus, vagus nerve, phrenic nerve, brachial plexus, recurrent laryngeal nerve, thoracic duct, thyroid, lung apex, spinal cord. In penetrating trauma, zone I injuries carry the highest mortality rate.
  ○ Testing/management: angiography vs CT angiogram, esophagram/esophagoscopy
- Testing and treatment for zone II injury
  ○ Inferior border: inferior border of cricoid
  ○ Superior border: angle of mandible
  ○ Structures at risk: internal jugular vein; common, external, and internal carotid artery; vertebral artery; trachea; larynx; pharynx; hypopharynx; vagus nerve; submandibular gland; phrenic nerve; accessory nerve; hypoglossal nerve; marginal mandibular nerve; spinal cord
  ○ Testing/management: somewhat controversial. If symptomatic, surgical exploration is indicated. If asymptomatic, consider surgical exploration vs angiography or CT angiogram.
- Testing and treatment for zone III injury
  ○ Inferior border: angle of mandible
  ○ Superior border: skull base
  ○ Obstacles to surgical access: mandible, mid face
  ○ Structures at risk: internal jugular vein, vertebral artery, internal carotid artery, branches of the external carotid artery, pharynx, parotid gland, facial nerve, cranial nerves, spinal cord
  ○ Testing/management: angiography vs CT angiogram
- Treatment points
  ○ If unstable (shock or evolving stroke), then consider immediate exploration.
  ○ Initially, bleeding should be controlled with direct pressure.
  ○ Manipulation and probing of the site of injury and removal of penetrating objects should be avoided until in a controlled environment and large-bore intravenous lines have been secured.
  ○ Surgical consultations
    – Vascular surgery for complex repair of the carotid system
    – Thoracic surgery for low zone I vascular injuries

– Neurosurgery for high zone III injuries that may require craniotomy for control
– Interventional neuroradiology for zone III vascular injuries that may benefit from embolization or stenting

6.5 Voice Emergencies

Vocal emergencies, although not life-threatening, can pose significant risk to those who use their voice for vocation. Untreated vocal emergencies are capable of causing significant scarring of the vocal folds or polyp formation, leading to decreased vibratory capacity and ultimately chronic voice alterations.

▶ **Etiology**
- Hemorrhage (often associated with sudden voice changes that occur during vocal strain, coughing, vomiting)
- Vocal fold tear
- Severe laryngitis (bacterial, fungal, or viral)
- Upper respiratory infections

▶ **Evaluation**
- History
  ○ Pain with phonation
  ○ Smoking history
  ○ Sudden onset versus progressive
  ○ Voice change
  ○ Vocal hygiene
  ○ Preexisting symptoms of chronic laryngitis
  ○ Upcoming vocal demands/performance obligations
- Physical examination
  ○ Dysphonia
  ○ Flexible laryngoscopy
  ○ Videostroboscopy if available

▶ **Treatment**
- Voice rest
- Supportive care (hydration, mucolytics, general rest, cessation of smoking)
- Treatment of underlying causative, contributing, or exacerbating factors
- Voice therapy after acute phase
- Avoidance of laryngeal irritants
- When indicated, consider
  ○ Antibiotics
  ○ Antifungals
  ○ Corticosteroids (oral or intramuscular)
  ○ Proton pump inhibitors
- Avoid blood-thinning agents
- Identify pending vocal engagements to determine how quickly the restoration of normal voice is needed. This will affect the aggressiveness of therapy and establish the need to cancel pending engagements.

7 Emergency Airway Management and Tracheotomy

Adam S. Jacobson and Joseph J. Rousso

7.1 Introduction

Airway control is the most critical component of emergency patient care and accordingly is the first step in cardiopulmonary resuscitation. Emergency airway management requires quick and decisive action, and a functional knowledge of anatomical landmarks. There are several methods of accessing the airway in both the emergent and controlled settings, including endotracheal intubation, cricothyrotomy, and tracheotomy.

7.2 Incidence of Disease

Several pathologic processes result in the need for airway management. The most common reason for tracheotomy and tube placement is respiratory ventilation for longer than 1 to 2 weeks.

7.3 Terminology

The term *airway* generally refers to the route of air passage from the upper aerodigestive tract into the tracheobronchial tree. The airway can be compromised anywhere along this route. A keen understanding of the airway anatomy allows the practitioner to have a clearer picture of interventions and procedures that can be used to access the airway.

Tracheotomy is a surgical opening made directly into the trachea, below the cricoid cartilage. *Cricothyrotomy* is a surgical opening through the cricothyroid membrane, which lies between the thyroid and cricoid cartilages.

7.4 Applied Anatomy

Inspired air enters the nasal cavity, where it is warmed and humidified. It continues through the nasopharynx, oropharynx, and endolarynx to enter the trachea via the subglottis, below the true vocal cords.

The anterior neck has palpable landmarks that assist in finding an entry point for a surgical airway. The sternal notch and cricoid cartilage serve as excellent indicators of the midline, the expected location of the normal trachea in its longitudinal course. The thyroid cartilage, often referred to as the Adam's apple, is typically a prominent surface landmark that reliably protects the structures of the deeper endolarynx. Below the thyroid cartilage lies the cricoid cartilage. The cricoid cartilage is the most important landmark in tracheotomy because it lies immediately above the superior tracheal rings.

In the emergent setting, in which exposure is not ideal, palpable anterior cervical landmarks are the most valuable tool available to the surgeon. When the neck is palpated, the first palpable prominence above the sternal notch typically represents the cricoid cartilage. The second, more superior and larger palpable prominence represents the thyroid cartilage. The slight indentation or valley between these two prominences represents the cricothyroid membrane, the entry point for emergent cricothyrotomy.

7.5 Disease Process

7.5.1 Etiology and Pathogenesis

Airway complications can arise from several causes, including trauma, anaphylaxis, cardiopulmonary arrest, infection, toxic exposure, congenital, neurologic insult, hypoventilation, and many others.

7.5.2 Natural History and Progression

In the hemodynamically unstable patient with acute obstruction, the airway must be secured immediately because anoxia results in death within 4 to 5 minutes. In the hemodynamically stable patient or the patient whose airway is secured, further evaluation can be afforded. Patients who are endotracheally intubated are at risk of several complications, including tracheal and laryngeal stenosis; the risk increases with prolonged intubation.

7.5.3 Potential Complications

Damage to the airway can lead to dysphonia, stridor, difficulty breathing, and potentially death.

7.5.4 Disease Grading

Airway grading systems are not generally used for the assessment of surgical airways.

However, thinner individuals with a full range of neck extension and palpable cricoid and thyroid cartilages are considered favorable surgical candidates.

The simplest and most common method of endotracheal intubation assessment is the Mallampati classification, which indicates how much of the posterior pharynx can be visualized with the mouth fully opened. The Mallampati system divides patients into four classes. Class I indicates full visualization of the pillars, fauces, soft palate, and uvula and is considered predictive of a relatively uncomplicated intubation. On the other end of the spectrum, class IV indicates visualization of the hard palate only because of a large tongue obscuring the view and is predictive of a difficult endotracheal intubation.

7.6 Medical Evaluation

7.6.1 Presenting Complaints

The presentation of a patient in respiratory distress can be highly variable. The presentation can range from a conscious patient who complains of "throat tightness" to an unconscious patient who is unable to be ventilated. Stridor, drooling, rapid breathing, shallow breathing, decreasing oxygen saturation, tachycardia, tongue swelling, dysphonia, globus sensation, and facial fractures are all signs of possible or pending loss of airway and should be assessed with urgency.

7.6.2 Acute Evaluation in the Unconscious Patient

Initial evaluation in the unconscious patient should include a chin lift and rapid assessment of breathing, with care taken not to manipulate the cervical spine in a trauma setting. After it has been established that the airway is compromised, further considerations should include the mechanism of injury, site of obstruction, overall hemodynamic stability, and possible immediate interventions. From the moment the patient arrives at a medical setting, a cardiac monitor with a functional pulse oximeter and large-bore intravenous access must be in place.

7.6.3 Acute Evaluation in the Conscious Patient

The urgency of airway evaluation should not be ignored in the conscious patient as several factors can lead to immediate instability. After the initial and secondary survey, the focused history should include an assessment of allergen exposure, medications, timing and onset of symptoms, mechanism of injury, associated symptoms, substance use, and medical and surgical histories.

Stridor is a very important symptom that may be elicited by the patient history and/or a sign that may be found on physical examination. The characteristics of the patient's stridor can give the physician a preliminary impression as to the level of anatomical disturbance. Inspiratory stridor is indicative of a disturbance at the level of the larynx, whereas expiratory stridor suggests obstruction more distally in the tracheobronchial tree. Biphasic stridor is a symptom of a glottic or subglottic cause of respiratory distress.

7.6.4 Physical Examination

A complete physical examination is invaluable in the clinician's decision-making process. Assessment of the neurologic status should include a Glasgow Coma Scale score. Examination of the head and neck, with complete evaluation of the eyes, ears, nose, throat, and face, is necessary, with particular attention given to traumatic injury. Furthermore, a dedicated head and neck examination should include thorough and careful neck palpation to evaluate for masses that could be causing airway compression. A cardiac and pulmonary examination should then be performed, with attention to respiratory effort and the use of accessory muscles of respiration. If the patient is stable, visualization of the endolarynx and airway via fiber-optic endoscopy is appropriate and extremely useful when available.

7.6.5 Laboratory Studies and Imaging

Imaging studies, particularly noncontrast computed tomography, present the physician with further information as to the structural integrity of the upper aerodigestive structures in patients who are sufficiently stable to undergo the tests. Arterial blood gas values assist in identifying the source of respiratory distress.

7.6.6 Differential Diagnosis

Several pathologic processes can present similarly to acute airway distress. Anxiety disorder can manifest as panic attacks, which often present with respiratory distress. The associated hyperventilation further aggravates the patient's sense of choking and impending doom.

Paradoxical vocal fold movement is another pathologic entity that in severe cases can manifest with acute respiratory distress and be mistaken for asthma.

Acute airway distress can have several causes. Any source of anatomical disruption or obstruction of the airway can lead to respiratory distress. Tumors, masses, traumatic injury, and foreign bodies at any level of the pharynx, larynx, or trachea can lead to profound respiratory difficulty. Direct compression of the airway from an extratracheal mass, such as an anaplastic thyroid carcinoma or thyroid goiter, can have grave airway consequences. True vocal cord immobility, particularly when bilateral, can lead to nearly complete airway obstruction.

7.7 Treatment

7.7.1 Endotracheal Intubation

Endotracheal intubation is the first step of achieving airway control in the acute setting.

Rapid-sequence intubation is the method of choice when time permits. This consists of preoxygenation with 100% oxygen via a non-rebreather mask for several minutes. If ventilation is necessary, bag gently while cricoid pressure is applied. The administration of either midazolam 0.2 mg/kg or etomidate 0.3 mg/kg can be used for induction in the hemodynamically stable patient. A paralytic, such as succinylcholine, can then be administered for easier access into the oral airway and will take effect within 30 seconds. Finally, the endotracheal tube is placed and secured. If the endotracheal tube cannot be placed, the patient should be ventilated with a bag valve mask. If the orotracheal intubation is unsuccessful, other options must quickly be considered. Nasotracheal intubation with visualization via the use of a fiber-optic nasopharyngoscope is helpful in obtaining a difficult airway. However, nasotracheal intubation is challenging and requires an experienced practitioner.

Complications of endotracheal intubation can be differentiated into immediate and postprocedural. Immediate complications include esophageal intubation, main bronchus intubation, tooth damage, mucosal tears, laryngospasm, and traumatic disarticulation or laceration of endolaryngeal structures. Postintubation complications include subglottic stenosis, pneumothorax, vocal cord granuloma, vocal cord paralysis, and tracheal edema.

7.7.2 Surgical Treatment: Cricothyrotomy

Cricothyrotomy is the procedure of choice for emergency establishment of an airway in a patient who is unable to be intubated. The procedure consists of identifying the cricothyroid membrane as a slight indentation in the skin inferior to the

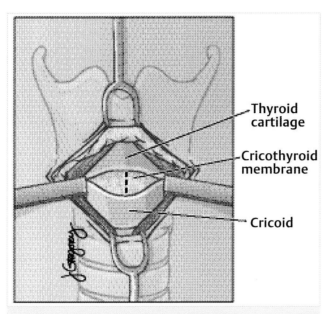

Fig. 7.1 The surgical landmarks for cricothyrotomy.

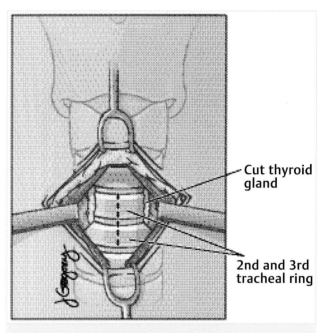

Fig. 7.2 The surgical landmarks for tracheotomy.

laryngeal prominence. The membrane is relatively superficial without any overlying large vessels or fascial layers, allowing easy access. A vertical skin incision is made from the thyroid cartilage to below the cricoid cartilage to increase exposure and minimize hemorrhage by avoiding the vertically coursing anterior jugular veins. Continuous palpation is necessary to feel the location of the cricothyroid membrane. Once the membrane is found, a stab wound is made and extended horizontally, and a small endotracheal tube or tracheotomy tube is placed. ▶ Fig. 7.1 demonstrates the anatomical landmarks for cricothyrotomy.

The major complication associated with cricothyrotomy is the increased rate of subglottic stenosis that occurs in comparison with tracheotomy. Therefore, it is recommended that cricothyrotomy be converted to formal elective tracheotomy as soon as safely possible.

7.7.3 Surgical Treatment: Needle Cricothyrotomy

A variation of a formal cricothyrotomy performed in dire emergencies is the needle cricothyrotomy. A large-gauge needle with a cannula is inserted into the cricothyroid membrane until air can be aspirated with the attached syringe. The cannula is then inserted into the airway and attached to a supply of oxygen. This allows the patient to be oxygenated for a short time, but the removal of carbon dioxide is not adequate and acidosis may ensue rapidly.

7.7.4 Surgical Treatment: Tracheotomy

Tracheotomy is a reliable procedure for access into the trachea. The modern procedure was described by Dr. Chevalier Jackson in 1909. Tracheotomy can be performed in the emergent setting ("slash trach") when other methods of airway control are not attainable. However, the majority of tracheotomies are performed electively under general anesthesia.

There is some discrepancy as to the preferred skin incision for an elective tracheotomy (vertical vs horizontal), although the consensus is that an emergent tracheotomy must have a vertical incision. ▶ Fig. 7.2 demonstrates the appropriate surgical landmarks for a tracheotomy. The incision should be placed below the cricoid cartilage, with anticipation of placing the tube between the third and fourth tracheal rings.

The incision is taken down below the platysma until the strap muscles are visualized. The strap muscles are separated at the midline raphe and retracted to reveal the isthmus of the thyroid. At this point, the isthmus can be retracted superiorly or transected to expose the underlying trachea. A window is made in the anterior wall of the trachea, with care taken not to insert the blade deeply enough to rupture the cuff of the endotracheal tube. A tracheal dilator is then inserted into the lumen of the trachea and the window expanded. At this point, the anesthesiologist is asked to deflate the cuff and slowly pull back the endotracheal tube until it lies immediately above the tracheotomy site. It is important that the endotracheal tube remain in the trachea at this point, in the event that the tracheotomy tube cannot be easily positioned through the window and into the trachea; should this occur, the endotracheal tube can be advanced below the tracheotomy site and the patient ventilated while the tracheotomy exposure is improved to allow easier placement of the tracheotomy tube. A cuff-tested and prepared tracheotomy tube (▶ Fig. 7.3) is then inserted into the lumen of the trachea. Auscultation of the lungs and end-tidal carbon dioxide detection are used to confirm placement of the tracheotomy tube into the trachea. Furthermore, a flexible fiber-optic endoscope can be placed through the tracheotomy tube to visually confirm placement. The endotracheal tube is then completely removed, and the tracheotomy tube is sutured into place and a tracheotomy tie placed around it for additional security.

In the first 24 hours after tracheotomy, the patient should be treated with the same level of urgency as a patient with pending respiratory distress. Postoperatively, the patient should be

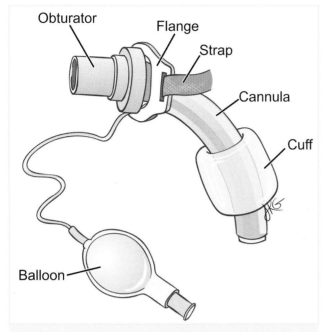

Fig. 7.3 A tracheotomy tube with the components labeled.

admitted to an observation unit with continuous cardiac and pulse oximeter monitoring and placed on humidified oxygen to prevent acute tracheal crust formation. The tracheotomy tube obturator should be kept by the bedside in an obvious but secure place. Any possible concerns that arise in these patients should be addressed immediately because tracheotomy tube replacement in a fresh surgical airway is extremely difficult. Suctioning should be performed frequently but only to the distal tip of the tube because excessive suctioning the tracheal lumen can cause irritation, granulation, and stenosis or erosion. If acute obstruction of the tracheotomy tube occurs, the inner cannula should be removed immediately and cleaned before it is replaced.

If the tracheotomy tube is displaced or falls out of place, the inner cannula should be removed and replaced by the obturator. The tracheotomy tube should be replaced immediately by manipulating it through the stoma. If the stoma has closed and the original tube cannot be passed, a smaller tracheotomy or endotracheal tube should be placed through the stoma. This can be facilitated (especially in patients expected to be difficult to reintubate, such as those with severe kyphosis or an obese neck) by the placement of stay sutures through the anterior trachea at the time of surgery that are taped to the patient's neck; these stay sutures are gently pulled laterally to aid in opening the tracheotomy track. If these measures do not allow fast access into the airway, the patient should be ventilated with a bag mask, and orotracheal intubation may be necessary. It is important to remember that a surgical airway does not necessarily preclude orotracheal intubation, if it becomes necessary.

As a rule of thumb, it takes about 7 days for a safe, well-formed track to form between the skin and the tracheal opening. Therefore, absolutely no unnecessary manipulation of a tracheotomy tube should be done until this time. Furthermore,

a new tracheotomy tube should remain secured with sutures as well as a tracheotomy tube tie. At postoperative day 7, the sutures can be removed. There is discrepancy between the timing and necessity of the first tracheotomy tube change. Some practitioners will routinely change the tracheotomy tube at postoperative day 7 for hygienic purposes, whereas others feel that this is unnecessary and unsafe. If the patient originally required a cuffed tracheotomy tube for ventilation purposes, the tracheotomy tube should be changed to an uncuffed one as soon as possible, as long as the tract is well formed. This prevents cuff-related tracheal ulceration, necrosis, and granulation tissue, which may otherwise result. If the patient is to have the tracheotomy tube in place for a long time, it should be replaced every 1 to 3 months. The peristomal skin should be cleansed meticulously to avoid irritation and breakdown from tracheal secretions.

Operative complications include injury to the esophagus, recurrent laryngeal nerves, and great vessels. Furthermore, pneumothorax, anesthetic complications, and perforation of the posterior tracheal wall can rarely occur intraoperatively. Postoperative complications include innominate artery erosion, tracheoesophageal fistula, tracheal stenosis, infection, and persistent stoma. The most severe complication that may arise from the placement of any form of surgical airway is death, most often resulting from tube displacement or hemorrhage. Complications in emergency tracheotomies are two to five times more frequent than when tracheotomy is done as an elective procedure.

7.8 Prognosis

After the airway has been secured, the patient's prognosis depends on overall hemodynamic stability and concomitant medical conditions.

Postoperative care of the surgical airway is vital to avoiding further airway complications. Frequent suctioning and pulmonary toilet prevent crusting and secretion buildup in the patient with a fresh tracheotomy. A patient with a tracheotomy tube should always have an obturator at the bedside to assist in timely replacement if the tracheotomy tube comes out of place.

7.9 Roundsmanship

- The airway is the physician's first priority in resuscitating a patient.
- Basic comprehension of the airway anatomy and cervical landmarks is vital to securing an airway in an unstable patient.
- The urgency of airway evaluation should not be ignored in the conscious patient as several factors can lead to immediate instability.
- Endotracheal intubation is the first step in accessing an airway in the emergent setting.
- If there is an immediate need for a surgical airway in the emergency setting, cricothyrotomy should be performed.
- Tracheotomy is a reliable procedure for airway access that is most successful when performed electively in a controlled setting.

7.10 Recommended Reading

[1] Goldenberg D, Bhatti N. Management of the impaired airway in the adult. In: Cummings C, Haughey B, Thomas JR, et al, eds. Cummings Otolaryngology: Head and Neck Surgery. 4th ed. Philadelphia, PA: Elsevier Mosby; 2005:2441–2452

[2] Lore JM, Medina JE. The trachea and mediastinum. In: Cohen JI, Clayman G, eds. Atlas of Head and Neck Surgery. Philadelphia, PA: Elsevier Saunders; 2005:1015–1068

[3] Margolis GS, American Academy of Orthopaedic Surgeons. Pharmocoligic aids in endotracheal intubation. In: Paramedic: Airway Management. Sudbury, MA: Jones and Bartlett Publishers; 2004:271–277

[4] National Institutes of Health, National Heart, Lung, and Blood Institute. What is a tracheostomy? http://www.nhlbi.nih.gov/health/dci/Diseases/trach/trach_all.html. Accessed October 10, 2013.

8 Head and Neck Anatomy

Ameet R. Kamat and Edward J. Shin

8.1 Face

8.1.1 Muscles of the Face

The facial muscles are subcutaneous, some in a plane continuous with the superficial muscular aponeurotic system (SMAS). Their unique attachments with the skin, fascia, and bone allow for a variety of facial expressions. The muscles of facial expression are all derived from the second pharyngeal arch and are innervated by the seventh cranial nerve (the facial nerve).

Muscles of the Forehead

The anterior belly of the occipitofrontalis muscle is known as the frontalis. It arises from the epicranial aponeurosis posteriorly and attaches to the skin of the eyebrows anteriorly without a bony attachment. It is responsible for elevating the brow and producing transverse wrinkles. The cutaneous attachment of the procerus muscle is continuous with frontalis and arises from the upper nasal dorsum. It is responsible for transverse forehead wrinkles over the bridge of the nose. The corrugator supercilii muscle arises from the nasal bones and orbital part of the orbicularis oculi and connects to the skin of the brow. It is responsible for oblique wrinkles of the bridge of the nose.

Muscles of the Mouth, Lips, and Cheeks

Several muscles allow the human mouth to exercise a myriad of movements. The sphincter of the mouth is the orbicularis oris muscle, with fibers that encircle the mouth and lie within the lip. The muscle is responsible for mouth narrowing (as during whistling) and lip tightening (as during speech and mastication). The buccinator muscle works in conjunction with the orbicularis to hold the cheeks against the molar teeth during mastication and whistling. It arises from the pterygomandibular raphe posteriorly and extends to the alveolar processes of the maxilla and mandible. The zygomaticus major and minor muscles originate from the zygomatic arch, insert on the skin of the nasolabial fold, and act to retract the upper lip. The levator labii superioris and levator labii superioris alaeque nasi are more medial and elevate the lip, as well. The depressor anguli oris originates from the mandibular border lateral to the mental nerve and everts the lower lip. The platysma muscle is broad and thin, lying in a subcutaneous plane. It arises inferiorly from the deltoid and pectoralis fascia to extend superiorly to the lower border of the mandible, where it is continuous with the SMAS. The platysma tenses the skin, depresses the mandible, and contributes to inferior retraction of the chin and lower lip.

Muscles around the Orbit

The orbicularis oculi is responsible for closing the eye gently during blinking and squinting, and also for wrinkling the forehead. Its fibers wrap around the eye concentrically, attaching to the medial orbital margin and palpebral ligament. It is divided into three parts: preseptal, pretarsal, and orbital.

8.1.2 Arteries of the Face

The face is known for its abundant blood supply with extensive anastomosis. The major arterial supply is from the facial artery, the fourth branch of the external carotid artery. After branching, the facial artery courses deep to the submandibular gland, then along the inferior border of the mandible in a superficial plane just deep to the platysma until it ascends over the mandible anterior to the masseter muscle attachment. It then travels superomedially, crossing the maxilla and buccinator muscle and finally ending at the medial canthus in an anastomosis with the dorsal nasal branch of the ophthalmic artery. During this ascent, it gives off the superior and inferior labial arteries, which supply the lips and nose. Distal to the superior labial artery, the facial artery is known as the angular artery (▶ Fig. 8.1).

The superficial temporal, occipital, transverse facial, and posterior auricular arteries also supply lateral or superior portions of the face, mainly the scalp. They also originate from the external carotid artery.

8.1.3 Veins of the Face

The retromandibular vein is formed by the union of the superficial temporal and maxillary veins. It runs deep and posterior to the ramus of the mandible, through the parotid gland, deep to the facial nerve. The anterior retromandibular vein and facial vein join to become the common facial vein, with subsequent drainage into the internal jugular vein. The posterior retromandibular vein joins with the posterior auricular vein to become the external jugular vein. The facial vein communicates with the superior ophthalmic vein near the medial canthus, with possible drainage into the cavernous sinus.

8.1.4 Nerves of the Face

Motor Innervation

All of the muscles of facial expression are innervated by the facial nerve (cranial nerve VII). The facial nerve exits the cranium through the stylomastoid foramen between the mastoid tip and styloid process. Before entering the parotid gland, it gives off the posterior auricular nerve, which passes posterosuperiorly towards the ear to supply both the occipital belly of the occipitofrontalis muscle and the posterior auricular muscle. The facial nerve then enters the parotid gland and divides into five terminal branches at the pes anserinus. The temporal branch courses superiorly over the zygomatic arch to supply the frontalis and orbicularis oculi muscles. The zygomatic branch further divides into several branches that supply the inferior orbicularis oculi. The buccal branch courses anteriorly to supply the buccinator muscle and orbicularis oris. The mandibular branch leaves the parotid at its inferior border, then crosses the mandible deep to the platysma within the submandibular gland fascia to innervate the depressor anguli oris. The cervical branch courses inferiorly to supply the platysma muscle. Other than the muscles of facial expression, the facial nerve is responsible for innervation

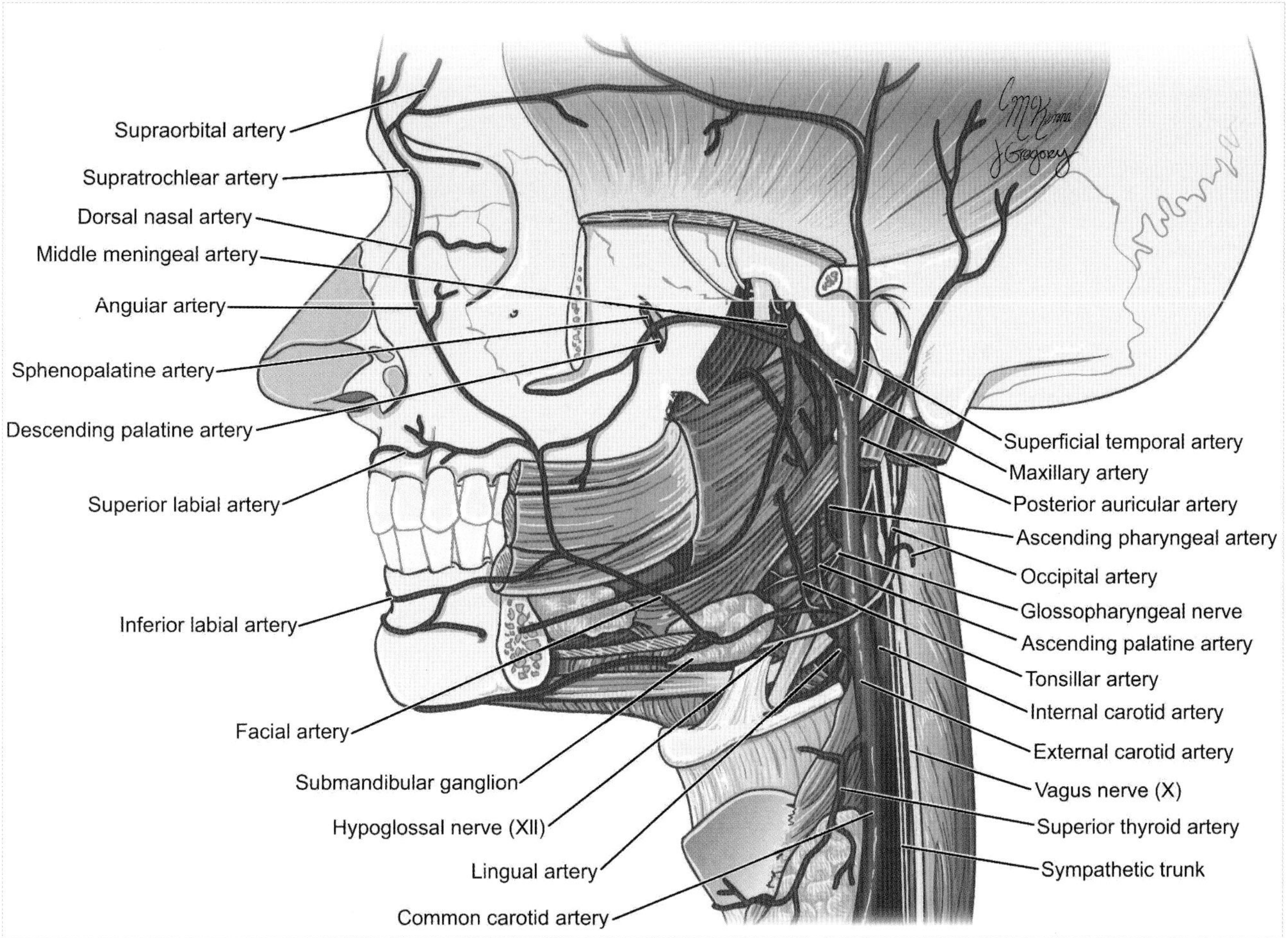

Supraorbital artery
Supratrochlear artery
Dorsal nasal artery
Middle meningeal artery
Angular artery
Sphenopalatine artery
Descending palatine artery
Superior labial artery
Inferior labial artery
Facial artery
Submandibular ganglion
Hypoglossal nerve (XII)
Lingual artery
Common carotid artery
Superficial temporal artery
Maxillary artery
Posterior auricular artery
Ascending pharyngeal artery
Occipital artery
Glossopharyngeal nerve
Ascending palatine artery
Tonsillar artery
Internal carotid artery
External carotid artery
Vagus nerve (X)
Superior thyroid artery
Sympathetic trunk

Fig. 8.1 Arteries of the face.

of the posterior belly of the digastric muscle and of the stylohyoid and stapedius muscles (▶ Fig. 8.2).

Sensory Innervation

The trigeminal nerve (cranial nerve V) is the primary sensory nerve of the face. Cranial nerve V has three branches after leaving the trigeminal ganglion: the ophthalmic nerve (V_1), maxillary nerve (V_2), and mandibular nerve (V_3). V_1 and V_2 are entirely sensory, whereas V_3 contains motor fibers for the muscles of mastication and smaller muscles. The ophthalmic nerve is the smallest and most superior of the three divisions. After leaving the trigeminal ganglion, it enters the orbit via the superior orbital fissure and divides into three terminal branches: nasociliary nerve, frontal nerve, and lacrimal nerve. These nerves supply the nose (via the external nasal nerve and infratrochlear nerve) and the skin of the forehead and upper eyelid (via the lacrimal, supratrochlear, and supraorbital nerves). The maxillary nerve is the intermediate division of the trigeminal ganglion and exits the cranium via the foramen rotundum to enter the pterygopalatine fossa. It gives off branches to the pterygopalatine ganglion and zygomatic nerve before passing into the infraorbital foramen. Before exiting the foramen as the cutaneous infraorbital nerve, it gives off the zygomaticotemporal and zygomaticofacial nerves. It is responsible for sensation of the skin of the temple, upper cheek, lower eyelid, upper lip, maxillary teeth, and mucosa of the maxillary sinus. The mandibular nerve is the most inferior and largest division of the trigeminal ganglion and exits the cranium via the foramen ovale. Its sensory branches include the auriculotemporal, buccal, and inferior alveolar nerves, which supply the lower portion of the face. The auriculotemporal nerve arises from two roots that pass around the middle meningeal artery, through the parotid gland, to the temporal region. It conveys secretomotor fibers to the parotid and sensation to the auricle, external auditory canal, and temporal skin. The buccal and inferior alveolar nerves supply the cheek, buccal gingiva, skin of the chin, lower lip, and labial gingiva (▶ Fig. 8.3 and ▶ Fig. 8.4).

8.2 Nasal Cavity and Paranasal Sinuses

8.2.1 Nasal Cavity

The nasal cavity is entered anteriorly through the nares and posteriorly from the nasopharynx through the choanae. The roof of the nasal cavity is narrow anteriorly, widens intermediately, and narrows posteriorly. The floor of the nose is formed by the palatine bone and maxilla. The medial wall is formed by

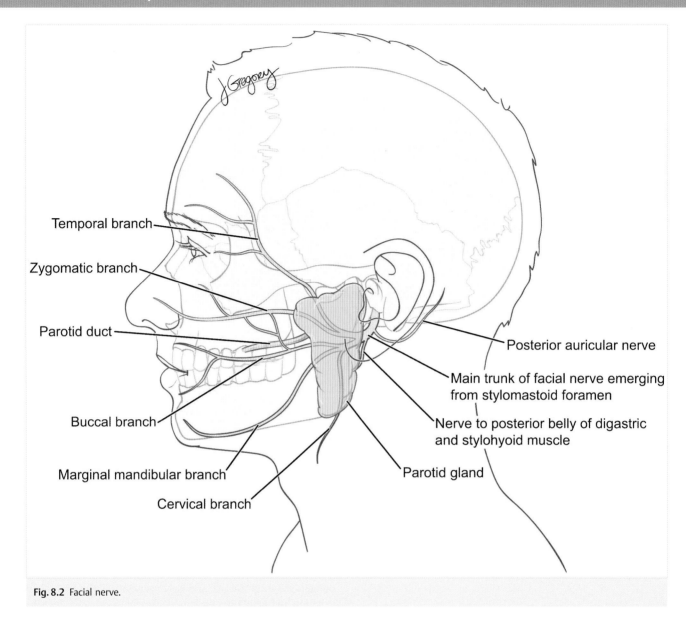

Fig. 8.2 Facial nerve.

the bony and cartilaginous nasal septum. The lateral wall is most intricate, consisting of three bony projections, each covered in respiratory mucosa. These conchae, also called turbinates, are most important for the structures lateral and inferior to them. The inferior turbinate is a separate bone and plays an important role in the nasal cycle, given the abundance of vascular sinusoids within its substance. The nasolacrimal duct opens inferolateral to the inferior turbinate in the inferior meatus. The middle turbinate is part of the ethmoid bone and is important as a landmark in endoscopic sinus surgery. Lateral to the middle turbinate, the bulla ethmoidalis is found bulging from the lateral wall. Inferior to this bulge rests an opening known as the hiatus semilunaris, which leads laterally into the ethmoid infundibulum. The frontal, maxillary, and anterior ethmoid sinus air cells also empty into this space. The superior turbinate contains both respiratory epithelium and olfactory mucosa along its upper surface. Posterosuperior to the superior concha lies the sphenoethmoidal recess, into which drain the sphenoid and posterior ethmoid cells.

8.2.2 Paranasal Sinuses

The paranasal sinuses are air-filled continuations of the nasal cavity and are typically named for the bone within which they exist. They are lined by ciliated respiratory epithelium, which allows them to pass secretions into a designated ostium for entrance into the nasal cavity. The frontal sinus lies between the anterior and posterior tables of the frontal bone and is not present at birth; it is usually detectable only after the age of 6 years. Each frontal sinus drains into a frontonasal duct that empties into the ethmoid infundibulum. The ethmoid sinus is actually made up of several smaller cells that pneumatize the ethmoid bone between the nasal cavity and orbit. The lateral wall of the ethmoid cells is an extremely thin bone known as the lamina papyracea. The ethmoid sinus is divided into anterior and posterior ethmoid air cells by the posterior bony attachment of the middle turbinate to the medial orbit, known as the basal lamella. The sphenoid sinuses are located in the body of the sphenoid bone and can be divided unevenly by a bony

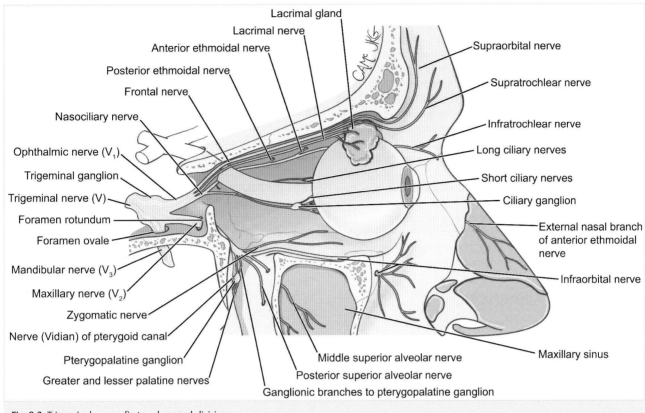

Fig. 8.3 Trigeminal nerve: first and second divisions.

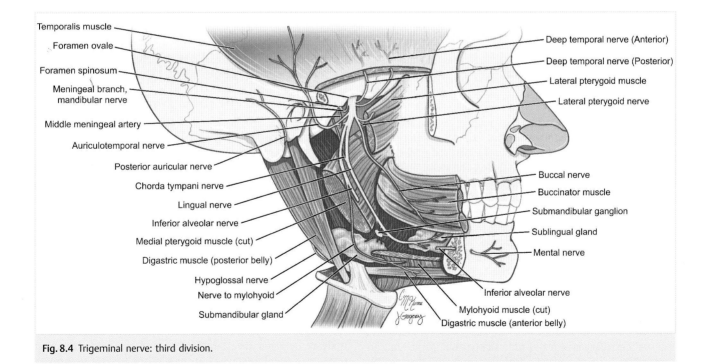

Fig. 8.4 Trigeminal nerve: third division.

septum. The sphenoid is bordered posteriorly by the sella turcica and laterally by the cavernous sinus (with associated nerves), optic chiasm, and internal carotid arteries. The maxillary sinuses are the largest sinuses. They are located within the maxilla below the orbit and above the alveolus.

8.2.3 Arteries and Veins of the Nasal Cavity and Paranasal Sinuses

The arterial supply of the nasal cavity comprises four main divisions. First, the sphenopalatine artery (branch of the internal maxillary artery) enters the nasal cavity on the lateral wall be-behind the middle turbinate via the sphenopalatine foramen. Once entering the nose, it typically divides into two branches supplying the posterior and lateral portions of the nasal cavity along with the septum. The anterior and posterior ethmoidal arteries are branches of the ophthalmic artery from the internal carotid system. They supply the superior and lateral nasal wall along with the superior concha and septum. The greater palatine artery is a branch of the internal maxillary artery that supplies the floor of the maxillary sinus. The superior labial branch of the facial artery supplies the anterior nasal cavity, including both lateral wall and septum. Anteriorly along the septum, the vessels anastomose to form the Kiesselbach plexus, the most common site for anterior epistaxis.

The venous drainage of the nose is through a rich plexus deep to the nasal mucosa that ultimately drains into the sphenopalatine, facial, and ophthalmic veins. These vessels are important for both thermoregulation and humidification.

8.2.4 Sensory Innervation

The anterosuperior part of the nasal cavity is innervated by the anterior and posterior ethmoidal branches of the nasociliary nerve (V_1). The posteroinferior and lateral part is innervated by the maxillary nerve (V_2). The septum is also innervated by the maxillary nerve (V_2) via the nasopalatine branch. The frontal sinuses are innervated by branches of the supraorbital nerve (V_1). The ethmoid and sphenoid sinuses are innervated by anterior and posterior ethmoidal branches of the nasociliary nerve (V_1). The maxillary sinuses are innervated by the anterior, middle, and posterior superior alveolar nerves, which are branches of the maxillary nerve (V_2).

8.3 Salivary Glands

8.3.1 Parotid Gland

The parotid gland lies between the ramus of the mandible and the temporal bone landmarks of the external auditory canal and mastoid tip. Anteriorly, it is found superficial to the masseter muscle, and posteriorly, it rests over the sternocleidomastoid muscle. Medially, the parotid gland can extend as deep as the pharyngeal wall. It is incompletely surrounded by parotid gland fascia, a continuation of the superficial or investing layer of deep cervical fascia. The parotid duct, or Stenson duct, passes over the masseter muscle, runs in close proximity to the buccal branch of the facial nerve, pierces the buccinator muscle, and empties into the oral cavity opposite the second maxillary molar. Within the parotid gland are several important structures. The facial nerve divides the parotid into superficial and deep lobes. The external carotid artery divides into its terminal branches—the superficial temporal and internal maxillary arteries—within the parotid gland. The retromandibular vein is formed from the union of the superficial temporal and maxillary veins within the gland. It travels deep to the facial nerve before dividing into anterior and posterior branches.

8.3.2 Submandibular Gland

The submandibular gland lies within the submandibular triangle of the neck, below the mylohyoid muscle and superior to the anterior and posterior digastric muscle. It is covered by the investing layer of deep cervical fascia, which also contains the marginal mandibular branch of the facial nerve. The submandibular duct, or Wharton duct, which arises from the portion of the gland that lies between the mylohyoid and hyoglossus muscles, travels anteriorly to open lateral to the frenulum in the anterior portion of the floor of the mouth behind the incisors. As it travels in a lateral to medial direction, the lingual nerve is found to loop under the duct. The arterial supply for the gland is the submental artery.

8.3.3 Sublingual and Minor Salivary Glands

The sublingual glands are located within the submucosal layer of the floor of the mouth between the mandible and the genioglossus muscle. There are numerous small sublingual ducts that open in the floor of mouth. The arterial supply of the sublingual glands comes from the sublingual and submental arteries. Minor salivary glands lie within the submucosal layer of the oral cavity, oropharynx, nasopharynx, and hypopharynx.

8.3.4 Parasympathetic Innervation

Parotid Gland

The preganglionic fibers begin in the medulla at the inferior salivatory nucleus. They travel along the glossopharyngeal nerve into the tympanic plexus (Jacobson nerve), then course through the lesser superficial petrosal nerve through the foramen ovale to synapse on the otic ganglion. From here, postganglionic parasympathetic fibers travel along the auriculotemporal nerve (branch of V_3) to reach the parotid gland.

Submandibular and Sublingual Glands

The preganglionic fibers begin in the pons at the superior salivatory nucleus. They travel along the facial nerve, then course with the chorda tympani nerve to join the lingual nerve. The fibers synapse on the submandibular ganglion, located near the submandibular gland. From here, postganglionic parasympathetic fibers travel to the submandibular gland directly and to the sublingual gland via branches of the lingual nerve.

8.4 Thyroid Gland

The thyroid gland is located deep to the sternohyoid and sternothyroid, anterior and lateral to the trachea, approximately midway between the sternal notch and thyroid cartilage. It consists of two lobes, which meet over the trachea to form an isthmus, usually over the second and third tracheal rings. The thyroid is surrounded by its own fibrous capsule, which is just deep to the visceral layer of the pretracheal layer of the deep cervical fascia. In approximately half of individuals, a small amount of thyroid tissue, known as a pyramidal lobe, extends superiorly from the isthmus or either lobe. The thyroid gland is supplied by the superior and inferior thyroid arteries, and occasionally by a thyroid ima artery. Venous drainage is typically from the superior, middle, and inferior thyroid veins. The important structures that lie immediately around the thyroid gland include the four parathyroid glands; these lie deep to the thyroid lobes and the paired recurrent laryngeal nerves, which course in the tracheoesophageal groove to reach the larynx (▶ Fig. 8.5).

8.5 Parathyroid Glands

The parathyroid glands usually lie external to the thyroid capsule on the medial half of the posterior surface of the each thyroid lobe. The superior parathyroid glands, which have a more reliable position, can usually be found at the level of the inferior border of the cricoid cartilage, approximately 1 cm superior to the entrance of the inferior thyroid artery into the thyroid gland. The inferior parathyroid glands, which are more unpredictable, are usually near the inferior pole of the thyroid lobe, approximately 1 cm inferior to the entrance of the inferior thyroid artery into the thyroid gland. Most people have four parathyroid glands; however, approximately 5% have more than four glands. In addition, the position of each parathyroid gland can be quite variable. The superior parathyroid glands arise from the fourth branchial pouch and descend with the thyroid gland, so they may be directly embedded within the thyroid gland. They can also be located in a retroesophageal, retropharyngeal, or retrolaryngeal position. The inferior parathyroid glands arise from the third branchial pouch with the thymus, so they can be located in the anterior mediastinum or within the thyroid. The parathyroid glands are supplied primarily by the inferior thyroid artery. The venous drainage is through the parathyroid veins, which empty into the thyroid venous plexus.

8.6 Oral Cavity

The oral cavity begins anteriorly at the lips and extends posterosuperiorly to the junction of the hard palate and soft palate, and posteroinferiorly to the circumvallate papillae of the tongue. The mylohyoid muscle forms the floor, and the buccinator muscles border the oral cavity laterally. The oral cavity can be broken down into several subsites, which include the lips, buccal mucosa, alveolar ridge, retromolar trigone, hard palate, oral tongue, and floor of the mouth.

8.6.1 Oral Tongue

The anterior two-thirds of the tongue develop separately from the posterior one-third. Whereas the anterior two-thirds are covered with foliate, filiform, and fungiform papillae, the posterior one-third is mostly lymphoid tissue.

Muscles of the Oral Tongue

The tongue itself is actually a mass of muscles covered by mucous membrane. The muscles of the tongue do not act in isolation; rather, a collaboration of many muscles gives the tongue its unique versatility. The musculature can be divided into intrinsic and extrinsic muscles. In general, the extrinsic muscles, such as the genioglossus, hyoglossus, styloglossus, and palatoglossus muscles, alter the position of the tongue. The intrinsic muscles, including the superior and inferior longitudinal, transverse, and vertical muscles, alter the shape of the tongue. The genioglossus contributes most of the bulk of the tongue and is responsible for protrusion, depression, and deviation of the tongue. The hyoglossus, acting with its attachment to the hyoid bone, is responsible for depression and retraction. The styloglossus, acting with its attachment to the styloid process, retracts and elevates the tongue. In conjunction with the genioglossus muscle, the styloglossus allows curling of the tongue sides to create a trough during swallowing. The palatoglossus arises from the palatine aponeurosis and acts more to depress the palate than to elevate the posterior tongue during swallowing.

Vasculature of the Oral Tongue

The arterial supply to the oral tongue comes mainly via branches of the lingual artery from the external carotid artery. The main branches include the dorsal lingual, deep lingual, and sublingual arteries. The lingual artery is unique in that it courses medial to the hyoglossus muscle rather than lateral like most of the other vessels and nerves. The venous drainage is mainly through the dorsal and deep lingual veins.

Innervation of the Tongue

Sensory innervation of the tongue is divided into general sensation and special sensation or taste. General sensation of the anterior two-thirds of the tongue is provided by the lingual nerve, a branch of the mandibular nerve (V_3). The posterior one-third and circumvallate papillae are supplied by the lingual branch of the glossopharyngeal nerve. For special sensation (taste), the anterior two-thirds is supplied by the chorda tympani nerve, a branch of the facial nerve. The posterior one-third of taste sensation is supplied by the glossopharyngeal nerve. All the muscles of the tongue except the palatoglossus muscle derive their motor innervation via the hypoglossal nerve or cranial nerve XII.

8.6.2 Floor of the Mouth

The floor of mouth is formed primarily from the mylohyoid and geniohyoid muscles. The mylohyoid extends from the anterior portion of the hyoid bone to the inner surface of the mandible. Its contraction elevates the hyoid bone, floor of the mouth, and tongue during swallowing and speaking. The sublingual gland and a portion of the submandibular gland lie above the mylohyoid muscle. The lingual nerve enters the oral cavity medial to the third mandibular molar. It initially lies superior and lateral to the submandibular duct but subsequently dives inferior then medial to the duct. The hypoglossal nerve enters the oral cavity lateral to the hyoglossus muscle then superior to the mylohyoid muscle below the submandibular duct.

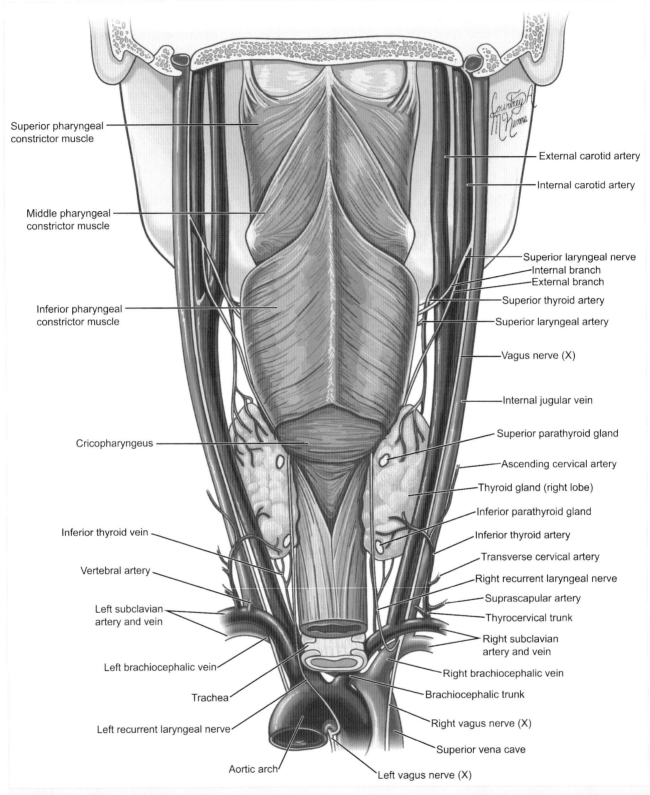

Superior pharyngeal constrictor muscle

Middle pharyngeal constrictor muscle

Inferior pharyngeal constrictor muscle

Cricopharyngeus

Inferior thyroid vein

Vertebral artery

Left subclavian artery and vein

Left brachiocephalic vein

Trachea

Left recurrent laryngeal nerve

Aortic arch

External carotid artery

Internal carotid artery

Superior laryngeal nerve
Internal branch
External branch
Superior thyroid artery

Superior laryngeal artery

Vagus nerve (X)

Internal jugular vein

Superior parathyroid gland

Ascending cervical artery

Thyroid gland (right lobe)

Inferior parathyroid gland

Inferior thyroid artery

Transverse cervical artery

Right recurrent laryngeal nerve

Suprascapular artery

Thyrocervical trunk

Right subclavian artery and vein

Right brachiocephalic vein

Brachiocephalic trunk

Right vagus nerve (X)

Superior vena cava

Left vagus nerve (X)

Fig. 8.5 Posterior aspect of the visceral compartment of the neck.

Table 8.1 Structures that pass into the pharynx between the pharyngeal constrictors

Gaps between pharyngeal constrictors	Structures that pass to the pharynx
Skull base to superior constrictor	Levator palatini muscle, eustachian tube, ascending pharyngeal artery
Superior to middle constrictor	Stylopharyngeus muscle, stylohyoid ligament, glossopharyngeal nerve
Middle to inferior constrictor	Superior laryngeal branch of superior thyroid artery, internal branch of superior laryngeal nerve
Below inferior constrictor	Inferior laryngeal branch of inferior thyroid artery, recurrent laryngeal nerve

Innervation of Floor of the Mouth and Rest of Oral Cavity

The lingual nerve (V_3) supplies sensation to the floor of mouth, lingual aspect of the lower alveolar ridge, and mucosa of the lip. The buccal nerve (V_3) supplies sensation to the buccal mucosa and buccal margin of the upper and lower alveolar ridges. The infraorbital nerve (V_2) carries sensation for the upper lip mucosa and the most anterior part of the upper oral cavity. The mental nerve (V_3) supplies the mucosa of the lower lip and the most anterior portions of the lower oral cavity. Motor innervation to the floor of the mouth muscles (mylohyoid and anterior belly of the digastric) is by the mandibular nerve (V_3). The geniohyoid is innervated by the cervical roots from C1 carried by the hypoglossal nerve.

8.7 Pharynx

The pharynx lies posterior to and communicates with the nasal cavity, oral cavity, and larynx. It extends from the skull base to the inferior border of the cricoid cartilage anteriorly and the inferior border of the C6 vertebra posteriorly. Posteriorly, the pharynx is bordered by the buccopharyngeal fascia and retropharyngeal space. This fascia and space allow the pharynx to move along the vertebral column. The buccopharyngeal fascia is continuous with the pretracheal layer of deep cervical fascia inferiorly. The pharynx is made up of mucosa (either ciliated columnar or stratified squamous) and pharyngeal muscles.

8.7.1 Muscles of the Pharynx

The muscles of the pharynx consist of an inner longitudinal layer and an outer circular layer. The inner muscular layer mainly consists of the palatopharyngeus, stylopharyngeus, and salpingopharyngeus muscles. These muscles are responsible for elevation of the larynx and shortening of the pharynx during swallowing and speaking. The outer circular layer consists of the three pharyngeal constrictor muscles: superior, middle, and inferior. The muscles are bordered internally by the strong pharyngobasilar fascia and externally by the thin buccopharyngeal fascia. The pharyngeal constrictor muscles contract involuntarily and in a sequential fashion to propel food into the esophagus. The superior constrictor originates from the pterygoid hamulus and pterygomandibular raphe. The middle constrictor originates from the stylohyoid ligament and hyoid bone. The inferior constrictor originates from the thyroid and cricoid cartilages. Posteriorly, the pharyngeal muscles insert into the median raphe of the pharynx. The muscles overlap so that the inferior fibers of one muscle are inside the superior fibers of the next (▶ Fig. 8.5). This allows food to be propelled more

efficiently. The structures that must pass between the pharyngeal constrictors to reach the pharynx are detailed in ▶ Table 8.1 and ▶ Fig. 8.6.

8.7.2 Innervation of the Pharynx

The nerve supply to the pharynx, motor and most sensory, derives from the pharyngeal plexus. The pharyngeal plexus is made up of branches of the glossopharyngeal nerve (IX), vagus nerve (X), maxillary nerve (V_2), and postganglionic sympathetic fibers from the sympathetic trunk. Motor fibers from the cranial root of the accessory nerve are carried by the vagus nerve via pharyngeal branches to supply all the pharyngeal muscles except the stylopharyngeus (IX) and tensor veli palatini (V_3). Sensory innervation of the upper part of the nasopharynx is derived from the maxillary nerve (V_2). Sensory innervation of the rest of the nasopharynx, oropharynx, and hypopharynx is derived from the glossopharyngeal nerve. The piriform sinus sensory innervaton is primarily from the vagus nerve through the internal branch of the superior laryngeal nerve.

8.7.3 Nasopharynx

The nasopharynx is the posterior extension of the nasal cavities through the choanae to the level of the soft palate. The roof and posterior wall of the nasopharynx lie inferior to the body of the sphenoid bone. The lateral wall of the nasopharynx is marked by the torus tubarius, a bulge created by the cartilage of the eustachian tube. Extending inferiorly from the medial end of the eustachian tube is a vertical fold of mucous membrane known as the salpingopharyngeal fold. Posterior to the torus tubarius and the salpingopharyngeal fold is a slitlike lateral projection known as the pharyngeal recess or fossa of Rosenmuller. Posteriorly and superiorly lie the adenoids, part of the Waldeyer ring.

8.7.4 Oropharynx

The oropharynx is bounded by the soft palate superiorly and the superior border of the epiglottis inferiorly. Anteriorly, the oropharynx extends to the sulcus terminalis and includes the posterior one-third of the tongue. The posterior one-third of the tongue is continuous with the epiglottis via the vallecula formed by the three glossoepiglottic folds. The lateral walls of the oropharynx are marked by the palatine tonsils, which reside between the tonsillar pillars, palatoglossus, and palatopharyngeus muscles. The blood supply to the tonsil is via branches of the lingual, facial, ascending pharyngeal, and internal maxillary arteries. The soft palate is composed of muscle that allows depression, elevation, and contraction during swallowing and phonation. The

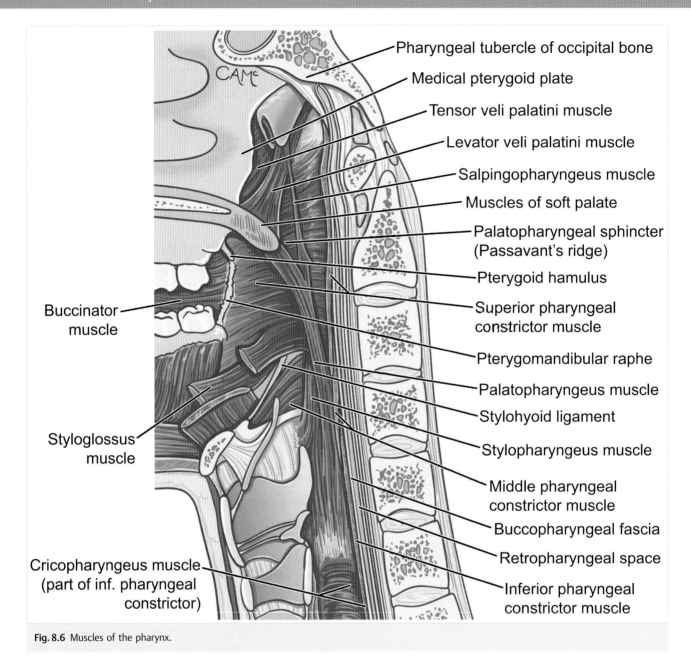

CAMc

Pharyngeal tubercle of occipital bone

Medical pterygoid plate

Tensor veli palatini muscle

Levator veli palatini muscle

Salpingopharyngeus muscle

Muscles of soft palate

Palatopharyngeal sphincter (Passavant's ridge)

Pterygoid hamulus

Superior pharyngeal constrictor muscle

Pterygomandibular raphe

Palatopharyngeus muscle

Stylohyoid ligament

Stylopharyngeus muscle

Middle pharyngeal constrictor muscle

Buccopharyngeal fascia

Retropharyngeal space

Inferior pharyngeal constrictor muscle

Buccinator muscle

Styloglossus muscle

Cricopharyngeus muscle (part of inf. pharyngeal constrictor)

Fig. 8.6 Muscles of the pharynx.

tensor veli palatini arises from the scaphoid fossa of the medial pterygoid plate and descends in the nasopharynx and nasal cavity to attach to the palatine aponeurosis. It is responsible for tensing the soft palate and opening the eustachian tube. The levator veli palatani muscle arises from the petrous portion of the temporal bone and passes between the superior and middle constrictors to attach to the palatine aponeurosis. It functions to elevate the soft palate during swallowing. The palatoglossus muscle arises from the palatine aponeurosis and extends inferiorly to attach to the side of the tongue. It is responsible for elevating the posterior part of the tongue and depressing the soft palate. The palatopharyngeus muscle arises from the palatine aponeurosis and hard palate and attaches to the longitudinal layer of lateral pharyngeal wall. It functions to tense the soft palate and pulls the pharyngeal wall superiorly, anteriorly, and medially during swallowing. The musculus uvulae arises from the posterior nasal

spine and palatine aponeurosis. It functions to shorten and elevate the uvula. The blood supply to the soft palate is mainly from the ascending palatine branches of the facial artery and palatine branches of the internal maxillary artery.

8.7.5 Hypopharynx

The hypopharynx is a continuation of the oropharynx and lies posterior and lateral to the larynx. It extends from the superior border of the epiglottis and pharyngoepiglottic folds to the inferior border of the cricoid cartilage. Its posterior and lateral walls are formed by the middle and inferior pharyngeal constrictors. The piriform sinus is a small pyramid-shaped depression on either side of the larynx, separated by the aryepiglottic folds. Laterally, the piriform sinus is bordered by the medial surface of the thyroid cartilage and thyrohyoid membrane.

Table 8.2 Intrinsic laryngeal muscles

Muscle	Attachments	Functions
Posterior cricoarytenoid muscle	Muscular process of the arytenoid, posterior surface of cricoid lamina	Sole vocal fold abductor
Lateral cricoarytenoid muscle	Muscular process of the arytenoid, cricoid arch (anterior)	Adducts vocal folds
Thyroarytenoid muscle	Muscular process of the arytenoid, posterior surface of thyroid cartilage	Decreases length and tension of vocal folds
Vocalis muscle (part of thyroarytenoid)	Vocal process of the arytenoids, vocal ligaments	Fine control of vocal fold tension
Interarytenoid muscle	Between the bodies of the two arytenoids	Adducts vocal folds
Cricothyroid muscle	Inferior margin and inferior horn of thyroid cartilage, anterior part of cricoid cartilage	Stretches and tenses vocal folds

8.8 Larynx

The larynx lies in the anterior neck at the level of the bodies of the C3 to C6 vertebrae. It extends internally from the superior border of the epiglottis to the inferior border of the cricoid cartilage. It is continuous with the trachea below the cricoid cartilage and with the hypopharynx through the laryngeal inlet. The supraglottis extends from the epiglottis to the apex of the laryngeal ventricle between the two infoldings of mucous membrane, the false (vestibular) and true vocal folds. The glottis extends from the apex of the laryngeal ventricle to 1 cm inferiorly. The space between the true vocal folds is known as the rima glottidis. Each wedge-shaped vocal fold is made up of squamous epithelium, superficial lamina propria, vocal ligament, and vocalis muscle. The subglottis begins 1 cm below the laryngeal ventricle and extends to the inferior border of the cricoid cartilage. Phonation and airway protection are mediated through a variety of muscles tethered to laryngeal cartilages.

8.8.1 Laryngeal Cartilages

The laryngeal skeleton consists of nine cartilages joined by ligaments and membranes. The thryoid, cricoid and epiglottic cartilages are singular while the arytenoid, corniculate, and cuneiform cartilages are duplicated bilaterally. The thyroid cartilage is the largest of these and is made up of two laminae that join in the midline to form the laryngeal prominence. The superior border of the thyroid cartilage attaches to the hyoid bone by the thyrohyoid membrane. It attaches inferiorly to the cricoid cartilage by the cricothyroid membrane and cricothyroid joint. The cricoid cartilage is a complete ring of cartilage that lies below the thyroid cartilage. It is made up of a tall posterior lamina and a shorter anterior arch. The arytenoid cartilages are pairs of three-sided pyramids that articulate with the posterior lamina of the cricoid cartilage. Each cartilage has an apex superiorly that articulates with the corniculate and cuneiform cartilages, an anterior vocal process that forms the posterior margin of the vocal fold, and a lateral muscular process where the posterior and lateral cricoarytenoid muscles attach.

8.8.2 Muscles of the Larynx

The muscles of the larynx can be divided into extrinsic and intrinsic muscles. The extrinsic muscles include the suprahyoid and infrahyoid muscles. The suprahyoid muscles include the mylohyoid, stylohyoid, geniohyoid, and digastric muscles. They act together to elevate the hyoid and larynx during swallowing and phonation. The infrahyoid muscles include the omohyoid, sternohyoid, sternothyroid, and thyrohyoid muscles. They act together to depress the hyoid and larynx. The intrinsic laryngeal musculature is detailed in ▶ Table 8.2.

8.8.3 Vasculature of the Larynx

The superior thyroid artery with its superior laryngeal branch supplies the superior part of the larynx and cricothyroid muscle. The inferior thyroid artery with its inferior laryngeal branch supplies the inferior part of the larynx. Laryngeal veins accompany the arteries to drain to the internal jugular vein or left brachiocephalic vein (▶ Fig. 8.7).

8.8.4 Innervation of the Larynx

Sensory innervation for the larynx above the vocal folds is carried by the internal branch of the superior laryngeal nerve of the vagus nerve. The sensory innervation below the level of the vocal folds is carried by the recurrent laryngeal nerve of the vagus nerve. Motor innervation for all intrinsic laryngeal musculature except the cricothyroid muscle is by the recurrent laryngeal nerve of the vagus nerve. The cricothyroid muscle is innervated by the external branch of the superior laryngeal nerve of the vagus nerve.

8.9 Neck

The neck extends from the inferior border of the mandible and skull base to the clavicles inferiorly. It is divided into anterior and posterior triangles by the sternocleidomastoid muscle and into smaller triangles by the omohyoid and digastric muscles. The anterior triangle is bordered by the anterior border of the sternocleidomastoid muscle laterally, the inferior margin of the mandible superiorly, and the clavicle inferiorly. The posterior triangle is bordered by the posterior margin of the sternocleidomastoid muscle medially, the anterior margin of the trapezius muscle laterally, the skull base superiorly, and the clavicle laterally (middle one-third). The anterior and posterior triangles can be subdivided into smaller triangles (▶ Table 8.3).

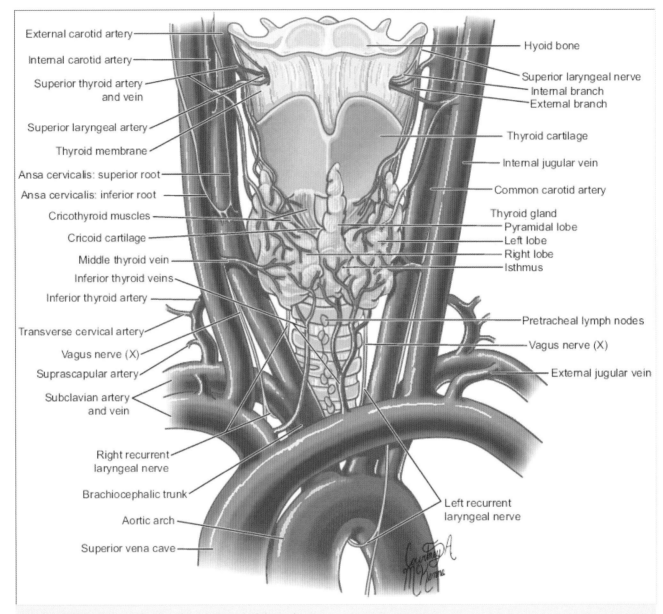

External carotid artery

Internal carotid artery

Superior thyroid artery and vein

Superior laryngeal artery

Thyroid membrane

Ansa cervicalis: superior root

Ansa cervicalis: inferior root

Cricothyroid muscles

Cricoid cartilage

Middle thyroid vein

Inferior thyroid veins

Inferior thyroid artery

Transverse cervical artery

Vagus nerve (X)

Suprascapular artery

Subclavian artery and vein

Right recurrent laryngeal nerve

Brachiocephalic trunk

Aortic arch

Superior vena cave

Hyoid bone

Superior laryngeal nerve
Internal branch
External branch

Thyroid cartilage

Internal jugular vein

Common carotid artery

Thyroid gland
Pyramidal lobe
Left lobe
Right lobe
Isthmus

Pretracheal lymph nodes

Vagus nerve (X)

External jugular vein

Left recurrent laryngeal nerve

Fig. 8.7 Anterior aspect of the visceral compartment of the neck.

8.9.1 Fascia of the Neck (▶ Fig. 8.8 and ▶ Fig. 8.9)

Superficial Cervical Fascia

The superficial cervical fascia is a thin layer of connective tissue that separates the dermis from the investing layer of the deep cervical fascia. Within this layer run cutaneous blood vessels and nerves surrounded by subcutaneous fat. Anterolaterally, it envelopes the platysma muscle.

Deep Cervical Fascia

The deep cervical fascia consists of three fascial layers: investing, pretracheal, and prevertebral. All three layers come together to form the carotid sheath around the common carotid arteries, internal jugular vein, and vagus nerve.

Investing (Superficial) Layer of Deep Cervical Fascia

The investing fascia lies below the superficial cervical fascia and surrounds the entire neck. It splits to form deep and superficial layers to invest the trapezius, sternocleidomastoid, submandibular glands, and parotid glands. Superiorly, the investing layer attaches to the superior nuchal line, mastoid process, zygomatic arches, mandible, hyoid bone, and spinous processes of the vertebrae. Inferiorly, it attaches to the manubrium of the sternum, the clavicles, and the spines of the scapulae.

Pretracheal Layer of Deep Cervical Fascia

The pretracheal layer is in the anterior part of the neck and is further divided into a visceral layer and a muscular layer. The visceral layer encloses the thyroid gland, trachea, and

Table 8.3 Neck triangles

Triangle	Borders	Contents
Posterior triangle		
Occipital	Trapezius, posterior border of sternocleidomastoid, inferior belly of omohyoid muscle	External jugular vein, posterior branches of cervical plexus, accessory nerve, trunks of brachial plexus, transverse cervical artery, occipital artery, lymph nodes
Supraclavicular	Inferior belly of omohyoid muscle, posterior border of sternocleidomastoid, clavicle	Third part of subclavian artery, suprascapular artery, lymph nodes
Anterior triangle		
Submental	Midline, anterior belly of digastric muscle, hyoid bone	Small veins en route to anterior jugular vein, lymph nodes
Submandibular or digastric	Mandible, anterior and posterior bellies of digastric muscle	Submandibular gland, hypoglossal nerve, mylohyoid nerve, facial artery (deep to submandibular gland) and vein (superficial to submandibular gland)
Carotid	Anterior border of sternocleidomastoid, posterior belly of digastric muscle, superior belly of omohyoid muscle	Carotid sheath (common carotid artery, internal jugular vein, vagus nerve), external carotid artery and branches, hypoglossal nerve, superior ansa cervicalis, accessory nerve, thyroid, larynx, pharynx, lymph nodes
Muscular	Superior belly of omohyoid muscle, anterior border of sternocleidomastoid, midline	Sternohyoid, sternothyroid, thyroid and parathyroid glands

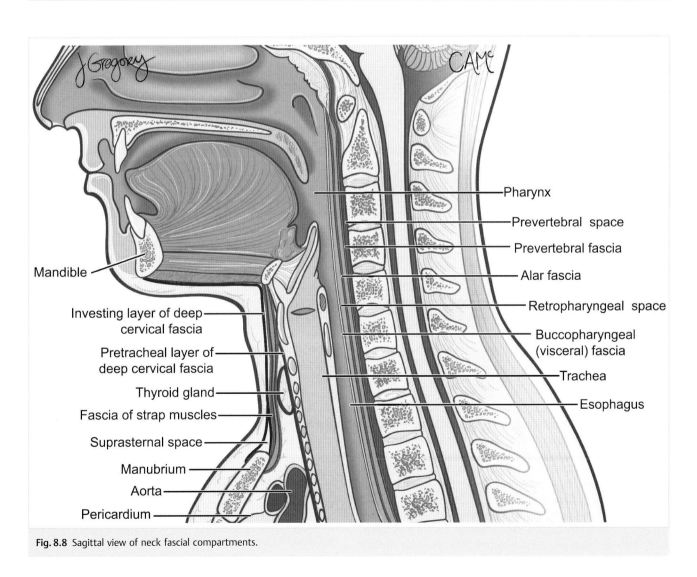

Fig. 8.8 Sagittal view of neck fascial compartments.

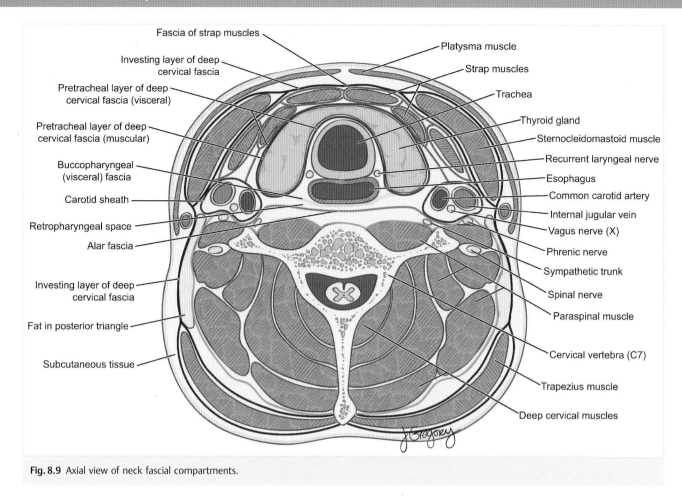

Fig. 8.9 Axial view of neck fascial compartments.

esophagus. It is continuous with the buccopharyngeal fascia of the pharynx. The muscular layer encloses the infrahyoid muscles and forms the tendons that divide the anterior and posterior bellies of the digastric and the inferior and superior bellies of the omohyoid.

Prevertebral Layer of Deep Cervical Fascia

The prevertebral layer envelopes the vertebral column and paraspinal musculature. It extends from the skull base to the T3 vertebra.

8.9.2 Muscles of the Neck

The superficial muscles of the neck include the platysma, sternocleidomastoid, and trapezius muscles. The platysma lies in the subcutaneous tissue to cover the anterolateral portion of the neck. Its fibers originate from the fascia covering the deltoid and pectoralis major muscles inferiorly. Superiorly, the platysma extends over mandible to blend with the fascial muscles and SMAS while leaving an anterior gap for the larynx. It acts to tense the skin and depress the mandible. The sternocleidomastoid is a straplike muscle that attaches superiorly to the mastoid process of the temporal bone and superior nuchal line. Inferiorly, it divides into two heads—sternal and clavicular (middle third)—which are named for their attachments. Each sternocleidomastoid muscle acts independently to flex and rotate the

head and neck so that the ear approaches the shoulder and the chin faces the opposite side. Acting together, the sternocleidomastoid muscles can flex the head and protrude the chin. The trapezius muscle is large triangular muscle located in the posterolateral aspect of the neck and thorax. Superiorly and medially, the trapezius attaches to the superior nuchal line, ligamentum nuchae, spinous processes of C7 to C12, and lumbar and sacral spinous processes. Inferiorly and laterally, the trapezius attaches to the lateral third of the clavicle, acromion, and spine of the scapula. It acts to elevate (superior fibers), retract (middle fibers), and rotate (inferior fibers) the shoulder via the scapula.

The muscles of the posterior triangle include the splenius capitis, levator scapulae, and scalene muscles. The scalene muscles (anterior, middle, and posterior) attach to the cervical spine and first rib. The roots of the brachial plexus and subclavian artery pass between the anterior and middle scalene muscles. The subclavian vein and phrenic nerve pass anterior to the anterior scalene (▶ Fig. 8.10).

8.9.3 Vasculature of the Neck

Arteries

The main arteries of the neck originate at the arch of the aorta. The three main branches are the left common carotid, left subclavian, and brachiocephalic arteries. The brachiocephalic artery gives rise to the right subclavian and common carotid

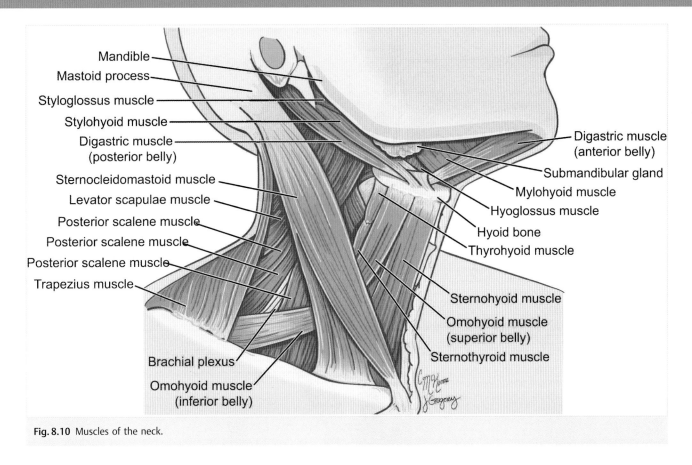

Fig. 8.10 Muscles of the neck.

arteries. The common carotid arteries course superiorly in the neck to approximately the level of the thyroid cartilage before dividing into the internal and external carotids. The internal carotid artery has no branches in the neck. It enters the skull through the carotid canals to supply the brain and orbital structures. A slight dilatation in the proximal portion of the internal carotid artery, the carotid sinus, contains blood pressure sensors. The carotid body, which lies at the bifurcation, has chemoreceptors sensitive to changes in oxygenation. The external carotid artery runs posterosuperiorly in the neck behind the mandible and anterior to the auricle before dividing into its two terminal branches: the maxillary and superficial temporal arteries. The branches of the external carotid artery and their distribution are detailed in ▶ Table 8.4 and ▶ Fig. 8.11.

The subclavian arteries supply the limbs, neck, and brain. In the neck, the four main branches include the vertebral artery, internal thoracic artery, thyrocervical trunk, and costocervical trunk. The vertebral artery arises from the first part of the subclavian and ascends along the scalene and longus muscles before entering the foramina of the transverse processes of C1 to C6 to enter the cranium via the foramen magnum. It is the main supply to the posterior part of the brain and brainstem. The internal thoracic artery passes into the thorax to supply the anterior chest wall and abdominal wall. The thyrocervical trunk has three main branches: the inferior thyroid artery (supplies thyroid), transverse cervical artery (supplies trapezius), and suprascapular artery (supplies scapula). The costocervical trunk arises from the posterior aspect of the second part of the

Table 8.4 Branches of the external carotid artery

Branch	Structures supplied
Superior thyroid	Supplies upper thyroid; superior laryngeal branch pierces thyrohyoid membrane to supply superior larynx
Ascending pharyngeal	Supplies pharynx
Lingual	Passes behind posterior edge of hyoglossus to supply tongue and floor of mouth
Facial	Passes deep to submandibular gland over the mandible to supply face
Occipital	Supplies scalp and back of head
Posterior auricular	Passes behind auricle to supply scalp
Superficial temporal	Crosses zygomatic arch, passes anterior to auricle to supply scalp
Internal maxillary	Passes medially into infratemporal fossa with several branches supplying deep face structures

subclavian to supply the first two intercostal spaces and the posterior deep cervical muscles.

Veins

The venous drainage of the neck is similar to the arterial supply in that each artery usually has a corresponding vein. For details, please refer to the section on venous drainage of the face.

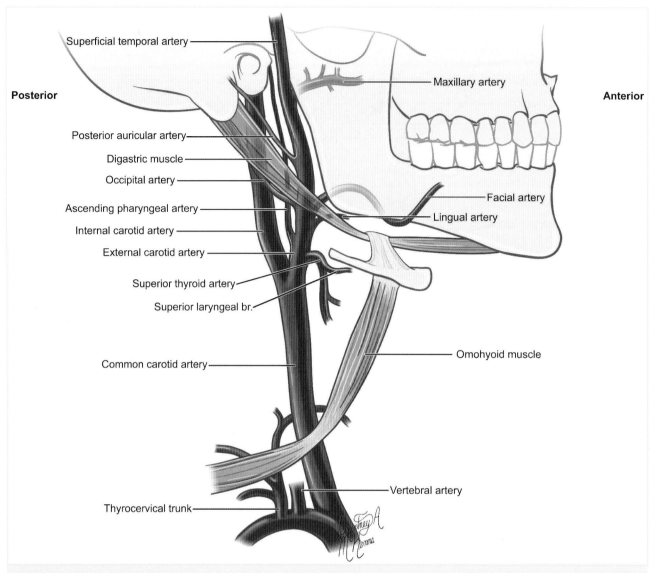

Fig. 8.11 Branches of the external carotid artery.

8.9.4 Innervation of the Neck (▶ Fig. 8.12)

Sensory Innervation

The anterior skin of the neck is supplied by various cutaneous branches originating from the ventral rami of the cervical spinal nerves (C2-C4) that form the cervical plexus. The posterior skin is supplied by cutaneous branches of the dorsal rami (C2-C5). Named branches include the greater auricular nerve, transverse cervical nerve, supraclavicular nerve, and lesser occipital nerve.

Motor Innervation

The sternocleidomastoid muscle and trapezius muscle are supplied by the spinal accessory nerve (XI), whereas the paraspinal muscles are supplied by direct branches of the cervical plexus. The mylohyoid and anterior belly of the digastric are supplied by the mandibular nerve (V₃), whereas the stylohyoid and posterior belly of the digastric are supplied by the facial nerve. The infrahyoid muscles are supplied by branches of the ansa cervicalis.

Vagus Nerve

The vagus nerve exits from the cranium via the jugular foramen and descends in the neck within the carotid sheath in the posterior angle between the common carotid artery and internal jugular vein. The right vagus nerve then passes anterior to the first part of the subclavian artery and posterior to the brachiocephalic vein to enter the thorax. The left vagus nerve passes between the common carotid and subclavian arteries and posterior to the sternoclavicular joint. The vagus nerve contains both sensory and motor fibers, with several branches to the larynx, pharynx, and heart. In addition, the vagus provides sensory innervation to the external ear and meninges. The branches to the larynx include the superior laryngeal nerve and recurrent laryngeal nerve. The superior laryngeal nerve, after

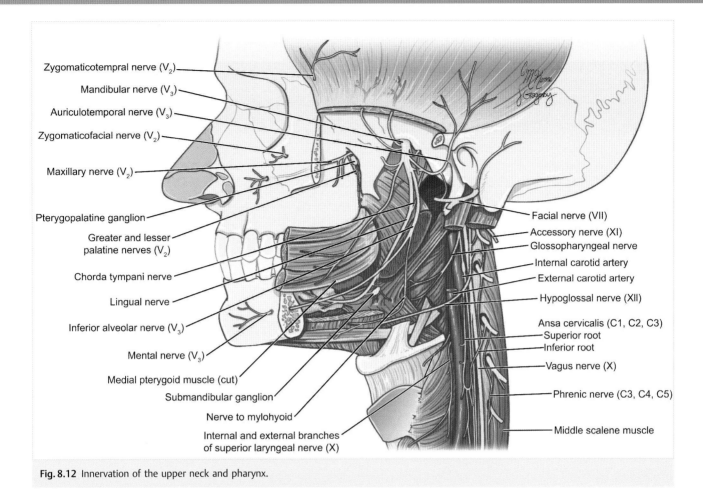

Zygomaticotempral nerve (V$_2$)
Mandibular nerve (V$_3$)
Auriculotemporal nerve (V$_3$)
Zygomaticofacial nerve (V$_2$)
Maxillary nerve (V$_2$)
Pterygopalatine ganglion
Greater and lesser palatine nerves (V$_2$)
Chorda tympani nerve
Lingual nerve
Inferior alveolar nerve (V$_3$)
Mental nerve (V$_3$)
Medial pterygoid muscle (cut)
Submandibular ganglion
Nerve to mylohyoid
Internal and external branches of superior laryngeal nerve (X)

Facial nerve (VII)
Accessory nerve (XI)
Glossopharyngeal nerve
Internal carotid artery
External carotid artery
Hypoglossal nerve (XII)
Ansa cervicalis (C1, C2, C3)
Superior root
Inferior root
Vagus nerve (X)
Phrenic nerve (C3, C4, C5)
Middle scalene muscle

Fig. 8.12 Innervation of the upper neck and pharynx.

leaving the vagus, divides into an internal and an external branch. The internal branch pierces the thyrohyoid membrane to supply sensation to the larynx above the vocal cords. The external branch passes inferiorly to supply motor innervation to the cricothyroid muscle. The recurrent laryngeal nerve travels in the tracheoesophageal groove on either side of the neck and carries motor and sensory fibers, as described previously. The right recurrent nerve, after branching from the vagus, loops inferior to the right subclavian artery at the T1–T2 level. The left recurrent nerve, after branching from the vagus, loops inferior to the aortic arch at approximately the T4–T5 level.

Phrenic Nerve

The phrenic nerves form superficial to the anterior scalene muscles, mainly from the ventral rami of cervical spinal roots C3 to C5. They descend into the thorax in the prevertebral fascia overlying the scalene muscles between the subclavian arteries and veins. Each provides both sensation and motor innervation to its respective half of the diaphragm.

Sympathetic Trunk

The cervical sympathetic trunk lies medial to the carotid sheath within the prevertebral layer of deep cervical fascia. There are three sympathetic ganglia—superior, middle, and inferior—which receive presynaptic sympathetic fibers from the superior

thoracic spinal nerves and associated white rami communicantes through the sympathetic trunk. The superior sympathetic ganglion lies at the skull base, the middle lies at the level of the cricoid cartilage, and the inferior lies at the level of the first rib. Postsynaptic sympathetic fibers leave the ganglion to pass onto cervical spinal nerves or direct visceral nerves or to run with arteries to their destination. Branches to the head and viscera of the neck run with the vertebral, internal, and external carotid arteries.

8.10 Orbit

The orbit is a pyramid-shaped bony cavity with four walls and an apex. The superior wall is formed by the frontal bone, which separates it from the anterior cranial fossa. Farther posteriorly, near the apex, the superior wall is formed by the lesser wing of the sphenoid bone. The medial wall is formed primarily from the ethmoid bone, along with smaller parts of the frontal, lacrimal, and sphenoid bones. The lateral wall is formed by the frontal process of the zygomatic bone and greater wing of the sphenoid. The inferior wall is formed by the maxilla, zygomatic, and palatine bones. The apex of the orbit lies within the lesser wing of the sphenoid just medial to the superior orbital fissure. The contents of the orbital fissures are detailed in ▶ Table 8.5. The orbit contains the eyeball (globe), optic nerve, ocular muscles, fascia, nerves, vessels, orbital fat, lacrimal gland (which lies

Table 8.5 Orbital fissures

Orbital fissure	Contents
Superior	Cranial nerves III, IV, V_1, and VI; superior ophthalmic vein; superior orbital vein; orbital branch of middle meningeal artery; sympathetic fibers
Inferior	Infraorbital nerve and zygomatic nerves (V_2), infraorbital artery and vein, parasympathetics to lacrimal gland, inferior ophthalmic vein
Optic canal	Optic nerve, ophthalmic artery, central retinal vein

Table 8.6 Muscles of the orbit

Muscle	Origin and insertion	Innervation	Action
Levator palpebrae superioris	Lesser wing of sphenoid, anterosuperior to optic canal to tarsal plate and skin of upper eyelid	Oculomotor (III) nerve, sympathetic fibers (superior tarsal muscle)	Elevates upper eyelid
Superior rectus	Common tendinous ring to sclera	Oculomotor (III) nerve	Elevates, adducts, and rotates eyeball medially
Inferior rectus	Common tendinous ring to sclera	Oculomotor (III) nerve	Depresses, adducts, and rotates eyeball laterally
Medial rectus	Common tendinous ring to sclera	Oculomotor (III) nerve	Adducts eyeball
Lateral rectus	Common tendinous ring to sclera	Abducens (VI) nerve	Abducts eyeball
Superior oblique	Body of sphenoid to sclera deep to superior rectus after its tendon passes through a fibrous ring laterally	Trochlear (IV) nerve	Abducts, depresses, and rotates eyeball medially
Inferior oblique	Anterior part of orbital floor to sclera	Oculomotor (III) nerve	Abducts, elevates, and rotates eyeball laterally

superorlaterally), and lacrimal sac. The muscles of the orbit are detailed in ▸ Table 8.6.

8.10.1 Innervation of the Orbit

Sensory Innervation

The sensory innervation of the orbit is derived primarily from the lacrimal, frontal, and nasociliary branches of the ophthalmic nerve (V_1). The lacrimal nerve carries sensation for the lateral aspect of the upper eyelid. It also carries secretomotor fibers for the lacrimal gland from the zygomatic nerve (V_2). The frontal nerve runs superiorly in the orbit to divide into the supraorbital and supratrochlear nerves, giving sensation to the skin of the forehead. The nasociliary nerve passes superomedially to the eyeball, providing sensation to the nasal cavity, external nose, ethmoid and sphenoid sinuses, lacrimal sac, eye, and cornea. The optic nerve enters the orbit through the optic canal and is surrounded by meninges. Visual stimuli from the retina are transmitted through the optic nerve.

Autonomic Innervation

The preganglionic parasympathetic fibers, which innervate the sphincter pupillae muscle and ciliary muscle, originate at the Edinger-Westphal nucleus. The fibers travel along the oculomotor nerve to synapse on the ciliary ganglion. From here, the postsynaptic fibers travel along short ciliary nerves of the nasociliary nerve (V_1) to reach the musculature. Contraction of the sphincter pupillae constricts the pupil, whereas contraction of the ciliary muscle relieves tension on the suspensory ligaments of the lens, increasing its power. The preganglionic sympathetic fibers, which innervate the dilator pupillae and superior tarsal muscles, originate in the thoracic spinal cord. The fibers travel along the sympathetic trunk and synapse in the superior sympathetic ganglion. From here, the postsynaptic fibers travel along the internal carotid artery to reach the orbit. The fibers then travel along the long ciliary nerves of the nasociliary nerve (V_1) to reach the dilator pupillae. The fibers also travel along the ophthalmic artery to reach the superior tarsal muscle. Contraction of the dilator pupillae dilates the pupil, while contraction of the superior tarsal muscle elevates the upper eyelid.

8.11 Pterygopalatine Fossa

The pterygopalatine fossa is a small pyramid-shaped space just inferior to the apex of the orbit between the posterior maxilla and the pterygoid process. It connects laterally with the infratemporal fossa through the pterygomaxillary fissure, medially with the nasal cavity through the sphenopalatine foramen, and inferiorly with the oral cavity through the palatine canal. Anterosuperiorly, it connects with the orbit through the inferior orbital fissure. Posterosuperiorly, it connects with the middle cranial fossa through the foramen rotundum and vidian canal. The pterygopalatine fossa contains the third part of the internal maxillary artery and its branches, maxillary nerve (V_2), vidian nerve, and pterygopalatine ganglion.

8.11.1 Maxillary Artery

The maxillary artery enters the pterygopalatine fossa through the pterygomaxillary fissure, where it lies anterior to the

Table 8.7 Muscles of the infratemporal fossa

Muscles	Attachments	Innervation	Actions
Temporalis	Floor of temporal fossa to coronoid process and anterior border of mandibular ramus	Mandibular (V_3) nerve	Elevates and retracts mandible
Masseter	Inferior border of zygomatic arch to lateral surface of mandibular ramus and coronoid process	Mandibular (V_3) nerve	Elevates and protrudes mandible
Lateral pterygoid	Superior head: greater wing of sphenoid Inferior head: lateral surface of lateral pterygoid plate to neck of mandible, articular disk and capsule of temporomandibular joint	Mandibular (V_3) nerve	Protrudes mandible and depresses chin, side-to-side movements
Medial pterygoid	Deep head: medial surface of lateral pterygoid plate Superficial head: maxillary tuberosity to medial surface of ramus of mandible	Mandibular (V_3) nerve	Elevates and protrudes mandible

pterygopalatine ganglion. Here, it gives off various branches that follow the similarly named branches of the maxillary nerve (V_2). These branches include the posterior superior alveolar artery, descending palatine artery, infraorbital artery, and sphenopalatine artery. The sphenopalatine artery divides into posterior lateral nasal branches and posterior septal branches.

8.11.2 Maxillary Nerve

The maxillary nerve enters the pterygopalatine fossa through the foramen rotundum. It then gives off the zygomatic nerve, which further divides into the zygomaticofacial and zygomaticotemporal nerves. These nerves supply sensation to the lateral part of the cheek and temple.

Secretomotor fibers to the lacrimal gland are also carried on the zygomaticotemporal nerve. Within the fossa, the maxillary nerve also gives off two pterygopalatine nerves that carry sensory fibers that pass through the pterygopalatine ganglion without synapsing to supply the nose, palate, tonsil, and gingiva. These sensory nerves include the greater and lesser palatine nerves, which travel through the palatine canal. The maxillary nerve then passes through the inferior orbital fissure, becoming the infraorbital nerve.

8.11.3 Autonomic Innervation

The preganglionic parasympathetic fibers of the vidian nerve originate from the facial nerve by way of the greater superficial petrosal nerve. After synapsing at the pterygopalatine ganglion, postsynaptic fibers join branches of the maxillary nerve to reach the mucus-secreting glands of the nasal cavity, paranasal sinuses, and palate. Postganglionic parasympathetic fibers also travel along the zygomaticotemporal nerve and its communicating branch to the lacrimal nerve to supply secretomotor fibers to the lacrimal gland. The preganglionic sympathetic fibers of the vidian nerve originate in the thoracic spinal cord before synapsing in the superior cervical ganglion. Postganglionic sympathetic fibers then travel along the internal carotid artery, where they branch off to become the deep petrosal nerve. After passing through the vidian canal, these fibers join branches of the maxillary artery.

8.12 Infratemporal Fossa

The infratemporal fossa lies deep to the zygomatic arch and ramus of the mandible. It is posterior to the maxilla, lateral to the lateral pterygoid plate, anterior to the mastoid and styloid process, and inferior to the greater wing of the sphenoid bone. The medial pterygoid muscle attachment to the mandible marks its inferior extent. The infratemporal fossa contains the inferior part of the temporal muscle, lateral and medial pterygoid muscles, maxillary artery and branches, mandibular nerve (V_3) and branches, otic ganglion, and pterygoid venous plexus. The muscles of the infratemporal fossa are detailed in ▶ Table 8.7.

8.12.1 Maxillary Artery

The maxillary artery is a terminal branch of the external carotid artery that gives off several branches as it courses through the infratemporal fossa. It passes either medial or lateral to the lateral pterygoid muscle before exiting the fossa through the pterygomaxillary fissure. The lateral pterygoid muscle divides the maxillary artery into three parts, the first two of which lie within the infratemporal fossa. Important branches of the first part include the middle meningeal artery, which courses superiorly, splitting the auriculotemporal nerve to enter the cranium via the foramen spinosum, and the inferior alveolar artery, which supplies the mandible, gingiva, and teeth. Important branches of the second part include the deep temporal arteries, pterygoid arteries, masseteric arteries, and buccal arteries.

8.12.2 Mandibular Nerve

The mandibular nerve, as described earlier, enters the infratemporal fossa through the foramen ovale. Here, it divides into both motor and sensory branches. The branches include the auriculotemporal nerve, inferior alveolar nerve, lingual nerve, and buccal nerve. The otic ganglion lies just inferior to the foramen ovale medial to the mandibular nerve.

8.13 Recommended Reading

[1] Hollinshead WH. Anatomy for Surgeons: The Head and Neck. Vol 1. 3rd ed. Philadelphia, PA: Lippincott Williams & Wilkins; 1982

[2] Moore K, Dalley A. Clinically Oriented Anatomy. 4th ed. Philadelphia, PA: Lippincott Williams & Wilkins; 1999:850–1062

9 The Complete Otolaryngology Physical Examination

James Azzi, Jean-Paul Azzi, Anthony P. Sclafani, and Edward J. Shin

9.1 Introduction

The proper evaluation and treatment of patients presenting to an otolaryngologist–head and neck surgeon require a thorough and complete history and physical examination. Establishing rapport with the patient is essential. Greet the patient with eye contact and a smile. Explain your role on the medical team, what you plan to do, and why you plan to do it. When patients are at ease and you have gained their trust, the evaluation can be the most productive.

Although a complete otolaryngologic examination should be performed on all patients, a thorough medical history is essential in determining the key portions of the examination. It is important to *listen* to patients and to guide them to a thorough description of their complaint, without interrupting them. As with any medical evaluation, a complete past medical/surgical history, a list of medications and any allergies to medications, social and family histories, and a review of systems will aid the clinician in making the correct diagnosis.

9.2 General Appearance

While donning gloves, observe the patient for any obvious abnormalities, noting behavior as well as physical appearance. For example, a gait disturbance may suggest cerebellar dysfunction, or brown stains on the teeth may signify heavy tobacco use. Next, evaluate the skin of the head and neck. Pay particular attention to areas that receive significant sun exposure. These include the nose, ears, scalp, and the back of the neck. Look for any irregular lesions that may indicate malignancy.

9.3 Face

Evaluate the patient for any facial asymmetry, paresis, or paralysis. Use the American Academy of Otolaryngology-Head and Neck Surgery facial nerve grading system or the House-Brackmann classification (▶ Table 9.1) to grade the severity of dysfunction. Palpate the face for any deformities or bony

irregularities. In patients with a history of trauma, pay particular attention to the periorbital areas, zygomatic arches, and dorsum of the nose, palpating any bony step-offs. Tap above and below the orbits to evaluate the frontal and maxillary sinuses; tenderness in these areas may indicate sinusitis. The temporomandibular joint is evaluated by placing two or three fingers anterior to the external auditory canal and having the patient open and close the mouth. Tenderness, clicking, or grinding may indicate temporomandibular joint dysfunction.

9.4 Neck

In the evaluation of the neck, the normal midline structures, including the trachea and the hyoid, thyroid, and cricoid cartilages, should be identified. With the examiner standing behind the seated patient, the cartilages of the larynx are palpated. The examiner places both thumbs behind the patient's neck and the remaining four fingers of each hand in the paratracheal grooves. Gentle alternating finger pressure should move the larynx to and fro; a fixed larynx is highly suspicious for malignant disease. The thyroid is located inferior to the cricoid cartilage and lateral to the trachea. While the patient swallows, each thyroid lobe rises and can be palpated separately. Any enlargement or nodule should be noted.

Systematically palpate levels I through VI of the neck (▶ Fig. 9.1) to assess for adenopathy. Any large lymph node (> 1 cm) or hard fixed lesion, especially in a patient with a history of tobacco use and/or alcohol abuse, warrants further investigation and a thorough mucosal examination of the upper aerodigestive tract. Alternatively, in the setting of fevers, night sweats, and weight loss, a diagnosis of lymphoma should be entertained.

Level I is defined by the body of the mandible, the anterior belly of the digastric muscle, and the stylohyoid muscle. Level I can be further subdivided into IA and IB. Level IA includes the submental nodes. Level IB contains the submandibular nodes. Level II contains the jugulodigastric lymph nodes and extends from the base of the skull to the hyoid bone, anterior to the sternocleidomastoid muscle. Levels IIA and IIB are located medial and lateral to the spinal accessory nerve, respectively. Level III begins superiorly at the level of the inferior hyoid bone and ends inferiorly at the level of the cricoid cartilage. The jugulodigastric nodal chain can be followed inferiorly to level IV, which extends from the cricoid to the clavicle. Levels III and IV are bordered anteriorly by the sternohyoid muscle and posteriorly by the lateral sternocleidomastoid muscle. Level V includes the lymph nodes from the lateral sternocleidomastoid muscle to the anterior trapezius muscle. Finally, level VI is defined by the hyoid superiorly, the sternal notch inferiorly, and the common carotid arteries laterally.

9.5 Ears

The auricle is examined for appropriate size, shape, definition, and location. The preauricular area is inspected for skin tags

Table 9.1 House-Brackmann scale of facial paralysis

Grade	Facial movement
I. Normal	Normal function
II. Mild dysfunction	Eye with complete closure, forehead and mouth with some asymmetry
III. Moderate dysfunction	Eye with complete closure, forehead and mouth with slight movement
IV. Moderately severe dysfunction	Eye with incomplete closure, no forehead movement, asymmetry of mouth with maximal effort
V. Severe dysfunction	Eye with incomplete closure, no forehead movement, mouth with slight movement
VI. Complete paralysis	No movement

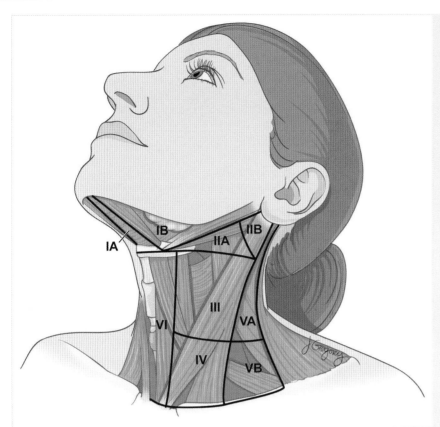

Fig. 9.1 Diagram of levels of the neck.

and pits; the postauricular area is also examined, especially for swelling, discoloration, or lesions. In the setting of acute otitis media, it is important to visually and manually inspect for mastoiditis. If mastoiditis is complicated by a subperiosteal abscess, the ear will often protrude. Postauricular ecchymosis, or the Battle sign, may indicate trauma and possible temporal bone fracture.

To evaluate the external auditory canal and tympanic membrane, use a pneumatic otoscope with the largest possible speculum to create an airtight seal without traumatizing the canal skin. The auricle is grasped and retracted posteriorly and superiorly to straighten the canal. The speculum is advanced beyond any hair in the external auditory canal but should not be passed into the bony portion of the external auditory canal. The fifth finger of the hand holding the otoscope is used to stabilize the hand against the patient's temple (▶ Fig. 9.2). This is particularly important when children, who may make sudden movements, are examined. If cerumen is obstructing visualization of the tympanic membrane, it is removed by suction, curet, or irrigation.

Tenderness, otorrhea, or edema can signal infection. Acute otitis externa typically will present with tenderness on examination, particularly with tragal manipulation. The external auditory canal will be edematous and may also contain purulent debris. Fungal otitis externa may present with white or brown spores in the external auditory canal. If the patient is diabetic or immunocompromised, be aware of the increased risk for malignant otitis externa, which presents with granulation tissue at the junction of the bony and cartilaginous portions of the canal. The external auditory canal may be narrowed by nodular growth, which may represent an osteoma or exostoses. A history of cold water exposure, such as with surfers, increases

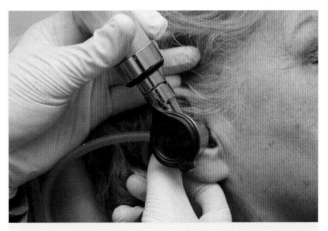

Fig. 9.2 Proper hand positioning in examination of the ear. The fifth finger of the hand holding the otoscope is braced against the temple, while the opposite hand draws the auricle posteriorly to straighten the external auditory canal.

the likelihood of exostoses. If severe, this narrowing can increase the risk for acute otitis externa.

The tympanic membrane (▶ Fig. 9.3) is inspected and all anatomical landmarks identified; any abnormalities should be documented. The mobility of the tympanic membrane is assessed with a pneumatic otoscope by gently insufflating air and observing the movement of the membrane. This will be effective, however, only if the speculum creates a seal with the external auditory canal, as described above. Common causes of immobility include improper use of the otoscope, perforation,

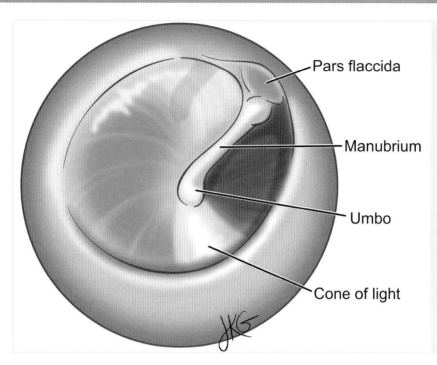

Fig. 9.3 Diagram of the right tympanic membrane.

Pars flaccida

Manubrium

Umbo

Cone of light

and middle ear fluid. Significantly better outward than inward movement of the tympanic membrane is suggestive of eustachean tube dysfunction. Masses, discolorations, or other abnormalities of the tympanic membrane are evaluated and described according to location by quadrant. Extension of any abnormality into the middle ear is carefully evaluated, and the visible margins of any lesions are described.

Basic tuning fork testing is best done in a quiet room, and the results are always reported with the frequency tested. To perform the Weber test, place a vibrating (512 or 1,024 Hz) tuning fork on the center of the patient's forehead. (Alternatively, the fork can be placed between the patient's central incisors). The patient is asked in which ear the sound is perceived as louder or if it is equal bilaterally. A lateralized Weber test may indicate ipsilateral conductive hearing loss or contralateral sensorineural hearing loss. The Weber test should be documented as "negative" for midline responses and as either "right" or "left" for lateralization.

To perform the Rinne test, a vibrating tuning fork is first placed over the mastoid process (bone conduction) and then held 2 to 3 cm from the external auditory canal (air conduction); the patient is asked which sound is perceived as louder. A conductive loss will cause the sound to be louder over the mastoid process. This is referred to as "Rinne negative." When the air conduction is louder than bone conduction, this is referred to as "Rinne positive." If the two positions have the same intensity, then this is referred to as "Rinne equal."

9.6 Oral Cavity, Oropharynx, and Nasopharynx

The oral cavity and oropharynx (▶ Fig. 9.4) are examined with an adequate light source (preferably a headlight to free both hands). The lips, dentition, and gums are evaluated, with

attention paid to dental occlusion, masses, or lesions that may require further investigation. The dorsal and ventral tongue, as well as the sides of the tongue and floor of the mouth, are examined by asking the patient to elevate and move the tongue from side to side. Palpate the lateral tongue and the floor of the mouth, and examine the buccal mucosa and hard palate. Bimanual palpation, with one finger of one hand in the oral cavity and oropharynx and the other hand on the corresponding areas of the external neck, can aid in palpating deeper lesions of the floor of the mouth and base of the tongue.

The posterior tongue, soft palate, tonsillar pillars, and vallecula are examined. Two tongue depressors are used to fully manipulate and expose all areas to be visualized (▶ Fig. 9.5). The tonsils are graded on a scale from 1 + to 4 + (1 + indicated tonsils barely visible in the tonsillar fossae and 4 + indicates tonsils that "kiss" in the midline). The nasopharynx can then be examined with a warm nasopharyngeal mirror suspended just behind and below the uvula while the tongue is depressed with a tongue blade for wider exposure. A flexible fiber-optic endoscope can also be used and may provide a superior examination. The patency of the posterior choanae should be assessed, and any obstruction from polyps or adenoid hypertrophy should be noted. The eustachean tube orifices should be unobstructed, and the posterior wall of the nasopharynx should be smooth and without masses.

9.7 Nose, Nasopharynx, and Larynx

9.7.1 Anterior Rhinoscopy

The anterior portions of the nasal cavity are easily evaluated with a nasal speculum and light source (▶ Fig. 9.6). Note any abnormal findings, such as a deviated septum or boggy,

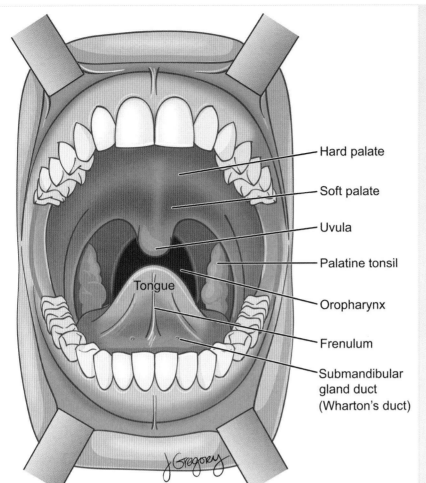

Fig. 9.4 Diagram of the oral cavity and oropharynx.

- Hard palate
- Soft palate
- Uvula
- Palatine tonsil
- Oropharynx
- Frenulum
- Submandibular gland duct (Wharton's duct)

Tongue

9.7.2 Endoscopic Examination

When indicated by history or physical examination, endoscopy can be performed to better visualize suspected pathologic processes. A topical anesthetic and decongestant (see Box Dr. Chodosh's Topical Airway Anesthetic/Decongestant Solution (p.47)) is applied to both sides of the nose before endoscopy to ensure patient comfort during the examination.

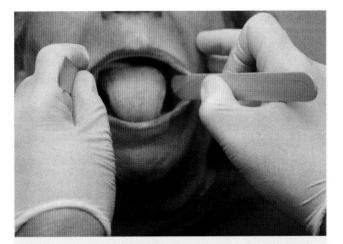

Fig. 9.5 With two tongue depressors, the cheeks are held laterally to fully visualize the entire oral cavity.

> **Dr. Chodosh's Topical Airway Anesthetic/ Decongestant Solution**
>
> - Lidocaine 1%
> - Phenylephrine
> - Peppermint oil

9.7.3 Nasal and Nasopharyngeal Endoscopy

The nose and nasopharynx can be evaluated with either a rigid or a flexible endoscope. Suctioning, biopsy, and manipulation are far simpler when a rigid endoscope is used. Generally, it is easier to pass the scope close to the floor of the nose, and each

edematous turbinates. Visualization can be improved by spraying a mist of nasal decongestant (oxymetazoline or phenylephrine) in the nose. An unobstructed nasal cavity should allow visualization of palatal elevation by anterior rhinoscopy while the patient pronounces the sound of the letter *K*.

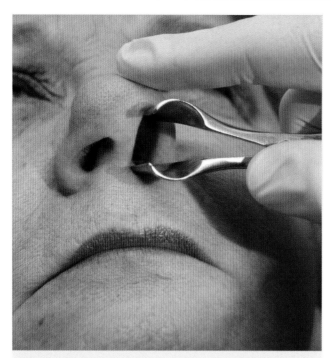

Fig. 9.6 Proper hand positioning during anterior rhinoscopy. The nasal speculum blades should be oriented vertically and the hand stabilized on the nasal tip with the index finger.

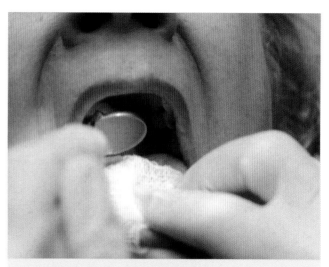

Fig. 9.7 Proper form for indirect laryngoscopy.

Table 9.2 Cranial nerves

Cranial nerve	Function
I	Sense of smell
II	Visual acuity and visual fields
III	Extraocular movements
IV	Superior oblique muscle
V	Corneal reflex and sensation to the face
VI	Lateral rectus muscle
VII	Motor and symmetry of facial muscles
VIII	Auditory and vestibular function
IX	Gag reflex and soft palate
X	Vocal fold mobility, gag reflex, and soft palate
XI	Sternocleidomastoid, trapezius muscles
XII	Tongue movement and symmetry

side is examined from anterior naris to nasopharynx. The size and color of the inferior and middle turbinates and middle meatus are noted, as are any polyps, crusting, purulent debris, or masses in these areas. The septum is inspected, again by examining the color and quality of the mucosa, as well as verifying septal integrity and assessing septal deflections, curvatures, and spurs.

The nasopharynx is examined by advancing the flexible endoscope beyond the posterior choanae on one side and turning the tip as needed to allow adequate assessment of the entire nasopharynx. The posterior and lateral nasopharyngeal walls, fossae of Rosenmüller, and eustachean tube orifices should all be evaluated and any masses, mucosal abnormalities, or adenoidal vegetation/hypertrophy noted.

9.7.4 Laryngoscopy

Ideally, indirect laryngoscopy should be performed on all patients. The seated patient leans forward with the chin slightly elevated (in a "sniffing" position), while the examiner sits just to the side of the patient. The examiner gently holds the patient's outstretched tongue with a gauze pad and places a warm laryngeal mirror to elevate the soft palate and uvula (▶ Fig. 9.7).

The patient is asked to say *EEE*, and the vocal folds should be observed for brisk symmetric movement and complete glottis closure during phonation. The piriform sinuses are better dilated for inspection while the patient pronounces a long-*A* sound. The vallecula, lingual and laryngeal surfaces of the epiglottis, aryepiglottic folds, arytenoid cartilages, and post-cricoid area should all be visualized; all should be smooth-surfaced, nonerythematous, and without masses or ulcerations.

The examination of patients with a strong gag reflex, or of patients who otherwise cannot tolerate indirect laryngoscopy, can be facilitated by spraying the oropharynx and tongue with a topical anesthetic. For patients who still cannot tolerate the mirror examination or in whom a more prolonged evaluation of the hypopharynx and larynx is necessary, flexible nasopharyngolaryngoscopy can be performed. The endoscope is introduced transnasally and passed into the nasopharynx; at this point, it is advanced beyond the soft palate as the patient gently inspires. While the same structures are inspected, the tip of the scope can be manipulated into the vallecula or piriform sinus for improved visualization. In compliant and well-anesthetized patients, the tip of the endoscope can be advanced to (and sometimes through) the glottis inlet to view the upper trachea.

Any significant erythema or edema (especially in the hypopharynx or larynx) warrants further investigation and airway control. Patients with laryngopharyngeal reflux may complain of hoarseness, globus sensation, throat irritation, and cough. They commonly have edema and erythema of various portions of the supraglottis and hypopharynx; however, the most common finding is erythema of the posterior larynx and diffuse pachydermia of the pharyngeal walls. As patients with infections, systemic diseases, or mass lesions may present with similar complaints, a thorough evaluation is warranted.

9.8 Cranial Nerves

Finally, perform an abbreviated neurologic examination, with particular attention given to the cranial nerves (▶ Table 9.2). Focal deficits may be suggestive of an underlying mass lesion or neurologic process requiring further work-up including, but not limited to, imaging and consideration of neurologic and/or ophthalmologic consultation.

9.9 Roundsmanship

- A thorough otorhinolaryngologic examination includes a detailed history and a complete head and neck examination.

- The otorhinolaryngologic examination should proceed in a structured and orderly fashion to avoid overlooking any portion of the examination.
- Resting the fifth finger of the hand holding an otoscope against the patient's temple braces the otoscope and prevents inadvertent injury if the patient (especially a child) moves suddenly.
- Warming mirrors prevents fogging during indirect nasopharyngoscopy or laryngoscopy.

9.10 Recommended Reading

[1] Bickley LS, Szilagyi PG. Bates' Guide to Physical Examination and History-Taking. 8th ed. Philadelphia, PA: Lippincott Williams & Wilkins; 2003
[2] Couch ME, Blaugrund J, Dario K. History, physical examination, and the preoperative evaluation. In: Cummings C, Haughey B, Thomas JR, et al, eds. Cummings Otolaryngology: Head and Neck Surgery. 4th ed. Philadelphia, PA: Elsevier Mosby; 2005:3–15

10 Radiology of the Head and Neck

Hasit Mehta and Ajay Hira

10.1 Introduction

Imaging plays a large role in the noninvasive diagnosis of head and neck pathology. In the following two chapters, we will briefly review the various imaging modalities available, as well as the relevant radiologic anatomy and pathology.

10.2 Imaging Modalities

10.2.1 Radiography

Radiographs are the oldest and most basic imaging modality. X-rays were discovered in 1895 by Wilhelm C. Roentgen, who produced the first X-ray (of his wife's hand) in the same year. Radiographs (better known as X-rays or plain films) have historically been the primary imaging modality for the diagnosis of head and neck pathology. In the past three decades, radiography has largely been replaced by computed tomographic, ultrasound, and magnetic resonance imaging. Radiography is performed by exposing a region of the body to ionizing radiation (X-rays); the X-rays are differentially absorbed or transmitted to varying degrees by the imaged body structures (depending on the density of the structures imaged). A detector (digital or film) placed in line with the X-ray generator and behind the imaged body part registers the transmitted X-rays and creates the radiograph. The radiograph contains varying shades of gray; the whitest structures represent the densest body structures (which attenuate the most X-rays), such as bone, and the darkest structures on the radiograph represent the least dense structures, such as air in the aerodigestive tract or lungs. The ability to detect pathology depends primarily on the density, size, and location of the pathologic process. Radiography is still in use (▶ Table 10.1), but its application in otolaryngology is primarily in the emergency department for quick evaluation of the upper aerodigestive tract, particularly in the pediatric population for the rapid evaluation of epiglottitis and croup (given the lower radiation exposure than with CT). Other clinical uses include exclusion of foreign body, evaluation of the upper airway (frontal and lateral views), and quick evaluation of the orbits, paranasal sinuses, and maxillofacial structures when other imaging modalities are unavailable (▶ Fig. 10.1). Virtually all other former indications of radiography have been replaced by alternative imaging modalities.

10.2.2 Computed Tomography

Computed tomography, better known as CT scanning, has revolutionized noninvasive head and neck imaging. CT has replaced radiography as the primary imaging modality for most acute head and neck pathology. A CT machine consists of a ringlike structure with multiple X-ray generators and detector arrays. The patient is placed on a movable gantry that traverses the center of the CT scanner; as the computer-controlled gantry moves the patient through the CT scanner, the X-ray generator and detector elements rotate around the patient, acquiring a large helical data set. Substantial computational hardware is necessary both to acquire and to post-process the data stream. The data set is analyzed with a variety of algorithms, traditionally filtered back projection, although currently more complex iterative methodology is used to produce the cross-sectional tomographic images from the data stream (▶ Fig. 10.2). Current modern CT scanners are capable of extremely high-resolution image acquisition and routine helical image acquisition, allowing three-dimensional/volumetric reconstruction (▶ Fig. 10.3) from the single data set. The helical data set is then post-processed by the CT technologist and/or radiologist to produce representative cross-sectional images in any plane (▶ Fig. 10.4). The fundamentals of CT and radiography are similar; CT images are also primarily dependent on the attenuation of X-rays by body structures, measured quantitatively in Hounsfield units. Qualitatively, denser structures will appear whiter on a CT image. The CT image can be viewed at various window widths and levels to accentuate various spectra of density. The three-window width and levels that would be typically used by the otolaryngologist include soft-tissue, bone, and lung window and level presets (▶ Fig. 10.5). Each of these presets accentuates different spectra of density.

CT of the head and neck can be performed with and/or without iodinated intravenous (IV) contrast material. IV contrast material is radiodense and produces a white appearance on the CT image because of its radiodensity. It can be administered to allow detailed imaging of the vascular compartment.

Table 10.1 Advantages and disadvantages of radiography

Advantages	Disadvantages
Inexpensive	Poor evaluation of submucosal lesion/mass
Quick	Ionizing radiation
Readily available, even in underserved regions	Variability with positioning of patient
Interpretation by non-radiology, non-ENT physicians possible	Poor assessment of salivary and endocrine glands
Medium-size and portable units available	Generally diminished sensitivity and specificity for detection of lesions compared with newer imaging modalities
> *Abbreviation: ENT, ear, nose, and throat.*	

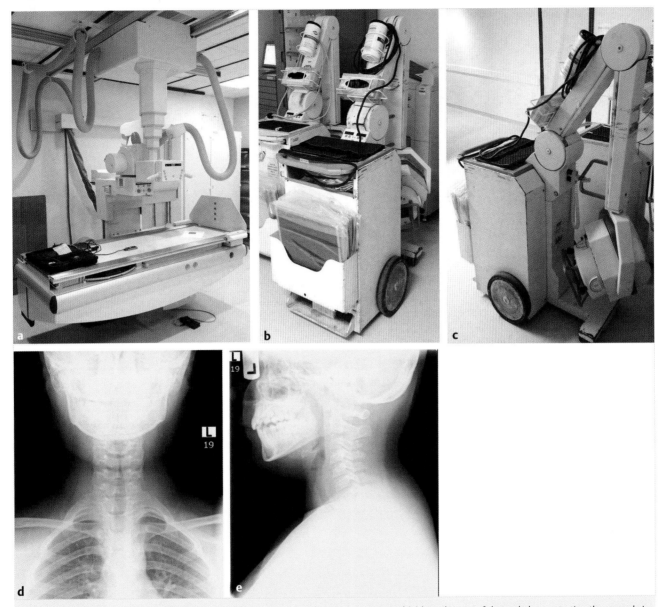

Fig. 10.1 (a) Fixed X-ray/fluoroscopy unit. (b,c) Portable X-ray units. (d) Posteroanterior and (e) lateral X-rays of the neck demonstrating the normal air column.

Additionally, contrast can help accentuate various pathologic processes, which may cause pooling of contrast either from hyperemia or tissue breakdown. Its application can dramatically improve the sensitivity of CT when administered in the appropriate setting. The primary limitations to the use of contrast material are renal dysfunction, cross reactivity with certain medications, and allergic reaction to contrast media. Various guidelines exist to screen patients at risk for contrast-induced nephrotoxicity, and premedication regimens are available. Contrast is typically indicated in the evaluation of head and neck neoplasms and most head and neck infections. It is not routinely necessary in the evaluation of the paranasal sinuses or temporal bone unless there is a suspicion of neoplasm or large soft-tissue extension of infection.

CT of every compartment of the head and neck is in active clinical use worldwide. It is the imaging modality of choice for

acute head and neck pathology, including trauma, acute infection, airway obstruction, and foreign body evaluation. It is the most sensitive examination to evaluate fine bony detail. CT is also an important adjunct in the evaluation of head and neck neoplasms. It is the imaging modality of choice for evaluation of the paranasal sinuses and is a critical component in planning for functional endoscopic sinus surgery. Three-dimensional reconstructions allow the pre- and postoperative assessment of complex trauma and reconstruction. CT is also routinely used for the minimally invasive image-guided biopsy of head and neck lesions (▶ Table 10.2).

10.2.3 Ultrasonography

Medical ultrasonography came into use around the period of World War II after advances made during wartime research.

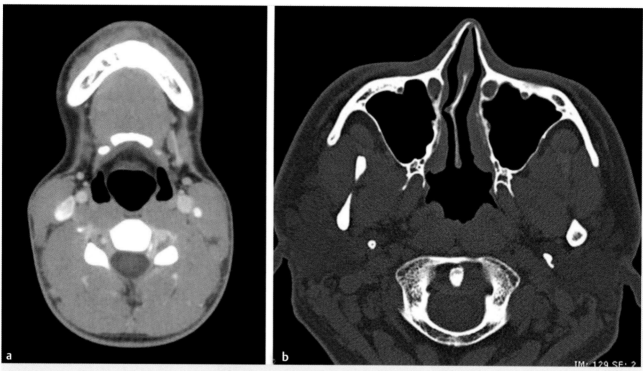

Fig. 10.2 (a) Axial soft-tissue window of the neck at the level of the hyoid and piriform sinuses on computed tomographic scan. (b) Axial bone window at the level of the maxillary sinuses demonstrating bony septal deviation to the right.

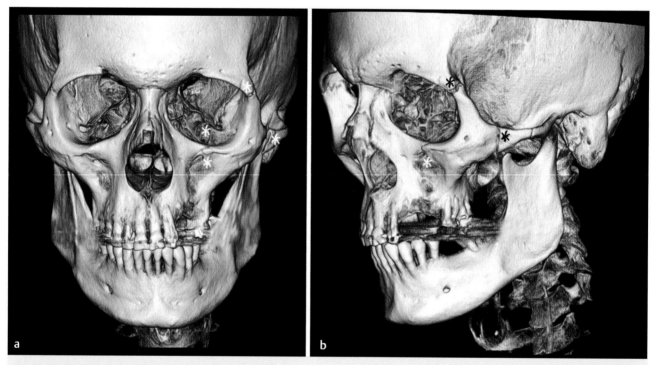

Fig. 10.3 Computed tomographic data can be reformatted to produce a three-dimensional image of selected tissue. (a) Frontal and (b) left oblique three-dimensional bone surface reconstructions of facial structures. Note fractures at the left infraorbital rim, zygomaticomaxillary suture/zygomatic arch, zygomaticofrontal suture, and orbital floor (*asterisks*).

Ultrasound uses sound waves that are beyond the range of human hearing. Sound waves are generated by a piezoelectric transducer probe (▶ Fig. 10.6), and echoes are reflected back to the probe depending on the echotexture of the tissue being ex-amined. A grayscale anatomical image representative of the tissue being imaged is generated. The time of the returning echo depends on the depth of the structure. The intensity of the returning sound wave encodes the brightness of the pixel on the generated image; more echogenic structures reflect more ultrasound energy and appear brighter on the image than do less echogenic structures. Typically bright (echogenic) structures include bony structures and calcifications. Muscle and soft tissue have intermediate echogenicity and are typically varying shades of gray. Fluid, gas, and aqueous material are extremely hypoechoic and thus very dark gray to black on the ultrasound image. Modern ultrasonography equipment can generate two-dimensional anatomical images in real time (▶ Fig. 10.7) and provide three-dimensional image acquisition and flow-

dependent velocity measurements within vascular structures (▶ Fig. 10.8).

Ultrasound is a rapid, noninvasive imaging technique that does not use ionizing radiation. This makes ultrasound an ideal imaging modality in the pediatric population. Ultrasound offers significant advantage in the pediatric population because imaging can routinely be obtained without sedation. Modern ultrasound equipment has evolved to the point of including extremely portable and mobile units that can be used in nearly any clinical environment. Some units are so small that they can be battery operated and carried in a handheld unit by a physician or technologist. However, the current typical medical-grade diagnostic ultrasound unit is of medium size, on wheels, and portable to most locations within a hospital or clinical setting. Ultrasound offers excellent soft-tissue detail for superficial lesions. In the head and neck, it is a primary imaging modality for evaluation of the thyroid gland, as well as evaluation of soft-tissue masses and infections of the neck in children. However, ultrasound typically cannot provide images of deep structures such as the aerodigestive tract, and radiography is still the imaging modality of choice for epiglottitis and croup. Real-time ultrasound imaging is also used for the image-guided intervention/biopsy of head and neck lesions typically performed by the otolaryngologist, radiologist, or pathologist (▶ Table 10.3).

10.2.4 Magnetic Resonance Imaging

Magnetic resonance (MR) imaging is a complex imaging modality that leverages the unique properties of the nucleus of an atom. Atoms have a magnetic field that is related to their nuclear spin. These nuclear magnetic fields will align with a strong, externally applied magnetic field. The atoms are then subjected to electromagnetic energy, which they can absorb. This boosts them to an excited state, and they subsequently release the energy as they return to a ground state. The energy is detected and formed into images with complex pulse sequences and image generation. The MR scanner consists of a large tubular structure that contains an extremely powerful, liquid helium–cooled superconducting magnet. Additionally, a series of radio-frequency coils are present within the tubular structure, as well as coils placed on the patient's body in the region of

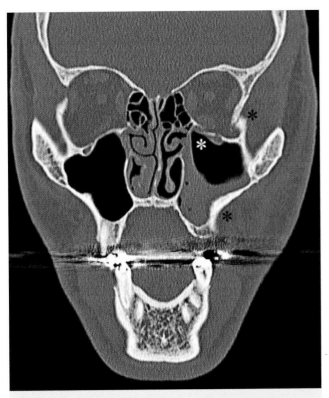

Fig. 10.4 Coronal projection computed tomographic scan of the patient in ▶ Fig. 10.3.

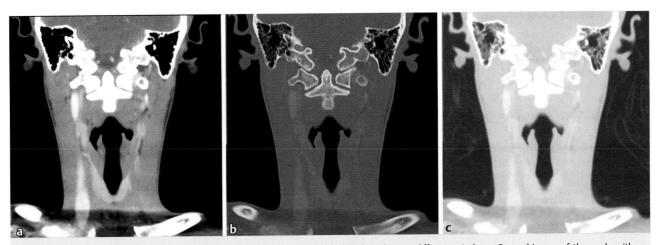

Fig. 10.5 Different details can be highlighted on a computed tomographic scan by selecting different windows. Coronal image of the neck, with images presented in (a) soft tissue, (b) bone, and (c) lung window widths and levels.

Table 10.2 Advantages and disadvantages of computed tomography

Advantages	Disadvantages
Excellent fine bony detail	Ionizing radiation exposure
Very good soft-tissue delineation	Moderately expensive
Cross-sectional imaging allows excellent detection of submucosal lesions and other lesions that may not be seen with endoscopy	Prone to artifact
Fast imaging modality, thus moderately impervious to motion artifact	Relatively more complex to interpret
Excellent delineation of airway	Large, complex imaging unit; typically fixed immovable imaging system
	Readily available in most developed nations but not necessarily in developing nations

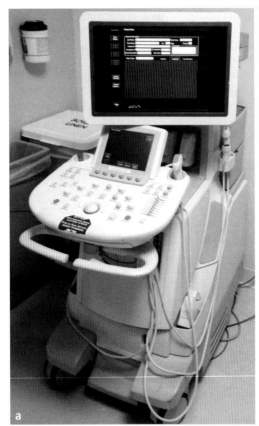

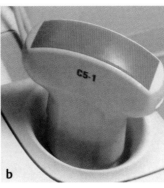

Fig. 10.6 Ultrasound (a) unit and (b) probe.

imaging interest. These coils generate radio-frequency energy to agitate species of atoms in precise computer-controlled patterns. The energy absorbed and emitted is also captured by the coils and processed by the computer system to generate MR images. MR imaging allows exceptional soft-tissue delineation and excellent delineation of deep structures. Various pulse sequences can be used to accentuate certain tissues. The major sequences used in head and neck imaging include T1-weighted sequences (▸ Fig. 10.9), T2-weighted sequences (▸ Fig. 10.10), and fat-suppressed T2-weighted or STIR (short tau inversion recovery) pulse sequences (▸ Fig. 10.11). T1 imaging may be performed with or without contrast material. T1-weighted imaging is most useful for imaging lesions that enhance, such as neoplasm and infection. Fat is extremely bright on T1 imaging and typically is suppressed during contrast administration to allow a more sensitive detection of enhancement (▸ Fig. 10.12). T2-weighted pulse sequences are fluid-sensitive and allow the visualization of edema and fluid-containing structures, including congenital cystic lesions of the head and neck.

MR imaging is the imaging modality of choice to evaluate soft tissues of the head and neck. It offers excellent delineation of the deep and superficial fascial planes of the neck. There are limitations to its use in patients with implanted metallic devices and/or foreign bodies, and these patients need to be assessed on a case-by-case basis. Additionally, MR imaging contrast agents may be contraindicated in patients with end-stage renal failure because of the risk for nephrogenic systemic fibrosis. MR imaging is not a primary modality used in the imaging of the paranasal sinuses and temporal bone because of the lack of free protons in calcium and air, which limits the ability to

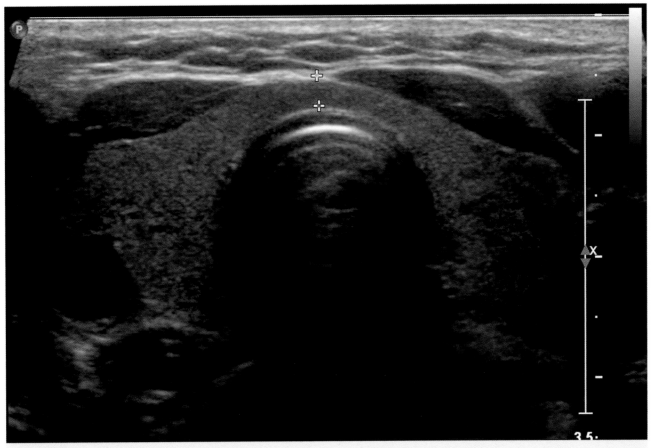

Fig. 10.7 Ultrasound image of thyroid gland. The plus signs indicate the thickness of the isthmus, which continues bilaterally to the lobes.

generate MR signal, although it can be used as an adjunct imaging technique to evaluate for soft-tissue and perineural spread of disease (▶ Table 10.4).

10.2.5 Positron Emission Tomography and Positron Emission Tomography–Computed Tomography

Positron emission tomography (PET) is unique in that it is a physiologic imaging modality and not strictly anatomical. A PET-CT unit consists of a large tubular imaging structure similar in appearance to a CT or MR imaging unit. Within the tubular structure are the components of both a CT scanner and a PET scanner. Typically, the patient is placed on the computer-controlled gantry, and a whole-body CT scan of the patient is performed, typically in less than 1 minute. Subsequently, the patient is slowly moved through the scanner over a period of approximately 30 minutes while the PET imaging portion of the examination is performed. The two imaging data sets are co-registered on a dedicated imaging workstation and interpreted by the radiologist.

In order to generate the PET image, the patient is injected with an IV dose of a radioactive material (radioactive tracer). The most commonly administered radiopharmaceutical agent is fluorodeoxyglucose F 18 (^{18}F-FDG). This agent is produced in a cyclotron near the imaging facility. With a half-life of approximately 1,010 minutes, the agents are usually ordered the day before an examination and delivered to the imaging facility on the day of examination. The ^{18}F-FDG is injected and taken up from the vascular compartment by GLUT receptors in cells in a similar fashion to glucose. Once in the cells, the ^{18}F-FDG undergoes phosphorylation to ^{18}F-FDG-6-phospate by hexokinase; the ^{18}F-FDG-6-phosphate is trapped in the cells and when measured can be an indirect indicator of the relative rate of glucose metabolism in the cells in the imaged tissue. The injection is given approximately 1 hour before imaging to allow time for tissue uptake of the radioactive tracer. Neoplastic processes tend to exhibit markedly elevated glucose utilization and thus take up more ^{18}F-FDG.

^{18}F undergoes radioactive positron decay (one proton decays into a neutron, with the release of a positron in the process). This positron will collide with its antimatter counterpart, an electron, in short order. The collision process (annihilation) of the electron and positron converts their mass into energy in the form of two 511-keV photons, which travel away from each other in opposite directions. The two photons are detected by scintillator detectors in the PET scanner via coincidence detection. The greater the number of photons emitted by the tissue, the more intense the image will appear. The amount of activity may be semiquantified with a standardized uptake value (SUV). SUV is the amount of activity in a measured region of interest that has been normalized for the injected dose and ratio of body weight to surface area. As a ratio, it is a unitless measure

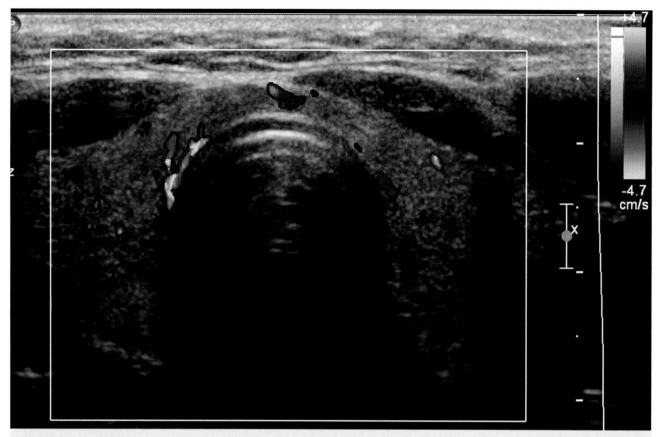

Fig. 10.8 The intensity and direction of blood flow in the thyroid gland can be assessed with ultrasound.

Table 10.3 Advantages and disadvantages of ultrasound imaging

Advantages	Disadvantages
Low cost, readily available	Low spatial resolution ("fuzzy" image)
Extremely portable imaging units; ability to perform scans in nearly any environment on any patient	Poor evaluation of deep structures of the head and neck
No ionizing radiation	Highly dependent on skill of ultrasonographer, which reduces test reproducibility compared with other imaging modalities
Excellent evaluation of the thyroid, parotid, and submandibular glands	Inadequate evaluation of the aerodigestive tract
Real-time imaging modality ideal for image-guided interventional procedures	

and should be used with caution because it is prone to error if all variables are not properly considered. The imaging data set can be constructed into a three-dimensional image and can be fused with the CT data set (▶ Fig. 10.13).

PET-CT imaging offers the best of two worlds: high-spatial-resolution anatomical CT imaging and excellent physiologic PET imaging to maximize the detection and staging of head and neck carcinoma. It is the imaging modality of choice for staging and following the treatment of head and neck carcinoma. PET-CT has greater sensitivity and specificity than MR imaging in the staging of head and neck neoplasm and is the imaging modality of choice for staging for nodal involvement. PET-CT is also excellent in the detection of a treatment response after head and neck resection and/or chemoradiation. PET-CT is of critical value in the detection of recurrent head and neck neoplasm and is especially useful for detecting distant metastasis. Local recurrence detection is more difficult because of uptake in inflammatory tissue in the postoperative bed; however, CT and MR imaging have similar drawbacks. If the PET scan is negative, a recurrence is unlikely, whereas a positive PET scan may necessitate a biopsy to distinguish granulation/scar tissue from recurrence.

Interestingly, PET-CT is not useful for distinguishing benign from malignant salivary gland neoplasms as both have similar uptake of ^{18}F-FDG (▶ Table 10.5).

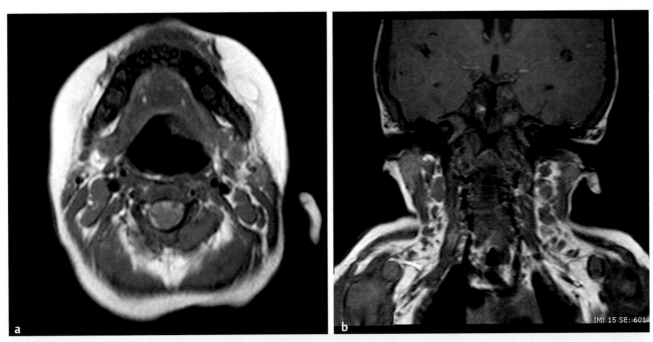

Fig. 10.9 (a) Axial and (b) coronal T1-weighted magnetic resonance imaging sequence of the neck.

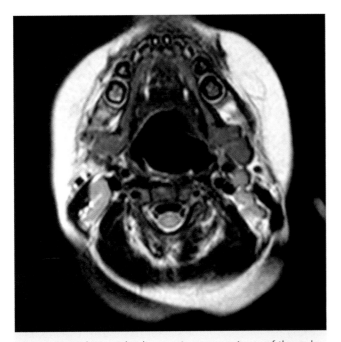

Fig. 10.10 Axial T2-weighted magnetic resonance image of the neck.

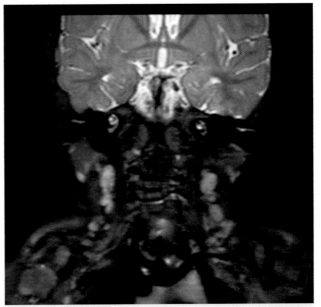

Fig. 10.11 Coronal fat-suppressed T2-weighted magnetic resonance image of the neck.

10.3 Imaging Anatomy

10.3.1 Skull Base

Temporal Bone

Middle Ear

The middle ear comprises three principal components: the epitympanum (above the level of the tympanic membrane and extending to the tegmen tympani, which separates it from the middle cranial fossa); the mesotympanum (at the level of the tympanic membrane); and the hypotympanum (below and medial to the tympanic membrane). The tympanic membrane attaches superiorly to the scutum, which is a sharp bony excrescence that is best seen on coronal images. The tympanic membrane will be seen as a thin wispy structure on CT. The tegmen tympani, or roof of the middle ear, is also best visualized on coronal imaging. It is a very thin structure, and close attention to its integrity is essential during the imaging of infectious, traumatic, and neoplastic processes of the middle ear. Erosion/

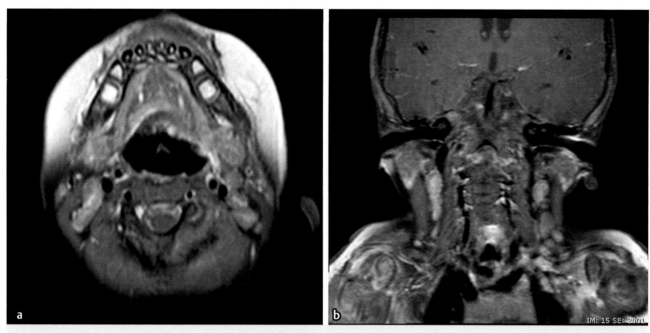

Fig. 10.12 (a) Axial and (b) coronal contrast-enhanced T1 image with fat suppression of the neck.

Table 10.4 Advantages and disadvantages of magnetic resonance imaging

Advantages	Disadvantages
No ionizing radiation	Long imaging time
Excellent soft-tissue and spatial resolution	Prone to artifact
Excellent delineation of soft tissue and perineural spread of disease	Confined imaging location/claustrophobia
	Extremely complex and expensive imaging modality
	Significant expertise needed to perform and interpret examination
	Limited availability
	Large fixed imaging unit

disruption of the tegmen may provide direct access to the central nervous system/intracranial compartment.

The Prussak space, just medial to the scutum, lies between the scutum and ossicles and is normally aerated. This is especially important because soft tissue seen on CT imaging in this space should raise the possibility of a cholesteatoma. All aerated structures in the middle ear are typically very dark on CT imaging. Any alteration in the uniformity of the dark black appearance suggests opacification of these spaces, possibly indicating infection, such as otitis media, or a mass lesion, such as cholesteatoma or other neoplasm. The scutum is best visualized on coronal imaging and should taper to sharp point (▶ Fig. 10.14a). Blunting or erosion of the scutum with opacification of the middle ear is a sine qua non of acquired cholesteatoma.

The malleus, incus, and stapes are evaluated well with thin-section CT imaging. The head of the malleus articulates with the incus. On imaging, the malleus and incus are frequently described as having an "ice cream on cone" appearance, with the malleus making up the ice cream portion and the incus the cone (▶ Fig. 10.14b). This is especially important in the setting of trauma because ossicular disruption is often visualized as a

loss of this classic "ice cream on cone" appearance. The lenticular process of the incus articulates with the head of the stapes. The stapes has a horseshoe appearance on imaging and comprises an anterior and posterior crus and footplate. The footplate covers the oval window. A quick way to ensure that CT imaging of the middle and inner structures is technically adequate is to determine whether you can easily and reliably identify the footplate of the stapes. This usually requires thin-section images that are less than 1 mm in thickness.

Within the middle ear, two muscles deserve special mention because these can be visualized on imaging. The tensor tympani muscle is seen extending along the eustachian tube and inserts onto the manubrium of the malleus. The stapedius muscle originates from the pyramidal eminence, an osseous mound that is found within the hypotympanum and attaches to the head of the stapes.

Inner Ear

The principal components of the inner ear include the cochlea and the vestibular apparatus. The cochlea, semicircular canals,

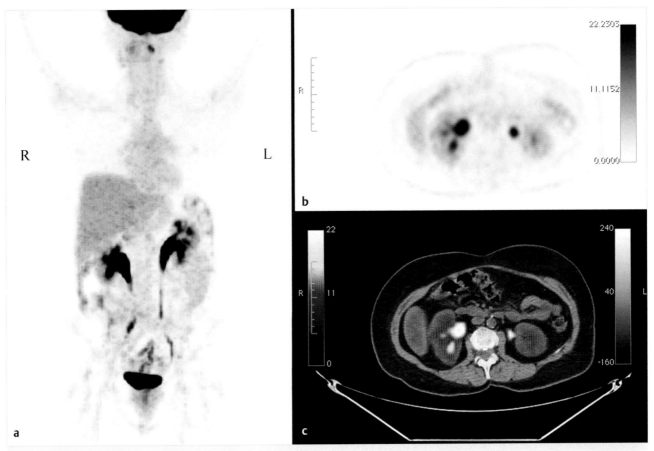

Fig. 10.13 A positron emission tomographic–computed tomographic (PET-CT) scan can provide anatomical detail and show the physiologic activity of tissues. **(a)** Three-dimensional volume-rendered image of the entire PET data set. This is shown in anteroposterior view but can be rotated on the workstation. **(b)** Axial PET image and **(c)** axial PET-CT fused image through the abdomen. PET-CT fusion clearly shows fluorodeoxyglucose F 18 excreted in the renal collecting system (normal), without a renal mass. The PET data (shown in color) are fused onto the CT image with a three-dimensional workstation.

Table 10.5 Advantages and disadvantages of positron emission tomography–computed tomography (PET-CT)

Advantages	Disadvantages
Physiologic and anatomical imaging	High dose of ionizing radiation
Fusion of CT improves spatial resolving power limitations of PET imaging	Significant expertise is needed to properly interpret examination
Excellent for staging and postoperative evaluation of head and neck carcinoma	Time-consuming examination, both in preparation and scan time
	Limited availability, large scanner, and requirement to be near cyclotron for production of radioactive tracer
	Confined imaging location/claustrophobia
	Very expensive
	Large, fixed imaging unit

and vestibule comprise the bony labyrinth. The cochlea has two and a half turns (apical, middle, and basal). The modiolus is the bony central portion of the cochlea seen on imaging. The lateral, superior, and posterior semicircular canals converge on the vestibule and are crucial for propagating information involved in balance. The cochlea and vestibular apparatus are very well visualized with CT and MR imaging. CT of the temporal bone is integral in the evaluation of congenital malformations of the inner ear. Additionally, multiplanar reconstructions of the temporal bone allow excellent evaluation of the semicircular canals for dehiscence. The vestibular aqueduct is an important inner ear anatomical structure that is well visualized on thin-section CT scans and can be reliably assessed for enlargement.

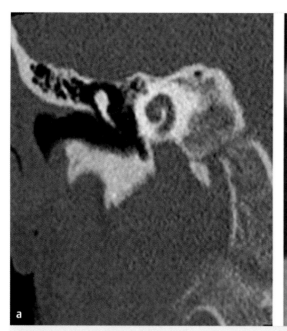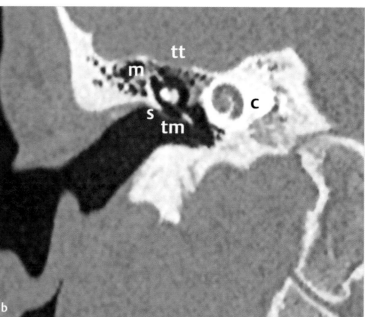

Fig. 10.14 **(a)** Coronal view through the external auditory canal shows a sharply defined scutum, head, and long process of the malleus; an air-filled Prussak space; ventilated mastoid air cells; an intact tegmen tympani; and 1.5 turns of the cochlea. **(b)** Another coronal view of the scutum (*s*), tympanic membrane (*tm*), mastoid air cells (*m*), tegmen tympani (*tt*), and cochlea (*c*). The incudomalleolar joint is seen between the tegmen and the tympanic membrane.

External Ear

The external auditory canal is bound anteriorly by the glenoid fossa and posteriorly by the mastoid air cells and extends medially to the tympanic membrane. The external auditory canal, meatus, and auricle are well visualized on routine CT imaging. CT allows excellent characterization of associated anomalies of the ossicles, inner ear, and facial nerve canal in cases of external ear anomalies.

Facial Nerve

The facial nerve is a complex cranial nerve that spans numerous anatomical compartments and spaces. The primary modalities used to image the facial nerve include CT and MR imaging. There are three primary components of the facial nerve: visceral motor component/parasympathetic component (autonomic control to the lacrimal, submandibular, and sublingual glands); branchial motor component (innervation to the muscles of facial expression); and special sensory component (taste from the anterior two-thirds of the tongue). The visceral motor and branchial motor components arise from nuclei within the brainstem at the pontine tegmentum. The root entry zone and cisternal segments of the facial nerve can be well visualized with high-resolution T2-weighted balanced fast field imaging of the brain stem. Cranial nerves VII and VIII (including the superior and inferior vestibular divisions and cochlear division) can be identified with high-resolution imaging. This is of importance during an evaluation for vestibular schwannoma or congenital aplasia of the cochlear nerve. Imaging of the proximal intracranial segments of cranial nerve VII and VIII is best done at high-field-strength, 3-tesla MR imaging. The motor fibers of the facial nerve course ventrally and laterally at the cerebellopon-

tine angle to exit as the more anterior nerve. The canalicular segment of the facial nerve is located in the anterior superior quadrant of the internal auditory canal. The facial nerve has a complex path in the temporal bone that is poorly visualized on MR imaging. However, the bony facial nerve canal is well visualized on CT scan of the temporal bone. The geniculate ganglion of the facial nerve may be visualized on MR imaging. On contrast-enhanced MR imaging of the facial nerve, no enhancement should be seen in the pre-geniculate portions of the facial nerve, but normal enhancement may be seen in the post-geniculate segments of the facial nerve because of the extensive perineural blood supply. Enhancement in the pre-geniculate portions of the facial nerve is suggestive of neuritis or neoplasm. The facial nerve exits the temporal bone at the stylomastoid foramen, which is best visualized on coronal and axial CT scans. The facial nerve then courses anteriorly into the parotid gland, running superficial to the retromandibular vein and dividing into peripheral branches, many of which cannot be resolved with current imaging technology.

Sinuses

It is prudent to discuss the sinonasal apparatus in terms of drainage pathways, centered on the ostiomeatal complex serving as the common pathway for drainage of the anterior ethmoid, frontal, and maxillary sinuses, with the sphenoethmoidal recess serving to drain the posterior ethmoid and sphenoid sinuses. The ostiomeatal complex comprises the maxillary sinus os, the uncinate process, the infundibulum, and the hiatus semilunaris, with drainage into the middle meatus. The cilia within the maxillary sinus serve to steer drainage toward the superomedial ostium within the sinus. A bony extension, the uncinate process, projects superiorly from the superomedial

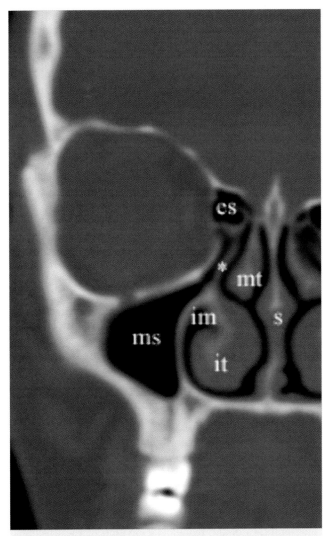

Fig. 10.15 Coronal view through the nose and sinuses, showing normal structures: maxillary sinus (*ms*), ethmoid sinus air cells (*es*), middle turbinate (*mt*), inferior turbinate (*it*), septum (*s*), uncinate process (*asterisk*), and inferior meatus (*im*). The middle meatus is located between the uncinate process and the middle turbinate, whereas the ethmoid infundibulum is located lateral to the uncinate process.

maxillary sinus wall. Lateral to the uncinate process, the hiatus semilunaris is the half-moon–shaped entry to the infundibulum, the trough lateral to the uncinate process, through which mucus drains into the middle meatus and eventually to the back of the nasal cavity. The osseous structures of the ostiomeatal unit are best assessed on coronal reformatted CT scans of the paranasal sinuses. The various bony landmarks and details are well appreciated on routine CT of the paranasal sinuses with coronal reconstructions (▶ Fig. 10.15).

The lateral attachment of the middle meatus to the medial orbit is termed the basal lamella and serves as the anatomical landmark dividing the anterior from posterior ethmoid air cells. The air cell lying just superior to the infundibulum is termed the ethmoid bulla. The frontal sinuses, as do the anterior ethmoid air cells, drain directly to the middle meatus via the frontal recess. The sphenoid sinuses and posterior ethmoid air

cells drain via the superior meatus and the sphenoethmoidal recess.

Ethmoid air cells of specific interest include agger nasi cells, Onodi cells, and Haller cells. Agger nasi cells are ethmoid air cells anterior and lateral to the frontal recess; they can obstruct frontal sinus outflow. Onodi cells are ethmoidal air cells that extend into the posterior orbit or sphenoid bone. Haller cells are anterior ethmoid air cells that are seen inferior to the orbit and extend into the maxillary sinus; they also can obstruct outflow.

The nasal cavity comprises the superior, middle, and inferior turbinates. Imaging of the nasal passage is straightforward. One must remain aware of nasal cycling, with alternating mucosal hyperemia in the nasal passages. This can lead the inexperienced imager to overcall nasal mass lesions. A simple rule of thumb in the evaluation of the nasal passages is that if a rim of air (no matter how thin) can be traced around the nasal mucosa, there is a low likelihood of a space-occupying mass lesion, and any asymmetry can be attributed to nasal cycling. Below the inferior turbinate, one finds the opening for the nasolacrimal duct, originating from the lacrimal sac; the bony canal for the nasolacrimal duct can often be identified on coronal images. The septum serves to divide the right and left nasal cavities and comprises an anterior cartilaginous portion and a posterior bony portion.

10.3.2 Head and Neck Mucosal Surfaces

Nasopharynx

The nasopharynx is bound by the mucosal surface that lies above the soft and hard palate. Posterolaterally, the eustachian tube orifice can be found. On either side of the eustachian tube are the tensor veli palatini and levator veli palatini. Deep to the mucosa of the nasopharynx, the buccopharyngeal fascia and pharyngobasilar fascia serve to prevent the spread of disease to the retropharyngeal and parapharyngeal spaces. Additionally, lymph nodes and minor salivary glands are found throughout the nasopharynx. The nasopharynx is well imaged with either CT or MR imaging. A rudimentary evaluation of the nasopharynx can be made with radiography. Close attention to the mucosa and submucosal fat planes may allow early detection of nasopharyngeal carcinoma. MR imaging may be particularly sensitive to evaluate for neoplasm. Sagittal reformatted images are a key component in the evaluation of the nasopharynx.

Oral Cavity

The lips, buccal and gingival surfaces, hard palate, anterior two-thirds of the tongue, and floor of the mouth comprise the oral cavity. The lingual space is the area between the mylohyoid muscle and the hyoglossus muscle; the lingual nerve and hypoglossal nerve and the sublingual gland are located in this space. The mylohyoid muscles define the floor of the mouth. The submandibular gland is found within the floor of the mouth and drains via the Wharton duct. Below the mylohyoid muscles, one finds the submental space. Determining the exact spaces involved by pathology is especially important because this greatly affects surgical approach. The oral cavity is an extremely difficult space to image. This is primarily because of extensive artifact that is generated by dental amalgam, and streak artifact on

CT scan will diminish its sensitivity and specificity. MR imaging results in magnetic susceptibility artifact, which appears as dark black holes on the image. These artifacts make evaluation of the oral cavity extremely challenging. A detailed history and any information from the physical examination help the interpreting radiologist to "read through the artifact."

Oropharynx

As in the oral cavity and nasopharynx, minor salivary glands are found in abundance within the oropharynx. The imaging modality of choice for most oropharyngeal lesions is CT or MR imaging. The exception to this would be the evaluation of epiglottitis and croup in pediatric patients, in whom radiography is the first imaging modality typically employed because of its accessibility, speed, and relatively low radiation exposure.

Hypopharynx

The hypopharynx is most typically attended to on imaging when there is extension of squamous cell carcinoma to this region. It is well assessed with multiplanar CT or MR imaging. PET-CT can be very useful is evaluating the degree of neoplasm extension to the hypopharynx.

Larynx

The larynx is subdivided into the supraglottis, glottis, and subglottis. The cricoarytenoid joint is the marker for the level of the true vocal fold; however, this is often difficult to visualize. Another marker that is used is the paraglottic space, found lateral to the laryngeal mucosa, which contains fat at the false vocal fold level but contains muscle at the true vocal fold level. Again, multiplanar CT and MR imaging are the typical imaging modalities of choice in evaluating the larynx.

10.3.3 Soft Tissues of the Neck

Parapharyngeal Space

The prestyloid parapharyngeal space is readily identified on CT. This region is bound posteriorly by the carotid space, laterally by the parotid space, anteriorly by the masticator space, anteromedially by the oropharynx, and posteromedially by the retropharyngeal space. This area contains fat, lymphatics, small branches of the external carotid artery, and the mandibular nerve. However, this area is especially important in placing pathology into the various spaces of the neck by determining the displacement of the parapharyngeal fat. For example, a mass within the masticator space will displace the parapharyngeal fat posteromedially, whereas a mass from the parotid gland will displace the parapharyngeal fat anteromedially. This point will continue to be illustrated throughout the following sections. Lesions in the parotid space can be visualized very clearly with CT or MR imaging techniques. The axial imaging plane is usually the most useful plane for visualizing the parapharyngeal space.

Carotid Space

This space is also known as the post-styloid parapharyngeal space and extends the entire length of the neck. It contains the carotid artery, internal jugular vein, cranial nerves IX through XII, and the sympathetic nerve plexus, as well as lymph nodes, which are found throughout its course. Lesions originating within the carotid space will displace the parapharyngeal fat anteriorly. The carotid space is best evaluated with mulitplanar CT or MR imaging. Axial and sagittal planes allow the best visualization and delineation of this space.

Parotid Space

The parotid space contains the parotid gland, cranial nerve VII, and branches of cranial nerve V, as well as vasculature including external carotid artery branches and the retromandibular vein. The deep portion of the parotid gland extends through the stylomandibular tunnel, found between the mandibular ramus and the digastric and sternocleidomastoid muscles. Most of the gland is superficial to the masseter muscle and the mandible. The Stensen duct drains the parotid gland passing over the masseter muscle and then pierces the buccinator muscle before terminating within the buccal mucosa. The parotid gland is relatively superficial and amenable to excellent visualization with ultrasound, CT, or MR imaging modalities. Lesions within the parotid gland are best characterized with CT or MR imaging; however, many solid lesions may require biopsy or surgical resection because the specificity of imaging in the delineation of benign versus malignant neoplasm of the parotid gland is poor.

Masticator Space

The muscles of mastication, including the temporalis and masseter muscle as well as the medial and lateral pterygoid muscles, are contained by the superficial layer of the deep cervical fascia in the masticator space. The mandibular ramus is centrally located in the masticator space and contains the inferior alveolar nerve, which traverses the masticator space. Other contents include branches of the mandibular division of the trigeminal nerve and the inferior alveolar vein and artery. The buccal space is often included in a discussion of the masticator space because of its close physical proximity to the masticator space and its lack of true fascia boundaries. The masticator space is ideally imaged with CT or MR imaging. The axial and coronal imaging planes are the most useful orientations to appreciate the relevant anatomy and spread of disease.

10.4 Roundsmanship

- Emergent imaging of the head and neck frequently will involve one of two entities: infection or airway obstruction. Contrast-enhanced CT of the neck is the examination of choice to evaluate for acute head and neck infection in most cases and will also adequately assess the airway. In the pediatric population, one may consider radiography to evaluate and exclude epiglottitis because of the decreased radiation dose.
- Reviewing your imaging studies with your interpreting radiologist will likely greatly improve the accuracy of the interpretations and allow the highest-quality medical care for your patients. Do not hesitate to consult your radiologist frequently. Head and neck imaging is challenging, even for many experienced neuroradiologists, and feedback from the

ordering otolaryngologist often leads to the most accurate interpretations.

- Be aware of radiation doses and possible side effects of IV contrast material when ordering imaging of the head and neck. If there is a risk–benefit question, always consult your radiologist.
- Remember that image-guided (CT or ultrasound) percutaneous needle biopsy of deep lesions of the head and neck is a service that is available at many institutions.

10.5 Recommended Reading

[1] American College of Radiology. Manual on Contrast Media v9. . Accessed October 11, 2013

[2] Curry TS, Dowdy JE, Murry RC Jr. Christensen's Physics of Diagnostic Radiology. 4th ed. Philadelphia, PA: Lippincott Williams & Wilkins; 1990

[3] Hasso A. Diagnostic Imaging of the Head and Neck: MRI with CT & PET Correlations. Philadelphia, PA: Lippincott Williams & Wilkins; 2012

[4] Som PM, Curtin HD. Head and Neck Imaging. 5th ed. St. Louis, MO: Mosby; 2011

[5] Mafee MF, Valvasorri G, Becker M. Valvasorri's Imaging of the Head and Neck. 2nd ed.New York, NY: Thieme; 2005

[6] Hashemi RH. MRI: The Basics. 3rd ed. Philadelphia, PA: Lippincott Williams & Wilkins; 2010

[7] Huda W. Review of Radiologic Physics. 3rd ed. Philadelphia, PA: Lippincott Williams & Wilkins; 2009

11 Radiographic Imaging of Common Clinical Presentations in Otolaryngology–Head and Neck Surgery

Hasit Mehta and Ajay Hira

11.1 Introduction

The radiologic imaging of a number of disorders of the head and neck can be highly distinctive and often diagnostic. A number of clinical scenarios and the characteristic radiologic appearance of each are described below. The reader is referred to the previous chapter for more detailed discussions of the various imaging modalities available.

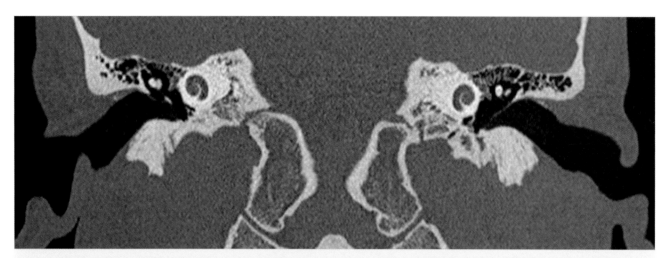

Fig. 11.1 Coronal computed tomography (CT) through the temporal bone demonstrates marked diastasis of the left incudomalleolar joint, compatible with ossicular dislocation. This is the appearance of the "ice cream scoop" falling off the "cone." The partially visualized right incudomalleolar joint demonstrates a tight joint space and no diastasis. CT of the temporal bone (with coronal and axial thin sections) is the ideal imaging modality to make this diagnosis.

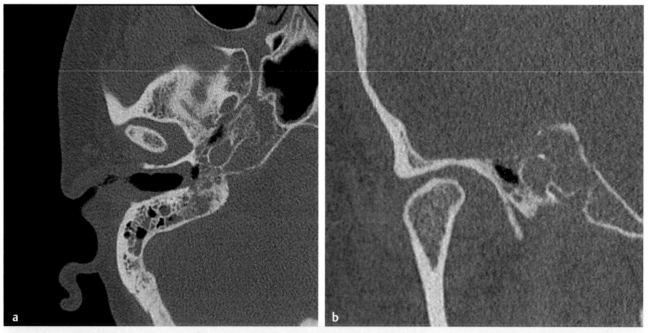

Fig. 11.2 Axial (a) and coronal (b) computed tomographic scans of the temporal bone demonstrate extensive otomastoiditis with associated petrous apicitis. There is erosion of the many septa within the mastoid air cells, as well as erosion into the middle cranial fossa. In this situation, magnetic resonance imaging of the brain would be useful to evaluate for possible intracranial extension of an infectious process.

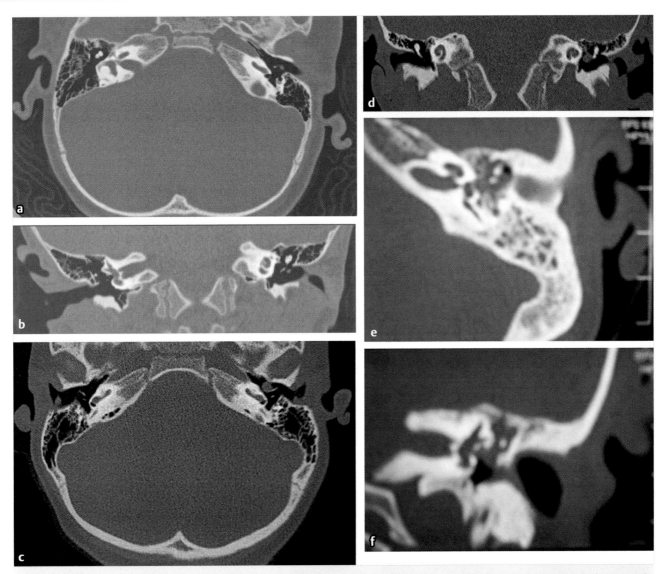

Fig. 11.3 (a) Axial and (b) coronal projections through the temporal bone. The scutum is sharp. There is a 2-mm ovoid soft-tissue-density lesion noted above the left tympanic membrane that may be contiguous with the tympanic membrane, compatible with a small primary congenital cholesteatoma. In another patient, (c) axial and (d) coronal views show a 4-mm ovoid soft-tissue mass in the left middle ear medial to the left ossicular chain, in close proximity to the expected location of the long process of the incus and stapes. These findings are compatible with congenital cholesteatoma. Other diagnoses to consider include facial nerve schwannoma (although there is no evidence of expansion of the bony facial nerve canal) and glomus tympanicum. Correlation with direct examination is useful. In another patient, soft tissue in the left middle ear and mastoid associated with bony erosion on (e) axial and (f) coronal computed tomographic scans is more suggestive of acquired cholesteatoma.

11.2 Disorders of the Ear

11.2.1 Ossicular Discontinuity (▶ Fig. 11.1)

The diagnosis of traumatic ossicular dislocation is best visualized on thin-section computed toographic (CT) scans of the temporal bone. Ossicular dislocation is often seen with traumatic temporal bone fracture. Ossicular injury and conductive hearing loss are more commonly seen with longitudinal and longitudinal oblique fractures of the temporal bone than with posterior transverse fractures the temporal bone, which may present with sensorineural hearing loss. The most common ossicular dislocation is dislocation of the incudomalleolar joint.

The incudomalleolar joint is a true joint with a joint capsule and is best visualized on high-resolution axial CT scans of the temporal bone. Diastasis of the head of the malleus and short process of the incus is characteristic of incudomalleolar dislocation and may also be appreciated on coronal imaging. Incudostapedial ossicular dislocation is less common and more difficult to visualize. This is typically best seen with coronal high-resolution sagittal imaging of the temporal bone. Careful attention must be given to the long process of the incus and the head of the stapes. Often, in the acute traumatic setting, with extensive blood product and debris within the middle ear, the diagnosis of ossicular dislocation may not be made. Follow-up CT of the temporal bone after resolution of the acute traumatic injury may be useful in this case. Occasionally, portions of the incus,

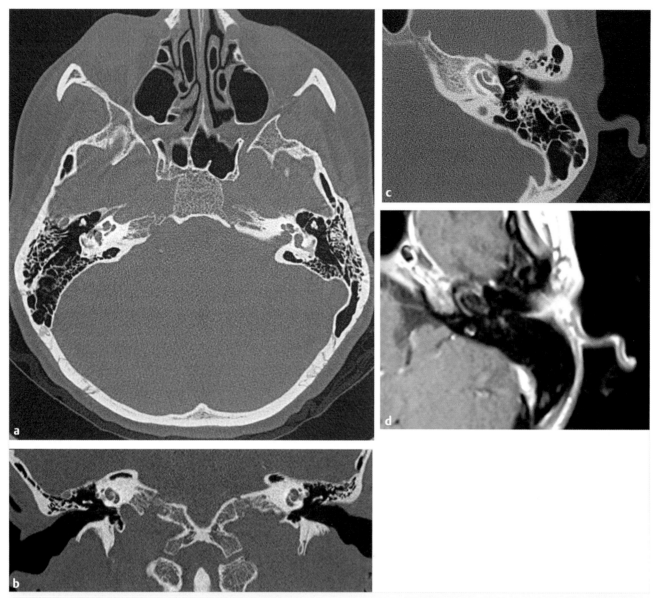

Fig. 11.4 Noncontrast thin-section computed tomographic (CT) scans of the temporal bone in the (**a**) axial and (**b**) coronal planes demonstrate small regions of lucency within the temporal bone just anterior to the oval window bilaterally in the region of the fissula ante fenestram, right greater than left. This finding is typically seen in early fenestral otosclerosis. The remainder of the otic capsule appears spared. (**c**) Axial CT scan demonstrating radiolucent appearence about the cochea, giving the appearance of an extra turn about the left chochlea. (**d**) Axial magnetic resonance image demonstrates enhancement around the left cochlea. Both of these imaging findings are characteristic of cochlear otosclerosis.

malleus, and stapes may be completely disrupted, with free-floating bone fragments in the middle ear; close attention to the osseous structures on coronal, axial, and sagittal planes is necessary to make this diagnosis.

11.2.2 Chronic Ear Disease, Mastoiditis, and Cholesteatoma (▶ Fig. 11.2)

Chronic otitis media demonstrates soft-tissue accumulation in the middle ear and mastoid cavities. Often, the ossicles are surrounded by a dense, sometimes calcific soft-tissue mass; bone erosion may be seen. The normal septa of the mastoid cavity may be broken down, creating a large central cavity filled with soft tissue. The disease can spread into an aerated pertrous

apex. Potential erosion into the middle cranial fossa should be examined.

Acquired cholesteatomas are collections of keratinous debris that lead to infection and inflammation. Soft tissue will be seen within the middle ear cavity, and erosive change can involve the mastoid air cells and inner ear structures. The most common type of cholesteatoma is the acquired pars flaccida subtype. The pars flaccida subtype begins in the Prussak space, between the scutum and the incus. On CT, soft tissue is seen within the Prussak space. This by itself is a nonspecific finding. However, larger lesions will be accompanied by osseous erosion, which is very characteristic of acquired cholesteatomas and can lead to ossicular chain disruption and erosion of the scutum. The more uncommon pars tensa subtype will begin

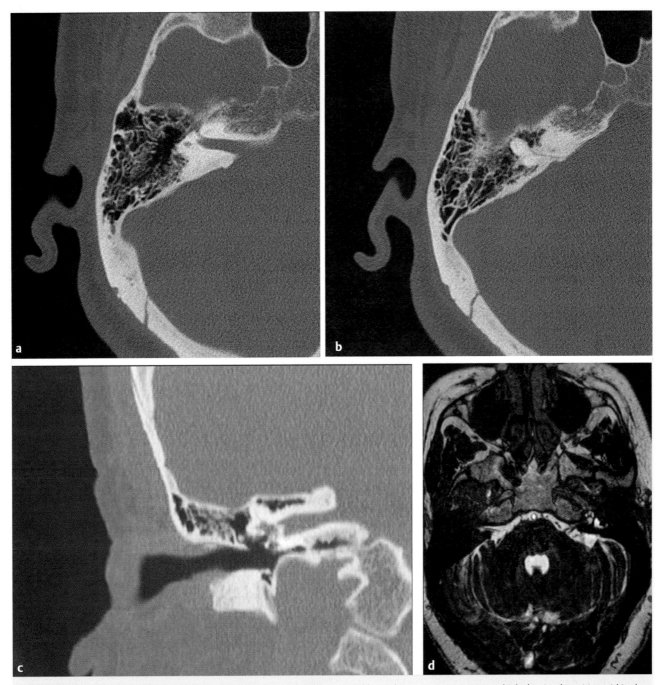

Fig. 11.5 (a,b) Axial and **(c)** coronal computed tomographic scans of the temporal bone demonstrate an extensive, high-density deposition within the membranous labyrinth. This may present with sensorineural hearing loss, often secondary to a traumatic or infectious insult to the inner ear. **(d)** Axial high-resolution T2 images through the region of the internal auditory canals demonstrate a paucity of expected endolymph in the right membranous labyrinth, compatible with labyrinthine ossificans. In severe cases, the cochlear nerve may be small.

with soft tissue within the posterior mesotympanum medial to the ossicles. The scutum is usually spared, unlike in the pars flaccida subtype. Extension of a cholesteatoma into the mastoid air cells in common. Additional complications include semicircular canal fistulas, erosion of the tegmen tympani, and dehiscence of the tympanic segment of the facial nerve. Noncontrast CT of the temporal bones is the imaging test of choice to assess for the aforementioned findings. Magnetic resonance (MR)

imaging can also be utilized to demarcate a nonenhancing cholesteatoma from enhancing granulation tissue, but this is generally unnecessary, with cholesteatomas appearing hypointense on T1, of intermediate intensity on T2, and nonenhancing. Congenital cholesteatomas (▶ Fig. 11.3) develop because epidermal rests reside in the middle ear cleft embryologically. These are typically more anteriorly located and may not have the same degree of bony erosion as acquired cholesteatomas.

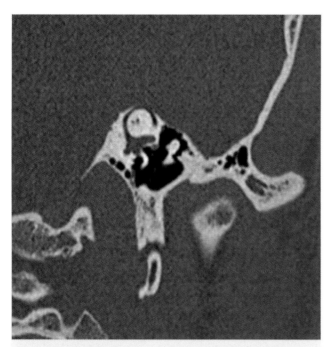

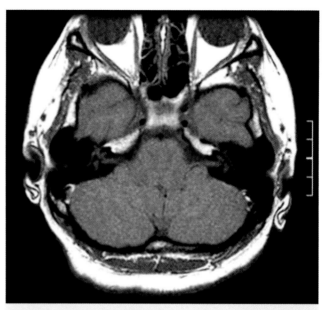

Fig. 11.6 The imaging of superior semicircular canal dehiscence requires high-resolution, thin-section (1-mm or smaller interval) temporal bone imaging; additionally, oblique multiplanar reformatted images are useful in demonstrating the entire course of the superior semicircular canal to adequately detect dehiscence. This image is an oblique coronal view through the inner ear structures. The roof of the left superior semicircular canal is dehiscent into the left middle cranial fossa, with marked demineralization.

Fig. 11.8 Axial T1 images through the cerebellopontine angle region (a) before and (b) after contrast demonstrate curvilinear enhancement involving the most distal segment of the right internal auditory canal and extending to the labyrinthine and geniculate segments of the right facial nerve, which appear enlarged. Portions of the horizontal segment of the right facial nerve also appear enlarged in a tapered fashion. This configuration is characteristic of facial nerve schwannoma. Other etiologies that could have a similar appearance include metastatic disease and lymphoma. Facial neuroma/schwannoma may occur along any segment of the facial nerve. The geniculate ganglion is often involved. The symptomology depends on which segment of the facial nerve is involved. In distinguishing between facial schwannoma and other etiologies, expansion of the facial nerve canal is highly suggestive of facial schwannoma, excluding inflammatory neuritis. When the lesion enters the internal auditory canal and cerebellopontine angle, it may be indistinguishable from vestibular schwannoma.

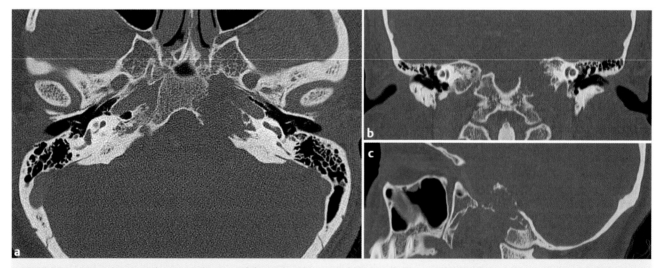

Fig. 11.7 Noncontrast computed tomographic scan of the temporal bone in the (a) axial, (b) coronal, and (c) sagittal planes demonstrates a large, destructive mass lesion involving the petrous portion of the left temporal bone. The mass extends to the clivus, involving portions of the basisphenoid. The lesion is centered in the region of the petroclival synchondrosis, characteristic of an aggressive skull base chondrosarcoma. Typically, these lesions contain extensive calcified chondroid matrix in a ring-and-arc type of pattern; however, this patient's lesion demonstrates minimal intratumoral calcified matrix, making the diagnosis more difficult. This diagnosis should be included in the differential of a large expansile lesion with regions of mixed osseous structures within the lesion. Other diagnoses to consider include metastatic lesions, plasmacytoma, petrous apex cholesteatoma, and chordoma.

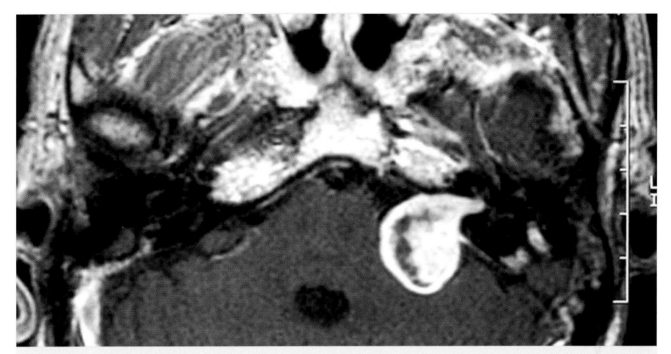

Fig. 11.9 Axial T1 postcontrast magnetic resonance imaging through the region of the cerebellopontine angle demonstrates a large enhancing lesion that extends from the internal auditory canal through the internal auditory meatus/porus acusticus into the cerebellopontine angle. The appearance of this lesion is that of an ice cream cone (with the scoop of ice cream melting off into the cerebellopontine angle) and is characteristic of vestibular schwannoma. With a large canal-to-cerebellopontine angle schwannoma, it is impossible to distinguish between vestibular and facial schwannoma. Schwannomas typically enhance homogeneously, although when they are large, the central portions may demonstrate heterogeneous enhancement, as in this case. Differential considerations include meningioma, lymphoma, and metastatic disease.

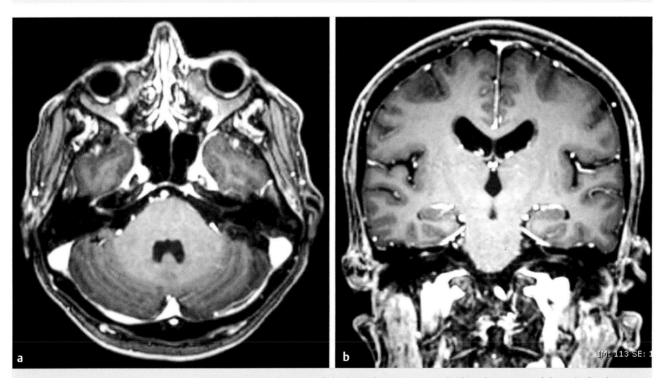

Fig. 11.10 Postcontrast T1-weighted (a) axial and (b) coronal images of the brain demonstrate canalicular enhancement of the right facial nerve extending to the labyrinthine segment as well as the geniculate ganglion. The differential diagnosis for this finding primarily includes facial nerve schwannoma, neuritis (e.g., Bell palsy), and metastatic cranial nerve lesion. Inflammatory processes, such as sarcoidosis or Lyme disease, may also present with cranial nerve enhancement. However, this patient was known to have lymphoma, which can present with cranial nerve enhancement. Additionally, more cephalic images demonstrated asymmetric abnormal enhancement of the right trigeminal nerve, compatible with lymphomatous involvement of cranial nerve V. Computed tomography of the temporal bones may be useful to differentiate cranial nerve mass lesions (e.g., schwannoma) from neuritis because a mass lesion typically will demonstrate remodeling and enlargement of the osseous structures when the mass is large enough.

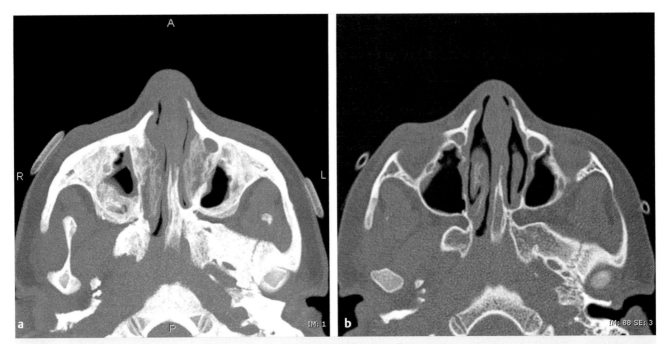

Fig. 11.11 (a) Soft-tissue and (b) bone axial window computed tomography (CT) is the imaging modality of choice for choanal atresia. Thin-section CT of the maxillofacial region as well as maximum-intensity-projection reconstructions may be obtained to evaluate more completely the nasal passage and nasal choanae. In this case, the posterior nasal cavity is narrow, with bony atresia of the left choana and a small membranous component inferiorly. The vomer is enlarged asymmetrically, left greater than right. The left maxillary sinus is rotated laterally. There is no significant air–fluid level in the nasal passage. These findings are typical for left choanal atresia.

11.2.3 Otosclerosis/Otospongiosis

Fenestral otospongiosis is more common than cochlear otosclerosis. Young and middle-aged patients often present with progressive conductive or with mixed conductive and sensineural hearing loss. Often, symptoms and findings are bilateral. In fenestral otospongiosis, radiographic findings begin at the anterior margin of the oval window, which is called the fissula ante fenestram. On CT, this begins as a hypoattenuating focus at the fissula ante fenestram (▶ Fig. 11.4a, b). However, with time, this often spreads to involve the additional margins of the oval and round windows. Over time, or in cochlear otosclerosis, demineralization can involve the middle and basal turns of the cochlea, resulting in an apparent double ring or halo appearance of hypoattenuation surrounding the cochlea (▶ Fig. 11.4c, d). In the late healing phase, new bone or increased sclerosis will be seen along the oval and round windows. MR imaging, often not needed in the evaluation, may demonstrate subtle enhancing foci within the medial portions of the middle ear in the regions of the oval and round windows.

11.2.4 Labyrinthine Ossificans (▶ Fig. 11.5)

Following trauma, infection, or inflammation, the activation of fibroblasts or osteoblasts may result in fibrosis or ossification within the cochlea. Most commonly, this follows meningitis in young children, resulting in bilateral sensorineural hearing loss. Less commonly, the semicircular canals or vestibule can be involved. On CT, dense sclerosis of the labyrinthine portion of the cochlea is seen. On T2 MR imaging, low-intensity foci will be

seen within the fluid-filled spaces of the inner ear, most often the cochlea. This can be seen as an apparently increased size of the modiolus, which is normally of low signal intensity on T2-weighted sequences.

11.2.5 Superior Semicircular Canal Dehiscence (▶ Fig. 11.6)

Semicircular canal dehiscence is best imaged with thin-section CT of the temporal bone. The coronal or paracoronal imaging plane is usually the best for evaluating the semicircular canal. To diagnose semicircular canal dehiscence on imaging, one must note extreme demineralization and thinning of the bony covering of the semicircular canal measuring 2 mm or greater, typically the superior posterior semicircular canal. If the region of dehiscence is less than 2 mm, it may represent a normal anatomical variant, with thinning rather than complete dehiscence of the bony covering of the semicircular canal. Semicircular canal dehiscence may present with vestibular disturbance. Typically, the region of dehiscent or thinned bone measures 2 to 5 mm. Semicircular canal dehiscence may also be visualized with high-resolution T2 MR imaging, typically with an internal auditory canal protocol of the brain.

11.2.6 Temporal Bone Chondrosarcoma (▶ Fig. 11.7)

Chondrosarcoma is included within the differential of skull base neoplasms and will be found off midline, most often at the petro-occipital fissure. CT is important in the evaluation of skull

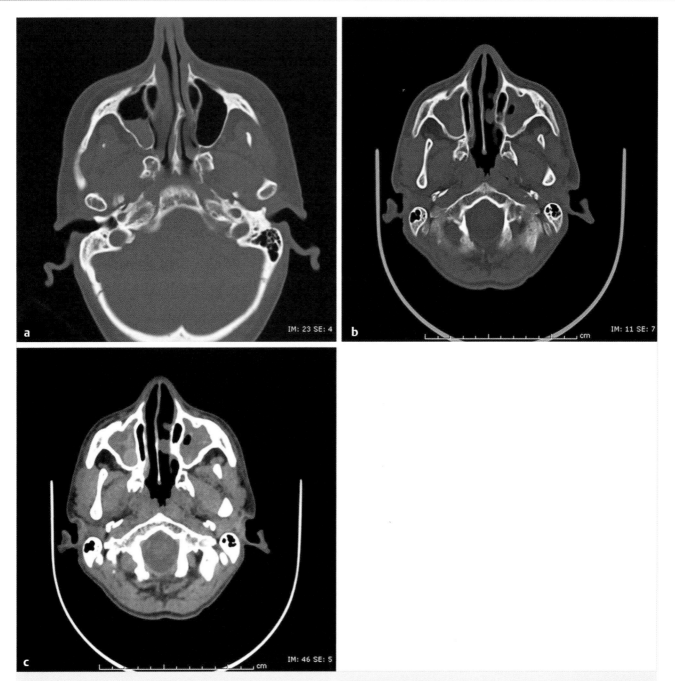

Fig. 11.12 Sinusitis. (**a**) Acute sinusitis. Axial noncontrast computed tomographic (CT) scan of the paranasal sinuses demonstrates an air–fluid level in the right maxillary paranasal sinus with a bubbly stranding at the medial aspect of the air–fluid level. These findings are suggestive of acute sinusitis. (**b,c**) Chronic sinusitis. Axial noncontrast CT scans through the paranasal sinuses demonstrate complete opacification of the maxillary paranasal sinuses. Severe bony hypertrophy, sclerosis, and thickening noted about the maxillary paranasal sinuses are compatible with chronic sinusitis, which is most easily appreciated on the axial image provided in (**b**) bone window width and level. Inspection of the maxillary paranasal sinus using (**c**) soft-tissue window demonstrates hyperdensity in the central portion of the opacified maxillary paranasal sinuses, which may represent inspissated secretions or fungal sinusitis change.

base masses and will best demonstrate the chondroid tumor matrix, which helps in distinguishing this tumor from other lesions involving the skull base. Chondroid matrix has been described as arclike or ringlike calcifications, or it may be amorphous, appearing as osteoid matrix that demonstrates cortical and medullary elements. The masses appear aggressive and will result in bone destruction and expansion. On MR imaging, the tumor will demonstrate low signal intensity on T1 and high signal on T2. Calcifications will appear dark on T1- and T2-weighted sequences. Enhancement will be heterogeneous on CT and MR imaging.

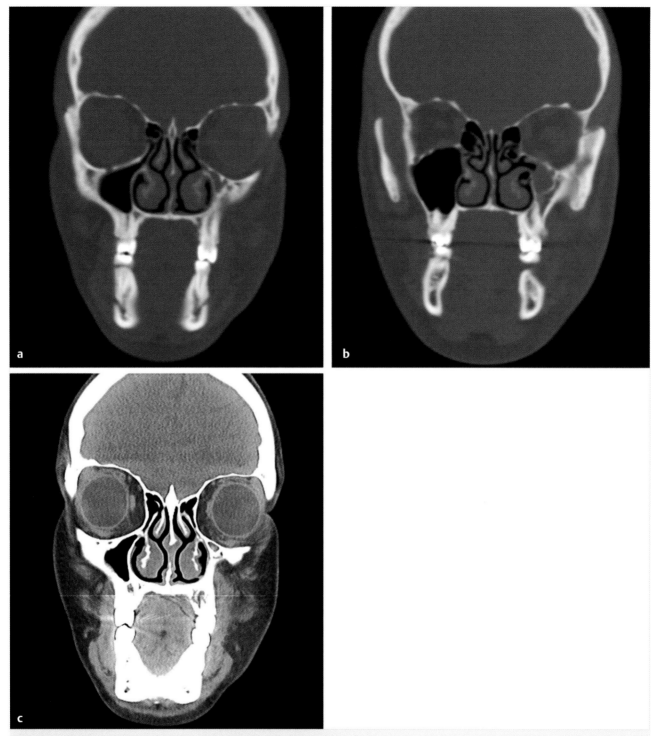

Fig. 11.13 Silent sinus syndrome. (**a**) Note the small left maxillary sinus with thickening of the lateral wall of the left maxillary sinus. There is associated enlargement of the left orbital contents. (**b,c**) Note the lateral position of the left uncinate process with narrowing of the infundibulum. These patients may present with enophthalmos and involution of the maxillary sinus after occlusion of the infundibulum. Coronal computed tomography is the ideal imaging modality to make this diagnosis.

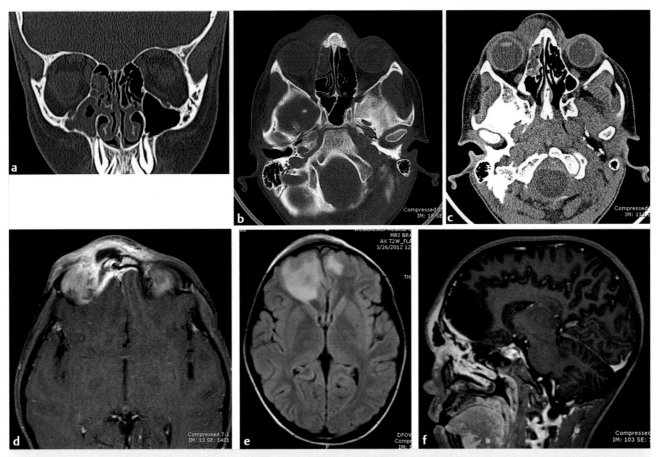

Fig. 11.14 (**a**) Coronal and (**b,c**) axial computed tomographic scans through the paranasal sinuses demonstrate extensive paranasal sinus opacification, particularly involving the right ethmoid and maxillary paranasal sinuses. There is associated extensive soft-tissue swelling and collection from the right medial canthus region to the soft tissues overlying the right nasal bridge, as well as both pre- and postseptal right orbital cellulitis. These findings are typical of sinusitis with the complication of Pott's puffy tumor and associated soft-tissue abscess. This patient subsequently underwent magnetic resonance imaging of the brain. (**d**) A soft-tissue abscess is seen in the right frontal to periorbital soft tissues. Multiplanar imaging of the brain demonstrates extensive intracranial extension of this infectious process with associated dural hyperemia (**d**), compatible with meningitis and associated subdural phlegmon/early empyema, as well as extensive edema within the right greater than left frontal lobes, compatible with cerebritis (**e,f**). This entity can lead to rapid central nervous system deterioration and death, particularly if there is thrombophlebitis of the intracranial cortical veins and/or intracranial dural venous sinuses.

11.3 Lesions of the Central Nervous System

11.3.1 Internal Auditory Canal Lesions (▶ Fig. 11.8 and ▶ Fig. 11.9)

Schwannomas of the facial nerve may arise anywhere along the course of the nerve. Given the proximity of the nerve to the vestibulocochlear nerve, patients will present with hearing loss more often than facial nerve palsy. On noncontrast temporal bone CT, expansion of the bony facial nerve canal will be seen. On MR imaging, nodularity of the facial nerve will be seen best visualized on thin-section, high-resolution T2-weighted images. However, fat-saturated T1-weighted imaging will demonstrate the extent of the mass most clearly (see ▶ Fig. 11.8). It is important to realize that the facial nerve can demonstrate enhancement normally distal to the anterior genu. However, the facial nerve should never demonstrate enhancement within the cisternal (cerebellopontine angle), meatal (internal auditory canal), and extracranial segments. Enhancement can been seen with a facial nerve schwannoma, perineural spread of another head and neck malignancy, or inflammation associated with idiopathic facial paralysis (Bell palsy).

Often, enhancing masses will be seen at the cerebellopontine angle. Diagnostic considerations for these masses include schwannomas, epidermoid cysts, meningiomas, arachnoid cysts, and metastasis, to name a few. Schwannomas on imaging will be avidly enhancing, similar to a meningioma or metastasis. However, enhancement and the mass will extend into the porus acusticus, unlike a meningioma, which will often demonstrate a dural tail of enhancement. Furthermore, a schwannoma will have a dumbbell appearance, with the waist of the mass at the porus acusticus, and will also expand the porus acusticus. Epidermoid and arachnoid cysts, on the other hand, will not enhance. Arachnoid cysts will follow the signal intensity of cerebrospinal fluid on all sequences, and epidermoid cysts will demonstrate restricted diffusion, evident as high signal on diffusion-weighted imaging and decreased signal on apparent diffusion coefficient (ADC) maps.

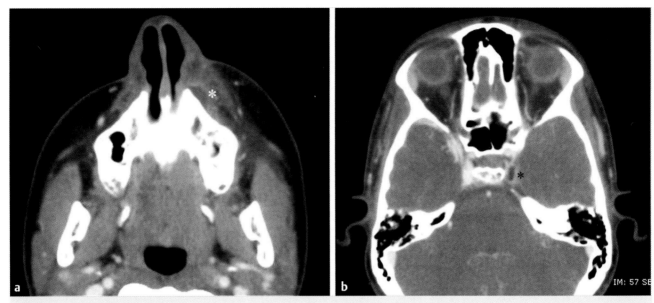

Fig. 11.15 Postcontrast axial images through the maxillofacial region (**a**) demonstrate extensive cellulitis and phlegmon in the left premaxillary tissues extending to the left nasal soft tissues. Additionally, abutting the left anterior maxilla there is a well-demarcated ovoid abscess (*asterisk*). A more cephalic image (**b**) demonstrates an ovoid hypoenhancement (*asterisk*) in the left cavernous sinus, consistent with left cavernous sinus thrombosis. Close attention to the cavernous sinus is necessary because this lesion can rapidly lead to death from sepsis or overwhelming intracranial central nervous system infectious involvement.

11.3.2 Central Nervous System Lymphoma (▶ Fig. 11.10)

Central nervous system (CNS) lymphoma can be separated into two major categories: primary CNS lymphoma and metastatic CNS lymphoma. For the purposes of this text, metastatic intracranial lymphoma will be briefly discussed. Metastatic intracranial lymphoma can involve any portion of the CNS structures; however, it is typically seen as a dural or leptomeningeal lesion. Metastatic CNS lymphoma may also affect peripheral nerves. MR imaging of the brain with contrast is the best imaging modality to evaluate for CNS lymphoma. CNS lymphoma is a great imaging mimicker and may appear in any fashion; however, multiple T2 isointense to hypointense lesions with avid enhancement are typical of CNS lymphoma. On the CT scan, lymphoma may be hyperdense because of its low cytoplasmic-to-nuclear ratio. When CNS lymphoma involves the dura, meninges, and cranial nerves, the primary differential considerations vary depending on the location. For the purposes of this text, when enhancement is seen about the trigeminal nerve, facial nerve, or vestibulocochlear nerve, one must consider the possibility of metastatic lymphoma as well as other etiologies, including a peripheral nerve sheath tumor from a phakomatosis such as neurofibromatosis or a primary peripheral nerve sheath tumor such as schwannoma. Other neoplastic processes may metastasize to the cranial nerves, such as breast or lung carcinoma. These neoplasms also have a propensity for leptomeningeal and dural spread with CNS metastases. The other major category of disease processes that may present with cranial nerve enhancement includes inflammatory or infectious processes that result in neuritis, such as Bell palsy or Lyme disease. Typically, these lesions do not have a masslike appearance.

11.4 Disorders of the Nose and Paranasal Sinuses

11.4.1 Choanal Atresia (▶ Fig. 11.11)

Choanal atresia is a narrowing of the posterior nasal apertures. Patients will present with respiratory distress during feeding, especially if the stenosis is bilateral. High-resolution noncontrast CT is used to characterize the stenosis and to assess for membranous or osseous obstruction. Before imaging, it is important to suction secretions from the nasal cavity. The choana will measure less than 0.34 cm, and the vomer will be thickened to more than 0.23 cm. Either soft tissue or bone may be seen obstructing the posterior choana. Additionally, the posterior walls of the maxilla may be bowed medially.

11.4.2 Sinusitis

Imaging may play a role in acute sinusitis in the setting of medically refractory sinusitis or when there is clinical concern for spread to adjacent orbital or cranial structures. Noncontrast CT of the paranasal sinuses is the typical modality of choice to evaluate for acute paranasal sinus disease. If there is a high degree of clinical suspicion for concomitant spread of infection into the orbit or cranial vault, MR imaging with and without contrast may be obtained. The imaging hallmark of acute sinusitis is an air–fluid level within a paranasal sinus, oftentimes seen with strandy or bubbly secretions, as well. These findings are most easily appreciated in the maxillary sinus. It may be difficult to appreciate an air–fluid level within the ethmoid and frontal paranasal sinuses because of their relatively small size. Mucosal thickening and polypoid lesions within the paranasal

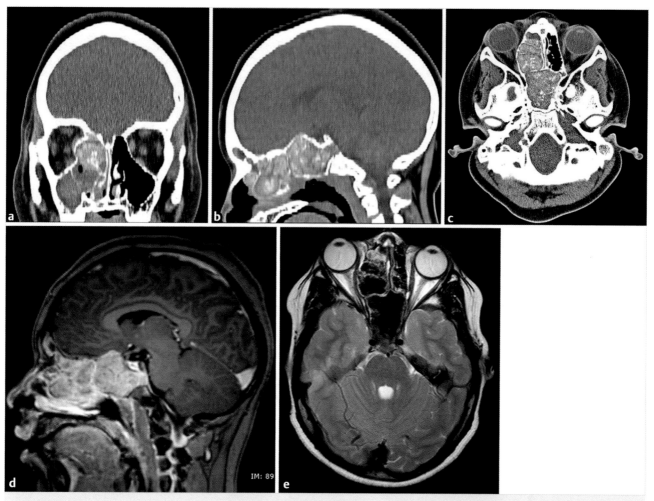

Fig. 11.16 Extensive opacification with hyperdensity and stippled calcifications is seen on computed tomographic scans (**a–c**) and sagittal T2 magnetic resonance (MR) imaging (**d**) within the entirety of the visualized right maxillary, ethmoid, sphenoid, and frontal sinuses. There is associated expansion and thinning of the sinus walls, including the posterior lateral wall of the right maxillary sinus, right lamina papyracea, and entire sphenoid sinus. On T2 axial MR imaging (**e**), thickened, inspissated secretions in the expanded right ethmoid sinuses are hypointense and can be missed. Although this lesion may appear to the inexperienced imager to mimic a neoplastic aggressive mass lesion, these findings are suggestive of chronic allergic fungal sinusitis in the correct clinical setting.

sinuses may mimic an air–fluid level. Conversely, nearly complete opacification of any of the paranasal sinuses with fluid may mimic a large polypoid lesion.

Imaging in the setting of sinusitis is often nonspecific. Radiologic reports will focus on descriptive comments regarding location, configuration, and the magnitude of mucosal thickening and opacification. In the differentiation of chronic from acute sinusitis, attention must be turned to the bony confines of the paranasal sinuses. With long-standing chronic paranasal sinus disease, there is often a periosteal reaction and thickening of the bony confines of the affected paranasal sinus. This may be termed *mucoperiosteal thickening*. The bony confines may become extremely thick and hyperdense. When chronic sinusitis is suspected, CT of the paranasal sinuses may be obtained to evaluate for anatomical variants of the paranasal sinuses that may predispose to the development of chronic sinusitis. CT is the imaging modality of choice to evaluate for chronic sinusitis because it allows the most complete assessment of the bony confines of the paranasal sinuses. Attention to the soft-tissue window when the paranasal sinuses are examined is important to evaluate for hyperdense paranasal sinus disease. On MR imaging, the appearance of secretions and the sinuses is related to the proteinaceous content of the secretions. In general, as the protein content increases, the appearance will become more intense on T1-weighted imaging and less intense on T2-weighted imaging; however, as the secretions become more solid or mineralized (as in fungal sinusitis), their appearance can be dark on T1- and T2-weighted imaging and can thus mimic an aerated sinus. If hyperdense material is appreciated in the paranasal sinuses, one must exclude fungal sinusitis. Other etiologies for hyperdense paranasal sinus disease are inspissated secretions, blood product, or hyperdense mass lesion.

The location of the mucosal thickening, as well as the presence of any anatomical variants, is essential in planning sinus surgery. Often, sinonasal disease is categorized into a number of patterns, including infundibular, ostiomeatal complex, sphenoethmoidal recess, sporadic, polyposis, frontal recess, and dental source. In the infundibular pattern, disease is limited to

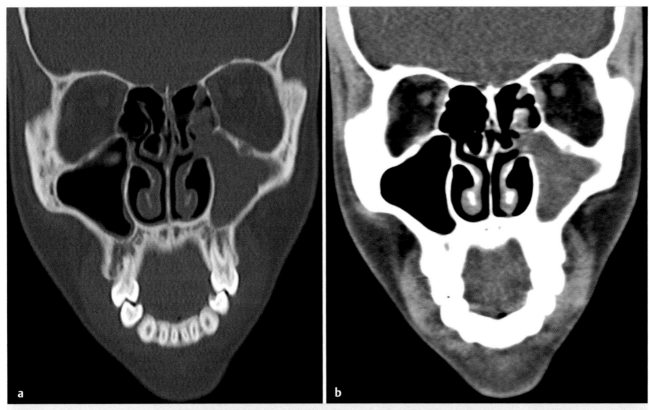

Fig. 11.17 (a) Coronal bone and (b) soft-tissue window computed tomographic scans demonstrating opacification of the left maxillary sinus with polypoid extension into the middle meatus and posterior nose without significant bone erosion, consistent with an antrochoanal polyp.

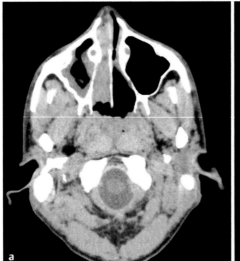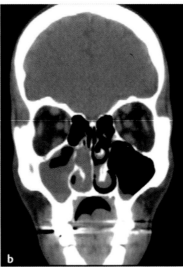

Fig. 11.18 (a) Axial and (b) coronal noncontrast computed tomographic scan of the paranasal sinuses demonstrates paranasal sinus opacification (most prominent in the right maxillary sinus), mucosal thickening, and partial opacification. There is a large polypoid component extending into the right nasal passage with extensive destruction of the right middle nasal turbinates and portions of the right inferior nasal turbinate. These findings suggest an aggressive polypoid lesion, and the extensive osseous destruction suggests malignant degeneration. Tissue pathology was consistent with a squamous cell carcinoma arising from an inverted papilloma.

the maxillary sinus, with obstruction of the ostium. In the ostiomeatal complex pattern, disease is often variable but involves the sinuses that drain via the ostiomeatal complex (anterior ethmoid, maxillary, and frontal sinuses). In the sphenoethmoidal recess pattern, disease involves the sphenoid sinus and posterior ethmoid air cells. The sporadic pattern is, as the name implies, more random in appearance and cannot be classified by a specific drainage pattern. The sinonasal polyposis pattern is characterized by polypoid-appearing lesions within

the sinuses. The frontal recess pattern is characterized by occlusion of the frontal recess, resulting in disease within the ipsilateral frontal sinus. The dental source pattern is characterized by maxillary disease, with lucent, cystic-appearing lesions involving the maxillary teeth (▶ Fig. 11.12 and ▶ Fig. 11.13).

Moreover, care should be taken to evaluate for potential complications of sinusitis. The visualized brain parenchyma should be carefully assessed to evaluate for the presence of an epidural or subdural abscess (▶ Fig. 11.14). This will appear as a

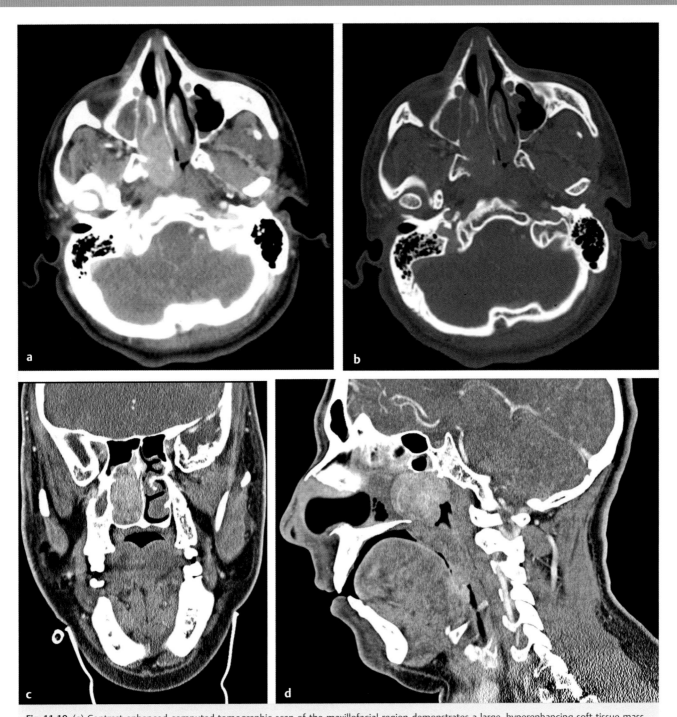

Fig. 11.19 (a) Contrast-enhanced computed tomographic scan of the maxillofacial region demonstrates a large, hyperenhancing soft-tissue mass arising from the region of the right sphenopalatine foramen that involves the right anterolateral nasopharyngeal wall and extends into the right nasal passage. (b,c) There is associated extension into the pterygopalatine fossa with mild osseous erosion of the base of the right pterygoid plate. The findings are compatible with juvenile nasopharyngeal angiofibroma. These lesions are often treated with endovascular embolization before surgical resection to aid hemostasis. (d) Note the large, extremely hypodense ovoid collection in the anterior right nasal passage; this represents hemostatic packing material and a balloon tamponade catheter.

hyperdense fluid collection resulting in mass effect and displacement of the underlying brain parenchyma. If contrast was administered, enhancement of the dura will make the empyema more conspicuous. On MR imaging, diffusion weighted sequences, if obtained, will demonstrate increased signal, indicating empyema. In the setting of ethmoid disease, infection will often spread to the adjacent orbit.

Additionally, in the setting of contrast administration, evaluation of the cavernous sinuses is important to evaluate for the presence of thrombosis. A thrombosed cavernous sinus will demonstrate enlargement, and a hypodense clot may be seen on CT (▶ Fig. 11.15). Secondary signs of cavernous sinus thrombosis include engorgement of the ipsilateral superior ophthalmic vein. On MR imaging, evaluation of the cavernous sinus for

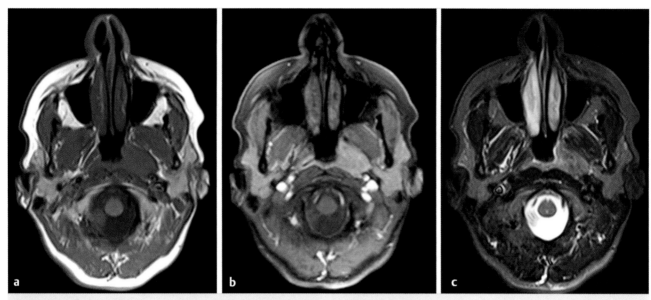

Fig. 11.20 Left nasopharyngeal carcinoma. **(a)** On T1 precontrast imaging, the lesion is isointense to muscle, but **(b,c)** it is hyperintense to muscle on postcontrast T2 imaging with fat suppression. The mass lesion is centered in the left nasopharynx with effacement of the left fossa of Rosenmüller and the left eustachean tube. These structures are preserved in the uninvolved right nasopharynx.

thrombosis is best performed with routine contrast-enhanced sequences. High-resolution three-dimensional gradient-echo sequences may be employed after the administration of contrast to interrogate the cavernous sinus. Alternatively, imaging performed with a sellar protocol allows evaluation of the cavernous sinus. It is important to note that MR venography will not allow adequate evaluation of the cavernous sinuses.

Allergic fungal sinusitis results in the opacification and expansion of multiple sinuses. On imaging, this can appear very aggressive, with diffuse involvement resulting in bony remodeling and apparent cortical thinning or erosion (▶ Fig. 11.16a–c). However, centrally within the sinuses, hyperdense secretions will be seen. On MR imaging, as described above, signal characteristics are variable depending on the proteinaceous content of the secretions. Typically, these secretions are hypointense on T2 sequences and variable on T1 sequences (▶ Fig. 11.16d, e).

11.4.3 Antrochoanal Polyp (▶ Fig. 11.17)

An antrochoanal polyp is an inflammatory polyp arising from the maxillary sinus antrum and herniating through the maxillary os into the nasal cavity. It is most often found in adolescents and young adults, who present with unilateral nasal obstruction. On imaging, the lesion is dumbbell-shaped, bridging the maxillary sinus and nasal passage and expanding the maxillary ostium. On CT, the mass will be of low density and demonstrate peripheral enhancement. Depending on the water or mucoid content, the mass will be of low intensity on T1 and of high intensity on T2. Of course, this can vary depending on the protein content of the lesion. Enhancement will be peripheral, as on CT.

11.4.4 Inverting Papilloma

Papillomas are most often centered in the middle meatus and may result in obstructive sinonasal disease. On CT, a soft-tissue

mass with nonspecific characteristics will be seen (▶ Fig. 11.18a, b). Calcifications will often be seen within the mass. On MR imaging, the mass will demonstrate isointensity on T1 and T2 sequences. The enhancement pattern has been described as curvilinear or "cribriform." It is important to note that squamous cell carcinoma often coexists with inverting papillomas.

11.5 Disorders of the Pharynx

11.5.1 Juvenile Nasal Angiofibroma

A juvenile nasal angiofibroma is a benign, highly vascular, locally aggressive tumor typically affecting young male adolescents, who present with nasal obstruction and recurrent epistaxis. On imaging, the mass will enhance intensely and often originates from the sphenopalatine foramen or the pterygopalatine fossa (▶ Fig. 11.19a, b). It is important to look for local spread of the mass. Common locations of local spread include the paranasal sinuses (most commonly the sphenoid sinus), or the tumor may spread via the pterygopalatine fossa, vidian canal, or foramen rotundum to extend into the orbit or infratemporal fossa, or intracranially. This is especially important to recognize to ensure proper surgical planning for a complete resection.

On CT, the mass is isodense to muscle and demonstrates marked enhancement (▶ Fig. 11.19c,d). The mass does demonstrate locally aggressive features, and imaging will show bony remodeling and destruction, including bowing of the nasal septum and posterior wall of the maxillary sinus and enlargement of the pterygopalatine fossa. As mentioned above, the mass is found within the nasal cavity; however, local spread must be evaluated thoroughly. MR imaging will demonstrate a heterogeneous mass that is isointense to skeletal muscle on T1-weighted and of intermediate to high intensity on T2-weighted images. Flow voids, often described as having a "salt and pep-

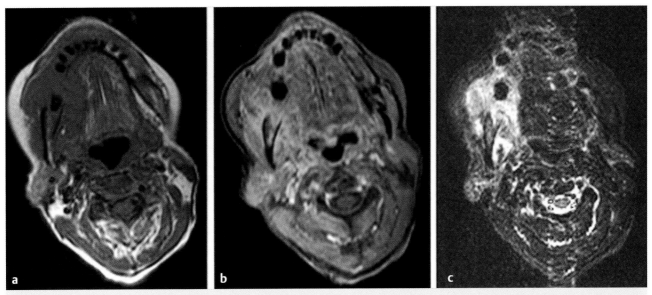

Fig. 11.21 Magnetic resonance (MR) imaging with (**a**) T1 precontrast, (**b**) T1 postcontrast, and (**c**) T2 with fat saturation sequencing of a right floor of mouth squamous cell carcinoma (SCCa) with extension and destruction of the right mandibular body. The neoplasm extends beyond the mandible into the right masticator space. MR imaging and CT are the best modalities to evaluate the extent of local disease in SCCa; positron emission tomography–computed tomography (PET-CT) is the imaging modality of choice for staging SCCa for both regional and distant metastasis.

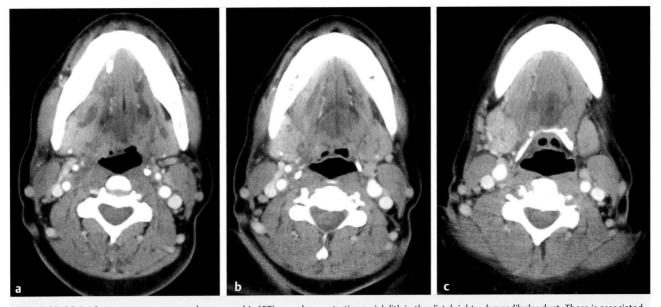

Fig. 11.22 (**a**) Axial postcontrast computed tomographic (CT) scan demonstrating a sialolith in the distal right submandibular duct. There is associated dilatation and likely infection within the right submandibular duct. (**b**) There are enlargment and enhancment of the right submandibular gland, compatible with sialadenitis (**c**). Note the small reactive lymph nodes at the right IB level. CT is the imaging modality of choice for the evaluation of salivary stone disease. If there is concern for very small stones, CT may be performed before and after contrast to avoid mistaking a small enhancing branch of the external carotid artery for a sialolith.

per" appearance, are often seen throughout the mass, illustrating its increased vascularity. Local extension is best evaluated with fat-saturated postcontrast imaging.

Before surgery, these patients will often be embolized to reduce intraoperative blood loss. On catheter angiography, the tumor will demonstrate a prominent capillary blush and is most often fed via branches of the internal maxillary and ascending pharyngeal arteries. Endovascular embolization is often accomplished with the use of particles. Alternatively, tumor emboliza-

tion may be accomplished percutaneously with the use of liquid embolic agents such as n-butyl cyanoacrylate (Onyx; eV3, Irvine, CA).

11.5.2 Cancer of the Pharynx

Most malignancies involving the mucosal surfaces of the head and neck are squamous cell cancer. The role of imaging is not to provide a histologic diagnosis, but rather to define the extent of

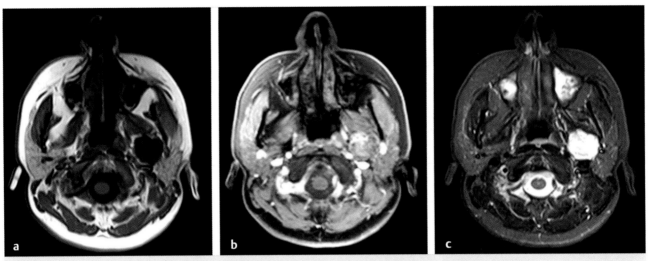

Fig. 11.23 Pleomorphic adenoma of the deep lobe of the left parotid gland. These lesions are usually smooth and ovoid in shape, with relatively homogeneous enhancement. (**a**) They have low intensity on T1, (**b**) enhance brightly with contrast, and (**c**) may have extremely high T2 signal, as in this case, which increases the specificity of the diagnosis of pleomorphic adenoma. The T1 signal varies depending on the presence of protein and/or blood products within the lesion. Larger lesions demonstrate a lobulated appearance and more heterogeneous enhancement. Computed tomography is adequate in sensitivity for the detection of parotid adenoma; however, its specificity is not as high as that of magnetic resonance imaging. Ultrasound should be used with caution because lesions in the deep lobe of the parotid may not be well visualized.

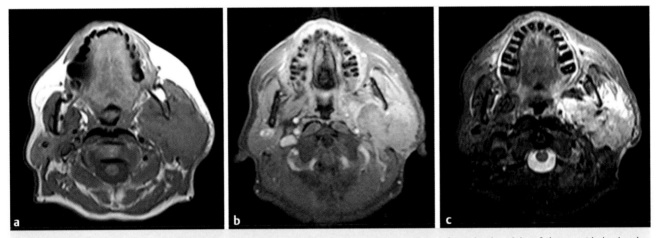

Fig. 11.24 Left parotid mucoepidermoid carcinoma. (**a**) T1 precontrast image shows a tumor arising from the deep lobe of the parotid gland and invading the left masticator space. (**b**) Image with contrast enhancement. (**c**) T2 signal abnormality extends to the left mandibular ramus, indicative of osseous extension, with likely perineural extension along the inferior alveolar nerve. Note the infiltration and involvement of the left pterygoid musculature.

disease to better stage the malignancy and aid in making treatment-related decisions. Squamous cell carcinoma is generally isodense to muscle on CT, isointense to muscle on T1-weighted images, and mildly hyperintense on T2-weighted images, and it will demonstrate modest enhancement. However, background enhancement of lymphoid tissue will often limit detection. The key to detection and defining extent is to be mindful of the fat planes and fatty architecture normally present within the muscles and spaces of the neck.

For example, replacement of the fat (bright on T1) in front of the prevertebral musculature may suggest invasion, making carcinoma potentially unresectable. Muscle invasion can also be suggested by increased T2 signal within the muscle or nodular

enhancement of the muscle itself. Another example is the use of fat to determine tumor spread at the eustachian tube orifice. The levator veli palatini and tensor veli palatini normally have an abundant amount of striated fat within the muscle bellies; if these areas are involved in spread of disease, this fatty architecture will be lost (▶ Fig. 11.20a–c).

Osseous invasion is also important to assess with imaging. Cortical involvement can be seen on CT as cortical thinning or destruction. On T1 MR imaging, cortex is normally hypointense. This linear hypointense signal will be lost if there is tumoral invasion. Medullary involvement is depicted well on MR imaging. The normal marrow is bright on T1 sequences and will become hypointense when involved with tumor. Bright signal

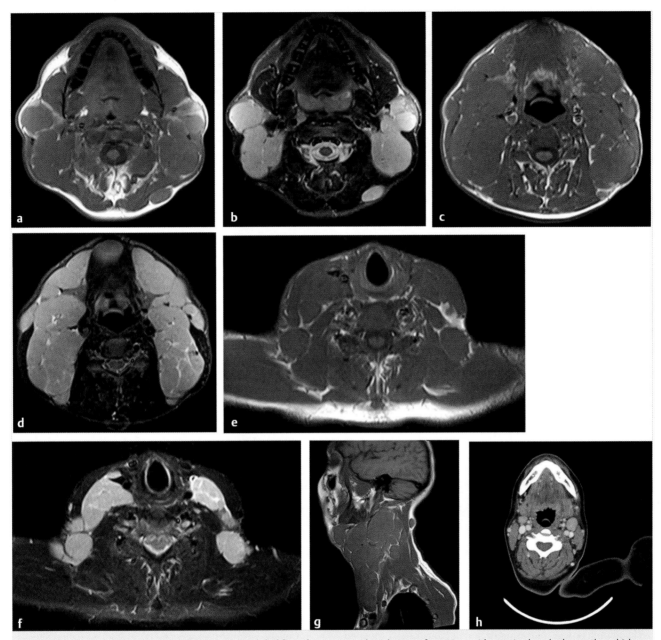

Fig. 11.25 (**a,c,e**) T1-weighted axial and (**g**) sagittal and (**b,d,f**) T2 fat-suppressed axial views of a patient with massive lymphadenopathy, which biopsy proved to be lymphoma. (**h**) More often, reactive lymph nodes are characterized by more modest enlargement and uniformity.

following gadolinium and hyperintense signal on T2 images are less specific evidence of medullary involvement with malignancy (▶ Fig. 11.21).

11.6 Disorders of the Salivary Glands

11.6.1 Sialolithiasis and Sialadenitis (▶ Fig. 11.22)

Imaging is often performed to evaluate for sialadenitis and assess for underlying stones. Radiography may be employed to detect large radiopaque stones. CT with or without contrast can be utilized to evaluate for obstructing stones resulting in upstream ductal dilatation with or without accompanying gland inflammation. On CT, a stone will be visualized as a hyperdense focus found within or along the draining ducts (▶ Fig. 11.22a), most often of the submandibular or parotid glands. Contrast allows better resolution of the soft tissues, as well as better evaluation for microabscesses, which may form within the gland. However, contrast does decrease sensitivity for the detection of small stones, which like contrast appear hyperdense. On imaging, glandular swelling, reticulation of the overlying subcutaneous fat, and skin thickening are signs of inflammation (▶ Fig. 11.22b, c). MR imaging can demonstrate similar findings,

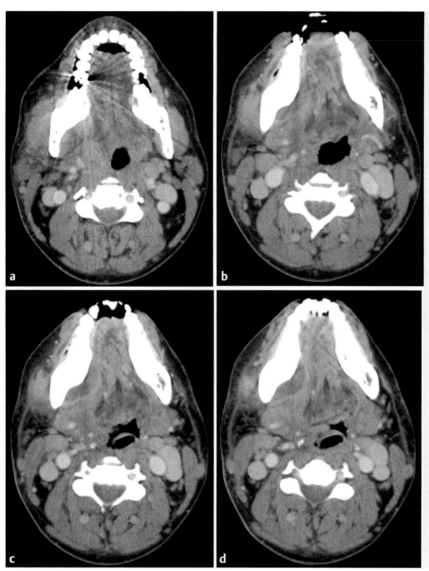

Fig. 11.26 (a–d) Multiple axial postcontrast computed tomographic scans through the region of the mandible demonstrate an ovoid, hypodense, peripherally enhancing abscess along the buccal surface of the distal body extending to the angle of the right mandible. There is associated extensive soft-tissue swelling and cellulitic change with phlegmon in the surrounding soft tissues. Additionally, reactive right greater than left cervical chain lymphadenopathy is present, with a markedly enlarged, partially enhancing right station IIA cervical chain lymph node.

with edema and inflammation best seen on T2 sequences with fat saturation. Stones will be visualized on T1 or T2 sequences as hypointense foci. Ultrasound can demonstrate a swollen gland and intra- and extraductal dilatation. However, stone detection is very operator-dependent. In general, contrast-enhanced CT is sufficient and offers optimized stone detection as well as the detection of complications.

11.6.2 Salivary Gland Masses

Salivary gland masses have considerable overlap on imaging, with most benign or malignant tumors appearing isodense to muscle on CT, and many malignant tumors can have bright signal on T2 sequences. Additionally, the margin of the lesion can be well defined or infiltrative in benign or malignant settings. Thus, imaging is focused on location so that appropriate decisions can be made in terms of surgical approach.

Pleomorphic adenomas are the most commonly seen tumor within the parotid gland. These masses are isodense to muscle on CT and of low signal intensity on T1 sequences

(▶ Fig. 11.23a), demonstrate avid enhancement following the administration of gadolinium (▶ Fig. 11.23b), and are very bright on T2-weighted images (▶ Fig. 11.23c). Occasionally, calcifications and cysts can be seen within pleomorphic adenomas. Warthin tumors are the most common bilateral tumors within the parotid gland. These tumors are dark on T1 sequences but can be very heterogeneous on T2-weighted images.

Mucoepidermoid carcinoma is the most common malignant tumor of the parotid gland (▶ Fig. 11.24). Low-grade mucoepidermoid carcinomas can have very bright signal on T2 sequences, whereas higher-grade tumors can be of low signal intensity. Adenoid cystic carcinoma is the most common malignant tumor of the submandibular, sublingual, and minor salivary glands. As with mucoepidermoid carcinoma, signal intensity on T2 sequences is highly variable. However, unlike mucoepidermoid carcinoma, adenoid cystic tumors have a propensity for perineural spread, so particular attention must be paid to cranial nerves V and VII. Other malignant tumors of the salivary glands include metastatic lesions, lymphoma, squamous cell carcinoma, and adenocarcinoma.

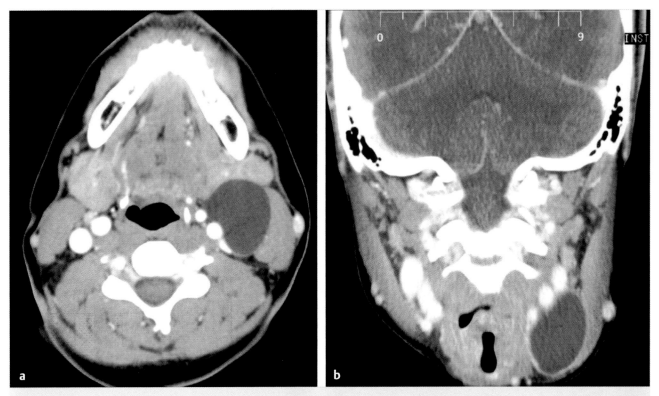

Fig. 11.27 (a) Axial and (b) coronal postcontrast computed tomographic scans through the neck demonstrate an ovoid homogeneous cystic lesion located posterior to the submandibular gland, medial to the left sternocleidomastoid muscle and anterolateral to the left carotid sheath. The appearance and location of this lesion are characteristic of a second branchial cleft cyst, with a typical appearance of homogeneous hypodensity and a thin, smooth wall (unless infected). Alternate diagnoses in the differential include submandibular gland neoplasm/cyst, venous or lymphatic malformation, abscess, and necrotic lymph node.

11.7 Disorders of the Neck

11.7.1 Lymph Nodes (▶ Fig. 11.25)

Lymph nodes within the neck have designated levels and are described elsewhere. Lymph nodes are isodense to muscle on CT and isointense to muscle on T1-weighted images. Nodes are well seen in patients with abundant fat. Nodes are normally hyperintense on T2-weighted images obtained with fat saturation. The fatty hilum is not always seen on imaging but when seen portends benignity. In the setting of infection, lymph nodes will often demonstrate avid reactive enhancement. Suppurative lymph nodes (in the setting of tuberculosis, fungal disease, or staphylococcal infections) will look like abscesses, demonstrating hypoattunation on CT and hyperintensity on T2 sequences with ring enhancement. However, necrotic lymph nodes may also be seen in the setting of head and neck malignancy (even occult lesions), and lymph nodes larger than 1 cm in greatest short-axis diameter should be considered pathologic.

11.7.2 Deep Neck Infections (▶ Fig. 11.26)

Imaging within the deep spaces of the neck is centered upon localizing pathology to a certain space in the neck. For example,

localization of a lesion to the carotid or masticator space will greatly aid the differential diagnosis. However, certain lesions, such as infiltrative neoplasms and infections, can be trans-spatial. Many infections within the extramucosal spaces of the head and neck have a dental origin; other possible etiologies for infection include antecedent trauma, often minor.

Infection is often evaluated within the emergency department setting with the use of CT. Phlegmonous changes on CT will demonstrate loss of the expected fat planes and architecture within the deep spaces of the neck. Secondary signs of infection include enlarged enhancing lymph nodes within the ipsilateral neck, which are reactive in nature. Sometimes, these lymph nodes may become necrotic secondary to superinfection. However, squamous cell cancer can also present with necrotic lymphadenopathy. Clinical data, including signs of infection, are especially important in making a proper diagnosis. Pharyngitis and tonsillitis may be visualized on CT, but imaging is not routinely performed in this setting unless there is concern for a complication such as abscess formation.

Abscesses will demonstrate fluid attenuation higher than that of water and a peripheral rim of enhancement following contrast administration. On MR imaging, signal characteristics will include low to higher signal intensity on T1 sequences (depending on the proteinaceous content of fluid), high signal on T2 sequences, and peripheral enhancement following gadoli-

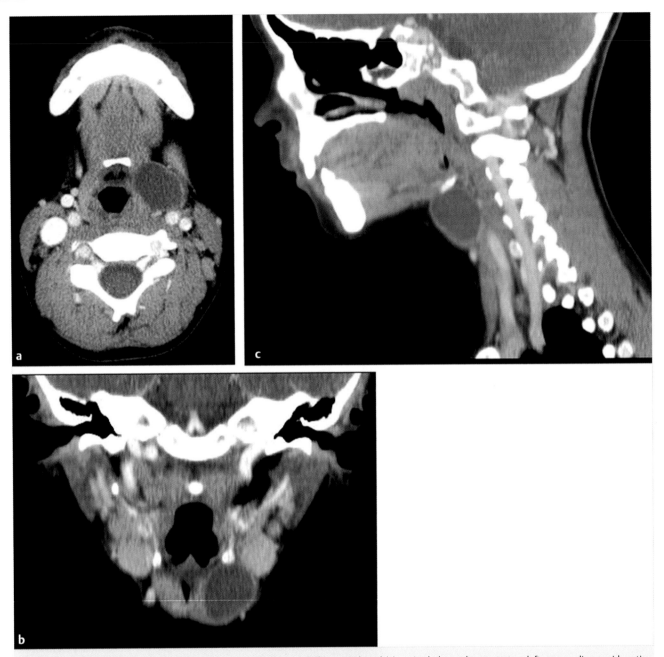

Fig. 11.28 Postcontrast computed tomographic scans in the (**a**) axial, (**b**) coronal, and (**c**) sagittal planes demonstrate a left paramedian ovoid cystic lesion deep to the infrahyoid muscles and abutting the undersurface of the left hyoid bone. These imaging characteristics are most suggestive of a thyroglossal duct cyst. Included in the differential diagnosis are venous or lymphatic malformations and necrotic lymph node. The uniformity and lack of multiloculation, as well as the anterior location, make the lymphatic malformation a less likely diagnosis.

nium administration. Diffusion sequences are especially helpful because abscess will demonstrate high signal intensity on diffusion-weignted images with low signal on ADC maps, in keeping with restricted diffusion. Imaging can also aid in localizing a source such as an infected tooth. Osteomyelitis or osteonecrosis of the mandible is often seen in conjunction with dental infections. It is especially important to identify infection within the retropharyngeal space, or the so-called "danger space." Infection in these locations allow a conduit into the mediastinum. Moreover, close inspection of the carotid space is important to exclude thrombosis and secondary thrombophlebitis.

11.7.3 Branchial Cleft Cyst (▶ Fig. 11.27)

The second branchial cleft cyst is the most commonly encountered branchial cleft remnant. It arises from incomplete closure of the cervical sinus of His, which is an ectodermal pit that arises from the second through fourth branchial clefts. It is most commonly found along the angle of the mandible and along the carotid sheath and most often lies posterolateral to the submandibular gland and anteromedial to the sternocleidomastoid muscle. The lesion has signal characteristics classic for cysts:

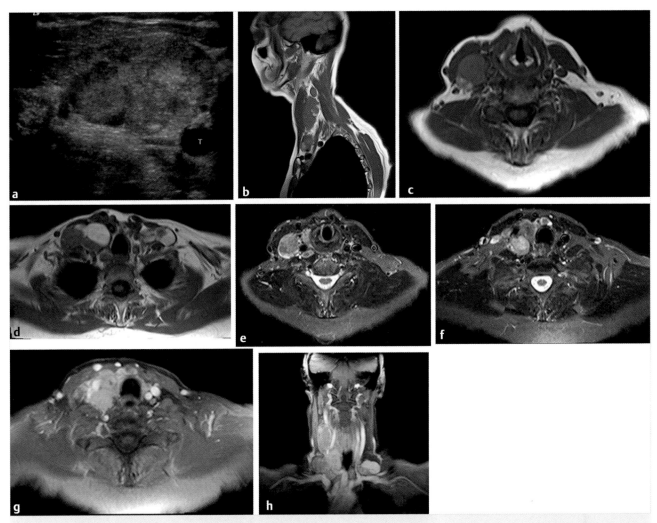

Fig. 11.29 (a) Ultrasound of the thyroid gland demonstrating a large right thyroid mass of mixed echogenicity, later proven on biopsy to be papillary thyroid carcinoma. *T*, trachea. Magnetic resonance images of the neck including (b) sagittal T1, (c,d) axial T1, (e,f) axial T2 fat-suppressed, and (g) axial and (h) coronal T1 fat-saturated postcontrast pulse sequences demonstrate the large carcinoma of the right thyroid, with extensive enlarged ipsilateral lymph nodes.

hypointense on T1 and hyperintense on T2 with thin peripheral enhancement and attenuation similar to that of fluid or possibly slightly hyperdense to water on CT. If infected, the wall may become thick and then become indistinguishable from necrotic or infected lymphadenopathy. As mentioned, differential diagnostic considerations for second branchial cleft cysts include cystic or necrotic lymphadenopathy and lymphatic malformations. However, lymphatic malformations are more often found posterior to the sternocleidomastoid muscle or may be trans-spatial within the neck, and they are often multilocular, containing fluid–fluid levels indicating intralesional hemorrhage.

11.7.4 Thyroglossal Duct Cyst (▶ Fig. 11.28)

Thyroglossal duct cysts are remnants of the thyroglossal duct, which forms along the pathway of descent of the thyroid gland from the foramen cecum to the thyroid bed. Most are found at the level of the hyoid bone or within the infrahyoid neck. Most,

but not all, are found within the midline. With that said, some can be seen embedded within the musculature. The relationship with the hyoid bone is important to recognize because the hyoid bone will be resected during the Sistrunk procedure. Imaging characteristics follow those of cysts—namely, fluid attenuation on CT, low intensity on T1-weighted images, and high intensity on T2-weighted images. If there is proteinaceous debris within the cyst, then high intensity can be seen on T1-weighted images. If the cyst is superinfected, enhancement of the cyst wall can be seen. Carcinoma is rare; however, it does occur in fewer than 1% of cases.

11.7.5 Thyroid Nodules (▶ Fig. 11.29)

Sonography remains an important tool to evaluate thyroid nodules. However, the vast majority of detected nodules are benign. Nodules can vary in shape, echogenicity, and internal architecture. Specific characteristics that have been associated with malignancy include nodules that have a solid component, are hypoechoic, contain microcalcifications, are taller than wide on

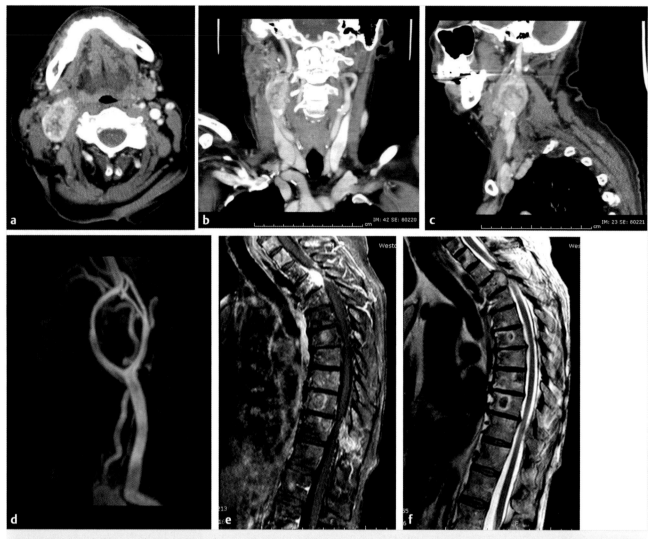

Fig. 11.30 (a) Axial, (b) coronal, and (c) sagittal postcontrast computed tomographic scans of the neck demonstrate an avidly enhancing, mixed-density lesion in the right carotid sheath splaying the right internal and external carotid arteries. This is best demonstrated on (d) magnetic resonance (MR) angiography, which shows marked splaying of the internal and external carotid arteries. The lesion demonstrates multiple early-filling arterial vessels. The finding is characteristic of paraganglioma/carotid body tumors. These can occur anywhere along the sympathetic chain. Typically, on imaging these lesions demonstrate a smooth contour with extensive enhancement because of their high vascularity. There may be a salt-and-pepper appearance on MR imaging due to the extensive flow voids. Catheter angiography will show extensive tumoral blush. This case is unique because there are multiple metastatic lesions (including an upper thoracic lesion resulting in thoracic spinal cord compression) seen on (e) sagittal T1 and (f) T2 images. The spinal lesions were histopathologically proven metastatic paraganglioma lesions.

transverse views, and have irregular margins. As the number of worrisome characteristics increases, the risk for malignancy increases. Nodules that are photopenic on iodine nuclear scans have a 20% risk of malignancy.

11.7.6 Paragangliomas

Carotid body tumors (▶ Fig. 11.30) arise from chemoreceptor cells derived from the primitive neural crest. These masses arise at the carotid bulb and splay the internal and external carotid arteries apart from each other. This is well seen on sagittal projections and helps distinguish these slowly growing vascular masses from schwannomas, which do not splay the internal and external carotid arteries. The masses are generally unilateral but can be bilateral in certain inherited conditions, such as

succinate dehydrogenase enzyme deficiency, multiple endocrine neoplasia, and Von Hippel-Lindau syndrome.

On CT, the mass will be isodense to muscle and demonstrate avid contrast enhancement. On MR imaging, the mass will be isointense to muscle on T1-weighted images and hyperintense on T2 and will demonstrate avid enhancement. Once again, as with other vascular head and neck tumors, a "salt and pepper" appearance on unenhanced MR images will be seen, with the flow voids representing the "pepper" and hemorrhage or slow flow representing the "salt." On angiography, a strong contrast blush will be seen, indicating the vascular nature of the mass. Before resection, embolization with particles is often used to limit blood loss during surgery.

Glomus jugulare and glomus vagale tumors may also be seen within the carotid space. However, glomus vagale tumors will

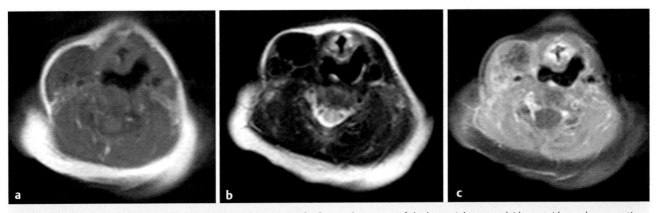

Fig. 11.31 (a–c) Multiple magnetic resonance images demonstrate fusiform enlargement of the lower right sternocleidomastoid muscle, suggestive of fibromatosis colli. However, given the presence of mild peripheral T2 hyperintensity and heterogeneous postcontrast enhancement, infectious myositis should also be considered. If further evaluation is necessary, fine needle aspiration may be performed. Signal abnormality and enhancement are confined to the sternocleidomastoid muscle, making malignant neoplasm (such as rhabdomyosarcoma) less likely.

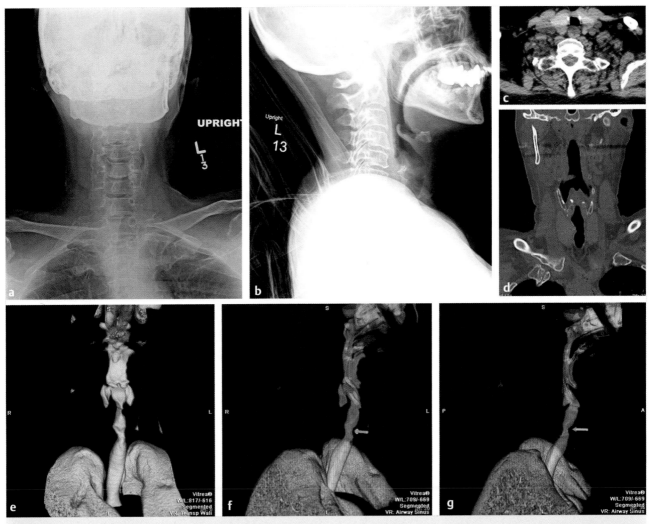

Fig. 11.32 (a,b) Radiographs of the soft tissue of the neck in this patient with prior tracheotomy demonstrate a suggestion of narrowing of the subglottic trachea at the level of the thyroid cartilage; however, this is poorly visualized because of the confluence of shadows and the limitations of radiography. The irregular contour is in better appreciated on a lateral as opposed to a frontal projection. Subsequent computed tomography (CT) of the neck without contrast was performed. (c) Axial and (d) coronal images, as well as (e–g) three-dimensional surface-shaded minimal-intensity-projection reconstructions, were performed to demonstrate and more clearly visualize the stenosis of the trachea at the level of the patient's presumed prior tracheostomy, with narrowing of the trachea by approximately 40 to 50%. There is also a slightly patulous appearance of the trachea distal to the stenosis and possible air trapping within the lungs. This entity and associated findings are much more clearly visualized on CT than on radiography in many cases.

not splay the internal and external carotid arteries but rather will displace the carotid arteries anteriorly and the jugular vein posteriorly. Additionally, these tumors are generally found about 2 cm below the jugular foramen and thus are much higher than carotid body tumors. Glomus jugulare tumors may extend into the carotid space; however, they also involve the skull base and jugular foramen. Erosion of the jugular spine is common, and a permeative destruction pattern is often seen on CT.

Glomus tympanicum originates from glomus cells in the cochlear promontory. Imaging characteristics are similar to those of other paragangliomas; however, location within the middle ear is the distinguishing feature of these masses. Clinical symptoms include a retrotympanic mass and pulsatile tinnitus. CT will demonstrate the characteristic location of these lesions along or about the cochlear promontory. Enhancement characteristics are generally visualized only with MRI; however, this is generally unnecessary if the clinical presentation and CT features are characteristic.

Indium-111 octreotide nuclear medicine scintigraphy will demonstrate increased activity with paragangliomas. Additionally, distant metastases can be evaluated utilizing whole body imaging. However, false negative scans do exist, especially for smaller lesions and lesions which do not express the proper somatostatin receptors.

11.7.7 Fibromatosis Colli (▶ Fig. 11.31)

Fibromatosis colli is a focal thickening and fibrosis of the sternocleidomastoid muscle, thought to be secondary to birth trauma. On imaging, thickening and fusiform enlargement of the sternocleidomastoid muscle are seen. On MR imaging, the muscle may be slightly hypoattenuating to other muscle and will be hypointense and hyperintense on T2-weighted images. It is important to recognize that changes will involve only the muscle, and adjacent tissues will lack inflammatory change.

11.7.8 Acquired Airway Stenosis

Acquired intrinsic airway stenosis is most often secondary to prolonged intubation or prior tracheostomy. Additional causes of intrinsic stenosis include prior trauma, laryngeal carcinoma, granulomatous diseases, inflammatory conditions involving the tracheal cartilage, tracheopathia osteochondroplastica, and prior radiation. Extrinsic compression secondary to thyroid malignancy and lymphadenopathy can also result in compression of the trachea. Thin-section CT allows accurate characterization of the length of stenosis, assessment of abnormal soft tissue, and assessment of calcification, which can provide clues to possible etiologies. Irregular posterior tracheal wall calcifications may be seen with amyloidosis, whereas tracheopathia osteochondroplastica will have regular-appearing calcifications that spare the posterior wall. Other etiologies, such as sarcoidosis, relapsing polychondritis, and Wegener granulomatosis, will usually not calcify. Three-dimensional images can be reformatted, and virtual bronchoscopy can allow luminal evaluation of the stenosis. One of the few current indications for radiography of the soft tissue of the neck is evaluation of the airway for patency (▶ Fig. 11.32a, b), in addition to evaluation of pediatric epiglottitis and croup. CT, with or without three-dimensional surface-shaded minimal-intensity-projection reconstructions, may be more helpful in planning surgery (▶ Fig. 11.32c–g).

11.8 Recommended Reading

[1] Benson MT, Dalen K, Mancuso AA, Kerr HH, Cacciarelli AA, Mafee MF. Congenital anomalies of the branchial apparatus: embryology and pathologic anatomy Radiographics 1992; 12: 943–960

[2] Capps EF, Kinsella JJ, Gupta M, Bhatki AM, Opatowsky MJ. Emergency imaging assessment of acute, nontraumatic conditions of the head and neck Radiographics 2010; 30: 1335–1352

[3] Hira A, Chao K. Direct endoscopic intratumoral injection of Onyx for the preoperative embolization of a recurrent juvenile nasal angiofibroma Interv Neuroradiol 2011; 17: 477–481

[4] Kwak JY, Han KH, Yoon JH et al. Thyroid imaging reporting and data system for US features of nodules: a step in establishing better stratification of cancer risk Radiology 2011; 260: 892–899

[5] Lee TC, Aviv RI, Chen JM, Nedzelski JM, Fox AJ, Symons SP. CT grading of otosclerosis AJNR Am J Neuroradiol 2009; 30: 1435–1439

[6] Lee YY, Wong KT, King AD, Ahuja AT. Imaging of salivary gland tumours Eur J Radiol 2008; 66: 419–436

[7] Madani G, Beale TJ. Sinonasal inflammatory disease Semin Ultrasound CT MR 2009; 30: 17–24

[8] Mafee MF, Tran BH, Chapa AR. Imaging of rhinosinusitis and its complications: plain film, CT, and MRI Clin Rev Allergy Immunol 2006; 30: 165–186

[9] Rao AB, Koeller KK, Adair CF. From the archives of the American Forces Institute of Pathology. Paragangliomas of the head and neck: radiologic-pathologic correlation Radiographics 1999; 19: 1605–1632

[10] Schubert MS. Allergic fungal sinusitis: pathophysiology, diagnosis and management Med Mycol 2009; 47 Suppl 1: S324–S330

[11] Som PM, Curtin HD, Mancuso AA. Imaging-based nodal classification for evaluation of neck metastatic adenopathy AJR Am J Roentgenol 2000; 174: 837–844

[12] Weis , sman JL, Tabor EK, Curtin HD. Sphenochoanal polyps: evaluation with CT and MR imaging Radiology 1991; 178: 145–148

12 General Anesthesia and Anesthetic Considerations for Otolaryngologic Surgery

Jason G. Lai and Andrew M. Malinow

12.1 Introduction

The anesthetic management of a patient undergoing surgery of the head, neck, ear, nose, or throat challenges the anesthesiologist to develop an anesthetic plan that will accommodate the needs of the surgeon, anesthesiologist, and patient. Optimally formulated before the surgical procedure and in consultation with the surgeon, the anesthetic plan should always allow modification to meet the ever-changing requirements encountered in the operating room. Just as a surgical procedure is divided into a series of steps, so is the delivery of a general anesthetic (see Box Steps of the Delivery of General Anesthesia). (p. 89)

Steps of the Delivery of General Anesthesia

1. Preoperative evaluation
2. Patient preparation
3. Induction of anesthesia
4. Airway management
5. Maintenance of anesthesia
6. Emergence from anesthesia
7. Recovery from anesthesia

12.2 Steps of the Delivery of General Anesthesia

12.2.1 Preoperative Evaluation

During the preoperative evaluation, the anesthesiologist:
- Summarizes the patient's general health, including new or ongoing medical conditions, allergies, and current medications. Patients presenting for otolaryngologic surgery often have a history of heavy smoking, alcohol abuse, obstructive sleep apnea, chronic upper respiratory tract infections, or chronic obstructive pulmonary disease, as well as a high incidence of coronary artery disease, hypertension, and chronic renal insufficiency. All of these factors impact the formulation of the anesthetic plan for each patient in an attempt to minimize perioperative morbidity and mortality.
- Performs a complete physical examination, focusing not only on the pulmonary and cardiovascular systems but also especially on the airway in an attempt to uncover anatomy that may make manual ventilation and the placement of a tracheal tube difficult. The steps of asking the patient to open the mouth and then assessing the visible anatomical structures have been widely adopted by anesthesiologists to determine the possibility of a difficult airway. The Mallampati classification system (► Table 12.1 and ► Fig. 12.1) has been developed to correlate the visual oropharyngeal anatomy, seen during a preoperative evaluation, with visualization of the glottic

aperture during direct laryngoscopy. Evaluation of the oropharynx is accomplished with the patient sitting upright, with the head in the neutral position, the mouth open as widely as possible, and the tongue protruded maximally. Other anatomical features that are often noted on preoperative examination include the patient's ability to actively flex the neck to achieve a "sniffing" position and the ability to anteriorly protrude the mandible ("upper lip bite"); both of these maneuvers are important in the process of direct laryngoscopy. A large tongue (relative to the capacitance of the oral cavity), protruding incisors, a small mandible, and a restricted mouth opening may all contribute to the inability of the anesthesiologist to visualize the glottic aperture during direct laryngoscopy.
- Requests and evaluates appropriate laboratory tests and studies (e.g., complete blood cell count, serum chemistries, coagulation studies, electrocardiogram, chest radiography, pulmonary function tests, echocardiography, myocardial stress test) to assess acute and chronic medical conditions as well as positive findings from the physical examination.
- Discusses with the patient any previous personal or familial adverse reactions to general anesthetics (e.g., allergies, family history of malignant hyperthermia), the available anesthetic options, and the relative risks and benefits of each.
- Obtains the patient's informed consent for anesthesia.
- Provides preoperative instructions as to medications to take or avoid on the day of surgery, and when to discontinue eating and drinking to reduce the risk for pulmonary aspiration, especially during the induction of and emergence from general anesthesia.
- Formulates an anesthetic plan that takes into consideration the proposed surgery, patient's medical condition, requirements of the surgeon, and wishes of the patient.

Once the preoperative evaluation is completed, the patient is assigned an American Society of Anesthesiologists (ASA) physical status (► Table 12.2). Among anesthesiologists, as well as other members of the perioperative team, the ASA physical status communicates anesthetic risk more efficiently than any individual patient characteristic. The ASA classification system ranges from physical status 1 through 6. The suffix "E" is added to the physical status for patients undergoing emergency surgery.

Table 12.1 Mallampati classification

Class	Visible oropharyngeal structures
I	Soft palate, fauces, uvula, tonsillar pillars
II	Soft palate, fauces, uvula
III	Soft palate, base of the uvula
IV	Hard palate only

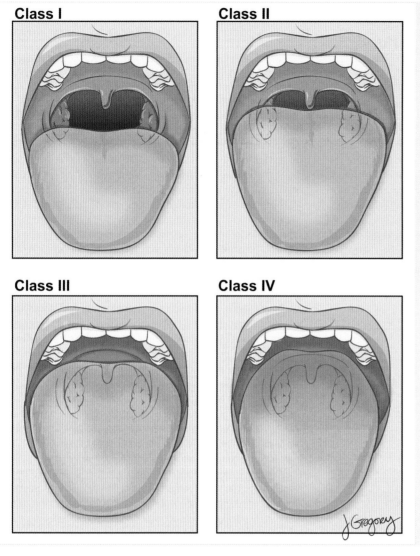

Class I **Class II**

Class III **Class IV**

Fig. 12.1 Mallampati classification.

Table 12.2 American Society of Anesthesiologists classification of physical status

Class	Description
1	Normal, healthy patient
2	Patient with mild systemic disease that results in no functional limitations (e.g., hypertension, smoking, diabetes without complications)
3	Patient with severe systemic disease that results in functional limitations but is not incapacitating (e.g., diabetes with vascular complications, stable angina, previous myocardial infarction, pulmonary disease that limits activity)
4	Patient with incapacitating systemic disease that is a constant threat to life (e.g., congestive heart failure; unstable angina; advanced pulmonary, renal, or hepatic dysfunction)
5	Moribund patient who is not expected to survive without the operation (e.g., ruptured abdominal aneurysm, pulmonary embolus, head injury with increased intracranial pressure)
6	A brain-dead patient whose organs are being removed for donor purposes

12.2.2 Patient Preparation

In the preoperative holding area, initial preoperative preparation begins with measurement of the vital signs, confirmation of nil per os status, placement of a peripheral intravenous (IV) line, and review of the anesthetic plan with the patient. Most, but not all, patients are given an "anxiolytic" dose of an IV sedative (e.g., midazolam). Larger, "sedative" doses of these medications should be avoided in patients with obstructive sleep apnea and patients with symptoms of upper airway obstruction. Premedication with an antisialagogue (e.g., glycopyrrolate, atropine), which improves the surgical exposure, is beneficial before endoscopy or surgery in the oral cavity.

After transferring the patient into the operating room and before inducing anesthesia, the anesthesiologist will attach appropriate monitors (e.g., electrocardiogram leads, noninvasive blood pressure cuff, pulse oximeter) and confirm that the peripheral IV line is "in situ" and patent.

12.2.3 Induction of Anesthesia

Before the surgeon can make an incision, the patient must enter an anesthetic state in which he or she has no awareness, feeling, or response to surgical stimuli. Induction of this anesthetized state begins with preoxygenation, during which the patient is allowed to breathe 100% oxygen through an anesthesia face mask attached to a breathing circuit. Oxygen thus replaces most of the nitrogen contained in the patient's lungs and lessens the chance of hypoxemia during the apnea associated with anesthetic induction. Loss of consciousness is then achieved with IV injection of induction agents, inhalation of anesthetic vapors (especially in children), or a combination of both (vide infra).

12.2.4 Airway Management

After the patient loses consciousness, the anesthesiologist will most often attempt to "open the airway" by lifting the chin and then ventilate the patient's lungs by manually applying positive pressure via the anesthesia machine circuit bag and mask. Once the airway is deemed "open" (e.g., observation of rise and fall of the chest with ventilation, detection of end-tidal carbon dioxide, auscultation of breath sounds), the immediate maintenance of anesthesia usually continues with the use of inhaled anesthetics, delivered to the lungs most commonly by tracheal intubation.

In certain patients, the anesthesiologist will instead choose to insert a laryngeal mask airway (LMA). The LMA consists of a wide-bore tube whose proximal end is connected to a breathing circuit and distal end is attached to an elliptical, inflatable cuff. Once properly placed in the patient's posterior oropharynx, the cuff is inflated to form a low-pressure seal around the glottic structures, providing a patent airway for ventilation.

Via the tracheal tube or the LMA, either the patient can spontaneously ventilate or the anesthesiologist can apply positive-pressure (usually manual) ventilation. The cuff on the tracheal tube creates a mechanical barrier, separating the distal trachea and main bronchi from the upper airway, which is potentially soiled with contents aspirated from the stomach or with blood/infection from surgery on the airway. Therefore, a tracheal tube provides a more "secure" airway than the LMA in preventing aspiration.

Designed as a compromise between a face mask and tracheal tube, the LMA has enjoyed a quarter century of novel application in the modern practice of anesthesiology. Routinely used to maintain ventilation under anesthesia, the LMA has also become a lifesaving adjunct routinely used (and suggested by ASA protocols) by anesthesiologists in any patient for whom manual bag and mask ventilation is ineffective and whose trachea cannot be intubated. Once effective (and lifesaving) ventilation and oxygenation have been established, the LMA can be used as a conduit for blind or even fiber-optic bronchoscope–guided insertion of a tracheal tube.

The otolaryngologic surgical patient often presents with difficult airway management problems, including the following: certain anatomical characteristics (e.g., decreased cervical spine range of motion, large tongue, receding jaw); history of stridor and hoarseness (e.g., airway narrowing and possible vocal cord dysfunction); history of neck surgery, trauma, or radiation therapy; history of difficult intubation; and infections (e.g., epiglottitis, retropharyngeal abscess, Ludwig angina). Neoplastic growths anywhere within the upper airway may achieve significant size with little evidence of airway obstruction in the nonanesthetized patient. However, airway compression can occur with the use of sedative medication, the induction of anesthesia, and the use of muscle relaxants. Moreover, these tumors are often friable, leading to unexpected hemorrhage. Attempts at tracheal intubation can induce hemorrhage and edema, causing severe compromise of the airway. In addition, patients with head and neck cancer often have had previous surgery or radiation therapy; these treatments may further impair airway management by decreasing tissue compliance and adversely affecting neck range of motion and mouth opening. Abscesses in the upper airway may be of sufficient size to mimic neoplasms, presenting the same problems of airway distortion, compression, and compromise. An additional problem is the potential for the abscess to rupture spontaneously or during tracheal intubation, potentially obscuring the anesthesiologist's view during laryngoscopy and causing pneumonia.

Radiologic evaluation of the airway (e.g., plain films of the trachea and larynx, computed tomography, and magnetic resonance imaging studies of the airway) may identify anatomical distortion and aid the anesthesiologist in developing a logical plan for "securing" the airway. If difficult upper airway management is anticipated, then an awake fiber-optic intubation of the trachea or even a tracheostomy under local anesthesia may be indicated.

In a patient with a Le Fort III fracture, nasotracheal intubation risks the introduction of foreign material from the nasopharynx into the subarachnoid space and the consequent development of meningitis. More importantly, nasotracheal intubation risks the introduction of the tracheal tube into the substance of the brain, causing direct mechanical trauma. Even positive-pressure bag and mask ventilation is contraindicated; the increase in volume and pressure of inhaled gas within the nasopharynx can force foreign material or air into the skull. In such patients, the airway is most often "secured" after tracheostomy with local anesthesia.

Several methods have successfully been used to provide oxygenation and ventilation during endoscopy (e.g., laryngoscopy, microlaryngoscopy, esophagoscopy, bronchoscopy). Most commonly, the trachea is intubated with a small-diameter (4.0 to 6.0 mm) tracheal tube through which conventional positive-pressure ventilation is administered. The advantages of intubation include protection against aspiration, the ability to administer inhalational anesthetics, and the ability to continuously monitor end-tidal carbon dioxide. When a tracheal tube is used, caution must be exercised during head and mouth gag manipulation; the tracheal tube may be inadvertently obstructed, disconnected, dislodged, or advanced into a main bronchus.

In some cases, tracheal intubation may interfere with the surgeon's visualization or performance of the procedure. An alternative approach to this is an intermittent-apnea technique, in which periods of ventilation with 100% oxygen by face mask, small catheter, or tracheal tube alternate with periods of apnea, during which time the surgery is performed. The duration of apnea, usually 2 to 3 minutes, is routinely determined by the peripheral oxygen saturation as measured by a pulse oximeter. Hypoventilation with hypercarbia and pulmonary aspiration are risks of this technique.

Jet ventilation is a more sophisticated technique of ventilation employing a manual jet ventilator connected to a side port of the laryngoscope. During inspiration, a high-pressure source of oxygen (but not volatile anesthetic) is directed through the glottic opening, entraining room air into the lungs; expiration is passive through the patent upper airway. It is important to constantly monitor chest wall motion and to allow sufficient time for exhalation so as to avoid air trapping and barotrauma. Jet ventilation is advantageous because it provides an unobstructed operating field and increased safety with laser use (vide infra); however, it poses an increased risk for gastric aspiration and distension, pneumomediastinum, pneumothorax, and hypoventilation.

12.2.5 Maintenance of Anesthesia

Once the airway has been established, most often the anesthesiologist chooses to continue the anesthesia by allowing the patient to inhale an anesthetic, thereby maintaining the state of unconsciousness and providing amnesia and analgesia. Maintenance of anesthesia can also be (totally or partially) achieved with IV anesthetics; an alternative to inhaled anesthetics sometimes is a necessity for certain procedures (e.g., oxygenation via intermittent-apnea or jet ventilation techniques; vide supra).

During the maintenance of anesthesia, the anesthesiologist

- Delivers inhaled anesthetic gases or IV anesthetic agents at levels that provide adequate depth of anesthesia for the surgical stimuli.
- Injects narcotic drugs, as needed, to lessen the requirement for inhaled/IV anesthetic agents and to provide analgesia during the emergence and recovery phases of anesthesia.
- Injects neuromuscular blocking drugs to maintain muscle paralysis, if required.
- Injects other drugs, if indicated (e.g., antibiotics, antiemetic agents).
- Monitors cardiorespiratory parameters, temperature, and urine output; intervenes with adjustments to the anesthetic technique (e.g., ventilator settings) or injects medication (e.g., vasopressors) when necessary.

12.2.6 Emergence from Anesthesia

As the surgery nears completion, the anesthesiologist executes the plan for emergence from anesthesia, transforming the patient's state from comatose and unresponsive to awake and alert. The usual emergence sequence routinely includes

- Reversal of any residual neuromuscular blockade with combinations of anticholinesterase and anticholinergic drugs so that the patient will have full muscle strength upon awakening.
- Discontinuation of the inhaled or IV anesthetics while the patient is allowed to breathe 100% oxygen.
- Extubation of the trachea after the patient has demonstrated adequate respiratory function and when full protective laryngeal reflexes return. In patients with reactive airway disease (e.g. asthma), a "deep" extubation may be warranted to minimize the risk for bronchospasm and laryngospasm.

- Monitoring of cardiorespiratory parameters.
- Continued administration of oxygen by face mask or nasal cannula after extubation and during transfer to the postanesthesia care unit (PACU).

Although never 100% possible, "smooth" emergence from anesthesia is the anesthesiologist's goal. Straining, bucking, or coughing during emergence will cause an increase in venous pressure that may lead to postoperative bleeding, disruption of delicate suture lines, and/or dislodgement of tympanic membrane graft following tympanoplasty. A "smooth" emergence will also minimize laryngospasm and the need for positive-pressure ventilation by face mask, particularly after nasal cosmetic surgery, when the nose is unstable and the application of a face mask is undesirable.

Excessive upper airway bleeding, edema, or pathology may preclude tracheal extubation in the operating room. If edema is a concern at the time of tracheal extubation, then the tracheal tube may be removed over a tube changer, gum elastic bougie, or fiber-optic bronchoscope, leaving a guide in case the tube needs to be immediately replaced. Even the spontaneously ventilating patient is often transported while breathing supplemental oxygen in an attempt to avoid hypoxemia if a period of hypoventilation occurs before admission to the PACU.

12.2.7 Recovery from Anesthesia

After leaving the operating room, the patient is admitted to the PACU, where the anesthesiologist is available for consultation and emergency airway management. In the PACU, the anesthesiologist commonly manages postoperative pain, nausea and vomiting, and cardiorespiratory compromise (e.g., hypoxemia, hypoventilation, hypertension, hypotension, tachyarrhythmias, bradyarrhythmias).

12.3 Anesthesia during Laser Surgery of the Airway

Laser light offers the surgeon excellent precision and hemostasis with minimal postoperative edema or pain; yet, it also introduces major hazards into the operating room. General precautions include evacuation of toxic fumes from tissue vaporization because these may have the potential to transmit microbacterial disease. All operating room personnel should wear eye protection gear, and the patient's eyes should be taped shut.

The greatest fear during laser airway surgery is a tracheal tube fire. This can be avoided by using a technique of ventilation that does not involve a flammable tube or catheter, such as intermittent-apnea or jet ventilation. However, some surgical procedures require a tracheal tube because of the expected duration of the case, location of the lesion, or preexisting lung problems that might warrant airway pressures unattainable with jet ventilation. In these cases, a tracheal tube resistant to laser ignition is used.

Nitrous oxide as well as oxygen supports combustion. If a volatile agent is chosen to maintain anesthesia, then consideration should be given to using a mixture of air/oxygen or helium/oxygen to decrease the inspired oxygen concentration, thus minimizing the risk for an airway fire. Cuffed tracheal tubes can be

Table 12.3 Levels of sedation/analgesia and general anesthesia

Function/structure affected	Minimal sedation (anxiolysis)	Moderate sedation/analgesia (conscious sedation)	Deep sedation/analgesia	General anesthesia
Responsiveness	Normal response to verbal stimulation	Purposeful response to verbal or tactile stimulation	Purposeful response following repeated or painful stimulation	Unarousable even with painful stimulus
Airway	Unaffected	No intervention required	Intervention may be required	Intervention required
Spontaneous ventilation	Unaffected	Adequate	May be inadequate	Frequently inadequate
Cardiovascular function	Unaffected	Usually maintained	Usually maintained	May be impaired

inflated with methylene blue–dyed sterile saline; not only would a laser-induced rupture of the cuff be readily detectable, but the spark might be extinguished by the saline before an airway fire occurred.

If an airway fire occurs, then ventilation is discontinued, and the tracheal tube is disconnected from the breathing circuit and removed from the patient. Saline is poured into the pharynx to absorb heat, and the airway is suctioned before ventilation resumes with 100% oxygen. The trachea is then reintubated with a new tube and the airway is examined by bronchoscopy. Complications of airway fires include airway edema, inhalation injury caused by heat and smoke, tracheal and laryngeal granulation tissue formation, and airway stenosis.

12.4 Intravenous Sedation and Analgesia

Sedation and analgesia comprise a continuum of states ranging from minimal sedation to general anesthesia (▶ Table 12.3). As an anesthetic technique, IV sedation and analgesia is attractive because it does not routinely involve supporting ventilation or manipulation of the airway, although chin lift, jaw thrust, or even insertion of a nasopharyngeal or oral airway may be required. IV sedation and analgesia, along with injection of local anesthetic by the surgeon, usually produces fewer physiologic perturbations than general anesthesia, making it an especially useful anesthetic technique for patients undergoing facial plastic surgery procedures (e.g., rhinoplasty, blepharoplasty, rhytidectomy). The drugs most commonly injected during IV sedation and analgesia include incremental doses or continuous infusions of benzodiazepines (e.g., midazolam), opioids (e.g., fentanyl, remifentanil), and sedative–hypnotics (propofol, dexmedetomidine, ketamine).

12.5 Analgesics

Pain control is an essential part of perioperative management. Two common classes of drugs used to provide analgesia are opioids and nonsteroidal anti-inflammatory drugs (NSAIDs). Commonly used opioids include morphine, hydromorphone, methadone, fentanyl, alfentanil, sufentanil, and remifentanil; side effects of opioids include respiratory depression, nausea, vomiting, constipation, biliary spasm, and pruritus.

NSAIDs are commonly used to treat postsurgical pain and work by inhibiting cyclooxygenase and the production of other

Table 12.4 Antiemetic medications

Antiemetic medication class	Examples
Serotonin (5-HT$_3$) antagonists	Ondansetron, granisetron
Dopamine (D$_2$) antagonists	Metoclopramide, prochlorperazine
H$_1$ antagonists	Diphenhydramine
Antimuscarinics	Scopolamine
Corticosteroids	Dexamethasone

chemical mediators of inflammation. Side effects of NSAIDs include gastrointestinal ulceration, inhibition of thromboxane synthesis and platelet aggregation, renal dysfunction, and hypersensitivity reactions. Ketorolac is an IV NSAID commonly used in clinical anesthesia.

12.6 Postoperative Nausea and Vomiting

Postoperative nausea and vomiting (PONV) is a common side effect caused by both anesthetic medications and the surgical procedure. During surgery, blood from the upper airway may passively drain into the stomach. The placement of a throat pack or suctioning of the stomach with an orogastric tube at the conclusion of surgery therefore may attenuate the severity of PONV. Minimizing the use of opioids and/or nitrous oxide while ensuring adequate IV hydration may also help decrease the incidence of PONV. The routine use of antiemetic medications has also significantly reduced the incidence of PONV (▶ Table 12.4).

12.7 Drugs for the Induction of Anesthesia

12.7.1 Intravenous Drugs

Thiopental, propofol, etomidate, and benzodiazepines exert their effects through specific interactions with γ-aminobutyric acid (GABA), the principal inhibitory neurotransmitter in the central nervous system. Ketamine exerts its anesthetic properties through antagonism of the excitatory N-methyl-D-aspartate (NMDA) receptor (▶ Table 12.5).

Table 12.5 Intravenous drugs for the induction of anesthesia

Intravenous anesthetic	Pros	Cons
Thiopental	Excellent brain protection, potent anticonvulsant, inexpensive	Myocardial depression, vasodilation, histamine release, possible precipitation of porphyria in susceptible patients
Propofol	Prevents nausea/vomiting; rapid, clear-headed recovery if used as sole anesthetic agent to maintain anesthesia	Myocardial depression; vasodilation; pain on injection; supports bacterial growth, which limits duration of safe use after it has been drawn up in a syringe; expensive
Etomidate	Intravenous anesthetic with fewest myocardial effects	pain on injection, adrenal suppression, myoclonus, nausea, vomiting
Ketamine	Minimal depression of cardiorespiratory system; analgesic and amnestic properties; can be given intravenously, orally, rectally, or intramuscularly	Dissociative anesthesia with postoperative dysphoria and hallucinations, increases intracranial pressure and intraocular pressure, increases airway secretions
Benzodiazepines (midazolam, diazepam)	Minimal depression of cardiorespiratory system; anticonvulsant, anxiolytic, sedative, and amnestic properties; reversible with flumazenil	Slow onset of unconsciousness, delayed awakening, pain on injection (diazepam)

Table 12.6 Inhalational drugs for the induction of anesthesia

Inhaled agent	Pros	Cons
Isoflurane	Inexpensive; renal, hepatic, coronary, and cerebral blood flow preservation	Relatively long time to onset/offset, irritating to airway so cannot be used for inhalation induction
Desflurane	Extremely rapid onset/offset	Expensive, stimulates catecholamine release, irritating to airway so cannot be used for inhalation induction
Sevoflurane	Extremely rapid onset/offset, nonirritating to airway so can be used for inhalation induction	Theoretical potential for renal toxicity from inorganic fluoride metabolites
Nitrous oxide	Extremely rapid onset/offset, nonirritating to airway so can be used with sevoflurane for inhalation induction	Diffuses freely into gas-filled spaces (bowel, pneumothorax, middle ear); increases pulmonary vascular resistance; nausea, vomiting; combustible

12.7.2 Inhalational Drugs

Inhaled agents fall into two categories: volatile anesthetics and nitrous oxide (▶ Table 12.6). Volatile anesthetics (e.g., isoflurane, desflurane, sevoflurane) are liquids at room temperature, and a vaporizer is required to convert the liquids to gases, which are then delivered to the patient through the anesthesia breathing circuit.

Nitrous oxide is a gas of low anesthetic potency that is commonly used in combination with volatile anesthetic agents to reduce the amount of volatile anesthetic required. The relative insolubility of nitrous oxide compared with nitrogen can cause the expansion of closed, air-filled compartments in the body, with adverse effects such as rupture of alveolar blebs (causing a pneumothorax) or further expansion of an existing pneumothorax. To avoid pressure-related disruption of the repair or displacement of the graft during tympanoplasty, nitrous oxide is discontinued before tympanic membrane graft placement.

In some circumstances, the anesthesiologist may choose to induce anesthesia by a purely inhalational method. The inhalation of pleasant-smelling sevoflurane is well tolerated by children, leading to a rapid and smooth loss of consciousness. Once the patient is anesthetized, the anesthesiologist can then painlessly and more easily insert an IV catheter for the remainder of the anesthetic.

12.7.3 Neuromuscular Blocking Drugs

Neuromuscular blocking drugs can be classified depending on whether or not they depolarize the postsynaptic membrane of the neuromuscular junction. Succinylcholine is the depolarizing neuromuscular blocking drug routinely used. Injected IV, succinylcholine works rapidly, although briefly, to produce conditions suitable for tracheal intubation. Common side effects noted after the injection of succinylcholine include skeletal muscle fasciculations (with resultant myalgia, increased intraocular pressure, and increased intracranial pressure) and hyperkalemia. Uncommon side effects after the injection of succinylcholine include malignant hyperthermia in genetically sensitive patients and prolonged paralysis in patients with abnormal or absent plasma cholinesterases.

Nondepolarizing neuromuscular blocking drugs (e.g., rocuronium, vecuronium, cisatracurium) bind competitively at the acetylcholine receptors in the neuromuscular junctions of striated muscle. Therefore, the blockade can be reversed by using anticholinesterase drugs (e.g., neostigmine, edrophonium), which increase the amount of acetylcholine present at the neuromuscular junction. Anticholinergic agents (e.g., glycopyrrolate, atropine) must be administered immediately before the reversal drugs to prevent profound muscarinic-mediated vagal effects on the cardiovascular system (e.g., bradycardia).

Table 12.7 Steps of Emergency Therapy for Malignant Hyperthermia

1	Call for help.
2	Discontinue administration of volatile anesthetics and succinylcholine.
3	Hyperventilate the patient with 100% oxygen at flows of 10 L/min or more.
4	Administer dantrolene 2.5 mg/kg; repeat every 5 minutes until signs of malignant hypertension are reversed; up to 30 mg/kg may be necessary.
5	Administer bicarbonate 1 to 2 mEq/kg to treat metabolic acidosis.
6	Institute cooling measures (e.g., gastric lavage, cooling blankets, cold intravenous solutions).
7	Administer inotropes and antiarrhythmic agents as necessary to treat dysrhythmias.
8	Treat hyperkalemia with: hyperventilation, calcium, bicarbonate, and glucose/insulin.
9	Promote urine output (2 mL/kg/h) with aggressive fluid therapy; mannitol and furosemide may also be required.
10	Monitor temperature, urinary output, electrolytes, glucose, blood gases, end-tidal carbon dioxide, and coagulation studies.
11	Consider invasive monitoring of arterial blood pressure and central venous pressure.
12	If necessary, consult on-call physicians at the 24-hour MHAUS (Malignant Hypertension Association of the United States) hotline: **1–800-MH-HYPER**.

Adequate muscle relaxation is often necessary to prevent swallowing during intraoral procedures and facilitate surgical exposure. However, in some surgical procedures (e.g., parotidectomy), nerve monitoring is used to identify and preserve specific nerves; therefore, neuromuscular blockade is contraindicated.

12.8 Recognition and Treatment of Malignant Hyperthermia

Susceptibility to malignant hyperthermia is inherited in an autosomal-dominant pattern. In genetically susceptible individuals, all of the volatile anesthetic agents as well as succinylcholine are capable of triggering malignant hyperthermia, a disorder of intracellular calcium regulation in skeletal muscle. Administration of a triggering agent(s) leads to a sudden release of calcium from the sarcoplasmic reticulum. The intense and sustained muscle contraction that follows results in signs of hypermetabolism, including tachycardia, metabolic acidosis, hypercarbia, hypoxemia, hyperthermia, ventricular dysrhythmias, hyperkalemia, rhabdomyolysis, muscle rigidity (even in the presence of neuromuscular blockade), and tachypnea in the spontaneously breathing patient. As soon as malignant hyperthermia is suspected, all triggering anesthetics are discontinued and the patient is hyperventilated with 100% oxygen. The IV injection of dantrolene, which inhibits calcium release from the sarcoplasmic reticulum, reverses the metabolic reaction taking place in the muscle cells by stabilizing intracellular calcium metabolism. In addition, adequate hydration, active diuresis, correction of metabolic abnormalities, cardiac monitoring, and active cooling are all part of the immediate management of this life-threatening condition (see Table ▶ Table 12.7 Steps of Emergency Therapy for Malignant Hyperthermia). The Malignant Hyperthermia Association of the United States (MHAUS) is a valuable clearinghouse for information about the familial inheritance, recognition, management, and patient follow-up of this disease and maintains a hotline (1–800-MH-HYPER) for health care providers to call with urgent questions.

12.9 Roundsmanship

- The goal of anesthesia is to provide the desired combination of analgesia, amnesia, and optimal operating conditions while ensuring physiologic homeostasis.
- Careful preoperative assessment of the patient and a cooperative relationship between the surgeon and anesthesiologist will improve the operative outcome, especially in more complex cases.
- The equipment and personnel required for an emergency tracheostomy must be immediately available when a difficult airway is being managed.
- If there is a chance of postoperative edema involving structures that could obstruct the airway, the patient should be carefully observed in the postanesthesia care unit or even remain intubated until a trial of spontaneous ventilation, perhaps around a deflated cuff, can be attempted.
- The earliest signs of malignant hyperthermia are tachycardia, hypercarbia, and muscle rigidity. Hyperthermia may be a late development.

12.10 Recommended Reading

[1] Barash P, Cullen B, Stoelting R, Cahalan M, Stock M, eds. Clinical Anesthesia. 6th ed. Philadelphia, PA: Lippincott Williams & Wilkins; 2009

[2] Jaffe R, Samuels S, eds. Anesthesiologist's Manual of Surgical Procedures. 4th ed. Philadelphia, PA: Lippincott Williams & Wilkins; 2009

[3] Miller R, ed. Miller's Anesthesia. 7th ed. Philadelphia, PA: Churchill Livingstone; 2010

13 Infectious Diseases of the Oral Cavity, Pharynx, and Larynx

E. Ashlie Darr and Edward J. Shin

13.1 Oral Cavity

The oral cavity extends from the skin–vermilion border to the junction of the hard and soft palate and includes the buccal mucosa, superior and inferior alveolar ridges and teeth, retromolar trigone, hard palate, floor of the mouth, and oral tongue. The normal oral flora consists of approximately 100 million organisms per milliliter of saliva, with 700 species of organisms represented. Odontogenic infections typically result from commensal oral flora; however, primary pathogens, such as herpes simplex viruses, *Candida albicans*, and human papillomavirus, may also lead to oral cavity infectious disease.

13.1.1 Odontogenic Infections

Odontogenic infections include dental caries, periapical abscesses, pulpitis, gingivitis, and periodontal disease. These infections are typically polymicrobial, with a large percentage of obligate anaerobes comprising the microflora. More than 80% of cultivated organisms consist of *Streptococcus, Peptostreptococcus, Veillonella, Lactobacillus, Corynebacterium,* and *Actinomyces* species, with *Streptococcus mutans* particularly notable for its role in dental caries. Commensal flora must be able to adhere to tooth or mucosal surfaces, evade mechanical disruption, penetrate tissues, and survive host responses in order to become pathogenic. Odontogenic infections have the potential for hematogenous dissemination to the heart and prosthetic devices, and they may provide a nidus for deep neck space infections. Broad-spectrum antibiotics with good coverage against gram-positive and aerobic organisms are appropriate therapy.

13.1.2 Oral Candidiasis

Candida may lead to infections on the mucosal surfaces of the upper aerodigestive tract. *Candida albicans* is most commonly identified as the causative organism; however, *Candida tropicalis, Candida glabrata,* and *Candida krusei* may also cause disease. Oral candidiasis is characterized by white curdlike material on mucosal surfaces that can usually be scraped off with a tongue blade to reveal a friable, painful, erythematous base. The white material is a pseudomembrane consisting of keratin, sloughed epithelium, food debris, leukocytes, and bacteria. Oral mucosal candidiasis may be found in association with angular cheilitis. Diagnosis is usually based on the history and physical examination; however, a potassium hydroxide preparation or Gram stain of a specimen scraped from the mucosa will reveal hyphae, pseudohyphae, and yeast forms. Oral candidiasis represents an opportunistic infection associated with poor cellular immunity, especially in patients whose CD4 + cell counts fall below 200 to 300/mm³. As such, it occurs most commonly in patients with cancer or AIDS, although it may also develop in asthmatic patients using inhaled steroids who are otherwise healthy. In the latter, the infection usually resolves spontaneously without the patient discontinuing the inhalant. For all other patients, treatment consists of triazole antifungals, although resistance to fluconazole is a developing problem.

13.1.3 Oral Herpes Simplex

Human herpes simplex virus type 1 is the most common cause of oral and oropharyngeal ulcerative lesions, with 600,000 new cases per year diagnosed in the United States. The virus is most commonly transmitted by contact with individuals who have active primary or recurrent disease. Infection is caused by viral attachment to the mucosal cell surface, where it undergoes endocytosis, replicates, and ultimately causes cell lysis. This releases viral particles and clinically leads to the formation of vesicles. Human herpes simplex virus type 1 is also taken up by neurons, where it becomes latent and will later replicate when recurrent infection is provoked. Diagnosis is primarily clinical, although viral culture, vesicle content analysis, and serum antibody titers may be used to confirm or follow disease. Multilobulated viral inclusion particles called Tzanck cells are pathognomonic.

Primary herpetic gingivostomatitis is characterized by the onset of tenderness and erythema of the oral and often oropharyngeal mucosal surfaces, followed by an eruption of small vesicles with inflammatory borders that quickly degenerate to ulcerative lesions. The onset of symptoms occurs 5 to 7 days after contact with an infected individual. Signs and symptoms are usually self-limited and resolve within 7 to 14 days with supportive treatment. Recurrent or "secondary" episodes of oral herpes simplex are caused by reactivation of the virus within dermatome-specific ganglia, leading to a prodromal period of altered sensation over the affected area followed by vesicular eruption. This occurs most commonly in the form of herpes labialis. The small vesicles may coalesce and persist for 1 to 2 days, after which ulceration and crusting may occur. Healing usually occurs within 5 to 7 days, and scarring is uncommon in immunocompetent individuals. Treatment with systemic antiviral agents is not required for most cases of oral herpes simplex; however, topical docosanol or penciclovir creams may be used to halt viral replication during labial recurrences.

13.2 Pharynx

The pharynx is subdivided into the nasopharynx, oropharynx, and hypopharynx and extends from the base of the skull to the esophageal inlet. The region predominantly affected by pharyngitis is the oropharynx, which extends from the junction of the soft and hard palate to the base of the tongue.

13.2.1 Bacterial Pharyngitis

Pharyngitis is inflammation of the pharynx, which presents as sore throat and involves predominantly the oropharynx. In adults, only 5 to 10% of cases of pharyngitis are caused by a

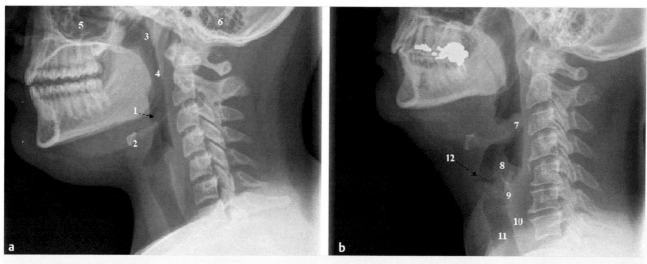

Fig. 13.1 (a) Normal lateral neck X-ray. *1*, Epiglottis; *2*, hyoid; *3*, nasopharynx; *4*, oropharynx; *5*, maxillary sinus; *6*, mastoid air cells. (b) Lateral neck X-ray in patient with epiglottitis. *7*, Enlarged epiglottis; *8*, thickened aryepiglottic folds; *9*, cricoid cartilage; *10*, esophagus; *11*, trachea; *12*, laryngeal ventricle.

bacterial infection. In children, the numbers of cases of bacterial pharyngitis are slightly higher, at 30 to 40%. The most common cause of bacterial pharyngitis in adults is group A β-hemolytic *Streptococcus pyogenes*, a gram-positive coccus that occurs in pairs and chains. Inflammation typically involves the soft palate, tonsillar pillars, posterior pharyngeal wall, and tonsils, which may be swollen and covered with a gray–white exudate. The oropharyngeal tissues are erythematous, the breath is foul-smelling, and soft palate petechiae may be present. Other signs and symptoms may include fever, anorexia, cervical lymphadenitis, odynophagia, and malaise. Rapid antigen tests or throat culture are used for diagnosis. Although the disease is usually self-limited within 3 to 7 days, treatment is recommended to decrease the odds of contagion and the development of rheumatic fever. Other possible sequelae of infection include scarlet fever, post-streptococcal glomerulonephritis, and distant infection due to hematogenous bacterial spread. Penicillin is the mainstay of treatment, and erythromycin or clindamycin may be used in penicillin-allergic patients. Other bacterial causes of pharyngitis include group C and G streptococci and *Arcanobacterium haemolyticum*. *Neisseria gonorrhoeae* may be sexually transmitted and cause pharyngitis concomitantly with genital infection.

13.2.2 Vincent Angina

Vincent angina is an acute necrotizing pharyngitis caused by *Spirochaeta denticulata* and the fusiform bacillus *Borrelia vincentii* (*Treponema vincentii*). These organisms similarly cause a form of gingivostomatitis known as trench mouth. Vincent angina presents with sore throat, high fever, and cervical lymphadenopathy, as well as a deep, friable ulcer of the tonsil that easily bleeds. Diagnosis is made by pharyngeal swab culture of tonsillar exudates. Appropriate antibiotic therapy includes penicillin or clindamycin, with resolution of infection occurring typically within 7 to 10 days.

13.3 Larynx

The larynx extends from the tip of the epiglottis superiorly to the inferior border of the cricoid cartilage. In general, infectious processes affecting the mucous membranes of the oral cavity and pharynx, such as mucocutaneous candidiasis, mucositis, and herpes simplex virus lesions, can also affect the mucosal surfaces of the larynx. A few unique infectious diseases of the larynx deserve special mention.

13.3.1 Epiglottitis (▶ Fig. 13.1)

Epiglottitis is bacterial cellulitis of the epiglottis, which causes supraglottic edema and can rapidly lead to upper airway obstruction. The disease has become rare since the development of the vaccine for *Haemophilus influenzae* type B, which was formerly the causative agent in more than 90% of cases. Today, the most common cause is group A β-hemolytic streptococci, although other organisms have been reported. The importance of epiglottitis lies in its potential for airway obstruction within hours and thus the need for prompt diagnosis and management.

The most common clinical signs of epiglottitis are fever and difficulty breathing. The classic description is the child with inspiratory stridor, retractions, severe sore throat, drooling, and dysphagia who may be sitting in a tripod or sniffing position to maximize airflow through an obstructed larynx. Diagnosis is made by direct visualization of the supraglottis in a controlled environment such as the operating room, where emergent airway interventions can take place in the event of complete obstruction due to further edema or laryngospasm. Although epiglottitis can be confirmed by the presence of the classic "thumbprint" sign on lateral neck X-ray, this study is not encouraged in a patient with potential airway compromise, and pharyngeal examination and other manipulations that may lead to obstruction should be avoided. In the operating room,

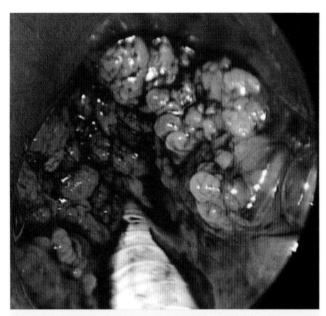

Fig. 13.2 Laryngeal papilloma. Intraoperative photograph of an intubated larynx with bilateral vocal fold papillomas.

cultures from the surface of the epiglottis, alongside blood cultures, should be sent. Ceftriaxone, cefotaxime, or ampicillin/sulbactam are appropriate initial antibiotic choice, and therapy should be further tailored based on culture results and clinical improvement. Extubation may be performed when epiglottic edema is adequately decreased as visualized by flexible or direct laryngoscopy or after a positive endotracheal tube leak test. Extubation can usually be achieved at 48 hours. Oral antibiotics should be continued to complete a 7- to 10-day course once peroral intake is accomplished.

13.3.2 Recurrent Respiratory Papillomatosis

Recurrent respiratory papillomatosis (▶ Fig. 13.2) is characterized by recurrent benign squamous papilloma of the aerodigestive tract caused by human papillomavirus types 6 and 11. Recurrent respiratory papillomatosis is the most common benign laryngeal neoplasm in children and the second most common cause of hoarseness in childhood. Two forms are known: an aggressive, juvenile form and a less aggressive adult-onset form, although disease in adults can also be aggressive. The disease primarily affects the larynx, where it may lead to airway compromise and the requirement for tracheotomy. Disease may also occur in the oral cavity, trachea, and bronchi. Recurrent respiratory papillomatosis affects patients of all ages and is notoriously difficult to treat because of spreading throughout the aerodigestive tract and recurrences that necessitate multiple surgeries. The course of the disease is variable, with some patients achieving full remission and others requiring lifelong treatment.

Human papillomavirus is a double-stranded DNA virus that infects epithelial cells, leading to the formation of benign or malignant neoplasms. To date, more than 100 types of human papillomavirus are known. Human papillomavirus infects mucosal basal layer stem cells, where it may become latent or actively express proteins that lead to cellular proliferation. The lesions of recurrent respiratory papillomatosis appear histologically as finger-like projections of squamous epithelium over a fibrovascular core. Grossly, recurrent respiratory papillomatosis it exhibits a cauliflower-like appearance, with white or pink sessile or pedunculated projections. These lesions have low malignant potential.

The mechanism of transmission has not been fully elucidated, but most cases are thought to involve vertical transmission from mothers with genital condylomas during transit through the birth canal. The most common presenting symptom is hoarseness, followed by inspiratory or biphasic stridor. Diagnosis is made by history and physical examination with nasopharyngolaryngoscopy or direct laryngoscopy. Various methods of surgical treatment have been described. Popular methods of microlaryngoscopic treatment include lesion excision with cold instruments, carbon dioxide laser ablation, and microdébridement. Adjuvant therapies are indicated for patients with rapid regrowth, with multiple-site disease, or requiring more than four surgeries per year. These include systemic therapies, such as interferon-α, ribavirin, acyclovir, and retinoids, as well as intralesional therapies such as cidofovir. Photodynamic therapy involves injection of a photosensitizing drug that is concentrated within papillomas, followed by argon pump dye laser ablation. This also shows potential as an effective therapeutic option.

13.3.3 Acute and Chronic Infectious Laryngitis

Most cases of acute laryngitis are caused by viral upper respiratory infections and are characterized by dysphonia and/or hoarseness. These symptoms may occur in association with sore throat, odynophagia, postnasal drip, malaise, cough, and other manifestations of upper respiratory illness. The most common agents include rhinoviruses, parainfluenza viruses, respiratory syncytial virus, adenoviruses, and influenza virus. Inhalation of humidified air and voice rest are recommended treatment, which is supportive.

Chronic laryngitis of infectious etiology may be caused by a variety of bacterial and fungal agents that commonly produce hoarseness or dysphonia, recurrent throat clearing, sensation of postnasal drip, or recurrent episodes of sore throat lasting for at least 3 months. Laryngeal tuberculosis, once a common sequela of severe pulmonary tuberculosis, now typically occurs in the absence of pulmonary disease. Examination of the larynx may reveal nonspecific inflammatory changes, superficial ulcerations, or exophytic lesions affecting any area of the larynx. Protein purified derivative testing is usually positive, and most patients do not have evidence of pulmonary infection on chest X-ray. Diagnosis is made by culture of sputum and/or laryngeal lesions, and treatment is medical. Fungal causes of chronic laryngitis include candidiasis, histoplasmosis, blastomycosis, cryptococcosis, and coccidioidomycosis. Diagnosis is made by clinical history and biopsy and culture of laryngeal lesions. Treatment is culture-based antibiotic therapy.

13.4 Roundsmanship

- Odontogenic infections typically result from commensal oral flora; however, primary pathogens, such as herpes simplex viruses, *Candida albicans*, and human papillomavirus, may also lead to oral cavity infectious disease.
- Multilobulated viral inclusion particles called Tzanck cells are pathognomonic for herpes simplex virus infection.
- In adults, only 5 to 10% of cases of pharyngitis are caused by a bacterial infection.
- Because of vaccination, the most common cause of epiglottitis is group A β-hemolytic streptococci.

13.5 Recommended Reading

[1] Bisno AL. Acute pharyngitis. N Engl J Med 2001; 344: 205–211

[2] Chow AW. Infections of the oral cavity, neck, and head. In: Mandell G, Bennett JE, Dolin R, eds. Mandell, Douglas, and Bennett's Principles and Practice of Infectious Diseases. 7th ed. Philadelphia, PA: Elsevier; 2009:855–873

[3] Haemophilus influenzae infections. Report of the Committee on Infectious Diseases. Chicago, IL: American Academy of Pediatrics; 1991

[4] Linder JA, Stafford RS. Antibiotic treatment of adults with sore throat by community primary care physicians: a national survey, 1989–1999. JAMA 2001; 286: 1181–1186

[5] Pichichero ME. Group A streptococcal tonsillopharyngitis: cost-effective diagnosis and treatment. Ann Emerg Med 1995; 25: 390–403

14 Antimicrobial Therapy for Head and Neck Infections

E. Ashlie Darr and Edward J. Shin

14.1 Antibacterial Agents (▶ Table 14.1)

14.1.1 Penicillins

Penicillins (PCNs) are a group of antibiotics that share a β-lactam ring and function by binding irreversibly to PCN-binding proteins in bacterial cell walls, leading to osmotic lysis and cellular death.

Natural Penicillins

Members of this class include oral penicillin V and parenteral formulations (e.g. aqueous, crystalline, procaine, and benzathine penicillin G).

Clinical Uses

The natural penicillins are active against *Streptococcus pyogenes* (group A β-hemolytic), most strains of *Streptococcus pneumoniae*, *Treponema pallidum*, *Actinomyces*, and some oral anaerobes. They are inactivated by a variety of enzymes produced by gram-negative and oral anaerobic organisms collectively known as β-lactamases, as well as by penicillinase produced by *Staphylococcus aureus*. Another mechanism of resistance is the alteration of PCN-binding proteins by certain strains of staphylococci and *S. pneumoniae*.

Penicillinase-Resistant Penicillins

Agents in this category include methicillin, oxacillin, cloxacillin, dicloxacillin, and nafcillin.

Clinical Uses

These agents are active against most forms of *S. aureus*, except for methicillin-resistant *S. aureus* (MRSA). They remain active against most streptococcal and pneumococcal infections. Nafcillin is metabolized by the liver, making it a good choice in patients with renal impairment. Among the oral agents in this group, dicloxacillin attains the highest blood concentrations.

Aminopenicillins

These include amoxicillin and ampicillin.

Clinical Uses

These agents are effective against certain gram-negative organisms, such as *Proteus*, *Haemophilus influenzae*, and *Escherichia coli*. They are inactivated by β-lactamases and are ineffective against *S. aureus*.

Table 14.1 Antibacterial agents

Class	Activity against	Adverse effects
Penicillins	Most streptococci, pneumococci, *Staphylococcus aureus* (except methicillin-resistant *S. aureus*)	Rash, gastrointestinal upset
Cephalosporins	Staphylococci, streptococci, and some gram-negatives	Rash, gastrointestinal upset
Macrolides	Gram-positive cocci, some upper respiratory gram-negatives	Nausea, abdominal cramping, elevated liver function tests
Clindamycin	Gram-positives and most anaerobes	Pseudomembranous colitis
Tetracyclines	*Chlamydia*, *Mycoplasma*, *Borrelia burgdorferi* (Lyme disease)	Nausea, photosensitivity, tooth enamel discoloration in children
Fluoroquinolones	*Pseudomonas*, some gram-positives	Nausea, central nervous system disturbances, rashes, phototoxicity
Vancomycin	Gram-positives, including methicillin-resistant *S. aureus*	Red man syndrome, nephrotoxicity, ototoxicity
Daptomycin	Gram-positives, including methicillin-resistant organisms	Skeletal muscle effects, gastrointestinal disturbances, increased liver function tests
Metronidazole	Anaerobes and some protozoa	Nausea, disulfiram-like reactions to alcohol, dysgeusia
Aminoglycosides	Gram-positive and gram-negative aerobes	Nephrotoxicity, ototoxicity
Mupirocin	Gram-positives, including methicillin-resistant *S. aureus*	Local itching, burning
Rifampin	Mycobacteria, combination therapy for methicillin-resistant *S. aureus*	Orange discoloration of body fluids, hepatitis, rash
Sulfonamides	Gram-positives and gram-negatives; some resistant *S. aureus*	Cholestatic jaundice, bone marrow suppression, severe hypersensitivity reactions
Oxazolidinones	Gram-positives, drug-resistant *S. aureus* and streptococci	Diarrhea, nausea, headaches, thrombocytopenia
Streptogramins	Resistant *S. aureus* strains	Arthralgias, myalgias, increased liver function tests

Augmented Penicillins

Members include amoxicillin/potassium clavulanate (Augmentin; Dr. Reddy's Laboratories), ampicillin/sulbactam (Unasyn; Pfizer), piperacillin/tazobactam (Zosyn; Pfizer), and ticarcillin/potassium clavulanate (Timentin; GlaxoSmithKline).

Clinical Uses

These agents combine a penicillin with an inactivator of β-lactamase. This confers effectiveness against *H. influenzae, M. catarrhalis*, anaerobes, and certain staphylococci (although not MRSA). Additionally, Timentin and Zosyn may be used to treat *Pseudomonas aeruginosa* infections. Ticarcillin and piperacillin, without the addition of β-lactamases, are not active against gram-positive bacteria.

Adverse Effects

Rashes occur in approximately 5% of patients using penicillins; however, this reaction recurs in only 50% of patients who go on to use the drug a second time. Anaphylaxis occurs in 0.05% of patients and is considered a contraindication to further penicillin use. Other potential adverse effects include interstitial nephritis, anemia, and leukopenia. Patients requiring prolonged high-dose therapy (for longer than 2 weeks) should be monitored with weekly serum creatinine levels and blood counts. Augmentin commonly produces unwanted gastrointestinal side effects. Amoxicillin, when taken in the setting of infectious mononucleosis, causes a maculopapular rash in 65 to 90% of patients. This is not indicative of a true PCN allergy. Oral PCNs, except for amoxicillin, are destroyed by gastric acid and should therefore be taken on an empty stomach. Any patient reporting a history of serious PCN allergy should undergo skin testing or desensitization before PCN use.

14.1.2 Cephalosporins

Cephalosporins are another family of β-lactam antibiotics, which are classified as first-, second-, third-, and fourth-generation. As a general rule, first-generation cephalosporins have the greatest activity against gram-positive organisms, whereas fourth-generation cephalosporins have the greatest activity against gram-negative species.

First-Generation Cephalosporins

These include cephalexin (Keflex; Shionogi) and cefazolin (Ancef, GlaxoSmithKline; Kefzol, Eli Lilly).

Clinical Uses

These agents are active against staphylococci, streptococci, and community-acquired species of *Proteus, Klebsiella*, and *E. coli*. They have limited activity against other enteric gram-negative organisms and anaerobes. Cefazolin is commonly used for its antistaphylococcal activity in surgical prophylaxis for infection at skin incision sites.

Second-Generation Cephalosporins

Members in this category include cefuroxime (Ceftin; GlaxoSmithKline), cefprozil (Cefzil; Bristol-Myers Squibb), and cefaclor (Ceclor; Eli Lilly).

Clinical Uses

These agents have slightly more activity than first-generation cephalosporins against gram-negative bacteria such as *Proteus, Klebsiella, Neisseria* species, and *Moraxella catarrhalis*. They have slightly less activity against gram-positive organisms.

Third-Generation Cephalosporins

These include cefpodoxime (Vantin; Pfizer), ceftriaxone (Rocephin; Genentech), ceftazidime (Fortaz; Covis Pharmaceuticals), cefdinir (Omnicef; Abbott Laboratories), and cefotaxime (Claforan; Sanofi-Aventis).

Clinical Uses

These agents are less active against *S. aureus* than the earlier generations, but they usually inhibit streptococci and have expanded coverage against gram-negative organisms. Ceftriaxone has good activity against pneumococci, *H. influenzae*, and *Neisseria meningitidis*, and it also effectively crosses the blood–brain barrier, making it a popular choice for treating meningitis as well as intracranial or intraorbital complications of sinusitis and otitis media. It is also useful for treating pharyngeal gonorrhea. Cefpodoxime and cefdinir are commonly used in treating acute otitis media and sinusitis because of their enhanced gram-positive activity relative to the other third-generation drugs. None of the oral cephalosporins are active against PCN-resistant pneumococci.

Fourth-Generation Cephalosporins

Cefepime (Maxipime; Elan Pharmaceuticals) is the only fourth-generation cephalosporin. It has the best activity of the cephalosporins against *P. aeruginosa* and thus may be used as a non-ototoxic and non-nephrotoxic alternative to aminoglycosides. It is effective against other often-resistant gram-negatives, such as *Enterobacter* and *Citrobacter*, as well as *S. aureus* and pneumococci.

Adverse Effects

Because of the molecular structural similarity between cephalosporins and PCNs, patients with a history of anaphylaxis after PCN use should not take cephalosporins. However, only 5 to 10% of patients who have a history of PCN rashes will develop a rash with cephalosporins. Mucocutaneous candidiasis or *Clostridium difficile*–induced pseudomembranous colitis may result from overgrowth of yeast or bacteria, respectively, primarily because of the broad-spectrum activity of cephalosporins. Ceftriaxone is associated with biliary sludging, especially in patients receiving total parenteral nutrition. Like PCNs, cephalosporins have been reported to cause interstitial nephritis, anemia, and leukopenia, and prolonged use indicates appropriate serologic monitoring.

14.1.3 Other β-Lactams

These include the carbapenems—imipenem (Primaxin; Merck), meropenem (Merrem; AstraZeneca), and ertapenem (Invanz; Merck)—and aztreonam (Azactam; Bristol-Myers Squibb), which is a monobactam.

Clinical Uses

Aztreonam is active only against aerobic gram-negative rods, such as *P. aeruginosa*. It has no known cross-reactivity with PCNs or cephalosporins and can therefore be used in PCN-allergic patients. Carbapenems are effective against most gram-positive, gram-negative, and anaerobic organisms, as well as against *P. aeruginosa* (except ertapenem). They are important antibiotics for polymicrobial and resistant bacterial infections.

14.1.4 Macrolides and Ketolides

Macrolides include erythromycin, azithromycin (Zithromax; Pfizer), and clarithromycin (Biaxin; AbbVie). Ketolides, such as telithromycin (Ketek; Sanofi-Aventis), are macrolide derivatives that have enhanced activity against *S. pneumoniae*. Both groups exert their antibacterial activity by binding to 50S subunits on bacterial ribosomes.

Clinical Uses

These agents are effective against respiratory infections caused by *Legionella, Mycoplasma, Chlamydia, Corynebacterium diphtheriae, Bordetella pertussis*, and susceptible streptococci. They are sometimes used to treat sinusitis and streptococcal pharyngitis, although less expensive and equally effective alternatives are available. Macrolides and ketolides are relatively ineffective against *H. influenzae*.

Adverse Effects

Erythromycin may cause nausea and vomiting and elevation of hepatic enzymes with prolonged use. Erythromycin and clarithromycin are inhibitors of cytochrome P-450, which may lead to increased levels of oral anticoagulants, theophylline, and other medications. Macrolides and ketolides can additionally prolong cardiac QT intervals, especially when used with other potentiating drugs.

14.1.5 Clindamycin

Clindamycin (Cleocin; Pfizer) works by inhibiting bacterial protein synthesis.

Clinical Uses

Clindamycin is highly active against most anaerobes, including most *Bacteroides fragilis*, as well as gram-positive organisms, including many strains of PCN-resistant pneumococci and MRSA. It penetrates well into abscess cavities and bone, making it ideal for the treatment of osteomyelitis and deep neck space abscesses caused by oral or dental infections.

Adverse Effects

Oral clindamycin may cause nausea or vomiting and should be taken with meals. It is also the most commonly implicated antibiotic in pseudomembranous colitis. Patients who develop diarrhea while taking clindamycin should immediately discontinue the medication. Pretreatment with metronidazole for several days before clindamycin is administered is sometimes employed to decrease the risk for colitis.

14.1.6 Tetracyclines

Tetracyclines include doxycycline, tetracycline, and minocycline. They exert bacteriostatic activity by binding to the 30S subunit of bacterial ribosomes, thus inhibiting protein synthesis. Tigecycline (Tygacil; Pfizer) is a derivative of minocycline.

Clinical Uses

Tetracyclines are popularly used to treat acne. They are also used as prophylaxis against traveler's diarrhea and against upper respiratory infections caused by *Legionella, Mycoplasma*, and *Chlamydia*. They may be used in Lyme disease and Rocky Mountain spotted fever. Oral preparations may relieve the pain of aphthous ulcers and may be effective against other oral infections, such as Vincent angina. Tigecycline is useful in skin infections with gram-positive bacteria, including MRSA, and is not susceptible to the tetracycline resistance mechanisms that commonly render other members of this class ineffective.

Adverse Effects

Tetracyclines are notable in causing brownish discoloration of teeth if taken during enamel formation and thus should not be given to pregnant or nursing women or to children younger than 10 years of age. Tetracyclines may also promote sunburn and esophagitis. Minocycline may cause transient vertigo.

14.1.7 Chloramphenicol

Chloramphenicol is effective against most gram-positives, including many PCN-resistant staphylococci, most anaerobes, and most gram-negatives. *Pseudomonas* and PCN-resistant streptococci are, however, not susceptible. Chloramphenicol readily crosses the blood–brain barrier. It is notable for causing bone marrow suppression, which can be fatal, and thus its use is reserved for life-threatening infections in patients who cannot tolerate alternatives. Chloramphenicol may also cause the "gray baby syndrome" in fetuses and neonates and thus should not be given during pregnancy.

14.1.8 Fluoroquinolones

This class includes ciprofloxacin (Cipro; Bayer HealthCare), levofloxacin (Levaquin; Janssen), gatifloxacin (Zymar; Allergan), gemifloxacin (Factive; Merus Labs International), and moxifloxacin (Avelox; Bayer HealthCare). Quinolones are broad-spectrum antibiotics that function by inhibiting bacterial DNA gyrase, which blocks DNA synthesis.

Clinical Uses

Members of this class are effective against most gram-negative infections, including those caused by *P. aeruginosa*. Topical preparations are thus commonly used in the treatment of otitis externa. They also have moderate activity against gram-positive organisms, *S. pyogenes*, and PCN-resistant pneumococci, as well as *H. influenzae, M. catarrhalis, Legionella*, and other atypicals. Of the quinolones, only moxifloxacin has significant activity against anaerobes.

Adverse Effects

Nausea, drowsiness, rashes, and photosensitivity are the most common adverse effects associated with fluoroquinolone use. Fluoroquinolones also may induce the prolongation of cardiac QT intervals. Pediatric and age-related arthropathy may also occur, so these agents should not be used in pregnant or lactating women and should be discontinued in patients who develop joint pain or tendinitis.

14.1.9 Vancomycin

Vancomycin (Vancocin; ViroPharma) is a parenteral antibiotic best known for its effectiveness against strains of resistant bacteria, including MRSA, PCN-resistant pneumococci, and enterococci, although resistant strains have emerged. It functions by interfering with gram-positive bacterial cell wall synthesis. Vancomycin may cause nephrotoxicity and/or ototoxicity, especially when administered together with aminoglycosides. Red man syndrome is upper body flushing and erythema caused by histamine release, which may occur with rapid vancomycin infusion. Because of its unique ability to combat highly resistant organisms, vancomycin should be used only in cases of severe infections that cannot be controlled with other medications.

14.1.10 Daptomycin

Daptomycin is a parenteral agent that works by inserting itself into the bacterial cell membrane, causing depolarization and cellular death. It is used to treat MRSA and methicillin-resistant *S. epidermidis* infections as a once-daily alternative to vancomycin. Its principal adverse effect is elevation of creatine phosphokinase levels and associated myopathy.

14.1.11 Metronidazole

Metronidazole (Flagyl; Pfizer) is active against anaerobes and some protozoa by promoting the accumulation of toxic metabolic byproducts. Metronidazole crosses the blood–brain barrier well and may be used to treat antibiotic-induced colitis. In the head and neck, metronidazole is useful in treating oral infections, or it may be employed in treating sinusitis, deep neck space infections, and chronic otitis media when used concomitantly with agents that have aerobic and gram-positive activity. Adverse effects include a disulfiram-like reaction with alcohol consumption and dysgeusia.

14.1.12 Aminoglycosides

Members of this class include gentamicin, tobramycin, amikacin, neomycin, and streptomycin. They interfere with the bacterial translation of messenger RNA into protein by binding to ribosomes. Aminoglycosides are effective against aerobic gram-positive and gram-negative bacteria, such as *P. aeruginosa*, and have a synergistic effect when used with PCNs, cephalosporins, or vancomycin. Resistance to one aminoglycoside does not necessarily imply resistance to the others in the group. Neomycin is a component of certain topical preparations used in the treatment of otitis externa; however, *P. aeruginosa* is often resistant. Gentamicin and tobramycin nasal irrigations may be used as antipseudomonal treatments in patients with cystic fibrosis. The use of aminoglycosides is limited by clinically significant oto- and nephrotoxicity. Because of its ototoxic effects, gentamicin has been used as a transtympanic therapy for refractory Meniere disease.

14.1.13 Mupirocin

Mupirocin (Bactroban; GlaxoSmithKline) is a topical ointment used to treat nasal carriers of *S. aureus*. It may be mixed with saline spray for deeper nasal penetration. It has a unique molecular structure and thus has no allergic cross reactivities.

14.1.14 Rifampin

Rifampin is most commonly used to treat mycobacterial infections; however, it is also active against *S. aureus* and *S. epidermidis* (including MRSA), streptococci, pneumococci, anaerobes (including *Bacteroides fragilis*), *Neisseria, H. influenzae*, and *Legionella*. Unless used for prophylaxis, rifampin should not be used as monotherapy because of the rapid resistance that may occur during treatment. Rifampin concentrates well in nasopharyngeal secretions and thus is useful for nasal carriers of *Neisseria* or *H. influenzae*. When combined with mupirocin, it is helpful in eradicating the *S. aureus* carrier state. Rifampin causes orange discoloration of body fluids and may be hepato- or nephrotoxic. It potentiates cytochrome P-450, which may lead to decreased serum levels of other medications.

14.1.15 Sulfonamides

Sulfonamides, such as sulfamethoxazole, are rarely used as monotherapeutic agents because of increases in resistance. Currently, sulfamethoxazoles are effective against about 75% of *H. influenzae* strains but are ineffective against most other respiratory pathogens. Trimethoprim/sulfamethoxazole (Bactrim; AR Scientific) produces a synergistic effect that is useful in treating *S. aureus* infections, including MRSA infections. It has also been used as adjuvant therapy in Wegener granulomatosis and in the treatment of *Pneumocystis carinii* infection.

14.1.16 Oxazolidinones

Linezolid (Zyvox; Pfizer) is an alternative to vancomycin for the treatment of MRSA infections and can even be used for infections with vancomycin-resistant strains of both *S. aureus* and enterococci. Unlike vancomycin, it is available in both parenteral and oral forms. At present, this medication is highly expensive. It may adversely lower platelet levels or lead to hypertension in those concomitantly using decongestant medications.

14.1.17 Streptogramins

Quinupristin/dalfopristin (Synercid; Pfizer) is a streptogramin. Streptogramins have a structure and function similar to those of macrolides. Synercid was developed to treat resistant gram-positive infections, such as those caused by MRSA, vancomycin-resistant enterococci (*Enterococcus faecium*, but not *Enterococcus faecalis*), and resistant pneumococci. It may cause arthralgias.

14.2 Antifungals

14.2.1 Amphotericin B

Amphotericin B (Amphotec; Alkopharma USA) is a broad-spectrum antifungal effective against systemic mycotic infections, including those caused by *Candida, Mucor,* and *Aspergillus.* It functions by interfering with fungal plasma membranes. Intravenous infusion is notable in producing several unpleasant side effects, including fevers, rigors, nausea/vomiting, hypotension, and tachypnea; however, lipid formulations may decrease these symptoms. Amphotericin B may also cause anemia or nephrotoxicity, both of which are reversible.

14.2.2 Triazoles

Triazoles interfere with ergosterol synthesis and are fungistatic. Fluconazole (Diflucan) is used in local and disseminated candidal infections and is a second-line agent against *Cryptococcus.* Unlike fluconazole, voriconazole (Vfend) and itraconazole (Sporanox) are effective against *Aspergillus.* Nausea, diarrhea, and rash are the most common adverse effects, although hepatotoxicity can be severe. Liver function tests should be monitored weekly. Voriconazole and itraconazole can both potentiate the effects of other medications, such as cyclosporin, warfarin, and digoxin, so serum levels should be monitored. Voriconazole may also produce visual disturbances, which are reversible.

14.2.3 Flucytosine

Flucytosine (Ancobon) may be used to treat *Candida* or *Cryptococcus* infection or as combined therapy with amphotericin B for *Aspergillus* infection. It may be taken orally and is better tolerated than amphotericin B, although resistance frequently develops during treatment. It may cause reversible bone marrow suppression.

14.2.4 Candins

Caspofungin (Cancidas) is a parenteral candin that may be used in refractory aspergillosis or candidal infections. It is relatively well tolerated, although it may cause flushing, fever, or a rash with infusion and may be hepatotoxic when used with cyclosporine.

14.2.5 Nystatin

Nystatin (mycostatin) is a topical preparation that is used for oropharyngeal and cutaneous candidiasis (thrush). No significant adverse effects or medication interactions are associated with its use.

14.3 Antivirals

14.3.1 Antiherpetic Agents

These drugs include acyclovir (Zovirax; GlaxoSmithKline), valacyclovir (Valtrex; GlaxoSmithKline), famciclovir (Famvir; Novartis), and penciclovir (Denavir; New American Therapeutics). They function as nucleotide analogues that inhibit DNA synthesis. Acyclovir is effective against herpes simplex and herpes zoster and comes in topical, oral, and intravenous forms. It may be used as prophylaxis against herpes simplex attacks; however, it functions only during the active phase of the viral life cycle, and thus recurrences can be expected. It may cause a nephropathy, especially in those with preexisting poor renal function. Valacyclovir is taken orally and is converted to high serum levels of acyclovir. It is effective in decreasing the symptoms associated with herpes simplex labialis attacks when taken within the first 2 hours of symptom onset. Some physicians treat idiopathic facial paralysis (Bell palsy) with antiherpetic agents because of the possibility of a viral cause.

14.3.2 Anti-influenza Agents

Amantadine (Symmetrel; Endo Health Solutions) and rimantidine (Flumadine; Forest Pharmaceuticals) block the entry of influenza A virus into cells. They are ineffective against influenza B. These agents are used within 48 hours of symptom onset and are continued for 7 to 10 days. They may be used as prophylaxis for patients who have been exposed but are known to be immune, or for patients in nursing homes or hospital staff during epidemics. Side effects include gastrointestinal distress or central nervous system symptoms, such as dizziness and confusion. Zanamivir (Relenza; GlaxoSmithKline) and oseltamivir (Tamiflu; Genentech) are both neuraminidase inhibitors that are effective against both influenza A and influenza B. Both may decrease symptom severity and illness duration when taken within 36 hours of initial symptom onset. Zanamivir is a dry inhalant that may cause nasal irritation or bronchospasm in patients with asthma, as well as gastrointestinal discomfort and headaches. Oseltamivir may cause nausea, vomiting, diarrhea, headaches, and dizziness.

14.4 Roundsmanship

- Rashes occur in approximately 5% of patients using penicillins; however, this reaction recurs in only 50% of patients who go on to use the drug a second time. Any patient reporting a history of serious PCN allergy should undergo skin testing or desensitization before PCN use.

- Because of its unique ability to combat highly resistant organisms, vancomycin should be used only in cases of severe infections that cannot be controlled with other medications.
- The use of aminoglycosides is limited by clinically significant oto- and nephrotoxicity. Because of its ototoxic effects, gentamicin has been used as a transtympanic therapy for refractory Meniere disease.

14.5 Recommended Reading

[1] Fairbanks DNF. Pocket Guide to Antimicrobial Therapy in Otolaryngology-Head and Neck Surgery. 14th ed. Alexandria, VA: American Academy of Otolaryngology-Head and Neck Surgery Foundation; 2007:1–24

[2] Ritchie DJ, Lawrence SJ. Antimicrobials. In: Green GB, Harris IS, Lin GA, Moylan KC, eds. The Washington Manual of Medical Therapeutics. 31st ed. Philadelphia, PA: Lippincott Williams & Wilkins; 2004:272–291

15 Evaluation and Management of Deep Neck Space Infections

Craig E. Berzofsky and Zhenqing Brett Wu

15.1 Introduction

Understanding the anatomy of the head and neck is important in the discussion of deep neck space infections. It is the relationship between the major structures in the neck and the fascial compartments that allows the infections to form and disseminate. The interconnecting lymphatic drainage of these areas also provides a means for infectious spread. The infections develop from tonsillitis, pharyngitis, trauma, and iatrogenic events. The incidence of deep neck space infections has dramatically decreased since the advent of antibiotics. However, delayed treatment of deep neck space infections can result in severe morbidity and mortality by causing respiratory distress, mediastinitis, vascular thrombosis/rupture, and cranial neuropathy.

15.2 Spaces and Infections

The deep cervical spaces can be divided into those existing above the hyoid bone, below the hyoid bone, and across the hyoid bone extending the entire length of the neck (▶ Fig. 15.1).

The spaces above the hyoid bone are the buccal, masticator, submandibular/sublingual, parotid, peritonsillar, and parapharyngeal spaces. The buccal space extends from between the teeth, buccal mucosa, and buccinator muscles medially; the superficial layer of the deep cervical fascia and muscles of facial expression laterally and anteriorly; and the mandible, parotid gland, and masseter and lateral and medial pterygoid muscles posteriorly; it contains the retromaxillary (buccal) fat pad. Infections here are usually odontogenic in origin and often arise from bicuspid and molar teeth.

The masticator space is surrounded by the superficial layer of deep cervical fascia extending from the skull base to the angle of the mandible. This space contains the muscles of mastication, mandibular nerve, ramus and body of the mandible, and pterygoid venous plexus. The source of infection is also typically odontogenic.

The parotid space is contained in the superficial layer of deep cervical fascia, which splits to envelop the parotid gland, lymph nodes, and branches of the facial nerve.

Abscess of this space may be multiloculate because of the septa from the superficial layer of the deep cervical fascia.

Peritonsillar space infections are associated with tonsillitis. This is a potential space between the tonsillar capsule and the palatoglossus, palatopharyngeus, and superior constrictor muscles.

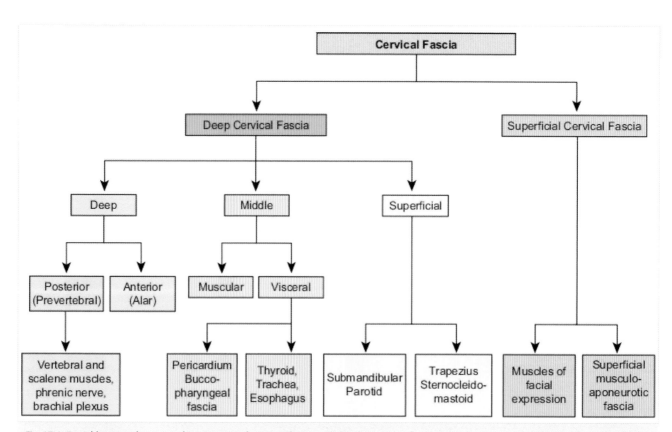

Fig. 15.1 Fascial layers and associated structures and spaces. The carotid sheath is made of superficial and deep cervical fascia.

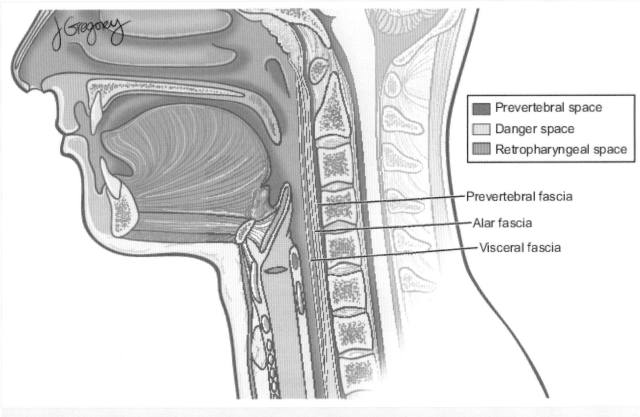

Legend:
- Prevertebral space
- Danger space
- Retropharyngeal space

Prevertebral fascia
Alar fascia
Visceral fascia

Fig. 15.2 Sagittal view of the deep neck spaces and fascial layers extending through the neck.

The submandibular and sublingal space is bordered by the mandible, floor of the mouth, superficial layer of the deep cervical fascia, and parapharyngeal space. The mylohyoid muscle originates from the mandibular line of the inner cortex of the mandible and separates the submandibular space below from the sublingual space above. Dental infections anterior to the second molar (above the mandibular line) usually result in sublingual space infections. Infections of the second and third molars (below the mandibular line) usually cause submandibular space infection and readily spread to the parapharyngeal space posteriorly.

The lateral pharyngeal or parapharyngeal space extends from the skull base to the hyoid bone. It is bounded by the ramus of the mandible, parotid, pterygoid muscles, and superior pharyngeal constrictors. It is divided into prestyloid and poststyloid compartments. The prestyloid space contains fat, the internal maxillary artery, and branches of the trigeminal nerve. The poststyloid space contains the carotid artery; internal jugular vein; cranial nerves IX, X, and XI; and the sympathetic chain. Because of its proximity to the peritonsillar, submandibular, masticator, and parotid space, the parapharyngeal space is readily involved.

The visceral space is the only space existing solely below the hyoid bone. It is bounded by the pharyngeal constrictors laterally and the alar fascia posteriorly. As the name suggests, it contains the pharynx, larynx, esophagus, trachea, and thyroid. Foreign body, trauma, and iatrogenic events are usually the causes of infections in this space.

The spaces that extend the entire length of the neck are the retropharyngeal space, danger space, and prevertebral space (▶ Fig. 15.2). The retropharyngeal space exists between the visceral division of the middle layer of the deep cervical fascia and the alar division of the deep layer of the deep cervical fascia. Between the alar and prevertebral divisions of the deep cervical fascia is the danger space. Clinically, infections in both these spaces typically arise from the nose, sinuses, and nasopharynx. They have the potential of causing mediastinitis by virtue of their location. The prevertebral space is posterior to the prevertebral division of the deep layer of the deep cervical fascia and contains the longus colli muscle. Infections here may travel farther below the diaphragm to the coccyx.

It is important to realize that although the fascial layers and spaces have distinct names and separate borders (▶ Fig. 15.3), infectious processes may readily spread through the boundaries. A simple manageable infection may become life-threatening unless prompt evaluation and treatment are instituted.

15.3 The Disease Process

15.3.1 Etiology

The etiology of deep space cervical infections varies widely. Parkiscar and Har-El reported that 43% of the infections are dental in origin, while the second most common cause is intravenous (IV) drug injection (12%). Other causes noted were pharyngotonsillitis, mandible fracture, skin infection, tuberculosis,

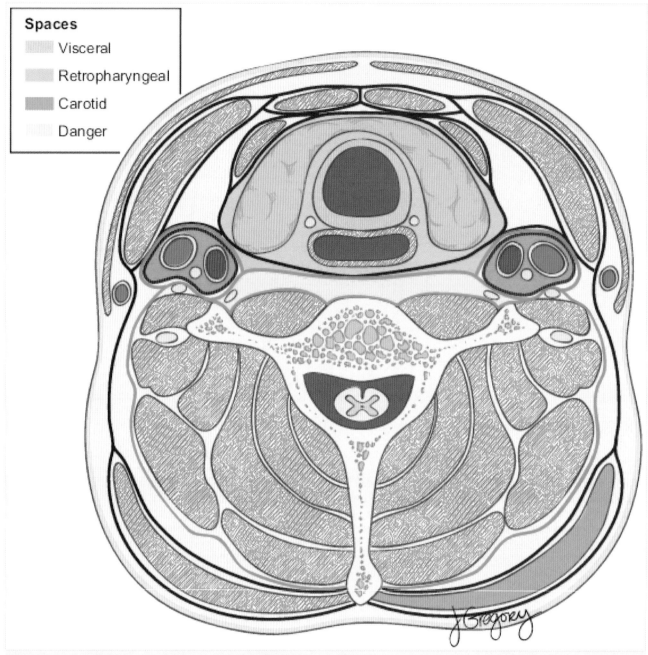

Fig. 15.3 Axial view through the lower neck demonstrating the fascial layers and deep neck spaces.

foreign body, trauma, peritonsillar abscess, sialolithiasis, and parotitis, together comprising the other 45% of infections.

15.3.2 Microbiology

Most of the deep space neck infections are polymicrobial in origin. Several studies have examined the culture results from these patient populations. The most commonly cultured bacteria are *Streptococcus viridans*, *Staphylococcus epidermidis*, *Staphylococcus aureus*, *Bacteroides* species, and β-hemolytic streptococci. Anaerobes were cultured in 35% of the infections. Gram-negative organisms were present in fewer than 4% of infections.

15.3.3 Potential Complications

Infections in each of these areas can lead to complications that can cause significant morbidity and mortality. The most urgent complication of deep neck space infection is airway compromise. Ludwig angina deserves special discussion. It is an extension of dental infection in the sublingual space. It is associated with necrotizing cellulitis, causing swelling of the floor of the mouth and base of the tongue. Airway compromise and death ensue if the condition is not promptly treated. Many of these patients require emergent airway establishment via tracheotomy followed by incision and drainage of the involved space.

Other notable entities include danger space and retropharyngeal space infections. The predominantly loose areolar tissue in these spaces affords little resistance to the spread of infection. The rapid development of mediastinitis may prove fatal.

Neurologic complications can occur through the irritation and compression of involved nerves, such as the cranial nerves and the sympathetic chains in the poststyloid compartment of the parapharyngeal space. They can also occur through the extension of infections from adjacent deep neck spaces. Pott abscess, for example, is a result of mycobacterial infectious extension posteriorly from a vertebral body.

Vascular compromise and septicemia can occur when the infection extends into the carotid sheath. Involvement of the internal jugular vein can lead to Lemierre syndrome, with associated pulmonary septic emboli. Carotid artery rupture preceded by sentinel bleeding is another feared complication with significant morbidity and mortality.

15.4 Medical Evaluation

15.4.1 Presenting Complaints

The presenting complaint for patients depends on the location of the infection. Systemic symptoms include fever, chills, pain, and loss of appetite. Symptoms and signs specific to the deep cervical spaces are listed in ▶ Table 15.1. When these patients are interviewed, it is important to obtain an accurate history of any recent infections, surgeries, dental care, or traumatic events. It is also important to gather a past medical history and social history, especially those pertaining to the immune status of the patient, such as HIV disease, diabetes, and IV drug use.

15.4.2 Physical Findings

A comprehensive head and neck examination should be performed. Special attention should be paid to any areas with edema, tenderness, and limitation of muscular or neural functions, which will help determine the deep neck space involved. Routine examination of the dentition will shed light on possible sources of infection in quite a number of cases. Trismus is a common finding in many of these deep neck space infections. Dyspnea is typically a significant finding, and the stability of the airway should be ensured before the patient is sent for any testing. Localized, tense swelling of the neck can help indicate the origin and location of a deep neck infection.

15.4.3 Testing

Diagnosing deep neck space infections may be obvious or require various imaging modalities. Maintaining a high index of suspicion is important. The patient should initially have a complete blood cell count, basic metabolic panel, coagulation profile, and blood and abscess cultures. When accessible, a fine needle aspiration can be performed at the bedside to obtain such a culture.

Imaging is usually performed in these patients to either localize or determine the presence of an abscess. Several studies have looked at the efficacy of different imaging modalities for this purpose. The original imaging modality because of its ease of use and low expense is the lateral neck X-ray. It is frequently used in retropharyngeal abscess. The results can be affected by head positioning, but the standard measurements for retropharyngeal soft-tissue thickness are 7 mm at C2 and 14 mm in children and 22 mm in adults at C6. A Panorex image can be

Table 15.1 Signs and symptoms of deep neck space infections

Space	Presenting symptoms	Clinical findings
Buccal	Cheek swelling, trismus	Gingival and/or buccal erythema and edema, facial edema and thickening of cheek, posterior teeth tenderness (usually the third molar)
Submandibular/sublingual	Submandibular/submental pain, oral dysphagia, odynophagia	Bulging of floor of mouth, restriction of tongue movement, submandibular/submental edema
Masticator	Trismus, cheek swelling, cheek pain, toothaches	External or internal cheek enlargement, trismus, posterior teeth tenderness (usually the third molar)
Parotid	Trismus, parotid pain	Swelling at angle of jaw, Stensen duct papillae, edema with or without pus drainage, trismus
Peritonsillar	Trismus, "hot potato" voice, dysphagia, drooling	Uvula deviation, soft palate swelling, tonsil displacement
Parapharyngeal	Prestyloid: trismus Poststyloid: neural compressive symptoms of cranial nerves IX, X, and XI and sympathetic chain	Prestyloid: swelling of angle of mandible, lateral displacement of pharyngeal wall and tonsil Poststyloid: swelling of posterior pharyngeal wall, cranial nerve and sympathetic chain deficits
Visceral	Dyspnea, dysphagia, hoarseness	Swelling and erythema of hypopharynx, subcutaneous emphysema, airway compromise
Carotid	Tenderness deep to sternocleidomastoid, torticollis to the opposite side, septicemia	Cyclic spiking fevers, septic hypotension and organ failure, neural deficits (cranial nerve X), carotid blowout
Retropharyngeal/danger	Dyspnea, dysphagia, odynophagia, neck pain and stiffness	Bulging of posterior pharyngeal wall, asymmetric enlargement of the neck masses, stridor
Prevertebral	Similar to those of retropharyngeal/danger space	Torticollis, decreased range of motion of the neck, neural involvement from compression of the cervical nerves

valuable in abscesses of dental origin. Proper dental evaluation and treatment can be promptly initiated.

Further testing is performed with computed tomography (CT) with IV contrast and magnetic resonance imaging. CT is by far the more commonly performed procedure given that it is rapid, widely available, and relatively inexpensive. An area of low density with a ring of enhancement on a contrast CT scan is diagnostic of abscess. Knowing the location, size, and relationship of the infection to surrounding structures is invaluable in the treatment of the disease. The extent of deep neck space infections may be underestimated in 70% of patients by physical examination, underscoring the importance of CT in aiding the evaluation of these patients.

15.5 Treatment

15.5.1 Initial Treatment

The patient's breathing should be assessed immediately; after the airway is secured, the circulation is assessed with blood pressure and physical signs of dehydration. Because of the incidence of dysphagia and sepsis, the patient may present with hypovolemia and shock. IV fluids are required for volume expansion. Occasionally, pressors may be necessary. Any metabolic derangement is corrected at the same time.

The initial treatment of deep neck space infections is the same for all patients, which is establishment a patent airway. Many of these patients can present with stridor due to soft-tissue swelling around the airway. This is further exacerbated by the frequent presence of trismus. Patients may require orotracheal or nasotracheal intubation; tracheotomy should be performed expeditiously if oral or nasal intubation cannot be performed. When dealing with a retropharyngeal abscess, the clinician must take special care to avoid rupturing the abscess during intubation. A Trendelenburg position may prevent aspiration.

15.5.2 Secondary Treatment

Once the patient is stabilized, attention is turned to treating the infection. In principle, cellulitis is managed with antibiotics, but abscesses require drainage combined with antibiotics. Sometimes, patients with a small abscess are given time to respond to IV antibiotics before surgery is pursued. In selected pediatric patients with retropharyngeal and parapharyngeal abscesses, antibiotics alone can achieve clinical resolution in many cases.

Conservative treatment with antibiotics is geared toward empiric coverage with antibiotics having broad-spectrum activity and β-lactamase resistance until cultures determine the causative organisms. The most common empiric antibiotics are clindamycin, ampicillin/sulbactam, cefuroxime, amoxicillin/clavulanate, metronidazole, and penicillin. These are used alone or in combination to cover the most common causative organisms. When a clinical response is observed, the parenteral antibiotics are usually continued for 48 hours before oral antibiotics are given.

If conservative antibiotic treatment fails, surgical drainage becomes necessary. Surgery usually requires incision and drainage followed by copious irrigation and placement of a drain.

Abscess cultures must be obtained to direct postoperative antibiotic therapy.

The surgical approach is different depending on the location of the abscess. However, the general surgical principle of an adequate exposure is key to evacuating an abscess without compromising the surrounding vital structures.

Buccal and peritonsillar infections can be accessed and drained through the oral cavity and allowed to drain freely. Buccal space abscesses can be drained through a mucosal incision above the Stenson duct, followed by blunt dissection of the buccinator muscle fibers and penetration of the buccopharyngeal membrane. Peritonsillar abscesses can be drained by incising the soft palate just above the superior tonsillar pole and bluntly dissecting the space above the tonsil with a fine curved clamp. Alternatively, peritonsillar abscesses can be aspirated with a 21-gauge needle. Care must be taken to avoid deep needle insertion into the peritonsillar space because of the proximity of the internal carotid artery. Parapharyngeal space abscesses are approached through a transcervical incision to allow identification and protection of the neurovascular structures. Submandibular/sublingual abscesses can be approached and drained through the oral cavity or an external incision. This is usually determined by the location of the abscess relative to the mylohyoid; abscesses superior to the mylohyoid can be drained through the oral cavity, whereas those inferior and posterior are drained through an external incision.

Retropharyngeal, danger, and prevertebral space abscesses can be drained through either an external or internal approach. This is determined by the extent of the infection. Localized infection can be drained intraorally with the patient intubated and in a Trendelenburg position. When the infection is large and life-threatening, a transverse cervical approach is used.

Treating immunocompromised patients with deep neck space infections requires a heightened suspicion for the involvement of atypical agents. *Pseudomonas*, methicillin-resistant *Staphylococcus aureus*, and fungal and mycobacterial agents must be included in the differential of offending organisms. Mycobacterial tuberculosis should be treated medically, not surgically, because of the increased risk for draining fistula after open surgical treatment.

15.5.3 Postoperative Care

Postoperatively, antibiotics are adjusted according to the culture results. Patients typically improve expeditiously, and surgical drains can be slowly advanced and removed as each patient's progress allows. Large abscess cavities sometimes require irrigation with saline. Lack of a response to the therapy should prompt a close examination for the persistence or reaccumulation of an abscess. Repeat imaging and drainage should be attempted.

15.5.4 Complications

Even after surgery, the airway should be closely monitored, as extrinsic compression and tissue edema take time to resolve. An endotracheal or tracheotomy tube is maintained until after a patent airway is confirmed with endoscopy. The aspiration of purulent fluid may have occurred before or during surgery, which can lead to pneumonia. Mediastinal extension with the development of mediastinitis is often preceded by unexplained tachycardia and fever. Chest X-ray shows a characteristic mediastinal widening. A thoracic surgery consultation should be sought promptly for possible drainage.

Other complications include internal jugular vein thrombosis with septic emboli, carotid rupture, and neurologic deficits of the involved cranial nerves and sympathetic chain. Necrotizing cervical fasciitis has a high morbidity and mortality rate due to a rapid, aggressive invasion of fascia and tissue with ensuing necrosis. Surgical débridement, parenteral antibiotics, and hyperbaric oxygen are usually indicated.

15.6 Roundsmanship

- In treating patients with deep neck space infections, airway control is the most important initial treatment decision.
- CT scan is the best imaging modality due to its cost, ease of access and diagnostic purposes.

- Treatment of deep neck space infections includes a combination of appropriate antibiotic and drainage.
- Antibiotics should be started empirically and specified to cultured bacteria, which is usually polymicrobial.

15.7 Recommended Reading

[1] Johnson J. Deep neck abscesses. In: Myers EN, ed. Operative Orolaryngology: Head and Neck Surgery. 2nd ed. Philadelphia, PA: Saunders Elsevier; 2008;671–678

[2] McClay JE, Murray AD, Booth T. Intravenous antibiotic therapy for deep neck abscesses defined by computed tomography. Arch Otolaryngol Head Neck Surg 2003; 129: 1207–1212

[3] Parhiscar A, Har-El G. Deep neck abscess: a retrospective review of 210 cases. Ann Otol Rhinol Laryngol 2001; 110: 1051–1054

[4] Daramola OO, Flanagan CE, Maisel RH, Odland RM. Diagnosis and treatment of deep neck space abscesses. Otolaryngol Head Neck Surg 2009; 141: 123–130

16 Evaluation and Management of Hearing Loss in Adults

Tina Qingxin He

Hearing loss affects approximately 28 million Americans. The prevalence increases with age, and it is estimated that a third of people age 65 and older have a significant hearing loss. Hearing loss can cause a major problem with communication, thereby affecting education, employment, and relationships.

16.1 Classification of Hearing Loss

Hearing loss is generally divided into three broad categories: conductive hearing loss (CHL), sensorineural hearing loss (SNHL), and mixed hearing loss. CHL is caused by an obstruction in the transmission of sound as the sound waves pass from the air through the auricle into the inner ear (▸ Fig. 16.1). The most common etiologies of CHL are cerumen impaction and middle ear infections. Conditions that alter ossicular stiffness, such as otosclerosis, produce predominantly low-frequency hearing loss, whereas changes in the mass of middle ear structures classically produce high-frequency deficit.

16.1.1 Selected Etiologies of Conductive Hearing Loss

- Congenital anomalies of the external and middle ear may be hereditary or sporadic in presentation and either syndromic or nonsyndromic. Patients usually present with a history of hearing loss since birth. Examples include aural atresia, microtia, and ossicular malformation.
- Foreign bodies of the external auditory canal and cerumen are common presentations of CHL. These can be easily removed if the patient is cooperative, the foreign body is small, and adequate tools are available. A microscope should be used

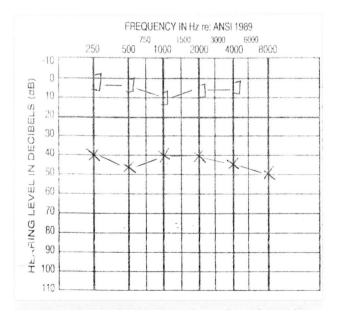

Fig. 16.1 Audiogram of mild conductive hearing loss with an air–bone gap. *ANSI*, American National Standards Institute.

when possible to prevent injury to the external auditory canal and tympanic membrane. In an uncooperative patient with a large occluding foreign body, removal of the foreign body under anesthesia may be the safest treatment.

- Inflammatory/infectious processes are one of the most common causes of CHL.
  - Otitis externa, either acute or chronic, is one of the most common problems causing CHL. Acute otitis externa can be caused by bacterial, viral, or fungal infections. The most common pathogens in acute otitis externa include *Pseudomonas aeruginosa*, *Staphylococcus*, and *Proteus*. Cleaning of the external auditory canal under the microscope and treatment with appropriate medication are usually all that is required. In cases of severe acute otitis externa in which the canal is extremely edematous, an ear wick is placed in the canal for several days to expand the canal and facilitate the administration of antibiotic drops deep into the canal. Necrotizing otitis externa (malignant otitis externa) is a rapidly progressive, potentially life-threatening infection involving the skin, cartilage, and bone surrounding the external auditory canal. This disease is usually found in elderly immunocompromised patients. *P. aeruginosa* is the most common causative agent. Hospitalization for the administration of intravenous antibiotics or prolonged oral antibiotics may be necessary for treatment.
  - Acute and chronic otitis media. The sequelae of chronic otitis media, including tympanic perforation, ossicular erosion, and tympanosclerosis, are major causes of hearing loss.
  - Cholesteatoma is an epidermal inclusion cyst of the middle ear and/or mastoid. It may be congenital or acquired. The cholesteatoma contains desquamated debris from keratinizing squamous epithelial lining. The expansion of a cholesteatoma can cause bone erosion of the ossicles and otic capsule.
- Trauma
  - Trauma to the auricle or external auditory canal is common. Poorly protected by surrounding structures, the external ear is vulnerable to blunt, sharp, and thermal injury. For example, athletes in sports such as boxing frequently present with auricular hematoma or laceration. Trauma can also result from frostbite or burn injuries.
  - The most common locations for traumatic tympanic membrane perforation are the anterior–inferior and posterior–inferior quadrants. Tympanic membrane perforation can be the result of a penetrating injury or blunt trauma. Whereas penetrating injury tends to present with a linear perforation, blunt trauma tends to present with a larger stellate defect.
  - Injury to the middle ear and temporal bone is much less common and requires much more intense force of trauma. The middle ear and temporal bone are protected by dense bones. Therefore, injuries to the middle ear and temporal bone rarely present in isolation; instead, temporal bone fractures are frequently the result of a motor vehicle accident, and patients may present with a constellation of injuries involving other major systems. Longitudinal temporal

bone fractures account for 70 to 90% of temporal bone fractures, are associated with bleeding from the external canal, and present with conductive hearing loss. SNHL is relatively uncommon in patients with longitudinal skull fractures. Transverse temporal bone fractures result from more severe occipital injury and present with SNHL and hemotympanum.

- Otosclerosis is a disease of the bone causing fixation of the stapes footplate in the oval window. Otosclerosis presents as progressive CHL in an otherwise normal-looking ear. It is an autosomal-dominant hereditary disease with variable penetrance and expression that affects more women than men.
- Neoplasms. Carcinomas and benign tumors of the external auditory canal and temporal bone are uncommon. Squarmous cell carcinoma is by far the most common malignant tumor of the external auditory canal, followed by basal cell carcinoma and adenoid cystic carcinoma. Carcinomas of the external auditory canal usually occur in older individuals.
- Systemic diseases
  - Wegener granulomatosis is a granulomatous disease associated with necrotizing vasculitis. It primarily affects the upper and lower respiratory tracts and kidneys. When the granulomatous process involves the eustachian tube, it will present as serous otitis media with CHL. Involvement of the inner ear will cause rapidly progressive SNHL.
  - Sarcoidosis commonly manifests with cough. Chest X-ray shows bilateral hilar adenopathy. Involvement of the temporal bone may cause facial, auditory, or vestibular nerve dysfunction.
  - Tuberculosis can rarely cause otitis media and tympanic membrane perforations. Patients who have this disease may present initially with painless multiple small perforations of the tympanic membranes that progress to form large tympanic membrane perforations. Otologic involvement occurs as a result of hematogenous or lymphatic spread to the middle ear.

SNHL is caused by problems involving sound processing after sound waves reach the inner ear (▶ Fig. 16.2). SNHL can occur at the level of the cochlea, cochlear nerve, central auditory pathways, or cerebral cortex centers. Noise exposure and presbycusis are the leading causes of SNHL.

16.1.2 Selected Etiologies of Sensorineural Hearing Loss

- Presbycusis is age-related hearing loss. This may affect more than 30% of persons older than 65 years of age. Patients commonly present with bilateral symmetric high-frequency SNHL and poor speech discrimination.
- Hereditary disorders. These can be divided into syndromic and nonsyndromic forms of hereditary hearing loss. An estimated 70 to 80% of cases of hereditary hearing loss are nonsyndromic. Although most cases of hereditary hearing loss present at birth, some persons inherit a tendency to develop hearing loss later in life. Some examples of syndromes associated with hereditary hearing loss include Waardenburg syndrome, Alport syndrome, and Usher syndrome.

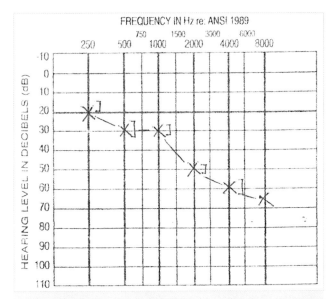

Fig. 16.2 Audiogram of sensorineural hearing loss in the left ear. *ANSI*, American National Standards Institute.

- Inner ear and temporal bone anomalies. Inner ear anomalies are classified as either membranous or combined membranous and osseous. These anomalies usually present as profound SNHL in children. In the case of large vestibular aqueduct syndrome, the SNHL can present in adulthood as progressive deterioration with a propensity for the sudden development of SNHL after head trauma.
- Infectious disorders
  - Labyrinthitis
    - Herpes zoster oticus or Ramsay Hunt syndrome is caused by reactivation of the varicella-zoster virus during a period of immunosuppression many years after the primary infection, which manifests as chickenpox. The cause appears to be a recrudescence of a latent varicella-zoster virus infection of the geniculate ganglion. The initial presentation includes painful vesicles on the pinna or along the external auditory canal. This is followed by facial paralysis in a couple of days. Auditory and vestibular symptoms develop in approximately 25% of these patients. The diagnostic work-up should include a Tzanck smear.
    - Serous and bacterial suppurative labyrinthitis generally presents with sudden severe SNHL and acute vertigo. The hearing loss is usually permanent, but the vertigo may improve with treatment.
  - Chronic otitis media and cholesteatoma. Paparella et al showed that in patients with chronic otitis media, permanent SNHL may result from the passage of toxic substances through the round window. When a large cholesteatoma expands to the otic capsule, it may result in SNHL, presumably secondary to suppurative labyrinthitis.
  - Syphilis can be classified as congenital or acquired. In congenital syphilis, hearing loss occurs in approximately one-third of patients. In acquired syphilis, the middle ear may be affected in late latent and tertiary forms. The symptoms may be sudden SNHL, fluctuating hearing loss, episodic vertigo, or progressive hearing loss and tinnitus. Otosyphilis can often be associated with the Hennebert sign and the

Tullio sign. The Hennebert sign is a positive fistula test in the absence of middle ear disease. The Tullio sign is vertigo and nystagmus elicited with exposure to a loud sound. A definitive diagnosis of syphilis requires a positive finding of *Treponema pallidum* on serology.

○ Lyme disease. *Borrelia burgdorferi* is the offending organism in Lyme disease. Facial nerve paralysis is the most common otologic manifestation. Auditory and vestibular manifestations such as SNHL, sudden hearing loss, and positional vertigo are less common.

○ Meningitis. This is a known etiology of acquired severe-to-profound SNHL.

- Pharmacologic toxicity
  ○ Aminoglycosides appear to affect the function of hair cells, some causing eventual cell death.
  ○ Loop diuretics alter metabolism in the stria vascularis. Hearing loss due to loop diuretics may be reversible.
  ○ Salicylates and aspirin may cause reversible SNHL. On discontinuation of the medication, hearing returns to normal within 72 hours. Ototoxicity due to nonsteroidal anti-inflammatory drugs is rare.

- Meniere disease is of unknown etiology. It results in endolymphatic hydrops and presents with episodic low-frequency SNHL, aural fullness, vertigo, and tinnitus. The hallmark of this disease is its variability and unpredictability. It is bilateral in 30 to 50% of cases.

- Systemic disease
  ○ Paget disease of bone is of unknown etiology. New bone formation or remodeling of temporal bone can cause hearing loss, tinnitus, and mild vestibular dysfunction.
  ○ Multiple sclerosis. Between 4 and 10% of patients with multiple sclerosis develop SNLH.
  ○ Wegener granulomatosis. When Wegener granulomatosis involves the ear, it usually causes CHL. Rarely, this disease involves the inner ear to cause SNHL.

- Neoplasm
  ○ Acoustic neuroma. This is a benign vestibular schwannoma that may account for 10% of patients who present with sudden SNHL.

- Trauma
  ○ Noise trauma is one of the most common adult hearing problems encountered. It is also one of the more easily preventable causes of SNHL. An estimated 10 million Americans have noise-induced hearing loss. The primary sites of damage are the inner hair cells and outer hair cells of the organ of Corti, with the outer hair cells most affected in the initial stages of hearing loss.
  ○ Labyrinthine injury can result from severe trauma to the head. Longitudinal temporal bone fractures mostly present with CHL but can also present with high-frequency SNHL. Transverse temporal bone fractures, however, almost always result in a complete loss of auditory and vestibular function.
  ○ Acquired perilymphatic fistula can result from barotrauma or as a complication of ear surgery. The fistula can occur at either the round or oval window. When barotrauma is the inciting etiology, the presenting history is acute hearing loss immediately following heavy lifting, straining, flying, or underwater diving. The fistula test may yield a positive Hennebert sign.

- Vascular disorders

○ Migraine. This is a common disorder that usually presents with headaches and an associated visual aura. Of patients with basilar migraine, 30 to 45% have been found to have low-frequency SNHL.

Mixed hearing loss is a combination of CHL and SNHL. It is often caused by a combination of the above etiologies.

16.2 Evaluation of Hearing Loss

When a new patient with hearing loss is evaluated, it is important to obtain a thorough history and physical examination before moving on to the audiogram.

16.2.1 History

Questions that should be asked in the work-up of hearing loss:
1. Age at onset.
2. Circumstances surrounding onset.
3. Unilateral or bilateral hearing loss.
4. Severity and speed of progression.
5. Duration of complaint; patients with sudden SNHL require a stat audiogram and need to be treated immediately.
6. Associating symptoms: tinnitus, vertigo, aural fullness, pain, otorrhea, or autophony.
7. Other ear-related history, including noise exposure, previous ear infections, and ear surgeries.
8. Personal and medical history, current medications, surgical history, social history, past head trauma, and exposure to ototoxic agents.
9. Family history of hearing loss.

16.2.2 Physical Examination

In addition to a complete head and neck examination, a thorough evaluation of the external and middle ear is essential. Keep in mind that patients with SNHL often have completely normal examinations. The removal of any obstructing foreign body or cerumen is absolutely essential. Many beginners make the mistake of looking for the light reflex only on the tympanic membrane. Make sure that the entire tympanic membrane is visualized. Some diseases can involve only a small portion of the tympanic membrane. For example, a middle ear cholesteatoma can manifest as a flattened crust on the posterior–inferior quadrant of the tympanic membrane. The mobility of the tympanic membrane is then checked with a pneumatic otoscope to determine the presence of retraction or fluid in the middle ear. In addition, an operating microscope can be useful for the removal of foreign bodies and for more detailed examination of the middle ear.

The Weber and Rinne tests can be performed to identify the side of hearing loss and to confirm the audiometric results. The Weber test is done by placing a vibrating tuning fork in the mid portion of the forehead and asking the patient which side he or she can hear more clearly. A normal Weber response occurs when the sound is heard equally in both ears or across the forehead. If the sound seems louder in one ear, this can indicate CHL in the ear with the louder response or SNHL in the contralateral ear. The Rinne test response is normal when the air conduction sounds louder than the bone conduction. The 512- and 1,024-Hz tuning forks are typically used for this purpose. A patient who has a recent history of acute pressure changes, such as a scuba diver, would benefit from a fistula test.

16.2.3 Audiometry

Audiometric testing is essential to verify and quantify the degree of hearing loss. Air conduction, bone conduction, speech audiometry, and tympanometry are the basic tests included in the audiogram. Speech audiometry, in addition to determining the nature of the SNHL, can provide prognostic information regarding the potential benefits of amplification. Tympanometry is essential for verifying any CHL and can confirm a retracted, stiff, or perforated tympanic membrane. Acoustic reflex testing can provide additional clues to the etiology of hearing loss. Auditory brainstem response (ABR) is useful for evaluating a retrocochlear etiology or for evaluating adult patients who are unable to respond to a normal audiogram. In offices where an audiologist is not readily available, therefore, the audiogram is ordered for a future date unless a sudden SNHL is suspected; in this case, the audiogram needs to be performed immediately so that the patient can be treated as soon as possible.

16.2.4 Laboratory Testing

For CHL, blood work is usually unnecessary; however, in unilateral or sudden SNHL, this can help determine the etiology in certain cases. The most useful test is the fluorescent treponemal antibody absorption (FTA-ABS) test.

16.2.5 Radiographic Testing

Most patients with CHL do not require radiographic examinations. Noncontrast computed tomography (CT) of the temporal bone can be used to visualize the middle ear and the mastoid. This can be useful for complicated middle ear pathology or persistent CHL despite treatment. On the other hand, CT is less useful in an adult with SNHL unless the hearing loss is congenital or secondary to recent trauma. Magnetic resonance imaging with gadolinium is used in patients with asymmetric or sudden SNHL to evaluate for a cerebral or retrocochlear cause of the hearing loss.

16.3 Treatment of Hearing Loss

16.3.1 Conductive Hearing Loss

Treatment of the underlying etiology is necessary to improve hearing loss. Some conditions are very easy to treat, such as cerumen impaction, acute ear infection, and foreign body, but others are much harder to correct. For conditions such as chronic serous otitis media, otosclerosis, tympanosclerosis, tympanic membrane perforation, canal stenosis, and ossicular chain abnormality, surgical intervention can be very beneficial. When surgery is discussed, the alternative of amplification with hearing aids must be presented. Patients with CHL have high speech discrimination scores and will experience significant improvement with hearing aids without the risks of surgery.

16.3.2 Sensorineural Hearing Loss

Most cases of SNHL are not reversible. The primary exception is sudden SNHL. This is defined as unilateral hearing loss not attributable to known causes that occurs in less than 3 days. Two-thirds of the patients recover to nearly normal hearing levels spontaneously and many improve with high-dose systemic corticosteroid treatment. Otherwise, treatment options for SNHL are limited. Even when the etiology of the hearing loss is corrected, the damage to the cochlea and auditory pathway is often permanent.

There are measures to mitigate the effects of SNHL on a patient's quality of life. Amplification devices such as hearing aids and assistive listening devices for telephones and televisions are a few examples. A hearing aid may be beneficial for patients with SNHL. When hearing aids are recommended, patient motivation and the perceived degree of handicap must be considered. Hearing aids have many limitations. Poor sound quality, discomfort, and the frequent need for battery change and cleaning are just a few of the common complaints. Many patients choose not to wear amplification simply because the social stigma of having a hearing aid. Many patients with SNHL have poor speech discrimination scores. Because hearing aids do not significantly improve speech discrimination, they often derive limited benefit. For patients with unserviceable hearing even with hearing aids, cochlear implantation should be considered.

16.4 Roundsmanship

- Conductive hearing loss is caused by an obstruction in the transmission of sound as the sound waves pass from the air through the auricle into the inner ear. Sensorineural hearing loss is caused by problems involving sound processing after the sound waves reach the inner ear. Mixed hearing loss is a combination of conductive and sensorineural hearing loss.
- Patients with hearing loss should be questioned about the timing and circumstances surrounding the onset of hearing loss, as well its progression and any associated symptoms of tinnitus, vertigo, aural fullness, otalgia, otorrhea, and autophony.
- The recent onset of sudden sensorineural hearing loss necessitates an audiogram as soon as possible.

16.5 Recommended Reading

[1] Chole RA, Cook GB. The Rinne test for conductive deafness. A critical reappraisal. Arch Otolaryngol Head Neck Surg 1988; 114: 399–403

[2] Kristensen S, Juul A, Gammelgaard NP, Rasmussen OR. Traumatic tympanic membrane perforations: complications and management. Ear Nose Throat J 1989; 68: 503–516

[3] National Institutes of Health, National Institute on Deafness and Other Communication Disorders (NIDCD). The NINCD Strategic Plan 2012–2016. www.nidcd.nih.gov/about/plans/strategic/Pages/Default.aspx. Accessed October 13, 2013

[4] Paparella MM, Brady DR, Hoel R. Sensori-neural hearing loss in chronic otitis media and mastoiditis. Trans Am Acad Ophthalmol Otolaryngol 1970; 74: 108–115

[5] Shuknecht JF. Pathology of the Ear. Cambridge, MA: Harvard University Press; 1974

17 Evaluation and Management of Otalgia

Michele M. Gandolfi and Christopher J. Linstrom

17.1 Introduction

Ear pain, or otalgia, reflects either localized otologic pathology (primary otalgia) or a problem within a periauricular or more distant source (referred otalgia) due to the complex sensory innervation of the ear. The physical examination usually reveals the source of the pain. Not uncommonly, however, a patient may have ear pain but no identifiable pathology within the ear, and the clinician should expand the differential diagnosis to include causes of referred otalgia. The source of otalgia can be as proximal and obvious as an acute otitis externa or as distant and occult as a laryngeal mass. The evaluation of patients with otalgia is aided by a detailed understanding of the innervation of the ear and knowledge of potential causes. Comprehension of the anatomy underlying shared neural pathways and the potential causes of referred otalgia arising from distant sites enables the physician to reach a diagnosis.

Sensory afferents from the trigeminal, facial, glossopharyngeal, and vagus nerves and the cervical plexus supply the auricle, periauricular region, external canal, and middle ear. All of these afferents can cause localized ear pain that is misleading; these nerves innervate distant sites that can harbor the culpable pathology. For example, the auriculotemporal branch of the mandibular division of the trigeminal nerve provides sensation to the tragus, anterior pinna, anterior lateral surface of the tympanic membrane, and anterosuperior external auditory canal. The vagus nerve similarly provides sensation to the larynx, hypopharynx, trachea, esophagus, and thyroid gland. The Arnold nerve (auricular branch of the vagus nerve) provides sensation to the concha, inferoposterior external auditory canal, tympanic membrane, and postauricular skin. Sensory innervation to the oropharynx, tonsils, and tongue base is provided by the glossopharyngeal nerve. The Jacobson nerve (tympanic branch of the glossopharyngeal nerve) provides sensation to the medial surface of the tympanic membrane, mucosa of the middle ear, eustachian tube, and mastoid air cells. The cervical roots C2 and C3 provide sensation to the postauricular region via the great auricular nerve. The facial nerve innervates the skin of the lateral concha and antihelix, lobule, mastoid, posterior external auditory canal, and posterior portion of the tympanic membrane. Pathology related to the distribution of these nerves can refer pain back to their afferent destination of innervation, leading to referred otalgia (▶ Fig. 17.1).

17.2 Differential Diagnosis

Otalgia can be separated into two types: primary and referred. Primary otalgia arises from local or regional pathology. The ear itself is the source of the pathology. Sources of primary otalgia include acute otitis externa, cerumen impaction, foreign body, inflammation or infection of the auricle, ear trauma, eustachian tube dysfunction, otitis media, and mastoiditis. Otalgia may be referred to the ear from pathology in an adjacent area, such as temporomandibular joint dysfunction, periauricular lymphadenopathy, and scalp or neck infections. Even more distant

sources should be suspected in cases of referred otalgia, such as periodontal or dental disease, parotitis, sinusitis, thyroiditis, tonsillitis, laryngitis, and hiatal hernia with gastroesophageal reflux. Referred pain is a manifestation of pathology in any region of the head and neck that shares a neural pathway with the temporal bone and periauricular region. In the initial assessment, examination of the ear indicates whether the otalgia is local or regional in origin. If the ear examination is completely normal, it is helpful to discern the exact focus of pain and redirect the physical examination to other areas that share neural pathways with the ear.

Referred otalgia is related to the wide distribution of the nerves that innervate the auricular area. The trigeminal nerve has a wide sensory distribution. Infection and neoplasms within the nasal cavity or paranasal sinuses, particularly the sphenoid or maxillary sinuses, can cause irritation of the vidian nerve. Nasopharyngeal surgery, neoplasms, and infections in this region are common sources of referred otalgia. In children, erupting dentition is the most common cause of referred ear pain. Similarly, an impacted molar in an adult may cause symptoms of ear pain. Dental malocclusion resulting in temporomandibular joint dysfunction can cause referred ear pain from masticator muscle spasms. A history of excessive gum chewing, malocclusion, and bruxism may suggest this diagnosis.

The facial nerve can be involved in referred ear pain in cases of geniculate neuralgia, Bell palsy, and herpes zoster oticus. The ear pain of herpes zoster oticus can occur even in the absence of a significant vesicular eruption, making the diagnosis even more difficult. The otalgia associated with Bell palsy frequently occurs before the onset of facial paralysis. The glossopharyngeal and vagus nerves can transmit referred ear pain as a result of pathology originating from anywhere within the upper aerodigestive tract. The glossopharyngeal nerve can be stimulated by pathology in the pharynx, such as tonsillitis, post-tonsillectomy inflammation, peri-tonsillar abscess, and neoplasms. Lingual tonsillitis and impacted foreign bodies within the tongue can also cause otalgia. Eagle syndrome (▶ Fig. 17.2) consists of ear pain secondary to stretching and irritation of the glossopharyngeal nerve resulting from elongation of the styloid process. Glossopharyngeal neuralgia is similar to trigeminal neuralgia. The pain is sharp and lancinating in quality; it originates in the tongue base, soft palate, or tonsillar fossa and radiates to the ear. Neoplasms within the larynx and esophagus have long been recognized as causes of referred otalgia. Ulcerations, foreign bodies, and reflux also can be seen in a similar manner. Chronic or subacute inflammation of the thyroid gland may cause referred ear pain through stimulation of the vagus nerve.

17.3 Evaluation: History, Physical Findings, and Testing

In order to define the specific etiology of otalgia, a thorough history is necessary, with detailed attention to the onset and duration of pain, quality of the ear pain, alleviating and exacerbating factors, and associated symptoms, such as fever, weight

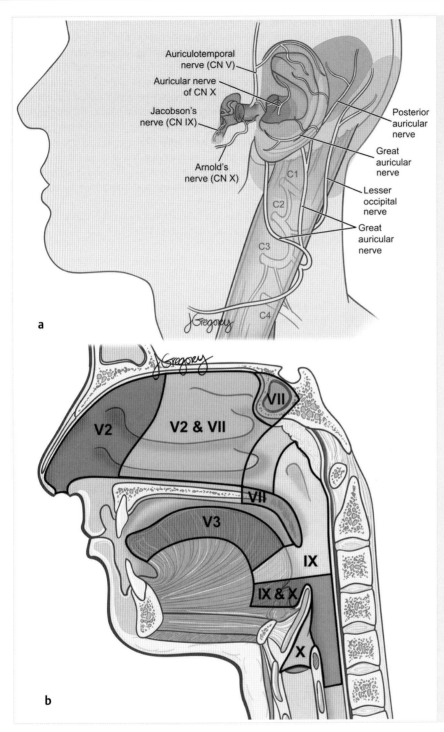

Fig. 17.1 Sources of referred otalgia. (a) The sensory innervation of the ear and periauricular area is from multiple nerves, including branches from cranial nerves V, VII, IX, and X, as well as C2 and C3 rootlets. (b) Multiple areas in the head and neck share sensory innervation with the ear. *CN*, cranial nerve.

loss, tinnitus, hearing loss, pruritus, vertigo, aural fullness, and other sources of pain. A careful initial examination of ear and pneumatic otoscopy (to test the movement of the tympanic membrane and see if this illicit any new symptoms) can help distinguish sources of referred pain. Fiber-optic nasopharyngolaryngoscopy should be performed to evaluate the pharynx and larynx if laryngitis, gastroesophageal reflux, or a mass is suspected because of associated symptoms. In patients with a significant history of tobacco and/or alcohol use, a mass in the oral cavity or laryngopharynx should be sought. Adults with a unilateral middle ear effusion detected on otoscopy should be presumed to have a nasopharyngeal mass until it has been proved otherwise by fiber-optic nasopharyngoscopy. A complete inspection of the nasopharynx, oral cavity, mandible, pharynx, larynx, and neck should be completed to find the source of otalgia.

If mastoiditis is suspected, computed tomography (CT) of the temporal bone without contrast is necessary to evaluate the extent of disease. If there is any suspicion of coalescent mastoiditis, a CT with contrast should be ordered. Audiography and

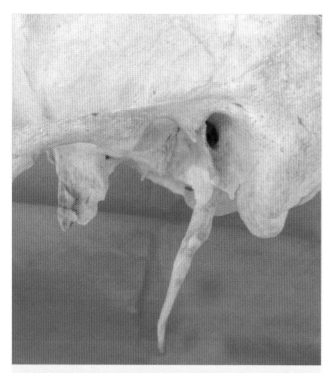

Fig. 17.2 Eagle syndrome from elongation of the styloid process or elongation of stylohyoid ligament.

electronystagmography/videonystagmography (ENG/VNG) should be ordered to evaluate the cause of otalgia if symptoms of hearing loss, tinnitus, or vertigo are also present. Magnetic resonance (MR) imaging or CT with contrast of the area involved should be ordered if any local head and neck masses are detected on examination.

17.4 Treatment

Infections such as acute otitis media, pharyngitis, and tonsillitis can be treated with broad-spectrum antibiotics such as amoxicillin, amoxicillin/clavulanate, or in the penicillin-allergic patient clindamycin to cover the more common head and neck pathogens, such as *Streptococcus pneumoniae*, *Haemophilus influenzae*, and *Moraxella catarrhalis*. If referred pain from a local site is suspected, treatment should be focused on the source. A patient with external tenderness over the temporomandibular joint, malocclusion, clicking, and teeth grinding should be referred to a dentist or oral surgeon who treats temporomandibular joint disease. In patients in whom an X-ray reveals an elongated styloid process, surgical shortening of the process can help relieve symptoms if other sources are ruled out. If nasal congestion or sinusitis is the cause of otalgia, treatment with antibiotics and nasal decongestants can help alleviate the symptoms. A unilateral peri-tonsillar abscess can also cause otalgia (although otalgia is not the most significant symptom in these cases). The peri-tonsillar abscess should be drained and the appropriate antibiotics should be given based on cultures and a steroid taper prescribed if there are no contraindications (immunocompromised, pregnancy etc.). Parotiditis can also cause otalgia, and the local infection should be treated with antibiotics, sialagogues, and massage. If a mass is found as a potential source, biopsy of the mass must be done; appropriate management and subspecialist referral should be based on the pathology results.

Otalgia is a vague symptom that can be the result of an extremely wide array of pathology. The physician must use the details of the patient's history and associated symptoms, as well as the physical examination findings, to tease out possible etiologies. In order to do so, a thorough knowledge of the innervation pathways that provide sensation to the ear is necessary. Localizing the pathology to a nearby anatomical structure is important for the treatment and resolution of referred otalgia. Diagnostic work-up and testing can help the physician discern whether audiography, electronystagmography, videonystagmography, CT, MR imaging, X-ray, fiber-optic nasolaryngoscopy, or other further studies are necessary.

17.5 Roundsmanship

- There are two types of otalgia. In primary otalgia, the ear is the direct source of pain, whereas in referred otalgia, the complex afferent innervations of the ear are the source.
- Intricate knowledge of the afferent innervation of the ear is necessary to discover the source of referred otalgia. Any location that shares innervation with the ear through branches of the trigeminal, facial, glossopharyngeal, or vagus nerve can be the source.
- Ear infections, sinusitis, tonsillitis, temporomandicular joint disorder, odontogenic sources, Bell palsy, nasopharyngeal mass, neck mass, or even thyroiditis can cause otalgia. A detailed documentation of associated symptoms is important to diagnose the cause of otalgia.
- A detailed history and physical examination with focused testing are helpful in determining the etiology of otalgia.

17.6 Recommended Reading

[1] Janfaza P, Nadol JB, Galla R. Surgical Anatomy of the Head and Neck. Cambridge, MA: Harvard University Press; 2011

[2] Myers EN. Operative Otolaryngology: Head and Neck Surgery. 2nd ed. Philadelphia, PA: Saunders Elsevier; 2008

18 Obstructive Sleep Apnea

Gene Ukrainsky and Boris Sagalovich

18.1 Introduction

Sleep is an essential part of our normal physiology. Profound changes occur during sleep, all of them part of the body's normal physiology. Although the exact nature and reason for sleep are not known, interruption of the physiologic processes and normally occurring sequences in sleep leads to a variety of pathologic conditions.

18.2 Incidence of Disease

Obstructive sleep-disordered breathing is probably one of the most common sleep-related disorders and includes obstructive sleep apnea (OSA). OSA is defined by the presence of the polysomnographic findings of upper airway obstruction and OSA syndrome, which is a combination of OSA, defined as presence of more than 5 upper ventilatory events per hour, and clinical symptoms.

In one of the most comprehensive studies undertaken, 24% of men and 9% of women had sleep-disordered breathing, defined as an apnea–hypopnia index (AHI) of 5 or higher. The prevalence of obstructive sleep-disordered breathing increases with age. Sleep apnea is characterized by partial or complete obstruction of the upper airway leading to episodic hypoxia, hypercapnia, and ultimately arousal with increased ventilatory effort. The arousals lead to sleep fragmentation and disruption of the normal sleep architecture. It is this disruption in the sleep architecture, as well as the tissue vibration and abnormal cardiovascular response during the hypoxic episodes, which explains patients' symptoms as well as the pathologic consequences of obstructive sleep-disordered breathing.

18.3 Terminology

Apnea is the cessation of airflow lasting 10 seconds or longer.

Hypopnia is a decline of at least 50% in airflow from baseline, associated with an electroencephalogram (EEG)-defined arousal or with a 4% drop in oxygen saturation.

A respiratory effort–related arousal is an arousal caused by an obstructive respiratory event.

The apnea–hypopnea index (AHI) is the sum of the number of apneic and hypopneic episodes per hour.

The respiratory disturbance index (RDI) may be synonymous with the AHI or may be a combination of the AHI and respiratory effort–related arousal.

18.4 Pathophysiology

Sleep is a reversible state of disengagement and unresponsiveness to the surrounding environment. It is subdivided into non–rapid eye movement (NREM) sleep and rapid eye movement (REM) sleep. NREM sleep is further subdivided into three stages that parallel the depth of the sleep continuum. NREM

sleep can be thought of as a period with relatively diminished brain activity, as demonstrated by brain waves registered on the EEG. REM sleep, by contrast, is characterized by EEG activation, muscle inactivity, and episodic bursts of rapid eye movements. It is not surprising, then, that most apneic episodes in adults occur during this stage of sleep, during which relative muscle atonia predominates. Abnormal upper airway structure is mostly responsible for obstructive sleep-disordered breathing. In children, this abnormality is most often caused by adenotonsillar hypertrophy. In adults, multiple anatomical and physiologic abnormalities along the upper airway can contribute to obstructive sleep-disordered breathing. It is useful to think of the upper airway as a series of conduits with both static and dynamic components. The dynamic components of upper airway collapse are tissue mass, tissue elasticity, and neuromuscular tone and airflow influencing airway diameter. The static determinants of airway size are the fixed skeletal and soft-tissue configuration of the nasal cavity, nasopharynx, oropharynx, and hypopharynx. Dilating forces reduce the potential for airway collapse as a result of increased negative inspiratory pressures. Hence, any decrease in neuromuscular tone increases the chance of airway collapse. Obesity (because of the increased fat deposition around the neck), upper airway soft-tissue hypertrophy (seen in adenotonsillar hypertrophy), and retrognathia increase extraluminal pressure and make upper airway collapse more likely.

Fujuita classified the patterns of obstruction according to anatomical location (▶ Table 18.1).

Nasal obstruction contributes to upper airway obstruction; however, it is not a sole cause but rather a contributor to OSA. Nasal obstruction contributes to increased upper airway resistance, and open-mouth breathing decreases the efficiency of the upper airway dilator muscles and promotes collapsibility of the upper airway.

18.5 Medical Evaluation

18.5.1 Presenting Complaints

Patients with OSA are rarely fully aware of the severity of their sleep-disordered breathing. Rather, a bed partner frequently insists on the evaluation. On questioning, however, patients with OSA will often have many of the symptoms listed in the Box Symptoms of Obstructive Sleep Apnea (p. 120).

Table 18.1 Fujita classification of airway obstruction

Type	Site of obstruction
I	Retropalatal area only
II	Retropalatal and retrolingual areas
III	Retrolingual area only

Symptoms of Obstructive Sleep Apnea

- Restless sleep
- Loud snoring
- Observed episodes of choking or gasping
- Excessive daytime sleepiness
- Morning fatigue
- Memory loss
- Gastroesophageal reflux disease
- Decreased libido and impotence
- Nocturnal sweating
- Depression

18.5.2 Physical Examination and Clinical Findings

The most common symptoms of OSA syndrome are fatigue and hypersomnolence. One of the most useful tools routinely used as a self-assessment for OSA is the Epworth Sleepiness Scale (▶ Table 18.2).

During the office visit of a patient with suspected OSA, it is important to measure the patient's height, weight, blood pressure, and neck circumference. More than 70% of adults with OSA are obese. Note the general body habitus and any facial characteristics, which may suggest the presence of retrognathia or maxillary hypoplasia. Keep in mind that daytime fatigue and loss of energy are the presenting symptoms of many medical conditions; these can both mimic and coexist with OSA. Patients with hypertension, cardiovascular disease, obesity, or diabetes mellitus should be screened for the presence of OSA.

Evaluate for specific signs of nasal obstruction: external or internal nasal valve collapse, nasal septal deviation, turbinate hypertrophy (mucosal or bony enlargement), sinusitis, polypoid nasal disease, and adenoid hypertrophy. The oropharynx

should be carefully examined. Note the type of dental occlusion; compared with persons who have a normal skeleton relationship, patients with class II occlusion are predisposed to OSA because the anatomical position of the tongue base may be displaced backward.

Cephalometric radiographs, although seldom used, may be very helpful in identifying underlying skeletal abnormalities. Note the size of the tongue, size of the tonsils, and length of the soft palate. An elongated soft palate, relative macroglossia, and tonsillar hypertrophy may give examiner a clue to the presence of sleep apnea and help to formulate treatment plan.

We use the Friedman classification to document and convey the relationships between the tongue, soft palate, and lateral pharyngeal wall as seen on direct intraoral examination (▶ Fig. 18.1 and ▶ Table 18.3). This classification allows an accurate and uniform description of the clinical findings and facilitates the development of a treatment plan.

Flexible endoscopy should be performed with the patient in both a sitting and a supine position; the latter allows visualization of the position of the tongue base against the epiglottis with the patient in a resting position. The Müller maneuver is performed during flexible nasopharyngoscopy. With the patient in a seated position and the tip of the endoscope positioned in the nasopharynx, the patient is asked to inhale against a closed mouth and nose. The negative pressure generated allows the examiner to observe palatal and lateral pharyngeal wall collapse.

This maneuver, together with other gathered information, can give examiner a clue to the major site of obstruction. There are several other examination techniques whose effectiveness has been clearly documented in the research setting but that are less widely used in clinical practice, including magnetic resonance imaging, drug-induced sleep video endoscopy, and somnofluoroscopy. All of these have been shown in clinical studies to be useful for planning surgical intervention; however, the technical difficulties and relative expense associated with these tests preclude their widespread use in clinical practice.

Nocturnal polysomnography has become the criterion standard in the diagnosis and treatment of OSA since it was first described in 1974 by Holland. Polysomnography provides objective data on sleep and respiratory status. Information gathered in the study includes pulse oximetry, electrocardiography, airflow, respiratory effort, extremity and submental electromyography, nasal and oral airflow, electro-oculography, and EEG evidence of arousal. After the information is gathered, it is then interpreted by a sleep physician. Nocturnal polysomnography gives precise information about the presence of sleep-disordered breathing and allows one to differentiate OSA from other sleep-related disorders. In a split-night study, a variation of nocturnal polysomnography, the first half of the night is devoted to standard polysomnography and the second part of the night is devoted to continuous positive airway pressure (CPAP) titration. In the interest of cost containment, other, less costly home studies have gained widespread acceptance as diagnostic tools. These studies usually measure overnight oxygen levels and respiratory effort. Studies have shown a good concordance between home-based polysomnography and studies obtained in the sleep ambulatory setting for the diagnosis of OSA. The main advantage of home-based studies is convenience for the patient

Table 18.2 Epworth Sleepiness Scale

Situation	Chance of dozing[a]
Reading	
Watching TV	
Sitting in a public place	
Driving a car, stopped at a traffic light	
As a passenger in a car for an hour without a break	
During a quiet time after lunch without alcohol	
Lying down to rest when circumstances permit	

[a]To derive the score, points are assigned according to the patient's answer for each situation and then totaled. 1, slight chance of dozing; 2, moderate chance of dozing; 3, high chance of dozing. Epworth score < 8, normal; Epworth score > 10, suspicion of sleep apnea.

Class I

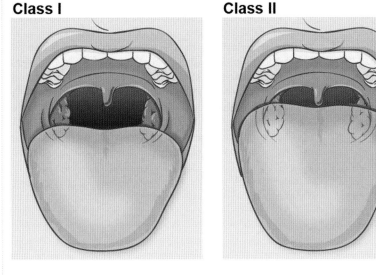

Class II

Class III

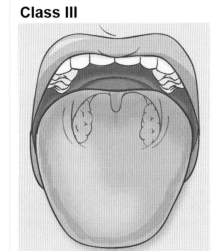

Class IV

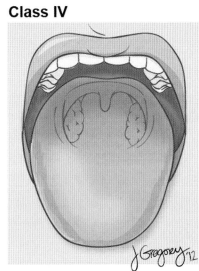

Fig. 18.1 Friedman classification of tongue position.

Table 18.3 Friedman classification

Friedman class	Tongue position	Tonsil size
I	1 or 2	+ 3 or + 4
II	1 or 2	0, + 1, or + 2
	3 or 4	+ 3 or + 4
III	3 or 4	0, + 1, or + 2
IV	Body mass index > 40	

and reduced costs. However, they fail to diagnose other sleep disorders that might be present together with OSA.

18.6 Potential Disease Complications of Obstructive Sleep Apnea

OSA, if left untreated, can lead to severe medical consequences. It is implicated in excessive daytime sleepiness and impaired mood, as well as impaired neurocognitive function. In one study, OSA was implicated as a causal factor in motor vehicle accidents. The prevalence of gastroesophageal reflux disease is much higher in patients with OSA than in the general population. OSA is an independent risk factor for the development of insulin resistance, and it is believed to lead to pulmonary and systemic hypertension. Mortality is increased in patients with an AHI higher than than 20.

18.7 Nonsurgical Treatment of Obstructive Sleep Apnea

Studies have documented significant improvement in the quality of life in individuals treated for OSA. The treatment of OSA should be tailored to the individual needs of the patient. Planning should include a consideration of the severity of the disease, the patient's weight and body habitus, medical comorbidities, and social demands. Often, weight reduction alone can significantly decrease or alleviate OSA.

The gold standard in the medical treatment of OSA is CPAP. After a diagnosis of sleep apnea, the patient is brought back to the sleep center and a second nocturnal polysomnography is performed while the patient uses a CPAP machine at various airway pressures. The pressure of the air applied acts to prevent collapse of the airway and, based on monitoring, is adjusted to the optimal minimal setting at which the recorded parameters normalize and apneic and hypopneic episodes disappear. The use of the CPAP machine alleviates most, if not all, of the medical sequelae of OSA. The most significant problem associated with CPAP use is compliance, which remains relatively low. Many patients are unable to tolerate the fit of the mask on the face or the rush of pressurized air, or they simply view it as a socially unacceptable treatment.

In general, the higher the positive airway pressure required to alleviate the obstruction, the less tolerable patients find CPAP treatment. To improve compliance with CPAP treatment, bilevel positive airway pressure (BiPAP) and autoadjustable positive airway pressure have been developed. These modalities deliver lower expiratory pressures and higher inspiratory pressures. Although the devices may be beneficial for individual patients, they have not been shown to improve overall compliance with the treatment. In recent years, oral appliances have gained widespread popularity in the treatment of snoring and mild to moderate OSA. The oral appliances are designed to shift the mandible forward, thereby increasing the diameter of the posterior oropharyngeal airway. They are usually composed of interlocking plastic molds that are placed on the maxillary and mandibular dentition so that the mandibular arch is in the protrusive position. Patients using dental appliances have a much higher compliance rate than those using CPAP devices.

18.8 Surgical Treatment of Obstructive Sleep Apnea

In 1981, Fujita and colleagues introduced uvulopalatopharyngoplasty (UPPP) as a surgical treatment option for patients with OSA. Together with tonsillectomy, UPPP is a procedure designed to alleviate oropharyngeal airway obstruction by removing redundant palatal and pharyngeal tissues. Despite its widespread use, the overall successes rate of this procedure for all patients is less than 50%, emphasizing the need for the use of a staging system and stepwise approach in the treatment of OSA. Available surgical procedures may be subdivided into four groups (▶ Table 18.4).

When a surgical treatment is chosen, it is necessary to take into consideration the patient's body mass index (BMI), severity of disease, tolerance of medical treatment, age, medical comorbidities, and anatomical sites of obstruction. The Friedman classification is a useful tool for determining the extent of surgical intervention necessary to achieve a good result. Patients with a low BMI, mild OSA, or snoring with obstruction limited to one anatomical site may be excellent candidates for an in-office procedure such as injection snoreplasty, palatal implants (designed to stiffen the soft palate and reduce the noise caused by palatal vibration with injection of a sclerosing agent or placement of a synthetic implant, respectively), or radio-frequency tongue base reduction. Most often, there are multiple sites of anatomical obstruction, so that several surgical procedures are required to achieve a successful outcome. It is essential to discuss the possibility of multiple procedures with the patient preoperatively, and to ensure that the patient realizes that the definition of surgical success most often used in the surgical literature is an RDI of less than 20 with at least a 50% improvement in the RDI; most studies of CPAP define success as an RDI of less than 5.

A patients undergoing surgery should meet the following criteria: has a BMI below 30; is noncompliant with or refusing medical therapy; is medically stable to undergo surgical procedures; 5 < AHI < 14; has upper airway resistance syndrome.

Planning for OSA surgery requires multidisciplinary approach. The anesthesiology team must be aware of the patient's difficult airway and potentially difficult intubation; often, when tongue base and hypopharyngeal procedures are needed, nasal intubation is helpful. Postoperative edema may compromise airway patency. Surgery in the hypopharyngeal area increases the risk for airway compromise; the patient should be counseled about the possibility of temporary tracheotomy. All patients should use CPAP in perioperative period because it has been clearly shown to reduce postsurgical airway compromise and the risk for postobstructive pulmonary edema (POPE). Admission to an intensive care unit for observation should be considered for patients who undergo multilevel surgical

Table 18.4 Types of surgical intervention for obstructive sleep apnea

Nasal surgery	Palatal surgery	Tongue base/hypopharyngeal procedures	Secure airway
Septoplasty	Injection snoreplasty	Lingual tonsillectomy	Tracheotomy
Inferior turbinate reduction	Palatal pillar implants	Radio-frequency reduction of tongue base	
Reconstruction of the nasal valve	Tonsillectomy	Midline posterior glossectomy	
Endoscopic sinus surgery to relieve obstruction from polyps	Uvulopalatopharyngoplasty and its variations	Hyoid myotomy and suspension	
Adenoidectomy	Transpalatal advancement pharyngoplasty	Tongue base suspension suture	
		Mandibular osteotomy and genioglossal advancement	
		Maxillomandibular osteotomy and advancement	

procedures. In trained hands, these surgical procedures can be quite safe, but temporary postoperative dysphagia is the rule. Bleeding may occur, either in the immediate postoperative period or 1 to 1.5 weeks after surgery. Nasopharyngeal reflux of liquids or, conversely, nasopharyngeal stenosis can occur after these surgeries.

18.9 Prognosis

It is essential to discuss the possibility of multiple procedures with the patient preoperatively, and to ensure that the patient realizes that the definition of surgical success most often used in the surgical literature is an RDI of less than 20 with at least a 50% improvement in the RDI; most studies of CPAP define success as an RDI of less than 5.

18.10 Roundsmanship

- Up to 24% of men and 9% of women have sleep-disordered breathing, defined as an apnea–hypopnia index (AHI) of 5 or higher.
- The prevalence of obstructive sleep-disordered breathing increases with age.
- Apnea is the cessation of airflow lasting 10 seconds or longer. Hypopnia is a decline of at least 50% in airflow from baseline, associated with electroencephalographically defined arousal or with a 4% drop in oxygen saturation.
- The AHI is the sum of the number of apneic and hypopneic episodes per hour. The respiratory disturbance index (RDI) may be synonymous with the AHI or may be a combination of the AHI and respiratory effort–related arousal.

- The gold standard for the medical treatment of obstructive sleep apnea (OSA) is continuous positive airway pressure (CPAP).
- Surgical success is most often defined in the surgical literature as an RDI of less than 20 with at least 50% improvement in the RDI; most studies of CPAP define success as an RDI of less than 5.

18.11 Recommended Reading

[1] Berger G, Finkelstein Y, Stein G, Ophir D. Laser-assisted uvulopalatoplasty for snoring: medium- to long-term subjective and objective analysis. Arch Otolaryngol Head Neck Surg 2001; 127: 412–417

[2] Cahali MB. Lateral pharyngoplasty: a new treatment for obstructive sleep apnea hypopnea syndrome. Laryngoscope 2003; 113: 1961–1968

[3] Carskadon MA, Dement WC. Normal human sleep: an overview. In: Kryer MH, Roth T, Dement WC, eds. Principles and Practice of Sleep Medicine. Philadelphia, PA: W. B. Saunders; 1994;16–25

[4] Coleman J. Overview of sleep disorders: where does obstructive sleep apnea syndrome fit in? Otolaryngol Clin North Am 1999; 32: 187–193

[5] Friedman M, Ibrahim H, Bass L. Clinical staging for sleep-disordered breathing. Otolaryngol Head Neck Surg 2002; 127: 13–21

[6] Friedman M, Ibrahim H, Joseph NJ. Staging of obstructive sleep apnea/hypopnea syndrome: a guide to appropriate treatment. Laryngoscope 2004; 114: 454–459

[7] Riley RW, Powell NB, Li KK, Guilleminault C. Surgical therapy for obstructive sleep apnea–hypopnea syndrome. In: Kryger MH, Roth T, Dement WC, eds. Principles and Practice of Sleep Medicine. Philadelphia, PA: W. B. Saunders; 2000:913–928

[8] Thatcher GW, Maisel RH. The long-term evaluation of tracheostomy in the management of severe obstructive sleep apnea. Laryngoscope 2003; 113: 201–204

[9] Walker-Engström ML, Tegelberg A, Wilhelmsson B, Ringqvist I. 4-year follow-up of treatment with dental appliance or uvulopalatopharyngoplasty in patients with obstructive sleep apnea: a randomized study. Chest 2002; 121: 739–746

19 Head and Neck Manifestations of Systemic Diseases

Edwin K. Chan

19.1 Introduction

The head and neck region is often the window into a disease process occurring throughout the rest of the body. The first clue for a clinician in diagnosing many systemic diseases may be revealed during the head and neck examination. Therefore with this in mind, otolaryngologists should approach their evaluation of the head and neck in a "global" manner, while general practitioners and physicians from other fields cannot neglect the head and neck evaluation before drawing up their differential diagnoses. This chapter reviews noninfectious inflammatory diseases that manifest in the head and neck and focuses on some of the more significant conditions in this category (▶ Table 19.1).

19.2 Wegener Granulomatosis

19.2.1 Pathogenesis

This systemic granulomatous disease may have an autoimmune in etiology and causes a vasculitis affecting the upper and lower respiratory tracts (chronic bronchitis) and kidneys (glomerulonephritis).

19.2.2 Types

- Limited form has only pulmonary involvement.
- Systemic form has pulmonary and renal involvement.

19.2.3 Histology

Necrotizing granulomas, multinucleated giant cells, and vasculitis of the upper/lower respiratory tracts and kidneys.

19.2.4 Head and Neck Presentation

Affects predominantly Caucasians.

Sinonasal

Chronic sinusitis is the most common head and neck manifestation of the disease; saddle nose deformity is due to severe septal perforation, epistaxis, nasal obstruction.

Otologic

Chronic serous otitis media, conductive hearing loss.

Laryngeal

Laryngeal ulcers, subglottic stenosis.

Oral

Mucosal ulcers, "strawberry" gingiva.

Ocular

Conjunctivitis, uveitis, keratitis.

19.2.5 Work-up

The most specific blood test is c-ANCA (antineutrophil cytoplasmic autoantibodies, cytoplasmic). Renal and/or pulmonary biopsies are most specific, showing necrotizing glomerulonephritis and vasculitis respectively. Nasal biopsy is frequently nondiagnostic, showing only nonspecific inflammation. Multiple nasal biopsies on the edges of the ulcers yield a higher success rate in finding the specific features of necrotizing granulomas and vasculitis. The erythrocyte sedimentation rate (ESR), urinalysis, blood urea nitrogen (BUN)/creatinine levels, and a chest X-ray may aid in the diagnosis.

19.2.6 Treatment

Immunosuppressive therapy with corticosteroids, cyclophosphamide, and/or methotrexate. Trimethoprim/sulfamethoxazole may be considered to prevent relapse and treat limited disease.

19.3 Sarcoidosis

19.3.1 Pathogenesis

This is a systemic granulomatous disease with an unknown etiology that affects the head and neck region and is also characterized by pulmonary, dermatologic, hepatic, renal, cardiac, osseous, and neurologic involvement.

19.3.2 Histology

Noncaseating epithelioid granulomas, giant cells, accumulation of T cells and mononuclear macrophages.

19.3.3 Head and Neck Presentation

Affects predominantly African-Americans and females.

Lymphatic

Cervical lymphadenopathy is the most common head and neck finding.

Sinonasal

"Cobblestoning" of the nasal mucosa, epistaxis, and dry crusting.

Laryngeal

Causes submucosal lesions that affect primarily the supraglottis. The epiglottis is the most commonly affected region of the larynx, and the aryepiglottic folds, false vocal folds, and subglottis are affected in descending order of frequency. The true vocal folds are rarely affected. Hoarseness due to vocal fold paralysis has been reported with this disease process.

Salivary Glands

An asymptomatic parotid mass may be part of a spectrum of symptoms in uveoparotid fever (Heerfordt disease), an extrapulmonary form of sarcoidosis that also causes uveitis, facial nerve palsy, sensorineural hearing loss, and fever.

19.3.4 Work-up

Most commonly presents when a chest X-ray incidentally reveals hilar adenopathy. Blood work may show an increased angiotensin-converting enzyme (ACE) level, abnormal liver function tests, and hypercalcemia. The electrocardiogram (EKG) may reveal an arrhythmia. Enlarged cervical lymph nodes, abnormal nasal mucosal lesions, laryngeal lesions, parotid masses, and subcutaneous nodules (Darier-Roussy nodules) found in the skin can be readily biopsied. Biopsy of any affected region may show the noncaseating granulomas.

19.3.5 Treatment

Systemic corticosteroids for exacerbations of pulmonary disease. Localized lesions may be treated with topical/injectable steroids, and supraglottic lesions are excised only if they are causing obstructive symptoms. Asymptomatic lesions are only monitored.

19.4 Lupus Erythematosus

19.4.1 Pathogenesis

A deposition of antibodies and immune complexes (type III hypersensitivity) underlies this autoimmune disease.

19.4.2 Histology

Inflammation and degeneration of the dermal–epidermal junction. Deposits of immunoglobulins (IgG and C3) in a bandlike pattern are seen in the subepithelial layer on direct immunofluorescence.

19.4.3 Types

Discoid Lupus Erythematosus

The least aggressive form of the disease that affects only superficial tissue and does not have visceral involvement.

Head and Neck Presentation

Affects predominantly affects young women.

Oral

Aphthous ulcers, superficial bullae, erythematous plaques with surrounding lacy, white strands.

Cutaneous

Raised erythematous plaques with hypopigmented edges and resultant alopecia and scarring.

Work-up

This is a clinical diagnosis because the antinuclear antibody (ANA) test and lupus erythematosus (LE) cell test are negative. Biopsy of the lesions may show immunoglobulin deposition on the basement membrane on immunofluorescence.

Treatment

Topical steroids and strict sunscreen use/avoidance of sun exposure.

Subacute Cutaneous Lupus Erythematosus

A mild systemic form of the disease with the same head and neck presentation as discoid lupus erythematosus but with cutaneous papulosquamous lesions that do not cause scarring. The diagnosis is also made from the clinical history and physical. Results of ANA, Sjögren syndrome A antibody (SS-A [anti-Ro]), and Sjögren syndrome B antibody (SS-B [anti-La]) blood tests are inconsistent.

Systemic Lupus Erythematosus

The most severe systemic form of the disease with widespread visceral involvement including polyarthritis, glomerulonephritis, anemia, pulmonary fibrosis, and endocarditis.

Head and Neck Presentation

Affects predominantly young women.

Oral

Similar to that of discoid lupus erythematosus.

Cutaneous

In addition to the lesions found in discoid lupus erythematosus, a pathognomonic malar "butterfly" rash is often present.

Laryngotracheal

Perichondritis of the laryngeal and tracheal cartilage and thickening of the vocal folds cause neck/throat pain and hoarseness, respectively.

Sinonasal

Nasal dryness, crusting, and septal perforation.

Otologic

Tinnitus with or without sensorineural hearing loss.

Work-up

Tests for nonspecific markers such as ANA, SS-A (anti-Ro), and SS-B (anti-La) are typically positive. Tests for specific markers such as anti–double-stranded (anti-DS) DNA and Sm antigen are positive. LE tests are typically positive, and positive immu-

Table 19.1 Noninfectious systemic diseases of the head and neck

	Pathophysiology	Histology	Symptoms and physical findings	Work-up	Treatment
Wegener granulomatosis	Vasculitis of the upper/lower respiratory tracts ± kidneys	Necrotizing granulomas, multinucleated giant cells	"Saddle nose," septal perforation, sinusitis, "strawberry gingiva," otitis media, subglottic stenosis	Positive c-ANCA, nasal biopsy, pulmonary/renal biopsy most diagnostic	Corticosteroids, immunosuppressants, trimethoprim/sulfamethoxazole may be considered
Sarcoidosis	Idiopathic granulomatous disease	Noncaseating granulomas	Cervical lymphadenopathy, epistaxis, nasal crusting, supraglottic submucosal lesions, parotid mass	Elevated ACE levels, biopsy of affected area	Corticosteroids
Lupus erythematosus	Type III hypersensitivity	IgG and C3 immunoglobulin deposition in subepithelium and basement membrane	Oral ulcers, cutaneous plaques, malar rash, nasal dryness, septal perforation, tinnitus ±sensorineural hearing loss in systemic form	Systemic form: positive ANA, SS-A (anti-Ro), SS-B (anti-La), anti-DS DNA, Sm antigen; positive LE test	Anti-inflammatories, corticosteroids, immunosuppressive agents
Sjögren syndrome	Autoimmune polyclonal B-cell activation affecting exocrine glands	Periductal exocrine gland lymphoid infiltration	Ocular, nasal, and oral dryness; fissuring of the tongue; parotitis, submandibular gland enlargement	Positive ANA, SS-A (anti-Ro), SS-B (anti-La), RF; minor salivary gland biopsy; Schirmer test	Topical eye and oral treatments, punctal plugging, pilocarpine hydrochloride
Relapsing polychondritis	Autoimmune inflammation of cartilage with high levels of glycosaminoglycans	Perichondrial infiltration with inflammatory cells	Auricular erythema/edema sparing lobule, saddle nose deformity, laryngeal collapse/stenosis	Elevated antibodies to type II collagen	Corticosteroids, nonsteroidal anti-inflammatory drugs, immunosuppressants, tracheotomy if airway collapse/stenosis
Langerhan cell histiocytosis	Idiopathic infiltration of dendritic cells (Langerhan cells) and histiocytes (macrophages) in affected tissue	Birbeck granules, CD1A- and S100-positive	Osteolytic bone lesions of the skull/mandible, mastoiditis, otitis media, gingival ulcers, alopecia, proptosis	Biopsy of a lesion (skin most accessible)	Excision of localized lesions, corticosteroids and chemotherapy for disseminated disease
Behçet disease	Idiopathic vasculitis, likely autoimmune, triggered by an infectious event; triad of aphthous ulcers, uveitis, and genital ulcers	Lymphocytic vasculitis with neutrophilic infiltrate, thrombotic clotting	Aphthous ulcers, uveitis, dysphagia, dysarthria, hearing loss	Elevated ESR, C-reactive protein; pathergy test	Topical oral steroids, sucralfate, and tetracycline for oral lesions; systemic corticosteroids and immunosuppressants for generalized disease
Cogan syndrome	Autoimmune reaction to a common antigen found in both the cornea and inner ear	Hydropic findings similar to those of Meniere disease, lymphocytic infiltration of cornea	Episodic vertigo; fluctuating hearing loss, tinnitus, and aural fullness; interstitial keratitis	Slit lamp examination, audiography and ENG	Systemic corticosteroids and immunosuppressants
Rheumatoid arthritis	Inflammatory disease affecting peripheral joints	Granulomatous lesions of the skin with small-vessel vasculitis, lymphocytic infiltration of synovium	Trismus, temporomandibular joint tenderness, hoarseness, conductive hearing loss	Elevated ESR, RF; audiogram; fiberoptic laryngoscopy; biopsy of cutaneous lesions	Corticosteroids, nonsteroidal anti-inflammatory drugs, DMARDs
Scleroderma	Autoimmune small-vessel vasculitis and fibrosis	Collagen deposition in affected tissue, smooth-muscle atrophy	"Pursed lip" appearance, gastroesophageal reflux, dysphagia, hoarseness, sicca syndrome	Positive ANA, barium esophagram, minor salivary gland biopsy	Proton pump inhibitors, corticosteroids, nonsteroidal anti-inflammatory drugs
Dermatomyositis/polymyositis	Autoimmune vasculopathy and myopathy of striated muscle	Inflammatory infiltrate in muscle and perivascular regions	Heliotrope rash, "shawl" sign, weakness in flexing neck, dysphonia, dysphagia	Elevated CK, LDH, AST, and ANA; barium swallow; biopsy of affected muscle	Proton pump inhibitors, systemic corticosteroids, immunosuppressants, IVIG

Table 19.1 *continued*

	Pathophysiology	Histology	Symptoms and physical findings	Work-up	Treatment
Giant cell (temporal) arteritis	Idiopathic vasculitis of medium-size and large arteries	Panarteritis, neovascularization, fragmentation of internal elastic lamina	Headache, jaw and tongue claudication, temporal tenderness, anosmia, dysphagia, hoarseness, vertigo, sensorineural hearing loss, amaurosis fugax	ESR, C-reactive protein, alkaline phosphatase elevated; temporal biopsy the gold standard test	Systemic corticosteroids
Churg-Strauss syndrome	Allergic granulomatous disease of small and medium-size vessels	Necrotizing granulomas with central eosinophilic core, giant cells	Nasal polyposis, nasal obstruction, sinusitis, allergic rhinitis	Eosinophilia on bloodwork, ESR and C-reactive protein elevated, p-ANCA positive, biopsy of involved tissue	Systemic corticosteroids
Kawasaki disease	Vasculitis, possibly infectious in origin, affecting predominantly medium-size vessels	Necrosis of smooth muscle causing aneurysms, fibrosis, and stenosis of vessels	Cervical lymphadenopathy, conjuctival injection, "strawberry tongue"	Elevated WBC count, ESR, C-reactive protein, cardiac enzymes (with myocardial infarction); EKG; CXR; echocardiogram	IVIG, salicylates/aspirin, close cardiovascular monitoring

Abbreviations: ACE, angiotensin-converting enzyme; ANA, antinuclear antibody; AST, aspartate aminotransferase; anti-DS, anti–double-stranded (DNA); c-ANCA, antineutrophil cytoplasmic autoantibody, cytoplasmic; CK, creatine kinase; CXR, chest X-ray; DMARD, disease-modifying antirheumatic drug; EKG, electrocardiogram; ENG, electroneurography; ESR, erythrocyte sedimentation rate; IVIG, intravenous immunoglobulin; LDH, lactic dehydrogenase; LE, lupus erythematosus; p-ANCA, antineutrophil cytoplasmic autoantibody, perinuclear; RF, rheumatoid factor; SS-A, Sjögren syndrome A antibody; SS-B, Sjögren syndrome B antibody; WBC, white blood cell.

nofluorescence testing of lesions may aid in the diagnosis. Complete blood cell count, urinalysis, and electrocardiography may detect other visceral involvement.

Treatment

Nonsteroidal anti-inflammatory drugs, corticosteroids, and immunosuppressive agents are used to control inflammation.

19.5 Sjögren Syndrome

19.5.1 Pathogenesis

This is an autoimmune systemic disease initially presenting with head and neck symptoms. Autoimmune destruction of the exocrine gland parenchyma with resultant atrophy, periductal lymphocytic infiltration, and polyclonal B-cell activation occurs with this disease process.

19.5.2 Histology

Foci of interstitial periductal lymphocytic infiltration of affected exocrine glands.

19.5.3 Types

1. Primary: disease is not associated with another autoimmune connective tissue disorder.
2. Secondary: disease is associated with another autoimmune connective tissue disorder, most commonly rheumatoid arthritis or systemic lupus erythematosus.

19.5.4 Head and Neck Presentation

Found primarily in peri- and postmenopausal women and may be the second most common autoimmune disease after rheumatoid arthritis. Sjögren syndrome can rarely progress to a non-Hodgkin lymphoma.

Ocular

Dry eyes most commonly described as a gritty or sandy sensation in the eyes, keratoconjunctivitis sicca, filamentary keratosis (mucinous threads adhering to damaged portions of the ocular surface).

Oral

Dry mouth manifested with dental caries, oral candidiasis, angular cheilitis, dysphagia, dysphonia, and/or dysgeusia. The oral examination reveals erythema and fissuring of the tongue with loss of papillae.

Sinonasal

Nasal dryness, epistaxis.

Salivary Glands

Bilateral parotitis with intermittent parotid swelling, but with atrophy occurring in advanced disease, submandibular gland enlargement may also occur.

19.5.5 Work-up

Positive SS-A (anti-Ro) and SS-B (anti-La), ANA, and rheumatoid factor blood tests. Polyclonal hypergammaglobulinemia on serum electrophoresis is often seen, and loss of a previous positive finding and/or development of a monoclonal gammopathy may indicate development of a lymphoma. Minor salivary gland biopsy from the inner lip showing lymphocytic infiltrates is the most definitive test. Sialography of the parotid gland shows a globular pattern of contrast collections throughout the gland described as an "apple tree appearance." The Schirmer test evaluates tear production by placing a strip of filter paper on the lower conjunctiva; a definitively positive result is less than 5 mm of wetting after 5 minutes (> 15 mm after 5 minutes is normal).

19.5.6 Treatment

Ocular dryness is treated with artificial tears, nighttime gels, cyclosporine drops, humidifiers, glasses with moisture shields, and plugging of the lacrimal puncta. Dry mouth is treated with artificial saliva, frequent sips of water throughout the day, a humidifier, and pilocarpine hydrochloride to stimulate saliva production.

19.6 Relapsing Polychondritis

19.6.1 Pathogenesis

A rare autoimmune condition causing inflammation of the cartilage and tissue containing high concentrations of glycosaminoglycans. Polyarthritis, pulmonary function compromise, renal disease, cardiac valve compromise, vascular aneurysms, and cutaneous nodules have been associated with the disease.

19.6.2 Histology

Perichondrial infiltration of inflammatory cells causing cartilage destruction and fibrosis.

19.6.3 Head and Neck Presentation

Occurs most frequently in Caucasians.

Otologic

Auricular chondritis in a relapsing pattern is the most common presenting symptom (erythema and edema of the auricle, sparing the lobule); conductive hearing loss caused by stenosis of the external auditory canal, eustachian tube chondritis, and/or serous otitis media; proposed vasculitis of the internal auditory artery may cause vestibular injury and sensorineural hearing loss.

Ocular

Ocular inflammation is most commonly manifested as episcleritis and scleritis.

Sinonasal

Nasal chondritis causing saddle nose deformity.

Oral

Aphthous ulcers are common.

Laryngotracheal

Chondritis of the laryngotracheal framework occurs more frequently in females, sometimes causing obstruction due to vocal fold paralysis, airway edema, airway collapse, and airway stenosis.

19.6.4 Work-up

Elevated antibodies to type II collagen (found in cartilage and the vitreous humor of the eye) is the most specific test; nonspecific tests include elevated ESR and C-reactive protein. Biopsy of cartilaginous structures is not performed unless necessary for diagnosis because of the possibility of infection and potential cosmetic deformity. Electrocardiogram, echocardiogram, chest X-ray, pulmonary function tests, urinalysis, and BUN/creatinine may detect the effect of the disease outside the head and neck region.

19.6.5 Treatment

Corticosteroids, nonsteroidal anti-inflammatory drugs, immunosuppressive chemotherapeutic agents. In patients with acute airway compromise, intubation may exacerbate the airway distress due to laryngotracheal edema and stenosis. Tracheotomy is the treatment of choice in securing the airway in these patients.

19.7 Langerhans Cell Histiocytosis (Histiocytosis X)

19.7.1 Pathogenesis

Infiltration and proliferation of eosinophils, T cells, dendritic cells (Langerhans cells), and histiocytes (macrophages) in the affected tissue without a primary cause.

19.7.2 Histology

Birbeck granules (which show a "zipper pattern") in the dendritic cells are pathognomonic. Nonspecific features include granulomatous lesions with a background of eosinophils, T cells, dendritic cells (Langerhans cells), and histiocytes (macrophages). CD1A- and S100-positive.

The disease occurs more frequently in Caucasians, and the incidence is higher among males.

19.7.3 Types

Eosinophilic Granuloma (Localized Form)

Head and Neck Presentation

Occurs in children 5 to 15 years old.

Osseous

Solitary, monostotic calvarial osteolytic bone lesion presenting with bone pain; can be found in mandible and also present with loose teeth.

Ocular

Periorbital osseous lesions may cause periorbital edema and proptosis.

Otologic

Mastoid involvement can cause chronic otitis media, mastoiditis, tympanic membrane perforations, external canal polyps, and facial paralysis.

Oral

Gingival erosions with bleeding.

Dermatologic

Scalp disease can cause scaling of the scalp with patchy lesions leading to alopecia; usually not pruritic, but may be tender.

Hand-Schüller-Christian Disease (Intermediate, Chronic, Disseminated Form)

Head and Neck Presentation

Occurs in children 2 to 10 years old. Classic triad of diabetes insipidus, exophthalmos, and polyostotic lesions, particularly of the skull. This disease has otologic, oral, and dermatologic findings similar to those of eosinophilic granulomas. It also may affect the lungs, liver, spleen, and lymph nodes.

Letterer-Siwe Disease (Severe, Acute, Disseminated Form)

Occurs in children younger than 2 years old. Presents with fever, anemia and thrombocytopenia, hepatomegaly and splenomegaly, and pulmonary infiltrates.

Head and Neck Presentation

Osseous

Osteolytic lesions are not common.

Otologic

The mastoid may be involved, causing chronic otitis media, otorrhea, postauricular edema, external canal polyps, and conductive hearing loss.

Lymphatic

Cervical lymphadenopathy may be present.

Work-up

Laboratory studies include complete blood cell count with differential, liver function tests, coagulation studies, and urine osmolality testing to rule out diabetes insipidus. Radiologic studies include chest X-ray and skeletal survey. Biopsy of a lesion (skin lesion is the most accessible) will establish the diagnosis.

Treatment

Localized/Single-Organ Disease

Monostotic bone lesions may be treated by curettage/excision. Polyostotic bone lesions can be treated with systemic steroids.

Skin lesions may be treated with topical steroids, and localized lymph node involvement can be addressed with excision.

Chemotherapy and radiation therapy are reserved for large lesions that may be causing severe pain, are difficult to access, or involve vital structures.

Disseminated/Multiple-Organ Disease

Systemic chemotherapy (methotrexate, vinblastine, etoposide) with or without systemic corticosteroids is standard. Diabetes insipidus is treated with desmopressin acetate. Rapidly progressive disease that is refractory to other treatment modalities may be treated with a bone marrow transplant for salvage.

19.8 Behçet Disease

19.8.1 Pathogenesis

The classic triad of symptoms includes recurrent oral aphthous ulcers, genital ulcers, and uveitis. However, this is a complex, multisystem disease affecting the skin; eyes; joints; cardiovascular, gastrointestinal, and urologic systems; kidneys; lungs; and central nervous system. The condition is an idiopathic vasculitis with a likely autoimmune component triggered by an infectious event

19.8.2 Histology

Lymphocytic vasculitis with a neutrophilic infiltrate; thrombotic clotting due to a hypercoagulable state may also be present. The histologic findings are nonspecific.

19.8.3 Head and Neck Presentation

The disease occurs predominantly in the Middle East, in particular Turkey, and in Asia, with a higher incidence especially in people of Japanese background. The gender prevalence depends on the country, but the disease is more prevalent in females in the United States.

Oral

Aphthous and herpetic lesions are the most common presenting symptom.

Ocular

Uveitis and retinal vasculitis causing blurry vision, scleral injection, eye pain, excessive lacrimation, photophobia, and possible blindness if the ocular symptoms develop early in the disease course. The ocular symptoms usually follow the oral symptoms.

Pharyngoesophageal

Dysphagia due to oropharyngeal and esophageal ulcers and neurologic impairment of the swallowing mechanism.

Otologic

Acute deafness due to neuro-otologic impairment.

Laryngeal

Speech difficulties due to neurologic impairment.

19.8.4 Work-up

Diagnosis is based on the clinical symptom and findings. Laboratory results show an elevated inflammatory state (elevated ESR, C-reactive protein, leukocytosis). Pathergy test: mild skin trauma induces the formation of an erythematous papule/pustule after 1 to 2 days.

19.8.5 Treatment

Topical steroids, tetracycline swish and swallow solutions and sucralfate for limited oral ulcerations, and systemic steroids for severe mucocutaneous disease. Immunosuppressive and immunomodulating agents such as azathioprine, colchicine, sulfasalazine, cyclosporine, and cyclophosphamide are indicated for more pervasive disease. Proper consultations as needed: surgery for possible gastrointestinal bleeds or perforation, neurosurgery for central nervous system thrombotic or aneurysmal events, cardiothoracic surgery for major vessel aneurysms/thrombosis, ophthalmology, dermatology, urology, gastroenterology, neurology, and nephrology.

19.9 Cogan Syndrome

19.9.1 Pathogenesis

Classic triad of nonsyphilitic interstitial keratitis, fluctuating vertigo/sensorineural hearing loss with tinnitus, and an associated autoimmune vasculitic condition (usually a large-vessel vasculitis). Autoimmune in etiology, likely in reaction to a common antigen found in both the cornea and inner ear.

19.9.2 Histology

Hydropic findings similar to those of Meniere disease in the inner ear, lymphocytic infiltration of the cornea with neovascularization.

19.9.3 Head and Neck Presentation

Predominantly in young adults and Caucasians.

Otologic

Symptoms similar to those of Meniere disease, with episodic vertigo, fluctuating sensorineural hearing loss associated with tinnitus, and possible aural fullness.

Ocular

Interstitial keratitis causing eye pain, redness, excessive lacrimation, blurry vision, and photophobia.

19.9.4 Work-up

Slit lamp examination reveals the anterior chamber findings of interstitial keratitis. Audiogram reveals a sensorineural hearing loss preferentially in the low and high frequencies. Electroneurography and rotary chair testing show a vestibular weakness.

19.9.5 Treatment

Systemic corticosteroids and immunosuppressants (azathioprine, cyclophosphamide).

19.10 Rheumatoid Arthritis

19.10.1 Pathogenesis

Systemic inflammatory disease affecting peripheral joints.

19.10.2 Histology

Neovascularization of synovium with lymphocytic infiltration. Rheumatoid skin nodules are characterized by a small-vessel vasculitis and granulomatous lesions.

19.10.3 Head and Neck Presentation

Female predominance with a high incidence in certain Native American populations.

Maxillofacial

Bilateral temporomandibular joint tenderness and swelling, trismus.

Laryngeal

Hoarseness due to cricoarytenoid joint inflammation/ankylosis.

Otologic

Conductive hearing loss due to ossicular chain fixation.

19.10.4 Work-up

Radiologic studies of the temporomandibular joint may show condyle erosion at the articular surface and obliteration of the joint space. Laryngoscopy may reveal arytenoid edema, impaired mobility of the vocal folds, and cricoarytenoid joint fixation. Rheumatoid nodules may appear on the vocal folds (bamboo nodules). Computed tomographic scan of the neck may show a soft-tissue swelling of the cricoarytenoid joint. Audiogram may show a conductive hearing loss. Laboratory studies show an elevated rheumatoid factor, ESR, and/or C-reactive protein. Biopsy of cutaneous nodules may be helpful in the diagnosis.

19.10.5 Treatment

Nonsteroidal anti-inflammatory drugs, glucocorticoids, and disease-modifying antirheumatic drugs (DMARDs): methotrexate, sulfasalazine, gold salts, penicillamine.

19.11 Scleroderma (Progressive Systemic Sclerosis)

19.11.1 Pathogenesis

A triad of processes including autoimmune activation causes a small-vessel vasculitis and progressive fibrosis due to excessive collagen deposition; smooth-muscle atrophy occurs in the gastrointestinal tract.

19.11.2 Histology

Extensive fibrosis of the skin and affected organs with collagen deposition, possible inflammatory infiltrates, and small-vessel vasculopathy with microthrombi.

19.11.3 Head and Neck Presentation

Cutaneous

Tight, fibrotic facial skin with thinning of the lips and reduction in the oral aperture ("pursed lip" appearance).

Esophageal

Gastroesophageal reflux (due to a patent lower esophageal sphincter); dysphagia from disease infiltration anywhere along the gastrointestinal tract but classically the lower two-thirds of the esophagus due to smooth-muscle involvement; oropharyngeal and esophageal cancers are more common in these patients.

Ocular and Oral

Xerostomia and dry eyes as part of a sicca syndrome may be present.

Laryngeal

Hoarseness due to gastroesophageal reflux or laryngeal fibrosis.

19.11.4 Work-up

Laboratory studies are positive for ANA. Barium swallow may show a dilated esophagus but incompetent lower esophageal sphincter (to distinguish from achalasia). Esophageal manometry will show normal upper esophageal pressures but the incompetent lower esophageal sphincter. pH probe studies can confirm the gastroesophageal reflux. Minor salivary gland biopsy will show extensive fibrosis but without the lymphocytic infiltrate seen in Sjögren syndrome.

19.11.5 Treatment

Gastroesophageal reflux precautions, proton pump inhibitors, nonsteroidal anti-inflammatory drugs, and corticosteroids may be considered. There are no FDA-approved therapies for scleroderma.

19.12 Dermatomyositis/Polymyositis

19.12.1 Pathogenesis

An autoimmune inflammatory vasculopathy and myopathy of striated muscle. When both skin and muscle are affected, it is termed *dermatomyositis*, and when only muscle is involved, it is called *polymyositis*. An inflammatory infiltrate is present in muscle and around vessels.

19.12.2 Histology

An inflammatory infiltrate is present in muscle (interfascicular in dermatomyositis and intrafascicular in polymyositis) and around vessels; affected skin has an inflammatory infiltrate at the dermal–epidermal basement membrane.

19.12.3 Head and Neck Presentation

More common in women.

Cutaneous

In dermatomyositis, the heliotrope rash—a reddish brown to purple discoloration around the eyelids with periorbital edema—is pathognomonic; an erythematous rash is prominent in the head and neck, sometimes in a V-shaped distribution on the neck ("shawl" sign); a psoriatic scalp dermatitis may lead to alopecia.

Musculoskeletal

Weakness in the neck flexors.

Pharyngoesophageal

Dysphonia and dysphagia are caused by oropharyngeal and esophageal striated muscle weakness (upper third of the esophagus).

19.12.4 Work-up

Blood work illustrates elevated creatine kinase (CK), lactic dehydrogenase (LDH), aspartate aminotransferase (AST), and ANA levels.

Radiologic studies may include a barium swallow showing esophageal dysmotility, and magnetic resonance imaging of an affected muscle may show an inflammatory myopathy. Electromyography of an affected muscle may be performed. Biopsy of an affected muscle reveals the histologic findings.

19.12.5 Treatment

Reflux precautions, systemic corticosteroids, immunosuppressive cytotoxic agents, intravenous immunoglobulin (IVIG).

19.13 Giant Cell (Temporal) Arteritis

19.13.1 Pathogenesis

Giant cell arteritis is the most common idiopathic vasculitis; it is a chronic vasculitis of medium-size and large arteries that causes concentric intimal hyperplasia of the vessel walls.

19.13.2 Histology

The intima, media, and adventitia of the vessel wall are affected (panarteritis); inflammation in the endothelium at the intima–media junction as well as the adventitia leads to neovascularization; giant cells may be present; fragmentation of the internal elastic lamina is often seen.

19.13.3 Head and Neck Presentation

Found predominantly in the elderly and more common in women and Caucasians. Headache is the most common presenting symptom.

Cutaneous

Erythema of the skin with facial pain and, if severe, necrosis of the skin.

Maxillofacial

Jaw claudication is pathognomonic; trismus, temporomandibular joint pain, tooth and gingival pain, tenderness over the scalp/temporal region.

Nasal

Edematous and inflamed nasal mucosa, anosmia.

Oropharyngeal

Dysphagia caused by edematous and inflamed oropharyngeal mucosa, necrotic lesions of the oral mucosa, tongue claudication due to ischemia, glottic ulcerations, ageusia.

Laryngeal

Hoarseness.

Otologic

Otalgia, tinnitus, vertigo, sensorineural hearing loss; lymphadenopathy and tonsillar hypertrophy may be present; salivary gland enlargement.

Ocular

Blindness is one of the most severe complications of the disease. Amaurosis fugax is the transient sensation of a "shade coming over the eye."

19.13.4 Work-up

Blood work includes elevated C-reactive protein and ESR (acute phase reactants), elevated alkaline phosphatase, normocytic normochromic anemia.

Temporal artery biopsy is the gold standard diagnostic test.

19.13.5 Treatment

Systemic corticosteroids are the first-line therapy.

19.14 Churg-Strauss Syndrome

19.14.1 Pathogenesis

An allergic granulomatous disease of small to medium-size vessels; closely related to Wegener granulomatosis. Six criteria (four or more criteria are highly sensitive and specific) for the disease include the following:
1. Asthma.
2. Eosinophilia of more than 10% in the peripheral blood.
3. Paranasal sinusitis.
4. Pulmonary infiltrates.
5. Histologic evidence of vasculitis with eosinophilic infiltrate.
6. Polyneuropathy.

19.14.2 Histology

Necrotizing granulomas with a central eosinophilic core and surrounding giant cells and macrophages; these findings are seen predominantly in the lungs.

19.14.3 Head and Neck Presentation

Sinonasal

Allergic rhinitis, nasal polyposis, chronic sinusitis, nasal obstruction.

19.14.4 Work-up

Blood work may illustrate the eosinophilia mentioned above and anemia. Elevated ESR and C-reactive protein are often present. BUN and creatinine and an abnormal urinalysis may indicate glomerulonephritis. Patients with this disease are often positive for p-ANCA (antineutrophil cytoplasmic autoantibodies, perinuclear).

Radiologic studies include chest X-ray to evaluate pulmonary involvement.

Tissue biopsy of an involved organ (lung, skin, muscle, nerve, kidneys) aids in the diagnosis.

19.14.5 Treatment

Systemic corticosteroids usually control the disease process.

19.15 Kawasaki Disease

19.15.1 Pathogenesis

Vasculitis that may be infectious in origin; it is most severe in medium-size vessels but may affect vessels of all calibers; the most common cause of acquired cardiac disease in children, followed by acute rheumatic fever.

19.15.2 Histology

Necrosis of smooth-muscle cells leads to splitting of the internal and external laminae, causing aneurysms. Fibrosis and stenosis of vessels subsequently occur as well, possibly leading to thrombosis and complete occlusion. Myocardial infarctions may occur and are due to coronary artery aneurysms and thrombosis.

19.15.3 Head and Neck Presentation

Most common in children younger than 4 years old and of Asian descent (Japanese in particular).

Systemic/Cutaneous

Fever and generalized erythematous, desquamating rash.

Ocular

Conjunctival injection.

Lymphatic

Cervical lymphadenitis; lymph nodes larger than 1.5 cm, not responsive to antibiotics.

Oral

Mucositis of the lips leading to fissuring and oropharyngeal erythema, "strawberry tongue" (glossal erythema and prominent papillae).

19.15.4 Work-up

Blood work includes elevated white blood cell count and acute phase reactants (ESR, C-reactive protein); elevated cardiac enzymes with myocardial infarction.

The EKG may shows signs of myocarditis or infarction; chest X-ray and echocardiography to evaluate cardiac disease.

19.15.5 Treatment

The mainstay of treatment is IVIG, salicylates/aspirin, and close cardiovascular monitoring.

19.16 Roundsmanship

- Multiple findings and symptoms across different areas of the head and neck should make the physician consider putting a systemic etiology higher on the list of differential diagnoses.
- A preliminary blood work-up that includes acute phase reactants, such as the erythrocyte sedimentation rate and C-reactive protein level, may be useful in diagnosing an inflammatory autoimmune disease presenting in the head and neck of a patient.

19.17 Recommended Reading

[1] Gubbels SP, Barkhuizen A, Hwang PH. Head and neck manifestations of Wegener's granulomatosis. Otolaryngol Clin North Am 2003; 36: 685–705

[2] Harris JP, Weisman MH. Head and Neck Manifestations of Systemic Disease. 1st ed. New York, NY: Informa Healthcare; 2007:3–117

[3] Mahoney EJ, Spiegel JH. Sjögren's disease. Otolaryngol Clin North Am 2003; 36: 733–745

[4] Schwartzbauer HR, Tami TA. Ear, nose, and throat manifestations of sarcoidosis. Otolaryngol Clin North Am 2003; 36: 673–684

20 Epidemiology of Head and Neck Cancers

Guo-Pei Yu and Stimson P. Schantz

20.1 Oral Cavity and Pharyngeal Cancers

20.1.1 Epidemiology

Almost all oral and pharyngeal cancers are squamous cell carcinomas with similarities in epidemiology, treatment, and prognosis. Oral cavity cancer is the 11th most common cancer in the world in terms of number of cases, while pharyngeal cancer ranks 20th. Oral and pharyngeal cancer, considered together, is the sixth most common form of cancer in the world. About 389,000 new cases occurred in the world in 2000, two-thirds of which were in developing countries. The rates of oral and pharyngeal cancer vary among countries. The highest incidence is observed in Australia, France, Hungary, South America (Brazil), and southern Africa, while the lowest incidence is seen in Mexico and Japan. Oral and pharyngeal cancers are responsible for about 200,000 deaths worldwide each year.

According to the estimates by the American Cancer Society, there were about 35,310 new cases (25,310 in men and 10,000 in women) of oral cavity cancer (22,900) and pharyngeal cancer (12,410)and about 7,590 people (5,210 men and 2,380 women) who died of these cancers in the United States in 2008. These cancers account for nearly 2.5% of all malignancies.

Of all squamous oral and pharyngeal cancers (excluding salivary gland and nasopharyngeal cancers), oral cavity cancers account for nearly 88% and pharyngeal cancers about 12%. In addition, most squamous oral cavity cancers occur in the tongue (43.1%), tonsillar fossa (23.4%), lip (9.1%), and floor of the mouth (7.8%). The rest occur on the gums, palate, and unspecified parts of mouth (▶ Table 20.1).

Oral and pharyngeal cancers can occur in young people. Of all patients, adults younger than 40 years of age account for 2.9%, and those younger than 50 account for 16.2%. The incidence of oral and pharyngeal cancers increases with age and reaches a peak at the ages of 70 to 79 years. The incidence declines after 80 + years except in women, in whom the incidence continues to rise (▶ Fig. 20.1). The incidence of oral and pharyngeal cancers is higher in men than in women, and the female-to-male ratio is 2:7 for oral cancer and 3:4 for pharyngeal cancer, respectively.

The incidence of oral cavity and pharyngeal cancers has gradually decreased over the past 30 years in the United States. The incidence of oral cavity cancer decreased 18.8% (from 8.7 per 100,000 to 6.5 per 100,000), and that of pharyngeal cancer decreased 44% (from 1.8 to 1.0 per 100,000; ▶ Fig. 20.2). In contrast to that of other oral cancers, however, the incidence of tongue cancer increased nearly 60% in American adults younger than 40 years of age during the same period. The increase continued until 1985, after which the incidence remained stable.

When patients with newly diagnosed oral and oropharyngeal cancers are carefully examined, about 15% will have another cancer in a nearby area, such as the larynx, esophagus, or lung. Of those who attain a complete cure of oral or oropharyngeal cancer, about 10% will develop a second cancer in one of these organs.

20.1.2 Risk Factors

Smoking and alcohol consumption are the major risk factors for oral and pharyngeal cancers. They are independent risk factors but produce a synergistic effect when combined. Smoking is estimated to be responsible for 41% of oral and pharyngeal cancers in men and 15% in women worldwide. In addition, both smoking and drinking account for approximately three-fourths of all oral cancers in the United States. Compared with nonsmokers, heavy smokers have a 4- to 10-fold increased risk after adjustment for alcohol intake. After control for smoking, moderate drinkers have a 3-fold increased risk for oral cancer, and heavy drinkers have an 8- to 9-fold increased risk. The combination of heavy smoking and drinking results in a greater than 35-fold excess risk. The significant decrease in cigarette smoking is considered a major factor responsible for the decreases in oral and pharyngeal cancers in the United States.

Smokeless tobacco use is another risk factor in some populations; it is associated with relative risks for oral cancers and oral leukoplakia as great as that for cigarette smoking. Among users of snuff, cancerous lesions typically arise at the site where smokeless tobacco, or quid, is held in contact with the buccal mucosa or gingiva. Chewing quid containing betel leaves and lime is thought to contribute to the majority of cases in parts of India and Southeast Asia. However, the rate of smokeless tobacco use is still relatively low in the United States.

Although tobacco use and alcohol consumption are considered major risk factors for oral and pharyngeal cancers, heritable familial factors may also play a role. Some studies have found a significantly higher proportion of cancer within the families of patients with oral and pharyngeal cancer(risk 3-fold higher than the risk in families of noncancer controls). The familial aggregation seems to be associated with defective DNA repair capability. After adjustment for potentially confounding factors, including tobacco and alcohol consumption, patients with both a family history of cancer and mutagen sensitivity

Table 20.1 Number of squamous oral cavity cancers by subsites, excluding cancers of the salivary glands and nasopharynx

Sites	Number	Percentage
Tongue	2,123	43.1
Tonsils	1,153	23.4
Lip	447	9.1
Floor of mouth	383	7.8
Gum	237	4.8
Palate	219	4.5
Other/unspecified parts of mouth	360	7.3
All oral cavity cancers	4,922	100.0

Source: Data are from the Surveillance Epidemiology and End Results program, 2006, which covers 17 cancer registry areas of the United States.

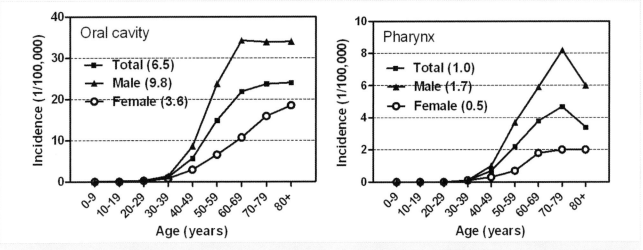

Fig. 20.1 Age-specific incidence of oral cavity and pharyngeal cancer, all races, Surveillance Epidemiology and End Results (SEER), 17 registry areas, 2006. The numbers in parentheses are age-adjusted incidence per 100,000.

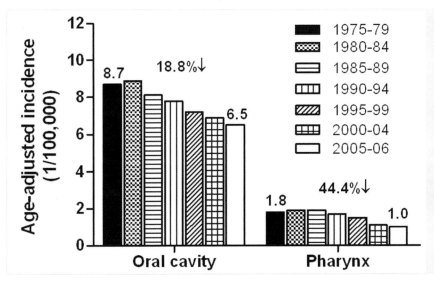

Fig. 20.2 Age-adjusted incidence of oral and pharyngeal cancers by time, Surveillance Epidemiology and End Results (SEER), 17 registry areas, 2006.

have a 7-fold or higher risk for oral and pharyngeal cancers in comparison with normal controls. The finding indicates the importance of genetic influence in the causation of the disease.

Oral human papillomavirous (HPV) infection is an additional risk factor for oral and pharyngeal cancers. Two types of HPV (types 16 and 18) seem to be the most carcinogenic and show a close correlation with *TP53* mutation. Overall estimates of HPV infection for oral neoplastic tissues are variable, ranging from 14 to 91%. Oral squamous carcinoma has an approximately 4-fold higher expression of HPV than normal oral mucosa. In addition, tumors of the oropharynx (in particular tonsillar tissue) have been found to be three times more likely to be HPV-positive than tumors at other sites in the head and neck. However, the exact relationship of HPV infection and carcinoma in the mouth and the role of cofactors are unknown. A low intake of fruits and vegetables is known to significantly increase the risk for oral and pharyngeal cancers.

20.2 Nasopharyngeal Cancer

20.2.1 Epidemiology

Nasopharyngeal cancer is a very rare malignancy in North America, Europe, and many regions of Asia, including Japan and Korea, where the incidence is less than 1 per 100,000. This cancer, however, is extremely common in southern regions of China, Southeast Asia, and North Africa. In Guangdong of China and in Hong Kong, the incidence of nasopharyngeal cancer is more than 20 per 100,000.

In 2002, roughly 80,000 new cases of nasopharyngeal cancer were diagnosed worldwide, and the estimated number of deaths exceeded 50,000. There are about 2,000 new cases each year in the United States. Most nasopharyngeal cancers are of the keratinizing type in the United States, whereas in Southeast Asia the undifferentiated type is most common.

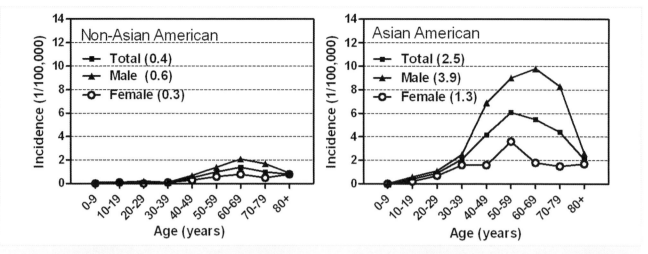

Fig. 20.3 Age-specific incidence of nasopharyngeal cancer by race, Surveillance Epidemiology and End Results (SEER), 17 registry areas, 2006. The numbers in parentheses are age-adjusted incidence per 100,000.

Nasopharyngeal cancer can occur in people younger than 40 years of age, suggesting a possible exposure to a common agent in early life. Young patients account for about 16% of all patients. The incidence of nasopharyngeal cancer increases with age, but the age peak is different in different races. In high-risk Asian Americans, the age peak is at 50 to 59 years, whereas in low-risk non-Asian Americans, the peak is at 60 to 69 years. The incidence of nasopharyngeal cancer is 2- to 3-fold higher in men than in women (▶ Fig. 20.3).

The incidence in descendants of Chinese who emigrate to the United States is significantly lower than that in native Chinese, but the rate remains six times higher than that in Caucasian Americans and African-Americans. Similarly high incidence rates have been observed among Chinese emigrants to the United Kingdom and Australia. The incidence risk for nasopharyngeal cancer seems to decrease with a longer duration of residence in Western nations.

The incidence of nasopharyngeal cancer has been high in Southeast Asia for several decades. However, the incidence of this cancer has declined gradually in Hong Kong since the 1970s, in Taiwan since the 1980s, and in Singapore Chinese since the late 1990s. A similar trend of decline has been noted in the United States between 1975–1979 and 2005–2006, during which time the incidence of the disease decreased 20% in whites, 38% in blacks, and 28% in other persons of races, such as Asians, Pacific Islanders, and Native Americans.

20.2.2 Risk Factors

Epstein-Barr virus (EBV) infection is a highly likely cause of nasopharyngeal cancer, and it distinguishes nasopharyngeal cancer from other oral cancers. EBV infection is a cause of the undifferentiated form of nasopharyngeal cancer recognized by International Agency for Research on Cancer (IARC). Many epidemiologic studies have observed that antibody titers and neutralizing antibodies against EBV-specific DNase are much higher among patients with nasopharyngeal cancer than among controls. In general, biopsy specimens of the undifferentiated form of this cancer are all EBV-positive and monoclonal

with regard to this virus. Specimens of severe dysplasia or carcinoma in situ of the nasopharynx are positive for EBV. However, the relationship between EBV infection and nasopharyngeal cancer is not entirely understood. An unexplainable fact is that all adults in areas of endemicity are infected with the virus, yet only a very small proportion of people develop nasopharyngeal cancer. In addition, it is unclear whether higher titers of EBV are a cause of or are caused by nasopharyngeal cancer—that is, whether EBV passively infects nasopharyngeal cancer cells or plays an active role in malignant transformation.

The intake of salt-preserved fish and other food is another risk factor. In southern China, boat-dwelling fishermen and their families consume a great deal of salted fish and other preserved foods, and the incidence of nasopharyngeal cancer in these people is extremely high. Traditionally, salted fish is used to wean infants in the Cantonese population, in which the incidence of nasopharyngeal cancer is as high as 20 per 100,000. The carcinogenic potential of salt-preserved fish is supported by experiments in rats, which develop malignant nasal and nasopharyngeal tumors after the consumption of salted fish. Salted fish contains varying amounts of volatile nitrosamines and bacterial mutagens. So far, however, the association of salt-preserved fish with nasopharyngeal cancer risk has not been proved by prospective studies.

Other suspected risk factors for nasopharyngeal cancer include genetic background; occupational exposures to fumes, dusts, or chemicals; low intake of fresh fruits and vegetables; tobacco smoking; use of herbal medicines; and previous chronic respiratory tract diseases. The familial aggregation of nasopharyngeal cancer has been widely reported. The risk is about 4- to 8-fold higher among first-degree relatives of patients with nasopharyngeal cancer than in those without a family history. Occupational exposure to wood dusts, fumes, or chemicals has also been noted to increase the risk for nasopharyngeal cancer. Individuals exposed to wood dust for 10 years or longer had an adjusted relative risk of 2.4; the risk was highest for those first exposed before the age of 25 years and in those seropositive for EBV.

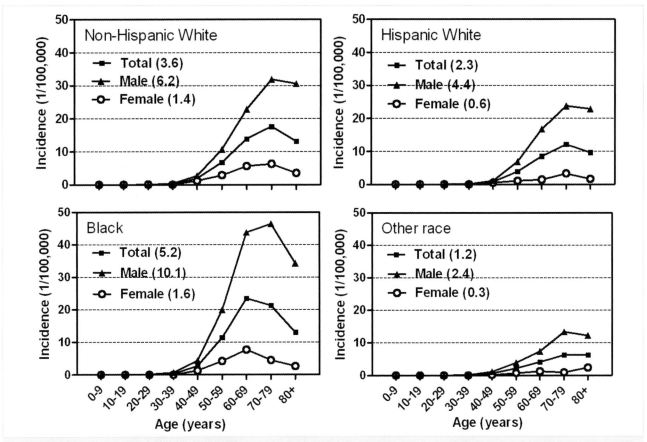

Fig. 20.4 Age-specific incidence of laryngeal cancer by race, Surveillance Epidemiology and End Results (SEER), 17 registry areas, 2006. The numbers in parentheses are age-adjusted incidence per 100,000.

20.3 Laryngeal Cancer

20.3.1 Epidemiology

More than 90% of cancers of the larynx are squamous cell carcinoma, and the majority originate from the supraglottic and glottic regions of the organ. Laryngeal cancer accounts for approximately 1 to 2% of all new cancer diagnoses, and its incidence varies by country. The incidence of laryngeal cancer is high in southern and central Europe, southern Brazil, Uruguay, and Argentina, whereas it is low in Southeast Asia and central Africa. A total of 140,000 new cases were diagnosed worldwide in 1990, of which 120,000 were in men. In the United States, the estimated number of new cases was 12,250 in 2008; 3,670 died of this disease.

Laryngeal cancer has an incidence pattern similar to that of cancers of the mouth and throat, occurring more often in men than in women, and more often in blacks than in whites. Rates among men range from a low of 2.4 per 100,000 in Asians, Pacific Islanders, and Native Americans to a high of 10.1 per 100,000 in blacks; rates for non-Hispanic whites and Hispanics are intermediate (6.2 per 100,000 and 4.4 per 100,000, respectively). Laryngeal cancer is much less common in women, with rates ranging from 0.3 per 100,000 in Asians, Pacific Islanders, and Native Americans to 1.6 per 100,000 in blacks. The male-

to-female ratios of disease incidence are 8:1 for Asians, Pacific Islanders, and American Indians; 7:1 for Hispanics; 6:1 for blacks; and 4:1 for non-Hispanic whites (▶ Fig. 20.4).

Laryngeal cancer is uncommon in patients younger than 40 years. The incidence of laryngeal cancer increases with age but decreases after the age of 70 years. The age-related peak incidence is as high as 46 per 100,000 in blacks, whereas it is about 32 per 100,000 in non-Hispanic whites, 22 per 100,000 in Hispanics, and 12 per 100,000 in other races.

As shown in ▶ Fig. 20.5, the age-adjusted incidence of laryngeal cancer significantly decreased between 1975–1979 and 2005–2006 in all racial groups (35% decrease in whites, 27% decrease in blacks, and 44% decrease in other racial populations). The incidence also significantly decreased with time in persons of all ages except for those 80+years of age. The magnitude of decrease varies by age, with larger decreases in younger age groups.

20.3.2 Risk Factors

As with cancers of the mouth, throat, and lung, smoking is the major cause of laryngeal cancer. Cigarette smokers have almost a 10-fold greater risk for laryngeal cancer than nonsmokers do, and risk increases with increased cigarette smoking. The smoking-related risk is also affected by alcohol use; the risk is highest

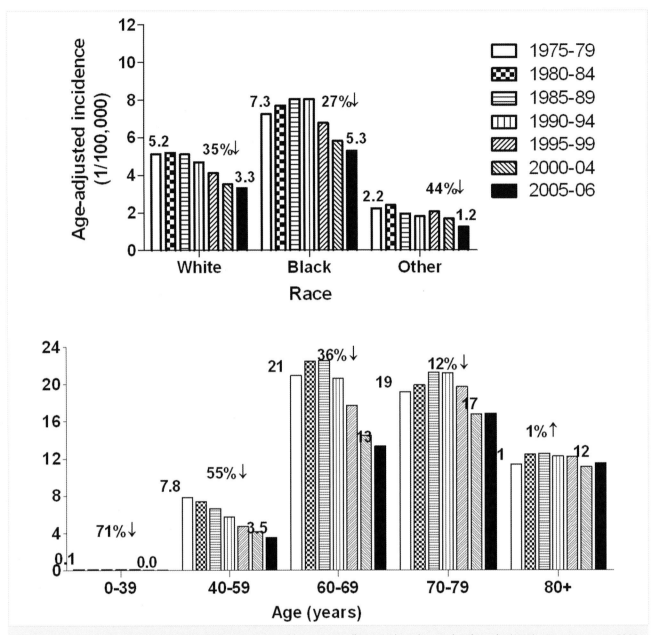

Fig. 20.5 Time trend of incidence of laryngeal cancer by race and by age, Surveillance Epidemiology and End Results (SEER), 17 registry areas, 2006.

among heavy smokers who are also heavy users of alcohol. The effect of tobacco is stronger for glottic than for supraglottic cancers. There is also a beneficial effect of quitting smoking. In addition, the effect of alcohol is stronger for supraglottic tumors than for tumors in other sites.

Additional risk factors for laryngeal cancer are occupational exposures to sulfuric acid, nickel, and asbestos; the link to sulfuric acid is best established. Occupational risk factors account for only a small fraction of all cases of laryngeal cancer.

HPV infection is also found to be associated with laryngeal cancer. Patients with laryngeal papillomatosis (associated with HPV-6 and HPV-11 infection) have an increased risk for laryngeal cancer. Herpes simplex virus type 1 is another virus with a possible causal role in laryngeal cancer.

20.4 Salivary Gland Cancer

20.4.1 Epidemiology

Salivary gland cancer is a rare malignancy, with an incidence rate of 1.5 per 100,000 people and 4,313 new cases in 2006 in the United States. Salivary gland cancer accounts for about 16% of all oral cavity cancers (squamous and nonsquamous). In contrast to other malignancies, salivary gland cancer shows very little international variation in incidence.

▶ Fig. 20.6 shows the incidence of salivary gland cancer among different races. The incidence is highest in non-Hispanic whites (1.6 per 100,000), whereas it ranges from 1.0 to 1.2 in other races. The incidence of salivary gland cancer increases

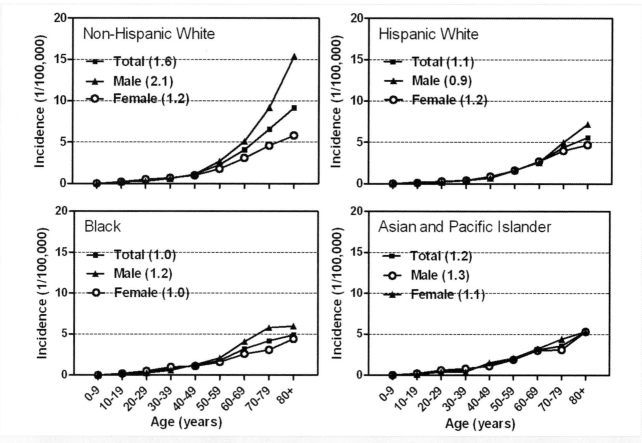

Fig. 20.6 Age-specific incidence of salivary gland cancer by race, Surveillance Epidemiology and End Results (SEER), 17 registry areas, 2006. The numbers in parentheses are age-adjusted incidence per 100,000.

with age. However, the age patterns of incidence differ between non-Hispanic whites and other racial populations; among people younger than 60 years old, the age patterns are similar in non-Hispanic whites and other races. However, the incidence of salivary gland cancer increases nearly 5 times (in non-Hispanic white males) and 2 times (in non-Hispanic white females) in persons 60 to 80 years old. Non-Hispanic male whites have a nearly 2 times higher incidence than non-Hispanic female whites, but there is no similar sex difference among other racial populations except for people who are 60 years of age or older.

The incidence of salivary gland cancer has increased 30 to 40% in the past 25 to 30 years in the United States in all ages and races (▶ Fig. 20.7). This trend has also been noted in other countries. The reasons for this increase are not well understood.

20.4.2 Risk Factors

Exposure to radiation is a well-established risk factor for salivary gland cancer. Strong evidence comes from the excess risk for salivary gland cancer among survivors of atomic bomb attacks. Additional evidence comes from the findings of exposure to prior dental radiography and therapeutic radiation, workplace exposure to certain radioactive substances, and exposure to ultraviolet B radiation.

Other risk factors for salivary gland cancer include smoking; alcohol drinking; EBV, HPV, and AIDS virus infections; certain occupational exposures; family history; low intake of vegeta-

bles; and cell phone use. However, the association of these risk factors with salivary gland cancer is relatively weak and sometimes controversial. For instance, smoking and heavy alcohol drinking are associated with a 1-fold higher risk for salivary gland cancer, whereas the risks of both factors are more than 2-fold higher when they are associated with other oral and pharyngeal cancers. As for viral association, EBV is found to be associated with lymphoepithelioma-like carcinoma of the salivary gland only among Asian patients. In addition, HPV does not appear to be associated with second cancers of the salivary gland. In occupational exposures, a high risk for salivary gland cancer has been observed among hairdressers and those working in beauty shops, indicating a possible hazard from dyes, sprays, and other inhaled chemicals. Moreover, an increased risk is also observed among workers who are exposed to nickel alloy dust or silica dust. However, these occupation-related links are still inconclusive because of the rarity of salivary gland cancer in those occupational populations. Although one study reported an increased risk for parotid gland tumors among heavy cell phone users, the link has been not proved by other studies.

20.5 Thyroid Cancer

20.5.1 Epidemiology

Thyroid cancer accounts for 2.6% of all malignancies. In the United States, 37,340 new cases of thyroid cancer were estimated

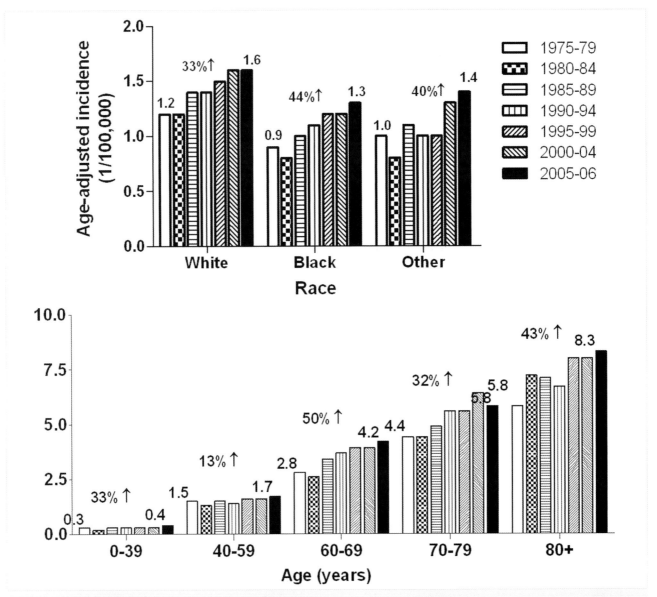

Fig. 20.7 Time trend of incidence of salivary gland cancer by race and by age, Surveillance Epidemiology and End Results (SEER), 17 registry areas, 2006.

in 2008, of which 28,410 were in women and 8,930 in men. About 1,590 people (910 women and 680 men) died of thyroid cancer in 2008. Thyroid cancer is one of the five most common cancers occurring among women ages 15 to 44 years. Most thyroid cancers are papillary (85%); the rest are follicular (9.6%), medullary (2.0%), or anaplastic (0.7%; ▶ Table 20.2).

Thyroid cancers occur in all age groups (▶ Fig. 20.8). Whereas the incidence of most other cancers increases markedly with age, the incidence of papillary thyroid cancer is highest in female adults 40 to 59 years of age and then decreases sharply as age increases. The age-related peak incidence of papillary tumor occurs later in males than in females. The incidence rates of other histologic types of thyroid cancer increase with age and reach a peak in the eighth decade.

In the United States, the highest age-adjusted incidence rate for thyroid cancer occurs in non-Hispanic whites (9.5 per

Table 20.2 Distribution of histologic type of thyroid cancer, all races, Surveillance Epidemiology and End Results (SEER), 17 registry areas, 2006

Histology	Number	Percentage
Papillary	7,042	85.1
Follicular	795	9.6
Medullary	163	2.0
Anaplastic	60	0.7
Others	215	2.6
Total	8,275	100.0

Source: Data are from the Surveillance Epidemiology and End Results program, 2006, which covers 17 cancer registry areas of the United States.

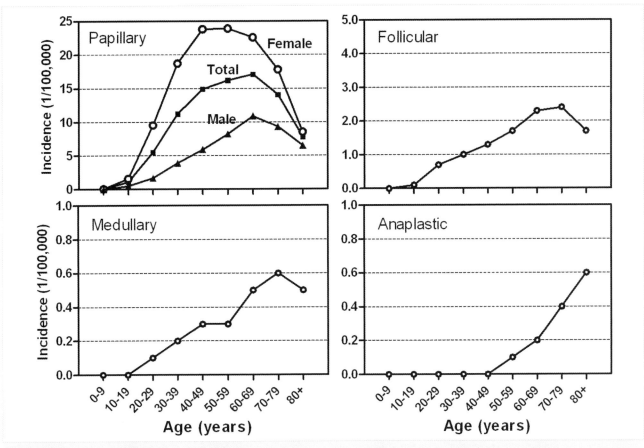

Fig. 20.8 Age-specific incidence by type of thyroid cancer, all races, Surveillance Epidemiology and End Results (SEER), 17 registry areas, 2006.

100,000) and Filipinos (9.3 per 100,000), whereas the lowest rates are seen in Native Americans (4.4 per 100,000) and African-Americans (5.0 per 100,000); moderate rates are noted in Asians and Pacific Islanders (8.6 per 100,000), Hispanic whites (7.7 per 100,000), and Chinese (5.5 per 100,000).

Thyroid cancer, mainly papillary thyroid cancer, has been increasing since the 1940s. The increase is characterized by continuity in time and significance in magnitude. From 1973 to 2006, the incidence of papillary thyroid cancer increased more than 2-fold in the United States (age-adjusted rates of 2.7 per 100,000 in 1973 and 9.4 per 100,000 in 2006). Medullary thyroid cancer showed a similar trend, but follicular and anaplastic thyroid cancers did not. The increase in papillary and medullary thyroid cancers has been observed in many other regions of the world, including Canada, the United Kingdom, Sweden, France, and Norway.

▶ Fig. 20.9 shows that papillary thyroid cancers other than microscopic tumors and tumors 5 cm in size or larger increased in frequency between 1992–1996 and 2000–2004 in all racial/ethnic groups in the United States other than Native Americans Indians/Alaska Natives.

20.5.2 Risk Factors

Radiation exposure is a well-known risk factor for thyroid cancer. Its effect was initially recognized in the 1930s and 1940s, when X-rays were often used in the treatment of skin diseases and other benign conditions, such as enlarged thymus or tonsils. Subsequently, an increased risk for thyroid cancer was observed in Japanese survivors of the atomic bomb, in persons exposed to fallout from atomic testing in the Marshall Islands, and in persons exposed to nuclear contaminations from the Chernobyl nuclear disaster. In general, the risk associated with X-rays is increased about 2- to 3-fold, but this increase rises to 10-fold or greater with exposure to nuclear radiation. In addition to therapeutic X-rays and nuclear radiation, some investigators also suspect that diagnostic X-rays (the most common human-made source of radiation exposure) may play a role in the occurrence of thyroid cancer. However, the effect of diagnostic X-rays remains controversial, and data appear weak.

Female hormones have been also considered a risk factor for thyroid cancer. Supporting evidence include that (1) females have 2- to 3-fold higher incidence of thyroid cancer than males; (2) the association is more pronounced for the papillary type than for the follicular type among young women; (3) the elevated levels of female hormones can promote thyroid hyperplasia; (4) pregnancy is associated with elevations in both estrogen and thyroid hormone levels; (5) pregnancy and early menopause appear to enhance the risk for thyroid cancer; and (6) risk is reduced for women who have never used oral contraceptives. However, the association between female hormones and thyroid cancer is still incompletely understood. For example, it remains unclear how female hormones influence thyroid carcinogenesis. In addition, there is no time consistency between

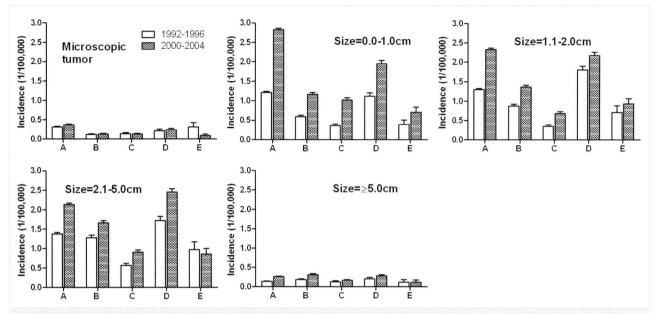

Fig. 20.9 Incidence of papillary thyroid cancer by race and two time periods: 1992–1996 and 2000–2004, Surveillance Epidemiology and End Results (SEER). *A*, non-Hispanic white; *B*, Hispanic white; *C*, black; *D*, Asian; *E*, American Indian/Alaska Native.

the increased use of female hormones and increased trend of thyroid cancer.

Iodine, which is essential in the synthesis of thyroid hormones, is an additional suspected risk factor for thyroid cancer. This is based on the positive correlation between either iodine deficiency (epidemic goiter) or iodine excess and the incidence and mortality of thyroid cancer. However, the findings also cannot explain the observed temporal trend of thyroid cancer. In general, iodine exposure is believed to have at most a weak effect on the risk for papillary thyroid cancer.

Cigarette smoking appears to have a protective effect for thyroid cancer; this may be a consequence of lowering the levels of endogenous thyroid hormones: thyroxine (T_4) and thyroid-stimulating hormone (TSH). In addition, smoking may have an anti-estrogenic effect.

Some have postulated that the increased incidence may be caused by enhanced diagnosis due to the increased use of new diagnostic techniques such as computed tomography, ultrasound, and fine needle aspiration biopsy. However, it is unlikely that new technologies would make a disease continuously increase year by year for decades. Second, many thyroid tumors can be detected by patients themselves when the tumor becomes symptomatic, including those tumors about 1 cm in size. Third, even though new diagnostic techniques can help find some subclinical tumors, the increase in cancer cases can be still explained by any of the following three scenarios: (1) Subclinical tumors do not increase, but diagnostic scrutiny increases; (2) subclinical tumors increase, but diagnostic scrutiny does not increase; and (3) both subclinical tumors and diagnostic scrutiny increase. Because one does not know whether there is a substantial increase in the number of nonlethal subclinical tumors hiding in the reservoir of the thyroid glands of the general population and whether the perceived increase via abnormal symptoms leads more patients to seek a clinical diag-

nosis, the possibility of a true increase of thyroid cancer cannot be excluded.

The thyroid is very sensitive to the stimulation of various factors. Because it is located superficially in the body, it may be more easily influenced by environmental carcinogenic factors. Suspected factors for the increased trend include the impact of nuclear fallout, increased use of hormone replacement therapy (HRT), increased use of diagnostic X-rays, and increased use of wireless phones. However, current data supporting the association of these factors with the increase of thyroid cancer are lacking. For instance, the incidence of thyroid cancer had already increased before nuclear fallout, and local atmospheric fallout is less likely to affect populations living in distant locations to the same degree. In addition, several large epidemiologic studies did not find any association between the use of exogenous estrogens and the risk for female thyroid cancer, and the factor of HRT cannot explain the increased trend of thyroid cancer in males. Although the increased uses of diagnostic X-rays and wireless phones are quite suspicious, evidence for both factors is lacking.

20.6 Roundsmanship

- Oral and pharyngeal cancer, considered together, is the sixth most common form of cancer in the world. Of all squamous oral and pharyngeal cancers (excluding salivary gland and nasopharyngeal cancers), oral cavity cancers account for nearly 88% and pharyngeal cancers about 12%. In addition, most squamous oral cavity cancers occur in the tongue (43.1%) and tonsillar fossa (23.4%). Smoking and alcohol consumption are the major risk factors for oral and pharyngeal cancers.
- Nasopharyngeal cancer is extremely common in southern regions of China, Southeast Asia, and North Africa. The incidence among the descendants of Chinese who emigrate to the

United States is significantly lower than that among native Chinese, but the rate remains six times higher than that among Caucasian Americans and African-Americans. Epstein-Barr virus infection is a cause of the undifferentiated form of nasopharyngeal cancer recognized by the International Agency for Research on Cancer (IARC). The intake of salt-preserved fish and other food is another risk factor. Other suspected risk factors for nasopharyngeal cancer include genetic background; occupational exposures to fumes, dusts, or chemicals; low intake of fresh fruits and vegetables; tobacco smoking; use of herbal medicines; and previous chronic respiratory tract diseases.

- More than 90% of cancers of the larynx are squamous cell carcinoma, and the majority originate in the supraglottic and glottic regions. Laryngeal cancer accounts for approximately 1 to 2% of all new cancer diagnoses and is more common in southern and central Europe, southern Brazil, Uruguay, and Argentina. It is seen less frequently in southeastern Asia and central Africa. As with cancers of the mouth, throat, and lung, smoking is the major cause of laryngeal cancer. Cigarette smokers have almost a 10-fold greater risk for laryngeal cancer than nonsmokers, and risk increases with as cigarette smoking increases. The smoking-related risk is also affected by alcohol use; the risk is highest among heavy smokers who are also heavy users of alcohol.
- Salivary gland cancer is a rare malignancy, with an incidence rate of 1.5 per 100,000 in 2006 in the United States. Exposure to radiation is a well-established risk factor for salivary gland cancer.

- Thyroid cancer accounts for 2.6% of all malignancies. Most thyroid cancers are papillary (85%), while the rest are follicular (9.6%), medullary (2.0%), and anaplastic (0.7%). Radiation exposure is a well-known risk factor for thyroid cancer.

20.7 Recommended Reading

[1] Adami HO, Hunter D, Trichopoulos D. Textbook of Cancer Epidemiology. 1st ed. New York, NY: Oxford University Press; 2002
[2] Bosetti C, Gallus S, Peto R et al. Tobacco smoking, smoking cessation, and cumulative risk of upper aerodigestive tract cancers. Am J Epidemiol 2008; 167: 468–473
[3] Chang ET, Adami HO. The enigmatic epidemiology of nasopharyngeal carcinoma. Cancer Epidemiol Biomarkers Prev 2006; 15: 1765–1777
[4] Herrero R, Castellsagué X, Pawlita M et alIARC Multicenter Oral Cancer Study Group. Human papillomavirus and oral cancer: the International Agency for Research on Cancer multicenter study. J Natl Cancer Inst 2003; 95: 1772–1783
[5] Sun EC, Curtis R, Melbye M, Goedert JJ. Salivary gland cancer in the United States. Cancer Epidemiol Biomarkers Prev 1999; 8: 1095–1100
[6] National Institutes of Health, National Cancer Institute. Surveillance Epidemiology and End Results. Surveillance Research Program, Cancer Statistics Branch. Released April 2009, based on November 2008 submission. . Accessed October 14, 2013
[7] Warnakulasuriya S. Global epidemiology of oral and oropharyngeal cancer. Oral Oncol 2009; 45: 309–316
[8] Yu GP, Li JC, Branovan D, McCormick S, Schantz SP. Thyroid cancer incidence and survival in the national cancer institute surveillance, epidemiology, and end results race/ethnicity groups. Thyroid 2010; 20: 465–473
[9] Yu GP, Zhang ZF, Hsu TC, Spitz MR, Schantz SP. Family history of cancer, mutagen sensitivity, and increased risk of head and neck cancer. Cancer Lett 1999; 146: 93–101

21 Head and Neck Histopathology

Codrin E. Iacob

21.1 Introduction

The relation between surgeon and pathologist has been masterfully described by Dr. Lauren V. Ackerman in an early edition of his surgical pathology textbook: "A good surgeon has not only technical dexterity (a fairly common commodity), but also, more importantly, good judgment and personal concern for his patient's welfare. The surgeon with a prepared mind and a clear concept of the pathology of disease invariably is the one with good judgment. Without this background of knowledge, he will not recognize specific pathologic alterations at surgery nor will he have a clear concept of the limitations of his knowledge, and therefore he will not know when to call the pathologist to help him. Without this basic knowledge, he may improve his technical ability but never his judgment. One might say that with him his ignorance is refined rather than his judgment."[1]

Rather than the memorization of specific microscopic images of certain pathologic processes, practicing head and neck surgeons are better served by an understanding of the general principles that guide tissue analysis in a pathology laboratory: the possibilities and limitations of tissue analysis; the advantages and possibilities of minimally invasive tissue examination techniques (e.g., fine-needle aspiration); the various special studies that can be conducted (e.g., microbiological cultures, frozen sections, molecular analysis of neoplastic tissues, conventional cytogenetics, molecular investigations for the identification of infectious agents, flow cytometry examinations, immunohistochemistry, histochemical techniques, immunofluorescence examinations, electron microscopy); the particulars of tissue submission (fresh, frozen, or fixed tissue); and the specific indications and time course of each test. Facing this vast and dynamic domain of laboratory analyses, head and neck surgeons can best help their patients by keeping in close contact with their pathologists via preoperative, intraoperative, and postoperative communication in an effort to integrate all clinical, imaging, and laboratory information into a comprehensive diagnostic and treatment plan.

21.2 Fine Needle Aspiration

Simple and cost-effective, fine-needle aspiration (FNA) is used as a tool for the initial screening of lesions of the glands (thyroid, salivary, and lacrimal), lymph nodes, and any neoplasm of the head and neck. There are no contraindications to FNA, although patients with a bleeding diathesis may be more susceptible to the development of a local hematoma. FNA of malignant lesions is frequently performed, and the likelihood of tumor implantation along the needle tract is considered negligible. FNA is done by palpation or under ultrasound or computed tomographic (CT) guidance. Immediate assessment of the adequacy of sampling (generally six clusters of five to 10 diagnostic cells)[2] is desirable. If the sample is adequate, part of the fresh tissue sample may be used for other ancillary studies (microbiology cultures, flow cytometry, immunohistochemistry), whereas the procedure should be repeated in case of an insufficient first sample. Smears should be prepared immediately after the procedure and rapidly fixed in 95% alcohol to avoid air drying. Tissue remaining in the syringe should never be discarded because it usually is sufficiently cellular for a cell block (solid deposit of spun-down fluid that is fixed in formalin and then processed like a tissue sample) to be formed, allowing serial sectioning of the paraffin block and further histochemical or immunohistochemical staining. Correlation among the clinical, imaging, and morphological findings significantly raises the accuracy of FNA interpretation.

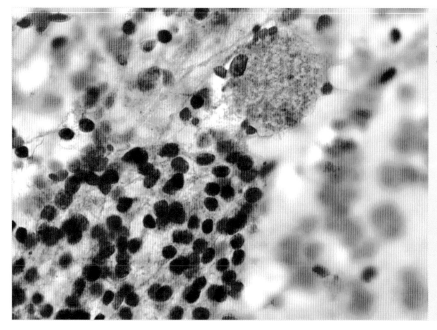

Fig. 21.1 Fine-needle aspiration biopsy of a goiter shows a flat sheet of benign follicular cells with a macrofollicular arrangement and hemosiderin-laden macrophages.

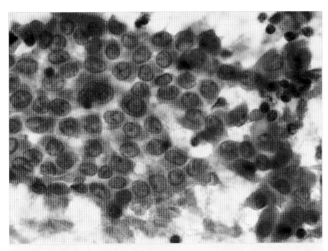

Fig. 21.2 This fine-needle aspiration biopsy is consistent with papillary carcinoma and demonstrates uniform, marked enlargement of nuclei with clear chromatin, irregular nuclear contours, nuclear grooves, and an intranuclear pseudoinclusion. Papillary carcinoma samples are usually hypercellular with solid or papillary architecture, enlarged nuclei with conspicuous nucleoli, and occasional intranuclear pseudoinclusions. Psammoma bodies (concentric calcium depositions), corresponding to sonographically identified microcalcifications, are very characteristic but rarely present in aspirates. Papillary carcinoma accounts for up to 80% of all thyroid malignancies

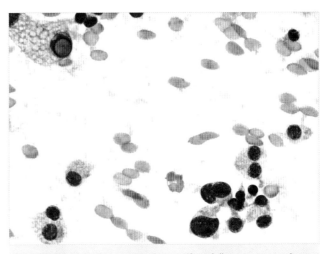

Fig. 21.3 Fine-needle aspiration biopsy of medullary carcinoma demonstrates round to elongated atypical nuclei with a stippled chromatin pattern (neuroendocrine type), occasional binucleation, and an intranuclear pseudoinclusion. Medullary carcinoma, a neuroendocrine malignancy arising from calcitonin-producing C cells of the thyroid, rarely has background amyloid.

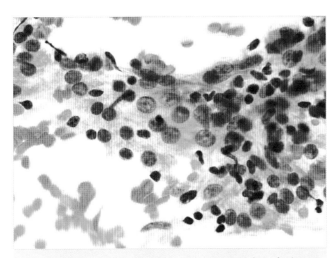

Fig. 21.4 Hashimoto thyroiditis (chronic lymphocytic thyroiditis) can be diagnosed on fine-needle aspiration biopsy when cytologically bland follicular cells with focal pink granular cytoplasm (oncocytic metaplasia) and diffuse lymphocytic infiltration are noted; occasional multinucleated histiocytes are seen.

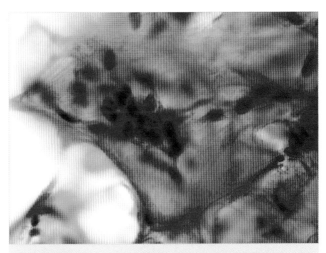

Fig. 21.5 Fine-needle aspiration (FNA) biopsy specimen from a pleomorphic adenoma shows a cluster of cytologically benign myoepithelial cells and ductal epithelial cells in a myxoid background with spindle mesenchymal cells. Pleomorphic adenoma, basal cell adenoma (monomorphic adenoma), and myoepithelioma may appear similar on FNA.

21.2.1 Fine Needle Aspiration of the Thyroid

FNA of the thyroid allows an assessment of the morphology of follicular cells and their nuclei, tissue architecture, colloid quality, and background (i.e., degenerative, inflammatory, neoplastic, necrotic). Benign follicular processes include follicular adenomas with macrofollicular architecture, as well as hyperplastic and colloid nodules in goiters. These are slowly growing lesions that can be clinically observed. They are all character-ized by moderately cellular samples with abundant colloid, variously degenerative background, and tissue fragments disposed in flat sheets with predominantly macrofollicular architecture (▶ Fig. 21.1). Suspicious follicular processes include follicular adenomas with a microfollicular growth pattern, follicular carcinomas, and follicular variants of papillary carcinomas, all of which yield hypercellular aspirates with microfollicular architecture, little or no colloid, and various tridimensional clusters; often, nuclear atypia is also present. Papillary carcinoma samples are usually hypercellular with solid or papillary architecture, enlarged nuclei with conspicuous nucleoli. Medullary carcinoma, a neuroendocrine malignancy, arises from calcitonin-producing C cells of the thyroid (▶ Fig. 21.2 and ▶ Fig. 21.3).

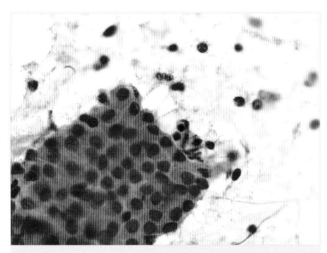

Fig. 21.6 Warthin tumor on fine-needle aspiration biopsy consists of a flat sheet of benign epithelial cells with oncocytic metaplasia in a lymphocytic background.

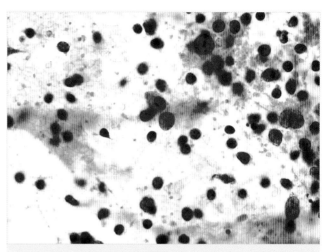

Fig. 21.7 Fine-needle aspiration biopsy of a reactive lymph node shows predominantly small lymphocytes (mainly B cells) but also a range of other lymphocytes, including cells of germinal center origin (centroblasts and centrocytes); in addition, tingible body macrophages (containing irregularly staining debris resulting from phagocytosis) and follicular dendritic cells are encountered. Occasional immunoblasts and plasma cells from the paracortex or medulla may also be present.

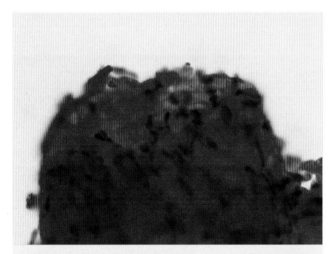

Fig. 21.8 Granulomatous lymphadenitis on fine-needle aspiration biopsy (FNA) is characterized by a dense cluster of spindle histiocytes with abundant pink cytoplasm and focal lymphocytic infiltration with occasional multinucleated giant cells in a necrotic background. All reveal clusters of histiocytes. A diagnosis of granulomatous lymphadenitis, such as cat-scratch disease or mycobacterial lymphadenitis, by FNA should be followed by microbiology cultures of the aspirate. By contrast, sarcoidosis lacks necrosis and harbors well-formed, compact gramulomas.

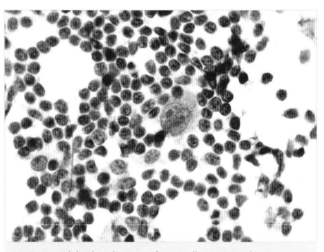

Fig. 21.9 Hodgkin lymphoma on fine-needle aspiration biopsy is diagnosed by the presence of Reed-Sternberg cells, which have a multilobed nucleus and prominent nucleoli, in a background of reactive lymphocytes. These cells are immunoreactive to CD30 and CD15.

Other malignancies, like poorly differentiated (insular) carcinoma, undifferentiated (anaplastic) carcinoma, lymphomas, and parathyroid tumors, can also be diagnosed on FNA, albeit with greater difficulty. The diagnosis of Hashimoto thyroiditis (chronic lymphocytic thyroiditis) can be made if bland follicular cells with focal pink granular cytoplasm (oncocytic metaplasia) and diffuse lymphocytic infiltration are noted (▶ Fig. 21.4).

Subacute granulomatous thyroiditis (de Quervain thyroiditis) on FNA displays frequent multinucleated giant cell histiocytes and benign follicular cells. A correct diagnosis on FNA avoids unnecessary surgery in these patients. Rare pathologic thyroid processes like Riedel thyroiditis and black thyroid (seen with the chronic use of tetracyclines, especially minocycline) are also rarely diagnosed on FNA.

21.2.2 Fine Needle Aspiration of the Salivary Glands

Chronic sialadenitis, frequently associated with sialolithiasis, usually shows acini and ductal epithelial cells with variable background lymphocytes. Salivary gland cysts (ranula and mucocele) show similar patterns of inflammatory cells in a proteinaceous background with more or less mucin. Pleomorphic adenoma is characterized by a cluster of cytologically benign

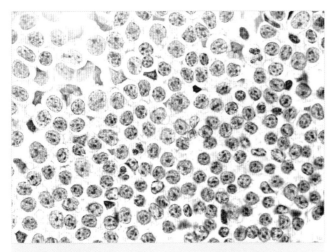

Fig. 21.10 Mantle cell lymphoma on fine-needle aspiration biopsy is characterized by monotonous, medium-size lymphocytes with vesicular nuclei and occasional conspicuous basophilic nucleoli.

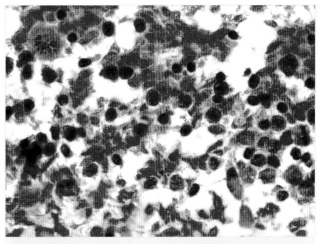

Fig. 21.11 Diffuse large B-cell lymphoma on fine-needle aspiration biopsy is recognized by large pleomorphic lymphocytes with irregular nuclear contours, hyperchromatism, frequent mitoses, and a "dirty" background comprising lymphoreticular bodies (cellular debris caused by the high turnover of neoplastic cells).

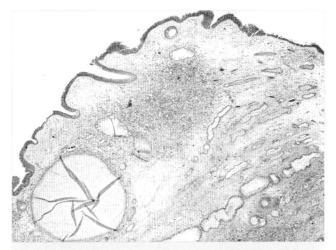

Fig. 21.12 Rhinitis and sinusitis are mostly of viral origin but sometime complicated by superimposed bacterial infections. Chronic sinusitis with inflammatory polyps demonstrates a diffuse chronic inflammatory infiltrate and eosinophilic infiltrate accompanied by lamina propria edema, focal mucus retention cyst formation, thickening of the basement membrane, and an unremarkable surface epithelium.

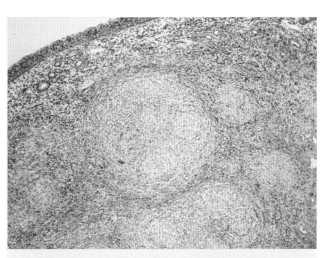

Fig. 21.13 Sarcoidosis affects the upper respiratory tract, lungs, and mediastinal lymph nodes. Histologically, there are well-formed, non-necrotizing granulomas with compact epithelioid histiocytes and occasional giant cells; note the unremarkable surface epithelium of the respiratory tract with underlying normal mucous glands.

myoepithelial cells and ductal epithelial cells in a myxoid background with spindle mesenchymal cell (▶ Fig. 21.5). By contrast, Warthin tumor displays a flat sheet of benign epithelial cells with oncocytic metaplasia in a lymphocytic background (▶ Fig. 21.6).

FNA biopsies of adenoid cystic carcinoma are usually hypercellular, with monotonous basaloid cells harboring angulated hyperchromatic nuclei and scant cytoplasm; microcysts and hyaline globules are frequently present. In mucoepidermoid carcinoma, FNA samples show large amount of mucin, intermediate cells (smaller uniform cells), and epithelial cells with epidermoid differentiation (intercellular bridging). Acinic cell carcinoma is composed of acinar cells with granular eosinophilic cytoplasm and various degrees of nuclear atypia.

21.2.3 Fine Needle Aspiration of the Lymph Nodes (▶ Fig. 21.7)

Acute lymphadenitis is characterized by excess neutrophils with scattered elements of a reactive lymphoid process; rarely, the etiologic agent (bacteria, fungi, or parasites) can also be identified (▶ Fig. 21.8).

Kimura disease is characterized by a dense eosinophilic background with reactive lymphocytic features and prominent vasculature. Kikuchi lymphadenitis is a subacute necrotizing condition with a large number of histiocytes and a complete lack of neutrophils. Sinus histiocytosis with massive lymphadenopathy (Rosai-Dorfman disease) harbors a reactive lymphoid pattern with numerous large, epithelioid background histiocytes that

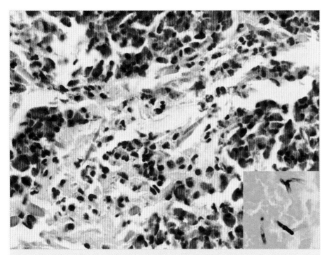

Fig. 21.14 Fungal disease of the sinonasal tract can be invasive (acute fulminant), noninvasive (mycetoma or "fungus ball"), or most frequently, as seen here, allergic. The specimen shows compact clusters of partially degenerated eosinophils, plasma cells, lymphocytes, cellular debris, and few spindled Charcot-Leyden crystals in a mucinous background. The inset shows fungal hyphae (Gomori methenamine silver stain).

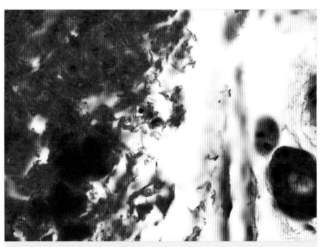

Fig. 21.15 Fungus ball (mycetoma) demonstrates noninvasive, dense, compact groups of fungal hyphae with neighboring unremarkable mucinous gland (periodic acid–Schiff stain). Cultures are recommended for identification of the causative fungus.

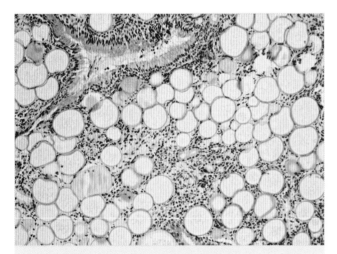

Fig. 21.16 Rhinosporidiosis has numerous thick-walled cysts or sporangia with a diameter of 100 to 300 μm containing numerous endospores in the mucosal lamina propria with a chronic inflammatory reaction.

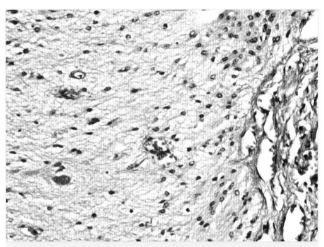

Fig. 21.17 Glial heterotopia, a congenital displacement of neuroglial tissue, can be found in the subcutaneous tissue of the nose (60%), in the upper nasal cavity (30%), and less frequently in the ethmoid sinus, palate, middle ear, tonsil, and pharyngeal area. Note the haphazardly distributed astrocytes with rare nucleolated large neurons in a generally fibrillary background (neuropil) and a fibrous reaction. An encephalocele is a developmental abnormality in which neuroglial tissue is present in the nasal cavity or middle ear and retains a connection to the central nervous system. Glial heterotopia and encephalocele both show a mixture of glial tissue, including astrocytes and neurons admixed with fibrovascular connective tissue, and are often distinguished by imaging studies only.

have specific immunohistochemical features (S-100–positive while CD1a- and Langerin-negative). Characteristically, foci of lymphocytes are engulfed in histiocytic cytoplasm (emperipolesis). Hodgkin lymphoma is diagnosed by the presence of Reed-Sternberg cells in a background of reactive lymphocytes (▶ Fig. 21.9).

Small lymphocytic lymphoma displays monotonous small lymphocytes with hyperchromatic nuclei and slight nuclear contour angulation; elements of a reactive lymphoid process are typically absent. Mantle cell lymphoma is characterized by medium-size lymphocytes with vesicular nuclei (▶ Fig. 21.10). Follicular lymphoma comprises cleaved cells (small, medium, or large). Aspirates of marginal zone B-cell lymphoma (MALT

lymphoma) contain small and intermediate-size lymphocytes with an increased number of monocytoid cells. Diffuse large B-cell lymphoma is identified by large pleomorphic lymphocytes with irregular nuclear contours, hyperchromatism and frequent mitoses (▶ Fig. 21.11).

For peripheral T-cell lymphoma and anaplastic large cell lymphoma, immunologic investigation is required to identify their T-cell origin. Plasmacytoma and multiple myeloma can yield hypercellular aspirates composed of seas of atypical plasma

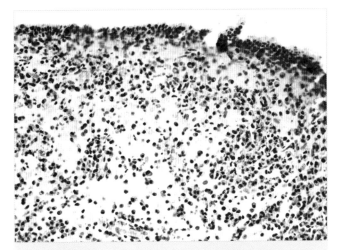

Fig. 21.18 Sinus histiocytosis with massive lymphadenopathy (Rosai-Dorfman disease) is an idiopathic disorder with significant lymphatic enlargement and secondary involvement of the nasal cavity, orbit, and other head and neck sites. Histologically, there are large infiltrating histiocytes (immunoreactive to CD68 and S-100 while CD1a- and Langerin-negative) with marked accompanying chronic inflammation in the mucosal lamina propria. Characteristically, the histiocytes show foci of emperipolesis (lymphocyte engulfment into histiocytic cytoplasm).

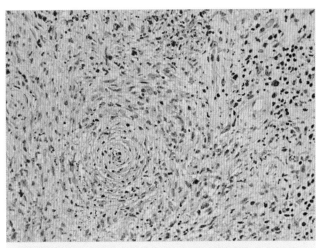

Fig. 21.19 Wegener granulomatosis is a systemic vasculitic process involving the upper and lower respiratory tract and kidneys. Note the vasculitis with complete vessel destruction and fibrinoid necrosis (center of image) surrounded by a granulomatous histiocytic reaction and eosinophilic infiltration.

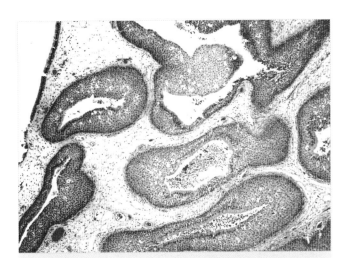

Fig. 21.20 Inverted papilloma histologically displays multiple islands of multilayered stratified epithelium proliferating inward in the mucosal lamina propria; note the overlying unremarkable, thin, respiratory type of epithelium.

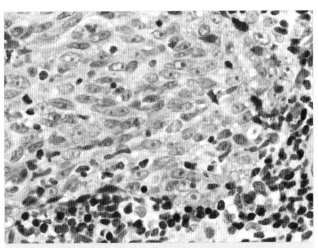

Fig. 21.21 Nasopharyngeal carcinoma, undifferentiated. Syncytial growth of undifferentiated malignant epithelial cells with indistinguishable cell borders and prominent nucleoli is seen. Nasopharyngeal carcinoma is most common in Southeast Asia and has a nearly constant association with Epstein-Barr virus. It affects both genders beyond the age of 30 years with a peak at 40 to 60 years. Its most frequent location is in the lateral wall of the nasopharynx (especially the fossa of Rosenmüller), followed by the superior posterior wall; it commonly presents with cervical metastases.

cells with binucleation, pleomorphic nuclei, and oftentimes visible nucleoli.

21.2.4 Fine Needle Aspiration of Cysts

Regardless of whether the source is a branchial cleft cyst, thyroglossal duct cyst, benign lymphoepithelial cyst of the parotid, or odontogenic cyst, these lesions as a group may show only nonspecific benign epithelial cells in an inflammatory background on FNA, and the results of FNA should be always correlated with the clinical findings.

21.3 Tissue Pathology

21.3.1 Nasal Cavity, Paranasal Sinuses, and Nasopharynx

Infectious/Inflammatory/Anatomic/Idiopathic (▶ Fig. 21.12 and ▶ Fig. 21.13)

Rhinitis and sinusitis are mostly of viral origin but sometime complicated by superimposed bacterial infections (▶ Fig. 21.12). Sarcoidosis displays e well-formed, nonnecrotizing granulomas

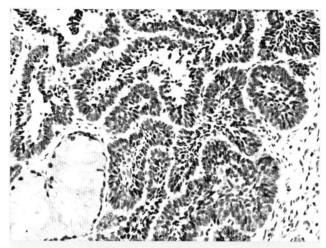

Fig. 21.22 Nonkeratinizing (cylindrical cell) carcinoma has a ribbonlike growth of atypical epithelial cells lacking maturation (no keratin production); note invasion by pushing border next to mucous gland of respiratory epithelium.

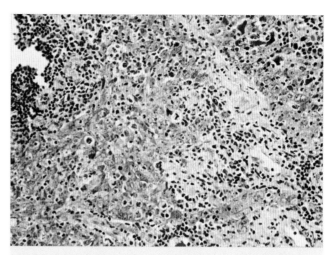

Fig. 21.23 Sinonasal undifferentiated carcinoma is a highly aggressive malignancy that typically presents with locally extensive disease and is typically negative for Epstein-Barr virus. It displays undifferentiated epithelial cells in small nests, trabeculae, or sheets, with a high nuclear-to-cytoplasmic ratio, frequent mitoses, and large areas of necrosis. Despite aggressive management, this tumor has poor prognosis.

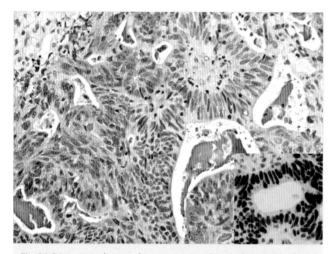

Fig. 21.24 Intestinal-type adenocarcinoma of sinus displays invading malignant epithelium with back-to-back irregular glands formed of columnar epithelial cells and occasional goblet cells with hyperchromatic nuclei. Inset shows nuclear labeling with CDX-2 immunohistochemical stain. Intestinal-type adenocarcinoma involves the ethmoid sinus (40%), nasal cavity (27%), and maxillary sinus (20%). Some of these tumors histologically simulate normal intestinal structures like Paneth cells, enterochromaffin cells, muscularis mucosae, and villi.

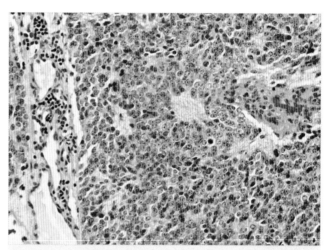

Fig. 21.25 Olfactory neuroblastoma (esthesioneuroblastoma) is a malignant neuroectodermal tumor arising from the olfactory membrane in the superior part of nasal cavity with intracranial and/or paranasal sinus extension. The tumors characteristically grow in the submucosa in circumscribed lobules or nests separated by richly vascularized fibrous stroma. Their cells harbor stippled nuclear chromatin ("salt and pepper") and scant cytoplasm. Some tumors show rosette formation (Homer-Wright pseudorosettes or Flexner-Wintersteiner real rosettes); some contain areas of necrosis. Based on the degree of differentiation, nuclear pleomorphism, necrosis, and mitotic activity, they are graded (patients with Hyam grades I and II tumors have better survival rates than those with Hyam grades III and IV tumors). The tumors are positive for neuroendocrine markers and negative for cytokeratin, and they display specific S-100–positive sustentacular cells at the periphery of tumor lobules.

with compact epithelioid histiocytes and occasional giant cells (▶ Fig. 21.13). Tuberculosis of the nasal cavity and paranasal sinuses demonstrates poorly formed caseating granulomas with a prominent fibrous and chronic inflammatory reaction. Acid-fast bacilli can be identified with special stains at the periphery of necrotic areas. Rhinoscleroma is a chronic granulomatous disease endemic in Central and South America.[3] It is caused by gram-negative *Klebsiella rhinoscleromatis* and affects primarily the nasal cavity and nasopharynx. The catarrhal phase has nonspecific tissue changes consisting of numerous neutrophils and cellular debris. The subsequent granulomatous phase shows pseudoepitheliomatous hyperplasia of the overlying mucosa with chronic inflammation that includes numerous macrophages with vacuolated cytoplasm (Mikulicz cells) containing Klebsiella organisms identifiable by special stains. The final phase is fibrotic with a few similar macrophages.[4] Fungal disease of the sinonasal tract can be invasive (acute fulminant),

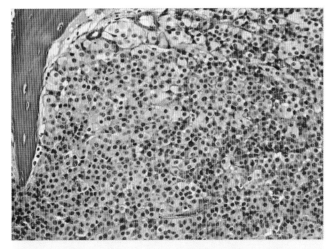

Fig. 21.26 Ectopic pituitary adenoma has polygonal, cytologically bland, small epithelial cells with distinct cell borders and various cytoplasmic tinctorial qualities. Ectopic pituitary adenomas arise in remnants of the embryonic adenohypophysis in the nasopharynx or sphenoid sinus. They contain polygonal epithelial cells that are positive for cytokeratin, neuroendocrine markers, and specific pituitary hormones.

noninvasive (mycetoma or "fungus ball"), or most frequently, allergic (▶ Fig. 21.14, ▶ Fig. 21.15). Rhinosporidiosis has numerous thick-walled cysts (sporangia) containing numerous endospores in the mucosal lamina propria (▶ Fig. 21.16).

Glial heterotopia, can be found in the subcutaneous tissue of the nose (60%), in the upper nasal cavity (30%), and less frequently in the ethmoid sinus, palate, middle ear, tonsil, and pharyngeal area (▶ Fig. 21.17). Dermoid cyst, a developmental abnormality related to midline closure of the face, can be encountered in the bridge of the nose and rarely in the nasopharynx.[5] It characteristically shows a cyst lined by epidermis with attached adnexal structures of the skin (hair follicles and/or sebaceous glands). Thornwaldt cyst is a cyst lined with ciliated epithelium located in the midline in the posterosuperior wall of the nasopharynx of young individuals.[6]Sinus histiocytosis with massive lymphadenopathy (Rosai-Dorfman disease) is an idiopathic disorder with significant lymphatic enlargement and secondary involvement of the nasal cavity, orbit, and other head and neck sites (▶ Fig. 21.18). Wegener granulomatosis is a systemic vasculitic process involving the upper and lower respiratory tract and kidneys (▶ Fig. 21.19).

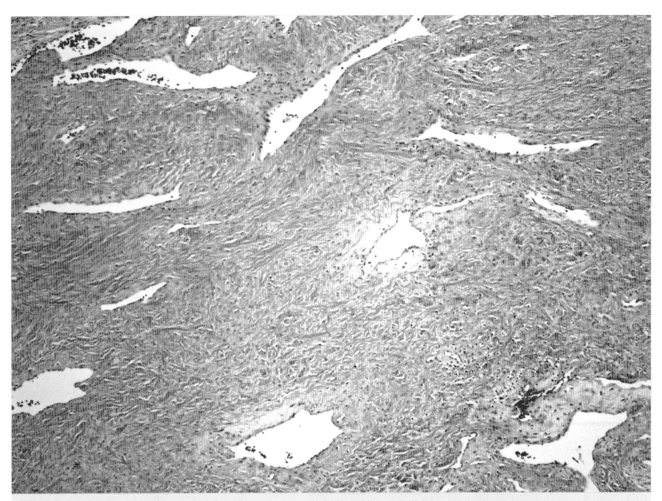

Fig. 21.27 Nasopharyngeal angiofibroma has thin-walled, irregular vascular spaces in a collagenized stroma with spindle-shaped and stellate fibroblasts. Nasopharyngeal angiofibroma is seen exclusively in young males, arises in the posterolateral nasal wall or nasopharynx, and demonstrates vascular proliferation in a fibrous stroma. The vessels are thin, slitlike, arborizing channels lined by endothelial cells and a discontinuous muscular layer. The rate of local recurrence can reach 20%.

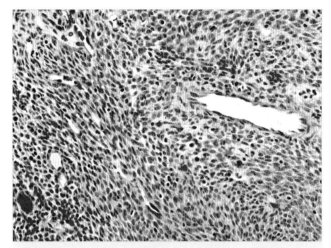

Fig. 21.28 Glomangiopericytoma (sinonasal-type hemangiopericytoma) is a sinonasal tumor demonstrating a proliferating perivascular myxoid phenotype, with ovoid nuclei, focal streaming, and neighboring irregular vascular spaces. It is a subepithelial unencapsulated tumor composed of closely packed cells growing in solid, fascicular, whorled, or storiform architecture with little intervening collagen and frequent branching vessels (staghorn vessels). It is immunoreactive to smooth-muscle actin, vimentin, and factor XIIIa but is specifically negative for CD34, Bcl-2, and CD99 (differing from soft-tissue-type hemangiopericytoma)

Pathologic features of Wegener granulomatosis include (1) mucosal ulceration with granulomas, (2) necrosis, and (3) vasculitis in the context of marked acute and chronic inflammation. Often, only some of these elements are present. Findings of necrosis, vasculitis, and granulomas are diagnostic if the patient has lung and/or kidney involvement. If two of these microscopic features are present, the biopsy is considered diagnostic only if both lungs and kidneys are involved; the diagnosis is considered probable if only one of lungs or kidneys is involved. In the presence of only one of the three microscopic features, the biopsy is considered suggestive if both lungs and kidneys are involved; it is considered suspicious if only one of lungs or kidneys is involved. Finally, if none of these microscopic features is identified, the biopsy is considered nonspecific even with clinical involvement of the lungs and kidneys.[7] Antineutrophilic cytoplasmic antibodies in a cytoplasmic pattern against proteinase-3 (c-ANCA) are specific for Wegener granulomatosis, but 10 to 50% of patients can be ANCA-negative.

Neoplasms

Schneiderian papillomas are benign epithelial tumors of adults associated in part with human papillomavirus (HPV) infection; they can be multifocal but usually are unilateral; three variants

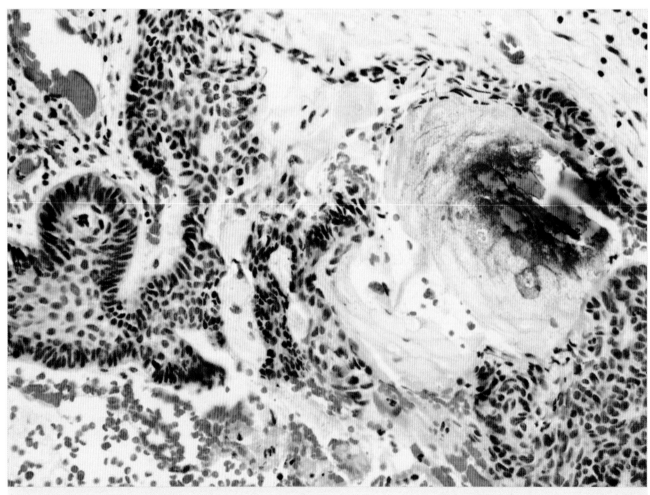

Fig. 21.29 Craniopharyngioma, usually a sellar tumor arising from Rathke pouch remnants, shows cords of multistratified squamous epithelium with nuclear peripheral palisading; note the compact accumulation of keratin (wet keratin) with focal dystrophic calcification.

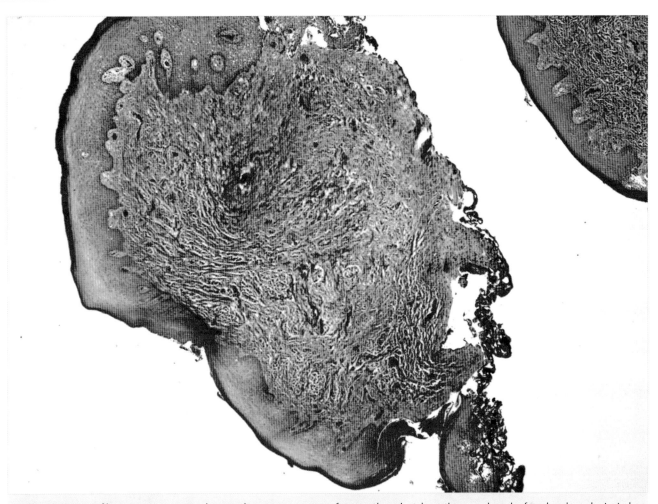

Fig. 21.30 Irritation fibroma is a common submucosal response to trauma from teeth or dental prostheses and can be found on buccal, gingival, labial, or lateral tongue mucosa. It presents as a polypoid growth with a densely collagenized core covered by stratified squamous epithelium showing reactive changes. Gingival fibromatosis and drug-induced fibrous hyperplasia have wide areas of gingival tumefaction showing rather avascular fibrous hyperplasia with scant chronic inflammation.

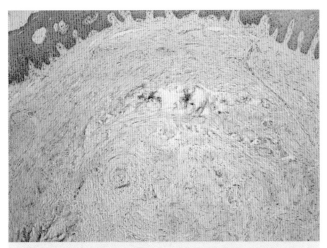

Fig. 21.31 Oral focal mucinosis occurs in young adults and shows irregular submucosal collections of myxomatous loose connective tissue on the hard palate or gingiva. Note the submucosal interstitial accumulation of mucoid material (Alcian blue stain) and the unremarkable surface epithelium. Pyogenic granulomas arise on the gingiva, lip, or tongue and harbor neovascularization with a fibrous reaction and mixed acute and chronic inflammation.

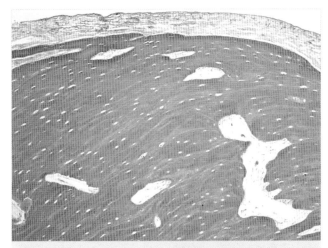

Fig. 21.32 Oral osteoma is a compact lamellar bone proliferation with few haversian canals. Bony exostosis and osteomas are histologically similar dense lamellar bone lesions on the mandible or maxilla that are reactive and neoplastic, respectively. Torus palatinus/mandibularis is a proliferation of mature lamellar bone on the hard palate/mandible.

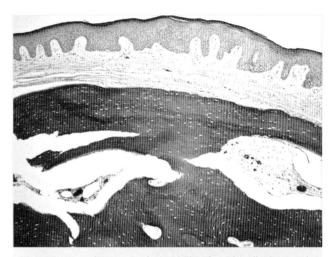

Fig. 21.33 Lingual osteoma (choristoma) is dense lamellar bone with occasional haversian canals proliferating in lingual soft tissue; note the unremarkable overlying epithelium. Heterotopic ossification is a reactive bone-producing soft-tissue proliferation of muscle or other connective tissue (in the masseter or other facial muscles). Soft-tissue osseous and cartilaginous choristoma is a histologically normal tissue (bone or cartilage) arising in an unexpected location, such as lingual muscle.

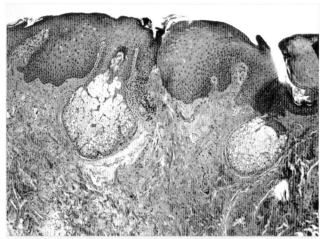

Fig. 21.34 Fordyce granules consist of normal sebaceous units without hair follicle attachment, aberrantly present in oral mucosa, with or without surface communication.

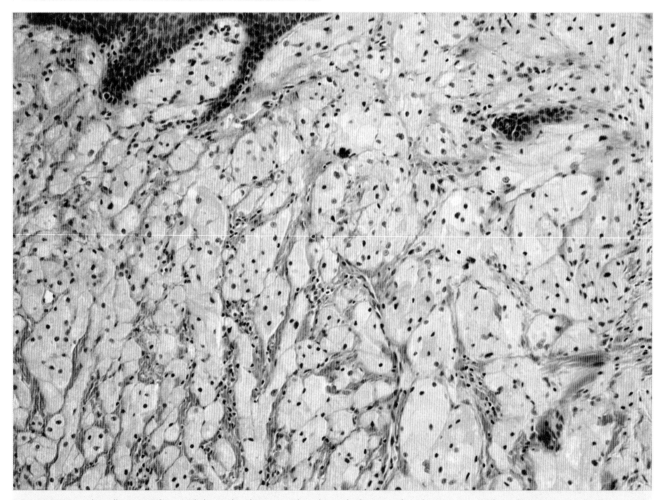

Fig. 21.35 Granular cell tumor is frequently located in the tongue, but also in the larynx and trachea. It consists of poorly circumscribed collections of round to spindle cells with small nuclei and a large amount of granular cytoplasm (numerous cytoplasmic lysosomes) that is positive for periodic acid–Schiff and immunoreactive to S-100.

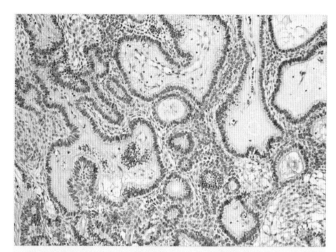

Fig. 21.36 Odontogenic tumors are derived from the tooth-forming apparatus. Ameloblastoma is a benign epithelial tumor of the enamel organ (producing dental enamel). Histologically, this tumor displays irregular islands of epithelium with characteristic palisading peripheral basal cells that have vacuolated cytoplasm and nuclei placed away from the basement membrane. The central epithelial cells are loosely arranged, with clear cytoplasm, and resemble stellate reticulum.

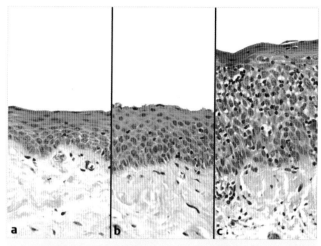

Fig. 21.37 Squamous dysplasia. (a) Mild. Architectural and cytologic changes are limited to the lower third of the epithelium. (b) Moderate. Changes extend into the middle third of the epithelium. (c) Severe. Architectural and cytologic changes occupy more than two-thirds of the epithelium.

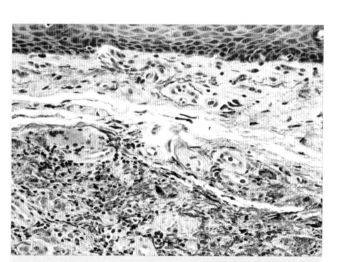

Fig. 21.38 Amalgam tattoo presents clinically as gray macules and is related to the epithelial implantation of heavy metal from dental filling material. Microscopically, dark brown or black particles are seen in the lamina propria with a haphazard and focally perivascular distribution.

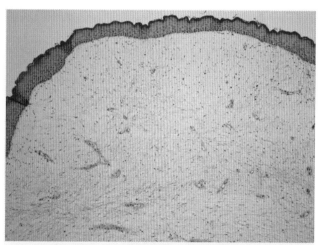

Fig. 21.39 Vocal fold polyps all harbor subepithelial myxoid, edematous, vascular, or hyaline changes in various proportions with a normal or mildly hyperplastic surface epithelium. Contact ulcers are posterior vocal fold lesions composed of granulation tissue with inflammatory infiltrates.

are described.[89] Exophytic papillomas are found almost exclusively found on the nasal septum; they show papillary fronds with central fibrovascular cores and thick, nonkeratinizing squamous epithelium. Inverted papillomas (▶ Fig. 21.20), probably the most frequent variant, affect the lateral nasal wall and sinuses (mostly maxillary) and display endophytic growth of similar nonkeratinizing squamous epithelium. Oncocytic papillomas (cylindrical cell papillomas), the least common type, are located similarly to inverted papillomas and are composed of multilayered columnar epithelial cells with eosinophilic and granular cytoplasm. Recurrence after surgical treatment is common because of incomplete initial excision. The rate of malignant transformation to squamous cell carcinoma reaches 11% in

inverted and in oncocytic papillomas, whereas malignant change is unusual in exophytic papillomas.[10]

The 2005 World Health Organization (WHO) classification distinguishes several types of nasopharyngeal carcinoma: (1) squamous cell carcinoma (with features of conventional keratinizing squamous cell carcinoma); (2) nonkeratinizing carcinoma with two subtypes, differentiated (retaining intercellular bridges and distinct cell margins) and undifferentiated (with indistinct cellular margins and a syncytial growth pattern); and (3) basaloid squamous cell carcinoma (similar to the tumor encountered in the larynx, ▶ Fig. 21.21). The mainstay of treatment is radiotherapy.[11]

Squamous cell carcinoma of the nasal cavity and paranasal sinuses is a rare tumor of adults arising in the maxillary sinus (60%), nasal cavity (12 to 25%), ethmoid sinus (10 to 15%), nasal

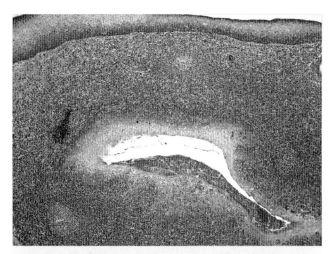

Fig. 21.40 Tonsillar cyst is lined by benign squamous epithelium with surrounding lymphoid hyperplasia.

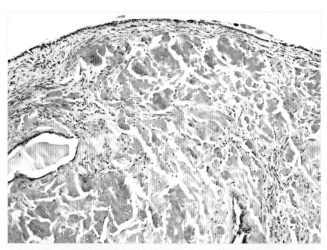

Fig. 21.41 Laryngeal amyloidosis displays dense subepithelial amorphous deposits of congophilic material (orange color on Congo red stain) with apple green birefringence under polarized light examination.

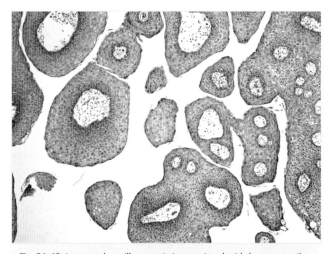

Fig. 21.42 Laryngeal papillomatosis is associated with human papillomatosis infection. The recurrence rate after excision is high, but malignant transformation is uncommon. Histologically, multiple papillary structures with fibrovascular cores and a squamous epithelial covering with occasional koilocytes are seen.

vestibule (4%), and frontal and sphenoid sinuses (each 1%).[12] It rarely metastasizes but is locally destructive. The majority are conventional squamous cell carcinomas with recognizable cellular margins, intercellular bridges, and an intracellular and extracellular accumulation of keratin. They can be well differentiated (forming numerous keratin pearls), poorly differentiated (lacking keratin pools), or moderately differentiated (harboring a few keratin conglomerates). A minority of cases are nonkeratinizing (cylindrical cell, transitional cell, ▶ Fig. 21.22). Rarely, verrucous carcinomas, papillary squamous cell carcinomas, basaloid squamous cell carcinomas, spindle cell carcinomas, or adenosquamous carcinomas are encountered.

Lymphoepithelial carcinoma is a rare undifferentiated carcinoma with a prominent lymphoplasmacytic infiltrate that affects the nasal cavity and paranasal sinuses. It has a morphology similar to that of its nasopharyngeal counterpart and a strong association with the Epstein-Barr virus (EBV). It responds favorably

to radiotherapy. Sinonasal undifferentiated carcinoma is a highly aggressive malignancy that typically presents with locally extensive disease and is typically negative for Epstein-Barr virus (▶ Fig. 21.23). Intestinal-type adenocarcinoma involves the ethmoid sinus (40%), nasal cavity (27%), and maxillary sinus (20%) (▶ Fig. 21.24).

Sinonasal non–intestinal-type adenocarcinoma (low-grade adenocarcinoma) displays glandular or papillary architecture with a single layer of cuboidal epithelium and locally invasive features. A variant, nasopharyngeal papillary adenocarcinoma, may have morphologic similarities to papillary carcinoma of the thyroid and must be distinguished from the latter by its negative immunohistochemical reaction to thyroglobulin and thyroid transcription factor-1 (TTF-1). Small-cell neuroendocrine carcinoma is a high-grade malignant tumor arising in the superior and posterior nasal cavity and extending to the paranasal sinuses and/or nasopharynx. It is composed of sheets or nests of small to intermediate-size cells with a high nuclear-to- cytoplasmic ratio, hyperchromatic nuclei with nuclear molding, and numerous mitoses. Immunohistochemically, the cells show reactivity to neuroendocrine markers (synaptophysin, chromogranin, neuron-specific enolase) and cytokeratin. Extremely uncommon, carcinoids of the sinonasal tract have also been described.

Olfactory neuroblastoma (esthesioneuroblastoma) is a malignant neuroectodermal tumor arising from the olfactory membrane in the superior part of nasal cavity with intracranial and/or paranasal sinus extension (▶ Fig. 21.25). Ectopic pituitary adenomas may arise in remnants of the embryonic adenohypophysis in the nasopharynx or sphenoid sinus. They contain polygonal epithelial cells that are positive for cytokeratin, neuroendocrine markers, and specific pituitary hormones (▶ Fig. 21.26).

Mucosal malignant melanoma is a rare tumor of the sinonasal tract seen in elderly patients. As in any other location, melanoma is considered the great mimicker and presents in a wide variety of cell types (epithelioid, spindle, plasmacytoid, rhabdoid, and/or multinucleated cells). Specific immunohistochemical markers, such as S-100, HMB-45, Melan-A, and microphthalmia

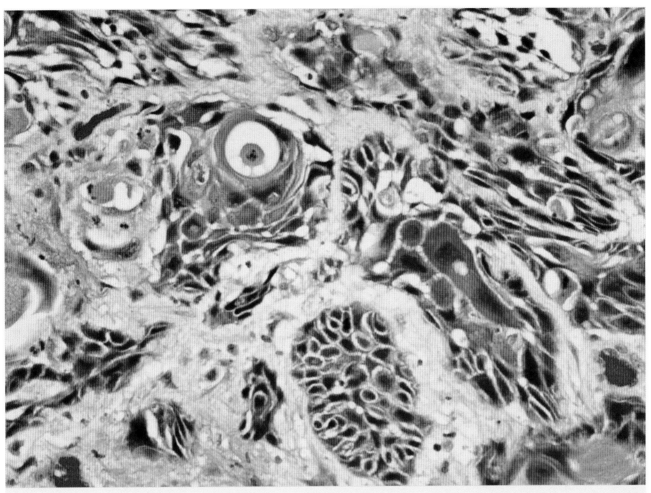

Fig. 21.43 Squamous cell carcinoma of the larynx is characterized by invading irregular islands or malignant squamous epithelium with well-preserved intercellular bridges and intra- and extracellular keratin accumulation.

transcription factor, help distinguish it. Other infrequent neuroectodermal tumors are Ewing sarcomas/primitive neuroectodermal tumors and paragangliomas. Hemangioma is a benign vascular tumor arising in the nasal septum, turbinates, and sinuses and is composed of benign proliferating capillaries with intervening fibrous stroma.

Nasopharyngeal angiofibroma is seen exclusively in young males in the posterolateral nasal wall or nasopharynx. Local recurrence rate is high (▶ Fig. 21.27).

Glomangiopericytoma (sinonasal-type hemangiopericytoma) is a subepithelial unencapsulated tumor composed of closely packed cells growing in solid, fascicular, whorled, or storiform architecture with little intervening collagen (▶ Fig. 21.28), branching vessels (staghorn vessels).

Solitary fibrous tumor is rare in the sinonasal tract and is composed of spindle fibroblasts with a dense vascular pattern. Cells are positive for CD34 and Bcl-2 and generally lack smooth-muscle actin reactivity.[13] Germ cell tumors of the sinonasal tract are rare. Mature teratoma shows a variable admixture of mature skin, skin appendages, neuroglial tissue, smooth muscle, bone, salivary glands, respiratory epithelium, and gastrointestinal epithelium. Ectodermal, mesodermal, and endodermal elements can be encountered in any distribution. Immature teratoma displays the same elements in their primitive, immature

variants, whereas teratoma with malignant transformation contains benign tissues of all three germinal layers and in addition a somatic malignancy, usually a carcinoma. If malignant epithelial and mesenchymal tissues are admixed, the tumor is called a teratocarcinosarcoma. Craniopharyngioma, is usually a sellar tumor which arises from Rathke pouch remnants (▶ Fig. 21.29).

21.3.2 Oral Cavity and Oropharynx

Infectious/Inflammatory/Anatomic/Idiopathic (▶ Fig. 21.30, ▶ Fig. 21.31, ▶ Fig. 21.32)

Peripheral giant cell granulomas are pyogenic granulomas with a prominent osteoclast-type giant cell component arising exclusively from the periodontal ligament enclosing the root of a tooth. The same periodontal ligament can produce a peripheral ossifying fibroma, which is a fibrous proliferation with scattered islands of woven or lamellar bone, usually with abundant osteoblastic rimming. Lingual osteoma (choristoma) displays dense lamellar bone with occasional haversian canals proliferating in lingual soft tissue, ▶ Fig. 21.33). Fordyce granules consist of normal sebaceous units without hair follicle attachment (▶ Fig. 21.34)

The juxtaoral organ of Chievitz is composed of nests of epithelial cells with an organoid pattern and a squamoid appearance

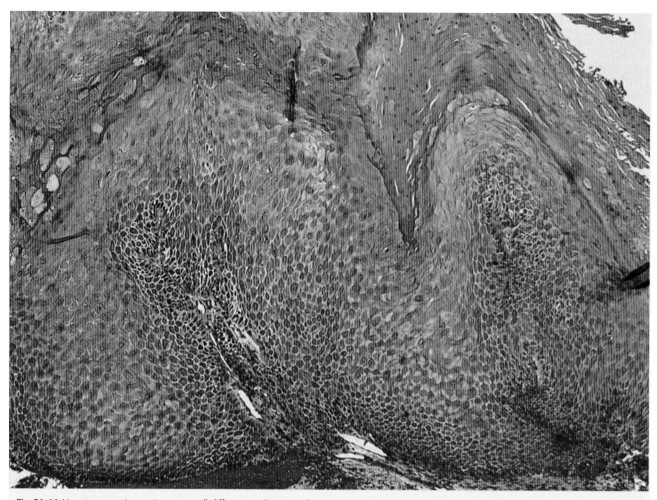

Fig. 21.44 Verrucous carcinoma is a very well-differentiated variant of squamous cell carcinoma. Histologically evident is the proliferation of atypical squamous cells with prominent hyperkeratosis without granular layer formation, as well as cellular dysplasia and rare mitoses; note the pushing base of the carcinoma without basement membrane violation.

devoid of keratinization arising in the buccotemporal fascia on the medial aspect of the mandible. Lingual thyroid is a vestigial rest of thyroid tissue at the upper end of the thyroglossal duct. Congenital epulis is a submucosal collection of cytologically bland histiocyte-like cells with granular cytoplasm that are S-100–negative. Median rhomboid glossitis is an area of pseudoepitheliomatous hyperplasia on the dorsal tongue accompanied by chronic inflammation and fungal organisms. Palatal and gingival cysts of the newborn have the appearance of epidermoid cysts arising from epithelial remnants of deeply budding dental lamina during tooth development. Nasolabial cyst (nasoalveolar cyst) arises from remnants of the embryonic nasolacrimal duct at the base of the nostrils just above the periosteum and is lined by respiratory-type, stratified columnar or pseudostratified columnar epithelium. Nasopalatine duct cyst arises from vestiges of the embryonal nasopalatine duct connecting the oral and nasal cavities. It arises on the anterior midline hard palate and is lined by squamous or cuboidal epithelium.

Neoplasms

Granular cell tumor is frequently located in the tongue, but can also be found in the larynx and trachea (▶ Fig. 21.35). Lipoma, a

mature adipose tissue tumor, can uncommonly be present in oral mucosa. Traumatic neuroma consists of moderately loose fibrovascular stroma admixed with irregular nerve fibers; it is usually related to tooth extractions or other forms of trauma. Mucosal neuroma is associated with multiple endocrine neoplasia syndrome and presents as multiple submucosal nodules composed of aggregates of nerves, often with thickened perineurium in a plexiform pattern. Palisaded encapsulated neuroma (solitary circumscribed neuroma) is a solitary, well-delineated nodule of proliferating Schwann cells (positive for S-100) with focal palisading nuclei and rare entrapped axons. Neurofibroma consists of a cellular proliferation of spindle Schwann cells with wavy nuclei and a variable amount of fibrous stroma with sparsely distributed axons.

Odontogenic tumors are derived from the tooth-forming apparatus. Ameloblastoma is a benign epithelial tumor of the enamel organ (▶ Fig. 21.36).

Ameloblastic fibroma is a benign tumor harboring ameloblastic epithelial islands in a myxoid cell–rich stroma with stellate fibroblasts resembling embryonic tooth pulp. Malignant counterparts of these tumors are ameloblastic carcinoma, in which ameloblastic epithelium shows cellular atypia, mitoses, necrosis, and invasive features, and ameloblastic fibrosarcoma, in

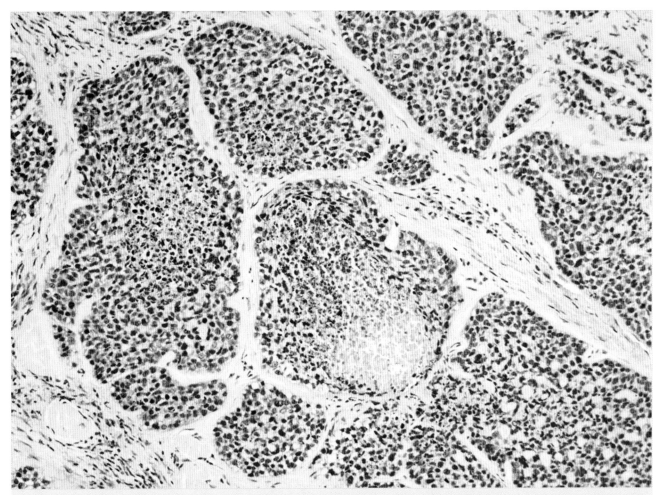

Fig. 21.45 Basaloid squamous cell carcinoma has a predilection for the hypopharynx, piriform sinus, and supraglottis and has a more aggressive clinical course. It characteristically has nests of basaloid tumor cells with large, hyperchromatic nuclei and scant cytoplasm (basaloid features), often accompanied by central necrosis (comedo-type necrosis) alternating with areas of regular squamous cell carcinoma.

which a benign ameloblastic epithelium is admixed with a malignant ectomesenchymal component. Keratogenic odonto-genic tumor (odontogenic keratocyst), mostly seen in the maxilla, is a cystic mass lined by parakeratinizing squamous epithelium with basal cells oriented away from the basement membrane and corrugated internal cystic surface.[14]

Epithelial Lesions

Squamous papillomas are benign epithelial tumors of the oral mucosa related to HPV infection. They have papillary architecture with central fibrovascular cores and a thickened squamous epithelial covering with some degree of keratinization. Verruca plana, also related to HPV infection, displays markedly thickened epithelium with hypergranulosis and hyperkeratosis including virally altered epithelial cells (koilocytes) in the upper layers; they are exophytic, showing epithelial folds, but no obvious papillary architecture is present. Condyloma acuminatum is caused by epithelial infection with HPV and displays short, blunt, rounded fronds of hyperplastic epithelium without keratinization and marked koilocytic changes. Focal epithelial hyperplasia is formed by multiple oral papillomas of buccal mucosa and tongue induced by HPV infection. Keratoacanthoma is

a keratinizing lesion of the mucosa of the skin and lip with rapid growth and clinically impressive craterlike center filled by hyperkeratosis. Histologically, there is a certain degree of squamous atypia without significant infiltrative features. Hairy leukoplakia is a well-demarcated verruciform hyperkeratotic plaque of the lateral tongue in HIV-positive patients related to EBV infection. Morphologically, the lesion displays superficial hyperkeratosis with parakeratosis and large collections of koilocytic intermediate cells with intracellular edema and basophilic viral nuclear inclusions. Frictional keratosis presents as a white hyperkeratotic line along the occlusal plane on buccal mucosa; it displays surface keratinization and mild inflammation. Leukoedema presents as bilateral semitranslucent gray or white plaques on buccal mucosa that typically have reticular streaks of thickened keratin with intracellular edema on microscopic examination. White sponge nevus shows white keratotic macules and plaques on buccal or labial mucosa with extensive and prominent intracellular edema in spinous layers on histologic evaluation. Actinic keilitis is related to excessive sun exposure and consists of atrophic squamous epithelium with underlying solar elastotic degeneration of the lamina propria and chronic inflammation.

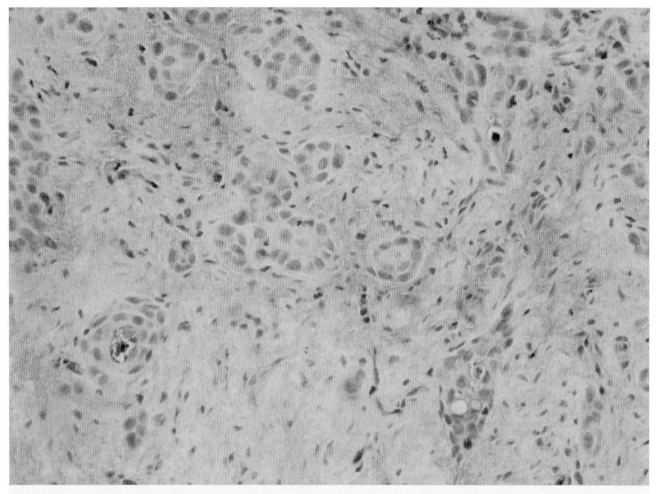

Fig. 21.46 Adenosquamous carcinoma displays invading islands of malignant epithelium with intercellular bridges (squamous cells) alternating with areas of columnar epithelial lining and mucin production (glandular differentiation), shown best with mucicarmine stain.

Squamous cell carcinoma is the most frequent malignancy of the upper aerodigestive tract. It affects adults of both genders with variable incidence rates worldwide according to local exposure to carcinogens (tobacco, alcohol, industrial pollution, and an unresolved role of HPV infection).

Oral cavity and laryngeal epithelial precursor lesions are clinically recognized as leukoplakia (well-delineated white elevated patch), erythroplakia (ill-delineated soft red patch), or a combination of the two, forming speckled leukoplakia. Although the histologic examination of leukoplakias frequently finds just hyperplasia of squamous epithelium, occasionally various degrees of dysplasia can be encountered. Erythroplakia most of the time harbors dysplastic changes and has a higher percentage of malignant transformation. Squamous cell dysplasia implies architectural changes (irregular stratification, loss of cellular polarity, increased mitoses, and dyskeratosis) and cytologic criteria (anisonucleosis, nuclear pleomorphism, anisocytosis, cellular pleomorphism, nuclear hyperchromasia, and increased nuclear-to-cytoplasmic ratio). The 2005 WHO classification of precursor lesions distinguishes several categories:

- Squamous hyperplasia: increased number of spinous cells (acanthosis) and/or basal and parabasal cells (basal cell hyperplasia) with regular stratification and maturation
- Squamous dysplasia, mild

- Squamous dysplasia, moderate
- Squamous dysplasia, severe
- Squamous cell carcinoma in situ: full-thickness epithelial involvement with abnormal superficial mitoses and not yet recognizable invasion

Simple hyperplasia has a likelihood of undergoing malignant progression of less than 1%, whereas severe dysplasia progresses to malignancy in 15 to 25% of cases[15] (▶ Fig. 21.37).

Inflammatory Epithelial Lesions

Lichen planus is an autoimmune mucositis with a subepithelial band of marked chronic inflammation and alterations of basal epithelial layers, including ballooning degeneration of epithelial cells and apoptotic single cells forming Civatte bodies. On immunofluorescence, there is a linear deposition of fibrinogen along the basement membrane.[16] Inflammatory mucosal ulcerations show granulation tissue with prominent inflammation surrounded by erythematous hyperplastic epithelium. Dysplasia or squamous cell carcinoma needs to be ruled out by histologic investigation. Pemphigus vulgaris is a bullous autoimmune inflammatory condition of the oral mucosa with a characteristic fishnet pattern of intercellular immunoglobulin deposits and

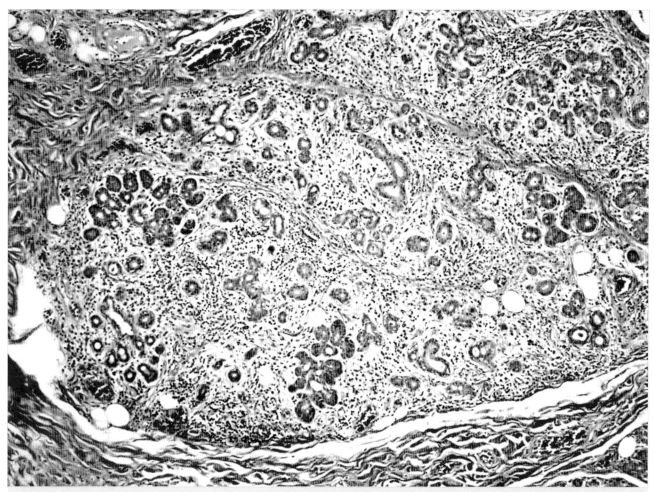

Fig. 21.47 Chronic sclerosing sialadenitis shows atrophic salivary gland parenchyma with edema, fibrosis, and chronic inflammation. Sialadenitis can be acute suppurative or, more frequently, chronic. The latter is associated with sialolithiasis and displays morphologically various degrees of glandular atrophy, fibrosis, and chronic inflammation with occasional intraductal mineralized concretions (lithiasis).

immune complement deposits on immunofluorescent examination. Intraepithelial blistering is seen with sparing of the basal epithelial layer (suprabasal bullae).[17] Mucous membrane pemphigoid, also an autoimmune mucositis, displays subepithelial blister formation and is characterized by immunoglobulin and complement deposits along the basement membrane. Amalgam tattoo presents clinically as gray macules and is related to the epithelial implantation of heavy metal from dental filling (▶ Fig. 21.38).

Other pigmented epithelial lesions include oral melanotic macule, the mucosal equivalent of the freckle on the skin. It displays otherwise normal epithelium with a basal intraepithelial deposition of melanin pigment. Mucosal melanocytic nevus is likewise the mucosal counterpart of the skin nevus and consists of well-delineated subepithelial clusters of cytologically benign melanocytes. Oral melanocytic neuroectodermal tumor of infancy (retinal anlage tumor) is a congenital tumor derived from neural crest cells and is located in the oral cavity, other craniofacial sites, brain, skin, mediastinum, epididymis, uterus, and so on. Microscopically, it displays small neuroblastic cells and larger melanin-containing epithelial cells in a vascularized, dense fibrous stroma. Immunhistochemically, the tumor displays a polyphenotypic expression of neural, melanocytic, and epithe-

lial markers.[18] Mucosal melanoma follows the same pattern described in the sinonasal mucosa.

21.3.3 Hypopharynx, Larynx, and Trachea

Infectious/Inflammatory/Anatomic/Idiopathic

Laryngeal tuberculosis, sarcoidosis, rhinosporidiosis, and rhinoscleroma have morphological changes identical to the ones described in the sinonasal location. Specific laryngeal infectious agents include *Treponema pallidum* (syphilis), *Actinomyces*, *Nocardia*, *Candida albicans*, *Coccidioides immitis*, *Paracoccidioides*, *Blastomyces*, *Cryptococcus*, *Histoplasma capsulatum*, cytomegalovirus, *Trichinella spiralis*, and others. Isolation of the etiologic agent requires a combined microbiological and histomorphologic effort.

Vocal fold polyps are characterized by subepithelial myxoid, edematous, vascular, or hyaline changes in various proportions with a normal or mildly hyperplastic surface epithelium (▶ Fig. 21.39). Contact ulcers are posterior vocal fold lesions composed of granulation tissue with inflammatory infiltrates.

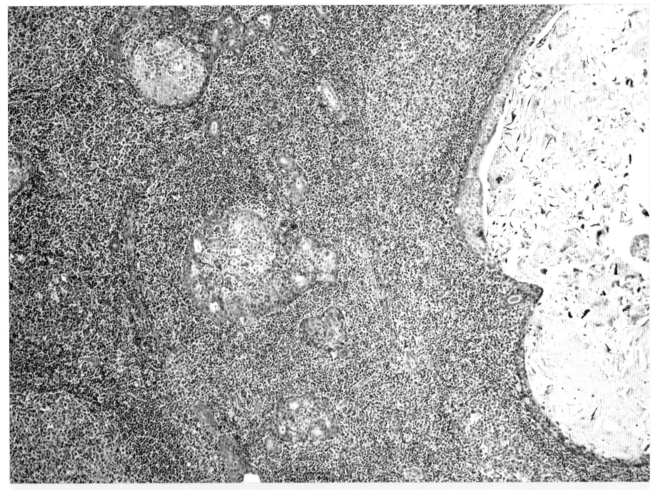

Fig. 21.48 Acquired immunodeficiency syndrome–related parotid gland cysts show multiple irregular lymphoepithelial islands with occasional lymphoepithelial cysts in a background of marked chronic inflammatory infiltrate.

Laryngeal cysts are of four categories: (1) laryngoceles, which are pulsion diverticula of the saccule (harbor full-thickness laryngeal wall structures, including respiratory-type epithelial lining); (2) saccular cysts, resulting from obstruction of the saccule (harbor mucus retention cysts that push on the thyrohyoid membrane and are analogous to the ones in the sinonasal tract); (3) ductal cysts (squamous, oncocytic, or tonsillar cysts), the most commonly encountered cysts, all mucin-filled and arising from minor salivary duct obstruction (squamous and oncocytic cysts are located in the glottis, ventricles, aryepiglottic folds, and epiglottis, whereas tonsillar cysts are located in the vallecula and show surrounding lymphoid hyperplasia, ▶ Fig. 21.40); (4) miscellaneous epithelial cysts (epidermal, dermoid, and branchial cleft cysts).[19]

Laryngeal amyloidosis displays dense subepithelial amorphous deposits of orange color on Congo red stain with apple green birefringence under polarized light examination (▶ Fig. 21.41). Wegener granulomatosis, pemphigus vulgaris, and mucous pemphigoid are similar to the lesions of the oral cavity and sinonasal tract previously described.

Neoplasms

Laryngeal papillomatosis is associated with human papillomavirus infection, and demonstrates a high recurrence rate but low potential for malignant degeneration (▶ Fig. 21.42). Squamous cell carcinomas of the larynx and hypopharynx account for 34% of upper aerodigestive tract carcinomas and are found (in decreasing frequency) in the supraglottis, glottis, hypopharynx, subglottis, and rarely the trachea.[20] Morphologically, these lesions range from well-differentiated tumors to poorly differentiated, undifferentiated, and spindle cell carcinomas, all with significant invasive features, especially perineurally, and lymphatic metastatic potential. The best outcome is noted with glottic tumors and the worst outcome with tumors in a hypopharyngeal, subglottic, or tracheal location. Several morphological features are of prognostic significance: involvement of the resection margins, lymphatic invasion (especially with extracapsular extension), perineural invasion, and invading front of the tumor (expansive pushing borders have a better prognosis, whereas infiltrative borders with isolated tumor islands at a distance from the main mass have a less favorable prognosis)[21] (▶ Fig. 21.43, ▶ Fig. 21.44, ▶ Fig. 21.45).

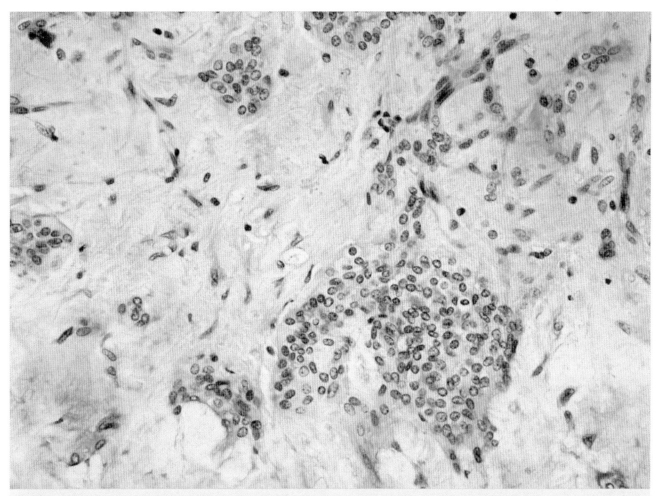

Fig. 21.49 Pleomorphic adenoma displays a proliferation of cytologically bland myoepithelial cells forming irregular nests in a myxoid mesenchymal background. The former component displays cuboidal, basaloid, squamous, spindle, plasmacytoid, or clear cells. The mesenchymal component shows myxoid changes, fibrosis, and rarely cartilaginous or osseous metaplasia. Recurrence after surgical treatment is encountered in 3.4% of cases after 5 years and in 6.8% after 10 years. Many recurrent pleomorphic adenomas are multifocal. Pleomorphic adenomas account for 60% of salivary gland neoplasms. Of these, 80% arise in the parotid gland, 10% in the submandibular gland, and 10% in minor salivary glands.

Papillary squamous cell carcinoma is frequently located in the supraglottis and has a better prognosis. It implies papillary architecture with a malignant squamous epithelial covering. Spindle cell carcinoma is most frequently present in the glottis and has a prognosis similar to that of regular squamous cell carcinoma. It is a biphasic tumor in which areas of regular squamous cell carcinoma alternate with sarcomatoid-appearing areas of spindle epithelial cells. Acantholytic squamous cell carcinoma, located in the hypopharynx and supraglottis, shows acantholytic detachments between squamous cells, creating the appearance of glandular differentiation. Adenosquamous carcinoma displays invading islands of malignant epithelium with intercellular bridges alternating with areas of columnar epithelial lining and mucin production (▶ Fig. 21.46).

Rare lymphoepithelial carcinomas are identical to the similar entity of the sinonasal tract. Neuroendocrine tumors of the larynx are similar to the carcinoid, atypical carcinoid, and small cell carcinomas described in the sinonasal tract. Laryngeal paraganglioma is morphologically identical to the one described in the middle ear. Malignant melanomas of larynx follow the same pattern as their sinonasal counterparts.

21.3.4 Salivary Glands

Infectious/Inflammatory/Anatomic/Idiopathic

Salivary gland heterotopia is commonly encountered as an incidental finding and consists of morphologically unremarkable serous and mucous acini with occasional ducts. The most frequent location is intranodal (in cervical lymph nodes); an extranodal location is described as high heterotopia (mandible, ear, palatine tonsil, mylohyoid muscle, pituitary gland, and cerebellopontine angle) or low heterotopia (associated with the branchial pouches of the lower neck and thyroid gland).[22] Polycystic (dysgenetic) disease is a rare developmental abnormality characterized by varying degrees of honeycombed cystic changes. Chronic sclerosing sialadenitis shows atrophic salivary gland parenchyma with edema, fibrosis, and chronic inflammation (▶ Fig. 21.47).

The microscopic hallmark of Sjögren syndrome is a lymphocytic sialadenitis present in minor salivary glands (frequently biopsied in the lip), in major salivary glands, and in lacrimal glands. Morphologically, there is chronic inflammation with lymphoid hyperplasia and focal lymphoepithelial islands

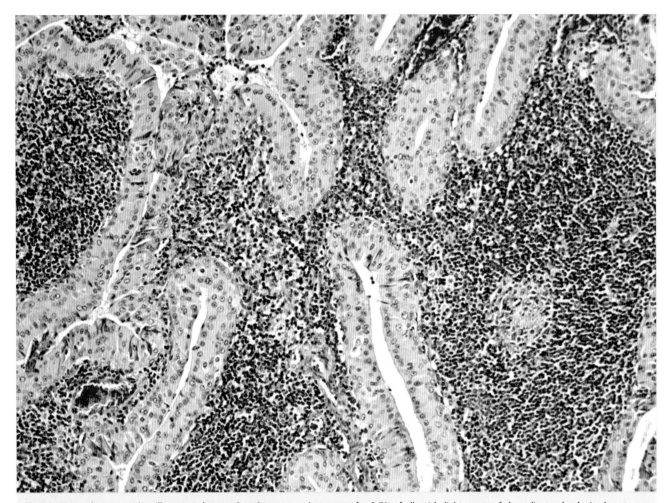

Fig. 21.50 Warthin tumor (papillary cystadenoma lymphomatosum) accounts for 3.5% of all epithelial tumors of the salivary glands, is almost exclusively found in the parotid gland, and can be multifocal or bilateral. Morphologically, it displays a characteristic cystic and papillary configuration in which epithelial cells with oncocytic metaplasia (high number of intracytoplasmic mitochondria, seen as large amount of pink, granular cytoplasm) arranged in double layers and forming papillary structures alternate with areas of lymphoid hyperplasia. A low recurrence rate is seen after resection.

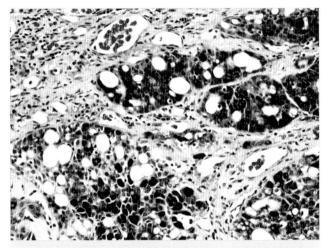

Fig. 21.51 Acinic cell carcinomas are malignant tumors, most commonly seen in the parotid gland, characterized by at least partial acinic differentiation (cytoplasmic zymogen secretory granules), as well as intercalated smaller cells and vacuolated and clear cells.

(compact clusters of epithelial and myoepithelial cells surrounded by inflammation). The risk for developing non-Hodgkin lymphomas is significantly higher in individuals with Sjögren syndrome than in age-matched control subjects. Mucocele and ranula show degenerative mucin-filled spaces without epithelial lining (mucus extravasation). Mucus retention cyst is an intraductal accumulation of mucin and is lined by stratified epithelium. Lymphoepithelial cyst is usually seen in major salivary glands and consists of a stratified squamous epithelial lining with surrounding lymphoid hyperplasia (▶ Fig. 21.48).

Necrotizing sialometaplasia is a reactive process of minor salivary glands in the palate or other oropharyngeal sites in which squamous metaplasia reaches into glandular acini, mimicking infiltrative islands of a squamous malignancy. Lack of mitotic activity and nuclear atypia help distinguish it from a squamous cell carcinoma.

Neoplasms

Pleomorphic adenomas account for 60% of salivary gland neoplasms. Of these, 80% arise in the parotid gland (▶ Fig. 21.49). Myoepitheliomas account for 1.5% of all tumors in salivary

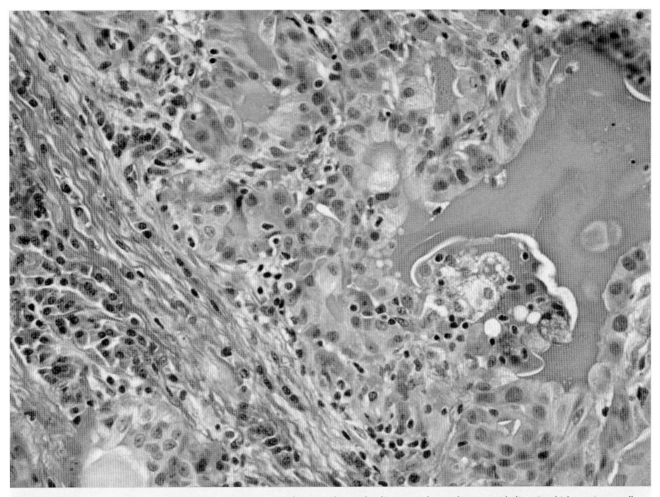

Fig. 21.52 Mucoepidermoid carcinoma is the most common malignant salivary gland tumor. It has malignant epithelium in which mucinous cells alternate with areas of epidermoid differentiation (large cells with visible intercellular bridges and no complete maturation to keratin production). A three-tiered grading system has good correlation with clinical outcome.

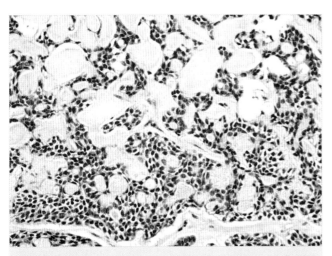

Fig. 21.53 Adenoid cystic carcinoma accounts for approximately 10% of salivary gland malignancies. Histologically, a cribriform pattern with mucopolysaccharide-filled spaces is seen; note the monotony of the proliferating myoepithelial cells with angulated hyperchromatic nuclei and scant clear cytoplasm. Histologic grading correlates well with clinical outcome

glands and are composed of proliferating myoepithelial cells with spindle, epithelioid, or plasmacytoid features. They are less prone to recur than pleomorphic adenomas. Basal cell adenomas are rare benign tumors of proliferating epithelial and myoepithelial cells with a basaloid appearance and trabecular growth pattern. They are like pleomorphic adenomas in which there is no mesenchymal part. Recurrence after complete excision is rare.

Warthin tumor (papillary cystadenoma lymphomatosum) accounts for 3.5% of all epithelial tumors of the salivary glands, is almost exclusively found in the parotid gland, and can be multifocal or bilateral (▶ Fig. 21.50).

Oncocytic adenoma (oncocytoma) is a rare salivary gland benign tumor composed of oncocytic epithelial cells that grow in a nesting and trabecular pattern. Canalicular adenoma frequently affects the upper lip and is composed of rows of columnar epithelial cells forming canaliculi. Sebaceous adenomas are benign salivary gland neoplasms with proliferating sebaceous units; some show intervening lymphoid tissue (sebaceous lymphadenomas). Ductal papillomas and cystadenomas are also rarely seen.

Acinic cell carcinomas are characterized by acinic differentiation, as well as intercalated smaller cells and vacuolated and

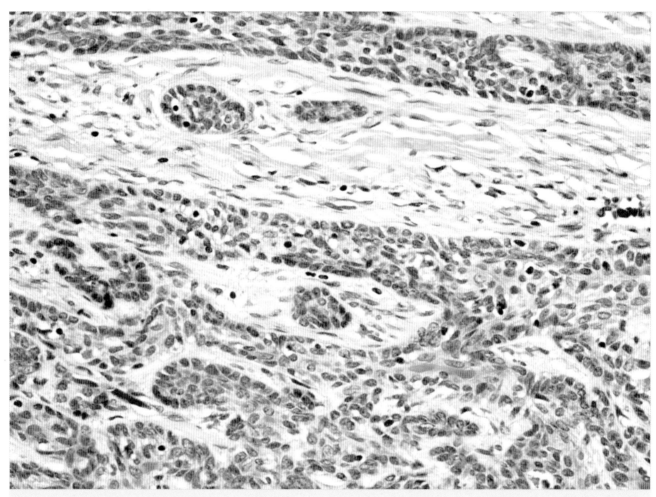

Fig. 21.54 Basal cell adenocarcinoma is the malignant counterpart of basal cell adenoma. These lesions have proliferating myoepithelial cells with frequent areas of ductal differentiation (epithelial and myoepithelial bilayering of lumina).

clear cells (▶ Fig. 21.51). Mucoepidermoid carcinoma has malignant epithelium in which mucinous cells alternate with areas of epidermoid differentiation (▶ Fig. 21.52). Adenoid cystic carcinoma accounts for approximately 10% of salivary gland malignancies and displays a cribriform pattern with mucopolysaccharide-filled spaces (▶ Fig. 21.53).

Polymorphous low-grade adenocarcinoma arises mostly in the palate and is characterized by cytologic uniformity, histologic diversity, and an infiltrative growth pattern. Epithelial–myoepithelial carcinoma, a rare malignant tumor, shows bilayered ductlike structures with an inner layer of cuboidal epithelial cells and an outer layer of myoepithelial cells with clear cytoplasm. A rare malignant tumor is clear cell carcinoma (hyalinizing clear cell carcinoma) arising mostly in intraoral minor salivary glands. It shows a monomorphic clear cell population with a high glycogen content. Basal cell adenocarcinoma has proliferating myoepithelial cells with frequent areas of ductal differentiation (▶ Fig. 21.54). Carcinoma ex pleomorphic adenoma is a mixed tumor in which the epithelial component has undergone malignant transformation (▶ Fig. 21.55).

Sebaceous carcinoma and sebaceous lymphadenocarcinoma are rare malignant tumors with sebaceous differentiation. Oth-er malignant tumors include cystadenocarcinoma, mucinous adenocarcinoma, oncocytic carcinoma, salivary duct carcinoma, adenocarcinoma not otherwise specified, carcinosarcoma, squamous cell carcinoma, small cell carcinoma, large cell carcinoma, and lymphoepithelial carcinoma.

21.3.5 Thyroid and Parathyroid Glands

Infectious/Inflammatory/Anatomic/Idiopathic

Thyroglossal duct cysts are the most common cystic developmental abnormalities of the neck, arising along a tract in the anterior midline between the tongue and thyroid gland (▶ Fig. 21.56). Subacute granulomatous thyroiditis (de Quervain thyroiditis) presents with neck pain following an upper respiratory tract viral episode. Microscopically, it presents as focal disruption of the thyroid follicles triggering a reactive chronic inflammation with granulomas and fibrosis. Palpation thyroiditis shows foci of histiocytic accumulation in disrupted thyroid follicles and is the result of frequent palpation of the thyroid gland. Hashimoto thyroiditis is characterized by lymphoplasmacytic infiltration of the thyroid parenchyma with focal lymphoid follicle

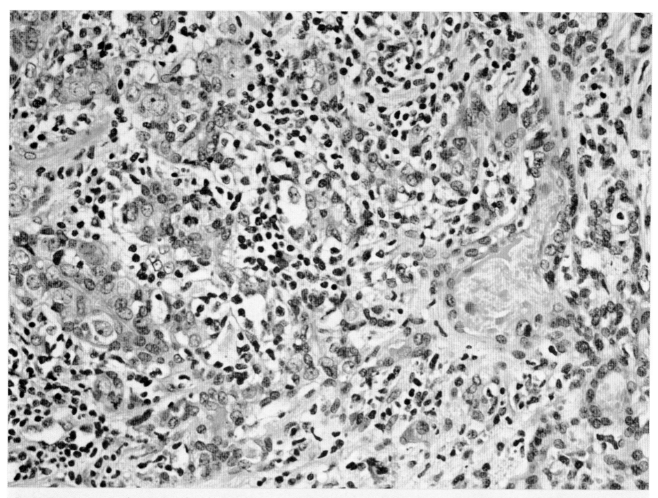

Fig. 21.55 Carcinoma ex pleomorphic adenoma is a mixed tumor in which the epithelial component undergoes malignant transformation, which can be only focally present and can be confined within the capsule of the benign tumor in which it arises. Note the large undifferentiated malignant epithelial cells (left side of image) arising in and invading the pleomorphic adenoma (right side of image).

formation. There is also reactive oncocytic changes in the thyroid epithelium Hashimoto thyroiditis is an autoimmune disorder affecting individuals with a genetic predisposition; it is associated with a variety of other autoimmune diseases (► Fig. 21.57).

In Riedel thyroiditis, hyalinized fibrosis replaces the normal parenchyma and extends into adjacent soft tissues of the neck. The mild inflammatory component is usually mixed and is also associated with occasional foci of venulitis. Amyloidosis (amyloid goiter) is a rare condition characterized by the massive interstitial deposition of amorphous congophilic deposits (apple green birefringent under polarized light). Hyperplasia of the thyroid gland may be associated with hyperfunction (Graves disease), hypofunction (endemic goiter, dysmorphogenic goiter), or normal function (multinodular goiter).[23] Graves disease shows diffuse and symmetric enlargement of the thyroid gland, which is beefy red on cut surfaces. Microscopically, there is preservation of the normal lobular architecture; follicles appear small and irregular, contain pale-staining colloid, and display numerous papillary epithelial infoldings with basally placed nuclei.

Dysmorphogenic goiter is usually present early in childhood and morphologically shows diffuse or nodular hyperplasia with irregular epithelial islands and foci of nuclear pleomorphism. Multinodular goiter (nontoxic, simple, adenomatoid, or colloid goiter) harbors asymmetric enlargement with incompletely encapsulated hyperplastic nodules undergoing partial degeneration with hemorrhage, calcification, fibrosis, cyst formation, and rarely ossification. There is variation in follicular size, areas of papillary hyperplasia, and occasional oncocytic changes (► Fig. 21.58).

Neoplasms

Follicular adenomas are benign thyroid tumor that are completely encapsulated by a thin rim of fibrous tissue and retain follicular architecture (► Fig. 21.59). Hyalinizing trabecular adenoma is another benign encapsulated tumor with a trabecular growth pattern and hyalinization. The proliferating follicular cells display nuclear enlargement and grooves; they are frequently misinterpreted as atypia or even papillary carcinoma on FNA biopsies.

Papillary carcinoma is the most common thyroid malignant tumor, typically presenting in adults; it is more common in

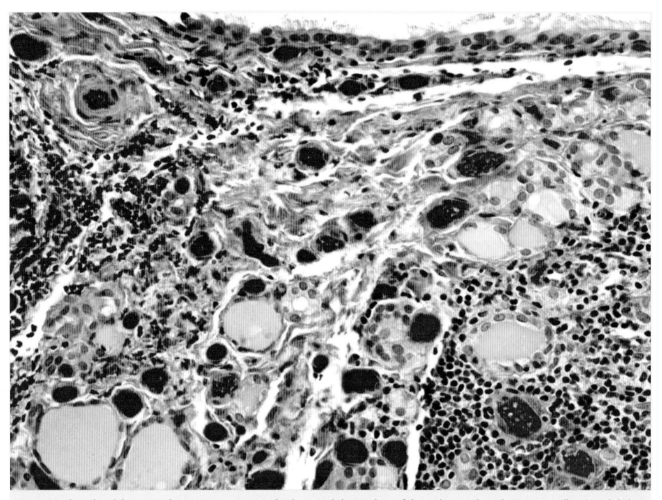

Fig. 21.56 Thyroglossal duct cysts, the most common cystic developmental abnormalities of the neck, arise along the anterior midline (mostly below and some above the hyoid bone, and very few in the tongue). Histologically, the cysts are lined by ciliated respiratory-type epithelium, squamous epithelium, or both and occasionally harbor attached vestiges of thyroid parenchyma.

women. Papillary carcinomas are usually diffusely invasive tumor and have high propensity for lymphatic invasion (▶ Fig. 21.60). Follicular carcinoma is usually a solitary large mass with a thick fibrous capsule and normal follicular or microfollicular architecture; follicular cells can be seen penetrating the thick fibrous capsule of the tumor) (▶ Fig. 21.61).

Poorly differentiated carcinoma (insular carcinoma) displays a solid growth pattern with poorly differentiated round epithelial cells, is highly invasive, and has metastatic potential. Undifferentiated (anaplastic) carcinoma is a rare and aggressive tumor harboring undifferentiated epithelial cells with areas of spindle cells, pleomorphic giant cells, or epithelioid cells. Distant metastases are usually present by the time of presentation. Medullary thyroid carcinoma arises from C cells (calcitonin-secreting cells) of the thyroid and is a neuroendocrine tumor; tumor cells are immunoreactive to calcitonin (▶ Fig. 21.62).

Spindle cell tumor with thymuslike differentiation (SETTLE) and carcinoma showing thymuslike differentiation (CASTLE) are rare malignant tumors in which there is co-expression of cytokeratin and CD5 (T cell marker). Other malignant thyroid tumors are squamous cell carcinoma, mucoepidermoid carcinoma, and mucinous carcinoma.

Parathyroid adenoma usually involves a single parathyroid gland, and areencapsulated neoplasms composed of solidly proliferating chief cells or oncocytes with clear cytoplasm forming solid and focally follicular arrangements without intervening adipocytes (▶ Fig. 21.63). Rare lesions are parathyroid cysts that are lined by a single layer of compressed cuboidal epithelial cells and show groups of chief or oxyphilic cells in neighboring fibrous tissue. Parathyroid carcinoma is diagnosed based on infiltrative features including desmoplastic reaction to invasion; cytologically, it displays cells identical to those of parathyroid adenoma. Primary chief cell hyperplasia is characterized by hyperplasia of all four parathyroid glands accompanied by hyperparathyroidism. Approximately 75% of cases are sporadic, whereas the rest are part of multiple endocrine neoplasia syndromes. Morphologically, there is nodular growth of chief cells with a normal number of oncocytes and transitional oncocytic cells and preserved intraglandular adipocytes.[24]

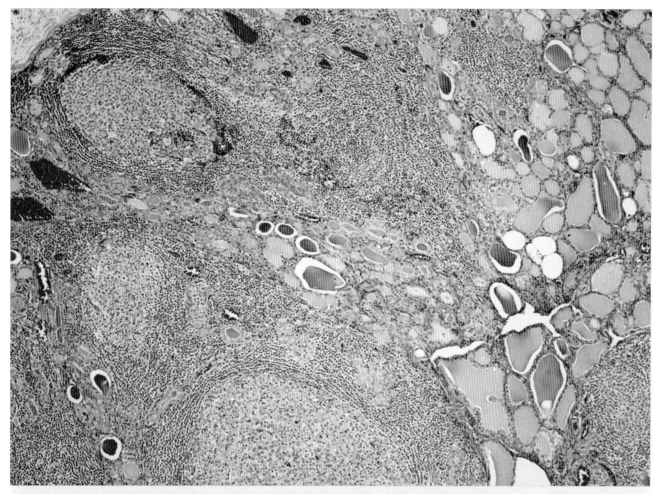

Fig. 21.57 Hashimoto thyroiditis harbors lymphoplasmacytic infiltration in the thyroid parenchyma with focal lymphoid follicle formation and surrounding reactive oncocytic changes in the thyroid epithelium (Hurthle cell metaplasia). Hashimoto thyroiditis is an autoimmune disorder affecting individuals with a genetic predisposition; it is associated with a variety of other autoimmune diseases, such as Graves disease, Sjögren syndrome, and rheumatic diseases. Patients with Hashimoto thyroiditis have a significant risk for the development of non-Hodgkin lymphomas; it is asserted that they also have a higher risk for the development of papillary carcinoma.

21.3.6 Soft-Tissue Tumors of the Head and Neck

Neoplasms

Juvenile hyaline fibromatosis is an extremely rare disorder characterized by the presence of subcutaneous tumorlike masses, predominantly in the head and neck. The nodules are composed of plump fibroblasts in a hyalinized collagen replacing normal tissues. Nuchal fibromas are benign, well-circumscribed but unencapsulated nodules in the posterior neck and upper back that harbor bundles of mature collagen with focal entrapment of nerve bundles, adipocytes, and skeletal muscle fibers. Desmoid-type fibromatosis shows poorly circumscribed soft-tissue masses composed of proliferating spindle cells with a uniform appearance in a collagenous background. Although no cytologic atypia or mitotic activity is seen, the lesion has infiltrative margins and is frequently incompletely excised, therefore showing a high recurrence rate. Dermatofibrosarcoma

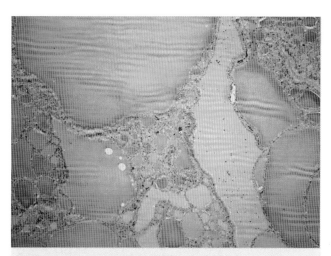

Fig. 21.58 An adenomatoid goiter has a large variation of hyperplastic thyroid follicles with cytologically benign follicular cells.

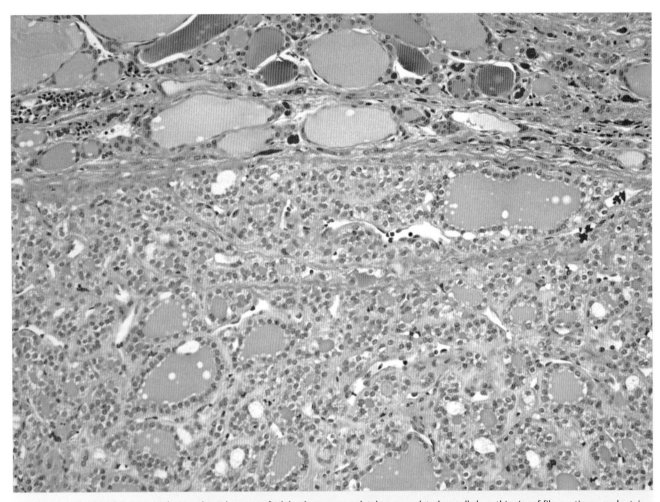

Fig. 21.59 Follicular adenomas are benign thyroid tumors of adults that are completely encapsulated, usually by a thin rim of fibrous tissue, and retain follicular architecture (follicular differentiation) with a normal amount of colloid. A follicular adenoma has proliferating follicular cells (lower part of image) that are larger than normal follicular cells of the thyroid (upper part of image). The cells have moderately enlarged nuclei in comparison with the normal thyroid. No tumor capsule or vascular invasion is found. Variants of follicular adenomas include oncocytic adenoma (Hurthle cell adenoma), follicular adenoma with papillary hyperplasia, signet-ring cell follicular adenoma, mucinous follicular adenoma, lipoadenoma (with included groups of adipocytes), clear cell follicular adenoma, atypical adenoma, and follicular adenoma with bizarre nuclei.

protuberans arises in the dermis and subcutis on the trunk and proximal extremities, with a certain percentage affecting the head and neck.[25] It displays a dense cellular proliferation of spindle fibroblasts with a honeycomb pattern, infiltrative margins, and little mitotic activity; neoplastic cells are immunoreactive to vimentin and CD34 while usually factor XIIIa– negative. Adult fibrosarcomas are diffusely infiltrating malignant tumors of soft tissues that are highly cellular and show hyperchromatic spindle nuclei with frequent mitoses; the growth pattern is storiform or herringbone-like. Tumor size and depth of invasion are prognostically significant. Pleomorphic malignant fibrous histiocytoma (undifferentiated high-grade pleomorphic sarcoma)is an aggresive tumor, invading widely and metastasizing; it has a poor prognosis (▶ Fig. 21.64).

Traumatic neuromas arise after trauma or surgery and are composed haphazardly arranged nerves and fibrous tissue. Neurofibromas and schwannomas are both benign tumors of the nerve sheath. The former arise in the substance of a nerve and entrap nerve fibers within the mass, whereas the latter grow attached to a nerve and do not harbor nerve fibers within the mass. Both contain proliferating Schwann cells (immunoreactive to S-100) with scattered fibroblasts and perineurial cells (▶ Fig. 21.65).

Perineuriomas are deep or superficially located soft-tissue nodules composed of small spindle cells. They derive from perineurial cells and are epithelial membrane antigen–positive while S-100–negative. Nuclear pleomorphism in a neurofibroma, a high degree of cellularity, increased mitotic activity, and tumor necrosis all suggest a malignant transformation (malignant peripheral nerve sheath tumor). Perineuriomas have an aggressive clinical courses and metastatic potential. Lipomas are collections of mature adipocytes and are frequently encountered in the head and neck; surgical excision is curative. Spindle cell lipoma and pleomorphic lipoma are

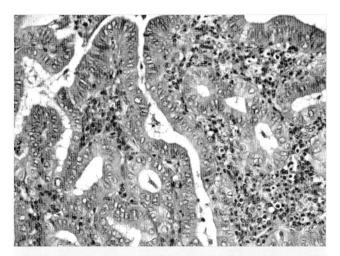

Fig. 21.60 Papillary carcinoma of the thyroid shows predominantly papillary (solid or follicular areas possible) architecture of the neoplasm with multilayered malignant epithelial cells that have distinct cytologic features (nuclear clearing, nuclear grooving, conspicuous nucleoli, and occasional intranuclear pseudoinclusions) and atypia. Psammoma bodies (concentric calcium deposits) are very characteristic but rarely encountered. Papillary carcinoma is by far the most common thyroid malignant tumor; it manifests in adult life and shows a female predilection. Papillary carcinomas can be encapsulated but are usually diffusely invasive tumors that break through the thyroid capsule and have high propensity for lymphatic invasion. Microscopic foci of papillary carcinoma smaller than 1 cm are described as papillary microcarcinomas. Variants of papillary carcinoma have been described (follicular, oncocytic, clear cell, macrofollicular, solid, diffuse sclerosing, tall and columnar cell), all with similar clinical outcomes.

the ends of a common histologic spectrum; they are well-circumscribed soft-tissue masses of bland spindle cells with various adipocytic components and scattered multinucleated giant cells with radially arranged nuclei in a floret-like pattern. Lipoblastomas are benign pediatric tumors composed of mature and immature adipocytes, the latter corresponding to lipoblasts in various stages of development. The lipoblasts are usually very scarce. Well-differentiated liposarcoma, an intermediate malignant mesenchymal tumor, is composed of mature adipocytes with significant variation in cell size, focal adipocytic nuclear atypia, and hyperchromasia. Dedifferentiated liposarcoma shows areas of fibrosarcoma or pleomorphic malignant fibrous histiocytoma. Myxoid liposarcoma shows primitive, round to oval, nonlipogenic mesenchymal cells and various numbers of lipoblasts in a myxoid stroma. Pleomorphic liposarcoma harbors bizarre cells and lipoblasts. Papillary endothelial hyperplasia is an intravascular clot organization and recanalization of a thrombosed vessel after a traumatic event; it shows pseudopapillae lined by plump, reactive endothelial cells. Capillary hemangiomas are irregular proliferations of thin walled capillaries with bland endothelial cells (▶ Fig. 21.66).

Kaposiform hemangioendothelioma is a locally aggressive, immature vascular neoplasm with a Kaposi sarcoma–like fascicular spindle cell growth pattern. Epithelioid hemangioendothe-

lioma is a vascular tumor that usually originates in a vessel. It shows centrifugal extension into neighboring soft tissue with partial vessel wall destruction by proliferating epithelioid endothelial cells with a low rate of mitotic activity and scattered nuclear pleomorphism. It is considered a vascular tumor of intermediate malignancy between hemangiomas and angiosarcomas. Angiosarcomas of the head and neck highly aggressive vascular tumors with metastatic potential and a high local recurrence rate (▶ Fig. 21.67).

Leiomyomas are benign smooth-muscle tumors arising from pilar smooth muscles or the muscularis of blood vessels. They are typically not well circumscribed and harbor interlacing fascicles of lightly eosinophilic spindle cells with cigar-shaped nuclei. The cells are positive for smooth-muscle actin and desmin. Leiomyosarcomas are rare in the head and neck. Microscopically, they show increased cellularity, nuclear pleomorphism and hyperchromasia, and frequent mitoses. Deep-seated leiomyosarcomas have a more aggressive clinical course. Adult rhabdomyomas arise in the pharynx, oral cavity, tongue base, and larynx. They are benign lobulated tumors of striated muscle, display large polygonal or round cells with abundant eosinophilic cytoplasm, and are immunoreactive to muscle-specific actin, desmin, and myogenin. Rhabdomyosarcomas are malignant striated muscle tumors of childhood. Embryonal rhabdomyosarcomas show primitive cells in various stages of myogenesis. Alveolar rhabdomyosarcomas show predominantly primitive cells with a high nuclear-to-cytoplasmic ratio. Pleomorphic rhabdomyosarcomas, arising exclusively in adults, consist of undifferentiated round to spindle cells with frequent pleomorphic nuclei. Epithelioid sarcoma is a tumor of young adults that seldom involves the head and neck. It is composed of epithelioid and spindle cells with nuclear atypia and frequent tumor necrosis. The cells are characteristically positive for both vimentin and epithelial markers, like cytokeratin and/or epithelial marker antigen. Alveolar soft-part sarcoma is a malignant tumor of young adults involving the tongue and orbit most frequently. It characteristically shows an organoid growth pattern with thin, fibrous septation. The cells are polygonal and show sharp cell borders and large nuclei with prominent nucleoli. Occasionally, there are rhomboid or rod-shaped crystalline inclusions that are positive for periodic acid–Schiff. Synovial sarcoma affects young adults. On histologic examination, it can be biphasic (epithelial cells and spindle cells), monophasic (usually spindle cells alone), or poorly differentiated. Epithelial cells are immunoreactive to cytokeratins, while vimentin is present in the spindle cells. Soft-tissue type hemangiopericytoma rarely affects the head and neck (▶ Fig. 21.68).

21.3.7 Bone Lesions of the Head and Neck

Neoplasms

Osteoma is a benign osseous tumor, almost exclusively present in head and neck, arising in the paranasal sinuses, mandible, bony part of the external auditory canal, and soft tissues (tongue, buccal mucosa, and nasal cavity); it is composed of a

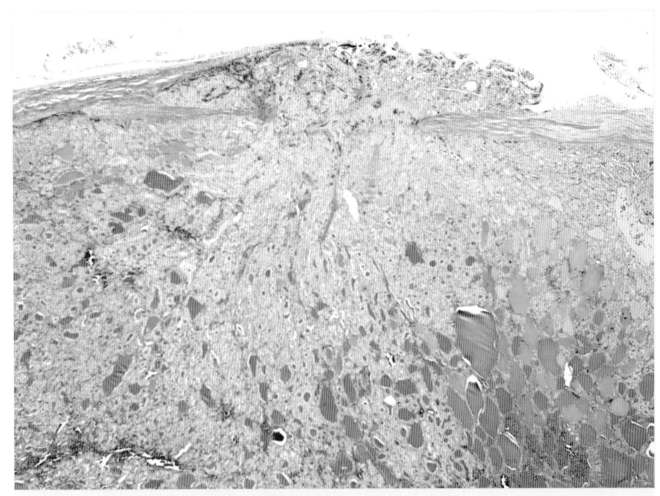

Fig. 21.61 Follicular carcinoma has neoplastic follicular cells breaking through the thick fibrous capsule of the tumor (mushrooming capsular invasion). Follicular carcinoma accounts for 10 to 15% of thyroid malignancies. It is mostly a solitary large mass with a thick fibrous capsule and normal follicular or microfollicular architecture. Invasiveness is identified along its capsule (complete capsular penetration with spread into neighboring thyroid tissue) or in vessels (most distant metastases are blood-borne). Minimally invasive follicular carcinoma shows few foci of vascular and capsular invasion but retains the general shape of an encapsulated neoplasm; its prognosis is excellent. Widely invasive follicular carcinoma shows multiple areas of invasion such that the initial capsule of the tumor can barely be recognized; distant metastases are usually present by the time of presentation.

proliferation of compact lamellar bone with a reduced number of haversian canals. Histologically identical is exostosis, which involves larger areas of the external auditory canals bilaterally and is distinguished from osteoma on clinical grounds. Osteoid osteoma is a rare benign bone tumor of young adults arising in the cervical spine, mandible, maxilla, and various skull bones; it characteristically presents with pain relieved by salicylates. It shows a central nidus with a peripheral denser rim on radiologic examination; this is matched on histologic examination by a central nidus with new bone formation and active osteoblastic rimming followed by mature bone formation at the periphery and balanced osteoclastic and osteoblastic activity.

Osteosarcoma is rare in the head and neck; typically affecting the mandible, maxilla, skull bones, and rarely the vertebrae of adults (▶ Fig. 21.69).

Chondroma is a benign cartilaginous tumor rarely seen in the skull base and other bones of the head and neck or in soft tissues. It shows lobules of hyaline cartilage with well-formed chondrocytes in unremarkable lacunae. Osteochondroma is a pedunculated benign tumor protruding from the parent bone that remains in direct continuity with the cortex of the affected bone; its distal part displays a cartilage covering. Chondroblastoma shows small, densely proliferating chondroblasts with well-defined borders and reniform nuclei with little mitotic activity. Chondrosarcoma can affect any area of

bone in the head and neck as well as the larynx in adults (▶ Fig. 21.70).

The general grading system of sarcomas (based on differentiation, mitoses, and necrosis) correlates well with clinical

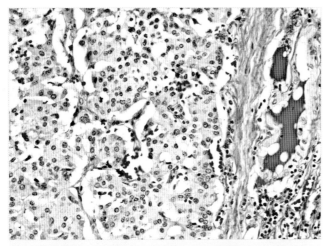

Fig. 21.62 Medullary thyroid carcinoma has neoplastic neuroendocrine cells with a stippled chromatin pattern (salt and pepper nuclei) and elongated, hyperchromatic nuclei, as well as amyloid deposition within the tumor and invasive features; note the unremarkable neighboring thyroid follicle. Medullary thyroid carcinoma arises from C cells (calcitonin-secreting cells), and the tumor cells are immunoreactive to calcitonin.

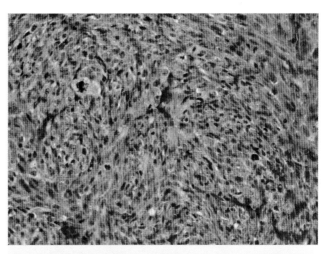

Fig. 21.64 Pleomorphic malignant fibrous histiocytoma (undifferentiated high-grade pleomorphic sarcoma) displays bizarre, pleomophic cells growing in a fascicular or storiform pattern with marked nuclear hyperchromasia and frequent mitoses. It invades widely, metastasizes, and has a poor prognosis.

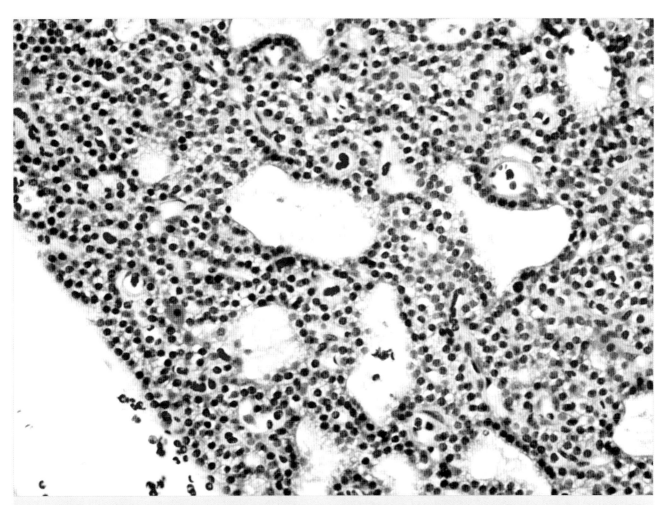

Fig. 21.63 Parathyroid adenoma usually involves a single parathyroid gland. The tumors are delicately encapsulated neoplasms composed of solidly proliferating chief cells or oncocytes with clear cytoplasm forming solid and focally follicular arrangements without intervening adipocytes; frequently, a rim of unremarkable parathyroid parenchyma is attached.

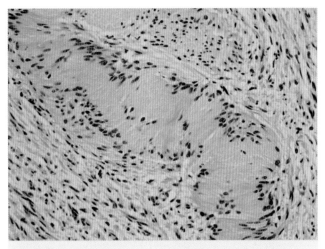

Fig. 21.65 Schwannoma is characterized by proliferating spindle Schwann cells with a fair amount of pink cytoplasm and indistinguishable cell borders; note the nuclear palisading around the acellular pink area (Verocay body).

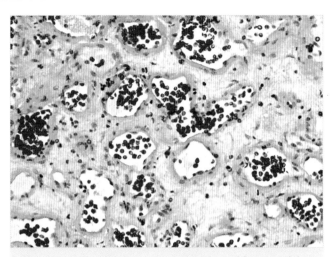

Fig. 21.66 Capillary hemangiomas are irregular proliferations of thin-walled capillaries with bland endothelial cells in a loose collagenous stroma.

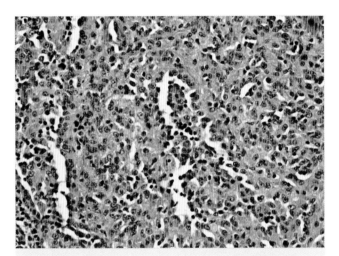

Fig. 21.67 Angiosarcomas demonstrate irregular and anastomosing vascular spaces with markedly pleomorphic endothelial cells and numerous atypical mitoses. The head and neck are the most common locations of cutaneous angiosarcomas. These are highly aggressive vascular tumors with metastatic potential and a high local recurrence rate.

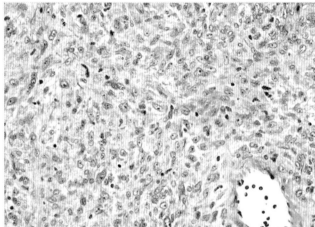

Fig. 21.68 Soft-tissue type hemangiopericytoma exhibits dense, proliferating pericytes with mitotic activity. It harbors densely cellular elongated cells with numerous intervening vessels with focal staghorn branching; a high number of mitoses is linked to a more aggressive clinical course, but the criteria for malignancy are ill defined. The tumor cells are immunoreactive to CD34 and CD99. Soft-tissue type hemangiopericytoma is generally deep-seated but rarely affects the head and neck.

outcome.[26] Some show primitive areas with undifferentiated cells (mesenchymal chondrosarcoma). Chordoma of the head and neck, an intermediate-grade malignant tumor that recapitulates notochord histology, affects the clivus (most chordomas generally arise in the sacrococcygeal area). It shows multivacuolated, physaliferous cells in a mucinous stroma; the cells are immunoreactive to S-100, epithelial markers, and vimentin (▶ Fig. 21.71).

Ossifying fibroma is an extraosseous neoplasm of fibrous tissue with central osteoid formation including some osteoclastic activity and mineralization. Aneurysmal bone cyst affects the mandible, maxilla, and midline bone structures of the head and neck in young adults (▶ Fig. 21.72).

21.3.8 Hematopoietic Lesions of Head and Neck

Infectious/Inflammatory/Anatomic/Idiopathic

Mononucleosis lymphadenitis affects adolescents and young adults. If a histologic diagnosis is necessary (unsuccessful serologic investigation), the excised lymph node shows partially effaced lymphoid architecture, an expanded paracortical T-cell zone, and occasional immunoblasts. Human immunodeficiency lymphadenitis shows three distinct morphological patterns

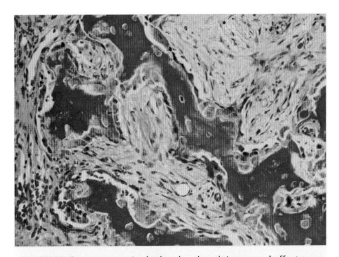

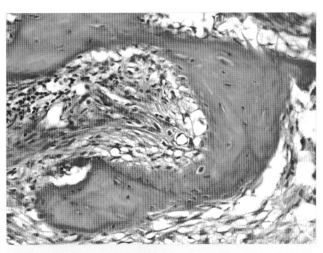

Fig. 21.69 Osteosarcoma in the head and neck is rare and affects mandible, maxilla, skull bones, and rarely the vertebrae of adults. On microscopic examination, it shows malignant mesenchymal cells with osteoid formation (immature bone with incomplete haversian system formation); in parallel, it can show fibroblastic, chondroblastic, or various mesenchymal differentiations. Seen here are trabeculae of woven bone with a single layer of osteoblastic rimming in a fibrous stroma.

Fig. 21.71 Fibrous dysplasia shows bone trabeculae with lamellar and woven bone, both devoid of osteoblastic rimming. It is well circumscribed and composed of bone replacement by fibroblastic stroma with irregular bone trabeculae arising directly from the fibrous tissue without the presence of osteoblasts. Fibrous dysplasia affects flat bones in the head and neck.

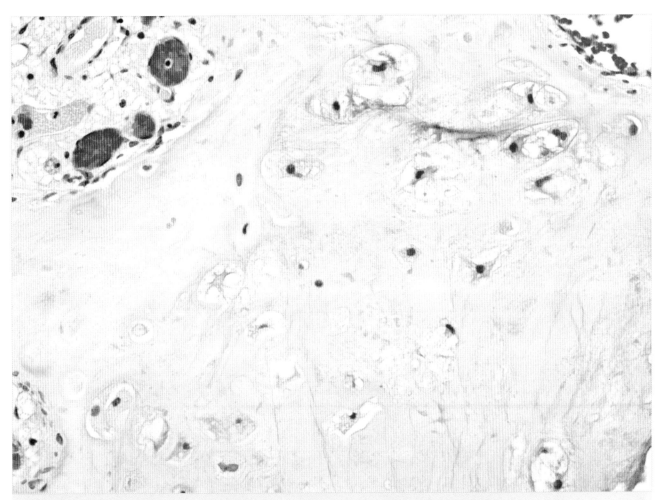

Fig. 21.70 Chondrosarcoma is characterized by irregularly distributed atypical chondrocytes with large, atypical, hyperchromatic nuclei and mitoses in irregular lacunae. Chondrosarcoma can affect any area of bone in the head and neck as well as the larynx in adults.

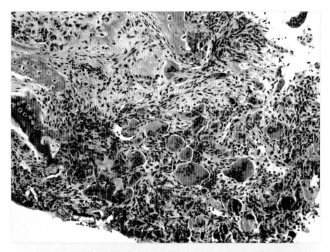

Fig. 21.72 Giant cell reparative granuloma (aneurysmal bone cyst) is a well-circumscribed, benign, variably cystic bone tumor with peripheral woven bone formation accompanied by osteoblastic rimming in a fibrous and focally hemorrhagic stroma with unevenly distributed multinucleated osteoclast-type giant cells. Note the neighboring bone trabeculae with reactive woven bone changes. It affects the mandible, maxilla, and midline bone structures of the head and neck in young adults.

based on stage of evolution. Pattern A displays enlarged lymph nodes with mildly disturbed lymphoid architecture and aggregates of monocytoid cells. Pattern B shows follicle effacement with lymphocytic depletion and vascular hyperplasia. Pattern C shows hyalinized germinal centers with transfixing, collagen-ensheathed arterioles and extensive angiogenesis.[27] Cat-scratch lymphadenitis usually presents with unilateral matted lympadenopathy showing necrotizing granulomas with central microabscesses (*Bartonella henselae*). *Toxoplasma* lymphadenitis reveals posterior cervical lymphadenopathy with well-preserved reactive lymphoid architecture, perifollicular and intrafollicular clusters of epithelioid cells, and patches of monocytoid cells without granulomas or necrosis. Mycobacterial lymphadenitis presents as caseating necrosis with granulomas in which rare bacilli can be found on special stains (acid-fast bacilli) (▶ Fig. 21.73). Sarcoidosis lymphadenopathy may be seen in multisystem sarcoidosis (▶ Fig. 21.74). Kimura lymphadenopathy, is common in young Asian males, usually seen in the neck and periauricular areas (▶ Fig. 21.75). Kikuchi lymphadenopathy, also seen predominantly in young Asians, can be found in unilateral cervical lymph nodes and generally resolves spontaneously (▶ Fig. 21.76). Sinus histiocytosis with massive lymphadenopathy (Rosai- Dorfman disease) is generally seen in

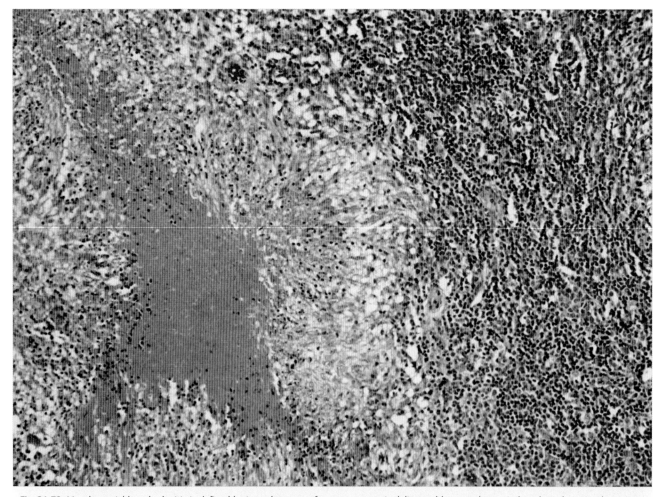

Fig. 21.73 Mycobacterial lymphadenitis is defined by irregular areas of caseous necrosis delineated by granulomas in lymph nodes. *Mycobacterium tuberculosis* lymphadenitis, the most common type of extrapulmonary tuberculosis, usually affects multiple lymph nodes. Histologically, it presents as caseating necrosis with granulomas in which rare bacilli can be found on special stains (acid-fast bacilli).

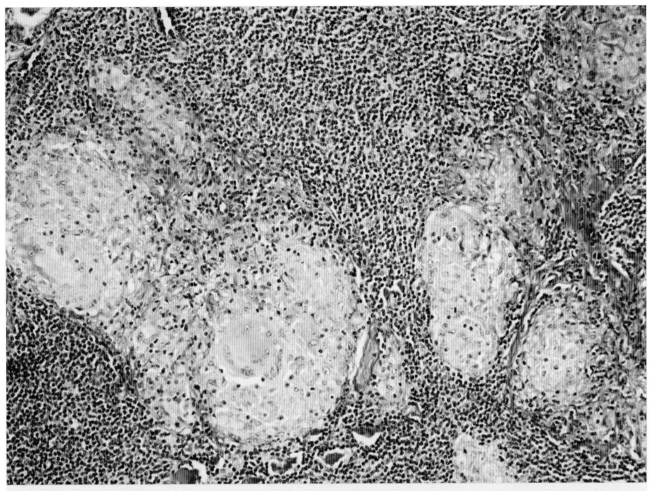

Fig. 21.74 Sarcoidosis lymphadenopathy accompanies multisystemic sarcoidosis. Histologically, it displays non-necrotizing granulomas with well-preserved lymphoid architecture.

children and adolescents, presenting with massive generalized lymphadenopathy of long duration (▶ Fig. 21.77).

Inflammatory pseudotumor shows enlarged, tumorlike lymph nodes and soft-tissue masses. It displays fascicles and whorls of spindle cells (fibroblasts and myofibroblasts) accompanied by vascular proliferation and moderate chronic inflammatory infiltration without evidence of monoclonality.

Neoplasms

Hodgkin lymphoma (classic type) shows four distinct variants. Nodular sclerosis Hodgkin lymphoma is the most common type in the United States and shows lymph node architecture effacement due to fibrosis. Lymphoid cells, with an eosinophilic background, harbor a large number of Reed-Sternberg cells and Hodgkin cells (immunoreactive to CD30 and CD15 but CD20-negative) (▶ Fig. 21.78). Lymphocyte-rich Hodgkin lymphoma shows few Reed-Sternberg cells in a largely lymphocytic background. Mixed-cellularity Hodgkin lymphoma is the most common type in underdeveloped countries and shows mixed

features of the first two. Lymphocyte depletion Hodgkin lymphoma affects elderly patients and shows severe lymphocyte depletion and few Reed-Sternberg cells with a diffuse fibrillary background.[28] Nodular lymphocyte–predominant Hodgkin lymphoma shows a nodular growth pattern, usually focal architectural replacement, and scattered neoplastic lymphocytic/histiocytic cells, which are in fact CD20-positive but CD30- and CD15-negative neoplastic B lymphocytes. No Reed-Sternberg cells are present. Marginal zone B-cell lymphoma (MALT lymphoma) is a low-grade lymphoma of adults arising in lymph nodes or extranodally. It harbors monotonous monoclonal small lymphocytes with slight nuclear angulation, very few mitoses, and B phenotype (CD20-positive with frequent CD43 coexpression and light chain restriction). Small lymphocytic lymphoma affects elderly persons and displays monotonous small lymphocytes with hyperchromatic nuclei and slight nuclear contour irregularity (immunoreactive to CD20, CD23, and CD5) with complete effacement of lymphoid architecture. Occasional proliferation centers populated by prolymphocytes are present. Mantle cell lymphoma is clinically aggressive and displays monotonous,

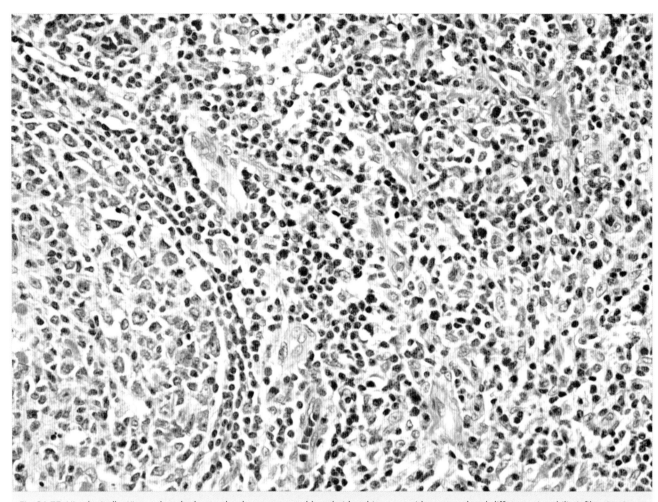

Fig. 21.75 Histologically, Kimura lymphadenopathy shows preserved lymphoid architecture with scattered and diffuse eosinophilic infiltration in a background of capillary endothelial hyperplasia in lymph nodes. Kimura lymphadenopathy, common in young Asian males, shows predilection for the neck and periauricular areas.

medium-size lymphocytes with vesicular nuclei, conspicuous basophilic nuclei, and a fair amount of mitoses (immunoreactive to CD20, CD5, and cyclin D1). Follicular lymphoma has high incidence in Western countries and affects elderly persons. It can show partial or complete nodal involvement with a follicular or diffuse growth pattern. It comprises cleaved cells (immunoreactive to CD20, CD10, Bcl-2, and Bcl-6) that can be small or large corresponding to a low or high histologic grade of follicular lymphoma, respectively. Diffuse large B-cell lymphoma is the most common lymphoma in Western countries and is high-grade. It can be nodal or extranodal and harbors large B lymphocytes (positive for CD20 with variable staining for CD10 and Bcl-6) with a high mitotic count and tumor necrosis. Burkitt lymphoma is a high-grade B-cell lymphoma

affecting young adults (▶ Fig. 21.79).

Myeloid sarcoma (extramedullary myeloid cell tumor) is the tissue counterpart of chronic myeloid leukemia in which circulating malignant myeloid cells (immunoreactive to CD13, CD15, CD33, CD43, and CD117) form tissue masses. Extranodal NK (natural killer)/T-cell lymphoma, nasal type, and peripheral T-cell lymphoma are the most frequent T-cell lymphomas of the head and neck. They are high-grade and display various T-cell antigen deletions in neoplastic lymphocytes. Plasmacytoma is a proliferation of atypical plasma cells with a high mitotic rate (▶ Fig. 21.80).

21.3.9 External, Middle, and Internal Ear

External Ear

Infectious/Inflammatory/Anatomic/Idiopathic

The most common congenital lesion of the external ear is the accessory tragus, which microsopically is a fragment of cartilage covered by unremarkable skin and subcutaneous tissue. Preauricular cysts and sinuses are derived from the first branchial arch and consist of spaces lined by squamous- or respira-

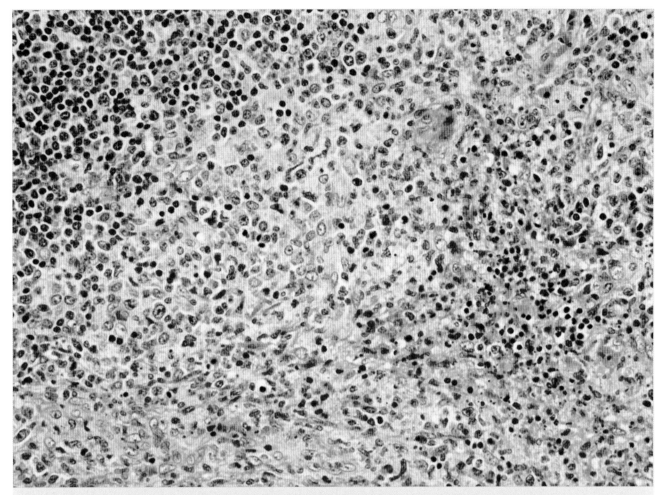

Fig. 21.76 Biopsied lymph nodes in Kikuchi lymphadenopathy display partially preserved lymphoid architecture with patchy areas of necrosis, nuclear debris, aggregates of histiocytes, apoptotic cells, and a total lack of neutrophils and eosinophils. Kikuchi lymphadenopathy, predominant in young Asians, affects cervical lymph nodes unilaterally and has a benign clinical course with spontaneous remission.

tory-type epithelium. Type I anomaly is cystic and entirely ecto-dermal, whereas type II also contains cartilage. Keloids are thick, irregular scars which grow beyond the limits of the origi-nal scar (▶ Fig. 21.81).

Chondrodermatitis helicis nodularis affects the external ear and consists of ulcerations with granulation tissue, necrobiosis of underlying cartilage, and surrounding hyperplasia of skin.

Neoplasms

Squamous cell carcinoma is associated with actinic injury and consists of atypical squamous cells with intercellular desmo-somes and various degrees of keratinization. It tends to invade widely into soft tissues and along perineural spaces. Basal cell carcinomas arise from the basal layer of the epidermis and in-vade the dermis as irregular nests of basaloid cells with periph-eral palisading. Some variants have irregular borders and are difficult to completely excise by standard methods (▶ Fig. 21.82). Malignant melanoma is characterized by nests of melanocytes with atypical nuclei and conspicuous nucleoli forming basal epidermal nests and spreading into the upper layers of the epidermis. Melanocytes are immunoreactive to S-100, MART-1 (Melan-A), and HMB-45 (▶ Fig. 21.83).

Undifferentiated epithelial cells with scant cytoplasm and large nuclei harboring stippled chromatin are seen in Merkel cell carcinoma, as are frequent mitoses, tumor necrosis, and dense core cytoplasmic granules (▶ Fig. 21.84). Dermatofibroma is a benign tumor of skin composed of proliferating spindle fi-broblasts), various amounts of deposited collagen, and inter-vening macrophages (▶ Fig. 21.85). Nodular fasciitis is a reactive growth secondary to trauma. Histologically, nodular fasciitis presents with a loosely arranged proliferation of myofibroblasts harboring occasional mitoses in a hypocellular or myxoid back-ground (▶ Fig. 21.86).

Kaposi sarcoma is a low-malignancy mesenchymal neoplasm of skin and subcutaneous tissue, but also with wide spread vis-ceral involvement; it is usually linked to immune deficiency.

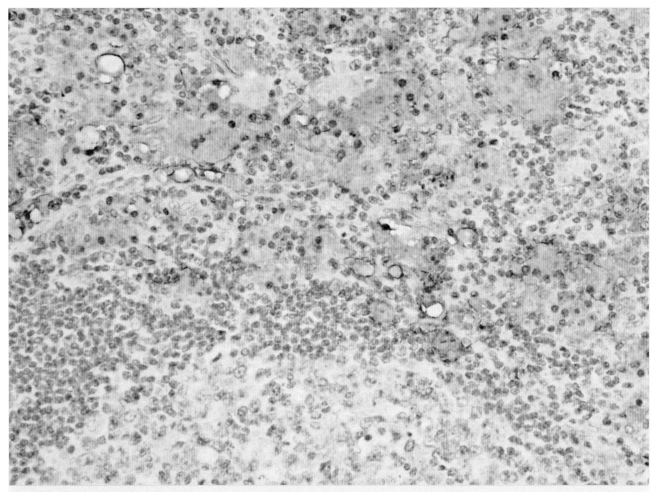

Fig. 21.77 Sinus histiocytosis with massive lymphadenopathy (Rosai-Dorfman disease) affects children and adolescents, presents with massive generalized lymphadenopathy of long duration, and can have a self-limited clinical course. Lymph node biopsies show effacement of lymphoid follicles with marked dilatation of interfollicular sinuses by an accumulation of histiocytes (S-100 immunohistochemical stain). Cells are CD68- and S-100–positive while CD1a- and Langerin-negative, devoid of necrosis, and capable of engulfing lymphocytes (emperipolesis).

Microscopically, it displays irregular vascular spaces lined by atypical endothelial cells with a low rate of mitotic activity and extravasated erythrocytes. Tumor cells show nuclear immunoreactivity for human herpesvirus 8 (HHV-8).[29] Angiolymphoid hyperplasia with eosinophilia is a chronic inflammatory condition presenting with swelling of skin and subcutaneous soft tissues in the head and neck, especially in the periauricular area; microscopically, it shows proliferating capillaries and various degrees of lymphocytic infiltrate with numerous eosinophils. External auditory canal cholesteatoma is a keratin-filled pearly expansion usually located in the inferior aspect of the canal. Long-standing lesions can be erosive/destructive of bone. Ceruminoma (adenoma of ceruminous glands) derives from transformed apocrine sweat glands of the external auditory cana (▶ Fig. 21.87).

Malignant tumors of the ceruminous glands can be adenocarcinomas (low- or high-grade) or have salivary gland tumor differentiation (adenoid cystic or mucoepidermoid carcinomas).

Middle Ear and Inner Ear

Infectious/Inflammatory/Anatomic/Idiopathic

Chronic otitis media, seen in all age groups, shows lymphoplasmacytic infiltration of the middle ear mucosa. Granulation tissue can be associated (forming aural polyps that hang into the external ear canal through tympanic perforations). Cholesterol granulomas are derived from intralesional bleeding. Fibrosis and calcification of the tympanic membrane can follow (tympanosclerosis), inflammation can affect the mastoid (chronic mastoiditis), and the tegmen can be eroded, allowing brain tissue to herniate into the middle ear (encephalocele).[30] Specific inflammatory processes of the nasal cavities and paranasal sinuses, like sarcoidosis, Wegener granulomatosis, tuberculosis, fungal infections, and others, can also occur. Cholesteatoma of the middle ear arises from retraction pockets of squamous epithelium in the tympanic membrane or from squamous metaplasia of the middle ear mucosa in long-standing inflammation and is istologically similar to its external auditory canal (▶ Fig. 21.88).

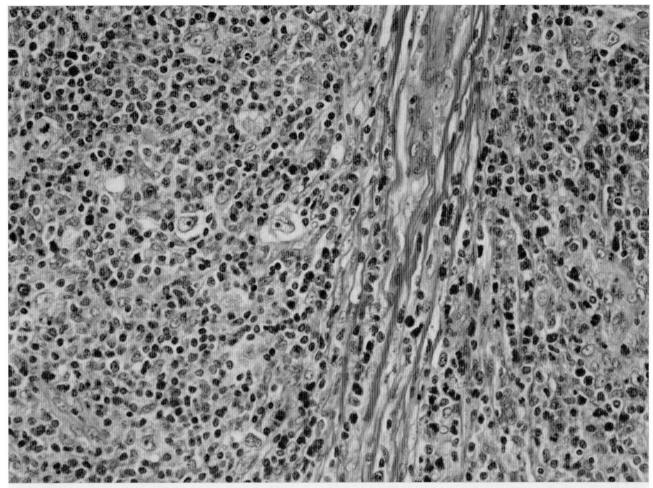

Fig. 21.78 Classic Hodgkin lymphoma, nodular sclerosing variant demonstrates fibrous bands separating nodules; a few Reed-Sternberg cells are seen with background eosinophilic infiltration.

Neoplasms

Adenomas of the middle ear are benign epithelial proliferations of packed small glands with single layer of cuboidal or columnar cells (▶ Fig. 21.89). The same epithelium can develop schneiderian-type papillomas of the middle ear (usually inverted papillomas), which are histologically identical to their nasal and paranasal sinus counterparts. Choristomas of the middle ear include salivary gland choristomas and glial heterotopias, in which benign salivary gland and glial tissue vestiges are found, respectively. Paraganglia are collections of neuroendocrine cells of neural crest origin that migrate during embryologic evolution in close association with cranial nerves, large vessels, and autonomic nerves and ganglia. We distinguish adrenal paraganglia (mainly secreting adrenalin) and extra-adrenal paraganglia, which can be sympathetic (mainly secreting noradrenalin) or parasympathetic (mainly secreting dopamine). Benign tumors derived from extra-adrenal paraganglia, all histologically identical, are found in decreasing order of prevalence at the bifurcation of the common carotid artery, middle ear, vagus nerve,

aortic arch, and other unusual locations, such as the larynx, orbit, cauda equina, nasopharynx, and others. The middle ear paragangliomas are most frequently attached to the jugular vein bulb (jugular paraganglioma) and less frequently to the tympanic nerve (branch of the glossopharyngeal nerve) in the area of the medial promontory wall (tympanic paraganglioma).[31] Collectively, they are called jugulotympanic paragangliomas (▶ Fig. 21.90).

Other benign tumors infrequently involving the middle ear are meningioma, schwannoma (acoustic neuroma; see ▶ Fig. 21.65), and lipoma of the internal auditory canal. Malignant tumors of the middle ear comprise squamous cell carcinomas, adenocarcinomas, and others. Considered to arise in the inner ear with possible secondary involvement of the middle ear is the endolymphatic sac tumor (aggressive papillary middle ear tumor), a neoplasm with low-grade malignant potential. It can occur sporadically but can also be associated with von Hippel-Lindau disease. On microscopic examination, it shows variable papillary, follicular, or glandular arrangement covered

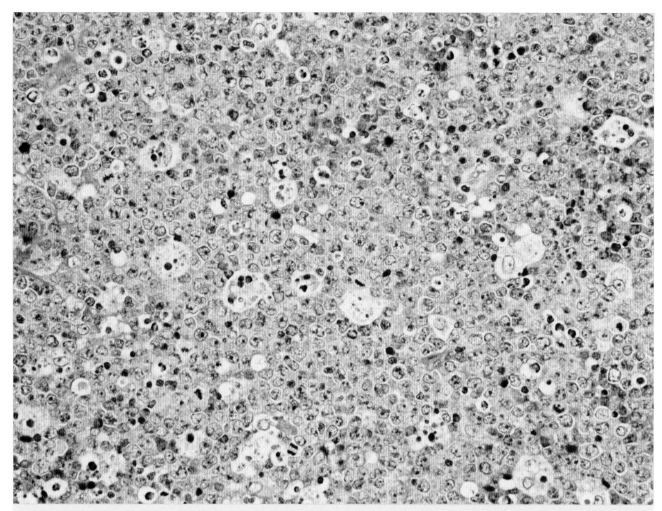

Fig. 21.79 Burkitt lymphoma is characterized by monotonous malignant large B lymphocytes with frequent scattered macrophages (starry sky appearance). Burkitt lymphoma is a high-grade B-cell lymphoma affecting young adults. It harbors large neoplastic B cells (immunoreactive to CD20, CD10, and Bcl-6 with Epstein-Barr virus positivity); the large numbers of macrophages attest to the high turnover rate of neoplastic cells.

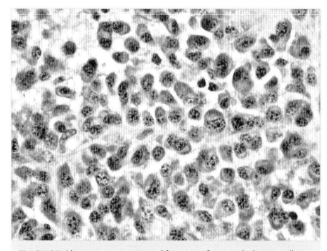

Fig. 21.80 Plasmacytoma is a proliferation of atypical plasma cells (immunoreactive to CD38 and CD138) with light- and heavy-chain restrictions, a high mitotic rate, and occasional necrotic foci with characteristic cartwheel nuclei, perinuclear hof (clearing at the nuclear concavity), and basophilic cytoplasm.

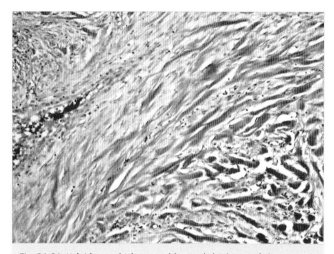

Fig. 21.81 Keloids are thick, extend beyond the limits of the original scars, and are raised with dense, irregular collagen bundles. The earlobes are frequently affected by keloid formation next to areas of piercing.

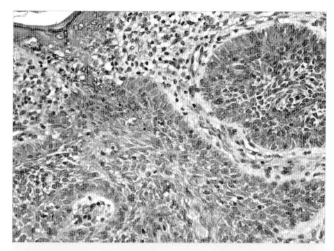

Fig. 21.82 Basal cell carcinoma displays invading islands of epithelial cells with large hyperchromatic nuclei and scant cytoplasm; note the connection to the basal layer of the epidermis (upper left corner). Basal cell carcinomas arise from the basal layer of the epidermis and invade the dermis as irregular nests of basaloid cells with peripheral palisading. Most are nodular and therefore easily excised; other variants (multifocal superficial and invading morphea type) have irregular borders and are difficult to completely excise by standard methods.

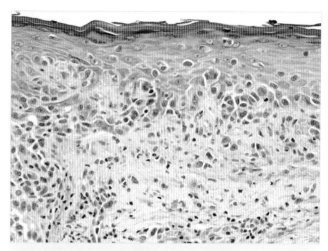

Fig. 21.83 Malignant melanoma is characterized by nests of melanocytes with atypical nuclei and conspicuous nucleoli forming basal epidermal nests and spreading into the upper layers of the epidermis. Malignant melanoma is one of the great mimics among neoplastic lesions; it can be pigmented or amelanotic, ulcerated or nodular, and histologically it displays an array of cytologic features ranging from large epithelioid cells to spindle and fusiform cells suggesting a mesenchymal lesion. Melanocytes are immunoreactive to S-100, MART-1 (Melan-A), and HMB-45. Proper margins of resection may be difficult to achieve on the skin of the external ear because of anatomical restrictions.

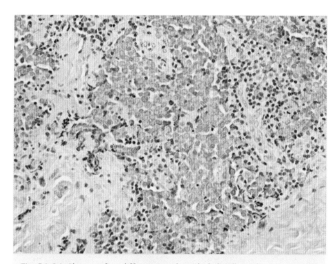

Fig. 21.84 Sheets of undifferentiated epithelial cells with scant cytoplasm and large nuclei harboring stippled chromatin are seen in Merkel cell carcinoma, as are frequent mitoses, tumor necrosis, and dense core cytoplasmic granules; note individual cell necrosis. Tumor cells react to neuroendocrine markers (synaptophysin, chromogranin, and CD56) and characteristically show paranuclear dotlike staining with CK-20 (a low-molecular-weight cytokeratin fraction).

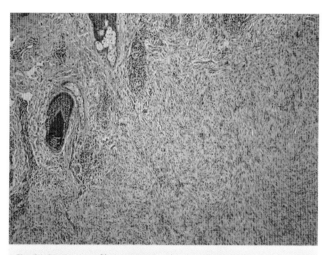

Fig. 21.85 Dermatofibroma is a poorly circumscribed benign tumor of skin composed of proliferating spindle fibroblasts (factor XIIIa–positive and CD34-negative), various amounts of deposited collagen, and intervening macrophages.

by cytologically bland epithelial cells in a single row; temporal bone invasion or middle ear infiltration is described.

21.4 Roundsmanship

- FNA as a screening test for thyroid nodules can subcategorize them as benign or suspicious, effectively preventing unnecessary surgery. A specific diagnosis may not always be possible.
- FNA as a screening test for salivary masses is efficient in distinguishing benign from malignant entities, thus facilitating preoperative planning.
- Submission of the FNA sample of a lymph node for flow cytometry analysis is essential if non-Hodgkin lymphoma is suspected; conversely, if Hodgkin lymphoma is high on the

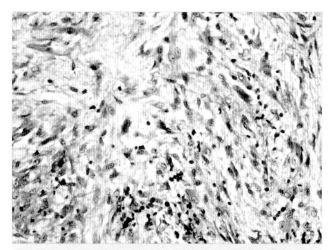

Fig. 21.86 Nodular fasciitis is a reactive rapid growth linked to a traumatic event. It presents with a loosely arranged proliferation of myofibroblasts harboring occasional mitoses in a hypocellular or myxoid background; note the occasional nuclear pleomorphism of fibroblasts.

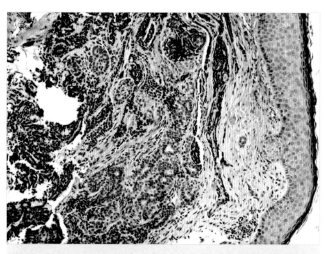

Fig. 21.87 Ceruminoma (adenoma of ceruminous glands) derives from transformed apocrine sweat glands of the external auditory canal. It is an unencapsulated subcutaneous glandular epithelial neoplasm with epithelial and myoepithelial cells (bilayered disposition) and an apocrine type of apical decapitation (apical snouting).

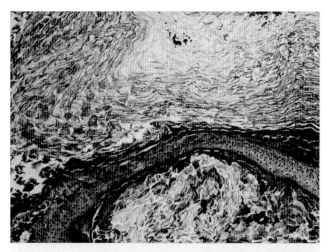

Fig. 21.88 Cholesteatoma of the middle ear arises from retraction pockets of squamous epithelium in the tympanic membrane or from squamous metaplasia of the middle ear mucosa in long-standing inflammation. Histologically similar to its external auditory canal counterpart, cholesteatoma of the middle ear shows an accumulation of flaky keratin with fragments of squamous epithelium.

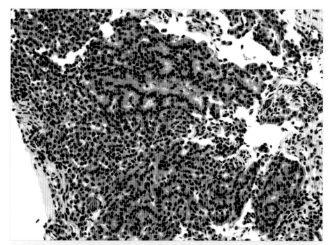

Fig. 21.89 Adenomas of the middle ear are unencapsulated benign epithelial proliferations of closely packed small glands with single layer of benign cuboidal or columnar cells.

differential diagnostic list, the entire sample should be saved for morphological examination.

- FNA of lymph nodes can reliably suggest a lymphoproliferative process and therefore justify an open biopsy (the gold standard for the histopathologic diagnosis of lymphoid lesions).
- The correlation of clinical, imaging, and cytologic findings is always desirable.
- In the head and neck, skin, epithelial, neural, respiratory, digestive, glandular, soft-tissue, bone, vascular, and lymphoid normal elements are combined in highly specialized structures within a relatively small anatomical area. The complexity of the pathologic processes here is unparalleled by that in any other area of the human body.
- The number of head and neck neoplasms with concomitant features of several different structures is high.
- Frozen sections in melanocytic skin lesions should be limited to surgical resection margins; the main lesion should be examined on permanent sections only after appropriate fixation.
- Malignant skin lesions of head and neck can be excised with only limited oncologic margins, and they should be excised with frozen section assessment of the surgical resection margins.

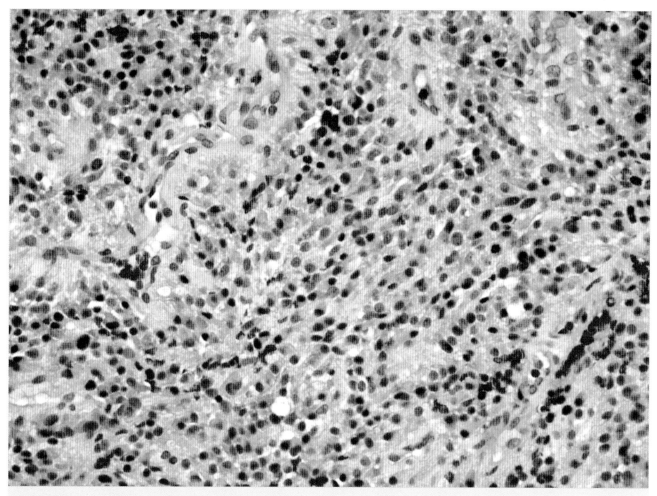

Fig. 21.90 On microscopic examination, paraganglioma shows polygonal neuroendocrine cells proliferating in clusters (zellballen) with intervening fibrous septa and scattered, flattened sustentacular cells (positive for S-100 and glial fibrillary acidic protein).

21.5 References

[1] Rosai J. Surgical Pathology. 8th ed. St. Louis, MO: Mosby; 1996:2–3

[2] Atkinson BF. Atlas of Diagnostic Cytopathology. 2nd ed. Philadelphia, PA: Elsevier; 2004:3–4

[3] Sedano HO, Carlos R, Koutlas IG. Respiratory scleroma: a clinicopathologic and ultrastructural study. Oral Surg Oral Med Oral Pathol Oral Radiol Endod 1996; 81: 665–671

[4] Prasad ML, Perez-Ordonez B. Nonsquamous lesions of the nasal cavity, paranasal sinuses, and nasopharynx. In: Gnepp DR, ed. Diagnostic Surgical Pathology of the Head and Neck. 2nd ed. Philadelphia, PA: Saunders Elsevier; 2009:115–116

[5] Stoll W, Nieschalk M. Kongenitale Fehlbildungen des pränasalen Raumes: Gliome, Fisteln, Epidermoidzysten. Laryngorhinootologie 1996; 75: 739–744

[6] Biurrun O, Olmo A, Barceló X, Morelló A, Condom E, Traserra J. [Thornwaldt's cyst. The experience of a decade] An Otorrinolaringol Ibero Am 1992; 19: 179–189

[7] Devaney KO, Travis WD, Hoffman G, Leavitt R, Lebovics R, Fauci AS. Interpretation of head and neck biopsies in Wegener's granulomatosis. A pathologic study of 126 biopsies in 70 patients. Am J Surg Pathol 1990; 14: 555–564

[8] Gaffey MJ, Frierson HF, Weiss LM, Barber CM, Baber GB, Stoler MH. Human papillomavirus and Epstein-Barr virus in sinonasal Schneiderian papillomas. An in situ hybridization and polymerase chain reaction study. Am J Clin Pathol 1996; 106: 475–482

[9] Lawson W, Ho BT, Shaari CM, Biller HF. Inverted papilloma: a report of 112 cases. Laryngoscope 1995; 105: 282–288

[10] Barnes L. Schneiderian papillomas and nonsalivary glandular neoplasms of the head and neck. Mod Pathol 2002; 15: 279–297

[11] Sze WM, Lee AW, Yau TK et al. Primary tumor volume of nasopharyngeal carcinoma: prognostic significance for local control. Int J Radiat Oncol Biol Phys 2004; 59: 21–27

[12] Pilch BZ, Bouquot J, Thompson LDR. Squamous cell carcinoma of nasal cavity and paranasal sinuses. In: Barnes L, Eveson JW, Reichart P, Sidransky D, eds. World Health Organization Classification of Tumours. Pathology and Genetics. Tumours of the Head and Neck. Lyons, France: IARC Press; 2005:15–17

[13] Thompson LDR, Fanburg-Smith JC, Wenig BM. Borderline and low malignant potential tumours of soft tissue. In: Barnes L, Eveson JW, Reichart P, Sidransky D, eds. World Health Organization Classification of Tumours. Pathology and Genetics. Tumours of the Head and Neck. Lyons, France: IARC Press; 2005:43–45

[14] Zwahlen RA, Grätz KW. Maxillary ameloblastomas: a review of the literature and of a 15-year database. J Craniomaxillofac Surg 2002; 30: 273–279

[15] Sakr WA, Gale N, Gnepp DR, Crissman J. Squamous intraepithelial neoplasia of the upper aerodigestive tract. In: Gnepp DR, ed. Diagnostic Surgical Pathology of the Head and Neck. 2nd ed. Philadelphia, PA: Saunders Elsevier; 2009:1–38

[16] Al-Hashimi I, Schifter M, Lockhart PB et al. Oral lichen planus and oral lichenoid lesions: diagnostic and therapeutic considerations. Oral Surg Oral Med Oral Pathol Oral Radiol Endod 2007; 103 Suppl: e1–e12

[17] Davenport S, Chen SY, Miller AS. Pemphigus vulgaris: clinicopathologic review of 33 cases in the oral cavity. Int J Periodontics Restorative Dent 2001; 21: 85–90

[18] Bouquot JE, Muller S, Nikai H. Pigmented mucosal lesions. In: Gnepp DR, ed. Diagnostic Surgical Pathology of the Head and Neck. 2nd ed. Philadelphia, PA: Saunders Elsevier; 2009:284–292

[19] Brandwein-Gensler MS, Mahadevia P, Gnepp DR. Cysts: laryngoceles, saccular cysts, and dermoid cysts. In: Gnepp DR, ed. Diagnostic Surgical Pathology of

the Head and Neck. 2nd ed. Philadelphia, PA: Saunders Elsevier; 2009:330–334

[20] Uzcudun AE, Bravo Fernández P, Sánchez JJ et al. Clinical features of pharyngeal cancer: a retrospective study of 258 consecutive patients. J Laryngol Otol 2001; 115: 112–118

[21] Cardesa A, Gale N, Nadal A, Zidar N. Squamous cell carcinoma. In: Barnes L, Eveson JW, Reichart P, Sidransky D, eds. World Health Organization Classification of Tumours. Pathology and Genetics. Tumours of the Head and Neck. Lyons, France: IARC Press; 2005:118–121

[22] Rosai J. Surgical Pathology. 9th ed. St. Louis, MO: Mosby Elsevier; 2004:874

[23] Cheung P-SY. Medical and surgical treatment of endemic goiter. In: Clark OH, Dub Q-Y, eds. Textbook of Endocrine Surgery. Philadelphia, PA: W. B. Saunders; 1997:15–21

[24] DeLellis RA. Primary chief cell hyperplasia. In: Atlas of Tumor Pathology. Tumors of the Parathyroid Gland. Washington, DC: Armed Forces Institute of Pathology; 1991:65–77

[25] Billings SD, Folpe AL. Cutaneous and subcutaneous fibrohistiocytic tumors of intermediate malignancy: an update. Am J Dermatopathol 2004; 26: 141–155

[26] Weiss SW, Goldblum JR, Eds. Enzinger and Weiss's Soft Tissue Tumors. 5th ed. Philadelphia, PA: Elsevier; 2008:4–10

[27] Ioachim HL, Medeiros LJ. Ioachim's Lymph Node Pathology. 4th ed. Philadelphia, PA: Lippincott Williams & Wilkins; 2009:99–104

[28] Swerdlow SH, Campo E, Harris NL, et al. World Health Organization Classification of Tumours. Pathology and Genetics. Tumours of Haematopoietic and Lymphoid Tissues. Lyons, France: IARC Press; 2008:326–334

[29] Weedon D. Skin Pathology. 2nd ed. Edinburgh, Scotland: Churchill Livingstone; 2002:1021–1025

[30] Davis GL. Ear: external, middle, and temporal bone. In: Gnepp DR, ed. Diagnostic Surgical Pathology of the Head and Neck. 2nd ed. Philadelphia, PA: Saunders Elsevier; 2009:905–906

[31] Barnes L, Tse LLY, Hunt JL, Michaels L. Tumours of the paraganglionic system. In: Barnes L, Eveson JW, Reichart P, Sidransky D, eds. World Health Organization Classification of Tumours. Pathology and Genetics. Tumours of the Head and Neck. Lyons, France: IARC Press; 2005:362–370

22 The Role of Radiation Therapy in the Management of Head and Neck Cancer

Kenneth S. Hu and Louis B. Harrison

22.1 Introduction

Radiation therapy is an integral component in the treatment of head and neck tumors. Machine-generated X-rays were discovered by William Roentgen in 1895. The first radioactive isotope (radium) was discovered in 1899 by Marie Curie and was first applied in the treatment of head and neck cancer in the early 1900s. Radioactive isotopes continue to be useful today in the form of brachytherapy. Machine-generated high-energy X-rays are the mainstay of treatment for the majority of head and neck tumors. Early orthovoltage and superficial voltage machines were limited in application because of skin injury during the treatment of subcutaneous tumors. Not until the development of the high-energy linear accelerator in the 1960s could external beam radiation be integrated into the treatment of head and neck cancer without prohibitive skin toxicity. Simulation, computed tomography (CT)–based treatment planning, field shaping with motorized multiple-leaf collimators, and intensity modulation of radiation represent important advances that have allowed the highly conformal delivery of radiation, optimizing the therapeutic ratio by concentrating the radiation around the tumor while sparing adjacent normal tissue such as salivary glands, pharyngeal muscles, and cranial nerves. Current radiation delivery systems allow millimeter precision and simultaneous differential dosing to areas at variable levels of risk. Such high levels of conformality increase the ability to integrate radiation in a multidisciplinary manner to provide excellent locoregional control and focus on organ function preservation.

22.2 Radiobiology

Radiation works primarily by causing reproductive cell death such that tumors are unable to replicate. The target of treatment is the tumor DNA, in which free radical formation from ionizing radiation therapy causes permanent double-strand breakage. Normal tissues have a greater capacity than tumor cells to repair themselves after radiation exposure. Fractionation exploits the repair differential such that doses high enough to kill tumors but that spare the function and integrity of normal tissue are used. In general, radiation doses of 50, 60, and 70 gray (Gy) are required for elective treatment, microscopic residual disease, and gross tumor, respectively. Advanced stage T3 and T4 tumors usually require the concurrent addition of a radiation sensitizer during radiation therapy to achieve a high probability of tumor control. Head and neck squamous cell carcinomas have the unique characteristic of delayed accelerated tumor repopulation during radiation therapy, which makes the total treatment time a vital aspect of optimal radiation delivery. The phenomena of on-treatment repopulation and differential repair ability underlie the rationale for several altered fractionated radiation regimens proven to improve locoregional control. Shortening the duration of treatment with accelerated radiation regimens from a conventional time of 7 to 6 weeks or less has yielded significant gains. Also, escalating the dose beyond the conventional dose of 70 up to 80 Gy with hyperfractionation and administering two treatments per day exploit the repair advantage of normal tissue over tumor such that long-term toxicity is no different but tumor control is improved.

22.2.1 General Approaches to Improving Locoregional Control with Radiation Therapy

Because of their location, cancers of the head and neck can severely impact speech, mastication, taste, swallowing, and cosmesis. Eradicating disease and preserving organ function are important goals of treatment. For early-stage disease, single-modality therapy is preferred, whereas a complex multidisciplinary evaluation is needed for locoregionally advanced disease. Important advances have been made, with altered fractionation and the incorporation of chemotherapy used to improve disease control. More recent advances include better targeting of tumor through improved imaging, radiation delivery, and biologic therapies. The preservation of quality of life and organ function is a crucial end point that guides the selection of an optimal treatment for individual patients.

22.2.2 Radiation Techniques and Particle Therapies

Multiple methods of delivering radiation therapy to optimize the therapeutic ratio have been developed. The mainstay of treatment has been with external beam techniques, which deliver photons generated by machine and shaped by blocks and collimation before the patient is treated. Brachytherapy is the direct placement of radioactive sources in the tumor and is most often used as a boost to augment a course of external beam radiation. Such an approach permits escalation of the dose to the primary site and decreased exposure of normal tissues to the dose.

External Beam Radiation

Two-Dimensional Technique

In the traditional two-dimensional technique, treatment fields are designed based on bony landmarks and wide margins up to 2 cm, with X-rays delivered to opposed lateral fields and a low anterior neck field. The target volume of the parallel opposed fields should include the primary site with margin plus draining lymph nodes of the upper neck, with a high match above the arytenoids for oropharynx lesions and a low match below the cricoid cartilage for laryngeal/hypopharyngeal lesions.

Radiation therapy has improved vastly from the initial use of orthovoltage/radium sources, block-shaped beams, and plain film–based imaging with large setup uncertainty to the use of high-energy linear accelerators with dynamic leaf collimation and CT-based treatment planning with precise setup and immobilization. The evolution in treatment planning has allowed the better-targeted delivery of radiation, with sparing of the structures important for salivation, hearing, swallowing, and chewing. Additionally, nausea can be prevented.

Intensity-Modulated Radiation Therapy

Recent efforts to improve radiation dose conformality and reduce toxicity have been made with three-dimensional and intensity-modulated radiation therapy (IMRT) techniques to treat complex, irregularly shaped head and neck tumors. IMRT has generated tremendous enthusiasm because it allows exquisite dose conformality with sparing of adjacent organs. Each radiation field is divided into a number of beamlets with the aid of an intensity modulator and inverse treatment planning. The different beamlets are added to form a cumulative dose distribution tailored to the shape of the tumor and respecting designated normal tissue tolerance constraints. IMRT also offers the possibility of differential dosing to the elective nodal basin, high-risk nodal areas, and primary tumor sites with resultant modestly accelerated radiation.

Cancers of the oropharynx and nasopharynx are ideal sites for IMRT because the tumors often present in close proximity to sensitive normal tissues such as the parotid glands or involve the pharyngeal wall/retropharyngeal nodes close to the spinal cord. Locoregional control of 87 to 89% appears similar and possibly better than that achieved with conventional techniques based on initial single-institution series. IMRT regimens of 70 Gy in 33 or 35 fractions are well tolerated, even with concurrent chemotherapy (▶ Fig. 22.1).

To date, the greatest benefit of IMRT in regard to toxicity has been the reduction of severe xerostomia compared with standard techniques. Eisbruch et al showed that stimulated salivary flow can be preserved if the mean dose to one parotid gland with IMRT is 26 Gy or less, with full recovery occurring up to 2 years after treatment. This is clearly an important advance because xerostomia is the primary quality-of-life complaint among long-term survivors of head and neck cancer treated with radiation.

IMRT may also be used to spare the cochlea, nausea center, constrictor muscles, carotid arteries, minor salivary glands of the oral cavity, submandibular gland, larynx, and pterygoid muscles.

Brachytherapy

Brachytherapy, or the implantation of radioactive seeds directly into the target volume, offers dose escalation to tumor and sparing of surrounding normal tissue by inverse-square attenuation, producing excellent dose conformality. Normal tissue toxicity is further lessened because the dose of external beam radiation is reduced, which is especially advantageous in those receiving concurrent chemotherapy.

Stereotactic Radiotherapy

Stereotactic radiation delivers highly focused radiation to tumors through the use of rigid immobilization techniques and non-coplanar beam arrangements. The foremost advantage of stereotactic radiation is that it delivers a single (stereotactic radiosurgery [SRS]) or hypofractionated (stereotactic radiation therapy [SRT]) dose of radiation having an ablative effect on the tumor with submillimeter margins of precision, allowing much smaller treatment volumes. The potential benefit of SRT over SRS is that the multiple fractions allow the repair of normal tissue, with the increased possibility of organ function preservation, an important consideration when tumors are adjacent to the optic nerve pathways, brain, and spinal cord. Both techniques require the use of a stereotactic frame, which creates a highly accurate three-dimensional localizing system orienting the treatment planning system to the precise location of the target. Stereotactic radiation is delivered by either of two methods: (1) a gamma knife device, which comprises 201 independently controlled cobalt sources arranged in a helmet, or (2) a linear accelerator, with conversion accomplished via a specialized collimating device. Stereotactic radiation is best applied to tumors that are less than 4 to 5 cm in size and well delineated on CT, magnetic resonance (MR) imaging, or angiography. It is most often used as a boost after a course of external beam radiation or as salvage therapy. It has proved particularly useful in malignant tumors of the skull base and paranasal sinuses, as well as benign tumors such as paragangliomas, meningiomas, pituitary adenomas, vascular malformations, and acoustic neuromas.

Particle Therapy

Radiation with heavy particles, such as protons and neutrons, offers unique advantages in dose deposition. Protons deposit radiation close to the tumor, with radiation falling off dramatically posterior to the target in a Bragg peak distribution. This allows the exquisite control of dose deposition. Traditionally, protons have been used to treat uveal melanomas and chondrosarcomas of the skull base, as well as adenoid cystic carcinomas of the parotid and lacrimal glands. Neutrons offer the high particle treatment of tumors thought to be resistant to radiation and destroy tumors without reliance on oxygenation because of their high linear energy transfer properties. They have been most successfully used in the treatment in suboptimally resected adenoid cystic carcinomas.

Altered Fractionated Radiation

Altered fractionated radiation therapy attempts to improve tumor control either by accelerating radiation treatment to overcome tumor repopulation or by dose escalation with hyperfractionation to make use of the radiation repair advantage of normal tissues over tumor. Radiation therapy can be successfully accelerated by delayed concomitant boost or a Danish regimen of six conventional treatments per week, whereas dose escalation is best accomplished by hyperfractionation. Meta-analysis has indicated a survival advantage of hyperfractionation with dose escalation compared with conventional fractionation.

A landmark trial conducted by the Radiation Therapy Oncology Group (RTOG 90–03) compared the leading U.S. altered fractionated regimens for cancers, primarily stages III and IV head and neck cancers or stage II hypopharynx or base of tongue cancers. At 8 years of follow-up, the results showed that hyperfractionated radiation therapy and accelerated radiation

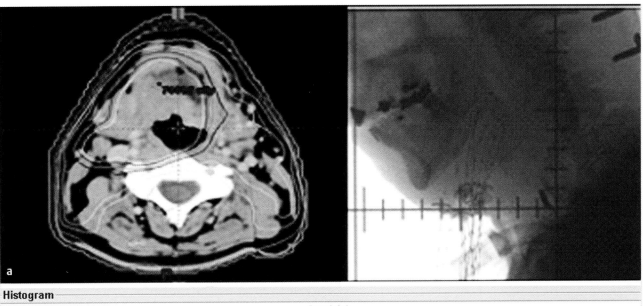

Histogram

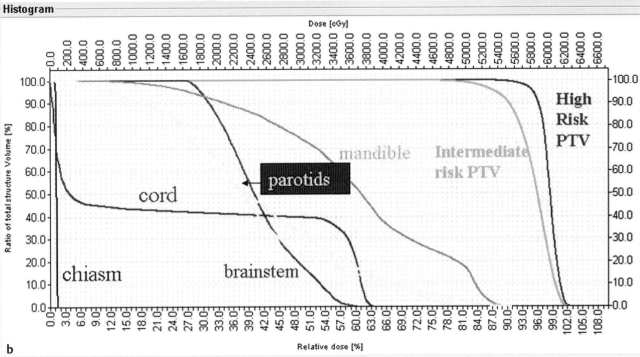

Fig. 22.1 (a) A 62-year-old man with a T2 N2b M0 base of tongue carcinoma treated with combined external beam radiation and concurrent chemotherapy, brachytherapy implant, and planned neck dissection. External beam radiation was delivered with intensity modulation in a reduced dose of 5,940 cGy to the involved primary site and nodes followed by a 20-Gy brachytherapy boost. (b) Dose–volume histogram demonstrating dose distribution from course of intensity-modulated radiation therapy.

by delayed concomitant boost improved locoregional control by 7 to 8% over conventional fractionation, with improved disease-free survival.

Concurrent Radiation and Chemotherapy

Numerous overviews demonstrate the advantage of adding chemotherapy to radiation. A meta-analysis by Monnerat et al concluded that concurrent chemotherapy offers an 8% survival benefit, induction chemotherapy a 2% benefit, and adjuvant therapy a 1% benefit. In general, there is a 10 to 20% improvement in locoregional control with concurrent chemotherapy.

The French Intergroup (GORTEC 94–01) Phase III randomized trial established concurrent chemoradiation as the standard treatment for locoregionally advanced oropharyngeal disease. Long-term follow-up demonstrated improved 5-year overall survival and disease-free survival and a locoregional control advantage with combined therapy (conventional radiation with three cycles of concurrent carboplatin/5-fluorouracil) over conventional radiation alone in patients with stage III and IV oropharyngeal carcinoma. Still, despite such intensive therapy, locoregional failure occurred in more than 50% of patients.

Chemotherapy Combined with Altered Fractionated Radiation

Efforts to further improve locoregional control and survival have explored combining concurrent chemotherapy with altered fractionated radiation because both approaches independently improve outcome for patients with head and neck cancer. The present challenge is to find the optimal chemoradiation regimen(s) that offer high rates of locoregional control and organ function preservation with acceptable morbidity and the possibility of integration with new biologic agents or additional chemotherapy.

The majority of Phase III trials show a benefit of the addition of concurrent chemotherapy to altered fractionated radiation with either hyperfractionation or delayed concomitant boost (DCB) compared with the same radiation regimen alone. Budach et al estimate a 2-year survival benefit of 12% with the addition of chemotherapy to either hyperfractionation or accelerated radiation.

Conventional versus Altered Fractionated Concurrent Chemoradiation

However, two recent randomized trials have shown no locoregional control or survival benefit of altered fractionated radiation over conventional fractionation in patients receiving concurrent chemoradiation. Thus, conventional fractionation is most commonly used in the setting of concurrent chemoradiation.

Role of Induction Chemotherapy

Induction chemotherapy has been used to reduce the tumor burden and increase the successful treatment of tumors with organ preservation therapy. This is particularly evident in patients with larynx and hypopharynx cancers. Multiple meta-analyses show only a minor survival benefit of induction chemotherapy. However, recent data show that the addition of docetaxel (Taxotere; Sanofi-Aventis) to induction chemotherapy with cisplatin/5-fluorouracil followed by radiation or concurrent chemoradiation improves survival and locoregional control.

A landmark trial randomized 202 selected patients with locally advanced hypopharyngeal cancer to radical resection with postoperative irradiation or to induction chemotherapy with two or three cycles of cisplatin/5-fluorouracil followed by conventional fractionated radiation (70 Gy for 7 weeks) if the patients had a clinical complete response after induction chemotherapy. At a median follow-up of 51 months, there was no statistical difference between the arms in rates of local and regional failure. At 5 years of follow-up, there was no significant survival difference (34% vs 29%). For all patients entered in the organ preservation arm, the 3-year organ preservation rate was 42%.

Most recently, the addition of docetaxel to induction cisplatin and fluorouracil (TPF) compared with induction PF alone increased larynx preservation. GORTEC 2000–01 randomized 220 patients with hypopharynx or larynx cancer for whom total laryngectomy would be required to either TPF or PF followed by conventionally fractionated radiation to 70 Gy. At a median follow-up of 35 months, larynx preservation at 3 years was improved by about 10% such that three-quarters achieved organ preservation.

Other induction chemotherapy trials with TPF before radiation or concurrent chemoradiation showed an improvement in overall survival versus induction PF. However, the benefit of induction TPF in the setting of standard cisplatin-based concurrent chemoradiation has not been established, and its role in the treatment of head and neck cancer continues to be defined.

Biologic Therapy: C225

Epidermal growth factor receptor (EGFR) is commonly expressed in head and neck cancer cell lines. Ang reported in a study of a cohort of RTOG 90–03 patients that patients who had tumors expressing a higher than median level of EGFR had a greater risk for 2-year locoregional relapse, lower 2-year disease-free survival, and lower 2-year overall survival compared with patients who had tumors expressing lower than median or median levels of EGFR. No difference in distant metastases were noted between the two groups.

A pivotal Phase III trial reported by Bonner et al demonstrated the benefit of adding cetuximab (C225), a monoclonal antibody targeting EGFR, to radiation. In this trial, 424 patients with stage III or IV head and neck cancer (primarily of the oropharynx/hypopharynx) were randomized to 7 weeks of C225 plus radiation (conventional fractionation or altered fractionation) or to radiation alone. At a median follow-up of 38 months, C225/radiation was superior to radiation alone with respect to 2-year locoregional control, 2-year overall survival, and median overall survival. With regard to toxicity, the addition of C225, unlike the addition of concurrent chemotherapy or the acceleration of radiation, did not significantly increase grade 3 or 4 mucositis but was associated with increased rates of dermatitis and infusion reaction.

22.3 Role of Radiation Therapy in Specific Sites of Disease

Radiation therapy has been used preoperatively or postoperatively in the definitive treatment of head and neck squamous cell carcinomas in conjunction with curative-intent surgical resection, and also as radical treatment to avoid surgical extirpation in an attempt to maintain organ integrity and preserve organ function. The site-specific roles and treatment outcomes are summarized in the following paragraphs.

22.3.1 Oral Cavity

In general, primary surgery with radical resection and selective neck dissection is recommended for oral cavity cancer as single-modality therapy in stage I and II. Adjuvant radiation therapy should be considered in the presence of perineural or lymphovascular invasion or in cases with close margins.

For stage III and IV disease, radical resection with adjuvant radiation alone or concurrently with chemotherapy should be considered. Factors warranting consideration for radiation therapy include lymphovascular or perineural invasion, level IV nodal involvement, and the presence of multiple nodes. Risk factors warranting the incorporation of chemotherapy concurrently with radiation are positive margins at the primary site and extracapsular nodal extension. In high-risk patients receiving adjuvant radiation, the total treatment time from the day of surgery to the end of radiation therapy is best kept to 11 weeks or less.

For patients with locoregionally advanced tumors of the oral cavity tumors who are not candidates for resection, concurrent chemoradiation remains the standard. If definitive radiation therapy is considered, the integration of brachytherapy with external beam radiation has yielded excellent outcomes in patients with oral cavity tumors.

22.3.2 Oropharynx

Early-stage oropharyngeal carcinoma is often treated with a single modality. This can be either a surgical resection or radiation therapy. The decision between these two modalities often depends on the expertise of the treating center and also the expected functional outcome. Chemotherapy is rarely used in treating early-stage oropharyngeal cancer. The overall outcome for patients with early-stage disease is excellent, with a cure rate that often exceeds 90%. Conventionally fractionated radiation therapy alone controls the majority of early-stage oropharyngeal lesions but may be suboptimal for T2 base of tongue and posterior pharyngeal wall cancers. For tonsil cancers, several large single-institutional series have shown excellent local control after conventional fractionated radiation alone (1.8 to 2.0 Gy per dose over 6.5 to 7 weeks to doses of 65 to 70 Gy), approximating 80 to 90% for T1 to T2 lesions and 63% to 74% for T3 lesions.

Ipsilateral External Beam Radiation Therapy for Early-Stage Tonsil Cancer

In general, most lateralized T1 to T2 lesions in patients with an N0 or N1 neck can be treated with ipsilateral radiation fields. Lesions that cross the midline, extensively involve the tongue base or soft palate, or are associated with N2 or more advanced neck disease should receive comprehensive bilateral neck therapy. Such an approach minimizes irradiation to the contralateral salivary glands and reduces the incidence of xerostomia. Eisbruch et al demonstrated that patients treated unilaterally experience less xerostomia and have a better quality of life than do those treated with bilateral IMRT with contralateral parotid sparing.

Many early-stage soft palate and pharyngeal wall cancers are near midline, leaving bilateral neck and retropharyngeal nodes at risk. Therefore, external beam radiation therapy is often preferable because of comprehensive nodal coverage with high rates of control for T1 and T2 lesions, similar to those for tonsil cancers. Also, functional deficits after surgery, such as uvulopalatal insufficiency requiring prosthetic obturators to prevent reflux into the nasopharynx/nasal cavity, can be avoided. Large single-institution series show similarly high rates of local control after external beam radiation therapy alone.

Treatment of Locally Advanced Resectable Disease: Stages III and IV

Radiation alone provides less optimal rates of local control in patients with resectable T3 and T4 lesions or with advanced N2 and N3 neck disease (because of high rates of persistent disease after treatment) compared with combined treatment but may be considered in patients with intermediate-stage cancers (T1/T2 N1 or T3 N0). However, the majority of patients with oropharyngeal cancer will present with stage III or stage IV disease and do require a multimodality approach that combines chemotherapy, radiation therapy, and surgery. The choice of the modality to be used often depends on the treating team and its experience. The options include the following: (1) Surgery followed by radiation therapy or chemoradiation. (2) Concurrent chemoradiotherapy, which is considered by many to represent the standard of care in the treatment of patients with locally advanced oropharyngeal cancer. The agent most studied is bolus cisplatin at 100 mg/m^2 given every 3 weeks during radiation. Patients who cannot tolerate this dose and schedule of platinum can be treated with weekly chemotherapy with paclitaxel/carboplatin, cisplatin, or cetuximab. (3) Sequential induction chemotherapy followed by radiation therapy or concurrent chemoradiotherapy. The induction chemotherapy regimen that is most widely used is TPF, given every 3 weeks for a total of three cycles, followed by radiation alone or radiation with weekly carboplatin.

For patients with T4 or N3 disease, chemoradiation therapy or sequential induction chemotherapy followed by concurrent chemoradiotherapy is considered. Sequential chemoradiotherapy is preferable for this group of patients if they have good performance status because they have a worse prognosis than the group with resectable disease, with a cure rate of 25 to 40% at 5 years.

Human Papillomavirus–Related Oropharyngeal Carcinoma

Recently, infection with the human papillomavirus (HPV), especially HPV-16, has been identified as the predominant risk factor in the Western world for developing oropharyngeal cancer. It is currently estimated that 50 to 60% of cases of oropharyngeal cancer are related to HPV-16. The major characteristics of this entity are the following:

- Patients are about 10 years younger than those with smoking- or alcohol-related oropharyngeal cancer. Many patients with HPV-related oropharyngeal cancer are in their forties and early fifties.
- Patients are often nonsmokers and nondrinkers.
- Patients typically present with a small primary lesion and bulky lymphadenopathy.
- The pathology specimen often has a "basaloid" appearance.
- The prognosis is excellent. Patients with HPV-related oropharyngeal cancer, even those with locally advanced disease, have excellent survival, with a cure rate that often exceeds 85 to 90%. This has led to the development of clinical trials targeted specifically toward this patient population. Until those trials are completed, treatment should not be modified based on HPV status.

HPV status can be checked via fluorescent in situ hybridization (FISH) or polymerase chain reaction (PCR). Alternatively, p16 immunohistochemistry can serve as a surrogate for HPV infection and be used to assess HPV status. These tests are all performed on the surgical specimen. It is strongly recommended that the HPV status of all patients with oropharyngeal cancer be assessed, given its prognostic implications.

Brachytherapy for Oropharyngeal Cancer

Brachytherapy has been a mainstay treatment for oropharyngeal cancers for decades, and excellent results have been reported. Brachytherapy, or the implantation of radioactive seeds directly into the target volume, allows escalation of the dose to the tumor and the sparing of surrounding normal tissue by inverse-square attenuation, producing excellent dose conformality. Normal tissue toxicity is further lessened because the dose of external beam radiation is reduced, which is especially important in those receiving concurrent chemotherapy.

Consistently excellent results with the use of this approach for base of tongue disease have been reported by multiple centers. Moreover, it has been demonstrated that such an approach improves the chance for swallowing preservation compared with conformal external beam radiation alone.

22.3.3 Nasopharynx

Nasopharyngeal carcinomas are located in a highly enriched lymphatic drainage area, which favors early regional spread to the retropharyngeal and cervical nodes (unilaterally and bilaterally). The primary tumor exists in an occult location with a propensity to invade the skull base, surrounding sinuses, nerves, and soft-tissue spaces before presenting clinically. Radiation therapy has been the mainstay treatment because it can cover the large areas of potential locoregional spread. Advances in radiation delivery with IMRT, imaging, integration of chemotherapy, standardization of an internationally agreed-upon staging system, multidisciplinary care, and scientific exchange have led to significant improvements in tumor control and quality of life.

In general, patients with early-stage tumors are amenable to treatment with radiation therapy alone with high rates of locoregional control, whereas those with T3 or T4 lesions or significant nodal disease require more intensive chemoradiation treatment because outcomes with radiation therapy alone have been associated with higher rates of locoregional failure and distant metastases.

Patients with early-stage disease account for fewer than 10% of all patients with nasopharyngeal cancer and may be treated with radiation therapy alone. Conventional fractionation and two-dimensional technique have shown generally good locoregional control rates for early-stage tumors but suboptimal outcomes for locoregionally advanced tumors. After conventional radiation, local control is obtained in 75 to 95% of T1/T2 tumors, compared with 44 to 80% of T3/T4 tumors. Improvement in early-stage disease control has been obtained by either dose escalation with brachytherapy or improved conformal technique. Moreover, with conformal techniques, improved preservation of salivary gland function, hearing, and overall quality of life has been demonstrated.

Although excellent outcomes are obtained in the treatment of early-stage disease with radiotherapy alone, 20 to 60% of patients with advanced-stage disease experience locoregional failure after radiotherapy only and high rates of distant metastases (50 to 70%), with 5-year overall survival rates of 28 to 56%.

In the United States, the standard of care is concurrent chemoradiation with cisplatin chemotherapy and radiation followed by three cycles of adjuvant chemotherapy comprising 5-fluorouracil and cisplatin. The basis for such treatment is the landmark Phase III randomized Intergroup Study 0099, which demonstrated that compared with radiation alone, the addition of three cycles of CDDP (*cis*-diamminedichloroplatinum) to radiation therapy followed by adjuvant CDDP/5-fluorouracil improved 3-year locoregional control and decreased the incidence of distant metastases, which translated into an approximate 10% increase in 3-year progression-free and overall survival. In the chemoradiation arm, there was a higher incidence of grade 3/4 leukopenia and vomiting. Compliance with the planned regimen was compromised because only two-thirds of the patients were able to complete all three cycles of concurrent cisplatin, with an additional one-fourth able to complete two concurrent cycles. Only 60% of patients received two to three planned cycles of adjuvant chemotherapy. Alternative schedules used outside the United States have included weekly cisplatin ($40\,mg/m^2$) with radiation alone without adjuvant chemotherapy and induction chemotherapy followed by chemoradiation.

22.3.4 Hypopharynx

Patients with early-stage disease constitute about 25% of all those who present with hypopharyngeal cancers. Important goals in patients with T1 or T2 resectable disease are to obtain local control while optimizing swallowing and voice preservation, which can be accomplished with either conservation surgery or radiation therapy. Neck management is indicated even in patients with N0 disease, who will have a 30 to 40% risk for occult neck metastases.

Early-stage lesions, including T1 or low-bulk T2 hypopharyngeal squamous cell carcinomas, may be effectively treated with external beam radiation therapy, especially when the tumors are exophytic and do not involve the apex. Radiation has the advantage of sterilizing occult and early cervical metastases, obviating the need for nodal dissection. The local control rates for T1/T2 lesions treated with radiation therapy alone vary widely depending on the series, radiation technique/dose, patient selection factors, and neck staging. Taken together, local control varies from 47 to 90%, and 5-year survival varies from 11 to 52%. In general, the best results have been obtained with conventional fractionation to doses higher than 65 Gy for T1 lesions and hyperfractionated radiation for T2 lesions in large single-institution series.

Primary resection is most often considered for advanced, bulky hypopharyngeal cancers because tumor control and organ preservation are suboptimal after nonsurgical therapy, and patients often have morbidity such as chronic aspiration due to the destruction of normal tissues by the tumor or treatment. In such a setting, total laryngectomy with partial or total pharyngectomy must be considered mandatory, followed by adjuvant radiation with or without chemotherapy.

For advanced-stage lesions, laryngopharyngectomy followed by postoperative radiation with or without chemotherapy is standard treatment. Small tumors with nodal involvement and nonbulky T3 lesions may be considered for management with radiation therapy and chemotherapy. In this setting, induction chemotherapy followed by radiation alone has been considered

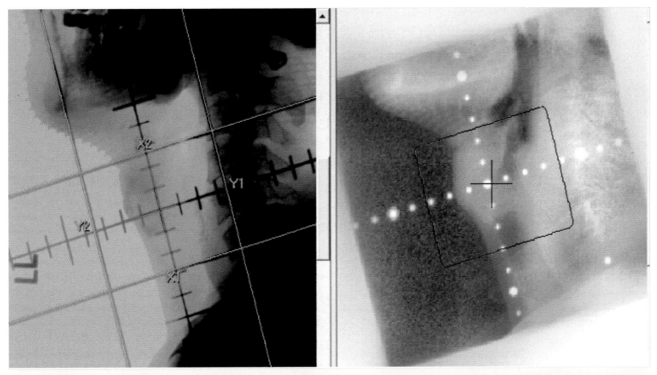

Fig. 22.2 Early-stage glottic larynx cancer treated with opposed lateral fields in the two-dimensional technique. The top and bottom borders are positioned to account for larynx motion during treatment. Note that the lymph nodes were not electively treated. *PTV*, planning target volume.

as well as an alternative to concurrent chemoradiation in an effort to minimize long-term swallowing complications resulting from fibrosis. Patients who are to be considered for induction up front should be evaluated for a three-drug regimen with TPF because this improves the chance for organ preservation compared with two-drug therapy. The addition of docetaxel to PF increases larynx preservation. Standard concurrent treatment consists of three doses of cisplatin with 7 weeks of radiation therapy.

For selected patients with advanced hypopharyngeal tumors who have good laryngopharyngeal function, combined-modality therapy with primary chemoradiation may be considered. Radiation alone results in suboptimal rates of local control in patients with T3/T4 lesions or with advanced N2/N3 neck disease because of high rates of persistent disease. Induction chemotherapy followed by radiation therapy or concurrent chemoradiation is the best treatment option.

22.3.5 Larynx

Glottic Larynx

Early-stage vocal fold lesions are highly curable because they have a low propensity for nodal metastasis and can be managed with single-modality treatment. Surgery or radiation is considered for early-stage lesions, whereas most often a combination of chemotherapy, surgery, and radiation is considered for advanced lesions. For advanced lesions, multidisciplinary treatment is designed to maximize tumor cure, preserve organ function, address regional spread, and be tailored to the patient's comorbidities and preferences.

Radiation therapy without chemotherapy offers an excellent chance for tumor control and organ function preservation in early-stage disease. Current techniques use simple opposed lateral fields to treat the larynx, typically prescribing 63 to 65 Gy in 28 or 29 fractions over 5 1/2 weeks (▶ Fig. 22.2). Treatment to the larynx alone without elective nodal coverage spares treatment of the major salivary glands, mandible, and oropharynx/oral cavity. The treatment time and total dose are important. The total duration of treatment is ideally less than 6 weeks. For patients with T2 lesions and impaired vocal cord mobility, a hyperfractionated radiation schedule can improve local control, albeit with increased acute toxicity. T2 lesions that invade areas of the supraglottic larynx may require elective nodal treatment. For T1 and T2 lesions, rates of local control are typically greater than 90% and 80%, respectively.

Total laryngectomy followed by postoperative radiation therapy once represented the standard of care for advanced glottic laryngeal cancers. However, in the Department of Veterans Affairs (VA) Laryngeal Cancer Study, organ preservation was achieved in two-thirds of patients undergoing induction chemotherapy with three cycles of 5-fluorouracil/cisplatin followed by radiation without compromise of survival in comparison with the control arm of total laryngectomy and postoperative radiation. A subsequent landmark randomized intergroup trial of patients with primarily T2/T3 tumors compared the VA regimen with concurrent chemoradiation with high-dose cisplatin or radiation alone and demonstrated that concurrent chemoradiation is superior to the VA regimen in improving larynx preservation (from 75 to 88%) and represents the current standard of care. No difference in overall survival was noted among all three arms because of high surgical salvage rates.

Thus, for patients with good performance status, 7 weeks of daily radiation to deliver 70 Gy given concurrently with high-dose cisplatin at 100 mg/m^2 for three cycles is recommended. More intensive induction regimens consisting of three drugs (TPF) followed by radiation alone have also improved organ preservation and may serve as an alternative to concurrent chemoradiation. The two approaches have not been compared in a randomized setting for larynx cancers.

In debilitated patients who are unable to tolerate standard chemotherapy, other options include radiation therapy alone or radiation therapy with a biologic therapy consisting of a monoclonal antibody targeting the EGFR.

For patients undergoing radiation therapy alone, a course of altered fractionated radiation therapy may be considered with either hyperfractionation or accelerated radiation by delayed concomitant boost, based on the outcomes favoring these two schedules over conventional once-daily treatment reported in RTOG 90–03.

The patients excluded from the above studies had tumors that invaded cartilage and/or extended outside the larynx into soft tissues. For these patients, total laryngectomy followed by adjuvant radiation with possible concurrent chemotherapy is the standard treatment.

Supraglottic Larynx

Patients with tumors located in the supraglottic larynx, even early-stage tumors, require management of the neck because regional involvement is likely regardless of stage. The primary tumor can spread into the paralaryngeal space and cause vocal cord fixation, into the pre-epiglottic space with extension into the tongue base, through the thyroid cartilage into the soft tissues outside the larynx, and laterally into the hypopharynx.

T1/T2 lesions of the supraglottic larynx require management of the primary site with elective treatment of the draining lymph nodes at levels II through IV. Like early-stage vocal cord cancers, these tumors may be managed with single-modality therapy. Radiation consists of 66 to 70 Gy to treat the primary site and elective neck therapy to a dose of 50 to 54 Gy. With conventional technique, the superior aspects of the parotid glands may be spared, in addition to the superior constrictor muscles.

For patients who have advanced supraglottic cancers, chemoradiation is recommended if they have an appropriate performance status and good baseline laryngopharyngeal function, whereas primary resection followed by adjuvant radiation is recommended for patients who have disease with extralaryngeal spread or poor baseline function.

Subglottic Larynx

Tumors located under the vocal cords are rare and clinically difficult to visualize, even with endoscopy, requiring examination under anesthesia. Because of their occult nature, they often present as advanced lesions invading the trachea and soft tissues of the neck. Such tumors may spread to the inferior cervical nodal chains as well as the superior mediastinal nodes. Radiation therapy may be considered to cover the tumor and extensive lymphatic drainage area, whereas a combined a surgical approach may best for T4 lesions.

22.4 Toxicity of Radiation Therapy: Optimizing Patient Outcomes

The major sequelae of radiation therapy can be divided into acute and chronic side effects. These depend on total dose, fraction size, fractionation, prior or concomitant therapy (i.e., surgery or chemotherapy), and target volume. Mucositis is the major dose-limiting toxicitiy of radiation. Severe mucositis can result in treatment breaks, which can compromise locoregional control and cause infection in patients compromised by chemotherapy. Xerostomia is the most pervasive chronic side effect of radiation therapy (▶ Table 22.1).

In order to optimize the chance for successful radiation therapy, patients must avoid smoking during treatment (smoking increases radiation resistance of the tumor) and be highly compliant with the radiation schedule, avoiding treatment delays totaling more than 5 days during the course of treatment, and they must be proactive with supportive measures to complete treatment. Patients should undergo a pretreatment evaluation with a speech/swallowing team, nutritionist, and pain management and psychosocial service team to help them cope with the acute and chronic effects of treatment. A pre-irradiation dental evaluation should include Panorex imaging, dental extractions if indicated, and provision of a fluoride tray, which may be useful for patients with fillings to wear during radiation therapy treatments as fillings may cause increased mucositis from radiation scatter.

22.4.1 Acute Side Effects

Patients usually begin to experience morbidity from radiation during the third week of treatment in the form of dermatitis, decreased mucus production, sore throat, hoarseness, dysphagia, fatigue, dysgeusia, and xerostomia. Rarely, within the first week of treatment, patients may develop a parotitis related to inspissated mucus from xerostomia. By the second half of the treatment, as symptoms intensify, most patients require creams/emollients for skin desquamation, mucolytics, narcotics for pain, antiemetics, and a change of diet soft solids and liquid nutritional supplements. Gastrostomy tube placement may be considered for patients not deemed strong enough to proceed through treatment, especially patients receiving concurrent chemoradiation. Patients may develop severe weight loss, which will impair their ability to heal and to complete treat-

Table 22.1 Complications of chemoradiation treatment

Complication	Incidence (%)
Dysgeusia	90
Chewing, eating difficulties	80
Xerostomia	78–95
Anorexia, weight loss, malnutrition	55–85
Dysphagia	40–65
Mucositis, stomatitis	35–75
Infection	14
Osteoradionecrosis	5–15

ment. It is important to minimize treatment breaks during therapy because impaired tumor control has been shown to occur, especially with treatment break days of more than 5 days.

22.4.2 Chronic Side Effects

Patients will recover for several weeks to several months after treatment and will typically be off medications by 4 to 6 weeks after treatment. Important long-term side effects include fibrosis of the neck and masticatory muscles, epilation, chondronecrosis, dysphagia, hypothyroidism, and xerostomia. Preventive swallowing exercises are important to minimize cricopharyngeal stricture and fibrosis of the swallowing muscles (which can lead to aspiration and feeding tube dependence). Dental decay and osteoradionecrosis may best be prevented by meticulous dental hygiene and avoidance of dental extraction/implantantion.

22.5 Directions for Future Research

The RTOG-H5022 randomized trial will test whether the addition of C225 to concurrent chemoradiation consisting of accelerated radiation by delayed concomitant boost with two cycles of CDDP improves outcome versus concurrent chemoradiation alone.

Given the excellent outcomes achieved with present regimens in HPV-positive patients who have oropharyngeal cancer, multiple institutions and cooperative groups are exploring the possibility of treatment deintensification. Lower doses of radiation and fewer cycles of chemotherapy may be used to obtain similar results but decrease toxicity.

For patients who require treatment intensification because of very aggressive disease, several approaches have been explored including the addition of induction chemotherapy, escalation of radiation dose, such as the application of a brachytherapy boost and integration of biologic therapies to concurrent chemoradiation. Other approaches include identifying radioprotectants to decrease mucositis and improving radiation treatment techniques to preserve organ function and allow patients to complete treatment and maintain quality of life. For example, dysphagia-oriented IMRT is being studied to reduce the risk for long-term dependence on tube feeding after chemoradiation by decreasing the dose to structures important in swallowing, such as constrictor muscles.

Incorporating imaging characteristics and molecular profiling represent important efforts to further individualize treatment to find the right balance of treatment intensity so as to eradicate disease with tolerated doses that best maximize organ preservation and cosmesis.

22.6 Roundsmanship

- Radiation works primarily by causing reproductive cell death such that tumors are unable to replicate. The target of treatment is the tumor DNA, in which free radical formation from ionizing radiation therapy causes permanent double-strand breakage.
- Normal tissues have a greater capacity than tumor cells to repair themselves after radiation exposure. Fractionation ex-

ploits the repair differential by using doses that are high enough to kill tumors but that spare the function and integrity of normal tissue.
- In general, radiation doses of 50, 60, and 70 Gy are required for elective treatment, microscopic residual disease, and gross tumor, respectively.
- Head and neck squamous cell carcinomas have the unique characteristic of delayed accelerated tumor repopulation during radiation therapy. The phenomena of on-treatment repopulation and differential repair ability underlie the rationale for several altered fractionated radiation regimens proven to improve locoregional control. Shortening the duration of treatment and escalating the dose with hyperfractionation have yielded significant gains.

22.7 Recommended Reading

[1] Al-Sarraf M, LeBlanc M, Giri PG et al. Chemoradiotherapy versus radiotherapy in patients with advanced nasopharyngeal cancer: phase III randomized Intergroup study 0099. J Clin Oncol 1998; 16: 1310–1317

[2] Bonner JA, Harari PM, Giralt J et al. Radiotherapy plus cetuximab for squamous-cell carcinoma of the head and neck. N Engl J Med 2006; 354: 567–578

[3] Budach W, Hehr T, Budach V, Belka C, Dietz K. A meta-analysis of hyperfractionated and accelerated radiotherapy and combined chemotherapy and radiotherapy regimens in unresected locally advanced squamous cell carcinoma of the head and neck. BMC Cancer 2006; 6: 28

[4] Denis F, Garaud P, Bardet E et al. Final results of the 94–01 French Head and Neck Oncology and Radiotherapy Group randomized trial comparing radiotherapy alone with concomitant radiochemotherapy in advanced-stage oropharynx carcinoma. J Clin Oncol 2004; 22: 69–76

[5] D'Souza G, Kreimer AR, Viscidi R et al. Case-control study of human papillomavirus and oropharyngeal cancer. N Engl J Med 2007; 356: 1944–1956

[6] Eisbruch A, Ten Haken RK, Kim HM, Marsh LH, Ship JA. Dose, volume, and function relationships in parotid salivary glands following conformal and intensity-modulated irradiation of head and neck cancer. Int J Radiat Oncol Biol Phys 1999; 45: 577–587

[7] Epstein JB, Robertson M, Emerton S, Phillips N, Stevenson-Moore P. Quality of life and oral function in patients treated with radiation therapy for head and neck cancer. Head Neck 2001; 23: 389–398

[8] Forastiere AA, Goepfert H, Maor M et al. Long-term results of Intergroup RTOG 91–11: a phase III trial to preserve the larynx—induction cisplatin/5-FU and radiation therapy versus concurrent cisplatin and radiation therapy versus radiation therapy. J Clin Oncol 2006; 24 18S: 5517

[9] Fu KK, Pajak TF, Trotti A et al. A Radiation Therapy Oncology Group (RTOG) phase III randomized study to compare hyperfractionation and two variants of accelerated fractionation to standard fractionation radiotherapy for head and neck squamous cell carcinomas: first report of RTOG 9003. Int J Radiat Oncol Biol Phys 2000; 48: 7–16

[10] Hall E, Giaccia A. Radiobiology for the Radiologist. 6th ed. Philadelhia, PA: Lippincott Williams & Wilkins; 2005

[11] Hammarstedt L, Lindquist D, Dahlstrand H et al. Human papillomavirus as a risk factor for the increase in incidence of tonsillar cancer. Int J Cancer 2006; 119: 2620–2623

[12] Harrison LB, Zelefsky MJ, Sessions RB et al. Base-of-tongue cancer treated with external beam irradiation plus brachytherapy: oncologic and functional outcome. Radiology 1992; 184: 267–270

[13] The Department of Veterans Affairs Laryngeal Cancer Study Group. Induction chemotherapy plus radiation compared with surgery plus radiation in patients with advanced laryngeal cancer. N Engl J Med 1991; 324: 1685–1690

[14] Lefebvre JL, Chevalier D, Luboinski B, Kirkpatrick A, Collette L, Sahmoud T EORTC Head and Neck Cancer Cooperative Group. Larynx preservation in pyriform sinus cancer: preliminary results of a European Organization for Research and Treatment of Cancer phase III trial. J Natl Cancer Inst 1996; 88: 890–899

[15] Monnerat C, Faivre S, Temam S, Bourhis J, Raymond E. End points for new agents in induction chemotherapy for locally advanced head and neck cancers. Ann Oncol 2002; 13: 995–1006

[16] Ogura JH, Biller HF, Wette R. Elective neck dissection for pharyngeal and laryngeal cancers. An evaluation. Ann Otol Rhinol Laryngol 1971; 80: 646–650

23 Diseases and Neoplasms of the Oral Cavity

Helen Yoo Bowne

23.1 Introduction

The oral cavity is the portal of entry for the aerodigestive tract, and its functions include taste, mastication, digestion of food, swallowing, and speech. Bordered anteriorly by the vermilion and posteriorly by the soft palate superiorly and circumvallate papillae inferiorly, the subunits of the oral cavity consist of the lips, buccal mucosa, upper and lower alveolar ridges, retromolar trigone, oral tongue (anterior two-thirds of the mobile tongue), hard palate, and floor of mouth (▶ Fig. 23.1).

23.2 Applied Anatomy

The mucosa lining the oral cavity is largely squamous epithelium interspersed by 1,000 minor salivary glands. The minor salivary glands are concentrated in the hard and soft palate. The alveolar ridge is composed of the osseous alveolar process and overlying gingiva lined by mucosa. The floor of mouth mucosa is supported by the mylohyoid, geniohyoid, and genioglossus muscles. The sublingual gland and numerous minor salivary glands lie between the mucosa and these muscles.

The anterior two-thirds of the mobile tongue are lined by squamous epithelium. The dorsum of the tongue is also lined by fungiform, filiform, and circumvallate papillae. The intrinsic muscles of the tongue, which include the superior longitudinal, inferior longitudinal, vertical, and transverse muscles, are sepa-rated at the midline by the median raphe, and their muscular functions produce speech and swallowing. The extrinsic muscles of the tongue (genioglossus, hyoglossus, styloglossus, and palatoglossus) also assist in the movement of the tongue backward, forward, upward, and downward.

The motor supply to the lips and cheek via the orbicularis oris and buccinator muscles is provided by the facial nerve. The hypoglossal nerve innervates the intrinsic and extrinsic muscles of the tongue. The muscles that control the movement of the mandible include the masseter, temporalis, and medial and lateral pterygoids, controlled by the second and third divisions of the trigeminal nerve. Sensory innervation of the oral cavity is supplied by the superior and inferior alveolar and lingual nerves (branches of second and third divisions of the trigeminal nerve). Taste is mediated by the innervation of the chorda tympani and secretomotor fibers to the submandibular salivary gland, which travel with the lingual nerve.

The vascular supply to the oral cavity consists of the branches of the external carotid artery. The lingual arteries supply the tongue, while facial arteries support the buccal mucosa and lips and the internal maxillary and inferior alveolar arteries supply the alveolar ridges. The lymphatics of the oral cavity drain to the submental, submandibular, and upper jugular–jugulodigastric lymph nodes. There is direct lymphatic drainage to the lower jugular lymph nodes from the tongue. The upper alveolar ridge and buccal mucosa also drain to buccinator lymph nodes.

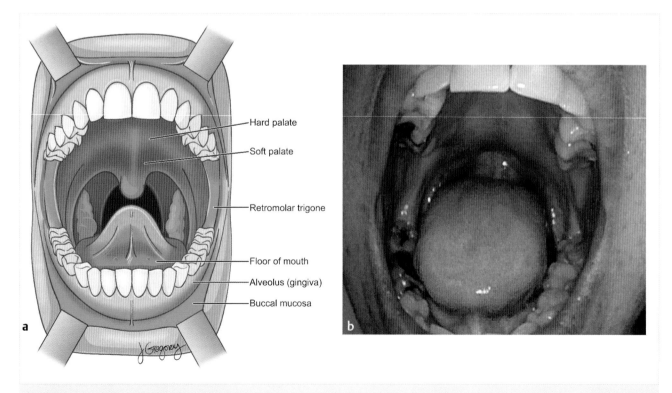

- Hard palate
- Soft palate
- Retromolar trigone
- Floor of mouth
- Alveolus (gingiva)
- Buccal mucosa

Fig. 23.1 (a) Drawing and (b) photo showing structures of the oral cavity, including the lip, alveolus (gingiva), hard palate, buccal mucosa, retromolar trigone, floor of mouth, and tongue.

23.3 Classification of the Disease Process

Diseases of the oral cavity may be classified into neoplastic and nonneoplastic processes. Benign and malignant neoplastic diseases may originate from the mucosa, salivary glands, or mesenchymal tissues, including bone, muscle, and fibroblastic tissues. Malignant neoplasms may be squamous cell carcinomas, adenocarcinomas, sarcomas, or other, less common cancers, such as mucosal melanomas, malignant peripheral nerve sheath tumors, or granular cell tumors. Benign neoplasms of the oral cavity may be pleomorphic or monomorphic adenomas, papillomas, fibromas, neurilemmomas, leiomyomas, pyogenic granulomas, benign melanonevi, or various benign odontogenic tumors. Nonneoplastic diseases consist of cysts (e.g., ranula and mucocele) and inflammatory conditions, which may be classified as (1) infections, (2) oral manifestations of systemic disorders, or (3) various medical conditions. Infectious diseases and head and neck manifestations of systemic disease affecting the oral cavity are covered in Chapter 13 and Chapter 19.

23.4 Malignant Neoplasms of the Oral Cavity

23.4.1 Incidence and Etiology

Oral cavity cancers account for 30% of all head and neck malignancies. Yearly, 22,000 new cases of oral cavity cancers (excluding lip cancers) are diagnosed, and oral cavity cancers are responsible for 6,000 to 7,000 deaths per year. The most common malignancy of the oral cavity is squamous cell carcinoma (95%). The most common location of carcinoma of the oral cavity is the oral tongue, followed by the floor of mouth. Risk factors associated with squamous cell cancer are the following:(1) tobacco exposure in any form (cigarettes, cigars, pipes, and chewing tobacco); (2) alcohol consumption (risk is increased when both tobacco and alcohol are consumed); (3) chewing betel quid (a common practice in south central Asia and Melanesia); and (4) infection with carcinogenic strains of human papillomavirus (HPV-16 and HPV-18), as well as sun exposure for lip carcinoma.

23.4.2 Pathogenesis

The carcinogenesis of squamous cell cancers is associated with mutagenic environmental exposure to tobacco, alcohol, betel products, and HPV, coupled with genetic susceptibility and predisposition. Progression to cancer is thought to occur in multiple steps, causing alterations in tumor suppressor genes and oncogenes. A variety of genetic changes have been reported in head and neck squamous cell carcinoma. They include p16 inactivation (70%) via deletion (predominantly) or promoter methylation and amplification, p53 mutation (50 to 80%), HPV integration (25% in oropharyngeal cancer), and epidermal growth factor receptor (EGFR) axis alteration (80 to 90%) via amplification, overexpression, and downstream activation.

Loss of 9p21 results in inactivation of the p16 gene, which inhibits cyclin-dependent kinase (CDK) involved in G1 cell cycle regulation, and inactivation of this protein enables cells to escape senescence. Loss of chromosome 9p21 occurs in the majority of invasive tumors and is also frequently present in dysplasia and carcinoma in situ. Loss of p16 appears to be necessary for the immortalization of keratinocytes.

When DNA damage is detected, p53 normally stops cell cycle progression. Loss of p53 function from mutations permits the progression of cancers from preinvasive to invasive lesions. A p53 mutation is prevalent in patients who smoke and drink alcohol. Squamous cell carcinoma induced by HPV-16 and HPV-18 is not associated with p53 mutations. Instead, the viral oncoprotein E6 promotes increased degradation of p53.

EGFR expression is normal in tissues of the dermis, gastrointestinal tract, and kidneys. However, dysfunction of this receptor occurs in 80 to 90% of head and neck squamous cell carcinomas. EGFR is related to multiple pathways controlling cellular proliferation, apoptosis, invasion, angiogenesis, and metastasis. There are numerous additional genetic alterations that play a role in carcinogenesis, proliferation, invasion, and metastasis. Research and technology advancement in the future will help elucidate and further clarify the pathogenesis of carcinoma and eventually lead to more specifically targeted therapies.

23.4.3 Natural History and Progression

Often, premalignant changes related to epithelial and subepithelial disturbances may appear as leukoplakia (white lesions; ▶ Fig. 23.2) or erythroplasia (red lesions). Histologically, this may represent hyperkeratosis, parakeratosis, and dysplasia as a result of keratin and/or cytoplasmic changes. The risk for the development of invasive carcinoma in leukoplakia is 4 to 6%, whereas the risk is as high as 30% in erythroplasia. Progression of the severity of dysplasia leads to carcinoma in situ, then frank invasion and subsequent metastasis to local and regional cervical lymph nodes. In some patients, progressive cytologic changes that are not apparent may develop into invasive squamous cell carcinoma. Eventually, distant metastasis to lung,

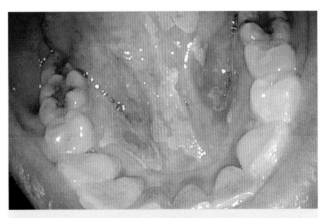

Fig. 23.2 Leukoplakia of the floor of mouth.

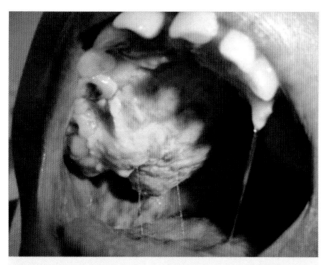

Fig. 23.3 Squamous cell carcinoma of the hard palate arising from squamous papilloma.

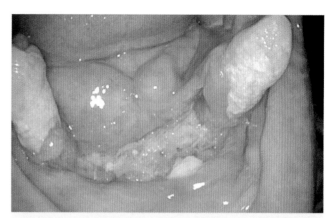

Fig. 23.4 Floor of mouth carcinoma with erosion of the mandible.

liver, and bone occurs. If left untreated, the disease is fatal. Treatment at earlier stages of disease is associated with improved survival and cure rates.

23.4.4 Potential Disease Complications

Complications of untreated oral tongue cancer include severe pain with impaired speech and swallowing, which can lead to aspiration pneumonia and significant morbidity. As a result of poor oral intake due to pain or dysphagia, malnutrition is a common problem. Invasion of the surrounding tissues, such as the nasal cavity, by cancers arising from the hard palate (▶ Fig. 23.3) or upper alveolus may cause nasal obstruction and bleeding. Involvement of the pterygoid muscles will cause severe pain and problems with mastication as well as trismus. Tumors of the buccal mucosa can perforate the skin, and lesions of the gingiva will erode the mandible (▶ Fig. 23.4).

23.4.5 Disease Staging: American Joint Committee Cancer Staging

Although invasion to a depth of more than 2 mm and higher histologic grade are associated with an increased risk for lymph node metastasis, the current tumor (T) grading system is based on the size of the primary lesion. T1 lesions are smaller than 2 cm, T2 lesions are 2 to 4 cm, and T3 lesions are larger than 4 cm. T4 lesions are more extensive; T4a disease includes invasion of underlying soft tissues, bone, or overlying skin, whereas T4b lesions are very advanced, with invasion of the masticator space, pterygoid plates, and skull base with or without internal carotid artery encasement.

Involved lymph nodes are classified by size and laterality. N1 nodal disease is involvement of a single ipsilateral lymph node 3 cm or less in size. N2 disease is more extensive; N2a disease is involvement of a single ipsilateral lymph node larger than 3 cm but smaller than 6 cm; N2b disease is involvement of multiple ipsilateral nodes (none larger than 6 cm), and N2c disease is involvement of bilateral or contralateral lymph nodes, none larger

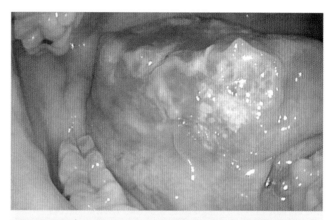

Fig. 23.5 Oral tongue cancer on the lateral surface with ulceration.

than 6 cm. Finally, any nodal metastasis larger than 6 cm is classified as N3 disease.

For the classification of oral cavity cancers, stage 0 is an in situ primary lesion with no nodal or distant metastases. Stage I disease is a T1 lesion and stage II is a T2 lesion, each with no nodal or distant metastases. Stage III disease is a T3 lesion with no nodal or distant metastases, as well as any T1–T3 lesion with N1 nodal disease and no distant metastases. Stage IV disease is divided in IVA, IVB, and IVC disease. A T1–T3 lesion with N2 nodal disease or a T4a primary lesion with N0–N2 nodal disease is stage IVA disease. Stage IVB disease includes any primary tumor with N3 nodal disease or a T4b lesion with any nodal state. Any distant metastasis establishes stage IVC disease.

23.4.6 Presenting Complaints and Clinical Findings

Presenting symptoms include persistent ulcers for more than 3 weeks, pain at the site of the lesion, pain on swallowing, referred otalgia, altered speech, and a lump in the neck. The clinical presentation of oral cavity malignancies may be ulcerative and endophytic with underlying firm and indurated soft-tissue components. Pain is usually severe with ulcerated lesions and with lesions located in the lateral border of the tongue (▶ Fig. 23.5) and adjacent floor of mouth. Carcinomas arising

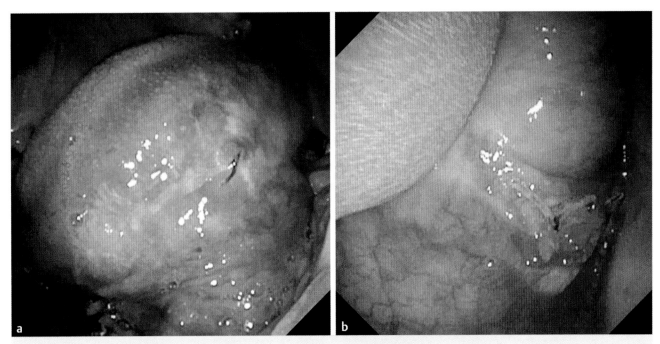

Fig. 23.6 (a) Lateral tongue and (b) lateral floor of mouth squamous cell carcinoma arising from leukoplakia.

from squamous papillomas may have papillary projections, and exophytic lesions may exhibit keratotic, verrucous, and cauliflower appearances. Occasionally, a superficial leukoplakic lesion presenting for a prolonged period of time with benign pathology may change and progress to carcinoma (▶ Fig. 23.6). Bleeding from the surface of these lesions is highly suggestive of friability and malignancy.

23.4.7 Medical Evaluation and Physical Examination

A comprehensive history, including the patient's social history and etiologic risk factors such as tobacco and alcohol use and a family history of cancer, should be obtained. A complete head and neck examination including fiber-optic nasopharyngolaryngoscopy is performed. Palpation of tumors to delineate the extent of the lesion and inspection of tumors in proximity to adjacent mandible and maxilla are essential. Occasionally, examination under general anesthesia with biopsy is indicated for severely painful tumors that cannot be thoroughly evaluated in the office. A wedge or punch biopsy of tissue including the periphery of the lesion and sufficient depth is needed to establish the diagnosis and detect invasion.

23.4.8 Testing

In addition to obtaining a diagnosis with a tissue biopsy, the examiner routinely has specimens assessed for the presence of HPV because this is associated with improved survival and favorable response to treatments. Although the guidelines for the treatment of HVP-positive tumors have not yet changed compared with those for tobacco- related squamous cell carcinomas, studies are under way to determine whether adjustments in the current standard of care with decreased side effects can be achieved.

Once the diagnosis is established by biopsy, imaging studies, including computed tomography (CT) with intravenous contrast or magnetic resonance (MR) imaging of the neck and positron emission tomography (PET)–CT, is recommended to complete the staging of cancer. CT is essential in determining bone invasion by tumor, and MR imaging is superior for soft-tissue details. PET-CT will provide advanced information regarding the patient's pulmonary status and occasionally second synchronous primary cancers or distant metastases.

23.4.9 Differential Diagnosis

The differential diagnosis of lesions of the oral cavity representing squamous cell carcinoma includes, in order of frequency, minor salivary gland malignancies and adenocarcinomas such as mucoepidermoid carcinoma, adenoid cystic carcinoma, and low-grade polymorphous adenocarcinoma. Mucosal melanomas (▶ Fig. 23.7) and other rare tumors such as lymphomas and sarcomas (including rhabdomysarcoma, liposarcoma, and malignant fibrous histiocytoma) should also be included in the differential. Although rare, granular cell tumors and metastatic disease from another primary site are also possibilities.

23.4.10 Medical and Surgical Treatments and Complications

The three main modalities of treatment of oral cavity cancer are surgery, radiation therapy, and chemotherapy. Early-stage cancers (stages I and II) can be treated effectively with one modality (either surgery or radiation alone). For advanced-stage cancers (stages III and IV), a minimum of two combined treatment options is required, and for very advanced cases, all three modalities are required. Even early-stage cancers with pathologic features suggestive of aggressive behavior, such as extracapsu-

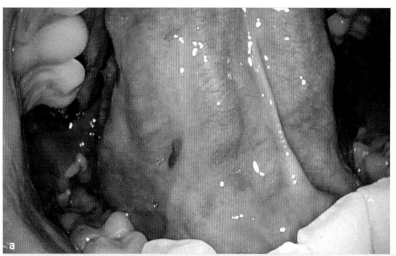
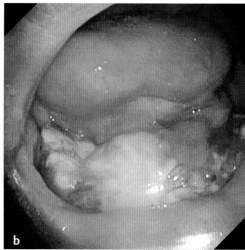

Fig. 23.7 (**a**) Invasive (early) mucosal melanoma of the ventral tongue. (**b**) Advanced mucosal melanoma of the floor of mouth.

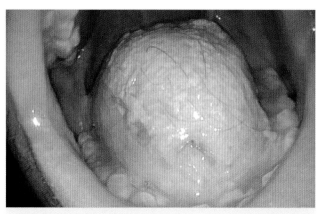

Fig. 23.8 Reconstruction of the oral tongue with lateral thigh free flap after nearly total glossectomy. This patient is able to eat and speak intelligibly.

lar extension and perineural and vascular invasion, warrant treatment with additional modalities.

Appropriate goals of treatment are (1) to cure the cancer, (2) to preserve or restore form and function, and (3) to minimize the side effects of treatment. Other factors to consider in formulating a treatment plan are anterior or posterior location of tumors, proximity to bone, depth of invasion, and histologic type. Small tumors in the anterior part of the oral cavity can be surgically excised intraorally with minimal functional deficit. Surgery rather than radiation is the treatment of choice for early oral cavity cancer because of the long-term sequelae of xerostomia and the risk for dental caries and osteoradionecrosis of the mandible. If surgery is chosen for the treatment of early lesions, elective neck dissection should be performed for tumors of the oral tongue and floor of mouth and for tumors with significant depth of invasion, which have a higher rate of lymph node metastasis in clinically N0 necks. In patients with clinically palpable neck disease, a minimum of comprehensive neck dissection including levels I through V is advised.

For most patients with large primary tumors, surgery with reconstruction followed by radiation or chemoradiation therapy is the treatment of choice. The location of the primary tumor will dictate the various surgical approaches described. Mandibulotomy, lower cheek flap, visor flap, and upper cheek flap approaches are some of the surgical techniques used to gain access to the primary tumor. Vertical or horizontal mandibulectomy or segmental mandibulectomy may be incorporated into the surgical plan, depending on the proximity and level of bone invasion by the tumor. Appropriate reconstruction with fibula, radial forearm, or anterolateral thigh free flaps is most commonly employed for the restoration of function and form in the oral cavity (▶ Fig. 23.8). Although not optimal, pedicled flaps, such as a pectoralis major myocutaneous flap, or rotation flaps with local tissue, such as tongue or cheek mucosa, may be required for reconstruction of the oral cavity defects in certain circumstances. Patients with significant concurrent medical disease may not be candidates for lengthy microvascular free flap procedures, and alternative reconstructions with a shorter operating time may be the option. Defects that require sufficient donor tissue to prevent functional compromise (such as tethering of the tongue) but are not large enough to require a microvascular free flap may benefit from local tissue transfer techniques and/or skin grafts.

Complications of surgery include bleeding, aspiration pneumonia, and fistula formation. Late complications are poor speech clarity, as well as mastication and swallowing dysfunction. Early complications of radiation therapy consist of mucositis and loss of taste. Late complications involve permanent xerostomia, dental caries, and osteoradionecrosis. Chemotherapy-associated complications include myelosuppression; nausea/emesis; alopecia; mucositis; pulmonary, renal, and hepatic dysfunction; and neuropathy, including ototoxicity manifested by nerve hearing loss and peripheral vestibular symptoms.

23.4.11 Prognosis

The most important factor determining prognosis and survival is the stage of disease at presentation. The overall 5-year survival rates for stages I and II are 80% and 70%, respectively. For patients with stages III and IV disease, the survival rates are 55% and 30%, respectively.

23.5 Benign Neoplasms and Cysts of the Oral Cavity

Benign tumors of the oral cavity originate from the various tissues (epithelium, salivary glands, muscles, fibrous tissues, nerve, and bone) of the oral cavity. Epithelial tumors such as *squamous papillomas* are caused by HPV-6 and HPV-11. They may occur on the oral tongue, lips, and buccal mucosa, usually closer to the lip. The surface of these lesions appears warty with papillary projections. Malignant changes in papillomas associated with HPV-6 and HPV-11 are rare. These lesions can be treated with surgical excision or carbon dioxide laser ablation with excellent control.

Fibromas of the oral tongue and buccal mucosa may develop as a result of local trauma and irritation. They are found in 1.2% of the adult population. They appear as smooth, well-delineated, submucosal masses that can be sessile or pedunculated. They are usually solitary and measure less than 1.5 cm. If symptomatic, these lesions can be locally excised. Otherwise, they can be clinically observed.

Fewer than 10% of salivary gland tumors arise from minor salivary glands, and 20 to 40% of minor salivary gland tumors are benign. The most common *adenoma* arising from minor salivary glands of the oral cavity is pleomorphic adenoma, most commonly found on the hard palate. Other benign salivary gland tumors include canalicular adenoma, papillary cystadenoma, oncocytoma, and myoepithelioma. These tumors generally present as smooth, painless, slowly growing masses. Complete surgical excision can usually be achieved transorally.

Mucoceles of the lips are cystic lesions that form as a result of the extravasation of glandular contents into the surrounding tissue, usually after local trauma. A *retention cyst* or *ranula* is caused by obstruction of the ducts with subsequent dilatation of the sublingual gland and formation of a cyst. A plunging ranula is a cyst that plunges under the mylohyoid muscle into the neck. Surgical excision or marsupialization is the treatment of choice for retention cysts.

Dermoid cysts, *enteric duplication cysts*, and *nasoalveolar cysts* are rare congenital conditions of the oral cavity. Dermoid cysts occur along embryonic fusion lines and form from trapped epithelial cells. They are lined by keratinizing squamous epithelium and may contain epidermal appendages such as hair follicles and sweat glands. Enteric duplication cysts contain gastrointestinal mucosa and are lined with columnar or stratified squamous epithelium. Both types can be found in the floor of mouth and tongue. These congenital cysts may enlarge to cause functional problems of the oral cavity. Complete surgical excision is curative. Nasoalveolar cysts may arise from trapped epithelial cells between the lateral and medial maxillary nasal processes. They become symptomatic later in life as the cysts increase in size and present as smooth, nontender, soft swellings in the nasolabial area. On examination, the cysts may cause submucosal elevation over the gingivolabial sulcus or floor of the nose, or displacement of the nasal alae. Excision can usually be achieved via the sublabial approach.

Granular cell tumors are of neural origin, as are *neurilemmomas (schwannomas)* and *neurofibromas*. Fifty percent of granular cell tumors occur in the oral cavity, and the tongue is most commonly involved. Up to 15% of patients have synchronous lesions. They present as firm, painless, pink, nodular, sessile masses. Granular cell tumors are malignant in about 1% of cases. Treatment requires surgical excision, with an overall recurrence rate of 10%. *Neurofibromas* are the most common peripheral nerve tumors found in the oral cavity and are derived from a combination of Schwann cells and perineural fibroblasts. Multiple neurofibromas may be associated with von Recklinghausen neurofibromatosis. In patients with this disorder, 70% of neurofibromas occur in the oral cavity and usually involve the tongue. They present as painless, slowly growing masses but are tender to palpation. Surgical excision is the treatment of choice, with a low risk for recurrence. Malignant transformation of a solitary neurofibroma is rare, but sarcoma may arise in 15% of patients with von Recklinghausen neurofibromatosis.

Pyogenic granulomas, or epulides (▶ Fig. 23.9), may occur in any part of the oral cavity but most commonly involve the gingiva or, in certain conditions, tissue that is prone to the development of an exuberant inflammatory reaction. Etiologic factors include repeated trauma and irritation, infections, dental eruption, and pregnancy. Histologically, pyogenic granulomas consist of proliferative vascular channels and fibrous tissues. They may appear as raised, red to purple lesions. Epulides gravidarum are self-limiting, but others require surgical excision.

Vascular tumors (▶ Fig. 23.10) of the oral cavity include hemangiomas and arteriovenous vascular malformations. Hemangiomas of the head and neck are common, with 14% occurring in the oral cavity, most frequently in the lip. They are

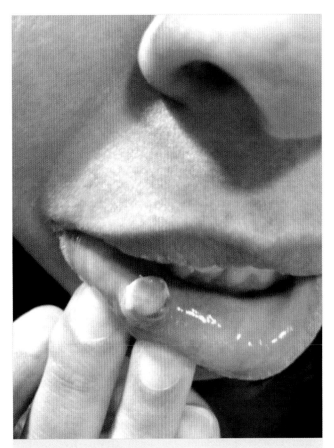

Fig. 23.9 Pyogenic granuloma.

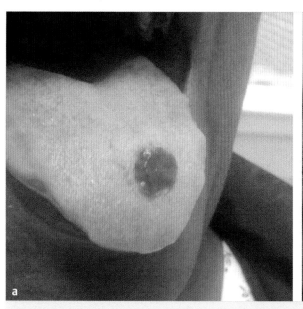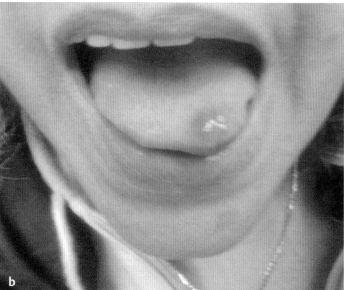

Fig. 23.10 (a) Hemangioma of the tongue. (b) Venous vascular malformation of the tongue.

usually present at birth and grow during a rapid proliferative phase, followed by spontaneous regression over years. Thus, intervention is recommended only for symptomatic lesions. Vascular malformations, on the other hand, become clinically apparent later in life and may progress over years. When they are symptomatic, surgical excision and/or sclerosing agents can be used for treatment, with variable results depending on the size and location of these malformations.

Torus palatinus (▶ Fig. 23.11) and torus mandibularis are benign, bony growths on the midline of the hard palate or on the lingual surface of the mandible. Tori of the oral cavity occur in 3 to 56% of the adult population and are more common in women. They can be pedunculated or broad-based, and they range from small to large (occupying almost the entire palate). They are usually asymptomatic, but when they cause problems with eating or pain from repeated trauma, a bur or osteotomes can be used to remove the bony masses. Tori are composed mostly of lamellar bone, with small marrow spaces that do not involve the deeper cancellous bone of the mandible or palate.

The following section on *odontogenic tumors* and *cysts* is a brief summary of the more commonly encountered lesions. For detailed information regarding odontogenic tumors and cysts, the reader is referred to the list of recommended reading at the end of this chapter.

Odontogenic cyst is a "pathologic cavity lined by epithelium of odontogenic derivation," usually nonkeratinized. Cyst expansion occurs as a result of the accumulation of inflammatory cells, fibrin, serum, and desquamated cells and/or mitotic activity of the cystic wall. Common odontogenic cysts include *dentigerous cyst (follicular cyst)*, *eruption cyst*, *keratinizing odontogenic cyst*, and *odontogenic keratocyst*. Eruption cyst is a subtype of dentigerous cyst that is confined by overlying alveolar mucosa. These cysts are associated with the crowns of unerupted teeth, developing teeth, and odontomas. Fluid accumulates between reduced enamel epithelium and tooth crown. Treatment is enucleation at the time of tooth extraction. Dentigerous cysts potentially have the ability to transform into true neoplasms.

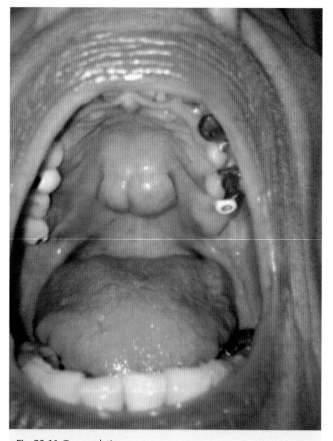

Fig. 23.11 Torus palatinus.

Associated ameloblastomas are noted in 17%, and rarely squamous cell carcinomas and mucoepidermoid carcinomas.

Keratinizing odontogenic cysts have an epithelial lining with thin keratinization. Keratinizing odontogenic cysts are usually asymptomatic and are not associated with basal cell nevus syndrome (Gorlin-Goltz syndrome). These cysts have a recurrence rate of 2% after removal with curettage. Odontogenic keratocyst is also defined as a *keratocystic odontogenic tumor*, a term that stresses the neoplastic nature of this lesion. Soft-tissue extension, extension into adjacent bones with bony destruction, and increased mitotic activity histologically have been reported. These lesions are more common in the mandible than in the maxilla. Patients are often symptomatic, with swelling, pain, and trismus, especially when the cysts are infected, athough odontogenic keratocysts are frequently identified as incidental findings on radiographs. Because the recurrence rate is as high as 62% with enucleation alone, additional curettage is recommended, which decreases the recurrence to 10%.

Malignant transformation of odontogenic cysts is rare but is considered to arise from residual cysts in an edentulous area. Malignant lesions are likely to present with pain, swelling, and dysethesia. The age at occurrence is the sixth or seventh decade, with a 2:1 male predominance. Treatment is based on size, histologic type, and histologic grade.

Ameloblastoma is the most common odontogenic neoplasm. Ameloblastomas arise from rests of primitive dental lamina related to the enamel organ in alveolar bone. These tumors generally present in the third decade of life as a painless, expansile mass in the mandible (85%) or maxilla. Radiography reveals unilocular or multilocular radiolucency with cortical bone expansion. Histologically, they are solid infiltrating tumors with a follicular or plexiform pattern. Standard *ameloblastoma* is the most aggressive of the benign odontogenic tumors. Ameloblastomas can readily infiltrate medullary bone, but compact bone such as the inferior border of the mandible or ramus provides some barrier protection. Resection with adequate margins (1 cm) beyond the radiographic evidence of tumor is the treatment of choice to prevent recurrence. The recurrence rate can be high as 22%, with one-half of recurrences occurring within 5 years. Rarely, malignant transformation can occur.

Unicystic ameloblastomas account for 15% of all ameloblastomas. Most are located in the posterior mandible. They occur in the second and third decades and are usually asymptomatic unless inflamed. Unicystic ameloblastomas are unilocular and unicystic, display no connective tissue invasion, and are considered prognostically distinct from the standard ameloblastomas. Histologic features involve only the luminal and intraluminal walls. The size of the lesion should be less than 2 cm. These lesions require only enucleation for treatment.

Malignant ameloblastomas are ameloblastomas with distant metastasis, which may occur many years following a delay in treatment or years after treatment. The lung is the most common site, with reported cases in the cervical lymph nodes as well. *Ameloblastic carcinoma* is rare but has histologic features associated with malignancy, such as increased mitoses, nuclear pleomorphism, and hyperchromatism.

23.6 Roundsmanship

- For malignant neoplasms, the stage at presentation predicts survival, with improved outcome for early stages.
- Early-stage cancers (stages I and II) may be cured with a single modality of treatment, whereas advanced cancers (stages III and IV) require a combined modality of treatments.
- Smoking and alcohol consumption are important risk factors associated with squamous cell carcinoma.
- Human papillomavirus–associated squamous cell carcinomas in nonsmokers have an improved clinical response to treatment.
- Benign oral cavity neoplasms and cysts are curable with local excision when symptomatic.
- Biopsy of uncertain characteristic lesions of the oral cavity should be performed to determine pathology.
- The difference between the biological behavior of unilocular ameloblastoma and that of standard ameloblastoma, which dictates appropriate surgery, must be recognized.

23.7 Recommended Reading

[1] Benjamin B, Bingham B, Hawke M, Stammberger H. A Color Atlas of Otorhinolaryngology. Philadelphia, PA: J. B. Lippincott; 1994

[2] Agrawal N, Califano J, Ha P. Head and Neck Cancers. In: DeVita VT Jr, Lawrence TS, Rosenberg SA, eds. Cancer: Principles and Practice of Oncology: Primer of the Molecular Biology of Cancer. Philadelphia, PA: Lippincott Williams & Wilkins; 2011:208–214

[3] Koch WM, O'Malley BB, Mendenhall WM. Cancer of the oral cavity. In: Harrison LB, Sessions RB, Hong WK, eds. Head and Neck Cancer: A Multidisciplinary Approach. Philadelphia, PA: Lippincott Williams & Wilkins; 2008:250–285

[4] Lenis M. Diseases of the Oral Cavity and Oropharynx. Slide Lecture Series. Philadelphia, PA: American Academy of Otolaryngology—Head and Neck Surgery Foundation; 2003

[5] Lip and oral cavity. In: Edge SB, Byrd DR, Compton CC, et al, eds. American Joint Committee on Cancer (AJCC) Staging Manual. 7th ed. New York, NY: Springer; 2010:49–61

[6] Smith EM, Rubenstein LM, Haugen TH, Pawlita M, Turek LP. Complex etiology underlies risk and survival in head and neck cancer human papillomavirus, tobacco, and alcohol: a case for multifactor disease. J Oncol 2012; 2012: 571862

[7] Carlson ER. Odontogenic Cysts and tumors: In: Miro M. ed. Peterson's principles of oral and maxillofacial surgery, 2nd ed. Hamilton, Ontario: B C Decker Inc. 2004

24 Diseases and Neoplasms of the Pharynx and Esophagus

Pat Colley and Stimson P. Schantz

24.1 Anatomy

24.1.1 Pharynx

The pharynx is the shared chamber of the respiratory and digestive tracts. It can be divided into three separate parts: the nasopharynx, the oropharynx, and the hypopharynx. The most superior of these structures is the nasopharynx, extending inferiorly from just posterior to the nasal choanae to the soft palate. Below the nasopharynx is the oropharynx, through which food and air pass into the hypopharynx, where food enters the esophagus and air enters the larynx. These three areas of the pharynx are discussed separately below.

Nasopharynx

The nasopharynx is the portion of the pharynx continuous with the nasal cavity. It begins at the nasal choanae. The lateral walls of the nasopharynx contain the eustachian tube orifices, each bounded posteriorly by the torus tubarius. Immediately behind the torus is the pharyngeal recess (fossa of Rosenmüller). The cribriform plate and sphenoid sinus form the superior portion of the nasopharynx, with the clivus making up the posterior border. Because the nasopharynx is contiguous with the nasal cavity, the mucosa of this region is made up mostly of pseudostratified columnar ciliated epithelium. The lymphoid tissue in the nasopharynx, the pharyngeal tonsil, is a midline structure that occasionally extends laterally to the eustachian tubes as Gerlach tonsils.

Oropharynx

The oropharynx is the largest of the areas within the pharynx. It extends from the border of the soft and hard palate inferiorly to the level of the hyoid and the vallecula. The mucosa of this region is mainly stratified squamous epithelium and is innervated by cranial nerves IX and X in the pharyngeal plexus. Notable subsites within the oropharynx are the tonsillar fossae (including the tonsils), soft palate (including the uvula), the base of tongue, and the pharyngeal wall.

The base of tongue is defined as the continuation of the lingual tongue from the circumvallate papilla to the vallecula. It contains muscles as well as the lingual tonsils. Blood supply to this area comes from the lingual arteries. This area is considered a midline structure, so that malignant involvement carries a high risk for metastatic spread to bilateral lymphatics.

The tonsillar fossa is an area formed by the palatoglossus (anterior tonsillar pillar) and palatopharyngeus (posterior tonsillar pillar) muscles; it houses the palatine tonsil itself. It receives its blood supply from the dorsal lingual branch of the lingual artery, tonsillar and ascending palatine branch of the facial artery, ascending pharyngeal artery, and descending palatine branch of the maxillary artery. The palatine tonsils are the most visible part of the Waldeyer ring, which includes the adenoids, palatine tonsils, and lingual tonsils.

The soft palate and uvula are directly posterior to the hard palate and are made up of stratified squamous mucosa overlying muscle. These muscles act in coordination to seal the nasopharynx and propel food down the oropharynx during swallowing. The pharyngeal wall has similar layers of mucosa with underlying muscle.

Hypopharynx

This area extends from the hyoid bone to the inferior border of the cricoid cartilage. The hypopharynx serves as a transit point for all substances entering the esophagus. It receives innervation from the superior laryngeal nerve.

Muscles of the Pharynx

The major muscles of the oropharynx are the superior, middle, and inferior constrictor muscles. These three overlapping muscles encircle the oropharynx, each inserting into the pharyngeal raphe posteriorly. The superior constrictor originates from multiple points, including the medial pterygoid plate, pterygoid mandibular raphe, alveolar process of the mandible, and lateral tongue. The muscle courses superiorly and posteriorly toward the skull base and inserts into the pharyngeal raphe just inferior to the base of the skull. The superior border of this muscle lies just inferior and posterior to the pharyngeal recess in the nasopharynx and forms the Passavant ridge during swallowing. The middle constrictor originates only from the cornua of the hyoid bone and fans out as it courses posteriorly to insert into the raphe. Lastly, the inferior constrictor muscle originates from the lateral side and inferior cornu of the thyroid cartilage as well as the cricoid cartilage. It courses posteriorly to insert into the raphe, with the most inferior fibers forming the cricopharyngeus muscle. All three of the pharyngeal constrictors are innervated by pharyngeal branches of the vagus nerve, with a small contribution from the recurrent laryngeal branch inferiorly.

In addition to the constrictor muscles, five smaller muscles in the pharynx play an important role in its function. The palatoglossus originates from the soft palate and inserts into the side of the tongue. It is innervated by the vagus nerve via the pharyngeal plexus and is the only muscle of the tongue that is not innervated by the hypoglossal nerve. The palatopharyngeus also originates from the soft palate but travels farther inferiorly to join the stylopharyngeus and insert onto the posterior border of the thyroid cartilage. It too is innervated by the vagus nerve via the pharyngeal plexus. Both the palatopharyngeus and palatoglossus are continuous with their counterparts on the opposite side of the pharynx via the soft palate. Fibers from the musculus uvulae intertwine with those of the palatopharyngeus and palatoglossus as this muscle courses from its origin on the posterior nasal spine inferiorly to form the uvula. The levator veli palatini and tensor veli palatini are the final two muscles of the pharynx. The levator veli palatini acts as an elevator of the soft palate and travels from its origin at the undersurface of the petrous portion of the temporal bone inferiorly and anteriorly to insert into the soft palate. The tensor veli palatini is just anterior and lateral to the levator and originates from the base of the medial pterygoid plate, the spina angularis of the sphenoid bone, and the lateral wall of the cartilage of the auditory tube. It passes inferiorly to insert near the midline of the soft palate. The tensor veli palatini plays an important role in proper functioning of the eustachian tube; contraction of this muscle opens the tube and allows middle ear pressure equalization. The tensor veli palatini is innervated by the medial pterygoid nerve, a branch of the third division of the trigeminal nerve. The levator veli palatini shares innervation with the other muscles of the soft palate and is innervated by the vagus nerve.

24.1.2 Esophagus

The esophagus begins at the inferior end of the hypopharynx and continues inferiorly for 38 to 40 cm before ending at the cardia of the stomach. The cricopharyngeus, or upper esophageal sphincter, forms the entrance to the esophagus. As stated above, the cricopharyngeus is made up of a portion of the inferior constrictor muscle and is therefore skeletal muscle. However, it is not under voluntary control. Relaxation of the upper esophageal sphincter is triggered by the swallow reflex and is therefore under control of the vagus nerve. The cricopharyngeus is the narrowest portion of the entire gastrointestinal tract and therefore the area at which a foreign body is most likely to become lodged. Inferior to the upper esophageal sphincter is the body of the esophagus, consisting of cervical, thoracic, and intra-abdominal portions. The esophagus ends at the cardia of the stomach, just below the lower esophageal sphincter. The lower esophageal sphincter is a 2- to 4-cm-long area of increased pressure just above the cardia of the stomach; it relaxes as a food bolus travels down the esophagus to allow entry into the stomach.

There are three distinct layers within the esophagus: the mucosal, submucosal, and muscular layers. The esophagus lacks a serosal layer, making perforation more likely, allowing the spread of malignancy, and making surgical repair significantly more challenging. The mucosal layer is composed almost entirely of stratified squamous epithelium except for the most distal 1 to 3 cm, which is lined by columnar epithelium similar to that of the stomach. The muscular layer of the esophagus is composed of outer longitudinal fibers and inner circular fibers. The upper third of these muscle fibers is striated muscle, whereas the inferior two-thirds is smooth muscle. These muscles receive innervation from the vagus nerve and the sympathetic chain. The blood supply to the esophagus comes from the inferior thyroid artery, thoracic aorta, and left gastric and inferior phrenic arteries.

24.2 Function

The basic functions of the pharynx are respiration and deglutition. During respiration, the pharynx must simply remain patent and allow air to pass from the oral and nasal cavities to the larynx and lungs. However, the act of swallowing is a complex sequence of events that requires precise timing and the proper functioning of multiple muscle groups as well as cranial nerves

V, VII, IX, X, and XII. The swallow is typically divided into three phases: oral, pharyngeal, and esophageal. The oral phase consists of mastication, addition of saliva to the oral contents, and assessment of the safety of the food. This entire phase is under voluntary control. When the decision is made to proceed with swallowing, the bolus is pressed against the anterior tonsillar pillar. This activates pressure receptors innervated by cranial nerves IX and X and initiates the involuntary pharyngeal phase.

The pharyngeal phase begins with contraction of the levator and tensor veli palatini in order to elevate the soft palate and create a seal against the posterior pharyngeal wall. This prevents regurgitation of the bolus into the nasopharynx. At the same time, the superior constrictor begins to contract, creating the Passavant ridge, just above its most superior border in the nasopharynx. Respiration pauses at this time, typically during expiration. Next, the true vocal folds close, followed by the false vocal folds. The arytenoids are pulled against the epiglottis, and the bolus is moved farther into the oropharynx by base of tongue elevation and contraction of the constrictor muscles. The larynx is elevated with the base of tongue causing rotation of the epiglottis posteriorly over the laryngeal vestibule. Elevation of the larynx causes dilation of the cricopharyngeus; this, when combined with active relaxation of the same muscle, allows passage of the bolus into the cervical esophagus, where the esophageal phase of swallowing begins. Primary peristalsis of the esophagus is initiated by bolus entry into the esophagus; the bolus is then propelled down the esophagus at a rate of 5 to 10 cm per second. Next, the lower esophageal sphincter relaxes and allows the bolus to pass into the stomach. Secondary peristalsis then clears the esophagus of any remaining food particles. In total, it takes 4 to 7 second for all three phases of swallowing to propel a bolus from the oropharynx through the esophagus into the stomach.

24.3 Infectious, Inflammatory Lesions of the Pharynx

Pharyngitis is one of the most common reasons why a patient visits his or her primary care physician and accounts for 15 to 20% of all office visits. It is defined as an inflammation of the mucosa and submucosa of the pharynx and can affect the nasopharynx, oropharynx, and hypopharynx. The introduction of bacteria or viruses into this area causes a significant reactive inflammatory response because of the high concentration of lymphatic tissue in the Waldeyer ring. In certain instances, infections in this area can lead to systemic disease, causing substantial morbidity and mortality.

24.3.1 Bacterial Pharyngitis

The normal bacterial flora of the pharynx is made up mostly of gram-positive aerobic organisms that live commensally until their environment is altered by outside forces or new organisms are introduced. These changes typically manifest clinically as pharyngitis. The most common cause of bacterial pharyngitis is infection by group A β-hemolytic streptococci. Patients with pharyngitis due to infection by group A β-hemolytic streptococci typically describe a sore throat, difficulty swallowing, and headache. Cough and rhinorrhea are not usually associated with group A β-hemolytic streptococcal pharyngitis. The onset of group A β-hemolytic streptococcal pharyngitis tends to be more sudden than that of viral pharyngitis. On examination, these patients can have a high-grade fever, soft palate petechiae, and exudative tonsils. Tender anterior cervical adenopathy is seen 60% of the time with group A β-hemolytic streptococcal pharyngitis. However, the history and physical examination often can be misleading in patients with acute pharyngitis. Centor et al created an algorithm for the management of group A β-hemolytic streptococcal pharyngitis based on clinical factors that incorporates the absence of cough, swollen anterior cervical lymphadenopathy, presence of fever and tonsillar exudate, and patient age. However, this algorithm still requires that the majority of patients undergo laboratory testing in order to confirm the diagnosis of group A β-hemolytic streptococcal pharyngitis. Laboratory testing typically consists of either rapid antigen detection testing (RADT) or traditional throat culture. The gold standard for the confirmation of group A β-hemolytic streptococcal pharyngitis remains throat culture because of its high sensitivity (90 to 95%) and ability to identify antibiotic sensitivities. However, throat cultures take a minimum of 24 hours to provide clinicians with accurate results. The RADT was developed as a more rapid means of providing similar data to the treating physician. With sensitivities ranging from 79 to 88% and specificities above 95%, RADT provides an excellent alternative to throat culture, and results are available immediately. Throat cultures are typically collected in addition to performing RADT because of the potential development of rheumatic fever as a result of not treating group A β-hemolytic streptococcal pharyngitis.

The treatment of group A β-hemolytic streptococcal pharyngitis typically consists of oral or intravenous antibiotic administration. Although group A β-hemolytic streptococcal pharyngitis is a self-limited disease, antibiotics are given to provide acute symptom relief, reduce suppurative complications, and reduce communicability. Penicillin is still the recommended first-line therapy in most areas of the country. However, if β-lactamase–producing organisms are present, treatment with clavulanate or another β-lactamase–inhibiting agent in addition to penicillin is required. Patients who are allergic to penicillin can be treated with erythromycin or a first-generation cephalosporin. Antibiotic treatment of group A β-hemolytic streptococcal pharyngitis reduces symptom duration by an average of 16 hours and significantly reduces rates of peritonsillar and retropharyngeal abscesses. The treatment of group A β-hemolytic streptococcal pharyngitis with antibiotics prevents rheumatic fever regardless of whether the group A β-hemolytic streptococcal pharyngitis has been fully eradicated or not. Antibiotic use does not have an effect on the development of acute poststreptococcal glomerulonephritis.

Rheumatic fever is a rare complication of untreated group A β-hemolytic streptococcal pharyngeal infection that develops after local invasion of bacteria causes the release of extracellular toxins and proteases. Group A β-hemolytic streptococci also release M proteins systemically that are similar in structure to myocardial sarcolemmal antigens. These proteins stimulate an inflammatory response against the patient's own cardiac muscle, joints, blood vessels, and subcutaneous tissues. The diagnosis is made with the American Heart Association modified

Table 24.1 American Heart Association's modified Jones criteria

Major criteria	Minor criteria
Carditis	Fever (101° to 102°)
Polyarthritis	Arthralgia without edema
Sydenham chorea (St. Vitus dance)	Prolonged PR Interval on electrocardiogram
Subcutaneous nodules	Acute phase reactants: increased erythrocyte sedimentation rate, presence of C-reactive protein or leukocytosis
Erythema marginatum	History of rheumatic fever or the presence of inactive rheumatic heart disease
	Evidence of preceding β-hemolytic streptococcal infection[a]

Note: The diagnosis requires two major criteria or one major and two minor criteria, along with evidence of a prior streptococcal infection.
[a]Evidence of preceding streptococcal infection: increased antistreptolysin O or other streptococcal antibodies, positive throat culture for group A β-hemolytic streptococci, positive result of rapid antigen detection testing (RADT), or recent scarlet fever.

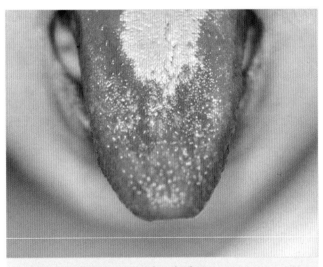

Fig. 24.1 "Strawberry tongue" of scarlet fever.

Jones criteria (► Table 24.1). The disease typically resolves after 6 weeks but can have lasting neurologic and cardiac effects. The patient must have a preceding streptococcal infection and two major criteria or one major and two minor criteria in order for the diagnosis to be made. Treatment involves antibiotics for the group A β-hemolytic streptococcal pharyngeal infection, nonsteroidal anti-inflammatory drugs, and corticosteroids, with possible treatment of cardiac complications.

Another complication of acute group A β-hemolytic streptococcal pharyngitis is scarlet fever. This condition manifests as a red, punctate, blanching rash that initially appears on the trunk but then quickly spreads to the entire body, sparing the face, palms, and soles. Patients will also have a swollen, red, and mottled "strawberry" tongue (► Fig. 24.1), along with perioral skin erythema and desquamation. The production of erythrogenic toxin and lysis of the bacteria by a bacteriophage is believed to be the mechanism behind this complication of group A β-hemolytic streptococcal pharyngitis. Before the advent of antibiotics, this condition carried a small but significant mortality risk that has all but disappeared since the discovery of penicillin.

Besides group A β-hemolytic streptococci, other bacteria can cause acute pharyngitis. The second most common cause of bacterial pharyngitis is *Staphylococcus* (*S. aureus* or *S. salivarius*). Infection by these bacteria tends to take place in patients who are dehydrated or are being treated with antibiotics. Patients may present with mucopurulent drainage, pharyngeal erythema, and edema as well as tonsillar pustules. Antistaphylococcal antibiotics, erythromycin, or first-generation cephalosporins are the antibiotics of choice for staphylococcal pharyngitis.

Another bacterial species known to cause pharyngitis is *Corynebacterium diphtheriae*. This gram-positive rod is found mostly in children younger than the age of 10 years in developing countries. After the bacteria gain access to the pharynx, bacterial exotoxin production causes local inflammation and tissue necrosis, resulting in the gray membrane classically associated with diphtheria. The local inflammation can affect the entire pharynx as well as the larynx, putting the patient at risk for airway obstruction. In addition, toxins released systemically can cause cardiomyopathy and dysrhythmias. The proper treatment of diphtheria includes management of the airway as well as antitoxin and antibiotic therapy. Widespread immunization programs have nearly eradicated diphtheria in developed nations.

Bordetella pertussis had been nearly eradicated in developed countries but is now having a strong resurgence because of waning immunity in adults vaccinated in childhood (as an increasing number of parents are choosing not to vaccinate their children). Infection by this gram-negative coccobacillus is characterized by a low-grade fever and upper respiratory symptoms. This marks the catarrhal phase of the disease. The paroxysmal phase follows, defined by the development of paroxysms of coughing followed by a loud inspiratory gasp that gives this disease its name, whooping cough. During this phase, *B. pertussis* produces an exotoxin that attacks ciliated epithelium and causes necrosis and mucopurulent exudate. The paroxysmal phase typically lasts 2 to 4 weeks and is followed by the convalescent stage, during which the coughing attacks slowly dissipate. The treatment of whooping cough is with a macrolide antibiotic in conjunction with supportive care. It is important to note that antibiotic therapy will not alter the course of the illness but will decrease infectiousness and spread of the disease.

Sexually transmitted diseases cause inflammation of the mucosal surfaces and can therefore affect the pharynx along with the genitals. *Neisseria gonorrhoeae* is a gram-negative diplococcus transmitted through sexual contact that can cause sore throat, tonsillar hypertrophy, and lymphadenopathy. Culture on chocolate or Thayer-Martin agar is required for identification of the organism. The treatment of gonococcal pharyngitis may be difficult because of a high incidence of antibiotic resistance, but ceftriaxone and doxycycline are recommended first-line agents. Infection by the spirochete *Treponema pallidum* may present as painless, dark red papules on the tonsils or pharyngeal wall, typically seen in secondary syphilis 2 to 3 months after primary infection. These lesions are highly contagious, and treatment with penicillin, tetracycline, or erythromycin is required.

24.3.2 Viral Pharyngitis

Viral pharyngitis is the most common cause of a sore throat. Patients tend to have a low-grade fever and other associated symptoms of an upper respiratory tract infection, such as coughing, sneezing, and rhinorrhea, as well as generalized adenopathy. The clinical course of viral pharyngitis is more indolent than that of bacterial pharyngitis and is not responsive to antibiotic treatment. Many viruses are associated with pharyngitis, including coronavirus, adenovirus, and rhinovirus. Clinically, it is difficult to distinguish which virus is responsible for a particular infection. However, certain viruses cause distinct physical findings and require special mention below.

Infection of the pharynx by herpes simplex virus (human herpesvirus, or HHV) presents with inflammation of the oral and pharyngeal mucosa as well as small vesicular lesions throughout the same area. It is caused by one of the two serologically distinct subtypes of HHV. Type 1 HHV is typically associated with oral or pharyngeal infection, whereas type 2 is seen more commonly in genital infections. However, both viruses can affect either area without restriction. The original infection by HHV can manifest symptoms for 7 to 10 days followed by quick resolution. Neonates or patients with compromised immune systems are at risk for disseminated infection by this virus and should be monitored for central nervous system involvement. The diagnosis of HHV infection is made through tissue culture, Tzanck preparation, or antigen detection. Tissue culture is the gold standard but can take up to 4 to 5 days to provide a result. Tzanck preparation and antigen detection tests are quicker but have a sensitivity rate between 50% and 70%. The treatment of HHV pharyngitis is with an antiviral, such as acyclovir or valacyclovir. However, this has not been shown to decrease the duration of illness or reduce symptomatology and may best be reserved for the immunocompromised patient.

Epstein-Barr virus (EBV) infection leads to infectious mononucleosis, an illness associated with exudative tonsillitis, fever, posterior triangle cervical lymphadenopathy, and malaise. Classically, patients also have splenomegaly on examination, although this has been shown to be present only in roughly 50% of patients with this disease. EBV infects B lymphocytes and has been linked to nasopharyngeal carcinoma and Burkitt lymphoma, although other factors are believed to be involved in the development of these malignancies. The diagnosis of this disease is based on clinical history and serum testing for heterophile antibodies with the monospot test. Complications associated with infectious mononucleosis include splenic rupture and acute airway obstruction due to pharyngotonsillar inflammation. However, in the large majority of patients, the symptoms resolve after 2 to 6 weeks of supportive care. Antibiotics should be avoided in these patients because they are ineffective in treating the disease, and patients given ampicillin or another penicillin develop a severe rash.

Pharyngitis caused by coxsackievirus A most often occurs in children younger than 5 years of age. It is characterized by vesicular or ulcerative lesions along the tonsillar pillars and buccal mucosa known as herpangina. This illness has a rapid course that includes high fevers and possible vesicular lesions on the extremities, including the palms of the hands and soles of the feet. The lesions on the extremities appear several days after the fever and pharyngitis begin. The diagnosis is made by clinical history and physical examination. The treatment of herpangina is supportive.

24.3.3 Fungal Pharyngitis

Although not a group of organisms commonly associated with pharyngitis, fungi can invade and damage the pharyngeal mucosa in individuals with compromised immune systems. *Candida* species are most commonly responsible for this condition. Patients with fungal pharyngitis will have a white, cheesy plaque along their oral or pharyngeal mucosa that is typically easily removed to reveal erythema below. The diagnosis is made by Gram stain or periodic acid–Schiff stain of a culture. Treatment is with topical nystatin or an oral azole. Individuals with no known history of immunosuppression should be sent for further immune testing once this diagnosis is confirmed.

24.3.4 Complications of Pharyngitis

Although infections of the pharynx are common, severe complications are rare. Most of these illnesses resolve spontaneously with few, if any, long-term sequelae. Occasionally, patients with pharyngitis will develop a condition that requires intervention beyond antibiotic treatment (e.g., peritonsillar abscess). The spread of infection beyond the tonsillar capsule allows purulent material to collect between the tonsillar capsule medially and the superior constrictor laterally. Patients have odynophagia, trismus, and soft palate swelling; uvular deviation away from the affected side and fullness in the superior soft palate are seen on physical examination. Symptoms of pharyngitis typically exist for at least 5 days before an abscess develops. The treatment of a peritonsillar abscess is incision and drainage with culture-directed antibiotic treatment for 7 to 10 days. Untreated, a peritonsillar abscess can spread to the parapharyngeal and retroesophageal spaces, causing airway obstruction, venous thrombosis, bacteremia; it may also spread to the mediastinum or even the central nervous system. However, these severe complications are rare now because of the effectiveness of antibiotic treatment. Patients with recurrent episodes of peritonsillar abscess are advised to undergo an elective tonsillectomy after resolution of their symptoms, with the goal of reducing or eliminating the risk for future infections.

24.4 Malignant Lesions of the Pharynx and Esophagus

24.4.1 Nasopharyngeal Cancer

Incidence and Background

Nasopharyngeal carcinoma (NPC) is a squamous cell carcinoma that develops from the epithelium of the nasopharynx. It is a rare cancer with an incidence of less than 1 per 100,000 in most countries. However, NPC occurs at a significantly higher rate in certain groups, such as ethnic Chinese in the southern part of China, Aleut Native Americans in Alaska, and Southeast Asians. The incidence in southern China has been documented to be as high as 30 per 100,000. The increased incidence is believed to be related to nitrosamines found in heavily salted fish in this area.

EBV is thought to play some oncogenic role in this tumor because of the high rates of EBV genome detection in NPC specimens. Nearly all patients with NPC also have EBV infection, and EBV RNA is found in almost all NPC cells. However, no substantial causative evidence has ever been found supporting the role of EBV in NPC development. The use of EBV serology has been proposed as a possible means of screening patients for NPC in regions where its incidence is high.

It is likely that genetic factors also play a role in NPC, based on the fact that first-degree relatives of patients with NPC are six times more likely to develop this cancer than are controls. Additionally, the incidence of NPC remains high among Chinese who have immigrated to the United States, although it decreases somewhat among Chinese born in North America. These North America–born Chinese should have NPC incidence rates similar to those of the general population, but their rates remain elevated despite removal of the causative environmental agents. To date, the only genetic associations made with NPC are HLA-BW46 and HLA-B17.

Classification

The World Health Organization (WHO) created a classification of NPC based on histopathology (▶ Table 24.2). Type I is the second most common type of NPC in North America and is referred to as sporadic NPC. Histopathologically, squamous differentiation is seen and is similar to that in other epidermoid carcinomas of the head and neck. Type I NPC is not associated with EBV but is related to tobacco and alcohol exposure. It carries a poor prognosis because of its lack of radiosensitivity. Type II NPC is the least common type. Together with type III NPC, it makes up the nonkeratinizing, or endemic, types of NPC. Type III NPC is the most common form. It includes a group of histopathologically similar forms of NPC, such as lymphoepithelioma and anaplastic and clear cell variants. Both type II NPC and type III NPC are associated with EBV and are radiosensitive.

Presentation

Nearly all patients with NPC are symptomatic at the time of diagnosis. One percent of NPCs are incidentally discovered on examination or imaging. The most common symptom of NPC at the time of diagnosis is a neck mass, followed by aural fullness and nasal obstruction. Neck masses typically present in level II or V and occur bilaterally in 20% of patients. Cranial neuropathies suggest infiltration of the skull base. Cranial nerves III through VI are the most commonly involved because of their location in relation to the skull base and cavernous sinus.

Table 24.2 World Health Organization classification of nasopharyngeal carcinomas

Type I	Keratinizing squamous cell carcinoma
Type II	Nonkeratinizing squamous cell carcinoma
Type III	Undifferentiated carcinoma

Evaluation

Computed tomography (CT) of the head and neck should be obtained, as well as magnetic resonance (MR) imaging, for all patients with NPC. CT provides information regarding cranial bone involvement and possible lymph node metastases. MR imaging allows better visualization of the soft tissues, including neural structures closely associated with the nasopharynx.

Differential Diagnosis

The differential diagnosis for NPC is limited but includes inflammation, infection, lymphoma, and Tornwaldt cyst. Individuals with Tornwaldt cysts have midline nasopharyngeal cysts that can mimic NPC lesions.

Staging

The staging of NPC is based on the 2010 American Joint Committee on Cancer (AJCC) staging guidelines. Both tumor and nodal staging are unique compared with that for the rest of the pharynx. The parapharyngeal space is a potential space shaped like an inverted pyramid, with its base at the skull base and extending inferiorly to the cornu of the hyoid bone. It is bordered medially by the constrictor muscle and laterally by the ramus of the mandible and deep lobe of the parotid. Involvement of this space portends a more locally advanced tumor.

A T1 lesion is confined to the nasopharynx or can extend to the oropharynx or nasal cavity without involvement of the parapharyngeal space, whereas a T2 lesion extends into this space. If the bony structures of the anterior skull base or sinuses are involved, the lesion is T3. T4 lesions have intracranial invasion and/or involvement of cranial nerves, hypopharynx, or orbit, or they extend into the infratemporal fossa or masticator space.

Unilateral cervical nodal metastasis above the supraclavicular fossa and/or uni- or bilateral retropharyngeal nodal involvement not larger than 6 cm represent N1 disease. N2 status is bilateral supraclavicular cervical nodal metastasis not larger than 6 cm. Nodal metastasis larger than 6 cm is classified as N3a, and nodal disease in the supraclavicular fossa is N3b. In situ disease is classified as stage 0, and T1 lesions with no nodal or distant metastasis are stage I. T1 disease with N1 nodal status or T2 primary lesions with N0 or N1 status are stage II disease. The combination of a T1 or a T2 primary lesion with N2 nodal status is stage III. T4 lesions with N0–N2 nodal disease are classified as stage IVA; any lesion with N3 nodal disease is stage IVB; any lesion with distant metastasis is stage IVC.

Treatment

Early-stage NPC is treated with radiation therapy; more advanced NPC is typically treated with combined chemoradiation therapy. Doses of 60 to 70 Gy are administered via external beam radiation to the nasopharynx and both sides of the neck. Accurate staging with precise pretreatment imaging by CT or MR imaging has allowed better dosimetry and a reduction in damage to adjacent tissue, reducing morbidity in such sensitive areas as the pituitary, eyes, ears, and surrounding neural structures.

Surgical resection of NPC is typically reserved for patients with tumor recurrence or radiation failure. Operating in the nasopharynx is technically challenging because of the lack of accessibility of this area. Contraindications for surgical intervention include carotid involvement, skull base erosion, and intracranial involvement. NPC can be approached from either an open or an endoscopic approach. Endoscopic treatment is rare and is used primarily for small recurrences in the central portion of the posterior nasopharyngeal wall.

There are multiple options for an open approach. A lateral rhinotomy with a medial maxillectomy can be used for recurrences limited to the nasopharynx or involving the pterygopalatine fossa. This procedure carries few side effects but provides limited access compared with other approaches, including the maxillary swing. In this approach, a Weber-Ferguson incision is made, and the outer maxillary wall is rotated laterally with the skin and soft tissue attached. Access to the pterygopalatine fossa is improved with the maxillary swing but at the cost of a larger incision than is used for the lateral rhinotomy.

The other indication for surgery in patients with NPC is residual neck disease. The surgery of choice for this situation is radical neck dissection, based on the fact that recurrent nodal disease is often along the chain of lymph nodes of the upper internal jugular vein as well as the accessory nerve. Also, metastatic lymph nodes have a higher propensity for extracapsular spread in NPC than in other squamous cell carcinomas of the head and neck. Because the areas involved in this surgery have been previously radiated, the risk for carotid blowout is higher; therefore, incisions should be planned carefully, and a pedicled flap (e.g., a pectoralis major flap) should be used for carotid coverage if there is a risk for this complication.

Outcomes

Local and regional control of NPC depends on the stage but in general ranges between 70% and 80% with combined therapy. Five-year survival is also between 70% and 80% depending on the stage. However, the risk for recurrence of NPC continues after 5 years, and 10-year survival ranges from 10 to 40%. This decrease in long-term survival is due partly to the high rate of distant metastases in NPC. Between 25% and 30% of patients with NPC will develop distant metastases, the highest rate of any head and neck cancer. This should be considered when a patient previously treated for NPC is being followed.

Complications of Treatment

Side effects of radiation for NPC include mucositis, xerostomia, sinusitis, otitis media with effusion, sensorineural hearing loss, trismus, pituitary dysfunction, and cranial nerve palsies.

24.4.2 Oropharyngeal Cancer

Incidence and Background

Cancers of the oropharynx make up 12% of all malignancies of the head and neck. More than 90% of all oropharyngeal cancers are squamous cell carcinoma (SCC). The overall incidence of oropharyngeal SCC had been declining because of decreased rates of smoking and alcohol intake. However, between 1973 and 2004, the incidence rate increased, especially in white males younger than 60 years old. In this same time period, the rate of oropharyngeal SCC that tested positive for human papillomavirus (HPV) nearly tripled, from a rate of 16.3% between 1984 and 1989 to a rate of 72.7% between 2000 and 2004. Oropharyngeal SCC had always been related to two main environmental factors, tobacco and alcohol intake; however, clinicians are now confronted with oropharyngeal SCC that lack the usual risk factors but are positive for HPV.

The oropharynx is composed mainly of mucosa, so it is clear why SCC accounts for the majority of malignant lesions in this region. However, the presence of the Waldeyer ring of lymphoid tissue in this area is the reason why the next most common malignancy seen in the oropharynx is lymphoma, typically involving the palatine tonsils or base of tongue. Lymphoepitheliomas also can develop from this ring of lymphoid tissue but are rare. Besides mucosa and lymphoid tissue, the oropharynx contains minor salivary glands that can undergo malignant transformation and lead to salivary gland carcinoma. Oropharyngeal malignancies can become very large before the onset of symptoms. For this reason, oropharyngeal SCC typically presents at an advanced tumor stage and with a rate of cervical lymph node involvement higher than 50% for all subsites. Lymph node metastases tend to occur in a stepwise progression, beginning at the superior lymph nodes in level II and proceeding inferiorly through levels III and IV. In addition, many oropharyngeal structures are midline, so both sides of the neck must be considered in treatment planning.

Evaluation

CT should be performed in all patients with oropharyngeal and hypopharyngeal SCC to assess for lymph node metastases and evaluate for invasion into surrounding structures. Patients with lesions in the inferior oropharynx and hypopharynx should undergo direct laryngoscopy and esophagoscopy in order to fully assess tumor involvement.

Differential Diagnosis

The differential diagnosis for an oropharyngeal lesion additionally includes infection, leukoplakia or erythroplakia, eosinophilic granuloma, pyogenic granuloma, giant cell tumor, papilloma, and verruciform xanthoma.

Staging

The staging of oropharyngeal cancer follows the TNM (tumor node metastasis) staging system and is based on the 2010 AJCC staging guidelines.

A T1 lesion is no larger than 2 cm. A T2 lesion is larger than 2 cm but smaller than 4 cm. Tumors that are larger than 4 cm or extend to the lingual surface of the tongue are classified as T3. T4a lesions invade the larynx, extrinsic tongue muscles, hard palate, pterygoid, or mandible. T4b lesions are very advanced locally, with invasion of the lateral pterygoid muscle, pterygoid plates, lateral nasopharynx, or skull base, or they encase the carotid artery.

N1 nodal disease is a single ipsilateral lymph node 3 cm or smaller. N2 disease is more extensive: N2a disease is a single ipsilateral lymph node larger than 3 cm but smaller than 6 cm; N2b disease is multiple ipsilateral nodes (none larger than 6 cm), and N2c disease includes bilateral or contralateral lymph

nodes, none larger than 6 cm. Finally, any nodal metastasis larger than 6 cm is classified as N3.

In situ disease is classified as stage 0, and T1 lesions with no nodal or distant metastasis are stage I. T2 primary lesions with N0 status are stage II disease. T3 primary lesions with no nodal involvement or T1–T3 lesions with N1 nodal status are stage III. T4a lesions with N0–N2 nodal disease or T1–T3 lesions with N2 nodal disease are classified as stage IVA; T4b primary lesions with any N status or any lesions with N3 nodal status are stage IVB; any lesion with distant metastasis is stage IVC.

Treatment

Tonsils and Lateral Pharyngeal Wall

The tonsils and surrounding pillars are the most common site of carcinoma in the oropharynx. Malignancies in this location can grow very large before detection. They most often present with dysphagia, odynophagia, otalgia, trismus, or a neck mass. Extension to adjacent structures is common, including the base of tongue, soft palate, retromolar trigone, and pterygoid muscles. At the time of diagnosis, clinically positive cervical lymphadenopathy accompanies 76% of tonsil carcinomas and 45% of tonsillar pillar carcinomas. Contralateral lymph node involvement is found between 5% and 11% of the time.

Early tonsillar cancer can be treated by either surgery or radiation therapy. Locoregional control rates and complications have been shown to be equivalent for both treatment modalities. Because it offers similar control rates, radiation therapy has become the treatment of choice for early tonsillar cancers.

Advanced tonsillar cancers can be treated with a variety of options, and a multidisciplinary approach is appropriate. Surgery is often a viable option but should be combined with postoperative radiation therapy or chemoradiation therapy. Advanced tonsillar cancer can also be treated with functional organ preservation therapy that combines chemotherapy and radiation. Several studies have shown that chemoradiation therapy achieves good locoregional control and has survival rates similar to those of surgery with postoperative radiation for advanced oropharyngeal SCC. However, no large randomized control trials that compare surgery plus radiation versus organ preservation therapy have been conducted at this time. Because of this, organ preservation therapy is often chosen as the initial therapy for tonsillar cancer, and surgery is used as salvage treatment after failure of the chemoradiation therapy.

In addition to treatment of the primary lesion, nearly all patients with tonsillar cancer require treatment of clinically present cervical metastases. Tonsillar SCC has a rate of nodal metastases higher than 20% for all T stages, and prophylactic treatment of a clinically negative neck is required. Lymph node metastases can be treated with neck dissection or radiation therapy, with both offering similar control rates; because of this, the method of neck treatment is typically the same method as is chosen to treat the primary lesion.

Tonsillar SCC can be approached transorally, but this is limited to the excision of very small lesions confined to the tonsillar pillar. Transoral robotic surgery may expand the number of lesions that can be approached through the mouth, but given the success of radiation therapy in treating small tonsillar lesions, the role of transoral robotic surgery may be limited. Another approach to tonsillar SCC is to use an anterior mandibulotomy with mandibular swing. This approach provides good access to tonsillar cancers without bony involvement. If bony involvement is present, a segmental mandibulectomy with en bloc resection encompassing the tumor and involved bone is used. Removing such a large piece of tissue carries significant morbidity and typically requires osteomyocutaneous flap reconstruction.

Patients with early tonsillar SCC have high 5-year survival and locoregional control rates—80% and 90%, respectively. However, both of these rates drop significantly with advanced tonsillar SCC. The 5-year survival and locoregional control rates range from 20 to 50% for stages III and IV disease.

Soft Palate

SCC of the soft palate is uncommon and accounts for fewer than 2% of all head and neck cancers. Because these lesions typically appear on the oral surface of the soft palate, they are easily detectable and frequently noted earlier than those at other oropharyngeal sites. Second primary lesions are found 13% of the time, and metachronous lesions are noted 26% of the time in patients with soft palate SCC. Rates of regional metastasis are higher than 20% for all T stages, with rates of bilateral spread as high as 15% for SCC of the soft palate. Tumor thickness of more than than 3 mm in this area has been associated with regional metastasis.

The treatment of soft palate SCC is by radiation therapy or combined chemoradiation. Small lesions on the soft palate can be surgically excised transorally, but the resection of larger tumors has a high rate of velopharyngeal insufficiency and is best avoided. In addition to treatment of the primary lesion, patients with soft palate SCC should receive bilateral irradiation of the neck or bilateral neck dissection depending on the initial stage.

The rate of locoregional control of soft palate SCC is higher than 75% for early through stage III lesions. The 5-year survival is higher than 65% for this same group of patients. However, locoregional control and survival both drop to below 40% for stage IV lesions.

Base of Tongue

This region stretches from the circumvallate papillae of the posterior tongue to the vallecula. SCC of the base of tongue is less common, but more aggressive, than that of the oral tongue. In addition to SCC of the base of tongue, this area can give rise to lymphomas because of the presence of the lingual tonsil. Patients with base of tongue SCC present most commonly with otalgia and odynophagia. The diagnosis is difficult because of challenges in examining this area. SCC of the base of tongue can invade other oropharyngeal subsites as well as the larynx. Cervical lymph node metastases are present in more than 60% of patients at the time of presentation. SCC of the base of tongue, which is a midline structure, involves bilateral cervical nodes in 20% of cases.

Radiation therapy or chemoradiation therapy is typically used for base of tongue cancer, with surgery reserved for superficial lesions and salvage after radiation failure. Both surgery and radiation therapy have similar survival outcomes, but operating in this area is classically associated with significant morbidity and functional disturbances. The cervical lymph node basins on both sides of the neck should receive treatment in patients with lesions of the base of tongue. If radiation therapy is used for the primary site, then it is typically used for the neck as well.

The surgery for base of tongue cancers is a hemiglossectomy and can be approached through methods similar to those used for tonsillar cancer. A mandibulotomy with a mandibular swing can be used to gain access to the base of tongue. Base of tongue lesions can also be treated surgically through the neck via a suprahyoid pharyngotomy approach. However, both of these approaches carry a moderate risk for postoperative functional morbidity. If a total or nearly total glossectomy is required for larger lesions, laryngectomy may be necessary to prevent chronic aspiration. Recently, the transoral approach has been advocated for appropriately selected patients with early base of tongue lesions. This operation can be performed with a handheld endoscope and a laser or robotically. Both endoscopic transoral surgery and transoral robotic surgery have been shown to have excellent locoregional control rates (higher than 85% for early base of tongue lesions).

Early base of tongue cancer is associated with a 5-year survival rate higher than 85% and a comparable locoregional control rate. However, advanced base of tongue carcinoma has a survival rate of less than 50% and is a particularly aggressive lesion.

Pharyngeal Wall

Lesions involving this subsite are rare but aggressive, with early invasion into surrounding structures such as the prevertebral fascia and hypopharynx. The metastatic potential is low for early pharyngeal wall cancers. Therefore, treatment of the lymphatic basins is often not required. Because most pharyngeal wall lesions cross the midline, lymph node metastases, when present, are often bilateral, and treatment of both sides of the neck is required. Lymphatic drainage is primarily to retropharyngeal and parapharyngeal lymph nodes but also may involve levels II through IV.

Pharyngeal wall cancers can be treated with surgery or radiation therapy. If surgery is performed, postoperative radiation therapy or chemoradiation therapy is typically incorporated. Because of its proximity to the spinal cord, administering radiation therapy to the posterior pharyngeal wall is challenging and requires precise planning. The treatment of lymph node metastases involves treating the retropharyngeal lymph nodes and therefore incorporates radiation therapy either as the primary treatment or as adjuvant therapy after neck dissection.

Pharyngeal wall lesions typically present at an advanced stage and carry a poor survival rate. One study noted a 5-year survival rate of less than 40% based on tumor staging.

Complications of Treatment

Side effects of radiation for oropharyngeal SCC include mucositis, xerostomia, sinusitis, osteoradionecrosis, dysphagia, laryngeal edema, and carotid artery rupture. Surgical complications depend on the approach used but include infection, malocclusion, and difficulty with speech and swallowing.

24.4.3 Hypopharyngeal Cancer

Hypopharyngeal cancer accounts for 6% of all head and neck cancers and has a worldwide incidence of from 0.8 to 5 cases per 100,000 persons. It is more common in well-developed countries. Of all hypopharyngeal cancers, 95% are SCC. These lesions are typically discovered late and are confined to the hypopharynx only 15% of the time. Regional lymph node metastases are noted at presentation in 65% of patients.

The main risk factors for hypopharyngeal SCC are tobacco and alcohol use, as for other head and neck cancers. In addition, hypopharyngeal cancer has also been associated with vitamin C deficiencies, exposure to asbestos and steel or coal dusts, and iron deficiency. Gastric reflux has been implicated in hypopharyngeal cancer, but no strong association has been discovered. Plummer-Vinson syndrome, however, has been associated with hypopharyngeal SCC, particularly in the postcricoid region. This syndrome affects mainly women and manifests with the triad of dysphagia, glossitis, and iron deficiency anemia. Improved nutrition and dietary fortification have reduced the incidence of Plummer-Vinson syndrome along with its role in hypopharyngeal SCC.

The hypopharynx is divided into three separate anatomical subsites: the piriform sinus, posterior hypopharyngeal wall, and postcricoid space. The piriform sinus is by far the most common subsite of hypopharyngeal cancer, accounting for approximately 75% of all lesions. The posterior pharyngeal wall accounts for 20%, and the postcricoid region accounts for the remaining 5%. The hypopharynx is a physically small space, so cancers tend to invade surrounding structures quickly. Lesions of the piriform sinus can spread to the subglottis, paraglottic space, and thyroid cartilage. Posterior hypopharyngeal wall lesions tend to spread superiorly into the lower oropharynx, whereas cancers of the postcricoid space often spread to the cervical esophagus. Submucosal spread underneath intact epithelium is frequently seen with hypopharyngeal cancers.

Presentation

The most common symptoms at presentation are odynophagia, referred otalgia, dysphagia, hoarseness, and neck mass.

Evaluation

See the earlier section on evaluation of the oropharynx.

Staging

The staging of hypopharyngeal cancer follows the TNM staging system and is based on the AJCC guidelines from 2010.

A T1 lesion is no larger than 2 cm and is limited to one subsite of the hypopharynx. A T2 lesion is larger than 2 cm but smaller than 4 cm without fixation of the hemilarynx, or it invades more than one hypopharyngeal subsite or an adjacent site. T3 tumors are larger than 4 cm or associated with fixation of the hemilarynx. T4a lesions invade the thyroid or cricoid cartilage, hyoid bone, thyroid gland, or prelaryngeal strap muscles or subcutaneous fat. T4b lesions invade the prevertebral fascia, encase the carotid artery, or involve mediastinal structures.

N1 nodal disease is a single ipsilateral lymph node 3 cm or smaller in size. N2 disease is more extensive: N2a disease is a single ipsilateral lymph node larger than 3 cm but smaller than 6 cm, N2b disease is multiple ipsilateral nodes (none larger than 6 cm), and N2c disease is bilateral or contralateral lymph nodes, none larger than 6 cm. Finally, any nodal metastasis larger than 6 cm is classified as N3.

In situ disease is classified as stage 0, and T1 lesions with no nodal or distant metastasis are stage I. T2 primary lesions with N0 status are stage II disease. T3 primary lesions with no nodal involvement or T1–T3 lesions with N1 nodal status are stage III. T4a lesions with N0–N2 nodal disease or T1–T3 lesions with N2 nodal disease are classified as stage IVA; T4b primary lesions with any N status or any lesion with N3 nodal status is stage IVB; any lesion with distant metastasis is stage IVC.

Differential Diagnosis

See the differential diagnosis for oropharyngeal cancer above. In addition, carcinoma of the larynx and esophagus should be included in the differential diagnosis for hypopharyngeal lesions.

Treatment

Early hypopharyngeal cancer is generally treated with radiation therapy because the disease-free survival rates are comparable and laryngeal and pharyngeal function is significantly better in patients treated with radiation than in those treated with surgery. Surgery is reserved for salvage after radiation failure or for lesions that are located in technically resectable areas, such as the upper piriform sinus and posterior pharyngeal wall. Transoral endoscopic resection with a laser is typically used for the surgical treatment of early hypopharyngeal cancers. Additional approaches for early lesions include partial laryngopharyngectomy and combined suprahyoid with lateral pharyngectomy. The partial laryngopharyngectomy can be used for cancers of the medial wall of the piriform sinus that are at least 1.5 cm from the apex. The combined suprahyoid resection with lateral pharyngectomy can be considered for early posterior hypopharyngeal wall cancers.

Advanced hypopharyngeal cancers involve surrounding structures, including the larynx and cervical esophagus, and therefore the treatment is similar to that for laryngeal or esophageal cancer. Organ preservation chemoradiation is commonly used as first-line therapy for advanced hypopharyngeal cancer. Surgery is reserved for poor responders and typically involves laryngectomy or laryngopharyngectomy. Esophageal involvement may require esophagectomy with gastric pull-up.

Hypopharyngeal cancer has a high rate of cervical lymph node metastasis, and the primary lesions often cross the midline. Because of this, both sides of the neck require treatment at all T stages. The decision whether to use radiation or surgery is typically based on the treatment of choice for the primary lesion.

Outcomes

Outcomes of the treatment of hypopharyngeal SCC depend on the subsite of the lesion. Pharyngeal wall SCC carries the worst prognosis, with a 5-year survival rate of 21%. Patients with piriform sinus lesions have the highest survival rate (approximately 50%). Postcricoid carcinoma has a survival rate of

35%. In addition, the rate of distant metastases is high for hypopharyngeal cancer, approaching 20% depending on the T stage.

24.4.4 Esophageal Cancer

Incidence and Background

In 2012, there were an estimated 17,460 new cases of esophageal cancer in the United States. More than 95% of these cases will be SCC or adenocarcinoma of the esophagus. Until recently, SCC accounted for the large majority of esophageal malignancies. However, in the past two decades, the incidence of adenocarcinoma has continued to rise while the incidence of SCC has fallen. Now, these two types of malignancy occur with roughly equal frequency in the esophagus; adenocarcinomas occur mostly in the distal esophagus, whereas SCC is more evenly distributed throughout all the levels of the esophagus.

Risk factors for esophageal cancer vary depending on the histologic type. The risk factors for esophageal SCC are smoking, alcohol, Plummer-Vinson syndrome, a history of radiation treatment to the mediastinum, and nonepidermolytic palmoplantar keratoderma. Risk factors for adenocarcinoma of the esophagus include Barrett esophagus, obesity, acid reflux, tobacco use, and a history of radiation treatment. Barrett esophagus is metaplasia of the squamous mucosa in the distal esophagus to columnar epithelium similar to that of the stomach. Metaplasia progresses to dysplasia, followed by malignant transformation at a rate of 0.5% per year.

Presentation

At the time of diagnosis, between 50% and 60% of patients with esophageal carcinoma have an unresectable primary tumor, making prompt diagnosis of this disease extremely important. The propensity for advanced disease is believed to be largely due to the lack of serosa around the esophagus and to the fact that esophageal cancer is usually asymptomatic in its early stages. Symptoms of esophageal cancer include dysphagia, odynophagia, and weight loss. Hoarseness may also occur and carries a poor prognosis because it is a sign of invasion of the larynx. Carcinoma of the cervical esophagus is rare and most often comes from the spread of hypopharyngeal cancer to the esophagus rather than an esophageal primary.

Evaluation

Patients with esophageal carcinoma require CT of the neck, thorax, and/or abdomen depending on the location of the primary lesion. Endoscopic ultrasound and barium esophagram also provide valuable information about esophageal carcinoma and are typically obtained. In addition to imaging studies, flexible or rigid esophagoscopy should be performed to visualize the mass and obtain a histopathologic diagnosis.

Staging

The staging of esophageal cancer follows the TNM staging system and is based on the 2010 AJCC guidelines. It includes tumor type, depth, and spread; nodal metastasis; distant metastasis; histologic grade; and tumor location.

A T1 lesion invades the lamina propria, muscularis mucosae (T1a), or submucosa (T1b). T2 lesions invade the muscularis propria, and T3 lesions invade the adventitia. T4 status implies invasion of adjacent structures: resectable tumors invading the pleura, pericardium, or diaphragm (T4a) or unresectable tumors invading other structures, including the aorta, vertebral body, and trachea (T4b).

N1 nodal disease implies the involvement of one to two regional lymph nodes, N2 three to six nodes, and N3 seven or more regional nodes.

Staging of Squamous Cell Carcinoma of the Esophagus

In situ disease (high-grade dysplasia) is classified as stage 0. T1 low-grade lesions with no nodal or distant metastases are stage IA; if the tumor is of intermediate or high grade, it is stage 1B, as are low-grade T2–T3 lesions of the lower esophagus (below the lower border of the inferior pulmonary vein). T2 primary lesions with N0 status (intermediate or high grade if in the lower esophagus, or low grade if in the middle or upper esophagus) are stage IIA disease. T2–T3 primary lesions with N0 status (intermediate or high grade in the upper or middle esophagus) or any T1–T2 lesions with N1 disease are classified as stage IIB. Any T1–T2 lesion with N2 disease, T3 lesion with N1 disease, or T4a lesion with N0 disease is stage IIIA; T3 lesions with N2 disease are stage IIIB. A T4a primary lesion with N1–N2 nodal disease, any T4b lesion, and any lesion with N3 nodal status is considered to be stage IIIC. Any lesion with a distant metastasis is stage IV.

Staging of Adenocarcinoma of the Esophagus

In situ disease (high-grade dysplasia) is classified as stage 0. T1 low- or intermediate-grade lesions with no nodal or distant metastases are stage IA; if the tumor is high-grade, it is stage 1B, as are low- or intermediate-grade T2 lesions. High-grade T2 primary lesions with N0 status are stage IIA disease. T3 primary lesions with N0 status or any T1–N2 lesions with N1 disease are classified as stage IIB. Any T1–T2 lesion with N2 disease, T3 lesion with N1 disease, or T4a lesion with N0 disease is stage IIIA; T3 lesions with N2 disease are stage IIIB. A T4a primary lesion with N1–N2 nodal disease, any T4b lesion, and any lesion with N3 nodal status is considered to be stage IIIC. Any lesion with a distant metastasis is stage IV.

Differential Diagnosis

The differential diagnosis for esophageal carcinoma includes achalasia, eosinophilic esophagitis, leiomyosarcoma, and peptic strictures due to reflux.

Treatment

The treatment options for esophageal cancer include surgery, radiation, and chemotherapy. The optimal treatment depends on the location and stage of the disease. Surgery is an option for a minority of patients with early-stage disease and typically consists of a partial or total esophagectomy. This can be accomplished through a transthoracic or trans-hiatal approach if the

213

tumor involves the thoracic or distal esophagus. Gastric transposition or pull-up is required for reconstruction of this defect. A transcervical approach can be used for access to cervical esophageal cancer lesions. However, most tumors have invaded the esophageal wall by the time they are diagnosed or have metastasized to regional lymph nodes, making complete surgical resection nearly impossible. For these patients, chemoradiotherapy is often chosen as first-line treatment. Chemoradiotherapy may also be used preoperatively to reduce tumor size and allow complete resection. However, no survival benefit has been demonstrated from preoperative radiation therapy, chemotherapy, or combined chemoradiotherapy.

Outcomes

The overall prognosis for esophageal cancer is poor. The 5-year survival rate for patients with stage II disease or worse is less than 15%. Stage I disease has a survival rate of more than 50%, but diagnosis at this stage is rare.

24.5 Roundsmanship

- NPC occurs at a significantly higher rate in certain groups, such as ethnic Chinese in the southern part of China, Aleut Native Americans in Alaska, and Southeast Asians.
- The proper evaluation of NPC includes CT and MR imaging.
- Between 25% and 30% of patients with NPC will develop distant metastases, the highest rate for cancer at any head and neck site.
- Plummer-Vinson syndrome (associated with hypopharyngeal SCC) affects mainly women and manifests with the triad of dysphagia, glossitis, and iron deficiency anemia.

- Hypopharyngeal cancers often cross the midline and have a high rate of cervical lymph node metastasis, so that treatment of both sides of the neck is required at all T stages.

24.6 Recommended Reading

[1] Esophagus and esophagogastric junction. In: Edge SB, Byrd DR, Compton CC, et al, eds. American Joint Committee on Cancer (AJCC) Staging Manual. 7th ed. New York, NY: Springer; 2010:129–144

[2] Al-Sarraf M, LeBlanc M, Giri PG et al. Chemoradiotherapy versus radiotherapy in patients with advanced nasopharyngeal cancer: phase III randomized Intergroup study 0099. J Clin Oncol 1998; 16: 1310–1317

[3] Pharynx. In: Edge SB, Byrd DR, Compton CC, et al, eds. American Joint Committee on Cancer (AJCC) Staging Manual. 7th ed. New York, NY: Springer; 2010:63–79

[4] Erkal HS, Serin M, Amdur RJ, Villaret DB, Stringer SP, Mendenhall WM. Squamous cell carcinomas of the soft palate treated with radiation therapy alone or followed by planned neck dissection. Int J Radiat Oncol Biol Phys 2001; 50: 359–366

[5] Law S, Wong J. Current management of esophageal cancer. J Gastrointest Surg 2005; 9: 291–310

[6] Lin DT, Cohen SM, Coppit GL, Burkey BB. Squamous cell carcinoma of the oropharynx and hypopharynx. Otolaryngol Clin North Am 2005; 38: 59–74, viii

[7] NCCN guidelines. http://www.nccn.org/professionals/physician_gls/f_guidelines.asp#site. Fort Washington, PA: National Comprehensive Cancer Network; 2013. Accessed October 16, 2013

[8] Takes RP, Strojan P, Silver CE et alInternational Head and Neck Scientific Group. Current trends in initial management of hypopharyngeal cancer: the declining use of open surgery. Head Neck 2012; 34: 270–281

[9] Wei WI, Sham JST. Nasopharyngeal carcinoma. Lancet 2005; 365: 2041–2054

[10] Centor RM, Witherspoon JM, Dalton HP, Brody CE, and Link K. The diagnosis of strep throat in adults in the emergency room. Medical Decision Making 1981, 1(3):239–246

25 Diseases and Neoplasms of the Larynx

Edward M. Stafford

25.1 Introduction

In the field of head and neck oncology, the evolution of the treatment of laryngeal cancer has followed the adage "everything old is new again." Although laryngeal cancer was once treated primarily as a surgical disease, advances in "organ preservation" protocols and intensity-modulated radiation therapy (IMRT) ushered in a new paradigm in its treatment. Now, partly because of treatment failures and sometimes poor functional outcomes in patients treated with primary radiotherapy or chemoradiotherapy, the pendulum has shifted again over the course of the last decade, with a reemergence of primary surgical therapy in the treatment of both early and advanced laryngeal cancer. With advances in transoral endoscopic techniques as well as a new-found appreciation for time-tested open conservation approaches to laryngeal surgery, the treatment algorithm for laryngeal cancer demonstrates the need for today's head and neck surgeons to have all the available tools, surgical and nonsurgical, at their disposal in treating this challenging malignancy. If there is one subsite in the head and neck where the surgeon's judgment is of paramount importance in choosing among a variety of treatment options, it is the larynx.

25.2 Incidence of Disease

Cancer of the larynx, compared with other malignancies, such as cancers of the breast or lung, is relatively uncommon. It accounts for fewer than 1% of all human malignancies. Within the head and neck, however, laryngeal cancer is much more common, representing roughly 25% of all head and neck cancers. According to the American Cancer Society, there will be an estimated 12,360 new cases of laryngeal cancer in the United States in 2012. There will also be an estimated 3,650 deaths attributable to laryngeal cancer. According to the Surveillance Epidemiology and End Results (SEER) database, the 5-year survival of patients with laryngeal cancer depends predominantly on the presence of regional and distant disease. From 1996 to 2004, overall survival for all T stages was 62.5%: the rates were 80.9% for patients with local disease, 50.2% for patients with metastatic disease in the neck, and 23.4% for those with distant disease.

25.3 Terminology

In order to understand the diagnostic and treatment algorithms in the treatment of laryngeal carcinoma, one must understand the associated terminology. First, when discussing the larynx as a functional unit, the surgeon will refer to the primary disease, or the site at which the carcinoma originates. The primary lesion is then described as occurring in the supraglottic larynx, glottic larynx, or subglottic larynx. As with other head and neck malignancies, when the carcinoma spreads outside the area of the primary lesion, the staging of the malignancy is affected. With regard to lymph node metastases, these are described as *regional* when they occur in the central and lateral neck compartments. When metastases occur outside the head and

neck, they are described as *distant.* Finally, particularly pertinent with cancer of the larynx, any extension of disease outside the boundaries of the larynx is categorized as *extralaryngeal* spread (▶ Fig. 25.1).

With regard to treatment, surgical therapies are divided into several categories. Surgery that employs endoscopic laser techniques to remove laryngeal carcinoma is categorized as transoral laser surgery. Techniques that employ robotic technology are categorized as transoral robotic surgery (TORS). Open surgical techniques that remove part but not all of the larynx are categorized as conservation laryngeal surgery. With regard to the use of radiation therapy, techniques that treat laryngeal cancer without surgical excision but with radiation and possibly the addition of chemotherapy are called organ preservation techniques. Finally, radiation therapy or chemotherapy given after surgical excision is described as *adjuvant* treatment, whereas *neoadjuvant* chemotherapy precedes surgical excision.

25.4 Applied Anatomy

As with all surgical disease, a thorough understanding of the underlying anatomy is indispensable for an understanding of the pathogenesis of laryngeal cancer. The larynx can be divided into three subsites: supraglottic, glottic, and subglottic. Each subsite of the larynx has a unique embryonic development and subsequently distinct lymphatic drainage patterns. The glottic larynx, or glottis, includes the paired true vocal folds, anterior commissure, and posterior commissure. The supraglottic larynx is that portion of the larynx superior to the glottis, including the false vocal folds, arytenoids, aryepiglottic folds, and epiglottis. The subglottic larynx begins 10 mm below the free margin of the true vocal folds and extends to the inferior border of the cricoid cartilage. With regard to the substance of the larynx, it consists of a bony and cartilaginous framework, fibroelastic ligaments, muscles, and mucosal and submucosal surfaces. The

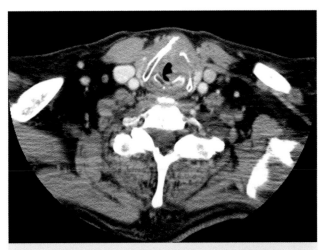

Fig. 25.1 Extralaryngeal spread as visualized in a patient with T4 glottic squamous cell carcinoma on computed tomography. Note the erosion of the outer table of the thyroid cartilage.

bony and cartilaginous framework includes the thyroid cartilage, cricoid cartilage, epiglottis, hyoid bone, and arytenoids.

Created by the various cartilages, ligaments, and membranes of the larynx are several distinct spaces that are of critical importance in evaluating the stage of laryngeal cancer, including the pre-epiglottic space, paraglottic space, and subglottic space. Of particular importance is a structure called the conus elasticus, which originates from the cricoid cartilage, attaches posteriorly to the arytenoid cartilages, and condenses medially to form the vocal ligament. Anteriorly, the conus elasticus attaches to the thyroid cartilage at the Broyle ligament, also known as the anterior commissure tendon. Because this area is devoid of an inner perichondrium (the thyroid cartilage normally has both an inner and an outer perichondrium), it is a frequent source of spread for lesions involving the anterior commissure. The anterior commissure is the area where the paired true vocal folds meet and is a frequent site of involvement in early larynx cancers. Other laryngeal ligaments and membranes of importance in delineating the potential spaces of the larynx include the thyrohyoid membrane, quadrangular membrane, and hyoepiglottic ligament.

The intrinsic muscles of the larynx control the movement of the true vocal folds. All intrinsic muscles of the larynx are innervated by the recurrent laryngeal nerve except the cricothyroid muscle. The cricothyroid muscle produces tension and elongation of the vocal folds and is innervated by the external branch of the superior laryngeal nerve. Other intrinsic muscles of note include the posterior cricoarytenoid, the only abductor of the vocal fold. The remainder of the intrinsic muscles of the larynx serve as vocal fold adductors to some extent.

25.5 The Disease Process

25.5.1 Etiology

The etiology of squamous cell carcinoma (SCC) of the larynx is typically multifactorial. As with other types of head and neck cancer, alcohol and tobacco intake have a synergistic effect in the pathogenesis of SCC, the most common pathologic type of squamous cell cancer. Other factors promoting carcinogenesis include asbestos, ionizing radiation, wood dust, gastroesophageal reflux disease, and nitrogen mustard. The role of the human papillomavirus (HPV) in the pathogenesis of SCC in many locations of the head and neck has been elucidated over the course of the last decade. Like disease in other subsites of the head and neck, HPV-associated disease may behave in a biologically distinct manner. Organ preservation approaches in the treatment of HPV-associated disease require less aggressive and toxic regimens, particularly in the choice of chemotherapy agents. Studies elucidating the role of "deintensification" in the treatment of HPV-related disease have yet to reach a consensus in this regard. Interestingly, laryngeal papillomatosis, which is a benign HPV-related condition of the larynx, is thought to undergo malignant transformation in up to 10% of adult patients with chronic disease.

25.5.2 Pathogenesis and Pathology

Laryngeal malignancies

Despite the variety of malignancies described in the larynx, SCC predominates. A few notes on the more common varieties of SCC. Carcinoma in situ is characterized as dysplasia that involves the entire thickness of the mucosa but does not involve the basement membrane. Microinvasive carcinoma is defined by malignant cells that do penetrate the basement membrane into the superficial lamina propria of the respiratory epithelium. Invasive SCC, the most common variety, accounts for 1% of all cancers and 95% of all laryngeal cancers. Invasive SCC, like microinvasive carcinoma, penetrates the basement membrane and extends through the lamina propria, but it also invades into the underlying tissues—in the case of the larynx, the underlying vocalis muscles (▶ Fig. 25.2 and ▶ Fig. 25.3a).

Table 25.1 Laryngeal malignancies

Epithelial	Neuroectodermal	Mesenchymal
Squamous cell carcinoma • Carcinoma in situ • Microinvasive carcinoma • Invasive squamous cell carcinoma	Neuroendocrine carcinoma • Carcinoid tumor • Atypical carcinoid tumor • Small cell undifferentiated neuroendocrine carcinoma	Chondrosarcoma
Papillary (exophytic squamous cell) carcinoma	Mucosal malignant melanoma	Synovial sarcoma
Verrucous carcinoma		Fibrosarcoma/malignant fibrous histiocytoma
Spindle cell squamous carcinoma		Malignant schwannoma
Basaloid squamous carcinoma		Liposarcoma
Adenosquamous carcinoma		Rhabdomyosarcoma
Lymphoepithelial-like carcinoma		Angiosarcoma/Kaposi sarcoma
Giant cell carcinoma		Leiomyosarcoma
Minor salivary gland tumors • Adenoid cystic carcinoma • Mucoepidermoid carcinoma		Hematolymphoid etiology

Source: Data from Wenig BM. Atlas of Head and Neck Pathology. Philadelphia, PA: Saunders Elsevier; 2008.

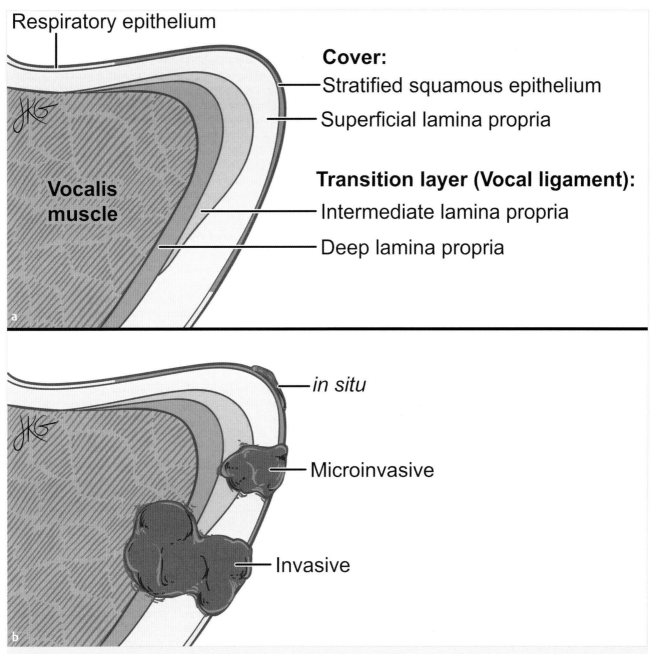

Fig. 25.2 (a) Layers of the glottic larynx, from superficial to deep. **(b)** Depth of in situ, microinvasive, and invasive carcinoma of the larynx.

25.5.3 Natural History and Progression of Disease by Site

Supraglottic SCCs account for roughly 25 to 40% of all laryngeal cancers and include carcinomas of the epiglottis, false vocal folds, aryepiglottic folds, ventricles, and arytenoids, in order of descending frequency. In fact, 50% of supraglottic carcinomas involve the epiglottis, with a majority of supraglottic lesions in other locations partially involving the epiglottis. The natural history of supraglottic tumors is to spread upward toward the free edge of the epiglottis and aryepiglottic folds, into the pre-epiglottic space, or outside the larynx into the piriform sinus mucosa or tongue base. In contrast to patients with carcinoma of the glottic larynx, those with early-stage supraglottic carcinomas may not have dysphonia. They often present with a globus sensation, cough, and exertional dyspnea, depending on the size of the lesion. Occasionally, a neck mass alone may be the presenting symptom. This is explained by a characteristic that distinguishes supraglottic carcinomas from glottic carcinomas: the rich lymphatic drainage of the supraglottic larynx. Up to 50% of patients with supraglottic carcinoma have a clinically positive lymph node metastasis. Additionally, as the T stage increases, the likelihood that regional lymph node metastases will be present at the time of diagnosis increases as well; similarly, as the size of clinically positive lymph node metastases increases, so does the likelihood that contralateral lymph node

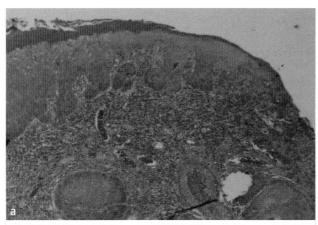

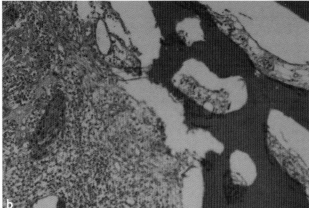

Fig. 25.3 (a) Squamous cell carcinoma with invasion through the basement membrane, indicating invasive disease. (b) Thyroid cartilage invasion at the microscopic level. Notice invasion of squamous cell carcinoma into the islands of cartilage.

extension (▶ Fig. 25.3b). As lesions that start in the supraglottis less commonly spread to involve the glottis, lesions that involve the glottis and epiglottis or other areas of the supraglottic larynx are typically staged as glottic primary lesions. Of note, involvement of the anterior commissure is an important prognostic consideration, particularly when a choice is made between organ preservation and primary surgical approaches. Multiple reports in the literature suggest that early-stage lesions that involve the anterior commissure are relatively less curable with radiation than with transoral laser, TORS, or open partial laryngeal surgery techniques. As mentioned previously, in contrast to the supraglottis, the glottic larynx has a relative paucity of lymphatic drainage. Routine treatment of the neck is not necessary for early-stage lesions (T1 or T2), whereas regional lymph node metastases are more common in T3 and T4 disease.

Cancers of the subglottic larynx are the least common type of laryngeal cancer. They account for between 1 and 8% of laryngeal cancers. Subglottic SCCs are defined as those lesions that begin 1 cm below the apex of the ventricle and extend to the superior margin of the cricoid cartilage. These are typically poorly differentiated and often have a prolonged asymptomatic period; patients will present late in the course of disease with airway obstruction. The natural history of spread is typically circumferential and anterior, with involvement of the cricothyroid membrane and thyroid. They can also spread posteriorly to involve the esophagus, inferiorly into the trachea, or into the framework of the larynx, including the thyroarytenoid muscle and cricoarytenoid joint. Regional lymph node metastases are less common than in supraglottic carcinomas but more common than in glottic carcinomas. When regional metastatic disease occurs, subglottic carcinomas tend to spread to prelaryngeal and pretracheal nodal basins. Because patients tend to present with advanced disease, the overall 5-year survival rate is a dismal 40%; many patients treated with total laryngectomy have early an recurrence with peristomal disease.

25.5.4 Potential Disease Complications

Disease complications of untreated carcinoma are typically respiratory, phonation-related, or digestive. Progressive airway obstruction is inevitable in untreated SCC of the larynx. This may begin as intermittent dyspnea with a ball valve lesion and progress to constant dyspnea with minimal exertion. Typically, the patient will develop stridor, which may be inspiratory or biphasic depending on the site of the primary lesion. Occasionally, the lesion may bleed, and the patient may notice mild hemoptysis. In addition, although supraglottic lesions do not necessarily cause vocal changes, lesions involving the glottic larynx invariably cause some measure of hoarseness and occasionally a breathy voice depending on the extent of disease. Finally, swallowing problems may develop because of simple tumor bulk, coexisting vocal fold paralysis, or extralaryngeal spread of disease in the piriform sinus or postcricoid mucosa. Complications of metastatic disease depend on the location of the metastases, which can occur in areas as varied as the lungs, liver, brain, and spine. Terminal events from untreated disease are often caused by catastrophic airway obstruction or hemorrhage from vascular sites adjacent to areas of primary disease (▶ Fig. 25.4).

metastases will be present. In particular, carcinomas of the epiglottis are prone to bilateral lymph node metastases. Even among patients with early-stage epiglottic lesions, up to 20% have occult bilateral lymph node metastases at the time of diagnosis. Clinically, supraglottic carcinomas range from exophytic to ulcerative. Patients with exophytic tumors present with more airway symptoms, often with a "ball valve" effect if the lesions are very bulky, as the lesions may intermittently cause obstruction during quiet respiration. Interestingly, those tumors that are very bulky and less ulcerative often tend to be less hypoxic and, accordingly, respond better to radiation therapy.

Accounting for 60 to 65% of all laryngeal SCCs, glottic carcinomas are the most common type of laryngeal carcinoma in the United States. These lesions commonly present with dysphonia in the early stages and with progressive airway complaints the later stages. Glottic carcinomas most commonly involve the anterior two-thirds of the vocal folds; involvement of the posterior one-third of the glottis is uncommon. The natural history of spread follows predictable patterns, including contralateral spread across the anterior commissure, anterior spread through the Broyle ligament with subsequent spread into the thyroid cartilage and soft tissues of the neck, extension to involve the posterior commissure and postcricoid mucosa, and supraglottic

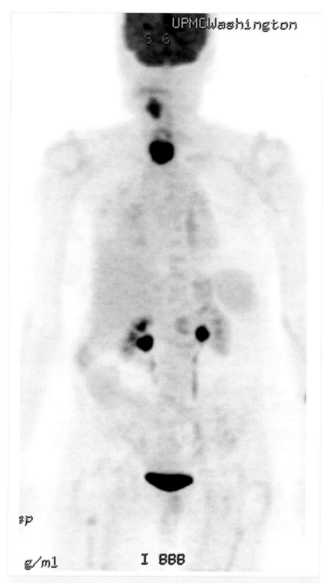

Fig. 25.4 Coronal positron emission tomography demonstrating primary disease at the level of the supraglottic and glottic larynx, as well as mediastinal pretracheal metastatic adenopathy. Terminal events can result from the direct extension of both primary and metastatic disease into vascular structures.

25.6 Disease Grading: American Joint Committee on Cancer Staging

The American Joint Committee on Cancer (AJCC) guidelines are based on the TNM (tumor node metastasis) system of staging. The T stage depends not on size but on extent of disease within the anatomical divisions of the larynx. The N and M staging criteria are similar to those used in other regions of the head and neck. Of note, disease in each division of the larynx (supraglottic, glottic, and subglottic) is staged separately because carcinoma in each region exhibits distinct biological behavior.

25.6.1 Supraglottis

Tumors that are confined to one subsite of the supraglottis and do not affect vocal fold mobility are classified as T1 lesions. T2 lesions involve the mucosa of more than one adjacent glottic or supraglottic subsite or region outside the glottis, such as the mucosa of the vallecula, medial wall of the piriform sinus, or base of tongue, without laryngeal fixation. A tumor limited to the larynx with vocal fold fixation and/or invasion of the post-cricoid region, pre-epiglottic space, paraglottic space, or inner cortex of the thyroid cartilage are considered T3 lesions. T4 status indicates moderately advanced (T4a) or very advanced (T4b) primary disease. T4a lesions invade the thyroid cartilage and/or invade tissues beyond the larynx, whereas T4b lesions invade the prevertebral space or mediastinum or encase the carotid artery.

25.6.2 Glottis

T1 lesions involve one (T1a) or both (T1b) vocal folds, which retain normal mobility. T2 lesions extend into the supraglottis and/or subglottis or impair vocal fold mobility. T3 lesions are limited to the larynx, with vocal fold fixation and/or paraglottic space and/or thyroid cartilage invasion. T4a lesions penetrate the outer thyroid cartilage cortex and/or invade tissues beyond the larynx. As with supraglottic lesions, T4b primary lesions invade the prevertebral space or mediastinum or encase the carotid artery.

25.6.3 Subglottis

T1 subglottic lesions are limited to the subglottis. T2 lesions extend to the vocal folds; mobility is either normal or impaired. T3 lesions are limited to the larynx and cause vocal fold fixation. T4a lesions invade the thyroid or cricoid cartilage and/or invade tissues beyond the larynx. As with supraglottic and glottic lesions, T4b primary lesions invade the prevertebral space or mediastinum or encase the carotid artery.

Regardless of the subsite within the larynx of the primary tumor, N1 status implies involvement of a single lymph node that is ipsilateral and smaller than 3 cm. N2a indicates involvement of a single ipsilateral lymph node larger than 3 cm but smaller than 6 cm. N2b disease describes the involvement of multiple ipsilateral nodes, none larger than 6 cm, and N2c describes the involvement of contralateral or bilateral nodes, none larger than 6 cm. N3 status is reserved for nodal disease larger than 6 cm.

Stage 0 indicates in situ disease. T1 lesions with no regional or distant metastases are classified as stage I; likewise, T2 disease without nodal or distant metastases is stage II. T3 disease with no nodal or distant disease, or T1–T3 disease with N1 disease, is considered stage III. T4a primary disease with N0 or N1 nodal status, and T1–T3 disease with N2 nodes, are considered stage IVA; T4b disease with any N disease, or any T disease with N3 disease, is considered stage IVB. Any distant metastasis implies stage IVC disease.

25.7 Pretreatment Medical Evaluation

As for other malignancies of the head and neck, a thorough history and physical examination are of paramount importance in the diagnosis and ultimate preoperative work-up of the patient with laryngeal cancer. Of particular importance are the presence of any progressive airway complaints and the presence of ear pain or dysphagia, which may indicate the possibility of extralaryngeal spread. Although indirect mirror laryngoscopy is entirely appropriate on a screening head and neck examination, fiber-optic laryngoscopy provides a panoramic view of the subsites of the larynx, as well as the oropharynx and hypopharynx. Fiber-optic laryngoscopy allows the examiner to determine the subsite(s) of involvement and assess the mobility of the true vocal folds and arytenoids, and it can provide evidence of extralaryngeal extension. For subtle lesions of the glottic larynx, video stroboscopy may provide additional detail, as well as determine the depth of invasion of glottic carcinomas. Palpation of both the central and lateral neck is critical to screen for regional lymph node metastasis. In addition, palpation of the thyroid cartilage should reveal normal laryngeal crepitus when the larynx is moved back and forth. The loss of normal laryngeal crepitus may indicate extension of a laryngeal primary into the prevertebral fascia. Occasionally, tumor extending through the thyroid lamina can be palpated.

25.7.1 Radiographic Imaging

Preoperative imaging modalities include computed tomography (CT), magnetic resonance (MR) imaging, ultrasound, and positron emission tomography (PET)–CT. The relative merits of each are discussed as follows. CT is particularly helpful in determining the presence of thyroid cartilage erosion. In a review of the bony windows of a noncontrast CT scan, a deossified appearance of the inner table of the thyroid cartilage can predict at least T3 and sometimes T4 disease. Furthermore, the addition of intravenous contrast is helpful in screening for regional lymph node metastasis. MR imaging, because it tends to provide better detail of soft-tissue planes, is often superior to CT in determining the extent of pre-epiglottic or paraglottic space involvement. Ultrasound of the central and lateral nodal basins, in the hands of a skilled ultrasonographer, can serve as an adjunct to the clinical examination in screening for regional lymph node metastasis. Finally, in the setting of laryngeal cancer, PET-CT probably has the largest role in the work-up of distant disease, although in the setting of biopsy-proven disease, it often does not add any information beyond that obtained from the clinical examination and traditional staging modalities, including chest radiography, liver function studies, and the previously discussed modalities of CT, MR imaging, and ultrasound.

25.7.2 Direct Laryngoscopy and Biopsy

There is no substitute for direct laryngoscopy in the staging of laryngeal cancer, although dynamic evaluation of the larynx with flexible laryngoscopy is critically important in determining vocal fold and arytenoid mobility. If no gross airway obstruction is present, an orotracheal intubation with anesthesia is entirely appropriate. The GlideScope GVL video laryngoscope (Verathon, Bothell, WA) can provide excellent visualization of the airway, which can assist in the placement of the endotracheal tube around an obstructing laryngeal lesion. Often, however, there is some degree of supraglottic or glottic airway obstruction beyond the comfort of the anesthesia team, and the otolaryngologist must take a leadership role in establishing the airway. In this circumstance, the table should be turned 90 degrees, with the otolaryngologist at the head of the table. For patients who have an airway that can safely accommodate a small-caliber (5.5 to 6 mm) endotracheal tube, the anesthesia team may provide sedation with propofol or a volatile anesthetic. If, with an oral airway in place, the patient can be safely ventilated with a bag mask, a short-acting paralytic will be administered. The otolaryngologist will then intubate through a Dedo laryngoscope. If the airway is marginally patent, an Eshmann stylet can be placed through the glottic airway, with the endotracheal tube then placed into the trachea over the stylet via Seldinger technique. In the event that the patient cannot tolerate a supine position or is not able to be safely ventilated with a bag mask, fiber-optic nasal intubation is an excellent option. Many anesthesiologists are trained in oral fiber-optic intubation or will attempt fiber-optic nasal intubation with the patient supine. This is inadvisable in the patient with laryngeal cancer and an obstructing lesion. Before the fiber-optic laryngoscope is placed into the glottic inlet, the topical application of 4% lidocaine can prevent laryngospasm during the intubation. After establishment of the airway via nasal fiber-optic intubation, a suspension microlaryngoscopy can commence. The orotracheal tube can then be placed through the vocal folds under direct visualization as the nasotracheal tube is withdrawn. Finally, for those patients with stridor, in whom a safe airway cannot be established by another method, an awake tracheotomy can be performed very quickly and safely immediately before staging direct laryngoscopy.

After establishment of the airway, direct laryngoscopy is performed. The Dedo and Hollinger laryngoscopes are used most commonly. The Hollinger, or anterior commissure, laryngoscope is particularly helpful in staging laryngeal carcinoma because it affords an excellent view of the anterior commissure. The Dedo laryngoscope is wider and easier to suspend for microlaryngoscopy, and the surgeon can pass instruments more easily through the lumen of this laryngoscope. Other laryngoscopes commonly used include the Lindholm laryngoscope, or supraglottiscope, which provides a more panoramic view of the supraglottic and glottic larynx. Finally, the Zeitels Universal Modular Glottiscope, like the Hollinger, has a tapered tip that affords an excellent view of the glottic airway and anterior commissure. In addition, like the traditional sliding Jackson laryngoscope, the Zeitels laryngoscope has a base that the surgeon can remove after suspension. This is helpful in situations in which the surgeon must intubate through a laryngoscope because one can withdraw the scope over the endotracheal tube more easily (▶ Fig. 25.5 and ▶ Fig. 25.6).

The anterior extent of tumor, involvement of the anterior commissure, and involvement of the false vocal folds, ventricles, postcricoid area, hypopharyngeal mucosa, and mucosa of the arytenoids are all factors of particular importance in staging a supraglottic or glottic carcinoma. Rigid angled endoscopes can be helpful in determining the inferior extent of a glottic lesion,

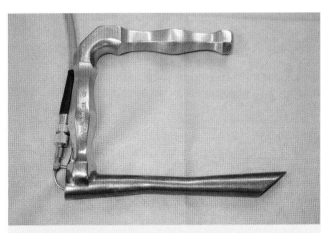

Fig. 25.5 Hollinger laryngoscope. This laryngoscope is ideal for difficult airways and the anterior larynx.

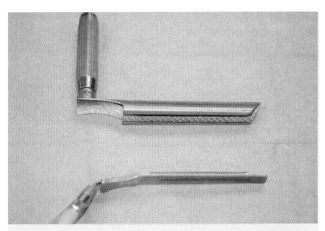

Fig. 25.6 Zeitels Universal Modular Glottiscope. It is beveled anteriorly and good for the anterior larynx, and like the sliding Jackson laryngoscope, it can be retracted around an endotracheal tube after intubation.

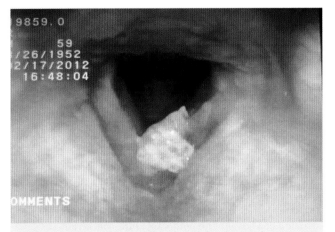

Fig. 25.7 Left glottic lesion, pedunculated. The ultimate diagnosis was papillary squamous cell carcinoma. The patient tested positive for human papillomavirus and was treated with transoral laser excision with negative margins.

as well as in determining subglottic extension in circumstances in which a transglottic carcinoma is present. When partial laryngeal surgery approaches are being considered, a thorough assessment of the arytenoids preoperatively and intraoperatively is of paramount importance. All partial laryngeal surgical excisions require at least one fully mobile and sensate cricoarytenoid complex with no involvement of the inter-arytenoid mucosa. Traditionally, palpation of the arytenoids at laryngoscopy was emphasized; however, with advancements in fiberoptic technology and "distal chip" fiber-optic laryngoscopes in common use, much of this information can be determined before staging laryngoscopy. Arytenoid fixation, when present, indicates involvement of the cricoarytenoid joint with tumor. This may preclude conservation approaches to laryngeal surgery. Of note, true vocal fold fixation is not the same as arytenoid fixation; vocal folds may be fixed because of tumor bulk or because of paraglottic space involvement.

The biopsy of a laryngeal lesion can be complicated by previous radiation therapy, and superficial biopsies may not yield enough evidence for a pathologist to render a diagnosis. Unfortunately, deep biopsies in the postradiation setting can precipitate laryngeal edema and sometimes chondronecrosis if cartilaginous structures are exposed. Diagnosing persistent disease early after treatment is particularly challenging in this regard because severe osteonecrosis of the larynx can mimic laryngeal cancer. Finally, for those obstructing supraglottic or glottic tumors diagnosed by intraoperative frozen section analysis, the use of a laryngeal microdébrider to reduce tumor bulk can improvee the airway in those patients who may ultimately be candidates for organ preservation therapy.

25.7.3 Differential Diagnosis

As mentioned previously, the vast majority of laryngeal carcinomas are SCCs, and although a great variety of pathologic lesions can develop in this area, a biopsy often only confirms what the surgeon has first strongly suspected. Nonetheless, there are several conditions to mention that can mimic laryngeal cancer. For example, collagen vascular diseases, such as sarcoidosis, amyloidosis, and Wegener granulomatosis, can all cause mass lesions of the larynx. Internal laryngoceles can give the appearance of significant glottic edema that may look suspicious for carcinoma. Of note, the head and neck surgeon should be wary of the internal laryngocele in a longtime smoker because an internal laryngocele can develop in the presence of a coexisting SCC. Certainly (HPV-related) laryngeal papillomatosis in an adult can mimic the appearance of SCC (▶ Fig. 25.7). Although rare, other benign epithelial lesions, such as minor salivary gland tumors, may be present in the larynx. A variety of benign mesenchymal and neuroectodermal lesions can present in the larynx, including granular cell tumors, rhabdomyomas, paragangliomas, lipomas, and hemangiomas, as well as numerous less common entities. These have variable appearances and less commonly mimic SCC. Finally, in the patient with suspected persistent or recurrent disease after definitive radiotherapy or chemoradiotherapy, one must consider the possibility of osteoradionecrosis of the larynx because profound posttreatment edema, although suspicious for malignancy, may be negative on serial biopsy despite the development of airway obstruction (▶ Fig. 25.8).

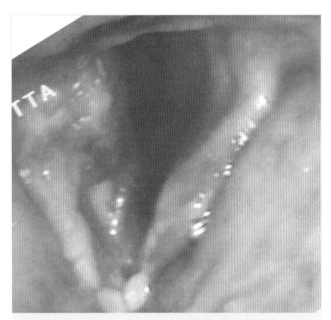

Fig. 25.8 Right glottic and false fold squamous cell carcinoma in an elderly woman who was treated with definitive radiotherapy. Persistent postoperative edema prompted repeat biopsy, which confirmed persistent disease.

25.8 Medical Treatment of Laryngeal Cancer

Part of the multidisciplinary evaluation of the patient with glottic carcinoma includes an assessment by a radiation oncologist. Early glottic malignancies are notable for a low incidence of occult nodal metastasis, and therefore single-modality treatment with curative radiotherapy alone is often an acceptable modality for many patients. Radiation therapy has many advantages, including its noninvasive nature, acceptable vocal outcomes, and excellent local control rates. For patients with early-stage lesions, functional outcomes are generally very good, with most experiencing only self-limited symptoms of mucositis, xerostomia, dysphagia, and local soft-tissue reactions. Advances in radiation therapy techniques, predominantly the use of IMRT, have allowed the radiation oncologist to provide treatment to the larynx alone while sparing other sites in the neck in settings where there is no clinical presence or little risk for regional lymph node metastasis. Although vocal quality does change after radiation therapy, most patients experience a return to nearly normal phonation 1 year after the treatment of early glottic cancer. With regard to outcomes, primary radiation therapy of early T1 glottic carcinoma results in excellent local control rates, typically around 90%. Local control rates for T2 glottic carcinomas are less impressive but are as high as 80% in reported series. Of note, in many published series, patients with involvement of the anterior commissure at diagnosis who were treated with primary radiotherapy generally fared worse in terms of local control.

The treatment of supraglottic malignancies with primary radiotherapy generally results in excellent control rates exceeding 90% for early-stage lesions. The supraglottic larynx has more substantial lymphatic drainage than the glottic larynx, so treatment volumes are generally higher because the radiation field must include the primary lesion as well as the regional lymph node basin. The specifics of radiation techniques vary with the institution and range from single-fraction once-daily treatments to twice-daily hyperfractionation and accelerated hyperfractionation schedules.

Although advanced (stage III or IV) laryngeal cancer had traditionally been managed with primary surgical therapy and possibly postoperative radiotherapy, a landmark study from the Department of Veterans Affairs Laryngeal Cancer Study Group in 1991 demonstrated that induction chemotherapy with definitive radiotherapy provides high larynx preservation rates without compromising overall survival. The past 20 years have seen a dramatic increase in the use of chemoradiation protocols in treating advanced laryngeal cancer. This paradigm shift has been controversial because chemoradiation protocols are associated with not-insignificant toxicity, including long-term dysphagia and xerostomia. Higher radiation treatment volumes can result in the devastating complication of osteoradionecrosis of the larynx, which can necessitate a tracheotomy or total laryngectomy, even in the setting of disease control. Coinciding with this paradigm shift, an overall survival decrease among patients with head and neck cancer was noted by Hoffman and others in a review of the National Cancer Data Base between the years of 1985 and 2001. The reasons for this change in survival are controversial. Current practice guidelines from the American Society of Clinical Oncology recommend a larynx preservation strategy, with surgery or radiation, for all patients who have T1 or T2 disease. For patients who have T3 or T4 disease without tumor invasion through cartilage into soft tissues, a larynx preservation strategy including chemoradiation therapy is an acceptable treatment option. These regimens may include neoadjuvant chemotherapy with concurrent chemoradiation, or alternatively concurrent chemoradiation. Choices among chemotherapeutic agents are diverse, ranging from traditional platinum-based agents such as cisplatin to newer agents such as cetuximab, a monoclonal antibody and epidermal growth factor receptor (EGFR) inhibitor.

With regard to postoperative radiotherapy or postoperative chemotherapy, many factors are considered. First, the extent of the disease is important to consider, including whether there is a close or positive margin, angiolymphatic invasion, or any extralaryngeal spread. With regard to the status of the neck, the presence of multiple positive lymph node metastases and extracapsular spread is considered when the need for adjuvant chemotherapy or radiation is determined. Adjuvant treatments are determined in conjunction with colleagues from medical and radiation oncology.

25.9 Roundsmanship

- The clinical examination is critically important in the preoperative evaluation of the patient with laryngeal cancer. Understaging a patient can result in treatment failures and intraoperative misadventures. Of particular importance in the staging of laryngeal carcinoma is anterior commissure involvement and subglottic extension (▶ Fig. 25.9).

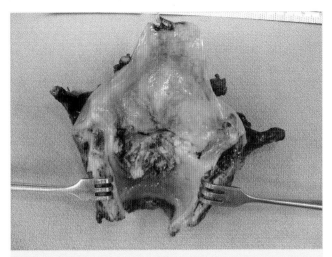

Fig. 25.9 Squamous cell carcinoma of the larynx. Transglottic lesion with extension into the subglottis.

- The supraglottic larynx lymphatic supply must be respected; elective treatment of the neck for patients with even early-stage supraglottic lesions should be considered.
- Many treatment modalities exist for the treatment of laryngeal cancer. Any treatment must be tailored to the individual patient, taking into account the biological behavior of the tumor as well as the ability of the patient to participate actively in recovery and rehabilitation. One size does not fit all.
- Although squamous cell carcinoma is far and away the most common type of laryngeal cancer, in the nonsmoking patient with few risk factors, conditions such as collagen vascular disease and other benign processes of the larynx can mimic laryngeal carcinoma. One should use caution in relying on an intraoperative frozen section results alone before undertaking definitive surgical extirpation.

25.10 Recommended Reading

[1] American Cancer Society. Laryngeal and Hypopharyngeal Cancer. Atlanta, GA: American Cancer Society; 2012

[2] Larynx. In: Edge SB, Byrd DR, Compton CC, et al, eds. American Joint Committee on Cancer (AJCC) Cancer Staging Manual. 7th ed. New York, NY: Springer; 2010:81–92

[3] Chiu RJ, Myers EN, Johnson JT. Efficacy of routine bilateral neck dissection in the management of supraglottic cancer. Otolaryngol Head Neck Surg 2004; 131: 485–488

[4] Hoffman HT, Porter K, Karnell LH et al. Laryngeal cancer in the United States: changes in demographics, patterns of care, and survival. Laryngoscope 2006; 116 Suppl 111: 1–13

[5] Pfister DG, Laurie SA, Weinstein GS et alAmerican Society of Clinical Oncology. American Society of Clinical Oncology clinical practice guideline for the use of larynx-preservation strategies in the treatment of laryngeal cancer. J Clin Oncol 2006; 24: 3693–3704

[6] National Institutes of Health, National Cancer Institute. Surveillance Epidemiology and End Results. 2012. . Accessed October 16, 2013

[7] Weinstein GS, Laccourreye O, Brasnu D, et al. The role of CT and MR in planning conservation laryngeal surgery. In: Yousem D, ed. Neuroimaging Clinics of North America. Philadelphia, PA: W. B. Saunders; 1996:497–504

[8] Wenig BM. Atlas of Head and Neck Pathology. 2nd ed. New York, NY: Saunders Elsevier; 2008:405–534

[9] Wolf GT et alThe Department of Veterans Affairs Laryngeal Cancer Study Group. Induction chemotherapy plus radiation compared with surgery plus radiation in patients with advanced laryngeal cancer. N Engl J Med 1991; 324: 1685–1690

[10] Wolf GT. Reexamining the treatment of advanced laryngeal cancer: the VA laryngeal cancer study revisited. Head Neck 2010; 32: 7–14

26 Surgery of the Laryngopharynx

Edward M. Stafford

26.1 General Types of Intervention, Rationale, and Goals

The goal of surgical therapy for laryngeal cancer, as for other malignancies in the head and neck, is the extirpation of all disease with negative margins. Although postoperative radiotherapy may be indicated in certain situations, regardless of the surgical modality chosen, negative margins should take priority. Certainly, with advances in organ preservation techniques and the morbidity added by postoperative radiotherapy, this principle should guide the surgeon's decision-making process, both in choosing among surgical modalities and in determining the appropriate extent of resection. Although the goal of negative margins is unambiguous, there are a variety of other considerations that inform the decision-making process. Of paramount importance, regardless of the surgical modality chosen, is the preservation of function. Therefore, included among the goals of therapy should be a plan to ensure voice rehabilitation, the adequacy and safety of the airway, and short- and long-term nutritional strategies.

26.2 Pertinent Anatomy

As was discussed in Chapter 25, the larynx is divided into subsites: the supraglottic, glottic, and subglottic larynx, each with its own unique embryonic development and lymphatic drainage. The supraglottic larynx is the portion of the larynx superior to the glottis, including the false vocal folds, arytenoids, aryepi-glottic folds, and epiglottis. The subglottic larynx begins 10 mm below the free margin of the true vocal folds and extends to the inferior border of the cricoid cartilage. Finally, the glottis includes the paired true vocal folds, as well as the anterior and posterior commissures. Of particular importance to the surgeon is an understanding of the anatomical spaces created by various cartilages, ligaments, and membranes of the larynx, including the pre-epiglottic, paraglottic, and subglottic spaces. Understanding these spaces is critically important in staging patients appropriately.

The pre-epiglottic space is an anatomical space with the following boundaries: anteriorly, the thyrohyoid membrane and the inner table of the thyroid cartilage; posteriorly, the epiglottis; superiorly, the hyoepiglottic ligament and mucosa of the vallecula; and inferiorly, the thyroepiglottic ligament. By definition, involvement of the pre-epiglottic space upstages a laryngeal carcinoma to at least a T3 lesion (▶ Fig. 26.1).

The paraglottic space borders the glottis laterally. This space extends both above and below the true vocal folds and is created by the following boundaries: medially, the quadrangular membrane, ventricle, and conus elasticus; laterally, the perichondrium of the thyroid lamina and cricothyroid membrane; anterosuperiorly, the pre-epiglottic space; and posteriorly, the mucosa of the piriform sinus. Extension into the paraglottic space often portends the transglottic and extralaryngeal spread of disease (▶ Fig. 26.2).

The subglottic space is a discrete anatomical space defined by the cricoid cartilage inferiorly and a distance of 5 to 10 mm inferior to the true vocal fold margin. When the extent of disease is not clear by physical examination alone, imaging modalities including computed tomography and in particular magnetic

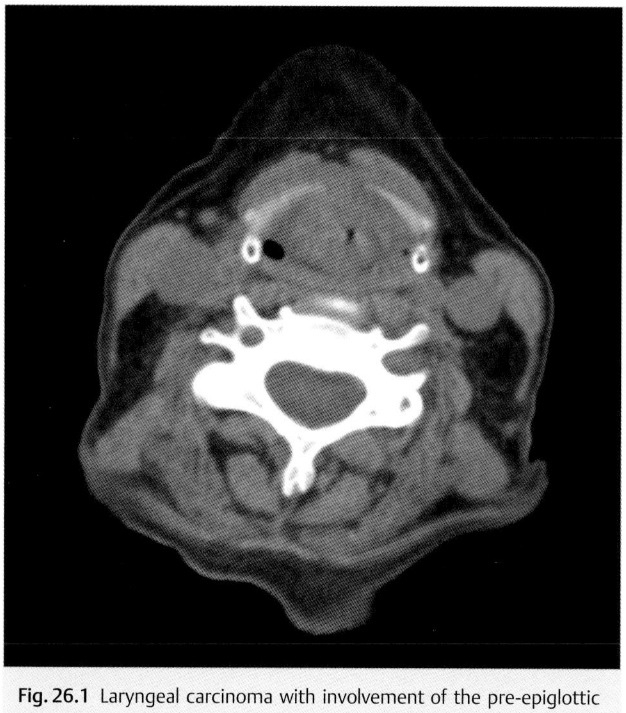

Fig. 26.1 Laryngeal carcinoma with involvement of the pre-epiglottic space.

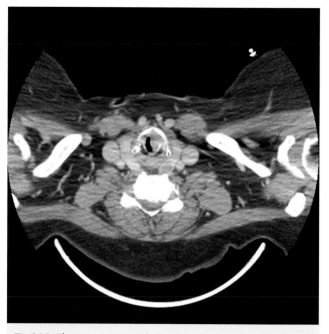

Fig. 26.2 Glottic carcinoma with extension into the paraglottic space.

resonance imaging can help elucidate it in the pre-epiglottic and paraglottic spaces, which often results in the upstaging of disease. This information is invaluable preoperatively or before the initiation of treatment if organ preservation techniques are employed.

A detailed description of the subsites of the larynx is included in the previous chapter, but a more detailed discussion of the glottic larynx is appropriate to review. The boundaries of the true vocal folds are the vocal processes of the arytenoids posteriorly and the anterior commissure anteriorly. The layers of the vocal folds, from superficial to deep, include the epithelium, followed by the lamina propria, followed by the vocalis muscle. The cartilaginous framework of the larynx at the glottic larynx is of particular importance in terms of how disease spreads locally. A structure called the conus elasticus, which originates from the cricoid cartilage, attaches posteriorly to the arytenoid cartilages and condenses medially to form the vocal ligament. Anteriorly, the conus elasticus attaches to the thyroid cartilage at the Broyle ligament, also known as the anterior commissure tendon. This area is devoid of an inner perichondrium and consequently is a frequent source of spread for lesions involving the anterior commissure. Understanding this anatomical relationship informs decision making when disease involves the anterior commissure because the extent of disease may be underestimated by flexible laryngoscopy alone.

26.3 Specific Techniques

26.3.1 Endoscopic Techniques (Including Specific Indications for Each Technique)

Transoral laser microsurgical approaches for treating squamous cell carcinoma of the larynx have improved significantly over the last 20 years, with advances in endoscopic instrumentation and laser technology. Advantages over primary radiation therapy or conservation laryngeal surgery include an abbreviated treatment time, potentially requiring only an outpatient surgical procedure. In addition, with transoral laser approaches, primary control is often attainable without adjuvant radiation therapy. Transoral laser techniques provide oncologic control rates roughly equivalent to those of organ preservation techniques, again typically exceeding 90% for early-stage lesions. Overall survival rates are also comparable. In addition, cost–benefit analyses argue in favor of transoral laser microsurgical approaches. Myers and colleagues from Pittsburgh demonstrated transoral laser surgery for T1 glottic lesions to be a cost-effective option compared with open conservation laryngeal surgery and radiation. A later report from the same group demonstrated equivalent quality-of-life outcomes and functional results when patients treated with endoscopic excision were compared with those treated with radiation, and the patients treated with radiation had an increased number of work hours missed and increased costs related to travel. Finally, although it has traditionally been accepted that vocal quality is better after radiation therapy than after transoral laser microsurgery for glottic carcinomas, many reports have questioned this assumption. Although the postsurgical patient tends to have a breathier voice and the postradiation therapy patient a harsher, raspy voice, vocal quality after laser cordectomy is overall comparable with voice quality after radiation therapy.

The carbon dioxide laser is indispensable in transoral endoscopic approaches. The wavelength of the carbon dioxide laser is 10,600 nm. The helium–neon (He-Ne) aiming beam allows excellent finesse and control of this laser. Typically, the laser is applied through an operating binocular microscope (400-mm lens) and controlled with a micromanipulator. Carbon dioxide laser fibers can be threaded through the distal aspect of rigid instruments and provide the surgeon with other options when exposure is challenging. The surgeon will select the spot size, power of the laser, and mode of the laser (i.e., continuous or pulse). The system is always tested on a tongue blade before use on the patient. Nd:YAG (neodymium:yttrium aluminum garnet) and KTP (potassium titanyl phosphate) lasers, in contrast to carbon dioxide lasers, are absorbed by red pigment and may be preferable with very vascular lesions. These lasers are helpful, for example, in the treatment of subglottic or vascular tracheal lesions, such as hemangiomas.

The lesion is always photographically documented before resection is begun. After a secure airway has been established with a laser-safe endotracheal tube, a rigid 0-degree endoscope is used to assess and document the extent of disease. An angled endoscope may be helpful in assessing the anterior commissure. Even when a small-caliber (5.0 or smaller) endotracheal tube is used, the posterior commissure is often obscured by the endotracheal tube. This can be displaced anteriorly to allow better visualization, but removing the endotracheal tube is necessary to fully assess the extent of the lesion.

Endoscopic approaches can address the vast majority of early-stage and some late-stage laryngeal carcinomas. These approaches, with or without robotic assistance, allow the successful treatment of lesions ranging from T1 to limited T3 disease. For a variety of glottic T1 lesions, including T in situ, T1a, and T1b lesions, endoscopic cordectomy is an effective (and cost-effective) approach associated with minimal morbidity, and it provides superior functional and oncologic outcomes. Mid-fold T1a lesions are among the most readily accessible for this approach. T1 lesions extending into the anterior commissure can be addressed with this technique as long as the exposure obtained permits an adequate anterior exposure. Of note, one of the long-held principles of oncologic resection is Halstead's principle of en bloc resection. For the surgeon using transoral laser techniques, it is often not possible, or advisable, to attempt en bloc resection.

Endoscopic management is often the best option for patients with early-stage supraglottic squamous cell carcinoma, particularly lesions of the suprahyoid epiglottis and aryepiglottic folds. As with glottic lesions, the traditional principles of en bloc resection are less relevant with these approaches because early epiglottic malignancies are often best addressed with the initial line of resection through the tumor, which facilitates lateral resection and adequate margins. As with patients who are candidates for open conservation laryngeal surgery, a preoperative pulmonary and speech–language pathology evaluation may be helpful, although patients treated with endoscopic approaches often recover more quickly than their counterparts undergoing open approaches (▶ Fig. 26.3, ▶ Fig. 26.4, ▶ Fig. 26.5, ▶ Fig. 26.6).

Finally, for patients with more extensive disease, including those with T3 disease, endoscopic approaches can be an appro-

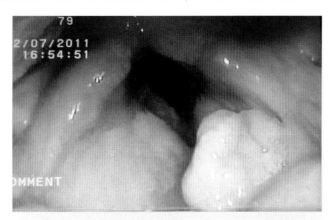

Fig. 26.3 Supraglottic carcinoma before treatment.

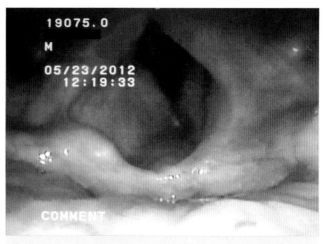

Fig. 26.4 Same patient as in ▶ Fig. 26.3 after treatment with transoral laser surgery.

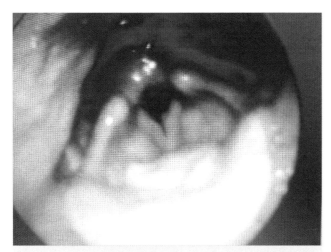

Fig. 26.5 Carcinoma of the laryngeal surface of the epiglottis before treatment.

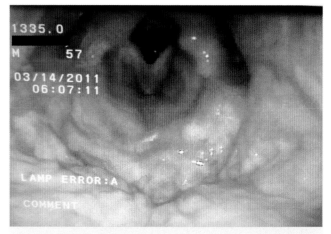

Fig. 26.6 Same patient as in ▶ Fig. 26.5 after transoral laser surgery.

priate primary strategy as long as the extent of pre-epiglottic space involvement has been evaluated by imaging and judged to be resectable. Robotic techniques are particularly appropriate for disease that is at a more advanced stage. Although these approaches are still in their infancy, early data are promising in terms of both feasibility and oncologic efficacy. Robotic techniques offer increased degrees of freedom, allowing more three-dimensional access to the larynx. A cautionary note in reviewing the literature for patients treated with transoral endoscopic techniques is that in some of the reports touting the superior oncologic effectiveness of these approaches, a significant percentage of the patients also have received postoperative radiotherapy.

26.3.2 Surgical Management

Open Management of Laryngeal Cancer: Techniques and Indications

The open management of glottic and supraglottic malignancies is time-tested and oncologically sound. In increasing level of complexity, these procedures range from laryngofissure with cordectomy and reconstruction, vertical partial laryngectomy,

open supraglottic laryngectomy, and supracricoid laryngectomy to total laryngectomy. All approaches that do not result in complete extirpation of the larynx are referred to as organ preservation techniques.

Cordectomy with reconstruction is ideal for T1 glottic lesions that would otherwise be amenable to transoral laser microsurgical excision. However, some patients (including patients with trismus or retrognathia, and possibly patients with prior radiotherapy) do not have sufficient anterior exposure for these lesions to be addressed endoscopically. This approach is not recommended for patients with disease involving the contralateral vocal fold. A tracheotomy is generally necessary with this technique. For a simple cordectomy, healing by secondary intention is an acceptable reconstructive strategy, followed by alloplastic medialization procedures if necessary. Intraoperative reconstruction based on use of the ipsilateral strap muscles to augment the neocord has also been described. Most commonly, patients who undergo open cordectomy with laryngofissure typically compensate well from a speech and swallowing standpoint, although they may have a breathy voice postoperatively.

Vertical partial laryngectomy is most commonly used to treat T1 and selected T2 lesions of the vocal folds. A tracheotomy is likewise required for this approach. Contraindications to this approach include T3 disease without cricoarytenoid joint involvement; this is better addressed with a supracricoid laryngectomy. A laryngofissure is performed; the thyrotomy location is determined by the location of the tumor as assessed endoscopically. In the standard vertical partial laryngectomy, the resection extends from the anterior commissure to include the full extent of one membranous vocal fold and the intrinsic musculature of the larynx posteriorly to the vocal processes of the arytenoids. Many "extensions" of this procedure have been described, including the frontolateral vertical hemilaryngectomy, posterolateral vertical laryngectomy, and extended vertical laryngectomy (▶ Fig. 26.7). In addition, as with simple cordectomy, a variety of local reconstructive techniques have been described to facilitate voice restoration.

Open supraglottic laryngectomy is appropriate for T1 and T2 lesions of the supraglottic larynx, with local control rates for T1 disease exceeding 90%. Contraindications include glottic level involvement, invasion of the cricoid or thyroid cartilage,

involvement of the tongue base to within 1 cm of the circumvallate papillae, and involvement of the deep muscles of the tongue base or pre-epiglottic space. The typical supraglottic laryngectomy preserves both true vocal folds, both arytenoids, the tongue base, and the hyoid bone (▶ Fig. 26.8). Pre-epiglottic space involvement necessitates resection of the hyoid, which can otherwise be left intact. Of particular importance when the hyoid is resected is preservation of the superior laryngeal neurovascular pedicle. This is likewise critically important in the supracricoid laryngectomy. Reconstruction is similar to that of the supracricoid laryngectomy.

The supracricoid laryngectomy has perhaps the most diverse utility because it can be used in T1b, T2, T3, and selected T4 supraglottic and glottic carcinomas. It can also be used in patients with decreased vocal fold motion or fixation, pre-epiglottic space invasion, glottic involvement at the anterior commissure or ventricle, or limited thyroid cartilage erosion without extralaryngeal spread. Excellent local control rates and 5-year survival data are typical in most large series. Contraindications to supraglottic laryngectomy include fixation of the arytenoids secondary to cricoarytenoid joint fixation, extrinsic laryngeal

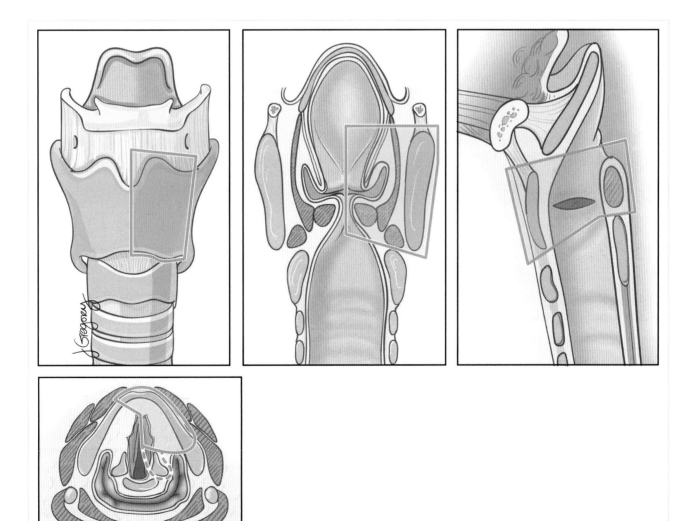

Fig. 26.7 Extent of vertical partial laryngectomies.

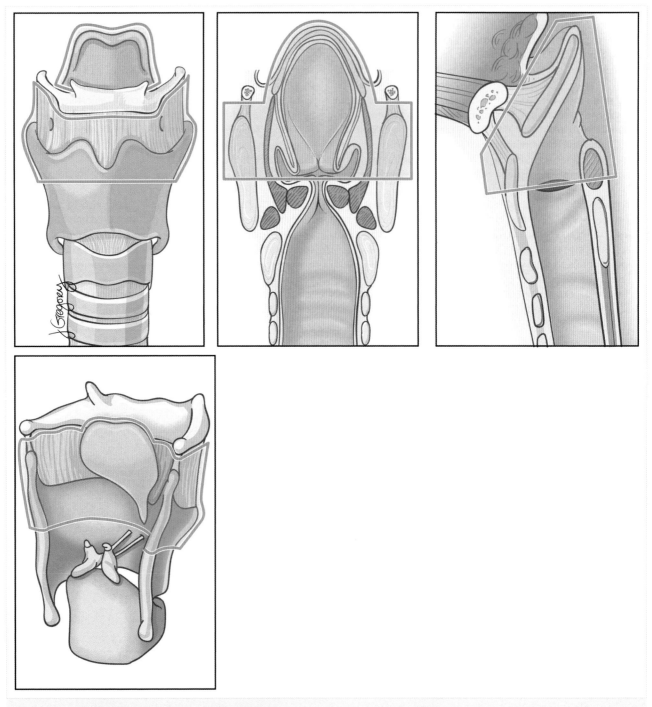

Fig. 26.8 Tissue resected in supraglottic laryngectomy.

muscle involvement, recurrent laryngeal nerve involvement, subglottic extension beyond 1 cm or direct invasion of the cricoid, posterior commissure involvement, extralaryngeal spread, or disease extension to the outer perichondrium of the thyroid cartilage. The surgical excision is en bloc and includes both true vocal folds, both false vocal folds, both paraglottic spaces, sometimes the epiglottis, and the entire thyroid cartilage, and it may include one partial or full arytenoid (▶ Fig. 26.9). Of particular importance in the surgical resection is preservation of the recurrent laryngeal nerve when the cricothyroid joint is disarticu-

lated. As mentioned previously, preservation of the superior laryngeal neurovascular bundle is of critical importance in ensuring postoperative rehabilitation of swallowing. The reconstruction is predicated upon impacting the hyoid bone and tongue base with or without the epiglottis to the cricoid cartilage with three symmetric 1–0 Vicryl submucosal sutures (▶ Fig. 26.10).

The complications of all conservative approaches to laryngeal surgery are very similar. Aspiration and postoperative dysphagia are common in the early postoperative setting but may

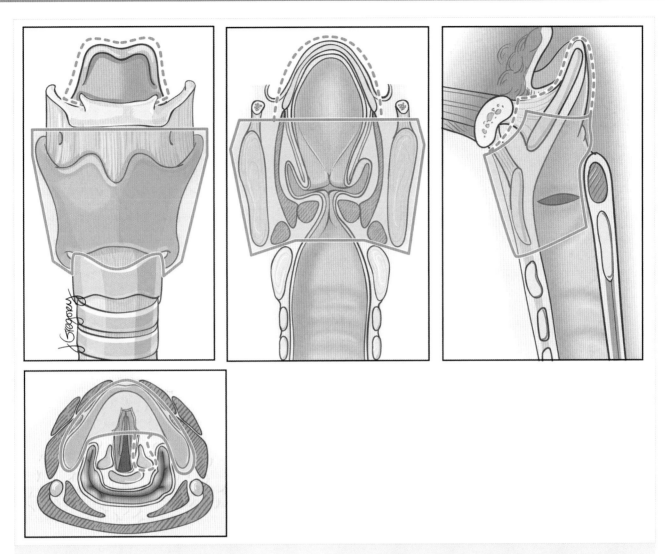

Fig. 26.9 En bloc resection in supracricoid laryngectomy.

be prolonged in some patients, resulting in the need for a percutaneous gastrostomy. Pharyngocutaneous fistula can occur, although the risk is much less than with total laryngectomy. Of note, it is critically important in open techniques such as supracricoid laryngectomy to separate the tracheotomy from the reconstructed neolarynx and remainder of the neck contents. Finally, an inability to decannulate the patient may result from an inadequate glottic airway secondary to reconstruction technique or recurrent laryngeal nerve injury.

Finally, total laryngectomy involves extirpation of the entire larynx as well as the hyoid and several tracheal rings, depending on the level of subglottic extension. Total laryngectomy creates a complete separation between the upper respiratory tract and pharyngoesophageal tract. It is a time-tested and oncologically sound procedure. The procedure typically begins with an awake tracheotomy if the patient has airway obstruction. Typically, a "high trach" is advisable to provide additional trachea that will be removed with the specimen. For lesions involving the supraglottic larynx, or in circumstances in which nodal metastases are present at diagnosis, bilateral neck dissections are performed first. In the N0 neck, a bilateral selective neck

dissection may be appropriate. Next, the suprahyoid and infrahyoid muscles are divided, and the inferior constrictors are divided at the lateral lamina of the thyroid cartilage. A freer elevator is used to mobilize the piriform sinus mucosa superiorly to preserve as much mucosa as possible for closure of the pharynx. The superior and inferior parathyroid glands should then be identified and lateralized on the side of the primary lesion while the inferior thyroid artery is preserved. On the side of the primary lesion, the thyroid lobe is typically included with the specimen. The contralateral thyroid lobe is mobilized off the trachea with Bovie cautery, leaving both the superior pole vascular pedicle and the inferior thyroid artery blood supply intact. Once the suprahyoid musculature has been divided, the hyoid bone is mobilized, typically with an Allis clamp, and the greater cornu of the hyoid is freed from the surrounding soft-tissue attachments. The hypoglossal nerve is identified and carefully preserved while the greater cornu is mobilized laterally (▶ Fig. 26.11). At this time, if a tracheotomy was previously performed, the trachea should be transected at the level of the tracheotomy. A 2–0 polypropylene suture should be placed in the distal trachea to prevent retraction of the trachea into the

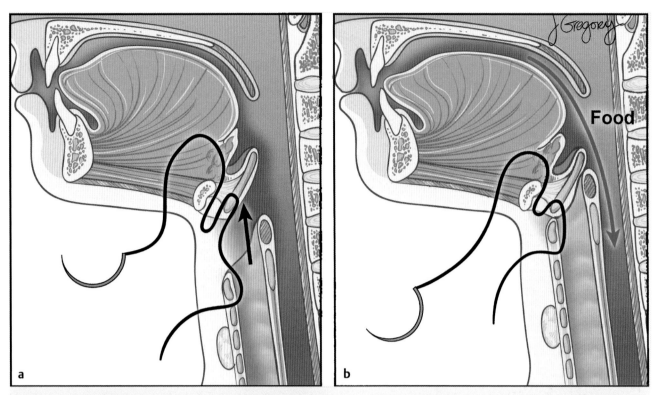

Fig. 26.10 (a,b) Reconstruction after supracricoid laryngectomy is facilitated by a cricohyoido(epiglotto)pexy, impacting the residual neoglottis superiorly near the base of the tongue. This allows food boluses to pass posteriorly behind the airway, preventing aspiration. The epiglottis can be sacrificed, if necessary, for oncologic reasons.

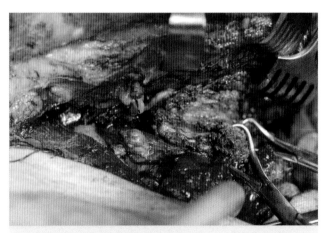

Fig. 26.11 During total laryngectomy, the hyoid is freed from the superior muscles and mobilized. The hypoglossal nerve is at risk during this dissection and should be preserved.

mediastinum. The back wall of the trachea may be divided with a No. 15 blade or Bovie cautery down to the "party wall" between the esophagus and trachea.

Deciding where to enter the pharynx is predicated upon the preoperative laryngoscopy or direct laryngoscopy at the beginning of the case. Generally, the surgeon should endeavor to enter the pharynx in an area uninvolved with tumor, which will allow extirpation of the larynx under direct visualization. This may be in the vallecula, piriform sinus, or postcricoid mucosa. The vallecula is generally the most expeditious route. Place-

ment of a Yankauer suction or small Deaver retractor into the vallecula of the patient's oropharynx will indicate an approximate location to enter. Once the pharyngeal mucosa has been incised, the epiglottis may be grasped with an Allis clamp. The surgeon, positioned at the head of the table, then uses curved Mayo scissors to incise the pharyngoepiglottic ligament, carefully leaving a healthy margin of tissue around the tumor. This continues inferiorly. One should endeavor to leave as much piriform sinus mucosa as is oncologically feasible. Inferiorly, the postcricoid mucosa will be incised, allowing removal of the larynx. When the margins of resection are unclear, intraoperative frozen section consultation is appropriate. Additional tracheal margins should be sent as well. A prophylactic stomaplasty is helpful in ensuring a patent tracheostoma, particularly if postoperative radiotherapy is contemplated. One option is a modified W-plasty. The midline trachea is incised through roughly two tracheal rings. A W-shaped wedge of skin is then excised from the peristomal skin. A 2–0 polypropylene suture is used, in a half-mattress technique, to bring each apex of the trachea to the bases of the W. Then, 2–0 polypropylene sutures with alternating 2–0 Polyglactin 910 sutures are used to create the lower half of the stoma (▶ Fig. 26.12). A cricopharyngeal myotomy should be performed before closure of the pharynx. If a tracheoesophageal puncture (TEP) is to be placed, a right-angle clamp should enter the posterior wall of the trachea 1 cm inferior to the proposed stoma. A 14F red rubber catheter is then placed through the puncture site into the esophagus. Some centers will place a nasogastric feeding tube as well for enteric nutrition during the early postoperative period; however, with appropriate care, the red rubber catheter will allow enteric

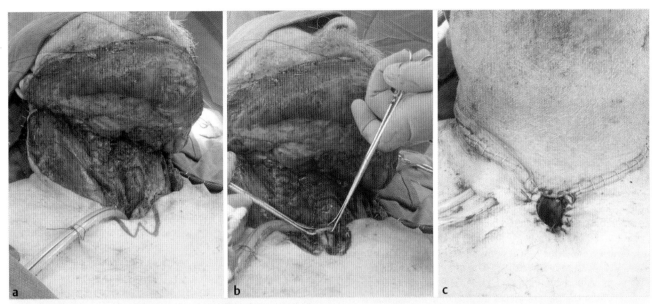

Fig. 26.12 (a) A W-stomaplasty planned to enlarge the tracheostomy. (b) The anterior trachea is split and mobilized to be sutured to the apices of the W-plasty. (c) Completed stomaplasty.

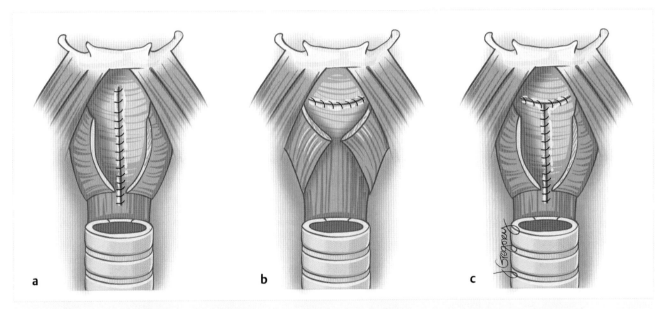

Fig. 26.13 (a,b,c) Pharyngeal closure can be in the shape of a T, vertical or horizontal.

nutrition and is less uncomfortable for the patient than a nasogastric feeding tube.

Closure of the pharynx depends on a variety of factors, including the amount of available piriform sinus mucosa, whether the patient has previously been treated with radiation, and surgeon preference. If adequate piriform sinus mucosa is available, a vertical closure with an inverted Connell suture is a reliable closure. This typically begins with an anchoring suture in the tongue base and extends inferiorly in the vertical plane. A reliable assistant should invert the edges of the piriform mucosa as the surgeon proceeds inferiorly with the closure. A horizontal closure is more challenging, particularly toward the center of the closure, because it is often under more tension at this point. Finally, a T closure has the disadvantage of a trifurcation at its

center, which is a natural point of weakness of the closure. When performed properly, however, all of these methods are acceptable choices (▶ Fig. 26.13). Imbricating sutures reinforcing the pharyngeal closure are appropriate, although closure of the constrictor muscles may result in postoperative dysphagia. Saline dyed with methylene blue is then placed into the neopharynx with a bulb syringe to rule out extravasation of saline. Focal areas of leakage may be addressed with imbricating sutures. To minimize the risk for pharyngocutaneous fistula, meticulous care is used when the pharynx is closed, regardless of the method employed. Fibrin glue along the closure may help minimize fistula rates.

Reconstruction in the postradiation setting may proceed as described. Other options, even in the setting of adequate piriform sinus mucosa, may include closure with a pectoralis major myocutaneous flap reconstruction, radial forearm free flap reconstruction, or anterolateral thigh free flap reconstruction. Advantages of these closures may include decreased risk for pharyngoesophageal stricture and decreased rates of pharyngocutaneous fistula. Several groups have described the use of prophylactic "muscle-only" pectoralis muscle flaps to augment the pharyngeal closure in the setting of salvage laryngectomy, with successful decreases in the incidence of postoperative pharyngocutaneous fistula formation.

Voice restoration techniques after total laryngectomy are diverse. TEP provides intelligible esophageal speech in appropriately chosen patients. Patients who are candidates for a TEP should have good or correctable eyesight and good hand–eye coordination, and they should be reliable in terms of follow-up because a TEP needs to be cleaned and changed on a regular basis. A variety of hands-free systems allow the patient to phonate without having to occlude the TEP opening digitally. An electrolarynx is another option, which provides robotic-sounding speech when the patient places the machine on the skin of the neck or in the mouth with an oral cavity adapter.

Finally, for selected patients who were formerly treated with primary radiotherapy or chemotherapy and who present with persistent or recurrent disease, although total laryngectomy traditionally has been the standard of care, transoral laser microsurgical and open conservational laryngeal surgery approaches are gaining acceptance. Steiner and colleagues have advocated transoral laser microsurgery as a surgical modality in the salvage setting. Holsinger and others have advocated conservation laryngeal surgical approaches, including supracricoid laryngectomy, in the salvage setting, although with an increased risk for postoperative aspiration, dysphagia, and airway obstruction secondary to neolaryngeal edema. Nonetheless, these strategies are useful tools in the armamentarium of the head and neck surgeon treating recurrent disease after radiotherapy.

Surgical Management of the Neck in Laryngeal Cancer

Factors influencing management of the neck in laryngeal cancer include the TNM (tumor node metastasis) stage of the primary lesion, the subsite of the larynx involved, and the modality chosen to treat the primary lesion. Patients with early-stage lesions of the glottic larynx have low rates of regional lymph node metastasis because of the paucity of lymphatic drainage from this area. For patients with early-stage lesions of the glottic larynx in an N0 neck, close observation is an acceptable management strategy. The supraglottic larynx, on the other hand, has an extensive bilateral network of lymphatics along the jugulodigastric nodal basin. Although conservative management of the neck in patients with selected T1 lesions treated with

transoral laser microsurgery may be appropriate, the majority of patients with higher-stage lesions will require elective treatment of the neck, regardless of the clinical stage of the neck on physical examination, through either routine bilateral selective neck dissection (levels II, III, and IV) or radiotherapy that includes at-risk nodal basins in the treatment field. In those patients whose primary lesions are treated with radiation, the central and lateral neck nodal basins will be included in the radiation field. Finally, those patients with N + disease at presentation should be treated with an appropriate neck dissection.

26.4 Roundsmanship

- Postradiation and postchemoradiation settings present challenges in terms of wound healing and functional outcomes. Organ preservation techniques in these patients, however, are not contraindicated.
- Early-stage disease involving the anterior commissure may be better managed with transoral laser microsurgical techniques or with open partial laryngeal surgical techniques than with radiotherapy alone.
- In the surgical management of glottic malignancies involving the supraglottic larynx and of supraglottic malignancies, the surgeon must address the bilateral regional nodal basins at risk with either surgery or radiotherapy.
- Although these reports are in their infancy, a careful review of the literature concerning newer techniques, including transoral laser microsurgical endoscopic techniques, should provide an understanding of which patients require postoperative radiotherapy or a tracheotomy, and of long-term oncologic efficacy.

26.5 Recommended Reading

[1] Farrag TY, Koch WM, Cummings CW et al. Supracricoid laryngectomy outcomes: The Johns Hopkins experience. Laryngoscope 2007; 117: 129–132

[2] Gil Z, Gupta A, Kummer B et al. The role of pectoralis major muscle flap in salvage total laryngectomy. Arch Otolaryngol Head Neck Surg 2009; 135: 1019–1023

[3] Holsinger FC, Funk E, Roberts DB, Diaz EM. Conservation laryngeal surgery versus total laryngectomy for radiation failure in laryngeal cancer. Head Neck 2006; 28: 779–784

[4] Holsinger FC, Nussenbaum B, Nakayama M et al. Current concepts and new horizons in conservation laryngeal surgery: an important part of multidisciplinary care. Head Neck 2010; 32: 656–665

[5] Myers EN, Wagner RL, Johnson JT. Microlaryngoscopic surgery for T1 glottic lesions: a cost-effective option. Ann Otol Rhinol Laryngol 1994; 103: 28–30

[6] Smith JC, Johnson JT, Cognetti DM et al. Quality of life, functional outcome, and costs of early glottic cancer. Laryngoscope 2003; 113: 68–76

[7] Tufano RP, Stafford EM. Organ preservation surgery for laryngeal cancer. Otolaryngol Clin North Am 2008; 41: 741–755

[8] Weinstein GS, O'Malley BW, Snyder W, Hockstein NG. Transoral robotic surgery: supraglottic partial laryngectomy. Ann Otol Rhinol Laryngol 2007; 116: 19–23

27 Transoral Robotic Surgery

Sumeet M. Anand and Adam S. Jacobson

27.1 Introduction

Minimally invasive techniques in surgery are being readily evaluated and endorsed among both surgeons and patients. In otolaryngology, two evolving areas of great interest include transoral laser microsurgery (TLM) and, most recently, transoral robotic surgery (TORS). In the treatment of head and neck cancer, the evolution of these advances has been influenced by a paradigm shift toward organ preservation and toward offering, when possible, a management option with less morbidity than conventional chemoradiation.

The first report of robotic surgery in the head and neck came in 2005, when a supraglottic laryngectomy was performed in a canine model by Weinstein et al. This was a significant moment for the application of robotics as a surgical treatment option in the upper aerodigestive tract. In that same year, McLeod and Melder were the first to describe the use of robotic surgery in a patient, to excise a vallecular cyst. Over the next year, the group led by Weinstein and O'Malley pioneered the introduction and application of the da Vinci robot (Intuitive Surgical, Sunnyvale, CA) to head and neck surgery, publishing a series of reports on the feasibility, safety, and use of the technique in human patients. In 2009, the FDA approved the use of the da Vinci surgical system in TORS for benign processes and early-stage T1 and T2 mucosal malignancies of the oropharynx, hypopharynx, and larynx. Since 2009, there has been a rapid expansion in the number of cancer centers that are now incorporating TORS into the management of head and neck cancer, with the goal to potentially deintensify adjuvant treatment and improve quality-of-life and functional outcomes, while maintaining survival.

TORS presents a novel change from conventional surgical management in many facets, in particular for oropharyngeal squamous cell carcinoma (SCC). The oropharynx is an area that has traditionally required a challenging and extensive surgical approach. Surgical access requires a lip-splitting incision and mandibular osteotomy in order to swing the mandible out of the surgical field. This radical approach requires a tracheotomy for airway protection. In comparison, in treating oropharyngeal SCC, TORS does not require a lip incision, mandibulotomy, mandibular swing, or tracheotomy for airway protection. Eliminating such invasive surgical maneuvers provides a patient with a far less morbid procedure and increases operative efficiency.

A second paradigm shift that TORS represents is that the surgical defect created during extirpation is usually not reconstructed and instead is allowed to heal by secondary intention. This is a significant change from the conventional surgical philosophy that when a mucosal barrier is violated, the surgical defect is reconstructed immediately with a local, regional, or free tissue transfer. Traditionally, the oropharyngeal or hypopharyngeal conduit is reconstituted with a hermetic reconstruction to prevent a communication between the upper aerodigestive tract and the neck and avoid a potential salivary fistula. If a fistula occurs, the patient is at risk for a carotid blowout. Additionally, a salivary leak can delay postoperative oral intake and the commencement of adjuvant treatment. In early-stage disease, the ability to avoid a reconstruction with TORS significantly reduces surgical time and the morbidity associated with the treatment of a cancer of the oropharynx. As the experience with TORS in head and neck surgery increases and the application expands to larger and more advanced lesions, the need for robotically assisted reconstructions will unquestionably become more significant. Recent reports have started to describe the role of robotically assisted local and free flap reconstruction for oropharyngeal TORS defects.

The da Vinci surgical robot provides several technical advantages in comparison with TLM and more traditional transoral suspension techniques. The visualization console of the robot is outfitted with two different three-chip cameras mounted within one integrated 12-mm stereoscopic endoscope. This optical system generates a wide-angle, high-definition illusion of a three-dimensional surgical field. The movable endoscope also offers a benefit of in-field optics, which can change viewing angles and position and so optimize visualization from unique perspectives. This technology overcomes the line-of-sight issue associated with TLM and traditional suspension approaches. Additional degrees of freedom, reduced natural hand tremor, and three-dimensional imagery allow a meticulous translation of larger hand movements at the operating console to small, highly dexterous movements of the robotic instruments at the surgical site. Collectively, these characteristics make possible a precise dissection of surgical tissue planes in the pharynx that was not attainable before application of the da Vinci robot to head and neck surgery.

The introduction of novel technology and operative equipment, plus a change in surgical philosophy, comes with an inherent learning curve. To date, establishing a TORS program has been shown to be a safe and efficient undertaking in a number of cancer centers. In most hospitals, head and neck robotic units are being initiated concurrently with da Vinci programs in urology, gynecology, general surgery, and cardiac and thoracic surgery. Moore et al reported that the learning curve for operative efficiency in TORS can be reached after approximately the first 10 patients. After preliminary experience of the operative team, the mean setup time for TORS is less than 30 minutes. In a review of seven studies reporting on feasibility, it was shown that the average operating time had decreased to less than 75 minutes for oropharyngeal SCC resections, a significant reduction in time from that required for traditional open oropharyngeal approaches.

There are differing opinions with respect to the management of neck disease in patients undergoing TORS. To permit healing of the surgical defect in advanced oropharyngeal SCC before the neck is entered, Weinstein et al advocate a separate staged neck dissection within 3 weeks of the initial TORS procedure. In adopting this algorithm, they theorize that the risk for creating a communication, with a resultant salivary fistula between the oropharynx and the neck, is reduced. Other studies advocating a concomitant neck dissection and TORS resection show that operating on the neck simultaneously does not increase the risk for a salivary fistula. Moore et al recently reported their retrospective data on 148 patients undergoing TORS with a concomitant neck dissection. A communication between the oropharynx and neck was noted in 42 patients (29%), which were managed conservatively in all cases. Of the 42 patients, 6 (14%) developed a cervical fluid collection that required a formal incision and drainage. In no instances was there a delay in starting adjuvant radiation therapy. These investigators concluded that performing an oropharyngeal TORS resection with a concomitant neck dissection offers patients a single operation with acceptable risks and no delay regarding potential adjuvant treatment. For patients with advanced oropharyngeal SCC, all surgeons appear to agree on the need for a neck dissection; however, there is as of yet no consensus on the timing of the procedure. An assessment of regional nodal disease in oropharyngeal SCC is essential to determine the need for adjuvant external beam radiation therapy or chemoradiation.

Data regarding long-term oncologic results and functional outcomes with TORS are now being reported. In 2010, Weinstein et al published their results with 47 patients who had advanced stage III or IV oropharyngeal SCC. The rates of local, regional, and distant disease control were 97.9%, 95.7%, and 91.5%, respectively, at a mean follow-up of 26.6 months. Overall survival rates at 1 and 2 years were 95.7% and 81.8%, respectively. Their data showed rates with TORS management similar to those with standard treatment protocols. They also looked at gastrostomy tube dependence as a marker of swallowing function and found a significantly lower rate of gastrostomy tube dependence in patients undergoing TORS than in those undergoing traditional nonsurgical management. In 2012, Moore et al published their results with 66 patients undergoing TORS after more than 2 years of follow-up. Nearly all patients (64 of 66; 97%) were consuming an oral diet within 3 weeks of surgery and before starting adjuvant therapy. Long-term gastrostomy tube use was required in 3 (4.5%) of the 66 and long-term tracheotomy in 1 (1.5%). The 3-year estimated local control and regional control rates were 97.0% and 94.0%, respectively. The 2-year disease-specific survival and recurrence-free survival rates were 95.1% and 92.4%, respectively.

One of the primary premises for undertaking a TORS procedure is that if negative margins are achieved and no other adverse prognostic factors are noted in the specimen—namely, lymphovascular invasion, perineural invasion, multiple positive lymph nodes, and extracapsular extension—then adjuvant chemotherapy and external beam radiation therapy can potentially be deintensified or withheld. In 2011, Hurtuk et al published their results with 64 patients who had T1–T3 oropharyngeal SCC. Among 64 patients, 50% of those with stage I or stage II disease were spared adjuvant radiation therapy or combined chemoradiation, and 34% of those with stage III or stage IV disease were spared chemotherapy. In 2009, Moore et al published a prospective study on 45 patients with T1–T4 oropharyngeal SCC treated with TORS. In all instances, the resection margins were negative, and as such, the adjuvant radiation therapy dose was reduced.

Despite of all its advantages, there are also practical and technical limitations to the use of TORS. At times, it may be difficult to gain adequate exposure of the lesion within the pharynx and larynx because of anatomical constraints. In our experience, it is imperative to individually select the correct retractor for each case to provide optimal exposure of the pharyngolaryngeal segment of interest. Reports have successfully described the Feyh-Kastenbauer (FK) retractor (Gyrus ACMI, Southborough, MA), the Crowe-Davis or Dingman mouth gag, and the LARS (Larynx Advanced Retractor System) retractor (Fentex, Tuttlingen, Germany) for different pharyngeal and laryngeal tumor sites. Adequate tumor visualization when there are anatomical constraints is a challenge in all transoral surgical approaches. Additional limitations of TORS include the thermal effects of monocautery, leading to a challenge in histopathologic margin analysis, and the lack of proprioception and tactile feedback. In selected reports, a flexible carbon dioxide laser and robotic bipolar forceps have been described. In future models, these may become more commonplace because they allow precise mucosal and muscular dissection with less peripheral tissue damage. It has been noted that the excellent three-dimensional imagery of the da Vinci robot can assist in partially offsetting the undeniable advantages of haptic feedback during an open operation.

In summary, TORS offers a novel surgical approach with less morbidity than conventional open surgery. This technology is feasible and safe, with an attainable learning curve for surgeons already familiar with transoral approaches. There are a growing number of reports suggesting that the short- and long-term functional outcomes of TORS are acceptable. Furthermore, the short- and long-term oncologic outcomes reported appear to be comparable with those of traditional nonsurgical management. As we move forward, patient outcomes with TORS must be critically evaluated and compared with those of current nonsurgical chemoradiation protocols. As this technology continues to evolve, there is emerging evidence for primary TORS resection and reconstruction in the upper aerodigestive tract, with a prospective opportunity for the deintensification of adjuvant treatment.

27.2 Roundsmanship

- TORS involves fewer invasive surgical maneuvers and provides the patient with a far less morbid procedure and increased operative efficiency.
- The surgical defect created during TORS extirpation is usually not reconstructed and instead is allowed to heal by secondary intention.
- Patients must be carefully selected for TORS because it may be difficult to gain adequate exposure of the lesion within the pharynx and larynx as a consequence of anatomical constraints.
- A growing number of reports suggest that the short- and long-term functional outcomes of TORS are acceptable.

27.3 Recommended Reading

[1] Desai SC, Sung CK, Genden EM. Transoral robotic surgery using an image guidance system. Laryngoscope 2008; 118: 2003–2005

[2] Dowthwaite SA, Franklin JH, Palma DA, Fung K, Yoo J, Nichols AC. The role of transoral robotic surgery in the management of oropharyngeal cancer: a review of the literature. ISRN Oncol 2012; 2012: Epub 2012 Apr 23

[3] Genden EM, O'Malley BW, Weinstein GS et al. Transoral robotic surgery: role in the management of upper aerodigestive tract tumors. Head Neck 2012; 34: 886–893

[4] Haus BM, Kambham N, Le D, Moll FM, Gourin C, Terris DJ. Surgical robotic applications in otolaryngology. Laryngoscope 2003; 113: 1139–1144

[5] Leonhardt FD, Quon H, Abrahão M, O'Malley BW, Weinstein GS. Transoral robotic surgery for oropharyngeal carcinoma and its impact on patient-reported quality of life and function. Head Neck 2012; 34: 146–154

[6] McLeod IK, Melder PC. Da Vinci robot-assisted excision of a vallecular cyst: a case report. Ear Nose Throat J 2005; 84: 170–172

[7] Moore EJ, Olsen SM, Laborde RR et al. Long-term functional and oncologic results of transoral robotic surgery for oropharyngeal squamous cell carcinoma. Mayo Clin Proc 2012; 87: 219–225

[8] Mukhija VK, Sung CK, Desai SC, Wanna G, Genden EM. Transoral robotic assisted free flap reconstruction. Otolaryngol Head Neck Surg 2009; 140: 124–125

[9] O'Malley BW, Weinstein GS, Snyder W, Hockstein NG. Transoral robotic surgery (TORS) for base of tongue neoplasms. Laryngoscope 2006; 116: 1465–1472

[10] Weinstein GS, O', M, alley BW, Hockstein NG. Transoral robotic surgery: supraglottic laryngectomy in a canine model. Laryngoscope 2005; 115: 1315–1319

[11] Weinstein GS, O'Malley BW, Cohen MA, Quon H. Transoral robotic surgery for advanced oropharyngeal carcinoma. Arch Otolaryngol Head Neck Surg 2010; 136: 1079–1085

28 Nonneoplastic Salivary Gland Diseases

Neha A. Patel and Stimson P. Schantz

28.1 Introduction

The salivary glands consist of the paired parotid, submandibular, and sublingual glands, as well as 600 to 1,000 minor salivary glands. Disease processes of the salivary glands are divided into nonneoplastic and neoplastic diseases. Nonneoplastic diseases of the salivary gland can be further divided based on etiology into inflammatory infectious, inflammatory noninfectious, and noninflammatory diseases (see Box Nonneoplastic Diseases of the Salivary Glands (p.236)).

> **Nonneoplastic Diseases of the Salivary Glands**
>
> **Inflammatory, infectious**
> - Acute bacterial sialadenitis
> - Acute viral sialadenitis
> - Granulomatous infection
>
> **Inflammatory, noninfectious**
> - Sialolithiasis
> - Radiation sialadenitis
> - Sjögren syndrome
> - Sarcoidosis
>
> **Noninflammatory**
> - Sialorrhea (ptyalism)
> - Xerostomia
> - Sialadenosis (sialosis)
> - Cysts
> - Mucoceles
> - Trauma

28.2 Applied Anatomy

The salivary glands play an important role in oral hygiene because saliva has antimicrobial properties and acts as a barrier to protect the oral mucosa from local irritants. In addition, as a lubricant, saliva aids in the functions of speech and swallowing. Therefore, manifestations of salivary gland diseases can range from simple aesthetic changes to debilitating functional morbidities. Understanding salivary gland anatomy (▶ Fig. 28.1) is critical in understanding the pathology of the salivary glands. During a physical examination of the salivary glands, it is important to palpate externally as well as intraorally.

28.2.1 Parotid Gland

The parotid gland is the largest salivary gland. It excretes predominantly serous secretions via the Stensen duct to the buccal mucosa at the level of the second maxillary molar. It lies lateral to the masseter and anterior to the ear from the zygomatic arch superiorly to the angle of the mandible inferiorly, with its posterior tail overlying the sternocleidomastoid muscle. The facial nerve divides the gland into superficial and deep lobes. Parasympathetic innervation to the parotid is from the glossopharyngeal nerve via the otic ganglion (by way of the auriculotemporal nerve). Sympathetic innervation of all the salivary glands is from the superior cervical ganglion.

28.2.2 Submandibular Gland

The submandibular gland is the second largest salivary gland and excretes seromucous secretions via the Wharton duct to the anterior floor of mouth. It sits on the mylohyoid muscle in the submandibular triangle between the anterior and posterior bellies of the digastric muscle. Parasympathetic innervation of the submandibular gland and sublingual glands is from the superior salivatory nucleus through the chorda tympani (by way of the lingual nerve) before it synapses in the submandibular ganglion.

28.2.3 Sublingual Gland and Minor Salivary Glands

The sublingual gland and minor salivary glands excrete more viscous mucinous secretions that tend to contain higher levels of lysozymes and have more antimicrobial properties. The sublingual gland is superficial to the mylohyoid and drains in the floor of the mouth via the ducts of Rivinus (some of which fuse to form the Bartholin duct, which drains into the Wharton duct). On the other hand, minor salivary glands are located throughout the upper aerodigestive tract and drain individually.

28.3 Inflammatory, Infectious Diseases

28.3.1 Acute Bacterial Sialadenitis

Pathogenesis

Acute bacterial sialadenitis is caused by decreased production/dehydration related to salivary stasis (as in obstruction caused by stones). Infection is most commonly caused by coagulase-positive *Staphylococcus aureus*, followed by *Streptococcus* species and other oral pathogens such as *Enterococcus coli, Haemophilus influenzae*, and anaerobes such as *Bacteroides*.

Evaluation

Acute bacterial sialadenitis usually presents with unilateral, tender glandular swelling and purulent drainage at the ductal orifice of the involved gland. The overlying skin may be warm, erythematous, and indurated. The disease may be seen in postoperative patients as well as in elderly patients, who often take medications that can cause dehydration. Patients may have

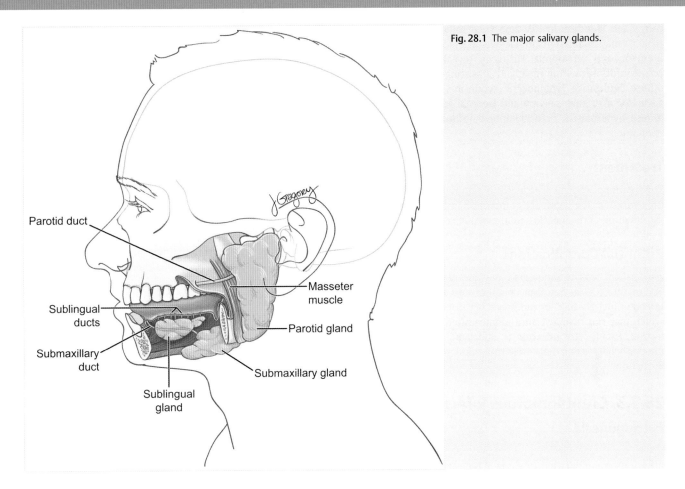

Fig. 28.1 The major salivary glands.

Parotid duct

Masseter muscle

Sublingual ducts

Parotid gland

Submaxillary duct

Submaxillary gland

Sublingual gland

fevers, and blood work may show neutrophilia. The parotid gland may be more prone to infection because its predominantly serous secretions have less antimicrobial activity than submandibular gland saliva, which contains more mucin. The diagnosis is based on the clinical examination findings, although ultrasound and computed tomography (CT) can confirm the presence of stones and collections.

Treatment

Antibiotic treatment should cover for β-lactamase activity and, depending on severity, include oral amoxicillin/clavulanate, clindamycin, oral or intravenous ampicillin/sulbactam, or intravenous vancomycin/metronidazole. Culture can guide treatment. A "sialadenitis regimen" should be offered to all patients; this includes hydration, sialagogues (lemon drops, orange juice, or sugar-free gum), warm compresses, bimanual massage, oral hygiene, and smoking cessation.

Potential Complications

Untreated acute bacterial sialadenitis may lead to abscess formation, which may require incision and drainage and placement of a drainage catheter. In the case of a parotid abscess, instruments are spread in the direction of the facial nerve branches to preserve nerve function in the setting of an inflamed gland. Untreated infection can also lead to sepsis. Repeated episodes can lead to chronic sialadenitis.

28.3.2 Acute Viral Sialadenitis

Pathogenesis

Acute viral sialadenitis can be caused by infection with viruses such as the mumps paramyxovirus, coxsackievirus, cytomegalovirus, echovirus, and influenza virus. Mumps virus is the virus most commonly involved in parotitis. Salivary gland disease in association with HIV infection in the pediatric population is AIDS-defining.

Evaluation

Viral sialadenitis tends to be bilateral and is usually accompanied by symptoms such as low-grade fever, pain with chewing, fatigue, headache, and, myalgia. The mumps virus is a paramyxovirus that affects children 4 to 6 years old. The incubation period for mumps is 2 to 3 weeks, and the systemic symptoms often resolve before parotitis. On history, it is important to ask about the patient's immunization history. On physical examination, the parotid glands will be swollen and firm but nonsuppurative. Imaging often shows diffuse bilateral enlargement of the glands. The diagnosis can be confirmed with a serum viral titer. The mumps virus is transmitted through contact with respiratory secretions and can be detected in a patient's saliva. Cytomegalovirus can specifically cause a rare salivary gland inclusion disease in newborns. This is diagnosed by its association with other physical findings, such as cerebral atrophy, hepatosplenomegaly, thrombocytopenia purpura ("blueberry muffin" baby), and jaundice. In HIV-associated salivary gland disease, patients may manifest glandular swelling, localized facial disfigurement, and xerostomia. Histology reveals periductal lymphatic infiltrates within the gland consisting of CD8 + T cells. In diffuse infiltrative lymphocytic syndrome, patients infected with HIV may have salivary and lacrimal gland swelling with diffuse hyperplastic, cystic lymphoid infiltrations throughout the body.

Treatment

The treatment of viral sialadenitis is symptomatic care, including hydration. The incidence of mumps has decreased since the introduction of the measles–mumps–rubella vaccine.

Potential Complications

Mumps can lead to meningitis and encephalitis, pancreatitis, and orchitis. Otolaryngologic complications of cytomegalovirus infection include mild or moderate sensorineural hearing loss, which may not manifest until months after the congenital infection. Finally, HIV infection is associated with benign lymphoepithelial lesions that rarely may undergo malignant transformation.

28.3.3 Granulomatous Infection

Pathogenesis

Infectious granulomatous diseases of the salivary gland include tuberculosis, infection with atypical mycobacteria, cat-scratch disease, toxoplasmosis (*Toxoplasma gondii*), and actinomycosis. Tuberculosis infection is thought to be spread from person to person when the glands are seeded from oral sites via the ductal system. Cat-scratch disease is caused by the gram-negative bacillus *Bartonella henselae* after a cat bite or scratch. Toxoplasmosis is spread by the ingestion of cysts in undercooked meats or cat feces. *Actinomyces* is a gram-positive branching anaerobe found in the oral cavity that can cause retrograde ductal seeding of the glands.

Evaluation: *Mycobacterium*

Tuberculosis infection is rare but presents primarily with acute unilateral parotid swelling. Secondary hematogenous or lymphatic spread of tuberculosis generally involves the submandibular and sublingual glands. In high-risk persons such as immigrants and patients with HIV infection, a purified protein derivative (PPD) test should be placed. The PPD test result can be negative in cases caused by atypical mycobacteria, more commonly seen in children 1 1/2 to 3 years old. Acid-fast staining may be sent with salivary cultures. Tuberculosis infection can also present chronically with a slowly growing tumor-like lesion that on fine-needle aspiration contains Langhans giant cells and acid-fast bacilli. On the other hand, lymphoid tissue involved in cat-scratch disease is positive for Warthin-Starry silver stain. Cat-scratch disease can present with cervical, submandibular, or periparotid erythematous and fluctuant lymphadenopathy near the site of the original papule formed at a

scratch site. On pathology, ultrasound, and CT, the lymph nodes are vascular with central necrosis. Serology can also help confirm cat-scratch disease. Actinomycosis can present with painless enlargement of the affected salivary gland and purulence that can cause cutaneous fistulas to form. The diagnosis is confirmed by the presence of sulfur granules in smears.

Treatment

The treatment of acute sialadenitis caused by tuberculosis is with a multidrug antituberculosis regimen and the excision of involved tumors. Lymphadenopathy caused by cat-scratch disease usually resolves in a few months; treatment is symptomatic with analgesics and warm compresses. Toxoplasmosis in immunocompromised patients, such as those with HIV infection, is treated with pyrimethamine and trisulfapyrimidines. Penicillin (doxycycline for penicillin-allergic patients) is the accepted treatment for actinomycosis.

Potential Complications

In patients with cat-scratch disease who are highly symptomatic, such as those with suppuration and severe fevers, ciprofloxacin and azithromycin have been used. Surgical excision may be necessary when actinomycosis is complicated by sinus tracts.

28.4 Inflammatory, Noninfectious Diseases

28.4.1 Sialolithiasis

Pathogenesis

Salivary calculi form in the context of stasis and consist predominantly of hydroxyapatite; 80% of calculi are in the submandibular gland. The submandibular duct is long, and flow through the duct is against gravity. Submandibular saliva is more alkaline, with a high concentration of calcium, phosphate, and viscous mucus. Gout-related calculi consist of uric acid.

Evaluation

Sialolithiasis presents with periprandial pain and swelling of the affected gland. Ultrasound, CT, and more recently magnetic resonance (MR) sialography (without contrast) has been used to detect calculi that are not palpable. On CT, about 90% of submandibular calculi are radiopaque, whereas 90% of parotid calculi are radiolucent.

Treatment

Superficial calculi can be removed intraorally, but acute obstructive sialadenitis can recur. For calculi in the hilum or for recurrent infections, surgical excision of the affected gland can be performed. With new, minimally invasive technology, conservative treatment, such as sialoendoscopy and laser intracorporeal lithotripsy, is an option. Surgery is avoided during episodes of acute inflammation to minimize ductal perforation.

Potential Complications

Sialolithiasis is often associated with chronic sialadenitis. It can also lead to ductal stricture and very rarely to sialocutaneous and sialo-oral fistulas.

28.4.2 Radiation Sialadenitis

Pathogenesis

During the treatment of head and neck cancer, exposure to more than 50 Gy of radiation can cause irreversible salivary gland damage and the loss of acinar cells. The parotid glands are most sensitive to damage. Salivary function can decrease by 60% with just 1 week of radiation therapy at 10 Gy. The treatment of thyroid cancer with radioactive iodine can also lead to radiation sialadenitis and xerostomia.

Evaluation

Radiation sialadenitis causes pain and swelling of the affected gland and is associated with xerostomia, oral infections, stomatitis, and increased dental caries.

Treatment

Hydration, sialagogues, and warm compresses can help with symptomatic management. Pilocarpine, a cholinergic secretagogue, may be used for postradiation xerostomia.

Potential Complications

Radiation sialadenitis can lead to xerostomia, taste alterations, and dental infections.

28.4.3 Sjögren Syndrome

Pathogenesis

Sjögren syndrome is an autoimmune disease that causes a lymphocytic infiltration and dysfunction of the salivary and lacrimal ducts. Patients may have primary Sjögren syndrome with xerophthalmia (keratoconjunctivitis sicca) and xerostomia alone, or they may have secondary Sjögren syndrome, in which another autoimmune disorder is also involved. There is a 9:1 female-to-male ration of those affected, and most patients present in their fifties. The presence of HLA-B8 and HLA-Dw3 has been linked to an increased predisposition to primary Sjögren syndrome, whereas HLA-DRw4 is linked to the secondary form. It is hypothesized that environmental triggers, such as a viral infection (e.g., with HTLV-1 [human T-cell leukemia/lymphoma/lymphotropic virus] or Epstein-Barr virus), may induce cell lysis, leading to the formation of autoantigens that cause a lymphocytic infiltration of gland tissue and thus a decrease in glandular secretion.

Evaluation

Patients with Sjögren syndrome may present with dry eyes, inflamed and red conjunctivae, and a foreign body or sandy sensation in their eyes. Oral manifestations include dry mouth; changes in taste, speech, and swallow function; dry lips; fissured tongue; and poor oral hygiene. Ductal obstruction by lymphocytic infiltrates can cause recurrent salivary gland enlargement, particularly of the parotid gland, that can be bilateral and aggravated by eating. Extraglandular manifestations include low-grade fevers, arthritis, dry skin, myalgia, and purpura. Lower lip minor salivary gland biopsies show lymphocytic infiltrates. Histologically, benign lymphoepithelial lesions as described by Godwin can be associated with Sjögren syndrome, although patients with benign lymphoepithelial lesions do not always have symptoms of Sjögren syndrome. Objective tests include sialometry and the Schirmer test (less than 5 mm eye moisture in 5 minutes). Serology should be performed to test for anti-SS-A/Ro and anti-SS-B/La. In addition, Sjögren syndrome is associated with other autoimmune disorders, so testing for rheumatoid factor, antinuclear antibodies, and anticentromere antibodies can be positive.

Treatment

Symptomatic treatment includes hydration, sialagogues, oral hygiene, salivary substitutes, and artificial tears. Pilocarpine, the muscarinic agonist, has been used as a sialagogue but has systemic side effects of perspiration, flushing, and micturition, and it is contraindicated in patients with asthma. Steroids and immunomodulators are used for severe systemic manifestations of Sjögren syndrome.

Potential Complications

MR imaging may be helpful because there is a 44-fold increase in the risk for non-Hodgkin lymphoma in those with Sjögren syndrome. Care must be taken to follow patients with recurrent gland swelling, lymphadenopathy, vasculitis, lung infiltrates and hepatosplenomegaly, pancytopenia, hypergammaglobulinemia, and an increased erythrocyte sedimentation rate.

28.4.4 Sarcoidosis

Pathogenesis

Sarcoidosis is a noninfectious, inflammatory granulomatous disease of unknown etiology.

Evaluation

Sarcoidosis is more common in African-American women and often presents with cervical lymphadenopathy, pulmonary manifestations, and cutaneous nodules. Heerfordt syndrome (uveoparotid fever) is a form of sarcoidosis that begins with a prodrome of fever, fatigue, and night sweats and later manifests with acute parotitis and uveitis. Diffuse bilateral involvement of the glands of the face is possible, so a labial biopsy may reveal noncaseating granulomas involving lymphoid tissue.

Treatment

Glandular swelling may be chronic and usually resolves spontaneously, although steroids have been used in the acute setting.

Potential Complications

Facial paralysis not infrequently accompanies uveoparotid fever, but it tends to resolve with or without steroid treatment.

Symptomatic care includes artificial tears, lubricating ointment, and securing the eyes closed at night. An ophthalmologic evaluation is important because uveitis can lead to glaucoma. Rare cases of sudden hearing loss from neurosarcoidosis and supraglottic sarcoidosis have been reported.

28.5 Noninflammatory Diseases

28.5.1 Sialorrhea (Ptyalism)

Pathogenesis

Ptyalism, or sialorrhea, is the oversecretion of saliva. Medications like pilocarpine or the antipsychotic clozapine can cause hypersecretion of saliva. Stroke, Parkinson disease, and motor neuron diseases such as amyotrophic lateral sclerosis can cause sialorrhea in adults. In children, rather than being due to overproduction of saliva, drooling can be caused by the involuntary escape of saliva through the mouth, as seen in cerebral palsy. Ptyalism can accompany dysphagia in inflammatory conditions, such as a peritonsillar abscess. Ptyalism gravidarum is of unknown origin and often associated with hyperemesis during pregnancy.

Evaluation

Patients with sialorrhea often report difficulty swallowing. The patient should be assessed for deficits in sensation or oral motor function that would compromise swallowing or lip competence. Concurrent neurologic deficits may suggest a cerebrovascular accident.

Treatment

Speech therapy targeting oral movements is recommended for those with motor dysfunction. Anticholinergics such as scopolamine patches and oral atropine can help decrease secretions, but they may also lead constipation, bradycardia, blurred vision, and urinary retention. Intraglandular botulinum toxin can temporarily treat sialorrhea. Surgical treatments include gland excision, ductal ligation, submandibular duct relocation, and the chorda tympani neurectomy.

Potential Complications

Sialorrhea has negative hygienic and social effects. It can also lead to skin maceration, infection, and aspiration.

28.5.2 Xerostomia

Pathogenesis

Inflammatory causes of dry mouth, or xerostomia, include radiation and autoimmune disorders like Sjögren syndrome, as described above. Other noninflammatory causes include dehydration, autonomic effects of stress, and medication side effects. Medications that can cause xerostomia due to anticholinergic side effects include antihypertensives, tricyclic antidepressants, antipsychotics, antihistamines, antiparkinsonian drugs, and anti-asthma bronchodilators. Diabetes has also been linked to xerostomia, presumably as a consequence of neuropathy, microvascular abnormalities, or metabolic dysfunction from inadequate control of diabetes.

Evaluation

Xerostomia is the subjective sensation of dry mouth, and this clinical finding does not correlate with objective measurements of salivary secretions. Patients who have xerostomia can present with a burning sensation in the mouth, dysphagia, speech and swallowing dysfunction, halitosis, and overall poor dental hygiene, including caries. On physical examination, patients may have cracked lips, pale oral mucosa, and dental decay.

Treatment

Hydration, sialagogues, stress management, and good oral hygiene should be encouraged. Changes in medication regimens can also help alleviate symptoms, especially in elderly patients taking numerous medications with anticholinergic side effects.

Potential Complications

Xerostomia can lead to oral infections such as candidiasis and to changes in taste, speech function, and swallow function.

28.5.3 Sialadenosis (Sialosis)

Pathogenesis

Sialadenosis, or sialosis, is a disease of the salivary glands characterized histologically by noninflammatory acinar enlargement. It has been linked to malnutrition and to metabolic and hormonal disturbances that may cause peripheral autonomic neuropathy. It is hypothesized that acinar enlargement is caused by neuropathy leading to impaired exocytosis of secretory granules and loss of myoepithelial mechanical support.

Evaluation

Sialadenosis typically presents with bilateral diffuse swelling of the salivary glands (typically the parotid glands). It is usually seen in association with a systemic condition such as diabetes, hypothyroidism, pregnancy, obesity, hypoproteinemia, alcoholic cirrhosis, or malnutrition. Imaging and biopsy are performed to establish a diagnosis.

Treatment

Partial or total gland excision has been performed in cases of pain and poor cosmesis despite conservative treatment and the management of systemic disturbances.

Potential Complications

Because sialosis may be related to systemic disturbances that lead to autonomic neuropathy, the remaining glands may become affected despite the surgical removal of one.

28.5.4 Cysts

Pathogenesis

Branchial cysts are true cysts with an epithelial lining and lymphoid tissue. Type I ectodermal first branchial cleft cysts arise from duplication of the membranous external auditory canal.

They run parallel to the external auditory canal toward the oropharynx and are lateral to the facial nerve. Type II first branchial cleft cysts are of ectodermal and mesodermal origin and have cartilaginous components. They can run medial or lateral to the facial nerve. Dermoid cysts can be congenital or acquired and are lined with epidermis. They contain trapped skin appendages such as sebaceous glands, hair follicles, and connective tissue. Acquired cysts may occur after trauma and inflammatory injury as described throughout this chapter.

Evaluation

Parotid branchial cysts usually present as slowly growing, painless, firm masses around the anterior and upper third of the sternocleidomastoid muscle. They tend to present in persons 10 to 30 years olds and can have sinus tracts. Type I sinus tracts can be in the region of the pinna. Type II sinus tracts tend to run from the external auditory canal and drain near the angle of the mandible. Dermoid cysts tend to present in orbital, oral, and nasal regions but rarely can present as a firm, rounded parotid mass.

Treatment

The treatment of branchial cysts is complete excision with cranial nerve preservation. Parotid dermoid cysts should be removed with a partial parotidectomy to prevent recurrence.

Potential Complications

Failure to completely excise a salivary gland cyst can lead to recurrent infections and abscesses.

28.5.5 Mucoceles

Pathogenesis

Mucoceles are collections of mucus that can be true cystic lesions lined with epithelium (retention cysts) or pseudocysts that are simply covered with granulation tissue (extravasation cysts). Mucus retention cysts form from ductal dilation secondary to obstruction and the accumulation of mucus. A simple ranula is a retention cyst of the sublingual gland at the floor of the mouth. Trauma to a salivary duct can lead to the extravasation of mucus. If an excretory duct of a minor salivary gland is damaged, the salivary collection can cause an inflammatory reaction in the neighboring connective tissue, causing a granulation tissue–lined extravasation cyst to form. A plunging ranula is an extravasation cyst of the floor of the mouth.

Evaluation

Mucoceles are commonly found in minor salivary glands of the lips, buccal mucosa, ventral surface of the tongue, and floor of the mouth. They present as a smooth swelling that tends to be painless but can be irritated by chewing or swallowing movements. Mucoceles can be pink or blue from vascular congestion and the cyanosis of tissue stretched by saliva accumulation. A plunging ranula presents as a mass in the submandibular space. Imaging can help visualize the extent of a ranula, and fine-needle aspiration biopsy can rule out other cystic lesions.

Treatment

The treatment of mucoceles is complete excision. A ranula can also be completely excised, or treatment may involve excision of the entire gland to prevent recurrence. If critical nerves are involved, marsupialization of the cyst may be performed, with the risk for recurrence. A combined intraoral and cervical approach may be necessary for excision of a plunging ranula.

Potential Complications

Mucoceles may rupture, reaccumulate, or become infected.

28.5.6 Trauma

Pathogenesis

Traumatic injury to the salivary glands is rare. The parotid glands are the most exposed and therefore more likely to be injured. Penetrating trauma is more likely to cause complications than is blunt trauma. Common causes of facial injury include knives, motor vehicle accidents, gunshots, and iatrogenic maneuvers.

Evaluation

Understanding the gland anatomy is key to recognizing the complications of trauma. The Stenson duct travels superior to the masseter in close proximity to the transverse facial artery and buccal branch of the facial nerve before piercing the buccinator muscle to enter the oral mucosa. Lacerations involving these structures should be repaired at the time of cheek laceration repair.

Treatment

Glandular trauma can be repaired by suturing the capsule, closing the laceration, and applying pressure dressings to prevent the formation of a sialocele. Hemostasis must be achieved, and facial nerve damage should be immediately addressed surgically. In the repair of ductal lacerations, intraoral probing of the ductal orifice or the retrograde injection of methylene blue can help identify the distal duct while the gland is milked, and an evaluation of salivary flow can help identify the proximal duct (this can be done more easily if atropine and glycopyrrolate, used to reduce secretions, have not been used during anesthesia). Three basic treatment options exist for ductal repair. Penetrating trauma is repaired with a microsurgical primary anastomosis, in which the duct is dissected off the neighboring tissue for a tension-free repair done over a stent. If primary repair is not possible, an autogenous vein graft can be interposed. Alternatively, saliva can be diverted by suturing the proximal duct to an opening in the oral mucosa. If damage to the gland is too extensive for diversion, salivary atrophy can be promoted by ligating the proximal duct, avoiding oral feeding, and administering antisialagogues and pressure dressings.

Potential Complications

Failure to identify and treat salivary gland injuries can lead to sialocele formation and cutaneous fistulas when ductal damage is not addressed appropriately. Amylase levels in sialoceles can be higher than 10,000 U/L. Sialoceles can be conservatively managed with botulinum toxin A injections, pressure dressings, antisialagogues, and aspiration. Similar conservative and surgical options are available for fistula treatment, but it is best to explore a suspicious wound initially before ductal injuries are missed and fibrosis occurs.

28.6 Roundsmanship

- During a physical examination of the salivary glands, it is important to palpate externally as well as intraorally.
- For acute sialadenitis, a "sialadenitis regimen" includes hydration, sialagogues (lemon drops, orange juice, or sugar-free gum), warm compresses, bimanual massage, oral hygiene, and smoking cessation.
- Salivary function can decrease by 60% after just 1 week of radiation therapy at 10 Gy. Radioactive iodine treatment of thyroid cancer can also lead to radiation sialadenitis and xerostomia.
- In cases suspicious for Sjögren syndrome, serology should be sent for anti-SS-A/Ro and anti-SS-B/La in addition to rheumatoid factor, antinuclear antibodies, and anticentromere antibodies.
- In repairing ductal lacerations, intraoral probing of the ductal orifice or the retrograde injection of methylene blue can help

identify the distal duct while the gland is milked, and the evaluation of salivary flow can help identify the proximal duct.
- Sialoceles resulting for trauma can be conservatively managed with botulinum toxin A injections, pressure dressings, antisialagogues, and aspiration.
- Mucoceles are collections of mucus that can be true cystic lesions lined with epithelium (retention cysts) or pseudocysts simply covered with granulation tissue (extravasation cysts).

28.7 Recommended Reading

[1] Benjamin B, Dalton C, Croxson G. Laryngoscopic diagnosis of laryngeal sarcoid. Ann Otol Rhinol Laryngol 1995; 104: 529–531

[2] Chiu AG, Hecht DA, Prendiville SA, Mesick C, Mikula S, Deeb ZE. Atypical presentations of cat scratch disease in the head and neck. Otolaryngol Head Neck Surg 2001; 125: 414–416

[3] Hoffman E. Branchial cysts within the parotid gland. Ann Surg 1960; 152: 290–295

[4] Hornibrook J, Cochrane N. Contemporary surgical management of severe sialorrhea in children. ISRN Pediatr 2012; 2012: 364875

[5] Lewkowicz AA, Hasson O, Nahlieli O. Traumatic injuries to the parotid gland and duct. J Oral Maxillofac Surg 2002; 60: 676–680

[6] Re Cecconi D, Achilli A, Tarozzi M et al. Mucoceles of the oral cavity: a large case series (1994–2008) and a literature review. Med Oral Patol Oral Cir Bucal 2010; 15: e551–e556

[7] Rice DH. Advances in diagnosis and management of salivary gland diseases. West J Med 1984; 140: 238–249

29 Benign Neoplasms of the Salivary Glands

Vikas Mehta and Stimson P. Schantz

29.1 Introduction

Benign neoplasms of the salivary glands usually present as slowly enlarging, painless masses arising in the face, oral cavity, or neck. However, despite their benign nature, differentiating these neoplasms from malignant tumors is difficult based on the history, physical examination, imaging, and fine-needle aspiration biopsy. Besides pleomorphic adenomas, which constitute the majority of all salivary gland tumors, many of the other benign neoplasms of the salivary gland are rarely encountered. Additionally, pleomorphic adenomas carry the potential for malignant transformation. All of these factors lead to the need for the surgical excision of these nonmalignant growths. Future research with molecular genetics and imaging may help head and neck surgeons tailor their treatment of these rare entities.

29.2 Incidence

Overall, salivary gland neoplasms are relatively rare, accounting for only 3 to 4% of all head and neck tumors. The incidence of salivary gland neoplasms as a whole is approximately 1.5 cases per 100,000 individuals in the United States. These tumors can be segregated into two major groups based on location: tumors of major salivary glands and tumors of minor salivary glands. The major salivary glands are the paired parotid glands, submandibular glands, and the sublingual glands. The minor salivary glands consist of approximately 600 to 1,000 small glands scattered throughout the upper aerodigestive tract.

Of all salivary gland tumors, 70 to 80% are located in the parotid gland, and 75% of these parotid neoplasms are benign. Submandibular neoplasms constitute 10 to 15% of all salivary gland neoplasms, and approximately half of these are malignant. The remaining tumors are situated in the sublingual and minor salivary glands, and 75% of these are malignant. In summary, as the size of the gland decreases, the overall incidence of tumors decreases and the incidence of malignancy rises by 25%. This is known as the 25/50/75 rule, referring to the percentages of malignant tumors in the parotid, submandibular, and sublingual/minor salivary glands, respectively.

In adults, approximately 60% of all tumors are pleomorphic adenomas, with Warthin tumors the second-most common benign neoplasm (12%). In general, 54% of salivary gland neoplasms in adults are benign, and 65% of all salivary gland neoplasms in children are benign. Hemangiomas are the most common salivary gland neoplasms in children, followed by pleomorphic adenomas.

29.3 Terminology

A list of benign tumors and their relative frequencies is provided in ▶ Table 29.1. In general, benign tumors are slowly growing, painless, firm masses that are well circumscribed and can be treated with surgical excision including a cuff of normal tissue. The most common of these rare neoplasms are listed in the table.

29.3.1 Pleomorphic Adenoma

Also referred to as benign mixed tumor, pleomorphic adenoma is the most common tumor of the salivary glands. Commonly presenting in the fifth decade of life, they affect men and women equally and present as an asymptomatic, solitary mass. Rare cases of multifocal primary disease have been described. These tumors are referred to as pleomorphic or benign mixed tumors because of their composition of epithelial and connective tissue components in varying proportions. As noted above, pleomorphic adenomas account for 75% of all benign salivary gland neoplasms.

In the parotid gland, pleomorphic adenomas arise lateral to the facial nerve 90% of the time. Rarely, these tumors will extend between the stylomandibular ligament and the mandibular ramus into the parapharyngeal space and create the characteristic "dumbbell-shaped" appearance seen on imaging. Only 10% of parotid gland pleomorphic adenomas originate from the deep lobe of the parotid. Pleomorphic adenomas are the most common tumors of the prestyloid parapharyngeal space. Of all submandibular gland tumors, 36% are benign mixed tumors. The most common locations of a minor salivary gland pleomorphic adenoma are the palate and upper lip.

Pathologically, pleomorphic adenomas are firm and round, and the color varies from whitish gray to yellow. They are usually well encapsulated in the parotid gland and nonencapsulated in the minor salivary glands. Histopathologic analysis can show areas of focally thin capsule with pseudopodia, which are microextensions of the tumor into surrounding tissue. It is therefore imperative to take a cuff of normal tissue when excising the tumor. Abiding by this principle can lead to a recurrence rate of less than 5%. A benign mixed tumor never invades the facial nerve, so the facial nerve should never be sacrificed during excision.

Recurrence of these tumors poses a particular challenge for the head and neck surgeon. They often recur in a multifocal fashion, and the cure rate after salvage resection can be 25% or less. Surgical excision remains the mainstay of treatment for recurrent tumors, but the risk for facial nerve paralysis is significantly higher. Radiation therapy is controversial but can be employed in cases of inadequate margins or multifocal disease. Malignant transformation of pleomorphic adenoma is rare but can occur in patients with long-standing tumors. The risk for malignant transformation to carcinoma ex-pleomorphic adeno-

Table 29.1 The most common benign salivary gland neoplasms and their relative frequencies among all salivary gland neoplasms

Benign salivary neoplasm	Relative frequency
Pleomorphic adenoma	45%
Warthin tumor	10%
Monomorphic adenoma	2%
Oncocytoma	<1%
Hemangioma and vascular malformations	<1%

ma is 1.5% within the first year of diagnosis, but this risk increases to 10% after observation for more than 15 years.

29.3.2 Warthin Tumor (Papillary Cystadenoma Lymphomatosum)

Warthin tumors are the second most common benign tumors of the salivary glands, accounting for approximately 10% of lesions. The more appropriate name for these tumors is papillary cystadenoma lymphomatosum because of their histopathologic characteristics. Warthin tumors occur almost exclusively in the parotid gland and affect men more often than women (male-to-female ratio, 5:1). This has been hypothesized to occur because of the role smoking plays in the pathogenesis of Warthin tumors. Warthin tumors are bilateral in 10% of cases and occasionally may be painful as a result of inflammation secondary to an immunologic response to the lymphoid component.

Pathologically, these tumors are spherical or ovoid, smooth or lobulated, and encapsulated. Upon sectioning, the tumors exhibit solid gray tissue encapsulating white lymphoid tissue and multiple papillary cysts containing a mucoid brown fluid, explaining the name papillary cystadenoma lymphomatosum. The recommended treatment is surgical excision with facial nerve preservation. Recurrence may occur because of the multifocal, bilateral nature of these lesions.

29.3.3 Monomorphic Adenoma

The most common monomorphic adenomas are basal cell adenomas and clear cell adenomas. These lesions account for 2% of all salivary neoplasms. They occur most commonly in the upper lip and parotid gland. They are the least aggressive of all salivary gland tumors, presenting as firm, well-encapsulated, slowly growing masses. They have an intact basement membrane without extracapsular extension. These tumors may be difficult to distinguish from the solid variant of adenoid cystic carcinoma, but certain characteristics help with the distinction; lack of invasion into surrounding tissues, peripheral palisading of the outer basaloid cells, lack of perineural invasion, and a vascular stroma are unique characteristics of basal cell adenomas.

29.3.4 Oncocytoma

Oncocytes are large epithelial cells with a granular eosinophilic cytoplasm. The granular appearance is due to the large number of mitochondria in these cells, which can be identified on electron microscopy. These unusual tumors account for 1% of all salivary gland neoplasms and occur later in life with an equal predilection for men and women. They present as painless, solitary masses. Oncocytomas are most commonly found in the superficial lobe of the parotid gland but can occur in all of the salivary glands, as well as the pancreas, respiratory tract, thyroid, parathyroids, pituitary, adrenal glands, and kidneys.

Oncocytomas are usually well-circumscribed and encapsulated neoplasms that are pink or rust-colored. However, in minor salivary glands, the capsule is not present, which allows the tumors to be locally destructive. They can erode cartilage or bone but rarely metastasize. Benign oncocytomas must be differentiated from malignant salivary tumors with oncocytic components (i.e., adenoid cystic carcinoma, mucoepidermoid carcinoma, adenocarcinoma, and malignant oncytoma), as well as metastatic renal cell and thyroid carcinoma. The treatment for benign oncocytoma is surgical excision.

29.3.5 Hemangioma and Vascular Malformations

As stated above, the most common benign salivary gland lesions in children are hemangiomas. A more detailed description of hemangiomas is described elsewhere in this text, but in general, hemangiomas present in infancy and undergo a growth phase from 1 to 6 months of age followed by an involution phase that can last up to 12 years. Hemangiomas are more common in girls and are usually asymptomatic, unilateral, compressible masses. They occur most commonly in the parotid gland and can cause changes of the overlying skin.

On pathologic examination, they are dark red, lobulated tumors without a capsule. Histopathologically, they are composed of capillaries lined with proliferative endothelial cells. A full discussion of the treatment of these complicated tumors is beyond the scope of this chapter, but surgery is traditionally reserved for tumors that continue to proliferate despite medical therapy (steroids and more recently propranolol) and cause significant compressive, vascular, and/or cardiac symptoms.

Vascular malformations are different from hemangiomas in that they are not true neoplasms. They may be one of three types: venous malformations, arteriovenous malformations, or lymphatic malformations. Generally, these lesions are congenital and present at birth, and they continue to enlarge throughout life. Surgery of these lesions can be tedious and treacherous because they often invade locally and can bleed excessively. However, surgery currently remains the mainstay of treatment for vascular malformations of the salivary glands.

29.4 Applied Anatomy

As mentioned previously, these tumors are preferentially located in the superficial lobe of the parotid, followed by the submandibular glands and finally the sublingual and minor salivary glands. Surgical excision of primary benign salivary gland tumors remains the treatment of choice, and a detailed understanding of the usually consistent anatomy can result in largely complication-free surgical procedures.

Embryologically, the salivary glands start to form at 6 to 9 weeks of gestational age. The major salivary glands arise from ectodermal tissue, while the minor salivary glands arise from either ectodermal or endodermal tissue. The submandibular gland becomes encapsulated earlier than the parotid gland, which allows lymph nodes to be trapped in the parotid gland. This embryologic difference explains why lymphatic metastases may manifest within the substance of the parotid gland but not the submandibular gland.

The excretory unit of the salivary gland consists of acini and ducts. The acini secrete saliva that is either mucinous or serous, or both. The acini cells drain into the intercalated ducts, then the striated duct, and finally the excretory duct. Myoepithelial cells surround the acini and intercalated duct and serve to expel

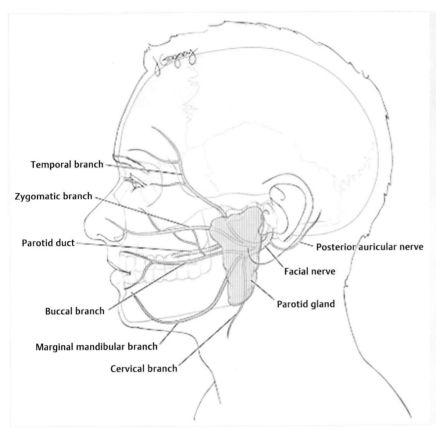

Fig. 29.1 Anatomy of the facial nerve as it exits the stylomastoid foramen and enters the parotid gland. The nerve is shown dividing into its various branches within the parotid parenchyma. Note that the Stensen duct travels with the buccal branch of the facial nerve.

Temporal branch

Zygomatic branch

Parotid duct

Buccal branch

Marginal mandibular branch

Cervical branch

Posterior auricular nerve

Facial nerve

Parotid gland

secretory products into the ductal system. The saliva from the parotid is predominately serous, the sublingual and minor salivary glands secrete mucinous saliva, and the submandibular gland has a mixed product.

29.4.1 Parotid Gland

The parotid gland is actually a single-lobe gland that is described as having a superficial and a deep lobe based on the surgical resection of glandular tissue lateral and medial to the facial nerve, respectively. The gland receives parasympathetic innervation from preganglionic fibers arising in the inferior salivatory nucleus, which travel with the glossopharyngeal nerve (cranial nerve [CN] IX) via the jugular foramen. Upon exiting the skull base, the preganglionic fibers leave CN IX to form the Jacobson nerve and reenter the skull via the inferior tympanic canaliculus. The fibers traverse the middle ear space over the cochlear promontory and exit the temporal bone superiorly as the lesser petrosal nerve. The lesser petrosal nerve exits the middle cranial fossa through the foramen ovale, where the preganglionic fibers synapse in the otic ganglion. The postganglionic fibers travel with the auriculotemporal nerve to supply the parotid gland.

The Stensen duct drains the parotid gland. It runs approximately 1 cm below the zygoma in a horizontal direction, often in close proximity to the buccal branch of the facial nerve (▶ Fig. 29.1). The duct penetrates anterior to the masseter muscle through the buccinator muscle, where it opens intraorally just opposite the second maxillary molar. The arterial

supply to the parotid gland is via the external carotid system, and it is drained by the posterior facial vein. As mentioned above, the parotid gland contains lymphatics within that drain to the jugular lymphatic chain.

The parotid gland is contained in what is termed the parotid compartment. The wedge-shaped parotid compartment is bounded superiorly by the zygomatic arch; anteriorly by the masseter muscle, lateral pterygoid muscle, and mandibular ramus; and inferiorly by the sternocleidomastoid muscle and posterior belly of the digastric muscle. The deep portion lies lateral to the parapharyngeal space, styloid process, stylomandibular ligament, and carotid sheath. The parotid fascia envelops the gland and suspends it from the zygoma. The parotid compartment contains the facial, auriculotemporal, and greater auricular nerves; the superficial temporal and posterior facial veins; and the external carotid, superficial temporal, and internal maxillary arteries.

The facial nerve (CN VII) exits the stylomastoid foramen and travels anterolaterally to enter the parotid gland. The nerve gives off motor branches to the posterior auricular muscle, posterior belly of the digastric muscle, and stylohyoid muscle before entering the gland (see ▶ Fig. 29.1). Immediately upon entering the gland, the facial nerve divides into two major branches (upper and lower) at the pes anserinus. Generally, the upper branch divides into the temporal and zygomatic branches, while the lower branch is subsequently responsible for the buccal, marginal mandibular, and cervical divisions. Knowledge of this anatomy is imperative for facial nerve preservation during parotid gland surgery.

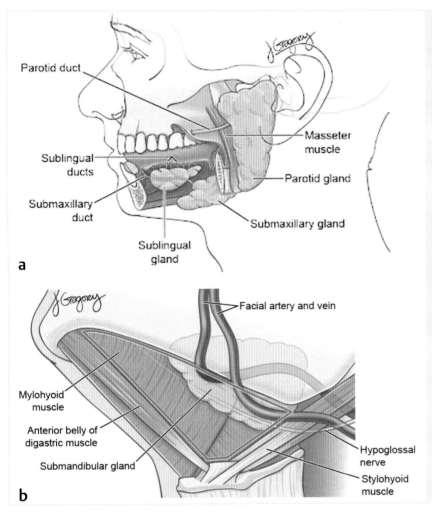

Fig. 29.2 (a) Major salivary glands. (b) Anatomy of the submandibular triangle and the important neurovascular structures in relation to the submandibular gland. The hypoglossal nerve is shown passing deep and inferior to the gland, while the facial artery and vein are deep and superior.

29.4.2 Submandibular Gland

The submandibular gland is located in the submandibular triangle, which is bound by the anterior and posterior bellies of the digastric muscle and the mandible. The gland receives preganglionic parasympathetic innervation from the superior salivatory nucleus. These fibers leave the brainstem and travel via the nervus intermedius to the facial nerve and then with the chorda tympani. The chorda tympani synapses in the submandibular ganglion and provides postsympathetic innervation. The submandibular ganglion is located just deep to the gland near the lingual nerve. The arterial supply is from the lingual and facial arteries, venous drainage is to the anterior facial veins, and lymphatic drainage is to the submandibular nodes. The Wharton duct, which drains the gland, passes between the mylohyoid and hyoglossus muscles along the genioglossus and enters the oral cavity just lateral to the frenulum of the tongue.

There are several important neurovascular structures surrounding the gland that must be preserved during removal (see ▶ Fig. 29.1 and ▶ Fig. 29.2). The marginal mandibular nerve lies superficial to the gland. The hypoglossal nerve is deep to the gland, inferior to the Wharton duct. The lingual nerve is superior to the gland and deep to the mylohyoid muscles. Finally, the facial artery sits deep to the gland, and only its branch to the gland should be ligated during excision.

29.4.3 Sublingual and Minor Salivary Glands

The sublingual gland is an unencapsulated gland that is situated medial to the mandible just above the mylohyoid muscle and deep to the floor of the mouth. The gland has 8 to 20 small ducts that penetrate the oral mucosa posterolateral to the Wharton duct. Innervation is via the same pathway as the submandibular gland, arterial supply is from the lingual artery, and lymphatic drainage is to the submental and submandibular nodes.

The minor salivary glands are scattered throughout the upper aerodigestive tract and number approximately 600 to 1,000. Each gland has a discrete opening into the oral cavity and functions as a separate unit.

29.5 The Disease Process

29.5.1 Etiology

The exact etiology of salivary gland neoplasms is not known. However, certain factors, such as radiation, smoking, and specific occupational exposures, have been shown to increase the risk for developing salivary gland tumors. A recent study found a 4.5-fold increase in the incidence of salivary gland cancer and a 2.6-fold increase in the incidence of benign tumors (especially

Warthin tumors) among persons exposed to head and neck irradiation. Warthin tumor is also strongly associated with cigarette smoking. Occupational exposure to silica dust and nitrosamines among rubber workers has been linked to an increased risk for cancer of the salivary glands.

29.5.2 Pathogenesis

There are two competing theories for the origin of salivary gland neoplasms: the bicellular stem cell theory and the multicellular theory. The multicellular theory implies simply that each tumor type arises from a specific, previously differentiated cell (e.g., pleomorphic adenomas arise from intercalated duct cells, oncocytomas from striated duct cells, and acinic cell carcinomas from acinar cells). The bicellular theory posits that tumors arise from either of two undifferentiated stem cells: the excretory duct reserve cell or the intercalated duct reserve cell. Intercalated stem cells give rise to pleomorphic adenomas, oncocytomas, adenoid cystic carcinomas, adenocarcinomas, and acinic cell carcinomas, whereas excretory stem cells give rise to squamous cell and mucoepidermoid carcinomas. The bicellular theory is supported by the presence of multiple cell types in pleomorphic adenomas and Warthin tumors.

29.5.3 Natural History and Progression

Overall, benign neoplasms of the salivary glands tend to enlarge slowly over a period of years. Despite their slow growth, patients may still report a "recent" growth. The vast majority are painless, with the notable exception of Warthin tumors, which will occasionally have an inflammatory component.

29.5.4 Potential Disease Complications

These neoplasms may cause cosmetic disfigurement, but functional obstruction generally develops only once they become very large. Deep lobe tumors may enlarge intraorally or into the parapharyngeal space and create dysphagia and/or trismus. Minor salivary gland tumors can also cause dysphagia and odynophagia in the oral cavity or oropharynx. If located in the nasal cavity or nasopharynx, they can cause obstructive sinusitis. Finally, laryngeal minor salivary glands can cause hoarseness and airway obstruction. If either the Stensen duct or Wharton duct is obstructed by a neoplasm, salivary backup and sialadenitis can develop in the parotid and submandibular glands, respectively. Oncocytomas may cause local destruction of cartilage or bone, and pleomorphic adenomas can undergo malignant transformation over time.

29.6 Disease Grading

There is no standard grading system for benign salivary gland tumors. See the earlier sections for discussion of the individual tumor types.

29.7 Presenting Complaints

Many diseases can affect the salivary glands, but most nonneoplastic causes can be excluded based on a thorough history. Autoimmune, inflammatory, and infectious diseases can all mimic neoplastic processes. Acute, diffuse painful swelling is usually associated with an infectious or inflammatory process. Bilateral disease is often associated with viral infection (i.e., HIV infection or mumps) or Sjögren syndrome. Infection is more common in those who are elderly, malnourished, immunocompromised, or dehydrated. Care should be taken not to assume, however, that a patient with these problems does not have a neoplasm because a salivary gland tumor, whether benign or malignant, can cause all of these symptoms.

Initial questioning should focus on the presentation of the mass, growth rate, changes in size or symptoms with meals, facial weakness or asymmetry, and associated pain. A firm, unilateral, slowly growing painless mass in the parotid is more often than not a benign neoplasm, whereas such a presentation in the submandibular gland is often due to chronic obstruction and inflammation. Questions about a history of smoking and toxin exposure should be asked, as well. Further description of possible patient complaints is discussed above.

29.8 Clinical Findings, Physical Examination

Patients with a salivary gland mass should undergo a thorough head and neck examination. Those with parotid neoplasms should undergo thorough palpation, including bimanual, intraoral palpation to ascertain involvement of the parapharyngeal space. A facial nerve examination should be performed and documented (even if normal) as part of the preoperative documentation. Submandibular gland neoplasms may sometimes be difficult to discern from diffuse gland enlargement but can be distinguished if freely mobile. Both submandibular and sublingual gland masses should also be assessed via bimanual palpation. The patient with a submandibular gland mass should also be assessed for any weakness or numbness of the tongue and weakness of the facial nerve, indicating perineural spread via the hypoglossal, lingual, and marginal mandibular nerves, respectively.

A benign neoplasm of the salivary gland will appear as a firm, well-circumscribed, freely mobile tumor on examination. Fixation to the surrounding structures or skin, nerve paresis or paralysis, regional lymphadenopathy, and local destruction are often associated with malignancies. Recall that minor salivary gland tumors are rarely benign, so these should be treated more aggressively.

29.9 Testing

Currently, the work-up for a salivary gland neoplasm can involve a combination of fine-needle aspiration biopsy and/or imaging. The use of these techniques is not disputed when the tumor occurs in an unusual location (i.e., parapharyngeal space) or where there is a high chance of malignancy. However, when a single, mobile, firm nodule presents in the superficial lobe of the parotid, the utility of these diagnostic procedures can be questioned.

29.9.1 Fine-Needle Aspiration Biopsy

Fine-needle aspiration biopsy is an extremely sensitive (86 to 99%) and specific (96 to 100%) tool when performed at an institution familiar with salivary gland neoplasms. The test is easily performed, safe, and relatively inexpensive. If the lesion is deep, the accuracy of the biopsy can be improved with the use of ultrasound. In general, fine-needle aspiration biopsy is a better test for benign lesions than for malignant ones because there are many lesions that can mimic malignancies on cytologic analysis.

Proponents of fine-needle aspiration biopsy state that the test can prevent surgery in patients with certain benign lesions (e.g., chronic inflammation, benign lymphoepithelial lesions), high-risk or elderly patients with benign lesions, and those with lymphoma. Also, the ability to plan preoperatively for an extensive cancer resection and counsel a patient regarding the potential morbidities and outcomes is a valuable asset that fine-needle aspiration biopsy provides. Opponents argue that if the patient's work-up is done properly, the test is not necessary on all lesions. Also, despite the general safety of the procedure when performed with a 25-gauge needle, Warthin tumors can become inflamed after the procedure, further complicating resection. Few would argue for the use of fine-needle aspiration biopsy in the submandibular gland or minor salivary gland areas because tumors in these glands are likely to be malignant or metastatic disease.

29.9.2 Imaging

When contemplating the use of imaging, a surgeon must consider how the use of this modality will alter the treatment plan. Although an argument can be made for fine-needle aspiration biopsy, a patient with a solitary, firm, mobile nodule of the parotid gland usually does not require any type of imaging study because this will rarely change the proposed surgery. If there is suspicion for a malignancy or the tumor involves any location other than the superficial lobe of the parotid, an imaging modality is clearly warranted.

The two most commonly used modalities for imaging salivary gland neoplasms are computed tomography (CT) and magnetic resonance (MR) imaging. CT should be performed with contrast, and the salivary glands are readily visualized with this modality. Encapsulated lesions can be identified easily with CT (▶ Fig. 29.3), but the various tumors cannot be distinguished from one another. Bilateral disease and cervical metastases are also readily appreciated on both MR imaging and CT, which can help with treatment planning. If readily available and not contraindicated, MR imaging is the study of choice for salivary gland neoplasms in any location. Dynamic contrast-enhanced MR imaging can be used to differentiate pleomorphic adenomas and Warthin tumors with a sensitivity of 100% and a specificity of 80%. Pleomorphic adenomas have a very high T2-signal intensity, whereas Warthin tumors display a highly characteristic necrotic, cystic component. MR imaging is also superior to CT in showing extraglandular extension, perineural invasion, parapharyngeal space involvement, and demarcation from the glandular tissue itself. Despite the accuracy of MR imaging, the only salivary gland neoplasm that can be definitively diagnosed via imaging is a lipoma. All others require a pathologic diagnosis.

Ultrasound is usually used for directing fine-needle aspiration biopsy in children and pregnant women. It can provide a quick, inexpensive evaluation of the tumor by helping to clarify whether the process is diffuse or isolated, cystic or solid, or vascular; identify margins; and potentially diagnose the tumor.

29.10 Differential Diagnosis

The differential includes all the lesions described above (see ▶ Table 29.1), the salivary gland malignancies discussed in the next chapter, and the various inflammatory processes discussed in the previous chapter.

29.11 Treatment: Surgical Excision

Currently, the only acceptable treatment for benign neoplasms of the salivary gland is surgical excision. Radiotherapy can be used for recurrent, multifocal disease. Observation is usually reserved for those patients who are high-risk surgical candidates. As a general principle, regardless of pathology, all benign tumors of the salivary glands require excision with a cuff of normal tissue to prevent recurrence.

29.11.1 Parotidectomy

A clear drape should be placed over the ipsilateral portion of the patient's face to allow adequate visualization to identify any intraoperative stimulation of the facial nerve muscles. The standard Blair parotidectomy incision is made in the preauricular crease, starting at the level of the root of the helix. The incision extends inferiorly around the lobule of the ear over the mastoid tip. It gently curves down along the sternocleidomastoid muscle and then slightly forward in a natural skin crease in the upper neck 1 to 2 finger breadths below the mandible. Skin flaps are elevated in the plane superficial to the parotid fascia in the preauricular region and in the subplatysmal plane in the cervical portion of the incision. The great auricular nerve and the external jugular vein are identified over the sternocleidomastoid muscle and may be divided to free the tail of the parotid gland.

Next, the posterior belly of the digastric muscle is exposed proximal to its attachment to the mastoid bone. The facial nerve will lie in the same plane superior to this muscle. The parotid gland is then dissected free of the auricular cartilage and retracted anteriorly. This exposes the tragal pointer; unless displaced by tumor, the facial nerve is usually located approximately 1 to 1.5 cm deep and inferior to the tragal pointer. A more constant landmark also used to identify the facial nerve is the tympanomastoid suture line, which runs approximately 6 to 8 mm superficial to the stylomastoid foramen. Finally, the facial nerve can also be identified by finding one of its peripheral branches and following it to the main trunk (see Box Methods of Facial Nerve Identification (p.248)).

Methods of Facial Nerve Identification

- Superior to the posterior belly of the digastric muscle
- 1 to 1.5 cm deep and inferior to the tragal pointer
- Deep to the tympanomastoid suture line
- Retrograde dissection along peripheral branch of facial nerve

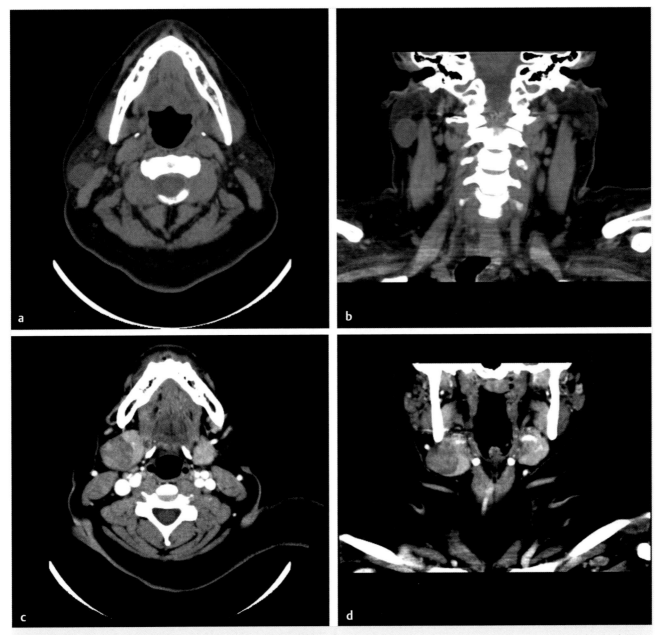

Fig. 29.3 (**a**) Axial and (**b**) coronal computed tomographic scans of the neck with intravenous contrast in a patient with a right-sided parotid pleomorphic adenoma. (**c**) Axial and (**d**) coronal slices in a patient with a right-sided submandibular pleomorphic adenoma. Note that the tumors are well encapsulated with clearly delineated borders and do not invade the surrounding structures.

Once the facial nerve is identified, the branches are traced peripherally, and the parotid tissue overlying it can be dissected free and resected. If the tumor abuts the facial nerve, the neoplasm should be meticulously dissected from the nerve with a scalpel. The facial nerve should never be sacrificed for benign disease. If the tumor extends to the deep lobe, a total parotidectomy may be indicated, requiring deep dissection between the peripheral branches of the nerve.

Complications

Facial nerve injury can range from neurapraxia to complete transection. Temporary dysfunction is fairly common (46%), but permanent paralysis is rare (4%) after parotid surgery. The transient weakness is usually due to traction on the nerve and will often resolve within days. However, it can take up to a few months, and proper eye care measures should be taken if complete weakness is noted. If a portion of the nerve or the entire nerve is transected and this is noted intraoperatively, a primary neurorrhaphy or nerve cable graft should be performed to optimize the outcome.

Frey syndrome occurs when the disrupted postganglionic, parasympathetic fibers to the parotid gland cross-innervate the sympathetic fibers to the sweat glands. This results in gustatory sweating, which is flushing and sweating of the ipsilateral facial skin during mastication. The exact percentage of patients in whom this actually occurs is unknown, but rarely are the symptoms severe enough to require treatment. A glycopyrrolate roll-on antiperspirant, botulinum toxin A injections, and tympanic neuronectomy have all been described to treat Frey syndrome. Placing an autologous or cadaveric acellular dermal graft or expanded polytetrafluoroethylene (e-PTFE) sheet under the skin after removal of the parotid gland has also been described to prevent postoperative gustatory sweating.

Other common complications are sensory deficits due to great auricular nerve sacrifice, hematoma, and sialoceles. Great auricular nerve sacrifice is overall well tolerated. Hematomas should be addressed immediately to prevent skin flap necrosis. Sialoceles can be managed conservatively with aspiration and pressure dressings.

29.11.2 Submandibular Gland Excision

A 3- to 4-cm incision is marked, preferably in a neck skin crease approximately 2 to 3 cm below the inferior border of the mandible overlying the gland. The incision is carried down through the platysma layer, and small subplatysmal flaps are created inferiorly and superiorly, with care taken to avoid injuring the marginal mandibular branch of the facial nerve. The nerve lies immediately beneath the deep cervical fascia and can be identified crossing the anterior facial vein. The vein is ligated well below the nerve, and upward retraction of the transected vein displaces the nerve superiorly, protecting it from injury. In managing bulky tumors or malignancy, positive identification and dissection of the marginal mandibular branch provide wider exposure and allow complete excision of the level I lymph nodes.

The facial artery is then divided as it approaches the mandible, freeing the superior portion of the gland. The submandibular gland is dissected free of its anterior attachment to the mylohyoid muscles. The mylohyoid muscle is retracted medially while the gland is pulled laterally and outward. This maneuver exposes the undersurface of the submandibular gland and reveals the hypoglossal nerve inferiorly, the lingual nerve superiorly, and the Wharton duct. These structures lie superficial to the hyoglossus muscle. The contributions of the lingual nerve to the submandibular gland and the Wharton duct are both ligated. The facial artery is ligated again near the external carotid, and the submandibular gland is removed.

Complications

The major complications of submandibular gland excision arise when either the lingual or hypoglossal nerve is injured or transected. Although rare, injury results in unilateral tongue paresthesia (lingual) and paresis/paralysis (hypoglossal). Hematoma and sialocele are also common complications and are dealt with as they are in the parotid gland.

29.11.3 Parapharyngeal Space Tumor Excision

The approach to the surgical excision of salivary gland tumors within the parapharyngeal space is based on the location and size of the tumor. For a smaller tumor in the deep lobe of the parotid or inferior part of the parapharyngeal space, a parotid incision with further cervical extension is made. First, a superficial parotidectomy is performed if the tumor involves the deep lobe of the parotid. If not, only the inferior portion of the facial nerve is identified and preserved. Further dissection involves identification and preservation of the internal and external carotid arteries, internal jugular vein, and CNs IX, X, XI, and XII. The stylomandibular ligament is divided, and the styloid process can be resected to deliver larger tumors. In patients with very large tumors or those located at the skull base, the addition of a mandibulotomy may be needed.

29.12 Prognosis

After surgical excision with a cuff of normal tissue, the patient with a benign salivary gland neoplasm can usually be considered cured. The recurrence rate for pleomorphic adenoma is less than 5%, with the other tumor types demonstrating similar responses to therapy. Recurrence of pleomorphic adenoma remains particularly troublesome, as mentioned previously. Overall, the prognosis of these patients is excellent.

29.13 Roundsmanship

- Of all salivary tumors, 75% are located in the parotid gland, and 75% of those are benign.
- The 25/50/75 rule: as the size of the gland decreases (parotid, submandibular, sublingual/minor salivary glands), the likelihood that a salivary neoplasm is malignant increases.
- Pleomorphic adenomas make up 75% of all benign lesions. They can become malignant over time, and postsurgical recurrence is difficult to treat.
- Warthin tumors can be bilateral and are the only benign tumors that can present with pain.
- Surgical resection is the mainstay of treatment for benign salivary gland neoplasms. Cranial nerves should never be sacrificed during excisions.
- Preoperative fine-needle aspiration biopsy is generally accepted as the standard of care. However, imaging is not necessary in a tumor that is isolated, superficial, mobile, and small. MR imaging is the imaging modality of choice.

29.14 Recommended Reading

[1] Hanna EY, Lee S, Fan CY, Suen JY. Benign neoplasms of the salivary gland. In: Cummings CW, Flint PW, Haughey BH, et al, eds. Cummings Otolaryngology: Head and Neck Surgery. 4th ed. Philadelphia, PA: Elsevier Mosby; 2005:chap 60

[2] Mendenhall WM, Mendenhall CM, Werning JW, Malyapa RS, Mendenhall NP. Salivary gland pleomorphic adenoma. Am J Clin Oncol 2008; 31: 95–99

[3] Sadetzki S, Oberman B, Mandelzweig L et al. Smoking and risk of parotid gland tumors: a nationwide case-control study. Cancer 2008; 112: 1974–1982

[4] Thoeny HC. Imaging of salivary gland tumours. Cancer Imaging 2007; 7: 52–62

30 Malignant Neoplasms of the Salivary Glands

Vikas Mehta and Stimson P. Schantz

30.1 Introduction

Malignant neoplasms of the salivary glands account for only 6% of all head and neck malignancies, with an incidence of 11.65 per 1 million people per year in the United States. There are more than 20 different histologic subtypes of malignant salivary gland tumors, not including the various cancers that can metastasize to the salivary glands. In the majority of patients, the presenting symptoms are exactly the same as in those with benign salivary gland disease. All of these factors contribute to the difficulty and confusion that exists in the treatment of these rare entities. This chapter will focus on the more common salivary gland malignancies and the currently accepted standards of care.

30.2 Incidence

Approximately 1 per 100,000 people per year will develop a salivary gland malignancy. The epidemiology of malignant salivary gland tumors varies based on age, sex, and tumor location. The majority of salivary gland carcinomas occur in the parotid gland (accounting for 25% of parotid gland neoplasms). Mucoepidermoid carcinoma is the most common malignant neoplasm of the salivary glands (29 to 43% of all salivary malignancies). Of mucoepidermoid carcinomas, 70% occur in the parotid gland, so that it is the most common malignancy in this location. Adenoid cystic carcinoma and adenocarcinoma are the second and third most common types, accounting for 20% and 14% of all salivary gland malignancies, respectively. However, adenoid cystic carcinoma is the most common malignancy of the minor salivary glands and submandibular gland.

Salivary gland malignancies occur much more often (3- to 5-fold higher frequency) in patients older than 50 years of age, but they are distributed equally in males and females. Of the more common tumor types, squamous cell carcinoma occurs more often in older patients and in males. Acinic cell carcinoma and adenoid cystic carcinoma are more common in female patients and younger patients. Risk factors for salivary gland malignancies include smoking, alcohol intake, irradiation, and certain occupational and environmental exposures, with the exact etiology to be discussed elsewhere.

30.3 Terminology

Salivary gland malignancies are classified according to histologic subtype. A list of the more common malignancies is provided in ▶ Table 30.1 with their relative frequencies. A full discussion of all tumor subtypes is beyond a scope of this chapter. As discussed in the previous chapter, if one subscribes to the bicellular theory of tumor origin, the tumors that arise from the intercalated duct (adenocarcinoma, adenoid cystic carcinoma) tend to be less aggressive than those arising from the excretory duct (squamous cell carcinoma and mucoepidermoid carcinoma).

30.3.1 Mucoepidermoid Carcinoma

Mucoepidermoid carcinoma occurs most commonly in the parotid gland, accounting for 8% of all parotid tumors. When it occurs in the minor salivary glands, the buccal mucosa and palate are the two most common sites. Mucoepidermoid carcinomas contain two different cell types: mucous cells and epidermoid cells. Based on the relative cellular composition of the tumors, they are classified into low-, intermediate-, and high-grade tumors. Low-grade tumors have a larger percentage of mucous cells, whereas epidermoid cells are much more prevalent in high-grade malignancies, which can be difficult to distinguish from squamous cell carcinoma. Only special staining for the few mucoid cells present will distinguish these two neoplasms.

On gross examination, low-grade tumors tend to be small and mostly encapsulated, with cystic components. High-grade tumors are large and infiltrative, lack a definitive capsule, and frequently have lymphatic metastases. On histologic examination, the presence of four or more mitotic figures per 10 high-power fields, perineural invasion, necrosis, a small cystic component, and cellular anaplasia indicate high-grade behavior.

The prognostic significance of tumor grade has been demonstrated in several studies. The 5-year survival rates for the three grades in one study were 95%, 72%, and 0%, respectively. At 10 years, the majority of patients with low-grade neoplasms remain free of disease (80 to 90%), whereas a much larger percentage of patients with high-grade disease either have died or have recurrence locally or in regional nodes. Likewise, the histologic grade determines the adjuvant treatment required for each patient. Despite the improved outcome, patients with low-grade tumors may have recurrence more than 15 years after initial treatment, so that significant long-term follow-up is required regardless of tumor grade.

30.3.2 Adenoid Cystic Carcinoma

Adenoid cystic carcinoma is the second most common malignancy of the salivary glands and the most common in the submandibular and minor salivary glands. Adenoid cystic carcinoma occurs most frequently in the oral cavity, with the palate

Table 30.1 Malignant salivary gland neoplasms and their relative frequencies

Malignant salivary gland neoplasms	Relative frequency
Mucoepidermoid carcinoma	34.4%
Adenoid cystic carcinoma	22.0%
Adenocarcinoma	17.6%
Carcinoma ex-pleomorphic adenoma	12.6%
Acinic cell carcinoma	6.6%
Squamous cell carcinoma	4.1%
Other	2.7%

the predominant subsite. Grossly, the tumors are nonencapsulated and infiltrate the surrounding tissues. There are three different histologic subtypes of adenoid cystic carcinoma: solid, cribriform, and tubular. Solid tumors demonstrate sheets of neoplastic epithelial cells with few cystic spaces. The tubular pattern is characterized by cells arranged in small ducts and tubules. The cribriform subtype has a many cystic spaces with basophilic mucus filling the spaces. Adenoid cystic neoplasms may contain all three subtypes, but usually one predominates. The solid pattern carries the worst prognosis, and the cribriform type usually has the best outcome.

Adenoid cystic carcinoma is known for its slow growth, perineural invasion, and distant metastasis. This tumor is notoriously difficult to eradicate and can recur locally or distantly (most often in the lungs) one to two decades after treatment. The 5-year survival rate is 65% because of the slow growth of the tumor, and patients can live for many years, even after recurrences are detected. However, adenoid cystic carcinoma does carry a 15-year survival rate of 12%. Regional node metastases are rare (12%), so there is often no need to address the cervical nodes. Treatment involves surgical resection, with postoperative radiation showing moderate benefit.

30.3.3 Acinic Cell Carcinoma

Acinic cell carcinoma is a rare form of malignancy comprising only 6 to 8% of all salivary gland malignancies. The tumor originates from serous cells, accounting for its high prevalence in the parotid gland. Acinic cell tumors are encapsulated, hard, gray–white tumors made up of lobules of round, uniform-appearing cells with abundant cytoplasm arranged in nests. Occasionally, they will have a clear cytoplasm, resulting in their alternative name—clear cell carcinoma.

Overall, acinic cell carcinomas tend to carry the best prognosis. Recently, evidence has demonstrated that there may be different grades of these tumors with varying prognoses. Facial pain or paralysis, deep lobe invasion, and/or multiple cervical metastases are all associated with a significantly worse outcome. The 5-, 10-, and 15-year survival rates are 83%, 76%, and 65% respectively. These tumors are treated with surgical resection and neck dissection if clinical nodes are evident.

30.3.4 Malignant Mixed Tumor

The term *malignant mixed tumor* refers to three distinct entities: carcinoma ex-pleomorphic adenoma, carcinosarcoma, and metastasizing mixed tumor. These tumors collectively account for 5 to 12% of all salivary gland malignancies and are distinct entities with unique behaviors. As mentioned in the previous chapter, pleomorphic adenoma carries a 1 to 1.5% per year chance of degeneration into carcinoma ex-pleomorphic adenoma. On gross examination, the tumor is firm, unencapsulated, and necrotic, with areas of hemorrhage. Patients report a long-standing, stable mass that has started to enlarge rapidly. The lesions are most often located in the parotid and microscopically show a malignant process within a pleomorphic adenoma. The 5-, 10-, and 15-year survival rates are 40%, 29%, and 19%, respectively, with a significant number of patients developing cervical and distant (especially bone and lung) metastases. Patients with submandibular or minor salivary gland disease often fare worse.

Carcinosarcomas, or true mixed tumors, are very rare and carry an even worse prognosis. One series showed a 5-year survival rate of 50%, which dropped to 30% over 10 years. Finally, metastasizing mixed tumors (metastasizing benign pleomorphic adenomas) are most common in the parotid gland and are unusual in that both the primary tumor tissue and metastatic (typically seen in bones and the lungs) tumor tissue appear benign on histopathologic examination. Patients can even develop distant metastasis, but few die of their disease. For all of these tumors, surgical resection remains the treatment of choice, and postoperative radiation is indicated for carcinosarcoma and carcinoma ex-pleomorphic adenoma.

30.3.5 Adenocarcinoma

Adenocarcinoma was traditionally described as any carcinoma arising from the salivary duct unit and accounted for almost 20% of all salivary gland malignancies. However, as the understanding of salivary gland tumors evolved, three distinct tumors within this larger group were identified and noted to behave differently clinically. What is now referred to as an adenocarcinoma (or adenocarcinoma "not otherwise specified") accounts for 1 to 9% of all salivary gland malignancies. This rare tumor (68% occur in the minor salivary glands) is quite aggressive, with a 50% recurrence rate; cervical metastases occur 17% of the time, and 5-year survival rates are less than 40%. Tumors have been subclassified into adenocarcinoma, mucinous adenocarcinoma, papillary adenocarcinoma, trabecular adenocarcinoma, and sebaceous adenocarcinoma.

Polymorphous low-grade adenocarcinoma (also known as terminal duct carcinoma) is the general exception to salivary gland malignancies in terms of clinical course. As the name suggests, patients with this indolent variant of adenocarcinoma demonstrate a 10-year survival rate of more than 90%. The tumors occur primarily in the oral cavity, with the palate and lip the most common locations. The rate of cervical metastasis is less than 5%, and the tumors rarely recur after wide local excision. Adjuvant therapy and neck dissection are rarely indicated and have not been shown to improve outcomes.

Salivary duct carcinoma is at the opposite end of the spectrum from terminal duct carcinoma. This highly aggressive malignancy predominantly affects males in their seventies and presents in the parotid with cervical metastases (50%). On histologic analysis, islands of tumor cells with comedonecrosis appear similar to mammary duct carcinoma. Salivary duct carcinoma tends to recur both locally and distally, so that patients require total parotidectomy, neck dissection, and adjuvant chemoradiation.

30.3.6 Squamous Cell Carcinoma

Squamous cell carcinoma of the salivary glands is almost always metastatic from the skin, external auditory canal, or upper aerodigestive tract. Additionally, high-grade mucoepidermoid carcinoma is difficult to distinguish from squamous cell carcinoma. These factors make true primary salivary gland squamous cell carcinoma a rare entity. It occurs most often in the parotid gland. Cervical metastasis is present in 46% of patients, and 30% have occult cervical disease. Patients often develop local and regional recurrences, and the 5-year survival is only

24%. Treatment should involve radical resection, neck dissection, and postoperative radiation.

30.3.7 Lymphoma and Metastatic Carcinoma

Neoplastic disease in the salivary gland does not always originate from the salivary gland itself. Lymphoma can arise primarily in the lymphatics surrounding the tissue or can represent systemic disease. This most often occurs in the parotid, and patients with Sjögren disease have a 40-fold increased risk for developing primary lymphomas in the parotid. Chemotherapy and/or radiation remain the mainstay of treatment except for MALT (mucosa-associated lymphoid tissue) lymphoma, which can also be treated with surgical excision.

Metastatic spread (lymphatic or hematogenous) to the parotid and submandibular glands may occur. The parotid is most at risk for lymphatic spread from cutaneous malignancies of the scalp and face, while metastases to the submandibular gland are likely to come from the oral cavity and oropharynx. The most likely culprits for distant metastasis to the salivary glands are kidney, lung, and prostate malignancies.

30.4 Applied Anatomy

See the previous chapter for anatomical descriptions of the salivary glands.

30.5 The Disease Process

30.5.1 Etiology

Little is understood about the exact etiology of salivary gland malignancies. However, several risk factors have been identified, with exposure to ionizing radiation the most common and often described. An increased risk has been demonstrated in atomic fallout survivors in Japan, patients treated with radiation for Hodgkin lymphoma, those imaged with full-mouth dental X-rays (while those imaged with Panorex X-rays did not), and those who received radiation in childhood for both benign and malignant conditions. The exact dose required to increase the risk is unknown, but the correlation is evident.

Other risk factors include working in the rubber industry, cooking with kerosene fuel, exposure to nickel alloy, exposure to silica dust, and use of hair dye. Tobacco and alcohol have not been shown to be specific risk factors for salivary gland malignancy but do increase the risk for salivary gland lesions. Finally, Sjögren disease drastically predisposes a person to developing primary lymphoma of the parotid gland. The most common location and type of induced malignancy among patients exposed to irradiation is a parotid mucoepidermoid carcinoma.

30.5.2 Pathogenesis

The competing theories for the origin of salivary gland tumors are the bicellular stem theory and the multicellular theory. Of these two, recent evidence has suggested that the bicellular theory is more likely to be correct. For a further in-depth discussion of these theories, the reader is referred to the preceding chapter.

30.5.3 Natural History and Progression

The most common initial presentation of a salivary gland malignancy is a firm, solitary, painless mass. Clinically, it is often difficult to distinguish a malignant from a benign lesion. Usually, the lesion has been enlarging slowly over time. In the parotid or submandibular gland, the lesion will be an asymptomatic mass. Minor salivary gland tumors can cause obstructive symptoms, depending on their location. If located in the oral cavity or oropharynx, they can cause dysphagia or dysphonia. In the nasal cavity, enlargement can lead to sinusitis or nasal obstruction. Laryngeal masses can cause airway obstruction, dysphonia, and dysphagia.

Malignant lesions of the salivary glands will cause specific symptoms in 25% of patients, and the presence of symptoms often indicates an advanced lesion. The most common symptoms are pain and nerve palsies. A parotid neoplasm can cause a facial nerve palsy, which dramatically decreases the chance of survival; the 10-year survival rate of patients with facial nerve palsies is 12%. The proximity of the submandibular gland to the lingual and hypoglossal nerves may result in specific neurologic tongue deficits. Constant pain is usually associated with a malignancy, whereas intermittent pain can be due to obstruction of drainage pathways with associated inflammation. Other common symptoms include bleeding, trismus, fixation, loosening of dentition, and paresthesias.

Malignant lesions will progress to regional and distant metastases, depending on their histology. In general, high-grade mucoepidermoid carcinoma, salivary duct carcinoma, carcinoma ex-pleomorphic adenoma, and adenocarcinoma all carry a significant risk for cervical metastases, and therefore treatment of the regional nodes is warranted. Distant metastasis is likely to occur in lung and bone. Spread to these tissues is possible with all types of salivary gland malignancy (especially in the long term) but most notoriously occurs in adenoid cystic tumors. More specific descriptions of the natural progression of each tumor type can be found in the respective sections on histology.

30.5.4 Potential Disease Complications

As previously mentioned, the possible complications of salivary gland malignancies depend on the location of the tumor and on the tumor type and grade. Despite aggressive treatment, many tumors recur, and patients die of their disease. Often, the sequelae occur years after treatment, and therefore these patients require life-long follow-up.

30.6 Disease Staging

The most recent American Joint Commission on Cancer (AJCC) staging system was released in 2010, and salivary gland malignancies are staged based on the TNM (tumor node metastasis) system.

T1 primaries are smaller than 2 cm and T2 lesions are between 2 and 4 cm, both without extraparenchymal extension. T3 lesions are larger than 4 cm and/or have extended beyond the gland. T4a lesions invade skin, mandible, external auditory canal, and/or the facial nerve, while T4b lesions invade the skull base or pterygoid plates and/or encase the carotid artery.

N1 status implies involvement of a single lymph node that is ipsilateral and smaller than 3 cm. N2a indicates involvement of a single ipsilateral lymph node that is larger than 3 cm but smaller than 6 cm. N2b disease is the involvement of multiple ipsilateral nodes, none larger than 6 cm, and N2c disease is involvement of contralateral or bilateral nodes, none larger than 6 cm. N3 status is reserved for nodal disease larger than 6 cm.

Stage I disease indicates T1 lesions, and stage II disease indicates T2 lesions, both without nodal or distant metastasis. A T3 lesion without metastasis and T1–T3 lesions with N1 disease are classified as stage III disease. T4a primary lesions with N0–N1 nodal status or T1–T3 or T4a lesions with N2 nodes are stage IVA. T4b primary lesions with any N status or any T status with N3 disease is stage IVB. Any distant metastasis is classified as stage IVC.

The 5-year survival rates are 85% for stage I tumors, 66% for stage II, 53% for stage III, and 32% for stage IV. These figures suggest the poor outcome associated with large nodal disease, nerve involvement, extraparenchymal or extracapsular spread, and distant metastasis. The major flaw of the AJCC staging system is that it does not include the histopathologic subtype, which, as discussed above, can vastly change the survival rate of patients with the malignancy. As more information is gathered about these rare malignant neoplasms, the survival data for each neoplastic subtype will be extrapolated and further clarified. It is hoped that, as was done with thyroid cancer, tumor subtype will be included in the next classification scheme.

30.7 Presenting Complaints

As discussed in the chapter on benign salivary gland tumors, many diseases can mimic a salivary gland tumor. Eliciting a thorough history can tease out many of these nonneoplastic forms of salivary gland pathology. However, every unilateral salivary gland mass should be treated as a possible malignancy unless proven otherwise, especially if it occurs in the sublingual or minor salivary glands. Seventy-five percent of patients with a malignant salivary gland neoplasm will present with a painless, firm, solitary mass, making it difficult to distinguish a malignant lesion from a benign one. Pain, fixation, cervical adenopathy, trismus, paresthesias, paralysis, bleeding, and loose dentition are all signs of advanced malignancy and warrant a more aggressive work-up and early intervention.

30.8 Clinical Findings, Physical Examination

A patient with a salivary gland mass should undergo a thorough head and neck examination. Those with parotid neoplasms should undergo thorough palpation, including bimanual, intraoral palpation. A facial nerve examination should be performed and documented because it is important not only for ruling out malignant disease but also for preoperative documentation. Submandibular gland neoplasms are difficult to discern from diffuse gland enlargement but can be distinguished if freely mobile.

Both submandibular and sublingual gland masses should also be assessed via bimanual palpation. In addition, the patient with a submandibular gland mass should be assessed for any weakness or numbness of the tongue and facial nerve weakness, indicating perineural spread via the hypoglossal, lingual, and marginal mandibular nerves, respectively. If the tumor occurs in the nasal cavity, an assessment of ocular function and visualization of the skull base are important. Any tumor of the pharynx or larynx mandates a fiber-optic examination and documentation of vocal cord function.

30.9 Testing

Fine-needle aspiration biopsy and imaging are the two modalities used to evaluate salivary gland tumors. Their use in patients with solitary, mobile, well-circumscribed, superficial parotid tumors is controversial. However, any other salivary gland lesion, especially those that are suspected malignancies, warrants preoperative testing to guide treatment properly.

30.9.1 Biopsy

Fine-needle aspiration biopsy is a highly sensitive and specific test that many argue is an essential preoperative tool. Tissue sampling is the only way to confirm a malignancy, and fine-needle aspiration is simple to perform and requires no anesthesia. Proponents of fine-needle aspiration biopsy state that its use helps in counseling patients before surgery if a malignancy is identified. However, most physicians would agree that major treatment decisions (i.e., deep lobe dissection, facial nerve sacrifice, chemoradiation vs surgical resection) should be made only after an open biopsy. Frozen section, although highly sensitive and specific, is not 100% accurate. It is therefore prudent to await the results of the permanent histologic diagnosis and appropriately discuss the expected surgical outcome with the patient. Tumors that are readily accessible (oral and nasal) can be biopsied with standard techniques.

30.9.2 Imaging

The two most commonly used modalities for imaging salivary gland neoplasms are computed tomography (CT) and magnetic resonance (MR) imaging. CT should be performed with contrast, and the salivary glands are readily visualized with this modality. Also, the interface between soft tissue and bone can be interpreted on CT. Encapsulated lesions can be identified easily with CT, but the various tumors cannot be distinguished from one another. Bilateral disease and cervical metastases are also readily appreciated on both MR imaging and CT, which can help with treatment planning. If readily available and not contraindicated, MR imaging is the study of choice for salivary gland neoplasms in any location. MR imaging is superior to CT in showing extraglandular extension, perineural invasion, parapharyngeal space involvement, and demarcation from the glandular tissue itself. MR imaging does not identify bony involvement as readily as CT but can show bone marrow extension. Despite the accuracy of MR imaging, the only salivary gland neoplasm that can be definitively diagnosed via imaging is a lipoma. All others require pathologic diagnosis.

In positron emission tomography (PET)–CT, the pattern of radionuclide uptake by cancerous tissue is superimposed on anatomical CT images, and PET-CT has become widely used in many different cancers. A recent article found PET-CT to be both highly specific and sensitive for salivary gland malignancy. However, CT alone was comparable in its ability to diagnose malignancy and distant metastasis. PET-CT was most useful in determining the resectability of high-grade malignancy and whether adjuvant or palliative treatment would be indicated.

30.10 Differential Diagnosis

The differential diagnosis for a salivary gland mass includes all of the malignant subtypes discussed above, the benign neoplasms mentioned in the previous chapter, and various nonneoplastic causes that are addressed elsewhere in this book. It is important to rule out a benign or nonneoplastic cause before any major resection of these rare entities is considered.

30.11 Treatment

Besides lymphoma, the current primary treatment modality for malignant tumors of the salivary glands is surgical excision. Adjuvant therapy and cervical node dissection may be implemented based on tumor stage and histology.

30.11.1 Surgical Excision

Based on the location of the tumor, the appropriate surgical excision with clear margins is indicated. For more detailed descriptions of salivary gland surgery, the reader is referred to the surgical descriptions in the chapter on benign neoplasms of the salivary glands. If facial nerve sacrifice is required, an attempt at primary anastomosis should be made. If the segment removed is too long to achieve a tension-free closure, a nerve graft should be attempted while the nerve is exposed. An in-depth description of all facial nerve rehabilitation techniques is beyond the scope of this chapter.

Cervical lymphadenectomy is reserved for those cases in which there is obvious disease, either palpable or seen on imaging, or in which the risk for regional metastasis of the tumor subtype is high. If an elective node dissection is to be performed, the surgeon can perform a selective node dissection and reserve more comprehensive cervical lymphadenectomy for those patients with nodal disease. In general, ipsilateral level I through III dissection is sufficient for tumors larger than 4 cm, squamous cell carcinoma, adenocarcinoma, undifferentiated carcinoma, and high-grade mucoepidermoid carcinoma of the parotid. Selective neck dissections for minor salivary gland tumors will differ depending on the location.

30.11.2 Adjuvant Therapy

Radiation and chemotherapy are reserved for those patients with stage III or IV tumors or those with aggressive histology or features. Radiation therapy has been shown to have a greater positive impact on locoregional control than on overall survival. However, better locoregional control has been shown to improve overall quality of life, making it an important factor to consider. Adenoid cystic carcinoma remains highly resistant to radiation treatment, although some promise has been shown with neutron-based irradiation. Chemoradiation has been shown to improve survival for advanced-stage salivary gland malignancies but increases the morbidity and mortality associated with treatment.

30.12 Prognosis

The long-term prognosis remains fairly dismal for patients with most salivary gland malignancies, depending on the tumor stage and histology.

30.13 Roundsmanship

- The most common salivary gland malignancy is mucoepidermoid carcinoma, and the most common location is the parotid gland.
- Adenoid cystic carcinoma is the second most common malignant neoplasm and the most common submandibular and minor salivary gland malignancy.
- High-grade mucoepidermoid carcinoma, squamous cell carcinoma, adenocarcinoma, and carcinoma ex-pleomorphic adenoma require elective neck dissection because of the high rates of cervical metastasis.
- Adenoid cystic carcinoma is notorious for lung metastasis and perineural spread, which can occur more than 15 years after treatment.

30.14 Recommended Reading

[1] Major salivary glands. In: Edge SB, Byrd DR, Compton CC, et al. American Joint Committee on Cancer (AJCC) Cancer Staging Manual. 7th ed. New York, NY: Springer; 2010:103–109

[2] Aro K, Leivo I, Mäkitie AA. Management and outcome of patients with mucoepidermoid carcinoma of major salivary gland origin: a single institution's 30-year experience. Laryngoscope 2008; 118: 258–262

[3] Boukheris H, Ron E, Dores GM, Stovall M, Smith SA, Curtis RE. Risk of radiation-related salivary gland carcinoma among survivors of Hodgkin's lymphoma: a population-based analysis. Cancer 2008; 113; (11): 3153–3159

[4] Simental A. Malignant neoplasms of the salivary gland. In: Cummings CW, Flint PW, Harker LA, et al. Cummings Otolaryngology: Head and Neck Surgery. 4th ed. Philadelphia, PA: Elsevier Mosby; 2005

[5] Thoeny HC. Imaging of salivary gland tumours. Cancer Imaging 2007; 7: 52–62

31 Diseases and Neoplasms of the Thyroid

Nisha Jayani and Monica Dorin Schwarcz

31.1 Thyroid Physiology

The thyroid gland regulates metabolism and thermogenesis within the body via thyroid hormones. Numerous spherical follicles (▶ Fig. 31.1) make up the thyroid gland, with parafollicular (or C cells) interspersed throughout the gland. The follicles are composed of a single layer of secretory epithelial cells called follicular cells, which secrete into their center proteinaceous colloid. Colloid contains thyroglobulin, which is the substrate involved in thyroid hormone synthesis. When the thyroid is actively synthesizing and secreting thyroid hormone, the follicles swell and increase in size.

31.1.1 Thyroid Hormone Production

At the follicular lumen, iodine is oxidized through an organification reaction with thyroid peroxidase and hydrogen peroxide. The reactive iodine atoms rapidly attach to tyrosyl residues in thyroglobulin to form iodotyrosines (mono- or diiodotyrosine). Thyroid peroxidase also joins iodotyrosine residues via an ether linkage, which produces T_3 or T_4, depending on the number of iodine atoms present in a reaction called coupling. Thyroid hormones may be released into the bloodstream, and thyroglobulin is taken back into the follicular cell. Thyroid hormone synthesis is summarized in ▶ Fig. 31.2.

31.1.2 Thyroid-Stimulating Hormone Action

Thyroid-stimulating hormone (TSH) regulates thyroid function via the TSH receptor, which is a 7-transmembrane G protein–coupled receptor on the basolateral surface of follicular cells. The TSH receptor is coupled to the α subunit of the G protein, which activates adenylyl cyclase, thereby increasing cyclic adenosine monophosphate (cAMP) production. This action leads to thyroglobulin resorption from the lumen of the follicle and proteolysis within the cells, allowing the release of produced thyroid hormones into the bloodstream. TSH also stimulates phospholipase C, causing increased phosphatidylinositol turnover. Thyrotropin-releasing hormone (TRH), from the hypothalamus, stimulates TSH release from the pituitary gland. Excess circulating thyroid hormone inhibits the release of TSH via T_3 receptors in the pituitary gland. Other molecules, such as insulin-like growth factor-1, epidermal growth factor, transforming growth factor-β, endothelins, and various cytokines, also regulate thyroid hormone synthesis.

31.1.3 Thyroid Hormone Transport and Metabolism

The thyroid secretes approximately 20 times as much T_4 as T_3. T_3 has a shorter half-life than T_4. Both are bound to plasma proteins, which increase the pool of circulating hormone, delay hormone clearance, and modulate hormone delivery to selected tissues. These plasma proteins include thyroxine-binding globulin, transthyretin, and albumin. Thyroxine-binding globulin has the highest affinity for the thyroid hormones, and although it is present at a low concentration in the plasma, it carries approximately 80% of the bound hormone. In contrast, albumin has a low affinity for thyroid hormones but has a higher concentration in the plasma. Transthyretin carries the smallest amount of the bound thyroid hormones.

There are several deiodinases that convert T_4 to T_3. Type I deiodinase has a lower affinity for T_4 and is found predominantly in the thyroid, liver, and kidneys. Type II deiodinase has a higher affinity for T_4 and it is found predominantly in the pituitary, brain, brown fat, and also in the thyroid. Type III deiodinase converts T_3 and T_4 to reverse T_3. Conversion of T_4 to T_3 can be impaired by a variety of conditions, including fasting, systemic illness, acute trauma, oral contrast, and medications.

31.1.4 Thyroid Hormone Action

Thyroid hormones may enter cells via specific transporters or by passive diffusion. They act primarily on nuclear receptors, although they may also stimulate plasma membrane and mitochondrial enzymatic responses. In the nucleus, thyroid hormones bind to α and β nuclear thyroid hormone receptors with high affinity, each having unique isoforms that are expressed at different levels in various organs. The nuclear thyroid hormone receptors bind to specific DNA sequences called thyroid response elements, which are found in promoter regions of target genes. The activated receptors can either stimulate or inhibit gene transcription. T_3 binds with greater affinity than T_4 to the thyroid receptors.

Thyroid disease is diagnosed with assessment of the hypothalamic–pituitary–thyroid axis and an understanding of its feedback mechanism (▶ Fig. 31.3). TSH secretion is very sensitive to the plasma concentration of free thyroid hormone, and

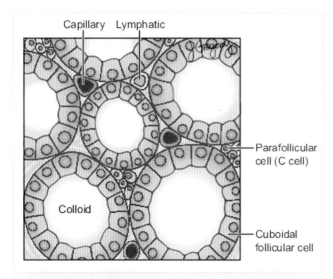

Fig. 31.1 Thyroid follicular structure.

Labels: Capillary, Lymphatic, Parafollicular cell (C cell), Colloid, Cuboidal follicular cell

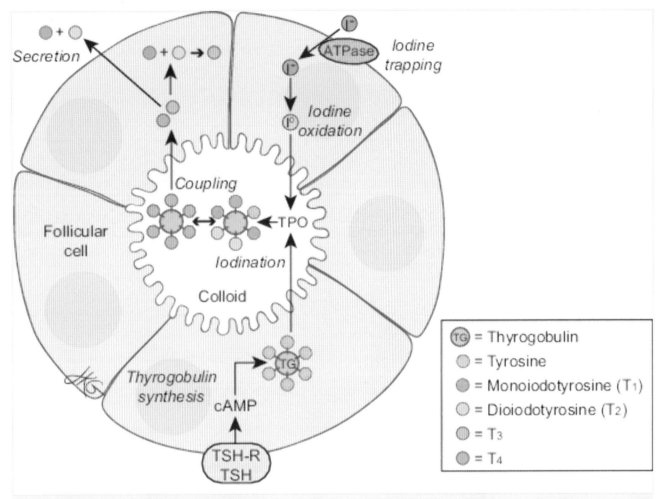

Fig. 31.2 Thyroid hormone production. *ATPase*, adenosine triphosphatase; *cAMP*, cyclic adenosine monophosphate; *TSH*, thyroid-stimulating hormone; *TSH-R*, thyroid-stimulating hormone–releasing hormone.

small changes in thyroid hormone production will produce large changes in TSH. Invariably, patients with hyperthyroidism and thyroid hormone overproduction will have suppressed TSH, whereas patients with primary hypothyroidism will have increased TSH and decreased T_3 and T_4 values. A suppressed TSH level with normal T_3 and T_4 levels is labeled subclinical hyperthyroidism; it is often asymptomatic but associated with an increased risk for atrial fibrillation in older patients. Subclinical hypothyroidism is characterized by slightly elevated TSH with normal T_3 and T_4 values. Hypothyroidism may also be secondary to decreased pituitary secretion of TSH resulting from a pituitary mass effect or damage.

The only direct measurement of thyroid function is with radioactive iodine uptake (RAIU), in which a radioactive isotope of iodine (^{123}I) is used. The rate of hormone synthesis and release can be inferred from the percentage uptake calculated within 24 hours as the plasma level of the tracer iodide decreases exponentially. A normal uptake is usually between 5% and 20% in an iodine-sufficient area. RAIU can be helpful in distinguishing hyperthyroidism caused by Graves hyperthyroidism from that caused by thyroiditis and toxic nodules.

31.2 Thyrotoxicosis

The term *thyrotoxicosis* refers to the physiologic manifestations of excessive thyroid hormone levels resulting from any source of thyroid hormone. The term *hyperthyroidism* also refers to overproduction of thyroid hormone by the thyroid gland but may present with few or no symptoms, only laboratory evidence of disease. Most patients with thyrotoxicosis have hyperthyroidism, but not all conditions are directly caused by increased thyroid hormone synthesis. Examples include silent subacute thyroiditis, exogenous thyrotoxicosis from excessive thyroid hormone replacement, and destructive thyroiditis from drugs such as amiodarone (see Box Rare Causes of Thyrotoxicosis (p. 257)).

Rare Causes of Thyrotoxicosis

- Thyroid-stimulating hormone–producing pituitary adenoma
- Struma ovarii
- Choriocarcinoma
- Thyrotoxicosis factitia
- Functional metastatic thyroid cancer

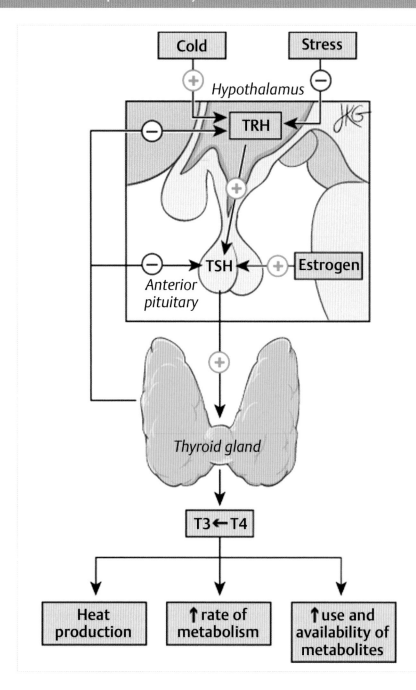

Fig. 31.3 Hypothalamic–pituitary–thyroid axis. *TRH*, thyrotropin-releasing hormone; *TSH*, thyroid-stimulating hormone.

Conditions producing hyperthyroidism commonly include Graves disease, toxic adenoma, and toxic multinodular goiter. Hyperthyroidism can also be induced by the ingestion of iodine or iodine-containing drugs. Iodine-induced hyperthyroidism (Jod-Basedow phenomenon) occurs in previously euthyroid patients with multinodular or endemic goiters after they have been given large doses of iodine, such as in imaging contrast medium. Subclinical hyperthyroidism is characterized by suppressed TSH concentration and normal serum T_3 and T_4 levels, which can occur in the setting of mild Graves disease, toxic multinodular goiter, or thyroiditis. The patient is usually asymptomatic or has mild symptoms of thyrotoxicosis.

Although toxic nodular goiter is less common than Graves disease, its prevalence increases with age and in the presence of iodine deficiency. Toxic multinodular goiter occurs when hyperthyroidism arises from autonomous thyroid hormone production in a long-standing multinodular goiter. Painless and subacute thyroiditis results in the inflammation of thyroid tissue with the release of preformed hormone into circulation. About 10% of hyperthyroid patients present with painless thyroiditis and can occur post partum, with certain medications such as lithium or cytokine therapy, and in 5 to 10% of amiodarone-treated patients. Subacute or de Quervain thyroiditis is characterized by pronounced thyroid tenderness and fever.

The typical signs and symptoms of thyrotoxicosis are easily evident in the young; but in the elderly, a masked or apathetic thyrotoxicosis may be present, with cardiac arrhythmias and weight loss as the only obvious markers of disease. Excess thyroid hormone affects almost every organ system, and manifestations can range from minimal to life-threatening cardiac arrhythmias. An increased metabolic rate causes many of the cardiovascular symptoms in thyrotoxicosis. The increase in sympathetic tone and decrease in vagal tone account for many of the manifestations. Peripheral vascular resistance is decreased, cardiac output increased, and stroke volume increased. There is a direct inotropic effect on cardiac contractions, causing tachycardia and widening of the pulse pressure. The "palpitations" often described are a result of this increased force of contraction. Atrial fibrillation may be present, and patients older than 60 years have an increased risk for developing this arrhythmia. Atrial fibrillation is one of the most serious consequences of hyperthyroidism and can lead to increased embolic events. The treatment of hyperthyroidism can often lead to a restoration of cardiac rhythms.

The elevated metabolic rate that accompanies thyrotoxicosis produce increased appetite, heat intolerance, and increased lipid metabolism. The increase in sympathetic nervous system activity is not due to an increase in plasma concentrations of epinephrine and norepinephrine; rather, the excess thyroid hormone exerts an additive effect and increases receptor sensitivity to catecholamines. Manifestations of hyperthyroidism include hyperkinesia, nervousness, hyperreflexia, and emotional lability. There is an association between Graves disease and myasthenia gravis, and they are coexistent in approximately 3 to 5% of patients. Eye changes seen in thyrotoxicosis are due to increased adrenergic sensitivity; patients often have a "stare" from retraction of the upper and lower eyelids. Additionally, some patients with Graves disease would benefit from receiving iodine for about 1 week and may have infiltrative and edematous changes in the eyes, leading to Graves orbitopathy. Patients also note increased sweating, with moist soft skin and fine hair. Frequent bowel movements and increased appetite may occur. Thyrotoxicosis affects the skeletal system by increasing the excretion of calcium and phosphorus, leading to bone loss and an elevated alkaline phosphatase level. Clinical symptoms of thyrotoxicosis involve most organ systems, as summarized in ▶ Table 31.1.

31.2.1 Graves Disease

Graves disease, the most common cause of hyperthyroidism, is caused by circulating autoantibodies specific to the TSH receptor, resulting in increased thyroid hormone production. It is most common in the third and fourth decades, often presents with a goiter and thyrotoxicosis, and can be accompanied by infiltrative orbitopathy and dermatopathy. The gland is characterized by a lymphocytic infiltration without follicular destruction. The natural course of the disease is unpredictable, with some patients having cyclic recurrences or persistent disease for many years. Approximately one-third of patients become hypothyroid after 20 years. Orbitopathy, characterized by inflammation of the orbit, proptosis, and exophthalmos, may occur before, during, or even after the diagnosis of hyperthyroidism.

The laboratory diagnosis of hyperthyroidism is initially made with a low (usually undetectable) TSH level, along with elevated T_4 and T_3 levels. Radioactive iodine scans (▶ Table 31.2) may be helpful in differentiating the hyperthyroidism caused by Graves disease and toxic goiter, which have elevated iodine uptake values (▶ Fig. 31.4), from the subacute, painless, and iodine-induced hyperthyroidism characterized by low iodine uptake (▶ Fig. 31.5).

Treatment

There are three main treatment types for Graves disease: antithyroid medications, radioactive iodine therapy, and surgical resection. Definitive treatment is tailored to the individual patient after an assessment of the likelihood of remission, pregnancy considerations, patient comorbidities, and patient preference.

Medical therapy includes β-blockade and thionamides. β-Blockers help relieve symptoms of tremulousness, palpitations, excessive sweating, eyelid retraction, and increased heart rate secondary to increased adrenergic sensitivity. Propranolol also weakly blocks the conversion of T_4 to T_3. Treatment with β-blockade can be continued until euthyroidism is restored by antithyroid drugs, unless it is contraindicated in patients with heart failure or asthma.

Thionamides, including propylthiouracil (PTU) and methimazole, inhibit oxidation and the organic binding of thyroid iodide and produce an intrathyroidal iodine deficiency, resulting in decreased thyroid hormone production. PTU also inhibits the conversion of T_4 to T_3. Because of possible increased adverse hepatic effects of PTU, the American Thyroid Association states that methimazole is currently the drug of choice, except during the first trimester of pregnancy. Antithyroid drugs can be used short term to prepare patients for radioactive iodine therapy or surgery and may even induce remission in a minority of patients. Frequent follow-up is required every 4 to 6 weeks until the levels of free T_4 have normalized. Adverse reactions include skin rashes, arthralgias, gastrointestinal upset, and abdominal pain. More severe side effects include hepatitis, cholestasis, and agranulocytosis; these adverse events are idiosyncratic. Agranulocytosis (0.2 to 0.5%) is often accompanied by fever and sore throat. Methimazole is contraindicated in the first trimester of pregnancy because of teratogenic effects. Other medications that have been used in hyperthyroidism include lithium and dexamethasone. Lithium inhibits thyroid hormone secretion; this effect is temporary because the blocking effect is lost over time. In patients who are allergic to thionamides, these agents may be used as temporizing measures.

Definitive therapy is required in most patients with hyperthyroidism, leading to treatment with radioactive iodine or surgical resection. Radioactive iodine for thyroid ablation is safe and effective and can be used as first-line treatment in Graves hyperthyroidism or toxic goiter. Contraindications include desired pregnancy within 6 months of dose, pregnancy, diagnosis of thyroid cancer, and failure to comply with safety precautions. Treatment usually involves a fixed or calculated dose of ^{131}I, with higher doses given for toxic adenoma and toxic multinodular goiter than for Graves disease. Thionamides interfere with radioactive iodine therapy and should be discontinued 3 to 7 days before treatment. The effects of treatment are seen within 8 weeks, with most patients becoming hypothyroid in 6 months. Standard precautions to minimize radioactivity exposure to others are taken after treatment. Active Graves ophthalmopathy is a relative contraindication to radioactive iodine because radioactive iodine has been associated with exacerba-

Table 31.1 Symptoms of hypothyroidism and hyperthyroidism

Organ system	Hypothyroidism	Hyperthyroidism
Hair	Coarse, thin hair	Hair loss
	Loss of outer third of eyebrows	
Brain	Mental slowing	Emotional lability
	Apathy	Fatigue
	Tiredness	Anxiety
	Psychosis	Restlessness
Face, ears, eyes	Myxedema features (i.e., puffy face, coarse features)	Exophthalmos
	Deafness	Lid retraction
		Lid lag
		Predisposition to keratitis
Neck	Goiter	Goiter
	Hoarse voice	
Heart	Bradycardia	Palpitations
		Tachycardia
		Atrial fibrillation
Bowel	Constipation	Diarrhea
		Increased appetite
Sexual organs	Amenorrhea	Menorrhagia
		Infertility
		Reduced libido
Muscles	Slowing of activity	Proximal myopathy
	Proximal myopathy	
Hands	Cold hands	Tremor
	Carpal tunnel syndrome	Warmth
		Sweating
Reflexes	Slow relaxation phase	Increased
Skin, bones, adipose tissue	Weight gain	Osteoporosis
	Cold intolerance	Heat intolerance
	Decreased sweating	Increased sweating
	Chronic edema (caused by increased capillary escape of albumin)	Weight loss
	Cold, dry skin	Pretibial myxedema

Table 31.2 Radioactive iodine uptake in thyroid disease

Etiology	Radioactive iodine uptake
Graves disease	Elevated
Toxic multinodular goiter	Elevated in nodules
Toxic adenoma	Elevated in nodules
Subacute thyroiditis	Low
Iodine-induced hyperthyroidism	Low

tion of disease, and pretreatment with glucocorticoids may be required.

Surgery is used less frequently for treating Graves disease in the United States and usually involves subtotal thyroidectomy leaving approximately 2 g of tissue. Indications include very large goiters, thyroid cancer, and uncontrolled disease despite treatment with thionamides. Surgery is also indicated for patients desiring pregnancy in the very near future, those who are pregnant and whose disease is not controlled with thionamides, and those with significant thyrotoxicosis who cannot be

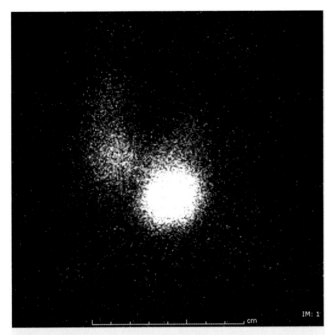

Fig. 31.4 Hot nodule in the inferior left lobe of the thyroid gland on ^{123}I scan.

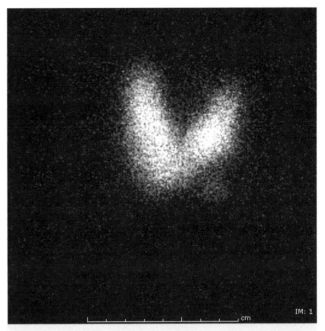

Fig. 31.5 Absence of radioactivity in the left lower lobe indicates a cold nodule.

treated with radioactive iodine and have had adverse reactions to thionamide therapy. To prevent thyroid storm, patients should be euthyroid if possible before surgery, preferably through pretreatment with thionamides. If thionamides are contraindicated, the patient can be prepared with β-blockers and high doses of iodine, such as Lugol solution, to block new thyroid hormone production. Iodine is used only in the short term because there is an iodine escape called the Wolff Chaikoff effect; after iodine loses efficacy, it can exacerbate hyperthyroidism. Additionally, all patients with Graves disease should receive iodine for about 1 week preoperatively to decrease thyroid vascularity. After surgery, patients are hypothyroid and will require thyroid hormone replacement.

31.2.2 Thyroid Storm

Thyroid storm is an extreme form of thyrotoxicosis that can be fatal if not promptly treated. It usually occurs abruptly in the setting of preexisting thyrotoxicosis that has been incompletely treated or undiagnosed. Precipitating factors such as infection and intercurrent illness are commonly involved. Before it became possible to control disease preoperatively, thyroid storm frequently occurred after thyroidectomy. The clinical picture is one of severe hypermetabolism, with fever, tachycardia, and possibly pulmonary edema or heart failure. Nausea, vomiting, abdominal pain, and extreme restlessness may also be present.

The diagnosis of thyroid storm is based on symptoms, and guidelines have been published. Treatment involves large doses of antithyroid drugs, iodine in form of Lugol solution or SSKI (saturated solution of potassium iodide), and glucocorticoids. Although it is preferable to start antithyroid drugs before iodine, in the setting of thyroid storm iodine treatment should not be withheld to rapidly decrease thyroid hormone release. Large doses of dexamethasone to support the stress response

and inhibit hormone release are also given. In the absence of cardiovascular insufficiency or asthma, β-blockade can be administered. Supportive measures to bring down fever should be instituted in febrile patients. Salicylates should be avoided because they compete with T_3 and T_4 for binding to thyroxine-binding globulin and transthyretin, increasing free hormone levels. If treatment is successful, improvement occurs within days and recovery within a week, at which point iodide and dexamethasone can be discontinued and plans for long-term treatment instituted.

Treatments for other forms of hyperthyroidism depend on the etiology. Subacute thyroiditis is treated symptomatically with β-blockers and nonsteroidal anti-inflammatory drugs, and with glucocorticoids for severe cases. Silent thyroiditis and postpartum thyroiditis may present with an initial hyperthyroid phase that resolves spontaneously, often leading to hypothyroidism. Amiodarone-associated thyrotoxicosis requires either medical management or rarely thyroidectomy, if feasible, if medical management is not successful in controlling a significant thyrotoxic state. Radioactive iodine treatment cannot be used in the short term, given the high iodine content of amiodarone and its prolonged half-life.

31.3 Hypothyroidism

Thyroid hormone deficiency causing hypothyroidism is common, with a prevalence of 2% of the population. In primary hypothyroidism, TSH is elevated and thyroid hormones are reduced. Hypothyroidism can be transient or permanent. Worldwide, iodine deficiency is the most common cause of hypothyroidism, but Hashimoto thyroiditis or chronic autoimmune thyroiditis is the most common cause in North America. Patients with autoimmune hypothyroidism will usually have elevated titers of antibodies to thyroid peroxidase and sometimes to thyroglobulin. Hashimoto thyroiditis is more common in women and increases in incidence with age. Elevated titers of antithyroid antibodies may also be present in patients with subacute thyroiditis. In these patients, the hypothyroidism is usually transient and follows a brief phase of thyrotoxicosis. In secondary hypothyroidism, TSH deficiency can occur in the setting of a pituitary or hypothalamic disorder, especially after surgery in the area of the pituitary. The presenting symptoms of hypothyroidism range from nonspecific and mild to severe and life-threatening. Common symptoms include cold intolerance, fatigue, weight gain, and constipation. Signs may include delayed tendon reflexes, bradycardia, hypothermia, and periorbital edema, summarized in the Box Rare Causes of Thyrotoxicosis (p. 257). An elevated TSH level is the best initial screening test for primary hypothyroidism. Treatment involves levothyroxine, usually dosed at 1.6 µg/kg daily. Replacement thyroid hormone is taken without food because foods, as well as calcium and iron supplements, interfere with thyroid hormone absorption. Drugs such as estrogen and anticonvulsants may increase dose requirements; estrogens increase thyroxine-binding globulin levels, and some anticonvulsants increase the metabolic clearance of thyroxine. Elderly patients who may have cardiac disease should initially be given lower doses of levothyroxine (25 to 50 µg) and monitored closely.

The goals of therapy are to bring the TSH levels into the normal range and lessen the symptoms associated with hypothyroidism. TSH should be measured about 6 weeks after treatment initiation. The T_4 level will usually exhibit change within 7 days and may also be used to monitor therapy. Liothyronine or T_3 has been used in conjunction with T_4 in some patients who have hypothyroidism. There are no convincing data that combination therapy is superior to treating with levothyroxine alone. Patients who require urgent surgery and have untreated hypothyroidism are usually not at increased risk for perioperative mortality, but elective surgery should be delayed until patients are euthyroid. In those patients undergoing surgery in whom thyroid hormone is adequately replaced, levothyroxine can be held for several days after surgery until the patients can eat. This does not result in hypothyroidism, given the 7-day half-life of levothyroxine.

Patients who are hospitalized may develop sick euthyroid syndrome, initially characterized by decreased total T_3, then decreased total T_4 and sometimes low free T_4 with TSH that may be normal, decreased, or sometimes elevated in the recovery phase. The syndrome is probably due to decreased conversion of T_4 to T_3, inhibition of T4 binding to plasma proteins, and central hypothyroidism, which can be seen in severe illness. Treatment is not indicated in these patients.

31.4 Thyroid Neoplasia and Carcinoma

Nontoxic goiter can be defined as thyroid enlargement. Goiter may be endemic in a region with iodine deficiency or sporadic. In an autopsy series, thyroid nodules were found in almost 50% of cadavers. The etiology of goiter appears to be multifactorial—both genetic and environmental. The TSH concentration is usually normal in patients with goiter, so the process may be TSH-independent. Nontoxic goiter is more common in females and

often clusters within families. Very large goiters can cause physical discomfort, but most are asymptomatic. The goiter may displace the trachea, esophagus, and neck vessels and can be associated with stridor and dysphagia.

The increase use of medical imaging, including computed tomography (CT) and magnetic resonance (MR) imaging of the neck and chest and carotid duplex scanning, has augmented the diagnosis of asymptomatic thyroid nodules and subsequently increased the diagnosis of thyroid carcinoma. Thyroid nodules are quite common, with epidemiologic studies showing the prevalence of palpable nodules to be 5% in women and 1% in men in iodine-sufficient areas. Thyroid "incidentalomas" that are nonpalpable and found on high-resolution ultrasound are detected in 19 to 67% of individuals. A minority, approximately 5 to 15%, are diagnosed as carcinomas, whereas the majority are benign thyroid nodules. Although the incidence of thyroid cancer has increased, the mortality has not, likely because of the small size and early stage of these incidentally discovered thyroid carcinomas. Differentiated thyroid cancer, including papillary and follicular cancer, accounts for almost 90% of all cases of thyroid cancer. The yearly incidence increased 2.4-fold from 1973 to 2002, primarily because of the increase in small papillary thyroid cancer.

The history and physical examination can often favor a benign versus a malignant nodule. Features that would make a physician concerned include a family history of thyroid cancer, male sex, and older age. A history of exposure to external ionizing radiation in childhood, such as acne therapy, treatment for Hodgkin lymphoma, or thymus irradiation, and of exposure to nuclear accidents such as the one at Chernobyl increases the risk for thyroid carcinoma. A rapidly growing mass, abnormal lymphadenopathy, and vocal cord paralysis are also concerning features. Given the high prevalence of thyroid nodules and the excellent prognosis of papillary microcarcinomas, nodules smaller than 1 cm are usually not investigated unless concerning features are present. In general, patients with thyroid carcinoma are euthyroid, but there may be a slightly increased risk for thyroid cancer in patients with Graves disease. ▶ Fig. 31.6 outlines the decision-making process in evaluating thyroid nodules.

31.4.1 Imaging

Ultrasonography (▶ Fig. 31.7) often detects even minute thyroid nodules, with one study showing 65% of patients having nodularity. Ultrasound can characterize the heterogeneous echotexture of the pseudonodules of Hashimoto thyroiditis (▶ Fig. 31.8) and demonstrate increased blood flow on Doppler in Graves hyperthyroidism. It is most useful in characterizing thyroid nodules and neck lymphadenopathy. Ultrasound is the imaging modality of choice in patients with nodules, and certain ultrasonographic features increase the suspicion of thyroid cancer. Benign indicators include a completely cystic nodule and hyperechogenicity. Criteria predictive of malignancy include solid hypoechoic nodules, especially with microcalcifications; irregular margins; absence of halo; and nodules taller than they are wide (▶ Fig. 31.9). If a ^{123}I scan is done to evaluate thyroid function and a nodule not concentrating radioactive iodine is found, further investigation, including ultrasound-guided fine-needle aspiration, is usually indicated.

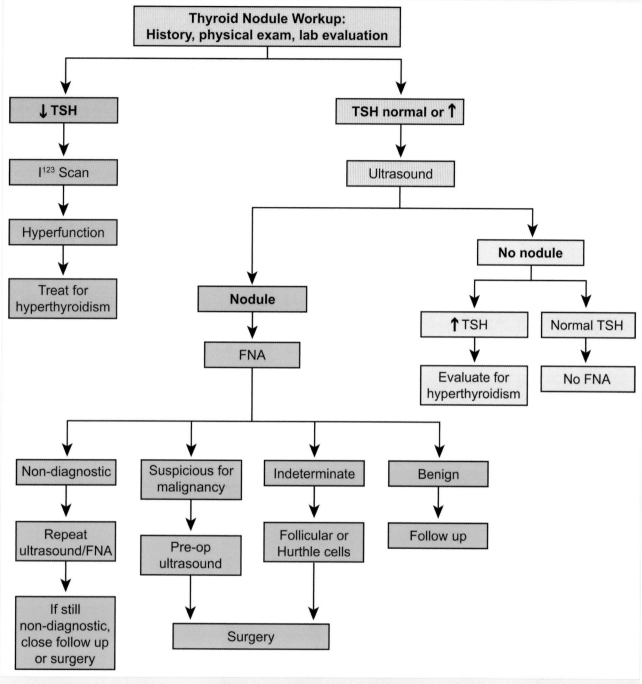

Fig. 31.6 Evaluation of a thyroid nodule. *FNA*, fine-needle aspiration; *TSH*, thyroid-stimulating hormone.

Nodules that are suspicious for malignancy should undergo fine-needle aspiration biopsy. This technique has excellent sensitivity and specificity of more than 90%, especially when performed under ultrasound guidance. It is easy to perform and safe, and it causes little discomfort. A satisfactory specimen needs to include at least six groups of 10 to 15 well-preserved cells obtained from three to six passes in the nodule. Generally, a 25- or 27-gauge needle is used for the aspiration. Fine-needle aspiration biopsy is extremely useful in diagnosing papillary thyroid cancer through the nuclear changes observed in cytology. The sensitivity and specificity approach 100%. Follicular neoplasms, by contrast, are more difficult to differentiate. Often, these aspirations are characterized as indeterminate, and surgical resection and lobectomy of the affected side are required for accurate diagnosis. At surgery, follicular neoplasms are commonly benign; the rate of finding carcinoma in suspicious nodules is approximately 20%. Recently, *BRAF* analysis has become commercially available. *BRAF* is a mutation commonly found in papillary and follicular cancers and may aid in the management of indeterminate nodules.

Patients with a multinodular thyroid gland have the same risk for malignancy as those with a solitary nodule. The Ameri-

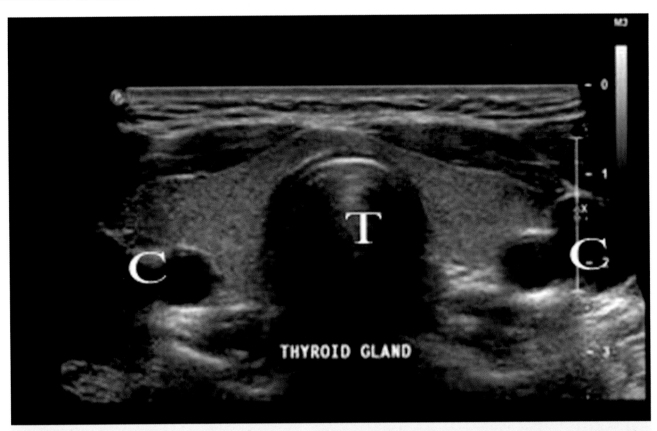

Fig. 31.7 Ultrasound of a normal thyroid gland. The gland lies over and around the trachea and abuts both carotid arteries. *T*, trachea; *C*, carotid artery.

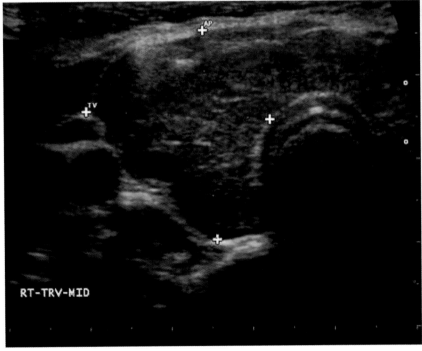

Fig. 31.8 Thyroid ultrasound demonstrating the heterogeneous echotexture and pseudonodules seen in Hashimoto thyroiditis.

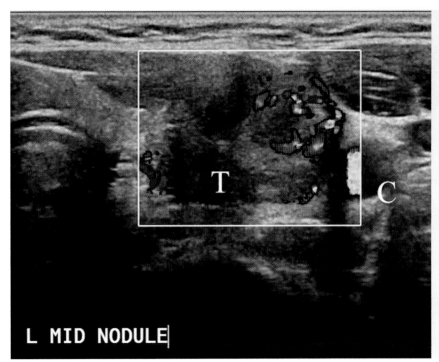

Fig. 31.9 Ultrasound demonstrating indistinct borders, microcalcifications, and increased vascularity on Doppler imaging in papillary carcinoma of the left lobe of the thyroid. *T*, trachea; *C*, carotid artery.

L MID NODULE

can Thyroid Association recommends aspirating those nodules that are larger than 1 cm and have a suspicious sonographic appearance. If a nodule is found to have benign cytologic findings, follow-up with serial ultrasound is recommended, with repeat fine-needle aspiration if there is a 50% increase in volume or an increase in size of 2 mm or more within two nodule dimensions.

31.5 Prevalence of Thyroid Carcinoma

Differentiated thyroid cancers are the most common malignant thyroid tumors, with papillary thyroid carcinoma accounting for more than 80% of cancers and follicular carcinoma comprising about 15% of cases. Medullary carcinoma, a neuroendocrine tumor of the calcitonin-producing thyroid cells, occurs 3% of the time and may be associated with multiple endocrine neoplasia type II. Anaplastic carcinoma, with an aggressive course, occurs in 1 to 2% of cases. Lymphoma of the thyroid can also rarely occur in a background of Hashimoto thyroiditis and may be diagnosed in a rapidly growing thyroid mass.

31.5.1 Staging of Thyroid Carcinoma

Thyroid carcinoma staging is based on tumor type and size, extension beyond the thyroid gland, lymph node status, and patient age. T1a lesions are 1 cm or smaller; T1b lesions are between 1 and 2 cm. T2 lesions are 2 to 4 cm in size without extrathyroid extension. T3 lesions are those larger than 4 cm and limited to the thyroid or any tumors with limited extrathyroid extension (sternothyroid muscle or perithyroid soft tissues).

T4a lesions are of any size but extend beyond the thyroid to invade the larynx, trachea, esophagus, recurrent laryngeal nerve, or subcutaneous tissues; T4b tumors invade the prevertebral fascia or encase the carotid artery. The above categories apply to all thyroid tumors except anaplastic tumors, which are all considered T4 lesions; T4a lesions are intrathyroid, and T4b tumors extend beyond the thyroid.

Level VI (pretracheal, paratracheal, and prelaryngeal) lymph node involvement is considered N1a disease; unilateral, bilateral, or contralateral involvement of cervical, retropharyngeal, or superior mediastinal nodes is classified as N1b.

Papillary and Follicular Carcinoma

For patients younger than 45 years of age, disease is considered stage I unless there is a distant metastasis, in which case is classified as stage II. In patients older than 45 years, T1 tumors are stage I and T2 lesions are stage II in the absence of nodal disease. T3 lesions without nodal disease or T1–T3 tumors with N1a nodes are graded as stage III. T1–T3 lesions with N1b nodes or any T4a lesion without metastasis is considered stage IVA. T4b lesions without distant metastases are considered stage IVB, and any distant metastasis is defined as stage IVC disease.

Medullary Carcinoma

T1 medullary carcinoma is considered stage I, and T2 and T3 lesions are considered stage II if there is no nodal involvement. T1–T3 lesions with N1a disease are considered stage III. T1–T3 tumors with N1b nodal status and any T4a lesion are classified as stage IVA. All T4b lesions are considered stage IVB, and any distant metastasis is classified as stage IVC disease.

Anaplastic Carcinoma

All anaplastic carcinomas are considered stage IV. T4a lesions are considered stage IVA, T4b tumors are stage IVB, and the presence of a distant metastasis implies stage IVC.

31.5.2 Management of Thyroid Carcinoma

Surgical resection is the mainstay of treatment in thyroid carcinoma, with total thyroidectomy and lymph node dissection if indicated. Subcentimeter tumors may also be treated with lobectomy provided no high-risk features are present. Total thyroidectomy is also indicated in patients with indeterminate nodules, marked atypical or suspicious cytology, or a family history of thyroid carcinoma or radiation exposure. Preoperative ultrasound of the neck for contralateral lobe findings and lymph node involvement is recommended. Ultrasound-guided fine-needle aspiration of sonographically suspicious lymph nodes should be performed to confirm malignancy. After surgical resection, the TNM (tumor node metastasis) classification system is used for prognostication and follow-up.

31.5.3 Postsurgical Treatment

If a patient undergoes total thyroidectomy, postoperative radioiodine may be required depending on pathology results. Patients at decreased risk for recurrence do not usually require radioactive iodine therapy, whereas patients with larger tumors and those with extrathyroidal spread usually benefit. Ablation of the small amount of residual normal thyroid remaining after total thyroidectomy may facilitate the early detection of recurrence based on serum thyroglobulin measurement. In addition, new data have indicated that lower doses of radioactive iodine may be as effective as higher doses in preventing recurrence in low-risk cancers. Higher doses may be appropriate in those patients with aggressive tumor histology (tall cell, insular columnar cell carcinoma). Patients undergoing radioactive iodine therapy require levothyroxine withdrawal to raise the TSH level above 30 mU/L and a diet low in iodine. Recombinant TSH can be used in some patients in lieu of withdrawal, and studies have shown short-term recurrence rates to be similar. One week after radioactive iodine remnant ablation, a scan is performed to evaluate for metastases.

Differentiated thyroid cancer expresses TSH receptor on the cell membrane and responds to TSH stimulation with increased expression of several thyroid-specific proteins and increased rates of cell growth. Suppression of TSH with levothyroxine therapy is used to decrease the risk for thyroid cancer recurrence. Suppression of TSH to below 0.1 mU/L is recommended for patients with high- and intermediate-risk thyroid cancer, while maintenance of the TSH level at the lower limit of normal or slightly below is appropriate for patients with low-risk disease (0.1 to 0.5 mU/L).

The long-term management of differentiated thyroid cancer includes surveillance for possible recurrence. In patients who have not undergone total thyroidectomy and those who have not undergone ^{131}I ablation, measurement of thyroglobulin and thyroglobulin antibodies and ultrasonography of the neck are the mainstays of follow-up. Anti-thyroglobulin antibodies, which are present in approximately 25% of patients with thyroid cancer, may falsely lower the thyroglobulin determination in immunometric assay. Approximately 20% of patients who are clinically free of disease, with serum thyroglobulin levels below 1 ng/mL during thyroid hormone suppression of TSH, will have a detectable serum thyroglobulin level after TSH stimulation at 1 year after initial therapy. One-third of these will have persistent or recurrent disease; the others will have stable or decreasing stimulated serum thyroglobulin levels over time. Patients who develop locoregional disease or tumors in the cervical lymph nodes or soft tissues of the neck will require surgical resection.

31.6 Roundsmanship

- TRH stimulates the pituitary secretion of TSH. Circulating thyroid hormone provides negative feedback, inhibiting TSH release via pituitary T_3 receptors.
- The thyroid secretes 20 times more T_4 than T_3, and T_3 has a shorter half-life than T_4. T_4 is also deiodinated peripherally to produce T_3.
- Graves disease is the most common cause of hyperthyroidism.
- Methimazole is the drug of choice in treating hyperthyroidism except in the first trimester of pregnancy.
- The treatment of thyroid storm includes antithyroid medication, iodine (Lugol solution or SSKI), glucocorticoids, and β-blockers if not otherwise contraindicated.
- Iodine deficiency is the most common cause of hypothyroidism worldwide, but Hashimoto thyroiditis is the most common cause in North America.
- Treatment of hypothyroidism includes 1.6 µg of levothyroxine per kilogram per day; patients with cardiac disease and elderly patients should be started at 25 to 50 µg/d. TSH measurement should be repeated 6 weeks after the initiation of treatment.
- Fine-needle aspiration biopsy is highly sensitive and specific for papillary thyroid carcinoma; only 20% of thyroid glands with follicular neoplasms diagnosed by fine-need aspiration are found to have follicular carcinoma at surgery.

31.7 Recommended Reading

[1] Thyroid. In: Edge SB, Byrd DR, Compton CC, et al. American Joint Committee on Cancer (AJCC) Staging Manual. 7th ed. New York, NY: Springer; 2010:111–122

[2] Cooper DS, Doherty GM, Haugen BR et alAmerican Thyroid Association (ATA) Guidelines Taskforce on Thyroid Nodules and Differentiated Thyroid Cancer. Revised American Thyroid Association management guidelines for patients with thyroid nodules and differentiated thyroid cancer. Thyroid 2009; 19: 1167–1214

[3] Bahn Chair RS, Burch HB, Cooper DS et alAmerican Thyroid AssociationAmerican Association of Clinical Endocrinologists. Hyperthyroidism and other causes of thyrotoxicosis: management guidelines of the American Thyroid Association and American Association of Clinical Endocrinologists. Thyroid 2011; 21: 593–646

[4] Burch HB, Wartofsky L. Life-threatening thyrotoxicosis. Thyroid storm. Endocrinol Metab Clin North Am 1993; 22: 263–277

[5] Escobar-Morreale HF, Botella-Carretero JI, Escobar del Rey F, Morreale de Escobar G. REVIEW: Treatment of hypothyroidism with combinations of levothyroxine plus liothyronine. J Clin Endocrinol Metab 2005; 90: 4946–4954

[6] Gharib H. Changing concepts in the diagnosis and management of thyroid nodules. Endocrinol Metab Clin North Am 1997; 26: 777–800

[7] Hegedüs L. Clinical practice. The thyroid nodule. N Engl J Med 2004; 351: 1764–1771

[8] Osman F, Franklyn JA, Holder RL, Sheppard MC, Gammage MD. Cardiovascular manifestations of hyperthyroidism before and after antithyroid therapy: a matched case-control study. J Am Coll Cardiol 2007; 49: 71–81

[9] Papini E, Guglielmi R, Bianchini A et al. Risk of malignancy in nonpalpable thyroid nodules: predictive value of ultrasound and color-Doppler features. J Clin Endocrinol Metab 2002; 87: 1941–1946

[10] Schlumberger M, Catargi B, Borget I et alTumeurs de la Thyroïde Refractaires Network for the Essai Stimulation Ablation Equivalence Trial. Strategies of radioiodine ablation in patients with low-risk thyroid cancer. N Engl J Med 2012; 366: 1663–1673

[11] Sherman SI. Thyroid carcinoma. Lancet 2003; 361: 501–511

[12] Spencer CA, LoPresti JS, Fatemi S, Nicoloff JT. Detection of residual and recurrent differentiated thyroid carcinoma by serum thyroglobulin measurement. Thyroid 1999; 9: 435–441

[13] Tan GH, Gharib H. Thyroid incidentalomas: management approaches to nonpalpable nodules discovered incidentally on thyroid imaging. Ann Intern Med 1997; 126: 226–231

[14] Tuttle RM, Brokhin M, Omry G et al. Recombinant human TSH-assisted radioactive iodine remnant ablation achieves short-term clinical recurrence rates similar to those of traditional thyroid hormone withdrawal. J Nucl Med 2008; 49: 764–770

32 Parathyroid Hormone, Vitamin D, and Bone Mineral Metabolism

Guy Valiquette

32.1 Introduction

The physiology of parathyroid hormone is so intricately inter-twined with vitamin D and bone mineral metabolism that these topics must be approached together if the discussion is to be cogent and comprehensive. These interactions are summarized graphically in ▸ Fig. 32.1. PTH primarily regulates the concentration of extracellular ionized calcium, whereas vitamin D regulates the absorption of calcium from the diet and, indirectly, bone mineralization, which accounts for 99% of the calcium reserves in the body.

"Bone is an organ?" Yes! Bone is very active metabolically and, as the primary repository of the body's calcium stores, is intimately involved in the regulation of the body's extracellular calcium and ionized calcium concentrations. The extracellular ionized calcium concentration is critical to multiple cellular functions, including intracellular signaling, hormone secretion, and muscle and neural functions, and it must be maintained within very tightly controlled limits. Hypocalcemia leads to neuromuscular hyperexcitability; milder degrees are manifested as hyperesthesia with positive Chvostek and Trousseau signs, whereas more severe hypocalcemia may lead to tetany, seizures, and death. Hypercalcemia leads to lethargy, weakness, and eventually coma and death. Approximately 50% of extracellular calcium is present as ionized calcium, but this is somewhat pH-dependent. Intracellular calcium concentrations are several orders of magnitude below the extracellular concentration, although some organelles, such as the mitochondria, have higher concentrations. Extracellular ionized calcium normally is regulated within a margin of less than ± 10%.

32.2 Physiology

32.2.1 Parathyroid Hormone

Human parathyroid hormone (PTH, hPTH) is an 84–amino acid polypeptide hormone; the amine-terminal 34–amino acid fragment of hPTH, hPTH 1–34, expresses the full classic biological activity of hPTH and is used clinically, particularly to treat osteoporosis. The classic PTH receptor has been sequenced; it is a G protein–linked, 7-transmembrane-spanning segments receptor that binds PTH and the PTH-related peptide (PTHrp) with equal affinity, although PTHrp does not stimulate 1-hydroxy-lase activity in the kidney to the same extent that PTH itself does. The PTH receptor is heavily expressed in bone and in the kidneys, although other organs also express the receptor at lower levels. More recently, a novel PTH receptor that binds the carboxyl-terminal fragments of PTH, present in the circulation and previously thought to be inactive, has been identified. This novel receptor does not bind PTHrp, and it is not yet clear what role, if any, it plays in bone mineral metabolism, or in any other function.

Parathyroid gland cells express a calcium-sensing receptor, another G protein–linked, 7-transmembrane-spanning segments receptor, that binds and responds to multiple cations, of which only the divalent cations calcium and magnesium are physiologically relevant. Lower levels of ionized calcium will stimulate PTH secretion, whereas higher levels of ionized calcium will suppress PTH secretion, thereby controlling PTH secretion and maintaining ionized calcium levels within narrow limits. Multiple mutations in this receptor, with both loss and gain in function, have been reported and are key to understanding familial hypocalciuric hypercalcemia (FHH; see below) and certain hypocalcemic syndromes, such as familial hypoparathyroidism.

PTH increases the resorption of calcium from the kidneys, increases bone resorption, and increases vitamin D 1-hydroxylase activity in the kidneys. All these actions contribute to restoring a normal ionized calcium level in the circulation.

32.2.2 Vitamin D

Pro-vitamin D (cholecalciferol) is synthesized in the skin from 7-dehydrocholesterol by photocatalysis in the presence of ultraviolet light in the 290- to 315-nm range (see ▸ Fig. 32.1). This wavelength is at the very limit of the atmosphere's transparency to ultraviolet light, and the synthesis of pro-vitamin D in the skin is seasonal at higher latitudes. Pro-vitamin D precursors are also photolabile, and prolonged exposure to sunlight does not lead to vitamin D intoxication. Therefore, the rate of pro-vitamin D production, with long-term irradiation, is not related to skin pigmentation, although it is reduced in darker-skinned individuals with short-term irradiation. Pro-vitamin D is bound to transcalciferin (vitamin D–binding protein) and is carried to the liver, where it undergoes 25-hydroxylation to become calcidiol.

The availability of vitamin D in our diet is limited, and very few foodstuffs provide us with vitamin D. Milk and dairy products in the United States and Europe are fortified with vitamin D, and they provide approximately 100 international units (IU) of vitamin D per portion. Unfortified dairy products and human milk are very poor sources of vitamin D. Eggs provide approximately 20 IU of vitamin D per yolk; egg whites do not contain any vitamin D. Fish are a major source of dietary vitamin D, which ranges from about 250 IU per portion of canned tuna up to 1,000 IU per portion of fresh wild salmon. No vegetable product contains vitamin D, but mushrooms may contain up to 1,500 IU/100 g if grown in the presence of sunlight.

Vitamin D is actually a pro-hormone; the active hormone is $1-25-(OH)_2$ vitamin D (calcitriol). Normally, calcitriol is produced in the kidneys from vitamin D, calcidiol, by 1-hydroxylation of this pro-hormone. The renal 1-hydroxylase activity is under the control of PTH, and therefore $1-25-(OH)_2$ vitamin D levels correlate with PTH levels. High PTH levels, generally in response to hypocalcemia, will therefore stimulate $1-25-(OH)_2$ vitamin D production and increase the intestinal absorption of calcium to normalize serum levels of ionized calcium. Some other tissues can express 1-hydroxylase activity, independently of PTH control, in some pathologic conditions (see below).

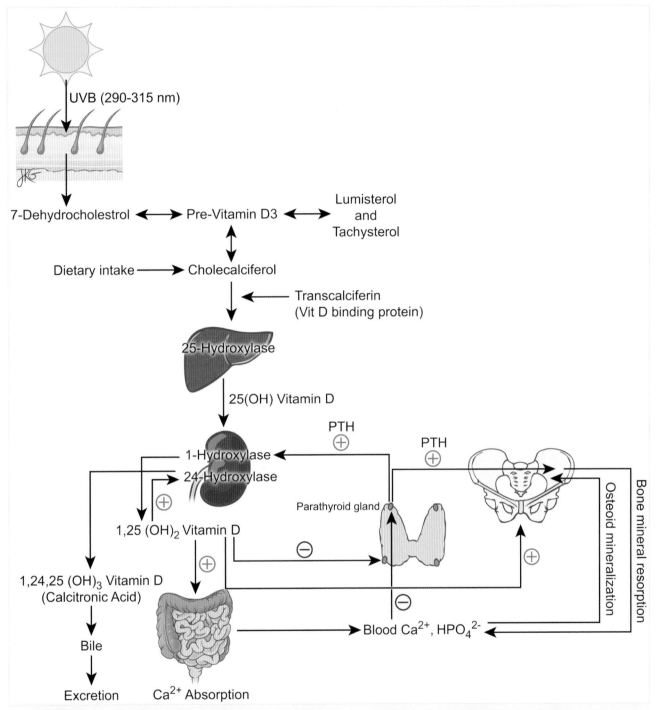

Fig. 32.1 Integration of vitamin D, parathyroid hormone, and bone mineral metabolism. Vitamin D precursors are produced in the skin from 7-deoxycholesterol by photocatalysis in the presence of ultraviolet radiation. The synthesis of 25-OH vitamin D, the storage form of the pro-hormone, to 1,25-(OH)$_2$ vitamin D, the active hormone, is under the control of parathyroid hormone. 1,25-(OH)$_2$ Vitamin D increases calcium absorption from the gastrointestinal tract. Serum calcium and phosphate levels allow the mineralization of new bone matrix and feedback on parathyroid hormone secretion. Higher levels of parathyroid hormone increase bone resorption when necessary to maintain normal serum calcium levels and stimulate the synthesis of 1,25-(OH)$_2$ vitamin D by the kidneys.

32.2.3 Bone Mineral Metabolism

Bone is generally thought of as a major structural component of the body. However, bone also has a significant metabolic function as a reservoir for calcium, phosphate, and carbonate, and it plays a significant role as a buffer in the body's acid–base balance. Bone is made of a matrix of connective tissue, which is mostly but not completely mineralized, and specialized bone cells. The skeleton is generally conceptually divided into the axial skeleton, which includes the skull, vertebrae, sternum, ribs, and pelvis, and the appendicular skeleton, which includes the long bones of the limbs down to the digits. Bone can also be divided into trabecular, or cancellous, bone, which is highly active metabolically, and cortical bone, which is denser and less active metabolically but can be recruited in severe or prolonged bone disease. The axial skeleton has a higher proportion of trabecular bone, whereas the appendicular skeleton has more cortical bone.

Specialized bone cells include the osteoblasts, osteocytes, and osteoclasts. Osteoblasts are derived from mesenchymal stem cells and produce the connective tissue matrix; this secondarily becomes mineralized, thereby producing new bone. Most osteoblasts undergo apoptosis, but a minority are integrated in the bone matrix to become osteocytes or remain on the surface of the bone to form the periosteum. In becoming osteocytes, these cells develop multiple long processes radiating from the cell bodies that form gap junctions with neighboring osteocytes and the periosteum. Osteocytes act as sensors of the mechanical stresses to which bones are subjected and play an important role in the modulation of bone remodeling. Osteoclasts are large multinuclear cells derived from the fusion of mononuclear cells of the macrophage lineage, stimulated mainly by nuclear factor-κB (RANKL), produced during the apoptosis of osteoblasts, and by macrophage colony–stimulating factor. Osteoclasts destroy both the mineral component of bone by dissolution and the collagenous matrix by proteolysis, thereby mediating bone resorption.

Normal bone is constantly being broken down through resorption by osteoclasts, and new bone is laid down by osteoblasts in what is described as the bone-remodeling cycle. Normally, bone resorption and bone formation are in balance. The bone-remodeling cycle is important in repairing microfractures resulting from the everyday stresses imposed on the skeleton and thereby maintaining its structural integrity.

32.2.4 Calcium-Sensing Receptor

As mentioned above, parathyroid cells express the calcium-sensing receptor. The calcium-sensing receptor was first identified in bovine parathyroid glands and later confirmed in human tissues. The calcium-sensing receptor is expressed in parathyroid glands, where it was first isolated, and also in kidneys, bone, intestine, lungs, brain, and other tissues.

Both mutations and acquired disorders of the calcium-sensing receptor can lead to clinically relevant disease, causing hypocalcemia as well as hypercalcemia. The clinical relevance of these disorders is discussed in detail further below.

32.3 Hypercalcemic Disorders

32.3.1 Pseudohypercalcemia

Pseudohypercalcemia is an elevation in the total serum calcium with a normal level of ionized calcium. It is generally due to an increase in serum proteins (mainly albumin) associated with severe dehydration or to the presence of abnormal proteins, such as the paraproteins of multiple myeloma. Note, however, that multiple myeloma can also cause true hypercalcemia through bone resorption (see below).

32.3.2 Primary Hyperparathyroidism

Primary hyperparathyroidism is by far the most common cause of hypercalcemia. The prevalence of hyperparathyroidism, as estimated in recent studies, is about 2% in women ages 55 to 75 years, with an annual incidence rate of 22 per 100,000. The etiology of the disorder is not clear but does not involve a mutation in the calcium-sensing receptor. Primary hyperparathyroidism is most commonly caused by a solitary parathyroid adenoma, and less frequently by parathyroid hyperplasia involving all four glands; most of these cases are sporadic, but a minority are secondary to hereditary syndromes. Cases of parathyroid carcinoma are rare, accounting for fewer than 1% of all cases.

Since the introduction of automated chemistry analyzers in the late 1970s, most cases of primary hyperparathyroidism have been asymptomatic at the time of diagnosis. The classic clinical presentation of symptomatic hypercalcemia, with nephrolithiasis and bone lesions or bone pain, is rarely seen today in the developed world, although a certain number of cases still present as nephrolithiasis. Most cases are diagnosed after a diagnostic work-up for incidental hypercalcemia.

Normocalcemic forms of primary hyperparathyroidism have been proposed but remain controversial. What is agreed upon is that causes of secondary hyperparathyroidism must be carefully excluded before a diagnosis of normocalcemic hyperparathyroidism is made. There are no guidelines for the management of normocalcemic hyperparathyroidism.

Clinical manifestations of primary hyperparathyroidism, when present, may include nephrolithiasis, fatigue, anxiety, and muscle weakness. Hypertension and cardiovascular disease are more common in patients with hyperparathyroidism than in the general population. Low bone mineral density in the appendicular bones, such as the distal third of the radius, is common, whereas bone mineral density in the axial skeleton, such as the spine, is more commonly normal.

Laboratory characteristics of primary hyperparathyroidism include hypercalcemia (generally mild), hypophosphatemia, and elevated or inappropriately normal PTH levels. Total serum calcium must be corrected for the albumin: corrected total serum calcium (mg/dL) = actual total serum calcium (mg/dL) + {[4.0 – serum albumin (g/dL)] x 0.8)}. Occasionally, it must also be corrected for other serum protein levels, and serum ionized calcium may be measured directly for confirmation or clarification. Urinary calcium levels, measured in a 24-hour urine collection, are usually normal or high despite the increased fractional resorption of calcium. It is also important to rule out hypercalcemia due to FHH before making a diagnosis of primary hyperparathyroidism because surgery is contraindicated in this syndrome (see below).

Relevant imaging studies include distal radius bone mineral density, renal ultrasound, and abdominal computed tomography (CT), to rule out nephrolithiasis or nephrocalcinosis, and a sestamibi nuclear scan (▶ Fig. 32.2). The sestamibi scan should

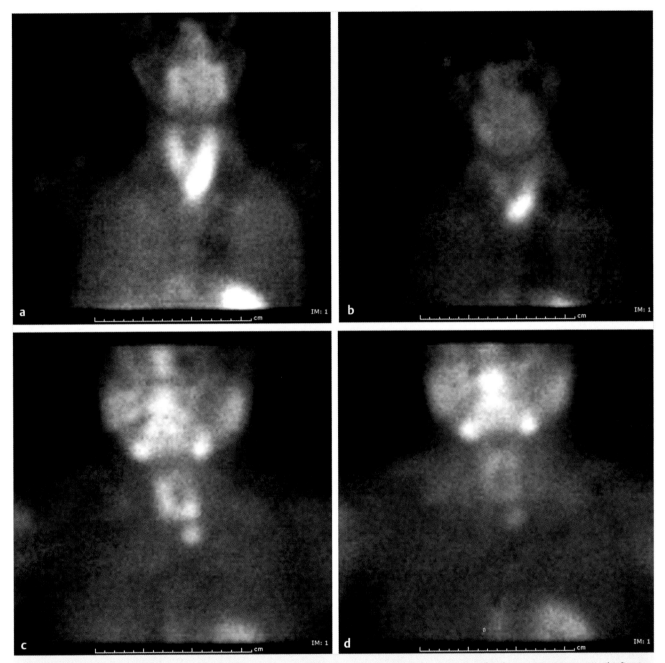

Fig. 32.2 For a sestamibi parathyroid scan, the neck is imaged with a gamma camera twice after an injection of technetium Tc 99 m sestamibi: first in an early-phase scan at 10 to 20 minutes after injection and then in a late-phase scan at approximately 2 hours. The early phase images the thyroid gland as well as the parathyroid glands; in the late-phase image, the thyroid gland "washes out" while the radioactivity in the parathyroid gland(s) persists better and so images the adenomatous parathyroid tissue. (**a**) Early and (**b**) delayed images show a strikingly obvious, but far from typical, parathyroid adenoma. (**c**) Early and (**d**) delayed images show a more typical (lower left) parathyroid adenoma.

not be used for diagnostic purposes, only for localizing purposes to assist the surgeon in preparing for the surgery. Ultrasound exploration of the neck (▶ Fig. 32.3) may also be useful in identifying a parathyroid adenoma, again to assist the surgeon, not for diagnostic purposes.

The natural history of primary hyperparathyroidism has been better defined by the study of one cohort of patients over 10 and 15 years. In this study, 37% of the patients who either did not meet criteria for surgery or initially declined surgery

developed symptomatic disease and eventually met these criteria. Although asymptomatic mild primary hyperparathyroidism can safely be observed for several years, the advisability of this approach is now being questioned.

The most recent guidelines developed by the Third International Workshop on the Management of Asymptomatic Primary Hyperthyroidism recommend surgery for asymptomatic patients that meet any of the following criteria: (1) total serum calcium more than 1 mg/dL above the upper limit of normal,

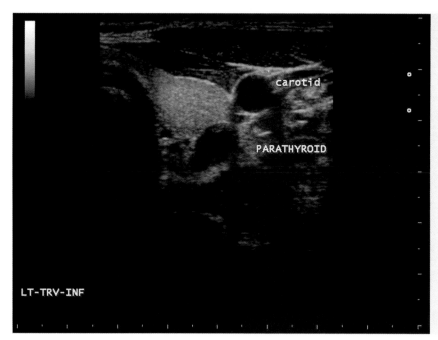

Fig. 32.3 Ultrasonographic view of a large parathyroid adenoma inferior and lateral to the thyroid gland.

(2) estimated creatinine clearance below 60 mL/min, (3) bone mineral density T score at any site of less than –2.5 or any fragility fracture, and (4) age younger than 50 years. The previous criterion of a urinary calcium excretion rate of more than 400 mg/d has been dropped, although many physicians still use it in their decision-making process.

Immediate postoperative care should include close monitoring for hypocalcemia, which is frequent but generally mild and transient. More severe hypocalcemia may require intravenous and oral calcium supplementation. Postoperative hypocalcemia is more common and more severe in patients with concomitant vitamin D deficiency, and vitamin D deficiency generally should be corrected preoperatively.

32.3.3 Tertiary Hyperparathyroidism

Tertiary hyperparathyroidism is parathyroid hypertrophy and hyperplasia in patients with end-stage renal failure on hemodialysis or patients who were previously on hemodialysis after renal transplant. Parathyroid hyperplasia and parathyroid adenomas develop as a result of prolonged stimulation of the parathyroid glands from uncontrolled hypocalcemia, calcitriol deficiency, or hyperphosphatemia. This parathyroid hyperplasia obviously persists after renal transplant, when the physiologic environment is dramatically changed. There are no clear guidelines for parathyroid surgery in tertiary hyperparathyroidism; however, most experts agree that surgery is indicated in cases of uncontrolled hypercalcemia or of hyperparathyroid metabolic bone disease or extraskeletal calcifications refractory to oral phosphate binders, and in the presence of a high PTH level, generally above 600 to 800 pg/mL. There is no consensus on the surgical approach; both subtotal parathyroidectomy and total parathyroidectomy with auto-transplant have their proponents.

32.3.4 Familial Hypocalciuric Hypercalcemia

FHH is a relatively rare cause of hypercalcemia, with a prevalence rate estimated to be between 1 per 10,000 and 1 per 100,000. This may actually be an underestimate because FHH is generally totally asymptomatic. The main reasons for surgeons to be well aware of this syndrome is that FHH had been identified as the cause of failed parathyroid surgery in patients misdiagnosed as having primary hyperparathyroidism; this misdiagnosis may account for nearly 25% of failed parathyroid surgeries. FHH is an autosomal-dominant disorder resulting from a loss-of-function mutation in the calcium-sensing receptor gene, which leads to a resetting of the PTH–calcium set point and a mild to moderate hypercalcemia; because the calcium-sensing receptor is present along most of the nephron, hypocalciuria is typical of this syndrome, in contrast to the hypercalciuria generally seen in primary hyperparathyroidism. The diagnosis is usually suggested by a calcium-to-creatinine urinary clearance ratio of less than 0.01 and is confirmed by a positive family history or genetic testing. Note, however, that there is significant overlap in the calcium-to-creatinine clearance ratios of FHH and primary hyperparathyroidism, in which the ratio is typically, but not always, above 0.01. Acquired cases of an FHH-like syndrome due to autoantibodies to the calcium-sensing receptor have also been described.

32.3.5 Other Causes of Hypercalcemia

There are many other causes of hypercalcemia, generally of interest more to the endocrinologist than to the surgeon. Nevertheless, these will be reviewed briefly here (see Box Causes of Hypercalcemia (p.273)). Generally, it is most useful to start the evaluation of a patient with hypercalcemia by measuring the serum PTH, PTHrp, and 1,25-(OH)$_2$ vitamin D levels.

Causes of Hypercalcemia

- Pseudohypercalcemia
- Primary hyperparathyroidism
- Secondary hyperparathyroidism
- Tertiary hyperparathyroidism
- Familial hypocalciuric hypercalcemia
- Paraneoplastic syndrome
  - Parathyroid hormone-related peptide (PTHrp)–mediated hypercalcemia
  - Parathyroid hormone (PTH)–mediated hypercalcemia
  - Tumor necrosis factor–, interleukin-1–, or RANKL-mediated hypercalcemia
- Vitamin D intoxication

Causes of hypercalcemia mediated by the PTH receptor include primary hyperparathyroidism, either sporadic or associated with a multiple endocrine neoplasia syndrome; tertiary hyperparathyroidism, typically in a patient with renal failure after renal transplant; and PTHrp-mediated hypercalcemia, a paraneoplastic syndrome. Rarely, some tumors may secrete PTH itself, rather than PTHrp. FHH-associated hypercalcemia, as discussed above, results from a reduced sensitivity of the calcium-sensing receptor to circulating ionized calcium levels. Finally, hPTH 1–34 (teriparatide) is approved for the treatment of osteoporosis; its use normally results in a transient hypercalcemia lasting only a few hours, but it may cause persistent hypercalcemia in some individuals.

Vitamin D intoxication can cause hypercalcemia, but hypercalcemia is generally seen only in patients with a 25-(OH) vitamin D level above 100 ng/mL. This cause of hypercalcemia was seen much more frequently before the development of histamine type 2 (H_2) receptor antagonists and proton pump inhibitors (PPIs), when calcium carbonate and milk were recommended in the treatment of peptic ulcers ("milk alkali syndrome"). Extrarenal sources of vitamin D 1-hydroxylase, not under the control of PTH, can also lead to hypercalcemia. This is generally seen in disorders, benign or malignant, involving cells of the macrophage lineage, such as lymphomas or chronic granulomatous diseases.

Tumors can cause hypercalcemia, as mentioned above, by secreting PTHrp or rarely PTH itself, but other tumors, including solid tumors with bony metastases and multiple myelomas, cause hypercalcemia by secreting various cytokines. These cytokines include tumor necrosis factor, interleukin-1, RANKL, and others.

32.4 Hypocalcemic Disorders

32.4.1 Pseudohypocalcemia

As noted above under the heading of hypercalcemia, pseudohypocalcemia is also possible if calcium-binding proteins in serum are decreased. This most commonly is the result of hypoalbuminemia due to hepatic or renal disease. Acidosis will also reduce total serum calcium by increasing albumin binding of calcium.

32.4.2 Hypocalcemia with Low Parathyroid Hormone Levels

The major cause of hypoparathyroidism is surgery. Surgical hypoparathyroidism can occur after thyroid, parathyroid, or other head and neck surgery. Transient hypoparathyroidism occurs in up to 50% of patients undergoing a total thyroidectomy for thyroid cancer, and permanent hypoparathyroidism in up to 20% of patients with neck dissections. Rates of permanent hypoparathyroidism can be as high as 1 to 3% in patients undergoing a total thyroidectomy for benign disease. Other causes include autoimmune hypoparathyroidism and other, more unusual disorders (see Box Causes of Hypocalcemia (p.273)). Autosomal-dominant hypocalcemia is the counterpart of FHH, in which a gain-of-function mutation in the calcium-sensing receptor gene results in a lower set point for serum calcium regulation.

Causes of Hypocalcemia

- Low parathyroid hormone Levels
  - Postoperative hypoparathyroidism
  - Autoimmune hypoparathyroidism
  - Autosomal-dominant hypocalcemia
- High parathyroid hormone levels
  - Acute pancreatitis
  - Severe vitamin D deficiency
  - Pseudohypoparathyroidism

The treatment of hypocalcemia in low-PTH conditions, except autosomal-dominant hypocalcemia, is based on increasing calcium absorption with calcium supplementation and supraphysiologic doses of vitamin D. Typically, these patients may require up to 6 g of calcium and 2 µg of calcitriol, or 1,25-$(OH)_2$ vitamin D, daily. Because these patients lack the calcium-retaining effect of PTH in the kidneys, urinary calcium must be monitored closely to avoid hypercalciuria, urolithiasis, and nephrocalcinosis. It may be necessary to add a thiazide diuretic to reduce the urinary excretion of calcium. Also, serum calcium does not need to be corrected completely into the normal range; a low normal or slightly low serum level of calcium is acceptable if the patient is asymptomatic. Although trials have shown that treatment with PTH itself is effective in treating hypoparathyroidism, this treatment is not approved by the FDA.

Autosomal-dominant hypocalcemia should not be treated with calcium supplements and vitamin D; fortunately, this syndrome is very rare and generally asymptomatic.

32.4.3 Hypocalcemia with High Parathyroid Hormone Levels

The treatment of high-PTH hypocalcemic states is more diverse. Secondary hyperparathyroidism is the normal response of the parathyroid glands to hypocalcemia, whatever the etiology. Therefore, acute pancreatitis, in which hypocalcemia is due to the sequestration of serum calcium in calcium soaps by released free fatty acids, and severe vitamin D deficiency, in which hypocalcemia is due to the decreased absorption of dietary calcium, both induce secondary hyperparathyroidism to maintain serum free calcium levels. Note, however, that most patients with vitamin D deficiency [levels of 25-(OH) vitamin D below 20 ng/mL] present with a high PTH level and a normal serum calcium level.

Pseudohypoparathyroidism, which is the result of loss of function of the PTH receptor, is treated with calcium supplements and vitamin D, just like hypoparathyroidism. Vitamin D deficiency is obviously treated by replenishing vitamin D, generally with 50,000 IU weekly for 6 to 8 weeks. The hypocalcemia associated with hypomagnesemia is completely reversible by correcting the hypomagnesemia. Generally, other conditions causing hypocalcemia respond to treatment of the underlying cause.

32.5 Osteoporosis

As we noted above, bone is constantly turning over, allowing the repair of damages from everyday stresses. Normally, bone resorption and bone deposition are tightly coupled, and bone mass remains constant. If bone deposition lags behind bone resorption, bone mass decreases, and the result is osteoporosis. This overview addresses the most common form of osteoporosis, postmenopausal osteoporosis. The management of osteoporosis in premenopausal women and in men does differ from that in postmenopausal women to a significant extent, and the reader is referred to recent relevant reviews.

Osteoporosis can be diagnosed only by a determination of bone mineral density. The "gold standard" technology for determining bone density is dual-energy X-ray absorptiometry (DEXA). Although other technologies, such as calibrated CT and quantitative ultrasound measurements of the calcaneus, have been proposed, either they have not gained universal acceptance (calibrated CT) or they measure parameters other than bone density that may predict fracture risk (ultrasound) but are not comparable with bone mineral density. Osteoporosis is defined as a bone mineral density that is more than 2.5 standard deviations below the mean of young adults (T score). The bone mineral density can also be compared with that of persons of the same age and sex (Z score), but this metric is used only for epidemiologic studies, not for fracture prediction or therapeutic decision making. Osteopenia is defined as a bone mineral density T score between –1.0 and –2.49.

The treatment of osteoporosis involves both nonpharmacologic and pharmacologic interventions. Nonpharmacologic interventions include diet, exercise, smoking cessation, and avoidance of drugs that may increase bone mineral loss, primarily glucocorticoids. The diet should include an adequate intake of calories and protein, in addition to calcium and vitamin D supplementation. Consuming a diet rich in calcium (mostly dairy products) is preferable to supplementation, but this may be difficult or may interfere with other dietary goals (e.g., reducing cholesterol intake). If necessary, calcium supplementation should consist of about 500 to 1,000 mg/d, taken in divided doses and with food. Recently, there has been some controversy over what daily intake of vitamin D should be recommended for the general population. However, there is no doubt that vitamin D deficiency is extremely prevalent in older adults and

carries an increased risk for mortality. Most osteoporosis experts recommend supplementing the diet with up to 2,000 IU of vitamin D. Exercise has been shown to reduce the risk for fracture and to slightly increase bone mineral density; generally, a minimum 30 minutes of weight-bearing exercise three times weekly is recommended for skeletal health.

Pharmacotherapy should be considered for postmenopausal women who have fragility fractures or osteoporosis or who are at high risk for osteoporosis. The World Health Organization has developed a fracture prediction tool, FRAX, to estimate the 10-year osteoporotic fracture risk and assist in treatment decision making. Pharmacotherapy regimens used for the treatment of osteoporosis can be classified as either antiresorptive or anabolic. Antiresorptive agents include bisphosphonates, selective estrogen receptor modulators (SERMs), postmenopausal estrogen replacement therapy, and denosumab. The only anabolic agents approved are teriparatide (PTH 1–34) and intact PTH (PTH 1–84).

Strontium ranelate is approved in Europe for the treatment of osteoporosis and appears to have both antiresorptive and anabolic properties, although its exact mechanism of action in humans is not clear.

Other therapeutic modalities have either been shown to be ineffective (calcitriol) or have mostly been abandoned because of the emergence of more effective modalities (calcitonin).

The treatment of osteoporosis is obviously quite complex, requiring careful decision making and balancing the risks and potential benefits of treatments designed to prevent serious complications of an asymptomatic condition over years, if not decades. This overview is therefore not designed to be a treatment guide, but rather a summary of the problem and various treatment options.

32.6 Roundsmanship

- Parathyroid hormone primarily regulates extracellular ionized calcium concentration, whereas vitamin D regulates the absorption of calcium from the diet and, indirectly, bone mineralization, which accounts for 99% of the body's calcium reserves.
- Approximately 50% of extracellular calcium is present as ionized calcium.
- Pro-vitamin D (cholecalciferol) is synthesized in the skin from 7-dehydrocholesterol during photocatalysis by ultraviolet light in the 290- to 315-nm range. This is further modified in the liver and kidneys to produce the active hormone.
- Pseudohypercalcemia is an elevation in the total serum calcium with a normal level of ionized calcium. It is usually due to an increase in serum protein concentrations seen in severe dehydration, or to the presence of abnormal proteins, such as the paraproteins of multiple myeloma.
- Primary hyperparathyroidism is most commonly caused by a solitary parathyroid adenoma, and less frequently by parathyroid hyperplasia involving all four glands.
- Tertiary hyperparathyroidism consists of parathyroid hypertrophy and hyperplasia in patients with end-stage renal failure on hemodialysis or in patients who were previously on hemodialysis after renal transplant.

32.7 Recommended Reading

[1] Bilezikian JP, Khan AA, Potts JT. Guidelines for the management of asymptomatic primary hyperthyroidism: summary statement from the third international workshop. J Clin Endocrinol Metab 2009;94(2):335–339

[2] Brown EM, Pollak M, Seidman CE et al. Calcium-ion-sensing cell-surface receptors. N Engl J Med 1995; 333: 234–240

[3] Brown EM. Mutations in the calcium-sensing receptor and their clinical implications. Horm Res 1997; 48: 199–208

[4] Cusano NE, Rubin MR, Sliney J, Bilezikian JP. Mini-review: new therapeutic options in hypoparathyroidism. Endocrine 2012; 41: 410–414

[5] Ferrari S, Bianchi ML, Eisman JA, et al. Osteoporosis in young adults: pathophysiology, diagnosis, and management. Osteoporos Int 2012;23(12):2735–2748

[6] Holick MF, Binkley NC, Bischoff-Ferrari HA et alEndocrine Society. Evaluation, treatment, and prevention of vitamin D deficiency: an Endocrine Society clinical practice guideline. J Clin Endocrinol Metab 2011; 96: 1911–1930

[7] Holick MF. Vitamin D deficiency. N Engl J Med 2007; 357: 266–281

[8] American Society for Bone and Mineral Research. ASBMR Bone Curriculum. http://depts.washington.edu/bonebio/ASBMRed/ASBMRed.html. Accessed October 19, 2012

[9] FRAX: WHO Fracture Risk Assessment Tool. http://www.shef.ac.uk/FRAX/. Accessed October 19, 2012

[10] Lew JI, Solorzano CC. Surgical management of primary hyperparathyroidism: state of the art. Surg Clin North Am 2009; 89: 1205–1225

[11] Marcocci C, Cetani F. Clinical practice. Primary hyperparathyroidism. N Engl J Med 2011; 365: 2389–2397

[12] Murray TM, Rao LG, Divieti P, Bringhurst FR. Parathyroid hormone secretion and action: evidence for discrete receptors for the carboxyl-terminal region and related biological actions of carboxyl- terminal ligands. Endocr Rev 2005; 26: 78–113

[13] Rosen CJ, Abrams SA, Aloia JF et al. IOM committee members respond to Endocrine Society vitamin D guideline. J Clin Endocrinol Metab 2012; 97: 1146–1152

[14] Rubin MR, Bilezikian JP, McMahon DJ et al. The natural history of primary hyperparathyroidism with or without parathyroid surgery after 15 years. J Clin Endocrinol Metab 2008; 93: 3462–3470

[15] Watts NB, Adler RA, Bilezikian JP et alEndocrine Society. Osteoporosis in men: an Endocrine Society clinical practice guideline. J Clin Endocrinol Metab 2012; 97: 1802–1822

33 Surgical Techniques for the Management of Thyroid and Parathyroid Diseases

Augustine L. Moscatello and Mike Yao

33.1 Thyroid

The four most common types of thyroid cancer are papillary, follicular, medullary, and anaplastic. Although the techniques described in this portion of this chapter are applicable to any of these pathologies, the indications for surgery and lymph node dissection pertain only to well-differentiated thyroid cancers (papillary and follicular). The management of anaplastic and medullary thyroid cancer is beyond the scope of this chapter.

33.1.1 History of Thyroid Surgery

Modern thyroidectomy is credited to Theodor Billroth and his pupil, Theodor Kocher. From 1860 to 1867, as professor in surgery at the University of Zurich, Billroth performed 20 thyroidectomies for compressive symptoms. Eight of 20 patients died perioperatively, causing him to suspend these operations. When he relocated to the University of Vienna in 1867, he applied new techniques of anesthesia, hemostasis, and antisepsis and decreased his mortality rate to less than 10%. Theodor Kocher was a student of Dr. Billroth and is often lauded as the "father of thyroid surgery" because of his contributions to making thyroid surgery safer. He improved techniques of hemostasis and asepsis to decrease the mortality rate to less than 0.2% by 1898. Kocher was a meticulous surgeon and was able to remove the thyroid with minimal disruption of the surrounding tissues. In this manner, he was able to preserve parathyroid function before a defined understanding of the presence and function of these glands had been acquired. Based on his work to understand the function of the thyroid gland and improve the safety of surgery, he was the first surgeon awarded the Nobel Prize in Medicine and Physiology, in 1909. Largely through his discoveries, the complications of hypothyroidism, hypoparathyroidism, and vocal cord paralysis were understood and avoided, making thyroid surgery a safe operation.

33.1.2 Indications for Thyroid Surgery

The three main indications for thyroid surgery are concern for cancer, goiter causing symptoms, and hyperthyroidism. Based on the American Thyroid Association (ATA) guidelines from 2009, most thyroid nodules 1 cm or larger should be biopsied by fine-needle aspiration. The results of fine-needle aspiration are divided into six categories based on The Bethesda System for Reporting Thyroid Cytopathology: nondiagnostic, malignant, benign, neoplasm (either follicular or Hürthle cell), suspicious for malignancy, and follicular lesion of undetermined significance. Thyroid surgery should be performed for a diagnosis of malignant, suspicious for malignancy, or neoplasm suspicious for Hürthle cell. Patients with biopsy categories of nondiagnostic, neoplasm suspicious for follicular lesion, and follicular lesion of undetermined significance may or may not undergo surgery depending on other factors, such as a family history of thyroid cancer, history of radiation exposure, and

patient preference. Some of these patients may undergo biopsy again or followed with ultrasound. Nodules that grow rapidly, are symptomatic, or cause vocal cord paralysis require surgical intervention.

33.1.3 Indications for Neck Surgery

Therapeutic lymph node dissection is the removal lymph nodes harboring cancer. Typically, an entire lymph node level is dissected if diseased lymph nodes are found in that level. Neck levels II, III, and IV are at the highest risk. There is controversy about the risk for disease in levels IIb and V. Elective lymph node dissection is the removal of lymph nodes with high risk for disease but without evidence of disease on imaging or physical examination. Elective lateral neck dissection is probably not indicated, and elective central neck dissection is controversial. The ATA guidelines recommend consideration of an elective central neck dissection for advanced primary tumors (T3 or T4), although we tend to perform only therapeutic lymph node dissections.

The ATA guidelines for central neck dissection have standardized the boundaries:
1. Superior: hyoid bone
2. Lateral: carotid artery
3. Anterior: superficial layer of the deep cervical fascia
4. Posterior: deep layer of the deep cervical fascia
5. Inferior: innominate artery on the right and the corresponding axial plane on the left

Careful dissection of the parathyroid glands and the recurrent laryngeal nerves is necessary during a central neck dissection. The recurrent laryngeal nerves need to be traced inferiorly with atraumatic techniques. For the parathyroid glands, the ATA consensus statement on central neck dissections reports that the "superior parathyroid gland is preserved in situ along with its primary blood supply from the superior branch of the inferior thyroid artery. The inferior parathyroid gland is usually reflected laterally along with its blood supply from the inferior thyroid artery." Glands that are devascularized can be autotransplanted after frozen section confirmation of parathyroid tissue.

33.1.4 Indications for Radioactive Iodine Treatment after Surgery

The ATA guidelines recommend postoperative radioactive iodine ablation in patients with known distant metastases, incomplete tumor resection, gross extra-thyroidal extension, and primary tumor larger than 4 cm. Radioactive iodine ablation is recommended for selected patients with tumors between 1 and 4 cm confined to the thyroid who have lymph node metastases, microscopic tumor invasion of tissues, aggressive tumor histology, or thyroglobulin levels out of proportion to the radioactive iodine uptake scan. Aggressive histologies include tall cell, columnar cell, diffuse sclerosing, trabecular, insular, and solid. Radioactive iodine ablation is not recommended for patients with tumors smaller than 1 cm without other high-risk features.

33.1.5 Procedure

Intubation

Laryngeal nerve EMG endotracheal tubes are widely available in many operating rooms. The standard EMG endotracheal tubes have contact electrodes that sense electrical activity in the laryngeal musculature. These contact electrodes are not as sensitive as the intramuscular electrodes typically used in facial nerve monitoring, and thus they do not give as much feedback during the dissection. We typically use the EMG endotracheal tube with a stimulator probe to confirm the identity of the recurrent laryngeal nerve and do not use it as a warning for excessive manipulation of the nerve; however, to use it to monitor excessive nerve damage, some practitioners increase the sensitivity of the nerve monitoring in an attempt to approximate the sensitivity of the intramuscular electrodes.

Skin Incision

The incision is typically made in a horizontal neck crease. From a visualization perspective, an incision at level of the thyroid isthmus or cricoid cartilage affords the easiest access to both the superior and inferior poles of the thyroid; however, this results in a scar that is in the middle of the neck. With this in mind, some surgeons displace the incision inferiorly to approximately 1 finger breadth above the sternal notch. In this low position, the scar is more easily hidden by clothing or jewelry. The disadvantage of a low incision is that dissection around the superior poles of the thyroid is more difficult. This visualization can be improved by using endoscopic video techniques. A scar placed inferiorly over the clavicles or sternum will tend to widen and become less cosmetically acceptable.

Dividing the Strap Muscles

In most cases, subplatysmal dissection is not necessary, and dissection beneath the strap muscles is adequate for visualization. Dissection is carried through the subcutaneous fat to the level of the anterior jugular veins and the strap musculature. The anterior jugular veins are ligated as necessary but can often be left intact unless there are communicating vessels that cross the midline. The sternohyoid and sternothyroid muscles are elevated off the thyroid gland carefully to avoid damage to the prominent blood vessels in the capsule of the thyroid gland. Electrocautery or the harmonic scalpel is used to ligate any small blood vessels that are encountered to keep the surgical field as dry as possible. Once elevated, the strap muscles are retracted laterally, and the thyroid gland is retracted medially. Sometimes, it is necessary to transect the medial aspect of the superior attachment of sternothyroid muscle to the thyroid cartilage to allow better exposure (▶ Fig. 33.1). The lateral aspect of the thyroid gland needs to be dissected carefully to avoid damage to the middle thyroid vein, which can bleed profusely if damaged or avulsed (▶ Fig. 33.2).

Identification of the middle thyroid veins requires enough medial and lateral retraction to stretch the veins slightly without enough traction to avulse them. Novice thyroid surgeons often will not retract the thyroid gland and trachea enough to develop the surgical space to identify these veins. Once identified, the middle thyroid vein(s) need to be ligated close to the thyroid capsule in order to medialize the gland. At this level, the common carotid artery can be seen and should be dissected laterally away from the thyroid gland.

Most surgeons approach the thyroid dissection from lateral to medial and either medialize the gland to identify the recurrent laryngeal nerve and parathyroid glands or dissect the superior pole and ligate the superior pole blood vessels. We tend to do whichever maneuver is easiest first. However, in this manuscript, we describe medialization first. In addition, sometimes dividing the thyroid isthmus initially can help to mobilize the gland when routine mobilization methods are not successful.

Medializing the Thyroid Lobe

The gland is retracted anteriorly and medially, and dissection is performed on the capsule of the thyroid gland to free it from the surrounding soft tissues, including the carotid artery, spine, and esophagus (▶ Fig. 33.3). The ease of this step depends on the size of the gland, the extent to which the gland wraps posterior to the esophagus, and the degree of inflammation. In most cases, this can be achieved by using careful and patient blunt dissection with a Kelly clamp or Kittner (peanut) sponges. Once the esophagus is freed from the gland, the tracheoesophageal groove is exposed.

The recurrent laryngeal nerve ascends in the tracheoesophageal groove. On the left side, it wraps around the aortic arch, and on the right, it wraps around the subclavian artery before ascending in the tracheoesophageal groove. Because of this anatomical difference from side to side, the right recurrent laryngeal nerve is typically more lateral and superficial in position than the left. Non-recurrent laryngeal nerves occur mostly on the right side and are associated with arteria lusoria (in which the right subclavian artery originates from the aortic arch and passes posterior to the esophagus). Left sided non-recurrent laryngeal nerves are associated with dextrocardia.

Some surgeons find the recurrent laryngeal nerve at the level of the inferior thyroid artery and trace it superiorly to the Berry ligament (posterior suspensory ligament; ▶ Fig. 33.5). In this region, the nerve is found in the recurrent nerve triangle bound by the carotid artery laterally, trachea medially, and thyroid gland superiorly. The branches of the inferior thyroid artery are not ligated until the recurrent laryngeal nerve and all of its branches are identified and protected. The location of the recurrent laryngeal nerve is more variable in this low position, and a longer segment of the nerve needs to be dissected when this technique is used.

Alternatively, careful blunt dissection in the tracheoesophageal groove can be performed to further medialize the thyroid lobe until the area of the Berry ligament is reached without finding the nerve in the low position. In the high region, the superior parathyroid gland is often overlying the recurrent laryngeal nerve (see ▶ Fig. 33.4). If this technique is used, great

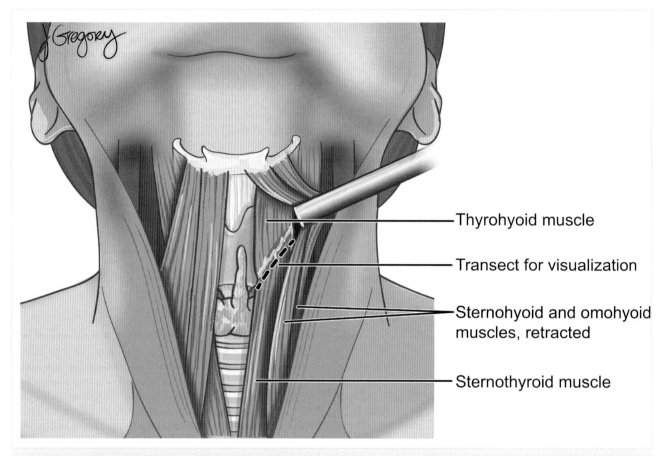

Thyrohyoid muscle

Transect for visualization

Sternohyoid and omohyoid muscles, retracted

Sternothyroid muscle

Fig. 33.1 Initial dissection of the strap muscles. The strap muscles are divided in the midline and dissected away from the thyroid gland. Sometimes, it is necessary to transect the medial aspect of the superior attachment of sternothyroid muscle to the thyroid cartilage to allow better exposure.

care must be taken to dissect the superior parathyroid gland away from the thyroid gland without devascularizing it and without damaging the recurrent laryngeal nerve. Even bipolar cautery must be used with great caution in this area because of the proximity of the parathyroid blood supply and the recurrent laryngeal nerve. Care must be taken to peel the parathyroid gland off the thyroid gland along its medial aspect to avoid damage to blood supply (▶ Fig. 33.5). The parathyroid gland is often identified and dissected free from the recurrent laryngeal nerve before the recurrent laryngeal nerve is identified. On occasion, the superior parathyroid gland is within the capsule of the thyroid gland, and dissection beneath the capsule is needed to free it. In all cases, the inferior thyroid artery is not ligated until the recurrent laryngeal nerve is identified and protected.

With either approach, once the recurrent laryngeal nerve is identified, it is traced superiorly and the Berry ligament is divided. The recurrent laryngeal nerve enters the larynx posterior to the cricothyroid joint, which can be identified on palpation as the region just below the inferior cornu of the thyroid cartilage. The nerve is dissected and protected all the way to its entrance into the larynx. The recurrent laryngeal nerve frequently branches before entering the larynx, and all of the branches need to be carefully protected. The fibers of the Berry ligament can be very adherent in the region of the cricothyroid joint, so great care is needed to divide these fibers without damage to the nerve. Often, there are small terminal branches of the

inferior thyroid artery that run superficial and parallel to the recurrent laryngeal nerve. These vessels can lead to troublesome bleeding and increased risk for recurrent laryngeal nerve injury if they are not ligated appropriately. Cautery cannot be used in this region, and some surgeons advocate the use of cotton pledgets soaked in epinephrine.

The recurrent laryngeal nerve is traced inferiorly, and the branches of the inferior thyroid artery are divided close to the inferior portion of the thyroid gland. Hugging the inferior pole of the thyroid gland minimizes the risk for damage to the blood supply to the inferior parathyroid glands.

Dissecting the Superior Pole

The superior pole of the thyroid and the trachea can be separated by using blunt dissection. Few blood vessels cross this area, and in most patients this is a bloodless plane (▶ Fig. 33.6). In this space, the external branch of the superior laryngeal nerve can be encountered (▶ Fig. 33.7). Most surgeons prevent injury to the external branch of the superior laryngeal nerve by avoiding it without identifying it. Some surgeons report identification of the external branch of the superior laryngeal nerve in 80% of cases and believe it is safer to attempt to identify it in every case. The external branch of the superior laryngeal nerve can run superficial to, through, or deep to the inferior constrictor muscle. When it is deep to the muscle, it cannot be identi-

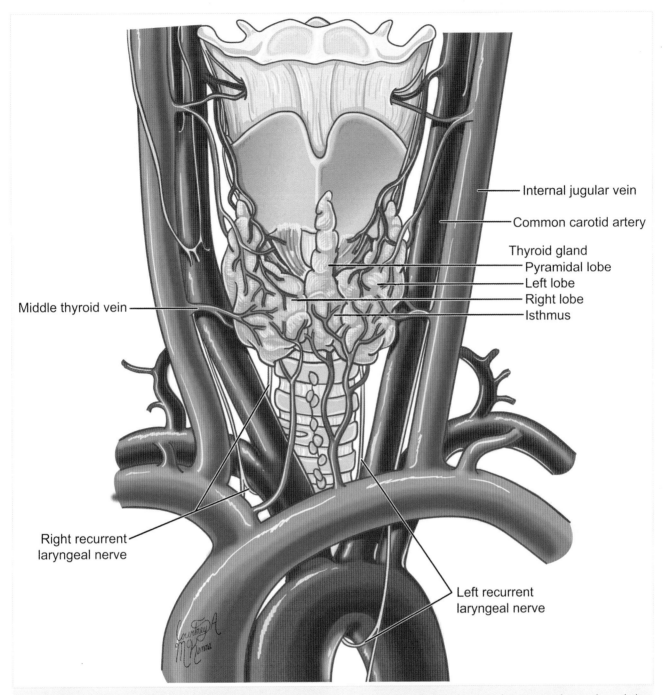

Fig. 33.2 Identification of the middle thyroid veins and dissection of the lateral aspect of the thyroid lobe. Once the strap muscles are elevated, the middle thyroid vein(s) need to be identified and carefully ligated close to the thyroid capsule. Identification of the middle thyroid veins requires enough medial and lateral retraction to stretch the veins slightly without enough traction to avulse them. Novice thyroid surgeons often will not retract the thyroid gland and trachea enough to develop the surgical space to identify these veins.

fied. When it is superficial or pierces the inferior constrictor muscle, it can be identified. Stimulation of the external branch of the superior laryngeal nerve provokes a brisk response in the cricothyroid muscle. We dissect the superior pole by hugging it closely and ligating only structures that are clearly entering the superior pole of the thyroid and appear vascular. Any structures that we think may be the external branch of the superior laryngeal nerve are stimulated and dissected away from the thyroid if possible, particularly any structures that cross toward

the larynx as they run inferiorly. Once the superior pole blood vessels are isolated and ligated, the remainder of the superior pole is freed with blunt dissection.

Removing the Thyroid Lobe

The medial portion of the thyroid lobe is dissected off the trachea, cricoid cartilage, thyroid cartilage, and cricothyroid muscle without damage to these structures. The pyramidal lobe

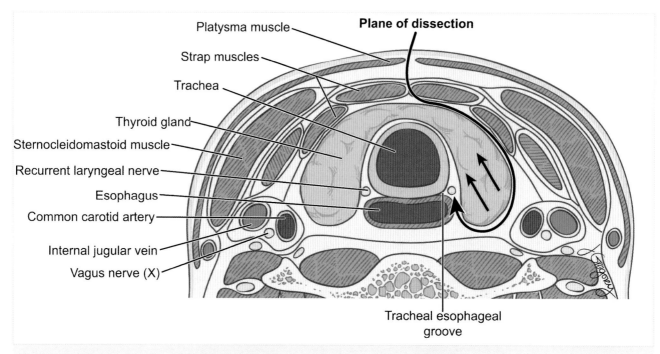

Fig. 33.3 Medialization of the thyroid lobe. The gland is retracted anteriorly and medially, and dissection is performed on the capsule of the thyroid gland to free it from the surrounding soft tissues, including the carotid artery, spine, and esophagus. The ease of this step depends on the size of the gland, the extent to which the gland wraps posterior to the esophagus, and the degree of inflammation. In most cases, this can be achieved by using careful and patient blunt dissection with a Kelly clamp or Kittner sponges (peanut). Once the esophagus is freed from the gland, the tracheal esophageal groove is exposed.

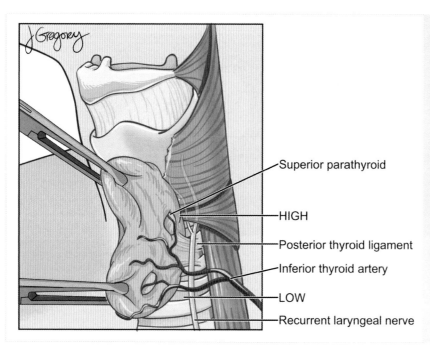

Fig. 33.4 Identification of the recurrent laryngeal nerve. The recurrent laryngeal nerve can be found at the level of the inferior thyroid artery (LOW) or in the region of the superior parathyroid gland and Berry ligament (HIGH). In the LOW region, the recurrent laryngeal nerve is found in the recurrent nerve triangle bound by the carotid artery laterally, trachea medially, and thyroid gland superiorly. To get to the HIGH region, careful blunt dissection in the tracheal esoph-ageal groove is performed to further medialize the thyroid lobe until the area of the Berry ligament is reached without finding the nerve in the LOW position. In the HIGH region, the superior parathyroid gland is often overlying the recurrent laryngeal nerve. If this technique is used, great care must be taken to dissect the superior parathyroid gland away from the thyroid gland without devascularizing it and without damaging the recurrent laryngeal nerve.

of the thyroid extends superiorly in the midline, and its extent varies from patient to patient.

For a total thyroidectomy, we typically place the dissected thyroid lobe back into the surgical bed and then proceed to the contralateral lobe and repeat the same dissection.

For a thyroid lobectomy, the isthmus is divided closer to the opposite side. When a lobectomy is planned, we do not elevate the strap muscles on the opposite side because if a completion thyroidectomy is ever needed in the future, that dissection in-creases scarring and the difficulty of a second surgery.

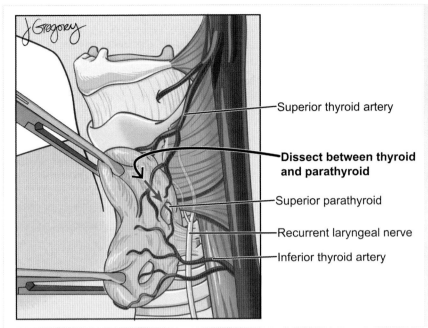

Fig. 33.5 Anatomical relationship of the superior parathyroid gland to the recurrent laryngeal nerve. Dissection of the superior parathyroid gland must be done along its medial aspect to avoid damage to the lateral blood supply. The parathyroid gland is often identified and dissected free from the recurrent laryngeal nerve before the recurrent laryngeal nerve is identified. On occasion, the superior parathyroid gland is within the capsule of the thyroid gland, and dissection beneath the capsule is needed to free it.

(Labels in Fig. 33.5: Superior thyroid artery; Dissect between thyroid and parathyroid; Superior parathyroid; Recurrent laryngeal nerve; Inferior thyroid artery)

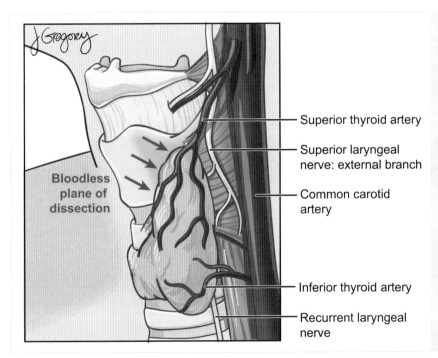

Fig. 33.6 Freeing the superior pole of the thyroid from the trachea. The superior pole of the thyroid and the trachea can be separated by using blunt dissection. Few blood vessels cross this area, and in most patients this is a bloodless plane. In this space, the external branch of the superior laryngeal nerve can be encountered.

(Labels in Fig. 33.6: Bloodless plane of dissection; Superior thyroid artery; Superior laryngeal nerve: external branch; Common carotid artery; Inferior thyroid artery; Recurrent laryngeal nerve)

33.2 Parathyroid Surgery

33.2.1 History

The parathyroid glands were first identified in 1850 by Richard Owen in an Indian rhinoceros at the London Zoo, and then in humans in 1887 by Ivar Sandstrom. Based on Sandstrom's work, Gley in 1890 noted that resection of the parathyroid glands in animals resulted in tetany, and MacCallum in 1909 explained the relationship of the parathyroid glands and calcium metabolism. Erdheim in 1907 reported the relationship of osteomalacia and parathyroid enlargement but explained this as being compensatory. Schlagenhaufer suggested in 1915 that parathyroid enlargement was the cause of bone disease, not a compensatory phenomenon, and recommended removal of the enlarged glands as treatment for bone disease. It was not until 1925 that Mandl reported the first resection of an enlarged parathyroid gland in a patient with severe bone disease, with dramatic results. Soon after, multiple centers reported success with the procedure.

33.2.2 Embryology

There are few surgeries in which an understanding of the embryology of the target tissue is more important than parathyroid surgery. Knowledge of the pattern of embryologic tissue

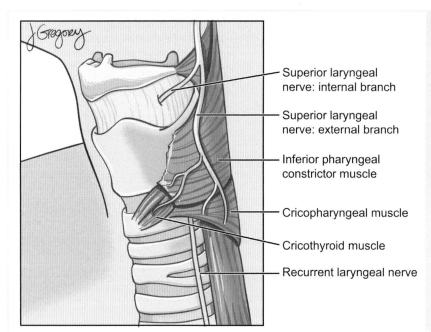

Superior laryngeal nerve: internal branch

Superior laryngeal nerve: external branch

Inferior pharyngeal constrictor muscle

Cricopharyngeal muscle

Cricothyroid muscle

Recurrent laryngeal nerve

Fig. 33.7 Avoiding the superior laryngeal nerve. The external branch of the superior laryngeal nerve can run superficial to, through, or deep to the inferior constrictor muscle. When it is deep to the muscle, it cannot be identified. When it is superficial or pierces the inferior constrictor muscle, it can be identified. When the blood vessels of the superior pole of the thyroid are ligated, the external branch of the superior laryngeal nerve must be avoided. Stimulation of the external branch of the superior laryngeal nerve provokes a brisk response in the cricothyroid muscle, and this can be used to determine the location of the nerve before vessel ligation.

migration is essential in predicting the possible location of normal and ectopic parathyroid glands. The glands arise from the endoderm of the third and fourth branchial pouches. Differentiation occurs at the 8- to 10-mm stage. The inferior parathyroid glands arise from the third branchial pouch, as does the thymic tissue. The superior glands arise from the fourth branchial pouch. The fourth and fifth pouches combine, forming the caudal pharyngeal complex from which the ultimobranchial bodies of the lateral thyroid gland arise. These structures then migrate inferiorly.

The inferior parathyroid glands separate from the thymus to rest at the inferior pole of the thyroid gland, and the superior parathyroid glands come to rest at the posterior–lateral aspect of the middle one-third of the thyroid gland. The longer migratory course of the inferior parathyroid glands compared with the superior glands explains the greater variability in the final location of the inferior glands. The inferior parathyroid glands can be found anywhere from the angle of the mandible to the pericardium (▶ Fig. 33.8). The inferior parathyroid glands are adjacent to the inferior pole of the thyroid gland 61% of the time, in the thyrothymic ligament or superior thymus 26% of the time, and bordering the middle one-third of the thyroid lobe 7% of the time; less frequently, they can be located more superiorly. The superior parathyroid glands are adjacent to or just above the superior one-third of the thyroid gland 85% of the time. If they are not in the typical location, they tend to descend in the retroesophageal space and can be as low as the posterior–superior mediastinum (▶ Fig. 33.9). Intrathyroidal parathyroid glands are seen in 0.7% of cases.

33.2.3 Hyperparathyroidism

Primary hyperparathyroidism is diagnosed based on elevated serum calcium and parathyroid hormone levels (PTH). It is caused by a single adenoma in 80% of cases and a double adenoma in 2 to 5% of cases. Parathyroid hyperplasia is the second most common cause of primary hyperparathyroidism. In secon-

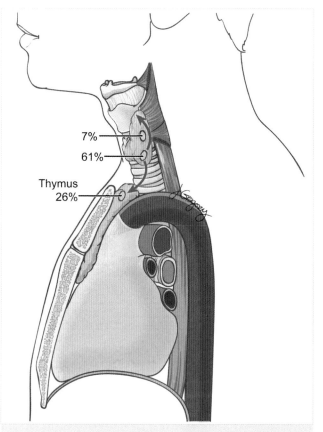

7%

61%

Thymus 26%

Fig. 33.8 Inferior parathyroid glands. The inferior parathyroid glands lie within 1 cm of the inferior pole of the thyroid gland in 61% of cases and in the thyrothymic ligament or superior thymus in 26% of cases.

dary hyperparathyroidism, an elevated serum parathyroid level is present in response to low serum calcium levels. This is most commonly due to chronic renal disease and often can be treated medically. Tertiary hyperparathyroidism results from

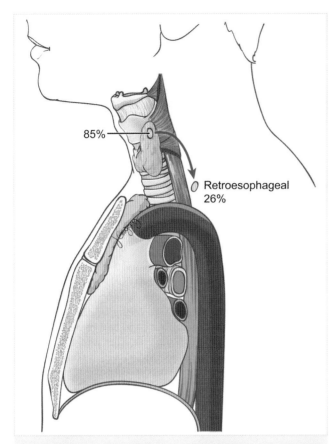

Fig. 33.9 Superior parathyroid glands. The superior parathyroid glands are adjacent to or just above the superior one-third of the thyroid gland 85% of the time. If they are not in the typical location, they tend to descend in the retroesophageal space and can be as low as the posterior–superior mediastinum.

the autonomous secretion of PTH related to long-term overstimulation in secondary hyperparathyroidism.

Traditionally, the complaints of patients with hyperparathyroidism included "stones, bones, and groans" secondary to nephrocalcinosis, osteitis fibrosa cystica, bone resorption, muscle weakness, and psychiatric disorders. Although neuropsychiatric abnormalities such as depression, anxiety, and cognitive disorders have been attributed to hyperparathyroidism, it has not been clearly shown that these conditions are relieved following surgical correction of the endocrinopathy. Although most patients today are asymptomatic at presentation, kidney stones are the most common clinical manifestation of the disease. The peak incidence is between 50 and 60 years of age, and women are three times more likely to be affected than men.

33.2.4 Indications for Parathyroid Surgery

Primary Hyperparathyroidism

The indications for parathyroid surgery are fairly well established based on workshop consensus statements, most recently from 2008:
1. Elevated serum calcium level to 1.0 mg/dL above the upper limit of normal

2. Creatinine clearance rate below 60 mL/min
3. T score below –2.5 for bone mineral density at any site and/or previous fragility fracture
4. Age younger than 50 years
5. Pregnancy (hyperparathyroidism can cause agenesis of the fetal parathyroid glands)
6. History of kidney stones
7. Symptoms: bone pain, neurocognitive disorder

Secondary Hyperparathyroidism

Surgery for secondary hyperparathyroidism is estimated to be needed in only 0.5 to 1.5% of patients based on improvements in medical management with calcimimetic medications like cinacalcet. For the few patients who fail calcimimetic therapy, the surgical guidelines are not well established. General indications for surgery are as follows:
1. Elevated PTH levels (500 to 800 pg/mL)
2. Severe osteoporosis
3. High bone turnover as demonstrated by bone metabolic markers, bone scintigraphy, or biopsy
4. Hypercalcemia
5. Enlarged parathyroid glands on ultrasound
6. Uncontrolled hyperphosphatemia
7. Ectopic calcification
8. Anemia resistant to erythropoietin

Tertiary Hyperparathyroidism

Renal transplant cures most patients of secondary hyperparathyroidism by correcting the metabolic abnormalities responsible for the disease. However, about 25% of patients have tertiary hyperparathyroidism with persistently elevated PTH levels at 1 year after transplant.

33.2.5 Localization Studies

The rate of failure to cure hyperparathyoidism after surgery has been stated to be as high as 5 to 10% in many series. Causes of failure include ectopic glands, multiple adenomas, and multiglandular hyperplasia. Preoperative localization studies to identify hypersecreting glands are performed in an attempt to decrease the incidence of surgical failure. The validity of the often-repeated aphorism that "the only localization study needed by a patient undergoing initial parathyroid surgery is to locate an experienced parathyroid surgeon" has been challenged by advances in parathyroid imaging and intraoperative rapid PTH monitoring. These advances have promoted the widespread acceptance of minimal access parathyroid surgery.

Technetium Sestamibi

Scanning with technetium Tc 99 m sestamibi is the most commonly used localization study. The radioactively labeled sestamibi is absorbed by both parathyroid and thyroid tissue. Parathyroid tissue is distinguished from thyroid tissue based on the higher rate of washout in the thyroid gland relative to the parathyroid glands. Persistent uptake 2 to 3 hours after injection of the sestamibi corresponds to parathyroid tissue.

Both normally located and ectopic adenomas can be localized. The reported sensitivity for single adenomas is between

85% and 100%, which drops to 37% for multiple adenomas. The sensitivity for hyperplastic glands is 62%. The sestamibi localizes in mitochondria, and the lower concentration of mitochondria-rich oxyphil cells in hyperplastic glands than in adenomas explains the decreased sensitivity in hyperplastic tissue. Multinodular thyroid disease also can confound the findings. The surgeon should always personally review the sestamibi scans, particularly negative scans, because the findings can be too subtle for the radiologist to make a definitive reading.

In addition to preoperative localization, ^{99m}Tc-sestamibi is used to determine the completeness of surgical resection without the need to wait for intraoperative PTH levels. Dr. James Norman and his associates inject patients with sestamibi just before surgery and use a gamma probe to quantify the amount of PTH each gland is producing. According to the "Norman rule," when the radioactivity in the resected gland is at least 20% of the excision site/background radioactivity, a solitary parathyroid adenoma is confirmed, with no further identification of other parathyroid glands necessary. Their data show that all solitary parathyroid adenomas contain radioactivity that is at least 18% of the excision site/background radioactivity, with the levels in most much higher. Hyperplastic glands always contain less than 16%. In 87% of patients, excised glands have radioactivity levels that are more than 20% of the excision site/background radioactivity, allowing the immediate confirmation of surgical cure.

Negative ^{99m}Tc-sestamibi scans occur with regularity and can deter endocrinologists and surgeons from pursuing surgical cure for parathyroid disease. Dr. Norman argues that negative scans are as useful as positive scans, if done well, and indicate that the abnormal gland is not outside the normal location for parathyroid glands. In his experience, the negative parathyroid scan almost always guarantees that the abnormal parathyroid gland is in a favorable location behind or around the thyroid.

Ultrasound

The accuracy of ultrasound is operator-dependent. In recent years, surgeon-performed ultrasound of the neck has gained widespread acceptance. The parathyroid glands are seen as a homogeneous, well-demarcated mass with lower echogenicity than that of thyroid tissue. Ultrasound has a reported sensitivity of 85% and a specificity of 94% for adenomas, and a sensitivity of 69% for hyperplasia. The identification of ectopic glands is limited because these often occur in areas that are not well visualized with ultrasound, such as the mediastinum and retroesophageal areas.

Ultrasound can be used to perform guided fine-needle aspiration biopsies to confirm the presence of parathyroid tissue. Aspirated samples can be sent for cytology, but a much more sensitive test for parathyroid tissue is PTH washout. The aspirated needle is washed with 2 mL of saline, and this is sent to the laboratory for a determination of PTH levels. Generally, a PTH level higher than the serum PTH level indicates parathyroid tissue.

Computed Tomography

This modality is particularly useful in the localization of ectopic glands. When used, the studies should be done with contrast and thin cuts (3 to 5 mm). For adenomas, the sensitivity is 50% and the specificity is 98%; the sensitivity for hyperplasia is 40%.

Magnetic Resonance Imaging

This modality is also useful in the identification of ectopic glands. Adenomas have increased T2 signal and are isointense on T1 sequences. Sensitivities of 78% for adenomas and 90% for ectopic mediastinal adenomas have been reported. The sensitivity is 71% for hyperplastic glands.

Single photon emission computed tomography (SPECT) and positron emission tomography (PET) have also been proposed as helpful localizing techniques but are not as widely used as the techniques discussed above.

Methylene Blue Injection

An intravenous injection of saline-diluted methylene blue given intraoperatively can help identify abnormal parathyroid glands as a result of absorption of the dye, which stains the glands blue. The recommended dose is 5 to 7.5 mg/kg. The mechanism of this action is not understood, but it can be a useful adjunct in the arsenal of a parathyroid surgeon. The administration of methylene blue should be avoided in patients taking selective serotonin reuptake inhibitors because neurologic side effects have been reported.

33.2.6 Surgical Considerations

The basic steps of a parathyroid exploration are the same as those for a thyroid lobectomy, as described earlier in this chapter. We generally use electrophysiologic monitoring of the recurrent laryngeal nerve and intraoperative PTH assays during all of our surgeries. Although some surgeons use a lateral approach to the parathyroid glands, dissecting between the anterior border of the sternocleidomastoid muscle and the lateral border of the strap muscles, we generally use a medial approach for an initial exploration. Meticulous hemostasis and strict adherence to the principle of dissection along natural tissue planes cannot be overstressed. Blood staining of tissue will complicate identification of the parathyroid glands, as well as other structures, such as the recurrent laryngeal nerves and the fine blood vessels that supply the glands. The parathyroid glands are often described as tan to reddish in color, with an oval shape. A normal gland weighs between 20 and 50 mg.

Once the thyroid lobe is dissected laterally, it is delivered into the wound. Occasionally, the superior pole vessels require suture ligation, and the superior medial aspect of the sternohyoid muscle may need to be incised to aid in lateralization of the strap muscles and delivery of the thyroid lobe. If preoperative localization studies have identified an enlarged gland, the exploration begins at that site. If not, the exploration begins with a search for the glands in their most common anatomical locations as part of the primary survey. Each surgeon should develop an algorithm for exploration that is methodical and complete, approaching each procedure with the goal of finding all four of the parathyroid glands, whether in normal locations or ectopic. Once an obviously enlarged gland is identified and removed, we do not continue exploring and base the need for further exploration on the results of the intraoperative PTH assay.

If the PTH levels drop 50% and into the normal range, the surgery is concluded. If not, the exploration for a second adenoma or additional hyperplastic glands continues.

In a patient with a nonlocalizing preoperative work-up, we generally begin the exploration at the superior thyroid pole. Although not essential, dissection of the recurrent laryngeal nerve is often helpful in locating the superior parathyroid gland. The superior gland will be within 1 cm of the point of entry of the nerve into the larynx 85% of the time, lateral and deep to the nerve (see ▶ Fig. 33.9). The inferior gland is within 1 cm of the inferior thyroid pole 61% of the time, commonly inferior and deep to the thyroid gland and medial to the recurrent laryngeal nerve (see ▶ Fig. 33.8). If two normal glands are identified or if an enlarged gland is excised and the PTH level does not normalize, the exploration proceeds to the opposite side. Double adenomas are present in 2 to 5% of patients, with the second lesion contralateral 80% of the time.

If only one normal gland and no enlarged gland is identified, a secondary survey is undertaken. The secondary survey involves a sequential exploration of the common locations of ectopic glands. An upper parathyroid gland is likely to be, in decreasing frequency, in the area posterior and lateral to the upper lobe of the thyroid, in the retrolaryngeal/retroesophageal space, or above the upper pole of the thyroid (see ▶ Fig. 33.9). On rare occasions, it may be found in the carotid sheath or scalene fat pad.

For the inferior gland, secondary areas to be explored are the thyrothymic ligament and upper thymus gland, the lateral neck at the level of the inferior thyroid pole, the area medial to the inferior pole along the trachea, the lower thymic tissue in the anterior mediastinum, and finally, although much less commonly, the upper neck from the mandible to the hyoid and carotid bifurcation (see ▶ Fig. 33.8). If at this point the involved gland has not been identified, termination of the procedure should be considered. A thyroid lobectomy on the side of the missing gland is not recommended unless preoperative imaging studies show the presence of a nodular lesion within the thyroid. If the exploration is unsuccessful, further localization studies including selective venous sampling should be done postoperatively to determine the likely location of the missed adenoma.

In the presence of hyperplasia in multiple glands, the surgical treatment can be total parathyroidectomy with auto-transplantation of parathyroid tissue in the forearm or subtotal parathyroidectomy with preservation of a 20- to 50-mg parathyroid remnant. in choosing one technique over the other, the risk for autograft failure should be weighed against the risk for recurrent hyperparathyroidism and need for reexploration in a previously dissected neck. If a parathyroid remnant is preserved, it should be marked with a surgical clip at the time of the original surgery to aid its identification if the need for reexploration should arise.

33.3 Roundsmanship

- The four most common types of thyroid cancer are papillary, follicular, medullary, and anaplastic.
- Theodor Kocher, the "father of thyroid surgery," won a Nobel Prize in Medicine and Physiology in 1909 for his work on thyroid and parathyroid physiology.

- The main indications for thyroid surgery are cancer, concern for cancer, symptomatic goiter, and hyperthyroidism.
- The Bethesda System for Reporting Thyroid Cytopathology divides the results of fine-needle aspiration aspiration biopsy of the thyroid into six categories: benign, malignant, nondiagnostic, neoplasm (either follicular or Hürthle cell), suspicious for malignancy, and follicular lesion of undetermined significance.
- The right recurrent laryngeal nerve is in a more lateral position than the left.
- Non-recurrent laryngeal nerves occur mostly on the right side and are associated with arteria lusoria (in which the right subclavian artery originates from the aortic arch and passes posterior to the esophagus).
- A left-sided non-recurrent laryngeal nerve is associated with dextrocardia.
- To preserve the blood supply to the superior parathyroid glands, the medial aspect of the parathyroid gland must be carefully peeled off the thyroid while the lateral blood supply is protected. Occasionally, the superior parathyroid gland is in the capsule or underneath the capsule of the thyroid.
- The external branch of the superior laryngeal nerve innervates the cricothryoid muscle, and it can lie in close proximity to the blood vessels of the superior pole of the thyroid.
- The superior parathyroid glands arise from the fourth branchial pouch and are typically adjacent to the upper one-third of the thyroid gland. They lie lateral and dorsal to the recurrent laryngeal nerve.
- The inferior parathyroid glands arise from the third branchial pouch and are typically adjacent to the inferior pole of the thyroid. They lie ventral and medial to the recurrent laryngeal nerve.
- For primary hyperparathyroidism, a drop in the PTH level of 50% into the normal range is indicative of surgical cure. Alternatively, with radioactivity-guided parathyroidectomy, radioactivity in the removed adenoma that is more than 20% of the excision site/background radioactivity indicates surgical cure.

33.4 Recommended Reading

[1] Bilezikian JP, Khan AA, Potts JT Third International Workshop on the Management of Asymptomatic Primary Hyperthyroidism. Guidelines for the management of asymptomatic primary hyperparathyroidism: summary statement from the third international workshop. J Clin Endocrinol Metab 2009; 94: 335–339

[2] Carty SE, Cooper DS, Doherty GM et alAmerican Thyroid Association Surgery Working GroupAmerican Association of Endocrine SurgeonsAmerican Academy of Otolaryngology-Head and Neck SurgeryAmerican Head and Neck Society. Consensus statement on the terminology and classification of central neck dissection for thyroid cancer. Thyroid 2009; 19: 1153–1158

[3] Cooper DS, Doherty GM, Haugen BR et alAmerican Thyroid Association (ATA) Guidelines Taskforce on Thyroid Nodules and Differentiated Thyroid Cancer. Revised American Thyroid Association management guidelines for patients with thyroid nodules and differentiated thyroid cancer. Thyroid 2009; 19: 1167–1214

[4] Murphy C, Norman J. The 20% rule: a simple, instantaneous radioactivity measurement defines cure and allows elimination of frozen sections and hormone assays during parathyroidectomy. Surgery 1999; 126: 1023–1028, discussion 1028–1029

[5] Norman J. Controversies in parathyroid surgery: The quest for a "mini" unilateral parathyroid operation seems to have gone too far. J Surg Oncol 2012; 105: 1–3

34 Soft-Tissue Tumors of the Head and Neck

Mark S. Persky and Theresa N. Tran

34.1 Introduction

Head and neck soft-tissue tumors comprise a diverse group of benign and malignant lesions, ranging from vascular tumors with indolent behavior to locoregionally destructive soft-tissue sarcomas with a high potential for distant metastases. This chapter highlights the wide spectrum of these tumors, with an emphasis on their natural history, evaluation, and treatment.

34.2 Paraganglioma

34.2.1 The Disease Process

Paragangliomas are vascular tumors that arise from the extra-adrenal paraganglia derived from the neural crest. They most commonly occur in the head and neck region. These tumors are closely associated with either blood vessels (carotid artery, jugular bulb) or nerves (vagus, tympanic plexus). Paragangliomas are usually slowly growing tumors in which the growth pattern may be described as biphasic because the growth rate of very small and very large paragangliomas is slower than that of intermediate-size tumors.

Paragangliomas may occur in patients with familial multiple endocrine neoplasia (MEN), both type IIA (pheochromocytoma, medullary thyroid carcinoma, and parathyroid hyperplasia) and type IIB (also includes mucosal neuromas). A familial history of paragangliomas may be present, and there is a significant incidence of multicentric tumors in both familial and sporadic cases. Familial or hereditary paragangliomas have been reported to account for 5 to 10% of all cases of head and neck paragangliomas, although some report that they may account for up to 25 to 50% of cases. Most (90%) cases of hereditary paragangliomas involve the carotid body. If a familial history is present, there is a 78 to 87% possibility of multiple paragangliomas. The most common multicentric combination is that of two carotid body tumors (▶ Fig. 34.1), which occurs in approximately 20% of patients with carotid body tumors.

Malignant paragangliomas are uncommon, and their diagnosis can be confirmed only by metastatic disease because histologic examination of the primary tumor is unreliable for establishing a diagnosis of malignancy. The prevalence of malignancy depends upon the site of the primary tumor, and there has been considerable variability in the reported frequency. The most common sites of distant carotid body tumor metastases are the bones, lungs, and liver. Malignancy is generally less common in familial paragangliomas than in sporadic cases. The most common sites of metastases for jugulotympanic paragangliomas are, in decreasing frequency, the lungs, lymph nodes, liver, vertebrae, ribs, and spleen. Although the reported rate of malignancy of vagal paragangliomas is as high as 19%, a 10% frequency is most frequently accepted. Vagal paragangliomas probably have the highest rate of malignancy (16 to 19%) among the more common types of head and neck paragangliomas. Primary orbital and laryngeal tumors demonstrate the highest rate of malignancy (20 to 25%) of all head and neck paragangliomas.

Carotid Body Tumor

As the carotid body tumor grows, it tends to splay the carotid bifurcation and progressively involves the carotid adventitia. Classically, the internal carotid artery is displaced posteriorly and laterally (▶ Fig. 34.2). With continued growth, the tumor extends superiorly along the internal carotid to the skull base and may cause bony erosion and/or affect adjacent cranial nerves, most commonly the vagus and hypoglossal nerves. Occasionally, the sympathetic chain is involved. Medial extension into the parapharyngeal space is reported in 20% of cases.

Jugular and Tympanic Paragangliomas

Tympanic paragangliomas arise from the paraganglia associated with the Jacobson and Arnold nerves. They may fill the middle ear cavity and extend posteriorly into the mastoid air cells or inferiorly to the jugular bulb. Jugular paragangliomas tend to spread along the paths of least resistance in multiple directions and gain access to various portions of the temporal bone and base of the skull neurovascular foramina. Progressive temporal involvement leads to posterior cranial fossa involvement. Intracranial extension can occur as posterior extension directly through the petrous bone, extension into and through the internal auditory canal, or infralabyrinthine extension. There is early intraluminal jugular extension into the sigmoid sinus and

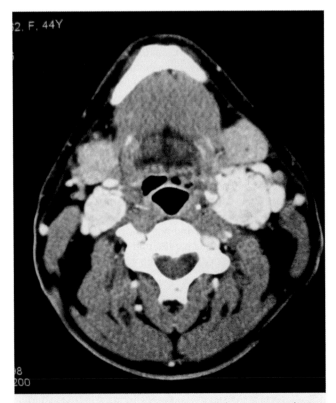

Fig. 34.1 Axial computed tomographic scan with contrast revealing bilateral, markedly enhancing carotid body tumors.

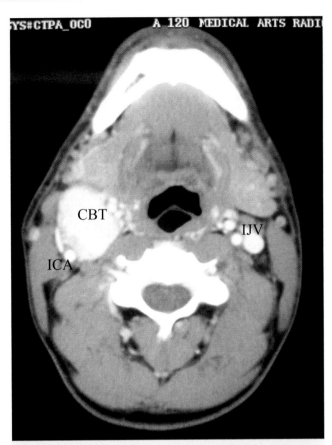

Fig. 34.2 Axial computed tomographic scan with contrast showing posterolateral displacement of the internal carotid artery by carotid body tumor. *CBT*, carotid body tumor; *ICA*, internal carotid artery; *IJV*, internal jugular vein.

internal jugular vein, with possible growth into the inferior petrosal sinus. Tumor can invade the middle ear cleft, petrous apex, or mastoid and retrofacial air cells. Inferiorly, jugular paragangliomas may extend through the infratemporal fossa and post-styloid parapharyngeal space into the neck.

Vagal Paragangliomas

Vagal paragangliomas most commonly arise from the nodose (inferior) ganglion, although they may also originate from the middle and superior ganglia, and less frequently anywhere along the course of the vagus nerve. Compared with the discrete carotid body, the vagal paraganglia are distributed more diffusely within the nerve or perineurium. Vagus nerve fibers "splay over" the surface of the vagal paraganglioma or, early in their development, enter the substance of the tumor; therefore, preservation of the vagus nerve is usually not possible with complete tumor resection.

Vagal paragangliomas have three basic patterns of spread. Because most vagal parangliomas originate at the nodose ganglion, they tend to spread inferiorly into the post-styloid parapharyngeal area. Extension superiorly toward the skull base in the area of the jugular foramen results in early involvement of the internal jugular vein and adjacent cranial nerves (IX, XI, XII). The tumor causes early anterior displacement of the internal carotid artery. Vagal paragangliomas

originating from the superior ganglion have a greater chance of assuming a "dumbbell" form with posterior cranial fossa tumor, in addition to extending into the parapharyngeal space inferiorly.

34.2.2 Evaluation

Carotid Body Tumor

The median age of patients at presentation for carotid body tumors is 45 to 54 years, with a range from 12 to 78 years. Most series report a female predominance of approximately 2:1. The most common presenting symptom of a carotid body tumor is a neck mass located at or superior to the carotid bifurcation and deep to the sternocleidomastoid muscle. On palpation, it is vertically fixed and laterally mobile because of its fixation to the carotid artery, and it may be pulsatile. Bruits have been reported in 10 to 16% of cases. Pain is present in approximately 25% of cases. Medial extension into the parapharyngeal space has been reported and may cause submucosal bulging of the lateral oropharynx and medial displacement of the tonsils. Cranial neuropathies are present in approximately 10 to 30% of cases at presentation.

Jugular and Tympanic Paragangliomas

Tympanic paragangliomas occur most commonly during the sixth decade of life, have a marked female preponderance, and usually present with a conductive hearing loss, pulsatile tinnitus, and a mass behind the tympanic membrane. On otoscopic examination, a red–blue middle ear mass that blanches on positive pneumatoscopic pressure (Brown sign) may be present. Perforation of the tumor through the tympanic membrane may occur, producing a vascular "polyp" that may bleed spontaneously. Within the middle ear, continued growth results in ossicular involvement and a subsequent conductive hearing loss. Continued growth with vestibular involvement produces a sensorineural hearing loss, vertigo, and occasionally pain from the associated inflammatory response.

Jugular paragangliomas most commonly occur in the fifth and sixth decades of life and demonstrate a female-to-male ratio of 4:1 to 6:1. Extension into the middle ear results in symptoms similar to those of tympanic paragangliomas and may result in a conductive or sensorineural hearing loss, depending on the extent of vestibular involvement. Hearing loss (55 to 77%) and tinnitus (56 to 72%) are the most common presenting symptoms. Symptoms related to lower cranial nerve (VII through XII) deficits are also common. Tumors of the skull base without extensive middle ear extension may present with isolated tongue weakness, hoarseness, dysphagia, or shoulder drop or with symptoms of multiple cranial nerve dysfunction. The jugular foramen syndrome (cranial nerve IX, X, and XI palsy, or Vernet syndrome) is occasionally encountered, and cranial nerve IX through XII palsy (Collet-Sicard syndrome) occurs in approximately 10% of patients with jugular paragangliomas.

Vagal Paragangliomas

Vagal paragangliomas most commonly present as an asymptomatic mass of the upper neck, typically more cephalad than carotid body tumors. Vagal paragangliomas are slow-growing, with a female-to-male preponderance of 2:1 to 3:1. As the tumor enlarges, it encroaches upon the lower cranial nerves and the adjacent sympathetic chain. Signs and symptoms include unilateral vocal cord paralysis, hoarseness, dysphagia, nasal regurgitation, atrophy of the hemitongue, shoulder weakness, and Horner syndrome. Hearing loss and pulsatile tinnitus are usually indicative of temporal bone extension.

Computed tomography (CT) and magnetic resonance (MR) imaging usually establish the diagnosis of paraganglioma. Imaging with indium In 111 pentetreotide (OctreoScan; Mallinckrodt Medical, Petten, The Netherlands) or fluorine F 18 dihydroxyphenylalanine (DOPA) positron emission tomography (PET) can also be used to evaluate paragangliomas, define multiple tumors, and detect the possible presence of metastatic disease. Angiography defines the vascular supply, may visualize vessel involvement (invasion), and paves the way for preoperative embolization, which is important if surgery is contemplated.

34.2.3 Treatment

Surgery

Traditionally, surgery has been the preferred method of treatment, especially with the evolution of more sophisticated approaches to the skull base, safer embolization protocols, and advanced vascular bypass procedures. However, postoperative cranial nerve dysfunction is anticipated in patients with those paragangliomas characterized by early neural involvement and skull base involvement, in whom surgery would require extensive rehabilitation efforts. The role of surgery should therefore be reevaluated as the primary treatment of choice for these slow-growing tumors. Some paragangliomas, especially very small ones, have been shown not to be progressive, and "wait and scan" management may be advisable. Relative contraindications to surgery include extensive skull base or intracranial involvement, advanced age of the patient, medical comorbidities, and bilateral or multiple paragangliomas for which surgery may result in the unacceptable postoperative morbidity of bilateral lower cranial nerve palsies.

If surgery is the chosen treatment course, preoperative embolization is often performed. There are major advantages in the use of combined endovascular embolization and subsequent surgery, assuming that certain criteria are fulfilled before embolization. Surgery is performed within 2 days of angiography and embolization in order to avoid recruitment of collateral tumor blood supply and before the onset of a significant postinflammatory effect. Short-term steroids are administered if there is concern about tumor edema that may compromise tumor dissection.

Radiation Therapy

Radiotherapy has traditionally been the treatment of choice for unresectable paragangliomas or those tumors in the medically infirm and elderly. However, radiotherapy has more recently been proved to be an effective therapeutic option and therefore should be considered as a form of primary treatment, especially in the setting of the significant potential morbidity that accompanies surgery for some tumors. Radiotherapy has been used primarily to treat jugular paragangliomas of the temporal bone and less frequently for the treatment of carotid body or vagal paragangliomas. Radiotherapy is the preferred treatment option for advanced tumors. Stereotactic radiosurgery offers the possibility of a single, highly focused, small-field treatment with a steep dose gradient to maximally spare the surrounding normal tissue.

34.3 Juvenile Nasopharyngeal Angiofibroma

34.3.1 The Disease Process

Juvenile nasopharyngeal angiofibroma (JNA) is a highly vascular, histologically benign, but locally aggressive and destructive tumor that exclusively affects boys of adolescent age. It accounts for approximately 0.5% of all head and neck neoplasms. The etiology and pathogenesis of the disease remain to be elucidated. The tumor appears to originate in the posterior nasal cavity rather than the nasopharynx. Specifically, it develops in the posterolateral wall of the superior aspect of the nasal cavity, at the junction of the sphenoid process of the palatine bone, the horizontal ala of the vomer, and the root of the pterygoid process of the sphenoid bone, near the superior margin of the sphenopalatine foramen. These tumors are unencapsulated and consist of proliferating, irregular vascular spaces lined by a single endothelial layer. The channels lack a complete muscular layer between the endothelial cells and stromal cells and are therefore subject to severe bleeding.

At diagnosis, most angiofibromas have extended beyond the nasal cavity and nasopharynx, with anterolateral erosion of the posterior wall of the maxillary sinus and lateral growth into the pterygomaxillary fossa. Extension into the pterygomaxillary fossa can erode the pterygoid process of the sphenoid bone. Further lateral extension via the pterygomaxillary fissure can fill the infratemporal fossa and produce the classic bulging cheek. Tumor can extend under the zygomatic arch and cause swelling above the arch. From the pterygomaxillary fossa, the angiofibroma can erode the greater wing of the sphenoid bone and the middle cranial fossa and invade both the inferior and superior orbital fissures. Posterior extension into the sphenoid sinus through the floor or ostium fills the sinus, and extension farther superiorly fills the sella turcica. Tumor in the sella or orbit can cause loss of vision. These tumors typically grow by centrifugal expansion, not by invasion; therefore, they may be intracranial but are usually extradural. The cavernous sinus may be compressed but not invaded. Cranial nerve palsies are rare, even with large tumors. However, particularly aggressive angiofibromas may invade the cavernous sinus and threaten multiple cranial nerves, the internal carotid artery, hypophysis, and optic chiasm.

Despite its tendency to be invasive, the rate of growth of JNA is thought to be slow. Because the tumor is rarely seen in young adults, it is believed to regress spontaneously. However, because regression cannot be assumed, these tumors should be treated. The prognosis for patients with JNA is good with early diagnosis; unfortunately, the diagnosis most often is made during later stages of the disease because of the nonspecific and innocuous presenting symptoms of JNA. JNA is characterized by

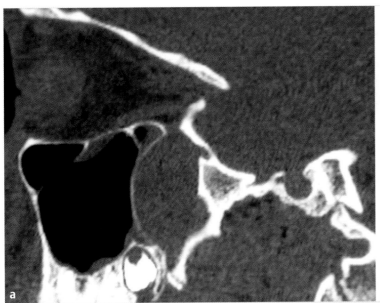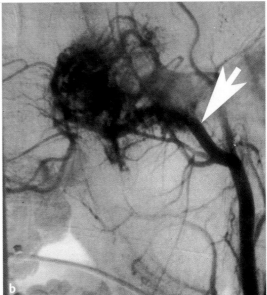

Fig. 34.3 (a,b) Sagittal computed tomographic scan displaying anterior bowing of the posterior wall of the maxillary sinus, known as the Holman-Miller sign, which is diagnostic for juvenile nasopharyngeal angiofibroma. (b) Lateral subtracted angiogram of internal maxillary artery (*arrow*) revealing tumor hypervascularity of the angiofiboma.

high recurrence rates, reportedly as high as 30 to 50%. It is a benign disease that is not multifocal; therefore, recurrence usually reflects persistent disease.

34.3.2 Evaluation

JNA is typically found in adolescent males; patients range in age from 7 to 29 years, with a median age of 15 years at diagnosis. They classically present with the triad of unilateral nasal obstruction, recurrent severe epistaxis, and nasopharyngeal mass; other common but nonspecific symptoms are purulent nasal discharge due to infection secondary to obstruction, hyponasal speech, and anosmia. Nasal obstruction and epistaxis occur in more than 80% of patients. Symptoms may be present for months to years before the diagnosis is made. Delay in presentation and/or diagnosis can be attributed to the tendency to associate the indolent symptoms of JNA with more common entities, such as rhinitis, sinusitis, and nasal polyposis.

Examination often shows a red–gray, smooth, lobulated mass in the nasopharynx and/or posterior aspect of the nose. The overlying mucosa is rarely ulcerated unless the patient has previously undergone biopsy or therapy. Other signs include facial deformity, proptosis, palate extension, serous otitis media, and visual or auditory impairment. Neurologic deficits may be seen in patients who have angiofibromas with significant intracranial extension.

The radiographic findings of angiofibroma are characteristic. On CT scan, there is anterior bowing of the posterior wall of the maxillary sinus, known as the Holman-Miller sign, and enlargement of the superior orbital fissure, which are considered diagnostic for JNA (▶ Fig. 34.3). CT is also ideal for localizing the tumor and useful in delineating the extent of the tumor. Magnetic resonance (MR) imaging is indicated in patients with intracranial extension. Angiography is not necessary in most patients but is useful in those whose diagnosis remains in question, usually those in whom previous treatment has failed. It

also is necessary for embolization, especially when surgery is anticipated.

34.3.3 Treatment

Surgery

The mainstay of treatment for JNA is surgery. The various surgical approaches are transpalatal, transnasal (including endoscopic), transantral, transmandibular, transzygomatic, combined craniotomy and rhinotomy, lateral rhinotomy, and midface degloving. Recurrence does not necessarily indicate the need for further treatment unless there are associated symptoms of bleeding, nasal obstruction, eye findings, or progressive growth as defined by radiographic studies.

The main blood supply of a JNA is from the internal maxillary artery; however, the thyrocervical trunk and the dural, sphenoidal, and ophthalmic branches from the internal carotid system can also contribute. Because of this extensive arterial supply, ligation of the external carotid artery before surgical excision does not help to decrease bleeding but instead may have the opposite effect by encouraging arterial collateralization from vessels that are less accessible or inaccessible. Techniques that have been used to decrease bleeding include preoperative embolization, ligation of the internal maxillary artery, electrocoagulation, and irradiation.

Radiation Therapy

Although surgery is considered to be the treatment of choice for JNA, the potential morbidity associated with the surgical resection of some extensive tumors makes radiation treatment a possible alternative. Radiotherapy is often considered an appropriate option for the treatment of recurrent angiofibromas. Lee et al reported 27 patients with extensive tumors who received radiation as the primary mode of treatment, with minimal

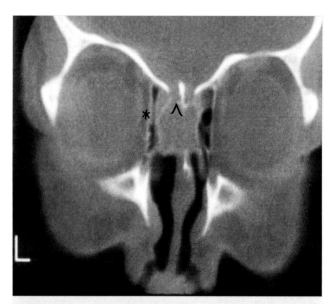

Fig. 34.4 Coronal computed tomographic scan demonstrating the usual location of olfactory neuroblastoma. *Caret*, intact skull base; *asterisk*, intact lamina papyracea.

complications and perhaps less risk for significant morbidity and mortality than that associated with surgical intervention. Long-term complications consist of growth retardation, panhypopituitarism, temporal lobe necrosis, cataracts, and radiation keratopathy.

34.4 Olfactory Neuroblastoma

34.4.1 The Disease Process

Olfactory neuroblastoma (also known as esthesioneuroblastoma) is an uncommon malignancy of neural crest origin arising in the olfactory epithelium of the nasal cavity. The cells of origin are presumed to be basal cells of the olfactory epithelium. Its histologic resemblance to undifferentiated small cell carcinoma can lead to a misdiagnosis. Neuroblastomas account for approximately 2 to 3% of all malignant nasal neoplasms and 0.3% of upper aerodigestive tract malignancies. No clear etiology for the development of olfactory neuroblastoma has been established.

Olfactory neuroblastomas are locally aggressive tumors that frequently invade the paranasal sinuses, skull base, and orbit. These tumors can be multicentric, with separate tumors above and below the cribriform plate and no gross or microscopic connection between the tumors. The location of this tumor, at the interface between the superior nasal cavity and anterior cranial fossa, leads to early involvement of the cribriform plate and allows rapid penetration into the anterior cranial fossa (▶ Fig. 34.4).

Metastasis to cervical lymph nodes can be found, either at diagnosis or at regional recurrence many years after treatment. Reports of the overall incidence of cervical metastasis range from 10 to 33%, and the incidence of distant metastasis ranges from 10 to 40% of patients, with the lungs, brain, and bones the most common sites. The overall 5- and 10-year survival rates for olfactory neuroblastomas are better than those for most

superior nasal vault malignancies and are estimated to be approximately 80% and 50%, respectively. Long-term endoscopic and MR imaging surveillance is mandatory because local, regional, and distant metastasis may be expected to occur for as long as 10 years or more after treatment.

34.4.2 Evaluation

Olfactory neuroblastomas can be found in patients ages 3 to 90 years. There is a bimodal distribution in age groups, with peaks at 11 to 20 years and at 51 to 60 years. Others have found a unimodal distribution concentrating in the fifth decade of life. There is no predilection for either gender. Early lesions are usually asymptomatic. Grossly, these tumors appear as soft, red–gray, polypoid masses located high in the nasal cavity. They present with symptoms of epistaxis and unilateral nasal congestion, which may be present for months to years. Additional symptoms include rhinorrhea, hyposmia or anosmia, headache, and serous otitis media. Other findings are related to sites of invasion and metastasis. Orbital symptoms, including proptosis, visual field defects, orbital pain, epiphora, and blindness, suggest orbital or intracranial extension and indicate a poor prognosis. The diagnosis is usually made late in the course of disease, and tumor extension may be extensive at presentation. A high index of suspicion is needed to diagnose olfactory neuroblastoma in patients presenting with unilateral nasal symptoms and epistaxis.

Radiographic findings are nonspecific, consisting of unilateral opacification of the ethmoid sinuses, with or without accompanying bone destruction, and a soft-tissue mass within the nasal cavity, with possible extension into the sphenoid and maxillary sinuses, orbit, and cranial vault. Bone expansion seen on radiographic imaging is consistent with slow progression of the tumor. MR imaging can aid in the initial diagnosis by differentiating neoplasm from obstructive disease and by identifying intracranial extension. MR imaging is also most useful for postoperative surveillance. CT is helpful in defining possible intracranial involvement in tumors with skull base erosion. Angiographic findings vary from definitive hypervascularity with early-draining veins to a faint but discrete tumor blush.

34.4.3 Treatment

Surgery

Surgical resection is the recommended treatment for olfactory neuroblastomas. The various surgical approaches used in the management of olfactory neuroblastomas include lateral rhinotomy or transnasal endoscopic resection, craniofacial resection, and combined endoscopic nasal and anterior craniotomy resection, depending on the size and extent of the tumor and the surgeon's expertise.

Adjuvant Therapy

Combined treatment with radiation, given before or after surgery, is often advocated to decrease the chance of local recurrence of olfactory neuroblastomas. Several investigators recommend surgery alone in low-grade or early-stage disease, whereas others advocate the addition of either preoperative or postoperative radiation, which has been demonstrated to significantly improve local control, even in early-stage disease. Furthermore, Koka et al showed improved outcomes with the addition of chemotherapy, but not radiotherapy.

No true consensus exists as to the best treatment approach; however, multimodality treatment regimens are currently the most frequently advocated interventions, with craniofacial resection the most commonly recommended surgical approach. Various sequences of surgery, radiation, and chemotherapy are used, depending on the extent of disease. Olfactory neuroblastomas are believed to be chemosensitive. Chemotherapy is usually given as neoadjuvant treatment for advanced disease. Several authors advocate preoperative chemotherapeutic treatment to reduce tumor size before surgical resection is attempted. Chao et al also advocate elective treatment, by either irradiation or radical neck dissection or both, of the upper neck in patients with more extensive disease, especially when the tumor has spread beyond the nasal cavity or paranasal sinuses.

34.5 Hemangiopericytoma

34.5.1 The Disease Process

Hemangiopericytoma of the head and neck is a rare neoplasm that originates from the pericytes, or cells of Zimmerman, surrounding normal vascular channels. It is considered by some to be a lesion with a low risk for malignant potential and by others to be a malignant lesion with high metastatic potential. Thus, it is known as a tumor that varies greatly in appearance and biological behavior. Hemangiopericytomas account for 3 to 5% of all soft-tissue sarcomas and 1% of all vascular tumors.

In the head and neck, the clinical behavior of a hemangiopericytoma may vary from a slowly enlarging rubbery mass to an infiltrating aggressive neoplasm. Distant metastasis to lung, liver, and bone may occur, but regional spread to lymph nodes has not been observed. The rate of metastasis varies significantly from 10 to 60% and is consistent with the observation that this tumor varies greatly in biological behavior. Gengler et al emphasize the difficulty of predicting the clinical behavior of hemangiopericytomas and patient outcomes; thus, close long-term follow-up is crucial for patients with hemangiopericytomas because of the high incidence of local recurrence and the potentially metastasizing course.

34.5.2 Evaluation

Hemangiopericytomas occur most commonly in the sixth and seventh decades of life and have no sex predilection. Many of these tumors may have been present for a long time before they are diagnosed, and patients typically present with a slowly growing mass that occasionally reaches a considerable size. Symptoms include facial pain, occasionally facial swelling, epistaxis, sinusitis, visual changes, and nasal obstruction, depending on the anatomical site of involvement. The facial skin overlying the tumor may be warm to the touch because of the rich vascularity of the hemangiopericytoma. In the oral cavity, its clinical appearance is that of a firm, usually well-circumscribed swelling of the mucosa. In the nose, it is usually described as soft, rubbery, pale gray or tan polypoid mass. Despite the pale, avascular appearance, these tumors bleed vigorously when biopsied. Because of their benign clinical appearance, they can be misdiagnosed as benign tumors or nasal polyps.

The diagnosis of hemangiopericytoma depends on an accurate pathologic assessment of the biopsied specimen. Radiographic imaging assists in the diagnosis. Hemangiopericytomas appear as rounded, sharply outlined or well-circumscribed, homogeneous masses that often displace neighboring structures on CT scan. CT can clearly demonstrate bone destruction within the nasal cavity, paranasal sinuses, and adjacent intracranial structures. Angiography shows a richly vascularized mass, dilated arteries, and diffuse capillary blush. Occasionally, early visualization of the veins suggests arteriovenous shunting. MR imaging reveals several characteristic features suggesting the diagnosis of a solitary fibrous tumor: isointensity on T1-weighted imaging and iso- to hypointensity on T2-weighted imaging.

The follow-up of patients with hemangiopericytoma should include regular clinical as well as radiologic examinations, especially patients with deep-seated tumors or those with suspicion of tumor recurrence and/or metastasis. Long-term follow-up of patients with these tumors should be maintained because some hemangiopericytomas, including histologically low-grade tumors, display late recurrence and metastasis, even beyond 5 years.

34.5.3 Treatment

The preferred treatment for hemangiopericytomas is wide surgical excision, usually performed via lateral rhinotomy, midface degloving, craniofacial resection, or endoscopic resection. Many advocate a craniofacial approach for patients with cribriform plate or base of skull involvement. Schlosser et al have demonstrated that endoscopic approaches can provide excellent visualization and tumor resection, even for tumors with skull base erosion, while avoiding the external facial incisions and complications associated with open techniques.

Preoperative Embolization

Perioperative embolization has been suggested as an adjuvant for decreasing tumor vascularity and size preoperatively, although most head and neck hemangiopericytomas are relatively small and amenable to en bloc resection without embolization. Several investigators encourage the use of routine angiography and preoperative embolization to delineate the extent of these tumors and their feeding vessels and to reduce intraoperative hemorrhage.

Adjuvant Therapy

Radiation therapy may decrease the size of the tumor, but cure is rare with radiation alone. Radiation therapy has been advocated as adjuvant treatment for hemangiopericytoma to reduce the rate of local recurrence. Some recommend adjuvant radiotherapy for patients when a hemangiopericytoma is larger than 5 cm or when the resection margins are inadequate. However, it is not clear whether the addition of radiotherapy improves survival. The role of adjuvant or palliative chemotherapy is not well defined for patients with hemangiopericytoma, even for those with advanced or unresectable disease.

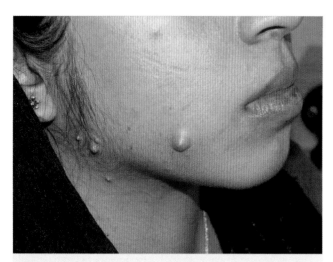

Fig. 34.5 Multiple facial neurofibromas in a woman with neurofibromatosis.

34.6 Nerve Sheath Tumors

34.6.1 The Disease Process

Nerve sheath tumors, most commonly referred to as schwannomas, neurilemmomas, or neurofibromas, are benign tumors that arise from Schwann cells in the nerve sheath.

Schwannoma

Head and neck schwannomas are most often solitary, slow-growing, well-encapsulated tumors associated with the nerve of origin (cranial nerves, cervical sympathetic chain, cervical sensory plexus, and brachial plexus). Rarely, schwannomas may be multiple. Approximately 25 to 45% of extracranial schwannomas occur in the head and neck. Schwannomas are the most common solitary neurogenic tumors in the neck and are usually seen in patients between 20 and 50 years of age.

Neurofibroma

Neurofibromas are unlike schwannomas in that they are not encapsulated; nerve fibers traverse and are frequently incorporated into the tumors. They are often multiple and are usually part of von Recklinghausen disease (neurofibromatosis; ▶ Fig. 34.5). The incidence of the latter is 1 in 3,000 births. The distinction between between schwannoma and neurofibroma is important clinically and prognostically. Schwannomas are not known to have malignant potential, but neurofibromas can give rise to malignant peripheral nerve sheath tumors.

34.6.2 Evaluation

Most patients with nerve sheath tumors are asymptomatic and present with a painless neck mass, although some may present with nasal obstruction, hearing loss, dysphagia, and hoarseness, depending on the location of the tumor. Schwannomas associated with cranial nerves or the sympathetic chain may present as a mass displacing the lateral pharyngeal wall.

CT and MR imaging are helpful in establishing the diagnosis of schwannoma, and MR imaging is superior to CT in its ability to differentiate schwannomas from other types of tumors with similar presentations. Histologic examination assists in the diagnosis of schwannoma by demonstrating the typical spindle cell features of elongated nuclei and alternating areas of organized, compact cells (Antoni type A) and loosely arranged, relatively acellular tissue (Antoni type B). In addition, immunohistochemical staining for the S-100 protein, a neural crest antigen present in the supporting cells of the nervous system, is helpful when classic morphological features are not obvious.

34.6.3 Treatment

Conservative local excision of the tumor with preservation of the nerve of origin is the treatment of choice. The relatively avascular nature of the tumor allows dissection of the tumor within the capsule and separation from the nerve of origin. However, if the nerve cannot be preserved during surgery, immediate reconstruction with postoperative rehabilitation should be undertaken.

34.7 Malignant Peripheral Nerve Sheath Tumors

34.7.1 The Disease Process

Malignant peripheral nerve sheath tumors are rare tumors that may arise sporadically or within a preexisting benign peripheral nerve sheath tumor, the latter usually in a patient with neurofibromatosis. They may be referred to as malignant schwannomas, neurofibrosarcomas, neurogenic sarcomas, neurilemmosarcomas, malignant fibrosarcomas, or malignant neurilemmomas. Malignant peripheral nerve sheath tumors comprise 2 to 6% of head and neck sarcomas. They arise in 13 to 29% of patients with neurofibromatosis; 20% of patients with malignant peripheral nerve sheath tumors have neurofibromatosis. Exposure to radiation is believed to play a role in the formation of malignant peripheral nerve sheath tumors, with a latency period of 10 to 20 years; therefore, some recommend that patients with neurofibromatosis who receive radiation treatment should be carefully monitored for the development of sarcoma. In a study by Loree et al, overall survival at 5 years approximated 52%, with improved survival in female patients and patients with low-grade tumors. The development of distant metastases correlated with tumor grade. Age, tumor site, and size had no impact on survival. Patients with neurofibromatosis had worse survival than those with sporadic forms of disease.

34.7.2 Evaluation

Patients with malignant peripheral nerve sheath tumors may present with mass lesions, and although some may be asymptomatic, others may present with pain, airway obstruction, or dysphagia, depending on the location of the tumor. In a study by Loree et al, the median age of these patients was 43 years, and 41% of them had a history of neurofibromatosis. CT and MR imaging assist in the diagnosis of malignant peripheral nerve sheath tumors, and immunohistochemical staining for p53, Ki-67, and MDM2 markers improves the accuracy of this diagnosis, although immunoperoxidase staining for S-100 has been the only reliable marker for a neurogenic tumor.

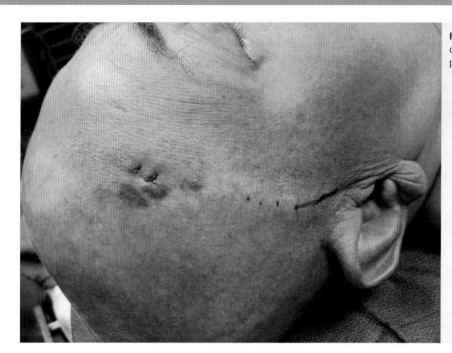

Fig. 34.6 Recurrent angiosarcoma seen as violaceous macules on the scalp of a patient who previously underwent wide local excisions.

34.7.3 Treatment

The mainstay of treatment of a malignant peripheral nerve sheath tumor is wide excision of the tumor. Clear margins are essential for achieving local control. Adjuvant radiotherapy is advocated to improve local control, including in patients with negative margins at the time of resection. Regional metastasis is rare; thus, elective neck dissection is not indicated.

34.8 Sarcoma

34.8.1 The Disease Process

Sarcomas of the head and neck comprise a heterogeneous group of tumors that range widely in biological behavior, from slowly growing tumors to aggressive lesions with metastatic potential. They affect numerous subsites within the head and neck and are classified by their tissue of origin. Malignant fibrous histiocytoma, also known as pleomorphic sarcoma, is the most common histologic subtype of soft-tissue sarcoma and includes tumors within a broad range of cellular origins. Angiosarcoma is an extremely rare type of vascular sarcoma (1 to 2% of all soft-tissue sarcomas), of which at least half occur in the head and neck region. It arises from cells of endothelial origin, and unlike most sarcomas, which tend to occur in deep locations, it commonly occurs in the skin or superficial soft tissues. Rhabdomyosarcoma is the most common form of sarcoma in children and arises in the head and neck in approximately 40% of cases. These tumors have a significant potential for metastasis to cervical lymph nodes as well as systemic metastases.

34.8.2 Evaluation

The clinical presentation is determined by the subsite of origin. Sarcomas arising in the neck usually present as a painless mass. However, deep tumors may impinge on vital structures, pro-

ducing symptoms of pain, paresthesias, dysphagia, or hoarseness. Malignant fibrous histiocytomas often present as subcutaneous or submucosal lesions in the parotid gland or neck and in the sinonasal tract. Angiosarcomas classically present as violaceous macules and plaques on the scalp or face (▶ Fig. 34.6) that can progress to nodular and ulcerated lesions. The diagnosis is often delayed because the lesion commonly mimics other dermatologic entities and is generally asymptomatic.

CT and MR imaging assist in establishing the diagnosis by accurately assessing the size and location of the sarcoma, as well as delineating bony involvement, intracranial extension, and regional metastasis. MR imaging offers much better soft-tissue resolution and is therefore better at evaluating the primary lesion, perineural extension, dural involvement, bone marrow replacement, and orbital invasion. Unfortunately, however, none of the imaging characteristics can be considered diagnostic, and thus a biopsy, which should be performed after the imaging, is necessary to definitively establish the diagnosis. Immunohistochemical stains and cytogenetic studies assist in confirming the diagnosis. Because sarcomas spread most commonly to the lungs, CT of the chest is also necessary to rule out pulmonary metastasis.

34.8.3 Treatment

In the absence of metastatic disease, surgical resection with wide margins provides the best chance of cure for sarcomas of the head and neck. The optimal treatment of angiosarcoma is not clearly defined because of the rarity of angiosarcomas and their poor prognosis, although several investigators have reported that the combination of surgery with postoperative radiation offers the best prognosis. The major challenges in the treatment of angiosarcomas include characteristics such as ill-defined borders, the frequency of multifocal disease, and a propensity to metastasize. The ability of these neoplasms to spread subcutaneously over large areas makes local recurrence a defining quality of these malignancies. Therefore, truly negative surgical margins are unlikely to be achieved, and frozen section analysis at the time of excision to ensure complete resection has little impact on outcome. Chemotherapy may have an emerging role in the management of sarcomas. However, its use is currently limited to unresectable tumors or nonsurgical candidates. The intralesional injection of cytokines has also been used for angiosarcomas in conjunction with surface irradiation, resulting in extended partial response. Recent literature supports the use of neoadjuvant chemotherapy, especially in patients in whom surgical treatment with or without radiation therapy can result in severe disfigurement.

34.9 Lymphoma

34.9.1 The Disease Process

Extranodal lymphomas of the head and neck constitute approximately 10% of all non-Hodgkin lymphomas and occur in the Waldeyer ring, most frequently the tonsils, paranasal sinuses, nasal cavity, larynx, oral cavity, salivary glands, thyroid, and orbit. Most are B-cell malignancies. Marginal zone lymphoma of the mucosa-associated lymphoid tissue (MALT) type is particularly associated with inflammatory conditions in the thyroid and salivary glands.

34.9.2 Evaluation

Patients with head and neck lymphomas may present with a variety of symptoms, depending on the subsite involved; these may include tonsillar swelling, nasal obstruction, sore throat, hoarseness, dyspnea, and neck mass. The diagnosis is most reliably made by open biopsy, although fine-needle aspiration biopsy is increasingly used. Radiographic imaging is used to assist in staging the disease. Chest X-rays are sufficient to evaluate for mediastinal or hilar adenopathy, and CT and MR imaging are useful in evaluating the extent of the primary lesion. More recently, PET-CT has become a major tool in the evaluation of lymphomas. Other tests performed in staging disease include complete blood cell count, liver function tests, lumbar puncture, and bone marrow biopsy.

34.9.3 Treatment

Surgery has a role only in the staging of head and neck lymphomas; the management of most extranodal lymphomas in the head and neck consists of radiation therapy and/or chemotherapy. For low-grade stage I or II lymphomas, the standard treatment has been involved field or extended field radiation therapy. For low-grade stage III or IV lymphomas, the standard treatment is chemotherapy. Interferon-α has been given after chemotherapy in selected patients and has been shown to prolong remissions, but not overall survival. For intermediate-grade stage I or II lymphomas, both radiation and chemotherapy are advocated, and for intermediate stage III or IV lymphomas, chemotherapy is the primary treatment. High-grade lymphomas, such as T-cell lymphoma, require combination chemotherapy including central nervous system prophylaxis. An exception is natural killer/T-cell lymphoma of the nasal type, which has a poor response to anthracycline-

based chemotherapy regimens; therefore, high-dose radiation is required. Intensity-modulated radiotherapy (IMRT) has been recommended for these cases to minimize risks to surrounding normal tissues. Thyroid and orbital lymphomas are commonly treated with radiation alone, although chemotherapy is often added for diseases with poor prognostic factors or high-grade histology. Stages III and IV disease is treated primarily with combination chemotherapy.

34.10 Malignant Melanoma

34.10.1 The Disease Process

Melanoma is a malignant neoplasm that arises in the melanocytic cells found in the basal layer of the epidermis. These cells are of neural crest origin and located predominantly in the skin but also in the eyes, ears, gastrointestinal tract, leptomeninges, and oral and genital mucous membranes. Melanoma frequently develops in a preexisting nevus. This chapter focuses on nonmucosal forms that occur within the head and neck. The behavior of head and neck melanoma is aggressive, and melanoma in this region has an overall poorer prognosis than that of melanoma in other skin sites. The prognosis of individuals affected with melanoma has been demonstrated to correlate with depth of invasion, which was initially reported as the *Clark level*, corresponding to varying regions of the epidermis and dermis. However, a more accurate measurement of tumor thickness, defined by the *Breslow level*, has become the standard to assess prognosis and is now used for tumor staging. The most important adverse prognostic factors are a high Clark level of invasion, increased tumor thickness, more than one mitosis per high-power field, clinical ulceration, a high degree of pleomorphism, the presence of microscopic satellites, a lack of tumor-infiltrating lymphocytes, primary site in the scalp, and regional lymph node metastasis. The incidence of distant metastasis is reported to be 50 to 85% in patients with involvement of the cervical lymph nodes. The incidence of occult nodal disease is approximately 4 to 23%.

34.10.2 Evaluation

Head and neck melanomas most often occur on the face, with the cheeks the most common site. Other common sites include the neck, scalp, and auricles. The most common physical finding is a new or changing nevus. Variation in color and/or an increase in the diameter, height, or asymmetry of the borders of a pigmented lesion are noted by more than 80% of patients with melanoma at the time of diagnosis. Other symptoms, such as bleeding, itching, ulceration, and pain in a pigmented lesion, are less common.

A full-thickness biopsy is crucial for an adequate diagnosis of the lesion and determination of the depth of invasion. Excisional biopsy is recommended for small lesions and for large lesions in a cosmetically favorable location. The biopsy should extend down to the subcutaneous fat, with a small (2 to 3 mm) peripheral margin. For large lesions and those in cosmetically unfavorable locations, and for those with a low suspicion of melanoma, an incisional or punch biopsy can be performed. Shave and curet biopsies are not recommended.

34.10.3 Treatment

The management of melanoma consists of wide local excision. Recommended margins of resection were determined based on the results of prospective randomized clinical trials organized by the World Health Organization Melanoma Group to evaluate the margins required to produce adequate local control. In general, for in situ lesions, the margin should be 0.5 cm; for lesions less than 1 mm in thickness, the margin of resection should be 1 cm; for lesions between 1.0 and 2.0 mm in thickness, the margins are generally accepted to be 1 to 2 cm. For melanomas thicker than 2 mm, 2-cm margins are required.

The risk for regional lymph node spread and distant metastatic disease is closely correlated with the depth of invasion, and the risk persists despite adequate excision of the disease at the primary site. It is believed that as the thickness of the primary melanoma increases to more than 1 mm, the likelihood of nodal metastases increases to more than 10 to 15%. Sentinel lymph node biopsy has been used to assess for presence of tumor cells in the lymphatics. However, the widespread use of sentinel lymph node biopsy in melanoma has been limited by several concerns, including potential damage to the facial nerve because 25 to 30% of the sentinel nodes are found within the parotid gland.

The role of elective neck dissection in the management of melanoma remains controversial because of the morbidity of the dissection without clear evidence of survival benefit. When elective neck dissection is contemplated, the site of the primary lesion must be considered. For primary lesions involving the parietal and frontal scalp, temple, lateral forehead, lateral cheek, or ear, superficial parotidectomy is performed in conjunction with neck dissection.

For patients with palpable cervical nodes, the likelihood of nodal metastases increases up to 80%, and a functional neck dissection is advocated. However, therapeutic neck dissection also has not been shown to have a survival benefit, although many favor the procedure for locoregional control. Survival drops to approximately 10% in the presence of a single positive lymph node. Thus, many feel that removal of the affected nodes would have a minimal effect on the already-poor survival. Nevertheless, there is a consensus among head and neck surgeons that surgical control of regional disease may improve patients' quality of life.

Numerous adjuvant therapies have been investigated for the treatment of melanoma. High-dose interferon alfa-2b has been approved by the FDA as an adjuvant treatment for high-risk melanomas. More recently, immunotherapy with a monoclonal antibody called ipilimumab has been approved by the FDA for patients with advanced or metastatic melanoma. No survival benefit has been demonstrated for adjuvant chemotherapy, nonspecific or passive immunotherapy, radiation therapy, retinoid therapy, vitamin therapy, or biologic therapy.

34.11 Roundsmanship

- Paragangliomas may occur in patients with type IIA familial multiple endocrine neoplasia (MEN) (pheochromocytoma, medullary thyroid carcinoma, and parathyroid hyperplasia) or type IIB MEN (also includes mucosal neuromas).
- Juvenile nasopharyngeal angiofibroma (JNA) typically presents in males 7 to 29 years of age (median age, 15 years) with the triad of unilateral nasal obstruction, recurrent severe epistaxis, and nasopharyngeal mass. Nasal obstruction and epistaxis occur in more than 80% of the patients.
- Radiographic anterior bowing of the posterior wall of the maxillary sinus (Holman-Miller sign) and enlargement of the superior orbital fissure are considered diagnostic for JNA.
- For malignant melanomas, in situ lesions are resected with a margin of 0.5 cm; for lesions less than 1 mm in thickness, the margin of resection should be 1 cm; for lesions between 1.0 and 2.0 mm in thickness, margins are generally accepted to be 1 to 2 cm; for melanomas thicker than 2 mm, 2-cm margins are required.

34.12 Recommended Reading

[1] Au A, Ariyan S. Melanoma of the head and neck. J Craniofac Surg 2011; 22: 421–429

[2] Batsakis JG. Paragangliomas of the Head and Neck. Baltimore, MD: Williams & Wilkins; 1979

[3] Bremer JW, Neel HB, DeSanto LW, Jones GC. Angiofibroma: treatment trends in 150 patients during 40 years. Laryngoscope 1986; 96: 1321–1329

[4] Colreavy MP, Lacy PD, Hughes J et al. Head and neck schwannomas—a 10 year review. J Laryngol Otol 2000; 114: 119–124

[5] Koch M, Nielsen GP, Yoon SS. Malignant tumors of blood vessels: angiosarcomas, hemangioendotheliomas, and hemangiopericytomas. J Surg Oncol 2008; 97: 321–329

[6] Levine PA, Gallagher R, Cantrell RW. Esthesioneuroblastoma: reflections of a 21-year experience. Laryngoscope 1999; 109: 1539–1543

[7] Loree TR, North JH, Werness BA, Nangia R, Mullins AP, Hicks WL. Malignant peripheral nerve sheath tumors of the head and neck: analysis of prognostic factors. Otolaryngol Head Neck Surg 2000; 122: 667–672

[8] Persky MS, Setton A, Niimi Y, Hartman J, Frank D, Berenstein A. Combined endovascular and surgical treatment of head and neck paragangliomas—a team approach. Head Neck 2002; 24: 423–431

[9] Rinaldo A, Ferlito A, Shaha AR, Wei WI, Lund VJ. Esthesioneuroblastoma and cervical lymph node metastases: clinical and therapeutic implications. Acta Otolaryngol 2002; 122: 215–221

[10] Spitz FR, Bouvet M, Pisters PW, Pollock RE, Feig BW. Hemangiopericytoma: a 20-year single-institution experience. Ann Surg Oncol 1998; 5: 350–355

[11] Sturgis EM, Potter BO. Sarcomas of the head and neck region. Curr Opin Oncol 2003; 15: 239–252

[12] Sykes JM, Ossoff RH. Paragangliomas of the head and neck. Otolaryngol Clin North Am 1986; 19: 755–767

[13] Witt TR, Shah JP, Sternberg SS. Juvenile nasopharyngeal angiofibroma. A 30 year clinical review. Am J Surg 1983; 146: 521–525

35 Principles and Techniques of Neck Dissection

Moustafa Mourad and Stimson P. Schantz

35.1 Introduction

The earliest documentation of head and neck cancer dates back to 3500 BC, in the Egyptian texts of the Ebers Papyrus. The papyrus describes the treatment of an "eating ulcer on the gums" with cinnamon, honey, gum, and oil. The importance of the presence of nodal disease in the prognostication of the disease was not fully appreciated or documented in the medical literature until 1790, and before the nineteenth century, no attempt at controlling metastatic nodal disease by surgery was made.

In 1837, John Collins Warren attempted to control metastatic spread to the cervical nodes with isolated, single-node excisions. With advances in antisepsis and antimicrobials, anesthesia, surgical technique, and perioperative management, the late nineteenth century saw an increase in the attempted management of nodal disease. En bloc resections of nodal disease were conducted in cases of advanced disease, pioneered by Europeans: Bernhard Rudolf Konrad von Langenbeck, Christian Albert Theodor Billroth, Richard von Volkman, and Theodor Kocher. Sir Henry Trentham Butlin introduced the concept of elective neck dissections in 1885, which brought about a dramatic improvement in local disease control and the survival rates of patients.

The early twentieth century saw a refinement in the surgical technique of nodal excisions, as well as the introduction by George Washington Crile of the radical neck dissection. Today, there are three major classifications of neck dissections, with a number of subtypes, all of which are a fundamental part of head and neck surgery and have drastically improved the outcomes of patients with head and neck cancer. A thorough understanding and appreciation of head and neck anatomy is essential in performing neck dissection.

35.2 Details of the Lymph Node Levels of the Neck

The lymph nodes within the neck maybe divided into seven anatomical subsites (▶ Fig. 35.1).

Level I: The nodes in this level can be subdivided into submental (IA) and submandibular (IB) nodes.

The submental (IA) nodes are contained within a triangular region bounded by the anterior belly of the digastric muscle and the hyoid bone. The submandibular (IB) nodes are found in the region bounded by the anterior belly of the digastric muscle, the body of the mandible, and the stylohyoid muscle.

Level II: Contains the upper jugular lymph nodes. The nodes in this level can also be subdivided into level IIA and level IIB nodes.

Level II lymph nodes are found in the region bounded posteriorly and laterally by the posterior border of the sternocleidomastoid muscle, superiorly by the skull base, inferiorly by the inferior border of the hyoid bone, and anteromedially by the stylohyoid muscle. The nodes in levels IIA and IIB are subdivided based on their relationship to the vertical plane created by the spinal accessory nerve in this region: level IIA nodes are anteromedial to this plane, whereas IIB nodes are posterolateral to the plane.

Level III: Contains the middle jugular lymph nodes. This region is defined as lying in an area bounded superiorly by the inferior border of the hyoid bone and inferiorly by the inferior border of the cricoid cartilage. Medially, these nodes are lateral to the lateral boundary of the sternohyoid muscle, and posteriorly and laterally they are bounded by the posterior border of the sternocleidomastoid muscle.

Level IV: Contains the lower jugular nodes. This level is defined as the area bounded superiorly by the inferior border of the cricoid cartilage, inferiorly by the clavicle, posteriorly by the posterior border of the sternocleidomastoid muscle, and anteriorly by the lateral border of the sternohyoid muscle.

Level V: Contains the posterior triangle lymph nodes and can be subdivided into levels VA and VB.

Level V nodes are found in the region bounded superiorly by the intersection point of the sternocleidomastoid muscle and the trapezius muscle, inferiorly by the clavicle, anteriorly by the posterior border of the sternocleidomastoid, and posteriorly by the anterior border of the trapezius muscle. Level V is divided into sublevels VA (above) and VB (below) by a horizontal plane created by the inferior border of the anterior cricoid arch.

Level VI: Contains the anterior compartment lymph nodes, including the prelaryngeal (delphian), pretracheal, and paratracheal nodes. This level is defined as an area with the superior boundary formed by the hyoid bone, the inferior boundary formed by the suprasternal notch, and the lateral boundaries formed by the common carotid arteries.

35.2.1 Details of Lymph Drainage

Understanding the patterns of lymphatic drainage in the various sites of the head and neck is critical to the performance of an appropriate neck dissection. ▶ Fig. 35.2 details the course of the lymphatics. Lymph nodes are commonly seen to course parallel to major venous pathways, as well as along selected neural pathways.

Afferent lymphatics from the submental and submandibular nodes drain the floor of the mouth, apex of the tongue, and lower lips. Subsequent efferent drainage courses to deep cervical nodes toward the internal jugular vein at the level of the hyoid bone (levels IIA and IIB), as well as to submaxillary nodes. The anterior cervical node afferents drain the subglottic and glottic larynx, apex of the piriform sinus, and cervical esophagus. Anterior cervical node efferent lymphatic drainage courses toward level II nodes, as well as upper mediastinal nodes. Level II nodes receive drainage from the oral cavity, nasopharynx, oropharynx, hypopharynx, and larynx, as well as the scalp, auricles, and back of the neck. Level II nodes also receive drainage from other nodal groups, particularly from the anterior cervical compartment, as well as the submental and submandibular group. Level II efferents subsequently drain into levels IV and V. Levels IV and V nodes receive drainage from the nasopharynx, oropharynx, and cutaneous structures of the posterior

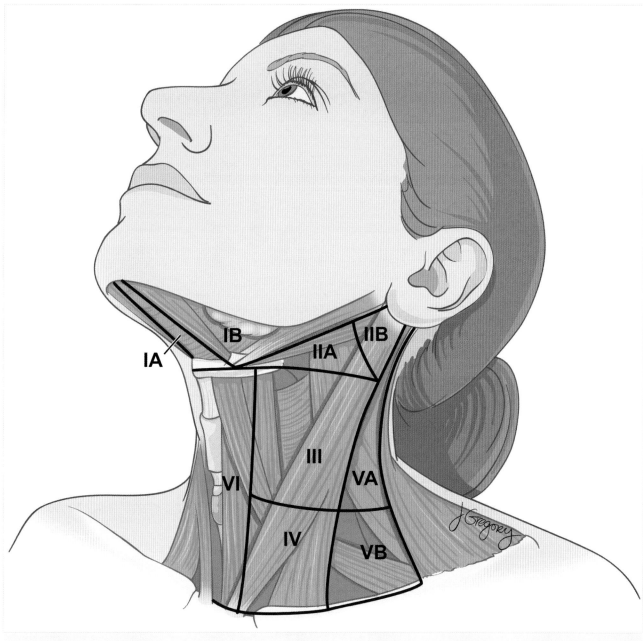

Fig. 35.1 Nodal levels of the neck.

scalp and neck. Efferents from this region join with efferents from levels II and III to form the jugular trunk. On the right side, the jugular trunk terminates at the branching point of the internal jugular vein from of the right subclavian vein. The jugular trunk on the left joins the thoracic duct.

35.2.2 Details of the Thoracic Duct

The thoracic duct originates in the cisterna chyli, a saclike structure located inferior to the right crus of the diaphragm at the level of L1 and L2. The duct enters the thorax lateral to the descending aorta and medial to the azygous vein. It continues to ascend through the thorax, crossing the arch of the aorta in the superior mediastium. The duct then courses laterally at the level of C7. The duct continues to run along the medial border of

the anterior scalene muscle, looping inferiorly and crossing the first segment of the subclavian artery anteriorly. The thoracic duct terminates at the junction of the left internal jugular vein and the subclavian vein, below the level of the clavicle. The thoracic duct drains the lower extremities (through the right and left lymphatic trunks) and abdomen.

35.3 Details of the Arteries of the Neck (▶ Fig. 35.3)

35.3.1 Details of the Subclavian Arteries

The right subclavian artery originates from the innominate artery posterior to the sternoclavicular joint and arches above the

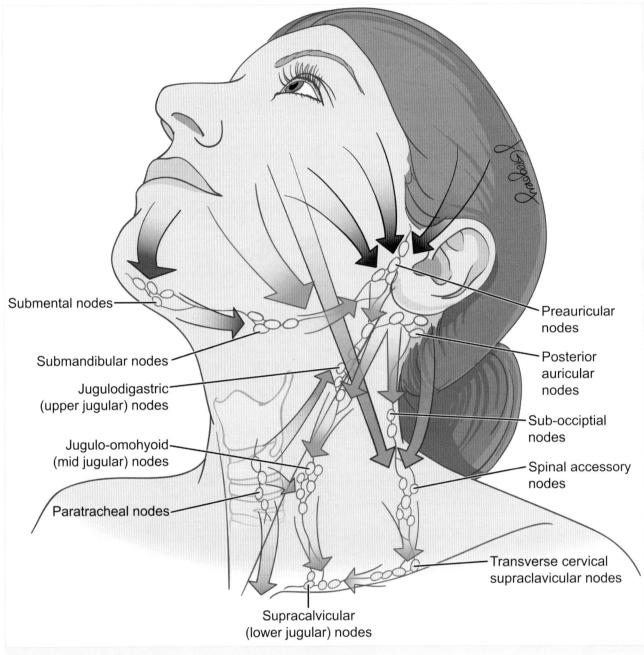

Submental nodes

Submandibular nodes

Jugulodigastric
(upper jugular) nodes

Jugulo-omohyoid
(mid jugular) nodes

Paratracheal nodes

Supracalvicular
(lower jugular) nodes

Preauricular
nodes

Posterior
auricular
nodes

Sub-occiptial
nodes

Spinal accessory
nodes

Transverse cervical
supraclavicular nodes

Fig. 35.2 Patterns of lymphatic drainage in the neck.

clavicle and subclavian vein. The right subclavian artery leaves the neck at the level of the first rib, becoming the right axillary artery. The left subclavian artery originates directly from the arch of the aorta and enters the base of the neck through the superior mediastinum. Similar to the right subclavian artery, the left subclavian leaves the neck at the level of the first rib to become the left axillary artery.

The subclavian artery can be subdivided into three segments based on its relationship to the anterior scalene muscle: the first segment lies medial, the second segment lies behind, and the third segment lies lateral to the muscle. The first segment on the right side is crossed by the internal jugular and vertebral veins and the vagus nerve. The first segment on the left side is crossed by the left common carotid artery, ansa

subclavia, vagus nerve, and internal jugular vein. Importantly on the left side, posterior to the first segment lie the esophagus, trachea, thoracic duct, and left recurrent laryngeal nerve. The third segment of the subclavian artery is crossed by the external jugular vein anteriorly and the middle scalene muscle posteriorly.

The branches of the subclavian artery arise predominantly from the first segment, although in some individuals the second and third segments may be the origin of the thyrocervical trunk. Branches of the subclavian artery include the vertebral artery, thyrocervical trunk, suprascapular artery, transverse cervical artery, inferior thyroid artery, internal thoracic artery, costocervical trunk, supreme intercostal artery, and deep cervical artery.

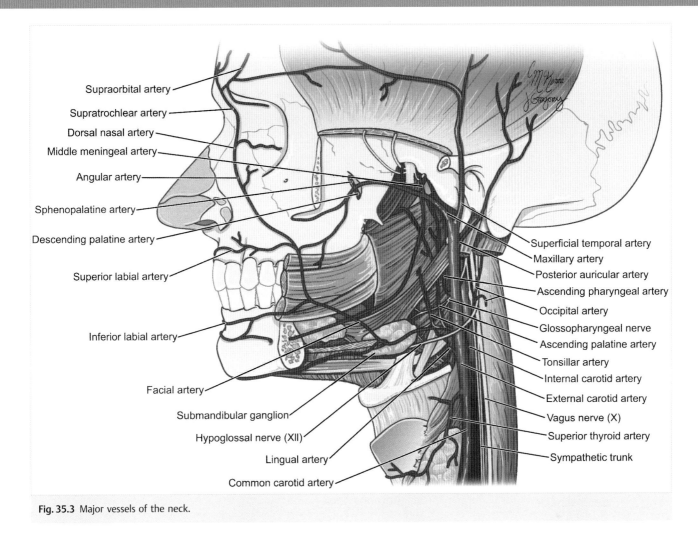

Fig. 35.3 Major vessels of the neck.

The transverse cervical artery originates from the thyrocervical trunk and is generally encountered in level V neck dissections. The artery crosses the anterior scalene muscle and brachial plexus and then penetrates the trapezius muscle, dividing into a superficial branch and a deep branch.

The inferior thyroid artery also originates from the thyrocervical trunk and ascends anterior to the vertebral artery, giving rise to the ascending cervical artery at C6. The artery passes behind the carotid sheath, arching downward, to reach the posterior pole of the thyroid gland.

35.3.2 Details of the Common Carotid Arteries

The right common carotid artery originates from the brachiocephalic artery at the level of the sternoclavicular joint, whereas the left common carotid artery is a direct branch of the aorta. Both common carotid arteries are protected by the sternocleidomastoid and the strap muscles of the neck. The carotid arteries bifurcate at the level of the thyroid cartilage, giving rise to the internal and external carotid arteries.

The internal carotid artery originates at the bifurcation of the carotid artery at the upper border of the thyroid cartilage. The internal carotid artery ascends superiorly under the sternocleidomastoid and posterior belly of the digastric before entering the carotid canal within the temporal bone without giving off any branches within the neck. Identification of the internal carotid artery, along with the internal jugular vein, cranial nerves IX through XII, and the sympathetic plexus, is aided by identification of the C1 transverse process immediately posteriorly.

The external carotid artery is formed at the bifurcation of the common carotid artery at the level of the thyroid cartilage and runs anteromedial to the internal carotid artery. The external carotid artery ascends posterior to the sternocleidomastoid muscle and deep to the posterior belly of the digastric muscle, penetrating the parotid behind the angle of the mandible before dividing into the terminal branches of the superficial temporal and maxillary arteries. The branches of the carotid artery include the superior thyroid artery, ascending pharyngeal artery, lingual artery, facial artery, and occipital artery.

The superior thyroid artery most commonly originates as the first branch of the external carotid artery, but it may be seen to arise from the common carotid artery. The artery passes anteroinferiorly to supply the intrinsic muscles of the larynx and the superior pole and isthmus of the thyroid gland just before terminating.

The lingual artery ascends deep to the digastric muscle in the lateral wall of the pharynx, coursing anteriorly until it reaches the hyoglossus muscle.

299

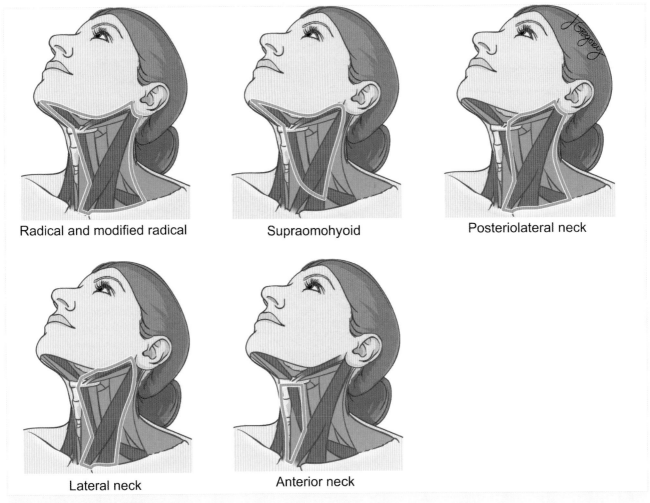

Radical and modified radical

Supraomohyoid

Posteriolateral neck

Lateral neck

Anterior neck

Fig. 35.4 Types of neck dissections.

The facial artery originates at digastric muscle near the level of the angle of the mandible. From its origin site, it ascends deep to the digastric and stylohyoid muscles to the submaxillary triangle.

35.4 Details of the Veins of the Neck

The veins of the neck can be subdivided into superficial and deep veins.

35.4.1 Superficial Veins

External Jugular Vein

The external jugular vein drains the external portion of the skull and deeper portions of the face. The retromandibular and postauricular veins unite to form the external jugular vein within the substance of the parotid gland at the level of the angle of the mandible. The external jugular vein courses along the sternocleidomastoid deep to the platysma. It continues its course into the posterior triangle, entering the deep fascia, where it terminates into the subclavian vein (two-thirds) or the internal jugular vein (one-third). The external jugular vein receives tributaries from the anterior and posterior jugular, transverse cervical, suprascapular, and cephalic veins.

Anterior Jugular Vein

The anterior jugular vein originates at the hyoid or suprahyoid level, formed by a confluence of veins from the parotid or retromandibular veins. Bilateral veins travel inferiorly over the sternohyoid and sternocleidomastoid muscles in a paired fashion, just off the midline of the neck. The right and left lines join above the sternum, forming a venous arch that descends to terminate in the subclavian or external jugular vein. Variations include the presence of only one midline cervical vein, absent venous arch, or absent anterior jugular vein.

35.4.2 Deep Veins

Internal Jugular Vein

The internal jugular vein receives venous drainage from the brain, face, and neck. The right internal jugular vein is usually larger then the left, and in 10% of individuals it is the predominant drainage of the head and neck. The internal jugular vein is

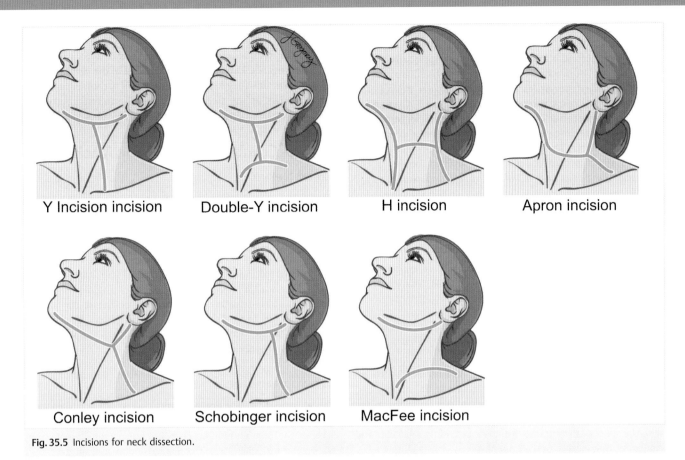

Fig. 35.5 Incisions for neck dissection.

formed by the union of the inferior petrosal sinus and the sigmoid sinus within the posterior compartment of the jugular foramen, exiting with cranial nerves IX, X, and XI. The vein also receives drainage from the lingual vein, facial vein, and retromandibular vein, forming a trunk below the level of the angle of the mandible.

The jugular bulb is the first portion of the vein as it descends into the floor of the middle ear space. The vein continues its course downward, crossing the transverse process of the atlas, with an anterolateral trajectory. The vein is encased within the carotid sheath, running lateral to the internal and common carotid arteries and anterior to cranial nerve X. At the level of the angle of the mandible, the vein is crossed by the posterior belly of the digastric muscle, stylohyoid muscle, occipital artery, and cranial nerve XI. In the right base of neck, the internal jugular vein crosses the first segment of the subclavian artery separated from the common carotid artery, while on the left side, the vein overlaps the artery. The subclavian vein joins the internal jugular vein, forming the brachiocephalic vein, inferior to the subclavian artery on the right and anterior to it on the left.

Subclavian Vein

The subclavian vein is a continuation of the axillary vein. It originates at the border of the first rib and continues to the medial border of the anterior scalene muscle. The subclavian veins courses anterior to the subclavian artery and anterior scalene muscle.

35.5 Details of the Nerves of the Neck

35.5.1 Spinal Nerves

The dorsal (posterior) rami of the cervical nerves (except for the rami of C1) innervate the muscles and skin of the neck. The dorsal rami contain medial and lateral branches; the medial branches innervate muscle and skin, and the lateral branches supply only muscle.

35.5.2 Cervical Plexus

The cervical plexus is formed by the anterior ventral rami of the C1 to C4 nerve roots and is located anterior to the levator muscle of the scapula and the middle scalene muscle. Anteriorly, it is covered by prevertebral fascia, which forms a barrier separating the plexus from the internal jugular vein. The cervical plexus can be subdivided into deep and superficial branches.

The deep branches of the cervical plexus contain the superior and inferior root of the ansa cervicalis. The superior root contains fibers originating from C1 and C2 that join with cranial nerve XII, providing innervation to the thyrohyoid and geniohyoid muscles. The inferior root of the ansa cervicalis contains fibers that originate in the C2 and C3 nerve roots. The superior and inferior roots connect to form the ansa hypoglossi, which provides innervation to the infrahyoid muscles.

The superficial (cutaneous) branches of the cervical plexus are formed by nerve roots C2 to C4 and include the lesser occipital, great auricular, transverse cervical, suprascapular, anterior (medial) supraclavicular, middle (intermediate) supraclavicular, and posterior (lateral) supraclavicular nerves. The lesser occipital nerve originates from C2 to C4, coursing around the posterior border of the sternocleidomastoid muscle and providing sensory innervation inferior and posterior to the auricle. The great auricular nerve originates from C2 to C3 and also courses behind the posterior border of the sternocleidomastoid muscle before running superiorly toward the ear; it provides sensory innervation to the skin overlying the parotid gland, the auricle, and the skin of the mastoid process.

35.5.3 Phrenic Nerve

The phrenic nerve originates from the C3, C4, and C5 nerve roots. It courses on the anterior surface of the anterior scalene muscle and is covered by prevertebral fascia.

35.5.4 Brachial Plexus

The brachial plexus is formed by ventral rami of the C5 through T1 nerve roots. The plexus originates between the middle and anterior scalene muscles and continues to run posterior to the inferior belly of the omohyoid muscle. The plexus continues with the subclavian vein into the axilla, providing muscular and cutaneous innervation to the upper limb.

35.5.5 Cervical Sympathetic Trunk

The cervical sympathetic trunk consists mainly of ascending preganglionic nerve fibers that travel through ventral roots of the upper thoracic nerves. The cervical sympathetic trunk includes the superior, middle, vertebral, and stellate (inferior) sympathetic ganglia; the vertebral and middle sympathetic ganglia are inconsistently found.

Superior Cervical Ganglion

The superior cervical ganglion is located at the level of C2 and C3 above the carotid bifurcation, posterior and medial to the beginning portion of the internal carotid artery. The ganglion sits along the longus capitis muscle. The ganglion branches into the external carotid and internal carotid nerve plexuses. The internal carotid nerve plexus is the major continuation of nerves from the superior cervical ganglion, providing fibers that supply the upper part of the face and the orbit.

Middle Sympathetic Ganglion

The middle sympathetic ganglion is located at the carotid tubercle (transverse process of the C6 vertebra) in close proximity to the inferior thyroid artery. It is the smallest of the cervical ganglia and is present in only 62.3% of cervical trunks. Branches of this ganglion communicate with rami of the fifth and sixth cervical nerves and also form thyroid branches that travel with the inferior thyroid artery to the thyroid gland.

Inferior (Stellate) Sympathetic Ganglion

The inferior sympathetic ganglion is located between the transverse process of C7 and the first rib, medial to the vertebral ganglion. Often, this may be fused with the first thoracic ganglion and is known as the stellate ganglion. The inferior portion of the ganglion lies inferior and posterior to the subclavian artery.

35.5.6 Cranial Nerves of the Neck

Facial Nerve

Within the neck, the cervical and mandibular branches of the facial nerve are commonly encountered. The mandibular branch appears along the anterior border of the parotid gland. This branch runs inferiorly below the lower border of the mandible, crossing the anterior facial vein and the superficial layer of the deep cervical fascia at the level of the submandibular gland. This branch innervates the depressor anguli oris muscle. The cervical branch runs at the inferior border of the parotid gland, coursing behind the angle of the mandible, providing innervation to the platysma. Terminal branches supply the depressor muscles of the lower lip.

Glossopharyngeal Nerve

The glossopharyngeal nerve (cranial nerve IX) is a combined motor and sensory cranial nerve that exits the brainstem at the level of the upper medulla. The glossopharyngeal nerve exits the jugular foramen lateral to the vagus nerve and the accessory nerve, medial to the internal carotid artery, and anteromedial to the jugular bulb. At the jugular foramen, cranial nerve IX gives off two branches—the tympanic branch (Jacobson nerve), which provides innervation to the middle ear, and the vagal communicating (auricular) branch, which provides innervation to the external ear. After exiting the foramen, the glossopharyngeal nerve continues to run between the jugular vein and the internal carotid artery, deep to the styloid process, providing its only motor innervation to the stylopharyngeal muscle. The nerve passes along the lateral border of the stylopharyngeal muscle and along the middle constrictor muscle. The nerve then turns anteriorly toward the tongue. The glossopharyngeal nerve divides into its tonsillar and lingual branches deep to the hyoglossal muscle.

Vagus Nerve

The vagus nerve (cranial nerve X) exits the jugular foramen medial to cranial nerves IX and XI, passing into the carotid sheath. As the nerve courses rostrally within the neck, the nerve is located between and posterior to the carotid artery and internal jugular vein. Branches of cranial nerve X within the neck include the auricular branch (Arnold nerve), pharyngeal branch, superior laryngeal nerve, external laryngeal nerve, internal laryngeal nerve, cervical cardiac branches, and recurrent laryngeal nerve.

The auricular branch (Arnold nerve) originates in the jugular fossa and exits from the tympanomastoid fissure, supplying skin of the back of the external auditory canal, skin of the lower part of the meatus, and inferior portion of the tympanic membrane. The pharyngeal branch runs along the lateral side of the internal carotid artery, providing motor innervation to the pharyngeal muscles. The superior laryngeal nerve is a branch of the vagus nerve that also has contributions from the superior sympathetic ganglion. The superior laryngeal nerve divides into the external and internal laryngeal nerves. The external laryngeal nerve provides innervation to the inferior constrictor muscles, terminating within the cricothyroid muscle. The internal laryngeal nerve courses anteriorly and pierces the thyrohyoid membrane along with the superior thyroid artery, innervating the laryngeal mucosa. The right recurrent laryngeal nerve branches off the vagus nerve anterior to the subclavian artery and courses upward posterior to the artery back toward the larynx. The nerve continues posterior to the trachea, crossing posterior or anterior to the inferior thyroid artery, and into the cricothyroid joint. The left recurrent laryngeal nerve branches off the vagus at the level of the aortic arch, looping posterior to the arch. The nerve then runs superiorly, within the tracheoesophageal groove, before terminating at the level of the cricothyroid joint.

Accessory (Spinal Accessory) Nerve

The spinal accessory nerve (cranial nerve XI) exits the jugular foramen along with the internal jugular vein, internal carotid artery, and cranial nerves IX and X. In two-thirds of individuals, the nerve crosses over the jugular vein, and behind the jugular vein in the remaining one-third. The jugular vein is crossed at approximately the level of the posterior belly of the digastric muscle. The nerve continues to run posteriorly and inferiorly toward the sternocleidomastoid. The nerve may run posterior to (18%) or through (82%) the sternocleidomastoid and then continues posteriorly, eventually terminating in the anterior muscular fibers of the trapezius muscle.

Hypoglossal Nerve

The hypoglossal nerve (cranial nerve XII) exits the skull base from the hypoglossal canal of the occipital bone. It travels toward the vagus nerve, running medial to the internal jugular vein and internal carotid artery. The nerve then runs deep to the posterior belly of the digastric muscle toward the submandibular fossa as it proceeds toward the tongue.

35.6 Types of Neck Dissections (▶ Fig. 35.4)

1. Radical neck dissection involves the resection of levels I through V nodes, as well as the spinal accessory nerve, internal jugular vein, sternocleidomastoid muscle, tail of the parotid, and submaxillary gland.
2. Modified radical neck dissection, like radical neck dissection, includes the removal of levels I through V nodes, with sparing of one or more of the following structures: spinal accessory nerve, sternocleidomastoid muscle, and internal jugular vein.
3. Selective neck dissections include the supraomohyoid neck dissection, posterolateral neck dissection, lateral neck

dissection, anterior neck dissection, and extended neck dissection.
   (a) The supraomohyoid neck dissection removes nodes from levels I through III lymph nodes.
   (b) The posterolateral neck dissection removes lymph nodes from levels II through V, including suboccipital lymph and retroauricular lymph nodes.
   (c) The lateral neck dissection removes levels II through IV lymph nodes.
   (d) The anterior neck dissection removes nodes from the anterior compartment of the neck.
   (e) The extended neck dissection includes a dissection of all structures resected in a radical neck dissection, in addition to lymphatic nodes in the retropharynx, superior mediastinum, buccinator space, and paratracheal space. Nonlymphatic structures that may be resected in an extended neck dissection include deep muscles of the neck; one or more segments of the carotid artery system; the hypoglossal, vagus, and facial nerves; and the hyoid bone and clavicle.

35.7 Types of Incisions

Factors to consider in determining a flap incision (▶ Fig. 35.5) include location of the primary lesion, exposure provided, flap viability, carotid artery protection, planned reconstructive procedures, history of prior radiotherapy, prior scars, and anticipated aesthetic results. Acute angles in flaps may produce narrow sections of skin that have an increased tendency to become necrotic because of compromised collateral circulation. Additionally, posterior cervical flaps have a higher tendency to flap failure than do superiorly and medially based flaps.

35.7.1 Y Incision

Advantages: Provides exposure of the mandible and upper neck; can provide oral cavity exposure if used in conjunction with a mandibulotomy.

Disadvantage: Produces an acute angle within the incision, with an increased likelihood for wound dehiscence and flap necrosis in the region covering the carotid artery.

35.7.2 Apron Incision

Advantage: Provides good exposure of the upper and lower neck.

Disadvantage: The large superior flap may become edematous in patients previously treated with radiation.

35.7.3 Schobinger Flap

Advantages: Provides excellent exposure as well as protection of the carotid arteries, with an improved cosmetic result due to decreased scarring in the middle neck.

Disadvantages: Produces a single acute angle below the angle of the mandible, at the posterosuperior tip of the flap. Exposure of the inferior sternocleidomastoid is limited, as well.

35.7.4 H Incision

Advantage: Provides excellent exposure of the anterior and posterior neck.

Disadvantages: There is strong potential for flap breakdown, particularly in the posterior flap. Flap breakdown over the superior flap may also result in carotid artery exposure.

35.7.5 MacFee Incision

Advantage: Provides an excellent cosmetic result.

Disadvantages: Compromised exposure, especially in shorter, fatter necks. There is also limited blood supply to the central segment and along the upper border of the flap. This may produce necrosis directly over the segment covering the carotid artery, especially in patients previously treated with radiation. There is also greater potential for seroma formation below the central flap.

35.8 Neck Dissection Technique (Authors' Preference: Right Modified Radical Neck Dissection)

The incision is marked extending from the mastoid tip on the right down in a Schobinger style fashion into the natural skin crease in the lower neck. The incision is then injected with 1% lidocaine and 1:100,000 epinephrine. The incision is made through the skin and subcutaneous tissue and down through the platysma muscle. Superior (up to the level of the horizontal ramus) and inferior (inferiorly to the level the clavicle) skin flaps are then raised in the subplatysmal plane. Flaps are raised anteriorly to the midline and posteriorly to the level of the posterior edge of the sternocleidomastoid. During the posterior dissection, care is taken not to injure the spinal accessory nerve as it emerges from the posterior border of the sternocleidomastoid. The anterior border of the sternocleidomastoid muscle is then dissected in an inferior to superior direction, taking care to gently apply pressure with a clamp to any tissue along the superior sternocleidomastoid muscle and checking for muscle twitching in order to prevent injury to the spinal accessory nerve. This dissection is carried posteriorly beneath the sternocleidomastoid to its most posterior edge.

As the anterior border of the sternocleidomastoid muscle is dissected superiorly, the spinal accessory nerve is identified running in an oblique fashion on the undersurface of the sternocleidomastoid muscle. It is generally found approximately 3 cm below the mastoid tip. It runs superiorly to the undersurface of the posterior belly of the digastric muscle, and at that point, it continues superiorly along the lateral border of the internal jugular vein. The carotid sheath structures are also identified at this point, and any fibrofatty tissue adjacent to the sternocleidomastoid muscle is elevated from the deep tissue, avoiding the rootlets of the cervical plexus. Once the spinal accessory nerve is identified, it is followed superiorly to identify the posterior belly of the digastric muscle, which is identified in its entirety. The submandibular fascia is then incised, and the fascia is raised off the submandibular gland in order to protect the marginal mandibular nerve. The submandibular gland is then separated inferiorly from the surrounding tissue.

The common facial vein is identified, as is the facial artery, as they cross the facial notch on the inferior edge of the midportion of the horizontal ramus of the mandible. The mylohyoid muscle is then identified and retracted medially with a loop retractor. The lingual nerve is identified superiorly and the submandibular ganglion is ligated, separating the submandibular gland from the lingual nerve. The submandibular duct is also identified and ligated. The hypoglossal nerve is identified inferiorly and protected as the submandibular gland and surrounding tissue are elevated in an anterior to posterior direction.

Perifacial lymph nodes within the submandibular triangle are also identified. These nodes are then dissected free from the surrounding tissue, respecting the submandibular fascia in order to preserve the marginal mandibular nerve. The tissues are retracted in a posterior direction and left in direct continuity with level II lymph nodes.

The level IIB lymph nodes are then dissected. An incision is created in the fascia surrounding the fibrofatty tissue down in level IIB, posterior to the spinal accessory nerve. The fibrofatty tissue is dissected free from the floor of the neck, with care taken to preserve the internal jugular vein, which enters this compartment. The tissue is then dissected free from the surrounding tissue and the tail of parotid, as well as the sternocleidomastoid muscle, and passed below the spinal accessory nerve and left in continuity with level IIA nodes. Once the entirety of the anterior border of the sternocleidomastoid muscle is separated from the fibrofatty tissue, the floor of the deep cervical fascia is incised. The fibrofatty tissue is then dissected free from the floor of the neck, superficial to the cervical rootlets, and dissected in a lateral to medial direction toward the internal jugular vein.

The omohyoid muscle is then identified inferiorly and left in continuity. The fibrofatty tissue along the floor of the neck is elevated and then dissected in a posterior to anterior dissection toward the carotid sheath structures. With a No. 15 blade, the cervical fascia investing the carotid sheath is separated from the internal jugular vein and elevated in continuity with the fibrofatty tissue medially. The vagus nerve and carotid artery are also identified at this point, and any fascia overlying these structures is separated and left in continuity with the fibrofatty tissue.

Once the remaining portions of the neck contents are elevated on the internal jugular vein, a No. 15 blade is used to separate them from the internal jugular vein and toward the sternohyoid muscle. This fibrofatty tissue is then dissected free from the sternohyoid muscle in a sharp fashion.

A thorough examination of the neck should reveal continuity of the spinal accessory, hypoglossal, and lingual nerves. The cervical rootlets should also be identified and continuity ensured. Finally, the internal jugular vein as well as the carotid artery should be inspected and found to be intact.

The wound is then copiously irrigated with normal saline, and blood and clots are cleared with suction. Hemostasis is achieved with bipolar cautery. After placement of a suction drain, the wound is closed by approximating the platysma with a running 3–0 chromic suture and the skin with staples.

35.9 Roundsmanship

- An understanding the lymphatic drainage patterns of the head and neck aids in the choice of proper neck dissection technique.
- Neck dissection incisions are chosen to provide adequate access for nodal dissection; the development of healthy, vascularized skin flaps, especially for carotid artery protection; and maximal cosmesis.
- Pertinent veins and significant arteries and nerves are preserved, if possible, during neck dissection; however, involvement by tumor generally requires that these structures be sacrificed.

35.10 Recommended Reading

[1] Gray H. Anatomy of the Human Body. Philadelphia, PA: Lea & Febiger; 1918. Illustrated at Bartleby.com;2000

[2] Janfaza P, Nadol J, Fabian R, Montgomery W, Galla R. Surgical Anatomy of the Head and Neck. 1st ed. Philadelphia, PA: Lippincott Williams & Wilkins; 2000

[3] Medina JE, Lore JM Jr. The neck. In: Lore JM Jr, Medina JE, eds. An Atlas of Head and Neck Surgery. 4th ed. Philadelphia, PA: Elsevier Saunders; 2005;780–817

[4] Onuigbo WI. Historical data on the dynamics of lymphatic metastasis. Oncology 1972; 26: 505–514

[5] Rinaldo A, Ferlito A, Silver CE. Early history of neck dissection. Eur Arch Otorhinolaryngol 2008; 265: 1535–1538

[6] Staffieri A, Sebastian P, Kapre M, Varghese B, Kazi R. Epidemiology, aetiology and natural history of head and neck cancer. In: Staffieri A, Sebastian P, Kapre M, Varghese B, Kasi R, eds. Essentials of Head and Neck Cancer. Delhi, India: Byword Books; 2011;1–15

36 Evaluation and Management of the Solitary Neck Mass

Ameet R. Kamat and Stimson P. Schantz

36.1 Introduction

The management of a solitary neck mass is an often-encountered dilemma for the otolaryngologist. However, a thorough history and physical examination, along with a concise differential diagnosis, usually will lead to the proper diagnosis. The treatment of a solitary neck mass is dictated by the clinician's confidence in that diagnosis. As in any other field of medicine, a step-by-step plan for diagnosis and treatment is imperative to helping the patient.

36.2 Terminology and Applied Anatomy

A concrete understanding of neck anatomy is essential to a timely diagnosis and the effective treatment of solitary neck masses. For convenience of localization, the neck can be divided into several triangles. The neck is first divided into anterior and posterior triangles. The anterior triangle is bordered by the posterior border of the sternocleidomastoid muscle laterally, the inferior margin of the mandible superiorly, and the clavicle inferiorly. The posterior triangle is bordered by the posterior margin of the sternocleidomastoid muscle medially, the anterior margin of the trapezius muscle laterally, the skull base superiorly, and clavicle laterally (middle one-third). For details of the smaller triangles that make up the neck, the reader is referred to Chapter 8 (Head and Neck Anatomy) and Chapter 35 (Principles and Techniques of Neck Dissection).

For purposes of localization, especially in the management of regional metastasis from upper aerodigestive tract carcinoma, the neck is divided into a series of levels as detailed in ▶ Table 36.1.

36.3 Medical Evaluation

36.3.1 Presenting Complaints

The differential diagnosis of a solitary neck mass is quite broad in comparison with that for other presenting symptomatology. A thorough and well-directed history and physical examination will allow the clinician to develop a concise differential diagnosis and guide further testing.

Focusing first on the neck mass itself, a clinician should elicit information regarding the onset and growth progression. Next, starting at the top of the head and proceeding to the base of neck, the clinician should elicit a thorough head and neck review of systems. The initial investigation should include a determination of the presence of constitutional symptoms, such as fever, weight loss, night sweats, loss of appetite, and fatigue. Symptoms such as trismus, decreased tongue mobility, dental pain, rhinorrhea, postnasal drip, sore throat, shortness of breath, hoarseness, dysphagia, and odynophagia should be duly noted. A history of recent upper respiratory tract infection, including recent sinusitis (facial pressure, pain, nasal discharge),

otitis media/externa (otalgia, otorrhea, aural fullness), and pharyngitis (sore throat, odynophagia), must also be included. Additional contributory factors include recent travel; exposure to pets, wild animals, or individuals with tuberculosis; and a history of immunodeficiency, including HIV infection, chemotherapy/radiation, steroids, and uncontrolled diabetes.

The age of the patient should guide further questioning because most pediatric neck masses are either inflammatory or congenital, and those in adults carry a higher risk for malignancy. A full social history should be elicited in an adult with a neck mass, including tobacco, alcohol, and illicit drug use.

36.3.2 Physical Examination

The character of the mass should be recorded with respect to size (larger or smaller than 3 cm); location; mobility; consistency (firm, soft, fluctuant, compressible); tenderness to palpation; and the presence of other lesions. Of these characteristics, location can help narrow the differential diagnosis in pediatric patients because most congenital or developmental masses tend to occur either midline or lateral neck at specific levels of the sternocleidomastoid (SCM) muscle or adjacent to other structures. Even in adult patients, the location of metastatic lymphadenopathy can help identify the primary site of a carcinoma in the upper aerodigestive tract. The character of the overlying skin is also significant in regard to erythema, induration, rash, blanching, audible bruit, palpable thrill, or fistula.

A systematic examination of all external and internal aspects of the head and neck should also be conducted. Especially with adult patients, attention should be paid to the external ear, nasal cavity, nasopharynx, oral cavity, oropharynx, hypopharynx,

Table 36.1 Neck node levels

Levels	Borders
IA	Symphysis of mandible, hyoid bone, medial aspect of anterior belly of each digastric muscle
IB	Body of mandible, posterior belly of digastric muscle, anterior belly of ipsilateral digastric muscle, stylohyoid
IIA	Skull base, level of hyoid bone, stylohyoid, spinal accessory nerve
IIB	Skull base, level of hyoid bone, spinal accessory nerve, posterior border of sternocleidomastoid
III	Hyoid bone, inferior border of cricoid cartilage, sternohyoid, posterior border of sternocleidomastoid
IV	Inferior border of cricoid cartilage, clavicle, sternohyoid, posterior border of sternocleidomastoid
VA	Convergence of sternocleidomastoid and trapezius, level of cricoid cartilage, posterior border of sternocleidomastoid, anterior border of trapezius
VB	Level of cricoid cartilage, clavicle, posterior border of sternocleidomastoid, anterior border of trapezius
VI	Hyoid bone, suprasternal notch, bilateral common carotid arteries

and larynx. The patient should be evaluated for skin or scalp lesions, and the palpation of other lymphatic sites (including axillary, supraclavicular, and occipital nodes) should not be forgotten. The palpation of all salivary glands and the thyroid gland, liver, and spleen can also provide important information.

36.4 Testing

36.4.1 Laboratory Testing

Laboratory testing may include simply a complete blood cell count with differential to identify markers of infection, such as an increased white blood cell count with a neutrophil predominance. For neck masses that may be a manifestation of systemic disease, the erythrocyte sedimentation rate levels of rheumatoid factor, antinuclear antibody, and HIV antibody can be diagnostic. In the case of specific infectious causes, serologic testing can provide definitive information, as with tuberculosis (purified protein derivative), infectious mononucleosis (monospot test or viral capsule antigen immunofluorescence), cat-scratch disease (antibody titers), and toxoplasmosis (antibody titers).

36.4.2 Pathological Testing

Fine-needle aspiration biopsy has become an essential tool in the diagnosis of neck masses. The procedure is quick and safe, and it can yield an abundant amount of information. A 22- to 25-gauge needle attached to a 10-mL syringe is inserted through the skin into the neck mass, and while the plunger is pulled and held back to maintain suction, multiple passes through the lesion are made. The aspirate is typically placed on a microscope slide for pathologic analysis. Although tissue architecture is generally not apparent, fine-needle aspiration biopsy can differentiate cystic from solid, benign from malignant, and lymphoid from squamous masses. Some controversy still exists regarding the timing of fine-needle aspiration biopsy before or after imaging. Nonetheless, the utility and ease of fine-needle aspiration biopsy cannot be discounted. If indeterminate, or if tissue architecture is needed for diagnosis and treatment such as with lymphoma, an excisional biopsy is frequently conducted in the operating room.

36.4.3 Imaging

Computed tomography (CT) and magnetic resonance (MR) imaging of the neck can be extremely helpful in the characterization of a solitary neck mass. They can define the actual size of a lesion and its effect on surrounding vasculature. It can also differentiate cystic, solid, vascular, and invasive characteristics. A mass can be further characterized by its relation to important head and neck structures. For example, a thyroglossal duct cyst can be identified by its close relation to the hyoid bone. With regard to head and neck cancer, CT can help delineate specific areas of possible local and regional involvement, with special attention to bone. MR imaging can aid the clinician in the definition of soft-tissue planes. Positron emission tomography (PET) can aid the diagnosis in the difficult scenario of a neck metastasis with an unknown primary. Ultrasonography can identify cystic masses and is especially useful with thyroid masses. It can also be used to aid accuracy during fine-needle aspiration of nonpalpable masses.

36.5 Differential Diagnosis

36.5.1 Inflammatory and Infectious Masses

Viral Lymphadenopathy

Reactive lymphadenopathy secondary to a viral infection is the most common type of cervical lymphadenitis to affect both children and adults. Typically, the reactive lymphadenopathy presents during or after a recent upper respiratory tract infection (URI). Common viruses include adenovirus, rhinovirus, coxackie virus A and B, Epstein Barr virus (EBV), cytomegalovirus, herpes simplex virus, and human immunodeficiency virus (HIV). Importantly, reactive lymph nodes can become secondarily infected by a bacterial agent causing suppurative lymphadenopathy. However, in most cases the lymph nodes are bilateral, symmetric, and regress in the 1–2 weeks following resolution of the URI. Treatment is typically supportive unless suppurative lymphadenopathy is suspected in an acutely enlarging, fluctuant, asymmetric, or exquisitely painful lymph node. Biopsy may be necessary if a lymph node persists several weeks beyond a cleared URI or if other alarming features discussed earlier arise.

Bacterial Lymphadenopathy

Bacterial lymphadenopathy, or suppurative lymphadenopathy, presents similarly to viral lymphadenopathy after an upper respiratory tract infection. However, these masses are often larger, more fluctuant, and accompanied by a sore throat, skin lesions, or high fever. The most common causative organisms are *Staphylococcus aureus* and group A β-hemolytic streptococci, although anaerobic and gram-negative bacteria can also be present. Treatment begins with a trial of antibiotics covering gram-positive and anaerobic bacteria. If this fails, intravenous antibiotics alone or incision and drainage with culture-directed antibiotic therapy is usually necessary. Other more common bacterial causes of lymphadenopathy include:

Cat-Scratch Disease

Cat-scratch disease typically is seen in patients younger than 20 years of age. Symptoms include tender submandibular or periauricular lymphadenopathy associated with fever, malaise, and a history of contact with cats. Parinaud (oculoglandular) syndrome can occur from inoculation near the eye or from eye rubbing. It presents with unilateral conjunctivitis and regional lymphadenitis. The causative bacterium is *Bartonella henselae*, which can be identified by Warthin-Starry staining. The diagnosis can also be aided by indirect fluorescent antibody testing for *Bartonella* DNA, which has been found to be both sensitive and specific. Treatment is typically supportive because the course is usually self-limited. However, antibiotic therapy with azithromycin or ciprofloxacin can expedite resolution. Incision and drainage should be avoided because of the potential for sinus formation.

Mycobacterial Infections

Atypical mycobacterial infections are typically caused by multiple mycobacteria including M. avium-intracellulare, M. scrofulaceum, and M. kansasii. They typically present as unilateral, anterior-superior cervical lymphadenopathy with overlying skin involvement. They are more common in children, immunocompromised patients, or those with recent foreign travel. The treatment of atypical mycobacterial infections can include complete excision or incision and drainage followed by antitubercular antibiotics.

In contrast, lymphadenopathy caused by M. tuberculosis is bilateral and not localized to a particular cervical region. While not as common with atypical infections, tuberculosis are associated with constitutional symptoms such as fever and weight loss. They are more common in adults, immunocompromised patients, recent foreign travel or exposure to an endemic population. The diagnosis of cervical tuberculosis (scrofula) is usually confirmed by acid-fast stain and culture after a lymph node biopsy, but can be suggested by positive tuberculin skin testing. Treatment of scrofula is simply antitubercular antibiotics.

Tularemia

Tularemia presents as an acute tonsillitis with fever, chills, and painful cervical lymphadenopathy. It is caused by the bacterium *Francisella tularensis* and transmitted to humans via rabbits, ticks, and contaminated water. The diagnosis is by serology and culture. The treatment is antibiotic therapy with intramuscular streptomycin.

Brucellosis

Brucellosis presents as a generalized lymphadenopathy with associated fever and malaise. It is caused by the bacterium *Brucella* and typically afflicts children after the ingestion of unpasteurized milk. The diagnosis is by serology and culture. The treatment typically includes antibiotic therapy with either trimethoprim/sulfamethoxazole or tetracycline.

Fungal Infections

Fungal infections are much less common than bacterial or viral infections in immunocompetent patients. However, their incidence rises dramatically in the immunocompromised population. Typical offending pathogens include *Candida*, *Histoplasma*, and *Aspergillus*. The diagnosis is typically by fungal smear with culture or by serology. The treatment is aggressive with agents such as intravenous amphotericin B and in some cases correction of the underlying immunocompromised state.

Protozoal Infections

One of the most common causes of protozoal lymphadenitis is toxoplasmosis. *Toxoplasma gondii* infection typically presents as a nonspecific cervical adenitis with an associated influenza-like illness. Inoculation typically occurs after the ingestion of uncooked meat or of oocytes from cat feces. The diagnosis is typically by serum titers or lymph node biopsy. The treatment includes antiprotozoal agents such as pyrimethamine or sulfonamides.

HIV–Associated Cervical Lymphadenopathy

Cervical lymphadenopathy in the patient with HIV infection may be due to idiopathic follicular hyperplasia. However, in immunosuppressed patients, other infectious or neoplastic conditions such as tuberculosis and lymphoma cannot be excluded without work-up. Typically, excisional biopsy is done for suspicious lesions that are rapidly enlarging or have failed antibiotic therapy. Patients with HIV infection patients may also be diagnosed with persistent generalized lymphadenopathy when no other identifiable cause is found. Typically, these patients will have adenopathy in both the axillary and inguinal regions for longer than 3 months. The treatment is typically observation with standard treatment of the HIV infection.

36.5.2 Noninfectious Inflammatory Disorders

Sarcoidosis

Sarcoidosis is an idiopathic granulomatous disease of unknown etiology. It is marked by the accumulation of mononuclear cells in affected organs with subsequent noncaseating granulomatous reaction and fibrosis. It most commonly presents in females and in the second decade of life; in the United States, African-Americans are more commonly affected, although worldwide Caucasians are more likely to be affected. Head and neck symptoms most commonly include cervical adenopathy, but nasal, orbital, and supraglottic masses are also possible. Heerfordt syndrome (uveoparotid fever) is the constellation of fever, parotid swelling, facial nerve palsy, sensorineural hearing loss, and uveitis. Systemically, sarcoidosis can be asymptomatic or present with progressive cough, dyspnea, and bone and joint pain. Pulmonary involvement is most common, but subcutaneous nodules, hepatosplenomegaly, cardiac arrhythmias, and cutaneous rashes can also be seen. The diagnosis is by chest radiography showing hilar adenopathy, biopsy of affected tissue showing noncaseating granulomas, and blood work showing increased serum angiotensin-converting enzyme (ACE) levels. The treatment includes steroids for acute exacerbations.

Rosai-Dorfman Disease

Rosai-Dorfman disease typically presents in children with massive, non-tender, bilateral cervical lymphadenopathy associated with constitutional symptoms such as fever and weight loss. It can also affect other nodal systems in the mediastinum, inguinal area or retroperitoneum. Extranodal locations include the skin, soft tissue, and upper aerodigestive tract (nasal cavity). Intracranial manifestations can also occur. Although the exact etiology is unknown, the disease is thought to result from an abnormal histiocytic response to a viral infection. The diagnosis is established by biopsy showing dilated sinuses, plasma cells, and histiocytic proliferation. The treatment is generally conservative because this disease has a self-limited course.

Kawasaki Disease (Mucocutaneous Lymph Node Syndrome)

Kawasaki disease initially presents in children younger than 5 years of age with fever lasting for at least 5 days in association with at least four of the following: acute, unilateral, nonpurulent cervical lymphadenopathy; rash; bilateral conjunctival injection; erythema of the lips and oral cavity; or erythema, induration, and desquamation of the hands and feet. The subacute and chronic phases are marked by thrombocytosis, the formation and enlargement of coronary aneurysms, and a risk for myocardial infarction. The diagnosis is by history and physical examination, with cardiac work-up more imperative in the later stages. The treatment is typically high-dose gamma globulin therapy in the acute phase. Aspirin and dipyridamole can be used for coronary aneurysms.

36.5.3 Congenital Neck Masses

These include branchial cleft cysts, thyroglossal duct cysts, dermoids and teratomas, laryngoceles, and sternocleidomastoid tumors. Lymphangiomas, hemangiomas, and vascular malformations are also within the differential diagnosis, but they will be discussed elsewhere.

Thyroglossal Duct Cysts

Thyroglossal duct cysts make up more than two thirds of all congenital neck masses and are the second most common pediatric neck masses. They are typically diagnosed before the age of 10, but can be seen as late as the third decade of life. They originate from a persistence of the tract followed by the thyroid diverticulum as it descends caudally from the foramen cecum of the tongue, just anterior to the hyoid bone, to its final paratracheal destination. Thyroglossal duct cysts present either as painless, cystic neck masses in the midline of the neck near the hyoid bone or as painful, cystic masses when acutely infected. However, they can be found anywhere between the tongue and thyroid gland, sometimes even within the tongue. A hallmark feature is the movement of these cysts when the patient protrudes the tongue or swallows. Treatment involves an excision not only of the dominant cyst but also of the medial portion of the hyoid bone and a cone-shaped cuff of tissue from the hyoid to the base of the tongue. This operation (Sistrunk procedure) is thought to reduce the risk for recurrence. Infected cysts often necessitate needle aspiration and antibiotic therapy; formal incision and drainage is not recommended.

Branchial Cleft Cysts

Branchial cleft anomalies account for roughly 30% of all congenital neck masses. While they present most commonly as cysts, they can also present as sinuses or fistulas to the aerodigestive tract. They typically present in childhood or early adulthood and do not have a sex predominance. The mechanism for their development is unclear, but some suspect they originate from the cervical sinus of His and become trapped, without an external (or internal) opening. Simply, they are thought to originate from a failure of obliteration of the branchial clefts and pouches. Others theorize that they develop from epithelial rests of tissue in the Waldeyer ring. A branchial cleft cyst typically presents as a fluctuant mass at the anterior border of the sternocleidomastoid muscle. The physical examination should include an evaluation of the upper airway, including the tonsillar fossae and piriform sinuses, for any evidence of connection. CT, MR

imaging, and ultrasound can be used to better characterize the mass. Fine-needle aspiration biopsy is contraindicated unless for drainage of an infected cyst because it makes surgical excision more difficult. However, in adults, FNA can be used to differentiate a branchial cleft cyst from cystic degeneration of a metastatic lymph node.

1. First branchial cleft cysts: These cysts make up fewer than 1% of all branchial cleft anomalies. They can involve the external auditory canal, parotid gland, or less frequently the middle ear. They are known to course close to the facial nerve, sometimes crossing between fibers. They are typically classified as type I or type II.
   a) Type I: These masses form as duplications of the membranous external auditory canal, contain ectoderm only, typically course lateral to the facial nerve, and may present as cysts near the auricle.
   b) Type II: These masses contain both ectoderm and mesoderm, can sometimes contain cartilage, and typically course medial the facial nerve. Their presentation is more variable than that of type I. They can present anywhere from the external auditory canal to the submandibular area. Most commonly, they present as cysts near the angle of the mandible, with tracts coursing superiorly through the parotid gland to end inferior to or in the external auditory canal.
2. Second branchial cleft cysts (▶ Fig. 36.1): These cysts are the most common, accounting for approximately 95% of all branchial cleft anomalies. They most typically present as solitary neck masses just anterior to the sternocleidomastoid muscle, separate from the carotid sheath. However, they can lie anywhere along a potential tract that passes deep to the sternocleidomastoid between the internal and external carotid arteries and pierces the tonsillar fossa.
3. Third branchial cleft cysts: These cysts are quite rare. Third branchial cleft cysts present at the lower, anterior border of the sternocleidomastoid (near the superior pole of the thyroid gland). The tract passes deep to the internal carotid artery and glossopharyngeal nerve and superficial to the vagus nerve, then enters the thyrohyoid membrane to enter the pharynx at the piriform sinus above the internal branch of the superior laryngeal nerve.

Treatment

Excision of first branchial cleft anomalies, especially type II anomalies, may include a superficial parotidectomy with facial nerve dissection. Unfortunately, recurrence is quite common, even after excision. Second branchial cleft anomalies can be resected through a standard transcervical incision. However, if a tract is noted, techniques that include cannulation, methylene blue injection, and stepladder incisions may be used to trace the entire length of the tract. Third branchial cleft cysts are treated similarly to second branchial cleft cysts. However, a thorough endoscopic examination is important to identify a piriform sinus opening.

Dermoid Cysts

Neck dermoid cysts comprise only 20% of all head and neck dermoids. They are thought to originate from the entrapment of

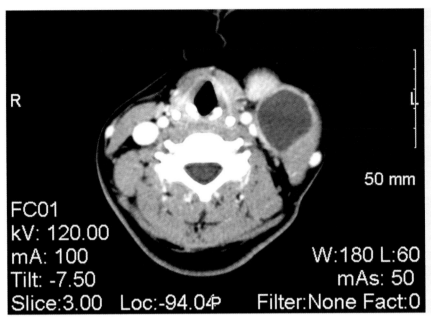

Fig. 36.1 Left-sided second branchial cleft cyst. Note the close relationship to the anterior border of the sternocleidomastoid muscle.

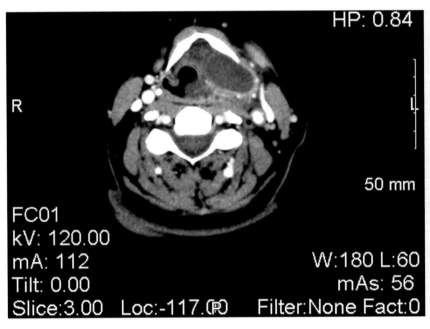

Fig. 36.2 Left-sided laryngopyocele. Note the origin medial to the thyroid cartilage, with extension externally through the thyrohyoid membrane.

epithelium along embryologic lines of fusion but can also occur from traumatic implantation. Dermoids contain both ectodermal and endodermal elements. They are lined by epithelium but can contain other elements, such as hair follicles and sebaceous glands. Dermoids present similarly to thyroglossal duct cysts, as midline (usually in the submental region), painless, slow-growing, superficial neck masses that can move during tongue protrusion and swallowing. However, infection is rare, and they can gradually increase in size. Surgical excision is the treatment of choice.

Teratomas

Head and neck teratomas comprise approximately 2% of all teratomas; aside from the neck, the other most common site in the head and neck is the nasopharynx. These teratomas form during the second trimester, are more common in females, and differ from dermoids in that they contain all three germ layers. Teratomas typically present at birth as firm, midline neck masses, with the CT/MR imaging finding of calcifications. They can sometimes be identified on prenatal ultrasound. If a teratoma is discovered prenatally, cesarean section may be necessary because of rapid growth and the potential for airway compromise and esophageal compression. Surgical excision is the treatment of choice.

Laryngoceles

A laryngocele is an air-filled dilatation or herniation of the laryngeal saccule that can also become infected (▶ Fig. 36.2). Laryngoceles are rare in children but can present in a congenital form as a remnant sac. However, typically they present in adults as an acquired form secondary to increased intraglottic pressure. There are three types of laryngoceles: internal, external, and combined. An internal laryngocele is a dilatation that does not extend beyond the thyroid cartilage. An external laryngocele extends beyond the thyroid cartilage through the thyrohyoid membrane and can present as a lateral neck mass. In addition to a lateral neck mass, all types of laryngoceles can present with hoarseness, dyspnea, and dysphagia. Endoscopic evaluation typically reveals a dilatation at the level of the ventricle or false vocal folds for an internal laryngocele. It is also important to rule out a laryngeal mass. CT is the diagnostic test of choice to differentiate laryngoceles from fluid-filled saccular cysts. Treatment is typically surgical: endoscopic excision for small internal laryngoceles or excision via an external approach for larger ones.

Thymic Cysts

Thymic cysts develop from the implantation of thymic tissue along the tract that the third branchial pouch takes as it descends into the mediastinum. They typically present as unilateral (more commonly left-sided), asymptomatic cystic neck masses. Like other congenital cysts, they can present after infection with pain and rapid enlargement. Surgical excision is the treatment of choice.

Sternocleidomastoid Tumors of Infancy

Sternocleidomastoid tumor of infancy typically presents 1 to 8 weeks after birth as a firm, painless, thickened mass confined to the muscle that slowly increases in size and then regresses. The infant usually holds its head and neck to the affected side and the chin to the opposite side. The tumors are thought to result from birth trauma, muscle ischemia, or intrauterine positioning. Their slow but typically complete regression allows conservative management with physical therapy and excision only for persistent cases.

36.5.4 Neoplastic Disorders

Metastatic squamous cell carcinoma from the upper aerodigestive tract, lymphoma, thyroid disease, paraganglioma, lipoma, and salivary gland neoplasms can all present as solitary neck masses. They are discussed in other chapters.

36.6 Treatment

The treatment of a solitary neck mass is dictated by the diagnosis. For congenital neck masses, the treatment is typically surgical excision. However, if the mass presents as an acute infection, then antibiotics, aspiration, and observation before excision are appropriate. Infectious and inflammatory neck masses are treated with either close observation or antibiotic therapy. However, the diagnosis of an infectious or inflammatory mass is often made with surgical excisional biopsy. Complications of treatment include bleeding, infection, and pain from surgical incisions. In addition, damage to surrounding structures such as nerves, arteries, and veins during surgical excision is a costly complication. There is also a high risk for recurrence, especially of surgically excised congenital neck masses. The prognosis for a patient with a solitary neck mass depends on the diagnosis and is improved by early evaluation and expeditious management.

36.7 Roundsmanship

- A thorough history and physical examination will lead to a concise differential diagnosis for the patient with an isolated neck mass.
- An understanding of the neck levels is important not only for localization but also for surgical management and an awareness of the potential complications associated with neck masses.
- Congenital neck masses can present during an acute infection. Incision and drainage is contraindicated in most instances.
- Virus-induced lymphadenopathy is the most common type of cervical lymphadenitis in both adults and children.
- Cervical lymphadenopathy in the patient with HIV infection is most commonly due to idiopathic follicular hyperplasia.

36.8 Recommended Reading

[1] Acierno SP, Waldhausen JH. Congenital cervical cysts, sinuses and fistulae. Otolaryngol Clin North Am 2007; 40: 161–176, vii–viii
[2] Al-Dajani N, Wootton SH. Cervical lymphadenitis, suppurative parotitis, thyroiditis, and infected cysts. Infect Dis Clin North Am 2007; 21: 523–541, viii
[3] Amedee RG, Dhurandhar NR. Fine-needle aspiration biopsy. Laryngoscope 2001; 111: 1551–1557
[4] Gross E, Sichel JY. Congenital neck lesions. Surg Clin North Am 2006; 86: 383–392
[5] Wetmore RF, Potsic WP. Differential diagnosis of neck masses. In: Cummings Otolaryngology: Head & Neck Surgery, 4th ed. Flint PW, Haughey BH, Lund VJ, Niparko JK, Richardson MA, Robbins KT, et al. Philadelphia: Mosby-Elsevier 2010, 184:4210–4222
[6] Lin DT, Deschler DG. Neck masses. In: Current Diagnosis and Treatment of Otolaryngology–Head and Neck Surgery. Lalwani A, ed. New York: Lange Medical Books/McGraw Hill 2004, 413–433

37 Blunt and Penetrating Neck Injuries

James Azzi, Jean-Paul Azzi, and Stimson P. Schantz

37.1 Penetrating Neck Injuries

Penetrating neck injuries are defined as any violation of the platysma. They comprise 5 to 10% of all traumas. Because the neck is a small, vulnerable area that houses a multitude of vital structures, trauma to this area can be emergent and life-threatening; hemorrhage is the most common cause of death in this group.

Air passages and vascular, gastrointestinal, and neurologic structures can all potentially be injured by penetrating neck trauma. Signs and symptoms can be divided among these groups of structures. Laryngotracheal injury may present with respiratory distress, stridor, hemoptysis, hoarseness, tracheal deviation, subcutaneous emphysema, or a sucking wound. Vascular injuries may present with a hematoma, persistent bleeding, neurologic deficit, absent pulse, hypovolemic shock, bruit, thrill, or change in sensorium. Neurologic injury may present with hemiplegia, quadriplegia, cranial nerve deficit, change in sensorium, or hoarseness. Pharyngoesophageal injury may be characterized by subcutaneous emphysema, dysphagia, odynophagia, hematemesis, hemoptysis, tachycardia, or fever. It is important to note that esophageal injuries are often subclinical.

To aid in decision making, the neck can be divided into three anatomical zones. Zone II lies between the cricoid and the angle of the mandible and is the zone most commonly injured. Zone I, the most caudal zone, lies between the cricoid and the sternal notch; injuries to this zone carry the highest mortality risk. Zone III lies between the mandibular angle and the skull base. Of great concern in the management of penetrating neck injuries is ease of surgical exposure. Zone II is the most easily accessed. Zones I and III are better protected by bone, so that surgical explorations are more difficult (▶ Fig. 37.1).

Patients presenting with penetrating neck injuries can be divided into three groups: unstable, stable, or asymptomatic. When this information is combined with knowledge of the neck zones involved, an algorithm for management can be established.

37.1.1 Mechanism

The mechanism of injury and velocity of the projectile are key factors influencing the risk for major injury. Gunshot wounds generally can be divided into low-velocity and high-velocity wounds. Most civilian handguns have a low muzzle velocity.

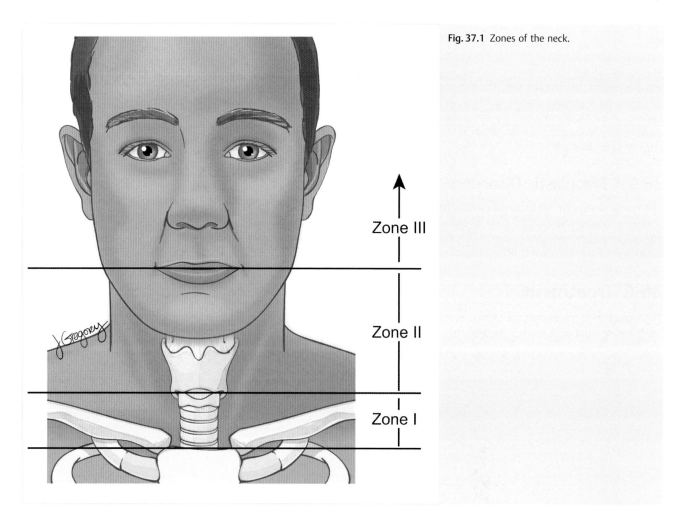

Fig. 37.1 Zones of the neck.

Zone III

Zone II

Zone I

These projectiles often will follow tissue planes, pushing aside vital structures and causing relatively less damage. High-velocity projectiles, like those of military rifles, cause greater destruction by transmitting energy to surrounding tissue after penetration. The path of destruction is more direct and the damaged cavity is wider, often deceptively so compared with the dimensions of the entry and exit wounds. Structures as far as two inches away from the cavity of a wound may be injured. Victims of these injuries to the neck often do not survive, and emergent surgical exploration often means the difference between life and death. In the event of a stable patient, selective surgical management is often an option.

Stab injuries take a more predictable path than gunshot wounds. One key difference is the risk for subclavian vessel injury. Gunshot wounds commonly run perpendicular to the neck, and the clavicles provide some protection to the subclavian vessels. Because the trajectory of a knife is often in a downward direction, penetration over the clavicle makes subclavian vessel lacerations more common than they are with gunshots.

37.1.2 Mandatory versus Elective Exploration

Penetrating neck injuries are managed according to the presentation. The first determination is whether or not an injury is immediately life-threatening. Signs of hemorrhage are key indicators, including expanding hematoma, hemodynamic instability, hypovolemic shock, hemothorax, and hemomediastinum. In these cases, immediate surgical exploration is mandatory.

In stable patients, imaging is often useful to determine the extent of injury and aid in the decision of whether or not to explore. To further aid in decision making, the neck may be divided into three zones, each with unique considerations.

Zone I injuries are particularly dangerous because of the presence of the great vessels. Although the bone cage of the thorax protects this region from injury, it also makes surgical exploration much more difficult. Zone I injuries have a mortal-

ity rate as high as 12%. Because of these factors, angiography is recommended to locate any possible injuries before surgical exploration.

Zone III includes structures above the angle of the mandible. High carotid artery and cranial nerve injuries are of great concern in this region. as in zone I, surgical exploration is difficult because of the narrow confines of the skull base and mandible. Therefore, in a stable patient with an intact airway and no signs or symptoms of hemorrhage, evaluation with angiography is appropriate. Furthermore, regular intraoral examinations are necessary because edema or hematoma formation can potentially compromise a once-stable airway.

Zone II, lying between the cricoid and the angle of the mandible, is the most frequently injured zone because it is the most exposed; for the same reasons, it is also the least difficult to explore surgically. There has been much debate regarding whether to make exploration mandatory in all zone II injuries or to use a more conservative approach of selective exploration with repeated examinations, endoscopy, and angiography. In favor of open treatment is that isolated venous and pharyngoesophageal injuries have been shown to be potentially difficult to detect preoperatively. However, clinically stable patients with zone II injuries can be admitted and evaluated with frequent, repeated physical examinations. These patients can undergo additional endoscopic and radiologic evaluation (▶ Fig. 37.2).

Patients with penetrating neck injuries, like all patients with trauma, first require management of the ABCs: airway, breathing, and circulation. Airway control is gained by intubation, cricothyroidotomy, or tracheostomy. In an airway with a direct injury, direct tracheal intubation is often the safest option. Care should be taken to avoid exacerbating an existing airway injury either by poor visualization during intubation or simply by extending the neck. Pneumothorax should be treated emergently with chest tube placement. Large-bore intravenous lines should be placed in all patients. Direct pressure should be placed to control hemorrhage or an expanding hematoma. Patients with major vessel hemorrhage should be surgically explored

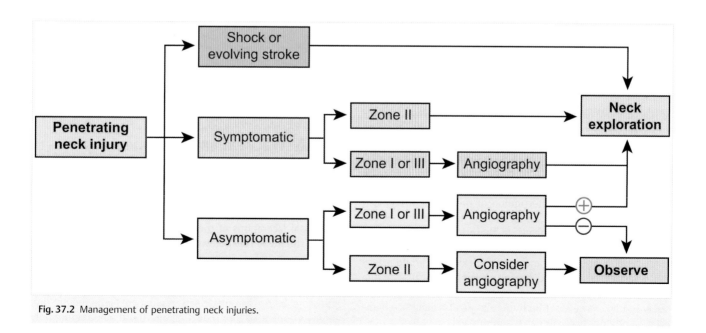

Fig. 37.2 Management of penetrating neck injuries.

emergently. Patients should be examined closely for vascular and neurologic signs because some findings can suggest the path of the projectile and additional injuries; for example, hypoglossal nerve deficit, hoarseness, or Horner syndrome would suggest possible concomitant carotid injury.

37.1.3 Diagnostic Evaluation

In a stable patient, a careful and thorough history and physical examination are performed. Particular attention should be paid to entrance and exit wounds and a comprehensive neurologic examination. Cervical spine radiographs should be obtained to rule out fractures, and chest X-rays will rule out hemothorax, pneumothorax, and pneumomediastinum; in some cases, subclavian injury can also be identified. Marking wounds with radiopaque objects can aid in the evaluation.

Some disagreement exists as to whether mandatory exploration is superior to selective management. Because prospective studies have not shown one approach to be better than the other, many centers employ selective management. This approach divides patients into three groups: unstable, which includes those with shock or evolving stroke; stable symptomatic; and stable asymptomatic. Unstable patients undergo emergent neck exploration. Stable patients with zone I or zone III injury are triaged to angiography, and subsequent exploration is performed as necessary.

Stable symptomatic patients with zone II injury undergo neck exploration. Asymptomatic patients with zone II injury can be considered for angiography or observed for 48 hours.

Penetrating zone II injury can be evaluated further to detect occult injury. The first consideration is whether the airway is compromised. If compromised, the patient is first stabilized, and then angiography, contrast gastrointestinal examination, and flexible and rigid endoscopy should be performed in order, with any positive finding warranting neck exploration. If the airway is adequate, attention is directed toward symptoms of the digestive, respiratory, vascular, and neurologic systems. Appropriate diagnostic evaluation is then done to determine whether exploration is necessary. Regardless of the results, all patients should be observed for 48 hours with frequent physical examinations.

37.1.4 Management of Vascular Injury to the Neck

Although a low cervical incision may suffice, zone I vascular injuries generally require thoracotomy, and early consultation with the thoracic surgery team is appropriate.

Zone II injuries can involve the common or internal carotid arteries. This zone is explored through an incision along the anterior border of the sternocleidomastoid muscle. A large hematoma or proximal interruption of the carotid artery can significantly decrease pulsation, making identification of the damaged artery more difficult. In these instances, it is often necessary to follow branches of the external carotid in a retrograde fashion. Injury to branches of the external carotid artery can generally be managed by suture ligation because of the abundant collateral circulation. Veins in the neck can also be safely ligated; however, if both internal jugular veins are damaged, an attempt to repair one is appropriate.

Zone III injuries may require a mandibulotomy. Injuries to this area often involve multiple vascular structures, including the internal carotid artery, internal maxillary artery, and external carotid artery. Consultation with an interventional radiologist should be considered when a challenging access at the skull base must be dealt with.

Several techniques for vascular repair have been described, including vessel wall repair, vessel ligation, vessel patch graft, autogenous vessel graft, and synthetic vessel graft. Autogenous grafting or end-to-end anastomoses are recommended when stenosis is evident on imaging studies. Ligation of the internal or common carotid arteries is not recommended and is considered only for irreparable injuries. Unrepaired vascular injuries may result in several delayed complications, including aneurysm formation, dissection, and arteriovenous fistulas.

37.1.5 Evaluation of the Digestive Tract

In the patient with a possible esophageal perforation, a thorough evaluation is paramount. Missed tears can progress to mediastinitis, which is associated with considerable morbidity and mortality. Studies have reported the use of flexible esophagoscopy to bypass the general anesthesia required for a rigid endoscopy; however, there have been reports of missed perforations in areas of mucosal redundancy.

Imaging can play a significant role in the diagnosis of esophageal perforations. Gastrografin swallow studies are performed initially because extravasated barium can cause a chemical mediastinitis; barium extravasation can also radiographically distort tissue planes. If this study is deemed to be normal and suspicion remains for a perforation, a barium swallow should be considered.

If suspicion of a perforation remains despite a normal examination, the patient can be observed while taking nothing by mouth. A widening mediastinum on serial chest radiographs, fever, or tachycardia will likely require repeated endoscopy or neck exploration.

Many surgeons perform direct laryngoscopy, bronchoscopy, and rigid esophagoscopy for penetrating injuries to the neck with air in the soft tissues, hemoptysis, or any other suspicious findings. When an esophageal perforation is found, management generally involves a primary, two-layer closure with débridement and adequate drainage. Some surgeons also advocate the placement of a muscle flap over the suture line for further protection. It is imperative, however, that definitive management of any airway compromise be a priority.

37.1.6 Tracheal and Laryngeal Injuries

Tracheal lacerations that do not encroach on the airway or detach a tracheal ring can usually be repaired without a tracheotomy. With more severe injuries, a tracheotomy, either through or below the injury, is prudent.

Mucosal lacerations of the larynx secondary to penetrating trauma should be repaired within 24 hours to decrease scarring and improve voice. Surgical approximation is necessary for significant glottic and supraglottic lacerations, as well as for displaced cartilage fractures. Computed tomography (CT) and endoscopy help differentiate between patients who require thyrotomy or open fracture reduction and those who require only observation. The reader is referred to Chapter 92 (Laryngeal Trauma) for further discussion.

37.2 Blunt Neck Trauma

Blunt trauma to the neck may occur following assault, sports injury, or a motor vehicle accident. The force may result in injury to any combination of airway, vascular, or digestive structures. Because the effects may be delayed in onset and therefore missed, close observation is recommended.

Patients with multisystem trauma are at risk for having their laryngotracheal injuries overlooked. These patients can have a slow progression of edema that may compromise the airway hours after the initial insult. CT can be helpful in determining the degree of injury to both the larynx and nearby vessels. Blunt trauma to the cervical vessels can result in tears, thrombosis, dissection, and possibly pseudoaneurysm. These injuries can be treated by observation, anticoagulation, or surgery. The treatment depends principally on the mechanism, type, and location of injury. Consultation with a vascular surgeon should be considered.

37.3 Roundsmanship

- Surgical exploration is necessary in patients with any penetrating neck trauma and life-threatening signs or symptoms.
- Hemorrhage is the leading cause of death in patients with penetrating neck injuries, and patients should be monitored for at least 48 hours.
- Classifying the injury by zone and mechanism can be helpful in determining the likelihood of major injury.

37.4 Recommended Reading

[1] Armstrong WB, Detar TR, Stanley RB. Diagnosis and management of external penetrating cervical esophageal injuries. Ann Otol Rhinol Laryngol 1994; 103: 863–871

[2] Beitsch P, Weigelt JA, Flynn E, Easley S. Physical examination and arteriography in patients with penetrating zone II neck wounds. Arch Surg 1994; 129: 577–581

[3] Jarvik JG, Philips GR, Schwab CW, Schwartz JS, Grossman RI. Penetrating neck trauma: sensitivity of clinical examination and cost-effectiveness of angiography. AJNR Am J Neuroradiol 1995; 16: 647–654

[4] McConnell DB, Trunkey DD. Management of penetrating trauma to the neck. Adv Surg 1994; 27: 97–127

[5] Noyes LD, McSwain NE, Markowitz IP. Panendoscopy with arteriography versus mandatory exploration of penetrating wounds of the neck. Ann Surg 1986; 204: 21–31

[6] Obeid FN, Haddad GS, Horst HM, Bivins BA. A critical reappraisal of a mandatory exploration policy for penetrating wounds of the neck. Surg Gynecol Obstet 1985; 160: 517–522

[7] Rao PM, Bhatti MF, Gaudino J et al. Penetrating injuries of the neck: criteria for exploration. J Trauma 1983; 23: 47–49

[8] Saletta JD, Folk FA, Freeark RJ. Trauma to the neck region. Surg Clin North Am 1973; 53: 73–86

[9] Sclafani AP, Sclafani SJ. Angiography and transcatheter arterial embolization of vascular injuries of the face and neck. Laryngoscope 1996; 106: 168–173

38 Facial Analysis

Alexander Ovchinsky

38.1 Introduction

Comprehensive facial analysis is a crucial element in the process of achieving a successful surgical outcome. A facial plastic surgeon, like an artist, should be able to envision the final result of his or her work, which depends not only on the surgeon's expertise but also on the anatomical characteristics of a given patient. Patients' characteristics may vary widely with ethnicity, age, gender, medical or surgical history, and history of facial trauma or prior surgery. Therefore, a thorough understanding of what is generally accepted to be the facial norm is essential in building a foundation for a successful result. Patients' expectations may sometimes be unrealistic because of certain anatomical limitations; it is of a paramount importance to communicate to the patient these limitations and how they will affect the final outcome in order to avoid an unhappy patient postoperatively.

38.2 Incidence of Disease

All humans eventually will exhibit aging-related changes in facial anatomy because of a combination of multiple factors, such as facial bony resorption, loss of soft-tissue support, soft-tissue atrophy, and age-related skin changes. Some patients will exhibit these changes earlier than others as a consequence of various factors, such as genetic predisposition (e.g., in progeria or Ehlers-Danlos syndrome); excessive sun exposure with resultant skin changes (wrinkling, pigmentation, loss of elasticity); body habitus; and certain medical conditions (e.g., skin changes in patients on long-term steroid therapy, facial lipodystrophy in patients on HIV antiretroviral therapy). Multiple syndromic conditions affect facial anatomy and will cause noticeable deviation from the norm at birth (e.g., Treacher Collins syndrome, Crouzon syndrome, Waardenburg syndrome).

38.3 Terminology

There are several important anatomical landmarks that greatly assist in facial descriptive analysis. Beginning superiorly, the trichion marks the superior extent of the forehead and corresponds to the level of the hairline. The glabella is the most prominent point of the forehead on the profile. The nasion is the depression at the root of the nose and corresponds to the nasofrontal suture line. The radix, incorrectly used interchangeably with the nasion, is the root of the nose and marks the deepest point of the nasofrontal angle. The rhinion corresponds to the bony–cartilaginous junction on the nasal dorsum. The subnasale is the junction of the columella and the upper lip at the base of the nose. The vermilion border of the lips is the mucocutaneous junction. The menton is the lowermost position of the soft tissues of the chin, while the pogonion marks the most anterior projection of the chin. The tragion is located at the supratragal notch and is an important landmark for determining the appropriate horizontal position, or Frankfort horizontal plane, which passes from the tragion to the inferior orbital rim (▶ Fig. 38.1).

38.4 Applied Anatomy

The face is commonly subdivided into horizontal "thirds" (▶ Fig. 38.2) and vertical "fifths" (▶ Fig. 38.3). The upper facial third is bounded by the hairline and the brows/glabella, the middle third spans the face from the glabella to the subnasale, and the lower third runs from the subnasale to the menton. This is a rough approximation, however, and the lower third of the face is generally slightly longer than the middle third (▶ Fig. 38.4). In addition, the lower face can also be divided into thirds, with the length of the upper lip equaling one-third and the lower lip and chin equaling two-thirds. Vertical fifths assist with the assessment of facial symmetry on the frontal view, in which each fifth approximates one eye width: helical rim to lateral canthus (two), lateral canthus to medial canthus (two), and intercanthal distance (one).

There are a number of facial angles that are used to define the relationships of the various facial structures to one another. Some of these angles are nearly constant for males and females, whereas others are variable depending on the sex of the patient (▶ Fig. 38.5 and ▶ Fig. 38.6). The nasofrontal angle measures the facial angle at the nasion or, in other words, the transition angle from the forehead onto the nasal dorsum. This angle ranges from 115 degrees (men) to 120 degrees (women). The nasolabial angle is the angle between the columella and the upper lip. It should be around 90 to 95 degrees in men and around 100 to 110 degrees in women. An increase in this angle results in an appearance of over-rotation of the nose, whereas a decrease leads to an appearance of under-rotation. The cervicomental angle measures the angle of transition of the neck into the inferior aspect of the chin; an increase in submental fat or a low-set hyoid bone leads to blunting of the cervicomental angle.

38.5 The Disease Process

38.5.1 Etiology

There are several theories of aging, all of which are concentrated around a common notion that facial aging is the result of progressive soft-tissue descent. Over time, the soft tissues of the face sag off bony structures, forming the distinctive wrinkles, folds, and skin and soft-tissue redundancy of the aging face. This descent is partially due to subcutaneous soft-tissue atrophy, leading to a proportional increase in the amount of skin and skin ptosis. Age-related loss of facial volume due to gradual bony resorption is also a contributing factor. This decrease in bony volume translates into a decrease in the amount of support for the soft tissues of the face, thus causing downward rotation of the soft tissues and ptosis. Sun-related skin damage, also known as actinic damage or solar elastosis, leads to a loss of skin elasticity, pigment changes, and a general appearance of aging.

38.5.2 Natural History and Progression

Superficial skin lines, or wrinkles, are discrete at first and over time become more numerous, deeper, and multidirectional.

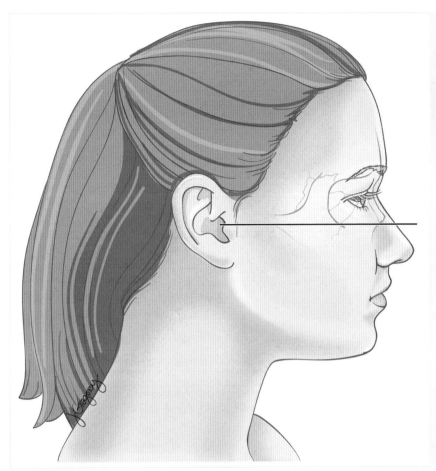

Fig. 38.1 The Frankfort horizontal plane is established by drawing a line from the tragion to the inferior orbital rim. Proper facial analysis is performed with the Frankfort horizontal plane parallel to the floor.

When wrinkles become associated with textural changes in the skin surface from photodamage and repeated muscular contraction, they become mimetic lines. The deepening of the mimetic lines into the dermis leads to the appearance of skin furrows. As skin redundancy worsens and skin ptosis continues, skin furrows slowly progress into skin folds.

38.6 Medical Evaluation

38.6.1 Clinical Findings, Physical Examination

It is important to consider the major aesthetic units of the face individually as well as in relationship to the rest of the face. These include the forehead, periorbital region, midface, nose, perioral region and chin, neck, and ears.

Forehead

Alopecia, or hair loss, may cause an elevation of the hairline, increasing the height of the upper face. Frontalis muscle hypertonicity and loss of skin elasticity can cause "worry lines" or horizontal forehead lines, which may range in severity from minor mimetic lines to deep, corrugated furrows. Procerus muscle action over time will cause the formation of horizontal nasal root wrinkles, while the action of the corrugator supercilii muscle forms the vertical glabellar lines.

Hypertonicity of these muscles also produces brow ptosis. Another factor contributing to brow descent is a decrease in the amount of supraorbital subcutaneous tissue, leading to "deflation" of the brow region. The brows should be examined for the degree of ptosis and for ptosis localization within the brow (i.e., medial, lateral, or generalized), as well as for any asymmetry accompanying bilateral brow ptosis. In the event of brow asymmetry, it is very important to bring this to the attention of the patient because it may not be corrected by browlifting procedures. When brow ptosis progresses, it may result in "lateral hooding" of the upper eyelid, causing a peripheral visual field deficit, a functional indication for brow ptosis correction.

Periorbital Region

The size, shape, position, and symmetry of the individual components should be assessed. The intercanthal distance, which should be equal to the width of one eye, may be increased in certain syndromes, as well as after facial trauma to the naso-orbital region, causing hypertelorism. Asymmetry of the palpebral apertures may be due to a unilateral upper lid ptosis, which should be documented and addressed during a corrective procedure. Other periorbital abnormalities, such as enophthalmos, exophthalmos, and lower lid laxity and ectropion, should be documented during the evaluation of the region. Signs of eyelid aging may be due to increased skin laxity (dermatochalasis),

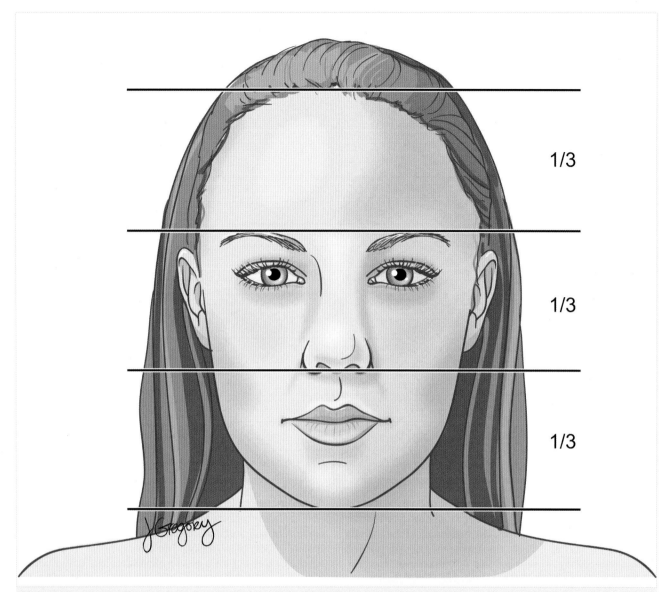

Fig. 38.2 The face can be divided roughly into vertical thirds, from the trichion to the glabella, the glabella to the subnasale, and the subnasale to the menton.

pseudoherniation of orbital fat through the orbital septum causing the development of the "eye bags," or a combination of the above. Hypertrophy of the orbicularis oculi muscle may lead to the formation of prominent wrinkles and muscular roll, seen mainly in the lower eyelids. Malar bags are thought to represent edema of the lateral infraorbital soft tissues.

Midface

The loss of midfacial ligamentous support results in anterior–inferior descent of the midfacial subcutaneous fat, causing a relative loss of the superior–lateral cheek fat and a relative increase in the inferior–medial cheek fat. The net effect of this fat redistribution is deepening of the nasolabial fold, the development of cheek skin folds lateral to the nasolabial fold, and skeletonization of the zygomatic region with the formation of submalar hollow and tear trough deformity.

Nose

If the cartilaginous nasal framework weakens with time or as the nasal skin thins and becomes less elastic, so will the support of the nasal tip, resulting in tip ptosis and a decreased nasolabial angle. The tip may also become broader because of weakening of the intercrural ligament and divergence of the domal regions of the lower lateral cartilages. A dorsal hump may become more prominent because of tip ptosis and thickening of the nasal skin.

Perioral Region and Chin

Atrophy of the soft tissues, or deflation of the perioral region, results in lengthening of the upper lip, thinning of the red lip portion, and the formation of perioral rhytids. "Marionette lines," which extend from the oral commissure inferiorly

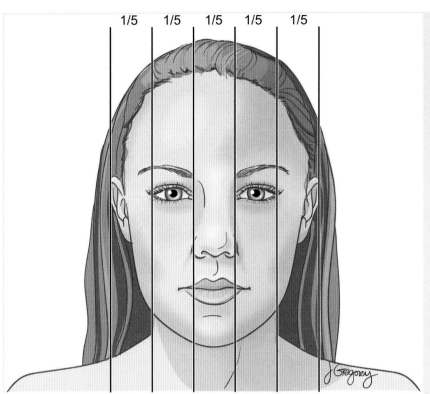

Fig. 38.3 The horizontals fifths of the face are bounded by the helical rims, lateral canthi, and medial canthi.

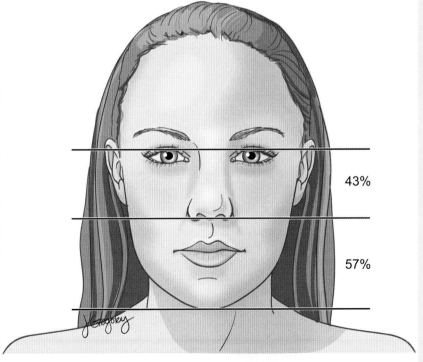

Fig. 38.4 The midface is generally shorter than the lower face.

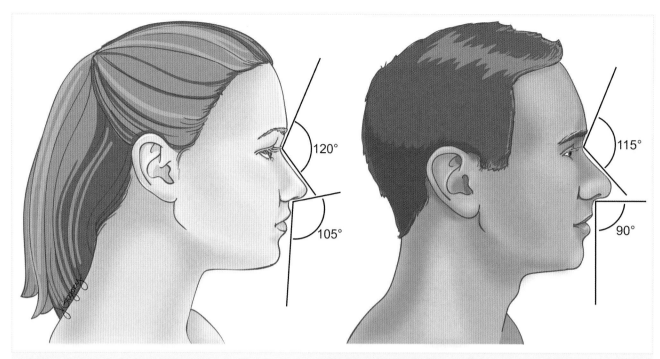

Fig. 38.5 Women tend to have wider nasofrontal and nasolabial angles than men.

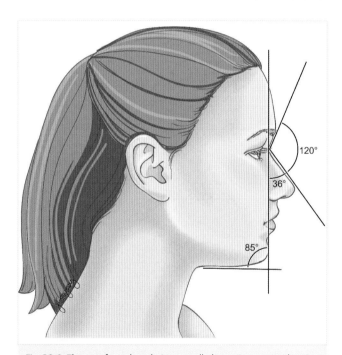

Fig. 38.6 The nasofrontal angle is generally larger in women than in men.

into the lower face, also become more prominent. Resorption of the mandible results in a decrease in chin projection, or microgenia.

Neck

Ptosis of the midfacial and lower facial soft tissues along the jawline causes the development of "jowls." Loss of elasticity of the skin with hypertonicity of the platysma muscle results in the formation of platysmal bands and blunting of the cervicomental angle. A congenitally low-set hyoid bone also makes the cervicomental angle more obtuse, and this should be noted before surgical correction is undertaken because it will affect the final outcome.

Ears

Ear malformations are most commonly developmental abnormalities but may also be acquired as a result of an infection, trauma, or surgery. Prominent, or lop, ears usually result from either a large conchal cartilage or maldevelopment of the antihelical fold. An increase in the size of the ear lobule is usually related to the aging process or heavy earring use.

38.6.2 Testing

The degree of a peripheral visual deficit due to brow ptosis and upper lid blepharochalasis can be assessed with visual field testing. The test compares the size of the peripheral visual field with and without correction of the upper eyelid hooding, which is done by taping the upper lids and brows in the elevated position.

Lower lid support is assessed with the use of a pinch or a snap test, in which the lower lid is manually pulled away from the globe or pulled downward, respectively, and then released; delayed return of the lid to the globe surface or return only after blinking is abnormal and generally indicates a need for lid tightening.

38.7 Prognosis

The final outcome of medical and surgical interventions depends not only on the expertise and knowledge of the physician but also (probably to the greater extent) on the physical characteristics of the patient. Patients' medical comorbidities, the degree of the problem in question, and social factors that include smoking, alcohol or drug use, and a history of sun exposure will profoundly affect the final result. Proper patient evaluation and a detailed facial analysis are of paramount importance in the process of achieving the best outcome possible.

38.8 Roundsmanship

- One needs to be thoroughly familiar with normal facial anatomy in order to fully apprehend the deviation from the norm and come up with the best possible corrective approach.
- It is helpful to break the face down into separate aesthetic subunits and analyze those individually as well as in conjunction with the rest of the face in order to conduct a thorough and comprehensive facial assessment.
- The changes of aging result from loss of skin elasticity, solar skin damage, decrease in the amount of the subcutaneous tissues, loss of fibrous soft-tissue support, attenuation of the muscles of facial expression, and resorption of the facial bony skeleton.
- Because the changes of facial aging involve multiple facial anatomical components, they commonly require multimodality therapy for an optimal result.

38.9 Recommended Reading

[1] Knize DM. An anatomically based study of the mechanism of eyebrow ptosis. Plast Reconstr Surg 1996; 97: 1321–1333
[2] Lemperle G, Holmes RE, Cohen SR, Lemperle SM. A classification of facial wrinkles. Plast Reconstr Surg 2001; 108: 1735–1750, discussion 1751–1752
[3] Pessa JE. An algorithm of facial aging: verification of Lambros's theory by three-dimensional stereolithography, with reference to the pathogenesis of midfacial aging, scleral show, and the lateral suborbital trough deformity. Plast Reconstr Surg 2000; 106: 479–488, discussion 489–490
[4] Powell N, Humphries B. Proportions of the Aesthetic Face. New York, NY: Thieme-Stratton; 1984

39 Wound Healing

Grigorly Mashkevich

39.1 Introduction

Wound healing is a complex process consisting of several overlapping phases: inflammatory, proliferative, and remodeling. Each phase serves a specific function and has defining characteristics at the molecular and tissue levels. Healing may occur by primary, secondary, or tertiary intention. Each type of wound healing has its own advantages and disadvantages, and selection depends on the presenting wound characteristics and various patient factors.

39.2 Incidence of Disease

Wounds can arise in multiple settings, most commonly trauma or surgery. Their incidence is not well enumerated because of the wide variety of presentations that lead to wound formation.

39.3 Terminology

The three phases of wound healing overlap one another (▶ Fig. 39.1). The inflammatory phase is the initial stage of wound healing, which begins immediately following tissue injury. This phase is characterized by sealing of the wound and the attraction of inflammatory immune system components. In the proliferative phase, a stable wound matrix forms, and granulation tissue is introduced into the healing wound. In the remodeling phase, which lasts up to 2 years, the scar matures and the wound is strengthened. Granulation tissue is newly forming tissue composed of fibroblasts and developing blood vessels.

Primary intention healing occurs in wounds repaired by direct closure. This results in elimination of the dead space and rapid re-epithelialization of the wound surface. Healing by secondary intention is a process in which wounds are allowed to heal on their own, without surgical intervention. Delayed primary closure, or healing by "tertiary intention," is typically used for infected wounds. Such wounds require daily care until the infection resolves, at which point the wound edges may be surgically approximated.

Wounds can affect all tissue layers. Soft tissues include the skin and subcutaneous tissues, such as fat, muscles, nerves, and blood vessels. More complex wounds involve trauma to the cartilage and bones comprising the facial skeleton.

39.4 The Disease Process

39.4.1 Etiology

The overwhelming majority of wounds arise from trauma or surgery.

39.4.2 Pathogenesis

Open wounds may fail to heal in a satisfactory fashion if appropriate wound care is lacking. Exposed wounds are at risk for becoming infected, leading to local tissue destruction and delayed healing. Dirty wounds and dry scabs interfere with healing by retarding epithelial migration across the surface of the wound. In addition to forming unfavorable scars, poorly healing

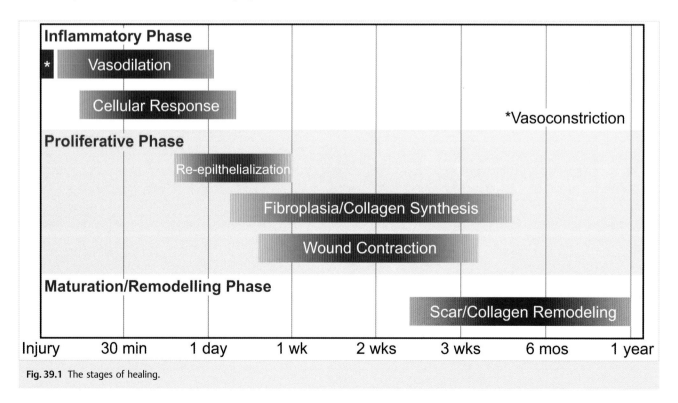

Fig. 39.1 The stages of healing.

wounds in the vicinity of the eye and nose may cause functional deficits, such as eyelid retraction and nasal obstruction.

39.4.3 Natural History and Progression

During the inflammatory phase, clot formed from bleeding tissues seals the wound. This process is accompanied by initial vasoconstriction followed by controlled vasodilation, which attracts platelets and fibrin into the wound. The clot also protects the wound from the environment and contamination. Inflammatory immune system components are attracted into the wound bed and release important cytokines and immune factors that regulate the remainder of the healing process. These include fibroblast growth factors (FGFs), platelet-derived growth factor (PDGF), and transforming growth factors (TGFs). A matrix consisting of fibronectin is eventually formed, creating the necessary mesh for cellular and protein deposition. Cellular immune components, such as neutrophils and monocytes, enter the wound bed and participate in phagocytosis. On the periphery of the wound, epithelial cells prepare to migrate as soon as 12 hours following injury. This process is marked by epithelial cell flattening and the formation of pseudopods. In sutured wounds, surface re-epithelialization can be completed within 48 hours. The inflammatory phase lasts from 5 to 15 days, depending on the size of the wound and degree of contamination. Clinically, edema and inflammation accompany the processes delineated above.

The proliferative phase guides regeneration of the cellular framework inside the wound. During this stage of wound healing, fibroblasts actively proliferate and deposit collagen, and granulation tissue, composed of inflammatory cells and regenerating blood vessels, is deposited. Clinically, a yellowish fibrinous exudate present during the inflammatory phase is gradually replaced by a cleaner, reddish granulation tissue.

The remodeling phase begins several weeks into the wound-healing process. This is the longest phase, lasting up to 2 years following tissue injury. Collagen fibers continue to be deposited and become thicker via cross-linking. Type III collagen is gradually degraded and replaced by type I collagen, which provides greater scar strength. The cellular components undergo changes that enhance long-term support of the healing wound. For example, fibroblasts differentiate into myofibroblasts, thereby promoting wound contracture. Blood vessels slowly regress, corresponding clinically to diminishing wound erythema and the white appearance typical of mature scars.

39.4.4 Potential Disease Complications

Untreated wounds may develop an infection and heal with cosmetically unacceptable scars. Significant bleeding may be encountered in open wounds with lacerations of the named vessels in the face and neck. Unrecognized facial nerve injury may lead to permanent paralysis. Lacerations of the parotid parenchyma or duct can cause a salivary cutaneous fistula or sialocele.

39.5 Medical Evaluation

The evaluation and management of wounds are covered in Chapter 41 .

39.5.1 Presenting Complaints

Patients' complaints related to healing wounds consist primarily of pain and discomfort. Deeper soft-tissue wounds in the head and neck may additionally involve nerve dysfunction or a salivary leak. These may not be obvious to the patient and require a thorough examination by the physician. Facial bony injuries may lead to additional complaints, such as diplopia in orbital blowout fractures or malocclusion in midfacial and mandibular fractures.

39.5.2 Clinical Findings, Physical Examination

Please see Chapter 41 .

39.5.3 Testing

In most patients with soft-tissue wounds, additional testing is unnecessary. Penetrating wounds of the head and neck should raise suspicion of deep vascular injury, requiring imaging with computed tomographic (CT) angiography. Any bony injuries require radiographic evaluation with facial bone CT. Basic blood testing (hemoglobin levels, electrolytes, and coagulation) is necessary in patients with wounds that require repair in the operating room.

39.5.4 Differential Diagnosis

The etiology of a wound is typically known at presentation. Just as pertinent in dealing with soft-tissue wounds is the physician's ability to formulate a "differential" for the treatment strategy. The reconstructive ladder is a conceptual paradigm for wound repair that starts with the simplest strategy and progresses to include more complex solutions. In order of increasing complexity, the reconstructive ladder includes the following steps:

1. Wound healing without surgical repair (secondary intention)
2. Wound healing with delayed surgical repair (tertiary intention)
3. Simple closure of the wound with sutures (primary intention)
4. Complex repair with local tissue rearrangement (primary intention)
5. Skin grafting
6. Complex repair with distant tissue (regional or free flaps)

39.6 Treatment

The medical and surgical management of wounds is covered in Chapter 41. Facial wounds best suited for healing by secondary intention are shown in ► Fig. 39.2.

39.7 Prognosis

Proper wound assessment and selection of the appropriate treatment strategy diminish the chance of unacceptable scarring and frequently lead to satisfactory outcomes. Certain wounds may require revision surgery for optimal results to

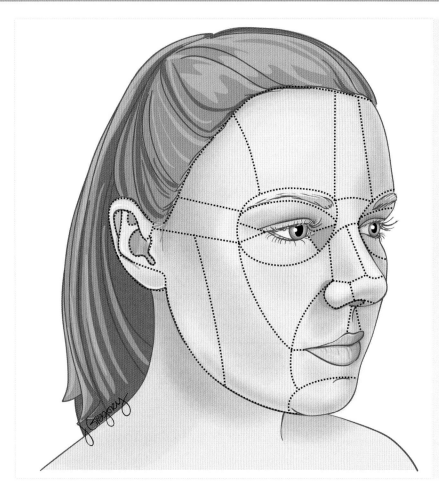

Fig. 39.2 The facial areas optimal for healing by secondary intention.

be achieved. Surgeon and patient commitment to the wound-healing process is a critical factor in influencing outcome and prognosis.

39.8 Roundsmanship

- The phases of wound healing phases consist of inflammatory, proliferative, and remodeling phases.
- The types of wound healing include primary, secondary, and tertiary.
- A reconstructive ladder helps formulate a treatment plan for healing wounds.

39.9 Recommended Reading

[1] Honrado CP, Murakami CS. Wound healing and physiology of skin flaps. Facial Plast Surg Clin North Am 2005; 13: 203–214

[2] van der Eerden PA, Lohuis PJ, Hart AA, Mulder WC, Vuyk H. Secondary intention healing after excision of nonmelanoma skin cancer of the head and neck: statistical evaluation of prognostic values of wound characteristics and final cosmetic results. Plast Reconstr Surg 2008; 122: 1747–1755

[3] Zitelli JA. Wound healing by secondary intention. A cosmetic appraisal. J Am Acad Dermatol 1983; 9: 407–415

40 Local and Regional Anesthesia for Facial Plastic Surgery

Alexander Ovchinsky and Anthony P. Sclafani

40.1 Introduction

The popularity of cosmetic surgery has increased significantly over the last decade, with facial plastic surgery procedures such as blepharoplasty, rhinoplasty, and facelift the ones most commonly performed. Although there is a tendency of patients and the media to minimize the risk of cosmetic procedures, most cosmetic surgeries are considered major surgeries from the perspective of anesthesia.

40.2 Incidence

Patients undergoing cosmetic surgery have traditionally received local anesthesia with or without sedation. Regional anesthesia (via nerve blockades), alone or to supplement other forms of anesthesia, can be used, as well. However, owing to the increasing complexity of facial plastic procedures and the increased duration of surgery, general anesthesia has become more popular with the advent of anesthetic agents that have rapid action and safe recovery profiles.

40.3 Terminology

Local anesthesia is achieved with numerous injectable local anesthetic agents (▶ Table 40.1) that have various onsets of action and durations of effect. The agents act locally and directly on peripheral sensory nerves.

40.4 Applied Anatomy

A detailed knowledge of facial anatomy in general, and of sensory innervation of the face in particular, assists greatly in the administration of good locoregional anesthesia.

Regional nerve blocks are commonly used for various facial plastic procedures. The supraorbital and supratrochlear nerves are the branches of the ophthalmic (V_1) division of the trigeminal nerve. The supraorbital and supratrochlear nerves emerge, respectively, from the supraorbital and supratrochlear foramina and supply sensory innervation to the forehead region. Supraorbital and supratrochlear nerve blocks allow good anesthesia of the upper third of the face and are generally adequate to carry out various procedures in the forehead/brow region, such as browlift, locoregional flaps, and scar revision. The infraorbital nerve, a branch of the maxillary (V_2) division of the trigeminal nerve, emerges from the infraorbital foramen and provides sensory innervation to the cheek/midface region. Infraorbital nerve block is commonly used for midface anesthesia. The mental nerve, a terminal branch of the inferior alveolar nerve (mandibular [V_3] division of the trigeminal nerve), emerges from the mental foramen, located near the lower border of the mandible between the first and second premolars. Mental block achieves anesthesia of the chin and lower lip and is used alone or in combination with other anesthetic modalities for the various procedures in this region (local flaps, repair of lacerations, chin implant placement, dermal filler use, excision of lesions, others). The dorsal nasal nerve is a branch of the anterior ethmoidal nerve and runs on the undersurface of the nasal bones, emerging 5 to 8 mm from the midline just below the caudal edge of the nasal bones. The dorsal nasal nerve supplies sensation to the lower nasal dorsum and the nasal tip. The zygomaticotemporal nerve, which innervates the skin lateral to the orbital rim and the zygoma, is a branch of the maxillary (V_2) division of the trigeminal nerve. The zygomaticofacial nerve is also a branch of the maxillary (V_2) division of the trigeminal nerve and innervates a quarter-size area of skin over the malar eminence.

40.5 The Disease Process

40.5.1 Etiology

Local anesthetics produce anesthesia by inhibiting the excitation of nerve endings or by blocking conduction in peripheral nerves. This is achieved by reversibly binding to and inactivating sodium channels. Two basic classes of local anesthetics exist, the amides and the esters, which differ in several respects (▶ Table 40.1). Esters are metabolized in the plasma by pseudo-

Table 40.1 Properties of local anesthetic agents

Drug	Onset	Maximum dose (with epinephrine)	Duration (with epinephrine)
Lidocaine	Rapid	4.5 mg/kg (7 mg/kg)	2 h (4 h)
Mepivacaine	Rapid	5 mg/kg (7 mg/kg)	3 h (6 h)
Bupivacaine	Slow	2.5 mg/kg (3 mg/kg)	4 h (8 h)
Ropivacaine	Medium	2–3 mg/kg	3 h (6 h)
Levobupivacaine	Medium	2.0 mg/kg or 400 mg/24 h	4–6 h (8–12 h)
Procaine	Slow	8 mg/kg (10 mg/kg)	45 min (90 min)
Chloroprocaine	Rapid	10 mg/kg (15 mg/kg)	30 min (90 min)
Prilocaine	Medium	5 mg/kg (7.5 mg/kg)	90 min (360 min)
Tetracaine	Slow	1.5 mg/kg (2.5 mg/kg)	3 h (10 h)

cholinesterase, whereas amides are metabolized in the liver. Esters are unstable in solution, but amides are very stable in solution. Esters are much more likely than amides to cause allergic hypersensitivity reactions. Commonly used amides include lidocaine, mepivacaine, prilocaine, bupivacaine, etidocaine, ropivacaine, and levobupivacaine. Commonly used amino esters include cocaine, procaine, tetracaine, chloroprocaine, and benzocaine. An easy way to remember which drug belongs in which category is that the names of all of the amides contain the letter *i* twice.

The physiologic activity of local anesthetics is a function of their lipid solubility, diffusibility, affinity for protein binding, percent ionization at physiologic pH, and vasodilating properties. All local anesthetics, with the exception of cocaine, are vasodilators. Vasodilation occurs via the direct relaxation of peripheral arteriolar smooth-muscle fibers. Greater vasodilator activity of a local anesthetic leads to faster absorption and thus a shorter duration of action. To counteract this vasodilation, epinephrine is often added to local anesthetic solutions. The maximum tolerable dose of lidocaine is 4.5 mg/kg; thus, for a 70-kg patient, the maximum dose is about 300 mg, or 30 mL of 1% lidocaine solution. The addition of epinephrine to the solution decreases the rate of local absorption of lidocaine, thus increasing the maximum tolerable dose, which then increases to 7 mg of lidocaine per kilogram. The maximal tolerable doses of other common local anesthetics are listed in ▶ Table 40.1.

40.5.2 Potential Complications

The two main manifestations of local anesthetic overdose are central nervous system (CNS) toxicity and cardiovascular toxicity. CNS toxicity usually precedes cardiovascular symptoms. The early signs of CNS toxicity are mild sedation, an abnormal metallic taste sensation, and (occasionally) tinnitus, which then may progress to seizures. Signs of cardiovascular toxicity included arrhythmias, heart block, and decline in cardiac contractility.

The treatment of early signs of CNS toxicity is aimed at the prevention of seizures by using medications to increase the seizure threshold, such as benzodiazepines (midazolam, diazepam) or barbiturates (thiopental, others). Significant cardiovascular toxicity may require a formal cardiovascular resuscitation; side effects related to epinephrine, such as anxiety and palpitations, are usually controlled with β-blockers.

40.6 Treatment

40.6.1 Supraorbital and Supratrochlear Nerve Blocks

Blockade of the supratrochlear nerve can easily be accomplished by injecting 1 to 2 mL of local anesthetic at the orbital rim above the medial canthus. The needle is then advanced along the supraorbital rim to inject an additional 1 to 2 mL along the orbital rim above the midpupil to block the supraorbital nerve.

40.6.2 Dorsal Nasal Nerve Block

The dorsal nasal nerve can be blocked by injecting approximately 1 mL of local anesthetic at the caudal edge of the nasal bones about 5 to 8 mm lateral to the midline.

40.6.3 Infraorbital Nerve Block

The infraorbital nerve is blocked by injecting local anesthetic just below the infraorbital rim in line with the medial limbus. This can be done directly through the skin or through a sublabial needle stick. The index finger of the nondominant hand is placed at the infraorbital rim to ensure protection of the globe.

40.6.4 Mental Nerve Block

The mental nerve is blocked by injecting anesthetic approximately 1 cm below the first and second premolars.

40.6.5 Zygomaticotemporal Nerve Block

The zygomaticotemporal nerve is blocked by introducing a needle alongside the lateral orbital rim until it is deep to and at the level of the middle of the zygoma. At this point, 1 to 2 mL of local anesthetic is injected.

40.6.6 Zygomaticofacial Nerve

To block the zygomaticofacial nerve, 1 to 2 mL of local anesthetic is injected over the bone at the junction of a line drawn along the zygoma and another line extending down from the lateral orbital rim.

40.7 Roundsmanship

- Local anesthetics work by reversibly inactivating neuronal calcium channels, blocking nerve impulse conduction.
- Epinephrine is added to local anesthetics to cause local vasoconstriction, which limits the diffusion and clearance of the local anesthetic and extends its duration of action.

40.8 Recommended Reading

[1] Nique TA. Ambulatory office general anesthesia. In: Anesthesia for Facial Plastic Surgery. New York, NY: Thieme Medical Publishers; 1993
[2] White PF, Freire AR. Ambulatory (outpatient) anesthesia. In: Miller RD, ed. Miller's Anesthesia. 6th ed. Philadelphia, PA: Elsevier Churchill Livingstone; 2005:2589–2635
[3] Zide BM, Swift R. How to block and tackle the face. Plast Reconstr Surg 1998; 101: 840–851

41 Facial Soft-Tissue Trauma

Grigorly Mashkevich

41.1 Introduction

Facial soft-tissue trauma may arise from motor vehicle accidents, physical altercations, work-related accidents, and other sources. Patients with facial trauma often present with concomitant injuries requiring a multidisciplinary evaluation. Most severe facial soft-tissue injuries resulting in open wounds may lead to significant scarring, facial nerve palsy, and parotid duct injury. In a setting of animal and human bites, facial penetration can be a source of communicable disease transmission. Although some wounds cannot be closed, the optimal management of most open wounds requires careful assessment and meticulous repair with the techniques discussed in this chapter.

41.2 Incidence of Disease

In 2006, emergency departments across the United States registered more than 5.4 million visits for all head and neck injuries. Although the specific breakdown is unknown, presumably many of these visits were for the treatment of facial soft-tissue trauma.

41.3 Terminology

Blunt trauma results in tissue injury without separation of the overlying skin. Penetrating injuries cause direct trauma to deep tissues via laceration of the skin. Animal and human bites are examples of penetrating trauma. Avulsion injury results in tissue loss. Primary closure is the approximation of wound edges, resulting in the elimination of dead space and rapid re-epithelialization of the wound surface. Healing by secondary intention is a process in which wounds are allowed to heal on their own. Delayed primary closure, or healing by "tertiary intention," is frequently utilized in infected wounds; such wounds require daily care until the infection resolves, at which point the wound edges are surgically approximated.

41.4 Applied Anatomy

The facial nerve traverses the substance of the parotid gland and exits at its periphery via several identifiable branches. The temporal branch of the facial nerve exits the superior aspect of the parotid gland and crosses the zygomatic arch at the junction of its anterior one-third and posterior two-thirds. An additional surface landmark is a line that begins at the inferior aspect of the ear lobule and bisects a line connecting the tragus and the lateral canthus (▶ Fig. 41.1). The buccal branch of the facial nerve closely follows the parotid duct, which runs along a line from the tragus to the midportion of the upper lip. The marginal branch of the facial nerve exits from the inferior aspect of the parotid gland, at the angle of the mandible, and descends up to 2 cm inferior to the body of the mandible before returning to innervate the mentalis and depressor anguli oris muscles (▶ Fig. 41.2).

41.5 The Disease Process

41.5.1 Etiology

Facial soft-tissue injuries may arise in multiple settings, most notably during motor vehicle accidents, physical altercations, and sports. These injuries may be blunt or penetrating.

41.5.2 Pathogenesis

The degree of facial soft-tissue damage is directly related to the shape of the striking object, the force with which it strikes, and the location of the impact. A greater depth of penetration places neurovascular and glandular structures at a higher risk for injury.

41.5.3 Natural History and Progression

Most open facial soft tissue wounds are "clean–contaminated." The head and neck region maintains a robust circulation, which helps prevent infection by maximizing wound oxygen tension and rapidly attracting immune system components. Untreated open wounds are at risk for delayed healing and significant scarring. Although no definitive rules exist on the timing of facial wound repair, most noninfected wounds can be closed primarily regardless of their duration. Conversely, any infected wounds, as judged by the presence of purulence and cellulitis, should be left open and treated with packing and antibiotics until all signs of infection are eliminated. Injuries to the facial nerve or parotid duct are not likely to heal without prompt surgical intervention with exploration and repair.

41.5.4 Potential Disease Complications

Untreated wounds may develop an infection and heal with cosmetically unacceptable scars. Significant bleeding may be encountered in open wounds with lacerations of named vessels in the face and neck. Unrecognized facial nerve injury may lead to permanent paralysis (▶ Fig. 41.3). Lacerations of the parotid

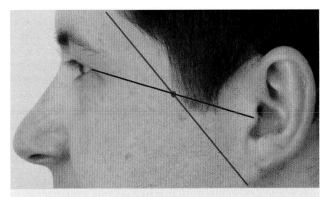

Fig. 41.1 Facial surface landmarks for the frontotemporal division of the facial nerve. See text for details.

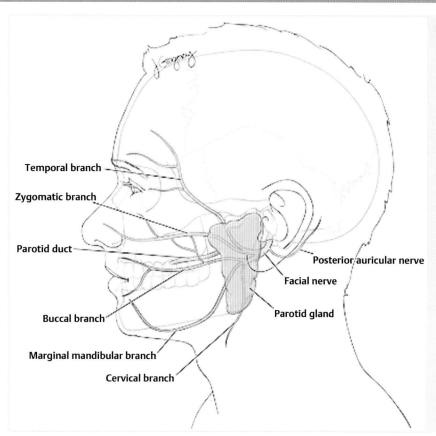

Fig. 41.2 Anatomy of the peripheral facial nerve.

Temporal branch

Zygomatic branch

Parotid duct

Buccal branch

Marginal mandibular branch

Cervical branch

Posterior auricular nerve

Facial nerve

Parotid gland

parenchyma or duct can cause a salivary cutaneous fistula or sialocele.

41.6 Medical Evaluation

A complete medical history and account of the traumatic event should be obtained from the patient. Witness descriptions may be of value in the case of patients with altered states of consciousness. Any suspected domestic abuse should be reported and investigated.

41.6.1 Presenting Complaints

Complaints related to soft-tissue trauma consist primarily of pain and discomfort. Patients may report difficulty with facial movement (cranial nerve VII involvement) or sensory deficits (cranial nerve V), both of which can arise from swelling alone. Any additional complaints indicating injury to adjacent structures (e.g., vision changes, trismus, malocclusion, breathing or swallowing difficulties) should trigger appropriate investigations.

41.6.2 Clinical Findings, Physical Examination

Any patients with trauma requires an initial evaluation of airway patency, breathing, and circulation. During the primary survey, all sites of injury are assessed, including the cervical spine.

The ENT (ear, nose, throat) evaluation consists of a complete examination of the head and neck. This includes a fiber-optic

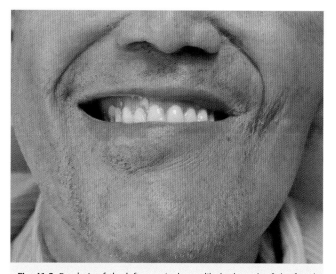

Fig. 41.3 Paralysis of the left marginal mandibular branch of the facial nerve.

assessment of the airway to rule out concomitant injuries to the upper aerodigestive tract. Palpation of the facial skeleton, with attention to trismus and bite abnormalities, should be performed to rule out fractures. Penetrating injuries of the head and neck require special protocols to exclude vascular or upper aerodigestive tract injury; these are discussed in Chapter 37 .

The soft-tissue evaluation relies on meticulous visual inspection and documentation of all abrasions and lacerations. Wounds may require cleaning for an adequate assessment of the depth of injury. Any suspected penetration of the neck should not be probed beyond the platysma muscle because doing so may disturb injured vessels and result in significant bleeding in an uncontrolled setting. Suspected penetrating injuries of the neck are best assessed with computed tomographic (CT) angiography. Facial injuries may be safely cleaned with half-strength peroxide diluted in saline or water. Cotton-tipped applicators are useful in separating wound edges and examining the extent of facial soft-tissue injury. Bleeding wounds may be temporarily packed with gauze to achieve hemostasis until a definitive treatment is undertaken. Head elevation, pressure dressings, and the placement of epinephrine-soaked gauze into the wound may further assist with hemostasis and visualization. Clamps in bleeding facial wounds should be used with caution because such action may inadvertently injure branches of the facial nerve.

Any patient with a laceration situated in the anatomical distribution of the facial nerve (see ▶ Fig. 41.2) requires a complete neurologic assessment of this structure. Deficiencies in brow elevation or eyelid closure, oral commissure excursion during smiling, and lip pucker indicate facial nerve injury. Any neurologic assessment of cranial nerve VII must occur before the use of local anesthetics. In sedated patients or those with altered mental status, a painful stimulus (such as chest rub) may induce a sufficient grimace to provide a baseline assessment of seventh cranial nerve integrity.

An assessment of the parotid duct may be difficult to perform at the bedside because of blood, debris, and poor lighting. Any presence of clear fluid, especially if expressed on manual compression of the gland, should raise suspicion of parotid duct injury. If available, lacrimal probes may be used intraorally to cannulate the orifice of the parotid duct to aid its identification in the wound.

41.6.3 Testing

Radiographic studies may include cervical spine X-rays and CT of the facial skeleton and cranium. Electrocardiography and basic blood tests for hemoglobin and electrolytes are important studies in patients presenting with suspected significant blood loss or any hemodynamic changes, or in those anticipated to undergo soft-tissue repair in the operating room. Photographic documentation of any open wounds before repair is critical from a medicolegal standpoint.

41.6.4 Differential Diagnosis

In addition to soft-tissue injury, the differential diagnosis includes concomitant skeletal injuries (orbital, maxillary, mandibular, and cranial fractures), vascular damage, and neurologic impairment. A specialist assessment may be necessary, especially in the areas of ophthalmology, neurosurgery, oral surgery, and vascular surgery.

41.7 Treatment

41.7.1 Medical Treatment

Soft-tissue bruising responds well to pain medications and the frequent application of ice in the first 48 to 72 hours. This diminishes inflammation, swelling, and discomfort. Beyond 72

hours, warm compresses and anti-bruising creams, such as *Arnica montana* (wolf's bane), can offer a quicker resolution of bruising and discoloration.

Superficial abrasions are best managed with daily cleaning (mild soap and water, with half-strength hydrogen peroxide for any crusts) and the application of antibiotic ointment (bacitracin) to hasten wound re-epithelialization in a moist environment. If an allergic reaction (itching, rash, or erythema) develops in response to bacitracin, a blander ointment such as petrolatum (Aquaphor, Vaseline) can be applied instead. Such treatment strategy results in healed abrasions in 5 to 14 days.

Bite injuries require antibiotic prophylaxis for potentially transmitted pathogens. Most common animal bites are from dogs, with a resultant multibacterial aerobic and anaerobic pathogen profile. The most common species include *Streptococcus*, *Staphylococcus*, *Pasteurella multocida*, and *Bacteroides*. Empiric antibiotics, such as amoxicillin/clavulanate, provide adequate coverage while culture identification is pending. Human bites are also multibacterial but may transmit viruses, as well. Any suspicion of possible HIV or hepatitis virus transmission should be brought to the immediate attention of the emergency department staff and infectious disease specialists. Hospital-specific protocols for testing, disclosure, and treatment should be closely followed.

Tetanus and rabies prophylaxis deserve consideration in appropriate cases. Wounds heavily contaminated with soil carry the highest risk for tetanus. Tetanus toxoid should be administered along with a booster injection, if one has not been given within 10 years. The need for rabies prophylaxis depends on the history (whether the offending animal is known to be ill), geographic rabies patterns, and examination of a captured rabid animal.

41.7.2 Surgical Treatment

Any manipulation of soft tissues requires informed patient consent. In a setting of soft-tissue trauma, this process may be complicated by patient's altered state of consciousness, resulting from either cranial involvement or sedative medications. Appropriate relatives and healthcare proxies, if designated, must be engaged in this process. In addition, photographic documentation must precede any attempted repair for medicolegal reasons.

Open wound repair requires a thorough assessment of tissue loss and preparation of the injured site by careful removal of debris and sharpening of the skin edges. This is made easier by introducing local anesthesia before any tissue manipulation, which diminishes oozing and improves patient comfort. The injection of 1% lidocaine with 1:100,000 epinephrine, buffered with 10% sodium bicarbonate (4:1 dilution), through a small (27- to 30-gauge) needle provides an effective means of achieving local anesthesia. Regional blocks of the supratrochlear, supraorbital, infraorbital, and mental nerves can be performed for larger wounds. Anesthetic agents with longer durations of action (such as bupivacaine) may be added if wound closure is expected to last several hours, or for prolonged postoperative pain control.

Local tissue rearrangement (advancement, rotation, and transposition skin flaps) may be necessary to achieve wound closure, especially in avulsion injuries. As much as possible, scars should be placed in existing wrinkles or within relaxed-skin tension lines. Sharp skin undermining and wound edge eversion are critical in achieving a tension-free closure and aesthetically pleasing scars. Sites of higher tension require the placement of permanent or long-lasting absorbable sutures (3–0 or 4–0 PDS [polydioxanone] or Vicryl), in some cases passed through the periosteum to counter unfavorable soft-tissue vectors. More quickly absorbed subcutaneous sutures (4–0 or 5–0 Monocryl) should be placed in areas with less tension. Nonabsorbable (5–0 or 6–0 Prolene or nylon) fine sutures are used for cutaneous closure. These cause minimal tissue reaction and are removed in 5 to 7 days.

Auricular Lacerations and Avulsions

Auricular lacerations can be challenging because of complex surface topography, the presence of cartilage, and a relative lack of tissue mobility. Through-and-through defects require meticulous approximation of all involved tissue layers. Skin eversion is particularly important in preventing external notching and contour irregularities. Any exposed cartilage should be identified and approximated with either permanent or long-lasting absorbable sutures.

The repair of composite auricular tissue loss relies on the preservation of native cartilage. In segmental auricular avulsions, a retroauricular pocket can be formed to store cartilage from the avulsed ear segment. Steps include de-epithelialization of the avulsed segment, reattachment of the cartilage stump to the remaining auricular cartilage, and placement of the avulsed segment under temporal skin coapted to the edge of skin on the auricular cartilage. After 6 weeks, the avulsed segment of the auricle is elevated along with the overlying temporal skin, and a skin graft is placed on its posterior aspect. The direct reattachment of avulsed segments, without pocket storage, is unpredictable and becomes especially unsuccessful with segments larger than 1.5 cm.

Subtotal avulsions with any remaining cutaneous attachments heal remarkably well following primary closure. An abundant blood supply to the ear provides an excellent circulation through the remaining attachments, allowing adequate perfusion of the auricle. In cases of total auricular avulsion, replantation with microvascular repair can be considered. Supportive measures for survival of the reconstructed auricle, such as hyperbaric oxygen, anticoagulation, and medicinal leeches, may be necessary adjunctive steps in most of these cases.

Lip Lacerations

The repair of lip lacerations must separately address all involved tissue layers. In the lip, these include skin, muscle, and mucosa. The cutaneous lip can be further divided into subunits, which consist of the philtrum medially, lateral segments laterally, and vermilion inferiorly. The vermilion–cutaneous junction is an important visual landmark. Even the slightest irregularities of this border can be highly noticeable because of the transition in color.

If possible, lip lacerations should be rearranged to allow final scars to fall into the borders between lip subunits. This optimizes scar camouflage. Additional incisions may be necessary to achieve adequate tissue advancement or rotation. If transected, the orbicularis oris muscle must be approximated with a 2–0 or 3–0 long-lasting absorbable suture. Superficial or small mucosal defects can heal inconsequentially by secondary intention. Larger or deeper mucosal wounds should be approximated with short-lasting absorbable suture material.

Eyelid Lacerations

All eyelid lacerations require work-up for concomitant ocular injuries. An ophthalmologist should be consulted to rule out damage to the cornea and retina. Physical examination of the periocular tissues must also exclude injuries to the levator muscle (ptosis), canthal tendons (displacement or rounding of the canthal angles), and canaliculi (epiphora).

Early eyelid repair is important in providing immediate corneal protection. Any particulate matter must be removed in order to avoid the development of a traumatic tattoo. Suspected injury to the canaliculi should be evaluated with lacrimal probes. The repair of duct walls requires loupe or microscopic magnification and is best accomplished with interrupted 9–0 permanent sutures placed over a Silastic stent.

Avulsion of the medial canthal tendon is addressed with a periosteal stitch to the lacrimal bone. Insufficient periosteum may require screw placement or transnasal wiring. Inadequate repair of this structure can lead to widening of the intercanthal distance, resulting in telecanthus.

Lacerations extending to the lid margin are best repaired with a 6–0 silk suture placed in a vertical mattress fashion to ensure eversion and prevent notching. Suture repair should begin at the gray line to properly align the lid edges. The tarsus and orbicularis oculi are approximated with 6–0 absorbable sutures. Lubricating ointment is applied liberally in the postoperative setting.

Facial Nerve Lacerations

Any suspected facial nerve injury requires immediate exploration and repair. The distal portion of the severed nerve continues to conduct and can be stimulated for up to 48 to 72 hours following transection. This greatly enhances identification of the nerve in the operating room with a nerve stimulator (0.5 to 1 mA). Nerve repair should be performed under loupe magnification (3.5x or higher) or microscopic magnification. Nerve ends must be exposed and mobilized for 1 to 2 cm for advancement and reduction of tension. Each nerve end must be cut clean, which removes about 1 mm of distance on each side. Adequate mobilization usually makes up for such a loss. In cases of missing nerve segments, grafting must be contemplated with one of several donor sources (great auricular, lateral antebrachial cutaneous, or sural nerve). This possibility needs to be discussed with the patient in advance of the operation. Nerve approximation requires the placement of three to seven interrupted 9–0 nylon sutures through the epineurium (▶ Fig. 41.4).

Parotid (Stensen) duct repair is determined by the extent of duct injury. For simple lacerations or transections, direct repair is performed over a stent placed intraorally. Small-caliber pediatric feeding tubes serve as excellent parotid duct stents and can be sutured intraorally to maintain the egress of saliva for 2 to 4 weeks. Injuries resulting in a loss of the parotid duct are

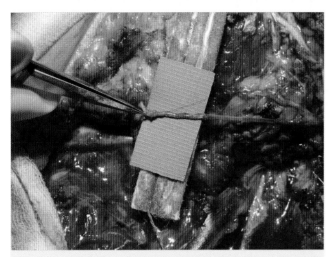

Fig. 41.4 Facial nerve repair under the microscope.

more difficult to repair. If both ends can be identified, an interposition vein graft (anterior or external jugular) is placed over a stent to replace the missing segment. In cases in which the distal parotid duct cannot be identified and the site of injury is anterior to the masseter, a diversion of the proximal duct intraorally can be performed. If the site of injury is posterior to the masseter, or if the proximal parotid duct cannot be identified, watertight closure of the parotid fascia to tamponade salivary flow should be performed with a permanent or long-lasting absorbable suture placed in a running locking fashion. In addition, 50 to 100 units of botulinum toxin can be injected into the parenchyma of the parotid gland to extinguish salivary production. This strategy rarely results in gland inflammation and/or infection.

41.8 Prognosis

Facial soft-tissue bruising, hematomas, and superficial abrasions resolve fully without major sequelae. Hyperpigmentation of abraded areas can be managed with sun protection and bleaching creams (2% or 4% hydroquinone). Repaired wounds may take 6 to 12 months to fully mature. Hypertrophic scars, keloids, and pincushioning may complicate wound healing. These respond to periodic steroid injections (triamcinolone acetate, 10 or 40 mg/mL). Cosmetically poor scars may require revision to improve appearance.

41.9 Roundsmanship

- Patients with facial soft-tissue trauma require a complete assessment for concomitant skeletal, upper aerodigestive, neurologic, and vascular injuries.
- Noninfected open wounds are optimally managed with tissue preparation and meticulous primary closure.
- Parotid duct and facial nerve injury must be considered in open wounds overlying these structures.
- Transected facial nerve branches are best repaired within 72 hours, when the distal ends can still be stimulated.

41.10 Recommended Reading

[1] Leach J. Proper handling of soft tissue in the acute phase. Facial Plast Surg 2001; 17: 227–238
[2] Pitts SR, Niska RW, Xu J, Burt CW. National hospital ambulatory medical care survey: 2006 emergency department summary. Natl Health Stat Report 2008; 7: 1–38

42 Maxillofacial Trauma

Alexander Ovchinsky

42.1 Introduction

Maxillofacial injuries remain serious clinical problems because of the high density of neural, vascular, digestive, and respiratory tissues in this area. In addition to these life-threatening issues, maxillofacial trauma can have significant psychological effects on patients because of the aesthetic deformities that they can cause.

42.2 Incidence of Disease

In the United States, trauma constitutes the third major cause of death among all age groups and the leading cause of death among the persons younger than 44 years of age. The major causes of trauma-related death are central nervous system injury and hemorrhage. In addition to fatal injuries, roughly 40 million people are treated in emergency departments each year, and the total cost associated with injuries is estimated to be more than $250 billion per year. Currently, more than 400 people in the United States die of injuries every day, and 50% of these deaths occur before arrival at the hospital. However, it is worth mentioning that the obligatory use of seat belts and the invention of air bag systems has resulted in approximately a 25% decrease in the frequency of injuries due to motor vehicle accidents

The incidence of facial trauma as a whole peaks in the first decade of life and slowly declines over the remaining decades of life. The incidence of facial bone fractures, in contrast, peaks in the third decade of life. Counter to the increasing incidence of facial bone fractures in the first three decades of life, the actual relative risk for facial bone fractures per accident increases with increasing age (4.4% per year of life) because of the associated decrease in bone density.

Most injuries in the first decade of life are isolated soft-tissue lacerations or dentoalveolar trauma (tooth impaction, alveolar process fractures, crown fractures, others), as opposed to the facial bone fractures seen in the adult population.

42.3 Classification of the Disease Process

The classification of maxillofacial trauma is usually related to the type of the injury sustained. Bruises or contusions are the result of soft-tissue blunt trauma followed by subcutaneous bleeding. The extent of bruising depends on the severity of the impact, the laxity of the tissues, the individual's predisposition to bruising, and the individual's age. Abrasions are superficial wounds that do not penetrate the full thickness of the dermis. Deeper abrasions, extending to the level of papillary and reticular dermis, frequently bleed, sometimes profusely. Abrasions are frequently associated with foreign bodies, such as wood splinters and road dirt. Lacerations are full-thickness wounds penetrating through the dermis and frequently extending into subcutaneous tissues and muscles; they are usually caused by a sharp object. If the length of the wound exceeds its depth, it is referred to as slash wound, and if the converse is true, a stab wound. Fractures are the loss of structural integrity of a bone resulting from mechanical overload and failure to resist deformation. Fractures may be further classified as closed fractures, in which there is no communication of the fractured bone with the outside environment, and open fractures, in which the fracture is exposed to the external environment via laceration or penetration of the fracture fragments through the overlying soft tissues and skin. Fractures are also categorized based on the region or bones involved.

42.4 Applied Anatomy

A thorough knowledge of normal facial anatomy is essential for the successful management of maxillofacial trauma. Although a detailed description of facial anatomy may be found in other textbooks, the surgical and anatomical considerations pertaining to patients with facial trauma are the basis of this discussion.

The frontal bone forms the anterior part of the skull and essentially the major portion of the upper face. It is connected to the zygoma laterally via the zygomaticofrontal process, and to the nasal bones medially via the nasofrontal suture line. These connections form three so-called vertical facial buttresses, two zygomaticofrontal and one nasofrontal, which serve as a major support mechanism for the facial skeleton. Inferiorly, the frontal bone articulates with the ethmoid, sphenoid, and lacrimal bones. Anterior pneumatization of the frontal bone forms the frontal sinus, with its anterior and posterior tables. Frontal sinus drainage is via the nasofrontal duct, which opens into the middle nasal meatus. The frontal bone is one of the strongest bones in the human body, and significant force is required to cause a fracture. Therefore, frontal sinus fractures are commonly associated with other significant injuries, such as cervical spine or brain injuries.

The nasal bones are paired rectangular bones that connect to each other in the midline to form the bony nasal dorsum. They articulate with the frontal bone superiorly, nasal processes of the maxilla laterally, and upper lateral cartilages inferiorly. On the undersurface, the nasal bones are connected with the bony and cartilaginous nasal septum. Because of their exposed location and relative fragility, the nasal bones are frequently injured.

The maxilla is formed by its alveolar, zygomatic, palatal, and nasal processes. The pyramid-shaped maxillary sinus occupies the midportion of the maxilla, draining into the middle nasal meatus. The anterior wall of the maxillary sinus is very thin and thus is easily fractured. The palatal processes merge in the middle, forming the larger portion of the hard palate; the alveolar process contains the dentition and forms the inferior portion of the maxilla. It joins the pterygoid plates of the sphenoid bones posteriorly; pterygoid plate fracture is the key component of all Le Fort-type fractures of the maxilla. The zygomatic and nasal processes are extensions of the maxilla that are important for facial form and function.

The zygoma forms the cheek eminence. It consists of a body and three processes—temporal, frontal, and maxillary—that connect the zygoma to the temporal and frontal bones and the maxilla, respectively. The zygoma also forms the part of the lateral orbital floor.

The mandible consists of the central symphysis and the bilateral mandibular bodies, rami, angles, and coronoid and condylar processes. The alveolar process of the mandible forms its superior portion and contains the lower dentition, which is innervated by the inferior alveolar nerve. The condylar process articulates with the glenoid fossa of the temporal bone, forming temporomandibular joint.

The orbit protects, supports, and maximizes the function of the eye. The orbit is shaped like a quadrilateral pyramid, with its base in a plane with the orbital rim. Seven bones join together to form the orbital structure. The orbital process of the frontal bone and the lesser wing of the sphenoid form the orbital roof. The orbital plate of the maxilla joins the orbital plate of the zygoma and the orbital plate of the palatine bones to form the floor. Medially, the orbital wall consists of the frontal process of the maxilla, the lacrimal bone, the sphenoid, and the thin lamina papyracea of the ethmoid. The lateral wall is formed by the lesser and greater wings of the sphenoid and the zygoma.

42.5 The Disease Process

42.5.1 Etiology

Maxillofacial injuries can be classified with respect to their etiology, including assaults, falls, sport-related injuries, animal or human bites, motor vehicle accidents, gunshot injuries, and burns. The etiology of facial fractures varies between urban and rural environments. Penetrating trauma and assault-related injuries are more common in cities, whereas injuries related to motor vehicle accidents, sports, and other recreational injuries are seen frequently in rural hospitals. In community emergency departments, fractures of the nose and mandible are the most common; in trauma centers, however, midface and zygomatic injuries are more frequent. Domestic violence and elder and child abuse are important causes of facial trauma. Facial injuries account for the majority of emergency department visits related to domestic violence. As many as one-fourth of women with facial trauma are victims of domestic violence.

42.5.2 Pathogenesis

The kinetic energy of a moving object is a function of its mass multiplied by the square of its velocity. The dispersion of this kinetic energy during impact produces the force that results in injury. High-impact and low-impact forces are respectively defined as those that are more or less than 50 times the force of gravity. These parameters determine the extent of the resultant injury because the amount of force required to cause damage to the facial bones differs regionally. A high-impact force is required to damage the supraorbital rim, mandible (symphysis and angle), and frontal bones, but a low-impact force is all that is required to damage the zygoma and nasal bone. Orbital blowout fractures are thought to occur when a sudden increase in the intraorbital pressure causes blowout of the thin medial wall and/or orbital floor.

42.5.3 Natural History and Progression

What the extent of the final deformity will be may not be very obvious immediately after the injury. However, with time, as the soft-tissue swelling subsides, the resultant facial asymmetry may become more pronounced. Later, the loss of structural support in uncorrected or poorly corrected facial fractures frequently translates into functional deficits. For example, telecanthus may gradually develop as the loose bony fragments of a naso-orbito-ethmoid (NOE) fracture lateralize because of the loss of medial canthal tendon stability. Enophthalmos may also be a late finding in orbital blowout fracture as the orbital contents slowly retract into the maxillary sinus. Diplopia may follow as the orbital contents herniate and become trapped within the fracture fragments.

42.5.4 Potential Disease Complications

The complications arising from maxillofacial trauma differ widely in severity, ranging from mild cosmetic deformity without any functional deficit, to significant functional disability related to orbital and neurovascular injury and malocclusion, to death in acute settings resulting from airway compromise, hemorrhage, and associated intracranial and spine injuries.

42.6 Disease Grading

Broadly speaking, maxillofacial injury can be classified as either blunt or penetrating trauma. Blunt trauma results from motor vehicle accidents, sports, falls, and occupation-related injuries. Penetrating trauma includes gunshot injuries, stab wounds, and injuries caused by impalement. The type and extent of injury and subsequent management depend on the region injured and the vital structures in proximity to the path of the penetrating object. With firearm injuries, the velocity, caliber, and presumed path of the bullet and the distance from the weapon provide important clues to the extent of the injury.

Maxillofacial fractures may be differentiated by their severity (displaced vs. nondisplaced, open vs. closed) and by the anatomical region involved. In nondisplaced fractures, the anatomical alignment of the fractured bone is maintained, whereas in displaced fractures, this alignment is lost, leading to specific findings on the physical examination such as loss of support and symmetry, palpable bony step-offs, and injury to vital structures by displaced bony fragments. Closed fractures do not have any communication with the outside environment, whereas open fractures communicate with the outside and so are more prone to infection or bleeding.

Based on the anatomical region involved, maxillofacial fractures are subdivided into the following categories:
- Frontal sinus fractures
- NOE fractures
- Zygomatico-orbital fractures
- Maxillary fractures
- Mandible fractures

Frontal sinus fractures may be further subdivided as follows:
1. Anterior table fractures
2. Posterior table fractures
3. Anterior and posterior table fractures

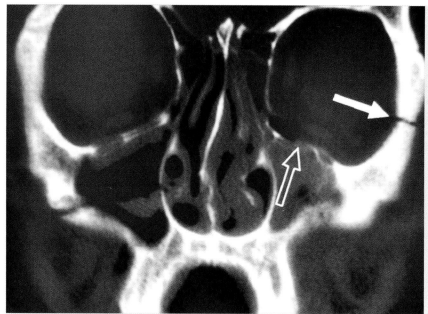

Fig. 42.1 Coronal computed tomographic scan of the facial bones depicting a mixed pattern of maxillary fractures, with Le Fort type I fractures on the right side and Le Fort type II fractures on the left side. The right-sided fractures involve the right piriform aperture and anterior–lateral wall of the maxillary sinus. The left-sided fractures involve the zygomaticofrontal process (*white arrow*) and inferior orbital wall/floor (*hollow arrow*).

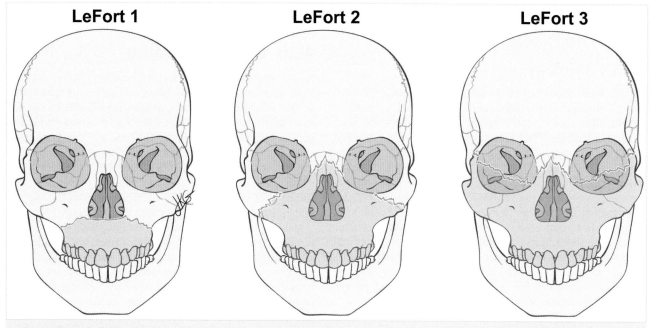

Fig. 42.2 Types of Le Fort fractures. The key distinguishing fractures are at the piriform aperture (Le Fort I), inferior orbital rim (Le Fort II), and zygomatic arch (Le Fort III).

NOE fractures may be type I, II, or III depending on the degree of disruption of the medial canthal region (see Box Naso-orbito-ethmoid (NOE) Fractures (p.334)).

Maxillary fractures (▶ Fig. 42.1), with the exception of alveolar and palate fractures, are commonly described according to the classification of René Le Fort published in 1901 (▶ Fig. 42.2; see also Box Maxillary Fractures (p.335)):

All three types of Le Fort fractures include fractures through the pterygoid plates.

Naso-orbito-ethmoid (NOE) Fractures

- Type I: minimal displacement of the whole NOE complex
- Type II: more comminution of the NOE complex with preservation of the medial canthal ligamentous attachment to a larger bony fragment, which can be plated
- Type III: severely comminuted fracture with disruption of the medial canthal tendon

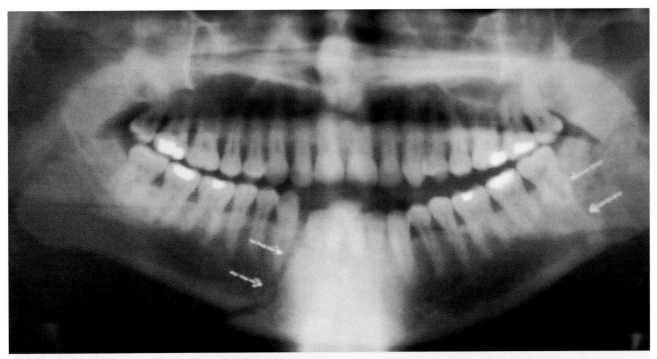

Fig. 42.3 Panorex film of the mandible showing bilateral mandible fractures: right body fracture and left ramus fracture (*arrows*).

Maxillary Fractures

- Le Fort I: fractures through the inferior portions of the medial and lateral maxillary buttresses and nasal septum; key fracture (differentiating this type from other types)—piriform aperture
- Le Fort II: fractures through the zygomaticomaxillary and frontomaxillary sutures; key fracture—inferior orbital rim
- Le Fort III: also known as craniofacial dissociation, involves fractures through the nasofrontal and zygomaticofrontal sutures and zygomatic arch; key fracture—zygomatic arch

Maxillary fractures rarely follow the classic bilateral Le Fort pattern and commonly present as a combination of Le Fort types. For example, one may see a type I pattern on the right side and a type II on the left.

Mandible fractures (▶ Fig. 42.3) are classified by the part of the mandible involved and include symphyseal, body, ramus, angle, and subcondylar fractures. Favorable fractures of the mandible are those in which the fracture edges tend to be drawn together by the forces of the masticator muscles; these edges are distracted in unfavorable fractures (▶ Fig. 42.4).

42.7 Medical Evaluation

42.7.1 Presenting Complaints

Patients with maxillofacial trauma usually present with swelling, ecchymosis, and pain in the area of injury. Open fractures are usually associated with hemorrhage from the wound. Patients with displaced fractures have associated facial asymmetry and deformity on examination. Frontal sinus and NOE fractures may present with cerebrospinal fluid (CSF) rhinorrhea, which should be differentiated from normal nasal secretions (see below). NOE fractures commonly present with flattening of the nasal bridge and telecanthus. Rounding of the medial canthus and excessive caruncular show are signs of medial canthal tendon disruption. Epiphora is frequently seen as a consequence of nasolacrimal duct obstruction. Patients with orbital fractures may have diplopia, pain on moving the eye, and/or decreased visual acuity. A swollen and tense globe may be the sign of intraorbital hematoma. Midface numbness is a common symptom and is secondary to infraorbital nerve injury. Displaced zygomatic fractures commonly present with trismus due to entrapment of the masseter and temporalis muscles by a fracture fragment. Flattening of the midface is seen as a result of displacement and rotation of the zygoma. Maxillary and mandibular fractures are usually associated with malocclusion, trismus, and pain on opening the mouth.

42.7.2 Clinical Findings, Physical Examination

Airway Management

Airway compromise in maxillofacial injuries can result from direct laryngeal injury, foreign bodies (including aspirated teeth and bone fragments), or active bleeding from an upper airway source. Treatment of the compromised airway is complicated by the likelihood that about 10% of patients with facial trauma have a cervical spine injury. Comminuted fractures of the mandible can lead to loss of support of the hyomandibular complex, with consequent ptosis and retroposition of the tongue. Manual anterior traction on the mandible symphysis often temporarily

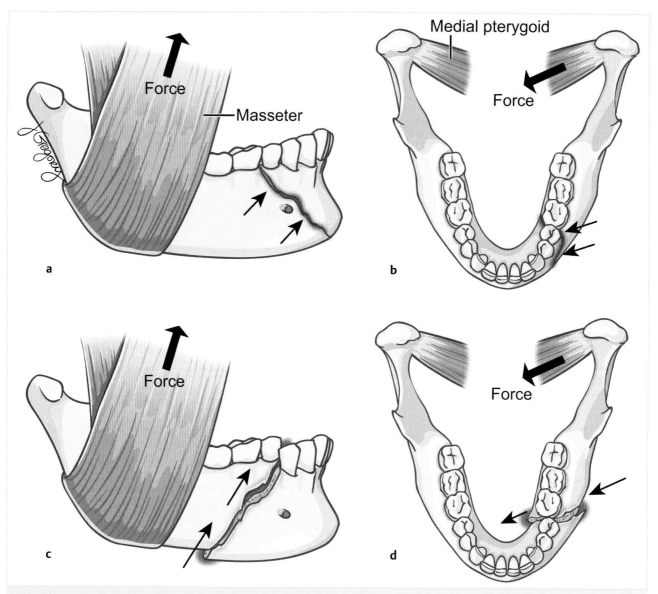

Fig. 42.4 (a,b) The medial pterygoid and masseter muscles bring the two segments of a favorable fracture together when they contract. (c,d) The fracture segments of unfavorable fractures undergo distraction when the masticator muscles contract.

resolves this obstruction until definitive control of the airway can be achieved.

Hemorrhage

The extensive vascularity of the head and neck can result in rapid, significant blood loss. The location of the injuries, however, allows sufficient access for direct pressure to control the hemorrhage. One must visualize the source of bleeding before suture ligature or cautery to avoid collateral damage to important adjacent structures.

Ocular Injury

Direct injury to the globe should be suspected in all patients with orbital fractures or lacerations to the periorbital region. Pain, decreased vision, and the appearance of spots before the eyes are all highly suggestive of globe damage. During the neurologic phase of the trauma assessment, a brief clinical ophthalmologic examination should be performed, including an assessment of visual acuity, pupillary response to light and accommodation, extraocular range of motion, and globe position. If there are any abnormal findings on the examination, an immediate ophthalmologic consult should be obtained for examination of the retina and ocular pressures. Injuries that may require immediate ophthalmologic treatment or result in permanent sequelae include corneoscleral lacerations, lens dislocation, major hyphema, acute glaucoma, and retinal detachment. Blindness at the time of presentation is rare but is an extremely poor prognostic factor for future sight. Patients who have light perception at the time of presentation but who then demonstrate progressive loss of vision during the trauma assessment must be treated aggressively. The most common cause of this presentation is traumatic optic neuropathy secondary to optic nerve compression from a retrobulbar hematoma, a bone fragment, or edema.

Disruption of the medial canthal ligament in type III NOE fractures leads to telecanthus (increase in interpalpebral distance). One may also see rounding of the medial canthus secondary to loss of support, or epiphora due to disruption of the nasolacrimal duct. A significant increase in the orbital volume due to a blowout orbital fracture may lead to the development of enophthalmos. Diplopia may be present as a consequence of the entrapment of extraocular muscles.

Cerebrospinal Fluid Leak

An active search for CSF leaks in patients with craniofacial or high maxillary fractures should be undertaken. Clear or serosanguineous nasal discharge, anosmia, or a salty taste in the mouth are highly suggestive of CSF rhinorrhea. A CSF leak into the nasal cavity implies abnormal communication between the subarachnoid space and the external environment. The thin bone in the anterior skull base and the close adherence of the dura to the anterior fossa and cribriform plate predispose to the penetration of fracture fragments into the subarachnoid space. Common associated fracture patterns include Le Fort II and III midface fractures, NOE fractures, orbital roof fractures, and displaced fractures of the posterior table of the frontal sinus. CSF is differentiated from normal nasal secretions on laboratory examination by its low protein concentration and by the presence of glucose (nearing plasma levels) but no mucin. The gold standard test for CSF is measurement of the β_2-transferrin levels, but it is more time-consuming than measurement of the glucose levels. Most traumatic CSF fistulas close spontaneously with bed rest. Fistulas that do not close spontaneously can be visualized on CT with metrizamide contrast, followed by surgical exploration and obliteration of the fistula.

Occlusion

Occlusion is contact of the posterior masticating (chewing) and anterior incising (cutting) surfaces of the maxillary and mandibular teeth. Malocclusion is an indicator of orthognathic fracture or dental injury. Angle's classification of occlusion refers to the relation of the first maxillary and first mandibular molars (▶ Fig. 42.5). In normal (class I) occlusion, the mesiobuccal (front lateral) cusp of the maxillary molar interdigitates with the mesiobuccal groove of the mandibular molar. In class II occlusion, the mandibular molar is shifted distally (posteriorly), and in class III occlusion, the mandibular molar is shifted mesially (anteriorly). Typical malocclusion patterns seen following fractures include an anterior open bite (gap between the upper and lower front teeth), which indicates that the fractured maxilla is impacted upward or that both condyles of the mandible have collapsed; a posterior open bite (gap between the upper and lower back teeth), often associated with a unilateral condylar fracture; or a posterior cross bite (back teeth lateral or medial to the normal arch form), which indicates either a mandible fracture or a comminuted fracture of the maxilla and palate. These malocclusive patterns indicate that surgical intervention is required.

Facial nerve injuries may result from penetrating trauma in the area of the main trunk or distal branches of the nerve, or from fracture of the temporal bone involving the intraosseous facial nerve canal. Parotid duct injury may result from penetrating facial trauma in the region of the superior aspect of the masseter muscle. This usually manifests as the absence of salivary flow or the presence of sanguineous secretions from the parotid duct on the involved side.

42.8 Testing

Laboratory testing in maxillofacial trauma should include a complete blood cell count to evaluate for possible blood loss, SMA (sequential multiple analysis) 12 to monitor for possible electrolyte imbalance and acidosis, and type and crossmatch in cases associated with significant blood loss.

Cervical spinal injury should be ruled out before any manipulation of the neck. Axial and coronal computed tomography (CT) is the gold standard in evaluating the majority of facial fractures. Three-dimensional CT reconstruction comes in very handy when complex panfacial fractures are being evaluated. Simple X-rays are still used in screening for facial fractures, but CT provides more detail. Panoramic dental X-rays (panorex) are a very useful adjunct for evaluating the fracture pattern and

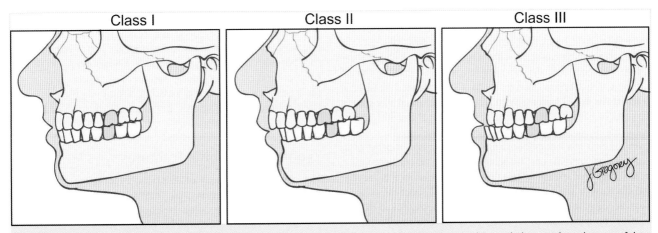

Fig. 42.5 In the Angle classification, normal occlusion (the mesiobuccal cusp of the first maxillary molar articulates with the mesiobuccal groove of the first mandibular molar) is class I. In class II occlusion, the cusp is positioned mesial to the groove by at least the width of a premolar. In class III occlusion, the cusp is shifted distally.

dentition status in patients with mandible fractures. Cervical spine series are required in patients with suspected cervical spine injuries or high-velocity trauma, or in unconscious patients. When vascular injury is suspected, CT angiography or standard angiography is indicated.

In all patients with maxillofacial fractures (other than isolated mandible fractures), an ophthalmologic examination is indicated to rule out orbital injury and retinal detachment, and to document visual acuity.

The traction test is used in patients with NOE fractures to evaluate for the integrity of the medial canthal tendon. The test involves grasping the edge of the lower eyelid and pulling it against its medial attachment. If an obvious "give" of the tendon occurs, a disruption of the medial canthus is likely.

The "tongue blade" test is used in patients with suspected mandible fracture. The patient is asked to bite down hard on a tongue blade. If the jaw is fractured, the patient cannot do this effectively and will experience pain.

42.9 Differential Diagnosis

Different fracture patterns may present with similar findings on physical examination. Therefore, it is very important to establish the correct diagnosis because the treatments may differ significantly. For example, both severe nasal bone fracture and NOE fracture may present with saddling of the nasal dorsum; however, in the case of NOE fracture, this finding may coexist with disruption of the medial canthus, which needs to be addressed to prevent telecanthus and/or a CSF leak. Open-bite deformity may result from both bilateral subcondylar fractures and palatine fracture, but the treatments obviously differ. Mandibular parasymphyseal fractures, routinely treated by rigid fixation alone, are frequently associated with contralateral subcondylar fracture, which requires additional closed or open reduction.

42.10 Treatment

42.10.1 Medical Treatment

The ABCDE (airway, breathing, circulation, disability, exposure) universal trauma protocol should be applied to all patients with maxillofacial trauma. For definitive control of the airway, an artificial oral or nasal airway is often possible, but blind nasal intubation should be carried out with caution. Nasal intubations can exacerbate bleeding from the nasal and nasopharyngeal regions, and the tube may be inadvertently placed into the cranial fossa in the obtunded patient with a comminuted skull base fracture. As for all patients with facial trauma, an airway should be secured early in the trauma assessment for those with significant maxillofacial injury. The secondary swelling that occurs over the first few hours following the trauma can impede, or in some cases prevent, oral intubation. Emergent tracheotomy is rarely indicated except in the unusual circumstance of laryngeal fracture or the inability to intubate orally because of massive bleeding or swelling. Semi-elective tracheostomy in the operating room is reserved for those patients requiring prolonged intubation because of massive soft-tissue and bony injuries or impaired consciousness.

Trauma patients are given intravenous fluids for volume replacement and packed red blood cells in cases of extensive blood loss. Intravenous antibiotics are given to prevent infection, especially in patients with significant soft-tissue trauma and open fractures. Tetanus prophylaxis is also indicated. Pain is usually controlled with intravenous or oral pain medications, depending on the patient's status.

The management of progressive vision loss remains controversial because it is unclear which patients benefit from emergent orbital decompression. If the eyeball is tense, then immediate lateral canthotomy and cantholysis is indicated to release the confining force of the lids. If a clear source of compression is visualized on CT, immediate operative decompression is indicated. All other patients are treated immediately with high-dose steroids; surgery is reserved for those with progression of vision loss.

42.10.2 Surgical Treatment

The facial stigmata of unreduced or poorly reduced fractures are fortunately rarely seen, but when present, they may be severe. Minor cosmetic changes after facial injuries are common; however, in modern society, "good" results are often not enough, and perfection is demanded. The common causes of poor outcomes include bad choice of surgical access, inability to operate early or operating too early, and poor reduction of fracture fragments.

The majority of facial fractures in adults with any significant displacement will require open reduction and internal fixation. Some fractures, such as nasal bone fractures and some mandibular fractures, may be treated with closed reduction techniques.

Frontal Sinus Fractures

Nondisplaced fractures of the anterior and posterior tables of the frontal sinus may be managed by observation. Displaced anterior table fractures (by more than the width of the anterior table) lead to noticeable cosmetic forehead deformity if left untreated and therefore need to be reduced. Displaced posterior table fractures frequently lead to complications such as CSF leak and intracranial hemorrhage. These fractures are managed either by open reduction and frontal sinus obliteration with abdominal fat, or by removal of the posterior table (which allows the brain to expand into the frontal sinus in a process known as cranialization) in cases of severe comminution. Frontal sinus fractures involving the nasofrontal duct are highly like to be associated with duct stenosis and mucocele formation, so that sinus obliteration is commonly required. Common surgical approaches include the use of existing lacerations for small, isolated anterior table fractures, but generally, bicoronal or hemicoronal incisions are used.

Zygomatico-Orbital Fractures

The standard treatment of displaced zygomatico-orbital fractures is open reduction and internal fixation (▶ Fig. 42.6). Ideally, three-point fixation is required to guarantee stability and proper reduction. Common plating areas include the following: the zygomaticofrontal suture line (accessed via an upper or lower blepharoplasty incision or via a hemicoronal

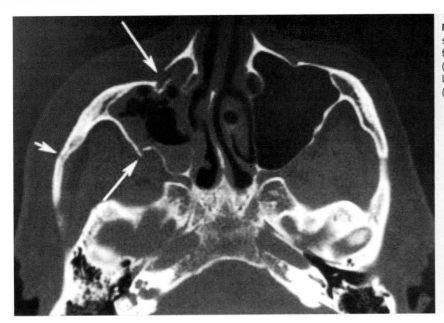

Fig. 42.6 Axial computed tomographic scan showing right zygomaticomaxillary complex fractures involving the anterior maxillary wall (*long arrow*), posterior–lateral wall of the maxillary sinus (*medium arrow*), and zygomatic arch (*short arrow*).

incision, if one is needed for other purposes); the infraorbital rim (approached via a transconjunctival or lower blepharoplasty incision); and the zygomaticomaxillary buttress (accessible via a transoral approach and a gingivobuccal incision).

Single, isolated zygomatic arch fractures are reduced via a Gillies approach, dissecting down from a temporal fossa incision in the plane below the temporalis fascia to place the elevator deep to the arch fracture. This approach is, by definition, an open reduction of the zygomatic arch fracture without internal fixation. Comminuted fractures require open reduction and internal fixation; exposure of the zygomatic arch is gained via a hemicoronal incision, and dissection is in a plane deep to the temporoparietal fascia.

Indications for the repair of isolated orbital floor fractures include large fractures (> 50% of the floor), posttraumatic enophthalmos, and diplopia due to muscular entrapment. The orbital contents that have herniated into the maxillary sinus are reduced into the orbit and supported by either a bone graft, cartilage graft, or alloplastic material. A transconjunctival approach is used.

Naso-Orbito-Ethmoid Fractures

Displaced NOE fractures require open reduction and internal fixation. A disrupted medial canthal tendon, as in type III NOE fractures, is repaired by suturing the tendon to a miniplate or wiring to the opposite nasal bone. Saddle nasal deformity is corrected with the use of an onlay graft (bone, cartilage, or alloplastic graft). Existing lacerations and bicoronal incisions are the most common approaches used in obtaining the access to the region.

Maxillary (Le Fort) Fractures

Proper occlusion must first be established by placing the patient into maxillary–mandibular fixation (MMF). The fractures are then sequentially reduced and fixed with the plates either starting at the most inferior fractures and going superiorly, or

vice versa. Common approaches include gingivobuccal incisions and midfacial degloving, which allows simultaneous bilateral exposure.

Mandible Fractures

The appropriate treatment of a mandibular fracture requires establishing proper occlusion with MMF. Nondisplaced or favorable fractures may be treated with MMF alone for 4 weeks or with rigid fixation. Displaced or unfavorable fractures are treated with open reduction and rigid fixation. Either miniplates or mandibular or reconstruction plates are used. Alternatively, a lag screw can be used to reconstruct the bony segments. Lag screw fixation (▶ Fig. 42.7) requires overdrilling the holes in the proximal bone, allowing the standard screw to glide through this segment of bone. When the threads of the screw engage the distal bone segment, this bone is drawn tightly against the proximal bone.

Ideally, a single plate in placed along the Champy line of ideal osteosynthesis (▶ Fig. 42.8), where the compressive forces along the lower mandible equal the distractive (tension) forces (▶ Fig. 42.9) along the dental border; however, in most locations along the mandible, this line lies along the course of the inferior alveolar nerve. An alternative treatment is to place a miniplate along the lower mandibular border and to use arch bars on the lower teeth to provide tension and maximally stabilize the bone segments.

Subcondylar fractures have commonly been treated with closed reduction (MMF); however, there has been a shift in paradigm in recent years toward the use of rigid fixation via an open or endoscopic approach. The surgical approach to the mandible fractures is generally intraoral via a gingivobuccal incision, but external (submental, submandibular, or preauricular) approaches are viable alternatives in certain cases. Generally, unstable or devitalized teeth along a fracture line are removed, but otherwise teeth, even if loose, are left in place to assist in alignment.

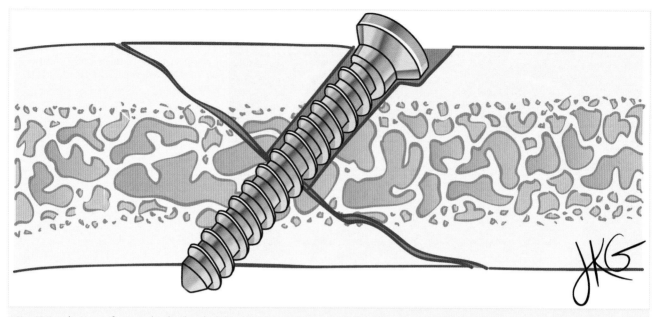

Fig. 42.7 In lag screw fixation, the distal end of the screw is used to engage and pull the distal bone segment into the proximal segment.

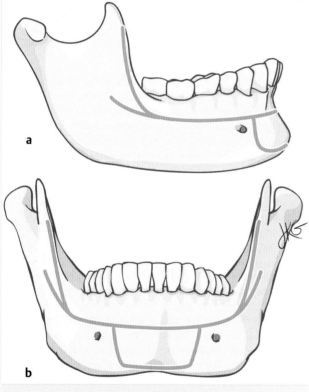

Fig. 42.8 (a,b) Ideal lines of osteosynthesis.

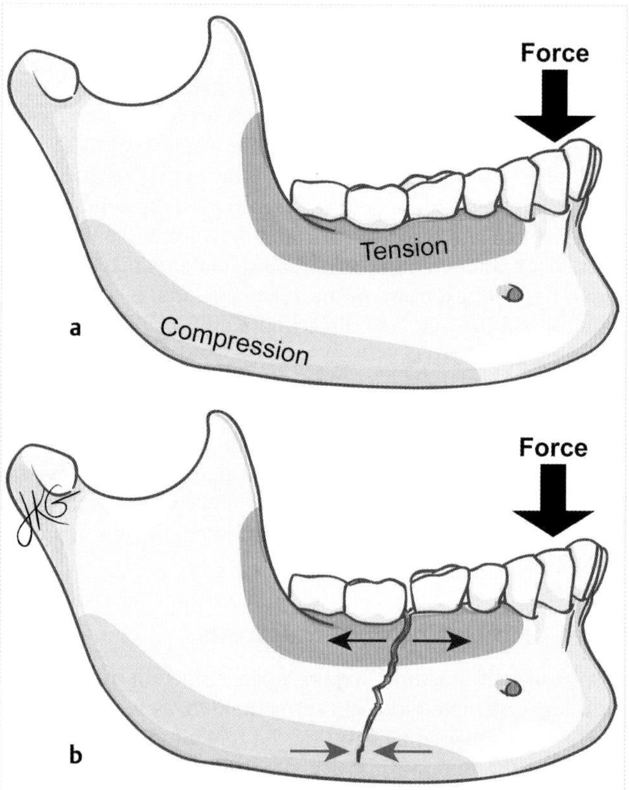

Fig. 42.9 (a,b) Tension and compressive zones of the mandible.

42.11 Complications

Potential complications of open reduction and rigid fixation of the facial fractures include poor reduction of the fracture segments leading to persistent deformity. Malunion or nonunion of the fracture due to improper alignment, infection, or insufficient immobilization commonly requires revision surgery. Iatrogenic injury to adjacent neural structures, such as facial nerve and the branches of the trigeminal nerve (inferior alveolar, infraorbital, mental, others), may lead to temporary and occasionally permanent motor or sensory deficit. Improperly reduced or missed mandibular fractures can lead to malocclusion. Injuries to the teeth due to the improper application of plating hardware have been described. Because the hardware used for rigid fixation is a foreign body, there is always a risk for infection (especially around carious or devitalized teeth).

Injury to orbital structures during the manipulation of fracture fragments and during the surgical approach to the fracture may result in diplopia, vision loss, and blindness.

42.12 Roundsmanship

- Maxillofacial trauma is frequently associated with life-threatening injuries, and patients should be assessed for concomitant airway, central nervous system, and orthopedic injuries.
- Initial management of maxillofacial trauma follows ATLS principles and involves airway management, control of hemorrhage, and rapid identification of injuries with significant morbidity, ocular injury, CSF leakage, neurologic damage, and malocclusion.
- A structured history, physical examination, CT-guided diagnosis, and reconstruction of the major facial buttresses with open reduction and internal fixation performed in a timely fashion are crucial for optimal functional and aesthetic outcome.
- Potential complications of open reduction and internal fixation include malunion or nonunion, poor fracture alignment, hardware infection, osteomyelitis, and injury to the surrounding vital structures.

42.13 Recommended Reading

[1] American Academy of Otolaryngology—Head and Neck Surgery Foundation. Resident Manual of Trauma to the Face, Head, and Neck (eBook format). 1st ed. Alexandria, VA: American Academy of Otolaryngology—Head and Neck Surgery Foundation; 2012

[2] Booth PW, Eppley BL, Schmelzeisen R. Maxillofacial Trauma and Esthetic Facial Reconstruction. New York, NY: Elsevier; 2003

[3] Fingerhut LA, Warner M. Injury Chartbook. Health, United States 1996–1997. Hyattsville, MD: National Center for Health Statistics; 1997

[4] Gassner R, Tuli T, Hächl O, Rudisch A, Ulmer H. Cranio-maxillofacial trauma: a 10 year review of 9,543 cases with 21,067 injuries. J Craniomaxillofac Surg 2003; 31: 51–61

[5] Hull AM, Lowe T, Finlay PM. The psychological impact of maxillofacial trauma: an overview of reactions to trauma. Oral Surg Oral Med Oral Pathol Oral Radiol Endod 2003; 95: 515–520

[6] MacKensie EJ, Fowler CJ. Epidemiology. In: Mattox KI, Feliciano DV, Moore EE, eds. Trauma. New York, NY: McGraw-Hill; 2000:2–22

[7] Tintinalli JE, Kelen GD, Stapczynski JS, Ma OJ, Cline DM. Tintinalli's Emergency Medicine: A Comprehensive Study Guide. 6th ed. New York, NY: McGraw-Hill; 2003: Section 22 (Trauma), Chapter 257 (Maxillofacial Trauma)

43 Scar Revision

Joseph J. Rousso and Anthony P. Sclafani

43.1 Introduction

When multiple layers of skin have been affected by an injury and the reticular dermis violated, the resultant healing process includes the inevitable formation of scar tissue. This can be a difficult and emotionally traumatizing process for even the least self-conscious of patients, particularly if the scar involves the face. The scarring process may also result in functional deficits if contracture forms in areas that limit movement of the eyes, mouth, nose, or neck. Scar revision refers to the various methods, both medical and surgical, to alter the appearance and form of the affected tissue. Scar revision can serve both cosmetic and functional purposes, depending on the site of scar formation. The human eyes' perception of scarring is based on anatomical locations and the orientation of the visible tissue. Therefore, a keen understanding of the geometric concepts of relaxed skin tension lines (RSTLs), aesthetic units, tissue healing, and general wound care is necessary to provide the patient with the best possible options for scar revision.

43.2 Incidence of Disease

Although scar revision is not associated with any "disease," several processes can lead to scar formation. Scar revision is performed in both the ambulatory and inpatient settings and accounts for a large percentage of procedures and treatments performed by various specialty practitioners, including facial plastic surgeons and dermatologists.

43.3 Terminology

A discussion of scar revision requires an understanding of the basic terminology used in describing wounds and an appreciation of the common nomenclature. Relaxed skin tension lines (RSTLs; ▶ Fig. 43.1) of the face refer to linear arrangements whose organization is based on the level of tension. These borderlines run in linear and curvilinear fashion perpendicular to the facial muscles underlying the subcutaneous tissue. Lines of maximal extensibility (LMEs) are oriented perpendicular to the RSTLs. Aesthetic units (▶ Fig. 43.2) and subunits (▶ Fig. 43.3) are units of the face contained within anatomical boundary lines. Aesthetic units contain tissue that is similar in color, texture, vascularity, density, and other qualities and may be bounded by skin transitions and folds. Furthermore, the human eye perceives the face in units based upon light reflections and shadows from these aesthetic boundaries.

43.4 Applied Anatomy

The aesthetic units of the face include the forehead, eyes, ears, nose, lips, chin, and neck. The subunits break the face down further into smaller, anatomically bounded areas. Specific areas of focus should be mentioned because of their unique characteristics and the challenges they present in scar revision. The cheek

is a facial subunit spanning an area extending from the malar eminence to the mandible, where a scar can draw much attention. RSTLs of the cheek are curvilinear—more horizontal medially and close to the lower eyelid, more oblique and vertical laterally and inferiorly. The forehead is vertically bounded by the trichion (hairline) cephalically and the glabella caudally. The RSTLs of the forehead are particularly prominent and run horizontally in most areas but obliquely in the region of the glabella and the temples. The eyebrows present a challenge because scars that affect hair-bearing areas can be very difficult to camouflage. The nose contains paired lateral nasal sidewall, lateral and medial alar, and soft-tissue facet subunits, and unilateral dorsal, tip, and columellar subunits. The ear's subunits correspond to identifiable anatomical landmarks.

43.5 The Disease Process

43.5.1 Etiology and Pathogenesis

Scar formation can result from any injury or trauma, including previous surgical incision. Inflammation and infection can lead to severe scarring. Acne can create crater-like and pitted marks; ice pick, rolling, and boxcar scars can result from the inflammatory process. Problematic scars are formed secondary to various factors, including configuration of the scar with respect to the location of RSTLs; extensive trauma; underlying medical conditions such as diabetes, smoking, nutritional deficiencies, and poor circulation; age; and sun-damaged skin.

Two specific forms of scarring that deserve particular attention are keloids and hypertrophic scars. The term *keloid* refers to a dense scarring process at an injured site, which results in a firm collagen mass that overgrows the boundaries of the wound. A hypertrophic scar, as its name would imply, is a form of overly thickened scar tissue, but it does not overgrow the boundaries of the injury site. Keloids are an exceptionally bothersome form of scarring because they do not regress spontaneously and are prone to recurrence after surgical excision. In contrast, a hypertrophic scar may undergo partial regression throughout its maturation course. Although hypertrophic scarring and keloids can occur in any patient population, white patients are less commonly affected than black and Hispanic patients.

43.5.2 Natural History and Progression

Tissue and wound healing is generally divided into three phases. The inflammatory phase occurs with the initial formation of a clot and subsequent inflammation mediated via chemotactic factors. The proliferative phase occurs within 24 to 72 hours and consists of the formation of granulation tissue, collagen production, and re-epithelialization. Finally, the maturation phase of wound healing produces collagen remodeling and wound contraction. Excisional wounds or injuries that create a large tissue defect are more likely to lead to substantial scarring on account of the more intense inflammatory reaction that

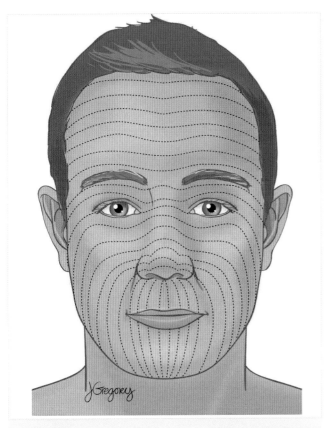

Fig. 43.1 Relaxed skin tension lines.

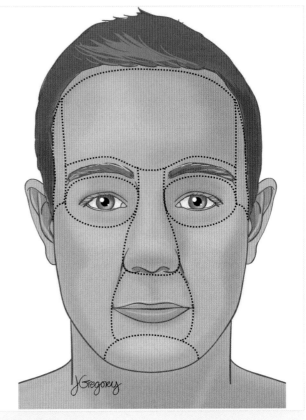

Fig. 43.2 Facial units.

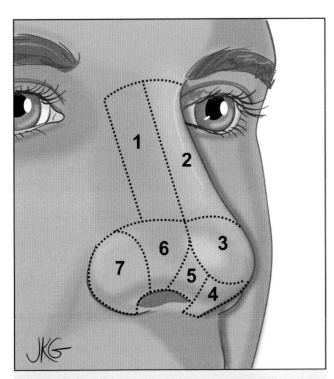

Fig. 43.3 Nasal subunits. *1*, Nasal sidewall; *2*, nasal dorsum; *3*, nasal tip; *4*, columella; *5*, soft-tissue facet; *6*, ala; *7*, lobule.

eventually leads to extensive collagen deposition. The single most important factor to delay healing is local infection due to the persistence of inflammation. Narrow and well-positioned scars continue to change and mature over the course of 12 to 36 months, and appearances may improve during this period.

43.5.3 Potential Disease Complications

Wound healing and scar formation can potentially lead to undesirable outcomes such as hypertrophic scars and keloids. Scar contracture may distort local tissues if located close (and especially perpendicular) to mobile structures such as the eyelids or lips. Scar revision procedures themselves can lead to further inflammation and continued collagen deposition. Psychological complications are a well-known morbidity associated with facial scar formation. Depression, unrealistic expectations, posttraumatic stress disorder, and anxiety are all considerations in the patient with facial scars. Accordingly, concomitant consultation with a mental health professional is warranted in patients who show signs of unrealistic expectations or psychological distress.

43.6 Medical Evaluation

43.6.1 Presenting Complaints

The presentation of patients can vary from simple dislike of their appearance to pain, restricted mobility, and decreased range of motion. It is important to emphasize to patients that scar revision can, at best, partially improve a scar's appearance.

Patients must have realistic expectations and should be informed that the scar will not be invisible but will be modified and camouflaged to appear less noticeable and bothersome.

43.6.2 Physical Examination

The physical examination is the most critical tool in the physician's arsenal for scar revision. The physician should present a detailed description of the affected area to the patient in terms that the patient can comprehend. This allows the physician and patient to have a common understanding of the most bothersome characteristics of the scar. As part of a detailed physical examination, photographs of the affected area should be taken in an area with appropriate lighting and a nonreflective background. These photos can be compared with photos taken after treatment to quantify changes in appearance. Specific features that should be described in the physical examination include size, shape, elevation, color, hair-bearing areas, consistency, geometric configuration, orientation to the RSTLs, and aesthetic unit(s) through which the scar runs.

43.6.3 Laboratory Studies and Imaging

Laboratory studies and imaging studies are dictated by the underlying cause of scarring or comorbid conditions.

43.6.4 Differential Diagnosis

Scarring can be diagnosed by physical examination alone; however, other pathologic entities can present similarly to scar tissue and include dermatofibromas, dermatofibrosarcomas, desmoid tumors, infection, granulomas, and foreign body reactions.

43.7 Medical Treatment

43.7.1 Cosmetology

Scar camouflage can be largely achieved with alterations in makeup and hairstyling. The assistance of a licensed cosmetologist is invaluable because this person can play a pivotal role in masking the appearance of a scar and accentuating other appealing features that may redirect visual focus away from the scar. Cosmetics can be particularly helpful in camouflaging dyspigmented scars or persistent erythema.

43.7.2 Intralesional Steroid Injections

Intralesional injections of corticosteroids are commonly used for keloids and other unfavorable scars. The injection should be placed within the substance of the scar or keloid and should avoid the unaffected dermis. Although noninvasive, intralesional injections generally must be repeated several times at intervals of 3 to 6 weeks before any benefit is appreciable. Side effects may include localized skin hypopigmentation and dermal or fat atrophy at the injection site.

43.7.3 Silicone Gel Sheeting

The topical placement of silicone gel sheets over sites of keloid formation and hypertrophic scars has shown significant benefit.

Although the mechanism is unknown (possibly related to scar hydration or direct interaction with silicone), patients are instructed to wear the silicone sheets for at least 8 hours per day for 6 to 12 months. Silicone gel sheeting is often attempted before surgical scar revision because the associated morbidity is minimal.

43.8 Surgical Treatment

43.8.1 Scar Excision with Primary Wound Closure

A scar that is appropriately oriented (within 30 degrees of RSTLs) and has formed secondary to improper wound closure may be treated by surgically with excision of the scar tissue and appropriate primary wound closure. The excision should remove all scar tissue and create fresh wound edges. The scar is removed by elliptical excision; if the central portion of the scar is depressed, the deep scar tissue is left in place to form a base for wound closure above it. Closure should be performed in layers, with absorbable sutures placed at a dermal level and minimally reactive, monofilament sutures placed at the external epidermal level. Closure should follow the tenets of Halsted: avoidance of tension, obliteration of dead space in the wound, and the use of fine, nonirritating sutures. In addition, wide undermining of adjacent tissue will assist in creating everted wound edges with minimal tension.

43.8.2 Serial Partial Excision and Tissue Expansion

In the case of extremely wide scars, closure after excision of the entire scar may either be impossible or require unacceptable wound closure tension. In this case, serial partial excision can be used. In this method, a portion of the scar is resected, with the incision placed along the edge or within the substance of the scar. The surrounding tissue is undermined and the wound is closed, effectively narrowing the scar. After wound healing and skin stretch by the process of biologic creep have been allowed to take place over a period of a few months, the remaining scar can be fully excised and the wound closed primarily. Alternatively, tissue expanders (see Chapter 50 for a discussion of tissue expansion) can be placed adjacent to the scar and the skin actively expanded over several weeks. The expanders can then be removed and the expanded skin used to fill the defect caused by removal of the scar tissue.

43.8.3 Irregularization Techniques

Scar revision is rooted in the principle of camouflaging visible scars so that they are less apparent to the human eye. Those scars that are most noticeable are linear and run perpendicular to RSTLs. Irregularization techniques achieve a more desirable appearance by breaking linear scars into zigzag lines adjusted to fall within the RSTLs and aesthetic subunits. The three most commonly used irregularization techniques are Z-plasty, W-plasty, and geometric broken line closure (GBLC).

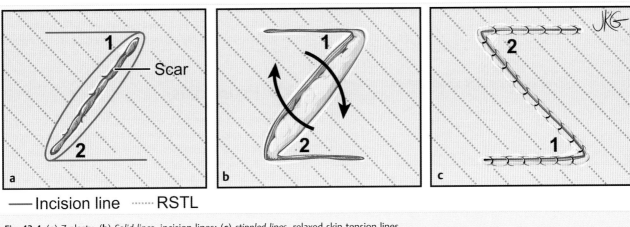

—— Incision line ········· RSTL

Fig. 43.4 (a) Z-plasty. (b) *Solid lines*, incision lines; (c) *stippled lines*, relaxed skin tension lines.

Z-plasty

Z-plasty creates a change in the direction and an increase in the length of the scar. The idea of the Z-plasty is to allow the new scar to fall closer to or exactly in the direction of the RSTL, as well as to break the forces of scar contracture. The scar is made longer, and the resultant tension is transposed and more widely distributed through the wound.

Z-plasty is performed by transposing triangles (▶ Fig. 43.4), in which the scar tissue lies in the central limb. The amount of scar lengthening that will be produced by this irregularization technique can be predicted based on the angles of the transposed triangle. As a rule of thumb, 30-degree Z-plasty angles will increase the length of a scar by 25%, 45-degree angles will lengthen the scar by 50%, and 60-degree angles will lengthen it by 75% (▶ Table 43.1). Multiple Z-plasties can be performed if necessary. Z-plasty is most useful for dealing with scars that cross RSTLs or distinct anatomical landmarks, or that create bands across concavities. Lengthening of the scar can improve function by releasing contracture.

W-plasty

W-plasty is an irregularization technique that is most useful around convex areas, including the nasal dorsum, border of the mandible, and dorsum of the nose. Unlike the aforementioned Z-plasty, W-plasty does not lengthen the scar. This technique essentially consists of regular, W-shaped complementary skin excisions on both sides of the existing scar (▶ Fig. 43.5). The scar tissue is excised and the surrounding tissue undermined. The triangular flaps are then interdigitated and the wound closed.

Geometric Broken Line Closure

GBLC is a powerful tool to reduce the visibility of long, unbroken facial scars, particularly those on convex areas. GBLC works well in areas that are large and flat, such as the forehead and cheek. Like W-plasty, GBLC does not increase the scar length; rather, it improves the scar appearance by creating an irregular scar pattern. GBLC is performed (▶ Fig. 43.6) by creating a series of irregular, small shapes that have equivalent counterparts on the opposite side of the scar edge. As with W-plasty, each limb of the GLBC should measure between 4 and 6 mm. The scar is

Table 43.1 Amount of lengthening of the central scar when Z-plasty is use for scar revision

Angles formed by central limb (scar axis) and lateral arms of Z-plasty	Percentage of lengthening of central limb
30 degrees	25%
45 degrees	50%
60 degrees	75%

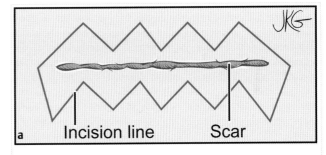

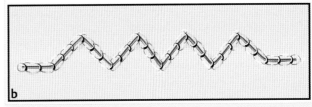

Fig. 43.5 (a,b) W-plasty.

excised, the surrounding tissue is undermined, and the geometric shapes are interdigitated. W-plasty and GBLC generally benefit from postoperative dermabrasion.

43.8.4 Dermabrasion/Laser Scar Resurfacing

Dermabrasion is not routinely used as a free-standing method for scar revision in the head and neck. However, it can be very

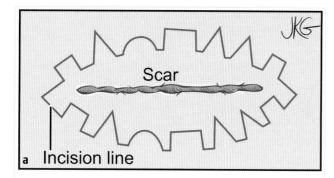

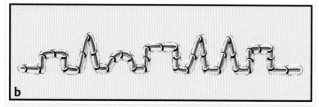

Fig. 43.6 (a,b) Geometric broken line closure.

useful as a complementary procedure to aid in wound healing after a scar revision procedure. Dermabrasion consists of removal of the superficial components of skin, allowing the stimulation of basal cells to achieve final wound closure. A rapidly rotating dermabrader (with a diamond-coated or wire brush wheel) is used to remove epidermal and superficial dermal layers, with injury to the underlying adnexal structures, which contribute to the regeneration of new epidermis, avoided. Passes are made at 45-degree angles to one another to avoid creating ridges, and the edges of the abraded areas should be feathered. Laser abrasion is performed similarly with carbon dioxide or Er:YAG (erbium-doped yttrium aluminum garnet) lasers (ablative or fractional); similar skin layers are removed, depending upon energy parameters and the number of laser passes. After skin abrasion, the wounds should be kept moist with hypoallergenic petroleum-based ointments (e.g., Vaseline; Unilever US, Englewood Cliffs, NJ; Aquaphor (Eucerin); Beiersdorf AG, Hamburg, Germany) until re-epithelialization is complete. Sun precaution is necessary until the erythema has faded, generally 6 to 12 weeks after treatment.

43.8.5 Laser Treatment of Telangiectasia/Scar Erythema

Telangiectasia around or on a scar will make the scar more noticeable as the observer's attention is drawn to the area of color difference. Even thin, flat, and well-healed scars will be visible if they are erythematous or surrounded by telangiectasia. Laser light at or near the wavelengths for peak hemoglobin absorption, such as 585 or 1,064 nm, can selectively cause blood vessels to constrict as the waves pass through the more superficial tissues without causing damage and are selectively absorbed by the hemoglobin in red blood cells. This absorbed energy is then converted to heat, lysing the red blood cells and initiating an in-

flammatory response in the vessel walls, eventually causing vessel constriction. This process, selective photothermolysis, reduces the red hues visible in the skin and helps fade the appearance of the scar.

43.9 Prognosis

Recovery after scar revision procedures is a multifactorial phenomenon. In addition to ensuring that patients have realistic expectations, it is imperative that the physician convey to them that the final appearance of the revised scar may not be appreciated until almost a year after the procedure is performed. Healing is a continuous process that is altered by factors such as smoking, diet, infection, and general overall health. In order to ensure the best outcomes after a scar revision procedure, meticulous wound care and frequent follow-up should be performed.

43.10 Roundsmanship

- When the reticular dermis has been fully violated, scar formation occurs.
- The ultimate perception of scarring depends upon the contours, anatomical location and orientation, width, and color of the scar.
- A keen understanding of the geometric concepts of relaxed skin tension lines (RSTLs), aesthetic units, tissue healing, and general wound care is necessary to provide the patient with the best-possible options for scar revision.
- It is important to ensure that patients have realistic expectations and are informed that the scar will not be invisible, but that it will be modified and camouflaged to appear less noticeable and bothersome.
- Wound healing and scar formation can potentially lead to complicated outcomes, such as hypertrophic scars and keloids.
- The three most commonly used irregularization techniques are Z-plasty, W-plasty, and geometric broken-line closure.
- Healing is a continuous process that is altered by factors such as smoking, diet, infection, and general overall health.

43.11 Recommended Reading

[1] Habif TP. Clinical Dermatology: A Color Guide to Diagnosis and Therapy. 5th ed. Maryland Heights, MO: Mosby Elsevier; 2009:226–234
[2] Kumar V, Abbas AK, Fausto N, Aster JC, eds. Robbins and Cotran Pathologic Basis of Disease. 8th ed. Philadelphia, PA: Saunders Elsevier; 2009:98–108
[3] Nouri K, Ballard CJ, Vejjabhinanta V. Essentials of tissue movement; http://emedicine.medscape.com/article/1130018-overview
[4] Thomas JR, Hochman M. Scar camouflage. In: Bailey BJ, Johnson JT, Kohut RI, et al, eds. Bailey's Head & Neck Surgery—Otolaryngology, 5th ed. Philadelphia, PA: J. B. Lippincott; 1993:2026–2033
[5] Thomas JR, Mobley SR. Scar revision and camouflage. In: Cummings C, Haughey B, Thomas JR, et al, eds. Cummings Otolaryngology: Head and Neck Surgery. Philadelphia, PA: Elsevier Mosby; 1998:572–581
[6] Thomas JR, Holt GR, eds. Facial Scars: Incisions, Revision, and Camouflage. St. Louis, MO: Mosby; 1989

44 Rosacea

Robert Deeb and Thomas C. Spalla

44.1 Introduction

Rosacea is one of the most common dermatologic conditions affecting the head and neck. It is characterized by persistent central facial erythema involving the convex areas of the face. Additional primary features are papules and pustules, transient flushing, and telangiectasia. Secondary features of the disease include burning or stinging, plaques, dryness, edema, ocular manifestations, peripheral locations, and phymatous changes. Given the prominent location of the disease pattern, individuals affected with this condition often feel a great deal of anxiety in both social and professional settings.

Although rosacea has readily identifiable characteristics, it remains a diagnosis of exclusion. This is due to the fact that there is no reliable laboratory test. Biopsies are often required to rule out other conditions that may mimic the clinical findings. A broad differential diagnosis must always be considered. Some diseases that must be considered include lupus erythematosus, chronic actinic damage, polycythemia vera, dermatomyositis, mixed connective tissue disease, carcinoid, mastocystosis, and allergic contact dermatitis.

44.2 Pathogenesis

The cause of rosacea remains unknown, although a large variety of mechanisms have been proposed. There is a great deal of debate as to whether or not the subtypes of rosacea all have a common underlying etiology. An alternate theory proposes that each subtype is a distinct disease entity and thus has a unique pathophysiologic mechanism. Given the heterogeneous nature of the disease presentation and the varied responses to treatment, it is likely each subtype represents a varied response to a combination of these purported factors.

Proposed etiologic mechanisms may be categorized according to the central trigger that activates the clinical symptomatology. These categories include vasculature, climate exposures, matrix degeneration, chemicals and ingested agents, pilosebaceous unit abnormalities, and microbial organisms. Each of these pathogenic theories has some supporting evidence, although none offers a comprehensive answer.

44.3 Classification

In 2002, the National Rosacea Society Expert Committee on the Classification and Staging of Rosacea developed a standardized classification system that divided rosacea into four distinct subtypes. Although the different subtypes have some manifestations in common, the committee emphasized the importance of recognizing each subtype as a somewhat distinct entity. The importance of this stratification lies in the fact that treatment options vary widely depending on the constellation of findings within the subtype. Additionally, this system provides uniform diagnostic criteria, which subsequently allow meaningful translational research.

The expert panel also made treatment recommendations for each subtype; these will be outlined, as well. It is important to emphasize that a progression from one subtype to another generally does not take place.

44.3.1 Erythemato-telangiectatic Type

The hallmark finding of the erythemato-telangiectatic rosacea (ETR) subtype is flushing and persistent erythema of the central face. There is characteristic sparing of the periocular skin. The stimuli that bring on the flushing may be emotional stress, hot drinks, alcohol, spicy foods, exercise, cold or hot weather, and hot baths or showers. These patients may also have telangiectasia, although this is not a diagnostic requirement. Common secondary features include burning and stinging sensations, edema, and roughness or scaling. Generally, patients with ETR are more sensitive to topically applied substances. The skin usually has a fine texture and lacks the sebaceous quality that is found in other subtypes.

This subtype of rosacea is often difficult to treat. No drugs have been approved to reduce flushing. As such, the mainstay of treatment is the avoidance of environmental and lifestyle triggers. Additionally, the use of nonirritating cosmetics may conceal the appearance of erythema and telangiectasia.

The telangiectasia and background erythema can also be treated with laser therapy. Most lasers used to treat the vascular components of rosacea have wavelengths in the 500- to 600-nm range. These are nonablative ranges and are thus not intended to destroy tissue. Options include long-pulsed dye, potassium titanyl phosphate, and diode lasers. Treatment with flashlamp pulsed dye laser has been shown to be effective, as well.

44.3.2 Papulopustular Type

Papulopustular rosacea (PPR) is considered to be the classic presentation of the disease (▶ Fig. 44.1). This subtype is characterized by persistent central facial erythema and transient central facial papules or pustules, or both. Secondary features of burning and stinging are sometimes reported. Flushing may occur, although this symptom is less severe than in the ETR subtype. Telangiectasia is often subtly present; however, the telangiectasia may be obscured by the erythematous background. Irritation from external stimuli or topical applicants is not a constant feature.

Like that of all subtypes of rosacea, the treatment of PPR depends on the severity of the condition. Mild cases may be treated with a topical therapy such as metronidazole, azelaic acid, or sodium sulfacetamide. The addition of oral therapy is indicated for more severe disease. A first-line option, which is FDA-approved, is a controlled-release formulation of oral doxycycline. Of note, the dose of this drug achieves low plasma levels that do not exert antimicrobial effects while retaining anti-inflammatory activity.

Refractory cases may require off-label oral trimethoprim/sulfamethoxazole, metronidazole, erythromycin, ampicillin, clindamycin, or dapsone.

347

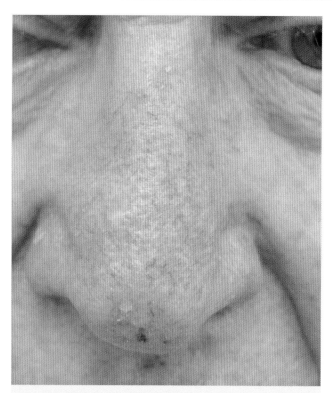

Fig. 44.1 Papulopustular type of rosacea.

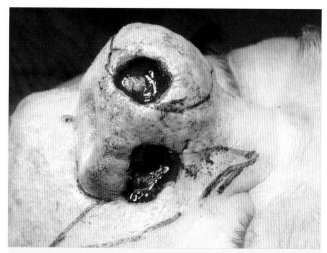

Fig. 44.2 Patient with rhinophyma after Mohs excision of two basal cell carcinomas. Note the extreme thickening of the skin.

44.3.3 Phymatous Type

Phymatous rosacea is characterized by many of the primary features of rosacea, including flushing, erythema, and papules or pustules. However, the presence of characteristic features of skin thickening, irregular surface nodules, and patulous follicles defines this subtype. Affected areas include the chin, forehead, cheeks, and ears; however, the nose is most commonly affected (i.e., rhinophyma).

As previously mentioned, a progression from one subtype to another generally does not occur. However, a possible exception is the progression of severe papulopustular rosacea to the phymatous type.

Management options for early-stage phymatous changes include topical and systemic antibiotics if inflammatory lesions are present. Isotretinoin therapy has been demonstrated to decrease nasal volume in rhinophyma, especially in younger patients with less advanced disease, although the volume may increase again after therapy is stopped. More severe forms of phymatous rosacea may require surgical intervention; these are detailed in the section below on the treatment of rhinophyma.

44.3.4 Ocular Type

The cardinal symptoms of ocular rosacea are blepharitis and conjunctivitis. The eyes generally have a watery or bloodshot appearance, and patients experience foreign body sensation, burning or stinging, dryness, itching, light sensitivity, and blurred vision. Patients may also have a history of recurrent chalazion. Telangiectasia of the eyelid margins or lids and periocular erythema may also be present. Inflammation of the mei-

bomian glands may be present. Ocular rosacea may precede the cutaneous signs by many years, and more than 60% of patients with cutaneous rosacea may also have ocular involvement.

Generally, patients with ocular rosacea should have regular interval evaluations by an ophthalmologist. Early-stage disease is treated with artificial tears, warm compresses, and regular cleansing of the eyelashes with baby shampoo. Antibiotic ointment may have benefit to decrease the presence of *Propionibacterium acnes*, *Staphylococcus epidermidis*, and *Staphylococcus aureus*. Severe disease may require treatment with a systemic tetracycline with or without a topical steroid. Cyclosporine ophthalmic emulsion may be used in severe cases, as well.

44.4 Rhinophyma

Phyma is a Greek word meaning "swelling," "mass," or "bulb." These growths typically occur about the face and ears. The most common form affects the nose and is thus termed *rhinophyma*. Rhinophyma is a slowly progressive dermatologic condition of the nose characterized by sebaceous hypertrophy, which leads to the appearance of a bulbous, greasy, and sometimes erythematous nose. With progressively increasing growth, the condition can lead to impaired breathing and severe cosmetic disfigurement. It occurs almost exclusively in men.

Rhinophyma is sometimes considered the end stage of acne rosacea because in many male patients with rhinophyma, the disease has slowly progressed from rosacea. This is not always the case, however. There is some thought that the inflammatory process may be triggered by a mite, *Demodex folliculorum*. There are four variants of rhinophyma.

44.4.1 Glandular Form

In this form of rhinophyma, the nose is enlarged primarily by lobular sebaceous gland hyperplasia. Superficially, the nose is characterized by pits and deep indentations. The tumor-like growths occurring on the nose are often asymmetric and when compressed yield a cheesy white discharge (▶ Fig. 44.2).

44.4.2 Fibrous Form

In this variant, the dominant characteristic is overgrowth of the connective tissue. Variable amounts of sebaceous gland hyperplasia are also present.

44.4.3 Fibroangiomatous Form

The fibroangiomatous form of rhinophyma causes the nose to become coppery red to dark red in appearance. Additionally, it is associated with pustules and a network of venous ectasia.

44.4.4 Actinic Form

In this variant, which is seen primarly in patients of Celtic origin (i.e., Fitzpatrick type I skin), the nose is distorted by nodular masses of elastic tissue.

44.4.5 Nasal Obstruction

With progressive disease, the tissue bulk can cause pressure on the upper lateral cartilages, restricting airflow through the internal nasal valve region. Additionally, the proliferation may result in excess bulk along the nasal ala and cause collapse of the external valve. In extreme cases, as reported by Lomeo et al, the sebaceous hypertrophy can become so significant as to block the nasal passages almost completely.

44.4.6 Treatment

Medical management of rhinophyma should be considered for patients who have mild disease or for those in whom surgery is best avoided or contraindicated. The modalities used to treat early-stage rhinophyma are similar to those employed in the management of rosacea. Additionally, topical forms of statins can be used in the treatment of acne, seborrhea, rosacea, and rhinophyma. When medical management of the disease is unsuccessful, and after appropriate counseling, surgical management of rhinophyma may be undertaken. As with all facial plastic surgery, photographic documentation is imperative. Several methods have been proposed to improve cases of rhinophyma.

Farrior has found that bulky disease can first be removed with a dermatome, and the edges may be blended with a wire brush dermabrader. Williams and Lam are in agreement; they also state that rhinophymatous tissue takes longer to heal and that a longer duration of the need for occlusive dressings and ointments is to be expected.

Electrocauterization and cryosurgery may also be used in the management of this disease. Seiverling found the Shaw scalpel helpful in relieving a patient of nasal obstruction secondary to rhinophyma. Additionally, coblation has been noted to yield acceptable outcomes, and Timms et al purport advantages due to the lower temperatures used with this technique. Radio frequency has been used successfully by Arikan et al, and the harmonic scalpel has also been employed.

Lasers offer another treatment modality to relieve rhinophyma. Ablative lasers allow tissue removal as well as new collagen formation, leading to tightening of the skin and an improved appearance. Carbon dioxide, Nd:YAG (neodymium:yttrium-aluminum garnet), and Er:YAG (erbium:yttrium-aluminum garnet) lasers have been used successfully for these purposes. Also, a diode laser has been found to yield acceptable results according to Tahery et al, and the Smoothbeam laser has been used to treat moderate rhinophyma.

Some authors recommend low-dose isotretinoin before and after surgical intervention to reduce the bulk of disease and maintain results. However, there is some concern that oral isotretinoin taken close to the time of surgery may result in hypertrophic scarring. This is the reason why many facial plastic surgeons will not resurface a patient's skin until the patient has refrained from using isotretinoin for 6 to 12 months.

44.4.7 Other Considerations

The excised tissue should be sent for pathologic examination. There are approximately 46 reported cases of malignancy within excised rhinophymatous tissue in the literature. In a study by Lazzeri et al, two cases of basal cell carcinoma and one case of squamous cell carcinoma were identified in the pathologic specimens.

44.5 Roundsmanship

- Rosacea is characterized by persistent central facial erythema involving the convex areas of the face, often in association with papules and pustules, transient flushing, and telangiectasia.
- Rosacea is divided into four distinct subtypes: papulopustular, erythemato-telangiectatic, phymatous, and ocular.
- Rhinophyma is a slowly progressive condition of the nose characterized by sebaceous hypertrophy that leads to the appearance of a bulbous, greasy, and sometimes erythematous nose.
- There are four variants of rhinophyma: glandular, fibrous, fibroangiomatous, and actinic.

44.6 Recommended Reading

[1] Arikan OK, Muluk NB, Cirpar O. Treatment of rhinophyma with radiofrequency: a case report. B-ENT 2010; 6: 209–213

[2] Borrie P. Rosacea with special reference to its ocular manifestations. Br J Dermatol 1953; 65: 458–463

[3] Crawford GH, Pelle MT, James WD. Rosacea: I. Etiology, pathogenesis, and subtype classification. J Am Acad Dermatol 2004; 51: 327–341

[4] Crawford GH, Pelle MT, James WD. Rosacea: II. Therapy. J Am Acad Dermatol 2004; 51: 499–512

[5] Gupta S, Handa S, Saraswat A et al. Conventional cold excision combined with dermabrasion for rhinophyma. J Dermatol 2000; 27: 116–120

[6] Irvine C, et al. Isotretinoin in the treatement of rosacea and rhinophyma. In: Marks R, Plewig G, eds. Acne and Related Disorders. London, England: Dunitz; 1989:301

[7] Jansen T, Plewig G. Clinical and histological variants of rhinophyma, including nonsurgical treatment modalities. Facial Plast Surg 1998; 14: 241–253

[8] Lazzeri D, Colizzi L, Licata G et al. Malignancies within rhinophyma: report of three new cases and review of the literature. Aesthetic Plast Surg 2012; 36: 396–405

[9] Odom R, Dahl M, Dover J et al. Standard management options for rosacea, part 1: overview and broad spectrum of care. Cutis 2009; 84: 43–47

[10] Rodder O, Plewig G. Rhinophyma and rosacea: combined treatment with isotretinoin and dermabrasion. In: Marks R, Plewig G, eds. Acne and Related Disorders. London, England: Dunitz; 1989:335

[11] Rohrich R, Griffin J, Adams W. Rhinophyma: review and update. Plast Reconstr Surg 2000; 10: 860–869

[12] Timms M et al. Coblation of rhinophyma. J Laryngol Otol. 2011 Jul;125 (7):724-8. Epub 2011 Apr 27

[13] Wilkin J, Dahl M, Detmar M et al. Standard classification of rosacea: report of the National Rosacea Society Expert Committee on the Classification and Staging of Rosacea. J Am Acad Dermatol 2002; 46: 584–587

45 Common Facial Skin Lesions

John A. Carucci and Joshua W. Trufant

45.1 Examining the Skin

The physical examination is an essential component of a thorough patient evaluation. Although dermatologists specialize in diseases of the skin, general internists and other medical specialists cannot help but examine the skin during a focused evaluation of their particular organ systems of interest. In addition to yielding important insights into internal disease states, the skin examination is an opportunity for physicians to screen patients for cutaneous malignancies. The early detection of skin cancers has been shown to decrease their associated morbidity and mortality. Otolaryngologists–head and neck surgeons are particularly well positioned to identify suspicious lesions for several reasons:

- Approximately 80% of nonmelanoma skin cancers—the most common malignancies worldwide—and 90% of cases of lentigo maligna—a form of malignant melanoma in situ—are located on the head, likely in part because of strong associations with exposure to ultraviolet (UV) light.
- Nonmelanoma skin cancers of the ears and central face have higher rates of local recurrence and metastasis in comparison with cutaneous cancers on the trunk or extremities.
- Invasive nonmelanoma skin cancers of the head and neck can result in cosmetic disfigurement that may be difficult if not impossible to conceal, causing patients significant psychological distress.
- Individuals receiving immunosuppressive therapies or ionizing radiation for internal malignancies, including head and neck cancers, are at increased risk for cutaneous malignancies.

It follows that in order to identify concerning lesions, the physician must also be able to identify common benign lesions of the head and neck. A working knowledge of benign facial lesions can also help the nondermatologist answer patients' questions and know when to refer them to a dermatologist for further evaluation. As in patient encounters across all specialties, the history can provide valuable diagnostic information. Lesion duration, the presence of symptoms such as pain, itching, bleeding, and discharge, and any changes in size, color, or appearance are particularly important. The ABCDE (*a*symmetry, *b*order irregularities, *c*olor variegation, *d*iameter larger than 6 mm, and *e*volving lesion that is changing in any way over time) acronym, initially devised to aid the lay public and primary care physicians in recognizing malignant melanoma, has been validated as a useful screening tool for evaluating pigmented lesions. Any of these characteristics may be cause for concern, although there are melanomas that do not have them (e.g., amelanotic melanoma) and benign lesions that do (e.g., seborrheic keratoses larger than 6 mm).

Proper lighting is critical to performing an adequate examination of the skin. Magnification can also aid in identifying smaller lesions or surface changes. Dermoscopy is an examination with a handheld device that combines magnification with polarized light or a fluid interface; it allows the visualization of structures in the epidermis or papillary dermis that are not visible to the naked eye.

45.2 Terminology

Familiarity with dermatologic terminology will also improve diagnostic accuracy and communication with physician colleagues. Although exact definitions vary, the following are useful working definitions of just a few of the most common primary lesions found on the head and neck. A *macule* is a circumscribed, flat lesion with color change that is *up to 1 cm* in size. A *patch* has similar characteristics but is *larger than 1 cm*. A *papule* is a circumscribed, elevated, superficial, solid lesion *up to 1 cm* in size. A *plaque* has similar characteristics but is larger *than 1 cm*. A *nodule* is also elevated and *up to 1 cm* in size, but it has more depth than a papule. A *mass* is a lesion with a depth of *more than 1 cm*.

When a confident diagnosis of benignity cannot be made by physical examination and history, or when a clinically malignant-appearing lesion is identified, a biopsy is required. Various techniques may be employed. *Shave biopsy* refers to shallow removal of a lesion to the depth of the dermis, typically performed with a scalpel or dermablade. *Saucerization* refers to a disk-shaped biopsy performed with a scalpel angled at 45 degrees, so that the subcutaneous fat is reached at the center of the sample. *Punch biopsy* refers to the use of a sharp, circular instrument ranging from 1 to 1.5 cm in diameter that removes tissue well into the subcutaneous fat. The resulting defect is typically closed with sutures. *Incisional biopsy* samples only a portion of a lesion and is frequently employed for larger lesions or those on cosmetically sensitive areas; it may be performed by punch biopsy or elliptical incision. *Full-thickness excisional biopsy* refers to total removal of a lesion with 1- to 3-mm margins; it can be performed with a punch biopsy instrument or by fusiform (elliptical) excision with a scalpel, followed by primary closure with sutures. Excisional biopsy has long been the recommended technique for lesions suspicious for malignant melanoma, although recent studies suggest that shave biopsy may be sufficient in some cases.

45.3 Common Facial Lesions

45.3.1 Seborrheic Keratosis

Among the most common benign epidermal tumors found on the head and neck, seborrheic keratoses (SKs) are characterized clinically by their stuck-on, waxy appearance (▶ Fig. 45.1). Lesions are typically tan to brown and may have a smooth or mammillated surface. Six subtypes have been described, most ranging in size from several millimeters to a centimeter in diameter, although "giant" lesions measuring nearly 10 cm have been reported. Dermatosis papulosa nigra, characterized by numerous 1- to 5-mm hyperpigmented papules on the face of darkly pigmented individuals, is considered by many to be an SK variant. SKs are commonly asymptomatic, but they may be associated with pruritus or more rarely with pain and bleeding, particularly more exophytic lesions prone to traumatization. Although their etiology is not well understood, genetic se-

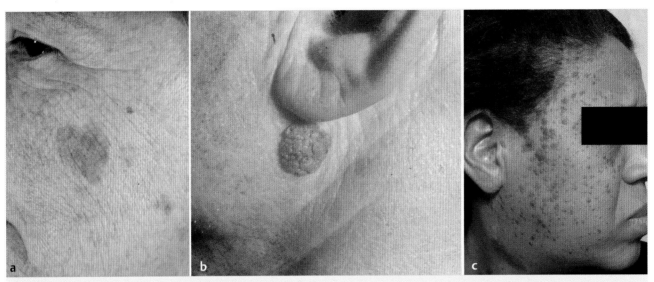

Fig. 45.1 (a,b) Seborrheic keratoses. (c) Multiple seborrheic keratoses on the face of an African-American woman, also known as dermatosis papulosa nigra.

quencing has revealed a number of associated oncogenic mutations. Advanced age is clearly a risk factor, but data regarding an association with sun exposure are conflicting. Human papillomavirus has been isolated in a subset of lesions. The sudden appearance of numerous SKs is widely thought to be a potential sign of internal malignancy, a paraneoplastic phenomenon known as the sign of Leser-Trelat, although recent studies have cast doubt on this association.

SKs can usually be diagnosed clinically based on their characteristic appearance. Biopsy is typically unnecessary. Dermoscopy can aid in differentiating SKs from melanocytic lesions by enhancing classic features such as comedo-like openings and milia cysts; however, cases of malignant melanoma mimicking SKs have been reported. Treatment of these benign neoplasms is elective, but patients may be bothered by symptomatic or cosmetically conspicuous lesions. A number of treatment modalities have been shown to be effective in removing SKs, including cryotherapy, electrodessication and curettage, and shave excision, although these methods are frequently complicated by scarring, pigmentary changes, and recurrence. Laser treatment with 532-nm diode, ablative carbon dioxide, Er:YAG (erbium-doped yttrium aluminum garnet), and Nd:YAG (neodymium-doped yttrium aluminum garnet) models is increasingly being used.

45.3.2 Sebaceous Hyperplasia

Sebaceous gland hyperplasia (SH) is characterized by yellow to flesh-colored papules, most commonly seen on the face (▶ Fig. 45.2). Although its incidence increases with age, it may occur at any age, including at birth. Subtypes include senile, linear, diffuse, functional familiar, juxtaclavicular beaded line variant, and giant lesions—plaques or cystlike lesions measuring up to 5 cm. SH represents an increased number of mature sebaceous lobules in the superficial dermis attached to a dilated central pore. Its etiology is unknown, but the incidence is increased in organ transplant recipients and in those taking cyclosporine. SH does not appear to be associated with Fitzpatrick skin type or solar elastosis, nor is it considered a part of the Muir-Torre syndrome, a rare autosomal-dominant genodermatosis characterized by rarer benign and malignant sebaceous tumors, keratoacanthomas, and internal malignancies.

The diagnosis of SH is typically made clinically. Particular care should be taken in evaluating lesions of the periocular region, the most common site of the rare sebaceous carcinoma. Magnification of SH by dermoscopy or other means typically reveals a central yellow to white ostium with surrounding linear telangiectasia. Successful treatment of SH has been achieved with photodynamic therapy; carbon dioxide, Nd:YAG, and pulsed dye lasers; cryosurgery; bichloracetic acid; electrodessication; and oral isotretinoin.

45.3.3 Trichoepithelioma

Trichoepitheliomas are benign follicular neoplasms most commonly found on the head and neck. Lesions typically appear in childhood or early adulthood as solitary, 2- to 8-mm, firm, flesh-colored papules. The desmoplastic variant, a plaquelike lesion with a central dell, is most often seen on the face of young women. Rarely, multiple lesions that tend to cluster about the central face may be inherited in an autosomal-dominant fashion, alone or in combination with other benign follicular neoplasms, as in Brooke-Spiegler syndrome (▶ Fig. 45.3). Inherited forms have been linked to loss-of-heterozygosity mutations in the cylindromatosis *CYLD* gene, whereas sporadic trichoepitheliomas have been linked to mutations in the *PTCH* tumor suppressor gene. The diagnosis can usually be made clinically, but biopsy may be required to differentiate a solitary lesion from basal cell carcinoma. Shave biopsy or curettage is also an effective treatment option for solitary trichoepitheliomas, but impractical for multiple lesions. Some have suggested that Mohs micrographic surgery is warranted for desmoplastic trichoepitheliomas because of their predilection for cosmetically sensitive areas and rare instances of local invasion. Other modalities for the treatment of multiple trichoepitheliomas that have been described with variable success include dermabrasion; electrosurgery; cryosurgery; ablation with Nd:YAG, Er:YAG, or carbon dioxide lasers; and photodynamic therapy. Medical treatments have included sodium salicylate and prostaglandin A$_1$, a combination of aspirin and adalimumab, and topical imiquimod.

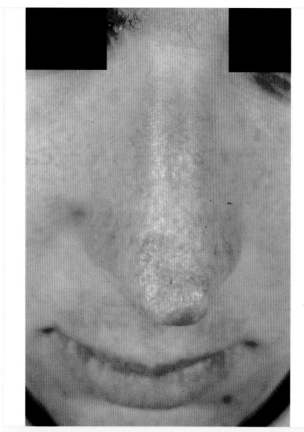

Fig. 45.2 Sebaceous hyperplasia.

45.3.4 Trichilemmoma

Trichilemmoma is a benign adnexal neoplasm believed to be derived at least partially from the outer root sheath of the hair follicle. Clinically, it appears as a flesh-colored papule or small nodule, most commonly on the central face. Sites of involvement include the cheeks, nose, upper cutaneous lip, and eyebrow, or less frequently the eyelid. Trichilemmoma, particularly the desmoplastic variant, may also arise within a nevus sebaceus (▶ Fig. 45.4). Solitary lesions tend to be sporadic, but multiple lesions should raise suspicion for Cowden syndrome, a multiple hamartoma syndrome associated with oral and gastrointestinal papillomatosis, as well as breast, thyroid, and gastrointestinal adenocarcinomas. Autosomal-dominantly inherited mutations of the *PTEN* tumor suppressor gene appear to underlie Cowden-associated lesions, but the pathogenesis of solitary trichilemmomas is less clear. Early suggestions based on histologic features that trichilemmomas represent old viral warts have not been borne out in more recent polymerase chain reaction–based studies looking for human papillomavirus DNA.

Biopsy may be necessary to differentiate trichilemmoma from basal cell carcinoma (BCC) or squamous cell carcinoma (SCC), or to differentiate Cowden syndrome from other genodermatoses characterized by facial adnexal neoplasms. Treatment is purely elective, and modalities are similar to those mentioned in relation to other adnexal neoplasms, including surgical excision, cryotherapy, electrodessication, and ablative laser treatment. Trichilemmal carcinoma, a rare low-grade malignant variant most commonly occurring on the face of elderly patients, is best treated with conservative local excision or Mohs micrographic surgery.

45.3.5 Hemangioma

Hemangiomas are vascular neoplasms that represent benign proliferations of endothelial cells. It is essential to proper management that they be differentiated from vascular malformations—a heterogeneous group of lesions that includes so-called

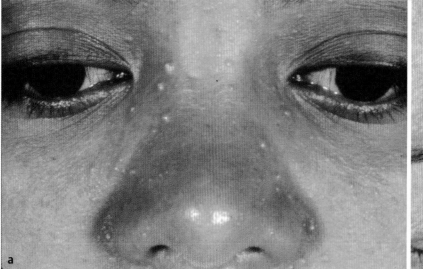
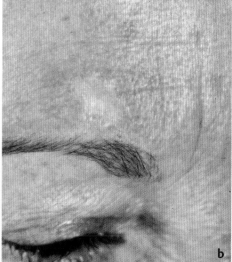

Fig. 45.3 (a) Multiple trichoepitheliomas. (b) Desmoplastic trichoepithelioma.

port-wine stains—which are composed of structurally abnormal vessels arising from errors of embryogenesis. Infantile hemangiomas are typically not present at birth; they appear within the first month of life, undergo a rapid proliferative phase for 6 months, and then, following a quiescent phase, undergo a more gradual involution beginning at roughly 1 year of age. In contrast, vascular malformations, which are nearly always present at birth, may grow slowly over time with the individual, and do not tend to involute. Both types of lesions—hemangiomas and vascular malformations—may be associated with distinct syndromes that require prompt systemic work-up to prevent or attenuate significant morbidity and mortality.

Infantile hemangiomas are the most common benign tumor of childhood, occurring in up to 10% of white infants, and among the most common vascular neoplasms encountered on the head and neck. Girls, children with light skin types, and premature infants are disproportionately affected. Although no formal classification system exists, a number of subtypes have been described based on characteristics such as as level(s) of skin affected (superficial, deep, or mixed) or on morphological characteristics (localized, segmental, multifocal). Superficial "strawberry" hemangiomas typically appear as solitary, bright red, well-demarcated papules or nodules, whereas deep or mixed tumors involving the dermis or subcutis tend to be more blue or flesh-colored (▶ Fig. 45.5). Focal hemangiomas are most often found on the central face at lines of developmental fusion. The presence of five or more focal lesions, or of larger solitary lesions, may indicate an increased risk for involvement of the gastrointestinal tract, particularly the liver. The segmental variety may appear as coalescing papules, a broad plaque, or a large tumor in a segmental, most commonly mandibular distribution.

Large or segmental hemangiomas are more frequently associated with extracutaneous manifestations. Up to one-third of cases may be associated with PHACE syndrome; PHACE is an acronym for a constellation of *p*osterior fossa anomalies, *he*mangiomas, *a*rterial anomalies, *c*ardiac anomalies (most commonly coarctation of the aorta), and *e*ye anomalies. Vascular tumors involving the lower face and neck may also affect the ororpharynx or larynx, potentially resulting in airway compromise. Two other rare vascular tumors distinct from true hemangiomas—the kaposiform hemangioendothelioma and the tufted angioma—can be associated with the Kasabach-Merritt phenomenon, a life-threatening consumptive coagulopathy associated with a decreased platelet count.

By way of contrast, a few well-known vascular malformations and other lesions that are not true hemangiomas bear mention here. The port-wine stain is a typically unilateral capillary malformation present at birth, most commonly in the ophthalmic or maxillary dermatome, that tends to become more prominent with time. Up to one-third of ophthalmic malformations, particularly bilateral lesions, may be associated with ipsilateral vascular malformations of the leptomeninges that can result in seizures and neurologic deficits (Sturge-Weber syndrome).

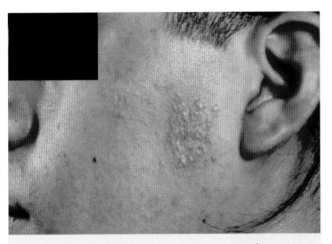
Fig. 45.4 Multiple tricholemommas arising in a nevus sebaceus.

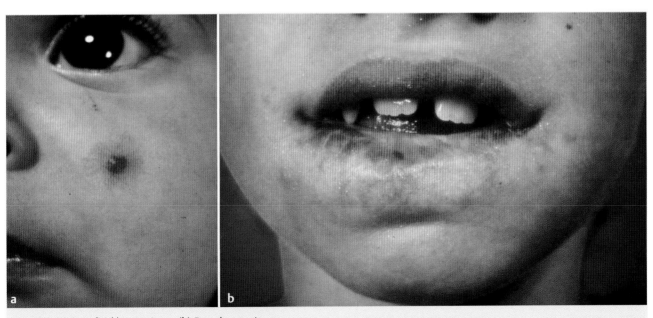
Fig. 45.5 (a) Superficial hemangioma. (b) Deep hemangioma.

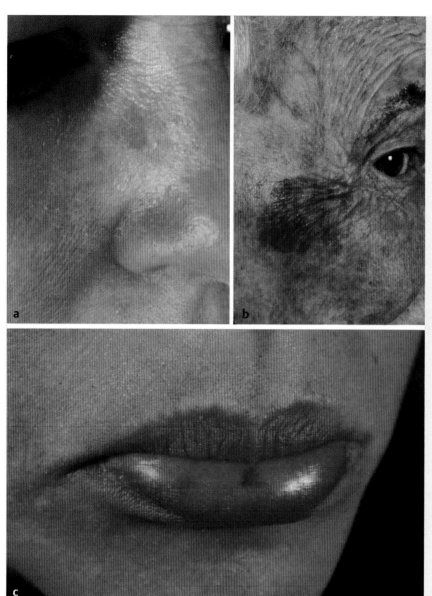

Fig. 45.6 (a–c) Lentigines.

Another, much more commonly encountered vascular malformation is the so-called salmon patch or stork bite, a capillary malformation present at birth on the central forehead or nape of the neck that tends to fade over the first few years of life. The cherry angioma is a 2- to 4-mm red papule representing a dilated and congested small vessel of the upper dermis that appears during adulthood; it is most frequently found on the trunk but also may appear on the head and neck.

The management of hemangiomas has changed dramatically in recent years. Although "watch and wait" is still an appropriate approach for the majority of focal infantile hemangiomas, β-blockers have joined, if not replaced, corticosteroids as the first-line treatment of severely disfiguring or complicated lesions. Since the first report of the successful treatment of severe infantile hemangiomas with intravenous propranolol, a number of case series and prospective trials have demonstrated the efficacy and relative safety of systemic β-blocker therapy. Treatment is generally well tolerated, but reported side effects have

included hypoglycemia, bronchospasm, and hypotension. In addition to corticosteroids, the use of interferon, vincristine, bleomycin, and cyclophosphamide has also been described. Topical propranolol and timolol, as well as topical corticosteroids, have demonstrated usefulness in hastening the regression of smaller, superficial lesions. Pulsed dye, long-pulsed Nd:YAG, and KTP (potassium titanyl phosphate) lasers are also effective in improving the cosmesis of patients with vascular neoplasms.

45.3.6 Lentigo

Solar or actinic lentigines, colloquially known as age spots or liver spots, are benign pigmented lesions, commonly found on the chronically sun-exposed skin of older, light-skinned adults (▶ Fig. 45.6). Their incidence increases with age, affecting 90% of whites older than 50 years of age. The face, neck, forearms, and dorsal hands are most frequently affected. Clinically, lentigines are tan to dark brown or black in color, may appear mottled, and range from a few millimeters to over a centimeter in diameter. Their borders are well defined but may be irregular. There are typically no surface changes such as scale or infiltration. Individuals who had ephilides (freckles) in adolescence or more than than two sunburns after age 20 are at increased risk for lentigines. Like ephilides, lentigines tend to darken in the sun, but they are much more likely to persist year-round.

The diagnosis of lentigines is usually made clinically, but biopsy may be necessary to differentiate them from lentigo maligna, a type of malignant melanoma in situ on chronically sun-damaged skin. Dermoscopy may aid in identifying features concerning for malignancy. Other lesions in the differential diagnosis include nevi and seborrheic keratoses. The treatment of solar lentigines is elective. Ablative cryotherapy is considered first-line treatment, but a wide variety of lasers have also demonstrated benefit. Combination treatment with hydroquinone and topical retinoids produces a less rapid response. The appearance in childhood of multiple facial lentigines, especially on the lips and oral mucosa, may occur as a benign isolated finding but should raise concern for rare familial cancer syndromes such as Peutz-Jeghers syndrome and Carney complex.

45.3.7 Intradermal Nevus

The intradermal nevus (IDN) is a benign melanocytic neoplasm most commonly seen in young children and the elderly. For years, it was widely believed that IDNs were mainly lesions of adulthood, representing the final stage of maturation of acquired melanocytic nevi that "drop down" from the epidermis over time. However, more recent epidemiologic and histologic studies of congenital and acquired nevi suggest that some IDNs may originate within the dermis. Congenital nevi, which are histologically dermal or compound (dermal and epidermal), are present at birth in 1 to 6% of neonates. They are commonly categorized by diameter—ranging from small (< 1.5 cm) to medium (1.5 to 20 cm) to large or "giant" (> 20 cm), which guides their management. Congenital nevi are typically tan to brown but may also appear blue, gray, or black. Acquired IDNs are usually 2 to 6 mm in diameter. They may be endo- or exophytic, dome-shaped, sessile or pedunculated, smooth or papillated papules (► Fig. 45.7). They range in color from flesh-colored to dark brown or black. The lesions may be firm or easily compressible. An older patient may relate a history of slow evolution from a flat, pigmented macule (junctional nevus). The variant most commonly found on the face, known as Miescher nevus, tends to be dome-shaped, firm, smooth, endophytic, and about 5 mm in diameter. Lesions may have overlying vessels or terminal hairs, particularly congenital IDNs. The differential diagnosis of endophytic varieties may include BCC, whereas more exophytic, pedunculated lesions may be mistaken for skin tags (acrochordons) or neurofibromas. Dermoscopy can aid in the diagnosis. Biopsy is often unnecessary but may be required to rule out malignant melanoma or nonmelanoma skin cancer in changing or otherwise clinically concerning lesions.

IDNs are benign, largely asymptomatic lesions, and as such they do not generally require treatment. If removal is desired, biopsy or simple surgical excision is effective for smaller lesions, whereas serial excisions, local, regional, or expanded flaps, and split-thickness or full-thickness skin grafts may be required for larger congenital nevi. Individual and combined laser treatments may improve cosmesis. Although it is well established that individuals with giant congenital nevi (> 20 cm) are at increased risk for developing malignant melanoma and neurocutaneous melanocytosis, an association between common acquired nevi or small congenital nevi and melanoma remains controversial.

45.3.8 Actinic Keratosis

Actinic keratoses (AKs), also known as solar keratoses, are common intraepidermal neoplasms with the potential to evolve into SCC. The prevalence in the United States in 2004 was estimated to be 39.5 million. AKs are generally held to exist in a continuum with SCC; however, the annual risk for malignant transformation of an individual AK is unknown, with reports ranging broadly from less than 0.025% to 16%; one recent prospective study puts the annual risk at 0.6%. Cumulative exposure to UV light, fair skin type, and immunosuppression—particularly in organ transplant recipients—are primary risk factors, as are genetic conditions that predispose to UV sensitivity. UVB-specific mutations of the *TP53* tumor suppressor gene identified in AKs provide molecular evidence of the pathogenic role of sunlight.

The most common clinical presentation of the AK is a pink to red, scaling papule or plaque on a sun-exposed area, most commonly the face, forearms, or dorsal hands. Lesions are typically

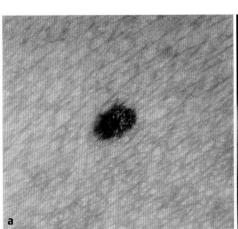
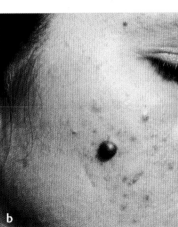

Fig. 45.7 (a) Intradermal nevus. (b) Blue nevus.

2 to 6 mm in diameter but may span several centimeters or occur as multiple discrete papules. The gritty, firmly adherent scale may be more easily felt than seen on a background of chronically sun-damaged skin. Lesions may become hypertrophic, occasionally producing a hyperkeratotic, cone-shaped protuberance known as a cutaneous horn. The differential diagnosis of AK includes SCC, seborrheic keratosis, and verruca vulgaris. The pigmented variant may be confused with BCC or malignant melanoma. Shave biopsy is typically sufficient to make a histologic diagnosis. Actinic or solar cheilosis (sometimes called cheilitis) is a related precancerous neoplasm that occurs on the lower lip. Risk factors are similar to those for AKs. A patient may complain of dry, rough, or painful lips, and physical examination may reveal scaliness, fissures, or ulcerations. Prompt identification of solar cheilosis is particularly important, given the greater risk for transformation into SCC and for metastasis from the lip than from other cutaneous sites.

The treatment of AKs prevents progression to SCC and its associated morbidity and mortality. It also relieves symptoms such as tenderness and pruritus. Cryotherapy is the most common treatment modality in the United States, particularly for solitary lesions. Biopsy, curettage, or surgical excision can each provide the benefit of a definitive diagnosis in addition to removing the lesion. Topical 5-fluorouracil—a chemotherapeutic agent that interferes with DNA synthesis—and imiquimod—a topical immune modulator—are both effective, generally well-tolerated, "field-directed" therapies that are especially useful for larger areas with multiple AKs. Photodynamic therapy, although expensive and not as widely available, is also effective. Systemic retinoids, lasers, chemical peels, and dermabrasion are less well-studied modalities.

Spontaneous remission of AKs occurs in 10 to 25% of lesions annually. This phenomenon, combined with the high prevalence of AKs, the relatively low annual risk that an individual AK will transform into SCC, and the high cost of treatment (estimated at $1.1 billion in the United States in 2004), has led some to suggest that clinical monitoring might be an acceptable management approach. However, given that most patients have multiple AKs and keep them for many years, their risk for SCC is considerably higher than the individual lesion annual progression rates might suggest. The significant morbidity and mortality associated with SCC, combined with the symptom relief provided, are sufficient to recommend treatment.

45.3.9 Basal Cell Carcinoma

BCC is the most common malignancy in the United States, with estimates of lifetime risk in fair-skinned individuals approaching 1 in 3. It accounts for more than 80% of the approximately 2 million nonmelanoma skin cancers diagnosed each year, and its incidence is rising. Exposure to UV light is the primary risk factor for the development of BCC. Related risk factors include fair skin type, occupations with greater outdoor exposure, and genetic disorders that increase sensitivity to UV light. Ionizing radiation, arsenic, and immune suppression are also established risk factors. The molecular pathogenesis of the majority of BCCs is thought to be associated with deregulation of the hedgehog signaling pathway, which is involved in cell proliferation.

Roughly 80% of BCCs occur on the head and neck, followed by sun-exposed areas of the trunk. There are three clinical BCC variants, each with a different presentation (▶ Fig. 45.8). The classic nodular BCC lesion appears as a firm, flesh-colored or "pearly" pink papule or nodule, 2 to 6 mm in diameter, with overlying telangiectasia and rolled borders. Central ulceration or crusting may be present. The differential diagnosis frequently includes hyperplasia of sebaceous glands and intradermal nevi. Amelanotic melanoma may have a similar appearance. Superficial BCC presents as an erythematous, scaly patch or thin plaque that is sometimes mistaken for SCC. Both nodular and superficial forms may be pigmented, mimicking melanocytic lesions. Morpheaform BCC, sometimes called fibrosing or infiltrative BCC, often appears as an indurated, scarlike plaque with poorly defined borders. Shave or punch biopsy is sufficient to make an accurate histologic diagnosis in most cases.

BCC is typically a slow-growing tumor. Metastasis is rare, occurring in 0.025 to 0.55% of cases, although larger tumors may have increased rates. However, neglected tumors can be locally invasive and result in significant disfigurement. Standard surgical excision with appropriate margins or electrodessication and curettage are generally thought to achieve 5-year cure rates of 95% for small, "low-risk" lesions on the neck, trunk, or extremities with nonaggressive histologic features. Radiotherapy can be an effective treatment modality for patients who are poor surgical candidates or who have inoperable tumors, or as adjuvant therapy for those with deeply invasive or metastatic tumors. Topical imiquimod is an option for the treatment of superficial BCC.

Mohs micrographic surgery is recommended for the treatment of "high-risk" BCC because of improved margin control and lower rates of recurrence. Characteristics of high-risk tumors include the following: tumor diameter larger than 2 mm, location on the ears or central face, neglected or long-standing tumor, incompletely excised or recurrent tumor, aggressive histologic subtype, previous irradiation, and perineural or perivascular invasion. The role of Mohs micrographic surgery in the treatment of low-risk tumors on the body remains controversial. Hedgehog pathway–inhibiting medications have shown promise for the treatment of inoperable and metastatic disease.

45.3.10 Squamous Cell Carcinoma

SCC is the second most common cutaneous malignancy after BCC, accounting for roughly 20% of all skin cancers. An estimated 250,000 new diagnoses are made each year in the United States alone, and evidence suggests that the incidence is rising worldwide, at least in the elderly population. Although not as common as BCC, it is much more likely to metastasize and is responsible for most nonmelanoma skin cancer–related deaths. Risk factors for development are similar to those for AKs— namely, genetic predisposition (fair skin type) and cumulative UV exposure. Men are disproportionately affected at a ratio approaching 3:1. Chronically immunosuppressed recipients of solid organ transplants are at a 65-fold increased risk for developing SCC in comparison with the normal population. SCC also has a propensity to develop in chronic ulcers or scars, or in

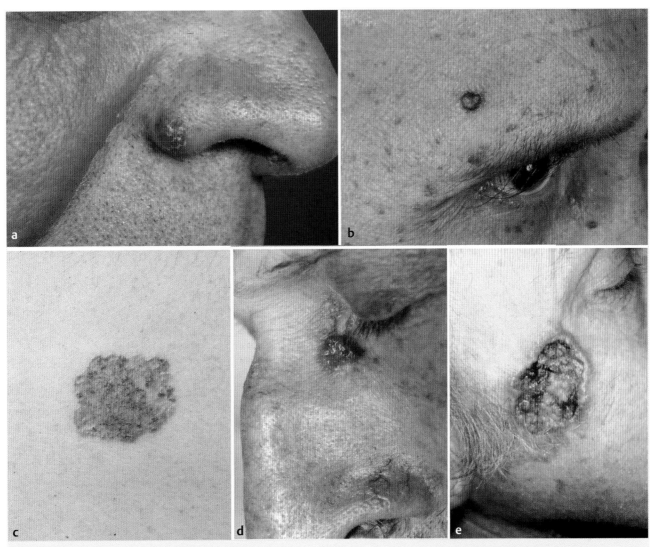

Fig. 45.8 (a) Nodular basal cell carcinoma (BCC). (b) Pigmented BCC. (c) Superficial BCC. (d) Nodular BCC, ulcerating. (e) Ulcerative BCC.

areas exposed to occupational or therapeutic irradiation. AKs are considered precursor lesions, although most AKs will never develop into SCC. SCC in situ, also known as Bowen disease, is confined to the epidermis but has the potential to develop into invasive SCC if left untreated.

SCC is most commonly found on the head and neck, especially the cheeks, nose, and ears (▶ Fig. 45.9). Clinically, SCC and AKs can be difficult to distinguish from each other. Both typically appear as nonhealing, 2- to 6-mm, pink to red scaling papules or plaques, although SCC is more likely to ulcerate. Lesions may be itchy or painful, or they may bleed with manipulation. The keratoacanthoma variant presents in the same distribution as a rapidly growing, symmetric, crateriform nodule with a central keratotic core. Verrucous carcinoma is rare variant that may present as a warty or cauliflower-like neoplasm within the oral cavity. The differential diagnosis of SCC includes AK, verruca vulgaris, and seborrheic keratosis. The nodular keratoacanthoma may be confused clinically with BCC. The diagnosis can often be made clinically but should be confirmed histologically. Shave biopsy yields adequate tissue in most cases.

Surgical excision is the treatment of choice for SCC. Standard excision with 4-mm margins has been suggested to achieve a 95% cure rate for small, primary, "lower-risk," invasive SCC of the trunk, extremities, or neck. Other physical modalities, such as electrodessication and curettage and cryotherapy, have demonstrated similar cure rates for low-risk tumors. Fractionated radiation monotherapy may be appropriate for early-stage lesions in patients who are unable to tolerate surgery. The authors, however prefer to use radiation therapy as an adjunct to surgery for SCC with perineural involvement. There is limited evidence supporting the use of topical 5-fluorouracil for the treatment of SCC in situ.

Reported recurrence rates following standard excision of low-risk primary SCCs range from 5 to 8% and are substantially increased in "high-risk" tumors (▶ Table 45.1). SCCs fulfilling any of following criteria are generally considered to be at high risk for recurrence or metastasis: diameter larger than 2 cm, depth to more than 2 mm, subcutaneous tissue invasion, previous recurrence, tumors arising in scars, or anatomical location on the scalp, ears, eyelids, nose, and lips. High-risk tumors,

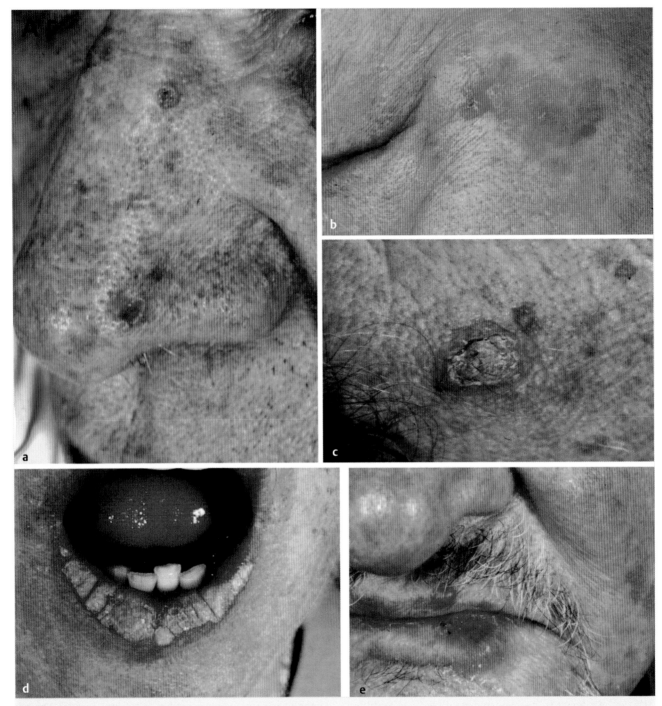

Fig. 45.9 (a) Bowen disease. (b) Squamous cell carcinoma. (c) Keratoacanthoma. (d) Actinic cheilitis. (e) Squamous cell carcinoma.

particularly those in cosmetically important areas, are preferably treated with Mohs micrographic surgery for improved margin control and tissue conservation. Perineural invasion, although it occurs in only 2 to 14% of patients with SCC of the head and neck, is associated with higher rates of recurrence and metastasis, most commonly to the parotid gland or regional lymph nodes. Nodal disease may occur in approximately 5% of cases, but reported rates vary widely. Postoperative radiotherapy, sentinel lymph node biopsy, and/or dissection of draining lymphatic basins may be required to achieve lasting local

control of SCC with perineural invasion. Radiotherapy alone may also be used to treat patients with significant medical co-morbidities that preclude surgical resection.

45.3.11 Lentigo Maligna

Lentigo maligna (LM) is a form of malignant melanoma in situ—that is, confined to the epidermis—that occurs on the severely sun-damaged skin of light-skinned, elderly individuals. It accounts for 4 to 15% of all melanomas, and 10 to 26% of all head and neck melanomas. Risk factors for the development of LM include light skin type, age, residence in locales with increased UV exposure, cumulative UV exposure, and a history of severe sunburns. LM is rarely seen in patients younger than 40 years or age, and its incidence increases with age, peaking in the seventh and eighth decades. The nomenclature surrounding this cutaneous malignancy can be a source of confusion. LM is to be differentiated from *lentigo maligna melanoma* (LMM), which invades the dermis and has a very different prognosis. LM is also distinct from the *solar* or *actinic lentigo*, sometimes referred to simply as *lentigo*, a nearly ubiquitous benign pigmented lesion on the sun-exposed skin of older white adults.

Approximately 90% of LMs occur on the face, with a predilection for the cheek. Clinically, LM is characterized by a slowly growing, asymmetric macule or patch with variegated color and an ill-defined, irregular border (▸ Fig. 45.10). Lesions may range in color from tan to dark brown or black. A rare amelanotic variant may present as an ill-defined, erythematous patch resembling SCC or BCC. The differential diagnosis includes solar or actinic lentigo, SK, melanocytic nevus, and LMM. A Wood lamp may aid in defining the lesion margins from the surrounding skin. Excisional biopsy of smaller lesions with 1- to 3-mm margins is ideal but is not feasible for larger lesions, particularly

those in cosmetically sensitive areas. In such cases, incisional or full-thickness punch biopsy of the darkest, most palpable, or otherwise clinically concerning area of the lesion is recommended. Sampling error can occur, however, and multiple punch biopsies may be required to make the diagnosis. Shave biopsy, although commonly practiced, is not traditionally recommended because it can obscure proper evaluation of the Breslow depth, the most important prognostic indicator in melanoma.

Surgical excision of LM is the gold standard of treatment. Complete excision is considered curative, but recurrence with standard excision is relatively common, with rates ranging from 7 to 20%. The 1992 National Institutes of Health consensus statement and the 2012 National Comprehensive Cancer Network clinical practice guidelines advise 5-mm margins for the treatment of malignant melanoma in situ. However, these recommendations are largely based on malignant melanoma in situ of the trunk and extremities. Studies of LM of the head and neck have shown the standard 5-mm margin to be inadequate in up to 50% of cases. Margins of more than 15 mm have rarely been required in studies of staged excisional techniques and Mohs micrographic surgery, which have demonstrated significantly lower recurrence rates. Nonsurgical treatment methods such as cryotherapy, laser ablation, irradiation, and topical imiquimod have much higher recurrence rates and should be used with caution as adjuvant therapy or monotherapy for patients who have unresectable lesions or are unable to tolerate surgery. Incompletely treated, lentigo maligna can progress to invasive LMM. Reported rates vary widely from 5 to 50%, but lesional size appears to be correlated with risk. LM that has progressed to LMM carries a prognosis similar to that of other invasive melanoma subtypes.

Table 45.1 Recurrence rates of squamous cell carcinoma after Mohs excision and standard excision

Scenario	Mohs excision	Standard excision
SCC of the lip	3.1%	10.9%
SCC of the ear	5.3%	18.7%
Locally recurrent SCC	10.0%	23.3%
SCC with perineural invasion	0%	47%
SCC larger than 2 cm	25.2%	41.7%
Poorly differentiated SCC	32.6%	53.6%

Abbreviation: SCC, squamous cell carcinoma.
Note: Recurrence rates are significantly lower after Mohs excision in certain circumstances.

45.4 Roundsmanship

- Approximately 80% of cases of nonmelanoma skin cancer and 90% of cases of lentigo maligna are found on the head and neck.
- A *macule* is a circumscribed, flat lesion with color change that is *up to 1 cm* in size. A *patch* has similar characteristics but is

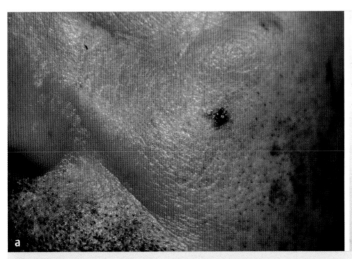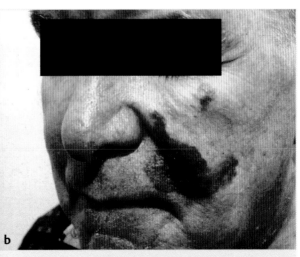

Fig. 45.10 (a) Lentigo maligna (melanoma in situ). **(b)** Lentigo maligna melanoma.

larger than 1 cm. A *papule* is a circumscribed, elevated, superficial, solid lesion that is *up to 1 cm* in size. A *plaque* has similar characteristics but is *larger than 1 cm.* A *nodule* is also elevated and is *up to 1 cm* in size, but it has more depth than a papule. A *mass* is a lesion with a depth *of more than 1 cm.*

45.5 Recommended Reading

[1] Berman B, Bienstock L, Kuritzky L, Mayeaux EJ, Tyring SK Primary Care Education ConsortiumTexas Academy of Family Physicians. Actinic keratoses: sequelae and treatments. Recommendations from a consensus panel. J Fam Pract 2006; 55: 1–8

[2] Bettencourt MS, Prieto VG, Shea CR. Trichoepithelioma: a 19-year clinicopathologic re-evaluation. J Cutan Pathol 1999; 26: 398–404

[3] Brownstein MH, Mehregan AH, Bikowski JB, Lupulescu A, Patterson JC. The dermatopathology of Cowden's syndrome. Br J Dermatol 1979; 100: 667–673

[4] Clark WH, From L, Bernardino EA, Mihm MC. The histogenesis and biologic behavior of primary human malignant melanomas of the skin. Cancer Res 1969; 29: 705–727

[5] Cohen LM, McCall MW, Zax RH. Mohs micrographic surgery for lentigo maligna and lentigo maligna melanoma. A follow-up study. Dermatol Surg 1998; 24: 673–677

[6] Dickie B, Dasgupta R, Nair R et al. Spectrum of hepatic hemangiomas: management and outcome. J Pediatr Surg 2009; 44: 125–133

[7] Elwood JM, Gallagher RP, Worth AJ, Wood WS, Pearson JC. Etiological differences between subtypes of cutaneous malignant melanoma: Western Canada Melanoma Study. J Natl Cancer Inst 1987; 78: 37–44

[8] Finn MC, Glowacki J, Mulliken JB. Congenital vascular lesions: clinical application of a new classification. J Pediatr Surg 1983; 18: 894–900

[9] Gallagher RP, Hill GB, Bajdik CD et al. Sunlight exposure, pigmentary factors, and risk of nonmelanocytic skin cancer. I. Basal cell carcinoma. Arch Dermatol 1995; 131: 157–163

[10] Glogau RG. The risk of progression to invasive disease. J Am Acad Dermatol 2000; 42: 23–24

[11] Headington JT, French AJ. Primary neoplasms of the hair follicle. Histogenesis and classification. Arch Dermatol 1962; 86: 430–441

[12] Holman CD, Armstrong BK. Cutaneous malignant melanoma and indicators of total accumulated exposure to the sun: an analysis separating histogenetic types. J Natl Cancer Inst 1984; 73: 75–82

[13] Holman CD, Armstrong BK, Heenan PJ. Relationship of cutaneous malignant melanoma to individual sunlight-exposure habits. J Natl Cancer Inst 1986; 76: 403–414

[14] Kasabach HH, Merritt KK. Capillary hemangioma with extensive purpura: report of a case. Am J Dis Child 1940; 59: 1063–1070

[15] Kopf AW, Bart RS, Hennessey P. Congenital nevocytic nevi and malignant melanomas. J Am Acad Dermatol 1979; 1: 123–130

[16] Léauté-Labrèze C, Dumas de la Roque E, Hubiche T, Boralevi F, Thambo JB, Taïeb A. Propranolol for severe hemangiomas of infancy. N Engl J Med 2008; 358: 2649–2651

[17] Lewis EJ, Dahl MV. On standard definitions: 33 years hence. Arch Dermatol 1997; 133: 1169

[18] McGuire LK, Disa JJ, Lee EH, Busam KJ, Nehal KS. Melanoma of the lentigo maligna subtype: diagnostic challenges and current treatment paradigms. Plast Reconstr Surg 2012; 129: 288e–299e

[19] Miller DL, Weinstock MA. Nonmelanoma skin cancer in the United States: incidence. J Am Acad Dermatol 1994; 30: 774–778

[20] Mulliken JB, Glowacki J. Hemangiomas and vascular malformations in infants and children: a classification based on endothelial characteristics. Plast Reconstr Surg 1982; 69: 412–422

[21] Newell GR, Sider JG, Bergfelt L, Kripke ML. Incidence of cutaneous melanoma in the United States by histology with special reference to the face. Cancer Res 1988; 48: 5036–5041

[22] Rubin AI, Chen EH, Ratner D. Basal-cell carcinoma. N Engl J Med 2005; 353: 2262–2269

[23] Smith MA, Manfield PA. The natural history of salmon patches in the first year of life. Br J Dermatol 1962; 74: 31–33

[24] Waner M, North PE, Scherer KA, Frieden IJ, Waner A, Mihm MC. The nonrandom distribution of facial hemangiomas. Arch Dermatol 2003; 139: 869–875

[25] Xu G, Lv R, Zhao Z, Huo R. Topical propranolol for treatment of superficial infantile hemangiomas. J Am Acad Dermatol 2012; 67: 1210–1213

[26] Ziegler A, Jonason AS, Leffell DJ et al. Sunburn and p53 in the onset of skin cancer. Nature 1994; 372: 773–776

46 Mohs Micrographic Surgery

John A. Carucci and Jesse M. Lewin

46.1 Introduction

Skin cancers are the most common human cancers. They can result in significant morbidity and even mortality when left untreated. Depending on histologic type and anatomical location, skin cancers may be amenable to excision or to destruction or ablation by radiation treatment. Skin cancers on the head and neck or selected aggressive or recurrent skin cancers at other anatomical sites may be best treated by Mohs micrographic surgery. Mohs micrographic surgery is the only technique that allows a complete evaluation of the entire peripheral and deep surgical margin. This in turn allows maximal conservation of normal tissue with optimization of function and cosmesis.

46.2 Historical Perspective

In the 1930s, Dr. Frederic E. Mohs, a general surgeon, developed a technique of excisional surgery in which a complete margin of skin cancer was plotted in three dimensions. The procedure was initially termed *chemosurgery* because it involved chemical fixation in situ before excision. Zinc chloride, used as a fixative, was combined with a permeant and an agglutinant, which were applied to the tissue in vivo while cytologic detail was maintained for microscopic evaluation. After this process, the tumor, along with a narrow margin of healthy tissue, was excised, and frozen sections were generated with the deep and peripheral margins in a single horizontal plane, allowing the tumor to be precisely mapped microscopically. In Mohs' original procedure, this process was repeated the following day until all residual tumor was removed, and the wounds were often left to heal by secondary intention. Later, the process was modified; zinc chloride fixation was replaced with local anesthesia and frozen section processing, which expedited the procedure while maintaining high cure rates. Eventually, in 1985, the term *chemosurgery* was replaced by *Mohs micrographic surgery* (MMS) to more accurately describe the process of fresh tissue fixation followed by the microscopic evaluation of layers of tissue. MMS was embraced by dermatologists and has become a technique performed only by dermatologic surgeons with special fellowship training in MMS.

46.3 Technique

Mohs surgeons for the most part perform MMS in an office setting with the patient under local anesthesia. At times, if a particular tumor requires an interdisciplinary approach (e.g., an aggressive tumor infiltrating vital structures in the orbit or involving the parotid gland or facial nerve), MMS may be performed in the operating room with the patient under general anesthesia and in conjunction with other surgical subspecialists, such as otolaryngologists or ophthalmologists.

In order to perform MMS and obtain an excellent repair, the surgeon must ensure that well-trained assistants and a laboratory equipped for processing and reading the fresh frozen sections are available. The tumor is initially identified based upon a prior biopsy site and preferably photographs and triangulation from the physician who initially performed the biopsy. The site is marked and infiltrated with local anesthesia. The tumor is then debulked with a curet, during which process macroscopically normal tissue can be further distinguished from malignant tissue by means of the surgeon's tactile sensation during curettage. Next, the specimen is excised tangentially, with a 45-degree angle initially. This beveled edge is in direct contrast to the 90-degree edge obtained with a standard excision. The beveled edge is crucial for evaluation of the entire surgical margin after the specimen has been mapped and processed via frozen section (▶ Fig. 46.1 and ▶ Fig. 46.2). Optimal margin control is obtained by examination of the entire perimeter of the specimen and contiguous deep margin. Meticulous mapping allows the directed extirpation of any residual tumor. A key defining feature of MMS is that the surgeon excises, maps, and reviews the specimen personally, minimizing the chance of error in

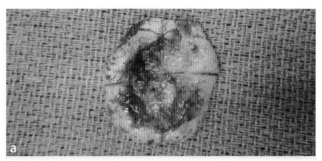
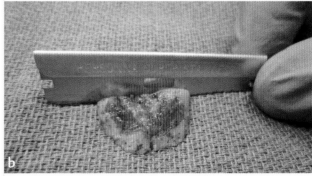
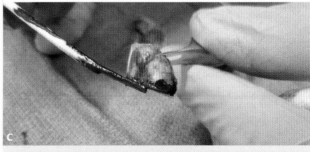

Fig. 46.1 (a) Specimen preparation. (b) The tumor and surrounding area of clinically normal skin are removed tangentially. (c) The tumor is sectioned before being marked with ink. Black and red ink are used to mark the deep aspect of each section, corresponding to a specified area of the Mohs map.

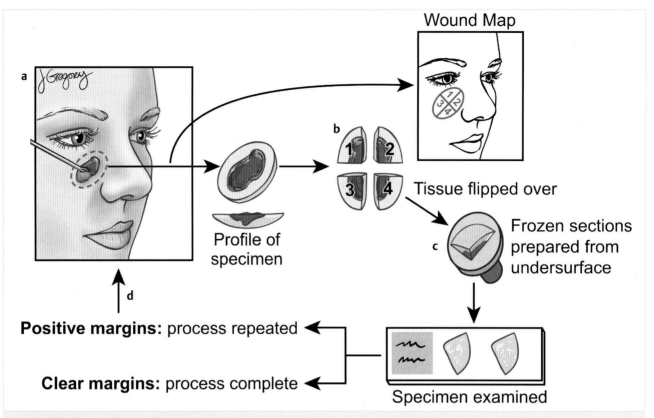

Fig. 46.2 Schematic representation of a Mohs procedure. (**a**) Initial debulking of the tumor by curettage is followed by tangential removal of the tumor with a margin of clinically normal-appearing skin. (**b**) The specimen is divided and inked to correspond to the map, allowing precise localization of the remaining areas of positivity. (**c**) Frozen sections are prepared, allowing visualization of the undersurface and peripheral margin ("worm's-eye view"). (**d**) Remaining areas of positivity are identified, localized, mapped, and excised until a clear margin is obtained.

tissue interpretation and orientation. If the Mohs surgeon, who is also acting as the pathologist, notes persistent tumor on the margins of a section, it is marked and excised tangentially in an additional stage limited to the area of persistent tumor. This process is repeated until the tumor margins are free of disease. The wound is then usually managed by the Mohs surgeon, who employs measures ranging from secondary intention healing to flaps and grafts, depending on the anatomical location, cosmetic subunits involved, and size of the defect. In some cases, a multidisciplinary approach may be used, and surgical subspecialists from otolaryngology, ophthalmology, and surgical oncology may be involved.

MMS has gained acceptance as the treatment of choice for recurrent skin cancers, as well as for primary skin cancers located at anatomical sites requiring maximal tissue conservation for the preservation of function and cosmesis. This is particularly relevant to dermatologic and head and neck surgeons approaching patients with facial cutaneous malignancies, for whom the desire to avoid disfigurement and functional impairment is paramount and can lead to the inadvertent performance of inadequate standard excisions. MMS allows the surgeon to be flexible in the setting of positive margins and to tailor the reconstruction in real time rather than having to bring the patient back for a second procedure if positive margins are identified by permanent section. As will be discussed in depth in the following sections, it is also crucial to respect the insidious

nature of certain subtypes of aggressive cutaneous malignancies and to approach them knowing the limitations as well as the strengths of MMS.

46.4 Indications

46.4.1 Nonmelanoma Skin Cancer

Each year, approximately 2 million cases of nonmelanoma skin cancer (basal cell carcinoma and squamous cell carcinoma) are diagnosed in the United States. There are more skin cancers in the population of the United States than there are all other cancers combined, and it is estimated that one in five Americans will develop skin cancer during their lifetime (more than 95% will be nonmelanoma skin cancer). As discussed above, MMS facilitates optimal margin control and the conservation of normal tissue in the management of nonmelanoma skin cancer. Although the detailed indications for MMS are beyond the scope of this chapter, the American Academy of Dermatology has outlined general guidelines, which include (1) high risk for local recurrence, (2) areas requiring tissue preservation, and (3) high risk for metastasis. Other treatment modalities, such as simple excision, electrodessication and curettage, cryosurgery, topical chemotherapy, and radiation therapy, may be used in other situations.

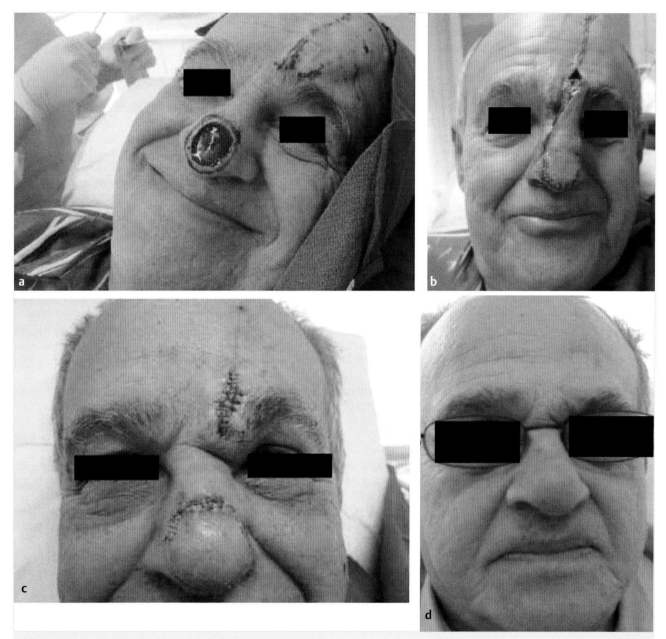

Fig. 46.3 Basal cell carcinoma (BCC) may extend far beyond what is expected on clinical examination. (**a**) BCC with perineural invasion involving most of the nasal tip. (**b**) Paramedian forehead flap repair. (**c**) Pedicle flap division. (**d**) Four-month follow-up.

46.4.2 Basal Cell Carcinoma

Basal cell carcinoma (BCC), a malignant neoplasm derived from nonkeratinizing cells that originate in the basal layer of the epidermis, is the most common cancer in humans. The pathogenesis of BCC involves exposure of the skin to ultraviolet (UV) light, particularly the UVB spectrum (290 to 320 nm), which induces mutations in tumor suppressor genes. A latency period of 20 to 50 years has been described between the time of UV damage and clinical onset of the tumor. Thus, in most cases, BCC develops on sun-exposed skin in elderly people, most commonly the head and neck, making it an entity that is often encountered by head and neck surgeons.

Clinically, BCCs may be recognized by their translucency, ulceration, telangiectasia, and rolled borders; however, it is important to note that features may vary for the different clinical subtypes, which include nodular (the most common subtype on the head and neck), superficial, morpheaform, and pigmented BCCs and fibroepithelioma of Pinkus.

For the most part, BCCs tend to be indolent tumors; however, when located on the ear, nose, eyelid, or lip, they are part of the "H" zone where MMS is indicated because of the high recurrence rate and potential to invade locally, resulting in substantial tissue damage to vital structures. One of the most common sites for BCC is the nose, where tumors may extend far beyond what may be expected based on clinical examination (▶ Fig. 46.3). In addition to the clinical subtypes of BCC, there are histologic subtypes that range from less aggressive patterns, such as nodular and superficial, to more aggressive patterns, such as infiltrative, micronodular, and sclerosing or morpheaform. The aggressive subtypes typically are more poorly defined clinically with less predictable radial growth patterns, leading to greater subclinical extension of tumor. When viewed during the traditional "bread loaf" processing of permanent sections, these areas of tumor extension can be missed, leading to a false-negative result.

When BCCs on the face are incompletely excised, these tumors recur between 12% and 41% of the time. It has been demonstrated that MMS has a 99% cure rate for primary BCCs, compared with 91.3% for other methods. In terms of recurrence, the rate of second recurrence of BBCs after treatment with MMS is 5.6%, as opposed to 17.6% after standard excision, 9.8% after radiation therapy, and 40% after curettage and desiccation. When the surgeon approaches the patient with a recurrent facial BCC, it is crucial to note that several recent studies have demonstrated greater efficacy of tumor clearance with MMS than with standard excision.

As mentioned briefly above, although most BCCs are indolent, slowly invading tumors, both perineural invasion and metastatic BCC can occur. The estimated incidence of metastatic BCC has been reported to be from less than 0.003% to 0.5%. Perineural invasion, which is defined as the observation of malignant cells in the perineural space of nerves, has been reported in fewer than 0.2% of cases. When perineural invasion is detected, every effort should be made to clear the tumor, preferably by MMS, at times employing an interdisciplinary approach. Patients with gross perineural invasion as indicated by neurologic symptoms will benefit from preoperative magnetic resonance imaging to assess the extent of tumor spread. Classic examples include brow paralysis due to involvement of the temporal branch of the facial nerve and midface paresthesias secondary to involvement of the trigeminal nerve. The estimated incidence of metastatic BCC has been reported to be approximately 0.0028% (28 cases per 1 million diagnoses of BCC) but has been cited to be as high as 0.5%. Relevant to otolaryngologists, more than 80% of metastatic BCCs originate from primary BCCs of the head and neck. Although the topic is beyond the scope of this chapter, studies are under way of molecular pharmacotherapy to target the hedgehog signaling pathway, thought to be responsible for the pathogenesis of BCC, and a new drug, vismodegib, has been approved by the FDA for the treatment of metastatic BCC.

MMS provides definitive surgical management of facial cutaneous malignancies. In addition, another factor to be considered is that the psychosocial implications of head and neck surgery and the resulting reconstruction and scarring cannot be underestimated. Given the morbidity associated with residual tumors after failed standard excisions and treatment with other modalities, and the rare recurrence after MMS, it is important for the surgeon to consider the psychological trauma and anxiety associated with multiple procedures in this region. One large prospective cohort study found that MMS was an independent factor for higher rates of long-term patient satisfaction when compared with standard excision or curettage and desiccation. In terms of guidance for patients following the surgical management of BCC, ongoing total-body skin cancer screenings by a dermatologist, sun protection measures, and skin self-examinations should be recommended because an estimated 40 to 50% of patients with primary BCC will develop at least one or more BCCs within 5 years.

46.4.3 Squamous Cell Carcinoma

Squamous cell carcinoma (SCC) is a neoplasm of keratinizing cells that shows malignant characteristics, including anaplasia, rapid growth, local invasion, and metastatic potential. More than 250,000 cases of SCC are diagnosed in the United States per year, making it the second most common human cancer after BCC. Whereas the behavior of BCC is determined by histologic phenotype, as described above, the risk for recurrence and morbidity in patients with SCCs is related to the cellular differentiation and depth of invasion of the neoplasm into the reticular dermis and subcutis.

As opposed to BCC, which is thought to arise de novo, SCC involving the epidermis alone (termed SCC in situ) tends to arise in association with preexisting actinic keratoses, most commonly on sun-damaged skin. Clinically, SCC often presents as an erythematous, scaling patch or a slightly elevated plaque; however, in the immunocompromised host, a more aggressive phenotype may be seen, including metastatic disease. Although SCC in situ is considered to have little to no risk for metastasis, invasive SCC can originate in neglected SCC in situ (▶ Fig. 46.4) and metastasize. The incidence of metastasis of invasive SCC is 3 to 5%. A higher incidence (10 to 30%) is associated with SCC arising on mucosal surfaces (lip, genitalia) and on sites of prior injury (scars, chronic ulcers). It is also important to note that immunosuppressed patients, such as those who have received organ transplants, are a special high-risk group in whom the incidence of SCC is increased more than 60-fold compared with that in the general population. Perineural invasion is associated with a high risk for recurrence and potential metastasis and may be observed in tumors thought to be otherwise low-risk on clinical examination (▶ Fig. 46.5).

For SCC on the head and neck, recurrence rates after MMS are lower than after traditional excisional surgery in primary SCC

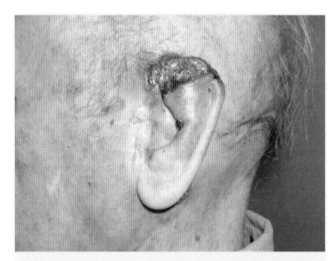

Fig. 46.4 Squamous cell carcinoma (SCC) may eventuate in local recurrence and metastasis. A patient with untreated SCC that continued to invade locally and subsequently metastasized to regional lymph nodes.

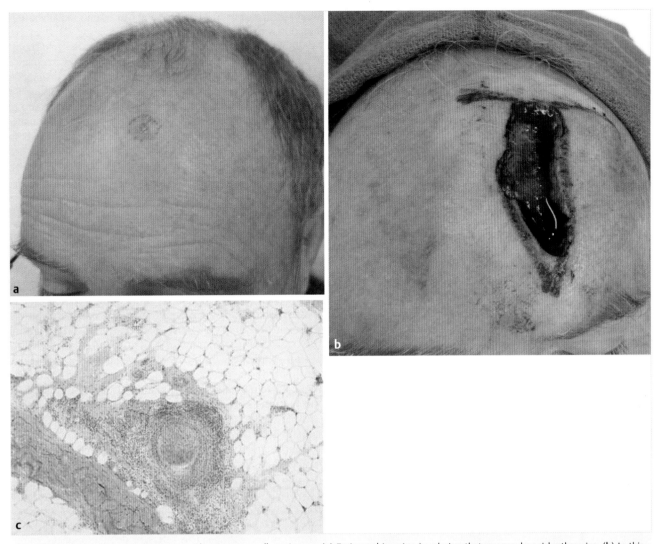

Fig. 46.5 Perineural invasion can occur with squamous cell carcinoma. **(a)** Perineural invasion in a lesion that appears low-risk otherwise. **(b)** In this case, perineural invasion involved the supratrochlear nerve, and multiple stages of Mohs surgery were required to achieve a tumor-free plane. **(c)** Microscopic view of perineural invasion from a Mohs section.

of the ear (3.1% vs 10.9%), primary SCC of the lip (5.8% vs 18.7%), recurrent SCC (10.0% vs 23.3%), SCC with perineural invasion (0% vs. 47%), SCC larger than 2 cm (25.2% vs 41.7%), and poorly differentiated SCC (32.6% vs 53.6%). The literature has reflected variations in the management of patients with SCC and perineural invasion, but several authors encourage interdisciplinary evaluation of these patients by a radiation oncologist for consideration of radiation therapy.

To highlight one anatomical site germane to head and neck surgeons, it is important to note that SCC of the scalp may be particularly aggressive and warrants careful management. This may be due to "field disease" or "field cancerization," which refers to the confluence of extensive actinic keratoses and SCCs with follicular involvement that is associated with higher-than-expected recurrence rates after superficially destructive measures leading to difficulty achieving negative margins. In addition, the extensive vasculature and lymphatic drainage patterns of the scalp permit penetration and spread of the tumor. One hazard of this lymphovascular network includes the potential for in-transit metastases or foci of cutaneous SCC. In-transit

lesions arise within dermal or subcutaneous tissue that is distinct from the primary tumor site. They occur between the site of the primary or recurrent tumor and the closest regional lymph nodes and are thought to represent local lymphatic metastases (▶ Fig. 46.6). It is critical to evaluate these patients for nodal and distant metastases. The in-transit lesions may be removed by either standard excision or MMS, followed by postoperative radiation therapy. MMS can be useful in cases in which there is difficulty distinguishing solitary in-transit metastasis from deep marginal recurrence.

46.4.4 Melanoma

Melanoma, a malignancy arising from melanocytes, is among the most common forms of cancer in young adults. The incidence of melanoma is rising worldwide; in the United States, the estimated lifetime risk for invasive melanoma is 1 in 1,500 for persons born in 1935, 1 in 600 for those born in 1960, and 1 in 62 for those born in 2006 (1 in 34 if in situ melanoma is included). Risk factors for developing melanoma include a history

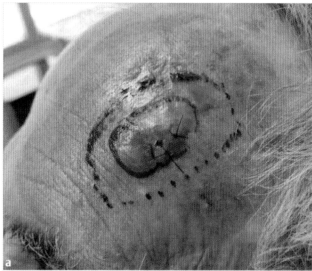

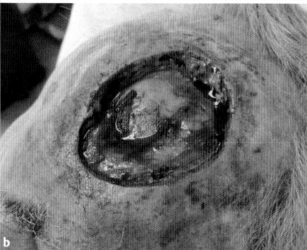

Fig. 46.6 (a) In-transit metastasis from primary cutaneous squamous cell carcinoma (SCC). (b) In-transit metastasis from SCC in a transplant recipient. Intraoperative view of removal before complete clearance was achieved.

of sunburns and/or heavy sun exposure, blue or green eyes, blonde or red hair, fair complexion, more than 100 typical nevi, any atypical nevi, prior personal or family history of melanoma, and certain genetic mutations. Melanoma has the potential to metastasize to regional lymph nodes and distant organs, including liver, bone, and brain. There are four major subtypes of primary cutaneous melanoma, listed in order of frequency of occurrence from highest to lowest: (1) superficial spreading melanoma (60 to 70%); (2) nodular melanoma (15 to 30%); (3) lentigo maligna melanoma (5 to 15%); and (4) acral lentiginous melanoma (5 to 10%). The prognosis for a patient with melanoma is proportional to the depth of invasion of the tumor; patients with malignant melanoma in situ (tumor confined to the epidermis) have an excellent prognosis and a high cure rate after excision. The term *lentigo maligna melanoma* refers to melanoma in situ occurring on sun-damaged skin; it is is most often encountered on the head and neck and may progress to invasive lentigo maligna melanoma. It is typically a slowly growing

tumor with a centrifugal pattern and thus grows radially as opposed to vertically.

Although wide local surgical excision remains the gold standard in the treatment of melanoma, there is growing acceptance and utilization of MMS for melanoma, particularly malignant melanoma in situ and thin melanomas. Excision margins for melanoma range from narrow (0.5 cm) for melanoma in situ to 2 cm for lesions of more than 2 mm in Breslow depth. For melanoma in situ, the commonly accepted 5-mm margin is based on the National Institutes of Health Consensus expert opinion and on data for melanomas on the trunk and extremities. However, with the growing utilization of MMS for melanoma in situ, new evidence may indicate that 5-mm margins are inadequate for achieving a tumor-free plane. A recent study of 1,120 malignant melanomas in situ excised with MMS followed by frozen section examination of the margins found that 86% of melanomas in situ were successfully excised with a 6-mm margin, whereas a 9-mm margin removed 98.9% of melanomas in situ. Although frozen sections have been shown to be 100% sensitive and 90% specific for detecting melanoma during MMS in some studies, these rates can vary significantly with surgeon ability and the processing technique of a given laboratory. It is important to note that special immunologic stains, including Melan-A/Mart-1, S100, Mel5, and HMB-45, have been used to enhance sensitivity in the detection of malignant melanocytes during MMS. Currently, rapid Mart-1 staining is most often used for this purpose.

Using MMS to accurately define tumor-free margins for melanoma is especially important on the head and neck, where recurrence rates have been shown to be high and function and cosmesis are important. Local recurrence rates after standard excision of melanoma on the head and neck approximate 9 to 13% but have been reported to be as high as 42% (▶ Fig. 46.7). For lentigo maligna melanoma after MMS, recurrence rates as low as 1.4% have been reported. Another treatment option is termed *staged excision*. This refers to debulking of the tumor with a narrow-margin standard excision to confirm depth combined with en face evaluation or peripheral margins. The peripheral specimens are divided and the margins are inked to maintain true orientation; however, tissue is sent for standard formalin fixation and paraffin embedding. A diagnosis of remaining areas of positivity is available within 24 to 36 hours, and any residual melanoma may be removed subsequently in a directed fashion. Once the surgical margins are confirmed to be clear, wound management may involve secondary intention healing, primary closure, skin graft, or flap repair. It is important for patients to be aware that the final size of the surgical defect after the staged excision of a lentigo maligna melanoma on the head and neck can be 2 to 10 times the original lesion size.

46.5 Conclusion

Mohs micrographic surgery is a tissue-conserving surgical technique for excising and mapping high-risk skin cancers. It allows a histologic assessment of the complete circumferential surgical margin with immediate frozen sections or special stains. In addition to the benefits that MMS offers in terms of margin control and conservation of tissue, it has proved to be cost-effective

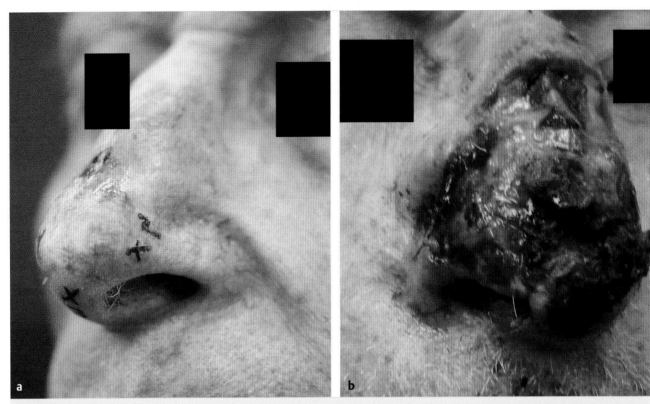

Fig. 46.7 Melanoma that recurred on the nasal tip after standard excision 4 years earlier. (**a**) Subtle appearance of recurrence. (**b**) Significant subclinical extension.

when compared with other modalities used to treat skin cancer. One study determined that the overall cost for MMS and immediate reconstruction by a fellowship-trained Mohs micrographic and reconstructive surgeon may be threefold less than the cost of surgery performed by a colleague from an allied surgical subspecialty in an ambulatory surgical center. In the correct clinical context, MMS provides patients with a treatment modality that leads to the highest cure rates and optimal functional and cosmetic results.

46.6 Roundsmanship

- Mohs micrographic surgery is the only technique that allows complete evaluation of the entire peripheral and deep surgical margin. This in turn allows maximal conservation of normal tissue with optimization of function and cosmesis.
- A key defining feature of MMS is that the surgeon excises, maps, and reviews the specimen personally, minimizing the chance of error in tissue interpretation and orientation.
- The American Academy of Dermatology general guidelines for MMS include (1) high risk for local recurrence, (2) areas requiring tissue preservation, and (3) high risk for metastasis.
- MMS achieves a 99% cure rate (compared with 91.3% for other methods) for primary BCC, and a 94.4% cure rate (compared with 82.4% for standard excision, 90.2% for radiation therapy, and 60% for curettage and desiccation) for recurrent BCC.
- For the following categories of SCC, MMS is associated with higher cure rates than traditional excisional surgery: primary

SCC of the ear (96.9% vs 89.1%), primary SCC of the lip (94.2% vs 81.3%), recurrent SCC (90.0% vs 76.7%), SCC with perineural invasion (100% vs 53%), SCC larger than 2 cm (74.8% vs 58.3%), and poorly differentiated SCC (67.4% vs 46.4%).

46.7 Recommended Reading

[1] Belkin D, Carucci JA. Mohs surgery for squamous cell carcinoma. Dermatol Clin 2011; 29: 161–174

[2] Bene NI, Healy C, Coldiron BM. Mohs micrographic surgery is accurate 95.1% of the time for melanoma in situ: a prospective study of 167 cases. Dermatol Surg 2008; 34: 660–664

[3] Carucci JA, Martinez JC, Zeitouni NC et al. In-transit metastasis from primary cutaneous squamous cell carcinoma in organ transplant recipients and non-immunosuppressed patients: clinical characteristics, management, and outcome in a series of 21 patients. Dermatol Surg 2004; 30: 651–655

[4] Carucci JA. Mohs' micrographic surgery for the treatment of melanoma. Dermatol Clin 2002; 20: 701–708

[5] Cascinelli N. Margin of resection in the management of primary melanoma. Semin Surg Oncol 1998; 14: 272–275

[6] Clark WH, From L, Bernardino EA, Mihm MC. The histogenesis and biologic behavior of primary human malignant melanomas of the skin. Cancer Res 1969; 29: 705–727

[7] Cohen LM. Lentigo maligna and lentigo maligna melanoma. J Am Acad Dermatol 1995; 33: 923–936, quiz 937–940

[8] Kunishige JH, Brodland DG, Zitelli JA. Surgical margins for melanoma in situ. J Am Acad Dermatol 2012; 66: 438–444

[9] Mahoney MH, Joseph M, Temple CL. The perimeter technique for lentigo maligna: an alternative to Mohs micrographic surgery. J Surg Oncol 2005; 91: 120–125

[10] Mohs FE. Chemosurgery: a microscopically uncontrolled method of cancer excision. Arch Surg 1941; 42: 279–295

[11] Mosterd K, Krekels GA, Nieman FH et al. Surgical excision versus Mohs' micrographic surgery for primary and recurrent basal-cell carcinoma of the face: a prospective randomised controlled trial with 5-years' follow-up. Lancet Oncol 2008; 9: 1149–1156

[12] Olhoffer IH, Bolognia JL. What's new in the treatment of cutaneous melanoma? Semin Cutan Med Surg 1998; 17: 96–107

[13] Rigel DS, Carucci JA. Malignant melanoma: prevention, early detection, and treatment in the 21st century. CA Cancer J Clin 2000; 50: 215–236, quiz 237–240

[14] Rigel DS, Friedman RJ, Kopf AW. Lifetime risk for development of skin cancer in the U.S. population: current estimate is now 1 in 5. J Am Acad Dermatol 1996; 35: 1012–1013

[15] Rogers HW, Weinstock MA, Harris AR et al. Incidence estimate of nonmelanoma skin cancer in the United States, 2006. Arch Dermatol 2010; 146: 283–287

[16] Rowe DE, Carroll RJ, Day CL. Prognostic factors for local recurrence, metastasis, and survival rates in squamous cell carcinoma of the skin, ear, and lip. Implications for treatment modality selection. J Am Acad Dermatol 1992; 26: 976–990

[17] Rowe DE, Carroll RJ, Day CL. Mohs surgery is the treatment of choice for recurrent (previously treated) basal cell carcinoma. J Dermatol Surg Oncol 1989; 15: 424–431

[18] Sekulic A, Migden MR, Oro AE et al. Efficacy and safety of vismodegib in advanced basal-cell carcinoma. N Engl J Med 2012; 366: 2171–2179

[19] Tierney EP, Hanke CW. Cost effectiveness of Mohs micrographic surgery: review of the literature. J Drugs Dermatol 2009; 8: 914–922

[20] Zitelli JA, Brown C, Hanusa BH. Mohs micrographic surgery for the treatment of primary cutaneous melanoma. J Am Acad Dermatol 1997; 37: 236–245

47 Grafts in Head and Neck Surgery

Thomas C. Spalla

47.1 Introduction

There will be times during head and neck surgery when reconstruction with one or more grafts becomes necessary. The graft may serve as the ideal reconstructive method for the defect; however, in some cases it may be a necessary, although not ideal, alternative. Regardless, the head and neck surgeon must have a firm understanding of the indications, surgical techniques, and complications that may arise from various grafting techniques.

As with any surgery, the surgeon must do his or her best to convey both the surgery and recovery periods to the patient and caregivers. In elective cases, the surgeon should have a good idea of whether or not grafts will be required for the surgery, although surprises do arise. The consideration of grafts preoperatively is necessary not only for informed consent (e.g., donor site morbidity); it also helps to have any additional instrumentation or personnel available in the operating room to facilitate a smooth operation. Preoperatively, conditions that may increase failure (smoking, diabetes, peripheral vascular occlusive disease, anemia, bleeding dyscrasias) must be examined and, if possible, their effects minimized. There should not be any hesitation to consult with other specialties (e.g., cardiology, endocrinology, hematology) so that the chance for the best possible outcome is maximized.

Grafts consist of numerous types of tissues, both native and foreign, and some of the most common will be discussed below. Each has its own unique indications, limitations, risks, and benefits, and a well-trained surgeon must have a firm comprehension of each of these.

47.2 Skin Grafts

Skin grafts play a large role in the repair of cutaneous defects in the head and neck. Some general principles must be kept in mind when a skin graft is considered as the means of tissue reconstruction. The skin graft is dependent on the recipient site for its blood supply. Ideally, the recipient site is well vascularized to provide a healthy bed on which the skin graft can survive. This tenet prohibits placing skin grafts over areas that are not vascularized, such as bone, cartilage, and bare tendon. However, there may be exceptions in which a small graft (i.e., one with fewer nutritional demands) successfully survives these conditions because of a robust blood supply delivered through the periphery via imbibition and neovascularization. It must also be kept in mind that because of the increased number of cells in the tissue and amount of tissue that is farther from the recipient bed (i.e., more superficial), full-thickness skin flaps require a greater blood supply for their survival. Also, the surgeon must try to match the skin tone and texture of the donor to the recipient site. This allows the best cosmetic result from a skin graft and helps to avoid the creation of a "patched" appearance.

Skin grafts are not limited to external indications. For example, skin grafts can be useful for intraoral defect coverage to decrease wound contracture and allow coverage of a large surface that might alternatively have been left to undergo a prolonged course of secondary intention healing.

47.2.1 Split-Thickness Skin Grafts

Split-thickness skin grafts (STSGs) include the entire epidermis and a variable amount of dermis. Varying thicknesses can be used depending on the recipient site requirements (▶ Fig. 47.1 and ▶ Fig. 47.2; ▶ Table 47.1). Thin grafts are often used when surveillance for tumor recurrence is important, and a thinner graft, although less cosmetically acceptable, allows an earlier detection of recurrence.

Keep in mind that the thinner the skin graft, the greater the chance for survival, but the greater the degree of contraction. The surgeon should thus harvest a graft that is larger (by approximately 25%) than the intended recipient site to allow for this contraction and a tension-free insetting.

47.2.2 Full-Thickness Skin Grafts

Full-thickness skin grafts (FTSGs) are helpful in situations in which the recipient site is not excessively large and the atrophic appearance of an STSG might be unfavorable (e.g., nasal tip). Additionally, FTSGs do not contract to the same degree as STSGs and therefore are appropriate in situations in which functional or significant cosmetic defects might result from significant contracture (e.g., eyelid defects).

Once the site of the defect is known and an FTSG is considered, the surgeon should examine the remainder of the patient's head and neck for an appropriate donor site. Ideally, the donor site should match in color and texture. Areas of prominent sun exposure often match well with recipient sites having similar exposure. Additional points must be kept in mind. The surgeon must ensure the following: Harvesting will not cause undue morbidity; harvesting will not create issues with immediate, or in the foreseeable future, reconstructions; and the selected donor site is free of cancer. Also, if there is concern for early cancer recurrence associated with an aggressive cutaneous malignancy, the surgeon may wish to use an STSG or FTSG as a temporary measure before more definitive reconstruction after an appropriate period of recurrence-free surveillance. Common donor sites include pre- and postauricular skin, upper eyelids, melolabial fold, and the supraclavicular fossae.

As with all surgery, a detailed discussion of the risks, benefits, and alternatives with the patient and/or caregivers is necessary before proceeding because multiple options are frequently available, and the patient's goals and expectations may not be in line with the surgeon's. Despite the surgeon's best attempts at color and texture match, the graft often ends up having some degree of "patchwork" appearance. This is usually most evident at first, while the blood supply is not yet strong, and becomes less noticeable over time (▶ Fig. 47.3). The patient must be made aware of this.

FTSGs require a robust blood supply in the recipient site to ensure complete healing, which is often referred to as "take."

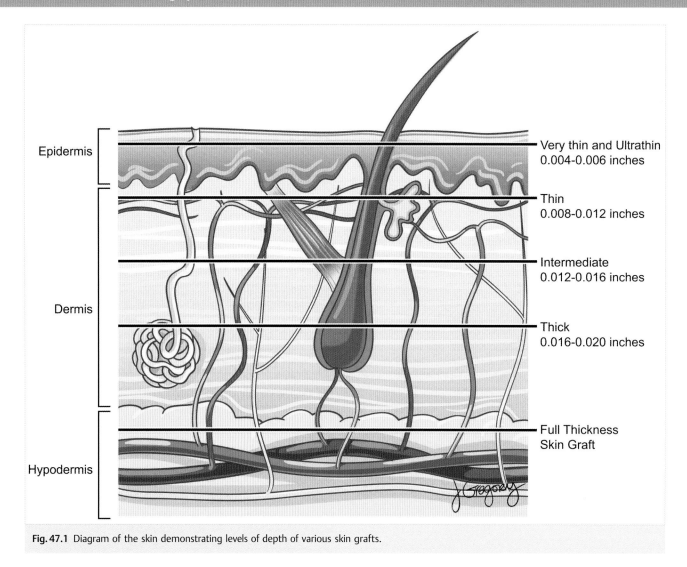

Epidermis

Dermis

Hypodermis

Very thin and Ultrathin
0.004-0.006 inches

Thin
0.008-0.012 inches

Intermediate
0.012-0.016 inches

Thick
0.016-0.020 inches

Full Thickness
Skin Graft

Fig. 47.1 Diagram of the skin demonstrating levels of depth of various skin grafts.

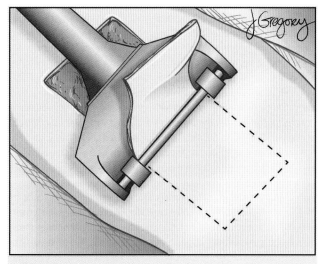

Fig. 47.2 It is essential to tent the split-thickness skin graft away from the dermatome as the harvest progresses.

Table 47.1 Split-thickness skin grafts

Graft	Thickness (in)
Thin	0.008–0.010
Medium	0.011–0.015
Thick	0.016–0.018

Bolstering the reconstruction (▶ Fig. 47.4), as detailed above, is necessary to ensure the best chance for a 100% take.

The potential for donor site morbidity is greater with FTSGs than with STSGs. Harvesting an FTSG requires layered closure of the donor site and almost always necessitates some degree of undermining to allow a tension-free repair. This creates some degree of dead space, which makes possible the development of a seroma or hematoma and, subsequently, infection. Meticulous surgical technique will keep this problem to a minimum and should not deter from the use of an FTSG. As with STSGs, additional procedures may be required to give the best possible final outcome.

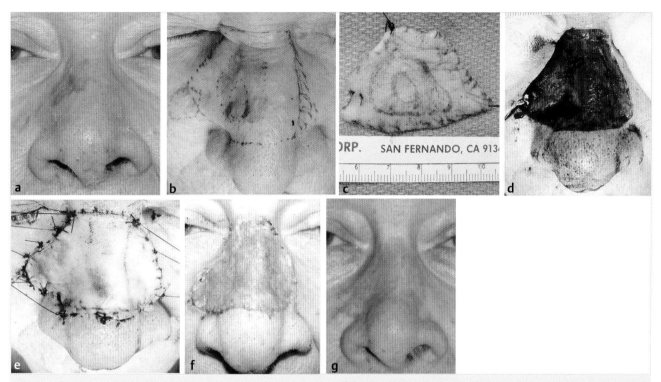

Fig. 47.3 Lentigo maligna melanoma excised from the nasal dorsum with appropriate margins. Remainder of violated nasal subunits also excised, and defect repaired with a full-thickness skin graft (FTSG). (**a**) Preoperative view. (**b**) Intraoperative view showing margins of the lesion and surgical margins extended to incorporate nasal subunits. (**c**) Surgical specimen. (**d**) Surgical defect. (**e**) Supraclavicular FTSG sutured in place. (**f**) Postoperative view at 5 days. (**g**) Two-year view shows mild hyperpigmentation of the FTSG.

47.2.3 Dermal Grafts

Dermal grafts are similar to FTSGs except that they lack an epidermal component. They are infrequently used as a way to bulk up the dermal layer. At times, they may be used to raise a depressed scar. Autologous dermal grafts are harvested by first raising an STSG (that is left pedicled to the skin at one end), then excising the dermis and covering with the STSG. The development of allograft dermis has supplanted this technique because it saves time and avoids any donor site morbidity.

AlloDerm (LifeCell, Branchburg, NJ) is cadaver-derived dermis that acts as a framework for tissue ingrowth and thus resists infection and extrusion. It is often used to aid in mucosal reconstruction (e.g., partial glossectomy) and also may be interposed between the parotid bed and superficial muscular aponeurotic system (SMAS) after a parotidectomy in the hope of decreasing the incidence of Frey syndrome. Another unique application of AlloDerm is as a tissue bed and scaffolding for donor site defects after radial forearm free flap harvesting. However, Wax et al did note its potential shortcoming of a prolonged healing time in comparison with an STSG.

47.2.4 Fat Grafts

Fat grafting can be used for improving a variety of soft-tissue deficits. It can be harvested by liposuction or the en bloc resection of subcutaneous fat. The fat in these situations relies on the recipient site for its blood supply. Some amount of loss is expected in the early healing phase, and therefore overcorrection is recommended. One of the difficulties encountered in fat transfer is resorption, which occurs with time. The timing and degree of resorption likely vary depending on technique, recipient site, graft preparation, and methods used to determine such lasting results. Despite these drawbacks, fat grafting has numerous applications in aesthetic (e.g., lip, nasojugal, malar, or full facial augmentation), functional (e.g., glottis insufficiency), and reconstruction (e.g., parotidectomy bed defect) settings.

47.2.5 Surgical Technique

Split-Thickness Skin Grafts

Most surgeons use a powered dermatome to harvest the STSG because this allows precise control over the thickness of the graft. The donor site is lubricated with mineral oil to prevent sticking and allow the dermatome to glide through the harvest, so that catching and tearing of the skin flap are avoided. Having an assistant gently grasp the ends of the skin with forceps as it passes through the dermatome is helpful to prevent bunching of the skin and subsequent tearing (see ▶ Fig. 47.2). Once the appropriate amount of skin is harvested, it should be stored in saline-moisted gauze. Do not immerse the graft in saline, or especially water, because this will promote edema within the graft and lead to maceration. Pinpoint bleeding is expected because the capillary loops in the papillary dermis will have been transected. Placing a gauze pad moistened with dilute epinephrine solution (1:100,000 to 1:300,000) is a simple way to slow the bleeding and facilitate the application of a dressing. The donor site may now be dressed with sterile bandaging in a

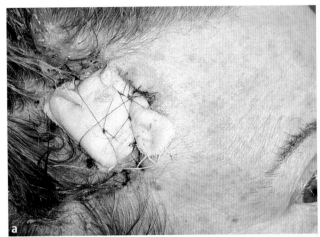

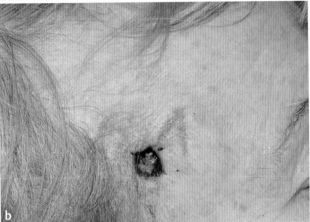

Fig. 47.4 **(a)** Skin defect of the right temple repaired with full-thickness skin graft, held in place with peripheral sutures and a tie-over bolster dressing. **(b)** Eight months later, at the time of repair of a second defect. Note mild hypopigmentation of the skin graft.

Preventing the accumulation of fluid (seroma or hematoma) beneath the graft is critical because its survival depends on the nutrition from the wound bed. Therefore, it may be wise to use interrupted sutures at the periphery to allow the egress of fluid beneath the graft. Some surgeons place tacking sutures in the central portion of the graft to help prevent it from lifting off the wound bed, thereby closing any dead space. This technique is particularly helpful with large grafts. Additionally, when larger grafts are used, creating a few fenestrations ("pie crusting") with a No. 15 blade may be helpful in allowing fluid egress. Drain placement is unnecessary, and the interposition of this foreign body prevents revascularization of the portion of the skin graft superficial to it.

No matter the size of the graft, bolsters are extremely helpful in promoting skin graft healing. Bolsters are usually created with fluffed gauze, or similar material, followed by a nonadherent dressing layer that is then coated with antibiotic ointment. This is then sewn over the graft with permanent monofilament suture. Bolsters serve two purposes. First, they eliminate dead space and prevent the formation of seromas beneath the graft; additionally, bolsters decrease the transmission of shear (laterally transmitted) forces across the graft. Shear forces disrupt the newly forming blood supply and may also traumatize the graft or recipient site, causing seromas or hematomas. Bolsters can be bulky and appear unsightly to the patient, but they are invaluable in graft survival and a favorable outcome. In general, bolsters are removed approximately 7 days after surgery unless the patient's clinical picture dictates otherwise. After bolster removal, the wound can be examined and local wound care applied.

Full-Thickness Skin Grafts

Because of the inherent definition of an FTSG, wound closure is necessary at the donor site. This is typically done in a fusiform fashion. Therefore, the surgeon must plan not only for the size of the necessary donor tissue but also for the excision of additional tissues around the donor site to prevent a standing cutaneous deformity.

Once the donor site is selected, a 10 to 15% overestimation of the recipient bed is wise because of the small amount of contracture that will occur. The skin is harvested and subcutaneous fat sharply trimmed away. This improves the chance for survival. The skin may be placed in saline-moistened gauze while hemostasis is obtained at the donor site and layered closure of this wound is performed.

The manner of insetting FTSGs is similar to that for STSGs, but "piecrusting" the graft is rarely indicated because these FTSGs are not generally much smaller than STSGs requiring this technique (e.g., coverage of a large scalp deficit).

Dermal Grafts

Autologous dermal grafts begin with the partial harvest of an STSG (thickness of 0.012 to 0.016 in). However, the STSG is left attached at the distal end. The dermatome width is reduced, and a deeper pass over the site is made (thickness of 0.012 to 0.014 in) to harvest the strip of dermis. The raised STSG may be tacked back down with a single layer of sutures, and a gentle dressing applied.

manner of the surgeon's preference. Some surgeons prefer a coating of antibiotic ointment followed by a nonadherent dressing and another layer of sterile dressing to act as padding and absorb the serous effusion, which is usually present for the first 48 to 72 hours. Other surgeons simply place a biosynthetic dressing, which permits re-epithelialization beneath its surface and avoids dressing changes in the early postoperative period.

Avoid the temptation to simply measure the recipient site and trim the graft accordingly on the back table. The error of excessive resection will force the surgeon to sew the "scraps" of this graft into the recipient site, fenestrate the remaining graft to allow it to reach the perimeter, or harvest a new graft. All of these situations should be avoided because they will not permit the best possible aesthetic outcome or will lead to additional donor site morbidity (which must be explained to the patient). An easy way to avoid this is for the surgeon to lay the oversized graft on the recipient site and place a tacking suture at the periphery before trimming the graft. Make incremental adjustments in graft size peripherally. Do not attempt to correct the entire graft size with one fell swoop of the knife. A few seconds of patience will pay off nicely in the end. Single-layered closure is all that is necessary at the periphery of the wound.

The dermal graft is then sutured into the recipient bed, typically with a dissolvable suture, with the dermal side facing superficially. In some situations, suturing is unnecessary, if migration is not an issue. AlloDerm is inserted in a similar fashion.

Fat Grafts

Fat grafts may be harvested through liposuction techniques or through open means. The surgeon's preference typically dictates the method chosen.

When liposuction is used, the abdomen is frequently chosen as the donor site because ample abdominal fat is usually present, and this remote site often allows a two-team approach to be used, thereby reducing operating time. During this technique, the surgeon must take care to stay in the subcutaneous tissues and avoid damaging the peritoneum. At the same time, the cannula opening must be directed away from the dermis. After harvest, a pressure dressing is sometimes used to decrease seroma and/or hematoma formation.

Open fat harvest may be performed similarly, with a small incision followed by scissor dissection of the skin away from the subcutaneous fat. The author generally prefers a semicircular umbilical incision if an abdominal fat harvest is being performed to prevent any additional abdominal scarring. If an abdominal lower quadrant incision is used, a left-sided incision is preferable to avoid confusing this scar with an open appendectomy incision. Also, marking the patient in an upright position with undergarments on is helpful to camouflage the position of the final scar.

47.2.6 Follow-up

If any sites of duskiness are seen, close follow-up is warranted. Local wound care (gentle cleansing with saline or peroxide to remove any crusting and the application of an antibiotic ointment) should be instituted, and any conditions that may contribute to this should be carefully reexamined and corrected. For example, seroma formation under the graft will decrease its ability to receive an adequate blood supply and therefore should be drained. Additionally, conditions such as tobacco use or uncontrolled diabetes may also lead to wound-healing issues and need to be managed post-operatively to maximize the chance for a successful outcome. Photography can be helpful in documenting and tracking the extent of the problem, and it serves as a means of future education for the surgeon and students. If sites of necrosis are seen, the aforementioned measures should be taken, but the area(s) of necrosis should be sharply excised so that they do not act as a growth medium for bacteria. Regrafting, or local tissue reconstruction, is not recommended at this time because the factors responsible for initial failure may still be present and lead to a repeat event, which is disheartening for both patient and surgeon. Rather, the area is reconstructed by allowing secondary intention healing of this site, and reconstruction at a later time is considered. An exception to this would be a moderate-size or large failure in an area where secondary intention would create functional impairment or a significant distortion of anatomical structures. In such situations, if the reasons for failure cannot be corrected or are unclear, then an alternative method of reconstruction should be considered to avoid a repeat situation.

As with all scars, the avoidance of ultraviolet light is critical in preventing long-lasting pigmentary changes. A sunblock or sunscreen of with a sun protection factor (SPF) of 30 or higher is recommended for the year after surgery. After successful healing, methods to improve the final aesthetic result can be considered. Camouflage with cosmetics is very helpful in both the short- and long-term management of residual aesthetic imperfections. A full discussion regarding dermabrasion is beyond the scope of this chapter, but dermabrasion to the periphery of the graft, as well as the facial subunit, can be considered to provide a better blending of color and texture. Also, certain laser and light applications may improve the final outcome by improving the surrounding skin. In general, these techniques are not covered by insurance companies, so they may not be a realistic option for many patients.

47.3 Cartilaginous Grafts

47.3.1 Nasal Cartilage

Septum

The quadrangular nasal septal cartilage is an invaluable source of graft material for the head and neck surgeon. The head and neck surgeon's familiarity with septoplasty makes the harvesting of this cartilage a rapid and low-risk procedure. In an otherwise normal and unoperated septum, the surgeon can expect to obtain a sheetlike piece of cartilage that is approximately 1 mm in thickness. It is easily cut into a desired shape and may be scored or morselized depending on the desired application.

One of the more common applications of the nasal septal cartilage graft is to improve a dysfunctional nasal valve. The size and shape of the cartilage allow it to be cut into rectangles (3 x 14 x 1 mm) easily and interposed between the upper lateral cartilages and the septum to widen the internal nasal valve. This technique can also be used to widen the middle vault of the nose and bolster upper lateral cartilages that may have been disrupted and have since collapsed into the nose. The nasal septal cartilage also is easily fashioned into batten grafts, which help resist external valve collapse.

Upper and Lower Lateral Cartilages

The upper and lower lateral cartilages of the nose are not generally considered primary autologous donor sites, primarily because of the aesthetic, and possibly functional, changes that may occur. However, during rhinoplasty, these cartilages may be trimmed (e.g., cephalic trim of the lower lateral cartilages). These remnants should be saved in moist saline gauze until the end of the case. In some instances, they can be crushed or morselized and used to camouflage minor irregularities, particularly of the nasal tip.

47.3.2 Auricular Cartilage

Auricular cartilage, generally harvested from the conchal bowl, is another frequently used source of graftable cartilage. Unlike nasal septal cartilage, auricular cartilage is bowl-shaped and therefore does not lend itself to certain applications. However, this shape is quite useful in nasal applications such as lower lateral cartilage reconstruction, alar rim grafts (in layered reconstruction), and butterfly grafts (to improve the internal nasal valves). The ability to simultaneously harvest auricular cartilage while the recipient site is being prepared is another advantage of this site. Unlike nasal septal cartilage, auricular cartilage is fairly weak. It is thinner and more flexible and is not suitable for situations in which resilience is required; in older patients, it may be quite brittle. The morselization of auricular cartilage may lead to its destruction and an appearance of moist, wet dust.

Pre- and postauricular harvest is possible (▶ Fig. 47.5). It is recommended that some form of bolstering technique (e.g., dental rolls or mattress sutures; see ▶ Fig. 47.5) be used when the donor ear is closed. This helps to reduce the possibility of a hematoma, which can lead to subsequent infection and chondritis, with a resultant "cauliflower" ear deformity.

47.3.3 Costal Cartilage

Costal cartilage is often used in situations of significant nasal and auricular reconstructions. It offers a reliably large piece of cartilage that can be carved to suit a host of reconstructive needs. One of the best-known uses for costal cartilage is in microtia repair. The creation of delicate features through cartilage carving requires expertise, and it is recommended that the surgeon practice this technique with substitute materials in his or her free time to gain mastery. However, no amount of ex vivo practice can reliably predict long-term postoperative results. The details of these techniques are covered in Chapter 52 .

Costal cartilage can be harvested simultaneously in a two-team approach, thereby decreasing operative time. Donor site morbidity must be considered when costal cartilage is used. A chest wall scar may become unsightly, and its placement in a female patient must be carefully considered. During harvest, the possibility of pleural injury is real and may lead to a pneumothorax. If one is identified during surgery, purse-string closure of the defect over a red rubber catheter under negative aspiration should lead to a safe outcome. As with any costal harvest, a postoperative chest X-ray is performed to detect a pneumothorax. If one is identified postoperatively, a chest tube should be placed and any appropriate consultation for management made. Other considerations include a possible unsightly chest scar, chest wall pain, atelectasis, and pneumonia. Therefore, thorough informed consent is especially stressed in cases of elective and cosmetic surgery.

47.3.4 Homografts

When the surgeon identifies a reconstructive situation in which the use of cartilage would be beneficial, another option remains a possibility. Irradiated cadaveric cartilage may be used, and its use depends on several factors. If the patient or caregiver will not consent to the harvest of autologous cartilage, or if the additional risks of autologous cartilage harvest outweigh the possible benefits, cadaveric cartilage may be used. Although some report significant resorption in long-term follow-up, others have not found the rate to be as high.

In addition to resorption concerns, there exists a concern for warping of the homograft cartilage, as well as the fear of viral

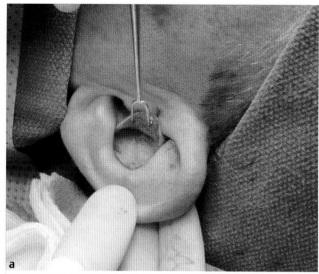

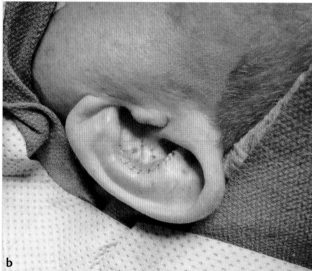

Fig. 47.5 (a) Anterior approach to concha cavum harvest. The surgeon is elevating beneath the perichondrium; dissection is aided through hydrodissection with 1% lidocaine and 1:100,000 epinephrine. (b) Closure of the anterior approach. Mattress sutures with 4–0 plain gut were used to close the dead space and prevent an auricular hematoma.

transmission (although the author is unaware of any reported cases). It is easy to see why many surgeons prefer to harvest autologous cartilage.

47.4 Composite Grafts

Composite grafts contain two or more layers of tissue, and therefore, even more so than FTSGs, require a robust recipient site blood supply. For this reason, proper patient selection and minimization of patient comorbidities (smoking, glucose control, blood thinners) are crucial for graft viability.

A common indication for the composite graft is in nasal ala reconstruction. The root of the helix offers a reliable and aesthetically pleasing source for this reconstruction. Graft placement is similar to that for the FTSG. Meticulous hemostasis and surgical technique cannot be overemphasized.

47.5 Osseous Grafts

Osseous grafts are useful in a variety of head and neck reconstructions. These grafts can be placed with vascularized or nonvascularized methods. Free tissue transfer is covered in Chapter 49 .

47.5.1 Nonvascularized Osseous Grafts

Split calvaria may be readily harvested for use in head and neck reconstruction, such as in a nasal cantilever graft for severe saddle nose deformities. An oscillating saw can be used to incise the outer calvaria, with care taken to prevent penetration through the inner calvaria and injury to the dura mater, which can result in an epidural or subdural hematoma. It is recommended that the surgeon, when harvesting calvaria, avoid suture lines to minimize the risk for dural injury.

Iliac crest offers a viable source of autologous bone. Oral surgeons frequently use the iliac crest for alveolar bone grafts when deficient native tissues preclude implant placement.

The ribs offer an alternative, although less often utilized, bone stock. As with cartilaginous rib harvest, the risks of this technique are real, and the bone stock at this site is generally less robust than that at the calvaria or iliac crest.

47.6 Implants

A variety of implant materials exist that offer flexibility in head and neck reconstruction without any donor site morbidity. No matter what the material, the risks for infection and rejection are greater than with any autologous material, and therefore the judicious use of foreign material and aseptic technique are mandatory.

47.7 Roundsmanship

- Split-thickness skin grafts (STSGs) include the entire epidermis and a variable amount of dermis, depending on the thickness.
- Full-thickness skin grafts contract less than STSGs.
- Dermal grafts can be used to raise a depressed scar. These grafts are harvested after an STSG has been raised. The STSG is left pedicled and then sutured back in position after the dermal graft has been taken.
- Composite grafts contain two or more layers of tissue, such as skin–cartilage or dermis–fat grafts.

47.8 Recommended Reading

[1] Donald PJ. Cartilage grafting in facial reconstruction with special consideration of irradiated grafts. Laryngoscope 1986; 96: 786–807

[2] Medina CR, Patel SA, Ridge JA, Topham NS. Improvement of the radial forearm flap donor defect by prelamination with human acellular dermal matrix. Plast Reconstr Surg 2011; 127: 1993–1996

[3] Mikhelson NM. Homogenous cartilage in maxillofacial surgery. Acta Chir Plast 1962; 4: 192–196

[4] Rowe NM, Morris L, Delacure MD. Acellular dermal composite allografts for reconstruction of the radial forearm donor site. Ann Plast Surg 2006; 57: 305–311

[5] Schuller DE, Bardach J, Krause CJ. Irradiated homologous costal cartilate for facial contour restoration. Arch Otolaryngol 1977; 103: 12–15

[6] Sinha UK, Saadat D, Doherty CM, Rice DH. Use of AlloDerm implant to prevent frey syndrome after parotidectomy. Arch Facial Plast Surg 2003; 5: 109–112

[7] Sinha UK, Shih C, Chang K, Rice DH. Use of AlloDerm for coverage of radial forearm free flap donor site. Laryngoscope 2002; 112: 230–234

[8] Toriumi DM, Larrabee WF. Skin grafts and flaps. In: Papel ID, Nachlas NE, eds. Facial Plastic and Reconstruction Surgery. St. Louis, MO: Mosby-Year Book; 1992

[9] Wax MK, Winslow CP, Andersen PE. Use of allogenic dermis for radial forearm free flap donor site coverage. J Otolaryngol 2002; 31: 341–345

[10] Welling DB, Maves MD, Schuller DE, Bardach J. Irradiated homologous cartilage grafts. Long-term results. Arch Otolaryngol Head Neck Surg 1988; 114: 291–295

48 Reconstruction of Facial Soft-Tissue Defects

Anthony P. Sclafani and James A. Sclafani

48.1 Introduction

The reconstruction of facial defects may be required after facial soft-tissue trauma or extensive infection, but it is most commonly required after the removal of skin cancers. Although any area of the body may be affected by these insults, the particular functional, psychological, and emotional significance of the facial appearance makes the seamless reconstruction of facial defects exceptionally important. The repair of such defects should (1) restore or maintain normal function of the affected and adjacent facial structures and (2) restore the integrity and appearance of the affected area (s) without (3) damaging or adversely affecting neighboring tissues.

48.2 Incidence of Disease

As noted, the most common reason for facial reconstruction is the repair of a defect caused by the removal of a skin cancer. In 2006, 3.5 million nonmelanoma skin cancers were diagnosed in the United States, affecting 2 million people. Basal cell carcinoma is the most common form, while squamous cell carcinoma accounts for approximately about one-fourth of cases. Nonmelanoma skin cancers were the fifth most common cancer in Medicare patients and accounted for 4.5% of Medicare costs for skin cancer in 2006. Approximately 100,000 cases of melanoma are diagnosed annually. Melanoma, by virtue of different treatment recommendations, typically generates larger defects. Approximately 80% of nonmelanoma skin cancers occur on the head, face, and neck, and 80% of these are on the nose. Other commonly affected areas in the head and neck are the auricles and upper lip.

48.3 Terminology

Soft-tissue defects of the face involve damage to or the destruction and loss of one or more parts of the facial envelope. A partial-thickness skin defect does not fully extend through the dermis (▶ Fig. 48.1); because there is a reservoir of basal cells, such a defect can generally be managed expectantly, although in some cases, excision of the remaining dermis (converting the defect to a full-thickness skin defect) with repair is a good option. If, especially in traumatic cases, the skin has been incised in an oblique fashion and one side of the laceration has been undermined more than the other side, a trapdoor deformity (in which the flap is depressed relative to the surrounding skin) may develop.

In order to camouflage facial scars maximally, it is helpful to align them, as much as possible, with relaxed skin tension lines (RSTLs). RSTLs (▶ Fig. 48.2) represent the facial skin's natural tendency to fold in a direction perpendicular to the dominant vectors of facial muscle contraction. Although RSTLs may fall within existing wrinkles, they exist in the absence of these and

can be best demonstrated by asking the patient to animate individually each part of the face.

The simplest of skin defect repairs is conservative care. As mentioned earlier, this may be appropriate in cases of partial-thickness injuries and includes cleansing and conservative débridement (when necessary); generally, occlusive or semiocclusive dressings are applied, which promote faster healing by speeding epithelial migration over the remaining dermis. In cases of small, inconspicuous full-thickness defects, healing by secondary intention may be acceptable. This relies on the natural contractile properties of the wound in addition to epithelial migration from the wound edges. In general, wounds healed by this method generate hypopigmented, depressed scars; however, small defects, especially in concave areas such as the alar crease or the region immediately adjacent to the medial canthus, can undergo healing by secondary intention with excellent cosmetic results. Healing by secondary intention should be avoided in areas of significant cosmetic importance and in areas of highly mobile aesthetic units, such as the eyelids and lips.

Primary closure, in which the wound edges are advanced together and all injured layers of the skin are sutured, is typically the preferred method of repair, if possible. Simple closure is reserved for situations of minimal dermal separation and is performed with a single layer of sutures. Layered closure includes multiple layers of sutures (epidermal and at least one dermal layer). Complex closure may require some undermining of the wound edge and/or deeper (e.g., facial or muscular) layers of sutures. Ideally, the closure should align with RSTLs (▶ Fig. 48.3).

Skin grafts (▶ Fig. 48.4) may be required to repair skin defects and are characterized by thickness. Split-thickness skin grafts (STSGs) include the epidermis and a portion of the dermis; thin STSGs are 0.005 to 0.012 inches thick, whereas thick STSGs are 0.018 to 0.030 inches in thickness. STSGs are generally more viable and leave less of a cosmetic defect because the donor site can be allowed to re-epithelialize. However, repaired areas may be thinner and depressed, and they may contract more than those repaired with full-thickness skin grafts (FTSGs). FTSGs, on the other hand, contain epidermis and the full thickness of dermis. FTSG donor sites are typically closed primarily with a resultant scar, so that they must be placed in inconspicuous areas with significant skin laxity/redundancy. However, wounds repaired with FTSGs undergo less contraction and are less likely to be depressed than are those repaired with STSGs.

Cartilage grafts are frequently used to rebuild or reinforce structure, especially in the nose or ear. Septal cartilage typically yields flatter cartilage grafts, whereas conchal cartilage grafts are often chosen to take advantage of the natural curve of the concha.

Other types of grafts include composite grafts, which contain two or more distinct tissue types, such as skin–cartilage or mucosa–cartilage grafts. Dermis–fat grafts, harvested by first removing the overlying epidermis (either by dermabrasion or by raising an STSG) and then harvesting the dermis and the

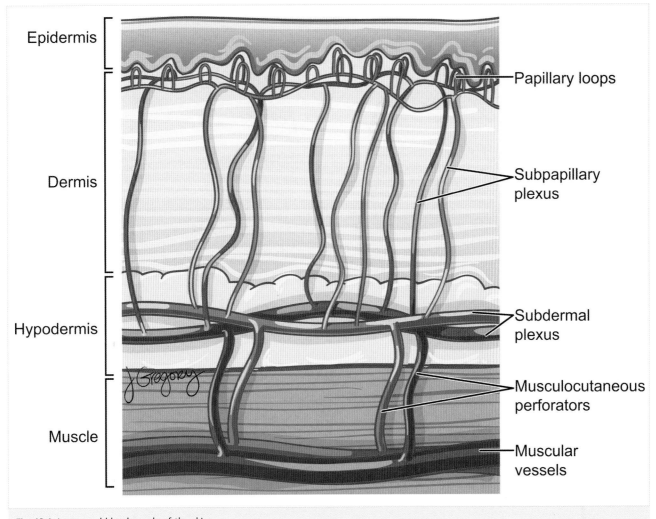

Fig. 48.1 Layers and blood supply of the skin.

underlying fat as a unit, can be used to add bulk volume to areas of tissue deficit. A skin–cartilage graft is typically harvested from the concha or helix of the ear.

All grafts are separated from their natural blood supply during harvesting and are nourished initially through a process of serum imbibition, in which nutrients present in the serum are transfer passively from the wound bed to the graft. Generally within 72 to 96 hours, microvascular connections between the recipient site and the graft develop (arterial connections slightly earlier than venous ones) to support the graft.

Skin flaps are partially elevated segments of skin that maintain an intact bridge to the surrounding skin through which blood supply flows. Skin flaps can be categorized as random skin flaps (relying on blood flow through the subdermal vascular plexus) or axial flaps (based over and fed by a specific artery). Flaps can also be described by the way they are moved to repair a skin defect. An advancement flap is moved unidirectionally into an adjacent defect, whereas a rotation flap pivots around a defect. A transposition flap is moved over surrounding intact skin to reach its intended recipient site, and an interpolation flap crosses under or over surrounding skin to reach its final location, leaving a pedicle.

48.4 Applied Anatomy

The repair of facial skin defects most commonly relies on random skin flaps. The subdermal plexus is the principal blood supply in random flaps. The extensive vascular interconnections found in the subdermis allow opening of choke vessels to shunt blood through the diminished flap base, or pedicle, toward the flap tip. Some flaps, such as the forehead flap (based over one or both supratrochlear arteries), are axial in nature.

48.5 The Disease Process

48.5.1 Etiology

Skin defects may be a result of trauma but are more commonly due to the excision of skin lesions. Traumatic injuries should be carefully prepared, ensuring the removal of any necrotic tissue or debris. Bite wounds should be treated cautiously with appropriate antibiotic coverage (amoxicillin/clavulanic acid); animal bites, if not grossly contaminated, can be closed, but injuries from human bites should be treated with antibiotics and undergo delayed closure to prevent infection.

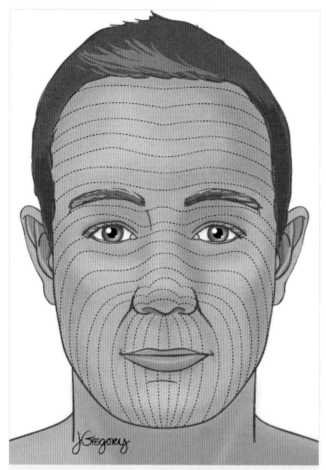

Fig. 48.2 Relaxed skin tension lines.

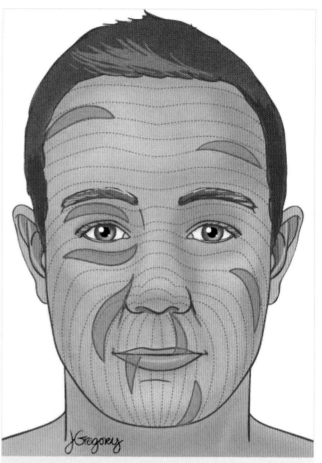

Fig. 48.3 Primary closures should be aligned as closely as possible to relaxed skin tension lines.

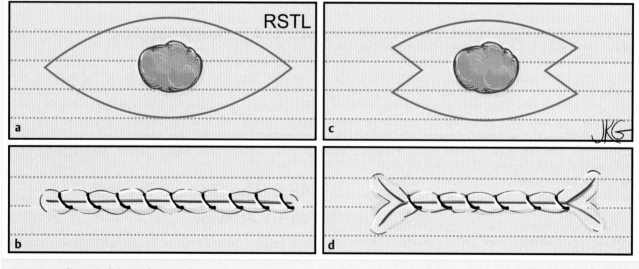

Fig. 48.4 (a–d) Types of skin grafts.

The majority of malignant skin lesions are nonmelanoma skin cancers. In the United States in 2006, more than 3 million nonmelanoma skin cancers were diagnosed. Melanomas are less common, occurring at a rate of approximately 100,000 per year.

48.5.2 Pathogenesis

The incidence of skin cancer among Medicare recipients increased from 1.1 million cases in 1992 to over 2 million in 2006. This tremendous increase is expected to continue. These numbers reflect cumulative skin damage induced by sun exposure. The role of the immune system is highlighted by the increased incidence of nonmelanoma skin cancers in patients with chronic immunosuppression.

48.5.3 Natural History and Progression

Skin defects, whether resulting from traumatic wounds or the removal of skin lesions, are typically best repaired as soon as possible. Open skin wounds of the head and face, if they are not contaminated and are treated with local wound care and antibiotics as appropriate, infrequently become infected because of the excellent blood supply of the skin in these areas. However, these wounds will undergo progressive contraction during healing by secondary intention, which may distort surrounding tissues; moreover, the resultant scars are usually thin, pale, and waxy and will appear noticeably different from the surrounding normal skin.

48.5.4 Potential Disease Complications

Unrepaired skin defects can distort surrounding facial structures if allowed to contract. This may be as simple as a stellate scar with mild puckering of the skin in its immediate area. More problematic is the contracted scar that causes eyelid malposition or ectropion, lip malposition generating asymmetry or a "snarling" appearance, or retraction/notching of the nasal ala.

48.6 Medical Evaluation

48.6.1 Presenting Complaints

Patients with skin defects typically present acutely, either in an emergent setting after a traumatic injury or semiemergently after a planned skin excision by a dermatologist or surgeon. A thorough history should be obtained, with specific inquiries regarding any conditions that would be expected to impair proper healing. The length of time between skin injury and presentation should also be determined; traumatic wounds of the face should ideally be closed within 12 hours of injury, although this time should be shorter in areas with less robust vascularity. The mechanism and instrument of injury should be determined, as well; grossly contaminated wounds should undergo delayed closure, and any foreign bodies expected (e.g., glass shards or road debris in cases of motor vehicle accidents) should be anticipated. Finally, intercurrent injuries (e.g., intracranial or cervical injuries) as well as existing medical conditions should be managed first.

48.6.2 Clinical Findings, Physical Examination

A careful examination of the wound is essential to determine both the timing and method of wound care. The area should be gently cleaned and any blood clots removed. Grossly contaminated, open wounds can be irrigated with a warm saline solution pulsed through a 20-mL syringe fitted with an 18- or 20-gauge plastic intravenous catheter. The wound should be evaluated for its depth, as well as the viability of remaining attached skin, laceration of any vascular structures, exposure of any underlying cartilage or bone, and proximity to vital or highly mobile structures. Sharp débridement can be performed at this point if needed to assess the wound, but in general, this should be minimized and restricted to the removal of obviously devitalized or necrotic tissues and grossly contaminated tissues. The proximity of the defect to mobile structures (e.g., margins of the lips or eyelids, nasal alae) should be noted. If a traumatic flap of skin has been created, the edges should be inspected because these cuts are typically beveled and are more likely to develop a pincushion deformity (in which the skin on the concave aspect of a curved skin cut contracts and is raised compared with the skin on the convex side of the cut). These margins should be resected to generate perpendicular wound edges and prevent pincushioning.

48.7 Treatment

48.7.1 Medical Treatment

In cases in which the wound will be allowed to heal secondarily, rapid wound healing affords optimal appearance and patient comfort. After the wound has been appropriately cleaned and appropriate hemostasis ensured, a moist dressing should be applied. In the face, gentle wound care and coverage with an antibiotic ointment is generally sufficient and acceptable to the patient. Based on the size of the defect, these wounds may take 6 to 10 weeks to fully heal, but as noted earlier, acceptable cosmetic results may be achieved.

48.7.2 Surgical Treatment

Before any defect is reconstructed, a number of conditions need to be met. A simple, common sense paradigm of wound closure should be employed in determining the best method of wound repair (▶ Fig. 48.5). The wound should be not infected; if infection is present (gross contamination should be assumed in cases of human bites), oral or intravenous antibiotics should be begun and antibiotic irrigation of the wound instituted for at least 48 hours before repair of the wound. If a tumor was removed, complete and proper oncologic resection should be ensured; if this is uncertain or if there is a high likelihood of recurrence, an STSG may be applied for wound coverage without impairing surveillance for recurrence. Partial-thickness wounds and small full-thickness wounds in cosmetically unimportant areas or in concave areas (e.g., the alar crease) can be allowed to heal by secondary intention with good cosmetic results, but they may take several weeks to heal. In other cases, the local tissue should be assessed for laxity; if sufficient, primary closure should be

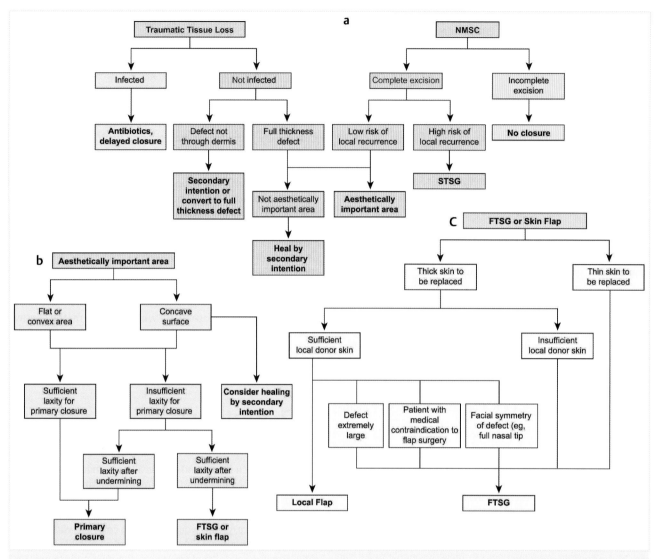

Fig. 48.5 Decision tree to determine the appropriate method of wound closure. (**a**) Traumatic lesion versus electively excised lesion. (**b**) Determining healing by secondary intention, primary closure, or full-thickness skin graft or local skin flap. (**c**) Choosing between FTSG and local flap. *FTSG*, full-thickness skin graft; *NMSC*, nonmelanoma skin cancer; *STSG*, split-thickness skin graft.

performed. Undermining in a subcutaneous plane peripherally from the defect can improve local tissue laxity, but care should be taken to avoid undermining too close to mobile structures (e.g., lower eyelid), which may be distorted by tissue movement. If primary closure is still not possible without producing unacceptable tension of the wound closure, either an FTSG or a skin flap may be used. Generally, the closer to the defect a graft is harvested, the closer the skin match. FTSGs for the face are most commonly harvested from the postauricular sulcus, but if sufficient laxity is present, they can also be harvested from the preauricular, non–hair-bearing area or (in patients with deep nasolabial folds) from the nasolabial crease. Contralateral eyelid skin can be used to repair eyelid defects, and this is often the best method of repair for eyelid defects. Larger FTSGs can be harvested from the supraclavicular fossa. On the nose, FTSGs are generally not used unless the defect is symmetrically located, especially on the nasal tip.

If there is sufficient adjacent donor tissue, a local skin flap (see Box Types of Facial Skin Flaps (p. 381)) can be used to repair the defect. The specific flap design is chosen based on the size, shape, and orientation of the defect and its proximity to aesthetic unit borders, where scars can be hidden. The simplest flap is the advancement flap (▶ Fig. 48.6), in which there is a unidirectional movement of the tissue. One or two relaxing incisions are made along or parallel to RSTLs, and the flap is moved in the same vector while the surrounding tissues are undermined to allow tissue movement. Advancement flaps are particularly helpful in the forehead, where the natural transverse creases are excellent places in which to hide the relaxing incisions. Near the base of the flap, the tissue adjacent to the flap may bunch into a "dog ear" or standing cone deformity, reflecting the shorter length of the flap than of the defect itself. A Burrows triangle, which in essence removes part or all of this skin excess, can be used to correct the deformity.

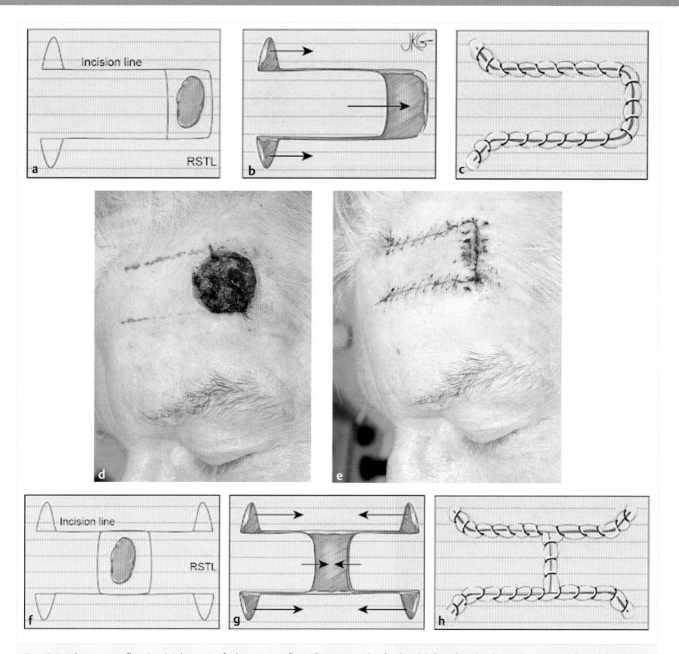

Fig. 48.6 Advancement flap. **(a–c)** Schematic of advancement flap. **(d)** Patient with a forehead defect closed with **(e)** advancement flap. **(f–h)** Bilateral advancement flaps can be used; Burrows triangles can be excised as necessary. *RSTL*, relaxed skin tension line.

Types of Facial Skin Flaps

- Advancement flap
  - Unidirectional movement into defect
- Rotation flap
  - Pivots around an axis
- Transposition flap
  - Transfer flap over normal intervening skin
- Interpolation flap
  - Flap with non-inset pedicle

A rotation flap (▶ Fig. 48.7) pivots around a point adjacent to its base after a curvilinear incision is extended to a length approx-

imately four times the distance from the pivot point to the distal aspect of the defect. Again, a Burrows triangle may be needed to correct the standing cone deformity. Rotation flaps are quite useful in the cheek, where the RSTLs are curvilinear. An O-T closure is essentially the use of bilateral rotation flaps when tissue rotational laxity is adequate and there is an aesthetic boundary or RSTL in which to hide the scars. O-T closures are very useful in the lips and the superior forehead (▶ Fig. 48.8).

In transposition flaps, such as rhombic and bilobed flaps, tissue is transferred across a bridge of intact skin to be inserted into the defect. Transposition flaps are based on geometric patterns. The classic rhombic flap (▶ Fig. 48.9) visualizes a rhombus with two 60-degree and two 120-degree angles. The

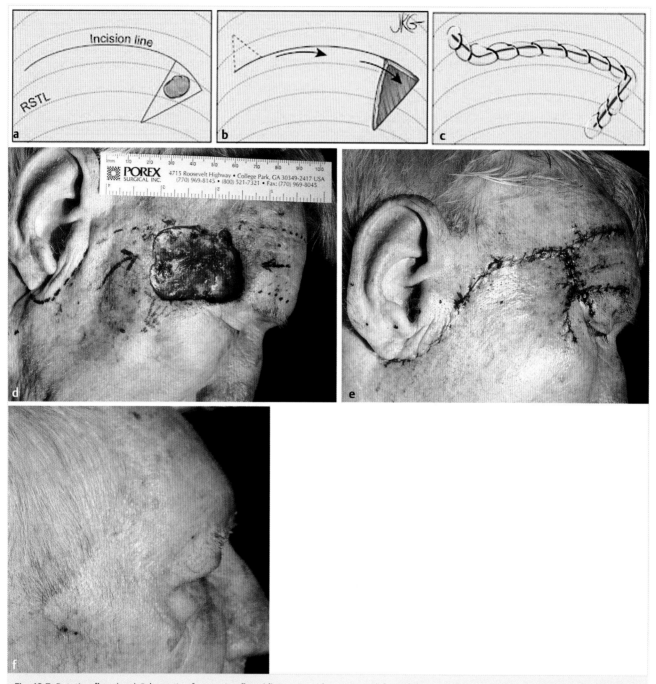

Fig. 48.7 Rotation flap. **(a–c)** Schematic of a rotation flap. **(d)** Patient with extensive defect of the temple repaired with **(e)** advancement flap above the brow combined with a temple rotation flap. This required excision of a Burrows triangle along the lateral orbital rim. **(f)** Patient 3 weeks after repair. *RSTL*, relaxed skin tension line.

rhombus is ideally oriented with its short axis parallel to RSTLs. An incision, equal in length to the short axis, is made from the defect margin as an extension of the short axis, and a back cut is then made equal in length and parallel to the side of the rhombus. The outlined flap is elevated, the donor site is advanced and closed primarily after wide undermining, and the flap is transposed into the defect. The Dufourmental modification (▶ Fig. 48.10) is used when the defect is relatively narrow and conversion to a rhombus would sacrifice a significant amount of normal skin. Instead, a narrow rhom-

boid is drawn around the defect. The first limb of the flap is angled to bisect the angle formed by the short-axis extension and the extension of the adjacent rhomboid side. The back cut is equal and parallel to the side of the rhombus. The flap generated is narrower than the standard rhombic flap; in order to facilitate closure, a Webster M-plasty is performed at the base of the defect, which serves to narrow the defect size. The rhombic flap allows alignment of the incisions with RSTLs fairly easily, but it leaves scars that are somewhat unnaturally sharp-angled.

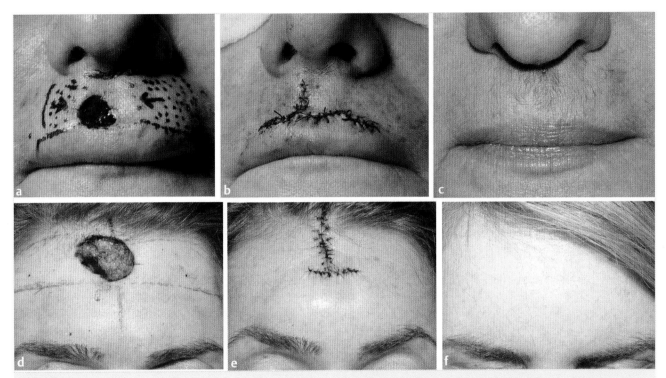

Fig. 48.8 O-T closures. (a) Preoperative markings around an upper lip defect indicate incisions along the vermilion border, undermining of the upper lip, and planned Burrows triangle along the right philtral column. (b) After closure, incisions lie along the vermilion border and on the right philtral column. (c) Two weeks after repair. (d) Forehead defect with transverse forehead rhytids marked. (e) Immediately after O-T repair, with Burrows triangle excised superiorly. (f) Four weeks after repair.

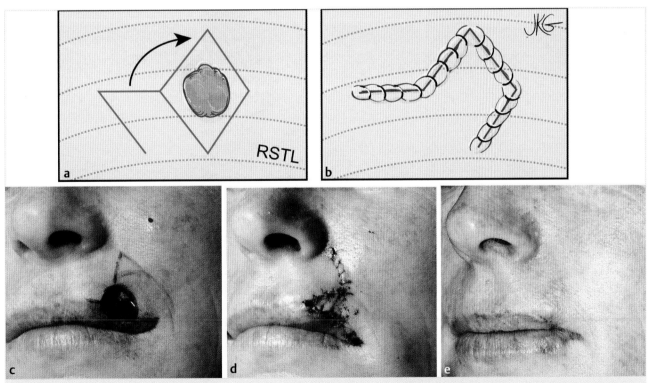

Fig. 48.9 Rhombic flap repair. (a,b) Schematic of a rhombic flap. (c) Defect of the right upper lip with rhombic flap drawn to lie in the nasolabial fold. (d) The rhombic flap is rotated clockwise into the defect, and the donor site closed primarily. (e) Three weeks after rhombic flap repair. RSTL, relaxed skin tension line.

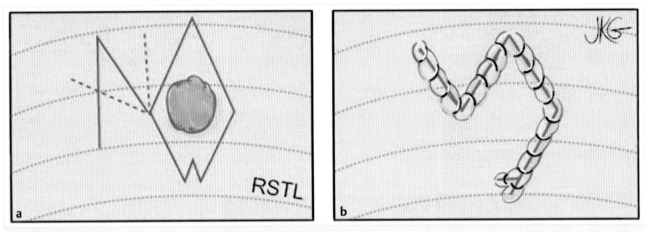

Fig. 48.10 (a,b) Schematic of a Dufourmental rhombic flap repair. *RSTL*, relaxed skin tension line.

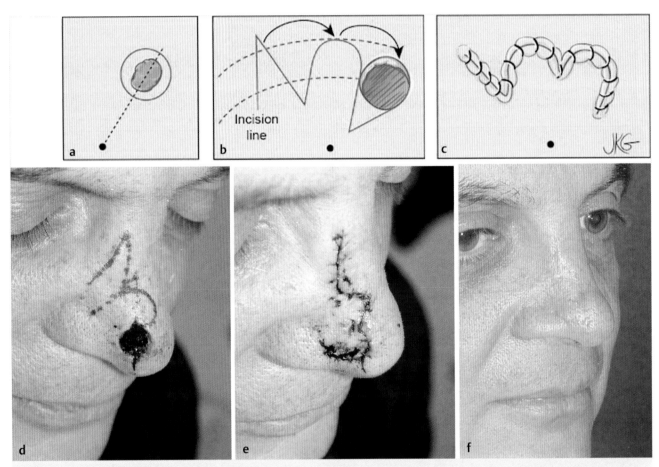

Fig. 48.11 Bilobed flap repair. (a–c) Schematic of a bilobed flap repair. The curvilinear lines represent arcs extending through the distal aspect of the defect as well as the center of the defect and curving around a defined pivot point. The first flap is drawn to be 80% of the width of the center of the defect, while the secondary flap is drawn to be 75% of the width of the center of the primary flap. The primary flap closes the defect, the secondary flap closes the primary flap donor site, and the secondary flap donor site is closed primarily. (d) Patient with nasal tip defect and bilobed flap drawn. (e) Bilobed flap rotated in place. (f) Four weeks after bilobed flap repair of nasal tip defect, with mild primary flap pincushioning that required subsequent intralesional corticosteroid injection.

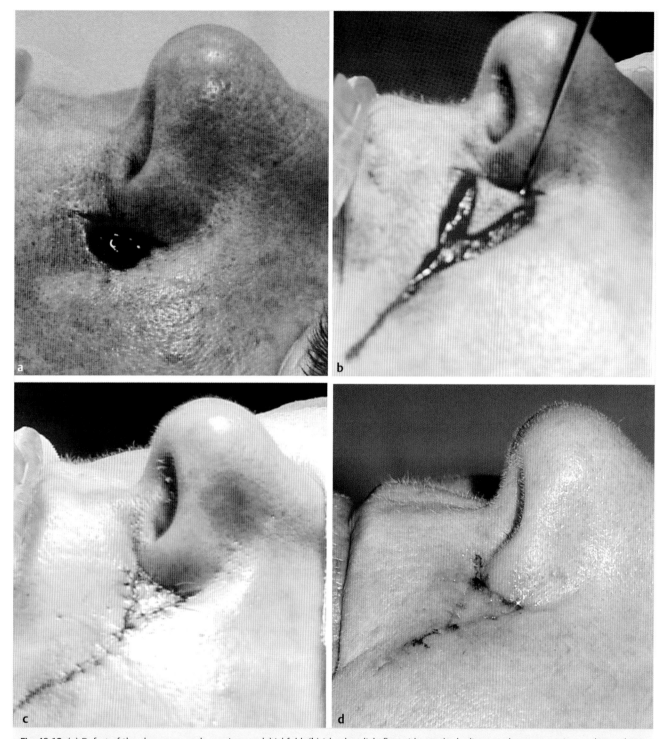

Fig. 48.12 (a) Defect of the alar crease and superior nasolabial fold. (b) Island pedicle flap with attached adjacent subcutaneous tissue advanced into defect. (c) Island pedicle flap advanced and sutured in place. (d) One week after repair of defect with island pedicle flap.

Bilobed flaps are most commonly used in lower nasal repairs less than 2 cm in diameter or in the occipital region. The bilobed flap (▶ Fig. 48.11) is aptly named because it is composed of a rotation/transposition flap with two lobes. A pivot point is chosen, and two arcs are drawn around this; the first extends through the center of the defect, and the second runs tangentially through the outer aspect of the defect. The first lobe is designed to be directly adjacent to the defect with its apex abutting the outer arc, and it should create no more than a 45-degree angle from the defect. The diameter of the primary lobe should be about 80% of the width of the defect. The second lobe also runs at less than 45 degrees from the first lobe, with a diameter that is approximately 75 to 80% the width of the first lobe. The surrounding tissues are undermined widely, and the

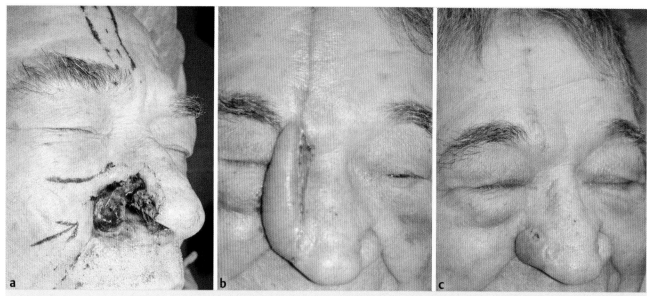

Fig. 48.13 Paramedian forehead flap. (**a**) Through-and-through defect of the right ala. Markings for cheek flap advanced into the alar crease and right paramedian forehead flap. Internal lining reconstructed with a septal flap and alar support re-created with a cartilage graft. (**b**) One week after paramedian forehead flap, with pedicle attached at the origin of the right supratrochlear artery. (**c**) One week after pedicle division (3 weeks after first stage of forehead flap).

donor site for the second lobe is closed primarily; this is facilitated by elevating the lobe as an extended flap with an angle of (no more than) 30 degrees at its distal end. The primary lobe is transposed into the defect while the second lobe is moved into the defect from the primary lobe. A bilobed flap allows the tissue to be shared over a wider area at the cost of a somewhat more complex scar. Rhombic and bilobed flaps are generally useful in closing defects up to 2 cm. Points of significant tension occur at the distal aspect of the flap, as well as at the point where the donor site meets the defect.

An island pedicle flap (▶ Fig. 48.12) transfers a segment of skin vascularized by a subcutaneous pedicle that can be tunneled under adjacent tissue and avoids removing or distorting tissue adjacent to the defect.

Facial defects larger than 2 cm may require larger flaps, including cervicofacial flaps. Incisions for these flaps can be hidden in the pre- or postauricular crease and along the anterior border of the sternocleidomastoid muscle. Large nasal defects can be repaired successfully with a forehead flap. A midline forehead flap is based over both supratrochlear arteries and consequently has a wide base, which limits its arc of rotation and reach. The paramedian forehead flap (▶ Fig. 48.13) is based on a single supratrochlear artery and has a much narrower pedicle; a narrower pedicle allows more effective rotation and a longer reach of the flap, and it can be used to reconstruct the nasal tip and columella. These flaps can be extended behind the frontal hairline, if necessary, but the use of hair-bearing skin for reconstruction often necessitates subsequent laser hair removal. The flap is turned and sutured to the distal aspect of the defect, while the pedicle from the brow area remains in place until blood supply to the distal end of the flap develops and crosses the scar from the surrounding skin. The donor site is generally closed primarily.

48.7.3 Complications (see Box Complications of Skin Defect Repair)

Contraction around areas allowed to heal by secondary intention can lead to tissue distortion if it occurs near mobile structures, such as the eyelids or lips. Repair of skin defects is generally quite successful, and although always possible, flap failure from arterial compromise or venous engorgement is uncommon. Because tissue has been lost, there is always some tension on the skin closure. Scars may become hypertrophic, widened, or hyperpigmented. With typical postoperative swelling, there may be some compromise to the superficial layers of skin of the distal flap (epidermolysis). The flap itself may stay swollen and raised (pincushioning) as excessive fibrosis develops (and may require corticosteroid injections), or less commonly, the flap may be depressed below the surrounding skin (trap door deformity). Finally, preexisting telangiectasia may become more prominent, or the scar may remain persistently erythematous after flap surgery and require laser treatment.

Complications of Skin Defect Repair

- Flap failure
- Scar issues (hypertrophy, keloid, dyspigmentation, depressed or widened scars)
- Dehiscence (secondary to excessive wound tension, infection, poor vascularity)
- Epidermolysis (if leads to deeper loss)
- Pincushioning/trap door deformity
- Scar retraction or distortion of surrounding skin

48.8 Roundsmanship

- Skin defects should be repaired with the method that most effectively fills the defect while generating the simplest scar.
- Repair should be performed only when there is no infection and complete resection of any malignancy is certain.
- Undermining of surrounding tissues facilitates tensionless closure.
- Incisions used to harvest flaps should be placed at the borders of aesthetic units and so that they blend maximally into relaxed skin tension lines.

48.9 Recommended Reading

[1] Baker SR. Local Flaps in Facial Reconstruction. Philadelphia, PA: Elsevier; 2007

[2] Chu EA, Byrne PJ. Local flaps I: bilobed, rhombic, and cervicofacial. Facial Plast Surg Clin North Am 2009; 17: 349–360

[3] Jackson IT. Local Flaps in Head and Neck Reconstruction. St. Louis, MO: Quality Medical Publishing; 2007

[4] Stucker FJ, Shaw GY, Boyd S, Shockley WW. Management of animal and human bites in the head and neck. Arch Otolaryngol Head Neck Surg 1990; 116: 789–793

49 Myocutaneous and Free Flap Reconstruction

Grigorly Mashkevich

49.1 Introduction

Complex defects of the head, neck, and upper aerodigestive tract often necessitate the transfer of regional or distant tissue in order to restore lost volume and function. Regional myocutaneous flaps and free flaps can provide the optimal bulk and three-dimensional configuration to match virtually any defect in the head and neck region. In previously irradiated patients with head and neck cancer, this method of reconstruction provides healthy, well-perfused tissue capable of withstanding the rigors of wound healing in a compromised tissue bed. Flap surgery requires meticulous planning with a targeted set of goals aimed at restoring volume and diminishing any functional impairment with respect to speech and swallowing.

49.2 Incidence of Disease

Regional and free flap repair is necessary in a small percentage of patients with head and neck cancer, trauma, or congenital anomalies. This method of reconstruction is typically reserved for large wounds, existing or anticipated, that are not amenable to primary closure.

49.3 Terminology

Free tissue or free flap reconstruction is a surgical procedure during which a segment of tissue, with its own intact vasculature, is harvested from a donor area and transferred to a recipient site. The artery and vein(s) perfusing the flap are cut in the donor region and sutured to recipient vessels in the head and neck via a process called microvascular anastomosis. In contrast, regional tissue transfer mobilizes healthy tissues from areas immediately adjacent to the head and neck. These areas include the anterior chest wall (pectoralis major flap) and posterolateral chest wall (latissimus dorsi flap). Regional flaps are most commonly transferred in a pedicled fashion. During pedicled transfer, the base of the flap at the site of perfusing blood vessels is progressively narrowed. This allows greater arching and mobilization of the flap while the connection of the perfusing blood vessels to their source is retained. The term *composite* refers to flaps containing multiple tissue types (skin, fat, muscle, and/or bone). Myocutaneous and osteocutaneous flaps are examples of composite flaps.

49.4 Applied Anatomy

The anatomy of the regional and free flaps most commonly used for head and neck reconstruction is outlined in ▶ Fig. 49.1 and ▶ Table 49.1. The salient points about each flap are discussed in the surgical section of this chapter. The pertinent head and neck anatomy includes recipient blood vessels, which are selected based on availability. In oncologic cases, tumor involvement, previous surgeries, and prior fields of radiation therapy determine vessel access. The facial and lingual arteries are most commonly used for arterial anastomosis. The facial artery can be readily identified on the posterior surface of the submandibular gland. The lingual artery has a close relationship with the hypoglossal nerve, which lies immediately superficial to it at the anterior aspect of the external carotid. The external jugular, common facial, and internal jugular veins are the largest-caliber veins in the neck. They are optimal for venous anastomosis owing to their location, length, and availability in the majority of cases. The anterior jugular veins should be avoided because of their proximity to the tracheotomy site (if one is needed). In a vessel-depleted neck, ipsilateral transverse cervical vessels or contralateral neck vessels are alternative choices. Transverse cervical vessels can be found in the lower portion of the neck, below the level of the omohyoid muscle (level IV). These vessels are commonly spared during neck dissections and lie outside most fields of radiation to the head and neck, making them less susceptible to radiation-induced intraluminal stenosis.

49.5 The Disease Process

49.5.1 Etiology

The extirpation of oncologic disease is the leading cause of large head and neck defects requiring reconstruction with regional and distal flaps. Trauma and congenital deficits are less common etiologies.

49.5.2 Pathogenesis

The evolution of surgical defects in the head and neck is determined by the tumor location and the need to obtain clear margins. Wounds may result in large losses of sensate skin or mucosa, cranial nerve damage, and impairment of critical functions such as speech and swallowing.

49.5.3 Natural History and Progression

Flap transfer to a recipient site leads to the gradual development of vascular interconnections between the flap and surrounding tissues. Initially, flap survival depends solely on perfusion through the vascular pedicle of the flap. At about 3 weeks, sufficient circulation is established across the flap borders such that transferred tissue may survive without its pedicle. This rule does not apply in settings of previous radiation therapy, in which the circulation in the recipient tissue bed is poor and longer periods of time are required for healing.

49.5.4 Potential Disease Complications

Flap failure can present as arterial or venous obstruction. The most common cause of each is thrombus formation. Multiple factors can lead to this event, including poor vessel geometry (kinking or twisting), a poorly executed anastomosis (insufficient vessel preparation and cleaning, or inadvertent placement of sutures spanning the vessel lumen), or underlying medical

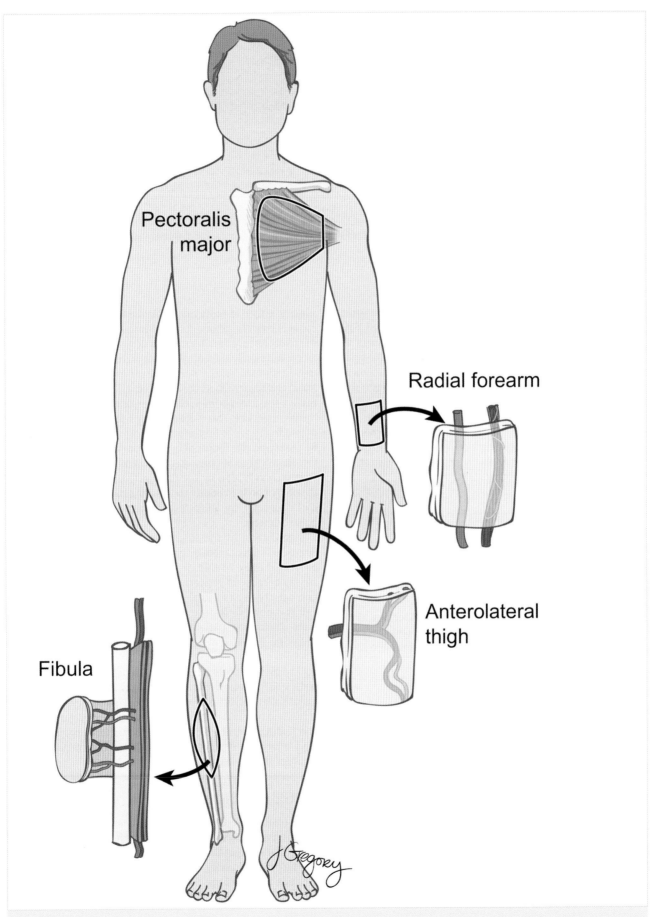

Fig. 49.1 The most commonly used flap donor sites for head and neck reconstruction.

Table 49.1 Regional and distal flap anatomy

Flap source	Flap type	Artery	Vein	Nerve	Defect
Pectoralis major	Pedicled, regional, or free flap	Pectoral branch of thoracoacromial and lateral thoracic	Venae comitantes	Lateral and medial pectoral nerves	Soft tissue[a]
Latissimus dorsi	Pedicled, regional, or free flap	Thoracodorsal	Thoracodorsal	Thoracodorsal (motor)	Soft tissue[a]
Radial forearm	Free flap	Radial	Cephalic vein and deep venae comitantes	Lateral antebrachial cutaneous	Soft tissue[a]
Anterolateral thigh	Free flap	Descending branch of lateral circumflex femoral	Venae comitantes	Femoral cutaneous	Soft tissue
Fibula	Free flap	Peroneal	Venae comitantes	Lateral sural cutaneous	Bony and soft tissue
Scapula	Free flap	Subscapular	Subscapular	Dorsal rami of spinal nerves	Bony and soft tissue

[a]Bone can be incorporated in rare circumstances.

problems predisposing to a hypercoagulable state. Clot formation is most common within 72 hours of the creation of a microvascular anastomosis. Insufficient arterial flow through the flap manifests as pale tissue, absent blood flow on needle pricking, and missing arterial Doppler signal. Venous obstruction results in engorged tissues, with continuous dark venous oozing on needle pricking and a single-phase "water hammer" signal on Doppler ultrasound in the initial stage of flap failure. Both scenarios necessitate urgent return to the operating room for reexploration of the blood vessels, clot evacuation, and revision of the anastomosis. If the revision is performed within 4 to 6 hours, the success rate approaches 50%.

49.6 Medical Evaluation

A patient undergoing regional and free flap transfer must receive a comprehensive medical evaluation, with specific emphasis on cardiovascular and pulmonary health. The patient's condition must be optimized to withstand long operative times under general anesthesia. Any risk factors adversely affecting wound healing should be assessed, including poor nutritional status, smoking, previous radiation therapy, connective tissue disorders, peripheral vascular disease, and diabetes.

49.6.1 Presenting Complaints

The presenting complaints revolve around the disease process requiring flap reconstruction. Flap-related preoperative concerns typically include the length of hospital stay, potential disfigurement of the donor site, and speech and swallow results following the operation. These must be addressed in sufficient detail in order to establish appropriate expectations and reduce preoperative anxiety.

49.6.2 Clinical Findings, Physical Examination

A general physical examination of all potential donor sites is required in order to assess any evidence of previous trauma or

surgery. Either of these may preclude flap harvest at a site because of concerns about potential vascular trauma. Particular to the radial forearm, an Allen test is done to ensure that the ulnar artery can supply the entire palmar arch on its own. During this test, performed on the nondominant hand of the patient, the radial and ulnar vessels are occluded and the patient is asked to make a fist several times, thereby exsanguinating the hand and thenar eminence. This is followed by release of the ulnar artery pressure and an assessment of the capillary refill time, judged by observing the return of a pink hue to the thumb. A time of less than 5 seconds indicates sufficient circulation and an adequate contribution by the ulnar artery to the distal aspect of the palmar arch. In poorly cooperating patients, or in those with dark skin color, the Allen test can be performed instead with a pulse oximeter.

Examination of the thigh focuses on skin laxity and the degree of subcutaneous tissue bulk. Excessive thigh fat may prevent the use of this site in soft-tissue defects around the airway because of concerns for potential compromise. In certain defects, such as total glossectomy, bulk may be desirable and is a positive feature of this site. A pinch test can determine whether a patient's thigh has sufficient laxity, with generally 8 to 10 cm of excess skin considered a desirable amount.

Examination of the leg focuses on palpation of the dorsalis pedis and posterior tibial pulses. Signs of peripheral vascular disease may consist of weak or absent pulses, cyanosis of the digits, and hair loss in the distal lower extremity. Any examination findings must be corroborated by vascular imaging (see below), which is the single most important determinant of suitability of the fibula as a donor location.

49.6.3 Testing

For a fibular free flap, magnetic resonance (MR) angiography can precisely assess the vascular anatomy of the leg. Certain congenital configurations or peripheral vascular disease involving the peroneal artery can be detected by MR angiography and preclude the use of this flap.

Table 49.2 Defect location and flap selection

Defect site	Location	Appropriate flap/reconstruction
Orbit	Orbital exenteration without eyelid preservation	Split-thickness skin grafting followed by osseointegrated implants and globe prosthesis
	Orbital exenteration with eyelid preservation	Orbit obliteration with RFFF followed by ocular prosthesis fitted into the upper and lower fornix
Maxilla	Superior maxilla with orbital exenteration	Orbit considerations as above; ALT or RAFF in cases of cavity obliteration; rib or split calvaria for infraorbital rim grafting
	Inferior maxilla and hard palate	Dental obturator or FFF
Oral cavity	Partial glossectomy	RFFF or thin ALT
	Hemiglossectomy	RFFF or thin ALT
	Near-total glossectomy	Bulky ALT or RAFF
	Buccal mucosa	RFFF or thin ALT
	Through-and-through cheek	RFFF or thin ALT for inner lining; cervicofacial rotation or folded portions of RFFF or ALT for external lining
Mandible	Anterior	FFF or serratus–rib free flap
	Lateral	FFF or spanning reconstruction plate covered by RFFF, thin ALT, or PMCF
Oro- and hypopharynx	Pharyngeal wall	RFFF or thin ALT
	Laryngopharynx	RFFF or thin ALT

ALT, anterolateral thigh free flap; FFF, fibular free flap; PMCF, pectoralis myocutaneous flap; RAFF, rectus abdominis free flap; RFFF, radial forearm free flap.

49.6.4 Differential Diagnosis

The determination of an optimal flap donor site depends on the location of the head and neck defect and the degree of missing tissue bulk. The majority of soft-tissue reconstructions in the head and neck can be achieved with radial forearm, anterolateral thigh, or rectus abdominis free flaps. A pectoralis major myocutaneous flap is an excellent second choice. It can become a primary option in patients who are poor candidates for free tissue transfer, for anatomical or health reasons. Bony reconstruction of the mandible is best achieved with a fibula free flap. Alternative flap choices include radial osteocutaneous, serratus–rib, scapula, and iliac crest flaps. Each has its pluses and minuses with respect to bone stock, length of the vascular pedicle, and ease of harvesting. Facial skeletal and palate defects are best repaired with prosthetics, obturators, or a combination of free bone and cartilage grafts with a soft-tissue flap cover.

49.7 Treatment

49.7.1 Medical Treatment

Several anticoagulants can be used for the prevention of thrombus formation in the postoperative setting. These include dextran and aspirin, which are equally efficacious. Aspirin at a dose of 81 mg is continued daily for 4 weeks following the operation to help maintain vessel patency. Broad-spectrum antibiotics, pain medications, and stool softeners are given in the immediate postoperative setting.

49.7.2 Surgical Treatment

Preoperative defect anticipation and intraoperative wound assessment are critical in assisting with flap selection and design. Potential flap choices, based on anticipated defect location and size, are listed in ▶ Table 49.2.

Each potential flap site has its advantages and disadvantages. The strengths of each site play an important role when one is planning to resurface a defect in the head and neck. The details of flap dissection are beyond the scope of this chapter; however, salient points about anatomy, flap design, and harvest are reviewed below for some of the flaps more commonly used in head and neck reconstruction.

The pectoralis major anatomy is shown in ▶ Fig. 49.2. Flap design takes into consideration the first two intercostal perforators emanating parasternally (▶ Fig. 49.3). These perforators supply the deltopectoral flap, which is a region of tissue extending from the sternum to the shoulder. This cutaneous flap can be used for coverage in cases of pectoralis major failure and should be preserved. Once incised, the pectoralis major muscle is identified and detached from the anterior chest wall. The pedicle (pectoral branch of the thoracoacromial artery) courses on the undersurface of the muscle and is easily identified. The lateral muscle attachments to the humerus, as well as the lateral thoracic vessels, are divided to improve the arc of rotation. A generous subcutaneous tunnel is then created under the deltopectoral flap, allowing passage of the pectoralis major into the neck. Care is taken to handle the skin paddle gently in order to avoid shearing the perforating vessels feeding it through the pectoralis major muscle. This flap can reach as high as the mid-

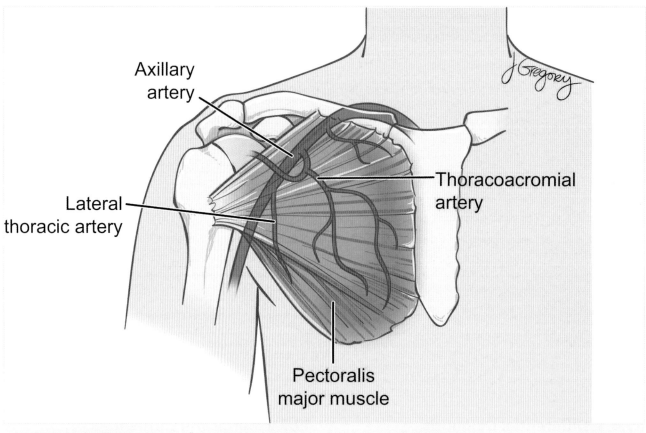

Fig. 49.2 Pectoralis major myocutaneous flap anatomy.

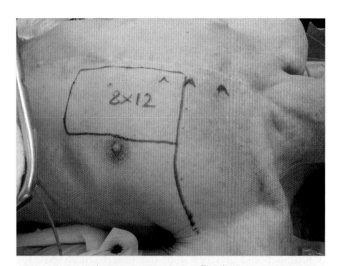

Fig. 49.3 Pectoralis major myocutaneous flap design.

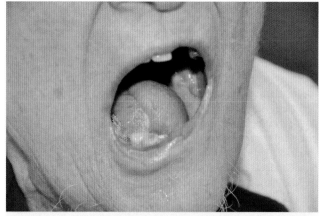

Fig. 49.4 Oral tongue reconstruction with a radial forearm free flap. The highly pliable skin paddle is able to conform to the original shape of the reconstructed left tongue and floor of mouth.

face; however, tension on the pectoralis major flap increases the risk for skin ischemia and breakdown. Partial skin loss can occur in as many as half of all pectoralis flaps. The resulting chest wall defect can be closed primarily in most situations.

The radial forearm free flap has several anatomical advantages that make it an ideal soft-tissue flap for numerous head and neck defects. The middle to distal skin of the forearm has a high degree of pliability, allowing it to conform to complex soft-tissue deficits in the head and neck. These commonly include

defects of the tongue (▶ Fig. 49.4) and pharynx (▶ Fig. 49.5). The other attractive feature of this flap is its long vascular pedicle and redundant venous drainage. In a vessel-depleted neck, the pedicle can reach to the opposite side for anastomosis with recipient vessels. The venous outflow through the cephalic vein and deep venous system, accompanying the radial artery, readily intercommunicates via a number of small vessels and a single large vein in the proximal forearm. The redundancy of the venous outflow allows the selection of either vein for the microvenous anastomosis. The skin paddle design is anatomically centered on the radial vasculature of the forearm (▶ Fig. 49.6). The medial border of the skin paddle is restricted at the palmaris tendon, to avoid potential exposure of the ulnar vessels. Important steps in flap elevation include early identification of the cephalic vein, preservation of the distal superficial branch of the radial nerve, and dissection of the communicating vein in the proximal forearm. Inclusion of the lateral antebrachial cutaneous nerve, which travels along the cephalic vein, provides a sensory nerve for reinnervation in the head and neck

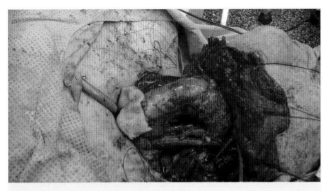

Fig. 49.5 Pharynx reconstruction with a radial forearm free flap. The skin paddle of the flap is tubed and sutured to itself to re-create the conduit between the oropharynx and esophagus. Part of the skin paddle is brought outside to provide coverage above the laryngectomy stoma.

region. A split-thickness skin graft is used for closure of the forearm wound. Long-term problems related to flap harvest may include sensory loss in the distribution of the superficial radial nerve, scar contracture with limitation of hand extension, and visible deformity. Grip strength and range of motion are rarely affected to any significant extent.

The main advantage of the anterolateral thigh flap over the radial forearm flap is reduced donor site morbidity. Most thigh defects following flap harvest can be closed primarily, thereby avoiding a skin graft. Flap design depends on identification of the perforating vessels from the flap pedicle—the descending branch of the lateral circumflex femoral artery. These perforators lie close to a line drawn between the anterior superior iliac spine and anterolateral patella. After redundant skin of the thigh has been pinched together, the medial and lateral borders of the flap can be marked (▶ Fig. 49.7). In older patients, skin paddles measuring 250 to 350 cm^2 can be elevated while primary closure in the thigh is achieved. Elevation of the anterolateral thigh flap requires meticulous dissection of the perforating vessels traversing the vastus lateralis muscle. Alternatively, this flap can be raised by keeping a portion of vastus lateralis muscle attached to the undersurface of the skin and fat, thereby eliminating tedious perforator dissection. The anterior lateral thigh flap pedicle is similar to that of the radial forearm flap, in that it is long and can reach to the opposite side of the neck if such need arises. Morbidity related to this flap is minimal, even in cases of muscle sacrifice. Gait disturbances are rare.

The fibula free flap is the optimal source of tissue for bony reconstruction of the head and neck, especially the mandible.

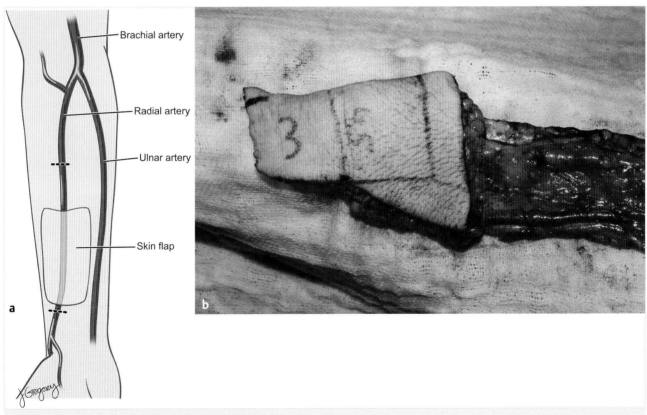

Fig. 49.6 (a) Radial forearm free flap design and (b) after harvest.

Favorable anatomical characteristics of this flap include an available bone length of up to 25 cm, strong cortical bone capable of supporting osseointegrated implants, and a reliable vascular pedicle. In addition, a large area of lateral leg skin can be harvested with this flap, up to 300 cm² (▶ Fig. 49.8). Harvesting beyond this amount risks partial skin loss. The fibular skin paddle can be used for resurfacing most tongue, cheek, and associated external defects. Fibular bone can precisely reconstitute any segmental mandible defect. Fibular contouring is performed with closing osteotomies. Each osteotomy segment, which relies on vascular supply from the periosteum, needs to be 3 cm or larger to preserve sufficient blood flow. Following the osteotomies, a reconstruction plate is applied to stabilize the fibula within the mandibular defect.

Complications of free flap transfer include flap failure (as previously discussed), bleeding (▶ Fig. 49.9), infection, wound

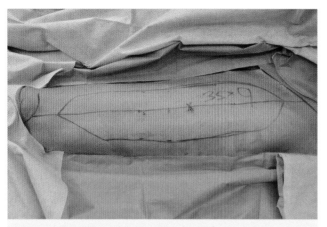

Fig. 49.7 Anterolateral thigh free flap design.

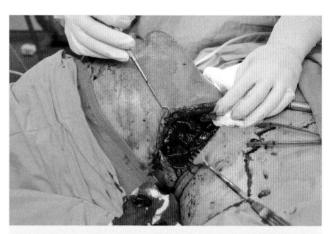

Fig. 49.9 Hematoma evacuation on the first postoperative day.

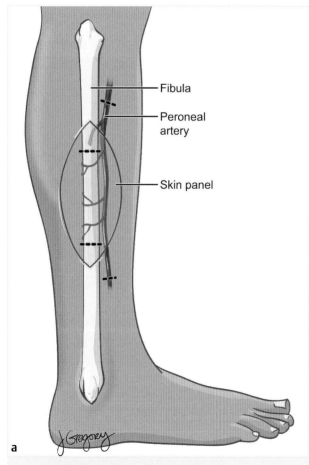

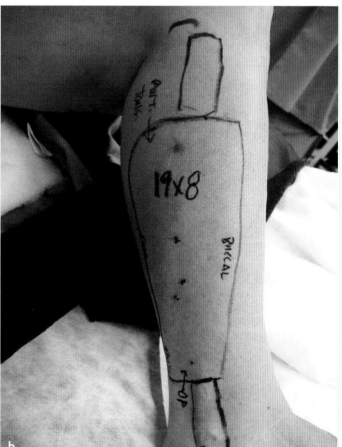

Fig. 49.8 (a,b) Fibula free flap design.

dehiscence, fistula formation, hardware exposure, excessive bulk, and several others. Soft-tissue flap revisions may be necessary to improve tissue contour and function. In applicable cases, revisions can be delayed until after the end of radiation therapy.

49.8 Prognosis

The overall success rate for free tissue transfer in the head and neck approaches 95% in several large series reported in the literature. The perioperative mortality is approximately 1%. The rate of medical complications, most commonly caused by cardiac and pulmonary manifestations, is about 20%. Surgical complications, such as wound infection, breakdown, and fistula formation, are significantly higher in patients with a history of previous radiation therapy.

49.9 Roundsmanship

- Flap selection depends on the missing tissues and the volume requirements of a head and neck defect.
- Free flaps are the optimal choice for the reconstruction of large head and neck defects.
- Free flap reliability approaches 95%.
- Effective elevation of a pectoralis major myocutaneous flap requires sectioning of the lateral thoracic artery and preservation of the first two intercostal perforators.

49.10 Recommended Reading

[1] Disa JJ, Pusic AL, Hidalgo DH, Cordeiro PG. Simplifying microvascular head and neck reconstruction: a rational approach to donor site selection. Ann Plast Surg 2001; 47: 385–389
[2] Suh JD, Sercarz JA, Abemayor E et al. Analysis of outcome and complications in 400 cases of microvascular head and neck reconstruction. Arch Otolaryngol Head Neck Surg 2004; 130: 962–966
[3] Urken ML, Cheney ML, Sullivan MJ, Biller HF. Atlas of Regional and Free Flaps for Head and Neck Reconstruction. New York, NY: Raven Press; 1995
[4] Wax MK, Kim J, Ducic Y. Update on major reconstruction of the head and neck. Arch Facial Plast Surg 2007; 9: 392–399

50 Tissue Expansion

Grigorly Mashkevich and Kenneth M. Wong

50.1 Introduction

Over the past 30 years, tissue expansion has become an increasingly useful adjunct in reconstructive surgery, especially in the region of the head and neck. Although the concept of tissue expansion has been known since ancient times, Neumann, using a rubber balloon gradually filled with air, first applied this technique in reconstructive surgery in 1957. Following publications by Austed and Radovan, tissue expansion gained wide acceptance during the 1970s and 1980s. Its safety and efficacy were well documented in the decades that followed. The technique of tissue expansion has been applied successfully to a wide range of clinical problems, including breast reconstruction, repair of burn wounds, pediatric plastic surgery, and head and neck reconstruction. Tissue expansion provides several distinct advantages, such as excellent color and texture match and the retention of cutaneous sensory function. For these reasons, tissue expansion continues to serve as a valuable tool for the reconstructive surgeon.

50.2 Incidence of Disease

Although exact data on the number of tissue expansion procedures performed are lacking, the use of tissue expansion has been well documented and published. In the head and neck region, the most frequent application has been for large scalp and neck wounds.

50.3 Terminology

A distinction should be made between long-term tissue expansion and intraoperative tissue expansion because they differ in technique and the process of expansion. Long-term tissue expansion involves placing an expander device under the skin in the appropriate area. The wound is allowed to heal for 2 weeks, and expansion is carried out in serial fashion over several weeks with sterile technique and saline injection. The expander is then removed in another surgical procedure and the wound reconstructed with the newly expanded tissue. Intraoperative tissue expansion, on the other hand, is performed synchronously with reconstruction of the wound. Intraoperative tissue expansion is carried out in cyclical fashion, with three cycles of expansion and deflation. A large Foley catheter or specific expander device is used. The balloon is inflated underneath the area to be expanded, left for 3 minutes, and deflated. The flap is then incised and used to reconstruct the wound in one setting.

50.4 Applied Anatomy

A thorough understanding of head and neck anatomy and the histologic layers of the skin is important in tissue expansion, especially when the expanders are placed. The skin comprises the epidermis and dermis, which are situated over the subcuta-

neous tissues. The dermis is further separated into papillary and reticular layers. All tissue components of the skin undergo physiologic changes during tissue expansion. Knowledge of the different layers in the head and neck is important in terms of the placement of expanders. In the scalp region, the tissue layers include the skin, connective tissue, galea aponeurosis, loose areolar tissue, and periosteum. An important layer in the facial region is the superficial musculoaponeurotic system (SMAS), which connects to the galea superiorly and platysma inferiorly.

50.5 The Disease Process

50.5.1 Etiology

Tissue expansion can address wounds in need of soft-tissue coverage, such as those resulting from burns, trauma, or cancer. In the head and neck region, tissue expansion can additionally be used for scar revision, the treatment of male pattern baldness, the release of contractures, and even the repair of cleft lip and microtia. In the pediatric population, tissue expansion can assist in the management of various disorders, including congenital nevi, hemangiomas, lymphangiomas, arteriovenous malformations, and congenital anomalies.

50.5.2 Pathogenesis

Although not a disease process, long-term tissue expansion results in mechanical, physiologic, and histologic changes ("biological creep") within the different tissue layers. The epidermis and dermis exhibit the most drastic changes.

Epidermal thickness remains the same or increases. Although the stratified layers remain intact, metabolic and mitotic activities increase. After expansion, the epidermis usually returns to normal, with hyperpigmentation and dryness the most common side effects.

Increased metabolic activity and physiologic changes are also observed in the dermis, which can lose 30 to 50% of its thickness. Fibroblast activity is enhanced, resulting in increased collagen synthesis. The basal layer of the dermis thickens and myofibroblasts increase in number, which can lead to flap contracture after flap transfer. The number of hair follicles remains the same, but the density decreases as the surface area increases. Adipose tissue and muscle tend to atrophy with tissue expansion. Adipose tissue can lose up to 50% of its thickness. Nerves lengthen with gradual expansion. One major advantage of long-term tissue expansion is neovascularization. Capillaries proliferate, leading to a lengthening of venules and arterioles. Increased vascularity improves flap survival and resistance to infection.

Tissue gain during intraoperative tissue expansion occurs via a different process. Intraoperative tissue expansion increases skin length through the process of mechanical creep, which involves the disruption and realignment of collagen and elastin fibers, displacement of adjacent tissue, and shifting of intersti-

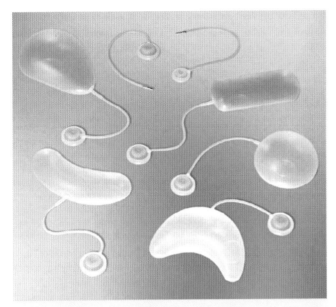

Fig. 50.1 Various shapes of tissue expanders. (Image provided courtesy of Mentor Corporation, Santa Barbara, CA.)

tial fluids. About 1 to 3 cm of additional flap length can be obtained through this approach.

50.5.3 Natural History and Progression

Many different shapes, sizes, and volumes of tissue expanders are used in long-term expansion (▶ Fig. 50.1). Common shapes include rectangular, crescent, and circular. Tissue expanders consist of an expandable chamber composed of silicone elastomers and an injection port. In the head and neck area, remote injection ports can be optimally placed away from sensitive areas of the face. In long-term expansion, progression occurs in a biphasic manner. There is a period of tissue resistance during the initial stages, which is followed by a rapid increase in compliance. Expansion should be continued until there is about twice the amount of tissue needed to cover a defect. On the other hand, intraoperative expansion, for reasons previously outlined, occurs much more rapidly and is performed in one setting.

50.6 Medical Evaluation

50.6.1 Presenting Complaints

Patient motivation is an important factor in the decision to proceed with tissue expansion. The patient should be prepared for multiple procedures and frequent office visits. The surgeon must counsel patients and caregivers with respect to the time course of expansion, expected physical appearance, and interim social functioning. During the later stages of the process, the physical appearance caused by the expanded tissue may interfere with work and social activities. Proper patient education before the process begins can help minimize expected anxiety. The surgeon should also inquire about any history of smoking, diabetes, or radiation because any of these may adversely affect wound healing and outcome.

50.6.2 Clinical Findings, Physical Examination

The wound should be measured, and the shape and size of the expander chosen appropriately. The shape of the expander should match the shape of the anticipated flap. If a large rotation flap is expected, then a crescent or circular expander is selected. Rectangular expanders are most commonly used for straight advancement flaps. The area of the base of the expander should be 2.5 to 3 times the area of the defect. The actual amount of tissue that can be used is only a fraction (about 35%) of the increased surface area.

50.6.3 Testing

Standard preoperative medical testing should be performed based on the patient's medical history, including electrocardiography, chest X-ray, and all necessary laboratory work. All required medical clearance should be obtained before any procedures are performed.

50.6.4 Differential Diagnosis

When dealing with a wound defect, the surgeon should weigh all the available reconstructive options. These include healing by secondary intention, primary reapproximation, local or regional flaps, split-thickness or full-thickness skin grafts, and microvascular free flaps. Tissue expansion can be an adjunct to any of these interventions by increasing the amount of available tissue. The advantages of tissue expansion include good color, texture and bulk match, minimal donor site morbidity, minimal scarring, and retention of sensory and adnexal function. Disadvantages include temporary cosmetic deformity during the expansion phase, prolonged period of expansion, need for multiple procedures, and complications associated with the implant and placement.

50.7 Surgical Treatment

Multiple procedures are needed for long-term tissue expansion. Once an expander with the appropriate size and shape has been selected, several technical considerations guide its insertion in the operating room. The incision is placed away from the site of expansion to minimize the chance of wound dehiscence and implant extrusion. The pocket for the expander should be large enough to accommodate it without resistance and folding. The injection port should be positioned in an optimal location, with patient comfort and visibility for the serial injections taken into account.

The area of expansion in the head and neck determines the tissue plane in which the expander is positioned. In the facial region, the expander is placed subcutaneously, superficial to the SMAS, to protect the facial nerve. In the neck, the expander can be placed either superficial or deep to the platysma muscle. When the expander is placed in the deeper plane, care must be taken to position the device away from the marginal branch of the facial nerve. The expander is placed between the galea and pericranium in the scalp and forehead. Superficial placement in the scalp region can lead to alopecia.

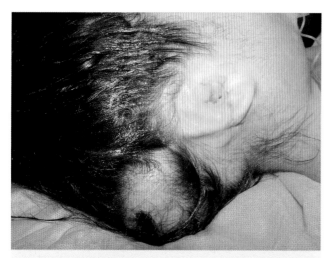

Fig. 50.2 Patient with bilateral microtia requiring long-term expansion of the postauricular tissue of the scalp to limit the need for skin graft. Impending necrosis developed at the end of the expansion cycle. The expander was removed and the expanded tissue successfully used for postauricular coverage after elevation of the auricular framework.

Complications associated with long-term tissue expansion occur in approximately 10% of adult patients and up to 30% of pediatric patients. These include hematoma, seroma, exposure or extrusion, infection, numbness due to neurapraxia, migration, and very rarely leakage of the device. Exposure and infection are the most common side effects. Their management depends on when they occur during the expansion process; if the device is exposed or infected early, implant removal is the most prudent course of action, whereas an implant can be left in place for an additional round of expansion and antibiotics con-tinued to prevent infection if the device is exposed near the end of the expansion process (▶ Fig. 50.2). Implant capsule formation can limit the pliancy of the expanded skin, and capsulectomy may be necessary.

50.8 Prognosis

When performed correctly, tissue expansion has excellent cosmetic and functional results. It has become a valuable tool, especially in the reconstruction of the head and neck region.

50.9 Roundsmanship

- There are two types of tissue expansion: long-term and intraoperative.
- Physiologic and histologic changes ("biological creep") occur during long-term expansion, whereas mechanical changes accompany intraoperative expansion, known as "mechanical creep."
- The size of expander should be approximately 2.5 to 3 times the size of the defect.
- Expanders should be removed if complications occur early in the expansion process. Expansion can be continued or shortened with late complications.

50.10 Recommended Reading

[1] Hoffmann JF. Tissue expansion in the head and neck. Facial Plast Surg Clin North Am 2005; 13: 315–324

[2] Hurvitz KA, Rosen H, Meara JG. Pediatric cervicofacial tissue expansion. Int J Pediatr Otorhinolaryngol 2005; 69: 1509–1513

[3] Motamed S, Niazi F, Atarian S, Motamed A. Post-burn head and neck reconstruction using tissue expanders. Burns 2008; 34: 878–884

51 Treatment of Facial Paralysis

Grigorly Mashkevich

51.1 Introduction

Facial paralysis is a challenging problem for both patients and physicians. This potentially disabling condition can arise from multiple causes, and a thorough understanding of the differential diagnosis and available treatment options is required. Optimal cosmetic and functional rehabilitation in patients with facial paralysis depends on an individualized treatment strategy performed in a multidisciplinary setting.

51.2 Incidence of Disease

The incidence of facial paralysis varies greatly based on its etiology. This information is provided in sections that follow.

51.3 Classification of the Disease Process

The House-Brackmann scale is a reliable tool for grading facial nerve dysfunction (▶ Table 51.1). This scale is not applicable to patients with facial nerve synkinesis. Other scales have been developed to help assess the physical and psychological impact of facial paralysis on afflicted individuals.

51.4 Applied Anatomy

The facial nerve enters the temporal bone via the internal auditory meatus and travels within the tight bony confines of the fallopian canal. Most inflammatory conditions cause pressure-induced paralysis in this portion of the nerve. Upon its exit from the stylomastoid foramen, the facial nerve penetrates the substance of the parotid gland, by which it is well protected in the preauricular region. Within the gland, it divides into five major branches, which exit the periphery of the gland deep to the superficial muscular aponeurotic system (SMAS). Anterior to the parotid gland, distal facial nerve branches substantially intercommunicate and innervate the midfacial musculature with redundancy.

51.5 The Disease Process

51.5.1 Etiology, Pathogenesis, Natural History, and Progression

Congenital

Birth Trauma

Several factors during the birth of a child may lead to facial nerve injury and associated paralysis. These include the use of forceps during the delivery, birth weight of more than 3.5 kg (7.7 lb), and first pregnancy. A contributing factor may be compression molding of the fetus while it passes through the birth canal. In this setting, the facial nerve is susceptible to stretch injury and requires time to regenerate. The overall prognosis is excellent, with up to 90% of children achieving complete recovery of their facial nerve function without surgical or medical intervention. In the rare instances in which transection injury is strongly suspected, surgical exploration may be warranted.

Mobius Syndrome

Mobius syndrome, first described in the 19th century, is characterized by concomitant facial and abducens nerve palsies. These may arise as a result of peripheral nerve underdevelopment or agenesis, as well as from poorly functioning brainstem nuclei. Additional cranial nerves may be affected in this syndrome. Clinically, patients struggle with facial movement and have extreme difficulty expressing emotion. Accompanying problems include oral incompetence, drooling, poor self-esteem, and social isolation—all of which exacerbate the challenges to persons with this condition. In this patient group, free muscle transfer has been successfully used for the rehabilitation of facial movement. Ideally, such intervention is performed before school entry in an attempt to avoid the psychological trauma caused by peer ridicule during the early formative years.

Melkersson-Rosenthal Syndrome

Melkersson-Rosenthal syndrome is the constellation of recurrent facial paralysis, facial swelling, and tongue fissures. Although the typical care of recurrent flare-ups includes steroid

Table 51.1 House-Brackmann grading scale for facial nerve dysfunction

Grade	Impairment	Deficits
I	Normal	Normal facial movement
II	Slight	Normal resting tone, complete eye closure, slight weakness with movement
III	Moderate	Mild facial asymmetry at rest, complete eye closure with effort, moderate weakness with movement
IV	Moderate–severe	Disfiguring asymmetry at rest, incomplete eye closure, some facial movement
V	Severe	Disfiguring asymmetry at rest, incomplete eye closure, slightly noticeable facial movement
VI	Complete	Absent facial movement

and anti-inflammatory medications, controversy remains over the management and prevention of facial palsy. Isolated case reports describing facial nerve decompression (opening its biologic bony confines to prevent nerve pressure during bouts of swelling) suggest that long-term resolution of facial nerve dysfunction is possible with this more aggressive approach.

Hemifacial Microsomia

Hemifacial microsomia comprises a spectrum of congenital facial anomalies arising from underdevelopment of one side of the face. This syndrome is marked by hemifacial soft-tissue deficiency and poor development of the lower jaw, maxilla, and external ear. In cases of accompanying facial weakness or paralysis, reconstructive surgery can be planned together with craniofacial repair directed at correcting jaw and ear abnormalities. The restoration of facial symmetry and smile can be especially effective with free muscle transfer because it provides a secondary benefit of facial augmentation.

Infectious

Bell Palsy

Bell palsy is also known as idiopathic facial paralysis. However, recent evidence suggests that herpes simplex virus is the most likely agent responsible for Bell palsy. The incidence of this condition approaches 30 per 100,000 people. Typically, the onset of paralysis occurs over a period of 24 to 72 hours and may be accompanied by other symptoms, such as pain around the ear, decreased taste, and diminished hearing on the affected side. Although the overwhelming majority of patients recover their facial nerve function, a small minority are left with a movement deficit, marked by aberrant facial movements (synkinesis). Steroids and antiviral medicines have been found helpful in improving functional recovery of the facial nerve in the acute stages of Bell palsy. In selected instances, in which electrical activity of the nerve is severely depressed during the first 2 weeks (see testing below), surgical decompression of the nerve's bony channel should be considered. In those with poor recovery and synkinesis, chemodenervation (paralysis) with botulinum toxin A and intensive physical therapy offer a promising rehabilitative option.

Ramsay Hunt Syndrome

Ramsay Hunt syndrome (herpes zoster oticus) is caused by reactivation of the varicella-zoster virus (human herpesvirus 3) within the facial nerve and is accompanied by vesicle formation and ear pain (zoster oticus). Other symptoms, such as hearing loss, tinnitus, vertigo, nausea, and vomiting, may be present, as well. These are thought to arise from irritation of the vestibulocochlear nerve, which is situated adjacent to the inflamed facial nerve in the temporal bone. Although no randomized studies exist on the treatment of this infrequent condition, a combination of steroids, antivirals, and pain medications can be used to control inflammatory injury of the facial nerve. This regimen is based on experience in the treatment of Bell palsy (with steroids), as well as the treatment of zoster infections in other parts of the body (with antiviral medications). The prognosis for facial nerve recovery is poor in Ramsay Hunt syndrome,

with chronic neuralgia (pain) commonly persisting following the resolution of infection.

Otitis Media/Mastoiditis

Otitis media/Mastoiditis is an acute infection of the middle ear and mastoid that in rare cases (fewer than 1%) may result in facial nerve paralysis. Swelling around the nerve and toxic substances released by bacteria are thought to be the causative factors behind facial nerve involvement. Successful treatment consists of the prompt recognition and eradication of infection. This includes broad-spectrum antibiotics and myringotomy with placement of a ventilation tube, so that a bacterial specimen can be obtained for culture. A mastoidectomy (removal of infection in the adjacent mastoid bone) may be performed in selected cases of associated mastoiditis. The prognosis for complete facial nerve recovery is excellent with the above interventions.

Cholesteatoma

Cholesteatoma is a slow-growing skin cyst that over time causes destruction in the ear by exerting pressure on surrounding structures and causing flare-ups of chronic infection. The incidence of facial paralysis in a setting of cholesteatoma approaches 3%. Prompt recognition of this disease process and surgical eradication are critical in successfully releasing pressure from the facial nerve and removing the source of chronic infection and inflammation. Poor prognostic factors for recovery include extension of a cholesteatoma into the petrous apex (deep portion of the temporal bone) and delayed surgical treatment. Patients who undergo early intervention are more likely to recover their facial nerve function completely.

Lyme Disease

Lyme disease is caused by *Borrelia burgdorferi*, a bacterium transmitted to humans through the bite of infected ticks. Typical symptoms and signs in acute stages of Lyme disease include headache, weakness, fever, and erythema chronicum migrans (a characteristic target-shaped rash that develops at the site of a tick bite). Although the incidence of accompanying facial paralysis reaches 11%, it completely resolves in 99.2% of patients. A high index of suspicion for Lyme disease should arise when a patient presents with a recent history of tick bites during the summer months in areas where the disease is endemic; the national risk map is available on the U.S. Centers for Disease Control and Prevention Web site (http://www.cdc.gov/lyme/stats/maps/interactiveMaps.html). Lyme titers should be obtained for confirmation and antibiotic therapy instituted, following guidelines published by the Infectious Diseases Society of America (http://www.idsociety.org/lymedisease.htm).

Other

A number of additional infectious processes can impair facial nerve function, including HIV infection, tuberculosis, infectious mononucleosis, and others. These conditions typically have other associated symptoms in affected individuals, and a high index of suspicion is required to make the diagnosis. Previous history and risk factors for exposure influence the decision to pursue these diagnostic possibilities in a setting of facial paralysis. The mainstay of management is targeted medical therapy, unless associated mastoiditis is identified on work-up. In this instance, mastoidectomy should be performed to control the infection and swelling around the facial nerve.

Systemic and Neurologic

Conditions in this category include autoimmune diseases, diabetes, sarcoidosis, Guillain-Barré syndrome, multiple sclerosis, and others. Infrequently, these can present with isolated facial paralysis. A correct diagnosis and prompt medical intervention form the initial treatment strategy, with anticipated recovery of facial movement in most cases.

Traumatic

Traumatic injuries to the head and cranium are one of the most common causes of acquired facial paralysis. In instances of blunt trauma, in which no lacerations or fractures occur, the facial nerve retains its continuity and is expected to recover. In a setting of suspected nerve laceration (penetrating trauma through facial skin and soft tissues), immediate surgical exploration with nerve repair is warranted. Ideally, this would take place within 3 days of injury, during which time the distal portion of the facial nerve can still be stimulated and thus identified during surgery.

When facial trauma results in a temporal bone fracture, accompanying facial nerve injury occurs in 10 to 25% of cases. Temporal bone fractures follow several patterns, defined with respect to the long axis of a temporal bone: longitudinal (80%), transverse (10%), and mixed (10%). Facial nerve paralysis occurs more frequently in transverse (50%) than in longitudinal (20%) fractures. Full recovery is expected in patients with a delayed onset of facial paralysis. In contrast, up to 50% of those with an immediate onset recover poorly. In many cases of significant facial trauma, concomitant acute conditions may delay examination and testing of the facial nerve. However, delayed surgical exploration, even months after the injury, can still be performed with reasonable success rates of functional improvement and recovery.

Iatrogenic injury to the facial nerve can occur during facial, bony, or intracranial surgery. The extent of nerve damage largely dictates the type of repair. In severe cases, nerve repair may not be possible, and other rehabilitative methods must be utilized (▶ Fig. 51.1).

Neoplastic

The extirpation of cancer invading or situated in the vicinity of the facial nerve may require significant nerve manipulation during surgery and possibly partial or complete transection. The most common tumors affecting the facial nerve are acoustic neuroma (vestibular schwannoma), glomus tumors, facial neuroma, and carcinoma of the parotid gland. When the facial nerve continuity is maintained during surgery, postoperative recovery is closely monitored. Stimulation of the nerve at the end of the procedure may provide useful prognostic data. Steroid medications are typically not given in this setting because several studies have clearly shown lack of benefit. Following

surgery, electromyography (EMG) can be utilized to assess reinnervation of the facial musculature. Depending on the stage of recovery, as well as individual challenges and concerns, several simple procedures are considered to aid with eye closure, facial symmetry, and oral competence (▶ Fig. 51.2).

51.5.2 Potential Disease Complications

In the setting of an intact or repaired facial nerve, the resolution of paralysis depends on axonal regeneration and regrowth into the facial musculature. Aberrant regeneration of facial nerve axons can be characterized by misdirection of fibers or sprouting of axons to innervate multiple facial muscles. This can result in synkinesis, which is an involuntary contraction of the facial muscles during facial mimetic movement (▶ Fig. 51.3). Other complications of facial paralysis include excessive globe dryness and exposure keratopathy, oral incompetence and drooling, and chronic cheek biting.

51.6 Medical Evaluation

In an acute setting, the medical evaluation should address a number of differential possibilities, as outlined in ▶ Fig. 51.4 and ▶ Fig. 51.5.

51.6.1 Presenting Complaints

Patients with facial paralysis experience a range of difficulties pertaining to appearance, speech, and swallowing. Periocular complaints may include blurry vision, excessive tearing, and discomfort or pain. Perioral deficits depend on the age of the patient and corresponding facial tone. These can include drooling, food spillage, and cheek biting. Facial asymmetry at rest and with movement can be a significant source of embarrassment and lead to social withdrawal.

51.6.2 Clinical Findings, Physical Examination

During the initial visit, a detailed examination of facial appearance at rest and with movement is photographed and videotaped. On physical examination, patients with facial paralysis display characteristic tissue sagging and lack of facial movement (▶ Fig. 51.6 and ▶ Fig. 51.7). The eye examination typically reveals lagophthalmos, or an inability to fully close the eye. The Bell phenomenon, which is an upward rolling of the globe on attempted eye closure, is an important finding denoting an added level of protection against dryness. Signs of excessive eye dryness and irritation include redness of the conjunctivae and mucoid or purulent drainage. Examination of the oral cavity may reveal drooling of saliva due to commissure incompetence and inner cheek trauma from biting.

51.6.3 Testing

In a setting of acute facial paralysis, electrodiagnostic testing can help identify patients who may benefit from surgical decompression of the facial nerve. Electroneurography of the facial nerve measures compound facial muscle action potential

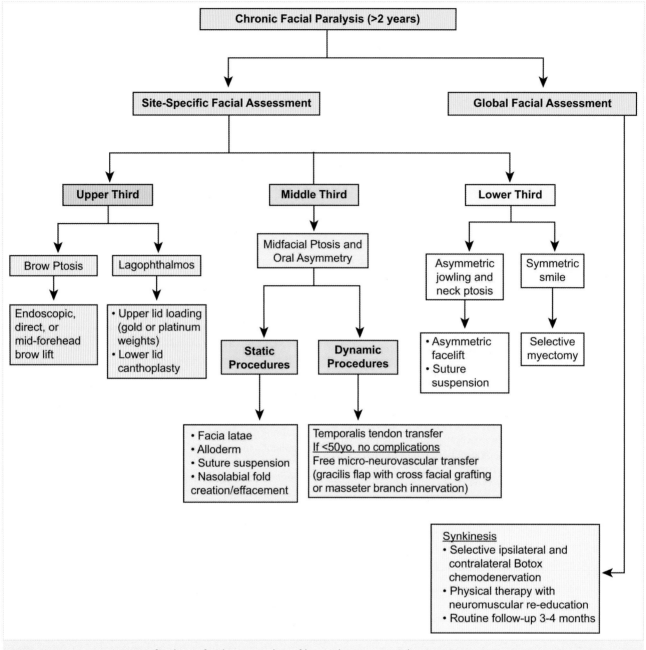

Fig. 51.1 Management strategies for chronic facial nerve paralysis of longer than two years' duration.

upon stimulation of the nerve at the stylomastoid foramen. Measurements from the paralyzed and healthy sides of the face are compared. In cases of more than 90% degeneration, decompression of the facial nerve may be indicated. In cases of paralysis lasting beyond 3 weeks, facial EMG can provide prognostic data. This test is performed by inserting a needle into one of several larger facial muscles, such as the orbicularis oculi and orbicularis oris, and recording action potentials. Polyphasic configuration of the action potentials indicates early reinnervation and impending return of facial function. Blood tests may be ordered depending on the level of suspicion for any number of infectious and systemic disease processes (see ▶ Fig. 51.4).

51.6.4 Differential Diagnosis

The differential diagnosis of facial paralysis is reviewed in an earlier section of this chapter (The Disease Process) and in ▶ Fig. 51.4 and ▶ Fig. 51.5

51.7 Treatment

51.7.1 Medical Treatment

The medical treatment of facial paralysis depends on the underlying etiology. Specific treatment guidelines are outlined in ▶ Fig. 51.4. All patients with facial paralysis receive

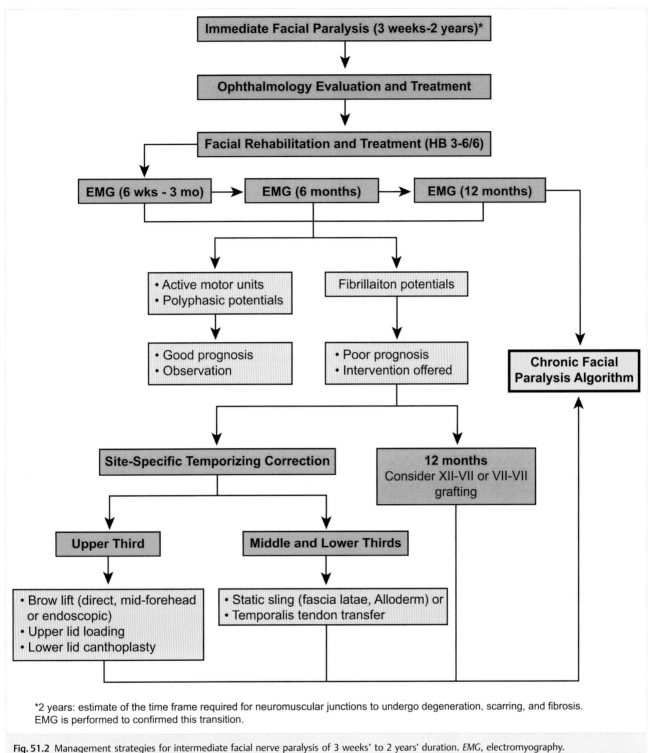

*2 years: estimate of the time frame required for neuromuscular junctions to undergo degeneration, scarring, and fibrosis. EMG is performed to confirmed this transition.

Fig. 51.2 Management strategies for intermediate facial nerve paralysis of 3 weeks' to 2 years' duration. *EMG*, electromyography.

eye care with natural tears and ointment until full resolution of lagophthalmos.

51.7.2 Surgical Treatment

The treatment options for facial paralysis and associated movement disorders are numerous and vary based on individual deficits, needs, and preferences. An individualized plan of care is formulated together with the patient. In many cases of facial paralysis, multiple treatments may be necessary in order to achieve optimal aesthetic and functional results. Specialty services, such as ophthalmology, otology, and physical therapy, are consulted on an as-needed basis.

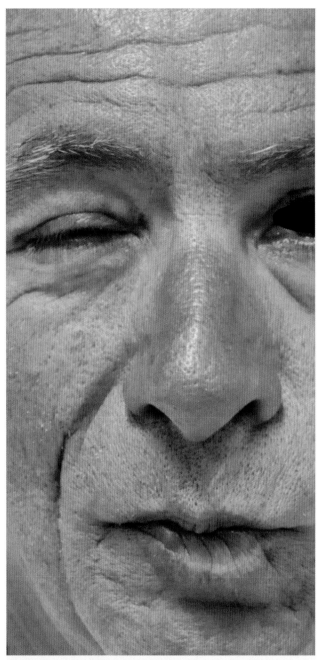

Fig. 51.3 Right facial synkinesis, or lip pucker. Note simultaneous contraction of the right orbicularis oculi, orbicularis oris, and platysma

Acute Facial Paralysis (0–21 Days)

Identifiable causes of acute paralysis are treated expediently with appropriate medical therapy, following proper identification of the cause (see ▶ Fig. 51.4). In rare instances, surgical intervention may be necessary to control infection and/or swelling around the facial nerve.

In a setting of facial nerve transection, several reconstructive options are available for immediate facial nerve repair, which minimize the sequelae of paralysis and promote the return of facial nerve function (see ▶ Fig. 51.5). Tension-free approximation is critical in achieving a successful neurorrhaphy. Identified

nerve ends can be mobilized for distances of several centimeters by releasing attachments to surrounding soft tissues. Larger gaps can be repaired with either regional (great auricular) or distal (lateral antebrachial cutaneous or sural) nerve grafts. Nerve stumps are approximated with fine, interrupted monofilament sutures (e.g., 9–0 nylon) placed under microscopic magnification.

Intermediate Facial Paralysis (21 Days–2 Years)

During this stage, facial nerve recovery is monitored with serial EMG examinations, which provide useful prognostic data. In the setting of a poorly recovering facial nerve, several procedures can be considered to restore facial appearance and rehabilitate function around the eye and mouth (see ▶ Fig. 51.2). In the early stages, at 6 weeks to 3 months, the placement of gold or platinum weights aids upper eyelid closure, and static sling suspension of the midface and lip can be performed with minimal associated downtime. These procedures do not interfere with the recovering facial nerve. In the later stages, if the facial nerve continues to display poor recovery on EMG, consideration is given to nerve transfer procedures designed to maintain neurologic input to the facial muscles. A graft from a nearby nerve, most commonly the hypoglossal nerve (cranial nerve XII), can provide such input. This ultimately allows the preservation of tone in the native facial musculature—usually, however, at the expense of causing synkinesis (involuntary simultaneous movement of multiple facial muscles). As an alternative, definitive reconstruction with a vascularized gracilis muscle transfer is also considered at this stage.

Chronic Facial Paralysis (More than 2 Years)

Paralysis

The management of chronic facial paralysis depends on numerous factors, including patient preferences and desires. Depending on the situation, medical considerations may limit available procedures. For example, older and frailer patients are poor candidates for nerve and muscle transfer procedures. Reconstructive options range from static suspensions to dynamic reanimation via muscle transfer to the paralyzed side (see ▶ Fig. 51.1). Both have their merits and serve a useful purpose in the aesthetic and functional rehabilitation of patients with facial paralysis.

Static slings are the simplest solution with the quickest recovery time. They reposition ptotic tissues of the face and aid in functional aspects, such as lip closure and the prevention of food spillage. Autologous fascia, homologous tissue (AlloDerm; LifeCell Corporation, Branchburg, NJ), sutures, and various manufactured materials (Gore-Tex; W. L. Gore & Associates, Newark, DE) can be used for this purpose. Static slings may relax and stretch over time, potentially requiring additional tightening.

Muscle transfer allows the restoration of symmetry and movement on the paralyzed side. These are more extended procedures with longer recovery times than those of static slings. Transfer of the temporalis muscle, however, requires the patient to bite down in order to activate the smile. The procedure of choice to regain involuntary smile is a two-stage transfer of the

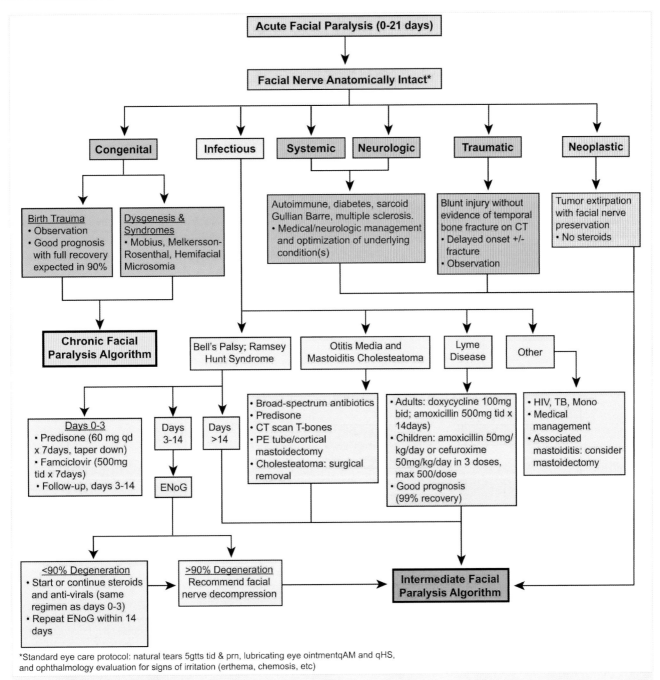

Fig. 51.4 Differential diagnosis and management of acute facial nerve paralysis with an intact facial nerve, 0 to 21 days' duration.

gracilis muscle. During the first operation, a smile-specific branch of the facial nerve is identified on the healthy facial side. This branch is then grafted across to the paralyzed side with a long nerve, such as the sural nerve (▶ Fig. 51.8, ▶ Fig. 51.9, ▶ Fig. 51.10). Approximately 6 to 9 months later, following axonal regeneration and the development of a Tinnel sign, a segment of the gracilis muscle is transferred to the paralyzed side and connected to the previously grafted nerve (▶ Fig. 51.11). In approximately 6 months, the transferred muscle becomes functional and provides movement on the paralyzed side. The gracilis transfer affords better precision with respect to the smile an-

gle and greater excursion (movement) of the commissure (corner of the mouth) in comparison with the temporalis transfer.

Synkinesis

Synkinesis is the poorly coordinated, simultaneous, and involuntary contraction of several facial muscles during purposeful movement of the face. For example, while eye closure is attempted, the corner of the mouth may move also, generating an unwanted smile (see ▶ Fig. 51.3). Such poor coordination results from random axonal regeneration within the recovering

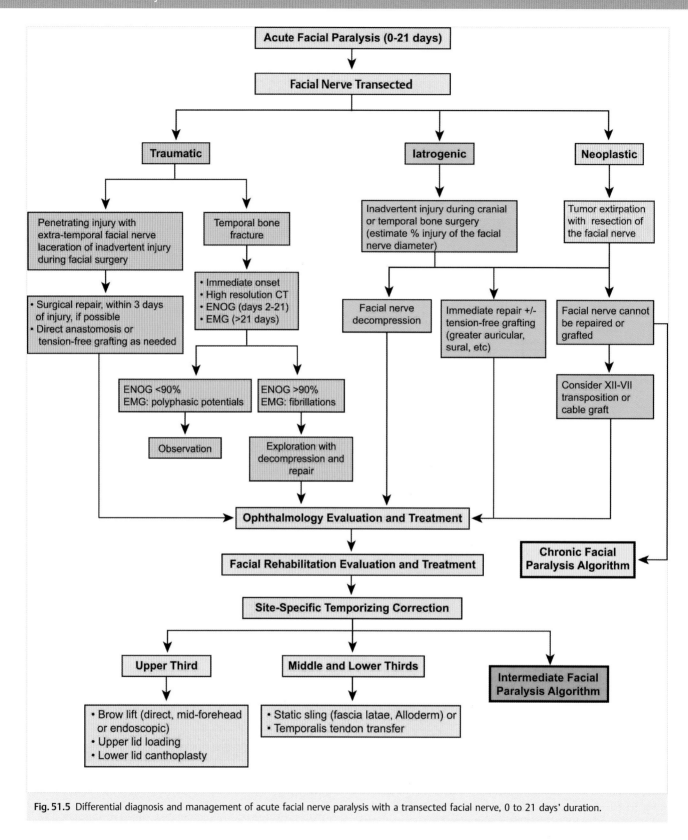

Fig. 51.5 Differential diagnosis and management of acute facial nerve paralysis with a transected facial nerve, 0 to 21 days' duration.

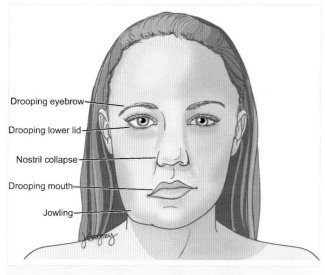

Fig. 51.6 Facial appearance in paralysis, frontal view.

Drooping eyebrow
Drooping lower lid
Nostril collapse
Drooping mouth
Jowling

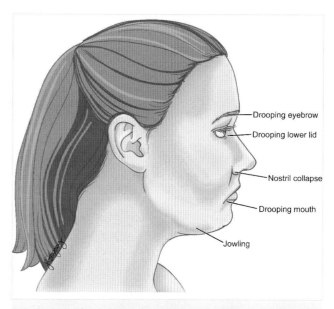

Fig. 51.7 Facial appearance in paralysis, lateral view.

Drooping eyebrow
Drooping lower lid
Nostril collapse
Drooping mouth
Jowling

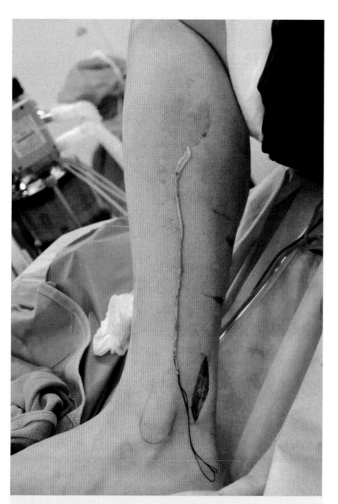

Fig. 51.8 Sural nerve harvest from the left leg. Note the length of the nerve and several small access incisions.

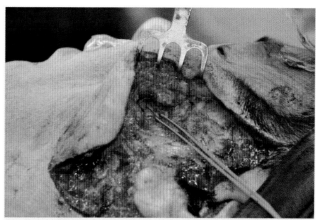

Fig. 51.9 Dissected facial nerve branch responsible for commissure elevation. This branch is cut and sutured to the sural nerve graft.

facial nerve. The successful management of synkinesis depends on selective chemodenervation with a paralytic agent (botulinum toxin A) in combination with facial physical therapy. The effects of botulinum toxin injections wear off, and the injections must be repeated every 3 to 4 months. Other therapies, such radio-frequency ablation, may reduce the required frequency of such injections but are still investigational at this juncture.

51.8 Prognosis

The prognosis for recovery of facial movement varies with the disease etiology and timing of presentation. Many patients with infectious or systemically based cases of facial paralysis recover fully with appropriate treatment. Outcomes in the surgical rehabilitation of chronic facial paralysis are more difficult to quantify and depend on numerous patient- and procedure-related factors.

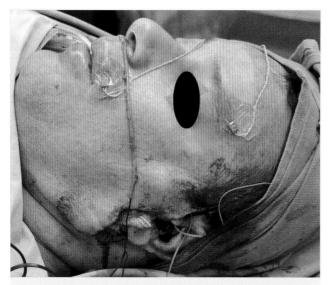

Fig. 51.10 The sural nerve graft is passed within the upper gingivo-buccal sulcus to the paralyzed side of the face.

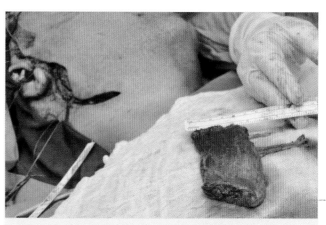

Fig. 51.11 Gracilis muscle graft, harvested and ready for inset. Note facial access incision for graft placement (upper left corner).

51.9 Roundsmanship

- Patients with facial paralysis require an individualized approach to achieve optimal cosmetic and functional outcomes.
- Recovering facial nerve can result in synkinesis. The optimal treatment of synkinesis includes chemodenervation with botulinum toxin A and physical rehabilitation.
- An assessment of the facial zones (forehead; periocular, perioral, and cervical regions) helps define the surgical goals in patients with chronic facial paralysis.

- Chronic facial paralysis can be managed with static repositioning or dynamic reanimation. The choice of surgery depends on the individual patient's presentation, needs, and goals.

51.10 Recommended Reading

[1] Hadlock TA, Greenfield LJ, Wernick-Robinson M, Cheney ML. Multimodality approach to management of the paralyzed face. Laryngoscope 2006; 116: 1385–1389

[2] Mehta RP, Hadlock TA. Botulinum toxin and quality of life in patients with facial paralysis. Arch Facial Plast Surg 2008; 10: 84–87

[3] Rosson GD, Redett RJ. Facial palsy: anatomy, etiology, grading, and surgical treatment. J Reconstr Microsurg 2008; 24: 379–389

52 Correction of Congenital Auricular Deformities

Anthony P. Sclafani and Anthony M. Sclafani

Congenital auricular deformities describe a wide range of anomalous auricular forms, from prominent to completely absent ears. These deformities may be associated with other congenital syndromes but most often are found in isolation. Although the correction of these deformities addresses the patient's physical appearance, they should not be considered *cosmetic*; these procedures are performed to restore a normal appearance of the ears and are rightly classified as *reconstructive* surgeries. The procedures can be performed at any age, but ear deformities are best corrected in childhood, before the patient has suffered psychologically from social stigmatization and has developed a sense of physical "self."

52.1 Incidence of Disease

The exact incidence of congenital auricular deformities is unknown, and this figure is most likely underreported because affected patients may simply style their hair to camouflage the deformity. Approximately 5% of Caucasians in the United States have protruding ears. The 2011 American Society for Aesthetic Plastic Surgery survey estimated that just slightly fewer than 27,000 "cosmetic" ear surgeries were performed; 59% of patients with prominent ears have a family history of the condition, and transmission is thought to be autosomal-dominant with variable penetrance. Cases of microtia/anotia, easily evident at birth, are more reliably reported, with a general incidence in the United States of approximately 1 in every 7,000 to 8,000 live births. Ethnic and national differences in incidence have also been described, with Hispanics, Asians, and Navajo Native Americans more commonly affected in the United States. Microtia is more common in boys (60 to 70% of cases) than in girls. More cases of microtia are noted on the right side (60%) than the on left (30%); approximately 10% of cases are bilateral.

52.2 Terminology

Terms to understand include those that refer to the structures of the normal auricle (listed below), as well as those pertaining to specific deformities and their associated abnormalities. The term *anotia* refers to the total absence of any external ear, whereas *microtia* describes an imperfectly formed auricle ranging from grade I (small but relatively normally shaped ear) and grade II (abnormally sized and formed auricle with some recognizable components of the auricle) to grade III microtia (skin and cartilage remnants only). Grade III microtia has been subdivided into lobule remnant and conchal remnant subtypes, in which only skin approximates a malpositioned earlobe (lobule remnant) or skin and malformed cartilage approximate an earlobe and inferior conchal bowl (conchal remnant). *Aural atresia* is to the absence of an external auditory canal, tympanic membrane, and intact ossicular chain and is frequently seen together with microtia. *Hemifacial microsomia* is a condition in which some or all parts of a hemiface are underdeveloped, also seen not infrequently together with microtia. *Cryptotia* refers to a mild auricular deformity in which the superior helical rim is tucked under temporal skin and does not project away from the head. A variety of common names have been used to phenotypically describe the prominent auricle, such as lop ear, bat ear, satyr ear, shell ear, and cup ear, among others. It is more valuable to identify the specific defects of the malformed ear because these features will be directly addressed during otoplasty.

52.3 Applied Anatomy

Surgeons performing procedures on the auricle should be familiar with the normal structures and forms of the natural auricle, such as the helix, antihelix, scaphoid fossa, fossa triangularis, conchal bowl, tragus, antitragus, lobule, helical root, cauda helicis, and postauricular crease (▶ Fig. 52.1). The auricle is composed of fibroelastic cartilage, and although flexible in youth, it becomes more rigid over time. The arterial supply to the auricle is from the posterior auricular artery and superficial temporal arteries, which are both terminal branches of the external carotid artery systems (▶ Fig. 52.2).

Rudimentary muscles help maintain the auricular position, and in some individuals they have a slight ability to move the auricle. Sensory nerves to the auricle are from the auriculotemporal nerve (from the mandibular division of the trigeminal nerve), the great auricular nerve (from C2 through C4 roots), the Arnold nerve (branch of the vagus nerve), and twigs of the facial nerve (▶ Fig. 52.3). Both the neural and vascular supply to the auricle follow a radial pattern, allowing a circumferential ring blockade around the base of the ear to anesthetize the entire auricle.

52.4 The Disease Process

52.4.1 Etiology

No specific causes of auricular malformation have been conclusively proved. Auricular prominence can occur sporadically, although about 60% of patients have a positive family history. Transmission between generations is as an autosomal-dominant trait with incomplete penetrance. Conversely, microtia appears to occur more commonly in certain countries (e.g., Finland and Equador) and cultures, suggesting some limited genetic role.

52.4.2 Pathogenesis

The external ear develops separately from the middle ear and inner ear. The auricle is formed from the tissues of the first and second branchial arch, with the first arch contributing the first three hillocks of His, while the fourth through sixth hillocks originate from the second arch; these are present by day 38 of gestation. The tragus and the root and body of the helix

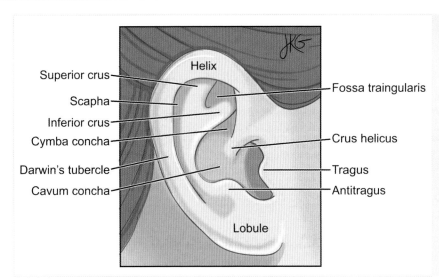

Fig. 52.1 Normal auricular landmarks.

Superior crus
Scapha
Inferior crus
Cymba concha
Darwin's tubercle
Cavum concha

Helix

Fossa traingularis

Crus helicus

Tragus

Antitragus

Lobule

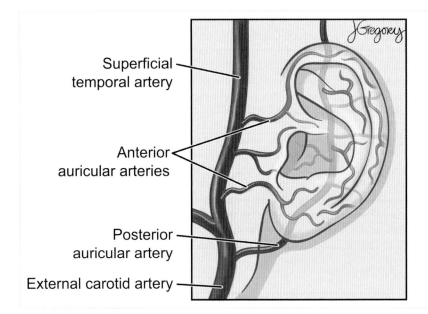

Fig. 52.2 Auricular blood supply.

Superficial
temporal artery

Anterior
auricular arteries

Posterior
auricular artery

External carotid artery

develop from first-arch tissue, while the remainder of the auricle originates from the second arch. The auricle develops between weeks 6 and 16 of gestation. The helix is believed to grow rapidly during weeks 8 through 12 and ultimately overhangs the rest of the auricle; during weeks 13 through 16, the antihelical curl develops and medializes the helix. It is thus reasonable to assume that the deformities seen in prominent ears form during weeks 10 through 16, whereas microtia deformities are a result of more significant, earlier gestational abnormalities and can be attributed to anomalous development of hillocks 2 through 5.

An alternative theory of auricular embryogenesis holds that the tragus and helical root develop from the first arch; the antihelix, conchal bowl, lobule, and antitragus develop from the second arch; and the remainder of the helix as well as the scaphoid fossa are derived from the free ear fold, a swelling just above and behind the developing arches. This theory relegates the hillocks of His to incidental findings.

52.4.3 Natural History and Progression

The auricle grows after birth and attains approximately 85% its adult size by 5 to 6 years of age. Without intervention, congenital auricular deformities do not improve over time.

52.4.4 Potential Disease Complications

Prominent ears do not progress or cause a physical debility. However, the social stigma of deformed ears can cause significant emotional distress. Children rarely suffer from teasing by peers before the age of 6 years, and surgery can be delayed until that time, when the patient will be more mature and cooperative. Microtia likewise does not worsen; however, microtia is typically associated with aural atresia and its associated maximal conductive (60 dB) hearing loss. In cases of bilateral microtia, auditory rehabilitation with bone-anchored hearing aids is essential to allow appropriate auditory cortical development.

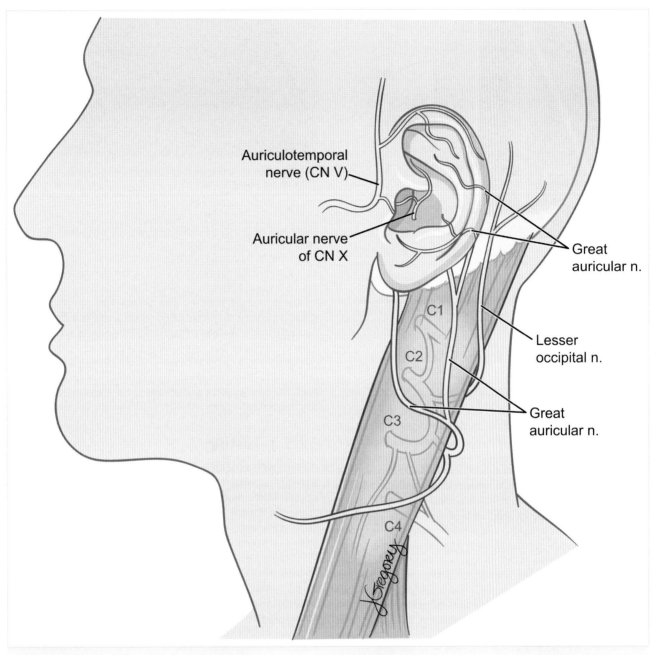

Fig. 52.3 Auricular sensory innervation. *CN*, cranial nerve.

52.5 Medical Evaluation

52.5.1 Presenting Complaints

Although microtia is immediately recognized at birth, patients frequently do not present until the age of 3 or 4 years because the family has been advised that no treatment is possible until the age of 5 or 6 years. Parents typically style the child's hair long to camouflage the deformity.

Patients with unilateral microtia, despite the maximal conductive hearing loss, rarely suffer from auditory deprivation because hearing in the contralateral ear is usually normal. The child should receive preferential classroom seating (front of class, unaffected ear toward the teacher). Aggressive and early treatment for even transient cases of childhood hearing loss (e. g., otitis media with effusion) is justified. By contrast, patients with bilateral microtia should be fitted with a bone stimulation hearing aid early to facilitate normal speech development. Patients with prominent ears have hearing loss no more commonly than do other patients.

Children with microtia younger than 5 years of age may be aware of the "different" appearance of their ears but typically are too young to demonstrate any anxiety about this difference. By 7 years of age, patients with microtia have become acutely aware of the abnormal appearance of their ears(s) and may have already suffered the taunts and teasing of classmates. In contrast, patients with prominent ears, despite a lesser degree of deformity, may present earlier with psychological issues and

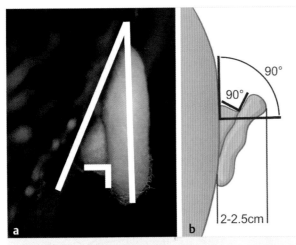

Fig. 52.4 Interrelations of auricular structures.

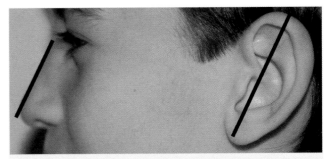

Fig. 52.5 The inclination of the auricle should be roughly parallel to that of the nasal dorsum.

by age 6 or 7 may be unwilling to participate socially because of embarrassment.

52.5.2 Clinical Findings, Physical Examination

Children with auricular anomalies should be assessed in a uniform manner. The anterior–posterior auricular position should be 5 to 6 cm lateral to the lateral canthus, and the top of the helix should be at the level of the eyebrow; deviations from these should be noted. Auricular position can be affected by craniofacial anomalies, including hemifacial microsomia. This may occur in as many as 40% of patients with microtia and can involve maxillary or zygomatic width, but it is most commonly is seen as mandibular asymmetry. This can be demonstrated by asking the patient to bite down on a tongue blade placed horizontally across the posterior teeth and observing the tilt of the blade. The basic outline of the auricle should be a smooth helical margin that extends from the helical root down into the earlobe. The shape and depth of the conchal bowl should be examined; the superior and inferior crura of the antihelix run into the common crus to form a gentle Y-shaped curve extending from the margin of the conchal bowl toward the helical rim. These basic structures thus define the scaphoid fossa and fossa triangularis; the tragus and antitragus define the incisura intertragica. The conchal bowl is separated into the cymba conchae and the concha cavum (see ▶ Fig. 52.1).

Furled auricles should manually be re-formed and the true height and width of the auricle noted. These dimensions should be 5 to 6 cm and 2.5 to 3.5 cm, respectively, and represent the amount of useable native cartilage available. The interrelation of the structures themselves should be evaluated: the auriculocephalic angle (between the head and the auricle, as seen from above) should be no more than 25 degrees; from the same vantage point, the conchomastoid angle should be about 90 degrees, while the antihelix should also turn away 90 degrees from the conchal bowl (▶ Fig. 52.4). Overall, the ear should protrude from the head no more than 10 to 12 mm superiorly, 16 to 18 mm in the midpoint of the helical rim, and 20 to 22 mm at the lobule. The inclination of the long axis is similar but not equal to that of the nasal dorsum (inclined about 20 to 30 degrees off vertical; ▶ Fig. 52.5).

Obviously, patients with microtia will have significantly fewer, if any, normal landmarks. The auricular remnant can be assigned a grade from I to III. Grade I microtia is a small ear with relatively normal features and proportions; an auricle with grade II microtia may have a few recognizable features of a normal auricle but is clearly "deformed." An auricle with grade III microtia typically has only a vestigial remnant, which can be categorized as a conchal remnant (mimicking a conchal bowl) or the more common lobule remnant (with a small, skin-covered, malformed block of cartilage at the superior end of a fleshy "lobule" remnant).

52.5.3 Testing

Patients with auricular deformities should be photographed before any surgical intervention. Standard frontal, lateral, and oblique views should be supplemented by posterior views (to assess the lateral projection of the ears) as well as close-up views of the ears. All patients should have a preoperative audiologic assessment for documentation as well as assistance in determining the need and feasibility of surgical aural rehabilitation (in cases of microtia/atresia). High-resolution computed tomography (CT) of the temporal bones should be obtained when the child is old enough to cooperate with the test to aid in further determining the candidacy of the patient for aural atresia repair. This is done preoperatively in our institution through the cooperative efforts of the facial plastic surgeon and the otologist. The patient with microtia should be assessed for evidence of other congenital deformities, especially hemifacial microsomia, congenital facial nerve impairment, and Goldenhar and Nager syndromes. Consultation with a geneticist and screening for cervical spine deformities (X-rays or CT of the neck) and renal anomalies (ultrasound) may be appropriate.

52.5.4 Differential Diagnosis

The diagnosis of microtia is fairly self-evident because the deformity is obvious and has been present since birth. Prominent ears also are simple to diagnose, but the surgeon should be aware that cranial anomalies can cause malposition and prominence of the ears; more commonly, postauricular inflammatory swelling may cause the ear to protrude.

52.6 Treatment

52.6.1 Medical Treatment

Although there is no medical treatment per se for an advanced-grade microtia, minor auricular deformities can sometimes be partially or fully corrected noninvasively. Especially within the first year of life, the auricular cartilage is quite soft and pliable. Taping and splinting prominent or folded auricles during the first several months of life can aid in correcting, or at least improving, the contour of the auricle.

A prosthesis can be made, with the contralateral ear used as a template, and be either glued in place or mounted with osseointegrated implants. A well-made prosthesis, although artificial and requiring maintenance, can look quite realistic.

52.6.2 Surgical Treatment

Otoplasty

Prominent auricles can be reshaped and repositioned by otoplasty. Ely described the first case of otoplasty in New York City in 1881, when he excised full-thickness portions of conchal bowl. In 1903, Morestin described many techniques currently in use, while Luckett used cartilage incisions and sutures to form the antihelix in 1910. Modern otoplasty maneuvers fall into two distinct categories: cartilage-cutting and cartilage-sparing techniques.

Cartilage-cutting techniques are powerful steps that can significantly remodel and reposition the auricle; however, these techniques can lead to unnatural, sharp edges when cuts through firm cartilage are seen through thin auricular skin. Cartilage-sparing techniques avoid sharp angles by relying mainly on sutures and postoperative fibrosis to bend, fold, and maintain the corrected shape and position of the auricular cartilage. The utility of this approach can be limited in adult patients, whose cartilage is stiffer and less pliable than that of pediatric patients.

Most otoplasty procedures use a postauricular approach, although an anterior approach can be used for anterior cartilage scoring. In this technique, a fine rasp or wire brush is used to make parallel longitudinal partial-thickness cuts through the cartilage of the lateral surface of the antihelix. Subsequent contractile forces, in addition to postoperative splinting, then promote cartilage warping and the creation of a more convex lateral surface. Again, cartilage irregularities are sometimes visible through thin lateral auricular skin.

Both cartilage-cutting and cartilage-sparing procedures access the auricular cartilage via a postauricular incision and fusiform skin excision. The skin on either side of the incision can be elevated and retracted for adequate exposure from the helical rim to the mastoid periosteum. Skin excision should be conservative and planned so as to allow the scar to fall into the postauricular sulcus.

Cartilage-cutting procedures may involve the exposure and removal of an overly convex conchal bowl cartilage that bows excessively and does not rest flat against the mastoid cortex. Other modifications include parallel incisions on either side of the apex of the antihelical curve, followed by sutures placed between the two larger segments; the strip of antihelical apex is allowed to ride over the sutured cartilage segments to camouflage the sharp angle formed by the junction of the two larger cartilage segments. Cartilage-sparing procedures are more commonly used. These are used to form a more defined antihelix, medialize the conchal bowl, correct prominence of the superior pole of the auricle, or correct earlobe prominence. Mustardé described mattress sutures placed between the sides of the antihelical fold and tied sufficiently tightly to better define the antihelix. The antihelix should be manually folded by the surgeon, and a 2–0 silk suture can be passed through the cartilage and across the antihelix about 1 cm below its apex (▶ Fig. 52.6) to mark the site for the two to four mattress sutures. The postauricular dissection is then exposed, and the entry and exit sites of the sutures as they pass through the cartilage are noted. These marking sutures are removed, and horizontal mattress sutures of a 3–0 or 4–0 braided, nonabsorbable suture material are placed at these sites (▶ Fig. 52.7) and tied while an assistant folds the antihelix appropriately. Three to five sutures are placed along the length of the common and superior crura of the antihelix. Suture bites should be wide enough to allow a gentle, rolling antihelical curve; however, sutures should not be placed too superiorly along the superior crus to avoid a "tent pole" deformity (in which the superior crus of the antihelix extends crisply up across the scaphoid fossa to the helix).

The conchal bowl can be sutured more medially to reduce its lateral extension in cases of prominence. If the mastoid surface of the conchal bowl is significantly rounded, partial-thickness cartilage excision is performed to "flatten" this surface of the cartilage. Horizontal mattress sutures are placed through the conchal cartilage extending away from the mastoid and tied to a suture bite of mastoid periosteum. It is important that the suture pull the conchal bowl *posteriorly* as well as medially; mastoid sutures placed too anteriorly will cause the anterior lip of the conchal bowl cartilage to move anteriorly and compromise the external auditory meatus.

Further contouring of the auricular position and shape can be performed with directed sutures for specific purposes. One

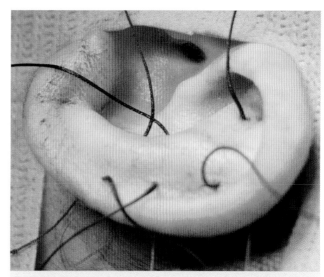

Fig. 52.6 Silk sutures placed to mark the sites for Mustardé sutures.

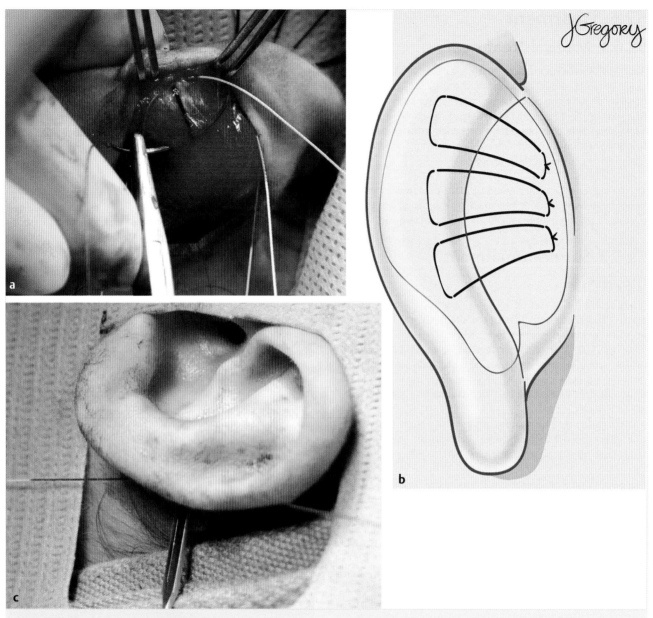

Fig. 52.7 Placement of conchohelical (Mustardé) sutures. Horizontal mattress sutures are **(a,b)** placed and then **(c)** tied while an assistant holds the antihelix in an appropriately folded position.

common finding after antihelical and conchal bowl correction is persistent prominence of the superior auricular pole. This can be fixed more medially with similar mattress sutures passed between the cartilage of the fossa triangularis and the temporalis fascia. Also, inferior pole prominence can occur, manifested by an overly lateral earlobe. This may be due to excessive soft tissue on the medial aspect of the earlobe (best treated by conservative skin excision from the medial surface of the earlobe) or to a prominent or laterally oriented cauda helicis. This can be treated either with conservative cartilage excision or with an additional mattress suture between the cauda helicis and conchal bowl.

It is important that both during and after placement of the cartilage sutures, the repositioned and re-formed cartilage not be stretched or pulled, but instead gently manipulated. Care should be taken to ensure that sutures do not tear through

cartilage. Once the auricle has been repositioned, the postauricular skin is redraped and any excess skin is conservatively excised. The wound may be drained with a sterile rubber band (if necessary), and the skin is closed with a running 4–0 chromic suture. A form-fitting, lightly compressive dressing is made from cotton soaked in mineral oil, packed lightly to fill the newly created concavities, underneath a mastoid dressing. The dressing and drain are removed on postoperative day 1, and an elastic athletic headband is worn over both ears constantly; after the first week, this is worn at nighttime only for the next 3 weeks (▶ Fig. 52.8).

Auricular Reconstruction

Most surgeons who treat microtia surgically generally follow the techniques described by Tenzer and Brent; Nagata has

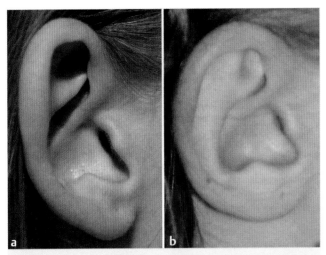

Fig. 52.8 (a) Before and (b) after otoplasty.

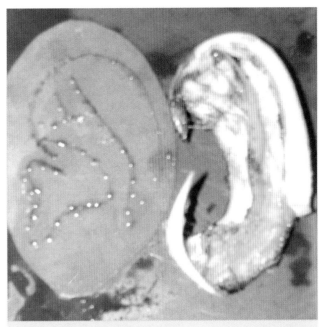

Fig. 52.9 Carved costal cartilage framework next to template based on the contralateral ear for microtia repair.

described a somewhat different technique but also used autologous rib cartilage to create the auricular framework. More recently, a synthetic material (Medpor; Porex Surgical, Newnan, GA) has been used, but management is problematic if it becomes infected after aural atresia repair is performed.

Stage 1

Reconstruction with autologous rib requires a staged approach. Surgery is generally begun after the patient is 6 to 7 years of age, so that adequate costal cartilage is available. A piece of clear X-ray film is placed over the normal ear, and the outline of the auricular structures is traced. The position and orientation of the normal ear relative to the temporomandibular joint, lateral canthus, and superior orbital rim are also drawn. Small perforations are made in the X-ray film with a needle along each of these marks to preserve them even after the template has been sterilized.

A 7- to 8-cm incision is made across the lower ribs approximately two finger breadths above the contralateral costal margin. The inferior oblique and rectus abdominis muscles are transected. The perichondrium over the seventh rib is incised and elevated, and this plane is followed medially until the synchondrosis of the sixth and seventh ribs is exposed. This entire section of the seventh rib with the synchondrosis and a portion of the sixth rib is then harvested en bloc after the deep perichondrium has been fully elevated; this will form the core of the auricular framework. An 8- to 9-cm segment of cartilage from the eighth rib is similarly harvested; this segment is used to form the helix. It is generally necessary to thin this segment to facilitate forming the convexity of the helical rim; the remaining cartilage can be used to form the tragus or to deepen the conchal bowl, or it can be "banked" subcutaneously in the temporal region and retrieved for use to provide additional auricular lateralization in the third-stage procedure.

During cartilage harvest, the perichondrium is carefully elevated circumferentially; although this is relatively simple to do on the anterior surface, particular care should be taken to remain between the cartilage and the perichondrium when working on the posterior surface. After the cartilage harvest, the integrity of the posterior perichondrium and parietal pleura

should be confirmed by filling the wound with warm sterile saline and noting the absence of any air leak (bubbles) during positive pressure ventilation. If these are present, the pleural violation should be identified and a soft red rubber catheter inserted into the pleural space while a purse-string suture is placed around the tear in the pleura. Suction should be applied and the suture tightened and tied as the catheter is withdrawn. Transected muscles are then reapproximated with an absorbable braided suture, and the wound is drained and closed.

The harvested cartilage pieces are then carved and sutured to form the auricular framework. Ideally, the synchondrosis between the fifth and sixth ribs forms the superior and inferior crura, fossa triangularis, and superior part of the scaphoid fossa; the remainder of the scaphoid fossa, common antihelical crus, conchal bowl, and inferior auricle are formed with the bulk of the seventh rib. The eighth rib is sutured to this inner-base framework to form the helix. Additional pieces of cartilage can be sutured to the framework to form additional bulk and support for a tragus. Clear, permanent monofilament 4–0 or 5–0 buried sutures are used to fix these cartilage segments in position based on the X-ray template (▸ Fig. 52.9).

Next, the template is again used to confirm the desired position of the constructed auricle. An incision is made in the skin so that a subcutaneous pocket for the framework can be developed and any malformed remnant cartilage removed. It is essential that this skin be elevated just below the dermis and any hair follicles to produce a thin flap that can wrap delicately around and highlight the curves of the framework. Clearly superfluous remnant skin is resected after proper placement and positioning of the framework. Another pocket is developed above the deep temporal fascia well superior to the planned position of the superior helix, and the unused cartilage segments are "banked" for use during auricular elevation and a resorbable suture placed to keep these segments away from the main pocket. The framework is placed, and then a small, flat,

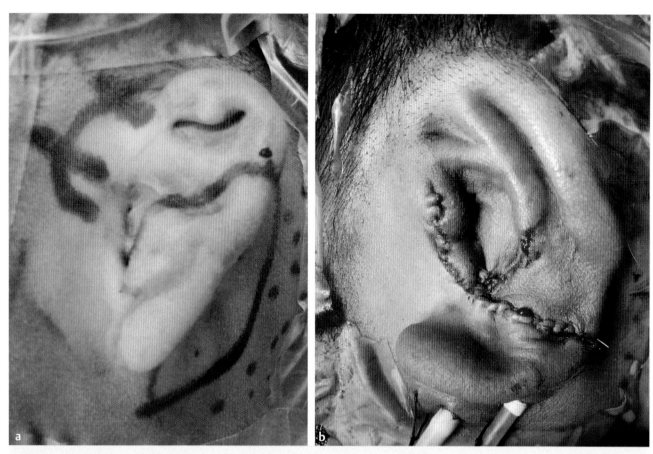

Fig. 52.10 (a) Before and (b) after framework placement and lobule transposition for microtia repair.

open-channel drain is placed to drain the area around the framework; once the framework has been placed on suction, the shape of the framework can be seen and checked for proper placement. Skin incisions are closed with resorbable monofilament sutures. A lightly compressive dressing is applied and maintained for 4 days while the drain is kept on low suction and is removed when the drainage decreases to less than 5 mL/d.

Stage 2

After 6 to 8 weeks, the earlobe is created. Remnant skin (in some cases, skin and cartilage) is generally located anteriorly, running vertically and crossing the desired conchal bowl position. A V-shaped incision is made based inferiorly around the microtia remnant, with the base kept as wide as possible inferiorly. A back cut is made extending up the lower part of the auricular framework. The most inferior portion of the framework is elevated, the remnant is transposed posteriorly and bivalved, and the framework is tucked into the flap. The skin incisions are then closed in layers with monofilament resorbable sutures. Alternatively, this stage can be performed at the same time as the framework construction and placement (► Fig. 52.10).

Stage 3

At 6 to 8 weeks after stage 2 (12 to 16 weeks after stage 1), the skin approximately 5 mm beyond the helical rim framework is incised. The auricular framework is then progressively elevated, while a generous cuff of soft tissue is left covering the medial aspect of the cartilage. The previously banked cartilage is retrieved and sutured to the medial–anterior aspect of the framework and covered with a soft-tissue flap elevated from the framework. Further wide undermining superiorly and posteriorly is performed and allows the occipital and temporal skin flap to be advanced anteriorly and inferiorly, respectively, to bring the edge of the flap up to the postauricular sulcus. A full-thickness skin graft is harvested from the inguinal region and used to cover the medial surface of the elevated auricle, and the donor site is closed primarily. An antibiotic/petroleum gauze bolster is sutured in place over the skin graft and removed after 1 week.

Additional Procedures

After the first three stages, patients who seek hearing restoration can undergo aural atresia repair. At that time or at a subsequent surgery, an anteriorly based skin flap can be raised from the conchal bowl (which can then be deepened) and wrapped around previously placed cartilage for tragus reconstruction, or simply used as the lateral tragal surface while a composite graft from the contralateral conchal bowl is used for tragal structure and medial surface coverage. Also, patients whose remnant skin was based too superiorly will have an elevated earlobe after stage 2; this can be transposed to a more symmetric, lower position if needed.

Complications

Otoplasty

In general, complications of otoplasty are fairly uncommon (see Box Complications of Otoplasty and Auricular Reconstruction (p.417)). Most are related to technique: cellulitis, chondritis, hypertrophic scar/keloid, suture failure, suture bridging, telephone ear, and recurrence. Cellulitis can occur and is generally caused by typical skin flora. Chondritis is marked by deep pain in addition to swelling and erythema that develop 3 to 5 days after surgery. Drainage, culture, and antibiotics (including coverage for *Pseudomonas* in cases of suspected chondritis) should be instituted as soon as the diagnosis is suspected. Excessive skin resection is generally the cause of "suture bridging," the visible span of sutures across the postauricular crease, whereas excessive skin closure tension may predispose to the development of hypertrophic or keloid scars. Uneven reduction of the auricular prominence can cause a "telephone ear" deformity, in which the superior and inferior poles project farther from the head than does the midportion of the auricle; careful inspection of the intraoperative result should identify this unwanted result. Recurrence of auricular deformity is uncommon (approximately 2%) and is generally a result of suture failure.

Complications of Otoplasty and Auricular Reconstruction

Complications of otoplasty
- Recurrence of deformity (2%)
- Telephone ear
- Suture bridging
- Hypertrophic scar/keloid
- Cellulitis
- Chondritis

Complications of auricular reconstruction
- Pneumothorax
- Atelectasis/pneumonia
- Cartilage exposure
- Blunting/loss of postauricular sulcus
- Hematoma
- Chondritis

Auricular Reconstruction

Pneumothorax is rare, and particular attention to remaining in the proper plane during cartilage harvest is essential. We routinely obtain a chest X-ray in the recovery room, as well as 6 hours later. Atelectasis is more common because patients splint postoperatively as a result of transection of the intercostal muscles. Patients should be given adequate analgesics, and early ambulation should be required. Skin breakdown and cartilage exposure can occur, generally early after placement of the framework. At this early stage, healing by secondary intention is rarely sufficient to close the wound; the cartilage should be conservatively débrided in order to remove devitalized tissue and covered with a local skin flap or (if there is minimal local skin laxity) a temporoparietal fascia flap. Loss of lateralization and blunting of the postauricular sulcus can develop if excessive skin graft contracture occurs; we prefer to advance the posterior skin flap into the apex of the postauricular crease and use the skin graft to cover only the medial surface of the auricle.

52.7 Roundsmanship

- The correction of prominent ears can be performed after the age of 6 years, by which time the ears have attained approximately 85% of their adult height.
- Cartilage-cutting techniques are more likely to produce sharp edges.
- Auricular prominence should be checked after each suture is placed, and even correction along the length of the auricle should be ensured.
- Methods of microtia reconstruction use cartilage segments of multiple ribs to construct different parts of the auricle.

52.8 Recommended Reading

[1] Brent B. Auricular repair with autogenous rib cartilage grafts: two decades of experience with 600 cases. Plast Reconstr Surg 1992; 90: 355–374, discussion 375–376
[2] Brent B. Technical advances in ear reconstruction with autogenous rib cartilage grafts: personal experience with 1200 cases. Plast Reconstr Surg 1999; 104: 319–334, discussion 335–338
[3] Furnas DW. Correction of prominent ears with multiple sutures. Clin Plast Surg 1978; 5: 491–495
[4] Janis JE, Rohrich RJ, Gutowski KA. Otoplasty. Plast Reconstr Surg 2005; 115: 60e–72e
[5] Mustarde JC. The correction of prominent ears using simple mattress sutures. Br J Plast Surg 1963; 16: 170–178
[6] Porter CJW, Tan ST. Congenital auricular anomalies: topographic anatomy, embryology, classification, and treatment strategies. Plast Reconstr Surg 2005; 115: 1701–1712
[7] Tanzer RC. Microtia—a long-term follow-up of 44 reconstructed auricles. Plast Reconstr Surg 1978; 61: 161–166
[8] Wellisz T. Reconstruction of the burned external ear using a Medpor porous polyethylene pivoting helix framework. Plast Reconstr Surg 1993; 91: 811–818

53 Primary Rhinoplasty

Anthony P. Sclafani and James A. Sclafani

53.1 Introduction

Rhinoplasty is the deliberate alteration of the form, shape, and often the function of the external nose. Although generally performed for cosmetic reasons, rhinoplasty can also be performed to improve nasal respiration or to repair congenital, traumatic, or otherwise acquired deformities. Each step in any procedure on the external nose should be performed with the dual effects on appearance and breathing kept in mind. Whereas an open reduction of a nasal fracture includes the creation of incisions in the nasal bones, which can then be repositioned, rhinoplasty includes additional contouring of the nose by altering the nasal bridge (by augmenting or reducing the size and/or width of the bones and cartilages) or the position, orientation, and shape of the nasal tip.

53.2 Incidence of Disease

Although it does not treat a specific "disease," primary rhinoplasty can be performed in a number of common scenarios: the dorsal "bump," the "large" nose, the deviated nose, the bulbous tip, and the overprojecting or underprojecting nasal tip are frequent indications for rhinoplasty. Rhinoplasty is the second most common facial plastic surgical procedure; more than 126,000 rhinoplasties were performed in 2011.

53.3 Terminology

In a discussion of the nose, movement from the glabella toward the nasal tip is described as *caudal*; movement in the opposite direction is *cephalic*. When the position of the nasal tip is discussed, *projection* refers to the degree the tip extends away from the face, whereas *rotation* denotes the upward (as viewed laterally) pivoting of the nasal tip (based at the nasal alae); *de-projection* and *de-rotation* refer to the opposite. The nose is often discussed in thirds; the upper third of the nose runs from the articulation of the nasal bones with the nasal process of the frontal bone and ends at the caudal margin of the nasal bones (▶ Fig. 53.1). The middle third of the nose continues caudally from the nasal bones to the anterior septal angle (the dorsal aspect of the most caudal portion of the septum). The lower third of the nose comprises the nasal tip.

There are two types of approach to rhinoplasty: *endonasal* rhinoplasty is performed solely through incisions placed within the nose, whereas an *open* or *external* rhinoplasty uses internal nasal incisions combined with one across the columella. Osteotomies are bony incisions through the dorsal or lateral bones of the nose in order to reshape, reduce, or reposition the nasal bones. Open reduction of a nasal fracture differs from rhinoplasty in that it is limited to osteotomy and repositioning of the nasal bones, whereas rhinoplasty involves active reshaping of the nose to a new form.

53.4 Applied Anatomy

The nasal bones extend inferiorly from the nasal process of the frontal bones and articulate laterally with the ascending process of the maxilla and with each other medially. Inferiorly, the paired upper lateral cartilages have a trapezoid shape and insert on the internal aspect of the lower (caudal) nasal bones for approximately 2 to 3 mm. Laterally, the upper lateral cartilages

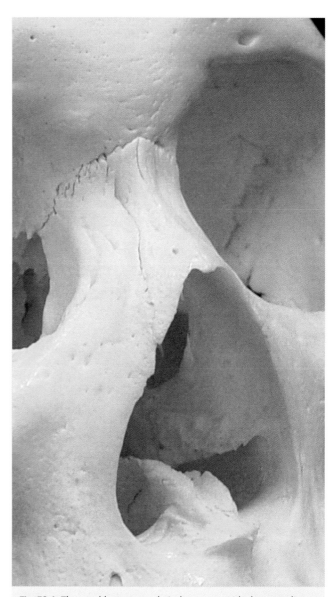

Fig. 53.1 The nasal bones are relatively narrow, with the ascending portion of the maxilla comprising significant portions of the nasal side walls. The maxillary crest sits along the nasal floor, upon which rests the quadrangular septal cartilage. The nasal process of the frontal bone articulates with the nasal bones superiorly.

are bound to the free margin of the piriform aperture (the caudal end of the bony nasal opening); they fuse with the dorsal nasal septum medially. The dorsal septum extends slightly more caudally than the lower aspect of the upper lateral cartilages, ending at the anterior septal angle (▶ Fig. 53.2).

Each lower lateral cartilage is an inverted V- or U-shaped cartilage, wider at the lateral crus, narrowing at the bend of the intermediate crus, and running inferiorly as the thinner medial crus. The most inferior part of the medial crus typically curves backward and has a fibrous attachment to the caudal septum, which serves as one of the three major tip supports. The cephalic end of the lateral crus extends for 1 to 3 mm over the caudal aspect of the upper lateral cartilage, and the fibrous attachment of these two areas forms the second major tip support, known as the scroll. The third major mechanism of tip support is the actual strength, integrity, and resilience of the lower lateral cartilages (▶ Fig. 53.3).

The shape, position, and orientation of the nasal tip are chiefly determined by the tip supports. The major and minor tip supports are listed in the Box Major and Minor Tip Support Mechanisms (p.419). These classifications may vary from patient to patient, and in certain cases, minor tip supports may be major ones, and vice versa; each patient should be assessed individually (▶ Fig. 53.4).

Major and Minor Tip Support Mechanisms

Major supports of the nasal tip
- Length and strength of the lower lateral cartilages
- Attachment of the upper lateral cartilages to the lateral crura of the lower lateral cartilages
- Attachment of the foot plates of the medial crura of the lower lateral cartilages to the caudal septum

Minor supports of the nasal tip
- Fibrous attachment of the domes of the lower lateral crura to each other (interdomal ligament)
- Nasal skin
- Membranous septum
- Anterior septal angle
- Posterior septal angle
- Sesamoid cartilage and fibrofatty tissue of the alae

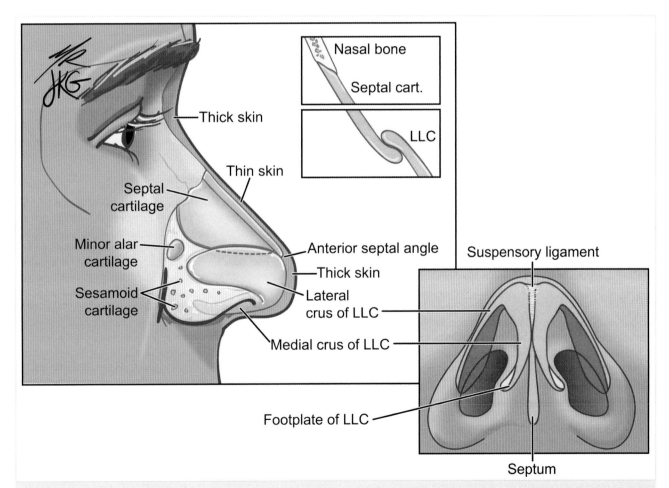

Fig. 53.2 The upper lateral cartilages insert on the undersurface of the nasal bones, fuse medially with the septal cartilage, and are attached to the lower lateral cartilages by fibrous tissue (*inset*). The lower lateral cartilages angle cephalically and do not run along the rim of the nostril. Fibrofatty tissue and sesamoid cartilage comprise the dense tissue of the nasal lobule. The nasal tip skin is thinnest over the rhinion. *LLC*, lower lateral cartilage.

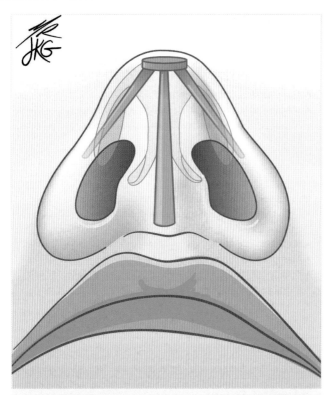

Fig. 53.3 The nasal tip support can be compared to a tripod, with each lateral crus of the lower lateral cartilages serving as one leg of the tripod and the fused medial crura serving as the third leg of the tripod.

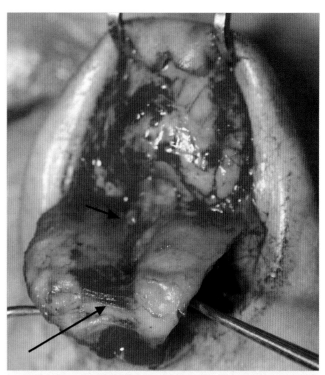

Fig. 53.4 The interdomal (Pitanguy) ligament (*long arrow*) and the anterior septal angle (*short arrow*) seen through an external approach rhinoplasty.

Functionally, an important area is the internal nasal valve. This is the cross-sectional area formed by the caudal end of the upper lateral cartilage, the nasal septum, the floor of the nose, and the inferior turbinate. This area serves as a variable resistor to nasal airflow. Excessive narrowing of this area by enlargement of the turbinate, septal deviation, or weakness or collapse of the upper lateral cartilage and/or the cephalic end of the lower lateral cartilage can lead to internal nasal valve collapse or stenosis.

53.5 The Disease Process

53.5.1 Etiology

Nasal deformity can be congenital, developmental, or acquired and may involve any or all of the areas of the nose. Dislocation of the septum during birth can, if left uncorrected, lead to deviated growth of the nose, and the septum should be gently repositioned as soon as possible. Cleft lip and cleft palate deformities are associated with typical patterns of distortion of the lower two-thirds of the nose. The onset of puberty is associated with significant nasal growth, and during this time subtle deviations may become more obvious. Most adults will recall at least one episode of "significant" nasal trauma during childhood. Adult nasal trauma may lead to malpositioning and subsequent malunion of the nasal bone and to fracture of the septum with displacement. Fractures of the caudal end of the nasal bone may weaken the attachment of the upper lateral cartilage, with subsequent collapse of the internal nasal valve. Injury of the nasal

septum (caused by traumatic, surgical, induced [e.g., intranasal cocaine abuse], or inflammatory/infectious [e.g., Wegener granulomatosis or syphilis] processes) can result in collapse of the nasal dorsum and subsequent nasal tip distortion. Unsuccessful rhinoplasty can also lead to an unacceptable nasal appearance.

53.5.2 Pathogenesis

Deformed noses lack a smooth contour, symmetry, and organic integration with the other facial structures. A complete discussion of facial aesthetics is beyond the scope of this chapter, but in general, the length of the nose should be appropriate for the rest of the face. The nose should begin superiorly at approximately the level of the upper eyelid crease and end at a nasal tip that projects away from the face by roughly 55 to 60% of the distance from the nasal root to the lateral alae. There should be a smooth and gentle sweep, beginning at the superomedial orbital rim and extending down along the side of the nose, that widens slightly at the ala (▶ Fig. 53.5). The ala should extend laterally to a point along a vertical line dropped from the medial canthus. From a basal ("worm's eye") view, the nasal tip should comprise approximately half of the width from ala to ala.

Asymmetry of the nasal bones, either from true asymmetry of the bones or from asymmetric malpositioning, will make the upper third appear deviated. Excessive bowing of the middle nasal third can make the nose look "crooked," even if the nasal bones are symmetrically placed (▶ Fig. 53.6). This may be due to medial collapse of the upper lateral cartilages or to a deviated dorsal septal cartilage. Lack of an appropriate "supratip break" (a visible step-off just above the midline of the cephalic edge of the nasal tip, where the nasal tip is seen to project 1 to 2 mm

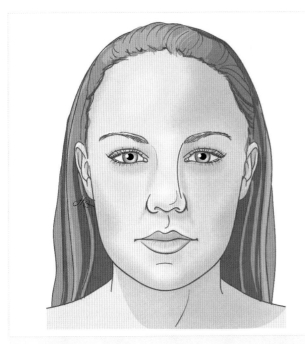

Fig. 53.5 A gentle sweep from the superior–medial orbital rim along the side of the nose widens at the ala in an aesthetic nose.

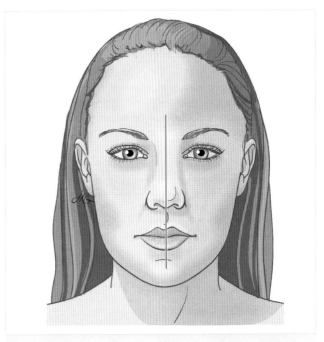

Fig. 53.6 The two nasal side walls course gently from the orbital rims to the alae in a symmetric fashion in the aesthetic nose.

above the nasal dorsum) will make the nose appear longer and will accentuate a dorsal hump. From the frontal view, the alar rims should approximate a "gull in flight" (▶ Fig. 53.7).

Viewed laterally, the rim of the ala should extend no more than 1 to 2 mm along a line bisecting the nasal opening; a greater distance is evidence of alar retraction. Similarly, the lower border of the nasal opening on this view should be no more than 1 to 2 mm below this line; greater distances indicate a hanging columella. An irregularity or bump along the nasal tip, referred to as a bossa, may be multiple and is frequently (but not always) an effect of a poorly performed rhinoplasty.

53.5.3 Natural History and Progression

Although most nasal deformities are fixed in nature, those that progress indicate some loss of structural integrity and support and should be investigated thoroughly. A collapsing bridge may indicate loss of dorsal septal support from an overly aggressive septal submucous resection, or indicate progression of a septal perforation or other significant septal process. Progressive widening of the nasal bones can occur in the presence of an enlarging neoplasm of the nasal cavity or of severe nasal polyposis. The nasal tip can become broader and more prominent in the setting of active rosacea. There is a natural tendency of the nose to appear longer with age as the nasal skin envelope loses elasticity. Especially in the setting of prior nasal surgery, the internal nasal valve may cause progressive nasal obstruction.

53.5.4 Potential Disease Complications

Nasal deformities and nasal obstruction are not life-threatening, nor will they typically worsen other conditions.

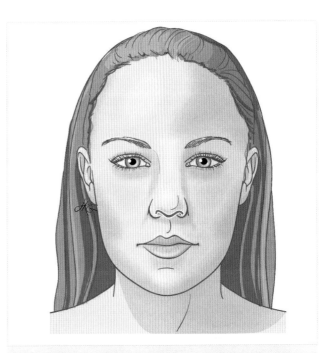

Fig. 53.7 On the frontal view, the alar rims together form a "gull in flight."

53.5.5 Disease Grading

Saddle nose deformity, which is a depression of the middle and upper thirds of the nose, is qualitatively described as major or minor. Otherwise, there is no universally accepted and used grading of nasal deformity. Much more important are a careful examination and description of the deformity and an understanding of the state of the underlying structures.

53.6 Medical Evaluation

53.6.1 Presenting Complaints

Whether a patient presenting for rhinoplasty requests specific changes to his or her nose or simply asks the physician to "make my nose look better," it is imperative to help the patient define the surgical goals. The patient should be asked to indicate precisely the changes desired while inspecting the nose in a mirror and using the end of a cotton applicator as a pointer. This simple exercise will help the patient develop a more precise surgical goal. The surgeon should assist the patient in this process by helping to define appropriate parameters for change, but the patient must be comfortable that thechoices and desires will be respected. Patients should be questioned about nasal obstruction (unilateral or bilateral), as well as any symptoms of sinusitis.

53.6.2 Clinical Findings, Physical Examination

A complete discussion of facial aesthetics can be found in Chapter 38. However, the surgeon should critically examine the patient's face and should assess the patient's general facial structure. Is there any facial bone deficiency or asymmetry? Is there underdevelopment of the cheeks or the chin, both of which will cause the nose to look larger? Is the nasal root at the appropriate height? Does the dorsum project sufficiently and smoothly, and is there a sufficient supratip break? Is the nasal length appropriate and is tip projection sufficient? This is easily assessed with the "3-4-5 right triangle" rule (▶ Fig. 53.8). The nose is viewed from the side, and a vertical line extending inferiorly from the low point of the nasal root is visualized. A horizontal line perpendicular to this vertical line and passing through the high point of the nasal tip is also visualized. These lines form two sides of a right triangle, while the third line connects the nasal root to the nasal tip and runs along the nasal dorsum. The vertical side of the triangle is assigned a value of 4; the horizontal side should be approximately three-fourths of the length of the vertical side, and the nasal tip projection (horizontal line) should be approximately three-fifths (55 to 60%) of the nasal dorsal length (third side).

The nasal tip, seen from a basal view (▶ Fig. 53.9), should approximate an equilateral triangle, with the nasal tip comprising about one-third of the width of the entire nasal base. The nasal alae should lie along or just within vertical lines dropped down from the medial canthi.

An important part of the examination of the nose is palpation. The nasal bones should be palpated for symmetry, contour, and angulation. The bridge of the nose should be assessed for incomplete contact of the nasal bones in the midline (an "open roof" deformity). The middle and lower thirds of the nose should be checked for adequate support, and the tip should be palpated for underlying symmetry.

The internal nose should also be examined by anterior rhinoscopy and (when appropriate) nasal endoscopy. The condition of the septum and inferior turbinates, including the nasal mucosa, should be noted.

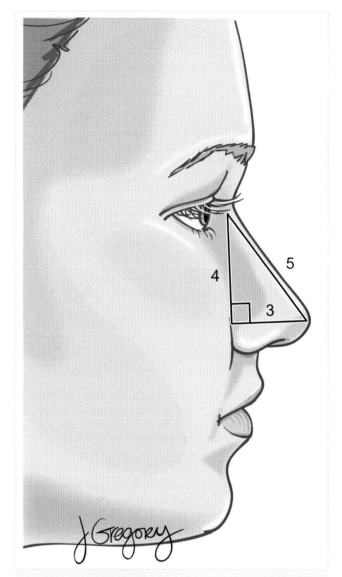

Fig. 53.8 The "3-4-5 right triangle" rule.

53.6.3 Testing

Although testing is generally not performed before rhinoplasty, those patients in whom nasal valve collapse or obstruction is suspected should undergo functional testing. To test nasal function and possible nasal valve collapse during respiration, a Cottle maneuver can be performed; the skin just lateral to the ala is stabilized (not drawn laterally) and the patient is asked to inspire deeply. Alternatively, a fine curet or the tines of a forceps can be placed inside the nose gently to stabilize the site of suspected collapse. If the nasal obstruction is decreased with either method of stabilization, the site of the collapse can be identified. Acoustic rhinometry or rhinomanometry can supplement the functional assessment of the nose. Radiographic assessment is rarely necessary, but computed tomography may be helpful in cases of suspected sinusitis.

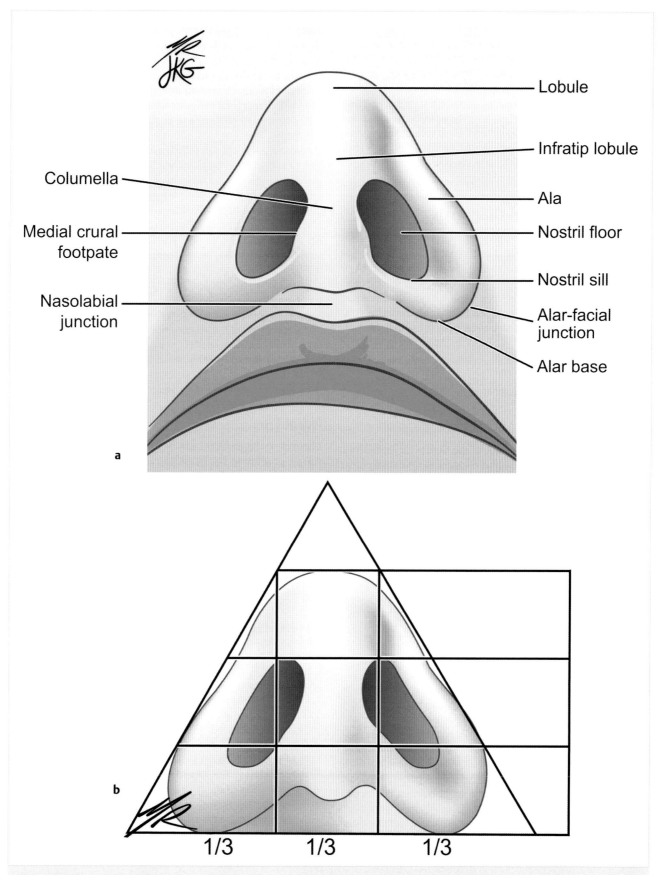

Fig. 53.9 (a) The structures of the nasal tip. (b) The lobule comprises one-third of the nasal tip height, and the nasal tip is approximately one-third the width of the nasal base.

53.6.4 Photography

Photographic assessment is imperative in rhinoplasty, as in all cosmetic interventions. Standardized photographs are invaluable in documenting the degree of preoperative deformity, as well as the postoperative changes. All photographs should be taken with the patient in front of a nonreflective background and in a "head neutral" position (with the gaze focused on a site at eye level). Right and left lateral and 45-degree oblique views, as well as a frontal projection, should be obtained; all views should include the top of the head to the thyroid notch. A close-up, "worm's eye" view should be taken of the nasal base.

53.6.5 Differential Diagnosis

One of the most significant preoperative duties of the surgeon is to assess the appropriateness of the patient for surgery. Patients who show inordinate concern for minor deformities or who attribute social, personal, financial, or employment difficulties to the appearance of their nose will be disappointed with even the best surgical results if these other concerns continue after surgery. It is essential to identify these patients preoperatively. In questionable cases, a preoperative psychiatric evaluation may be helpful.

53.7 Treatment

53.7.1 Medical Treatment

There is no way to alter the shape of the nose with medication. However, it is essential that a trial of nonsurgical management of nasal obstruction be made with topical nasal corticosteroid sprays. If nasal allergies contribute to nasal obstruction, these should be appropriately managed, as well. Confirmed cases of sinusitis should be treated with antibiotics and all evidence of sinusitis eliminated before rhinoplasty. In the case of chronic sinusitis that fails to resolve with appropriate antibiotic therapy, endoscopic sinus surgery can be performed at the same operative setting before the rhinoplasty. However, rhinoplasty should be deferred to another time if there is any concern for significant sinus bleeding, orbital penetration, or cerebrospinal fluid leak.

53.7.2 Surgical Treatment

Rhinoplasty can be performed through either an endonasal or an external approach. An endonasal approach keeps all incisions within the nasal vestibule. Simple access to the nasal dorsum is accomplished by making an intercartilaginous incision that is placed at the intersection of the caudal upper lateral cartilage with the lateral crus of the lower lateral cartilage (▶ Fig. 53.10a). Blunt or sharp undermining is performed above the upper lateral cartilage until the nasal dorsum is reached. When minimal changes to the nasal tip are planned, a transcartilaginous incision can be used. This approach moves the intercartilaginous incision more caudally and is located directly above the planned incision in the lateral crus. After the lateral crus is incised, the cephalic portion of the lateral crus is excised; generally, this provides a modest increase in definition of the nasal tip (▶ Fig. 53.10b). As an alternative, a retrograde dissec-

tion can be performed after an intercartilaginous incision is made and the same cephalic portion of the lateral crus is excised (▶ Fig. 53.10c). Finally, a delivery approach to the tip can be used; this combines an intercartilaginous incision that connects to a transfixion incision (a through–and–through incision of the membranous septum directly in front of the caudal septum) with a marginal incision (which follows the caudal margin of the lower lateral cartilage beginning near the foot plate of the medial crus, extends into the dome, and then follows the caudal margin of the lateral crus; ▶ Fig. 53.11). Once these incisions are made, the nasal tip and alar skin are dissected off the perichondrium of the lower lateral cartilage. The skin of the nasal margin is retracted with a hook cephalically, while a hook placed at the intercartilaginous incision retracts the lateral crus caudally until it can be delivered up and onto the caudal nasal margin. This approach provides wider exposure of lower lateral cartilage for more aggressive resection or suturing (▶ Fig. 53.12). Regardless of the treatment of the tip, these approaches all use the intercartilaginous incision to access the nasal dorsum.

An external approach ("open rhinoplasty") differs from these approaches in that it uses marginal incisions in each nasal vestibule, which are then connected by a broken-line incision across the midportion of the columella. This allows the skin and soft tissue of the nasal tip to be elevated off the perichondrium of the nasal tip cartilages (see ▶ Fig. 53.4).

Nasal Tip

Changes to the nasal tip can be made by incising, excising, suturing, or grafting the nasal tip cartilages. The changes can be predicted by understanding the concept of the nasal tip tripod (see ▶ Fig. 53.3). The nasal tip is visualized as a tripod, with the apex at the nasal tip. Each lateral crus serves as a leg of the tripod, and the two medial crura (together) serve as the third leg. Changes to any leg of the tripod will affect the tip position and projection in a predictable way.

Typical contouring changes to the tip include resection of a cephalic strip (a portion of the cephalic edge of the lateral crus), sutures to sharpen the angle of the cartilage in the area of the dome or to bind the two domes, and complete splitting of the cartilage (in a cephalic–caudal direction) at or near the dome. Cephalic strips are resected by carefully incising the cartilage of the lateral crus, with care taken to preserve an intact strip of caudal lateral crus; 5 to 8 mm of width of remaining crus should generally be left in place, although the precise amount necessary is determined by the resilience of the cartilage and its relative impact on tip support in the individual patient. After the cartilage is incised, it is dissected free of the underlying vestibular mucosa. It is essential to respect any natural asymmetries of the alar cartilages and leave symmetric portions of cartilage remaining. The resection of cephalic strips will weaken the lateral limbs of the tripod, and the apex will rotate cephalically; conversely, the resection of a portion of the medial crura will not only decrease tip projection but also rotate the tip downward. Further narrowing of the nasal tip can be effected with an interdomal suture, a mattress suture through both domes to narrow the domal angles (▶ Fig. 53.13).

More aggressive management of the tip can include vertical dome division, in which the lateral crus is divided from the

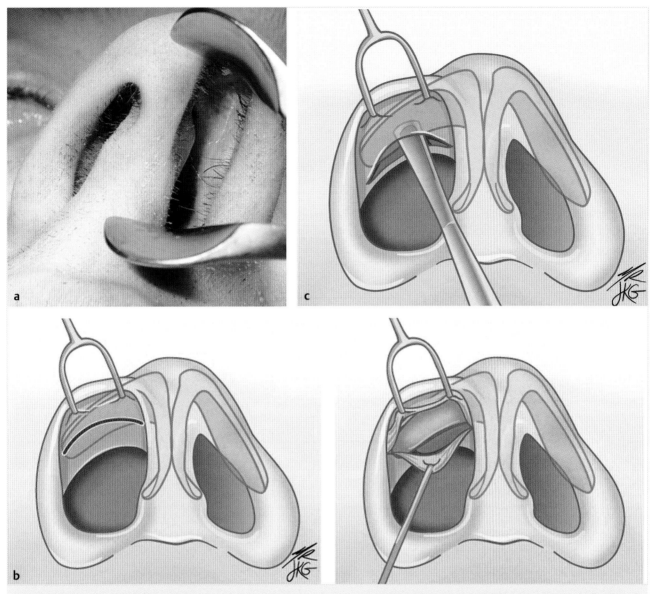

Fig. 53.10 (a) The site of the intercartilaginous incision can be demonstrated by opening a nasal speculum and pressing gently cephalically. This will bring the caudal edge of the upper lateral cartilage into relief. (b) A transcartilaginous incision transects the mucosa over the midportion of the lateral crus; the mucosa is dissected off the cephalic portion of the crus, the cartilage is transected at the level of the mucosa and cut, and the cephalic portion is removed. (c) Alternatively, an intercartilaginous incision is used, and retrograde dissection is performed to excise a cephalic portion of the lateral crus.

medial crus just lateral to the dome. Sutures are placed to secure the two medial segments and also to stabilize the lateral crura to the medial crura (▶ Fig. 53.14). Postoperative healing in the nasal tip will cause more significant narrowing and rotation of the nasal tip due to a weakened alar arch.

A powerful technique that both narrows the nasal tip and increases projection and rotation is the lateral crural steal procedure. The vestibular mucosa is dissected free from the alar cartilage at the dome and for a distance lateral to it, and the desired additional tip projection is measured lateral to the existing dome and marked. This area of cartilage is then lightly crushed with a forceps to allow further contouring. A mattress suture is placed, spanning this new dome symmetrically; as the suture is tightened, additional lateral crus is "stolen" and added

to the medial limb of the tripod. The tip is narrowed, and the shift of cartilage from the lateral to the medial segment leg increases projection and rotation. With or without cartilage shifting or resection, mattress sutures at the nasal tip can be placed to narrow the angle at each dome and/or to narrow the space between the domes.

Cartilage grafts (harvested from septal, conchal, or rib cartilage) can be used to add support to the nasal tip structures. A columellar strut can be carved and placed between the medial crura for additional medial tripod support of the tip; if needed, the graft can be wider at the posterior septal angle to correct a retracted columella. In patients who have severe nasal tip asymmetry or deformities of the alar cartilages at the domes, or in patients who require additional tip definition, a shield graft

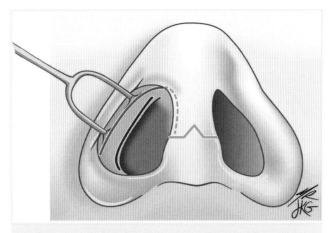

Fig. 53.11 Incisions to access the nasal tip. Marginal (*blue*), intercartilaginous (*red*), and transcolumellar (*green*) incisions.

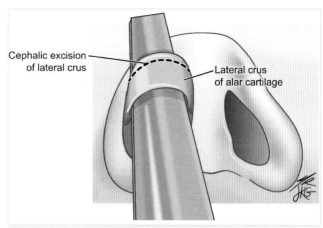

Fig. 53.12 Delivery of the lateral crus.

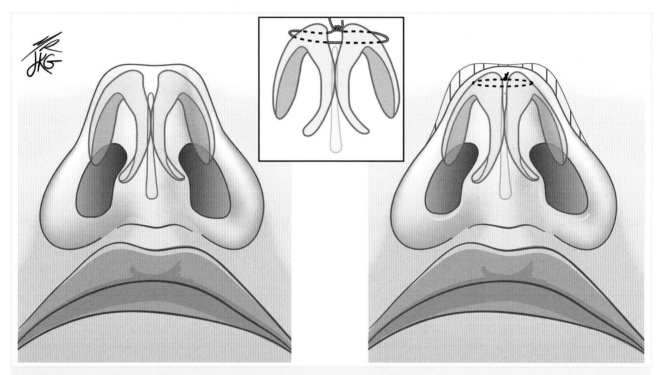

Fig. 53.13 A mattress suture though both domes narrows each domal angle and brings the domes together to refine the nasal tip.

can be placed in a precise pocket caudal to the medial and intermediate crura (endonasal approach) or sutured directly to the medial and intermediate crural segments (external approach). The nasal tip skin then will redrape over this additional cartilage, accentuating the contours of the tip; depending on how much above or below the natural dome the shield graft is allowed to extend, projection and apparent rotation can also be affected.

Spreader grafts (▶ Fig. 53.15) are rectangular grafts that can be placed between the dorsal upper lateral cartilages and septum unilaterally or bilaterally (through either an endonasal or an external approach) after the upper lateral cartilages have been separated from the dorsal septum. These grafts can help open the internal nasal valve and are useful in addressing middle nasal vault asymmetries caused by deviation of the dorsal septum. An alar batten graft can be placed from the piriform aperture to the septum over the junction of the lateral crus and the upper lateral cartilage; the lateral crus can be sutured to this graft to stabilize it and prevent valve collapse. Occasionally, a rim graft can be placed caudal to the lateral crus to extend the alar margin in cases of alar retraction. Premaxillary grafts are sometimes placed in front of the premaxilla to treat a deep nasolabial angle. Many other grafts can be placed for specific regions.

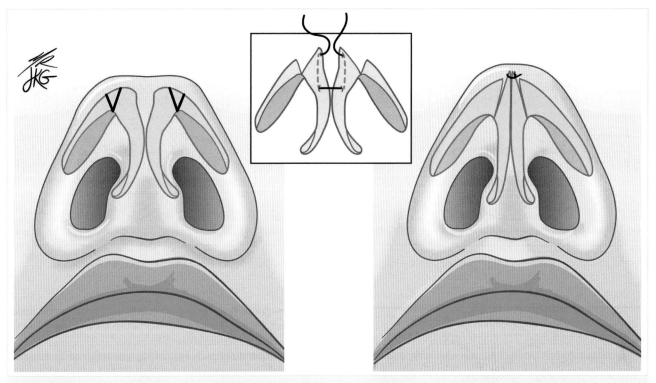

Fig. 53.14 Vertical dome division with resuturing of the cephalic ends of the cartilage segments can significantly narrow the nasal tip.

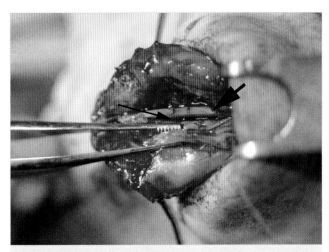

Fig. 53.15 The nasal tip and dorsum as seen from above (caudal on left, cephalic on right). Spreader grafts (held in the forceps) can be placed (unilaterally or bilaterally) into discrete pockets (*long arrow*) lateral to the septum (*short arrow*).

Nasal Dorsum

After the nasal tip has been exposed and treated, the nasal dorsum is fully addressed. Sharp or blunt undermining elevates the soft tissues above the perichondrium of the upper lateral cartilages and the dorsal septum. When the caudal edge of the dorsal nasal bones is reached, a periosteal elevator is used to elevate the periosteum off the dorsal aspect of the nasal bones. Cartilaginous dorsal humps are resected sharply (▶ Fig. 53.16), and violation of the underlying nasal mucosa is avoided when possible to prevent valvular stenosis. Larger bony humps can be

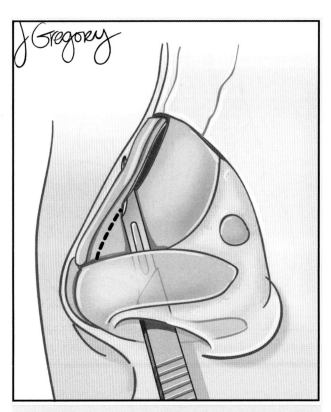

Fig. 53.16 Cartilaginous dorsal excess is excised incrementally with a No. 11 blade.

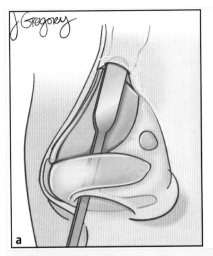
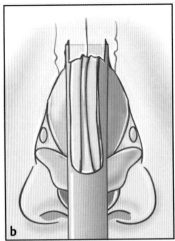
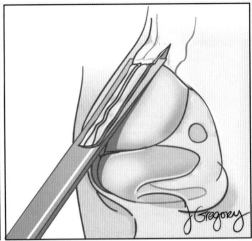

Fig. 53.17 (a) After the periosteum is elevated from the midline nasal bones, (b) an osteotome is used to remove larger dorsal humps.

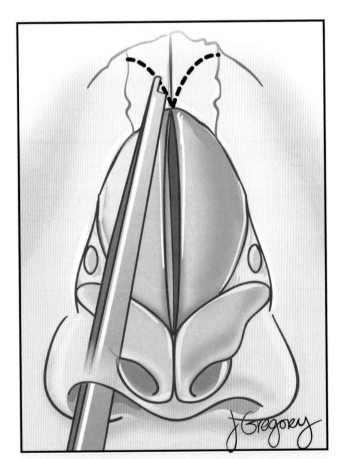

Fig. 53.18 Medial oblique osteotomies facilitate complete medialization of the nasal bones.

removed with an osteotome (► Fig. 53.17), whereas smaller humps can be filed down incrementally with rasps. Typically, removal of a bony hump creates an "open roof" (incontinuity of nasal bones across the bridge) almost to the root of the nose; if not, single-guarded osteotomes can be used to complete bilateral osteotomies separating the nasal bones medially (► Fig. 53.18). When a large cartilaginous hump is removed,

spreader grafts may be placed bilaterally between the upper lateral cartilage and the dorsal septum to prevent the development of internal nasal valve collapse.

Lateral osteotomies (► Fig. 53.19) are required to close an open roof or narrow a nasal bridge. These are performed by incising the mucosa just lateral to the anterior insertion of the inferior turbinate, elevating the soft tissues along the nasomaxillary junction and then performing the osteotomy. A triangle of bone ("Webster triangle") is preserved at the inferolateral aspect of the piriform aperture to prevent medial alar collapse postoperatively. The osteotomy progresses superiorly until it communicates with the medial osteotomy (► Fig. 53.20).

An inward rotation of the osteotome will help connect the two osteotomies if the medial osteotomy remains in the paramedial position. The nasal bones are then freely mobile and can be manipulated into the appropriate position. In cases of asymmetrically shaped or excessively wide nasal bones, an intermediate osteotomy can be performed after the medial osteotomy but before the lateral osteotomy by sliding the osteotome medially from the piriform aperture incision along the caudal edge of the bone. A unilateral osteotomy of this kind can adjust a misshapen nasal bone, whereas bilateral intermediate osteotomies can help narrow an overly wide nasal bridge.

Alar Base Modifications

The alar width should harmonize with both the nasal tip width and dorsal width, and it roughly should fall between vertical lines dropped from the medial canthi; from a basal ("worm's eye") view, the nasal alae and tip should form an equilateral triangle. Widened alae may be a result of thickened alar walls, rounded and widened alar apertures, or both (see ► Fig. 53.17). Alar base reductions are typically performed after tip-plasty and dorsal narrowing. Incisions are made along the nasal crease and into the vestibule. Triangular or wedge-shaped excisions are made to reduce the inner size or outer size (or both) of the ala, with the incision carried into the nasal vestibule or along the alar crease as needed. Deep absorbable sutures are placed to align the segments, and the vestibular incision is also closed with absorbable sutures; the external closure is performed with

5–0 or 6–0 monofilament permanent sutures (▶ Fig. 53.21 and ▶ Fig. 53.22).

Postoperative Care

After internal nasal incisions are closed with resorbable sutures and columellar incisions are closed with permanent monofilament sutures, a cast is applied to the nasal dorsum. Columellar sutures and the nasal cast are removed in 7 days, and the nasal tip and dorsum are further taped for an additional 7 days.

Complications

Complications (see Box Complications of Rhinoplasty) are infrequent but may occur. Bleeding should occur in fewer than 2 to 5% of cases, and infection is rare. Incomplete osteotomies may leave an open roof deformity. Excessively high lateral osteoto-

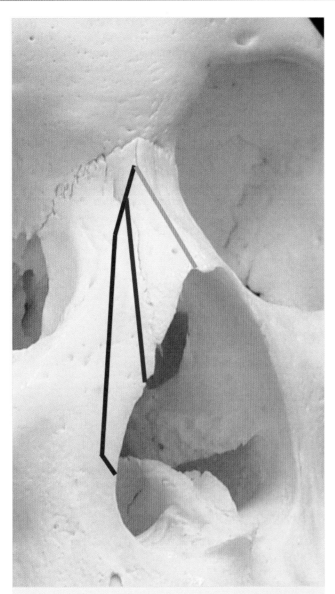

Fig. 53.19 Osteotomies are used to reshape or reposition nasal bones. Medial osteotomies are paramedian in location, whereas lateral osteotomies run mainly through the ascending portion of the maxilla and typically preserve a bone triangle at the lateral caudal piriform aperture. Intermediate osteotomies run between these two and can be used in cases of excessively wide or misshapen nasal bones.

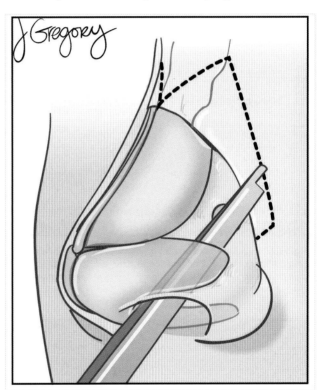

Fig. 53.20 A lateral osteotomy incises the nasal bone from the piriform aperture to the medial osteotomy.

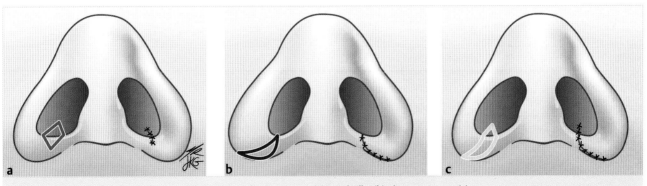

Fig. 53.21 Alar base reductions can be performed to reduce excessive (a) nasal sills, (b) alar margins, or (c) nares.

mies can lead to a "rocker deformity," in which the upper portion of the nasal bones protrudes when the lower portions are medialized because the lateral osteotomy has been carried across the concave portion of bone above the nasal root. Nasal obstruction can be a result of excessive dorsal narrowing, an untreated septal deviation or turbinate enlargement, or an internal or external nasal valve collapse/stenosis. Soft-tissue thickening in the nasal tip, excessive bony dorsal reduction, inadequate cartilaginous dorsal resection, or loss of tip support all can lead to a "pollybeak" deformity. Irregularities of the tip may develop early or late because of excessive cartilage resection or damage and postoperative fibrosis, especially in patients with thin skin, and these bossae will visible. Disruption of the internal nasal valve, failure to address septal deformity or turbinate enlargement, and even overly narrowing the nose can cause nasal obstruction. In general, rhinoplasty is a successful operation, and patient satisfaction rates should be in the 90% range (see ▸ Fig. 53.22; ▸ Fig. 53.23 and ▸ Fig. 53.24). Revision surgery, because of the prior surgery, may be successful in only 80% of cases.

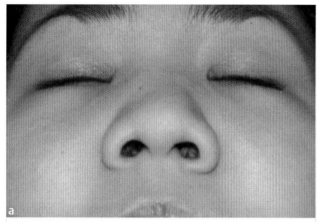

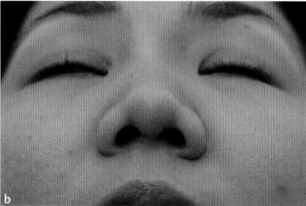

Fig. 53.22 (a) Preoperative and (b) postoperative views of rhinoplasty with dorsal augmentation in addition to increased tip projection and definition. Alar base reduction was necessary to restore appropriate balance to the nasal tip.

Complications of Rhinoplasty

- Septal hematoma
- Septal perforation
- Saddle nose deformity
- Residual hump
- Deviated nose
- Open roof deformity
- Rocker deformity
- Bossa
- Pollybeak deformity
- Nasal tip overrotation/underrotation/projection
- Nasal obstruction
- Epistaxis
- Nasal valve collapse/stenosis
- Alar retraction
- Hanging columella

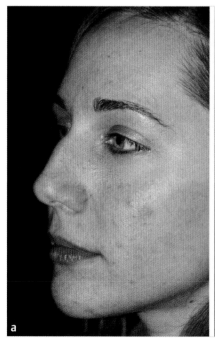

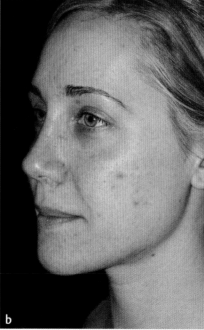

Fig. 53.23 (a) Preoperative and (b) postoperative views of rhinoplasty with dorsal reduction and conservative refinement of the nasal tip.

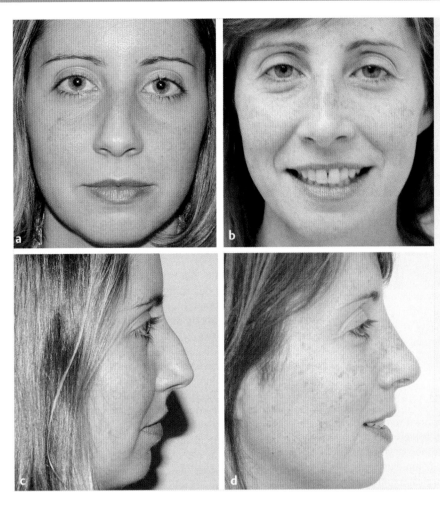

Fig. 53.24 Preoperative (**a,c**) and 7-year postoperative (**b,d**) views of external rhinoplasty to straighten and reduce the nasal dorsum and refine the nasal tip.

53.8 Roundsmanship

- Major and minor tip supports maintain the position of the nasal tip. Know them.
- Understand the tripod concept.
- Rhinoplasty should never sacrifice function for form.
- The height of nose (nasal root to nasolabial angle) is generally not changed. The position of the nasal tip and dorsum are generally based on the nasal height.
- Remember the 3–4-5 right triangle view of the nose.

53.9 Recommended Reading

[1] Adamson PA, Funk E. Nasal tip dynamics. Facial Plast Surg Clin North Am 2009; 17: 29–40, vi

[2] Dyer WK, Yune ME. Structural grafting in rhinoplasty. Facial Plast Surg 1997; 13: 269–277

[3] Johnson CM, Toriumi DM. Open Structure Rhinoplasty. Philadelphia, PA: W. B. Saunders; 1989

[4] Sclafani AP, Schaefer SD. Triological thesis: concurrent endoscopic sinus surgery and cosmetic rhinoplasty: rationale, risks, rewards and reality. Laryngoscope 2009;119(4): 778– 791

[5] Sheen JH, Sheen AP. Aesthetic Rhinoplasty. St. Louis, MO: Quality Medical Publishing; 1998

[6] Tebbets JB. Primary Rhinoplasty. 2nd ed. St. Louis, MO: Mosby; 2007

54 Revision Rhinoplasty

Alexander Ovchinsky

54.1 Introduction

Rhinoplasty is rightfully considered by many to be one of the most difficult facial plastic procedures. The tridimensional anatomy of the nose, involving multiple tissue layers with various anatomical properties (skin, bone, cartilage, and nasal mucosa), and the central location of the nose in the face make rhinoplasty a technically demanding task with variable final outcomes. These factors undoubtedly account for a fairly high revision rate of rhinoplasty surgery compared with other surgical cosmetic procedures.

In cases of dissatisfaction after rhinoplasty for aesthetic and/or functional reasons, revision rhinoplasty may be indicated to improve the patient's nasal appearance and function. Compared with primary rhinoplasty, revision rhinoplasty is an even more challenging operation because the main goal of this procedure is to modify functional and/or cosmetic defects or complaints after a previous procedure that was unsuccessful according to the patient's estimation.

54.2 Incidence of Disease

The revision rate of rhinoplasty surgery is known to be in the range from 10 to 15% nationwide. This fairly high incidence of revision surgery compared with that of other facial plastic procedures may be due to the intricacy and complexity of the nasal anatomy, requiring a high level of surgical expertise to consistently achieve good results. In addition, involvement of various tissues with very different physiologic and anatomical properties, such as bone, cartilage, skin, and mucosa, makes the healing process less predictable and more difficult to fully control.

54.3 Terminology

The terminology used in the description of normal nasal anatomy has been presented in earlier chapters. The term *saddle nasal deformity* describes a nasal dorsal height that is lower than normal, whereas *dorsal hump* indicates an excessive height of the nasal dorsum. *Polybeak deformity* indicates excessive fullness in the supratip region, which creates a beaklike appearance of the nasal profile. *Inverted*-V *deformity* is excessive narrowing or pinching of the cartilaginous midvault caudal to the bony–cartilaginous junction and may indicate the presence of internal nasal valve collapse. A Cottle maneuver is the test for internal nasal valve collapse, in which the upper lateral cartilage is manually supported on the undersurface while change in the patient's nasal breathing is assessed.

There exist multiple descriptions for postoperative nasal tip deformities, such as tip bossa and boxy, bifid, or bulbous tip. A bossa of the nasal tip is a knuckling of the lower lateral cartilages (LLCs) at the nasal tip due to contracting healing forces acting on overly weakened cartilages. Certain types of patients, especially those with thin skin and strong tip cartilages that are widely placed, are especially at risk. *Columellar show* describes the length of the columella visible on the profile view (normally 2 to 4 mm).

54.4 Applied Anatomy

An overview of nasal anatomy may be found elsewhere in the body of this text.

54.5 The Disease Process

54.5.1 Etiology

The dorsal abnormalities frequently necessitating revision surgery are saddle nasal deformity, persistent dorsal hump, and persistent dorsal asymmetry and deviation. The most common etiologies for saddle nasal deformity include overly zealous reduction of the nasal dorsum during primary surgery (▶ Fig. 54.1), inward collapse of flail nasal bones after osteotomy, and overly aggressive septoplasty with excessive resection of the bony and cartilaginous septum, leading to the loss of dorsal support (▶ Fig. 54.2). Overly zealous reduction of the bony dorsum relative to reduction of the cartilaginous dorsum leads to the polybeak deformity (▶ Fig. 54.3). Other etiologies of polybeak deformity include insufficient reduction of the cartilaginous dorsum, as well as extensive postoperative fibrosis in the supratip region (more common in patients with thick skin).

Insufficient cartilaginous midvault support due to overly reduced upper lateral cartilages (ULCs) or inadvertent detachment of the ULC from its attachment to the undersurface of the caudal nasal bone during dorsal hump reduction may lead to the inverted-V deformity and internal nasal valve collapse with resultant nasal airway obstruction.

Nasal tip deformities can occur after overly aggressive LLC reduction leading to a loss of cartilage strength and gradual deformity due to forces of postoperative scarring and fibrosis, after division of the LLC leading to a loss of continuity and weakness, or after poor surgical technique with asymmetric reduction or suturing (see ▶ Fig. 54.3). Excessive columellar show commonly results from the placement of a disproportionally large columellar strut or tip graft, buckling of the medial crura, or an excessively long caudal septum pushing the columella out. Additionally, columellar show should be distinguished from alar retraction, which, albeit occasionally an anatomical variant, most commonly results from inadequate alar support or excessive scarring.

54.5.2 Pathogenesis

Although some post-rhinoplasty deformities are purely cosmetic in nature, others may result in significant functional problems. Inverted-V deformity and saddle nasal deformity may result in internal nasal valve collapse and nasal obstruction. Significant nasal tip irregularities and weakness of the LLCs may cause alar stenosis and collapse, especially on inspiration, thus resulting in external nasal valve compromise (see ▶ Fig. 54.3).

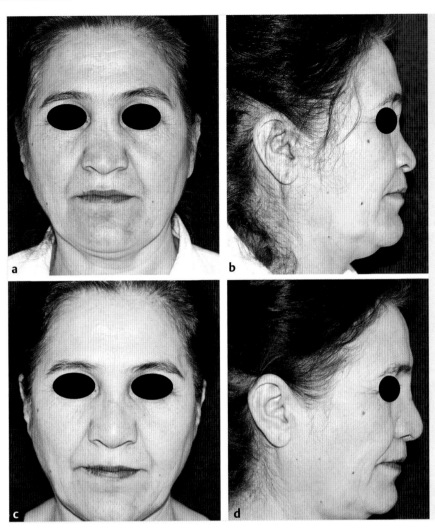

Fig. 54.1 (a,b) A patient with a history of prior nasal trauma and rhinoplasty who presented with saddle nose and open roof deformities, irregular and widened nasal bones, a ptotic nasal tip, and pinched lower lateral cartilages with external nasal valve stenosis. **(c,d)** Twelve months after revision rhinoplasty with dorsal costal cartilage graft, bilateral batten grafts, columellar strut, and lateral osteotomies.

Excessive resection of the nasal septum during primary septorhinoplasty results in a gradual loss of nasal support, progressive dorsal saddling, and nasal obstruction. Alternatively, insufficient correction of a preexisting septal deviation or failure to perform septoplasty during primary rhinoplasty when indicated will leave the patient with persistent nasal airway obstruction.

54.5.3 Natural History and Progression

The postoperative nasal appearance and function may initially be normal in patients with underlying structural deficits. With time, however, weakened, overresected cartilages buckle under the influence of subcutaneous fibrosis and scarring. Progressive subcutaneous fibrosis in the supratip region leads to the polybeak deformity, whereas progressive alar soft-tissue scarring, if not resisted by strong cartilaginous support, causes alar notching and collapse in more severe cases (see ▸ Fig. 54.3). Incorrectly performed osteotomies (i.e., incomplete osteotomies or osteotomies carried too far superiorly beyond the nasofrontal junction) commonly fail to correct nasal bony deviation. Failure to perform osteotomies to close an open roof after dorsal hump reduction results in open roof deformity and progressive scarring of the dorsal skin into the gap between the nasal bones (see ▸ Fig. 54.1). Onlay grafts placed during the primary surgery

(bone or cartilage autografts or allografts) may warp, shift, become infected, or be resorbed.

Because many postoperative changes occur gradually over time as a consequence of progressive bony–cartilaginous remodeling and the forces of scar contracture and fibrosis, the "final" result of rhinoplasty is typically described at 1 year or more after surgery. However, even after that, some (generally subtle, but possibly dramatic when significant structural integrity has been compromised) changes in nasal appearance and function may still take place over the following months to years.

54.5.4 Potential Disease Complications

As already discussed, the potential complications of rhinoplasty are primarily of two types: functional due to nasal obstruction and cosmetic due to persistent or worsened nasal deformity.

54.6 Medical Evaluation

54.6.1 Presenting Complaints

Patients evaluated for revision rhinoplasty most commonly present with aesthetic and/or functional nasal complaints that can be broadly subdivided into two categories: uncorrected or

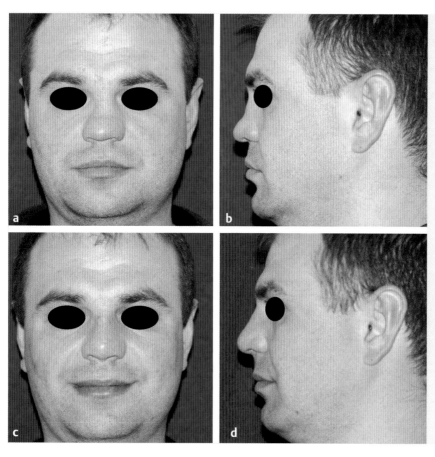

Fig. 54.2 (a,b) Patient with complaints of persistently deviated nasal dorsum, "low-set" nasal profile, and ptotic tip after rhinoplasty. (c,d) Fourteen months after revision rhinoplasty with costal cartilage dorsal graft, columellar strut, lateral and medial osteotomies, and tip refinement.

poorly corrected problems that were present before the original surgery and new problems that have occurred as a result of the previous rhinoplasty. The former include persistence of a dorsal hump because of insufficient reduction, persistence of a nasal dorsal deviation and an uncorrected septal deviation resulting in persistent nasal obstruction, and persistent tip irregularities that were insufficiently addressed or not addressed at all. The latter include open roof deformity, saddling of the nasal dorsum, inverted-V deformity, tip asymmetry and bossa, excessive columellar show, alar notching and retraction, internal and external nasal valve collapse, and various deformities due to poorly placed, designed, shifted, or warped nasal grafts.

54.6.2 Clinical Findings, Physical Examination

A thorough examination of the external nasal anatomy, which includes an evaluation of the nasal appearance on frontal, lateral, oblique, and base views, and careful palpation of the nasal bony–cartilaginous framework are performed. This commonly allows an accurate assessment of the existing problems and gives the surgeon an idea about what was done during the primary surgery. In a cephalic to caudal direction, the nasal bones and cartilaginous midvault are examined for deviation, excessive width or pinching, asymmetry, step-offs, and the presence of a dorsal hump or inverted-V deformity. The Cottle maneuver assists in confirming internal nasal valve collapse. The nasal tip is examined for adequacy of projection, rotation, and support, as well as for the presence of tip asymmetry, deviation, or alar

weakness. Anterior rhinoscopy and nasal endoscopy are routinely performed, particularly in patients with nasal obstructive symptoms, to better evaluate the internal nasal anatomy and rule out other potential causes of nasal obstruction, such as nasal polyps, sinusitis, and nasopharyngeal lesions.

54.6.3 Testing

Standard preoperative photography is always required before revision rhinoplasty. It should document the frontal and basal views, and the right and left 90-degree lateral and 45-degree oblique views. Rhinomanometry, an objective test for nasal airway resistance and obstruction, may be helpful in some instances to diagnose and document the degree of obstruction but is not routinely performed. This test, however, may come in handy when a patient reports significant nasal obstruction and there is no objective evidence of the cause of obstruction on examination. Computer imaging is frequently used as preoperative consultation tool; it greatly facilitates communication between surgeon and patient but should never be considered to be a guarantee of surgical outcome.

54.6.4 Differential Diagnosis

Nasal deformities are multifactorial in etiology, and they may be congenital or arise from prior surgery or trauma. The surgical planning is largely based on the deformity at hand rather than its possible etiology. However, revision rhinoplasties are usually more time-consuming and technically demanding

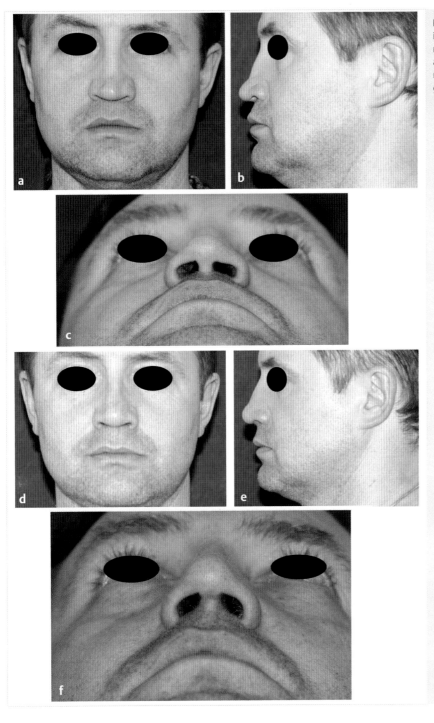

Fig. 54.3 (a–c) Progressive saddle nose deformity, tip ptosis, and alar notching with internal nasal valve stenosis developed in this patient after prior rhinoplasty. (d–f) Six months after revision rhinoplasty with dorsal costal cartilage graft, columellar strut, and bilateral batten grafts.

because of the altered nasal anatomy and scarring from the primary procedure. Patients should always be asked for their consent to the possible harvest of a cartilage (auricular or rib) and/or calvarial bone graft because there may not be any suitable or sufficient septal cartilage remaining after the original surgery.

54.7 Treatment

54.7.1 Medical Treatment

Medical treatment has limited application in cases in which the main problem is structural (i.e. loss of support, deviation,

other). However, there is a role for medical therapy in attempts to decrease nasal mucosal edema and hyperreactivity. Intranasal, as well as oral, steroids and antihistamines may be used in various combinations for this purpose. Steroid injections into the areas of excessive scarring (most commonly in the supratip region) assist in improving nasal appearance; injectable triamcinolone is commonly used, administered no more frequently than every 3 weeks.

Nasal alloplastic implants placed during the primary surgery may become infected, necessitating treatment with oral or intravenous antibiotics. Although unlikely to salvage the implant,

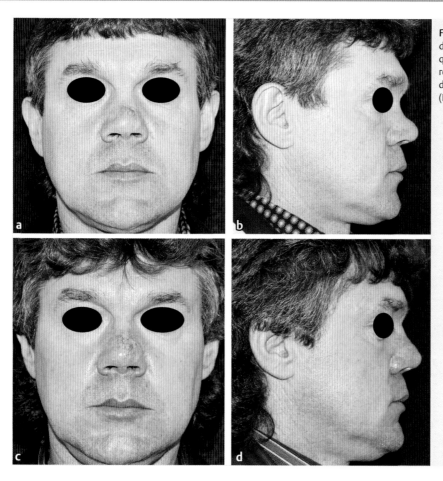

Fig. 54.4 (a,b) Severe bony–cartilaginous saddle deformity after prior nasal trauma and subsequent rhinoplasty. **(c,d)** Eighteen months after revision rhinoplasty with a dorsal onlay graft of diced costal cartilage wrapped in AlloDerm (LifeCell Corporation, Branchburg, NJ).

these help reduce the infectious load and optimize the patient for a revision procedure.

54.7.2 Surgical Treatment

Revision rhinoplasty is an indicated treatment for most of the nasal conditions, whether functional or cosmetic, that arise as a result of or that persist in spite of a prior rhinoplasty. Revision rhinoplasty surgery is usually a more demanding and difficult procedure from the surgeon's perspective because of the altered nasal anatomy, obliteration of the normal tissue planes by postoperative fibrosis, and frequently insufficient donor septal cartilage after prior septoplasty. The use of alloplastic materials, such as e-polytetrafluoroethylene (e-PTFE), silicone, and porous high-density polyethylene implants, remains a viable albeit controversial option in revision rhinoplasty and thus should be discussed with patients preoperatively. In secondary or tertiary revisions, when the defect is mainly cosmetic and not functional, many surgeons advocate a "minimalistic" approach by using various onlay grafts to camouflage the defect rather than undertaking a formal reconstructive rhinoplasty, which would be much more-time consuming and less predictable.

It is important to consider preoperatively whether the revision surgery is appropriate. Some post-rhinoplasty patients become so obsessed with their nasal appearance that they may desire revision after revision in the pursuit of perfection and an unrealistic goal. It is the responsibility of a surgeon to discuss all surgical limitations with patients and to carefully select operative candidates by excluding those with unrealistic expectations, psychiatric problems, or body dysmorphic disorder.

A persistent dorsal hump due to underreduction during a primary surgery can be corrected by further dorsal reduction with dorsal rasps or an osteotome for bony humps and a scalpel for cartilaginous reduction.

Correction of a persistent nasal deviation commonly requires revision osteotomies. Lateral osteotomies alone are frequently adequate; however, medial and/or intermediate osteotomies may be necessary in cases of thick, severely deviated, or asymmetric nasal bones (see ► Fig. 54.2). One should determine the reason for the failure to correct the nasal deviation during the primary surgery because failure to correct this during a revision procedure will likely lead to persistent dorsal deformity. Several common reasons for persistent dorsal deviation after a primary rhinoplasty include incorrectly performed osteotomies (either incomplete osteotomies or asymmetric osteotomies), failure to correct bony septal deviation (so that midline positioning of the nasal bones is not possible), and uncorrected deviation of the cartilaginous dorsum. Open roof deformity results from a failure to perform osteotomies after dorsal hump reduction and is usually corrected by lateral osteotomies.

Saddle nasal deformity is usually corrected by the placement of dorsal onlay grafts, which may be autografts, homografts, or allografts (see ► Fig. 54.1, ► Fig. 54.2, ► Fig. 54.3, ► Fig. 54.4). Autologous materials, which include septal, auricular, or costal cartilage grafts and calvarial bone grafts, are usually the preferred option; however, there are several inherent problems related to the use of autologous grafts, such as donor site morbidity, resorption, and warping (with most cartilage grafts, especially costal cartilage). Homografts (including irradiated cadaveric rib cartilage grafts) have been used with variable success because of reported resorption of the graft. The use of allografts, such as e-PTFE, silicone, and porous high-density polyethylene, avoids donor site morbidity and issues of insufficient graft availability; however, alloplastic materials are prone to migration, extrusion, foreign body reaction, and infection, which may exacerbate the nasal deformity and necessitate implant removal.

Asymmetries of the cartilaginous dorsum are commonly due to uncorrected deviation of the dorsal septal cartilage, asymmetric or weak ULCs, or asymmetrically placed onlay grafts during the primary surgery. Dorsal septal deviations are difficult to correct because simple excision of the deviated septal cartilage will undoubtedly lead to a loss of nasal support and saddle nose deformity. Numerous surgical techniques exist for the reconstruction of dorsal septal deviations, including spreader graft placement to brace and straighten the deviated cartilage (with or without prior cartilage scoring), complete removal of the cartilaginous septum and extracorporeal reconstruction of the cartilage pieces over a resorbable polydioxanone mesh that is then placed in the anatomical position and secured to the ULCs, or replacement of the septal cartilage with a costal cartilage L-shaped graft. In some instances, a simple detachment of the ULCs from the septal cartilage allows the release of septal tension forces and correction of the septal deviation. Asymmetry of the ULCs is usually corrected by the placement of a ULC onlay graft or a unilateral spreader graft; occasionally, an oversized ULC may be trimmed conservatively without sacrificing the support. Weakness of the ULC, either congenital or secondary to ULC overresection or detachment from the bony–cartilaginous junction, commonly leads to midvault weakness, inverted-V deformity, and internal nasal valve collapse. This can be corrected by the placement of spreader grafts, which are cartilaginous grafts placed between the ULCs and dorsal septal cartilage. Spreader grafts provide additional support to the cartilaginous midvault and increase the cross-sectional area of the internal nasal valve, thus improving its patency and relieving nasal obstruction. An asymmetric or shifted dorsal onlay graft may be repositioned or replaced altogether.

Polybeak deformity, or excessive fullness in the supratip region, results from excessive postoperative fibrosis in the supratip, underreduction of the cartilaginous dorsal hump, overresection of the bony dorsum, or progressive nasal tip ptosis postoperatively. Thus, a polybeak deformity should be corrected based on the primary causative factor with the cautious excision of subdermal scar and fibrosis, addition of structured tip grafts to provide a more substantial base upon which the skin and soft-tissue envelope can be draped, further reduction of the cartilaginous dorsum, and augmentation of the bony dorsum or correction of the nasal tip ptosis.

Nasal tip deformities usually result from excessive weakness of the LLCs from overresection, disruption of continuity, asymmetric LLC suturing, extensive scarring of the nasal tip skin, or a combination of these. The end result may be a bifid tip, bossae, alar collapse, excess or deficiency of columellar show, severely overrotated tip creating the appearance of a foreshortened nose, or an underprojected or droopy tip.

Tip bifidity, or divergence of the dome areas of the LLCs, usually results from the failure to properly secure the domes as a single unit; the domes are then pulled apart by the forces of scar contracture. The correction of a bifid tip requires resuturing the domes together with a nonabsorbable suture (Ethilon [Ethicon, Somerville, NJ] or polypropylene). There exist multiple techniques to correct nasal tip bossae, including direct excision of the bossae and reestablishment of the continuity of the LLCs with sutures and camouflage of the bossa with either an onlay or a tip graft. Alar collapse commonly occurs because of excessive weakening of the lateral crura of the LLCs secondary to overresection (i.e., excessive cephalic trim) or loss of continuity (in cases of LLC division). Occasionally, weak LLCs may collapse under the forces of scar contracture as a result of marginal incisions alone. Alar collapse usually leads to external nasal valve stenosis, in which the alar soft tissues collapse during inspiration under negative pressure, causing nasal obstruction. Reestablishing the strength of the LLC lateral crura with alar strut grafts (cartilage grafts placed on the undersurface of the lateral crura between the crura and the vestibular mucosa) or with alar batten grafts (onlay cartilage grafts placed over the lateral crura) improves alar support and usually corrects external nasal valve stenosis (see ▶ Fig. 54.1).

Excessive columellar show is caused by buckling of the medial crura, poor placement of the columellar strut or tip graft, or an overly long caudal septum. Alar retraction will make the columella more visible on the profile view. Buckled medial crura may be corrected with sutures or with excision of the buckled segment and the reestablishment of medial crural continuity with a permanent suture. Another option is to suture the medial crura onto the caudal septal cartilage, as in the so-called tongue-in-groove technique, which usually corrects medial crural deformity and adds to tip support. Poorly placed columellar strut or tip grafts need to be replaced or repositioned. Alar retractions are more difficult to correct; mild retraction may be corrected with an alar rim cartilage graft, whereas more severe retraction may require a composite graft (usually from the contralateral auricle). Insufficient columellar show is corrected by adding volume caudal to the medial crura with either a columellar strut or a tip graft. A premaxillary plumper graft, a diced cartilage graft placed into the pocket created at the base of the columella and in front of the anterior nasal spine, can also improve columellar show and creates an illusion of increased tip rotation.

An overrotated nasal tip and a foreshortened nose are the stigmata of unsuccessful rhinoplasty, or multiple rhinoplasties (▶ Fig. 54.5). They commonly result from the combination of overresection of the caudal septal cartilage, overly aggressive cephalic trim of the LLC lateral crura, and excessive lateral repositioning of the domes combined with skin contracture forces pulling the tip cephalad. The correction of a foreshortened nose requires de-rotation of the nasal tip, lengthening of the supratip region, the creation of an illusion of lengthening by placing a columellar strut or a tip graft, or a combination of the above techniques. Extended spreader grafts, which extend from the bony–cartilaginous junction to beyond the caudal extent of the septal cartilage and are connected to the columellar strut, recreate a new L-shaped nasal support structure upon which the final tip position is set. The addition of a tip graft assists with lengthening the nose, thus creating an illusion of more de-rotation, and can aid in camouflaging tip irregularities.

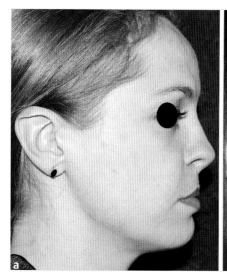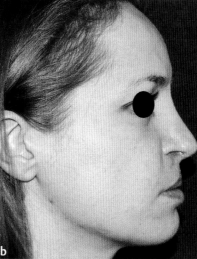

Fig. 54.5 (**a**) Patient with cleft lip nasal deformity who previously underwent two rhinoplasty surgeries, with overrotated nasal tip and "short nose." (**b**) Six months after revision rhinoplasty with bilateral extended spreader grafts, columellar strut, and tip refinement.

Underrotated or ptotic nasal tips occur from weakening and failure to reconstruct tip support structures during the primary surgery. Thick and heavy nasal tip skin and weak LLCs are the predisposing risk factors for postoperative tip ptosis. The ptotic tip needs to be resupported either with a strong columellar strut or by suturing the LLCs to the caudal septal cartilage, as in the tongue-in-groove technique.

54.8 Prognosis

As for primary rhinoplasty, there is a definitive revision rate for secondary rhinoplasty that averages about 15%. Proper patient selection is the key factor to a successful revision rhinoplasty; only patients with realistic expectations of the surgical outcome and with nasal deformities that are deemed correctable on preoperative evaluation should be offered a revision surgery. It is a universally recommended and accepted practice not to embark on a revision surgery too soon after the primary rhinoplasty; a year should be allowed to elapse before revision surgery is attempted, particular if the tip needs to be revised. This amount of time allows most of the postoperative changes to mature and gives the patient enough time to get used to the new nose; this latter factor alone helps significantly decrease the number of patient requests for a revision procedure.

54.9 Roundsmanship

- Revision rhinoplasty surgery is required in 10 to 15% of patients after primary rhinoplasty. This high revision rate is

mainly due to the intricacy of the nasal anatomy, complexity of the surgical technique, and difficulty of controlling the healing process in various tissues with different anatomical characteristics, such as bone, cartilage, mucosa, and skin.
- Alteration of the nasal anatomy during primary rhinoplasty surgery makes revision rhinoplasty a more technically demanding procedure with a less predictable final outcome.
- Only patients with correctable deformities and realistic expectations should be offered a revision procedure.
- An accurate assessment of the problem in question and careful surgical planning, which frequently includes auricular or costal cartilage or calvarial bone graft harvest, is imperative for optimizing the surgical outcome.
- All major structural revisions should be delayed for at least 1 year after the primary surgery. This allows enough time to elapse for scar maturation and for the nose to acquire its final shape.

54.10 Recommended Reading

[1] Chand MS, Toriumi DM. Treatment of the external nasal valve. Facial Plast Surg Clin North Am 1999; 7: 347–356
[2] Daniel RK, Sajadian A. Secondary rhinoplasty: management of the overresected dorsum. Facial Plast Surg 2012; 28: 417–426
[3] Davis RE, Bublik M. Psychological considerations in the revision rhinoplasty patient. Facial Plast Surg 2012; 28: 374–379
[4] Park SS, Hughley BB. Revision of the functionally devastated nasal airway. Facial Plast Surg 2012; 28: 398–406
[5] Tardy ME. Rhinoplasty: The Art and Science. Philadelphia, PA: W. B. Saunders; 1997

55 Special Considerations in Rhinoplasty

Grigorly Mashkevich

55.1 Introduction

Rhinoplasty changes the shape and/or function of the nose. In several clinical scenarios, special considerations are required for the planning and execution of this operation. These include patients with cleft lip/palate deformities and those of ethnic extraction, particularly of Middle Eastern, African, Asian, or Hispanic descent. Some of the nuances of rhinoplasty surgery pertinent to these groups of patients are addressed in detail in the sections that follow.

55.2 Incidence of Disease

The incidence of cleft lip and palate deformity varies depending on the population. In Caucasians, the incidence reaches 1 in 1,000 live births. The rate in the African population is approximately half of that, and the rate among Asians is twice as high.

55.3 Terminology

Cleft rhinoplasty is designed to restore appropriate height and symmetry to the affected side of the nasal tip in patients with history of cleft lip deformity. Ethnic rhinoplasty reflects a surgical modification of the nasal appearance in patients of ethnic extraction. Ethnic rhinoplasty has an implicit goal of maintaining the ethnic nasal appearance and avoiding "Westernization rhinoplasty."

55.4 Applied Anatomy

A cleft nose is marked by deformity limited to the nasal tip and affecting the lower lateral cartilage on the side of the cleft. This cartilage is typically flattened and lowered in comparison with the contralateral lower lateral cartilage (▶ Fig. 55.1). Because of the underlying cleft defect, the base of the nostril is widened; the columella and ala are situated farther apart on the cleft side, while the nasal septum is deviated to the noncleft side. The premaxilla is also frequently deficient.

Within each ethnic group, patients undergoing rhinoplasty display consistent external nasal features. These nasal features are listed for persons of Middle Eastern and African descent in ▶ Table 55.1.

55.5 The Disease Process

55.5.1 Etiology

The etiology and evolution of cleft deformity are outlined elsewhere in this textbook. Ethnic nasal structure and appearance represent variations of normal and occur because of inherent genetic differences between clustered populations.

55.5.2 Pathogenesis

If not surgically corrected, a nasal cleft deformity will lead to persistent flattening of the lower lateral cartilage on the affected side. This configuration can result in nasal obstruction at the level of the vestibule and external nasal valve. Despite growth and development, an obvious tip deformity will persist on the cleft side.

The external nasal appearance of persons of non-Caucasian lineage exhibits several defining characteristics, which are listed for selected groups in ▶ Table 55.1. For instance, persons of Middle Eastern extraction commonly have large dorsal humps and underrotated nasal tips. On the other hand, persons of African descent may have weak and underprojecting nasal bones, with large and thick nasal tips.

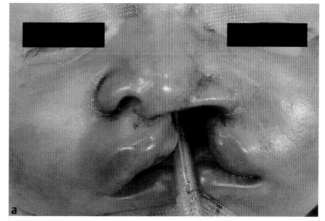
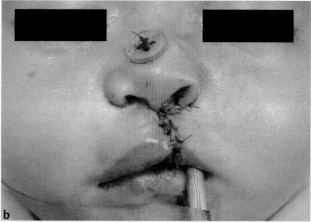

Fig. 55.1 Cleft lip and nose deformity (a) before and (b) after cleft lip and nose repair.

Table 55.1 Characteristics of the external nasal appearance in patients of Middle Eastern or African extraction

Nasal appearance	Middle Eastern	African
Skin and soft-tissue envelope	Thick skin and subcutaneous tissues of the tip	Thick skin and subcutaneous tissues of the tip
Upper third	Overprojecting bony dorsum and radix, dorsal widening	Underprojecting bony dorsum and radix, dorsal widening
Middle third	Widening of the osseous and cartilaginous vaults	Widening of the osseous and cartilaginous vaults
Nasal tip	Amorphous and hanging nasal tip, variation in width	Amorphous and wide nasal tip
Nostrils	Variable degree of alar flaring	Alar flaring

55.5.3 Natural History and Progression

The growth and development of ethnic nasal appearances are genetically driven, resulting in the unique features listed for selected groups in ▶ Table 55.1.

55.5.4 Potential Disease Complications

Potential complications in cleft noses include persistent external deformity and nasal airway obstruction at the level of the external nasal valve. Ethnic noses are not a form of disease and are without inherent structural problems that can lead to complications such as nasal obstruction. Most commonly, patients of ethnic extraction desire nasal surgery to improve their external appearance.

55.6 Medical Evaluation

The complete evaluation of children with cleft deformity is reviewed elsewhere in this textbook.

The initial consultation for an ethnic rhinoplasty allows the surgeon to discuss the patient's concerns and goals for surgery. The concept of maintaining an ethnic identity should be clearly communicated during the initial and subsequent visits. A surgeon should be cautious with patients requesting drastic changes in their nasal appearance because this may lead to unnatural results and "Westernization" changes. Such results may become a strong source of dissatisfaction in such patients.

Digital photography and morphing are used to convey proposed changes. These are shown and discussed as a point of reference, without implicit guarantees of the result. If needed, before and after photographs of previous surgical patients can be used to clarify differences in rhinoplasty goals between Caucasian and ethnic noses.

55.6.1 Presenting Complaints

Children with a cleft nose present primarily with cosmetic and functional deficits related to lip and palate clefting. The accompanying nasal deformity, although not a primary complaint of parents, must be noted, documented, and addressed during cleft surgery.

Patients who seek ethnic rhinoplasty present with complaints related to their appearance, which may include concerns

about any of the features listed for the selected groups in ▶ Table 55.1.

55.6.2 Clinical Findings, Physical Examination

The clinical findings and examination of the child with a cleft deformity are reviewed in thepathogenesis section of this chapter. The findings pertaining to patients undergoing ethnic rhinoplasty are listed in ▶ Table 55.1. As in all patients, nasal palpation should be performed to determine the inherent strength of the lower lateral cartilages, document any evidence of previous nasal surgery, and assess potential cartilage grafting sites, such as the septum and ear. Any reports of nasal obstruction should be evaluated during the physical examination by assessing valve competence and nasal allergies.

55.6.3 Testing

No special testing is required for patients with a cleft deformity beyond documenting appropriate growth and development in the first several months of life.

55.7 Treatment
55.7.1 Medical Treatment

The medical treatment of a child with a cleft deformity is discussed elsewhere in this textbook and is not applicable for the cleft nose defect. Ethnic patients with valve obstruction due to inherently weak lower lateral cartilages may benefit from external stents, such as Breathe Right nasal strips (GlaxoSmithKline, Philadelphia, PA). Patients with nasal obstruction due to underlying allergies should undergo allergy testing and be treated with corticosteroid sprays.

55.7.2 Surgical Treatment

The main goal of cleft rhinoplasty is reconfiguration of the lower lateral cartilage with restoration of nasal symmetry and projection on the affected side. Cleft rhinoplasty should accompany cleft lip repair in children at about 3 months of age. Infants are judged to be surgical candidates based on the "rule of 10s":

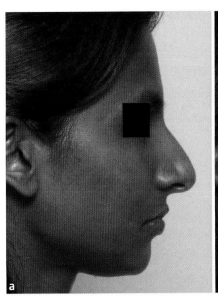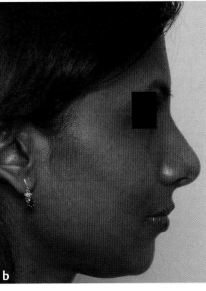

Fig. 55.2 Patient of Middle Eastern extraction (**a**) before and (**b**) 6 months after rhinoplasty. Note the maintenance of a strong radix and dorsum, with only a partial dorsal reduction and concomitant tip rotation.

Table 55.2 Surgical maneuvers commonly performed in Middle Eastern and African ethnic rhinoplasty

Surgical maneuvers	Middle Eastern	African
Skin and soft tissue envelope	Conservative removal of fat in the supratip region; postoperative monitoring and conservative steroid injections	Moderate–aggressive removal of fat in the supratip region; postoperative monitoring and conservative steroid injections
Upper third	Maintenance of high radix during dorsal hump reduction; elevation of the tip to enhance a visual illusion of dorsal hump reduction	Augmentation grafting of the radix and dorsum
Middle third	Osteotomies for dorsal narrowing; placement of spreader grafts to avoid internal valve collapse and an inverted-V deformity	Osteotomies for dorsal narrowing
Nasal tip	Cartilage-sparing maneuvers; preferential use of suture techniques for the dome region; placement of strong supports (columellar strut or septal extension graft, shield or cap grafts)	Cartilage-sparing maneuvers; preferential use of suture techniques for the dome region; placement of strong supports (columellar strut or septal extension graft, shield or cap grafts)
Nostrils	Alar base reduction in some cases	Alar base reduction in the majority of cases

weight over 10 lb, hemoglobin level over 10 g/dL, and age over 10 weeks. During cleft rhinoplasty, the skin overlying the deformed lower lateral cartilage is undermined, and a suspension suture is placed through the dome region. The lower lateral cartilage is sutured in a more cephalic and medial position (see ▶ Fig. 55.1). This suture is bolstered for several weeks with a silicone button. Definitive cleft rhinoplasty can be offered starting at age 16 for those patients with persistent nasal deformity and/or airway obstruction. An open rhinoplasty approach via a transcolumellar incision affords the best visualization of the lower lateral cartilages. These can be modified with suture and cartilage-grafting techniques to achieve desired tip symmetry and airway patency.

Ethnic rhinoplasty (▶ Fig. 55.2) addresses some of the visual characteristics particular to the ethnic nasal appearance. Native nasal harmony must be kept in mind when ethnic rhinoplasty is performed. This surgery has a goal for appearance that differs from what is desirable in Caucasian rhinoplasty. Like any other rhinoplasty operation, ethnic nasal surgery must incorporate the patient's goals and concerns. However, one of the primary objectives of ethnic rhinoplasty is the avoidance of surgical "Westernization." Excessive reshaping of the nose to match the ideal Caucasian nose creates an unnatural appearance in ethnic patients. Such a result generates a relative discord between the nose and the face. The surgical goals of ethnic rhinoplasty for Middle Eastern and African patients are listed in ▶ Table 55.2.

Several undesirable outcomes may complicate ethnic rhinoplasty. These include the same problems seen in Caucasian rhinoplasty, which are discussed in detail in a different section of this textbook. Particular to ethnic nasal surgery is surgical "Westernization," which is best avoided by understanding the native visual characteristics of ethnic noses.

55.8 Prognosis

Favorable outcomes are expected in most properly executed cleft and ethnic rhinoplasties. Errors leading to complications are best avoided by meticulous planning and precise execution. An understanding of native visual characteristics in ethnic noses should help avoid surgical "Westernization."

55.9 Roundsmanship

- Special considerations are important in the planning and execution of rhinoplasty surgery in patients with cleft deformities and in those of ethnic extraction.
- Cleft rhinoplasty should accompany cleft lip and palate repair at 3 months of age.
- Ethnic rhinoplasty addresses important visual characteristics in patients of Middle Eastern, African, Hispanic, and Asian backgrounds.

- The avoidance of surgical "Westernization" in ethnic patients is an important goal of ethnic rhinoplasty.

55.10 Recommended Reading

[1] Azizzadeh B, Mashkevich G. Middle Eastern rhinoplasty. Facial Plast Surg Clin North Am 2010; 18: 201–206

[2] Sykes JM, Tollefson TT. Management of the cleft lip deformity. Facial Plast Surg Clin North Am 2005; 13: 157–167

56 Surgical Treatment of the Aging Face

Anthony P. Sclafani and James A. Sclafani

56.1 Introduction

Modern surgery of the aging face was first reported in the early 1900s and was clouded in secrecy, with patients seeking to maintain anonymity and surgeons attempting to keep their techniques to themselves. Over the past 100 years, these procedures have become better designed, defined, and described by surgeons and accepted by the public at large. The procedures have become increasingly refined, with better and longer-lasting results, as well as smaller, less conspicuous scars and less morbidity.

56.2 Incidence of Disease

In 2008, 132,000 facelifts and 44,000 forehead lifts were performed in the United States. These procedures can be performed individually or in concert, depending upon the aesthetic needs of the patient.

56.3 Terminology

Browlift and *foreheadplasty* are distinct and separate terms. The browlift procedure elevates the brow only, whereas the fore-headplasty additionally treats rhytids of the forehead. Neither *facelift* nor *rhytidoplasty* is an accurate description of the procedure, which neither "lifts" the face nor solely treats wrinkles (rhytids). A better description is *facialplasty*, but the term *facelift* is used herein because of its common use. Similarly, a *midfacelift* rejuvenates and recontours the midface (the area between the lower eyelids and the nasolabial folds) and does not simply "lift."

56.4 Applied Anatomy

The soft-tissue anatomy of surgical facial rejuvenation includes the skin, superficial musculofascial layer, facial muscles, and nerves.

56.4.1 Skin

Elevation of the skin, when performed, in done by elevating the skin flap with a small amount of subcutaneous fat on the flap. This provides protection to the subdermal plexus of vessels. Elevation of this plane is relatively easy in the midface and lower face but is more difficult in the forehead, where the muscles are more intimately attached to the skin. Similarly, the skin is fairly firmly attached to slips of muscle from the sternocleidomastoid (SCM) muscle laterally and often requires sharp dissection.

56.4.2 Musculofascial Layers

Beginning in the forehead, the fascial layer of the galea aponeurotica covers and envelops the frontalis muscle. Posteriorly, this layer continues into the occipitalis muscle fascia; inferiorly, the galea fuses with the periosteum about 2 cm above the orbital rim, while laterally the galea fuses with multiple layes of fascia just medial to the superior temporal line (most superior attachment of the temporalis muscle). Anatomically, the galea becomes contiguous with the SMAS (superficial musculoaponeurotic system), a fascial tissue that covers and envelopes the facial muscles, at the zygomatic arch, where they fuse with the periosteum. Inferiorly, the SMAS is contiguous with the platysma muscle, whereas medially it sends fibrous slips superficially to the overlying skin. Laterally, this tissue is less mobile than medially and covers the parotidomasseteric fascia.

56.4.3 Facial Muscles

Important muscles encountered or modified during forehead-plasty include the paired frontalis muscles (brow elevators that originate posteriorly from the galea and course inferiorly to intermingle with each other in the midline and with the orbicularis oculi muscles more laterally); orbital portion of the orbicularis oculi muscles (brow depressors); paired corrugator and depressor supercilii muscles (brow medializers and depressors, respectively, originating from the superomedial orbital rim); and the midline procerus muscle (brow depressor originating from the nasal bones).

In the midface, most muscles are out of the immediate surgical field; however, the zygomaticus major muscle, coursing from the midportion of the zygomatic arch to the nasolabial fold and modiolus, is a landmark in the deep plane facelift. Similarly, the orbital portion of the inferior orbicularis oculi muscle, depending on the surgical approach, may require mobilization or modification.

In the lower face, the platysma is the inferior extension of the SMAS and runs from the clavicle to interdigitate with the facial muscles and SMAS just above the mandibular border. Starting in the lateral neck, this muscle extends to meet the muscle from the opposite side in the midline. Generally, these are fibrously bound together near the chin but dehisce more inferiorly, a state that worsens with age. Laterally, the SCM muscle runs from the mastoid inferomedially; especially superiorly, slips of fascia and muscle extend from this muscle to insert on the skin.

56.4.4 Nerves

Motor Nerves

The facial nerve is the only motor nerve within the surgical field of forehead, face, and neck rejuvenation procedures. After the nerve emerges from the stylomastoid foramen and branches at the pes anserinus, five main branches innervate the facial muscles. These branches become increasingly more superficial medially, where in particular the temporal and buccal branches have significant interconnections. The temporal branch runs superiorly to innervate the forehead and lateral orbicularis and corrugator muscles. The temporal branch crosses the zygomatic arch, usually in one to three branches, within the fusion of the SMAS and periosteum, and then runs on the undersurface of the galea into the forehead. Often, an upper and a lower buccal branch of the facial nerve run medially, parallel to the Stensen duct, to innervate the midfacial muscles from their deep surface. More inferiorly, the marginal mandibular nerve extends medially in the area of the mandibular border, usually dipping below the mandible before ascending over it to innervate the depressor anguli oris muscle. The temporal and marginal mandibular nerves are the motor nerves most at risk for injury during surgery.

Sensory Nerves

The supraorbital and supratrochlear nerves (branches of the ophthalmic division of the trigeminal nerve, V_1) supply sensation to the brow and forehead posteriorly to the crown. These nerves emerge from notches or foramina along the superior orbital rim accompanied by arteries and veins, run posteriorly, and branch and become more superficial peripherally. The supratrochlear nerve is generally found between 15 and 20 mm lateral to the midline, while the supraorbital nerve emerges approximately 23 to 26 mm from the midline. The infraorbital nerve (branch of the maxillary division of the trigeminal nerve, V_2) emerges from a foramen in the maxilla just below the orbital rim, accompanied by associated arteries and veins; this foramen is generally near the midpupillary line. The mental nerve (branch of the mandibular division of the trigeminal nerve, V_3) exits a bony foramen in the mandible below the canine tooth and is generally not encountered during a facelift unless a chin implant is being placed. The great auricular nerve (from C2 and C3) emerges around the Erb point (a point on the posterior aspect of the SCM muscle 6.5 cm below the external auditory canal) and crosses the middle one-third of the SCM muscle with multiple branches to innervate the lower portion of the auricle and mastoid area. The great auricular nerve is the most commonly injured nerve during facelifts.

56.5 The Disease Process

56.5.1 Pathogenesis

Facial aging is a complex concert of multiple processes that occur at different times and rates and to different degrees in individual patients. Skin aging occurs and is characterized by collagen loss, disorder, and degradation; loss of elasticity; dermal thinning; decreased integrity of the dermal–epidermal bond; and dyschromia (age spots, or mottled pigmentation). Fat in the face is organized in discrete compartments that undergo differential descent and/or atrophy with aging; midfacial fat is more likely to atrophy and descend as the fibrous support in this fatty tissue degrades, while fat accumulation in the submental region further ages the face. In addition to contributing to facial wrinkles because of repetitive contraction (e.g., "smoker's lines" around the mouth), some muscles may have an elevated tone (e.g., horizontal forehead lines that resolve when the patient's eyes are closed and the patient is no longer subconsciously elevating the eyebrows). Finally, facial bony resorption can occur and contribute to facial aging.

Each patient must be critically examined and the factors contributing to the undesirable appearance identified. Treatments should be designed to address these specific causes of facial aging.

56.5.2 Etiology

As our bodies age, our appearance is affected. Genetics clearly plays a major role in aging, and a full discussion of this topic is beyond the scope of this chapter. Disorders such as cutis laxa and Ehlers- Danlos syndrome produce a prematurely aged appearance due to a loss of normal elastin or collagen integrity, respectively. Clearly, several exogenous factors contribute to aging, as well. Tobacco use, excessive sun exposure, fluctuations in weight, and poor nutrition all lead to premature aging.

56.5.3 Natural History and Progression

It is self-evident that over time, our faces and bodies will continue to age. Patients frequently present asking, "It is *time* for a facelift?" When to undergo a facial rejuvenative procedure is an intensely personal decision for patients, but the surgeon can aid them in this decision by asking them to consider the similarity of their appearance to that of older relatives, as well as understanding that the overall sum of the multiple aging processes ongoing will determine the progression of aging. For example, in the study of Guyuron et al, the maintenance of facial volume was associated with a younger appearance in older patients; conversely, younger subjects with more facial fat appeared older.

56.6 Medical Evaluation

56.6.1 Presenting Complaints

A complete history and physical examination should be completed for every patient seeking facial rejuvenation. A frank and unpressured discussion with the patient should elicit from the patient the specific features he or she seeks to improve. It is important to discuss the patient's motivation for this surgery because proper patient selection is key to success. Patients who choose surgery to improve their personal life, win the approval or love of a spouse or significant other, or gain a promotion at work seek results that surgery cannot give. Patients with body dysmorphic disorder will express dissatisfaction with their appearance out of proportion to their actual deformity. These patients should be identified preoperatively, and a referral for psychiatric evaluation is appropriate. Patients with body dysmorphic disorder suffer from an unrealistic body image and will not be satisfied with the results of even the most skillfully performed surgery. Appropriate patients express a reasonable dislike of noticeable signs of aging and seek to improve their appearance to bolster their self-esteem or to "just look better." A complete medical and surgical history should be obtained; the surgeon should specifically inquire about any history of facial trauma, prior facial surgery, peripheral vascular disease, bleeding disorder, or collagen vascular skin disorder. A list of prescription, over-the-counter, and homeopathic medications used by the patient should be obtained, and tobacco and alcohol use should be assessed.

56.6.2 Clinical Findings, Physical Examination

The patient seeking rejuvenation of the face should undergo a comprehensive facial examination in a systematic way. Although patients may request treatment of a specific area, other parts of the face will impact the appearance of that area, and treatment should be planned in a way that achieves maximal improvement. For example, a patient who desires treatment of fat deposits of the neck may benefit from a chin implant if the projection of the chin is weak.

The patient should be assessed while seated upright with the head in a neutral position and eyes closed. Rhytids of the forehead and glabella should be noted, as should the position of the frontal hairline, which should be no more than 5 to 6 cm above the brows. Hair density should also be evaluated. The position of the eyebrows should be noted relative to the orbital rim and then lifted to an aesthetically pleasing position, and the amount of elevation required should be noted. Ideally, the male brow runs fairly horizontally at or slightly below the orbital rim, whereas in women the brow should arch and peak a few millimeters above the rim at or just medial to the lateral canthus. The medial and lateral brow should lie on the same horizontal plane. The medial brow should begin along a vertical line drawn from the nasal ala through the medial canthus, and the lateral brow should end on a line running tangentially from the ipsilateral ala through the lateral canthus.

The midface should show smooth contours, rising from a slight concavity below the lower eyelid, then falling to blend into the lower face. Ideally, there is only minimal depression inferiorly at the nasolabial fold, defining the boundary between the cheek and the perioral area; this depression is more defined superiorly as an extension of the alar crease but then ideally fades inferiorly. The ideal point of highest prominence of the midface should be at a point identified at the intersection of the extension of the lateral orbital rim and the zygomatic arch. Slight definition may be present below the malar arch, but a severe depression imparts a gaunt appearance.

The lower face extends below the oral commissure and ideally has a defined, smooth jawline extending from the mandibular angle to the chin. The neck should be smooth, without "bands" or "cords." The cervicomental angle (formed by the intersection of a line from the chin running along the submental area and a second line running along the anterior aspect of the neck on a lateral view) ideally should be 90 degrees but can be blunted by a low hyoid bone, an accumulation of submental fat, and platysmal bands.

56.6.3 Testing

As patients undergoing facial rejuvenative procedures are generally older, a complete medical evaluation should be performed, preferably by the patient's primary care physician. The surgeon should describe the planned procedure to the primary care physician and discuss the required perioperative care. Before surgery, a complete series (full-face frontal and bilateral oblique and lateral views) of photographs should be obtained.

56.6.4 Differential Diagnosis

Although the changes addressed with this surgery are generally self-evident, it is important to rule out conditions that may either mimic aging or cause compensatory changes that in turn will age the appearance of the patient. Patients with upper eyelid ptosis will use frontalis muscle contraction to provide additional upper eyelid lift at the expense of heavy horizontal wrinkles of the forehead. Likewise, enlargement or ptosis of the submandibular gland will mimic jowling. The facial skeleton should be addressed in older patients with bony facial aging or patients with congenitally hypoplastic bony features who demonstrate premature aging.

56.7 Medical Treatment

The surgeon best serves patients by presenting them with a range of options, from subtle to dramatic changes with minimal to extensive procedures, and allowing them to choose the procedure(s) that most suit their needs. Although minimally invasive treatments cannot remove redundant skin or elevate soft tissues, some changes can be sufficient for the patient who is not prepared to undergo more involved procedures. Botulinum toxin A, a neurotoxin approved by the FDA for treatment of glabellar lines in 2002, acts by blocking acetylcholine release at the neuromuscular junction. Treatment of the brow depressors, in the face of moderately increased tone of the frontalis muscle, with help elevate the brow. Botulinum toxin A can be used to reduce platysmal banding. Although it is generally safe and associated with minimal bruising, complications of botulinum toxin A result from its spread to and effect on nontarget muscles, such as the levator palpebrae muscle; its effect on this muscle causes ptosis (when it is injected around the eyes). Serious complications are generally limited to inappropriate use of the neurotoxin, the use of adulterated or unapproved toxin, or its use by inadequately trained injectors.

Soft-tissue fillers, such as autologous fat, hyaluronic acid derivatives, poly-L-lactic acid, porcine collagen, and calcium hydroxylapatite, have been used to fill both folds and wrinkles, as well as to restore facial volume. These "volume lifts" can smooth areas of the face and restore a more youthful appearance. Adverse effects associated with soft-tissue fillers include bruising, lumpiness or palpability, granuloma formation, and infection.

56.8 Surgical Treatment

56.8.1 Forehead

Multiple procedures are used currently to raise the eyebrows and smooth the forehead. The most predictable technique, the direct browlift, is the simplest and quickest to perform but can leave visible scars, and it addresses only brow position. A mid-forehead lift can additionally smooth the forehead but requires a visible scar. The coronal foreheadplasty hides the scar at or within the hairline and allows smoothing of the forehead as well as brow repositioning, but it requires a long incision and an increased recovery time. An endoscopic foreheadplasty can yield similar results with smaller scars and a much shorter recovery, but it requires dedicated endoscopic equipment and is less effective in cases of severe brow ptosis. Finally, a temporal lift, performed either through a limited open approach or endoscopically, can reposition the lateral brow and easily be combined with a facelift, but it has limited benefit in the midbrow and medial brow.

Direct Browlift

The direct browlift is a simple procedure that can be performed under local anesthesia to reposition the lateral two-thirds of the eyebrows. It is best reserved for patients with severe brow asymmetry, such as those with unilateral facial paralysis (▶ Fig. 56.1). The best candidate for this procedure is a fair-skinned man with thick eyebrows to provide maximal camouflage for the scar. The amount of brow elevation is directly marked as an ellipse resting on the upper brow hairs. This skin is then excised; the exposed orbicularis oculi muscle fibers inferiorly are then sutured superiorly to the fibers of the frontalis muscle. A layered skin closure is then performed. A modification of this technique, the indirect browlift, places the excisions in preexisting horizontal forehead creases 1 to 2 cm above the brows.

Midforehead Lift

The midforehead lift uses a broken line incision in an upper forehead crease between the midpupillary lines. The frontalis

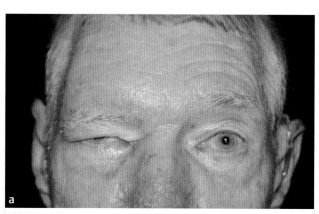

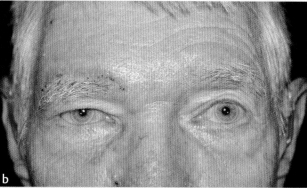

Fig. 56.1 (a) Patient with a right brow paralysis after tumor resection (note lack of rhytids on the right side of the forehead). The severity of the brow ptosis caused significant visual field reduction. (b) One week after direct browlift, there is improved symmetry of the brows and no visual field cut.

muscle is incised, and inferior dissection below the galea is performed until the corrugator supercilii and procerus muscles are identified; these can then be divided to smooth the glabella. The frontalis muscle is redraped superiorly, excess muscle is excised, and the muscle/galeal layer is closed. The skin is then redraped and the excess excised, followed by layered dermal and epidermal closure. The midforehead lift is a good option in patients who are bald or have severely thinning or receding hairlines and also have a deep forehead crease in which the scar can be hidden; however, its effectiveness in lifting the brow lateral to the midpupillary line is limited.

Coronal Foreheadplasty

The coronal foreheadplasty uses a much more significant incision, which runs from the top of one helical root over the crown to the other helical root. Laterally, the skin is elevated below the temporoparietal fascia (which is contiguous with both the SMAS and the galea), through which runs the temporal branch of the facial nerve, whereas between the temporal crests the plane is subgaleal. The dense periosteal attachments of the temporoparietal fascia and the galea are divided sharply at the temporal line. The dissection transitions to a subperiosteal plane approximately 2 cm above the orbital rim (where the galeal leaves fuse densely with the periosteum), and dissection proceeds to the orbital rim. The forehead flap can be "turned down" to expose the corrugator and procerus muscles inferiorly, which are then divided. The frontalis muscle is scored below the deepest transverse crease. The flap is then advanced superiorly, redundant skin is excised, and the galeal and skin incisions are closed after the wound is drained. The midforehead lift and the coronal foreheadplasty require a certain degree of overcorrection because the point of fixation is at the galeal closure (at the coronal incision), not at the brow (point of interest), and there is some "stretch back" of the flap over time. Midforehead lift requires elevation to about 150% of the desired elevation, and the coronal foreheadplasty typically requires 200 to 250% overcorrection.

Temporal Lift

The temporal portion of the coronal foreheadplasty can be performed in isolation to elevate the lateral brow. An open incision within the hair-bearing temple, supplemented by inferior dissection under direct vision or assisted with endoscopes, is performed inferiorly to the orbital rim. The attachments at the superior temporal line are divided down to the orbit, with release of the orbital retaining ligament in this process. The lateral brow is then elevated, and extra skin is removed and closed in layers under tension.

Endoscopic Foreheadplasty

Endoscopic foreheadplasty combines a number of features of these procedures but relies on a more functional understanding of brow dynamics. A number of 1- to 2-cm sagittal incisions (two to four, typically) are made in the hair-bearing scalp between the temporal lines. One additional incision is made in each temple, as in the temporal lift. The central incisions are used to develop a subperiosteal (less commonly, subgaleal) plane down to the orbital rim and glabella, while the temporal incisions allow a sub-temporoparietal fascia dissection medially to the superior temporal lines and inferiorly to the zygomatic arches and lateral orbital rims. During this dissection, care must be taken to protect the temporal branches of the facial nerve, which runs in the overlying temporoparietal fascia. This plane is relatively avascular, but a bridging vein (zygomaticotemporal vein, the so-called "sentinel" vein) crosses between the temporoparietal fascia and temporalis muscle and pierces the underlying deep temporal fascia in close proximity to the temporal branches. Cautery is best avoided, but if necessary (because of bleeding or for the enhanced exposure required during a midface lift; see below), it should be done at the deep origin of the vein. The dense fibrous attachments at the superior temporal line are divided down to the orbital rim. The periosteum is opened at the orbital rim (after the arcus marginalis, the periosteum of the rim of the superior orbit, has been identified). This incision should extend across the midline continuously between one lateral canthus to the other. In the glabella, the corrugator and depressor supercilii and the procerus muscles are identified and divided while the branches of the supraorbital and supratrochlear nerves are protected. With this release, the forehead flap is freely mobile and can be advanced superiorly as needed. Early failures of the endoforeheadplasty were most likely due to failure to provide sufficiently long (> 6 weeks) brow support to allow the periosteum/galea to become sufficiently adherent to the deep structures to resist gravitational descent. Moreover, residual corrugator and depressor supercilii and procerus muscle function will also pull the brow inferiorly. However, with bone-anchored sutures or resorbable fixation devices, which can provide this needed long-term support, the postoperative brow position is quite predictable, and significant overcorrection is unnecessary. Temporally, the elevated temporoparietal fascia is advanced superiorly and sutured to the deep temporal fascia and the wound closed. Recovery is quite quick, with patients often returning to work within a week (▶ Fig. 56.2).

Midfacelift

The endoscopic foreheadplasty can be extended by incising the periosteum of the superior edge of the zygoma and continuing subperiosteal elevation along the zygoma to the inferolateral orbital rim, then inferiorly into the midface. Special elevators allow dissection around the infraorbital nerve and inferiorly to just above the tooth roots. A suture is then passed through the midfacial fat and fixed superiorly to the deep temporal fascia at the temporal incision. The provides superolateral elevation of the midface.

An alternative approach to the midface is through the lower eyelid. Either by a transconjunctival or a transcutaneous approach, the periosteum is incised at the infraorbital rim (similar to the approaches used for midfacial fractures) and elevated on both sides of the infraorbital nerve to just above the maxillary tooth roots, between the nasal side walls medially and the masseter muscle laterally. After the periosteum and the lower end of the dissection have been incised, bone-anchored fixation devices as well as sutures to the orbital rim are used to mobilize and secure the periosteum and midfacial fat superiorly. Lateral

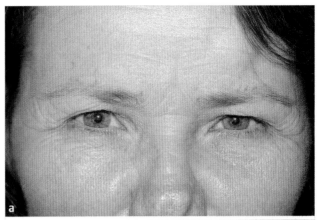
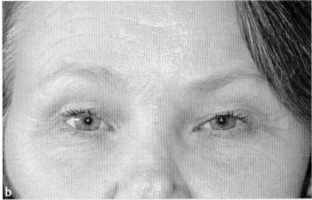

Fig. 56.2 (a) Moderate brow ptosis with lipoma of the left forehead. (b) After endoscopic browlift (with resection of the forehead lipoma), the forehead is notably smoother, and the brows are in a more relaxed position.

canthal suspension is important in these cases to avoid causing an ectropion.

Although the endoscopic approach requires no eyelid incision and has a low incidence of post operative lid malposition, there is a 1 to 2% risk for injury to the frontal or buccal branches of the facial nerve. Moreover, correction of a "tear trough" deformity (hollowing and concavity of the lower eyelid below the medial orbital rim) is not possible with this approach. Conversely, lid malposition at a rate of up to 19% has been reported in the transpalpebral approach, although this should be considerably lower with the use of bone-anchored fixation. The choice of approach depends upon surgeon preference and the specific needs of the patient.

56.8.2 Lower Face

Submental Liposuction

Many surgeons combine submental liposuction with other, more invasive procedures, such as facelift, neck lift, and platysmaplasty, to achieve maximum contouring of the neck and lower face. The aesthetic goals of younger patients with elastic skin and isolated submental or jowl fat deposits can be met with submental liposuction alone. Postoperative contraction of the skin in patients with good skin tone can provide subtle yet satisfying definition of the cervicomental angle. Older patients with increased laxity will likely benefit from submental liposuction in combination with another, more invasive procedure.

The procedure involves small stab incisions in the submental and subauricular regions. Pretunneling with progressively larger blunt-tipped cannulas without the use of suction elevates the subcutaneous plane before insertion of the liposuction cannula. A wetting solution of 0.1% lidocaine with 1:1,000,000 epinephrine can be injected before or during the pretunneling procedure. Aspiration liposuction is then conducted with 1 atm of negative pressure. The open face of a blunt-tipped, single-port cannula is oriented away from the dermis and a bimanual technique is used; the surgeon's nondominant hand guides the cannula through the subcutaneous fat layer in skin rolled and compressed by the dominant hand. Liposuction is performed conservatively, with a small amount of fat left on the flap to protect the subdermal plexus blood supply. The aspiration is typically done between the two SCM muscles laterally and as far inferiorly as the thyroid notch. Overlapping subauricular and submentally based fan patterns are used to avoid visible ridges and achieve a smooth contour. Care is taken to ensure uniform fat removal so that the flap redrapes naturally with peripheral tapering. After closure of the incisions, an elastic neck garment with fluff is applied for proper compression.

SMAS Facelift

The SMAS facelift is typically conducted after submental and subjowl fat deposits have been addressed with liposuction, as discussed above. An incision beginning in the temple, wrapping around the ear, and ending in or at the occipital hairline is made and may incorporate the previously made liposuction incisions. In women, the incision can be hidden behind the tragus (▶ Fig. 56.3). A subcutaneous dissection over the cheek and lateral neck is then performed, extending 4 to 10 cm from the tragus and preauricular incision. With scissors, a skin flap can be elevated in the occipital region while care is taken to avoid injury to the great auricular nerve. After the earlobe has been freed, the scissors can be directed toward the lower neck through the superficial subcutaneous plane. A vertically oriented strip of SMAS is incised approximately 2 cm anterior to the skin incision, exposing the parotidomasseteric fascia, and may curve around the earlobe. The SMAS is elevated (▶ Fig. 56.4) below the zygoma inferiorly to the junction of the platysma. Anterior to the parotid, if dissection is performed it must remain superficial to the masseter to avoid facial nerve branches. Inferiorly, the lateral aspect of the platysma is then identified and a minimal subplatysmal elevation is conducted. The SMAS–platysma flap is then secured with a superoposterior vector of traction and multiple sutures. After the SMAS–platysma flap has been realigned and sutured, excess SMAS and skin can be excised, with care taken not to put undue tension on the flap. This superolateral traction typically affects the lower cheek, jowl region, and anterior–superior neck. The incisions are then closed in a two-layer fashion, with careful attention paid to the hair-bearing skin. Improvements in the jawline and neck contour are seen relatively quickly.

Rhytidectomy with Lateral SMASectomy

Rhytidectomy with lateral SMASectomy was described as an alternative to the SMAS flap rhytidectomy, which required discrete elevation of the SMAS. Before the introduction of rhytidectomy with lateral SMASectomy, extensive SMAS dissection anterior to the parotid gland was thought necessary to effect significant change in the overall facial contour. However, this dissection was known to put facial nerve branches at higher risk. Advocates of the lateral SMASectomy approach argued that extensive SMAS dissection was not necessary in most patients and that its risks outweighed the long-term benefits. Lateral SMASectomy is essentially the removal of a portion of the SMAS overlying the anterior edge of the parotid gland. The direction of the SMASectomy is oriented so that the vectors of SMAS closure lie perpendicular to the nasolabial fold (▶ Fig. 56.5). This closure effectively brings the mobile medial SMAS up to the level of the more fixed lateral SMAS. Care is taken to remain below the malar eminence and in a plane superficial to the deep fascia and the parotid parenchyma, in order to minimize the risk for injury to the facial nerve branches. This rapid and relatively safe technique produces contouring of not only the nasolabial fold, but also the jowl and jawline. The lateral SMASectomy also generates a more superiorly oriented vector of lift.

Deep Plane Facelift

For the deep plane facelift, standard temporal, preauricular, and postauricular incisions are made that may extend into the temporal hairline and over the occiput. A short subcutaneous flap is elevated that extends up to about 3 cm anterior to the tragus and remains posterior to a line drawn from the angle of the mandible to the lateral canthus. A J-shaped vertical strip of SMAS is then excised, with care taken to stay posterior to the course of the temporal branch of the facial nerve. The sub-SMAS plane is entered and elevated inferiorly, and the osseocutaneous and fasciocutaneous ligaments are divided down to the subplatysmal plane approximately 3 to 5 cm below the margin of the mandible. The division of these ligaments allows complete mobilization of the deep plane flap. The flap is also elevated over the medial extent of the zygomaticus major muscle in a superior to inferior fashion to avoid injury to the zygomatic branch of the facial nerve. The subplatysmal flap can be elevated far medially, but it does not have to be carried across midline (▶ Fig. 56.6). Traction is then applied to the platysma–SMAS flap in a superolateral direction, and suturing is done to create an initial vector parallel to the mandibular ramus. Redundant skin may be excised at this point without creating tension in the flaps. Closure is conducted in multiple layers.

Corset Platysmaplasty

Platysmaplasty is considered to be particularly useful in patients with platysmal banding in order to establish a more defined cervicomental angle and jawline. Ideal candidates include those with good skin elasticity, moderate neck ptosis, and thin skin. The procedure can be conducted under local anesthesia in qualified patients, removing the morbidity associated with general anesthesia. Like many other techniques, platysmaplasty is often employed in conjunction with submental liposuction. This union not only allows improved defatting of the neck but also also aids in undermining the cervical skin in a relatively atraumatic fashion. Corset platysmaplasty can be used in concert with laterally based facelift techniques.

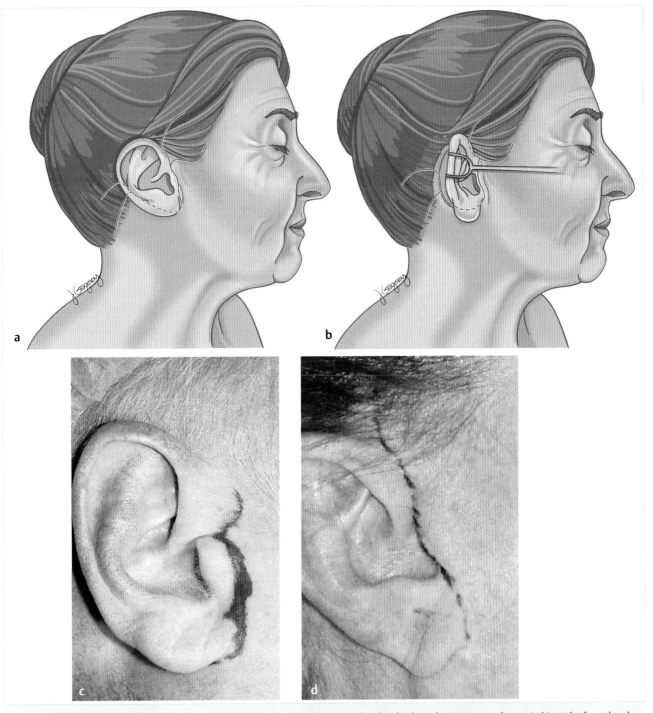

Fig. 56.3 (a) The standard facelift incision wraps around the ear. For a patient with a low hairline, the incision can be carried into the frontal and occipital hairline; for a patient with a higher hairline, the incision runs along the hairline. (b) The postauricular portion of the incision runs along the posterior conchal bowl when the ear is reflected forward, so that when the ear is in its normal position, the scar will fall into the postauricular sulcus. (c) In a male patient or a patient with a laterally displaced tragus, the incision is positioned in the pretragal crease to avoid draping beard hair onto the tragus or pulling the tragus more laterally, respectively. (d) When possible, the preauricular incision is placed on the inner aspect of the tragus to better camouflage the scar.

With the patient in the upright position, the anterior borders of the SCM muscles and the jawline, jowls, left and right bands of the platysma muscle, and thyroid cartilage are identified and marked out on the skin. The classic submental stab incision used during submental liposuction is extended approximately 4 cm after the completion of liposuction. After soft-tissue bridges have been divided between the dermis and underlying platysma, the medial edges of the platysma are identified and skeletonized. Each side of the muscle can then be horizontally transected at the level of the hyoid, and a running suture is used to bring the two edges of the platysma together in the midline from the submental zone down to the thyroid notch.

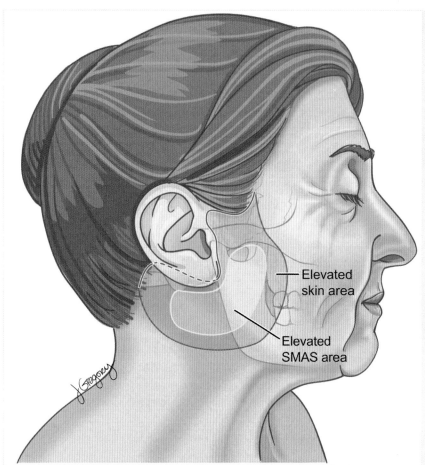

Elevated
skin area

Elevated
SMAS area

Fig. 56.4 In an SMAS facelift, a skin flap is raised toward the nasolabial fold and in the lateral neck; an incision is then made in the SMAS, and an SMAS flap is elevated in the same direction. The SMAS flap is then advanced posterosuperiorly and sutured. *SMAS*, superficial muscular aponeurotic system.

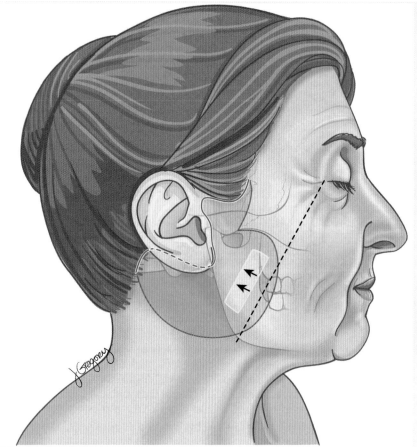

Fig. 56.5 A lateral SMASectomy is better reserved for patients with mild cervical skin laxity. A skin flap is raised, and a 1-cm strip of SMAS is excised from the angle of the mandible to the malar arch (directed toward the lateral canthus). The SMAS is sutured is a mostly superior direction.

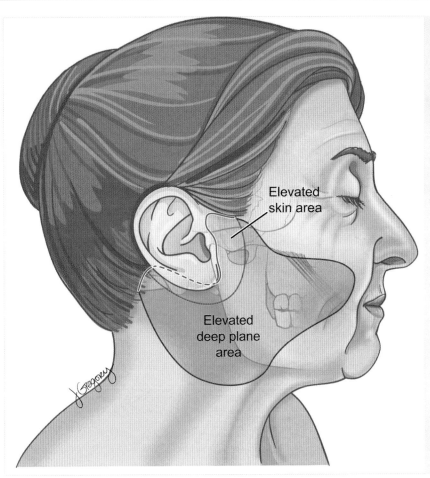

Fig. 56.6 A deep plane facelift relies on a relatively small skin flap, which allows access to the preauricular SMAS. The SMAS is incised and an SMAS flap is elevated as the surgeon identifies and progresses medially over the zygomaticus major muscle. The composite flap is then advanced posterosuperiorly.

The running suture is then returned superiorly with wider tissue bites and tied in the submental region (▶ Fig. 56.7).

Submental W-Plasty

Submental W-plasty is a technique employed in patients with significant skin laxity who are not candidates for a traditional facelift and neck lift procedure. It is typically reserved for older men with severe cervical skin laxity who are committed to maintaining a beard to camouflage the scar. The procedure involves the direct vertical excision of redundant submental skin and subcutaneous fat and closure of the vertical scar with a running W-plasty. The platysma is then plicated in the midline, allowing the skin to redrape properly. Tension is also removed by closing the incision with alternating deep dermal buried absorbable sutures at the midpoints of the limbs. The epidermis can be closed with eversion of the edges with interrupted nonabsorbable sutures (▶ Fig. 56.8).

Significant bleeding is uncommon in any of these procedures (rare in surgery of the forehead and midface), but as with any surgical procedure, it is possible. Patients should be specifically warned to avoid anticoagulants such as aspirin and nonsteroidal anti-inflammatory drugs for at least 2 weeks before surgery and for 1 week after surgery. Male gender, use of general anesthesia, intraoperative hypertension, and postoperative nausea and vomiting all increase the risk for hematoma. Hemostasis should be meticulously ensured before wound closure, and sealants such as platelet gel should not be relied upon to control bleeding. Drains are often used to ensure the adequate evacuation of any serum or small amounts of blood after a coronal or endoscopic forehead procedure or facelift. Hematomas typically present with pain out of proportion to the surgery and may be associated with external bruising and swelling or buccal ecchymosis. Active bleeding (expanding hematoma) requires reoperation to achieve hemostasis. Large, stable hematomas can be managed in the operating room or at the bedside by opening the facelift incision in the postauricular area and evacuating the clots (▶ Fig. 56.9). Small (< 1 cc) hematomas can be watched for 7 to 10 days and aspirated with a needle as the clot begins to break down. Hematomas are more common in men (7 to 9%) than in women (1 to 2%).

Complications of Facelift and Forehead-plasty

- Hematoma (1–7%)
- Sensory nerve injury (7%)
- Motor nerve injury (0.5–2.6%)
- Alopecia (1–2%)
- Infection (< 0.2%)
- Poor scarring
- "Pixie ear" deformity
- Skin slough

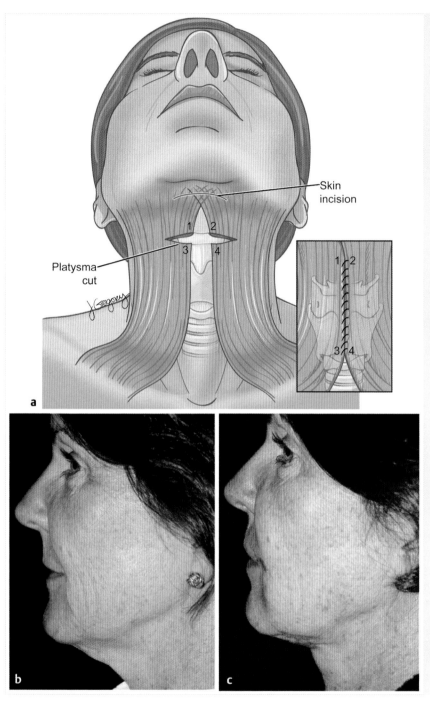

Fig. 56.7 (a) Platysmaplasty is performed through a submental incision and involves identification of the medial edges of the platysma and transverse platysmal transection at the level of the hyoid. The platysmal edges are sutured together. (b) Patient before platysmaplasty. (c) One week after platysmaplasty.

56.8.3 Infection (< 0.2%)

Infection after a facelift or browlift is rare but is more is more common in patients with poorly controlled diabetes or on immunosuppressive therapy. Untreated hematomas provide an excellent environment for the development of infection, and they should be evacuated as soon as possible. Patients with small hematomas that are being observed for clot lysis before aspiration should be treated with prophylactic antibiotics selected to cover the predominant bacteria, staphylococci. Obvious abscesses should be drained and cultured.

56.8.4 Motor Nerve Injury (0.5–2.6%)

Motor nerve injury is uncommon; the nerve most commonly affected is the marginal mandibular nerve. This nerve loops down below the mandibular margin and then ascends again medially to innervate the depressor anguli oris muscle. Injury to this nerve will result in an inability of the patient to evert the lower lip when smiling. The nerve may be injured directly or during liposuction contouring of the lateral jawline. Injuries to the temporal branch of the facial nerve can occur during the superior dissection of a facelift or the temporal dissection of a forehead procedure. Injury is best avoided by remaining in the appropriate surgical plane: below the temporoparietal fascia

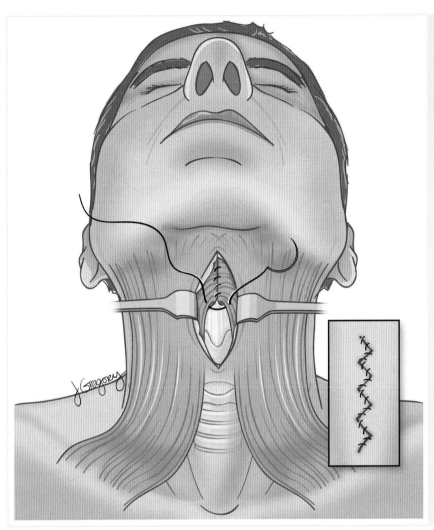

Fig. 56.8 Submental W-plasty involves direct skin excision, platysmal tightening, and W-plasty skin closure.

during dissection above the zygomatic arch and above the SMAS/temporoparietal fascia during the facelift dissection. The buccal branch of the facial nerve can be injured (▶ Fig. 56.10) during anterior dissection in deep plane facelifts or during midfacelifts. Even when the proper plane is maintained, these nerves may be injured by excessive traction, clamping, or cautery; hemostasis is best avoided because attempts to control bleeding may cause nerve injury.

If nerve transection is identified intraoperatively, tensionless microscopic neurrorrhaphy with 7–0 nylon sutures should be performed and can be expected to maintain tone and some active (but diminished) muscular function. If paralysis is noted postoperatively, adequate time for the resolution of all anesthesia must be allowed before a motor nerve paralysis is diagnosed. If persistent, it is important to remember that most of these injuries are transient and related to blunt nerve trauma or traction, and they often recover spontaneously. The injuries should be observed serially, and electrical stimulation should be used for monitoring. Nerve exploration and neurorrhaphy are indicated for cases in which there is an absence of electrical activity. Supportive care, such as gold weight placement and ophthalmic lubricants, is provided as indicated.

56.8.5 Sensory Nerve Injury (7%)

The great auricular nerve is the most commonly injured nerve, with injury in up to 7% of cases. After emerging from the Erb point, the nerve runs deep to the platysma posterior to the external jugular vein, and it can be injured during inferior facelift dissection. Injury to this nerve will cause anesthesia of the earlobe and the inferior half of the auricle. Although total transection of either the supraorbital or supratrochlear nerve is uncommon during forehead procedures, focal areas of hypesthesia may be noted over the forehead and frontal scalp after endoscopic foreheadplasty. These are typically small (<1 cm) areas that may be permanent but generally become smaller over time.

56.8.6 Alopecia

Alopecia after surgery for an aging face can be a disconcerting but transient effect of shock to the hair follicles (telogen effluvium). Patients generally recover in 3 to 4 months. More problematic is permanent alopecia.

Alopecia after facelift may occur in 1 to 2% of patients. When hair-bearing skin is incised, the blade of the knife should be

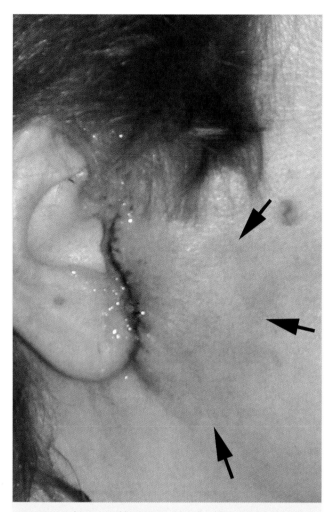

Fig. 56.9 Early pretragal hematoma after facelift (*arrows*).

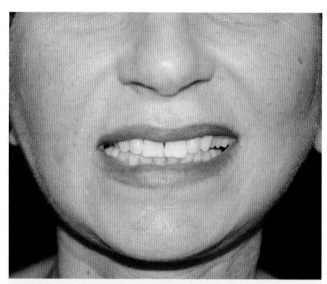

Fig. 56.10 Mild right upper lip weakness indicating buccal branch weakness.

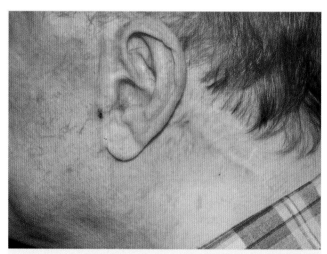

Fig. 56.11 Treatment of hypertrophic scars after a facelift complicated by the poor placement of incisions.

angled parallel to the angles of the hair shafts to avoid injury to the follicles. Flaps should be redraped, and continuity of the hairline should be restored when the flap is replaced and closed without excessive tension. Widened scars, even if properly positioned, will cause obvious alopecia. Small areas of postoperative alopecia may be treated with microfollicular hair grafts, whereas large areas may require excision and flap repair.

Alopecia after foreheadplasty depends upon the specific procedure. Most problematic is alopecia after a coronal foreheadplasty, and it is important to maintain the angle of the scalpel parallel to the hair follicles to avoid transecting hair roots and to preserve maximal postoperative hair density. Alopecia can occur around the incisions of an endoforeheadplasty; this was more common (6 to 10%) with the use of transcutaneous fixation screws, but the use of permanent bone-anchored devices has reduced the rate considerably (1 to 3%).

56.8.7 Poor Scarring

Scars that are too wide or hypertrophic will be obvious. They are more common in the postauricular area and are best prevented by a tensionless closure after SMAS support. Layered closure also reduces tension on the epidermal closure. Proper scar placement is essential for maximal camouflage (▶ Fig. 56.11).

Hypertrophic scars are treated with intralesional corticosteroid injections, which may be supplemented with the use of topical silicone gel sheeting. Widened scars, if the surrounding skin is lax, can be excised and the local skin advanced for closure. Inferior traction of the flap can distort the earlobe, pulling its insertion inferiorly and blunting its normally rounded shape. The risk for this pixie ear deformity, a telltale sign of facelift surgery, can be reduced by suturing the dermis of the inferior facelift flap superiorly to the conchal bowl perichondrium for support, as well as ensuring adequate SMAS support to the skin flap.

56.8.8 Skin Slough

Facelift surgery generates a large, medially based skin flap on each side of the face. The distal flap is located at the wound closure in the periauricular area, and this is the area of the flap with the most tenuous blood supply. Patients with compro-

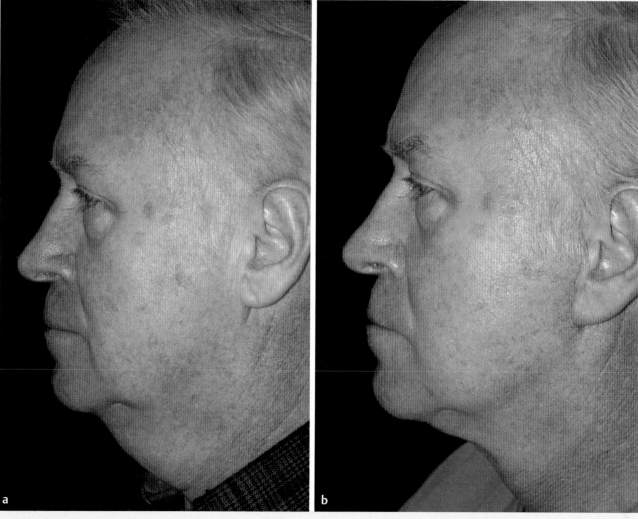

Fig. 56.12 (a) Before and (b) after SMAS facelift.

mised vasculature are at increased risk for skin slough in these areas; the most common precipitating factor is tobacco use. Patients undergoing facelift surgery must stop all tobacco use at least 6 weeks in advance of the surgery to reduce the vasoconstrictor effects of nicotine; in cases in which the surgeon suspects that the patient has been smoking, a blood or urine test for cotinine, a nicotine metabolite, can be performed. Evidence of recent tobacco use is an indication to delay the surgery. Additionally, a hematoma or other fluid collection may impair revascularization of the flap and lead to flap necrosis. In patients in whom impaired vascularity of the flap is suspected, a deep plane facelift should be strongly considered because the flap is more robust. The treatment of a skin slough is conservative, with expectant wound care and judicious débridement. Healed areas of skin slough are more likely to develop a hypertrophic scar. After full healing of the skin slough, the surgeon should consider revision of the scars.

56.9 Prognosis

The longevity of an aesthetic facial procedure depends not only upon the specific procedure and expertise of the surgeon but also upon the patient's ability to heal, skin care, lifestyle (e.g., smoking), and state of skin aging.

Forehead procedures maintain their effect over a longer period of time if the brow depressor muscles (corrugator supercilii, depressor supercilii, procerus, and orbital portion of the orbicularis oculi) are neutralized (e.g., by transection or the continued use of botulinum toxin A). However, brow procedures rarely "need" to be repeated because most of the cosmetic benefit is maintained over time.

Midfacial procedures performed subperiosteally rely on readherence of the periosteum to bone, a dense bond that stretches little and so maintains midface elevation. However, atrophy of the midfacial fat may prompt additional treatment (autologous fat transfer or injection of fillers) of the area to maintain an appropriate proportion of midfacial volume.

Facelift procedures, which rely on soft tissue–soft tissue adhesion, do have a limited "lifespan" because this scar tissue will soften and stretch over time. As a rule of thumb, deeper procedures "last" longer than those performed more superficially. The benefits of a subcutaneous facelift may be lost after a year or two, whereas an SMAS procedure may not need to be revised for 7 to 10 years in younger patients or for 5 to 7 years in older patients (▶ Fig. 56.12).

56.10 Roundsmanship

- In forehead rejuvenation procedures in general, greater elevationis required the more distal the point of fixation is from the brow.
- Modern facelift procedures rely on the SMAS to maintain elevation.
- The most commonly injured nerve during a facelift is the great auricular nerve; the most commonly injured motor nerves are the marginal mandibular and temporal branches of the facial nerve.
- The temporal branch of the facial nerve runs within the temporoparietal fascia; maintaining dissection below this fascia protects the nerve from injury.

- Brow elevation during endoscopic browlift depends on adequate myotomies of the muscles that depress the eyebrows.

56.11 Recommended Reading

[1] Guyuron B, Rowe DJ, Weinfeld AB, Eshraghi Y, Fathi A, Iamphongsai S. Factors contributing to the facial aging of identical twins. Plast Reconstr Surg 2009; 123: 1321–1331

[2] Rohrich RJ, Pessa JE. The fat compartments of the face: anatomy and clinical implications for cosmetic surgery. Plast Reconstr Surg 2007; 119: 2219–2227, discussion 2228–2231

[3] Williams EF, Vargas H, Dahiya R, Hove CR, Rodgers BJ, Lam SM. Midfacial rejuvenation via a minimal-incision brow-lift approach: critical evaluation of a 5-year experience. Arch Facial Plast Surg 2003; 5: 470–478

57 Blepharoplasty

YuShan L. Wilson and Grigorly Mashkevich

57.1 Introduction

The eyes are often the focus of attention of many patients seeking facial rejuvenation. Periocular aging manifests as a combination of brow descent, excess skin formation in the upper and lower lids, and orbital fat herniation. These processes are influenced by both heredity and age. Blepharoplasty is an operation designed to reduce redundant skin and fat in the aged periocular region. This surgery is most often performed for cosmetic reasons, but it can also correct functional deficits associated with reduced visual fields.

57.2 Incidence of Disease

Periorbital aging affects all individuals starting in their late twenties and early thirties. Blepharoplasty is one of the most frequently requested aesthetic facial procedures.

57.3 Terminology

Dermatochalasis is an acquired condition of excessive eyelid skin laxity that is related to genetic predisposition, natural aging, and environmental factors. Dermatochalasis is accompanied frequently by prolapsed orbital fat (▶ Fig. 57.1). *Steatoblepharon* denotes the prolapse of orbital fat through either true herniation or pseudoherniation from behind a weakened orbital septum. Aesthetically, this manifests as fullness of the eyelids, or "bags." *Blepharochalasis* is a disorder of the upper eyelids characterized by recurrent attacks of unilateral or bilateral lid edema, ultimately resulting in loss of skin elasticity and atrophic changes. Mainly young or middle-aged women are affected. *Festoons* are redundant folds of the orbicularis oculi

muscle in the lower lid that drape onto themselves, creating a hammock-like baggy appearance. *Malar bags* are soft-tissue prominences on the lateral edge of the infraorbital ridge and zygomatic prominence. They typically remain stable with facial animation but may worsen during smiling.

57.4 Applied Anatomy

The eyelids are composed of an outer and an inner lamella (▶ Fig. 57.2). The outer lamella consists of the skin and orbicularis oculi muscle, while the inner lamella includes the tarsus and conjunctiva (often, the orbital septum and tarsus are considered a middle lamella). The upper eyelid extends superiorly to the eyebrow, while the lower lid extends below the inferior orbital rim to join the cheek. The skin of the eyelids is the thinnest in the body, often less than 1 mm in thickness. The upper eyelid skin crease (superior palpebral sulcus) is formed by the insertion of the levator muscle aponeurotic fibers into the skin (8 to 9 mm in men and 9 to 11 mm in women).

In the midpupillary line, the upper lid margin should be situated more than 2 mm above the light reflex in the pupil, with smaller distances denoting upper lid ptosis. This distance is also referred to as margin reflex distance. The lower eyelid margin should rest at the level of the lower limbus.

The tarsus is composed of thick fibrous tissue and is present in both the upper and lower eyelids. It provides integrity and stability to the eyelids and contains sebaceous meibomian glands. The tarsus is an important landmark in eyelid surgery because incisions are often marked in comparison to its position.

The levator palpebrae superioris muscle is the major elevator of the upper eyelid. It originates from the superior orbital apex

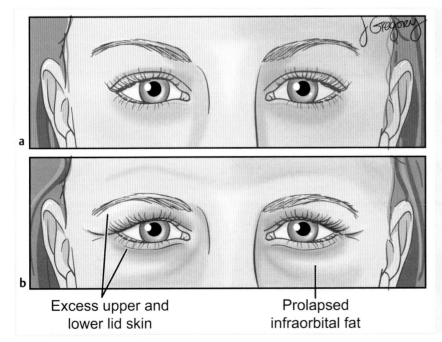

Fig. 57.1 (a,b) Aging-related changes in the periorbital region.

Excess upper and
lower lid skin

Prolapsed
infraorbital fat

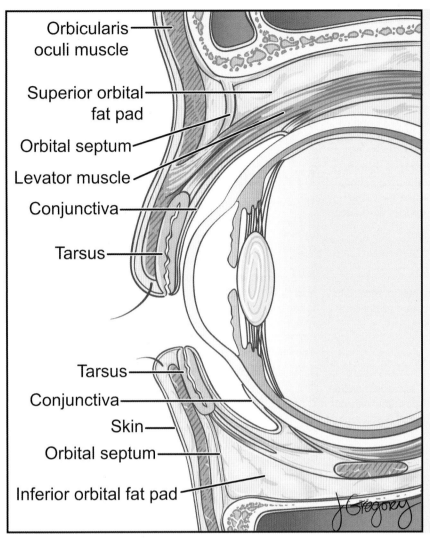

Fig. 57.2 Cross-sectional eyelid and orbital anatomy.

- Orbicularis oculi muscle
- Superior orbital fat pad
- Orbital septum
- Levator muscle
- Conjunctiva
- Tarsus
- Tarsus
- Conjunctiva
- Skin
- Orbital septum
- Inferior orbital fat pad

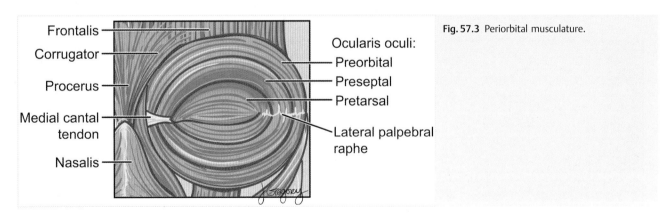

Fig. 57.3 Periorbital musculature.

- Frontalis
- Corrugator
- Procerus
- Medial cantal tendon
- Nasalis
- Ocularis oculi:
- Preorbital
- Preseptal
- Pretarsal
- Lateral palpebral raphe

and inserts into the upper lid. This attachment results in the superior eyelid crease that is a nearly ubiquitous feature in Caucasian eyelids.

The orbicularis oculi muscle is one of the muscles of facial expression, innervated by the temporal and zygomatic branches of the facial nerve. These branches are orientated horizontally and innervate the muscle from its undersurface. The muscle (▶ Fig. 57.3) is composed of orbital and palpebral segments, with the latter further subdivided into preseptal and pretarsal components. The palpebral segment is primarily responsible for blinking and voluntary winking, while the orbital segment generates forced closure. Medially, muscle heads of the pretarsal orbicularis unify to form the medial canthal tendon, which inserts into the anterior lacrimal crest. Laterally, these muscle fibers condense to become the lateral canthal tendon, which attaches to the Whitnall tubercle.

Immediately beneath the surface of the preseptal orbicularis lies the orbital septum. The orbital septum is a connective tissue structure that attaches peripherally to the periosteum of the orbit at the arcus marginalis. It serves as a boundary retaining the orbital contents. There are two upper eyelid fat pads—medial and central—with the lateral compartment occupied by the lacrimal gland. The lower eyelid fat pads are divided into medial, central, and lateral compartments. The inferior oblique muscle separates the medial and central fat compartments.

The Asian eyelid has distinct anatomical differences from the Caucasian eyelid. In the Asian upper eyelid, the lower insertion point of the levator aponeurosis leads to a smaller or absent upper lid fold. An upper eyelid skin crease is absent in approximately 50% of Asian persons. This variant is viewed as less desirable in the Asian culture because of the appearance of a heavier eyelid. Absence of the crease is often associated with medial epicanthal hooding.

57.5 The Disease Process

57.5.1 Etiology

The upper eyelid is one of the first facial features to exhibit signs of aging, typically starting in the late twenties. A combination of genetic predisposition and environmental influences contributes to this process, which results in eyelid skin laxity, weakening of the orbital septum, and fat atrophy and herniation.

57.5.2 Natural History and Progression

The youthful eyelid is smooth and free of rhytids or redundant folds. The lateral orbital rim is free of skin draping or hooding. The lower eyelid exhibits a smooth gentle convexity and blends seamlessly into the skin of the upper cheek. With aging, excessive skin forms in the upper and lower lids. The orbital septum weakens, allowing variable amounts of orbital fat to bulge. With the descent of the malar fat pad and sagging of the orbicularis oculi muscle, the bony outline of the infraorbital rim becomes more prominent. These changes give rise to a fatigued and aged periocular appearance.

57.5.3 Potential Disease Complications

Advanced dermatochalasis may result in superior and lateral visual field disturbances, secondary to obstruction by redundant upper eyelid skin.

57.5.4 Disease Grading

There is no formalized disease grading system for dermatochalasis and steatoblepharon. Emphasis is placed on description of the deformity and photographic evaluation of the aging-related changes.

57.6 Medical Evaluation

57.6.1 Presenting Complaints

As with any aesthetic procedure, it is imperative to establish a reasonable and rational motivation for the treatment. Patients who request eyelid surgery with the goal of attaining a more youthful appearance are good candidates. The most common complaint voiced by patients is a tired appearance. Patients with significant dermatochalasis may complain of difficulty seeing, especially when looking up.

57.6.2 Clinical Findings, Physical Examination, Testing

Medical conditions that would contraindicate any facial rejuvenation surgery should be elicited. Medications, vitamins, and herbal supplements that might interfere with clotting must be identified. These need to be discontinued at least 7 days before any planned eyelid procedure. A thorough ophthalmologic history, with attention to vision, dry eye, and recurrent ocular infections such as conjunctivitis, styes, chalazia, and herpes, must be obtained.

Eyelid evaluation begins with a general examination of the skin type—dry or oily, thin or thick. Any preexisting asymmetries or concomitant brow ptosis should be noted and discussed with the patient. Brow elevation surgery may be necessary to achieve the optimal cosmetic outcome.

Upper lid redundancy is best evaluated with the patient's eyes closed. The skin may be grasped with forceps in a medial to lateral direction to estimate the amount of skin that can be resected safely. Medial and central fat pseudoherniation can be evaluated while gentle pressure is applied to the globe. Excessive lateral fullness should alert the examiner to the possibility of a ptotic lacrimal gland.

Testing the lower lid tone determines the vulnerability of this structure to postoperative malposition. Tone may be assessed with the "snap" test (▶ Fig. 57.4), during which the lower lid is grasped gently between the thumb and forefinger, pulled away from the globe, and released. A normal lid will "snap" back to

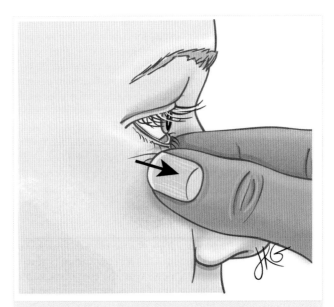

Fig. 57.4 The lower lid skin is grasped between the thumb and forefinger and pulled away from the globe. The time and ease with which the lid returns to its normal position indicate the lower lid tone.

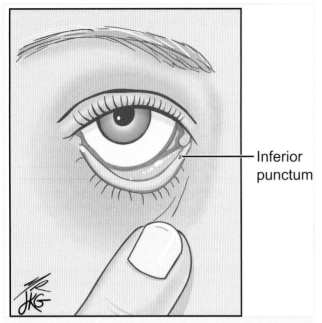

Fig. 57.5 Lower lid laxity can be assessed by distracting the lid inferiorly and allowing it to recoil.

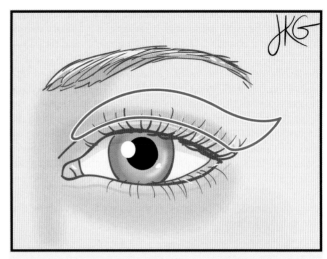

Fig. 57.6 The lower limb of the upper blepharoplasty incision runs in the supratarsal crease, while the upper limb is determined by the amount of redundant skin.

contact the globe like a spring. Slower returns indicate a poor lid tone. Similarly, a lid distraction test (▶ Fig. 57.5) can be performed, in which the lid is pulled inferiorly; the return of the lid to its normal position should be brisk. The worst response is failure of the eyelid to return until the patient blinks.

Pseudoherniation of fat in the lower lid can be ascertained by having the patient gaze upward and then to the right and left. Grasping the skin with forceps while the patient is looking upward identifies the amount of lower lid laxity.

The Schirmer test, which determines the level of tear production, is obtained in all patients interested in blepharoplasty. This test is performed by placing a strip of filter paper in the conjunctival sac of the lower eyelid for 5 minutes. The wet portion of the paper is then measured. Values above 15 mm denote a normal level, whereas readings below 5 mm indicate severe dryness. Blepharoplasty is relatively contraindicated in patients with severe dryness because such a procedure may precipitate a dry eye syndrome (persistent ocular pain and discomfort, with the potential for corneal ulceration). For patients in the intermediate category (5 to 15 mm), correlation of the Schirmer test result with the potential development of eye dryness after surgery is less clear. In this group, conservative skin excision may be undertaken.

57.6.3 Photography

As with all aesthetic surgery, preoperative photographic documentation is essential. Close-up 1:5 ratio photographs should include the following: frontal views with the eyes open, gazing upward, and closed; oblique and lateral views with the eyes open. These close-up photographs should include the eyebrow superiorly and the nasal ala inferiorly. A 1:10 full-face view is also appropriate. Pictures should be taken in good lightning without flash because flash photography may wash out finer details.

57.6.4 Differential Diagnosis

Upper eyelid ptosis may present concomitantly with dermatochalasis. This eyelid rim malpositioning cannot be treated with an upper lid blepharoplasty. Depending on the etiology, appropriate ptosis repair should precede blepharoplasty surgery.

57.7 Treatment

57.7.1 Medical Treatment

Although a multitude of facial rejuvenation products are available on the market, a discussion of their proposed mechanisms and efficacy is beyond the scope of this chapter. In general, superficial rhytids respond well to chemical peels and laser resurfacing, whereas redundant skin and prolapsed fat are best managed by surgical means.

57.7.2 Surgical Treatment

Blepharoplasty can be performed safely as an outpatient procedure with local anesthesia and with or without intravenous sedation. The procedure begins with marking of the eyelids. All makeup is removed, and the skin is cleansed with alcohol to remove natural skin oils. With the patient in the supine position, the brow is gently pushed toward the orbital rim to counteract the effect of gravity. The upper lid skin is then gently grasped with forceps, with one blade at the superior lid crease and the other grabbing just enough redundant skin to smooth the lid. The upper medial incision should not pass more medially than the nasal–orbital junction. Laterally, it is extended into a natural crease between the orbital rim and eyelid. Medially and laterally, the sinuously shaped markings join at 30-degree angles (▶ Fig. 57.6). A 30-gauge needle is used to infiltrate 1 to 2 mL of 1% lidocaine with 1:100,000 epinephrine, buffered with 8.4% sodium bicarbonate, subcutaneously. At least 10 minutes is allowed to pass for maximal anesthesia and vasoconstriction. Following the incisions, the redundant skin is removed sharply

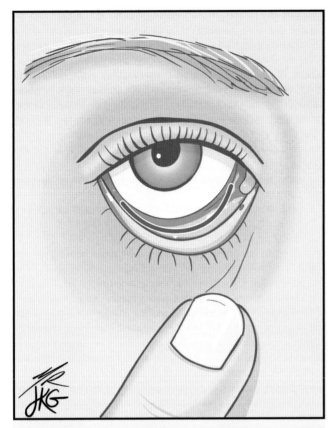

Fig. 57.7 The transconjunctival lower blepharoplasty incision is placed just below the lower border of the tarsus, dividing the capsulopalpebral fascia and lower lid retractors and allowing exposure of the orbital septum.

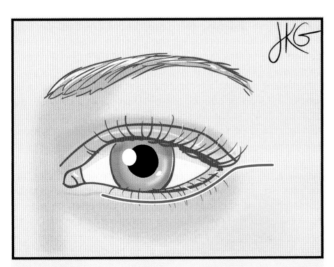

Fig. 57.9 Transcutaneous lower blepharoplasty with a subciliary incision.

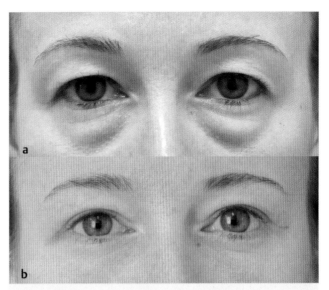

Fig. 57.8 Upper blepharoplasty with transconjunctival lower blepharoplasty. (a) Before and (b) after the surgery, at 6 months.

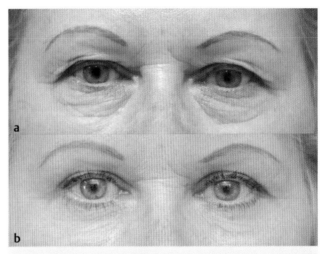

Fig. 57.10 Upper blepharoplasty and transcutaneous lower blepharoplasty, with skin–muscle flap. (a) Before and (b) after the surgery, at 6 months.

with Stevens scissors. The lateral aspect of the orbicularis can be trimmed for additional debulking and to induce lateral brow elevation. The excision exposes the orbital septum.

Redundant pseudoherniated fat is trimmed conservatively through buttonhole incisions in the orbital septum. Excessive fat removal may result in retraction of the lid and a pronounced overhang of the orbital rim, thereby producing the effect of an aged appearance. Each excised segment of fat is set aside so that a comparable amount can be removed from the contralateral eyelid.

Meticulous hemostasis before closure significantly reduces the risk for postoperative bleeding. Wound closure begins at the lateral edge of the incision, which is the area of greatest tension. This part of the incision is reapproximated with several interrupted mattress sutures. The rest of the wound is closed in a subcuticular fashion with a 6–0 nonabsorbable monofilament suture.

Lower lid blepharoplasty can be performed via either of two surgical approaches: (1) transconjunctival (see ▶ Fig. 57.2; ▶ Fig. 57.7 and ▶ Fig. 57.8) or (2) transcutaneous with a skin–muscle flap (▶ Fig. 57.9 and ▶ Fig. 57.10). The transconjunctival approach avoids an external scar and carries a lower incidence of ectropion. For the transconjunctival approach, the conjunctiva and cornea are first anesthetized with 0.5% tetracaine hydrochloride ophthalmic solution. Subsconjunctival injection with local anesthetic solution follows. Corneal protectors are placed to protect the eye from injury. A Desmarres retractor is then introduced to retract the lower lid margin, and an incision is made 3 to 4 mm below the tarsus. A preseptal plane is identified and developed via blunt dissection with cotton-tipped applicators. Fat pads are visualized while gentle pressure is applied to the globe. As with the upper eyelids, care should be taken to avoid aggressive fat removal because this may result in a hollow, or skeletonized, appearance. For patients with a tear trough deformity, repositioning and suturing of the orbital fat can also be performed though this exposure. The transconjunctival incision is approximated with several 6–0 fast-absorbing gut sutures. External skin redundancy can be addressed with a "pinch excision." One to three millimeters of redundant skin inferior to the ciliary margin is pinched with forceps and sharply excised with Iris scissors. The orbicularis muscle is not excised during this maneuver.

During a transcutaneous approach, a subciliary incision is made parallel and approximately 2 to 3 mm below the palpebral margin. A skin–muscle flap is then lifted to expose and incise the orbital septum. Depending on the individual needs, all three fat pads can be addressed in a similar manner as during the transconjunctival approach. The inferior oblique muscle, which separates the medial and central fat compartments, is identified to help prevent inadvertent injury. Following fat excision, any redundant skin is trimmed conservatively. If surgery is performed with the patient under conscious sedation or local anesthesia, asking the patient to gently open the mouth while gazing upward helps prevent cutaneous overresection. Lower lid support is reestablished by placing a vertical suspension suture in the lateral aspect of the orbicularis muscle, tied to the lateral orbital rim periosteum at the region of the lateral orbital tubercle.

57.7.3 Postoperative Care

Wounds are left uncovered and are lubricated with an antibiotic ophthalmic ointment. During the first two postoperative days, cold compresses are placed at hourly intervals for 20 minutes while the patient is awake. Acetaminophen with or without codeine is often sufficient to relieve discomfort. Patients are instructed to avoid any medications that can produce vasodilation (including alcohol) or increase the risk for bleeding, such as aspirin-containing products and nonsteroidal anti-inflammatory drugs. In addition to analgesics, antibiotic eye drops and lubricants are given. Sutures are removed on the fifth postoperative day, at which point makeup can be applied to the lid skin. Contact lenses may also be used at this time. Most patients are able to return to their normal level of activity by the seventh postoperative day. Light exercise can start 2 weeks after surgery, with full exercise resumed at 6 weeks.

57.7.4 Complications

Fortunately, serious complications of blepharoplasty are uncommon; however, several lesser complications and minor sequelae may occur following this procedure. The eye can sustain injury at any time during an eyelid procedure. Trauma from excessive pressure, cautery, or ill-positioned sutures can occur. The transconjunctival approach carries a greater risk for corneal abrasion. These injuries are extremely painful and can lead to ulcers. Abrasions are treated conservatively with ophthalmic drops or ointment, with ophthalmologic consultation. Postoperative problems that generally resolve after the second postoperative week include eyelid ecchymosis, tearing, contact lens difficulty, contact dermatitis, and a sensation of tightness. Long-dormant chalazia may be reactivated in the first few weeks following surgery. This relatively painless swelling is localized to the upper lid margin and is best treated with warm compresses and antibiotics.

Orbital hematoma after blepharoplasty remains rare. When encountered, it constitutes a true surgical emergency because increasing pressure within the orbit can damage the optic nerve and result in blindness. Any sudden increase in pain during the immediate postoperative period should raise suspicion of this possibility. Surgical intervention should be timely, with opening of the wound, removal of clots, and achievement of hemostasis. If the patient experiences decreasing vision or if the ocular pressure approaches 80 mm Hg, lateral canthotomy and inferior cantholysis are urgently performed to decompress the orbit and preserve vision. The development of lid hematoma in the immediate postoperative period also necessitates reopening the wound and establishing hemostasis. If discovered at a later time, the hematoma should be allowed to liquefy and can be aspirated with a needle in 7 to 9 days. If the clot is not removed, a firm nodular scar may form in this area.

The most common functional problem after blepharoplasty is dry eye syndrome. This is often preventable by obtaining a thorough history and identifying complaints of ocular itching, foreign body sensation, and burning. All patients undergo an ophthalmologic evaluation before blepharoplasty, which includes a Schirmer test. If despite these precautions a patient develops dry eyes following blepharoplasty, attention should be directed toward maintaining corneal protection with artificial tears, a nocturnal lubricant, and lid taping.

Persistent diplopia after blepharoplasty usually indicates injury to the inferior oblique muscle. Diplopia as a consequence of mild trauma to the muscle is often temporary, but transection may cause permanent ocular dysmotility requiring surgical intervention.

Problems of lid position may also arise after blepharoplasty. Typically, the lower lid margin rests at the corneal limbus, but minimal scleral show may be a normal variant. Postoperative displacement of the lower lid by 1 mm can often be seen. If moderate scleral show is noticed postoperatively, initial treatment consists of upward massage and closed-eye squints to strengthen the orbicularis oculi. More extensive scleral show, ectropion, or lateral lower lid rotation ("hound dogging") requires a more aggressive approach with horizontal lid shortening and potentially skin grafting.

Blepharoptosis, or upper lid ptosis, can be noticed postoperatively. Often, this is secondary to unrecognized preoperative lid ptosis or due to levator injury during blepharoplasty. Lagophthalmos, or inability to close the palpebral fissure after blepharoplasty, is usually a temporary phenomenon. After the completion of blepharoplasty, it is normal to see palpebral separation of up to 4 mm. Greater distances substantially increase the postoperative risk for lagophthalmos. If this is noticed intraoperatively, a strip of resected skin can be replaced before conclusion of the procedure.

At times, aesthetic concerns after blepharoplasty are not viewed as complications by the surgeon, but they may be considered as such by the patient. Patients may voice complaints of persistent malar bags and animated lateral wrinkling. Because these are not correctable by blepharoplasty, such misunderstanding is best avoided by adequate preoperative awareness, patient education, and realistic expectations.

57.8 Roundsmanship

- Blepharoplasty targets excessive periorbital skin and fat.

- Lower blepharoplasty approaches include transconjunctival and transcutaneous approaches.
- The inferior oblique muscle separates the medial and central fat compartments of the lower eyelid.
- Aggressive fat excision may result in orbital hollowing, accentuating an aged appearance.

57.9 Recommended Reading

[1] Fagien S. A critical analysis of the current surgical concepts for lower blepharoplasty. Plast Reconstr Surg 2004; 114: 794–796

[2] Pastorek N, Bustillo A. Blepharoplasty. In: Azzizadeh B, Murphy MR, Johnson CM, eds. Master Techniques in Facial Rejuvenation. Philadelphia, PA: W. B. Saunders; 2007; 59–89

[3] Rohrich RJ, Coberly DM, Fagien S et al. Current concepts in aesthetic upper blepharoplasty. Plast Reconstr Surg 2004; 113: 32e–42e

58 Facial Implants

Alexander Ovchinsky

58.1 Introduction

Alloplastic materials have long been used for the correction of functional and aesthetic facial problems. The recent development of new, biocompatible materials has further broadened the application of implants in facial plastic surgery. The major advantages of alloplasts are the following: abundance of implant materials; lack of need for a donor site, with related morbidity; and ease of customizing the implant according to the individual patient's needs by selecting from numerous sizes and shapes or by generating, with computer assistance, a custom implant based on the patient's anatomy.

The disadvantages are based on the fact that all alloplastic implants are foreign bodies with all the potential complications of such.

Thus, an ideal implant should be (1) nontoxic; (2) nonantigenic; (3) noncarcinogenic; (4) biocompatible with the host tissues; (5) infection-resistant; (6) easily shaped, molded, and carved and able to maintain its form and volume permanently; and (7) cost-effective.

58.2 Incidence

Alloplastic implants are commonly used in midfacial augmentation procedures as malar, submalar, shell, or tear trough implants (▶ Fig. 58.1); in rhinoplasty surgery for dorsal augmentation or as L-shaped structural implants; and in mandibular augmentation (▶ Fig. 58.2). A total of 8,789 malar implant procedures were done in 2009, comprising 0.6% of all cosmetic surgeries; 73% of the malar implant procedures were in women. Nearly $23 million was spent on malar implant surgery in 2009. A total of 13,000 chin implant surgeries were performed in 2009, which accounted for 0.9% of all cosmetic surgeries; 52% of these were in women and 48% in men. The total annual spending on chin augmentation surgery in 2009 was nearly $27 million.

58.3 Terminology

Facial implants are differentiated based on their application (malar, submalar, mandibular, other) or their composition. Various synthetic materials have been used for facial implants. Silicone implants have been used in clinical practice since the middle of the 20th century; silicone has a fairly high degree of chemical inertness and stability, and it is not allergenic. Tissue reaction to solid silicone implants is characterized by the formation of a fibrous tissue capsule without tissue ingrowth into the implant. Expanded polytetrafluoroethylene (Gore-Tex; W. L. Gore Associates, Flagstaff, AZ) has found wide application in facial augmentation because of its limited soft-tissue ingrowth

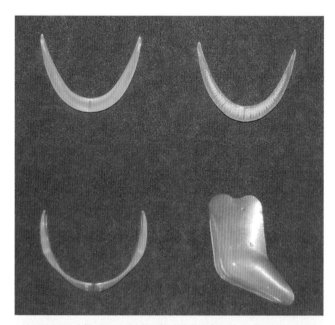

Fig. 58.1 Mandibular implants (silicone). Top left: extended anatomical chin implant. Top right: extended conform anatomical chin implant. Bottom left: prejowl implant. Bottom right: mandibular angle implant.

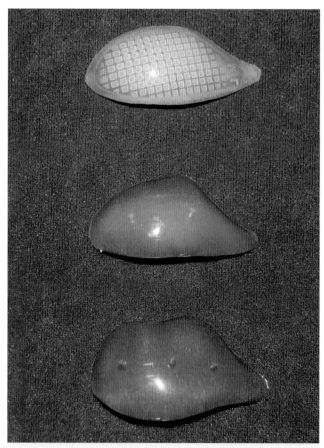

Fig. 58.2 Malar implants (silicone). Top: conform malar shell implant. Middle: malar shell implant. Bottom: combined submalar shell implant.

and minimal inflammatory reaction. The material allows for partial incorporation of the host's soft tissues, thus making it less susceptible to infection or migration, while not significantly compromising the ease of implant removal, if necessary. Porous polyethylene (Medpor; Porex Surgical, Newnan, GA) permits extensive tissue ingrowth into the implant pores, which provides additional stability but may make implant removal very difficult. Medpor is a very rigid material and therefore tolerates thin soft-tissue coverage poorly. Mesh polymers include Marlex, a high-density polyethylene (Marlex Pharmaceuticals, New Castle, DE); Mersilene, a polyester fiber mesh (Ethicon, Somerville, NJ); and Dacron, a condensation polymer obtained from ethylene glycol and terephthalic acid (Dow Corning, Midland, MI). Mesh polymers are easily folded and shaped and allow extensive soft-tissue ingrowth through the mesh network. This minimizes the risk for migration and infection but may make removal of the implant more difficult.

58.4 Applied Anatomy

Nasal dorsal implants are placed over the paired nasal bones (bony dorsum) and paired upper lateral cartilages (cartilaginous dorsum). An implant is placed directly over the bony–cartilaginous framework, underneath dorsal soft tissues. Nasal implants that are L-shaped are placed over the nasal dorsum (longer part of the L) and into the columella between the medial crura of the lower lateral cartilages (shorter part of the L).

The mandible consists of the central symphysis and the bilateral mandibular bodies, rami, angles, and coronoid and condylar processes. The alveolar process of the mandible forms its superior portion and supports the lower dentition, which is innervated by the inferior alveolar nerve. The condylar process articulates with the glenoid fossa of the temporal bone to form the temporomandibular joint. The mental nerve, the terminal branch of the inferior alveolar nerve, exits through the mental foramen, located between the first and the second premolars about 1 cm above the lower mandibular border. Mandibular implants are used to augment many of these anatomical areas and may be used unilaterally in cases of mandibular asymmetry or hemifacial microsomia. For example, anatomical chin implants are used to augment the symphysial area primarily, whereas extended anatomical chin implants augment both the mandibular symphysis and the parasymphysial and body regions. Prejowl implants provide augmentation to the area of the mandibular body just medial to the jowl without adding any volume to the symphysial region. Mandibular angle implants serve to augment the body and ramus of the mandible and are commonly used in patients with hemifacial microsomia.

The anatomy of the midface is primarily defined by the relationship between the zygoma and the soft tissues of the cheek and infraorbital region. The zygomatic bone is a tetrapod and consists of the body of the zygoma with four articulating processes: the zygomaticotemporal, zygomaticofrontal, zygomaticomaxillary, and zygomatico-orbital processes. The zygoma defines the cheek prominence and plays an important role in achieving the triangular shape of a youthful face. The masseter muscle is attached to the inferior aspect of the zygoma body and zygomatic arch. The zygomaticus major and minor muscles

of facial expression also originate from the inferior aspect of the zygoma and insert into the area of the upper lip and oral commissure. Several fat compartments have been described in the area of the midface; the malar, buccal, and suborbicularis oculi fat pads are the most important ones. Various important anatomical structures, such as branches of the facial and trigeminal (infraorbital and zygomaticofacial) nerves, parotid duct, and branches of the facial artery are located in the midface region.

58.5 The Disease Process

58.5.1 Etiology

Saddle nasal deformity is usually a result of nasal trauma or prior nasal surgery (secondary to overzealous reduction of the nasal dorsum or aggressive septoplasty leading to the loss of nasal dorsal support); some Asian and African-American patients may have a congenitally low dorsum, as well. Systemic diseases, such as Wegener granulomatosis and syphilis, and illicit drug use (cocaine snorting) may lead to the loss of nasal support and dorsal saddle deformity.

Mandibular deformities necessitating the use of implants are usually of developmental etiology. Microgenia and micrognathia lead to a small-appearing chin on the frontal view, and the profile may be improved with a mandibular implant. Hemifacial microsomia may be an isolated finding or a component of a syndromic condition (e.g., Treacher Collins syndrome, Crouzon syndrome) and commonly requires unilateral augmentation of the affected parts of the mandible.

A hypoplastic zygoma, either developmental or due to trauma, frequently benefits from augmentation. Soft-tissue voids in the infraorbital region due to midfacial ptosis and atrophy may also be improved with malar implants.

58.5.2 Pathogenesis and Natural History

Most facial deformities necessitating augmentation are cosmetic in nature, and their correction is aimed primarily at improving of the overall facial balance. Saddle nasal deformity, when severe, may result in symptoms of nasal obstruction.

58.5.3 Potential Complications

Complications related to facial implants can be broadly subdivided into two main categories. Immediate complications are related primarily to the surgical placement of an implant and include hematoma, bleeding, and neural injury leading to either motor or sensory deficits. Later complications, related mainly to the foreign body nature of the implant, include infection, foreign body reaction, implant migration or extrusion, and poor scarring of the access incisions.

58.5.4 Disease Grading

Most facial implants come in a variety of sizes, depending on the degree of augmentation needed. The selection of implant size is based primarily on the patient's needs and the surgeon's expertise. Many manufacturers offer implant sizers, which are sterilizable rubber replicas of the various implant sizes. Sizers provide good visual assistance during preoperative patient consultations and during selection of the correct implant size for a given patient.

58.6 Medical Evaluation

58.6.1 Presenting Complaints

Patients may feel that certain areas are disproportionly small or deficient (e.g., a small or "weak" chin, flat cheekbones, or a "low" nasal dorsum). Patients with microgenia frequently dislike a poorly defined or blunted cervicomental angle; they may also complain of a "big nose," not realizing that a disproportionally small chin may be the main underlying etiology.

58.6.2 Clinical Findings, Physical Examination

Midfacial hypoplasia may be secondary either to an insufficiently developed malar bone (type I) or to atrophy and ptosis of the midfacial soft tissues (type II). The former requires a malar shell implant to augment the zygoma and create a higher arch of the cheekbone. The latter may be corrected with a submalar implant, which augments soft-tissue deficiency below the malar arch without additional augmentation of the zygoma. The combined bony–soft tissue deficiency (type III) requires placement of a malar–submalar implant to address both problems simultaneously.

Saddle nose deformities present as a low, wide nasal dorsum and may be bony, cartilaginous, or a combination of bony and cartilaginous. The nose appears widened because of the lack of dorsal height.

Patient with micrognathia have class II occlusion on physical examination and are best treated with orthognathic surgery. However, patients with normal occlusion and microgenia are best served with a chin implant. In patients with hemifacial microsomia, the degree of mandibular asymmetry may vary. Isolated mandibular angle–ramus deficiency is common, but in some cases the whole hemimandible may be hypoplastic.

58.6.3 Testing

No specific testing is required except for a routine preoperative work-up. Computer imaging may be a useful consultation tool to communicate the proposed changes to the patient.

58.6.4 Differential Diagnosis

Saddle nasal deformity may be a result of prior trauma, surgery, or loss of septal support due to inhaled drug use or a systemic condition (i.e., Wagener granulomatosis, neoplasm, or syphilis). Midfacial and mandibular hypoplasias are usually developmental conditions, whether isolated or part of a craniofacial syndro-me, or may result from the aging process. Soft-tissue aging of the neck may exacerbate a mild chin deficiency.

58.7 Surgical Treatment

The basic principles of malar, nasal, and mandibular augmentation are in fact very similar. Selecting an implant of appropriate shape and size is very important in achieving a pleasing facial contour. Nasal dorsal implants can be placed via closed or open rhinoplasty approaches, depending on the particular problem at hand and the surgeon's preference. Surgical access for malar augmentation is usually through a gingivobuccal incision; however, transconjunctival or subciliary approaches may also be used. Mandibular implants can be introduced intraorally through a gingivobuccal incision or through the open approach via submental incision. With all implants, the dissection is carried on top of the bone in the subperiosteal plane. In the chin, a small strip of periosteum over the symphysis may be left intact, thus making the central portion of the implant supraperiosteal and the lateral portion subperiosteal. It is of paramount importance to create a precise pocket to fully accommodate the implant without undue tension or buckling, but at the same time to avoid excessive undermining to minimize the risk for implant migration and shifting. One should be aware of the location of the mental and infraorbital nerves in order to avoid injury during the dissection or introduction of the implant.

The implant is typically soaked in an antibiotic solution and then placed into the pocket. The area is evaluated for symmetry and the presence of palpable edges, and all needed adjustments are carried out. The wound is thoroughly irrigated with saline or an antibiotic solution, hemostasis is verified, and the incisions are closed. If the implant pocket is precise, it is usually not necessary to suture the implant. However, some surgeons prefer suturing implants either to the periosteum (mandibular implants) or to the overlying skin (malar and nasal dorsal implants) for additional security. A compression dressing is placed to minimize the chance of hematoma and to further stabilize the implant in the immediate postoperative period.

Surgical complications usually involve injury to the sensory (infraorbital and mental) nerves with resultant hypesthesia, which may be transient or permanent depending on the degree of injury. Weakness of the marginal mandibular nerve may occur during mandibular implant placement as a consequence of overzealous retraction and nerve compression; this is almost always a temporary problem. There is a potential for injury to the facial nerve branches during dissection over the masseter muscle and malar implant placement. Other surgical complications include hematoma, seroma, infection, and bad scarring. Long-term complications related to implants themselves were discussed earlier in this chapter.

58.8 Prognosis

The surgical success rate is universally good, with only small percentage of patients developing postoperative complications necessitating implant removal. Although challenging, facial implant procedures provide the patient with improved facial harmony that is long-lasting.

58.9 Roundsmanship

- Many different types of facial implants are available to create a variety of changes.
- Long-term implant-related complications include infection, foreign body reaction, migration, and extrusion.
- Detailed facial analysis and proper implant selection lead to optimal surgical outcome.

58.10 Recommended Reading

[1] Binder WJ. Submalar augmentation. An alternative to face-lift surgery. Arch Otolaryngol Head Neck Surg 1989; 115: 797–801

[2] Cuzalina L A, Hlavacek MR.. Complications of facial implants. Oral Maxillofac Surg Clin North Am; 21: 91–104

[3] Terino EO. Complications of chin and malar augmentation. In: Peck G, ed. Complications and Problems in Aesthetic Plastic Surgery. New York, NY: Gower Medical Publishers; 1991

59 Management of Aging Skin

Tova Fischer Isseroff and Alexander Ovchinsky

59.1 Introduction

As the "Baby Boom" generation ages and genetic breakthroughs uncover the etiology of many disease mechanisms, aging has come to be considered a disease process that can be treated, rather than the inevitable final pathway of all humans. Physicians have occupied themselves with discovering ways to help their patients live longer and feel better about themselves, all the while modifying chronic diseases and affecting lifestyle choices. The social renaissance in the 1960s and 1970s brought with it a surge in the acceptance and willingness of physicians to perform and of patients to request cosmetic surgery. The search for the fountains of youth generated an outpouring of new surgical techniques and dialogue. In addition, nonsurgical approaches to facial rejuvenation have peaked as the sale of over-the-counter and specialty products to reverse the signs aging has reached a market high, and as the offerings of aesthetic surgeons, dermatologists, and aestheticians in the realm of facial resurfacing have burgeoned.

59.2 Incidence of Disease

The incidence of aging is directly proportional to the lifespan of a given population; the specific appearance of an aged individual depends on a host of factors, including but not limited to genetic predisposition, diet, and environment.

59.3 Terminology

When analyzing a face, the physician observes for rhytids (skin wrinkles) and other obvious changes in the skin. Dynamic wrinkles are amenable to treatment with a neuromodulator because they are produced by mimetic musculature and can be reduced by weakening the underlying muscle. Static wrinkles need to be addressed separately because they may overlie areas of actinic keratosis, premalignant warty lesions that occur on the sun-exposed areas of the face. Skin tone and color are graded with standardized grading scales, such as the Fitzpatrick Scale (▶ Table 59.1) and the Glogau Wrinkle Scale (▶ Table 59.2). Skin rejuvenation techniques, which may be ablative or nonablative, are all aimed at improving the quality, texture, and appearance of the skin and are usually performed on skin that has aged or undergone actinic damage, acne scarring, or hypertrophic scarring. The ablative modalities employ different mechanisms of skin injury: chemical peels cause caustic injury, dermabrasion causes mechanical injury, and lasers cause thermal injury. Each rejuvenation procedure has its own vocabulary and instructions, which are essential for the operator to understand and use in communication.

59.4 Applied Anatomy

The skin is composed of three basic layers. The outermost later of skin is the epidermis; the dermis is deeper and is composed of the superficial papillary layer and the deeper reticular layer (▶ Fig. 59.1). Injury limited to the epidermis and papillary dermis, the end-product of most resurfacing procedures, results in a wound that heals without scarring, whereas injury to the deeper reticular layer usually heals with scar formation.

59.5 The Disease Process

59.5.1 Etiology and Pathogenesis

Multiple theories have been proposed to explain the aging process. The free radical theory is the basis of many over-the-counter serums, creams, and dietary supplements. This theory postulates that free radicals, routinely produced during cell metabolism, build up as the body ages and then interfere with

Table 59.1 Fitzpatrick Scale of skin types

Type I	White or freckled skin; blue or hazel eyes; blond or red hair; always burns, never tans
Type II	Fair skin; blond, red, or brown hair; usually burns, tans less than average
Type III	White to olive skin; sometimes burns mildly, tans average
Type IV	Brown skin; rarely burns, tans with ease more than average
Type V	Intermediate brown-colored skin; Asian, Latin, or Indian; brown skin; tans easily
Type VI	Black skin; never burns

Source: Data from Table 29.1. In: Cummings C, Haughey B, Thomas JR, et al, eds. Cummings Otolaryngology: Head and Neck Surgery. Philadelphia, PA. Elsevier Mosby; 1998:693–713 AND Mandy SH, Monheit GD. Dermabrasion and chemical peels. In: Papel ID, ed. Facial Plastic and Reconstructive Surgery. New York, NY: Thieme Medical Publishers; 2009:301–320.

Table 59.2 Glogau Wrinkle Scale

Group I: mild	Group II: moderate	Group III: advanced	Group IV: severe
Few wrinkles	Wrinkles with muscle contraction	Wrinkles at rest	All wrinkles
Little wrinkling or scarring	Early wrinkling; mild scarring	Persistent wrinkling; moderate acne scarring	Wrinkling; photoaging gravitational and dynamic
No keratosis	early actinic keratosis	Discoloration, telangiectasias, actinic keratosis	Actinic keratosis ± skin cancer or acne scars
28–35 y[a]	35–50 y[a]	50–65 y[a]	60–75 y[a]

Source: Adapted from Table 29.2. In: Cummings C, Haughey B, Thomas JR, et al, eds. Cummings Otolaryngology: Head and Neck Surgery. Philadelphia, PA: Elsevier Mosby; 1998:693–713.
[a]Approximate age range; severity of wrinkles depends upon other factors in addition to age.

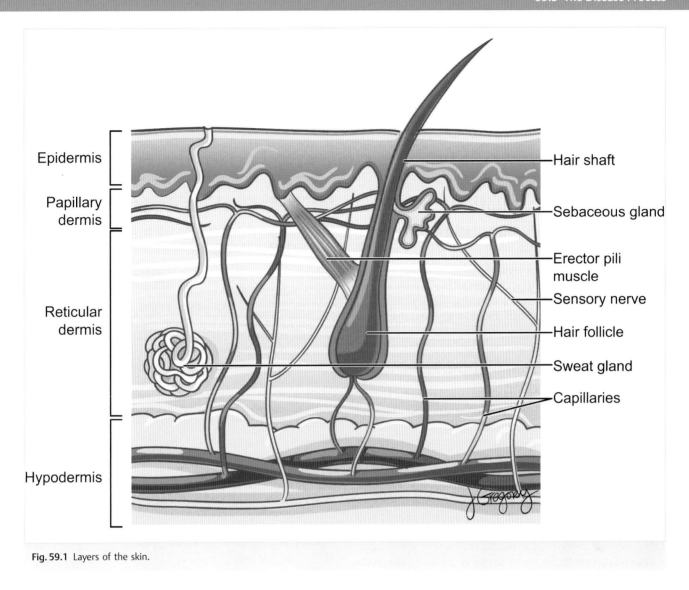

Fig. 59.1 Layers of the skin.

cellular respiration and energy production in the mitochondria, damaging the cell. A second theory centers on the decline in hormonal levels that naturally occurs as one ages. Female menopause and male andropause both lead to a decline in sexual hormone levels, which give the characteristic appearance of youth to those in their peak reproductive years. The cell senescence theory states that cells have a finite ability to replicate and with each replication lose a telomere protein. The telomere sequence determines the cell's age capacity. Yet another theory involves inflammation and an increase in cellular stress that occurs as certain chemicals and hormones naturally build up in the body. Histologically, aging skin shows a loss of epidermal call differentiation and degeneration of the underlying elastic network. The amount of collagen in the dermis decreases, dermal fibers degenerate, and the dermal–epidermal junction flattens. Lymphocytes infiltrate the dermis, and melanocytes become unevenly distributed, causing mottled pigmentation.

59.5.2 Natural History and Progression

A common end point for all humanity is aging. As hormone levels begin to decline, the body and face begin to show signs of aging. Wrinkles develop in dynamic and static locations, areas that are dependent or have been damaged by the sun. Smoking, diet, skin care, and genetics can alter facial appearance, as well.

59.5.3 Potential Disease Complications

Aging skin can cause physical and psychological distress. Skin laxity around the eyes can result in visual changes by affecting the palpebral fissure. Patients can become very distressed about their cosmetic appearance and the loss of their youthful glow.

59.5.4 Disease Grading

Grading systems and classifications are used to standardize and provide interphysician reliability with regard to physical examination and treatment, as well as guidance in determining an appropriate treatment modality for a specific patient (see ► Table 59.1 and ► Table 59.2).

Table 59.3 Brody relative and absolute contraindications to chemical peels

Relative contraindications	Darker skin type (Fitzpatrick IV–VI); history of keloid formation; history of herpes; history of cardiac abnormality; history of facial radiation therapy; marked quantity of vellus hair; telangiectasia
Absolute contraindications	Unrealistic patient expectations; physical inability to perform adequate postoperative care; significant renal and hepatic dysfunction; HIV infection; significant immunosuppression; emotional instability/mental illness; Ehlers-Danlos syndrome; scleroderma; collagen vascular disease; recent isotretinoin treatment; anticipation of inadequate photoprotection

Source: Adapted from Table 29.3. In: Cummings C, Haughey B, Thomas JR, et al, eds. Cummings Otolaryngology: Head and Neck Surgery. Philadelphia, PA: Elsevier Mosby; 1998:693–713.

59.6 Medical Evaluation

59.6.1 Presenting Complaints

Patients seeking a consultation for facial rejuvenation have complaints related to their aged appearance, whether a specific area with noted physical changes or the overall appearance. Changes in skin texture and laxity, pigmentation, and susceptibility to bruising and blemishing can also cause dissatisfaction.

59.6.2 Physical Examination, Laboratory Studies, and Imaging

A thorough social and medical history must be obtained from a patient seeking any cosmetic procedure. Any history of previous surgery, previous facial treatments, or trauma, medication use, allergies, and the likelihood of scar formation must all be taken into account when a specific treatment modality is considered. A history of sun exposure, whether remote or recent, is crucial in evaluating the degree of photodamage to the skin. Chronic medical conditions may preclude the use of certain treatment modalities, such as collagen vascular diseases and scleroderma, which are absolute contraindications to the use of chemical peels (▶ Table 59.3). A history of immunosuppression indicates a poor prognosis for healing after treatment, as does active smoking. A patient's expectations, functional status, and ability to care for himself or herself, and to comply with follow-up after a treatment, will also affect the readiness of a clinician to perform a certain procedure.

Examination of the face should be performed consistently, in a systematic and meticulous fashion. Careful attention must be paid to skin laxity, texture and coloration, and blemishes; the location of wrinkles; and the strength of bony structures. The face must be observed when active and in repose to study the movement of individual muscle groups. Photographic documentation, important for both consistency and postoperative comparison, should use standardized lighting and poses. No crucial laboratory tests are needed before intervention, other than preoperative screening.

59.6.3 Differential Diagnosis

Rare medical conditions, such as Hutchinson-Guilford syndrome (Progeria) appear as premature aging; however a simple history and physical exam will make this diagnosis evident.

59.7 Medical Treatment

The medical treatment of aging skin is divided into three basic categories. Skin resurfacing is discussed here; neuromodulation and injectable fillers are covered separately. Chemical peels chemically ablate differing thicknesses of the skin to reduce the effects of aging and sun damage.

Although the technique itself is easy to learn, experience is necessary to predict how different skin types and areas of the face will respond to peels. The concentration of the solution used and the length and number of applications determine the depth of peel. Peels work by causing protein precipitation or keratolysis.

When compared with photoaged, nonrejuvenated skin, skin that has undergone chemical peeling exhibits new bands of dermal collagen and ordered cellular differentiation in the epidermis, free of irregularities and actinic keratosis. Melanin granules are evenly distributed and bleached. The dermal–epidermal matrix is linearly oriented, with elastotic fibers paralleling the new collagen. There is decreased lymphocytic infiltration. Wrinkles are effaced by the new layers of connective tissue. Chemical peeling can decrease precancerous skin lesions.

Pretreatment with tretinoin is applied for 2 to 4 weeks before the peel; this thins the epidermis (allowing deeper penetration of the chemical peel) and increases the rate of dermal collagen production (speeding improvement and recovery after the peel).

A superficial chemical peel is generally suitable for all Fitzpatrick skin types and Glogau category I skin. Low concentrations of chemical agents are used to exfoliate the stratum corneum and epidermis to stimulate regrowth and temper superficial photodamage; these include 40 to 99% glycolic acid; 10 to 20% trichloracetic acid; Jessner solution (a mixture of salicylic acid, lactic acid, ethanol, and resorcinol); and salicylic acid. A medium-depth chemical peel (▶ Fig. 59.2) causes controlled injury down to the papillary dermis in a single application; it uses 35% trichloracetic acid combined with Jessner solution, solid carbon dioxide, or glycolic acid. It is appropriate for patients with Glogau category II skin, actinic keratosis, or mild acne scarring. A deep chemical peel wounds the skin down to the midreticular dermis and is effective in rejuvenating severely photoaged skin with deep rhytids; it is used for patients with Glogau category III or IV skin. A Gordon-Baker peeling solution (a combination of 88% phenol, septisol, croton oil, and distilled water) is most commonly used because it reliably and consistently produces the expected result. The phenol produces rapid denaturization and irreversible coagulation of the keratinocytes. It is this keratinocyte coagulation that limits the depth of penetration of the

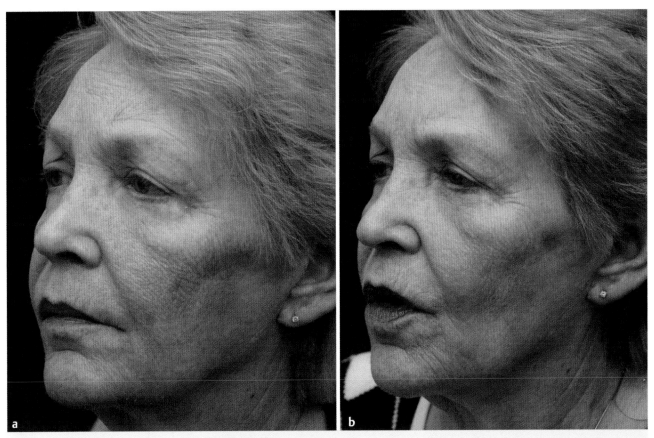

Fig. 59.2 Patient (**a**) before and (**b**) after 35% trichloracetic acid peel. Note the smoother and more even complexion and the effacement of fine lines after treatment.

peel; pure phenol penetrates less deeply because it has a greater coagulative effect.

Before application of the solution, the face is first cleansed to remove oils and exfoliate desquamated cells, and then the solution is applied with saturated gauze or a brush. A deep peel is a major surgical procedure, and both preoperative medical clearance and intraoperative intravenous sedation and hydration are necessary, as well as intraoperative monitoring and oxygen support. Phenol is cardiotoxic, nephrotoxic, and hepatotoxic, so hydration and extension of the application time to more than 1 hour for the entire face limits the toxic side effects of the preparation. Deep peels can be occluded (zinc oxide tape is applied to cover the phenol solution immediately after application in order to increase penetration of the solution in deeply wrinkled faces) or nonoccluded (which involves more skin cleansing and the application of greater amounts of peel solution, but no taping).

The skin heals within slightly different time frames depending on peel depth. After a deep peel, healing of the skin occurs in four phases. Inflammation is evident immediately, with erythema occurring as the epidermis separates and gradually sloughs off with the use of soaks and compresses. Coagulation then follows, and re-epithelialization begins on day 3 and continues into days 10 to 14, at which point fibroplasia commences and new collagen is formed. This phase lasts until about 4 months postoperatively. Patients must be informed that there is a higher potential for pigmentary disturbance and textural damage from chemical peels. All patients are advised to wear sunscreen at all times after the peel, and makeup may be necessary to camouflage certain areas, as well.

Dermabrasion is a mechanical method of removing the epidermis and regenerating the collagen of the papillary layer without injuring the underlying reticular layer. The new collagen that is produced supports a new epidermis. This technique is best used for skin with actinic damage, aging, or scarring. Dermabrasion wounds, just like chemical peels or laser wounds, heal by re-epithelialization from the wound margins and epidermal appendages that remain (such as pilosebaceous glands). Because the skin of the face is rich in sebaceous glands, it is an excellent skin surface for this procedure. The preoperative application of tretinoin, as in chemical peels, has been shown to shorten healing time by approximately 3 days. Additionally, chilling the skin before abrasion creates a rigid surface that can then be abraded evenly. Dermabrasion may use wire brushes or wheels covered with diamond chips. Microdermabrasion, in which small aluminum or glass particles are blown over the skin, produces an effect similar to that of superficial chemical peels.

Dermabrasion is done in an outpatient setting, and preoperative and intraoperative anxiolytics and painkillers are administered to make the patient more comfortable, as well as local anesthesia. Once the skin is solidified by the cooling agent or distended by the injection of a dilute anesthetic, abrasion is performed. Adequate depth through the epidermis is made evident by the loss of pigmentation, and depth to the papillary dermis is identified by punctate bleeding. Once the papillary dermis is entered further, faint bands of collagen become visible, and when this is destroyed, abrasion down to the reticular layer is complete. Postoperative occlusive dressings, especially biosynthetic dressings, speed healing time by keeping wounds moist and allowing wound fluid and growth factors to have maximum contact with the skin. Steroids reduce edema and discomfort, and as with any other procedure that removes epidermis, antiviral prophylaxis should be started 2 days before treatment and continued until epithelialization is complete. Patients are restarted on tretinoin at that time and are advised that they must use sunscreen when going outside. Most patients are able to resume daily activities after 7 to 10 days; however, it takes approximately 4 to 6 weeks for erythema to fade fully.

Light-based skin rejuvenative therapies depend upon the different effects caused by different levels of absorbed energy. The energy delivered is affected by the wavelength (▶ Fig. 59.3) used; shorter wavelengths impart more energy (▶ Fig. 59.4). Once in contact with a surface, the energy is differentially absorbed, reflected, scattered, or transmitted, according to the tissue qualities and the presence of chromophores in the skin corresponding to the wavelength of the light (▶ Fig. 59.5). The light energy absorbed by the tissue will cause photodynamic, electromagnetic, and thermal effects to differing degrees (▶ Fig. 59.6).

Laser resurfacing can be ablative or nonablative. Ablative laser resurfacing is accomplished with the carbon dioxide laser or the erbium:yttrium-aluminum garnet (Er:YAG) laser. Lasers produce effects by a process of photothermolysis, in which the laser's specific wavelength corresponds to a peak in the absorption curve of the chromophore. Unwanted effects are limited by choosing an absorption peak well separated from the absorption curve of other chromophores, such as hemoglobin and

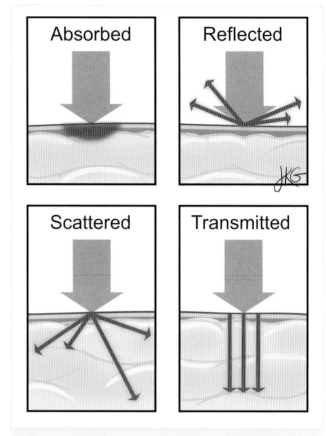

Fig. 59.5 Light energy striking a surface can be absorbed, reflected, scattered, or transmitted.

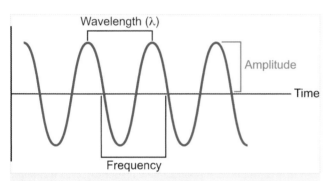

Fig. 59.3 Wavelength, frequency, and amplitude of light. The energy delivered increases as frequency increases.

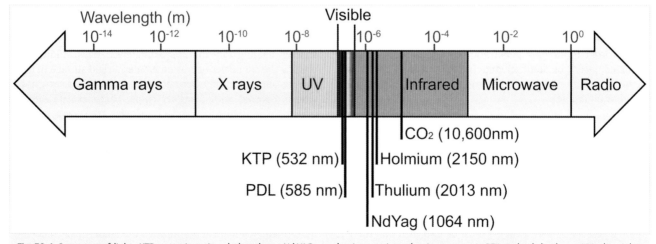

Fig. 59.4 Spectrum of light. *KTP*, potassium titanyl phosphate; *Nd:YAG*, neodymium:yttrium-aluminum garnet; *PDL*, pulsed dye laser; *UV*, ultraviolet.

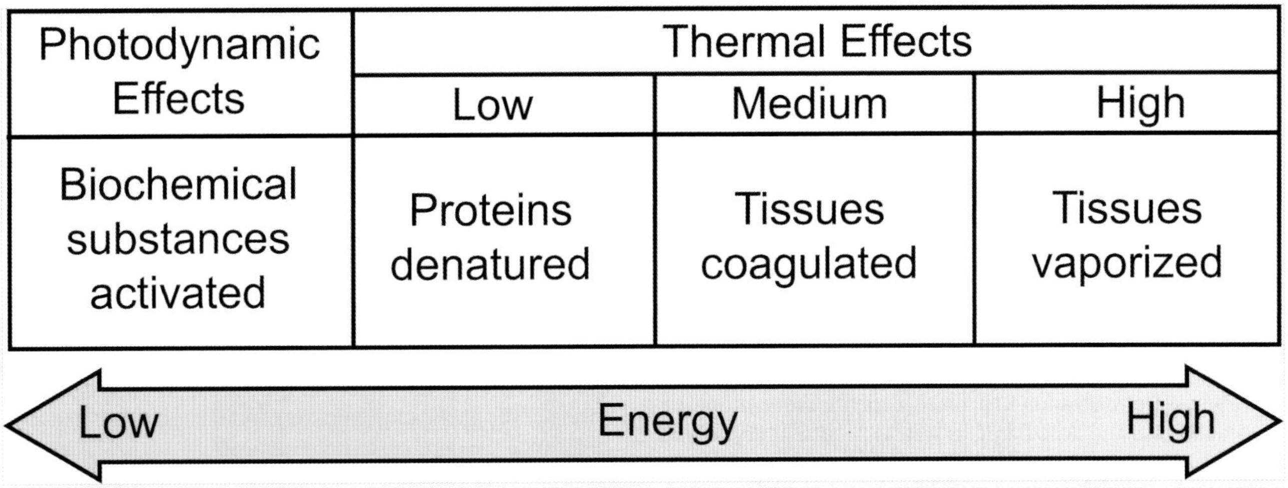

Photodynamic Effects	Thermal Effects		
	Low	Medium	High
Biochemical substances activated	Proteins denatured	Tissues coagulated	Tissues vaporized

Low ◄———— Energy ————► High

Fig. 59.6 Low levels of energy may affect biological systems in a nonlethal way, whereas higher levels may destroy, coagulate, or simply vaporize tissues.

melanin. Both the carbon dioxide and Er:YAG lasers use water as the selected chromophore because more than 90% of the epidermis is water. When the laser hits the target tissue, laser energy is absorbed by water molecules, where it is then converted to heat, vaporizing water and tissue alike. Ideally, only a limited amount of heat is transferred to the adjacent collagen-containing tissue, preventing unwanted tissue injury. Laser safety is of the utmost importance for the operator, support staff, and patient. This includes the use of protective eyewear, nonflammable drapes, laser masks, and a smoke evacuator, in addition to the removal of alcohol-based makeup and moisturizers. Intravenous, regional, or topical anesthesia is used.

The carbon dioxide laser uses a continuous wavelength of 10,600 nm. Over the past half century it has been reconfigured to provide a short pulse duration, ideal for resurfacing. The water absorbance of the Er:YAG laser is 10 times that of the carbon dioxide laser, owing to a wavelength of 2,940 nm. This causes more precise tissue thinning and less adjacent thermal injury, coupled with a faster healing time. However, less tissue tightening occurs with this laser because there is less thermal effect on adjacent tissue. Postoperative edema, recovery time, resultant hyper- and hypopigmentation, and scarring are significantly less when the erbium laser is used. Owing to the inherent differences and advantages of these two laser types, some combine both laser wavelengths in order to provide the benefit of the pooled result.

Many surgeons pretreat the skin with tretinoin, and all should advise patients to avoid sun exposure before resurfacing because it exacerbates postoperative hyperpigmentation due to melanocyte activation. As the laser vaporizes the epidermis, the tissue appears pink when the papillary dermis is entered; after more laser passes, the tissue color changes to a chamois yellow, which indicates reticular dermis and the need to stop skin ablation. Postoperatively, the use of occlusive dressings shortens healing time to 5 to 7 days. Strict sun avoidance is necessary for approximately 2 to 3 months until all of the postoperative erythema has subsided in order to decrease the risk for hyperpigmentation.

Nonablative lasers selectively affect the dermis and spare the epidermis. Minimal recovery is needed, which makes it a preferred choice for many patients. However, multiple treatment sessions are necessary, and the results are not as dramatic as those with ablative lasers or deep peels. The 1,320-nm neodymium:yttrium-aluminum garnet (Nd:YAG) laser provides the optimal wavelength for specifically targeting the dermis. It has been effective in wrinkle reduction and in treating acne scars through a process of stimulated dermal collagen deposition. The 1,450-nm diode laser has good dermal penetration, as well, and has achieved good results in reducing rhytids. Fractionated lasers work by creating multiple microscopic areas of thermal injury, around which the uninjured tissue promotes rapid healing. Re-epithelialization occurs within 24 hours, and erythema usually resolves within a week.

Intense pulsed light (IPL) is a noncoherent, polychromatic filtered light source used for photothermolysis. Initially approved by the FDA in 1995 for the treatment of leg telangiectasia, its benefits were soon noted in the treatment of photoaging and vascular lesions and in hair removal. Specially designed filters in the treatment head manipulate the wavelengths emitted in order to provide selective thermolysis based on the target tissue's absorption (e.g., vasculature vs epidermis). Multiple pulses to a given area allow thermal relaxation of the target tissue between pulses; relaxation time depends on tissue and skin type (Fitzgerald skin type, ethnicity). IPL is effective in treating facial telangiectasia and poikiloderma of sun-exposed areas, as a photorejuvenation modality, and for hair removal. Treating the entire face can reduce mottled pigmentation and freckling and can smooth the skin. Studies have shown an increase in the transcription of types I and III collagen and of elastin following IPL treatment.

Photodynamic therapy (PDT) is a nonablative photorejuvenation technique that employs the combination of a light source and the creation of reactive oxygen to biologically damage and change the underlying skin. A photosensitizing agent, such as aminolevulinic acid (5-ALA), is applied topically and penetrates abnormal keratin in cutaneous tissue and creates endogenous protoporphyrin IX, an activated oxygen intermediate. When an appropriate light source is then applied, the activated photosensitizer causes cell destruction and death. The damage inflicted must surpass the cellular repair mechanisms in order for destruction to be complete, known as the photodynamic response. The effectiveness of PDT depends on the photosensitizer used, the light source, and the oxygen status of the target tissue. PDT uses include the treatment of selected nonmelanotic skin cancers, acne and sebaceous hyperplasia, various infectious and inflammatory skin conditions, and actinic keratosis, in addition to cosmetic photorejuvenation.

The side effects of all of the above procedures include hypo- and hyperpigmentation, poor cosmesis, scarring, and infection. Patients with a history of herpesvirus infection are required to take prophylaxis after the procedure in order to prevent reactivation of the infection. Phenol is cardiotoxic, nephrotoxic, and hepatotoxic, and certain groups of patients are not eligible for deep peels. Dermabrasion can make patients more prone to milia outbreaks and acne flares, as well as persistent erythema, all of which can be managed with topical or oral agents. After laser resurfacing, patients frequently develop contact dermatitis in reaction to certain ointments; in this case, the use of those ointments should be stopped and the face treated with a corticosteroid cream. The development of scattered purpura is a unique side effect of both PDT and IPL treatment, although the incidence is low and it usually resolves on its own. Stinging pain is also a side effect of IPL, which can be reduced with the application of topical anesthetic cream before treatment.

59.7.1 Prognosis

Superficial chemical peels do not penetrate the epidermis and have no clinically noticeable recovery time. Medium-depth peels, superficial dermabrasion, and ablative laser resurfacing have a healing time of approximately 5 to 7 days. Repetitive peeling is often necessary to produce the full desired effect. Re-sults from deep and medium peels usually last for over 1 year. Barring the occurrence of side effects, the peels are effective in rejuvenating photoaged and actinic skin. Use of the Nd:YAG nonablative laser has been shown to be most effective in patients who have Fitzpatrick type I or II skin with mild, moderate, or severe rhytids.

59.8 Roundsmanship

- Skin resurfacing can be performed chemically with chemical peels, mechanically with dermabrasion, or thermally with ablative lasers.
- The strength (concentration) of the peeling solution, the duration of the application, and the condition of the treated skin determine the depth of a chemical peel.

59.9 Recommended Reading

[1] Beer K, Beer J. Overview of facial aging. Facial Plast Surg 2009; 25: 281–284
[2] Carniol PJ, Harmon CB, Hamilton MM. Ablative laser facial skin rejuvenation. In: Papel ID, ed. Facial Plastic and Reconstructive Surgery. New York, NY. Thieme Medical Publishers; 2009:321–330
[3] Cole PD, Hatef DA, Kaufman Y, Pozner JN. Laser therapy in ethnic populations. Semin Plast Surg 2009; 23: 173–177
[4] Fabbrocini G, De Padova MP, Tosti A. Chemical peels: what's new and what isn't new but still works well. Facial Plast Surg 2009; 25: 329–336
[5] Goldman MP, Weiss RA, Weiss MA. Intense pulsed light as a nonablative approach to photoaging. Dermatol Surg 2005; 31: 1179–1187, discussion 1187
[6] Koch RJ. Nonablative facial skin rejuvenation. In: Papel ID, ed. Facial Plastic and Reconstructive Surgery. New York, NY: Thieme Medical Publishers; 2009:331–336
[7] Mandy SH, Monheit GD. Dermabrasion and chemical peels. In: Papel ID, ed. Facial Plastic and Reconstructive Surgery. New York, NY: Thieme Medical Publishers; 2009:301–320

60 Facial Soft-Tissue Fillers and Neuromodulators

Anthony P. Sclafani and Anthony M. Sclafani

60.1 Introduction

Facial wrinkles may be a result of skin laxity, subcutaneous muscular contraction, volume loss, or dermal atrophy. Skin fillers were developed to help correct volume deficiency and focal dermal thinning. Other procedures, such as facelift and chemical or laser skin peel, address these issues only partially, and if performed overly aggressively, they may lead to a "tight," "surgical" appearance. Silicone oil injections have had a lengthy if poorly controlled history as a facial treatment, in terms of both material and technique used. Beginning in 1981, a number of materials were introduced in the United States as facial wrinkle fillers, such as collagen, hyaluronic acid (HA) derivatives, calcium hydroxylapatite (CaHA) and poly-L-lactic acid (PLLA); many more materials are available worldwide, but reliable clinical evidence is somewhat lacking.

The neurotoxins commonly in use in the United States are all toxins isolated from *Clostridium botulinum* bacteria. Originally isolated in 1895, botulinum toxin A (BTxA) was first used in the 1970s for the treatment of strabismus. In 1992, its use for the treatment of periocular wrinkles was first described; since then, BTxA has acquired a $2 billion market worldwide.

Soft-tissue fillers and neurotoxins offer the potential to significantly rejuvenate the face with a minimally invasive approach, but they have risks and must be administered properly by adequately trained medical professionals.

60.2 Incidence of Disease

Skin aging due to dermal or soft-tissue atrophy or to hyperkinetic lines will occur to varying degrees, and each patient needs to be addressed individually. Generally, facial aging worsens with age. Hyperkinetic lines and shallow rhytids due to dermal atrophy may become noticeable during a person's thirties, whereas soft-tissue atrophy and more severe rhytids may become noticeable only in a patient's forties or fifties. Hyperkinetic lines, such as crow's-feet (▶ Fig. 60.1), may develop because of patterns of facial expressivity or involuntary muscle contraction. Patients with fair skin are more prone to these changes. Women, smokers, and individuals with frequent significant fluctuations in weight are also more likely to develop these signs of premature aging.

60.3 Terminology

The term *rhytid* refers to any skin wrinkle. *Dermal atrophy*, or *thinning*, usually is a result of repeated skin folding during animation and will manifest as a fine etched line. *Skin folds*, such as nasolabial folds, are due to an overhang of skin and soft tissue above a fixed point and may be due to skin and soft-tissue descent or to subdermal atrophy below the fold. *Hyperkinetic lines* (see ▶ Fig. 60.1) occur because elevated muscle tone prevents full relaxation of the overlying skin; over time, dermal atrophy may result from this, even in the absence of muscle contraction. *Facial soft-tissue atrophy* refers more broadly to the differential loss of soft-tissue (mainly fat) volume in the face. This volume loss will alter the shape of the face, lead to a loss of the gentle convexities of youth, skeletonize parts of the face (most notably the infraorbital rim), allow the facial skin to sag, and generally age the face. Soft-tissue fillers are generally categorized as either volumizers (effecting beneficial action by occupying space), stimulators (increasing facial volume by stimulating collagen deposition), or both.

60.4 Applied Anatomy

Clinically relevant muscles in the upper face include the frontalis, corrugator and depressor supercilii, procerus, and orbicularis oculi muscles; see Chapter 56 (Surgical Treatment of the Aging Face) for a more complete discussion. An important midfacial muscle is the zygomaticus major, originating from the medial malar arch and inserting on the modiolus. The levator labii superioris alaeque nasi muscle originates from the nasomaxillary junction and inserts on the dermis of the lateral ala and upper lip. The orbicularis oris muscle runs circumferentially to serve as the sphincter of the mouth. It interrelates with other perioral muscles at the modiolus and is attached to the dermis of the lips intimately, although a potential space exists between muscle and dermis at the vermilion border. In addition to the orbicularis muscle in the lower face, the mentalis originates from the mentum and inserts (often with a midline cleft) into the chin pad, while the depressor anguli oris originates from the medial mandible and assists in depressing and everting the lateral lower lip.

There are multiple fat compartments in the face that are separated by delicate septa and may undergo atrophy or descent at different times and rates. Most significantly, the deep midfacial fat compartment may undergo early atrophy and produce significant facial aging.

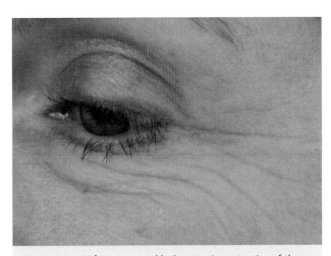

Fig. 60.1 Crow's-feet are caused by hypertonic contraction of the lateral orbicularis oculi muscle with folding of the overlying skin.

60.5 The Disease Process

60.5.1 Etiology

Dermal atrophy may be caused by genetic disorders such as cutis laxa or Ehlers-Danlos disease, but most dermal atrophy is a result of chronologic aging and photoaging. As the skin ages, the dermal collagen thins and loses its organization; the dermal rete pegs become more blunted. Photoaging, caused by damaging ultraviolet light, demonstrates elastin breakdown and can cause chronic heliodermatitis, marked by perivascular inflammation and extracellular pigment accumulation. These changes are clearly exacerbated by excessive sun exposure, tobacco use, and weight fluctuation. The exact mechanism of fat atrophy is unknown.

60.5.2 Disease Grading

The Glogau Wrinkle Scale can be used to classify the severity of facial wrinkles (see Box The Glogau Wrinkle Scale (p. 476)).

The Glogau Wrinkle Scale

- I: No wrinkles
- II: Wrinkles in motion
- III: Wrinkles at rest
- IV: All wrinkles

60.6 Medical Evaluation

Before treatment, the skin should be evaluated. Treatments should not be performed in areas of active infection. New, noninflammatory skin lesions should be examined, and referral to a dermatologist should be considered. A thorough medical history should be elicited, especially any medications taken or history of bruising or bleeding.

60.6.1 Presenting Complaints

Patients requesting treatment of facial rhytids and folds may complain about specific lines and folds but more commonly ask that "laugh lines," "crow's-feet," or frown lines be treated. Alternatively, patients may be even less specific, requesting that a "sad," "tired," "angry," or "gaunt" appearance be treated. The physician should help the patient to determine the specific deformities he or she finds most bothersome before initiating treatment.

60.6.2 Clinical Findings, Physical Examination

A complete aesthetic analysis is appropriate for each patient, even when the patient requests specific nonsurgical treatment. It is important for the physician to appreciate and point out to the patient the limitations of minimally invasive treatments. Rhytids should be assessed with the patient in animation as well as at rest; lines present at rest represent areas of dermal

and subdermal thinning, will not respond completely to neurotoxin treatment, and should be considered for soft-tissue augmentation.

60.7 Medical Treatment

60.7.1 Soft-Tissue Fillers

Most facial soft-tissue fillers are approved for the correction of facial wrinkles and folds, such as the nasolabial folds. Other common problems treated include forehead wrinkles and glabellar lines between the brows; so-called marionette folds (lines running from the mouth corners down the sides of the chin) and the prejowl sulcus (relative depression between the chin and jowl along the lower mandibular border) are also commonly treated. Lip volume augmentation was an early use for soft-tissue fillers; an expanding area of use now is for general facial (especially midfacial) volume restoration. Larger volumes can be injected into the cheek or temples and lateral brows (below or within the normal soft tissue) to restore facial fullness. Additionally, deeper injections can be placed at the posterior edge of the mandibular angle to better define the jawline.

Each filler has its own particular qualities and risks, and the specific material used should always be tailored to the intended site and application. In general, fillers with larger particles require deeper placement; a filler placed more superficially provides a greater degree of correction than a similar volume of a more deeply placed filler (▶ Fig. 60.2).

Collagen

Zyderm and Zyplast, when available, were based on bovine collagen. Individual collagen fibers were treated to remove the most immunogenic peptide portion and then suspended in saline with (Zyplast) or without (Zyderm) chemical cross-linking to increase persistence of the effect. Patients treated with these bovine collagen–based fillers required allergy skin testing beforehand. Human collagen–based products (Cosmoderm and Cosmoplast) obviated the need for skin testing. Zyderm and Cosmoderm were injected into the mid dermis, whereas Zyplast and Cosmoplast required injection into the deep dermis or subdermis. Because the collagen fibers were suspended in saline, significant overcorrection was necessary to achieve the desired result after resorption of the water. The clinical effect of these materials persisted for 2 to 4 months. Porcine collagen, cross-linked into a three-dimensional matrix, was more recently introduced and provided a volumizing effect for up to 12 months, but all of these materials were removed from the market by their manufacturers.

Hyaluronic Acid Products

HAs were first approved in 2003 and have become the predominant class of soft-tissue filler. HA is a naturally occurring polysaccharide that gives resilience to the skin, but levels decrease with age. HA is highly conserved evolutionarily, and commercially available HA, produced by streptococci, is identical to human HA. This HA is treated to cross-link the polysaccharide chains and increase persistence of the clinical effect. As the thickness and viscosity of these materials increases, the depth

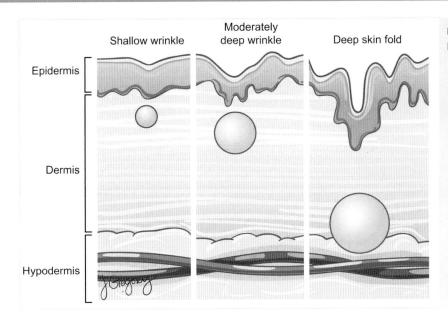

Shallow wrinkle | Moderately deep wrinkle | Deep skin fold

Epidermis

Dermis

Hypodermis

Fig. 60.2 Larger-particle soft-tissue fillers require placement in the deep dermis or subdermis.

of placement also increases, with thicker fillers placed at the dermal–subdermal junction to avoid vascular compromise and palpability. HAs can maintain a clinical effect for up to 12 months (▶ Fig. 60.3). These fillers are predominantly "volumizers," but there is some experimental evidence of the induction of neocollagen formation around the implants, which may explain subtle increases in persistence of the effect after multiple treatments.

Calcium Hydroxylapatite

Originally introduced as a bulking agent for the bladder neck, CaHA was later used for augmentation of the paralyzed vocal fold. CaHA was approved in 2006 by the FDA for the treatment of facial wrinkles and folds. CaHA microbeads are suspended in a gel carrier. After a subdermal injection, the gel carrier is resorbed and replaced over time by a small amount of fibrous tissue around the individual microbeads. Over time, the microspheres dissolve and are resorbed, but CaHA produces a clinical effect for 12 to 15 months.

Poly-L-Lactic Acid

PLLA was approved by the FDA in 2004 for patients with facial lipoatrophy as a result of highly active antiretroviral therapy (HAART) for HIV infection and was approved in 2009 for cosmetic facial uses. PLLA is provided as a sterile powder, which must be suspended and thoroughly mixed to avoid clumping. This is then injected subdermally, stimulating a fibrous response and thickening the dermis. Generally, three to six treatments, separated by intervals of 4 to 6 weeks, are necessary to produce clinically significant effects. Clinical benefit has been shown to persist for at least 24 months, at which time the PLLA beads are substantially resorbed and metabolized.

Silicone Oil

Silicone oil injections were popularized, and in some cases abused, from the 1940s to the 1960s. Currently, no silicone oil is FDA-approved for cosmetic indications, and any treatments performed are so-called off label (see below). A large-scale review of silicone treatments by Webster et al showed that an appropriate microdroplet technique (injecting minute amounts in multiple sites and avoiding large deposits of material) could provide permanent correction of facial wrinkles safely and effectively. However, as a permanent filler, silicone oil injections are more prone to delayed complications, even several years or decades after treatment.

Injection Techniques

Soft-tissue fillers should be injected safely, with the compliance of the treated skin always taken into consideration and excessive injection as well as intravascular injury (especially in the glabella) avoided. Intradermal injections meet greater resistance and cause more immediate and visible skin change than do subdermal injections. In general, blanching of the skin or visibility of the needle through the skin indicates an injection that is too superficial. Injections can be done either with a series of individual skin punctures or by linearly threading the needle in the correct plane and injecting upon withdrawal. The edges of injected material should be "feathered" to blend in with the surrounding tissues and generally can be massaged to produce a smooth effect.

60.7.2 Neuromodulators

Currently, three commercially available botulinum toxin A (BTxA) products are approved for cosmetic facial indications: onabotulinum toxin (Botox Cosmetic; Allergan, Irvine, CA); abobotulinum toxin (Dysport; Medicis Pharmaceutical Corporation, Scottsdale, AZ); and incobotulinum toxin (Xeomin; Merz Pharmaceuticals, Greensboro, NC). All are BTxA preparations, but they differ slightly in associated properties and in how they are dosed. Botox, Dysport, and Xeomin units are different and not interchangeable. However, once injected, all associated proteins are released and the "naked" BTxA protein is liberated (Xeomin has no associated hemagglutinins). BTxA is composed of a

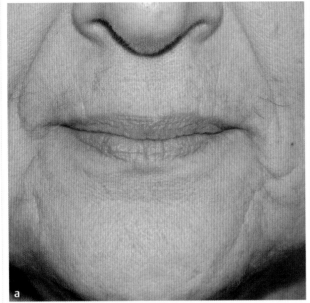

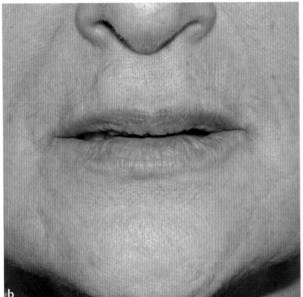

Fig. 60.3 (a) Deep nasolabial folds, marionette folds, and thin lips age the perioral area. (b) After treatment with a hyaluronic acid product, the lines have been smoothed and the mouth area rejuvenated.

heavy and a light chain joined by a disulfide bond. The heavy chain facilitates entry into the nerve ending; once it is internalized, a conformational change occurs, and the light chain of the molecule cleaves a portion of and inactivates soluble NSF attachment protein (SNAP)-25, a molecule essential for vesicle binding and acetylcholine release, as well as synaptobrevin and syntaxin. The process inactivates this particular synapse (▶ Fig. 60.4). Over time, additional neural sprouting will allow the resumption of neuromuscular transmission. A number of points along the target muscle are treated, eliminating or decreasing muscle tone and eliminating muscle contraction. Weakening of the treated muscle generally becomes apparent

in 2 to 7 days, and the full effect may take up to 14 days (▶ Fig. 60.5). Clinical effects typically last 3 to 4 months.

In the face, it is especially important to consider the effect of both target muscle tone and voluntary action, as well as the now-unopposed action of the target muscle's antagonist. The treatment of glabellar furrows (the only FDA-approved cosmetic use of BTxA) by injecting the depressor and corrugator supercilii and procerus muscles, or the effacement of crow's-feet by treating the lateral orbicularis oculi, will reduce or eliminate wrinkles in these areas but will allow frontalis contraction to alter the shape and position of the eyebrows; this can be done selectively to raise the brows and improve brow shape. The frontalis itself can be treated to eliminate transverse forehead rhytids; however, the frontalis muscle within 2 cm of the brows should not be treated to avoid a brow ptosis. Other muscles and areas treated include the levator labii superioris alaeque nasi to reduce an overly "gummy" smile, the depressor anguli oris to reduce the depth of marionette folds, the mentalis muscle to reduce wrinkles on the chin, and the paramedian platysma muscle to relax and efface platysmal bands.

60.8 FDA Considerations

It is important to remember that all soft-tissue fillers and neurotoxins approved by the U.S. Food and Drug Administration are indicated for specific purposes and locations. Properly trained physicians may use these materials in ways not specifically addressed by the FDA, but these uses are considered "off label." It is the physician's responsibility to be well trained, take proper precautions, use the materials in a way consistent with general medical practice and based on sound scientific reasoning, and discuss with the patient that the treatment is "off label." Common practice does not replace the need to discuss potential risks with each patient.

60.9 Postoperative Care

The soft-tissue fillers and neurotoxins described in this chapter are all considered minimally invasive treatments. These procedures are easily performed in the office with (at most) local or regional anesthesia. They are generally associated with little to no discomfort afterward. Typically, cold compresses are applied to the treated area for 30 minutes to a few hours after treatment. Generally, patients are advised to avoid manipulating the treatment area for 3 to 4 hours afterward. Patients treated with a neurotoxin are additionally advised to avoid head hanging or lying down for the same time period to avoid excessive spread of the toxin. Patients treated with PLLA are asked to massage the treated area several times a day for several weeks to minimize lumpiness.

60.10 Complications
60.10.1 Soft-Tissue Fillers

The injection of any material across the skin barrier may cause infection. Materials with a longer persistence of effect present

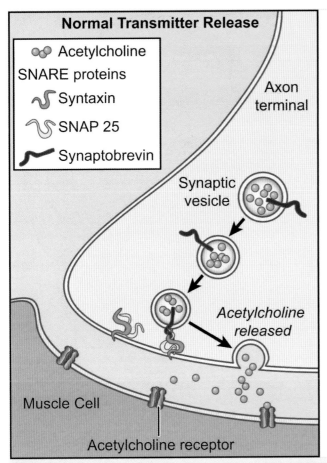
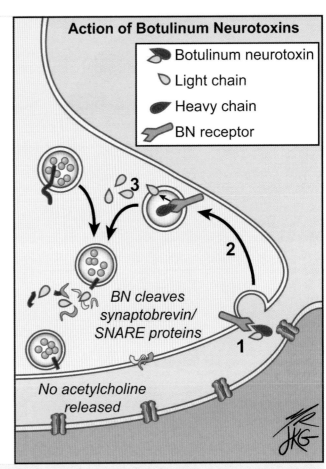

Fig. 60.4 Botulinum toxin A works at the motor end plate, inhibiting the release of acetylcholine by cleaving SNARE proteins. *BN*, botulinum neurotoxin; *SNAP*, soluble NSF attachment protein; *SNARE*, SNAP receptor.

greater problems when colonized by bacteria because a foreign body is present for a longer time; in these cases, treatment with antibiotics, often for several months, may be required. Allergic reactions to commonly used fillers (except bovine collagen) are rare. Migration of material is uncommon, but particulate fillers like CaHA and PLLA may form localized accumulations secondary to muscle contraction (especially in the lips) and should not be used in these areas. Intravascular injection or injections causing the constriction of arterial or venous flow in a localized area can lead to skin necrosis, most commonly seen in the glabella. Arterial occlusion causes immediate blanching of the skin. The injection should be stopped immediately if this is noted. Hyaluronidase should be injected to dissolve the injected material (if HA is being used). Warm compresses, topical nitroglycerin, and hyperbaric oxygen may be used to limit the degree of skin and soft-tissue necrosis if vascular occlusion is noted. Venous obstruction may also occur if the injected material compresses the venous outflow from a particular area. Venous occlusion is typically characterized by prolonged edema and ecchymosis with later (2 to 5 days) wound breakdown. Conservative wound care and patient support are essential to minimize tissue damage and patient anxiety if vascular occlusion occurs. Good technique and

aesthetic judgment are needed to ensure proper placement of the filler. Other potential complications include localized acne eruptions, cold sores, nodule formation, and asymmetry.

60.10.2 Neurotoxins

BTxA treatment is contraindicated in patients who are pregnant or breastfeeding and in those with preexisting neuromuscular disorders, such as myasthenia gravis. Inadvertent action on nontarget muscles can lead to facial distortion, asymmetry, or disability. Most commonly seen is eyelid ptosis (1 to 2%) as toxin injected into the glabella diffuses through the orbital septum to affect the levator palpebrae superioris. Eyelid ptosis typically lasts for only 2 to 3 weeks, even without treatment, but (if not contraindicated) the application of α-adrenergic eyedrops, such as 0.5% apraclonidine or 2.5% phenylephrine, will stimulate contraction of the Müller muscle to compensate for the loss of levator function. Excessive treatment of the medial frontalis with inadequate paralysis of the lateral frontalis can lead to the laterally overly arched "Mephisto" brow (▶ Fig. 60.6). This is easily managed with supplemental BTxA treatment to the lateral frontalis, which will allow the lateral brow to drop into a

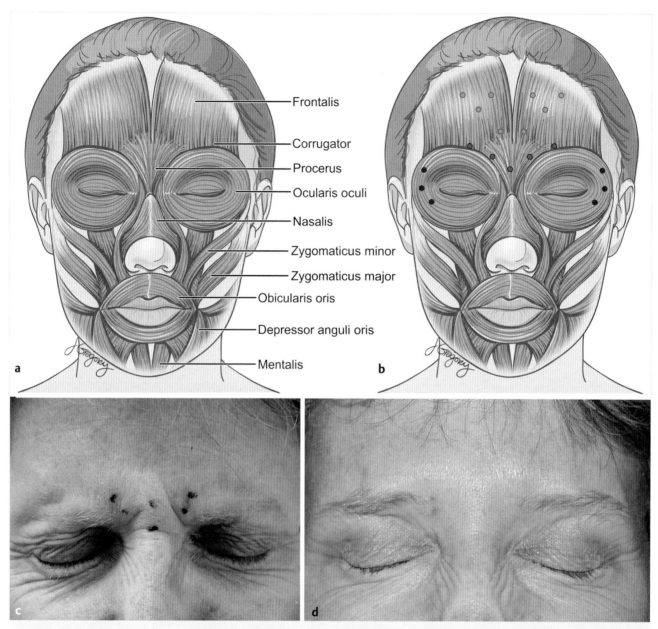

Fig. 60.5 (**a**) The facial muscles run in predictable, discernible areas in close proximity. Specifically targeting certain muscles can reduce hyperkinetic lines without altering resting facial expression. (**b**) Botulinum toxin A injections sites for horizontal frown lines (*green dots*), glabellar furrows (*blue dots*), and crow's-feet (*red dots*). (**c**) Hyperkinetic lines in the glabella and crow's-feet are created by contraction of the depressor and corrugator supercilii and procerus muscles and the orbicularis oculi muscle, respectively. (**d**) After treatment with botulinum toxin A in the glabella and the areas with crow's-feet, despite maximal effort the patient is unable to create rhytids. The patient declined treatment for "bunny lines" at the sides of the nose.

more appropriate position. The treatment of inferomedial crow's-feet may also paralyze the zygomaticus major muscle and alter the patient's smile. Dysphagia may occur if platysmal injections affect deeper muscles. Anti-BTxA antibodies may develop (generally associated with the much larger doses required to treat cervical dystonia) but do not seem to alter the clinical effect. Allergic reactions are uncommon.

60.11 Roundsmanship

- Soft-tissue fillers can smooth lines and change relative volumes in different facial units.
- Smaller-particle, less viscous fillers are appropriate for intradermal injections, whereas larger, more viscous fillers (typically longer-lasting) should be injected just below the dermis.

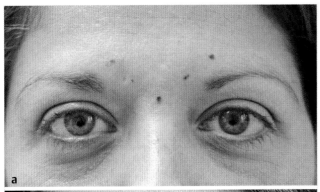
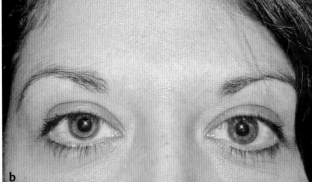
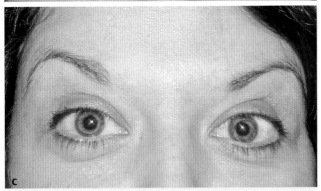

Fig. 60.6 (a) Before treatment with botulinum toxin A to the glabella at indicated sites. (b) Good result at rest after treatment of the glabella and forehead. (c) "Mephistopheles" brow due to an imbalance of medial and lateral frontalis muscle activity, which allows the lateral brow to be elevated disproportionately; correction is by treatment of the lateral frontalis muscle.

- Soft-tissue fillers can achieve volume augmentation by volumizing directly, by stimulating a fibrous response that augments dermal thickness, or both.
- Botulinum A toxin acts by inhibiting presynaptic acetylcholine release and produces a localized flaccid paralysis.
- Recovery after botulinum toxin A treatment occurs by the sprouting of additional neuronal twigs.

60.12 Recommended Reading

[1] Kelly PE. Injectable success: from fillers to Botox. Facial Plast Surg 2007; 23: 7–18, discussion 19–20

[2] Rohrich RJ, Pessa JE. The fat compartments of the face: anatomy and clinical implications for cosmetic surgery. Plast Reconstr Surg 2007; 119: 2219–2227, discussion 2228–2231

[3] Sclafani AP, Fagien S. Treatment of injectable soft tissue filler complications. Dermatol Surg 2009; 35 Suppl 2: 1672–1680

[4] Webster RC, Gaunt JM, Hamdan US, Fuleihan NS, Smith RC. Injectable silicone for facial soft-tissue augmentation. Arch Otolaryngol Head Neck Surg 1986; 112: 290–296

61 The Evolution of Pediatric Otolaryngology–Head and Neck Surgery

Robin A. Dyleski

The specialty of otolaryngology encompasses the medical and surgical management of diseases and conditions involving the head and neck. In recent years, the specialty has branched out into various areas of interest, such as facial plastic and reconstructive surgery, otology and neurotology, otolaryngic allergy, voice and laryngology, rhinology, head and neck cancer, and pediatric otolaryngology. Each of these subspecialties evolved to fill a niche created by various advances in technology and the need for dedicated specialists with distinct areas of expertise to care for certain subsets of patients.

Pediatric otolaryngology is a relatively new subspecialty, formally recognized for the last 25 to 30 years. It is a field dedicated to providing care mainly to infants and children younger than 18 years of age. Fellowship training in pediatric otolaryngology has been available in a formal manner for the last two to three decades; previously, this training was available only as an apprenticeship or as a focused interest. Although there has been interest in the care of otolaryngologic problems in children for decades (with pediatric patients comprising a large component of the typical general otolaryngologist's practice), pediatric otolaryngology took hold as a recognized subspecialty as a consequence of technologic advances in the survival of preterm newborns. These paralleled the development of dedicated children's hospitals providing subspecialized pediatric care in anesthesiology, cardiothoracic surgery, pulmonary medicine, critical care medicine, neonatology, and genetics to address the unique problems of sick children. Advances in neonatal medicine have saved the lives of many children who would not otherwise have survived but have left them with secondary problems.

Pharmacologic and technical advances have been instrumental in the development of pediatric otolaryngology as a subspecialty. The introduction of mechanical ventilators and advanced monitoring equipment for use in children in the early 1960s was an important step leading to the development of pediatric intensive care units. This progress in pediatric critical care led to the use of prolonged oral and nasotracheal intubation in infants and children instead of the then-standard tracheotomy with mechanical ventilation. As a result, otolaryngologists specializing in pediatric care became indispensable to physicians specializing in pediatric critical care for managing their patients' airways. The rising use of prolonged endotracheal intubation in the 1960s and 1970s was associated with increased rates of subglottic stenosis in these sick children.

The management of children with subglottic stenosis was radicalized with advances in endoscopic evaluation technology. In the mid 1960s, Harold H. Hopkins in England and Karl Storz in Germany collaborated to devise a unique rod–lens optical system in which fiber optics were used to transport light. A series of glass rods improved resolution and provided a brighter illumination system, resulting in a smaller-diameter instrument with a wider viewing angle. Hopkins and Storz introduced the new illumination system into pediatric bronchoscopy in 1968.

One of the pioneers in endoscopy in the United States, Dr. Sylvan Stool, was given a set of these new endoscopic instruments by Dr. C. Everett Koop (later to become the U.S. Surgeon General) in Philadelphia. Soon afterward, airway endoscopy in children was revolutionized by these instruments, and the development of accessories such as specialized endoscopic scissors and forceps (including optical forceps in which a telescope was incorporated) made possible procedures and interventions that could not have been performed previously. Advanced light sources, endoscopic cameras (allowing video and digital capture of the procedure and digital photo documentation), and microinstruments have permitted improvements in care and are routinely used today. Today's modern laryngoscopes, bronchoscopes, forceps, and cameras have brought pediatric otolaryngology to its current level.

62 The Otolaryngologic Examination of Children

Robin A. Dyleski

62.1 Introduction

As in all areas of otolaryngology, an appropriately detailed and focused history and examination are the basis of an accurate diagnosis and the subsequent treatment of pediatric illnesses and diseases. Because of the inability of many young children to readily and accurately communicate their symptoms and reliance upon their caregivers for this information, this information may be difficult to acquire. In addition, although the pediatric patient's examination is basically similar to the head and neck examination in older children and adults, there are a number of ways in which the examination of young children can be facilitated to make the process easier for the child, caregiver, and examiner.

62.2 Approaching the Young Patient

Many children are frightened by a visit to a doctor's office, and an otolaryngologist's office is no different, especially given the amount of unfamiliar equipment and instruments that are often visible in the otolaryngologist's examining room. Engaging the young child and gentle reassurance at the outset of the encounter is often calming and leads to great rewards during the examination phase.

With some children, no special approach will be needed, whereas others will favorably respond to explanations of what each of our diagnostic tools is and how they work. When a nonthreatening approach is used, the child can be fully examined without the examination becoming a traumatic event for all.

62.3 The Examination

Many physicians will proceed with the examination after obtaining the history, review of systems, and related family and social histories. The examination of the pediatric patient begins during the verbal parts of the encounter. Important facets of the child's condition should be observed, such as the following: presence and quality of the child's speech, the child's interactions with others, his or her breathing pattern while awake or asleep, the presence of stridor and other airway noises, possible swallowing functions for liquids and/or solids (snacks), and gait. These components sometimes can be observed only in a clandestine manner because children are highly likely not to speak when you need to hear their voice or speech, diminishing the information obtained in the examination.

62.3.1 Conducting the Examination

Although many children will readily sit in the examination chair themselves, others will require assistance from their caregiver. Many children will have to be held on the parent's lap for reassurance, and the parent's assistance may be needed for restraining them, so that the examination can proceed and the

children will be prevented from becoming injured if they are unable to remain still. There are a number of ways that children can be held to facilitate their examination.

The basic position for a child during examination is seated across one parent's thigh. If necessary, the child's legs can be restrained by the parent's thighs by having the parent cross his or her ankles; at the same time, the child's torso and arms are held with one hand and the head is steadied against the parent's chest by the parent's other hand. This technique can be used for infants and relatively calm children until the age of 4 or 5 years during many therapeutic maneuvers (cerumen removal) and diagnostic evaluations (fiber-optic laryngoscopy). When a child who is completely uncooperative with the examination is much older than 4 or 5 years, it becomes increasingly difficult to "hold" him or her in this way.

Other, more constraining apparatus is available for children who cannot be suitably held with the "parent lap hold" technique. In one method used for smaller children, a sheet is used to wrap their arms and legs close to the body in "papoose" style. This device consists of a board on which the patient is placed with the arms by the sides; strong Velcro straps are wrapped over and immobilize the patient. The papoose maneuver gives ready access to the head, which is carefully stabilized by a parent or nurse to allow the uncooperative child to be treated or examined. Wrapping the child snugly in a sheet often can provide similar results. With the child stabilized, the examination or even minor procedures may proceed safely without inadvertent injury to the moving child.

62.3.2 Otologic Examination

Most pediatric otolaryngologic examinations include a thorough examination of the outer ear, ear canal, and tympanic membrane with a hand-held otoscope—either an operating otoscope or a pneumatic otoscope with an insufflation bulb. Regardless of which is chosen, the otoscope is held with the first three fingers, while the fourth and fifth finger are braced against the child's temple (▶ Fig. 62.1). Should the child move suddenly, the instrument cannot penetrate more deeply into the canal.

The insufflating otoscope is the preferred instrument because it allows evaluation of the mobility of the tympanic membrane and enhances the detection of middle ear effusions. A tuning fork evaluation of hearing and the Weber and Rinne tests are performed in older children with suspected hearing impairment, as indicated. Microscopic examination is performed when indicated.

62.3.3 Nasal Examination

The nasal examination is usually performed via anterior rhinoscopy; often, the otoscope with either the nasal tip or the large ear speculum is used. Attention to the size, color, and contour of the turbinates, septum, secretions, and nasal airway patency are important facets of the nasal examination in children. The

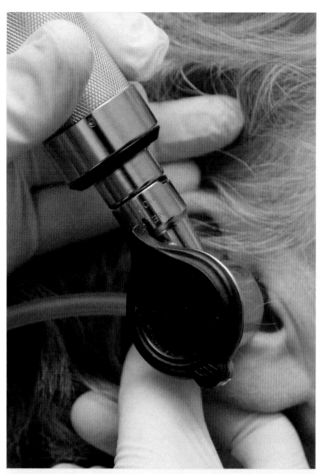

Fig. 62.1 The hand holding the otoscope is braced against the temple, maintaining the distance between the instrument and the ear.

examination may include a comparison of nasal examinations in the decongested and nondecongested states. Observation for intranasal secretions, prominent blood vessels, polyps, masses, and foreign bodies is made. In some children, flexible nasopharyngoscopy may be needed to visualize completely the nasal and nasopharygeal structures.

62.3.4 Oral Examination

The oral examination includes inspection of the lips, mucosal surfaces, tongue, floor of the mouth, and oropharynx. This may be performed with a flashlight or headlight. Generally, children are cooperative with this part of the examination and readily open the mouth in anticipation of the "tongue stick." Tongue shape and movement, the floor of the mouth, palatine tonsil size, uvula shape, and soft palate contour and mobility are noted. The superior aspect of the epiglottis is often seen during the normal oral examination in children.

62.3.5 Neck Examination

The neck examination in children focuses on the presence of any swellings, masses, or asymmetries. The location, firmness, mobility, and size of any mass are noted. Lymph node size, consistency, and position are compared with those in the opposite side of the neck. The thyroid gland is palpated for enlargement and masses. The neck skin is inspected for any congenital lesions, pits, or sinus tracts.

62.3.6 Airway Examination

The laryngeal and hypopharyngeal airway is examined when indicated with flexible fiber-optic laryngoscopy. This is safely accomplished in children in the office setting through either an anesthetized nostril or the oral cavity (in infants without teeth). The flexible fiber-optic laryngoscope may also be used to inspect the nose and nasopharynx for masses, polyps, and adenoid size. The procedure usually will require the child to be restrained by the parent, papoose board, or a sheet wrapped around the child. This is the most invasive portion of the head and neck examination and will require that older children be able to remain still during the examination. An explanation of the process and the adequate use of topical nasal anesthetics are usually all that is necessary for older children to permit the examination to proceed.

The entire airway from the nostrils to the subglottic area can be visualized with the fiber-optic laryngoscope. The color and condition of the mucosal membranes, the presence of any masses, and the configuration and appearance of the nasal structures, adenoids, eustachian tube orifices, oropharynx, hypopharynx, and larynx should all be assessed in this examination.

62.4 Roundsmanship

- The pediatric ear, nose, and throat (ENT) examination should include observation of the child while the history is being elicited, when details of the patient's speech, apparent hearing, gait and coordination, swallowing, and breathing can be assessed.
- The pediatric ENT examination should be performed in a calm, nonthreatening manner.
- An uncooperative patient can be restrained by the caregiver or a papoose to prevent inadvertent injury to the patient and allow the examination to proceed.
- Parts of the examination requiring restraint should be reserved for the end of the evaluation.

62.5 Recommended Reading

[1] Cook SP. Examination room design for the pediatric otolaryngology practice. Laryngoscope 1996; 106: 1049–1050

63 Special Considerations in Pediatric Anesthesiology

Rebecca L. Bagdonas

63.1 Introduction

Pediatric anesthesiology encompasses the pre-, intra-, and postoperative care of neonates through adolescence. Although many anesthetic techniques and pharmacologic agents are the same in both pediatric and adult populations, there are many differences with regard to their use and application. Children differ from adults in many respects, including anatomy, physiology, and most commonly seen diseases. In the care of a child, consideration of the concerns of the parent plays an important role because the interaction with the child's parent can be even more complex than the interaction with an adult patient.

63.2 Preoperative Concerns

The immune system of the young child is not fully developed, making children more susceptible to communicable diseases such as upper respiratory infections, strep throat, conjunctivitis, and otitis media. Often, these diseases are the very reason for the operative procedure (e.g., tonsillectomy or the placement of tympanostomy tubes).

Upper and lower respiratory tract infections, even 2 to 4 weeks before surgery, often lead to an increase in airway secretions, hypoxemia, and airway hyperreactivity, raising the risk for intraoperative laryngospasm and bronchospasm. The duration and symptoms of these common viral infections must always be evaluated because the severity of the upper respiratory symptoms may mean the difference between proceeding with and postponing the surgery. Additionally, an assessment of the child's birth history, including method of delivery (vaginal vs cesarean delivery, with reasons for the latter), prematurity versus full-term gestation, birth weight, perinatal hospitalization (including neonatal intensive care), and any genetic, cardiac, or pulmonary conditions, is of the utmost importance in planning safe anesthesia. It is important to determine if the patient has had any problems with prior anesthetics or if there are familial problems with anesthesia, especially symptoms compatible with malignant hyperthermia.

63.3 Pediatric Airway Anatomy, Metabolism, and Anesthetic Agents

The general shape of the pediatric airway is different from that of the adult airway. The pediatric airway is more conical than the adult airway, which is more cylindrical. In children, the airway is positioned more anteriorly and cephalad. The pediatric larynx and epiglottic cartilage are thinner and more collapsible. The narrowest point in the larynx of a child is at the cricoid cartilage (until the age of 5 years), as opposed to the vocal cords in an adult. Infants have a relatively large tongue for the size of their mouth and a relatively larger occiput, which can make positioning for airway support more difficult. In addition, neonates have fewer lung alveoli, decreased lung compliance, and increased chest wall compliance, which lead to decreased lung functional residual capacity (FRC) and resultant decreased oxygen reserves, culminating in hypoxemia and atelectasis during periods of apnea.

Alveolar ventilation in neonates, infants, and toddlers is greater than in adults. This, combined with increased blood flow to vessel-rich organs such as the brain and heart, leads to faster induction with inhaled anesthetics and a more rapid emergence from anesthesia. The minimum alveolar concentration (MAC) of inhaled anesthetics is at a peak in the infant period. The MAC decreases from infancy onward.

Cardiac output in neonates and infants relies on the heart rate, as opposed to the stroke volume. The pediatric patient has a relatively immature and noncompliant left ventricle that is unable to increase the cardiac output. The heart rate is more significant than the mean arterial blood pressure. The heart rate peaks in the neonatal period; rates of 120 to 160 beats/min are normal. The normal heart rate decreases as the child ages, with heart rates of 100 to 120 beats/min observed in infants and of 80 to 100 beats/min in 3- to 5-year-olds.

Temperature regulation is extremely important in children. The ratio of body surface area to weight is increased in neonates, and they have few fat stores; these characteristics, combined with the cold environment of the operating room and unheated anesthetic gases, render them more susceptible to hypothermia. It is important to monitor the body core temperature with a temperature monitor, to use body-warming devices like the Bair hugger blanket (Arizant, Eden Prairie, MN), and to warm the ambient operating room temperature for these patients. Hypothermia results in respiratory depression, delayed emergence/awakening from anesthesia, and increased pulmonary vascular resistance. The anesthesiologist must also monitor the patient for hyperthermia, or unexpected increase in body core temperature. Hyperthermia is an important indicator of malignant hyperthermia (although it is usually a late sign in the development of the disease).

Separation anxiety and generalized fear of the operating room are common in the pediatric population. Thus, many hospitals and ambulatory surgery centers permit the child's parent to be present during the induction of general anesthesia ("parent-present induction"). The parent's role is to reassure the child in the unfamiliar operating room environment, which permits a calmer and smoother anesthetic experience for the child. In some cases, a preoperative sedative may be used, such as midazolam (0.5 mg/kg orally 30 minutes before the procedure), to calm the child. This is commonly done for children with a high level of anxiety or for those with certain medical conditions, such as congenital heart disease. Another option is intramuscular ketamine for highly anxious children.

63.4 Intraoperative Management

Standard anesthesia monitoring is applied for all pediatric patients and includes three- or five-lead electrocardiography, pulse oximetry, noninvasive blood pressure monitoring, capnography, and temperature monitoring. Inhalational induction is administered by face mask with a combination of oxygen, nitrous oxide, and anesthetic gas. Sevoflurane is the most commonly used volatile anesthetic; it provides a smoother induction because it is less likely to cause airway irritability and cough than the other volatile anesthetics. After the child is asleep, the intravenous (IV) line is placed (especially in ambulatory patients), and other medications, such as atropine, analgesics/narcotics, and propofol, are administered before endotracheal intubation.

It is important to use the proper size of endotracheal tube in children because airway irritation and swelling from the use of an oversized tube leads to increased airway resistance after extubation. Uncuffed endotracheal tubes are often used in pediatric patients for this reason. The leak around the endotracheal tube is confirmed and optimally is between 18 and 24 cm H_2O. General formulas for endotracheal tube size include $(4 + age)/4$ or a size similar to the size of the distal phalanx of the pinky finger. After the endotracheal tube is secured, the patient's eyes are taped closed, the stomach is decompressed with a catheter, and all pressure points are padded.

A commonly used neuromuscular relaxant, succinylcholine, is much less frequently used in pediatric than in adult patients. Although it is a reliable depolarizing muscle relaxant and can quickly terminate laryngospasm, it is much more likely in children to cause hyperkalemia, rhabdomyolysis, muscle/masseter spasm, and cardiac arrhythmias (including bradycardia leading to cardiac arrest). It is also known to be a triggering agent in malignant hyperthermia.

The maintenance of anesthesia involves IV fluid management, the administration of inhalational gases, and the IV administration of medications such as antibiotics, steroids, antiemetics, and narcotics. Fluid management is crucial in pediatric cases because there is a slim margin of error in pediatric fluid balance. The calculation of maintenance fluids in children is based upon the patient's weight. The 4–2–1 rule is followed for all cases of standard pediatric fluid maintenance and for determining the fluid deficit incurred while the child's status is NPO (nil per os): 4 mL/kg/h for the first 10 kg + 2 mL/kg/h for the next 10 kg + 1 mL/kg/h for weight over 20 kg.

In neonates, hypovolemia manifests as hypotension, but without concurrent tachycardia. Neonates also require dextrose in their IV fluids, whereas older infants and children can receive isotonic fluids, such as lactated Ringer solution or normal saline. Excess free water, associated with hypotonic fluids, can easily led to hyponatremia, seizures, coma, and death if liberally administered, especially when there is a protracted loss of electrolyte-rich fluids (e.g., prolonged emesis).

As the surgical procedure nears completion, preparations are made for emergence and extubation. Narcotics may be titrated; the patient is weaned off the ventilator, spontaneous ventilation resumes, and reversal agents for muscle relaxation agents are given (if appropriate). It is extremely important to extubate the patient while either deeply anesthetized or in the fully awakened state to decrease the risk for laryngospasm (spasm of the laryngeal musculature that can lead to total airway obstruction). The in-between stage of anesthesia, often referred to as "stage II," is a dangerous time for extubating the patient because the airway is the most reactive at this time. IV lidocaine (1 mg/kg) is also beneficial to decrease the likelihood of laryngospasm.

If laryngospasm occurs, positive-pressure ventilation via mask is applied and will frequently cause the episode to cease. If the laryngospasm is refractory to positive pressure, succinylcholine may be given as a rescue drug. Once the airway patency is reestablished and ventilation restored, the patient is observed as oxygen saturation is maintained without support and taken to the postanesthesia care unit (PACU). In the PACU, the monitors are replaced, supplemental oxygen is given, and the vital signs are closely monitored.

Children undergo ambulatory surgery more commonly than in the past, when inpatient stays were frequent. Postoperative discharge criteria include adequate pain control, absence of nausea and vomiting, ability to void and ambulate, and adequate oral intake of fluids. Special consideration is given to premature and very young infants. Premature children who are less than 46 weeks past conception age are at increased risk for central apnea after general anesthesia because of the immature neurologic development of premature children. These patients require airway monitoring for at least 12 hours after anesthesia. When the child is between 46 and 60 weeks past conception age, the required monitoring period is at least 6 hours unless there are coexisting significant neurologic, cardiac, or pulmonary conditions, which require at least 12 hours of observation.

63.5 Pain Management

Many drugs in the pain management arsenal for adults may be used in the pediatric population. These medications include fentanyl, morphine, codeine, and oxycodone. Oxycodone is an excellent oral medication for children who require postoperative pain management. Acetaminophen is frequently given as a rectal suppository (30 to 40 mg/kg) at the time of induction and is noted to reduce narcotic requirements postoperatively. Codeine may be administered either orally (with or without acetaminophen) or rectally at a dose of 1 mg/kg every 6 hours as needed. Up to 10% of people lack the enzyme required to convert codeine into morphine, so that the effectiveness of codeine is not uniform, and this must be considered in patients whose pain is inadequately controlled with codeine. Conversely, an estimated 1 to 7% of patients are "ultra-high metabolizers," with DNA mutations in cytochrome P-450 2D6 that enhance the conversion of codeine to morphine and lead to elevated blood levels of morphine; the minimum doses of codeine should be used, especially in patients undergoing adenotonsillectomy for obstructive symptoms.

63.6 Fasting and NPO Guidelines

The preoperative fasting status (nil per os, or NPO) is very different in children than in adults. In general, patients are kept NPO to decrease the risk for aspiration and pulmonary complications during anesthesia. Neonates and infants up to 3 years old are physiologically more prone to dehydration and hypovolemia than older children are, and therefore their NPO requirements are shorter to reduce the risk for significant dehydration during the fasting period. Babies may be given clear liquids such as water, Pedialyte (Abbott Laboratories, Columbus, OH), or clear apple juice up to 2 hours before the onset of general anesthesia; this has been demonstrated to increase gastric

Table 63.1 NPO guidelines for children undergoing general anesthesia

Patient age	Clear liquids	Breast milk	Formula/full liquids
Birth–6 months	2 h	4 h	6 h
6–36 months	2 h	6 h	6 h
>36 months	2 h	6 h	6–8 h

emptying, leading to a lower gastric residual volume and lower risk for aspiration. Human breast milk is also quickly absorbed and moved from the stomach into the small intestine; it requires a 4-hour fasting period. Infant formula and nonhuman milk require a 6-hour NPO period in children up to 36 months old. At 36 months and older, children are expected to fast for a minimum of 8 hours for all full liquids (such as milk) and all solids; however, clear liquids (in limited quantities) may be given up to 2 hours before the anesthetic (▶ Table 63.1).

63.7 Complications of Anesthesia

The most commonly seen complications in the pediatric population are respiratory in origin, with laryngospasm encountered most often. Other potential perioperative problems in children undergoing anesthesia include bronchospasm, "postintubation croup," and negative-pressure pulmonary edema (also called postoperative pulmonary edema, or POPE). Bronchospasm is an abnormal spasm or constriction of the bronchi and bronchioles. Bronchospasm is often seen in persons who have hyperreactive irritable airways, with patients who have asthma and those who have had a recent viral respiratory illness at greatest risk. It manifests with wheezing, hypoxemia, and poor ventilation despite an adequate airway because it is due to spasm in the bronchi and larger bronchioles. Bronchospasm is treated with inhaled bronchodilators and the subcutaneous injection of terbutaline, a β_2-agonist. In refractory cases, an isoproterenol infusion can be used to break the airway spasm, in addition to the continued administration of inhaled anesthetic agents, which have potent bronchodilator properties.

"Postintubation croup" predominantly affects children ages 1 to 4 years and manifests as inspiratory stridor and a harsh cough following intubation for a surgical procedure. It is caused by localized edema or mucosal swelling in the airway, primarily subglottic, resulting from the presence of the endotracheal tube. In most cases it is self-limited and may respond to nebulized racemic epinephrine or IV steroids. The risk for postintubation croup increases with the use of inappropriately large endotracheal tubes, repeated attempts at intubation with subsequent airway trauma, repeated manipulation of the endotracheal tube, relatively long surgical procedures, and certain head and neck procedures.

Negative-pressure pulmonary edema (POPE) is an uncommon, potentially life-threatening condition caused by upper airway obstruction. POPE occurs most often during the induction of or emergence from anesthesia and affects mostly healthy patients without underlying cardiopulmonary pathology. It is estimated to occur in up to 10 to 15% of patients who have an episode of upper airway obstruction requiring intervention.

Risk factors for upper airway obstruction include a history of obstructive sleep apnea, the presence of known airway lesions, and anatomically difficult intubations, as well as nasal, oral, and laryngeal surgical procedures. POPE results from the generation of a highly negative intrathoracic pressure by forceful inspiration against an obstructed airway or closed glottis (sometimes from laryngospasm). The result of the negative intrathoracic pressure is a transudation of pulmonary interstitial fluid into the alveolar space. Signs and symptoms of respiratory distress include oxygen desaturation, hypoxemia, and chest retractions. Copious pink, frothy secretions and sputum are the hallmark of POPE and are seen in the endotracheal tube. Rales and wheezing are heard on auscultation, secondary to the fluid-filled airways. Tachycardia, bradycardia, hypertension, and diaphoresis are also often present. A chest X-ray demonstrates diffuse, bilateral interstitial and alveolar infiltrates and areas of "whiteout" in the lung fields. POPE is treated with supplemental oxygen, positive-pressure ventilation using positive end-expiratory pressure (PEEP) in intubated patients, or continuous positive airway pressure (CPAP) in extubated patients. The routine administration of diuretics has not been proved to correct POPE, but it may aid in the management of systemic fluid overload. The main goals are to reverse hypoxemia and decrease the fluid in the lungs. Resolution is usually rapid after diagnosis and the start of treatment, and most cases resolve within 24 hours or sooner. Prompt diagnosis and treatment are essential to avoid long-term sequelae.

63.8 Surgery-Specific Anesthesia Concerns

Tonsillectomy and adenoidectomy: Although it is such a common operation, children undergoing tonsillectomy and adenoidectomy (T + A) are at high risk for perioperative airway problems. The T + A procedure is best performed when the child is as free from respiratory symptoms as possible, and postponement is recommended if the patient has an acute infection or upper respiratory infection. Major complication of T + A include postoperative bleeding, laryngospasm, and POPE. Postoperative bleeding from the tonsillar fossa is a true emergency, and control of the hemorrhage is mandatory, with general anesthesia usually required. Patients with oropharyngeal hemorrhage are treated as though they have a full stomach and undergo rapid-sequence induction to minimize the risk for aspiration. After the airway is secured and the hemorrhage controlled, the stomach is suctioned to reduce the risk for aspiration at extubation.

Tympanostomy tubes: The induction of anesthesia via inhalation and the maintenance of anesthesia with a face mask comprise the technique usually used for the placement of tympanostomy tubes in children. Depending upon the presence of comorbid conditions and the ease or difficulty of face mask ventilation in the child, the placement of an IV line may be needed for the administration of medication.

Emergence delirium: Emergence delirium is seem in the pediatric population and is a side effect of sevofluorane administration. Studies have shown that the administration of IV propofol at the end of the case after the termination of sevofluorane will reduce the likelihood of emergence delirium.

63.9 Roundsmanship

- The normal neonatal heart rate is 120 to 160 beats/min; in infants, the normal rate is between 100 and 120 beats/min, while the normal heart rate of 3- to 5-year-olds is 80 to 100 beats/min.
- Endotracheal tube selection for children is approximated by the formula $(4 + age)/4$.
- Standard pediatric fluid maintenance for children with NPO status is calculated as follows: 4 mL/kg/h for the first 10 kg + 2 mL/kg/h for the next 10 kg + 1 mL/kg/h for weight over 20 kg.
- Premature children who are less than 46 weeks past conception age are at increased risk for central apnea after general anesthesia and require airway monitoring for at least 12 hours after anesthesia. Children between 46 and 60 weeks past conception age should be monitored postoperatively for at least 6 hours unless they have coexisting significant neurologic, cardiac, or pulmonary conditions, which require at least 12 hours of observation.
- Bronchospasm is treated with inhaled bronchodilators and the subcutaneous injection of terbutaline. In refractory cases, isoproterenol infusion can be used to break the airway spasm.
- Postoperative pulmonary edema (POPE) is treated with supplemental oxygen, positive-pressure ventilation using positive end-expiratory pressure (PEEP) if the patient is intubated, or continuous positive airway pressure (CPAP) if patient has been extubated.

63.10 Recommended Reading

[1] American Society of Anesthesiologists Committee. Practice guidelines for preoperative fasting and the use of pharmacologic agents to reduce the risk of pulmonary aspiration: application to healthy patients undergoing elective procedures: an updated report by the American Society of Anesthesiologists Committee on Standards and Practice Parameters. Anesthesiology 2011; 114: 495–511

[2] FDA Drug Safety Communication. Codeine use in certain children after tonsillectomy and/or adenoidectomy may lead to rare, but life-threatening adverse events or death. http://www.fda.gov/Drugs/DrugSafety/ucm313631.htm. Accessed October 28, 2013

[3] Hippard HK, Govindan K, Friedman EM et al. Postoperative analgesic and behavioral effects of intranasal fentanyl, intravenous morphine, and intramuscular morphine in pediatric patients undergoing bilateral myringotomy and placement of ventilating tubes. Anesth Analg 2012; 115: 356–363

[4] Pieters BJ, Penn E, Nicklaus P, Bruegger D, Mehta B, Weatherly R. Emergence delirium and postoperative pain in children undergoing adenotonsillectomy: a comparison of propofol vs sevoflurane anesthesia. Paediatr Anaesth 2010; 20: 944–950

[5] Morgan GE, Mikhail MS, Murray MJ. Pediatric anesthesia. In: Lange clinical anesthesiology, 4th ed. New York: McGraw-Hill, 2005

64 Common Genetic Syndromes in Otolaryngology

Morgan R. Bliss, Harlan R. Muntz, and Alan F. Rope

64.1 Introduction

A syndrome is a nonrandom pattern of anomalies that can be attributed to an identifiable genetic or environmental etiology or is heritable. A syndrome may have more than one etiology, with dozens of genes identified that are connected to that syndrome. No single feature is ever pathognomonic for a syndrome because syndromes are characterized by variable expression. The human genome consists of 46 human chromosomes containing approximately 23,000 protein-encoding genes, and knowledge of the pathophysiology of genetic syndromes is rapidly improving. Some syndromes have yet to be named. The initial definition of a syndrome requires astute observers to publish case series or reports of individuals with multiple anomalies. Most consider an anomaly to be associated with a syndrome if it occurs in 10 to 15% of individuals with the syndrome.

One study showed that in 119 infants with multiple congenital anomalies involving otolaryngologic defects, 51% were due to an unknown cause, 25% to a chromosomal anomaly, 10% to an identified mendelian condition, 3% to a known exposure to a teratogen, and 10% to a recognized pattern of defects of unknown cause. In mendelian inheritance, monogenic dominant or recessive traits are inherited from parents in a predictable manner. Recessive traits require two alleles for expression, whereas dominant traits are expressed if one allele is inherited. X-linked traits may be dominant or recessive, but they will be expressed in males regardless of whether they are dominant because males have a single X chromosome. The trait will be expressed in females with two recessive X-linked alleles.

Most genetic disorders are polygenic and multifactorial and do not demonstrate mendelian inheritance patterns. Another reason for alterations in expected mendelian inheritance is incomplete penetrance. Penetrance is the proportion of individuals carrying a specific genotype who demonstrate the expected phenotype. Incomplete penetrance may be due to environmental factors or to other genes that regulate the expression of one gene. Variable expression of genes also complicates the picture of genetic heritability. Variable expression can cause differing phenotypes in individuals with the same genotype.

The otolaryngologist is an integral part of the multidisciplinary team required to optimally treat patients with genetic syndromes. Up to 3% of infants are born with a major anomaly that is diagnosed in the first year of life. Of infants with a syndrome, 84% will have an otolaryngologic anomaly. Some of the genetic syndromes associated with the most prominent anomalies of the head and neck include the following: Down syndrome (trisomy 21), 22q11 deletion syndrome (velocardiofacial syndrome), Treacher Collins syndrome, Beckwith-Wiedemann syndrome, and ocular–auricular–vertebral spectrum (OAV). An understanding of the pathophysiology, associated anomalies, and new developments in treatment avoids delays in diagnosis and leads to optimal outcomes.

64.2 Down Syndrome (Trisomy 21)

Down syndrome (trisomy 21) is the most common chromosomal syndrome (▶ Fig. 64.1). The incidence is considered to be about 1 in 700 to 1 in 1,000 live births, although Resta reports that it would affect 1 in 629 births without any prenatal intervention. Of the cases, 94% are due to trisomy of chromosome 21, which occurs during meiosis I, but occasional cases are due to translocation or mosaicism. The major risk factor for Down syndrome is advanced maternal age; whereas the risk is only 1 in 1,500 for mothers younger than 25 years of age, the risk increases to 1 in 10 for mothers older than 45 years of age. Other risk factors include a previous pregnancy complicated by trisomy and chromosomal translocations, inversion, or aneuploidy in either parent.

Typical features of Down syndrome (see ▶ Fig. 64.1) include characteristic craniofacial features: flat occiput, brachycephaly, upward-slanting palpebral fissures, hypertelorism, flat nasal bridge, stenotic external auditory canals, macroglossia, narrow palate, hypotonia, developmental delay, intellectual disability, excessive skin at the nape of the neck, hypertrophic tonsils, xerodermia, and single palmar creases with short metacarpals

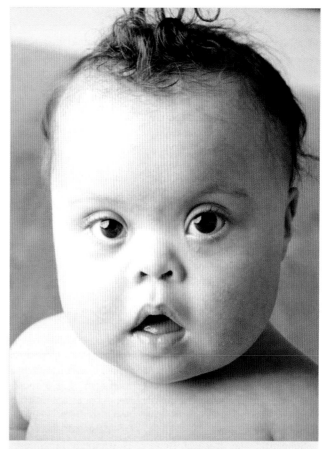

Fig. 64.1 Down syndrome.

and phalanges. Up to 60% of patients have associated cardiac anomalies. Affected individuals have an increased incidence of duodenal atresia, Hirschsprung disease, and imperforate anus, and 5% of patients have some type of gastrointestinal anomaly.

Hearing loss in individuals with Down syndrome is common; it may be conductive or sensorineural. A recent study of 432 children with Down syndrome in Utah found that 46.1% of the children had a conductive hearing loss. Past reports have found up to a 60% rate of conductive hearing loss in patients with Down syndrome. This is often due to serous otitis media, although up to 40% of children will have a persistent conductive hearing loss after the placement of pressure equalization (PE) tubes. The treatment and diagnosis of serous otitis media are complicated by stenotic external auditory canals, which are present in 40 to 50% of cases. A study from 2001 conducted at Cincinnati Children's Hospital found that 83% of children with Down syndrome younger than 2 years of age required PE tubes for chronic ear disease and persistent middle ear effusions. A study from 2003 showed that children with Down syndrome had a 3.6 times greater chance of having normal hearing when PE tubes were in place than when they were not. Eustachian tube dysfunction is common and may lead to the need for several tympanostomy procedures. Dysfunction of the eustachian tube is due to the poor quality of its cartilage and narrow diameter, and to hypotonia of the tensor veli palatini. Congenital sensorineural hearing loss also occurs in 3.6% of affected individuals.

Children with Down syndrome should have a newborn hearing screen with auditory brainstem response (ABR) and otoacoustic emission (OAE) testing and follow-up testing every 6 months up to the age of 3 years. Frequent examination under the microscope until 2 to 3 years of age is recommended in children with stenotic external auditory canals. Individuals with Down syndrome and any degree of hearing loss benefit from early intervention with hearing aids in order to improve the development of speech and cognition.

There are many anatomical sites that can lead to obstruction and airway difficulties in individuals with Down syndrome. Infants and young children with Down syndrome have difficulty controlling the tongue, resulting in tongue thrusting. This leads to problems with latching on during feeding and to glossoptosis; macroglossia is occasionally seen. Mandibular and maxillary hypoplasia, hypertrophic tonsils and adenoids, and general hypotonia may contribute to obstructive sleep apnea. Sleep apnea affects the majority of individuals with Down syndrome and increases the risk for pulmonary hypertension, even in the absence of cardiac anomalies. Parental observation is not a sensitive test for sleep apnea in this patient population. Adenotonsillectomy is the first-line treatment for children with sleep apnea, but 50% of children with Down syndrome will continue to have an abnormal sleep study after this surgery. Children with persistent apnea should begin continuous positive airway pressure (CPAP) therapy or should undergo further studies, such as cine sleep magnetic resonance (MR) imaging and sleep endoscopy, to evaluate the precise airway level of persistent obstruction. Further surgeries can then be tailored to the problematic anatomical location.

Subglottic and tracheal stenosis is common in children with Down syndrome, and an endotracheal tube two sizes smaller than expected should initially be used to size the airway. Intraoperatively, pulmonary hypoplasia can lead to difficulties with ventilation. Atlantoaxial instability is another factor complicating management of the airway in children with Down syndrome. Cervical flexion and extension spine films are helpful but are not entirely reliable predictors of this anomaly in young children because of incomplete calcification of bone. For this reason, hyperextension of the neck should never be performed, and overall movement of the head during surgical procedures should be minimized. Furthermore, a complete neurologic examination should be conducted in the preoperative period to obtain a baseline.

Ideally, the approach to caring for a patient with Down syndrome begins prenatally. Screening may take place in the first or second trimester of pregnancy with serum testing and ultrasound. Prenatal diagnosis allows the medical staff to prepare for possible complications at delivery, and the family and caregivers to prepare for early aggressive interventions to optimize outcome. Echocardiography at birth is essential to detect congenital cardiac anomalies and plan possible cardiac procedures that may prevent long-term sequelae of undetected cardiac anomalies. Other screenings at birth should include a newborn hearing screen and screening for hypothyroidism. Up to 30% of children with Down syndrome will ultimately develop thyroid dysfunction; hypothyroidism is more common than hyperthyroidism. The thyroid-stimulating hormone and free T_4 levels should be checked at birth and 6 months of age, and then annually.

Patients with Down syndrome may require a psychological or psychiatric evaluation for the diagnosis and treatment of coexisting depression, anxiety, autism, or attention deficit. Developmental delay and intellectual disability are typical of the diagnosis, and children require regular evaluation to determine placement in appropriate educational classrooms and activity groups. Diet should be managed with consideration for the increased incidence of constipation and obesity.

Aggressive intervention is required not only at the time of initial diagnosis but also throughout the life of a person with Down syndrome. Even in the absence of other congenital anomalies, many individuals with Down syndrome will develop problems later in life: cardiac valve anomalies; autoimmune disorders; neoplastic processes such as leukemia, lymphoma, and testicular tumors; cataracts; and an increased rate of infections. The close surveillance required to detect multiple possible disease processes highlights the importance of a primary care provider who is able to coordinate care throughout the child's life and ensure that all appropriate tests and specialist consultations are carried out. Epidemiologic and outcomes research is rapidly expanding in this area, and dedicated physicians will ensure that individuals with Down syndrome are monitored and treated according to the most current evidence-based practices.

64.3 Chromosome 22q11.2 Deletion Syndrome (Velocardiofacial Syndrome)

Chromosome 22q11.2 microdeletions are responsible for what is commonly called DiGeorge syndrome, velocardiofacial

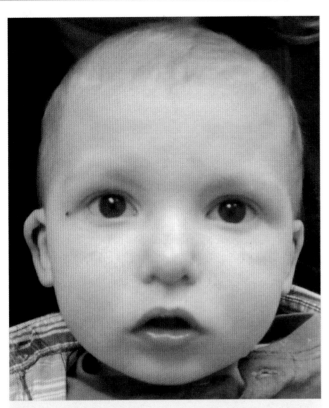

Fig. 64.2 Velocardiofacial syndrome in a patient with a bulbous nasal tip; narrow nares; small, cupped ears; and short, upward-slanting palpebral fissures.

syndrome, and a number of other well-characterized phenotypes (▶ Fig. 64.2). This is due to the highly variable expression of the same genotype. DiGeorge syndrome classically manifests with conotruncal cardiac anomalies, varying degrees of immune dysfunction/immunodeficiency, and distinctive facial features. Immunodeficiency may be seen with either a normal or an absent thymus, but some children without a thymus may have a normal immune system. Velocardiofacial syndrome is characterized by velopharyngeal insufficiency and/or incompetence, conotruncal cardiac anomalies, learning disabilities, and characteristic facial features. The incidence of the 22q11.2 microdeletion is 1 in 4,000 to 5,000 live births, and 85 to 90% of cases are due to a spontaneous deletion. This results in aberrant development of the third and fourth pharyngeal arches and pouches. The diagnosis is confirmed by fluorescence in situ hybridization (FISH) testing of targets in the critical region of chromosome 22q11.2.

In general, DiGeorge syndrome and velocardiofacial syndrome are actually the same entity, although some consider DiGeorge syndrome to be a worse phenotype. The 22q11.2 microdeletion causes a wide range of phenotypes, but approximately 50% of patients will have some major cardiac anomaly. Although this is easily diagnosed in infancy, other phenotypic traits are more difficult to detect until later in life. Velopharyngeal insufficiency and incompetence, as well as speech and language delay, may not be recognized until the child begins to attend school or day care. Chronic middle ear disease may also be present. A retrospective review from Children's Hospital of Philadelphia found that 76% of cases with 22q11.2 microdeletion had velopharyngeal insufficiency. In the absence of cardiovascular malformations or the Robin anomaly, this condition is very challenging to ascertain in the neonatal period. Affected individuals may demonstrate only abnormal palpebral fissures, hypertelorism, unusual ears, and a small mouth, but these are not specific for 22q11.2 deletion syndrome, and a high index of suspicion is required for early and accurate diagnosis. Hypocalcemia secondary to hypoparathyroidism in infancy can be a particularly important trait that allows a clinician to fit the clinical picture together.

Other otolaryngologic manifestations are variably expressed. Typical nasal anomalies include a bulbous nasal tip, a thickened nasal bridge, narrow nares, and a prominent nasal root. The most common auricular abnormality is an overfolded helix. The ears may also be small, posteriorly rotated, and protuberant, with a thickened helix or cupped shape. Common eye abnormalities include hooded eyelids, epicanthal folds, hypertelorism, and short, upward-slanting palpebral fissures. There are over 180 reported symptoms of 22q11 microdeletion, so this list is not exhaustive. Currently, there is no proven explanation for the large degree of variability in the expression of this genotype.

Sensorineural hearing loss is not a typical manifestation of 22q11.2 deletion syndrome, but conductive hearing loss is common. This is often due to chronic otitis media resulting from the palatal abnormality. Chronic otitis media is present in 40 to 75% of patients with 22q11.2 deletion syndrome.

Delayed speech and language development is one of the most pervasive features of 22q11.2 deletion syndrome and is due to a combination of overall developmental delay, velopharyngeal insufficiency/incompetence, and conductive hearing loss. Velopharyngeal insufficiency/incompetence is detected by hypernasality on perceptual analysis and by constant nasal air loss during phonation. In individuals with 22q11.2 deletion syndrome, velopharyngeal insufficiency/incompetence is most often due to a short velum, atonic velum, and/or a deep cavum, resulting in the inability of the soft palate to touch the posterior pharyngeal wall during speech. Other speech-related symptoms include poor articulation and overall unintelligibility. Overt cleft palate is present in a minority of cases, but a submucous or occult cleft may also contribute to difficulties in speech and swallowing.

Behavioral problems range from isolation to impulsiveness, hyperactivity, anxiety, and emotional lability. It is postulated that the inability to communicate effectively exacerbates these behavioral characteristics. Patients benefit from intervention with tympanostomy tubes and speech therapy.

Surgical procedures of the palate should be tailored to individual needs. Medially displaced carotid arteries are more common in 22q11.2 deletion syndrome than in the general population, and MR imaging of the neck has been suggested before pharyngoplasty, although this is controversial. Pulsation of the posterolateral pharyngeal wall is not sensitive or specific for abnormal orientation of the vasculature. Surgical options for the correction of velopharyngeal insufficiency include pharyngeal flap, sphincter pharyngoplasty, augmentation pharyngoplasty, and palatoplasty. Symptom improvement can be achieved nonsurgically with a palatal obturator or lift.

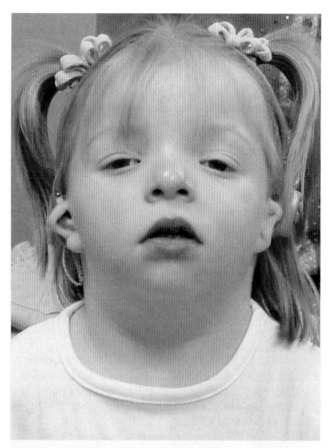

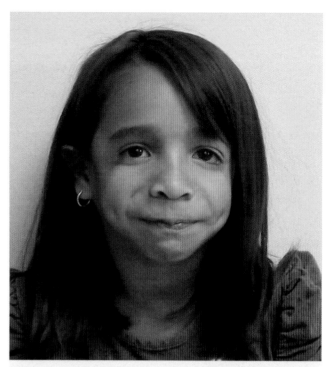

Fig. 64.4 Mild cases of Treacher Collins syndrome may manifest only mild depression of the zygoma and downward-slanted palpebral fissures.

Fig. 64.3 Some classic features of Treacher Collins syndrome are mandibular hypoplasia with retrognathia, downward-slanting palpebral fissures, and auricular deformities.

The outcomes of pharyngeal flap in a small group of children who had 22q11.2 deletion were compared with outcomes in a small group of children who had nonsyndromic, noncleft velopharyngeal insufficiency, and both groups were found to have excellent results 2 years after surgery, with no significant difference in quality of outcome. The patients with 22q11.2 microdeletion took longer to achieve excellent postoperative results than the nonsyndromic patients. Other studies have found that children with 22q11.2 deletion syndrome tend to require more revision procedures than nonsyndromic cases.

Velopharyngeal insufficiency may also affect the ability to swallow, and failure to thrive is common in infancy. A poor suck reflex and nasopharyngeal regurgitation may be due to the shortened or hypotonic palate. Airway anomalies are not a major manifestation of 22q11 microdeletion, although the degree of retrognathia should be considered in planning intubation and sedation/anesthetic procedures. Other laryngotracheal anomalies are more common in this population than in the general population, and any signs of airway obstruction or respiratory distress merit endoscopy for further evaluation.

Deaths in early childhood are almost always due to severe congenital heart disease or associated complications. This highlights the importance of lifelong aggressive medical monitoring and interventions to optimize overall health.

64.4 Treacher Collins Syndrome

Treacher Collins syndrome occurs in 1 in 25,000 to 1 in 50,000 live births and is inherited in an autosomal-dominant pattern with variable penetrance. Spontaneous gene mutations are the cause in 57% of cases. Deformities are due to the dysfunction of neural crest cells, resulting in the abnormal development of bone, cartilage, and connective tissue. Classic features include malar and mandibular hypoplasia with retrognathia, coloboma of the lateral one-third of the lower eyelid, sparse or absent eyelashes of the lower eyelid, and downward-slanting palpebral fissures. Auricular deformities are present in 85% of patients, as are middle ear deformities (▶ Fig. 64.3). Mild phenotypes may be detectable only by mild depression of the zygoma and by subtle downward slanting of the palpebral fissures. Some cases are detected only when computed tomography demonstrates the malar anomaly (▶ Fig. 64.4).

The airway requires special attention in individuals with Treacher Collins syndrome. Airway compromise is present at birth in 47% of cases. In most mild cases, the airway can be managed conservatively in infancy without tracheostomy. Positive-pressure mask ventilation, placement of a nasopharyngeal airway, and prone positioning may be sufficient to relieve symptoms of mild airway obstruction due to retrognathia and mandibular hypoplasia. Choanal atresia is also present in 11% of patients with Treacher Collins syndrome and complicates the already-difficult airway. A retrospective review of 30 individuals with Treacher Collins syndrome found that only 13% required tracheostomy in infancy and only 7% required emergent tracheostomy later in childhood. A smaller, earlier study from a different institution reported a 41% rate of tracheotomy in patients with mandibulofacial dysostosis, including individuals with Treacher Collins syndrome or Nager syndrome.

Obstructive sleep apnea is common in individuals with Treacher Collins syndrome, and polysomnography is suggested to obtain a baseline and evaluate severity. Adenotonsillectomy is an effective intervention for many individuals with Treacher Collins syndrome affected by obstructive sleep apnea, but many will continue to require the use of CPAP, and severe cases may require tracheostomy. Mandibular advancement with distraction osteogenesis may be performed before 10 years of age and enables decannulation in some children with airway obstruction and tracheostomy. Choanal atresia or stenosis also requires early repair. Genioplasty and hyoid advancement are reserved for refractory airway obstruction in children older than 12 years.

Conductive hearing loss is common, and one study of 46 cases found that the severity of hearing loss correlates with the degree of auricular deformity. Individuals with Treacher Collins syndrome should be counseled regarding the risks and benefits of auricular reconstruction versus an auricular prosthesis such as a bone-anchored hearing aid or a conventional hearing aid. Reconstructive surgery has typically achieved poorer outcomes for hearing in patients with Treacher Collins syndrome than in those with nonsyndromic cases of microtia. Prompt intervention for hearing loss within the first year of life enables children to begin to develop language. Speech and articulation are a challenge in almost 75% of children with Treacher Collins syndrome. Hyponasality occurs in most children with Treacher Collins syndrome because of the small size of the nasopharynx and oropharynx. However, almost one-third of affected children also have a cleft palate or velopharyngeal insufficiency and will instead demonstrate hypernasal speech. The timely repair of a cleft palate is more complicated in this population because of the coexisting difficult airway. The average age of children undergoing cleft palate repair is 2.1 years. Articulation problems also occur and are due to malocclusion and the posterior position of the tongue.

Individuals with Treacher Collins syndrome require multistage surgical treatment. Correcting the malar hypoplasia is one of the most challenging aspects of reconstruction because of the partial or complete resorption of grafts. Eyelid coloboma is corrected with a transposition flap from the upper to the lower eyelid, and downward-slanting palpebral fissures are corrected with bone grafting and lateral canthopexy at the time of the malar reconstruction. Rhinoplasty is performed in the teenage years to correct the prominent dorsal hump. Counseling affected individuals about realistic expectations for surgical outcomes is important. Many will require revision procedures to obtain an acceptable result, and some individuals have some residual dysmorphic features despite a full course of aggressive surgical treatment.

Affected individuals who are treated by a multidisciplinary team do well and are able to participate in all aspects of society into adulthood. Intellectual impairment is not expected with this disease process. Individuals with Treacher Collins syndrome may benefit from early diagnosis and airway management, foresight in overall surgical planning, and therapy to improve speech and manage the psychosocial aspects of coping with a rigorous treatment process.

64.5 Beckwith-Wiedemann Syndrome

Beckwith-Wiedemann syndrome (▶ Fig. 64.5) occurs in approximately 1 in 13,700 live births. The diagnosis is suggested clinically by the presence of three major features or of two major features and one minor feature of the syndrome. Major features include abdominal wall defects, macroglossia, macrosomia, anterior ear lobe creases or postauricular pits, visceromegaly, omphalocele, Wilms tumor, hepatoblastoma, hemihyperplasia, and specific renal abnormalities. Children are at risk for tumors, with an estimated 7.5% risk of tumor development within the first 8 to 10 years of life. Minor features include polyhydramnios, preterm delivery, neonatal hypoglycemia, nevus flammeus, cardiac anomalies, midface hypoplasia, suborbital creases or prominent mandible, diastasis recti, and advanced bone age. Other notable manifestations in the head and neck include prominent occiput, flattened nasal dorsum, and downward-slanting palpebral fissures.

Many features of the syndrome are attributed to the altered expression of genes located at chromosome 11p15.5, and 85% of cases are due to a spontaneous mutation. The diagnosis may be suspected during pregnancy by an increased rate of growth in the second half of pregnancy. Infants are typically in the 97th percentile for height and weight and the 50th percentile for head size. The presentation of some affected infants is similar

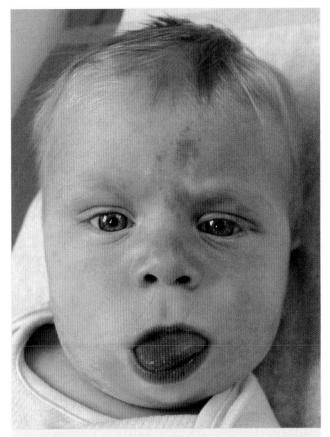

Fig. 64.5 Macroglossia and macrosomia are major features of Beckwith-Wiedemann syndrome.

to the presentation of infants affected by maternal diabetes (large for gestational age, hypoglycemia). Dysmorphic features are more prominent during infancy and childhood and gradually normalize in most cases throughout adulthood. The most common associated tumors are Wilms tumor, hepatoblastoma, rhabdomyosarcoma, adrenocortical carcinoma, and neuroblastoma.

There is a great degree of variability in expression, and some cases may not be diagnosed until adulthood. Affected individuals without obvious major features of the syndrome are still at increased risk for tumor development, and a high index of suspicion is needed to reach a diagnosis in children with atypical phenotypes so that effective tumor surveillance can be initiated. Tumor surveillance consists of detailed physical examinations coupled with serial abdominal ultrasound examinations (every 6 to 12 weeks until the age of 8 years) and the measurement of alpha fetoprotein levels (every 6 to 12 weeks until the age of 5 years). Rhabdomyosarcoma is the most common malignant tumor of the head and neck in individuals with Beckwith-Wiedemann syndrome, but fortunately these are rare, even in this population.

Acute management is often needed in infancy for several associated features. Abdominal wall defects are present in 60 to 75% of cases, and severe defects are repaired soon after birth. Severe hypoglycemia is present in 30% and must be controlled tightly to avoid complications. Macroglossia is present in more than 80% of affected individuals, and infants with significant macroglossia occasionally require tracheostomy. Macroglossia is due to hypertrophy/hyperplasia of both the anterior tongue and the base of tongue. Because of the diffuse tongue involvement, anterior tongue reduction may not be adequate to relieve symptoms. Affected individuals who are less symptomatic from macroglossia may benefit from a period of observation before surgical management because spontaneous resolution has been reported as the facial skeleton grows to accommodate the large tongue. In some patients with macroglossia and upper airway obstruction, the upper airway symptoms may be relieved with adenotonsillectomy alone. The surgical correction of severe upper airway obstruction in Beckwith-Wiedemann syndrome is essential to prevent the long-term sequelae of cor pulmonale, failure to thrive, and premature death.

Macroglossia causes additional speech and articulation problems. Children with Beckwith-Wiedemann syndrome typically have a normal IQ, but speech therapy may not be enough to help them to communicate effectively unless a tongue reduction is performed. Macroglossia resulting in constant anterior protrusion of the tongue can trigger teasing, and tongue reduction is indicated to achieve a better cosmetic outcome. Feeding difficulties due to macroglossia may be managed conservatively with changes in dietary consistency or the use of a nipple with a larger aperture.

Hearing loss is not a common feature of Beckwith-Wiedemann syndrome, but several cases of conductive hearing loss have been reported. These cases have been associated with the intraoperative finding of stapedial foot plate fixation, but more research is needed to determine whether this disease process is affected by 11p15.5 dysregulation. Hemihypertrophy/hemihyperplasia occurs in some patients with Beckwith-Wiedemann and is due to mosaicism of the dysregulated genes. Facial asymmetry may require surgical reconstruction in severe cases, but most cases are mild and will gradually improve throughout childhood.

64.6 Ocular–Auricular–Vertebral Spectrum

Hemifacial microsomia is part of the ocular–auricular–vertebral (OAV) spectrum. Goldenhar syndrome is the most specific phenotypic variant of this association. Cardinal features include auricular anomalies, typically located on the side of the face affected by microsomia; epibulbar dermoids; vertebral anomalies; coloboma of the upper eyelid; preauricular skin tags; unilateral parotid agenesis; and congenital facial nerve palsy (▶ Fig. 64.6). The severity of the mandibular microsomia correlates with overall disease severity. The estimated incidence is 1 in 5,600 live births, and the etiology is unknown. Males and females are equally affected. One-third of patients demonstrate dysmorphic features on both sides of the face, and the other

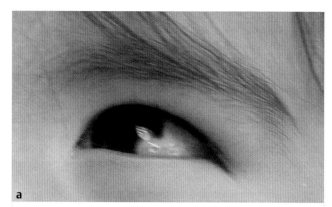
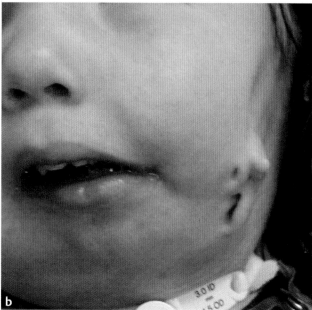

Fig. 64.6 (a) Epibulbar dermoids are seen in patients with Goldenhar syndrome. (b) Microtia, often with an anomalous course of the facial nerve, is common in Goldenhar syndrome, as is hemifacial and hemimandibular microsomia.

two-thirds are affected on only the right or left side, with equal rates noted for the two sides. The OAV spectrum is a genetically heterogeneous disorder. Although several cases of Goldenhar syndrome have been associated with chromosomes 5p15 and 14q32 deletions, other cases with similar phenotypes have been identified in patients with trisomy 18, trisomy 7, trisomy 9, and terminal deletion of 22q, but there is no localization to any region. Although most cases are spontaneous, family pedigrees have supported autosomal-dominant and autosomal-recessive patterns of inheritance. Maternal factors, including a diabetic state and the use of retinoic acid, thalidomide, or cocaine, are associated with the phenotype, as well. Because most anomalies involve first and second branchial arch derivatives, hemorrhage from the stapedial artery during the course of development results in the typical features. The overlapping features of the OAV spectrum and CHARGE (*c*oloboma of the eye, *h*eart defects, *a*tresia of the nasal choanae, *r*etarded growth, genital and/or urinary abnormalities, *e*ar abnormalities and deafness) syndrome have led to speculation that the aberrant development of neural crest cells plays a role in pathophysiology.

Extracraniofacial anomalies occur in more than half of patients with hemifacial microsomia, and affected individuals with more severe craniofacial manifestations are more likely to have anomalies of the skeleton, heart, lungs, central nervous system, or gastrointestinal tract. Extracranial skeletal findings are common in patients with hemifacial microsomia, and 40 to 60% of patients will have a skeletal anomaly. The most common skeletal deformities are of the vertebrae and ribs. The most common extraskeletal association is cardiac, and 25 to 50% of patients with hemifacial microsomia have a cardiac anomaly. The most common reported cardiac anomalies are ventricular septal defects.

Conductive or mixed hearing loss is the most common type of hearing loss associated with OAV spectrum and occurs in 70 to 75% of patients. Affected individuals may present with microtia, atretic auditory canals, malformed or fused ossicles, and absence of the round window. There is an increased incidence of chronic otitis media, and individuals may benefit from the placement of longer-lasting ventilation tubes. Occasionally, affected individuals have profound sensorineural hearing loss due to malformations of the inner ear, and they may have findings of dysplastic cochleas and semicircular canals. Ear surgery should never be performed on patients with OAV spectrum before a radiologic evaluation of the course of the facial nerve has been obtained because the location of the facial nerve is often atypical. Individuals with OAV spectrum have poorer outcomes overall than do patients with nonsyndromic cases of microtia or atresia after surgical reconstruction of the ear. The complex abnormal anatomy and growth of the surrounding facial skeleton are important factors.

Speech development is typically not affected by the auricular anomalies because hearing is usually preserved on one side. Rare patients who have bilateral hearing loss benefit from a conventional hearing aid or a bone-anchored hearing aid, and patients with profound bilateral sensorineural hearing loss benefit from a cochlear implant. Asymmetric weakness of the tongue musculature often causes articulation problems, and speech therapy is an important component of treatment. Coordination problems with the tongue also can affect feeding. Affected neonates who cough or choke during feeds should be evaluated for tracheoesophageal fistula because this is more common in individuals with OAV spectrum.

Craniofacial reconstruction is indicated only in severe cases and may be limited to mandibular distraction osteogenesis. Le Fort I repositioning of the maxilla and free flap reconstruction of the mandible have also been described. Reported outcomes of all of these procedures are variable, and some cases require multiple revision surgeries to obtain a cosmetically and functionally acceptable result.

64.7 Conclusion

The common theme among all of these described syndromes is phenotypic variability, and a thorough physical examination and history are required to make an accurate diagnosis and initiate appropriate treatment and screening. Patients require more frequent visits to primary care providers and specialists, and coordination with a multidisciplinary team ensures that all appropriate tests are done while redundant and excessive tests and procedures are avoided. Early intervention for hearing, speech, and airway management may optimize individual outcomes.

Affected individuals may benefit from psychosocial counseling to manage the stresses of dealing with a disfigurement, as well as neurocognitive testing to diagnose behavioral disorders or developmental delay that requires special attention. Prenatal diagnosis helps families to begin learning about the disease process and necessary interventions, and it helps caregivers to plan for potentially life-saving interventions at the time of delivery.

This overview only touches on some of the most common syndromes of interest to the otolaryngologist. In practice, the otolaryngologist must be well versed in the full spectrum of genetic syndromes because patients with myriad syndromes will require evaluation and treatment by this specialist. Consultations are commonly needed for individuals with genetic syndromes to manageme the difficult airway, chronic upper airway infections, and hearing loss and to treat speech and swallowing problems. A thorough knowledge of the anatomical anomalies and associated features of a variety of syndromes will help the otolaryngologist to avoid the pitfalls of inappropriate management.

Human genome mapping and the field of proteomics are rapidly changing what is known about the pathophysiology of syndromes. Advances in radiology and surgical technology are also constantly evolving and leading to improved outcomes. Clinicians should be up to date on the recent literature in order to provide the best outcomes, which a multidisciplinary approach helps to ensure.

64.8 Roundsmanship

- No single feature is ever pathognomonic for a syndrome because syndromes are characterized by variable expression.
- An otolaryngologic anomaly will be found in 84% of syndromic infants.
- An endotracheal tube two sizes smaller than expected should initially be used to size the airway of a patient with Down syndrome.
- Hemifacial microsomia is part of the ocular–auricular–vertebral (OAV) spectrum.

64.9 Recommended Reading

[1] Dyce O, McDonald-McGinn D, Kirschner RE, Zackai E, Young K, Jacobs IN. Otolaryngologic manifestations of the 22q11.2 deletion syndrome. Arch Otolaryngol Head Neck Surg 2002; 128: 1408–1412

[2] Enklaar T, Zabel BU, Prawitt D. Beckwith-Wiedemann syndrome: multiple molecular mechanisms. Expert Rev Mol Med 2006; 8: 1–19

[3] Horgan JE, Padwa BL, LaBrie RA, Mulliken JB. OMENS-Plus: analysis of craniofacial and extracraniofacial anomalies in hemifacial microsomia. Cleft Palate Craniofac J 1995; 32: 405–412

[4] Losken A, Williams JK, Burstein FD, Malick DN, Riski JE. Surgical correction of velopharyngeal insufficiency in children with velocardiofacial syndrome. Plast Reconstr Surg 2006; 117: 1493–1498

[5] Online Mendelian Inheritance in Man. OMIM®. McKusick-Nathans Institute of Genetic Medicine, Johns Hopkins Medicine, and National Human Genome Research Institute. . Updated October 28, 2013. Accessed October 29, 2013

[6] Park AH, Wilson MA, Stevens PT, Harward R, Hohler N. Identification of hearing loss in pediatric patients with Down syndrome. Otolaryngol Head Neck Surg 2012; 146: 135–140

[7] Rimell FL, Shapiro AM, Shoemaker DL, Kenna MA. Head and neck manifestations of Beckwith-Wiedemann syndrome. Otolaryngol Head Neck Surg 1995; 113: 262–265

[8] Rouillon I, Leboulanger N, Roger G et al. Velopharyngoplasty for noncleft velopharyngeal insufficiency: results in relation to 22q11 microdeletion. Arch Otolaryngol Head Neck Surg 2009; 135: 652–656

[9] Sculerati N, Gottlieb MD, Zimbler MS, Chibbaro PD, McCarthy JG. Airway management in children with major craniofacial anomalies. Laryngoscope 1998; 108: 1806–1812

[10] Shott SR. Down syndrome: common otolaryngologic manifestations. Am J Med Genet C Semin Med Genet 2006; 142C: 131–140

[11] Swillen A, Vogels A, Devriendt K, Fryns JP. Chromosome 22q11 deletion syndrome: update and review of the clinical features, cognitive-behavioral spectrum, and psychiatric complications. Am J Med Genet 2000; 97: 128–135

[12] Tewfik TL, Kaloustian VM. Congenital Anomalies of the Ear, Nose, and Throat. New York, NY: Oxford University Press; 1997

[13] Thompson JT, Anderson PJ, David DJ. Treacher Collins syndrome: protocol management from birth to maturity. J Craniofac Surg 2009; 20: 2028–2035

[14] Weksberg R, Shuman C, Beckwith JB. Beckwith-Wiedemann syndrome. Eur J Hum Genet 2010; 18: 8–14

65 Congenital Malformations of the External and Middle Ear

David J. Crockett and Jeremy D. Meier

65.1 Introduction

Throughout the evolutionary process, the ear has developed into a complex organ with many structures necessary for the transmission of sound. This chapter discusses the embryology and the most common congenital malformations of the external and middle ear. The primary responsibility of these structures is to assist with the transmission of auditory information from the environment to the inner ear. Malformations or deformities can lead to functional and aesthetic complications for the patients affected.

65.2 Embryology

The embryology of the external and middle ear is a complex process. Malformations of these structures usually occur from genetic or environmental influences during embryologic development. For this reason, appreciating the embryologic process will aid in understanding the malformations discussed in this chapter.

All structures of the ear develop concurrently with one another and with other head and neck structures. Development of the inner begins first, at around the end of the third week of gestation, and the inner ear develops independently of the middle and external ear. Sometime in the fourth week of gestation, the external and middle ear start to form. The first pharyngeal pouch (endodermal) principally forms the tubotympanic recess. Throughout the remainder of the developmental process, the tympanic cavity continues to expand, eventually surrounding the ossicles and their support structures. The ossicles generally lie completely within the tympanic cavity by the eighth month of development.

Neural crest mesenchyme of the first (Meckel cartilage) and second (Reichert cartilage) branchial arches is principally responsible for the development of the ossicles. The head of the malleus and the short and long processes of the incus are formed from Meckel cartilage. The long process of the incus, handle of the malleus, and stapes superstructure are formed from Reichert cartilage. The vestibular surface of the stapes footplate and the annular ligament are formed from mesoderm of the otic capsule.

The first branchial cleft (ectodermal), between the first and second branchial arches, forms the external auditory canal. This epithelium invaginates, and by approximately the 28th week of gestation the core has canalized, creating the external auditory canal and allowing access to the tympanic membrane. The tympanic membrane is composed of ectoderm from the first branchial cleft laterally, endoderm from the first pharyngeal pouch medially, and a central layer composed of neural crest mesenchyme.

The auricle begins development at around the fifth week of gestation. Three hillocks are noted to arise from the first branchial arch and three from the second branchial arch. The six hillocks are associated with the formation of distinct auricular structures in the adult: hillock 1, tragus; hillock 2, helical crus; hillock 3, ascending helix; hillock 4, horizontal helix and portions of the scapha and antihelix; hillock 5, descending helix and portions of the scapha and antihelix; hillock 6, antitragus and portion of the helix (▶ Fig. 65.1).

65.3 Common Malformations of the External Ear

As previously discussed, the external ear and middle ear develop separately from the inner ear because their embryologic origins are different. Alterations in the normal embryogenesis, through genetic and environmental agents, will lead to various malformations of the external and middle ear. A few of the common malformations are discussed.

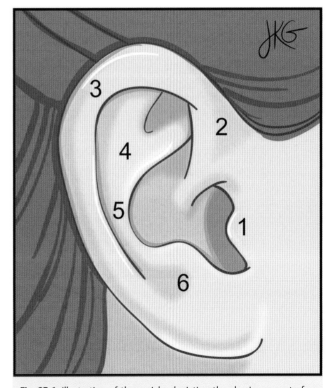

Fig. 65.1 Illustration of the auricle, depicting the classic concept of particular development from specific hillocks of His: hillock 1, tragus; hillock 2, helical crus; hillock 3, ascending helix; hillock 4, horizontal helix and portions of the scapha and antihelix; hillock 5, descending helix and portions of the scapha and antihelix; hillock 6, antitragus and portion of the helix.

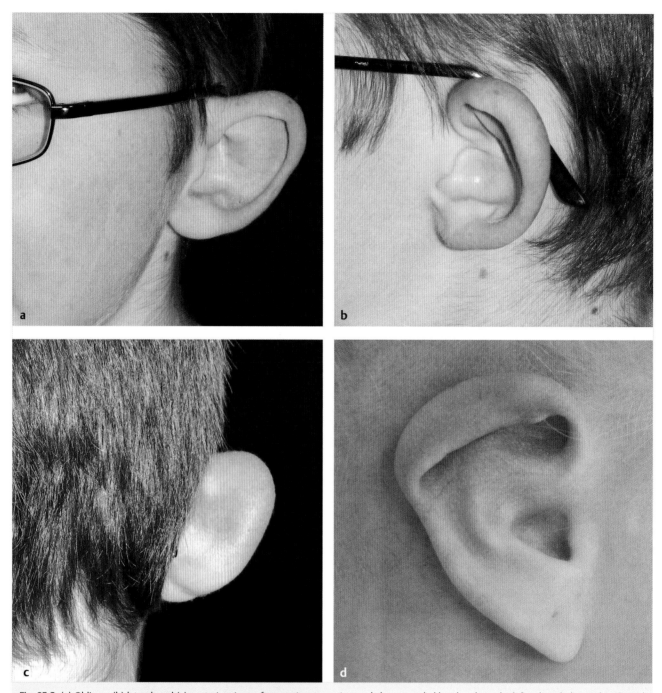

Fig. 65.2 (a) Oblique, (b) lateral, and (c) posterior views of a prominent ear. An overly large conchal bowl and poorly defined antihelix produce lateral prominence and pseudoptosis of the auricle. (d) Lop ear with abnormal folding of the superior helix.

65.3.1 Anomalies of the Auricle: Prominent Auricle and Lop Ear

Varying degrees of severity of auricular malformation have been discussed in the literature. Anotia, microtia (auricular hypoplasia), and prominent ear (▶ Fig. 65.2) are common anomalies of the auricle. The functional and aesthetic concerns resulting from these malformations can cause significant distress to a patient.

A prominent or protruding ear is a fairly common defect. If the antihelix fails to unfold during the embryologic develop-

mental process, the helix will continue to overhang and protrusion will persist, resulting in a lop ear. Various minor auricular anomalies can also occur. The most common abnormalities include increased angle between the auricle and the scalp (the normal angle between the ear and the head is between 15 and 25 to 30 degrees), underdevelopment of the antihelix, excessive conchal cartilage, and earlobe deformity (mainly protrusion).

Otoplasty is defined as the surgical repair, restoration, or alteration of the auricle. The auricle nears completion of growth in childhood, and it is safe to correct deformities of the external ear during this stage of life. Multiple surgical techniques have

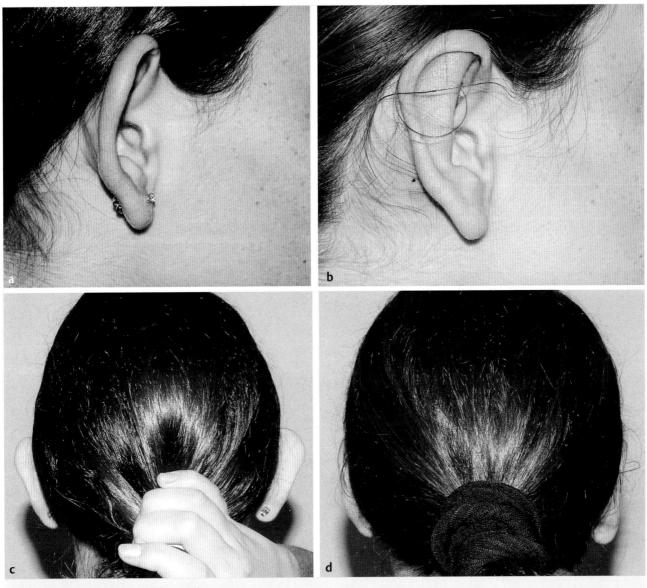

Fig. 65.3 (a, c) Before and (b, d) after otoplasty.

been described to correct such deformities (▶ Fig. 65.3). The Mustardé suturing technique is used to create an antihelical fold and involves placing several horizontal mattress sutures along the scapha. The Furnas technique involves placement of a conchomastoid suture that reduces the conchal bowl and allows retraction of the auricle. More aggressive techniques that include cartilaginous incisions have been developed by Pitanguy and Farrior. Common complications of otoplasty include inadequate correction, chondritis, hematoma, and "telephone ear" deformity (caused by too much flexion of the midportion of the antihelix and inadequate flexion of the superior and inferior poles). Otoplasty is discussed in more detail in Chapter 52 (Correction of Congenital Auricular Deformities).

65.3.2 Preauricular Pits and Skin Tags

Preauricular cysts, fistulas, and sinuses (also called "pits") commonly occur in the pediatric population. It is thought that these

arise from developmental defects of the first branchial cleft and first branchial arch. The location of these defects is usually anterior to the auricle close to the anterior border of the ascending limb of the helix. Sinuses are usually intimately associated with the adjacent helical cartilage, and inadequate excision may result in recurrence. The standard technique involves an elliptical cutaneous incision around the pit followed by dissection of the tract near the root of the helix. The elliptical incision can be extended to allow a supra-auricular approach, which improves access and so allows a more adequate excision.

Preauricular skin appendages are also common. These are small tags that occasionally contain cartilage. They are often found anterior to the auricle at the level of the supratragal incisura (▶ Fig. 65.4). Presumably, these preauricular appendages arise as a consequence of excessive growth during the developmental process. Simple excision, if desired by the patient or family, may be performed.

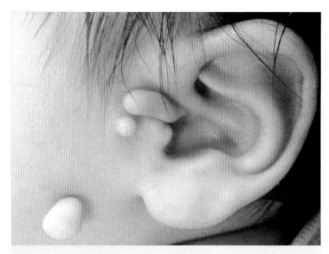

Fig. 65.4 Multiple preauricular skin tags.

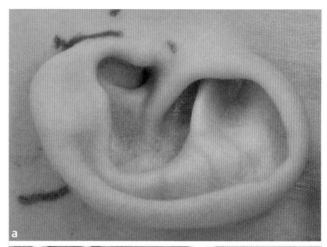

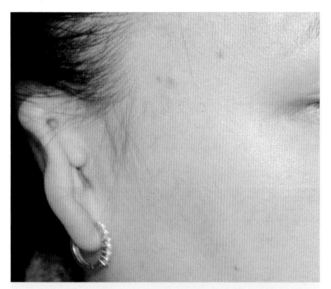

Fig. 65.6 Aural atresia is frequently associated with microtia. What appear to be a small conchal bowl and external auditory meatus end in a blind pouch.

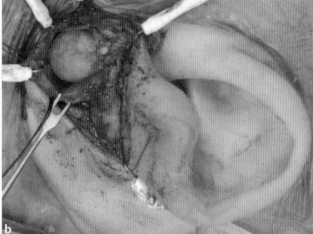

Fig. 65.5 (a) Pre- and (b) intraoperative views of a type I first branchial cleft cyst.

65.3.3 First Branchial Cleft Anomalies

As previously discussed, the first branchial cleft develops into the external auditory canal and the outer layer of the tympanic membrane. Maldevelopment may lead to cystic lesions, sinus anomalies, and fistulas. Sinuses arising from the first branchial cleft are of two major types. Type I lesions (▶ Fig. 65.5) are duplications of the external auditory canal; they exist as fistulous tracts and usually lie in close association with the lower pole of the parotid gland. Type II lesions are superficial sinuses or cysts in the anterior neck below the angle of the mandible. They are usually noticed earlier in childhood than type I lesions. Recurrent infection can be associated with both lesions. If aural discharge persists in the absence of middle ear disease, this anomaly should be suspected, especially if there is a history of a neck lump or abscess. If surgery is indicated, complete excision is recommended because of high recurrence rates. There is often

an intimate relationship of the cyst or sinus with branches of the facial nerve, requiring tedious dissection with possible partial parotidectomy.

65.3.4 Aural Atresia

Congenital aural atresia has a reported incidence of 1 in 10,000 to 1 in 20,000 births. Approximately one-third of these children will have bilateral aural atresia to some degree. Atresia of the ear canal with middle ear anomalies can occur in isolation or may be associated with other anomalies, such as microtia (▶ Fig. 65.6). As mentioned previously, the ear canal is formed from the first branchial groove. If canalization is arrested during the developmental process, a stenotic or membranous atretic canal may result. Atresia of the bony canal is secondary to malformation of the tympanic bone during development.

The evaluation and treatment of aural atresia include a detailed hearing assessment to determine the need for immediate amplification. Computed tomography (CT) of the temporal bone is indicated to evaluate the middle ear and facial nerve anatomy when surgical reconstructive options are being discussed and to identify potential cholesteatoma. In unilateral atresia, a maximal conductive hearing loss is present, but immediate intervention is unnecessary if there is normal hearing in the

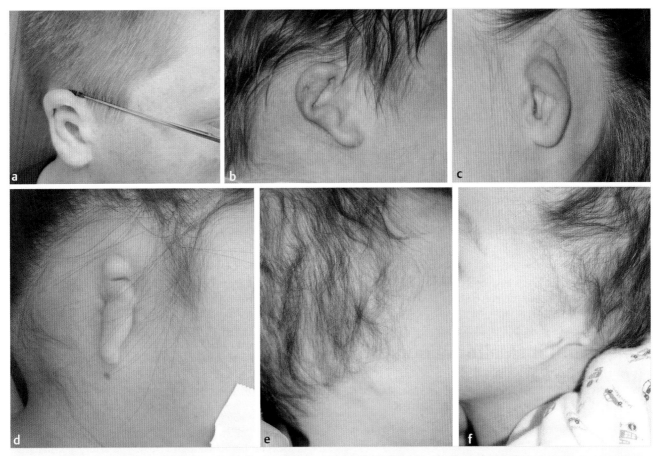

Fig. 65.7 Various degrees of microtia and anotia. (a) Grade I. (b,c) Grade II. (d) Grade III. (e) Anotia. (f) Nearly complete anotia.

contralateral ear. A hearing aid may be used in canal stenosis. Complete canal atresia requires a bone conduction hearing aid. Early amplification is necessary in bilateral atresia. A bone conduction hearing aid can be fitted after the first few months of life.

Should surgery be desired, it can be done as early as 6 to 7 years of age, generally after microtia repair so that the reconstructive procedure can be performed in unscarred tissues. Although it is difficult, the objective of the atresia surgery is to create a pathway that allows sound to reach the cochlea in a functional manner. Not all children are candidates for canal atresia repair. Jahrsdoerfer proposed a 10-point grading scale to predict the likelihood of a good hearing outcome after canalplasty. This scale assesses for the following: stapes present, middle ear space adequate, facial nerve position normal, malleus–incus complex present, mastoid well pneumatized, incus–stapes connection present, round window normal, external ear appearance normal, and oval window patent. Each parameter is awarded 1 point, except for stapes present, which is awarded 2 points. Children with a score of 8 points or more are considered to have the best chance of a good outcome.

65.3.5 Microtia

Microtia is graded based on the severity of the malformation of the external ear (▶ Fig. 65.7a–d). Anotia (▶ Fig. 65.7e, f) is complete absence of the pinna. Meurman classified the severity of

microtia on a three-grade scale. Grade I indicates a small, malformed auricle with most of the characteristic components present. Grade II indicates an auricle with a vertical remnant of cartilage and skin and a smaller anterior hook. Grade III denotes an auricle that is almost entirely absent except for a misplaced lobule and a smaller skin and cartilage remnant; a grade III auricle is often described as a "peanut ear."

Repair of the microtia and concomitant atresia requires coordination between an otologist and a facial plastic surgeon. Most physicians generally agree that 6 years is an appropriate age at which to proceed with microtia reconstruction because the normal contralateral pinna has reached about 85% of full adult size and can be used as a model. At this age, the patient has adequate donor cartilage for the surgery and is usually more prepared from a psychological standpoint. If the microtia is unilateral, waiting for additional growth is sometimes preferred because the harvested cartilage is thicker and more amenable to sculpting. Construction of an ear with autologous rib cartilage is discussed in more detail in Chapter 52 (Correction of Congenital Auricular Deformities).

In addition to reconstruction with autogenous cartilage, certain implants, such as porous high-density polyethylene (Medpor; Porex Surgical, Newnan, GA) implants, have been used to create the framework structure for the auricle. These implants are placed under a temporoparietal fascial flap and covered with a skin graft. The choice of reconstructive material is discussed preoperatively with the patient and family.

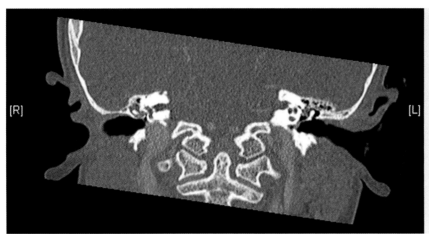

Fig. 65.8 High-riding jugular bulb of the right temporal bone.

Surgery is not the only reconstructive option for these patients. Auricular prosthetics have been found to be an adequate reconstructive option. Hearing can be improved with the use of a bone-anchored hearing aid in patients with canal atresia.

65.4 Common Malformations of the Middle Ear

65.4.1 Ossicular Chain Anomalies

The ossicles are derived from the first and second branchial arches. Deviation from normal embryologic processes will result in aberrant development of the ossicles. Anomalies vary widely, from minor morphological defects to rudimentary ossicular masses. Although ossicular deformities often occur simultaneously with deformities of the external auditory canal or tympanic membrane, they may occur alone because the ossicles develop through a different embryologic process.

Children who have ossicular chain anomalies often present with a unilateral conductive hearing loss in the range of 40 to 60 dB. These children frequently are identified during routine school audiometry. In a child without a history of trauma, middle ear effusion, or infection, the clinician should suspect a congenital ossicular malformation. Many surgical techniques have been developed to improve the hearing of these patients, and the overall prognosis is good. Because it is difficult to determine the exact deformity before surgery, the surgeon must be prepared to perform various ossicular reconstructive techniques depending on the findings during middle ear exploration. The most common abnormalities include fixation of the stapes, abnormalities of the stapes superstructure, ankylosis of the incudostapedial joint, and fixation of the malleus head to the tympanic ring.

65.4.2 Vascular Anomalies

Multiple vascular anomalies may occur within the middle ear. These anomalies are especially important to any surgeon operating on the ear in order to avoid inadvertent injury to the vessel. The internal carotid artery may assume an anomalous course and enter the middle ear in the hypotympanum.

Patients may present with pulsatile tinnitus, conductive hearing loss, and otalgia. The vessel may appear as a reddish mass medial to the inferior portion of the tympanic membrane. In a similar manner, the sigmoid sinus and the jugular bulb can present in abnormal locations. A high-riding or enlarged jugular bulb may present as a bluish mass medial to the inferior portion of the tympanic membrane (▶ Fig. 65.8). Failure to identify an anomalous carotid artery or high-riding jugular bulb during middle ear surgery or even a myringotomy can lead to devastating consequences.

Another rare congenital vascular anomaly is a persistent stapedial artery. The stapedial artery is the embryologic remnant of the second branchial arch artery. The artery normally regresses at approximately the 10th week of gestation. A persistent stapedial artery arises from the internal carotid artery in the hypotympanum and courses through the crura of the stapes to the fallopian canal, geniculate ganglion, and dura. Like other vascular anomalies, a persistent stapedial artery can cause difficulties with surgery involving the middle ear, especially the stapes.

65.4.3 Congenital Cholesteatoma

Cholesteatomas are expansile lesions composed of stratified squamous epithelium and desquamated keratin that may develop within the temporal bone. They may be acquired or congenital. Multiple complications may arise as a result of the presence of a cholesteatoma. Infection, facial nerve paralysis, hearing loss, bone destruction, and intracranial complications can all occur.

Congenital cholesteatoma has been defined as an embryonic rest of epithelial tissue in the middle ear in a patient without tympanic membrane perforation and without a history of otorrhea or prior ear procedures. On physical examination, congenital cholesteatomas often appear as a white mass in the anterior–superior quadrant of the tympanic membrane. CT is used to characterize the size, location, and extent of the cholesteatoma for surgical planning (▶ Fig. 65.9). The mean age of patients at presentation is 4.5 years, and a 3:1 male-to-female preponderance has been noted. The pathogenesis of these lesions is not fully understood. Treatment is similar to that for acquired cholesteatomas.

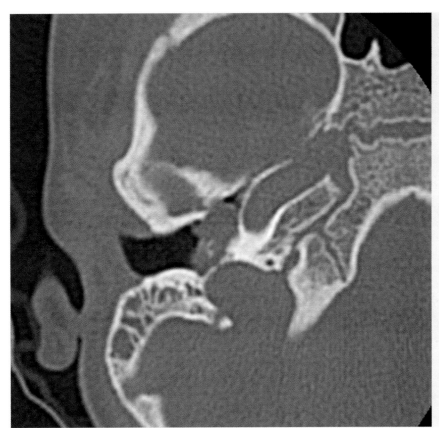

Fig. 65.9 Congenital cholesteatoma of the right temporal bone.

65.5 Conclusion

When the clinician is evaluating patients with malformations of the external or middle ear, a thorough understanding of the embryology and developmental processes is necessary. These malformations can lead to functional and aesthetic complications and concerns for the patients affected. Multiple procedures and therapies have been developed to address these complications. An improved understanding of congenital anomalies will assist in the diagnosis and treatment of those affected.

65.6 Roundsmanship

- The head of the malleus and the body and short processes of the incus are formed from Meckel cartilage, whereas the long process and lenticular process of the incus, handle of the malleus, and stapes superstructure are formed from Reichert cartilage. The vestibular surface of the stapes foot plate and the annular ligament are formed from mesoderm of the otic capsule.
- Type I first branchial cleft cysts are duplications of the external auditory canal and run lateral to the facial nerve. Type II cysts run inferiorly toward the angle of the mandible and may be lateral or medial to the facial nerve.
- Meurman classified microtia into three grades based on the presence or absence of normal external auricular landmarks. Know these!
- The most common congenital ossicular abnormalities include fixation of the stapes, abnormalities of the stapes superstruc-

ture, ankylosis of the incudostapedial joint, and fixation of the malleus head to the tympanic ring.

65.7 Recommended Readings

[1] Bauer BS. Reconstruction of microtia. Plast Reconstr Surg 2009; 124 Suppl: 14e–26e
[2] Bellucci RJ. Congenital aural malformations: diagnosis and treatment. Otolaryngol Clin North Am 1981; 14: 95–124
[3] Brent B. Technical advances in ear reconstruction with autogenous rib cartilage grafts: personal experience with 1200 cases. Plast Reconstr Surg 1999; 104: 319–334, discussion 335–338
[4] Chandler JR, Mitchell B. Branchial cleft cysts, sinuses, and fistulas. Otolaryngol Clin North Am 1981; 14: 175–186
[5] Farrior RT. Modified cartilage incisions in otoplasty. Facial Plast Surg 1985; 2: 109–118
[6] Jahrsdoerfer RA, Yeakley JW, Aguilar EA, Cole RR, Gray LC. Grading system for the selection of patients with congenital aural atresia. Am J Otol 1992; 13: 6–12
[7] Levenson MJ, Michaels L, Parisier SC. Congenital cholesteatomas of the middle ear in children: origin and management. Otolaryngol Clin North Am 1989; 22: 941–954
[8] Maniglia AJ. Embryology, Teratology, and arrested developmental disorders in otolaryngology. Otolaryngol Clin North Am 1981; 14: 25–38
[9] Meurman Y. Congenital microtia and meatal atresia; observations and aspects of treatment. AMA Arch Otolaryngol 1957; 66: 443–463
[10] Nofsinger YC, Tom LW, LaRossa D, Wetmore RF, Handler SD. Periauricular cysts and sinuses. Laryngoscope 1997; 107: 883–887
[11] Prasad S, Grundfast K, Milmoe G. Management of congenital preauricular pit and sinus tract in children. Laryngoscope 1990; 100: 320–321
[12] Work WP. Newer concepts of first branchial cleft defects. Laryngoscope 1972; 82: 1581–1593

66 Evaluation, Management, and Special Techniques in Pediatric Otology

Robin A. Dyleski, Nancy King, and Christopher J. Linstrom

66.1 Eustachian Tube Development

The eustachian tube (ET) is an organ that runs between the middle ear and the nasopharynx. It regulates pressure in the middle ear while protecting the middle ear from nasopharyngeal sounds and secretions and clearing middle ear secretions into the nasopharynx.

The ET lumen widens at both ends and narrows in its midsection (isthmus). The distal cartilaginous portion ends in the nasopharynx at a prominence known as the torus tubarius. The proximal osseous portion opens onto the anterior wall of the superior portion of the middle ear about 4 mm above the floor. The osseous portion is open at all times. The fibrocartilaginous portion is closed at rest but opens during swallowing or Valsalva maneuver. Muscles associated with the ET include the tensor veli palatini, levator veli palatini, salpingopharyngeus, and tensor tympani; these aid in opening and closing the cartilaginous portion of the ET.

The ET in children is immature and therefore less functional than it is in adults. The length of the pediatric ET averages about 18 mm, about half the length of the adult ET. Perhaps more importantly, the direction of the tube varies from horizontal to 10 degrees from horizontal in the child. Additionally, the tensor veli palatini is less efficient. This combination of anatomical differences leads to a decreased ability to clear middle ear secretions, appropriately ventilate the middle ear, and protect the middle ear from the bacterial flora migrating from the nasopharynx. This has been theorized to account for the increased incidence of pediatric otitis media. The ET reaches full size by the age of 7 years, and the incidence of otitis media generally decreases after this age.

66.2 Acute Otitis Media and Otitis Media with Effusion

Otitis media (inflammation of the middle ear and mastoid space) is the most common reason for sick visits in pre-school-age children. Otitis media can be described, based on duration, as follows:

Acute: 0 to 3 weeks
Subacute: 3 to 12 weeks
Chronic: longer than 12 weeks

Acute otitis media (AOM) is defined as the presence of fluid in the middle ear accompanied by acute symptoms such as otalgia, fever, and irritability. Recurrent AOM is defined as three or more episodes within 6 months, or four episodes within 12 months.

Otitis media with effusion (OME) is the presence of fluid in the middle ear space without signs or symptoms of an acute ear infection. OME is considered a separate entity from AOM; it is characterized by an acute onset of signs and symptoms, the presence of middle ear effusions, and signs and symptoms of middle ear inflammation.

OME can occur as a postinflammatory response to AOM, viral infection, or ET dysfunction. The persistent fluid collection can result in multiple sequelae, most commonly a conductive hearing loss due to decreased mobility of the tympanic membrane (TM).

Chronic suppurative otitis media is the persistence of purulent fluid behind the TM that is unresponsive to medical therapy.

66.2.1 Epidemiology

Children in the 7- to 36-month age range are most likely to develop AOM. Children with multiple episodes of AOM tend to have their first episode within the first year of life. Children who have not had AOM by the age of 3 years are unlikely to develop severe or recurrent otitis media.

OME will occur in 50% of children in the first year of life and persist in 30 to 40%, usually in an asymptomatic manner. The incidence of OME peaks in the second year of life during the winter months, in association with an upper respiratory infection; full resolution occurs within a few months without any medical or surgical intervention.

Children with craniofacial abnormalities affecting the ET are at greater risk for developing otitis media, including those with cleft palate, midface deformities, skull base deformities, or nose and paranasal sinus abnormalities. Other craniofacial abnormalities associated with otitis media include Down syndrome, Apert syndrome, and mucopolysaccharidoses.

Other children who may be more prone to otitis media include those with immunodeficiencies or nasal obstruction (e.g., chronic allergies, adenoid hypertrophy, sinonasal tumors).

66.2.2 Pathophysiology

Otitis media in the child is related to dysfunction of the ET. The immature ET is more horizontally aligned than the adult ET, leading to less effective drainage of the middle ear space. Edema of the ET due to an upper respiratory infection or allergies only compounds the problem. Congenital abnormalities of the palate musculature may also affect ET function.

66.2.3 Microbiology

The most common pathogens responsible for pediatric otitis media in descending order are *Streptococcus pneumoniae* (30 to 50%), *Haemophilus influenzae* (20 to 30%), *Moraxella catarrhalis* (10 to 20%), and group A streptococci (1 to 5%). One-third of *H. influenzae* and 100% of *M. catarrhalis* bacteria are β-lactamase–positive.

66.2.4 History

Common signs of AOM include otalgia, fever, irritability, and otorrhea (indicating a ruptured TM). Additional symptoms, such as facial paralysis, vertigo, and swelling behind the ear, may be indicative of a complicated AOM, and computed tomography (CT) may be required to determine if further intervention is required (see later section on complications of otitis media). Most children also have hearing loss. A child with OME may simply have hearing loss. A child with a ruptured TM secondary to AOM may have little to no pain, some hearing loss, and low-grade fevers.

66.2.5 Physical Examination

External Ear Examination

If the auricle is rotated forward and is erythematous and edematous with obliteration of the posterior auricular sulcus, there is concern for coalescent mastoiditis (see later section on acute coalescent mastoiditis)

Pneumatic Otoscopy

A normal TM (▶ Fig. 66.1) should be translucent, with the middle ear landmarks clearly visible. The TM can be in normal position, retracted, or bulging. AOM and OME can be present with a retracted or bulging TM. The color of the TM may be yellow, opaque, or bluish, indicating fluid in the middle ear. Hyperemia is not specific for infection and may simply be a sequela of crying or coughing. An air–fluid level can often be seen, or air bubbles that indicate the presence of fluid in the middle ear. Effusions can be categorized as serous (thin and watery), mucoid (thick and viscous), or purulent (presence of pus). Pneumatic otoscopy should show the TM to be mobile. Decreased motility

of the TM with positive or negative pressure can be an indication of fluid sitting behind the TM, limiting its motion.

A TM perforation can be a result of increased pressure caused by persistent fluid in the middle ear. In this case, fluid is often seen coming from the perforation (otorrhea). Clinically, the patient generally describes some relief of symptoms after the perforation occurs because the pressure behind the TM is released and the effusion is allowed to drain.

66.2.6 Management of Acute Otitis Media

AOM has a spontaneous resolution rate of 60% within 24 hours and of 80% within 48 to 72 hours. Once a diagnosis of AOM has been confirmed, an appropriate course of action is determined. The American Academy of Pediatrics and the American Academy of Family Physicians, together with experts in otolaryngology, have created guidelines for the evidence-based management of AOM.

Observation

In selected children with dependable follow-up, watchful waiting for 48 to 72 hours with only pain management is an option. Children between the ages of 6 months and 2 years with mild to moderate symptoms, uncomplicated AOM, or an uncertain diagnosis would be appropriate candidates for this strategy.

Medical Treatment

If medical treatment is appropriate, amoxicillin is the first-line medication for most children, dosed at 80 to 90 mg/kg/d. Other options include cefdinir and clindamycin. Symptomatic relief should occur within 48 to 72 hours of the initiation of antibiot-

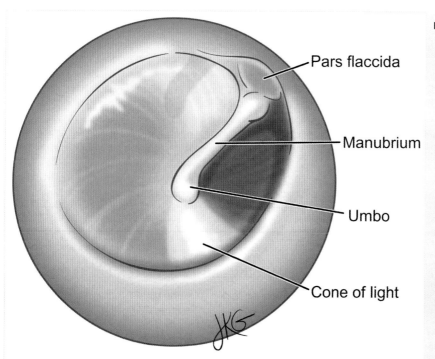

Fig. 66.1 Normal right tympanic membrane.

Pars flaccida

Manubrium

Umbo

Cone of light

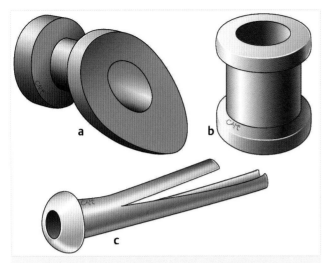

Fig. 66.2 Types of tympanotomy tubes. (a) Armstrong grommet. (b) Mini-grommet. (c) Feuerstein split.

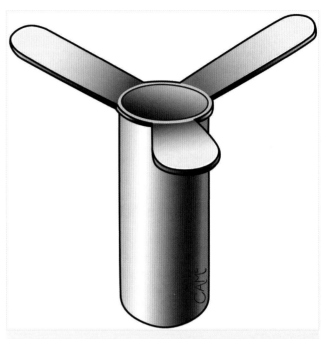

Fig. 66.3 Triune tube (Grace Medical, Memphis, TN).

ics. If no improvement is seen, the diagnosis of AOM should be reconfirmed. For AOM refractory to amoxicillin, the guidelines recommend amoxicillin/clavulanate for additional coverage. For patients who are allergic to penicillin, a cephalosporin (penicillin-allergic patients show 10 to 15% cross reactivity when treated with cephalosporins), trimethoprim/sulfamethoxazole, or a macrolide is recommended. Levofloxacin, azithromycin, or clarithromycin can also be tried in penicillin-allergic patients.

66.2.7 Management of Otitis Media with Effusion

In May of 2004, the American Academy of Otolaryngology-Head and Neck Surgery, the American Academy of Family Physicians, and the American Academy of Pediatrics revised the guidelines for the management of OME. The highlights are reviewed here.

- OME should be differentiated from AOM. OME is defined as the presence of fluid in the middle ear without signs or symptoms of AOM.
- Pneumatic otoscopy should be the primary diagnostic method, with confirmation by tympanometry. The laterality of OME, duration of the effusion, and any associated symptoms should be documented.
- Watchful waiting for 3 months after the onset of the effusion or the diagnosis is appropriate in most children because 75 to 90% of cases of residual OME after AOM resolve spontaneously within 3 months.
- If OME persists for 3 months or longer, significant hearing loss with associated speech or language delay is noted, or learning problems are suspected, a hearing test should be performed.
- If no hearing loss is found, children with OME should be reexamined every 3 to 6 months until the effusion disappears.
- If hearing loss is present, placement of a pressure equalization tube should be the initial procedure. Repeated tube insertion should be accompanied by adenoidectomy. Surgical candidates include children who have OME lasting 4 months or more with persistent hearing loss, children with persistent OME who are at risk regardless of hearing status, and children who have OME and structural damage to the TM or middle ear.
- In children at risk, such as developmentally delayed children with Down syndrome or children with cerebral palsy, who are more likely to have baseline speech or language delay, OME should be addressed earlier.
- Antibiotics, antihistamine decongestants, and steroid medications have not been shown to aid in the resolution of OME.

Tympanostomy Tube Selection

Tubes can be separated into three categories: short-term, mid-term, and long-term. For most normal children with chronic serous otitis media, a short-term tube is sufficient to ventilate the middle ear until ET function improves with age. Mid-term and long-term tubes are reserved for children who are expected to be tube-dependent for a long period of time. Children who fall into this category include those who have Down syndrome, are receiving their second or third set of tubes, or have long-standing ET dysfunction.

Short-term tubes generally reside in the TM for 6 to 24 months. Some popular types are shown in ▶ Fig. 66.2.

Mid-term tubes typically remain in place and function for 18 to 20 months and are shown in ▶ Fig. 66.3.

Long-term tubes are placed when there is a greater likelihood of recurrent disease and generally provide effective function for 2 to 3 years (▶ Fig. 66.4).

The incidence of complications, such as chronic TM perforation and granulomas, increases the longer a tube is left in place.

Myringtomy and Tube Placement Technique

1. Position the microscope and patient appropriately.
2. Place the largest ear speculum that will fit atraumatically into the external auditory canal.
3. Cerumen in the external auditory canal is removed, and visualization of the TM is maximized.

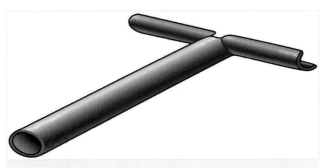

Fig. 66.4 T-tube.

4. Examine the eardrum and note the normal landmarks and any abnormalities in the drum.
5. If the patient is not under general anesthesia:
   a) Ear canal injection:

A solution of 1% lidocaine with 1:100,000 epinephrine can be injected at the cartilaginous–bony junction at 12 o'clock, 3 o'clock, 6 o'clock, and 9 o'clock through a 25-gauge needle. Inject slowly to prevent infiltration into the middle ear. Anesthetic in the middle ear can cause delayed vertigo if the solution crosses the round window or temporary facial paralysis if the patient has a dehiscent facial nerve canal.
   a) Topical phenol:

A wisp of cotton saturated with 100% phenol and applied discretely to the TM at the proposed myringotomy location produces excellent anesthesia with no postoperative complications. Alternatively, phenol can be administered with a phenol applicator (straight-handled otologic instrument with a "forked" tip that, when dipped, holds a small amount of phenol between the tines and allows discrete and focused application). The myringotomy is then made through the white coagulum created.
1. The myringotomy knife is inserted through the TM, and the incision is created in the location of choice. The length of the myringotomy incision should be about the diameter of a No. 5 suction vent to ensure easy tube insertion.
2. a) Myringotomy location:
   1. Epithelial migration of the squamous portion of the drum is believed to be responsible for tube extrusion. Migration begins at the umbo and radiates outward.
   2. Migration is fastest in the anteroinferior and posteroinferior quadrants.
   3. As the posterosuperior quadrant contains the ossicles, the anterosuperior quadrant is the ideal place for myringtomy and tube placement.
   4. The inferior quadrants are more easily accessible and are often used.
   b) Myringotomy direction:
   1. Radially oriented incisions parallel epithelial migration.
   2. Circumferential incisions run perpendicular to epithelial migration, leading to a faster extrusion rate.
   c) Hemostasis can be achieved with oxymetazoline-soaked pledgets, if necessary.
   d)
3. Suction the middle ear contents with a No. 5 suction vent through the myringotomy.

a) Mucoid secretions are sometimes difficult to evacuate; saline irrigation may be of value. Alternatively, a second counter-incision can be made through the TM to allow air to enter the middle ear space.
b) The tympanostomy tube is grasped with an alligator forceps, and the anterior edge of the inner flange is inserted into the myringotomy incision. The tube is then released. With either an alligator forceps or a Rosen pick, the lagging edge is gently pushed until it "pops" through the myringotomy incision (▶ Fig. 66.5).
4. Ensure patency of the tube by gently suctioning it with the thumb off the suction vent.
5. Administer otic antibiotic drops.

Tube Management

An audiogram should be obtained after tympanoplasty and compared with the pretreatment test to ensure improvement in hearing. The patient should be seen every 3 to 6 months and then yearly in order to visually examine the tubes and determine their location (in place, extruded, in the external auditory canal), their patency, and the status of the middle ear. Audiography is repeated as clinically necessary.

If the tubes persist longer than they are clinically needed and have shown no signs of spontaneous migration from the TM, removal of the tubes can be considered.

Factors to consider before tube removal:
- Recurrent/chronic drainage: Drainage from the ears is an indication that the tubes are clinically necessary. In this case, the tubes should be left in place.
- ET function: In the case of unilateral tube persistence, the contralateral ear can be examined to determine the maturity of the ET. If the contralateral TM is retracted, indicating continued poor ET function, the tubes are still clinically needed.

Complications of Tubes

Persistent Tympanic Membrane Perforation

After tube removal, the patient should observe water precautions and return for an examination in 3 months. In most cases, the perforation will be smaller or healed. If the perforation persists, repair of the TM is necessary.

Paper Patch Technique (▶ Fig. 66.6)

For dry perforations smaller than 3 mm, a paper patch is sufficient.
1. Position the patient reclining in the chair.
2. Examine the external auditory canal and TM, documenting the size and location of the perforation.
3. The edges of the perforation are de-epithelialized with a myringotomy knife or otologic needle. Make sure to remove only a minimal amount to avoid enlarging the perforation.
4. Use a right angle hook to sweep circumferentially around the medial portion of the perforation margin.
5. Rice (cigarette) paper or paper tape (Micropore strip tape; 3 M, St. Paul, MN) is used. The paper patch is trimmed to approximately twice the size of the perforation. The underside of the paper patch is moistened with sterile water or a nonsteroidal antibiotic drop.

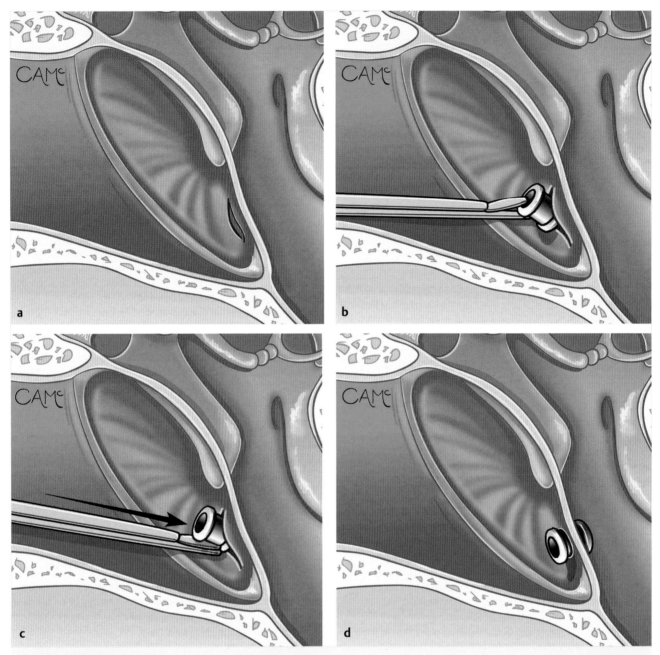

Fig. 66.5 Myringotomy with placement of a tympanotomy tube. (**a**) A radial incision is made in the tympanic membrane. (**b**) The anterior flange is placed through the myringotomy and then released. (**c**) A forceps or a pick is used to "pop" the posterior flange of the tube through the myringotomy until (**d**) the tube is in an appropriate position.

6. Place the paper patch over the perforation with an alligator forceps.
7. Smooth it against the TM with a cerumen curet.

For larger perforations, a formal tympanoplasty is needed.

66.2.8 Complications of Otitis Media

Facial Paralysis

The facial nerve, as it travels through the middle ear and mastoid bone, may be affected by adjacent infection. Facial paralysis can occur as a complication of AOM and should be addressed immediately to prevent permanent facial paralysis. It often resolves after myringotomy and tube placement, along with intravenous (IV) antibiotics. Should facial paralysis occur in the setting of acute coalescent mastoiditis (see below), a mastoidectomy should be performed urgently.

Acute Mastoiditis

Technically, all cases of AOM are accompanied by an acute mastoiditis because the mastoid cells are simultaneously inflamed. This process does not carry any additional symptoms beyond those of an AOM. The condition improves with improvement of the otitis media.

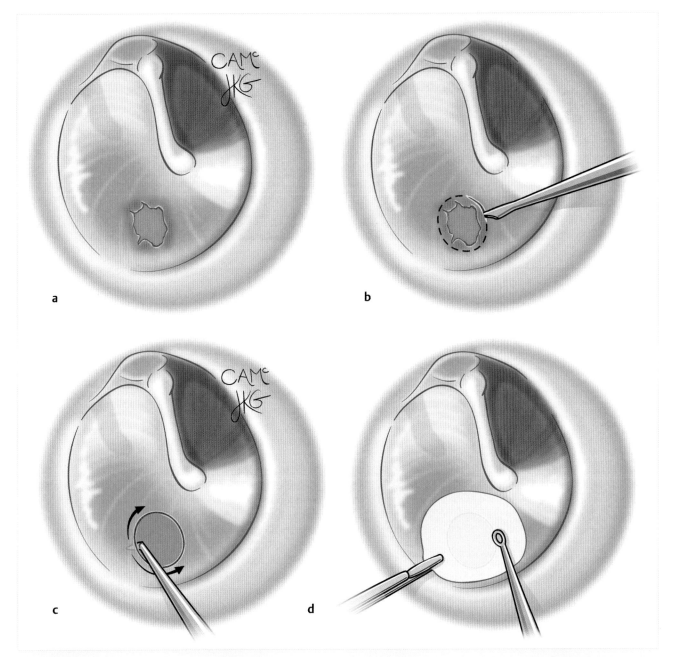

Fig. 66.6 (a) Small, dry tympanic membrane perforations may be closed effectively with a paper patch technique. (b) The perforation edge is de-epithelialized with a myringotomy knife or otologic pick, with minimal tissue removed. (c) The undersurface of the perforation edge is abraded with a right angle hook. (d) The moistened paper patch is applied directly over the perforation.

Acute Mastoiditis with Periosteitis

Acute mastoiditis with periosteitis involves inflammation and infection of the mastoid air cells extending to the periosteum, but without involvement of bone. Findings include inflammation and erythema of the postauricular area, displacement of the pinna inferiorly and anteriorly, and fluid in the middle ear (▶ Fig. 66.7). The postauricular crease may or may not be absent. Treatment with IV antibiotics and tube placement to facilitate drainage of the middle ear leads to resolution.

Acute Coalescent Mastoiditis

Also known as acute mastoid osteitis, acute coalescent mastoiditis is an infection that causes bony destruction. This usually presents in children 4 years of age or younger (mostly boys) who have had unrelieved symptoms of AOM and/or mastoiditis for 2 to 4 weeks. Coalescent mastoiditis tends to develop in children with well-developed mastoid air cells and children with no prior otologic disease. Pain may be localized to the posterior auricular area. The mastoid may be tender to percussion, there may be overlying erythema, and the posterosuperior external

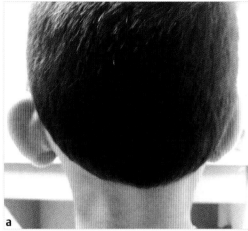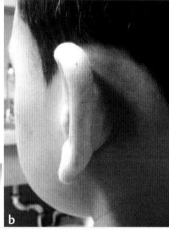

Fig. 66.7 (a) Posterior and (b) oblique views of the postauricular sulcus in a patient who has acute mastoiditis with periosteitis show protrusion and inferior displacement of the auricle, along with erythema of the postauricular sulcus.

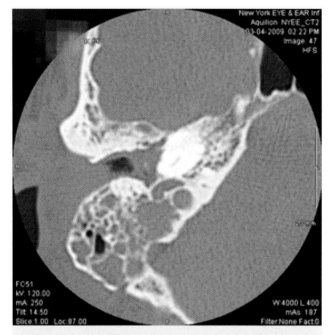

Fig. 66.8 Temporal bone computed tomographic scan showing loss of septa between the mastoid air cells, suggesting coalescent mastoiditis.

auditory canal may be sagging. These signs are usually present, but not always. The children look toxic with persistent high fevers. CT of the temporal bone should be obtained to clarify the extent of the disease (▶ Fig. 66.8).

Early acute coalescent mastoiditis may respond to tube placement and IV antibiotics. However, a simple mastoidectomy may be required. If acute coalescent mastoiditis is found in the setting of facial nerve paralysis, mastoidectomy should be performed urgently and 3 to 6 weeks of IV antibiotics initiated.

Acute coalescent mastoiditis may be accompanied by acute petrositis, indicating that infection has spread to the petrous portion of the temporal bone. *Gradenigo syndrome* is a triad of suppurative otitis media, ipsilateral ocular pain, and sixth cranial nerve paralysis.

Simple Mastoidectomy Technique

A safe technique for mastoidectomy in children is informed by an understanding of the differences between the adult and pediatric temporal bone. In children 2 years of age or younger, pneumatization has not progressed to the mastoid tip, resulting in a more superficially located stylomastoid foramen (▶ Fig. 66.9 and ▶ Fig. 66.10). This puts the facial nerve at increased risk for surgical injury in the pediatric patient. Unless it is impossible to obtain in a gravely ill patient, preoperative audiography should be performed to document conductive and sensorineural hearing.

1. The patient is placed in a supine position with the head turned away from the affected ear. The postauricular crease is infiltrated with local anesthetic (▶ Fig. 66.11).
2. Because of the more superficial location of the stylomastoid foramen in children, the postauricular incision is not carried down as far inferiorly as in adults. The incision is also made 6 to 8 mm posterior to the postauricular sulcus (▶ Fig. 66.12).
3. The incision is carried down to the loose areolar tissue over the temporalis fascia and mastoid periosteum (▶ Fig. 66.13a).
4. The superior boundary is the linea temporalis. A T incision is made along the linea temporalis from the zygomatic root to the occiptomastoid suture and from the linea temporalis to the mastoid tip with a monopolar cautery. An elevator is used to elevate the soft tissue off the bone (▶ Fig. 66.13b).
5. Self-retaining Weitlander retractors are placed to improve exposure, and key landmarks are identified: spine of Henle, cribriform area, and linea temporalis.
6. The MacEwen triangle is identified, which serves as a landmark for locating the mastoid antrum. The MacEwen triangle is bounded by the posterior border of the external auditory canal, the anterior line of the zygomatic arch, and a line that connects the two (▶ Fig. 66.14). The antrum is 15 mm medial to this. Under a 200- to 250-mm microscope, a cutting bur is used to remove the outer cortex of the mastoid beginning at a line along the linea temporalis. Copious irrigation is used to prevent excessive heat transfer to underlying structures. The tegmen is identified by a pinkish color seen through a thin bony covering and carefully respected. Posteriorly, as the cortex is removed, the bluish tint of the sigmoid sinus can be

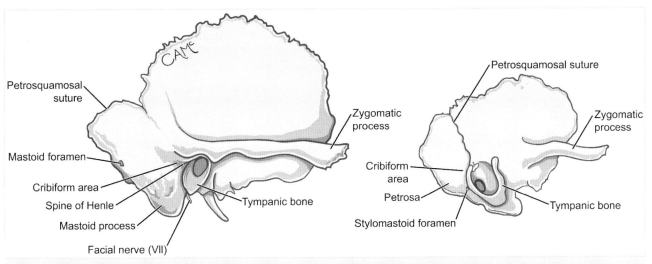

Fig. 66.9 Differences between the adult and pediatric mastoid bone. In children, the mastoid is far less pneumatized and the tympanic ring is much less developed.

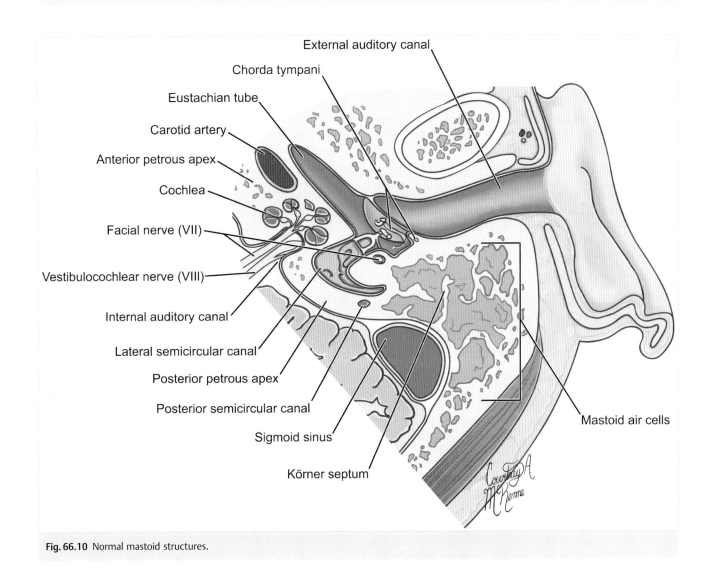

Fig. 66.10 Normal mastoid structures.

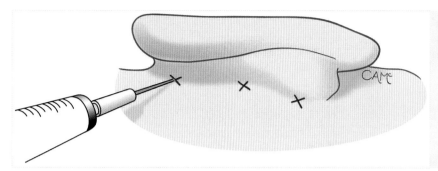

Fig. 66.11 Mastoidectomy. The postauricular sulcus is infiltrated with 1% lidocaine with 1:100,000 epinephrine.

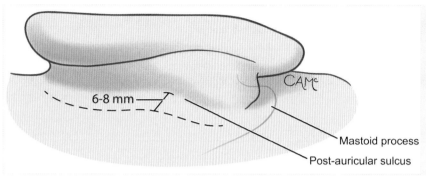

Fig. 66.12 Mastoidectomy. The postauricular sulcus incision is moved 6 to 8 mm posteriorly, and the incision does not extend as far inferiorly as in the adult to avoid facial nerve injury.

6-8 mm

Mastoid process

Post-auricular sulcus

seen as the bowl is progressively developed from the mastoid tip to the posterior aspect of the linea temporalis dissection. Anteriorly, bone is removed up to a few millimeters posterior to the spine of Henle. More air cells are opened as the bowl is progressively saucerized (▶ Fig. 66.15).

7. The Körner septum, a thin plate of bone of bone representing the petrosquamous lamina, is penetrated to fully open the mastoid antrum. Once this is done, the aditus ad antrum is inspected, identifying the lateral semicircular canal, fallopian canal, chorda tympani, and short process of the incus (▶ Fig. 66.16).

8. A tympanostomy tube should be placed in a patient with acute coalescent mastoiditis.

66.3 Evaluation and Management of Speech Delay in Children

The development of normal speech and language is evaluated as a component of the developmental milestones that are monitored by pediatricians during routine well-child visits. Early intervention to determine the nature and cause of speech delays is important in children who have either normal hearing or impaired hearing to help them reach their full potential. When hearing impairment is identified and treated before 6 months of age, there is a greater likelihood of normal speech and language development.

In the United States, nearly all states have legislated newborn hearing screening programs that test the hearing of newborn children before discharge from their birth hospital. The few states without legislated programs have voluntary programs to screen for hearing loss in infants. The Year 2007 Position Statement of the Joint Committee on Infant Hearing stresses the following points:

1. The definition of hearing loss has been expanded to include neural hearing loss (e.g., "auditory neuropathy/dyssynchrony").
2. Separate protocols are recommended for neonatal intensive care units (NICUs) and well-infant nurseries. NICU infants admitted for more than 5 days are to undergo auditory brainstem response (ABR) testing as part of their screening, so that neural hearing loss will not be missed.
3. Referrals from the NICU should be made directly to an audiologist for rescreening and comprehensive evaluation, including ABR testing.
4. For rescreening, a complete screening of both ears is recommended, even if only one ear failed the initial screening.
5. For all infants (NICU infants and well infants) readmitted during the first month of life with a condition associated with potential hearing loss (e.g., severe hyperbilirubinemia or culture-positive sepsis), a repeat hearing screening is recommended before discharge.
6. Only audiologists with expertise in evaluating newborns should provide audiology diagnostic and auditory habilitation services (selection and fitting of amplification device).
7. For infants in whom hearing loss is diagnosed, amplification should be fitted within 1 month of the diagnosis.
8. For infants with confirmed hearing loss, a genetics consultation should be offered to their families.
9. Every infant with confirmed hearing loss should be evaluated by an otolaryngologist with knowledge of pediatric hearing loss and should have at least one examination to assess visual acuity performed by a pediatric ophthalmologist.
10. All infants with any degree of bilateral or unilateral permanent hearing loss should be eligible for early intervention services.

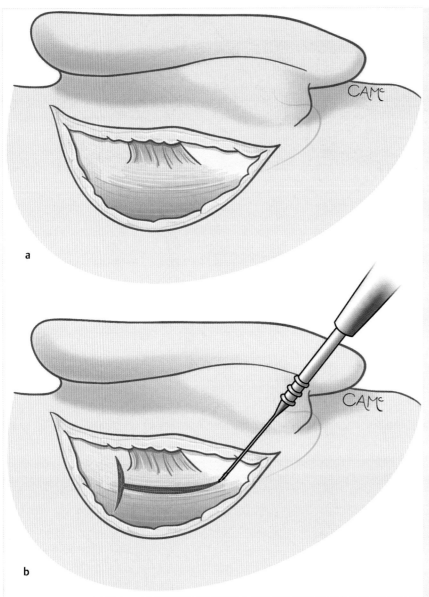

Fig. 66.13 Mastoidectomy. (**a**) The dissection proceeds down to temporalis fascia, which is (**b**) split and elevated until the bone is exposed.

11. Early intervention services for infants with confirmed hearing loss should be provided in home and center-based environments by professionals who have expertise in hearing loss.
12. For all infants, regular surveillance of developmental milestones, auditory skills, and middle ear status, as well as parental concerns, should be performed, consistent with the American Academy of Pediatrics (AAP) Periodicity Schedule (well-child care visits).
13. Families should be made aware of all communication options and available hearing technologies (presented in an unbiased manner).

Universal newborn hearing screening has allowed the early identification and treatment of children with impaired hearing. Early intervention programs vary from state to state but are instrumental in providing ongoing audiologic and speech therapy services for participating children and their families.

66.3.1 Speech Delay

Children who pass the newborn hearing screening (NBHS) evaluation at birth and in whom the onset of speech development is delayed are considered to be "speech-delayed." Regular and routine well-child visits should determine whether babies and children are reaching the recognized developmental milestones for their age (▶ Table 66.1). Normal hearing is essential for the normal development of speech and language.

Children with significant delays in speech acquisition and language development require careful evaluation of their ears and hearing. When a child presents with delayed speech acquisition, a careful history should assess for possible risk factors for speech delay. The history should include information about the pregnancy, with attention to prenatal infections associated with hearing loss. Other important considerations are the birth history and perinatal course, including hyperbilirubinemia, the use of mechanical ventilation and NCPAP (nasal continuous

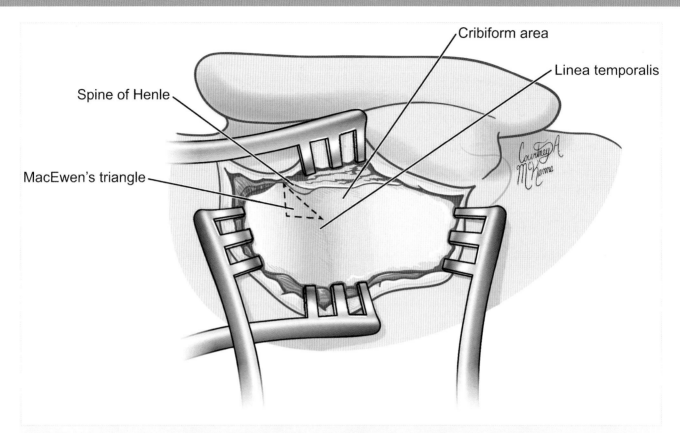

Cribiform area

Linea temporalis

Spine of Henle

MacEwen's triangle

Fig. 66.14 The MacEwen triangle serves as a landmark for identifying the mastoid antrum, which lies approximately 15 mm medial to it.

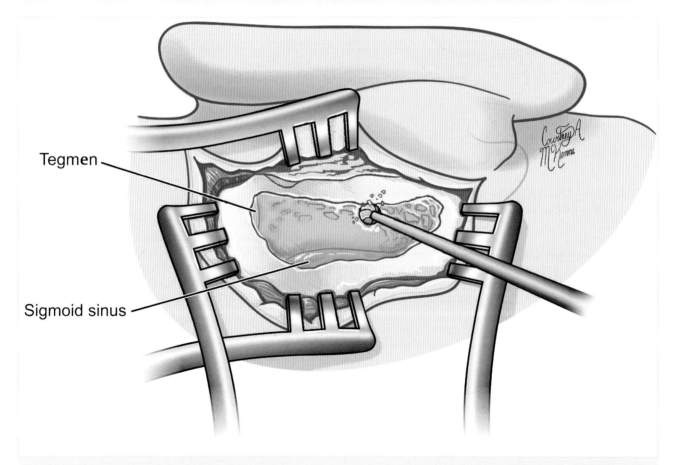

Tegmen

Sigmoid sinus

Fig. 66.15 The mastoid bowl is progressively opened. The pink gleam of the tegmen through a thin layer of bone forms the superior boundary of the dissection. Posteriorly, the bluish tone of the sigmoid sinus forms another boundary of dissection. Identification of the antrum aids in gauging the depth of dissection.

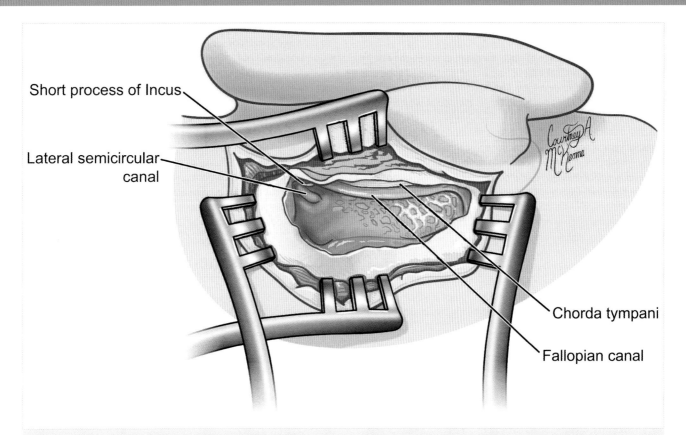

Short process of Incus

Lateral semicircular canal

Chorda tympani

Fallopian canal

Fig. 66.16 At the completion of the mastoidectomy, the aditus ad antrum is inspected, and the lateral semicircular canal, fallopian canal, chorda tympani, and short process of the incus are all visualized.

positive airway pressure), ototoxic drug exposure, and birth weight. Questions should evaluate for the presence of frequent ear infections and any other otologic history. A family history of hearing loss should be included.

The evaluation includes a complete head and neck examination, with particular attention to the ears and a search for middle ear effusions, and a complete audiologic examation, with audiography, OAE (otoacoustic emissions) or ABR tests, and tympanometry.

When hearing loss is identified by audiometric testing or a positive clinical finding is noted during the physical examination, such as a middle ear effusion, treatment is directed toward correction of the abnormality. For example, middle ear effusions would be treated with the placement of tympanostomy tubes and the hearing retested following the procedure to determine if it has been satisfactorily improved to normal.

In the case of a child with normal hearing test results and physical examination findings, a referral to speech therapy is made. The speech therapist will provide a variety of exercises for the patient to improve speech production and language development. Parents can participate in the child's therapy by continuing specific exercises with the child between the therapy sessions to reinforce the therapy goals. In most cases, speech therapy is able to help the child to "catch up" with speech development and production.

Table 66.1 Milestones for speech and language development

Age	Milestones
Birth–3 mo	Reacts to loud sounds Recognizes caregiver's voice Coos in response to pleasure
4–6 mo	Looks toward sounds and follows Babbles and makes different sounds Laughs, listens to music Knows when toys make sounds
7–12 mo	Turns head to listen to sounds Knows simple words like "milk," "juice" Makes long strings of sounds while babbling Has a few words by 12 mo ("mama," "dada")
12–24 mo	Acquires 50 or more words Puts two words together ("want milk") Points to body parts, pictures in books Uses a variety of consonants at the beginning of words
2–3 y	Makes short sentences Has a large variety of words Can be understood by caregivers and friends
3–4 y	Is able to tell a short story and relate activities Uses sentences with four or more words Hears and responds when called from another room

66.4 Roundsmanship

- The increased incidence of otitis media in children may be attributed to anatomical differences in the eustachian tube that resolve as the child develops. The eustachian tube generally reaches maturity by age 7, and this is the age at which otitis media decreases.
- *Acute otitis media* is defined as the presence of fluid in the middle ear accompanied by acute symptoms of otalgia, fever, and irritability of 0 to 3 weeks' duration. *Recurrent acute otitis media* is defined as three or more episodes within 6 months, or four episodes within 12 months. *Otitis media with effusion* is the presence of fluid in the middle ear space without signs or symptoms of an acute ear infection. *Chronic suppurative otitis media* is the persistence of purulent fluid behind the tympanic membrane that is unresponsive to medical therapy.
- The most common pathogens responsible for pediatric otitis media are *Streptococcus pneumoniae*, *Haemophilus influenzae*, *Moraxella catarrhalis*, and group A streptococci. One-third of *H. influenzae* and 100% of *M. catarrhalis* bacteria are β-lactamase–positive.
- Common signs of acute otitis media include otalgia, fever, irritability, and otorrhea. More concerning symptoms, such as facial paralysis, vertigo, and swelling behind the ear, may be indicative of a complicated acute otitis media and may require additional imaging.
- Management options for acute otitis media include observation for children between the ages of 2 months and 2 years with mild or moderate symptoms, an uncomplicated acute otitis media, and dependable follow-up. Medical treatment can be administered with amoxicillin as the first-line medication. For patients who are allergic to penicillin, a cephalosporin, trimethoprim/sulfamethoxazole, or a macrolide is recommended. Penicillin-allergic patients show 10 to 15% cross reactivity when treated with cephalosporins. Azithromycin or clarithromycin may also be used.
- Candidates for tympanostomy tube placement include children who have persistent otitis media with effusion for longer than 4 months with hearing loss, children who have otitis media with effusion and structural damage to the tympanic membrane or middle ear, and children who are at risk, defined as developmentally delayed children more likely to have a baseline speech or language delay.
- Complications of tympanostomy tube placement include persistent tympanic membrane perforation and tube retention.
- Complications of otitis media include facial paralysis, acute mastoiditis, acute mastoiditis with periosteitis, and acute coalescent mastoiditis.
- Acute coalescent mastoiditis can be identified on a CT scan by bony destruction and loss of septa between the mastoid cells. An early coalescent mastoiditis may be addressed with tympanostomy tube placement and IV antibiotics, but a simple mastoidectomy may be required. In the setting of a coalescent mastoiditis with facial nerve paralysis, an urgent mastoidectomy is required in addition to 3 to 6 weeks of IV antibiotics.

66.5 Recommended Reading

[1] American Academy of Family PhysiciansAmerican Academy of Otolaryngology-Head and Neck SurgeryAmerican Academy of Pediatrics Subcommittee on Otitis Media With Effusion. Otitis media with effusion. Pediatrics 2004; 113: 1412–1429

[2] Auinger P, Lanphear BP, Kalkwarf HJ, Mansour ME. Trends in otitis media among children in the United States. Pediatrics 2003; 112: 514–520

[3] Bluestone CD, Stool SE, Alper CM, et al, eds. Pediatric Otolaryngology. 4th ed. Philadelphia, PA: W. B. Saunders; 2003:487

[4] Burke P, Bain J, Robinson D, Dunleavey J. Acute red ear in children: controlled trial of non-antibiotic treatment in general practice. BMJ 1991; 303: 558–562

[5] Casselbrant ML, Mandel EM. Evidence-Based Otitis Media. 2nd ed. Hamilton, ON: B. C. Decker; 2003

[6] Graves GO, Edwards LF. The Eustachian tube: review of its descriptive, microscopic, topographic, and clinical anatomy. Arch Otolaryngol 1944; 39: 359–397

[7] American Academy of Pediatrics, Joint Committee on Infant Hearing. Year 2007 position statement: principles and guidelines for early hearing detection and intervention programs. Pediatrics 2007; 120: 898–921

[8] Mygind N, Meistrup-Larsen KI, Thomsen J, Thomsen VF, Josefsson K, Sørensen H. Penicillin in acute otitis media: a double-blind placebo-controlled trial. Clin Otolaryngol Allied Sci 1981; 6: 5–13

[9] Piglansky L, Leibovitz E, Raiz S et al. Bacteriologic and clinical efficacy of high dose amoxicillin for therapy of acute otitis media in children. Pediatr Infect Dis J 2003; 22: 405–413

[10] Rosenfeld RM, Kay D. Natural history of untreated otitis media. Laryngoscope 2003; 113: 1645–1657

[11] Teele DW, Klein JO, Rosner BA. Epidemiology of otitis media in children. Ann Otol Rhinol Laryngol Suppl 1980; 89: 5–6

67 Pediatric Nasal Disorders

Robin A. Dyleski

67.1 Introduction

Nasal and sinus complaints are among the most common reasons why children are brought to the primary care physician and to the otolaryngologist for medical attention. Because the etiology of the presenting problem may range from a simple upper respiratory infection to a life-threatening illness, it is important to be able to distinguish these illnesses by using the history, physical examination, and confirmatory testing to make an accurate diagnosis.

67.2 Embryology of the Midface

67.2.1 Nasal Development

Development of the nose and paranasal sinuses is a multifactorial process that begins early in embryonic development and continues until the face has reached maturity in the teenage years. The nose and sinuses originate in the fetus around the third to fourth week of life. A swelling on the lateral aspect of the head, the nasal placode, develops from a thickening of the ectoderm. Just above the oral stoma in the anterior portion of the developing head is a midline structure, the nasofrontal process. Simultaneous development of the nasofrontal process and the nasal placodes shape and form the midface, nose, and sinus portions of the face and head within the first months of life.

At the fifth week, the nasal placode extends into the underlying mesenchyme, transforming into the medial and lateral nasal processes, which results in the development of the nasal pit. As this occurs, the maxillary process of the first branchial arch enlarges and the nasal pit and orbit move anteriorly, with the nasal processes between and below the future orbits. As the nasal processes migrate medially and anteriorly, they ultimately fuse in the midline, creating the precursor of the nose. At this early period of nasal development, the nasal pit intrudes into the future nasal cavity minimally; the deep end of the nasal pit, called the nasobuccal membrane, separates the nasal opening from the oral cavity. The nasobuccal membrane usually canal-izes between the fifth and sixth weeks of life, creating an opening at the depth of the nasal pit. Choanal atresia is seen when the nasobuccal membrane fails to perforate.

The medial nasal processes ultimately form the nasal septum, the philtrum of the upper lip, and the premaxilla (upper maxillary ridge containing the four central incisors). The lateral nasal processes form the nasal alae, most of the nostrils, and the nasal floor (▶ Fig. 67.1).

Within the seventh week of embryogenesis, the medial nasal process, lateral nasal processes, and maxillary processes modulate and transform, with the development of the upper lip and upper alveolar ridge. The two lateral maxillary processes develop into the lateral palatal shelves (becoming the future hard and soft palates). These lateral palatal shelves fuse with the septum and premaxilla at the alveolar ridge bilaterally by the seventh week of development. Aberrations at this time in the development of the lip and palate result in the formation of cleft lip and cleft palate.

The two lateral palatal shelves then fuse in the midline between weeks 7 and 10, beginning anteriorly and extending posteriorly toward the future uvula. This process results in the separation of the oral cavity from the nasal cavity.

Simultaneously, the intranasal tissues are developing into the future lateral nasal structures and sinuses. Around day 40 of embryogenesis, a swelling develops in the anterolateral portion of the nasal wall, called the maxilloturbinate, and soon afterward another swelling, the ethmoturbinate, develops just superior to it; these will become the inferior and middle turbinates, respectively, with the middle meatus forming between them. The superior and supreme turbinates develop from ridges on the superior aspect of the ethmoturbinate around the fourth month of fetal development.

67.2.2 Sinus Development

At approximately 60 days of life, the initial differentiation of the sinuses begins with thickening and intrusion into the mesenchyme laterally from the lateral nasal wall. The maxillary sinus begins to be identifiable around 70 days as a dilatation in

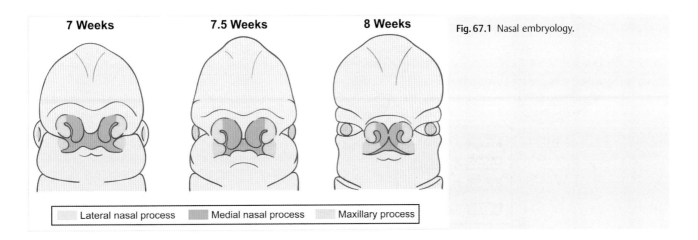

7 Weeks   **7.5 Weeks**   **8 Weeks**

Fig. 67.1 Nasal embryology.

Lateral nasal process   Medial nasal process   Maxillary process the infundibular groove of the middle meatus region. This dilatation deepens and enlarges into the rudimentary maxillary sinus.

Around the middle of the fourth month, the frontal recess develops just posterior to the anterior attachment of the middle turbinate, and the process of development of the frontal sinus begins. The ethmoidal bulla begins to develop around this time and is recognizable by the day 120, with continued development of the ethmoidal air cell lattice proceeding from that point.

The sphenoid sinus develops within the sphenoid bone, in contrast to the other paranasal sinuses. It is directly invaded by an outpouching from the posterior nasal cavity into the bone. This is noted to have occurred in most fetuses by the fourth month. The development of the sphenoid sinus is variable, and in some individuals, a sphenoid sinus does not develop at all.

The maxillary, ethmoid, and frontal recess buds and sphenoid paranasal sinuses are present at birth but continue to develop and mature well into the teenage years. It is important to consider the relative size and position of the sinuses of the child at various ages (▶ Fig. 67.2 and ▶ Table 67.1).

67.3 Congenital Nasal Anomalies

Derangements of embryologic development result in various congenital nasal anomalies. These congenital anomalies include choanal atresia, nasal dermoids and gliomas, proboscis lateralis, and various types of cleft lip and palate. The majority of these conditions are noted at birth, either by direct observation or because of symptoms directly related to the anomaly.

67.3.1 Choanal Atresia
Presenting Symptoms

Choanal atresia is a congenital malformation of the nasal region that can present as either a unilateral or bilateral condition. It is caused by failure of the nasobuccal membrane to perforate on one or both sides, preventing normal formation of the choanae. Choanal atresia occurs in approximately 1 in 35,000 live births. Children with bilateral choanal atresia usually present at or soon after birth with cyanosis relieved by crying. The atretic plate causes total nasal obstruction and prevents nasal respiration in newborns, who are obligate nasal breathers and in whom apnea and cyanosis develop if they are unable to breathe via the nose. (Oral breathing is a learned behavior that occurs within the first year of life.) The degree of respiratory distress varies among babies; however, bilateral choanal atresia is considered an urgent situation because of the repeated episodes of apnea and cyanosis in affected individuals.

Unilateral choanal atresia is more difficult to diagnose and may be missed in the infant because affected children are able to breathe through the unaffected side. These patients typically

Table 67.1 Sinus size at various ages

Age	Maxillary	Frontal	Sphenoid
Birth	5 mm	4 mm	3 mm
4 y	11 mm	5 mm	5 mm
10 y	18 mm	9 mm	10 mm
Adult	30 mm	25 mm	20 mm

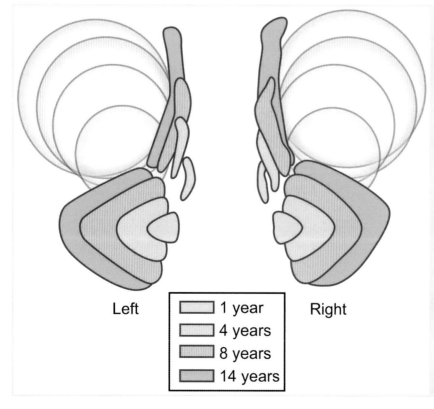

Left   Right

1 year
4 years
8 years
14 years

Fig. 67.2 Growth of the sinuses during childhood. (Adapted from Maresh MM. Paranasal sinuses from birth to late adolescence: I. Size of the paranasal sinuses as observed in routing posteroanterior roentgenograms. Am J Dis Child 1940;60(1):55–78.)

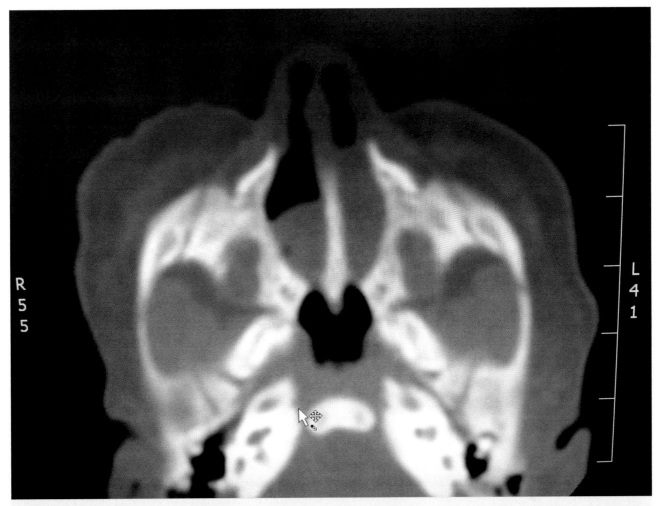

Fig. 67.3 Computed tomographic scan of bilateral choanal atresia.

present as toddlers with chronic unilateral nasal discharge that does not respond to medical therapy; they rarely complain of nasal obstruction.

Examination and Diagnosis

The diagnosis is usually suspected by the neonatologist in a newborn child with repeated episodes of cyanosis and apnea. Physical examination and anterior rhinoscopic examination of the newborn will often reveal normal external nasal features. A fiber-optic intranasal examination will often reveal a small intranasal cavity, and the examiner will encounter difficulty in passing the endoscope into the nasopharynx. Inability to pass a 5F feeding tube through the nasal cavity into the oropharynx strongly suggests the diagnosis of choanal atresia. Nasal airflow can be evaluated by simply holding a strip of tissue paper in front of the nares and observing movement of the paper during breathing.

Patients suspected of having choanal atresia should undergo axial computed tomography (CT) of the midface so that the diagnosis can be made definitively. In a patient with choanal atresia, the CT scan will distinguish between complete atresia of the choanal opening (▶ Fig. 67.3) and stenosis (narrowing) and determine the extent of the bony plate causing the obstruction.

The majority of patients with choanal atresia have a complete bony plate or a combination of bony and membranous obstruction. CT is instrumental in treatment planning and should not be supplanted with other studies.

Evaluation and Testing

Choanal atresia, when bilateral, is associated with other anomalies in about 50% of cases. The most common associated condition is the CHARGE syndrome (coloboma, congenital heart malformations, choanal atresia, retardation of growth, genitourinary tract malformations, and ear malformations and hearing loss). Before they undergo general anesthesia and correction of the choanal atresia, babies with bilateral choanal atresia should undergo genetic, cardiac, and renal evaluations to assess for the CHARGE association because of the significant possibility that they will have a congenital heart malformation.

Treatment

Bilateral choanal atresia is a life-threatening condition in the newborn until recognized because of the risk for apnea leading to cyanosis. An affected infant may initially be treated with an oral airway (bypassing the nasal obstruction) or intubation

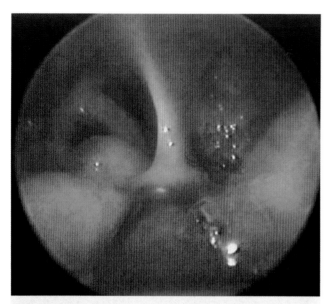

Fig. 67.4 Nasopharyngeal view of unilateral choanal atresia.

when an oral airway is not tolerated. Choanal atresia is definitively corrected by the creation of choanae. The procedure can be carried out via a transnasal endoscopic approach with drilling out of the bony atretic plate and posterior bony vomer plate, or via a transpalatal approach with drilling out of the posterior hard palate and atretic plate.

Stenting with transnasal tubes may be necessary. The procedure is carried out in infants as soon as they are stable and have been evaluated for cardiac malformations.

In the case of unilateral choanal atresia (▶ Fig. 67.4), treatment is deferred until the child is at least 2 years of age, even if the condition has been diagnosed in infancy. Correction at an older age is associated with improved success rates and a decreased need for revision surgery. Most cases of unilateral choanal atresia are corrected via the transnasal endoscopic approach. This approach incorporates drilling out of both the lateral wall bone and a portion of the posterior septum/vomer. In this procedure, stenting is not usually necessary. Transpalatal correction is reserved for patients with restenosis.

Complications

Bilateral choanal atresia, if unrecognized, can be a life-threatening condition in the newborn because of the development of hypoxemia and apnea in a baby who is unable to breathe nasally. After the diagnosis, the child should be assessed for the presence of associated medical syndromes. Unilateral choanal atresia is not typically a serious problem and rarely presents with complications before correction. Surgical complications include risk for injury to the brain and brainstem during initial perforation of the atretic plate. This rare complication can be reduced by using a 120-degree nasopharyngeal endoscope to observe the posterior aspect of the choanae during initial puncture of the atretic plate. The most common complication of choanal atresia correction is stenosis at the repair site. This may be caused by the inadequate removal of bone from the choana or septal edge, or the development of excess scar tissue in the posterior nasal cavity. Revision surgery may be per-

formed either transnasally or transpalatally. Transnasal endoscopic surgery has higher rates of stenosis and the need for revision surgery.

Prognosis

Children with choanal atresia have an excellent prognosis for satisfactory nasal breathing with adequate repair, particularly if they have unilateral choanal atresia and do not have the CHARGE association. Most children, even those who require revision surgery, are able to breathe well through the nose once they have healed from reconstruction of the choana.

When the CHARGE association is present, there is an increased risk for restenosis and the need for secondary procedures, yet these children usually fare well after correction of their choanal atresia.

67.3.2 Piriform Aperture Stenosis

Etiology, Pathophysiology, and Pathogenesis

Piriform aperture stenosis is a rare bony congenital malformation characterized by narrowing at the entry of the piriform aperture of the nose. It develops during embryologic formation of the nose and nasal cavity and often is associated with other craniofacial conditions, such as holoprosencephaly, congenital central maxillary incisor, and malformations of the sinuses. There is no known etiologic agent that causes nasal piriform aperture stenosis.

Presenting Symptoms

The most common symptom of piriform aperture stenosis is nasal obstruction in the neonatal period. Children with piriform stenosis may experience significant respiratory distress because they are obligate nasal breathers, and they usually demonstrate loud, stertorous breathing with snorting, chest retractions, and poor nasal airflow.

Medical Evaluation and Testing

Piriform aperture stenosis will have a congested nasal appearance on anterior rhinoscopy. In many cases, the nose will be so narrow that even a flexible fiber-optic nasopharyngoscope cannot be passed into the nasal cavity through the nostril. Choanal atresia can be excluded by visualizing air bubbling from the nostril at times; however, choanal stenosis is not excluded. The exterior of the nose usually appears normal.

The diagnosis is made when typical piriform aperture narrowing is seen on axial CT (▶ Fig. 67.5). An aperture width of less than 8 mm confirms the diagnosis. When piriform stenosis is present, other neurologic malformations should be excluded with imaging of the brain.

Treatment

Mild cases of piriform aperture stenosis can be successfully managed with careful observation, nasal steroids, and the suctioning of secretions with a bulb syringe. Babies who have the mildest cases of stenosis should be followed expectantly for growth of the piriform aperture.

Children who have considerable respiratory distress will usually benefit from surgical enlargement of the piriform aperture with removal of the obstructing bone. This is accomplished via a sublabial degloving approach with elevation of the piriform

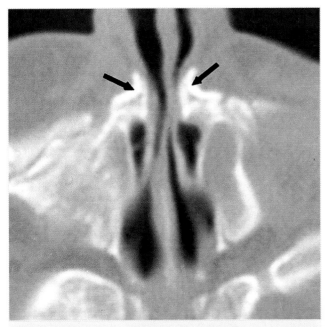

Fig. 67.5 Computed tomographic scan demonstrating piriform aperture stenosis (*arrows*).

aperture periosteum and careful drilling of the bone. The nasal opening is then stented to reapproximate the periosteum to the bone.

Prognosis

The prognosis is favorable for children who have mild piriform stenosis treated with conservative measures of saline lavage and frequent suctioning. In those babies undergoing surgical enlargement of the piriform aperture for severe symptoms, the prognosis depends upon the degree to which the stenosis can be enlarged. Children should be followed for growth and the maintained relief of nasal obstruction for at least 1 to 2 years.

67.3.3 Rare Congenital Nasal Anomalies

Derangements in embryologic formation of the nose can result in various abnormalities of the nasal structure. These conditions are rare and infrequently reported in the medical literature, but they can be highly alarming to the baby's parents.

Proboscis lateralis is a rare condition in which a tubelike formation either replaces the entire nasal structure (often in association with cyclopia, or single midline eye) or is located to the side of the nose. If the proboscis is on the side, the ipsilateral nostril is often absent or markedly smaller than the contralateral normal nostril (▶ Fig. 67.6). The ipsilateral nasal cavity may be smaller than normal, and the attachment point of

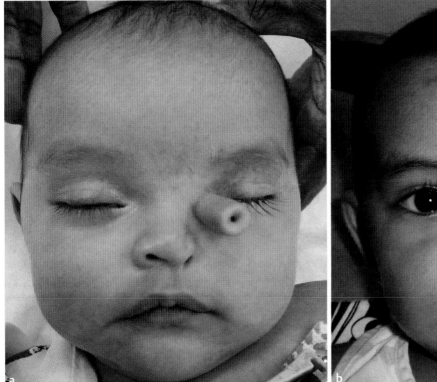
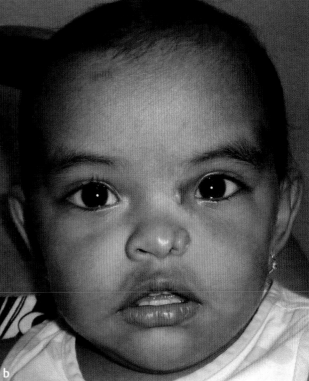

Fig. 67.6 (a) Proboscis lateralis with ipsilateral stenotic nostril. (b) After removal of the proboscis and left-sided reconstruction of the nostril with a portion of the proboscis.

67.3.4 Congenital Midline Nasal Masses: Dermoids, Gliomas, and Encephaloceles

Etiology, Pathophysiology, and Pathogenesis

Congenital midline nasal masses are uncommon and comprise a spectrum ranging from dermoid cysts through gliomas to encephaloceles; nasal dermoids are the most common. These masses are caused by errors in the development of the nasal space and are found in 1 per 20,000 to 1 per 40,000 live births. A child with a dermoid, glioma, or encephalocele may present with an external or internal nasal mass. Before nasal development, the foramen caecum of the developing neuropore normally closes by the third week of embryologic development, with ultimate separation of the intracranial and extracranial structures. When the foramen caecum fails to close, a tongue of prolapsing dura may extend into this space and extracranially into the developing nose and septum. If brain tissue is contained within the protruding dura and remains attached to the fully developed brain by a tubelike stalk, an encephalocele is present. When the dura or brain tissue inside the mass is isolated from the brain (85 to 90%) or attached only by a fibrous stalk (10 to 15%) in the region of the foramen cecum, the mass is defined as a glioma (▶ Fig. 67.8). Gliomas are most commonly extranasal (up to 60%) and affect males three times as frequently as females. Nasal dermoid cysts are considered to form similarly to gliomas and encephaloceles because the dura is closely approximated to the nasal skin around the time of neuropore closure and foramen caecum closure. It is felt that the proximity of the nasal skin to the dura at this time (approximately the third or fourth week of development) results in some of the skin cells being drawn up into the developing nasal cavity, with resultant formation of the dermoid cyst. Dermoid cysts consist of ectodermal and mesodermal embryonal germ layers, in contrast to teratomas, which also have an endodermal layer and are lined by skin with hair and sebaceous glands. Encephaloceles are often associated with other congenital abnormalities and are seen evenly in males and females.

Nasal Dermoid Cyst

Presenting Symptoms

Dermoid cysts are slowly growing, smooth masses that are firm and do not transilluminate in or around the nasal area. Often, a pore (with or without a tuft of hair) is present on the external skin, which is characteristic of dermoid cysts only. Dermoids are not compressible, nor do they enlarge with crying or Valsalva maneuvers. They are found anywhere from the glabella to the nasal tip, as well as intranasally or within the septum. Because of the unique embryologic development of dermoid cysts, there can be a fibrous connection intracranially through a patent foramen caecum. There may be deformation and lateral splaying of the nasal bones, depending upon the location of the cystic portion of the dermoid (▶ Fig. 67.9a and ▶ Table 67.2). Intranasal dermoids may present with nasal congestion and/or nasal obstruction. There may be widening of the nasal septum if the cyst is within the septal cartilage. When the mass is relatively small, the lesion may not be identified until the patient is older.

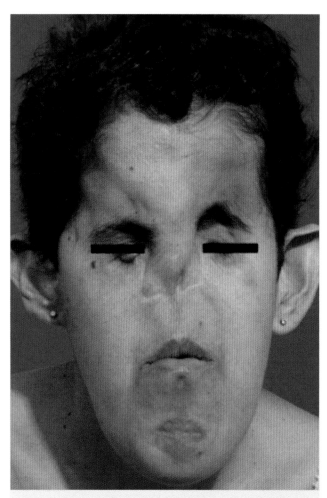

Fig. 67.7 Arrhinia with anophthalmia. Note the lack of a nasal opening.

the proboscis may indicate derangement of the tear duct system. Surgical management includes excision of the proboscis, evaluation of the continuity of the tear duct system, and reconstruction of the hypoplastic or absent nostril. These children have an excellent prognosis for appearance and nasal and tear duct function when the nostril and nasal cavity are less severely affected.

Supernumerary nostrils are duplication anomalies of the nose. Although rare, they are easily identified by their characteristic appearance at birth. The extra nostril is often superior to the true nostril and may, but not always, exist in continuity with the true nasal cavity. The treatment is surgical excision of the duplicate nostril; local flaps may be needed to restore normal contour to the perinasal crease.

Arrhinia is an extremely rare congenital condition in which the nose is absent. In this case, there is no nostril or nasal opening, and the nasal cavity is not present or patent. This condition results when the nasal placode fails to canalize during embryologic development. Treatment is aimed at maintaining an adequate airway, and early mouth breathing is mandatory. Surgical construction of an exterior nose is performed in multiple stages, and nasal passages are difficult to construct (▶ Fig. 67.7).

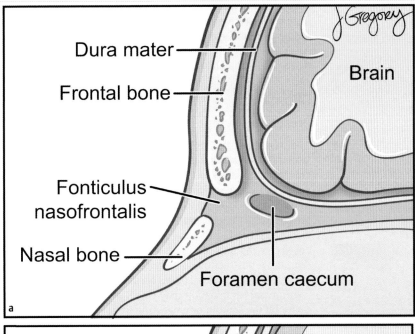

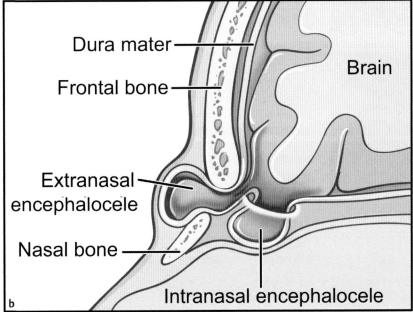

Fig. 67.8 (a) Normal anterior skull base. (b) Anterior skull base and foramen caecum location with encephalocele.

Medical Evaluation and Testing

After the mass is identified, radiographic imaging is obtained. CT in the axial and sagittal planes will not only demonstrate the mass but also delineate the bony confines and surrounding structures. There may be a bifid crista galli or widening of the foramen caecum in the anterior cranial fossa with the suggestion of a possible intracranial communication. Magnetic resonance (MR) imaging is very helpful in determining if a suspected intracranial communication is present and is felt to be more sensitive and specific for this component of the diagnosis; the T1-weighted MR image is hyperintense in dermoid cysts.

Treatment

The treatment for dermoid cysts is complete surgical excision when the lesion is diagnosed. There is a risk for infection in dermoid cysts, and if infection occurs with rupture of the cyst, complete excision is difficult. Incompletely excised dermoid cysts generally recur, with revision surgery even more complex than primary excision. Usually, an external approach (e.g., direct incision, external rhinoplasty, lateral rhinotomy) is used for lesions external to the nasal bones (▶ Fig. 67.9b). Intranasal cysts may require midfacial degloving or endoscopic approaches. Neurosurgical consultation is required for dermoids with intracranial extension, and craniotomy may be necessary for safe, complete removal.

Complications and Prognosis

Dermoid cysts may become infected, making definitive excision more difficult. Spread of infection to the paranasal tissues may occur. A cerebrospinal fluid (CSF) leak may occur in lesions with

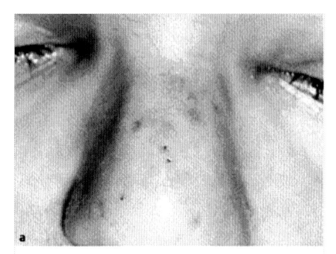

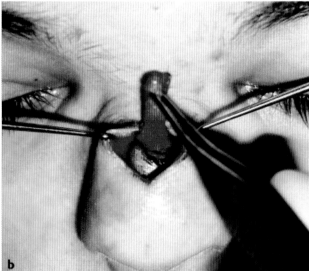

Fig. 67.9 (a) Nasal dermoid with hair protruding at midline. (b) Excision of a nasal dermal sinus cyst with the sinus tract passing through the nasal bones.

intracranial communication. Late complications include scars from external approaches, loss of septal cartilage integrity with saddle nose deformity, and cosmetic complications when the nasal bones are affected. The prognosis is excellent when the dermoid is completely excised.

Glioma

Presenting Symptoms

Gliomas present as external masses in the glabella region (about 60% of all gliomas) but may occur anywhere within or around the nasal region. When they are external, they are firm, nontender, and noncompressible masses. They do not transilluminate, and if close to the skin surface, they may have a purplish discoloration. Gliomas are usually diagnosed at birth when external, but the diagnosis of intranasal gliomas may be delayed. Symptoms of intranasal gliomas include nasal congestion, nasal obstruction, and stertorous snoring. Hypertelorism and splaying of the nasal bones occur with larger lesions.

Intranasal examination may reveal a mass high in the nasal cavity by the septum or emanating from the lateral nasal wall. The mucosa-covered mass usually will be smooth and firm to palpation.

Diagnostic Testing

The presence of an intranasal mass requires radiologic evaluation. MR imaging is the most specific and sensitive study. MR imaging can determine whether there is an intracranial stalk communication and helps to differentiate glioma from encephalocele. Gliomas are hyperintense on T2-weighted images; on T1-weighted images, they are variable in intensity. CT is complementary to MR imaging. Gliomas are isodense on CT. CT reveals important relationships to the intranasal anatomy and is useful for surgical planning (▶ Fig. 67.10).

Treatment

Once a glioma is diagnosed, consultation with a pediatric neurosurgeon is recommended because of the risk for intracranial

Table 67.2 Comparison of findings in congenital midline nasal masses

	Dermoid	Glioma	Encephalocele
Age at diagnosis	Infants and children	Infants and children	Infants and children
Location of mass	Intranasal + extranasal	Intranasal + extranasal	Intranasal + extranasal
Cranial defect	Rare	Up to 15%	All
Pulsation	No	No	Yes
Transillumination	No	No	Yes
Appearance	Firm ± pore or hair	Purplish, firm, smooth	Purplish, soft
Compressibility	No	No	Yes
Cerebrospinal fluid connection	Rare	Rarely	Yes
Possible infection	Local infection	Possible meningitis	Meningitis

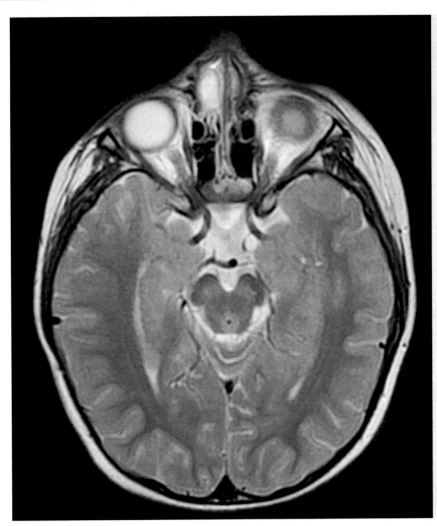

Fig. 67.10 Intranasal glioma on T2-weighted magnetic resonance image.

communication. Biopsy for diagnosis is not advised because of the risk for infection and the creation of a CSF leak if there is an intracranial communication. Surgical treatment is recommended with complete excision. External lesions may be removed in a manner similar to that used for nasal dermoids. Intranasal gliomas without intracranial extension may be removed endoscopically with or without a combined neurosurgical craniotomy for total resection. This may be accomplished in a single stage or in two procedures. Endoscopic techniques have evolved recently, and the use of intraoperative stereotactic image guidance systems increases the likelihood of complete excision (including gliomas with intracranial communication) and repair of the anterior cranial fossa defect.

Complications and Prognosis

Excision of a glioma carries a specific risk for CSF leak, particularly when an intracranial communication has not been anticipated. Endoscopic removal of the glioma increases the risk for CSF leak and fistula, which must be repaired as soon as it is discovered.

The prognosis is excellent with complete removal of the glioma, regardless of the resection technique. Recurrence rates are very low (< 10%), even if the lesion is incompletely removed.

Encephaloceles

Presenting Symptoms

Most encephaloceles, like gliomas, are diagnosed at or soon after birth, particularly when they are extranasal. Because encephaloceles contain brain tissue and CSF, they are compressible masses that readily transilluminate. They are smooth, slightly firm masses within or around the region of the nose. When intranasal, they tend to cause symptoms of nasal congestion, nasal obstruction, or stertor. Other physical findings may include hypertelorism and splaying of the nasal bones, similar to that seen in gliomas.

Diagnostic Testing

MR imaging and CT are recommended for reasons similar to those for gliomas. The foramen caecum is patent with a variably sized defect in the anterior skull base on CT scans. The MR image may show brain, meninges, or dura within the mass and intracranial communication. The MR image will demonstrate CSF within the mass and connecting stalk, which can help to distinguish an encephalocele from a glioma (▶ Fig. 67.11).

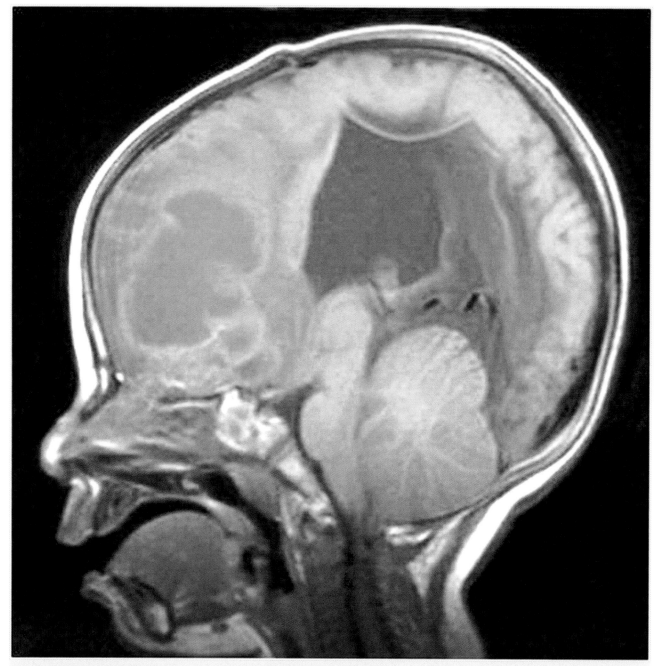

Fig. 67.11 Magnetic resonance image demonstrating brain tissue in a nasal encephalocele.

Treatment

The treatment options are similar to those for glioma. Biopsy for diagnosis is not performed on encephaloceles, for reasons similar to those for glioma. The need for neurosurgical consultation and collaboration is increased in cases of larger encephaloceles. Endoscopic management is possible for smaller masses, with the expectation of performing CSF and anterior cranial floor repairs.

Complications and Prognosis

The prognosis is excellent when a careful resection is planned and performed. The correction of associated deformities, such as hypertelorism, is often planned concurrently with the resection or as a later, staged procedure.

67.4 Epistaxis

67.4.1 Anatomy

The nose and nasal area have a rich blood supply from both the external and internal carotid arteries. The main arterial supply to the nose and septum comes from branches of the anterior and posterior ethmoidal arteries (superior), sphenopalatine artery (posterior), and greater palatine and superior labial arteries

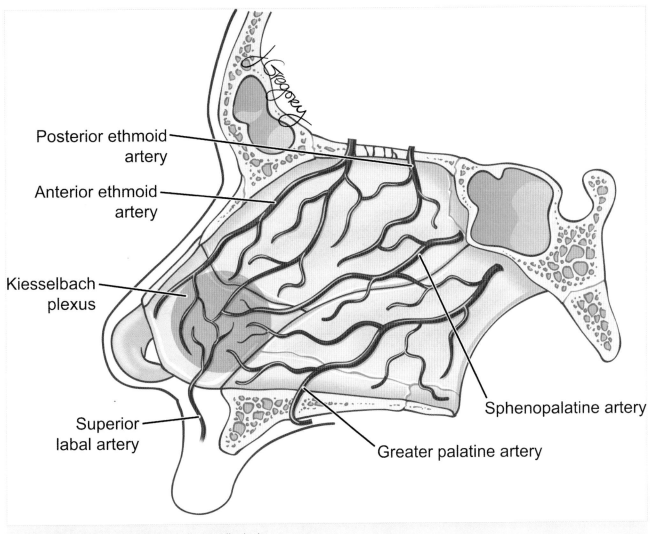

Fig. 67.12 Nasal septal vessels forming the Kiesselbach plexus.

(inferior). The anterior and posterior ethmoidal arteries are branches of the ophthalmic artery, an intracranial branch of the internal carotid artery. The sphenopalatine artery and the greater palatine artery are end branches of the internal maxillary artery, one of the main branches of the external carotid artery. The internal maxillary artery and its branches also supply the sinuses and lateral nasal wall. The greater palatine artery is a sub-branch of the internal maxillary artery and supplies the inferior septum and nasal floor. The superior labial artery is a sub-branch of the facial artery and supplies the anterior nasal floor and anterior septum. A rich vascular plexus, the Kiesselbach plexus, is formed from contributions of these arteries, particularly in the anterior septum (▶ Fig. 67.12). The Kiesselbach plexus is the most common location for epistaxis in young children because of its location in the anterior septal region and highly vascular nature.

67.4.2 Etiology and Pathogenesis

There are myriad causes of epistaxis in children. Common causes of epistaxis include trauma, abnormal airflow through the nose, dry air, and inflammation. Trauma to the delicate anterior nasal septal mucosa, especially if it is already inflamed, is the most common cause. Trauma to the nasal mucosa can be digital trauma ("nose picking"), direct blunt trauma (nasal fracture), or innocent rubbing of the nose. Injury to the mucosal integrity leads to excoriation and thinning of the mucosal surface over the blood vessels.

Inflammation plays a significant role in epistaxis in children. Children are predisposed to viral upper respiratory infections with associated nasal secretions. They are more likely to develop secondary bacterial infections of the nostril skin and nasal mucosa, which may increase the vascularity of the nasal tissues. The risk for epistaxis increases when infection is accompanied by drying of the mucus and crusting at the anterior septum and nares, compounded by digital trauma.

Abnormalities of airflow through the nose, often due to various types of nasal obstruction, may cause inflammatory changes to the mucosa of the nasal cavity, with increased vascularity. In addition, the nose serves to humidify the ambient air during respiration. When the humidity of the air is excessively low (in certain geographic regions, during the winter, or in heated environments), the mucosa will dry (especially in the anterior septal area), increasing the risk for microfissures and cracks, which result in epistaxis.

Children with tumors or systemic conditions may be at increased risk for epistaxis. Any medical condition resulting in a coagulation abnormality (e.g., hemophilia, von Willebrand disease) or thrombocytopenia (e.g., idiopathic thrombocytopenia, complications of chemotherapy, initial presentation of certain leukemias), as well as certain medications (e.g., aspirin, nonsteroidal anti-inflammatory drugs), can result in epistaxis that may be difficult to control.

67.4.3 Presenting Symptoms and Examination

Although epistaxis can be a life-threatening condition in children, most cases are mild episodes of bleeding from one or both nostrils. Most children seen in a medical office will present with a history of repetitive episodes of nose bleeding. The duration and frequency of the episodes should be determined. In girls and prepubescent boys, the most common finding on anterior rhinoscopy is multiple visible blood vessels on the anterior septum and nasal floor or shallow excoriations in this area. Care must be taken to evaluate the entire nasal cavity to exclude intranasal masses, especially in postpubescent boys, because juvenile angiofibroma may be a cause in this group.

67.4.4 Treatment

The treatment of epistaxis in children depends upon whether the child is actively bleeding at the time of evaluation. When the child is actively bleeding, the situation is more urgent, and the severity of bleeding and degree of blood loss must be rapidly determined and measures taken to halt the epistaxis. Maintaining a calm composure while dealing with the child and parents is essential to control a nosebleed, and if a child is unable to cooperate, restraints may be required.

If the nose contains blood and clots on first inspection, either having the child blow the nose or applying gentle suction is necessary. The nose is then inspected, either with an otoscope or with a nasal speculum and headlight. The nasal cavity is sprayed with a decongestant (either oxymetazoline or phenylephrine) and a topical anesthetic (usually 4% lidocaine). Often, the decongestant will stop the nosebleed. The nasal and septal mucosa is inspected for the bleeding site, and if it is identified, it may be cauterized (with silver nitrate or electrocautery), or a gelatin hemostatic sponge may be placed at the intranasal site. Antibiotic ointment should be placed on the site and may be used as the only treatment in mild epistaxis with efficacy similar to that of cautery.

More severe nosebleeds may require intranasal packing. Common materials include hemostatic balloons (although they are often too large for most young children), nasal packing with hemostatic agents (such as gelatin collagen sponges or other, similar dissolvable materials), or standard strip gauze packing. In some cases, general anesthesia may be required to evaluate and control severe epistaxis in children. The use of dissolvable agents is preferred in children whenever possible. A search for the cause of the epistaxis must be made, with correction of those underlying factors to reduce future episodes of epistaxis. Any clotting disorder (hemophilia, von Willebrand disease) or thrombocytopenia must be corrected in severe epistaxis for the maintenance of hemostasis.

67.4.5 Complications of Treatment

Complications from the management of epistaxis are uncommon when certain precautions are taken. Nasal packing, particularly with strip gauze, is a known risk factor for the development of toxic shock syndrome. Toxic shock syndrome is a severe, life-threatening condition resulting from toxin produced by *Staphylococcus aureus* or *Streptococcus pyogenes* suprainfection in the nasal packing material. Toxic shock syndrome consists of high fever (over 39°C), hypotension, a diffuse erythematous rash with desquamation, and severe organ system involvement. Although the risk for toxic shock syndrome cannot be eliminated, it is substantially reduced by the use of systemic antibiotics while nasal packing is in place.

Nasal septal perforation is a complication of extensive bilateral septal mucosal cauterization. This complication is reduced by limiting cauterization to one side of the septum with interval treatment of the opposite side. In many cases of bilateral bleeding from nasal septal vessels, treatment of the worse side may result in improvement in the opposite side, decreasing the need for treatment of the second side.

67.4.6 Prognosis

Children with epistaxis have an excellent prognosis, especially those with mild cases. Recurrent epistaxis can usually be substantially decreased with a reduction of the conditions resulting in digital trauma, an increase in humidification, and the use of daily topical antibiotic ointments. Patients whose epistaxis does not improve should undergo hematologic evaluation for a bleeding or clotting disorder. The control of underlying conditions is essential to reduce the impact of epistaxis in this group of patients.

67.5 Foreign Bodies in the Nose

67.5.1 Etiology and Pathogenesis

Children are prone to explore their bodies and will often place foreign objects into their nose or ears. The most common pathway children use to introduce foreign objects into their nose is via the nares, although foreign bodies may enter the nasal cavity via the nasopharynx and choanae. After the foreign body is placed into the nasal passage, it is unusual for children to complain about the discomfort the foreign body causes. Most foreign body insertions are not witnessed by caregivers.

67.5.2 Presenting Symptoms and Examination

Unless someone has seen the child place a foreign body into the nose or the child admits the act to a caregiver, the child will present with symptoms or complications caused by the presence of a foreign body in the nose. The nasal complaint will usually be unilateral (more rarely bilateral) chronic nasal discharge lasting days to weeks or longer. The nasal discharge is a direct effect of the foreign body on the nasal mucosa and possible obstruction of the nasal cavity by the foreign body.

The nasal examination will usually show thick mucus or mucopurulent discharge in the affected side of the nose, which may prevent the foreign body from being initially visualized. The unaffected side is usually normal in appearance. After the mucus has been suctioned, the foreign body is usually seen lodged between the septum and turbinates in the anterior or middle region of the nasal cavity. The mucous membrane may exhibit marked inflammation and irritation, with easy bleeding in the area of the object. Disc batteries are readily available in toys and common household objects that are accessible to children, and special attention and intervention are required if these are suspected as foreign bodies. When moistened with nasal secretions (electrolyte-containing fluids), the disc battery will begin to leak and cause a severe chemical burn to the nasal mucosa. The child will complain of severe pain, and nasal discharge will begin much sooner than with other foreign bodies. Disc batteries placed in the nose should be treated as an urgent matter.

67.5.3 Diagnostic Testing

Clinical examination is usually all that is needed to detect the vast majority of foreign bodies found in children's noses. If a foreign body is seen on a radiograph, it is usually an incidental finding on sinus series films or lateral neck films, such as those obtained for the evaluation of sinusitis or adenoid size.

67.5.4 Treatment

Most foreign bodies found in a child's nose can be removed safely in the office with the proper equipment and restraint of the child. Although older children may tolerate removal of a foreign body from the nose under topical anesthesia, younger children rarely are willing to cooperate. Proper restraint of the child is essential to safe removal. Often, a papoose board is needed to control the child during the treatment. The first attempt to remove a nasal foreign body is the one most likely to succeed, and the otolaryngologist is the health provider most likely to succeed.

After topical anesthesia and decongestion of the nasal cavity, a headlight or the microscope can be used to illuminate the nasal cavity. Using a nasal speculum and an appropriate tool, such as a Hartmann or bayonet forceps, right angle hook, or curved wire loop, the physician grasps the object or places the instrument behind the object. The object is then pulled forward and out of the nostril. The nasal mucosa is reinspected following the extraction. Care is taken to note any injuries to the mucosa caused by the foreign body or the removal, and care should be taken to ensure that only one foreign body was in the nose. Minor injuries to the mucosa can be expected to heal completely.

If the foreign body is a disc battery, it is most likely to have already leaked, causing a chemical burn of the nasal mucosa. Disc batteries can cause a direct septal perforation. If septal perforation has occurred, it is recommended to flush the area with saline to dilute the battery alkaline contents and cleanse the mucosa. Following foreign body removal, care of the nose includes the use of saline sprays and rinses.

67.5.5 Complications and Prognosis

Foreign body removal is usually successful as an office procedure; however, some children have been so traumatized by prior attempts that it is impossible to remove the foreign body without general anesthesia. Arrangements should be made to remove the foreign body as soon as possible, with NPO (nil per os) status and type of foreign body in mind. The removal of chronic foreign bodies, except for disc batteries, can wait until appropriate NPO status is possible.

Children, after successful removal of an intranasal foreign body, have an excellent prognosis. Although most foreign bodies do not cause sequelae, some foreign bodies can result in stenosis, synechiae, or perforation of the nasal septum. Saddle nose deformity may result if the septal cartilage has been damaged.

67.6 Nasal Trauma in Children

67.6.1 Etiology

Accidental nasal trauma frequently occurs in active young children during play and sports. Most commonly, there is minimal to mild swelling of the nasal soft tissues with possible self-limited epistaxis. When there is significant impact to the nose, nasal bones, or midface, the pediatric skeleton is unable to absorb the impact, and fracture of the affected area may occur.

67.6.2 Pathogenesis

The pediatric facial skeleton is capable of absorbing minor impacts because of the flexibility and somewhat elastic nature of the developing bones. The central facial area is prone to impact, especially the nasal area. The thin nasal bones are particularly at risk for injury from trauma, especially the inferior and lateral aspects of the nasal bones. Direct impact can result in fracture of the bone or cartilage of the nasal septum, as in the adult. However, in the younger child, the cartilage and bone are more pliable and elastic, and so are more likely to flex than to fracture. As children age into their teens, the nasal structures lose these elastic properties and become more prone to fracture, as in the adult.

67.6.3 Presenting Symptoms

Children with facial trauma present soon after the injury. The history must include the details of the incident and the mechanism of injury, as well as the presence of epistaxis or new nasal obstruction. An examination performed immediately after the injury may reveal the presence or absence of a deformation of the nasal bones; however, most patients present with moderate to severe facial soft-tissue edema, precluding an assessment of nasal bone displacement. Intranasal examination is very important, with particular attention to the septum. Complaints of nasal obstruction, combined with swelling of the septal mucosa (unilateral or bilateral) that is soft and compressible, are compatible with a septal hematoma, a relative emergency. The patient must be evaluated for possible associated ocular or orbital injuries, and ophthalmic consultation should be promptly obtained if indicated.

The examination should be repeated about 5 or 6 days after the injury if there is a question of nasal bone fracture. The delayed examination allows time for a reduction of perinasal edema and an easier assessment of displacement of the nasal bones. Periorbital ecchymosis may be seen days after the injury when a nasal fracture has occurred.

67.6.4 Diagnostic Testing

Clinical examination is usually all that is needed to make a diagnosis of nasal bone fracture and/or septal hematoma. Nasal bone radiographs are unlikely to provide information beyond what a careful evaluation of the position, symmetry, and contour of the nasal region will yield. In older children with prior episodes of nasal trauma, it may be difficult to differentiate current findings from prior injuries. When adjacent trauma is present, CT is recommended to evaluate the orbit or maxilla for associated fracture or trauma.

67.6.5 Treatment

Nasal fractures are usually treated with closed nasal bone reduction under local or general anesthesia. The optimal time for reduction of a nasal fracture in children is between 5 and 8 days. Children heal much more quickly than adults, and a fixation of the malpositioned fracture will develop in just a few days, so that the timing of treatment is more urgent in children. Septal hematoma requires urgent treatment with either aspiration or incision and drainage with packing as soon as the diagnosis is made to prevent the formation of a septal abscess or the late complications of septal cartilage loss and saddle nose deformity.

Closed nasal bone reduction in children is commonly performed with general anesthesia because of patient anxiety. The nasal cavity is prepared with the application of a topical decongestant (oxymetazoline) on cottonoid pledgets. The Goldman elevator is typically used to disimpact, elevate, and mobilize the displaced nasal bone. First, pressure is applied in the direction of the displaced bone, and the elevator is then used to elevate and replace the bone into the proper position. Finger pressure is applied to assist in the use of the elevator. When the procedure is successfully performed, the surgeon can often feel the displaced bone "pop" into its normal position. The symmetry of the nose should be evaluated from the frontal and bird's-eye position. A splint is applied for 5 to 7 days; in children, intranasal packing is rarely needed.

67.6.6 Complications

The main risk of nasal fracture and its treatment is unsuccessful reduction. If the displaced bone cannot be reduced, too much time may have elapsed between the injury and fracture reduction. Often, this is due to patient delay in seeking treatment. Inadequate fracture reduction may be the result of a greenstick type of fracture, with slow relapse of the bone to its pretreatment position. In addition to the nasal bone, the septum may sustain a fracture or become deviated, with resultant nasal obstruction.

When closed nasal reduction is unsuccessful, formal rhinoplasty can be considered once the child has achieved facial maturity. This is generally around the age of 15 to 16 years in girls, and 16 to 17 years in boys. Extensive nasal surgery, especially septal surgery, in younger children risks injury to the nasoseptal growth center, and midfacial and nasal growth

deficiencies may result. As previously mentioned, untreated septal hematoma may progress to septal abscess. The organisms most commonly encountered are *Staphylococcus* species. Septal hematoma or abscess may result in septal cartilage destruction and ultimate saddle nose deformity.

67.6.7 Prognosis

Most children who sustain a nasal fracture will have an excellent prognosis after prompt medical treatment. Successful closed nasal reduction is expected to restore the patient's preinjury cosmetic appearance. However, unrecognized and untreated septal trauma, when present, may become noticeable only as the child matures and a deviated cartilaginous dorsum becomes apparent. When treatment is delayed or unsuccessful, later rhinoplasty in the late teen years has an excellent outcome.

67.7 Nasal Obstruction

Nasal obstruction can be difficult to diagnose in children. Children do not usually reliably complain of an inability to breathe through the nose, and therefore other associated symptoms and signs must be considered to make the diagnosis of nasal obstruction. Nasal obstruction itself is a symptom of other conditions that may originate within the nose or in the nasopharynx. Symptoms of chronic mouth breathing, snoring, chronic runny nose, and a decreased sense of smell all indicate possible nasal obstruction and are important components of the medical history.

67.8 Rhinorrhea

67.8.1 Etiology

Rhinorrhea is frequent in childhood. It is a nonspecific state caused by many conditions affecting the nose, including foreign bodies and allergic, infectious, inflammatory, and obstructing conditions. The nose responds to various insults by increasing its output of nasal secretions. When the volume of the nasal secretions is increased over basal rates, rhinorrhea is seen. Rhinorrhea may occur as a unilateral or bilateral problem, be episodic or constant, and have an acute or a gradual onset.

67.8.2 Infectious Rhinitis

Viral Infection

Viral upper respiratory infections occur frequently in children and are the most common reason for health care visits in children. Until the age of 6 years, children have between six and 10 viral upper respiratory infections per year on average, with each lasting between 10 and 14 days. Although the upper respiratory infection may have resolved, some of the symptoms, such as cough, may persist for several more weeks. The viruses frequently implicated include rhinovirus, adenovirus, coxsackieviruses A and B, respiratory syncytial virus, and influenza viruses. Respiratory syncytial virus is an important cause of severe respiratory illness in children, especially children younger than 12 months of age, and premature children. Children in day care environments are known to be at increased risk for acquiring viral infections and have more upper respiratory infections. Rhinorrhea is seen in the prodromal stage in many viral infections, including measles, mumps, rubella, and roseola.

67.9 Treatment of Viral Infections

The treatment of viral nasal infections is symptomatic and aimed at reducing the impact of congestion and nasal obstruction. Nasal decongestants may be carefully used in the most severe cases. Nasal saline sprays and irrigations with frequent suctioning (with bulb syringe) are helpful in the youngest children and may reduce the possibility of bacterial superinfection.

67.9.1 Bacterial Infection

Bacterial infections of the nose are frequently seen in children and may result as a secondary infection after an upper respiratory infection. They are noted when discolored nasal discharge persists longer than 10 to 14 days or is associated with high fever or worsening symptoms of the upper respiratory infection. Purulent nasal discharge frequently may be caused by *Haemophilus influenzae*, *Moraxella catarrhalis*, *Streptococcus pneumoniae*, and other species of *Streptococcus* and *Staphylococcus*. Bacterial infection in the nose causes mucosal edema (particularly in the turbinates), a foul smell, halitosis, postnasal drip, and nasal obstruction.

Persistent nasal discharge lingering past the time when the symptoms of an upper respiratory infection should have resolved should be considered a bacterial suprainfection. It is recommended that cultures be obtained for long-standing nasal discharge and antibiotic therapy selected based upon the organism or proven sensitivities. Pending the culture results, antibiotic treatment with a β-lactamase–resistant or augmented penicillin, macrolide, or (usually second-generation) cephalosporin may be initiated; this can be adjusted, if necessary, based on the culture reports.

Rhinitis neonatorum is a bacterial nasal infection of infants. This condition deserves special mention because infants are still usually within the phase of obligate nasal breathing, and this nasal infection may cause considerable respiratory distress. The child usually presents with chronic watery or purulent rhinorrhea of some weeks' duration, nasal congestion, partial or complete nasal obstruction, and snorting or snoring. Some babies will demonstrate retractions, indicating more severe nasal obstruction. Infants are particularly susceptible to bacterial infections of the nose. Although they receive transplacental maternal antiviral antibodies during fetal life, their natural resistance against bacterial pathogens is weaker. Bacteria usually found on culture include *H. influenzae*, *Staphylococcus* species, and *Streptococcus* species, among others. Because of increased antibiotic resistance patterns, the administration of a culture-driven antibiotic for 7 to 14 days is recommended. Symptomatic care, including saline and suctioning, is recommended adjuvant treatment.

67.9.2 Complications and Prognosis

Although rhinitis and rhinorrhea are common conditions in childhood, most children are only mildly affected and recover well from these illnesses. Complications of rhinitis are rare, but untreated and persistent rhinitis may develop into rhinosinusitis with its potential complications.

Allergic Rhinitis
Etiology

Allergic rhinitis is the response of the nasal organ to antigen exposure in a sensitized individual. As in adults, allergic rhinitis in children is usually due to sensitization to an environmental agent or allergen that is present either seasonally (e.g., pollens and grasses) or year-round (e.g., human dust mites, molds, cockroaches, dander).

The allergic individual is not born with an allergic response to an allergen; rather, an allergic reaction develops following one or multiple exposures to the allergen. The nose is frequently affected because of the airborne nature of many potential allergens.

The development of an allergy requires an individual tendency (often familial) to develop the allergy *and* exposure to the actual allergen. Allergen-sensitized individuals will exhibit allergic symptoms after exposure to that specific allergen. Individuals may be sensitized to a single or multiple unrelated allergens. The most common allergens are pollen from trees, grasses, and other flowering plants; house dust; dander (cat and dog); mold spores; and peanut dust. Children who exhibit atopy, with eczema and asthma, are at the highest risk for allergic rhinitis.

Pathophysiology and Pathogenesis

Allergic rhinitis is a type of immediate hypersensitivity reaction to an allergen and is typically mediated by immunoglobulin E (IgE) antibodies to the allergen. Upon previous exposure to an allergen, the allergic individual produces IgE antibodies to that specific allergen. When the sensitized individual is again exposed to the specific allergen, the allergen combines with IgE antibodies on the cell membranes of mast cells in the submucosa of the nasal mucous membranes. A cascade is initiated that results in degranulation of the mast cells, with a mediator-regulated reaction and histamine release. This immune reaction results in tissue edema due to increased vascular permeability, increased nasal secretions rich with eosinophils, and concomitant congestion and nasal obstruction. Associated symptoms of itching, sneezing, and tearing frequently occur.

Presenting Symptoms, Medical Evaluation, and Testing

The diagnosis of allergic rhinitis is suggested by the symptoms of nasal congestion and obstruction; thin, clear, watery rhinorrhea; itchy nose; and increased sneezing after exposure to specific environmental agents. In some cases (particularly in perennially occurring allergies), the symptoms have been present so consistently and for so long that the patient is unable to identify specific environmental agents.

Examination of the nose will often reveal congestion of the mucosa; clear, watery rhinorrhea; and pale, boggy, bluish turbinates obstructing the nasal cavity. In long-standing cases, the physical examination findings may be less obvious: general congestion and typical rhinorrhea without significant turbinate pathology.

Collection of the nasal discharge may demonstrate a marked increase in the number of eosinophils on histologic smear. Although helpful by indicating the presence of allergy, eosinophil counts do not assist with identifying the allergen. More commonly used studies to determine specific allergens are serum IgE titers or skin prick (intradermal) testing. RAST (radioallergosorbent testing) is frequently used to identify specific titers, and the results are compared with norms. RAST is often used because it may test for many allergens in one serum sample, provides quantitative data, and carries no risk for the patient. On the other hand, skin prick testing is also an excellent test for allergens, albeit with an increased risk to the patient of an acute reaction. Skin tests are less expensive, available for a large number of potential allergens, and allow the detection of allergic reactions that are not IgE-mediated. The results of skin prick testing are nearly immediately available. Both RAST and intradermal skin testing should be performed after antihistamine drugs have been discontinued for 72 hours.

Treatment

Successful treatment for allergic rhinitis includes (1) elimination of environmental exposure when possible; (2) symptom control with medications (including antihistamines, topical steroids, and nasal decongestants); and (3) immunotherapy. For children afflicted with mild seasonal allergies, control of environmental exposures and pharmacologic therapy are most likely to succeed.

Control of environmental exposures is a critical component of the management of allergic rhinitis. Items likely to initiate allergic attacks, such as carpets, rugs, and stuffed toys in the case of dust mite allergy, must be removed from the environment. The use of HEPA (high-efficiency particulate air) filters on forced central air vents is helpful to reduce the circulation of dust in the home.

The pharmacologic control of allergic rhinitis has been revolutionized in the last 25 years by the development of nonsedating antihistamines (which do not cross the blood–brain barrier) and intranasal topical steroids. Diphenhydramine, a widely used antihistamine, is an excellent allergy medication, but its use is limited by its sedative side effect, as is the use of hydroxyzine. Although it is still used in the treatment of severe allergic reactions, diphenhydramine is not desirable for the treatment of allergy in children because they may be adversely affected by drowsiness.

Newer antihistamines commonly given to children include loratadine, cetirizine, and fexofenadine. These medications have the benefit of being administered once daily for 24-hour control, and they do not have sedating side effects because they are unable to cross the blood–brain barrier. They are preferred for school-age children and have excellent efficacy.

In addition to systemic antihistamines, the newer topical antihistamine sprays are useful when patients have only nasal or ocular symptoms. Topical antihistamine nasal sprays include Astelin (azelastine, Meda Pharmaceuticals), Omnaris (ciclesonide, Sunovion Pharmaceuticals), and Patanase (olopatadine, Alcon Laboratories). Astelin and Omnaris are approved for use in children 5 to 6 years of age and older, and Patanase is approved for children 12 years of age and older.

Topical intranasal corticosteroid sprays are highly effective for treating and inhibiting the symptoms of allergic rhinitis. The intranasal sprays typically contain steroids that are inactivated at pH levels typically found in gastric secretions and thus are minimally absorbed systemically. The sprays stabilize inflammatory cells and cell membrane permeability.

Topical nasal corticosteroid sprays are typically well tolerated by children as young as 2 years of age. Growth inhibition from the long-term use of intranasal corticosteroids is not seen, even after years of use.

Patients with long-standing allergies and incomplete symptom control with antihistamines and topical nasal steroids frequently experience symptom relief with the leukotriene receptor antagonist montelukast (Singulair; Merck). This agent also effectively treats asthma and perennial allergic rhinitis by modulating leukotrienes in the immune response. Excellent control of allergies may be seen with this once-daily agent.

Decongestants may be added to the regimen periodically to treat exacerbations of allergies, or at the onset of therapy with other agents. Oral pseudoephedrine is an excellent nasal decongestant without rebound, whereas topical oxymetazoline and phenylephrine both exhibit rebound effects following continuous use for 3 days or longer. These agents are recommended when symptoms are severe and intolerable. All three agents have the potential side effect of systemic hypertension.

Immunotherapy is used when symptoms cannot be controlled with the above pharmacologic measures. It involves the preparation of weak mixtures of the specific allergens that cause the patient's most significant symptoms and attempts to induce the formation of IgG blocking antibodies to the allergens, resulting in competition between IgG and IgE for the allergen receptors. Immunotherapy can provide excellent results in carefully selected patients with high levels of IgE antibodies to specific allergens.

Complications

The most common complication of allergic rhinitis is the impact of undiagnosed or undertreated allergic rhinitis on the patient's quality of life. Allergic rhinitis can affect sleep quality and efficiency. The effect of sleep disturbance in combination with the use of sedating antihistamines can have a profound impact on school performance in young children. Rarely, allergic rhinitis may progress to allergic nasal/sinus polyposis, which is a generalized swelling of the sinus mucous membranes with protrusion from their sinus confines into the nasal cavity through the sinus ostia. Allergic rhinitis is the underlying etiology of nasal polyposis, and medical management is mandatory.

67.10 Roundsmanship

- Newborn children have very small maxillary and ethmoid sinuses. The frontal and sphenoid sinuses begin to develop at about 4 to 6 years of age.
- Choanal atresia may be bilateral or unilateral. When it is bilateral, babies may present with cyanosis because newborns are obligate nasal breathers. In cases of bilateral choanal atresia, surgery must be performed after the baby is stabilized and the cardiology evaluation completed.

- Choanal atresia is found in about 1 in 35,000 live births. It is frequently seen in children with the CHARGE (coloboma, congenital *h*eart malformations, choanal *a*tresia, *r*etardation of growth, *g*enitourinary tract malformations, and *e*ar malformations and hearing loss) association.
- Choanal atresia may be corrected via a transnasal endoscopic approach or via a transpalatal approach. The endoscopic transnasal approach is less invasive but carries a higher risk for revision surgery for choanal stenosis.
- An intranasal mass in a young child may be a dermoid cyst, glioma, or encephalocele. Biopsy of any midline or superiorly located intranasal mass is not recommended until imaging studies are performed to evaluate for these congenital lesions.
- Epistaxis is a common ailment in children. Most frequently, nosebleeds occur from the disruption of superficial blood vessels in the anterior septum. Treatment with topical silver nitrate helps to substantially reduce most nosebleeds from this region.
- Severe nosebleeds may be from a juvenile nasal angiofibroma in teenage boys. A complete nasal examination is necessary to exclude this disease in pubescent males.
- Unilateral purulent nasal discharge is the most common presenting sign of intranasal foreign body.
- Nasal bone fractures heal much faster in children than in adults. Closed nasal reduction is most successful if performed within 10 days of the injury.
- The management of septal deviations in children is problematic. Facial growth centers are found in the septal/vomer region; disruption from septal surgery risks damage with possible resultant midface growth disturbances. Septoplasty for nasal obstruction is usually postponed until children are past the pubertal growth period.
- Allergic rhinitis is a common problem in children. The common treatments include topical steroid nasal sprays, antihistamines, leukotriene receptor antagonists, and immunotherapy. The prognosis is good when the specific allergen is identified.

67.11 Recommended Reading

[1] Belden CJ, Mancuso AA, Schmalfuss IM. CT features of congenital nasal piriform aperture stenosis: initial experience. Radiology 1999; 213: 495–501
[2] Hanikeri M, Waterhouse N, Kirkpatrick N, Peterson D, Macleod I. The management of midline transcranial nasal dermoid sinus cysts. Br J Plast Surg 2005; 58: 1043–1050
[3] Lelli GJ, Maher EA, Milite JP, Dyleski R. Proboscis lateralis. Ophthal Plast Reconstr Surg 2008; 24: 499–501
[4] Maresh MM. Paranasal sinuses from birth to late adolescence: I. Size of the paranasal sinuses as observed in routing posteroanterior roentgenograms. Am J Dis Child 1940; 60: 55–78
[5] Pinheiro-Neto CD, Snyderman CH, Fernandez-Miranda J, Gardner PA. Endoscopic endonasal surgery for nasal dermoids. Otolaryngol Clin North Am 2011; 44: 981–987, ix
[6] Rahbar R, Resto VA, Robson CD et al. Nasal glioma and encephalocele: diagnosis and management. Laryngoscope 2003; 113: 2069–2077
[7] Ramsden JD, Campisi P, Forte V. Choanal atresia and choanal stenosis. Otolaryngol Clin North Am 2009; 42: 339–352, x
[8] Rontal M. Embryology and anatomy of the paranasal sinuses. In: Bluestone CD, Stool SE, Alper CM, et al, eds. Pediatric Otolaryngology. 4th ed. Philadelphia, PA: W. B. Saunders; 2003
[9] Turner PJ, Kemp AS. Allergic rhinitis in children. J Paediatr Child Health 2012; 48: 302–310

68 Pediatric Sinus Disorders

Robin A. Dyleski

68.1 Acute Sinusitis

68.1.1 Etiology

Inflammatory infections of the nose in young children may progress to sinusitis. It is difficult to distinguish between purulent rhinitis and sinusitis in children, and the term *rhinosinusitis* is frequently used to describe an inflammatory condition affecting both the nose and paranasal sinuses.

Young children have approximately six to 10 viral upper respiratory infections per year, and up to 5% of these are complicated by bacterial rhinosinusitis. The otolaryngologist faces the dilemma of determining which child requires increased medical treatment for bacterial sinusitis as opposed to symptomatic care of an upper respiratory infection.

68.1.2 Pathophysiology and Pathogenesis

In order to maintain a healthy state in the paranasal sinuses, patent ostia, normal mucociliary function and flow, and secretions of normal composition are required. Derangements in any of these basic requirements impact the sinuses and result in various disease states.

The inflammatory effects of viral and bacterial pathogens on the nasal and sinus mucosa cause edema and congestion. The mucosal linings of the sinus ostia are similarly affected, resulting in obstruction of the sinus outflow tract. With obstruction, the sinus mucous secretions are prevented from exiting the sinus ostia, resulting in fluid buildup in the sinus; similarly, the flow of fresh air into the sinus is blocked, resulting in a hypoxic state within the sinus. The presence of stagnant secretions in a hypoxic sinus establish conditions favorable for bacterial supra-infection and the development of sinusitis (▶ Fig. 68.1).

In very young children, the ethmoid sinuses are the most developed and the most commonly affected. The ethmoid sinuses have tiny communicating ostia between the air cells and therefore are the most prone to mucosal inflammatory swelling during viral or bacterial infections. The maxillary sinuses are also frequently affected by sinusitis, but because of their location, they are less often sources of the complications of sinusitis.

68.1.3 Presenting Symptoms

Upper respiratory infection is the most common condition resulting in sinusitis. Acute sinusitis is usually diagnosed in children with purulent rhinorrhea persisting longer than 10 to 14 days after the onset of an upper respiratory infection (▶ Table 68.1). In most cases of acute sinusitis, the symptoms of an upper respiratory infection will persist without improvement past the usual 7 to 10 days; these include postnasal drip, daytime cough, purulent nasal discharge with nasal congestion, and continued (usually low-grade) fever with generalized irritability. When a high fever (> 38.5°C), facial swelling, or pain is present, the child must be monitored closely for potential development of the complications of sinusitis. The symptoms of acute sinusitis resolve spontaneously in 60% of patients in about 3 to 4 weeks.

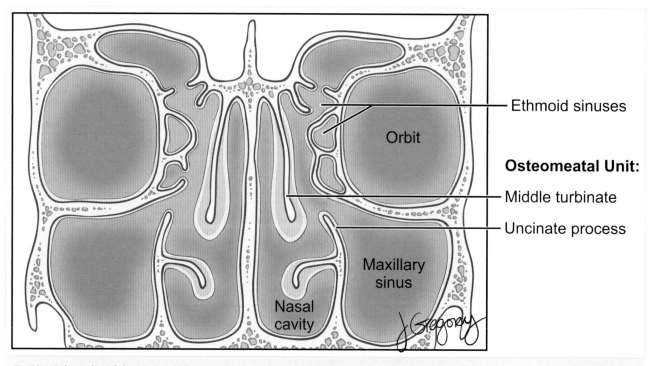

Fig. 68.1 Relationship of the osteomeatal unit to the turbinate and nasal structures.

Table 68.1 Major and minor features of acute sinusitis

Major features	Minor features
Purulent nasal discharge or postnasal drip	Fever (chronic)
Intranasal purulent discharge	Headache
Facial pain or pressure	Halitosis
Fever (acute)	Dental pain
Nasal obstruction or blockage	Cough
Hyposmia or anosmia	Ear pain or pressure
Facial congestion or fullness	Fatigue

Table 68.2 Common bacterial pathogens in acute sinusitis

Bacteria	Incidence (%)
Streptococcus pneumoniae	25–30
Haemophilus influenzae	15–25
Moraxella catarrhalis	15–25
Streptococcus pyogenes	<5
Anaerobes	<5
Sterile culture (no growth)	~ 20

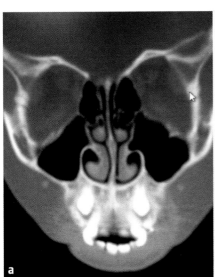 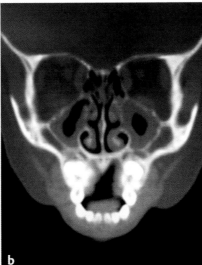

Fig. 68.2 (a) Coronal computed tomographic (CT) scan of normal sinuses. (b) Coronal CT scan of acute sinusitis with mucosal thickening.

Recurrent acute sinusitis, defined as repetitive episodes of acute sinusitis with full and complete resolution of symptoms between episodes, may occur in children.

68.1.4 Medical Evaluation and Testing

The examination will confirm the presence of nasal discharge or a purulent postnasal drip. Purulence in the middle meatus is a strong indicator of sinusitis. The nasal tissues often will be congested, and in compliant patients, the intranasal application of decongestants will permit a more thorough evaluation of the middle meatus. Facial or periorbital swelling is a sign of a potential complication of sinusitis. Purulent secretions should be cultured, especially if the patient has already received antibiotics and shows no improvement.

A clinical diagnosis is made in uncomplicated cases of acute sinusitis and treatment provided. In patients with altered mental status, severe headache (rare in young children), facial or orbital swelling, or severe facial pain, computed tomography (CT) is mandatory. CT (with contrast for suspected complications of sinusitis) is the preferred study for evaluating the bony confines of the sinuses, as well as inflammatory processes when sinusitis extends past the sinuses (▶ Fig. 68.2). Plain X-ray films, magnetic resonance (MR) imaging, and ultrasound are radiographic modalities of limited value in diagnosing and planning the treatment of sinusitis.

68.1.5 Treatment

The most common bacterial pathogens in acute sinusitis are the same bacteria that cause acute otitis media. *Streptococcus pneumoniae*, *Haemophilus influenzae*, and *Moraxella catarrhalis* are the most commonly cultured bacteria in pediatric acute sinusitis (▶ Table 68.2). Although antibiotic selection for these pathogens may seem straightforward, antibiotic resistance is increasing in these bacteria. In most cases, a 10- to 14-day course of an augmented penicillin, second-generation cephalosporin, or macrolide is used, but it is important to consider specific antibiotic resistance patterns within the patient's community.

Adjuvant therapy is aimed at diminishing symptoms. In addition to the use of systemic or topical nasal decongestants, nasal saline lavage is highly effective in relieving the symptoms of nasal congestion and improving the clearance of nasal secretions.

68.1.6 Complications

Sinus infection and inflammation that extend beyond the boundaries of the sinus into adjacent regions are serious complications of acute sinusitis and mandate immediate medical evaluation.

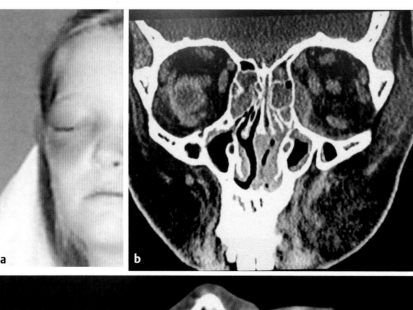

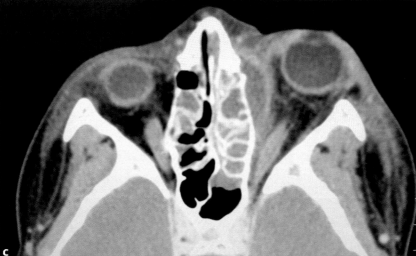

Fig. 68.3 (a) Patient with periorbital swelling from subperiosteal abscess. (b) Coronal computed tomographic (CT) scan of subperiosteal abscess, an orbital complication of acute sinusitis. (c) Axial CT scan of subperiosteal abscess with rim enhancement.

Orbital Complications

The most common complication of acute sinusitis is the spread of infection and inflammation to the orbit through the lamina papyracea of the ethmoid bone, either directly or hematogenously. The lamina papyracea is an eggshell-thin bone defining the lateral extent of the ethmoid complex. When an acute ethmoiditis erodes this bone or travels through preformed pathways, or if infection spreads hemotogenously, the infection may spread into the orbit. There are defined stages in the development and severity of the orbital complications of acute ethmoiditis, each carrying an increasingly worse prognosis: preseptal cellulitis, orbital cellulitis, subperiosteal abscess (▸ Fig. 68.3), orbital abscess, and cavernous sinus thrombosis (▸ Table 68.3).

Intracranial Complications

Intracranial complications of acute sinusitis in young children may occur by direct extension of the infection through a dehiscence of the bone of the sinus or preformed pathways, or by hematogenous spread of the infection (particularly the venous system). Spread may lead to the development of a subperiosteal abscess (either extracranial or intracranial), meningitis, or a subdural or parenchymal brain abscess. The incidence of intra-

cranial complications increases as patients approach puberty and the facial skeleton matures, with growth and development of the frontal sinus. Patients with a history of nondisplaced frontal sinus fracture managed conservatively are at increased risk for a complication of frontal sinusitis.

The management of these infections requires the administration of intravenous (IV) antibiotics, neurosurgical and infectious disease consultations, and appropriate treatment of the underlying sinus disease after patient stabilization.

Potts Puffy Tumor

Frontal sinus infection that spreads to the surrounding bone may result in osteomyelitis of the frontal bone, known as a Potts puffy tumor; this infection may spread intracranially or externally and result in abscess formation (▸ Fig. 68.4). Surgical drainage of the sinus and associated infection is necessary, with the administration of appropriate IV antibiotics to treat the osteomyelitis.

Prognosis

Most patients with sinusitis have an excellent prognosis, and infections resolve without the development of complications.

Table 68.3 Orbital complications of acute ethmoiditis

	Location	Cellulitis versus abscess	Proptosis	Vision	Extraocular muscle status	Mental status
Preseptal cellulitis	Edema anterior to eyelid septum	Cellulitis	No	Normal	Normal	Normal
Orbital cellulitis	Orbital space posterior to septum	Cellulitis	Yes	Normal	Impaired	Normal
Subperiosteal abscess	Under periosteum of the lamina papyracea	Abscess	Yes	Normal to mildly impaired	Impaired	Normal
Orbital abscess	Orbital soft-tissue abscess	Abscess	Yes	Severely impaired	Severely impaired	Normal
Cavernous sinus thrombosis	Abscess in cavernous sinus	Abscess	Yes	Severely impaired (bilateral)	Severely impaired (bilateral)	Impaired, meningeal signs

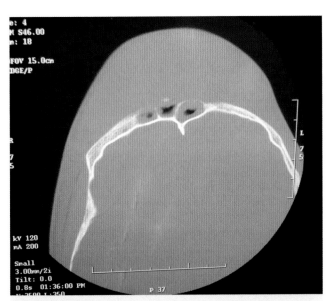

Fig. 68.4 Axial computed tomographic scan of frontal sinusitis with dehiscence of the anterior table and soft-tissue abscess.

Some children may have frequent episodes of acute sinusitis with their upper respiratory infections. As the children get older, they have fewer upper respiratory infections and fewer episodes of acute sinusitis.

68.2 Chronic Sinusitis

68.2.1 Etiology

Chronic sinusitis is defined by the presence of low-grade symptoms and findings of sinusitis lasting for longer than 3 months without improvement, the occurrence of six or more episodes of recurrent acute sinusitis in a 12-month period, or the persistence of some sinusitis symptoms with acute exacerbations for longer than 3 months. Children in whom these diagnostic criteria are met often have abnormal sinus anatomy—particularly a lack of osteomeatal unit patency, chronically inflamed mucous membranes, polyps, abnormalities of ciliary transport, or alterations in immunity. In some cases, children with chronic sinusitis simply have such frequent and severe upper respiratory

infections that they are unable to recover fully between infections, increasing the likelihood of rapid progression to sinusitis.

68.2.2 Presenting Symptoms

Symptoms will vary depending upon which criteria for the diagnosisof chronic sinusitis the patient has met. In patients in whom chronic sinusitis is diagnosed because of the persistence of sinusitis symptoms for 3 months or longer, the main complaints are chronic nasal obstruction, nasal discharge, and nasal congestion. Older children may also have facial pain, pressure, or headache; these symptoms are infrequent in younger children, even when all sinuses are affected.

Most pediatric patients are significantly affected by their chronic sinusitis and often report a poor quality of life as measured on validated scales. They experience sleep disruption caused by nasal congestion and obstruction, and they frequently have persistent nighttime cough. They often snore and are mouth breathers. Examination reveals intranasal findings similar to those previously described, and the patients may have large, congested turbinates and visible nasal or postnasal discharge.

68.2.3 Treatment and Diagnostic Testing

Children suspected by history and examination to have chronic sinusitis are usually treated in a specific, systematic manner. Children with chronic sinusitis are divided into two general treatment categories, based on age younger than or older than 6 years.

Children Younger Than 6 Years of Age

The initial management of children younger than 6 years of age with symptoms of chronic sinusitis who fail medical management with antibiotics and other symptomatic care is adenoidectomy. The rationale behind adenoidectomy is twofold: (1) The adenoids may be enlarged in children younger than 6 years and physically obstruct the nasopharynx and the normal drainage pathway of nasal secretions, thus increasing stasis within the nasal cavity. (2) Bacterial biofilms have been discovered on the surface of the adenoids. Bacterial biofilms are aggregations of bacteria and accretions that adhere to biological or nonbiological surfaces (e.g., indwelling catheters and tracheotomy tubes) without specifically causing an invasive infection of the biological surface. The presence of such biofilms on otherwise normal tissue creates a reservoir of bacteria; the bacteria are not usually eradicated with standard antibiotic treatment, and their presence in a biofilm may increase the antibiotic concentration necessary for eradication by a factor of 1 million. The presence of biofilm on the adenoids has no relationship to adenoid size or to whether the patient has recently been treated with antibiotics.

Many children with chronic sinusitis who undergo adenoidectomy experience improvement of their nasal symptoms and sinusitis. Complete cures are not usually obtained because the children are still predisposed to the initiating event, the upper respiratory infection, of their sinusitis. Generally, the children are free of symptoms for longer periods and have less severe symptoms during later upper respiratory infections.

Children Older Than 6 Years of Age

In patients who have chronic sinusitis without polyps, the initial treatment of chronic sinusitis is carried out with maximization of medical therapy before imaging studies are obtained. This involves total medical treatment with an appropriate antibiotic effective against the typical sinus bacteria (for up to 3 weeks) with topical nasal steroids, decongestants, and antihistamines (only if the patient has allergies) for a total of 4 to 6 weeks. After treatment, CT of the sinus is obtained, the patient is reevaluated, and the resolution of any symptom or finding is noted. Abnormalities on the CT scan, such as sinus mucosal thickening, opacification, and osteomeatal unit obstruction, are also noted (see ▶ Fig. 68.2b). These abnormalities represent sinus disease resistant to maximum medical therapy. Depending upon the degree of persistent sinus disease, either surgical management or observation may be considered.

68.3 Polyposis

In patients with visible nasal polyps, either in the nasal cavity or in the middle meatus (▶ Fig. 68.5), optimization of treatment of the underlying allergies is important. The spontaneous regression of polyposis in children is unusual, and most children will require surgical removal of the polyps in addition to ongoing medical management of the underlying allergies causing the polyposis. CT of the paranasal sinuses is obtained in axial and coronal planes for surgical planning at the time of diagnosis.

68.4 Special Surgical Considerations in Pediatric Sinus Surgery

Surgery for the management of pediatric sinus disease is generally similar to sinus surgery in adults, albeit with some differences. Pediatric sinus disease may be surgically managed with endoscopic intranasal techniques or via traditional external direct approaches with trephination or Lynch incisions. More often in children, traditional external approaches are used after failure of endoscopic sinus management. Under endoscopic magnification, the nasal structures are accessed similarly, after

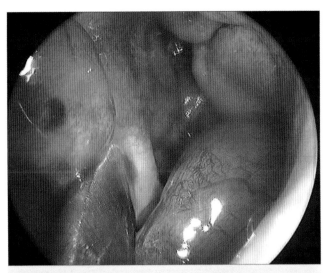

Fig. 68.5 Endoscopic image of a sinonasal polyp in the middle meatus.

decongestion of the mucosa. Although cocaine is popularly used in adult sinus surgery, it is *not* advised for use in children because of its dramatic effects on the cardiovascular system. Pediatric telescopes and small surgical forceps, scissors, and punches are available that allow access into even the smallest noses and sinus spaces.

Technically, pediatric endoscopic sinus surgery is challenging because of the much smaller intranasal space and limited options for the use of surgical forceps and powered instrumentation. In general, it is more important to improve and widen the affected sinus ostia than to remove all diseased mucosa within the sinus. The goal of pediatric sinus surgery is to improve affected sinus ostia patency and to remove tissue obstructing the middle meatus and ostia.

Intraoperative stereotactic image guidance is more important for sinus surgery in children, particularly when the frontal, ethmoid, and sphenoid sinuses are accessed (▶ Fig. 68.6). Although there is no substitute for technical familiarity with the paranasal sinus anatomy, intraoperative image guidance is particularly beneficial in pediatric patients with anatomical bony anomalies. In general, image guidance improves the likelihood of accessing all affected (especially the frontal and sphenoid) sinuses and increases safety by preventing intracranial and orbital penetration.

Absorbable sinus packing may be used, instead of packing that requires removal, in children younger than 10 to 12 years of age. In addition, postoperative débridement is often impossible without general anesthesia, and a "second-look" débridement may be needed 1 to 2 weeks following initial sinus surgery in some children.

68.4.1 Complications of Medical or Surgical Management

Complications of the disease process, when untreated, have been described in the preceding section. Complications of the surgical management of sinusitis involve traversing the bony confines of the sinuses into the orbit or cranium. Immediate detection of the penetration, prompt consultation with neuro-

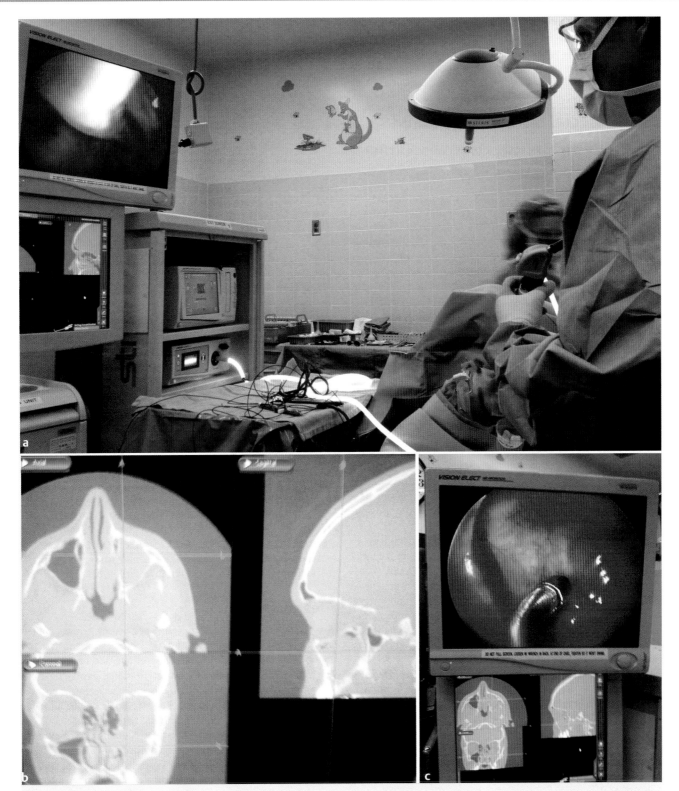

Fig. 68.6 (a) Stereotactic navigation image guidance system in use during pediatric endoscopic sinus surgery. (b) Image guidance provides three-dimensional localization of the surgical probe relative to the preoperative computed tomographic scans. (c) Stereotactic navigation image guidance localization is viewed alongside the endoscopic image during surgery.

surgery and ophthalmology, and repair of the dura and cerebrospinal fluid leak are necessary.

Children are at greater risk than adults for postoperative synechiae and scarring in the middle meatus because postoperative care is often difficult in children without general anesthesia.

68.5 Special Sinus Conditions

68.5.1 Cystic Fibrosis (Mucoviscidosis)

Etiology and Pathophysiology

Cystic fibrosis (CF) is a chronic multisystem genetic disease that primarily affects the respiratory and gastrointestinal systems. CF is caused by several mutations of the gene encoding the exocrine gland chloride channel receptor, transmembrane conductance regulator glycoprotein (*CFTR* gene, located on the long arm of chromosome 7). CF is transmitted in an autosomal-recessive pattern and is seen in approximately 1 in 3,500 Caucasian live births in the United States. Caucasians have the highest incidence, as noted; the incidence in Hispanics is 1 in 9,500 births, and the condition is very uncommon in Asian or African groups. Males and females are affected evenly. CF is usually diagnosed in infancy because of manifestations of pancreatic gland and pulmonary dysfunction. The diagnosis of CF is confirmed with a sweat chloride skin test; a sweat chloride concentration above 60 mEq/L is diagnostic.

The target of the CF DNA mutation is the cyclic adenosine monophosphate (cAMP)–mediated chloride channel on the apical surface of the epithelial lining of exocrine glands, which results in the secretion of abnormally viscid mucus. CF primarily affects the lungs and pancreas, with the production of thick mucus and the development of chronic lung disease, bronchiectasis, exocrine pancreatic insufficiency, rhinorrhea, nasal obstruction, and sinusitis.

Nasal secretions are noted to be very thick and difficult to clear from the nose, resulting in stasis and secondary bacterial colonization/infection of the nose and sinuses with *Staphylococcus aureus*, *Pseudomonas*, *Proteus*, and the other usual nasal bacterial pathogens. Nasal polyposis is commonly found in patients with cystic fibrosis. The frequent symptom of nasal obstruction is produced in these children by the combination of chronic nasal mucosal inflammation, thick viscid secretions, and the presence of nasal polyps.

The lifespan of patients with CF has increased recently, with patients living into their forties because of advances in the management of their lung disease.

Presenting Symptoms

Most children with CF have previously received medical attention when they are referred for the management of nasal symptoms of obstruction, secretions, and polyps. The specific aim is to reduce the nasal symptoms, particularly postnasal drip and obstruction, and improve the patient's quality of life.

Medical Evaluation and Testing

Typically, patients have thick, purulent (often greenish) nasal secretions that are difficult to suction and clear from the nasal

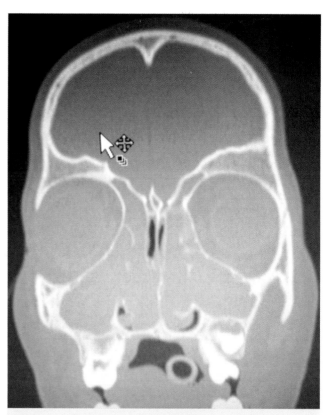

Fig. 68.7 Coronal computed tomographic scan of sinusitis with polyposis in a patient with cystic fibrosis.

cavity. The mucosa is hyperplastic, and polyps may be visualized in the middle meatus on rhinoscopy.

If not already performed by the patient's other medical caregivers, CT should proceed without the usual prior medical treatment of chronic sinusitis. CT scans usually demonstrate complete opacification of the sinuses, and possible hypoplasia of the frontal sinus in older children (▶ Fig. 68.7).

Treatment

Treatment is offered to patients with symptoms. The goal of the management of sinusitis in CF is to relieve nasal obstructive symptoms, reduce and thin nasal secretions, and improve quality of life. The initial use of tobramycin–saline nasal irrigations may thin and clear viscid nasal and sinus secretions and help control bacterial suprainfection. Endoscopic surgery is aimed at removing obstructive polyps and enlarging the sinus ostia to the greatest extent possible. Most patients with CF require increased treatment of their pulmonary problems, with a "tune-up" to improve their pulmonary status, before a general anesthetic is administered. Postoperatively, the tobramycin–saline nasal irrigations are resumed as soon as possible and are continued daily as maintenance treatment for the nasal manifestations of CF.

Prognosis

Because of the underlying genetic etiology of CF, it not possible to cure sinusitis in patients with CF. However, it is possible to control symptoms in a substantial number of children. Repeated hospitalizations and sinus procedures are not uncommon as the patients age.

68.5.2 Primary Ciliary Dyskinesia (Kartagener Syndrome)

Etiology

Primary ciliary dyskinesia, also known as immotile ciliary syndrome or Kartagener syndrome, is a rare, inherited autosomal-recessive disease in which abnormal cilia are present in the respiratory tract (including the nasal cavity and sinuses), ear, and genital organs.

Mutations on two genes are responsible for structural defects in the outer dynein arms, resulting in immotile cilia with abnormal function. Structural defects of the dynein arms, identified with electron microscopy, are diagnostic of this disorder.

Embryologic development is affected by the defective ciliary movement, resulting in situs inversus (reversed laterality of the internal organs) in children with primary ciliary dyskinesia. Situs inversus occurs randomly and is seen in about 50% of cases. It can occur with or without dextrocardia (right-sided heart).

Pathophysiology and Pathogenesis

The abnormal cilia in the respiratory epithelium result in the impaired clearance and stasis of lung, nasal, and sinus mucus. The result is chronic and recurrent episodes of pneumonia, bronchiectasis, and sinusitis.

Presenting Symptoms

Although primary ciliary dyskinesia is a rare condition, it may be suspected in children who present with a history of recurrent pneumonia in addition to the typical symptoms of recurrent sinusitis. Chronic nasal discharge, obstruction, and congestion are typical in these patients. Prolonged antibiotic therapy may have previously been unsuccessfully attempted.

Medical Evaluation and Testing

A high index of suspicion is required to make a diagnosis of primary ciliary dyskinesia because specialized testing is needed. Chest X-ray may demonstrate dextrocardia, which, although it raises suspicion for primary ciliary dyskinesia, is in itself not diagnostic. The diagnostic test for primary ciliary dyskinesia is biopsy of ciliated epithelium and the observation of dynein arm abnormality on electron microscopy. The most common sites for biopsy of the mucosa are the nose, bronchial tubes, and trachea. The nose and lungs may have areas of mucosa with a deficient quantity of cilia as a result of chronic bacterial infection. An alternative, and preferred, method of obtaining an adequate cilia sample is to use a bronchial brush in the nasal cavity. This method has a higher likelihood of obtaining a sufficient sample for electron microscopic analysis and may be performed in the office without the need for general anesthesia. Electron microscopy demonstrates typical dynein arm abnormalities and establishes the diagnosis, along with a history of recurrent pneumonia and chronic sinus infections.

Treatment

Treatment is aimed at the medical control of symptoms and surgical enlargement of the sinus ostia to permit postural drainage of the sinuses.

68.5.3 Tumor of the Sinonasal Tract: Juvenile Nasopharyngeal Angiofibroma

Etiology

Juvenile nasopharyngeal angiofibroma (JNA) is a rare benign tumor of the posterior nasal cavity and nasopharynx. It is seen only in boys at the onset of or during puberty. It initially occurs at the junction of the middle turbinate with the sphenopalatine foramen. Its exact etiology is uncertain, but growth of the tumor is influenced by androgen and estrogen hormones. JNAs account for fewer than 0.05% of all head and neck tumors and are more common in Middle Eastern and Indian boys.

Pathophysiology and Pathogenesis

JNAs originate in the area of the posterior nose at the sphenopalatine foramen. The tumors then slowly grow to occupy the ipsilateral nasal cavity with extension into the nasopharynx. Large tumors frequently extend into the pterygopalatine fossa, as well, and develop a "dumbbell" shape. The tumors enlarge by expanding the surrounding tissues, with erosion of the bony constraints into the maxilla, sphenoid, and skull base seen with very large tumors. In some cases, the JNA will have extended to the orbit. The blood supply to a JNA is usually based on the internal maxillary artery and its branches.

JNA is a benign vascular tumor composed of thin-walled blood vessels that have absent or incomplete smooth muscle within their walls. This accounts for the difficulty encountered in controlling epistaxis originating from a JNA.

Presenting Symptoms

Prepubescent and teenage boys present with a history of nasal obstruction (unilateral or bilateral, depending upon the size and location of the tumor) and epistaxis, sometimes reported as extreme with significant blood loss. Alteration of the speech resonance and bulging of the soft palate may be seen as the tumor grows.

Medical Evaluation and Testing

The tumor appears on physical examination as a reddish, smooth, mucosa-covered mass in the nasal cavity. It may cause septal deflection into the opposite nasal cavity, and if it is located in the nasopharynx, it may cause obstruction. This intranasal mass should not be biopsied because of the risk for significant epistaxis.

CT with contrast is often the initial radiographic study, showing excellent detail of the bony anatomy. MR imaging is complementary to CT and provides excellent detail of the soft-tissue extent of the tumor. The diagnosis is usually made through a combination of the clinical history, examination, and imaging studies (▶ Fig. 68.8).

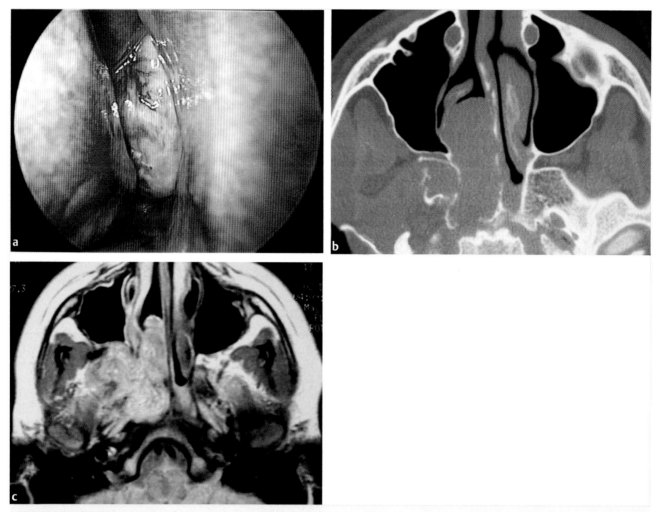

Fig. 68.8 (a) Endoscopic appearance of juvenile nasopharyngeal angiofibroma (JNA) in the nasal cavity. (b) Computed tomographic scan of JNA. (c) Magnetic resonance image of JNA.

Treatment

JNA is staged by its extent, particularly its orbital and intracranial extent; this information is useful in determining the techniques required for tumor removal.

Preoperative embolization allows complete removal of a JNA with reduced blood loss. The approach to complete tumor resection varies depending upon the stage and extent of the specific tumor, but many are resected endoscopically, with good a success rate for complete tumor removal. Other approaches include transpalatal lateral rhinotomy and combined otolaryngologic–neurosurgical procedures.

Radiation therapy is another option that is usually reserved for severe cases in which there is tumor recurrence or a tumor that cannot be entirely removed.

Complications

JNA is a benign tumor that can cause pressure-related damage to adjacent organs, such as the eyes. The vascular nature of a JNA can result in life-threatening epistaxis, and blood transfusion is not uncommonly required. Surgical complications are specifically related to the structures in the region.

Prognosis

The cure rate for JNA approaches 100% with complete resection of the tumor. This is reduced in cases of large, lobulated lesions, particularly with intracranial extension. There have been rare reports of malignant transformation of a JNA, but most of them had previously been treated with radiation therapy.

68.6 Conclusion

Children have numerous sinonasal conditions that can easily be confused, but the patient's history will soon point toward the diagnosis. Concern and a consideration of the patient's age and the impact of the condition on his or her quality of life will assist in the management of the pediatric patient.

68.7 Roundsmanship

- Most children have between six and 10 upper respiratory infections annually, but acute rhinosinusitis develops in only 5%.

- *S. pneumoniae, H. influenzae,* and *M. catarrhalis* are the most commonly cultured bacteria in pediatric cases of acute sinusitis.
- In most children, acute rhinosinusitis can be diagnosed by the observation of worsening symptoms of an upper respiratory infection or purulent discharge in the middle meatus. CT may be needed in special cases.
- Acute ethmoiditis and acute frontal sinusitis may present with intraorbital or intracranial complications. Treatment is a combination of appropriate antibiotic therapy and often surgical drainage.
- Adenoidectomy is often recommended as first-line surgical treatment for uncomplicated recurrent or chronic sinusitis in young children to reduce symptoms.
- Endoscopic sinus surgery, often with intraoperative stereotactic navigation guidance, is used in refractory cases, with improved outflow drainage from the sinus ostia as the goal of the procedure.
- "Second-look" endoscopic examinations with the patient under general anesthesia is sometimes needed following endoscopic sinus surgery.
- Children with special medical conditions, such as cystic fibrosis and primary ciliary dyskinesia, often require endoscopic sinus surgery to improve outflow drainage from the sinuses. These patients also require special management for their pulmonary problems.
- Juvenile nasopharyngeal angiofibroma is a serious, potentially life-threatening tumor seen only in peripubescent boys. The tumor should not be biopsied in the office setting because of the risk for severe hemorrhage. Imaging studies with a clinical history are diagnostic. Complete excision is recommended.

68.8 Recommended Reading

[1] Arnaoutakis D, Collins WO. Correlation of mucociliary clearance and symptomatology before and after adenoidectomy in children. Int J Pediatr Otorhinolaryngol 2011; 75: 1318–1321

[2] Becker SS, de Alarcon A, Bomeli SR, Han JK, Gross CW. Risk factors for recurrent sinus surgery in cystic fibrosis: review of a decade of experience. Am J Rhinol 2007; 21: 478–482

[3] Bedwell J, Bauman NM. Management of pediatric orbital cellulitis and abscess. Curr Opin Otolaryngol Head Neck Surg 2011; 19: 467–473

[4] Campbell R. Managing upper respiratory tract complications of primary ciliary dyskinesia in children. Curr Opin Allergy Clin Immunol 2012; 12: 32–38

[5] Mandal R, Patel N, Ferguson BJ. Role of antibiotics in sinusitis. Curr Opin Infect Dis 2012; 25: 183–192

[6] Pagella F, Colombo A, Gatti O, Giourgos G, Matti E. Rhinosinusitis and otitis media: the link with adenoids. Int J Immunopathol Pharmacol 2010; 23 Suppl: 38–40

[7] Parikh SR, Cuellar H, Sadoughi B, Aroniadis O, Fried MP. Indications for image-guidance in pediatric sinonasal surgery. Int J Pediatr Otorhinolaryngol 2009; 73: 351–356

[8] Piatt JH. Intracranial suppuration complicating sinusitis among children: an epidemiological and clinical study. J Neurosurg Pediatr 2011; 7: 567–574

[9] Rogers DJ, Bevans SE, Harsha WJ. Endoscopic resection of juvenile nasopharyngeal angiofibroma. Adv Otorhinolaryngol 2012; 73: 132–136

[10] Zuliani G, Carron M, Gurrola J et al. Identification of adenoid biofilms in chronic rhinosinusitis. Int J Pediatr Otorhinolaryngol 2006; 70: 1613–1617

69 Pharyngeal and Esophageal Disorders in Children

Joshua R. Bedwell and Robin A. Dyleski

69.1 Introduction

Problems concerning the oral cavity and throat are among the most common reasons why children visit an otolaryngologist. These conditions vary in cause, severity, and length of illness, and they may have a large impact on the well-being of a child. This chapter addresses the most common conditions affecting the oral cavity and throat in children.

69.2 Mucosal Conditions

69.2.1 History

A variety of infectious and inflammatory disorders may lead to mucosal changes in the oral cavity. Important historical points to elicit include age at onset, history of trauma to the region or exposure to chemicals, vaccination history, recently started medications, presence or absence of pain, and any systemic symptoms, such as fever. An immune-compromised state widens the differential diagnosis to include opportunistic pathogens not seen in otherwise healthy children. Any associated symptoms should be noted in a complete review of systems.

69.2.2 Physical Examination

A detailed oral and oropharyngeal examination should be performed, and the appearance of any lesions described in detail. Palpation will demonstrate any induration and/or tenderness. Exudates should be tested for adherence to the underlying mucosa and sent for culture. Any regional adenopathy should be noted.

69.2.3 Infectious Disorders

Several viral agents can cause oral mucosal lesions. Herpes simplex virus (most commonly type 1) can cause a stomatitis in which small, painful vesicles are typically seen on the gingivae, palate, lips, or tongue. The lesions rupture and leave ulcerations in which a gray exudate covers an erythematous base. Systemic symptoms such as fever and malaise may also be present. Treatment consists of oral acyclovir. Herpangina, caused by coxsackievirus A, manifests as an intensely painful pharyngitis associated with small vesicles in the posterior oral cavity and pharynx. Hand-foot-and-mouth disease, also due to coxsackievirus A, is similar to herpangina, with the addition of a papular rash on the palms and soles. The treatment of these infections is supportive. Koplik spots are red lesions with a light bluish center that are seen on the buccal mucosa in measles (rubella); they typically appear 24 to 48 hours before the generalized maculopapular rash, fever, and coriza generally observed in this infection.

There are a few rare but notable bacterial causes of oral lesions. Acute necrotizing ulcerative gingivitis (also known as Vincent gingivitis, or trench mouth) is an infection caused by multiple organisms, including the spirochete *Borrelia vincentii*.

Patients present with widespread inflammation and necrosis of the gingivae, with gray exudate and hemorrhage. This condition is most often seen in malnourished, immunocompromised, or otherwise debilitated patients. Treatment consists of oral hygiene and antibiotics, typically a penicillin. Primary syphilis, caused by *Treponema pallidum*, presents as a painless ulcer, or chancre, with surrounding induration; it is treated with penicillin.

The most commonly encountered fungal infection in the oral cavity is candidiasis, or thrush, caused by *Candida albicans*. Candidiasis presents with white plaques that when scraped off reveal a friable, erythematous mucosa that bleeds. Although thrush is often seen as a benign infection in infants and patients on antibiotics, it should serve as an alert for a possible underlying immune-compromised condition (e.g., diabetes, HIV infection). Treatment typically consists of topical antifungal agents (nystatin, clotrimazole lozenges), although systemic fluconazole can be used for more severe cases.

69.2.4 Inflammatory and Idiopathic Disorders

Aphthous stomatitis accounts for the most common oral ulcers. Patients present with a painful, white ulceration of the mucosa and surrounding erythema. Ulcers are categorized as minor (< 1 cm), major (> 1 cm), or herpetiform (multiple small ulcers). Major and herpetiform ulcers carry a risk for scar formation. Treatment is supportive, although topical steroids such as Kenalog in Orabase (triamcinolone oropharyngeal, Bristol-Myers Squibb) may bring some relief. Recurrent or chronically nonhealing ulcers should be biopsied to rule out carcinoma. Behçet disease is an autoimmune disorder in which patients present with painful oral and genital aphthous ulcerations, ocular inflammation (e.g., uveitis, iritis), and a host of other symptoms. Immunosuppressive therapy is the standard treatment.

Oral mucosal lesions may accompany the classic target-shaped cutaneous lesions of erythema multiforme. Erythema multiforme is an acute vasculitis that may occur spontaneously or as part of a hypersensitivity reaction. Patients will present with an abrupt onset of symptoms, along with fever. Stevens-Johnson syndrome is a serious form of erythema multiforme. The treatment of both is with corticosteroids and supportive care.

There are a number of autoimmune disorders in which antibodies are directed against various aspects of the attachments of epithelial cells to the underlying basement membrane. These disorders present as painful ulcerations that form with minor trauma. Pemphigus vulgaris is caused by the formation of autoantibodies to intracellular bridges and is the bullous disease most frequently presenting with oral mucosal lesions. The diagnosis hinges on skin biopsy showing intraepithelial deposits of immunoglobulin G. Corticosteroids are the mainstay of treatment.

69.2.5 Neoplastic Disorders

Oral neoplasms are rare in children, and the majority are of vascular or salivary origin. Rhabdomyosarcoma is a malignant tumor of skeletal muscle origin that can present in the oral cavity (most frequently on the tongue, palate, or cheek) as a nontender, firm, enlarging intramuscular mass. The diagnosis is made by biopsy of the mass with complete excision at the biopsy procedure if possible. Rhabdomyosarcoma is staged following pathologic diagnosis on the basis of the disease remaining in the patient, and thus a complete excision may affect staging of the disease. Chemotherapy with or without radiation is the mainstay of treatment, with surgical excision or debulking performed when it is possible to do so without creating a large cosmetic or functional defect.

69.3 Salivary Disorders

Most salivary disorders in children are acute, infectious, and self-limited. There are, however, a number of other important causes of salivary gland pathology that must be considered.

69.3.1 History

Patients will most often present with enlargement of one or more salivary glands. One should delineate the onset of symptoms (acute, insidious), the presence of pain, and any fluctuations in symptomatology (e.g., exacerbation with eating). A history of trauma, animal bites or scratches, recent dental procedures, and any recent illnesses should be elicited. Systemic complaints such as fever, chills, and malaise should be noted. A complete review of systems is important, as is an understanding of any coexistent medical conditions (especially immunodeficiency).

69.3.2 Physical Examination

The examination should focus on the degree and nature of glandular enlargement. Any overlying skin erythema or discoloration should be noted. Bimanual palpation of the affected gland can aid in differentiating between a diffusely enlarged gland, a discrete intraparenchymal mass, and a mass separate from the salivary gland (e.g., enlarged lymph node, branchial cleft cyst). Any discrete mass should be carefully characterized (firm or fluctuant, mobile or fixed, tender or nontender). An intraoral examination should note the amount, consistency, and appearance of saliva expressed from the duct orifice (scant, clear, purulent). Any palpable stones along the course of the duct should be noted.

69.3.3 Diagnostic Evaluation

In cases with a suspected infectious etiology, a leukocyte count and differential may be helpful. Other markers of systemic inflammation, such as the C-reactive protein level and erythrocyte sedimentation rate, may also be of value. Specific bacterial tests (*Bartonella henselae* titers, purified protein derivative [PPD] test) and viral titers (Epstein-Barr virus, HIV, mumps virus) can be obtained when appropriate. Salivary fluid should be sent for aerobic and anaerobic culture.

Imaging tests commonly employed to evaluate the salivary glands include ultrasound, plain X-ray, computed tomography (CT), and magnetic resonance (MR) imaging. More invasive studies, such as sialography, in which the salivary ducts are directly injected with contrast, are infrequently used. Ultrasound is useful in differentiating between solid and cystic lesions and between intrinsic and extrinsic salivary masses, and in directing fine-needle aspiration (FNA) biopsy. Advantages of ultrasonography include lack of a need for sedation and avoidance of radiation exposure. Plain films are primarily useful for identifying radiopaque salivary calculi (up to 80% of parotid stones and 20% of submandibular stones are radiolucent). CT and MR imaging are both useful for providing anatomical context to a mass. MR imaging is superior for providing soft-tissue detail, although the longer scan time often requires using sedation or even general anesthesia in young children and infants.

FNA biopsy of salivary gland lesions is controversial but can be of help in differentiating benign from malignant processes up to 93% of the time. Furthermore, FNA can aid in differentiating masses arising in salivary gland tissue from adjacent or intraglandular lymphoid tissue. FNA may need to be performed under sedation or general anesthesia in young children.

69.3.4 Infectious Sialadenitis

Acute Bacterial Sialadenitis

The majority of cases of infectious sialadenitis are bacterial in nature. Patients present with an acutely enlarged, painful gland and systemic signs of infection. Massage of the gland often expresses purulent discharge from the duct orifice. The parotid gland is more commonly involved than the submandibular gland. It is believed that the more mucinous saliva produced by the submandibular gland has more antibacterial activity than the serous saliva of the parotid gland. In either gland, infection is thought to arise because of salivary stasis due to obstruction by a stone or an extrinsic mass or to dehydration. Saliva from the affected gland should be expressed and sent for Gram stain and culture. The bacteria most commonly identified in acute bacterial sialadenitis are *Staphylococcus aureus* and *Streptococcus viridans*. Antibiotic treatment with a penicillinase-resistant penicillin (e.g., amoxicillin with clavulanate) is combined with glandular massage, warm compresses, hydration, and sialagogues (e.g., sour candy, lemon juice). The persistence or progression of fever and pain despite antibiotic therapy should raise concern for an intraglandular abscess, which can be evaluated with CT or ultrasound. An abscess requires incision and drainage under general anesthesia.

Chronic Bacterial Sialadenitis

Several bacterial agents forming granulomas can affect the lymph nodes adjacent to and within the salivary glands. Tuberculous mycobacterial infections are often associated with hilar and mediastinal lymphadenopathy and can be diagnosed with a positive PPD test. Treatment consists of systemic antituberculous drugs. Atypical mycobacterial infections are most commonly seen in children and frequently manifest in the head and neck. Violaceous discoloration of the overlying skin can be a clue to such infections. *Mycobacterium avium-intracellulare* is the most common causative agent. The PPD test may be weakly positive and cultures may be positive, but a long incubation is required. As a result, the diagnosis is often based on clinical suspicion or pathologic analysis. Because systemic antibiotic therapy is rarely successful, treatment consists of surgical excision of the lesion.

Cat-scratch disease, caused by *Bartonella henselae*, may result in chronic enlargement of the periparotid or intraparotid lymph nodes, mimicking a salivary neoplasm. A remote history of an animal scratch or bite may be elicited. FNA biopsy may show the non–acid-fast, gram-negative bacillus on a Warthin-Starry stain. Treatment is symptomatic, and macrolide antibiotics may be required to hasten resolution of the mass.

Viral Sialadenitis

Although extremely uncommon since the introduction of mandatory vaccination, mumps (caused by a paramyxovirus) may be a cause of sialadenitis. Patients who have mumps present with painful, diffuse swelling of the major salivary glands following a prodromal period of systemic complaints of fever, malaise, and symptoms of an upper respiratory infection. Associated findings include painful inflammation of the meninges, testicles or ovaries, and pancreas. The diagnosis can be made by the measurement of acute viral titers. The treatment is supportive in nature. Complications include sensorineural hearing loss and infertility due to orchitis/oophoritis.

HIV infection may cause chronic enlargement of the salivary glands, most often presenting as lymphoepithelial cysts within the parotid parenchyma. Diffuse enlargement due to lymphoid hyperplasia is also seen frequently, often as an initial presentation of the disease. Cysts should be managed conservatively, with needle aspiration employed for cosmetic deformity or discomfort. Parotidectomy is not advised because of the risk for injury to the facial nerve.

Sialadenitis may be seen as part of infectious mononucleosis (caused by the Epstein-Barr virus). Additional findings will include sore throat, posterior cervical lymphadenopathy, and possibly hepatosplenomegaly.

69.3.5 Obstructive Salivary Conditions

Salivary stones, or sialoliths, form from the deposition of calcium salts around an organic matrix. The submandibular gland is involved in 90% of cases and the parotid in 10%. The increased incidence in the submandibular gland is attributed to the more alkaline and viscous saliva produced, as well as the course of the Wharton duct, through which saliva travels against gravity. The calculi obstruct salivary flow, causing pain and intermittent salivary gland enlargement that is exacerbated with eating. Sialadenitis often results from salivary stasis. Palpation often reveals calculi near the Wharton duct orifice or along its intraoral course. Parotid calculi may be more difficult to palpate. Plain radiographs or noncontrast CT scans will show radiopaque calculi. Eighty percent of submandibular stones are radiopaque, as opposed to only 20% of those arising in the parotid. If the calculus is found near the ductal orifice, it may be either milked out or removed with a small incision intraorally. Patients who have stones within the glandular parenchyma require either submandibular gland excision or superficial parotidectomy.

Recurrent bouts of acute sialadenitis can lead to chronic glandular inflammation and distortion of the ductal architecture. Strictures can form, obstructing salivary outflow. Over time, the proximal duct can dilate (sialectasis), causing persistent glandular enlargement.

Obstruction of minor salivary glands can lead to two related but distinct entities. Mucous retention cysts are true, epithelium-lined cysts. A ranula is a mucous retention cyst that forms in the floor of the mouth as a consequence of obstruction of the sublingual gland. Ranulas can become quite large and extend into the neck deep to the mylohyoid muscle, a condition known as a "plunging" ranula. Mucoceles, in contrast, are not true cysts in that they represent the extravasation of mucus into surrounding tissue and lack an epithelial lining. Both mucous retention cysts and mucoceles are managed by marsupialization or complete excision. This can typically be accomplished via an intraoral approach, although a plunging ranula may require an external excision.

69.3.6 Congenital Masses of the Salivary Glands

A variety of congenital cysts may present in the salivary glands. Dermoid cysts most often present within the parotid gland, and complete excision is required to prevent recurrence. First branchial cleft anomalies can be found in the parotid region. Work type I anomalies are simple duplications of the membranous external auditory canal. Work type II anomalies involve duplication of the membranous and cartilaginous external canal. These are typically found posteroinferior to the angle of the mandible and can be closely related to the facial nerve. Congenital retention cysts may be seen in infants. These will typically regress spontaneously, and observation is appropriate.

69.3.7 Salivary Neoplasms

Salivary neoplasms are rare in children; however, a neoplasm in a child is more likely to be malignant than a neoplasm in an adult. In fact, if the vascular tumors are set aside, up to 50% of salivary gland masses in children will prove malignant. As in the adult population, the parotid is the most frequently involved gland.

Vascular Tumors

Unlike in adults, the most common neoplasms in children are vascular tumors; of these, hemangiomas are the most common. Hemangiomas appear shortly after birth, and their course is one of proliferation and growth over several months to a year, followed by a period of involution of variable duration. Because the majority of lesions will involute, observation is appropriate, barring complications. Complications include ulceration and hemorrhage, functional impairment, infection, incomplete involution with cosmetic deformity, and rapid growth with Kasabach-Merritt syndrome (platelet trapping within the tumor leading to a consumptive coagulopathy). Treatments range from medical therapy with propranolol or corticosteroids to more invasive techniques such as laser ablation and surgical excision.

Lymphatic malformations, also called lymphangiomas, present as compressible masses that consist of dilated, malformed lymphatic channels. They are classified as microcystic, macrocystic, or mixed based on the size of the cystic areas. These malformations can become quite large and may compromise the airway. Treatment is by complete resection when possible, although the use of sclerosing agents such as OK-432 has been gaining in popularity, especially for macrocystic lesions.

Finally, vascular malformations may present in the salivary glands. In contrast to hemangiomas, these malformations are present at birth and grow as the child grows, with no involution.

Benign Tumors

Pleomorphic adenoma is the most common benign epithelial neoplasm found in the salivary glands of children. As in adults, a pleomorphic adenoma presents as a slowly growing, firm nodule. FNA is often sufficient for diagnosis, and excision with a superficial parotidectomy is the treatment of choice.

Malignant Tumors

Mucoepidermoid carcinoma is the most common malignant salivary gland neoplasm in children. These tumors are designated as low- or high-grade based on their histologic characteristics, and staging is similar to that in adults. Low-grade lesions are treated very successfully by surgical excision with adequate margins of normal parotid. High-grade lesions require total parotidectomy, neck dissection, and possibly adjuvant radiotherapy. In either case, as long as it is not involved with tumor, the facial nerve should be preserved.

Acinic cell carcinoma is the next most common malignant salivary tumor. These tumors are most often low-grade, and the treatment is similar to that for low-grade mucoepidermoid carcinoma, with complete surgical excision and attempted preservation of the facial nerve.

69.3.8 Sialorrhea

Sialorrhea, or excessive saliva production, should be distinguished from ptyalism, or drooling. Ptyalism is often multifactorial, with components of excessive production and impaired clearance of secretions due to dysphagia. Conservative management with speech and swallowing therapy should be the initial step. Medical therapy includes an antihistamine such as scopolamine or glycopyrrolate. Surgical management should be used only in cases of medical failure. Various options include injection of botulinum A toxin into the salivary gland parenchyma under ultrasound guidance, submandibular gland excision, Wharton duct rerouting, intraoral duct ligation, and chorda tympani/tympanic neurectomy.

69.4 Tonsils and Adenoids

69.4.1 Anatomy and Physiology

The palatine tonsils, adenoids (pharyngeal tonsils), and lingual tonsils make up a ring of lymphoid tissue known as the Waldeyer ring. The lymphoid component consists primarily of B cells and T cells, with a small percentage of plasma cells. The tonsils are involved in secretory immunity (immunoglobulin production and regulation) and are situated in a prime location for sampling inhaled and ingested antigens. The tonsils and adenoids increase in size and immunologic activity in early childhood and involute after puberty.

The palatine tonsils are situated in fossae along the lateral oropharyngeal wall between anterior and posterior muscular pillars. The palatoglossus forms the anterior pillar, and the palatopharyngeus is present within the posterior pillar. The lymphoid tissue of the tonsil is tightly adherent to a fibrous capsule that lies adjacent to the pillars and the underlying pharyngeal constrictor muscle. The surface of the tonsil is marked by numerous invaginations or crypts lined with stratified squamous epithelium. The main arterial supply enters at the inferior pole, with contributions from the facial (tonsillar branch of the ascending palatine) and lingual (tonsillar branch of the dorsal lingual) arteries. The ascending pharyngeal and lesser palatine arteries enter at the superior pole. The venous drainage feeds into lingual and pharyngeal veins, which drain eventually into the internal jugular vein. Lymphatic drainage is to the jugulodigastric and superior deep cervical nodes.

The adenoids lie on the superior and posterior nasopharyngeal walls and project into the nasopharynx. This lymphoid tissue is covered by a pseudostratified ciliated columnar epithelium. The ascending pharyngeal branches from the internal maxillary and facial arteries supply the adenoids. As with the tonsils, pharyngeal veins drain into the internal jugular vein.

69.4.2 Infectious Disorders

History

Patients who have a tonsillar/pharyngeal infection most commonly present with a sore throat and odynophagia. Dysphagia can result from hypertrophy of the lymphoid tissue of the tonsils during acute infection. Otalgia may be present, caused by concomitant otitis as part of an upper respiratory tract infection; alternatively, the otalgia may be "referred pain," due to innervation of both the pharynx and the middle ear by the glossopharyngeal nerve. Fever and other systemic signs of infection are often part of the clinical picture.

One should evaluate the patient's ability to tolerate oral intake, and intravenous hydration and admission should be considered for patients who have signs of dehydration or are unable to maintain adequate oral intake. Any history of similar infections and the frequency of episodes of tonsillitis are important to know in counseling patients on the need for eventual surgical management. Finally, any history of immune suppression is important to know because opportunistic pathogens not seen in normal hosts may be encountered.

Physical Examination

The patient's general appearance, with special attention paid to signs of airway compromise, sepsis, and dehydration, must be noted. Examination of the pharynx will demonstrate enlarged, erythematous tonsils that may be covered in purulent exudate. The tonsil size should be rated on a scale of 0 to 4+ based on the degree of projection into the oropharyngeal airway. A designation of 0 is used to describe prior tonsillectomy. Grade 1+ tonsils are within the fossa and project into the airway, reaching less than 25% of the distance to midline; grade 2 + tonsils extend 25 to 50%, grade 3 + tonsils up to 75%, and grade 4 + tonsils more than 75% and often meet in the midline, nearly completely obstructing the oropharynx. The tonsils should be symmetric. Asymmetry should prompt concern for malignancy. Cervical lymphadenopathy is typically present. Unilateral bulging of the soft palate and/or medial displacement of a tonsil is seen in peritonsillar abscess. Severe odynophagia (as evidenced by refusal of oral intake and drooling), high spiking fevers, and a stiff neck raise suspicion of a retropharyngeal abscess.

Patients with acute adenoiditis will demonstrate purulent rhinorrhea and postnasal drip. Fiber-optic examination will reveal enlarged, erythematous adenoids covered in purulent exudate. Like the size of the tonsils, the size of the adenoids is rated based on the degree of obstruction of the choanae. Grade 1 + indicates 25% obstruction, grade 2 + indicates 50%, grade 3 + indicates 75%, and grade 4 + indicates complete obstruction.

Diagnostic Evaluation

Typically, the diagnosis can be made on clinical examination, often paired with a rapid strep test and throat culture to direct antimicrobial therapy. A monospot test may be useful in differentiating between infectious mononucleosis and bacterial pharyngitis. CT is helpful if a retropharyngeal or parapharyngeal abscess is suspected.

Viral Infections

Viral tonsillitis is often present along with other symptoms of an upper respiratory tract infection (cough, rhinorrhea, sneezing). Viruses responsible include rhinovirus, adenovirus (often with associated conjunctivitis), respiratory syncytial virus, influenza viruses, and parainfluenza viruses. Herpes simplex virus infection may demonstrate painful vesicular lesions, as will herpangina (coxsackievirus).

Pharyngitis caused by Epstein-Barr virus can be part of a complex of symptoms known as infectious mononucleosis. The tonsils may be greatly enlarged and are often covered with a fibrinous gray exudate. In addition, palatal petechiae may be noted. Associated findings include posterior triangle cervical lymphadenopathy, hepatosplenomegaly, fever, malaise, and rash. The diagnosis can be made based on a positive monospot test, the presence of heterophil antibodies, and a lymphocytosis with more than 10% atypical lymphocytes on a complete blood cell count, or EBV antibody titers.

Viral pharyngitis is most often self-limited, and supportive management is all that is required. Failure to improve or a worsening of symptoms should raise suspicion of a bacterial superinfection. The marked tonsillar enlargement seen in mononucleosis may lead to airway compromise requiring systemic steroids, a nasal airway trumpet, or in extreme cases endotracheal intubation.

Bacterial Infections

The most common culprits in acute bacterial tonsillitis are group A β-hemolytic streptococci. In comparison with viral infections, streptococcal pharyngitis tends to present with a more abrupt onset and higher fevers. Aside from erythematous ton-

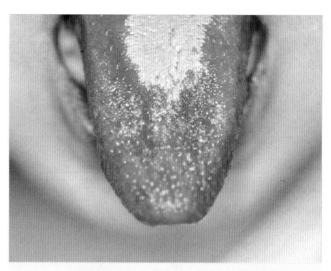

Fig. 69.1 Strawberry tongue.

Table 69.1 Jones criteria for the diagnosis of rheumatic fever

Major criteria	Minor criteria
Carditis	Fever
Aschoff bodies (subcutaneous nodules)	Elevated erythrocyte sedimentation rate or C-reactive protein level
Migratory polyarthritis	Elevated streptococcal titer
Chorea	Prolonger PR interval on electrocardiogram
Erythema marginatum	

sils and pharyngeal walls, one may find purulent exudates, tender lymphadenopathy, and palatal petechiae. Infection of the adenoids presents with similar symptoms and signs, as well as purulent rhinorrhea and postnasal drip. Group A β-hemolytic streptococci produce an endotoxin that may cause a complex of secondary effects known as scarlet fever, including rash, strawberry tongue (▶ Fig. 69.1), and perioral erythema and desquamation. The diagnosis is aided by rapid antigen tests and throat culture.

Treatment is aimed at preventing potential sequelae. Acute post-streptococcal glomerulonephritis presents 1 to 3 weeks after the pharyngitis with gross hematuria, fever, generalized edema, and hypertension. The nephritis is thought to arise from the deposition of antigen–antibody complexes and is typically self-limited. Rheumatic fever is a potentially more severe complication of group A β-hemolytic streptococcal infection that may have lasting consequences. Rheumatic fever arises because of the formation of antibodies against bacterial M-protein that cross-react with antigens in connective tissue of the heart, joints, and central nervous system. The diagnosis is based on the presence of two major or of one major and two minor Jones criteria following a group A β-hemolytic streptococcal infection (▶ Table 69.1).

Penicillin and amoxicillin are appropriate antibiotics for uncomplicated cases and should be continued for 10 days. Clindamycin is a good alternative in penicillin-allergic patients. Failure to respond within 48 to 72 hours should prompt escalation to amoxicillin with clavulanate.

A variety of other bacteria can cause pharyngeal and tonsillar infection, including *Moraxella*, *Haemophilus influenzae*, *S. aureus*, and *Escherichia coli*. Cases of diphtheria caused by *Corynebacterium diphtheriae* are rare and present with gray, adherent pharyngeal exudate. Laryngeal involvement can lead to airway compromise and exotoxin-induced shock. Treatment includes antitoxin and penicillin. The sexually transmitted infections syphilis and gonorrhea can cause pharyngitis. Syphilis, caused by the spirochete *T. pallidum*, can cause oral chancres in the primary phase or exudative pharyngitis in the secondary phase. As with the other manifestations of syphilis, treatment is with penicillin, tetracycline, or erythromycin. Infection with *Neisseria gonorrhoeae* may present as exudative pharyngitis and is treated with doxycycline or ceftriaxone, or a quinolone in older patients.

Fungal Infections

Candida albicans is the most frequent fungal pathogen in pharyngeal infections. Oropharyngeal candidiasis, or "thrush," is often seen in patients who are immunocompromised or undergoing antibiotic therapy. Physical examination will show white, cottage cheese–like plaques adherent to the underlying mucosa, which bleeds upon removal of the exudate. Depending on the severity, treatment can be topical (clotrimazole lozenges, nystatin swish and swallow) or systemic (fluconazole).

Chronic Infection

In contrast to acute bacterial tonsillitis, chronic infection is often polymicrobial, including both aerobic and anaerobic bacteria. Chronic adenoiditis and tonsillitis are treated with extended antibiotic therapy with β-lactamase–stable antibiotics and/or adenotonsillectomy. Chronic tonsillitis or adenoiditis may be a cause of halitosis, an otherwise rare complaint in children. Tonsiliths, or beige-colored granules, may be seen in the tonsil crypts. Tonsiliths are foul-smelling concretions of *Actinomyces* bacteria and are difficult to treat medically. Prolonged penicillin therapy or tonsillectomy is advised for this cause of chronic tonsillitis.

Complications

A peritonsillar abscess occurs when infection extends beyond the tonsillar capsule, with pus collecting in the potential space between the capsule and the surrounding pharyngeal musculature. Patients present with fever, severe odynophagia, trismus, and a muffled "hot potato" voice. They are often dehydrated and unable to tolerate oral intake because of pain. Examination will reveal a bulging soft palate and medially displaced tonsil on the affected side. Trismus may make the examination difficult. The diagnosis is confirmed with needle aspiration, and the abscess is treated definitively with incision and drainage and 10 to 14 days of antibiotics. In some cases, tonsillectomy is performed to drain the abscess and prevent recurrence. Interval tonsillectomy is recommended by many otolaryngologists and also prevents recurrence of peritonsillar abscess.

In severe cases, the abscess may extend beyond the immediate peritonsillar space or into the parapharyngeal space. Fiber-optic examination reveals lateral pharyngeal swelling extending inferiorly to the hypopharynx and potentially causing significant airway obstruction. Contrast CT should be obtained to determine the extent of the abscess. Management should begin with airway control and continue with drainage of the abscess in the operating room and a course of intravenous antibiotics. Spread into the retropharyngeal space is also possible and is managed like a parapharyngeal abscess, with localizing imaging and surgical drainage. Parapharyngeal or retropharyngeal space abscesses may be drained either transorally or through an external neck incision, depending upon the location of the abscess in relation to the carotid artery and jugular vein and the proximity of the abscess to the pharynx.

69.4.3 Tonsil and Adenoid Hypertrophy

The adenoids and tonsils are lymphoid tissue and can enlarge in response both to bacterial colonization with normal flora and to chronic or recurrent infections. Significant hypertrophy can cause pharyngeal airway obstruction, presenting as hyponasal speech, nasal obstruction, rhinorrhea, snoring, chronic mouth breathing, poor feeding, and obstructive sleep apnea (OSA). Enlarged, chronically inflamed adenoids may interfere with the normal function of the eustachian tubes, leading to recurrent otitis media. Patients may exhibit a characteristic "adenoid facies," consisting of an elongated face, flattened midface, high arched palate, short upper lip, and open-mouth breathing. Adenoid hypertrophy can be identified with either fiber-optic examination or lateral neck X-ray. Medical management with nasal steroid sprays may be attempted. Adenotonsillectomy is the definitive treatment for refractory or severe obstructive symptoms.

69.4.4 Neoplastic Disorders

Lymphoma and squamous cell carcinoma are the most common malignancies encountered in the tonsil. Unilateral tonsillar enlargement should raise suspicion for a neoplastic process, and tonsillectomy is performed for biopsy. The likelihood of malignancy increases with the presence of constitutional symptoms (weight loss, night sweats), cervical lymphadenopathy, and a rapidly progressive course. Nasopharyngeal carcinoma is a rare malignancy that may present in the nasopharynx in children. It often presents as a painless neck mass or enlarging neck lymph node in the posterior triangle (level V). The staging of these malignancies is similar to that in the adult and should prompt an oncologic consultation for treatment.

69.4.5 Indications for Tonsillectomy and Adenoidectomy

Indications for tonsillectomy include OSA; suspected malignancy; recurrent tonsillitis (more than five to six episodes in 1 year, four episodes per year for 2 years, or three episodes per year for 3 years); tonsillitis with febrile seizures; chronic tonsillitis unresponsive to antibiotic therapy; and peritonsillar abscess with a history of frequent tonsillar infection. Tonsillectomy may

Table 69.2 Indications for tonsillectomy and adenoidectomy

Indications for tonsillectomy	Indications for adenoidectomy
Recurrent acute tonsillitis	Recurrent adenoiditis
Tonsillitis with febrile seizures	Chronic sinusitis
Chronic tonsillitis	Recurrent acute otitis media
Peritonsillar abscess	Chronic middle ear effusion
Suspected malignancy	Suspected malignancy
Obstructive sleep apnea	Obstructive sleep apnea
Sleep-disordered breathing	Sleep-disordered breathing
Dysphagia	

Table 69.3 Differences in the presentation of obstructive sleep apnea in adults and children

Adults	Children
Daytime somnolence	Hyperactivity/behavioral disturbances
Frequent obesity	Underweight/failure to thrive

also be considered if significant hypertrophy is seen in association with significant dysphagia that has no other apparent cause or with speech abnormalities.

Indications for adenoidectomy include OSA, suspected malignancy (as a biopsy procedure), recurrent infection, chronic or recurrent sinusitis, and recurrent acute otitis media (▶ Table 69.2).

The risks of adenotonsillectomy should be well understood by the patient and family. They include bleeding (1 to 2% of children, typically 5 to 7 days postoperatively), odynophagia with poor oral intake and dehydration, and infection. Adenoidectomy may lead to velopharyngeal insufficiency (manifesting as hypernasal speech and nasal regurgitation of food and liquid), especially in the setting of a submucous cleft palate. Such situations are avoided by routinely examining the palate for evidence of a bifid uvula or diastasis of the palatal musculature. Patients with Down syndrome present a special case. These children are prone to atlantoaxial subluxation and should be evaluated with flexion–extension neck radiographs before surgery. Children who have velocardiofacial syndrome may have aberrant carotid arteries with an abnormally medial location, placing them at risk during routine tonsillectomy and adenoidectomy. Preoperative CT angiography will demonstrate such vascular anomalies.

69.5 Sleep-Disordered Breathing and Obstructive Sleep Apnea

69.5.1 History

Pediatric patients may present with nighttime symptoms that include snoring, witnessed episodes of apnea, gasping for breath, sweating, restless sleep, and enuresis. The frequency of the episodes of gasping or apnea should be elicited, as should the length of the apnea episodes. Unlike adults, who exhibit daytime somnolence, children with OSA are often hyperactive and inattentive, and they may have behavioral problems and a learning disability (▶ Table 69.3). Various medical conditions put children at greater risk for OSA, including craniofacial abnormalities (e.g., Treacher Collins syndrome or Pierre Robin syndrome) and neuromuscular disorders leading to decreased tone in the pharyngeal musculature (especially cerebral palsy and Down syndrome).

69.5.2 Physical Examination

The patient's height and weight should be plotted and compared with established norms. Any craniofacial abnormalities (retrognathia or micrognathia, cleft lip and/or cleft palate, macroglossia) should be noted. The size of the tonsils should be rated, as previously described. A fiber-optic examination should be performed to evaluate for nasal obstruction, adenoid hypertrophy, or other airway anomalies (e.g., laryngomalacia). The appearance and length of the soft palate are important to note, especially in children whose tonsils and adenoids are somewhat small.

69.5.3 Diagnostic Evaluation

A lateral neck film may be helpful in evaluating adenoid size in the uncooperative child. Polysomnography is discussed below.

69.5.4 Sleep-Disordered Breathing

Sleep disorders in children encompass a continuum, ranging from relatively benign primary snoring to potentially life-threatening OSA. The diagnosis and treatment of sleep disordered-breathing differ significantly between children and adults. Although apnea in adults is generally defined as the cessation of breathing for 10 seconds, the duration in children is shortened to two or more consecutive breaths. Hypopnea is variably described as a 50% reduction in airflow or respiratory effort, or an increased end-tidal CO_2 level (normally ~ 40 mm Hg).

Up to 10% of children snore during sleep. Those whose snoring is not accompanied by obstructive symptoms are given the diagnosis of primary snoring and require no further treatment. Children who snore and display evidence of partial airway obstruction, including frequent arousals due to increased respiratory effort, but who do not experience true apnea or hypopnea as defined above are classified as having upper airway resistance syndrome. Because of their frequent arousals, they may present with many of the daytime symptoms of children with OSA.

69.5.5 Obstructive Sleep Apnea

OSA is seen in 1 to 3% of children and is defined as airway obstruction (apnea and/or hypopnea) leading to hypoxemia and/or hypercarbia. As in adults, severe OSA can lead to pulmonary hypertension and cor pulmonale. Although it is true that obese children are at a greater risk for developing OSA, most children with OSA are not overweight, and they may, in fact, present with poor growth or failure to thrive.

The diagnosis of OSA is typically made by obtaining an appropriate history of sleep disturbance and obstructive symptoms.

Polysomnography provides information on a variety of parameters measured while the child sleeps. The accepted standard polysomnography includes electroencephalography to measure sleep stage, electromyography to measure limb movements and arousals, electrocardiography, measures of chest wall and abdominal movements with respiration, pulse oximetry, end-tidal CO_2, and oronasal airflow. Polysomnography will give information about the number of apnea and hypopnea episodes per hour (the respiratory disturbance index, or RDI); the degree of hypoxia (defined as arterial oxygen saturation [SaO_2] < 92%) and hypercarbia (peak end-tidal CO_2 > 50 mm Hg); and sleep architecture (non–rapid eye movement [NREM] vs rapid eye movement [REM] sleep). Although there are no widely accepted standards for stratifying the severity of OSA in children, an RDI above 1.5 is considered abnormal.

Although polysomnography is the gold standard for diagnosing OSA, it is not practical for every patient. Polysomnography should be used for high-risk patients (those with craniofacial abnormalities, neuromuscular disorders, or significant comorbidities that could complicate surgical management) and for patients whose history and physical examination findings are inconsistent.

The treatment of OSA in children typically consists of adenotonsillectomy to relieve pharyngeal airway obstruction when it is caused by large tonsils and adenoids. In patients with mild OSA, one can expect a resolution of obstructive symptoms after surgery, although patients with severe apnea may have persistent problems. Aside from the resolution of airway complaints, numerous studies have shown improvements in quality of life and in behavior and school performance.

More complex treatment may be required in children with craniofacial anomalies. In patients with severe OSA that is refractory to standard management, tracheotomy is indicated. Patients who have significant nasal obstruction related to allergy may benefit from medical therapy with nasal steroid sprays. Finally, patients who are poor surgical candidates or have persistent issues postoperatively can be managed with continuous positive airway pressure (CPAP) or bilevel positive airway pressure (BiPAP) as an alternative to tracheotomy.

69.6 Dysphagia and Gastroesophageal Reflux

Pediatric dysphagia encompasses an immense range of eating and/or swallowing disorders. An in-depth discussion of each of the possible causes of dysphagia in children is beyond the scope of this chapter; rather, the aim here is to present a framework for evaluating a patient, based on an understanding of the normal swallow mechanism, knowledge of the salient historical clues and physical examination findings, and an awareness of the broad categories in which the majority of diagnoses can be placed.

The normal swallowing mechanism can be separated into three phases: oral, pharyngeal, and esophageal. The oral phase involves the ingestion of food, mastication, and then posterior propulsion of the food into the oropharynx. The pharyngeal phase is reflexive and requires the coordination of multiple cranial nerves (including cranial nerves V, IX, X, and XII) to close the nasopharynx, elevate the larynx while closing the airway, and propel the food into the hypopharynx. The esophageal phase begins with relaxation of the cricopharyngeus, which allows the food bolus to enter the esophagus, where peristaltic contraction propels it to the stomach.

69.6.1 History

In the newborn, the prenatal and birth history take on extreme importance. A history of polyhydramnios may point toward esophageal malformation or neurologic compromise. Perinatal respiratory compromise requiring intubation should prompt concern for traumatic injury to the pharynx and/or larynx, or it can indicate a period of significant hypoxia leading to central nervous system damage. Prior surgical procedures should be noted, especially those that put cranial nerves at risk (ventriculoperitoneal shunt, patent ductus arteriosus ligation). A detailed family history is important in ruling out genetic, neurologic, and neuromuscular disorders.

In older children, the onset of the dysphagia (abrupt vs progressive) and the time course of the symptoms (constant vs episodic) deserve special attention. One should determine whether the patient has dysphagia to solids, liquids, or both. A history of the sudden onset of dysphagia in an otherwise normal child is concerning for foreign body ingestion, whereas a worsening dysphagia progressing from solids only to liquids points toward esophageal obstruction. Odynophagia points toward an infectious/inflammatory etiology, a foreign body, or caustic ingestion. Vomiting is an important associated symptom and should be characterized by timing with regard to feeding (during, immediately after) and by the nature of the food regurgitated (digested or undigested). Airway symptoms such as stridor and cyanosis with feeding may indicate airway obstruction as a cause of dysphagia; alternatively, they may result from aspiration.

A detailed review of systems is important in ruling out systemic issues such as autoimmune, endocrine, and neurologic disorders, as well as immunocompromised states and infection.

69.6.2 Physical Examination

The patient's height and weight should be noted and plotted over time to document adequate growth and development. Weight loss and failure to thrive (as indicated by weight below the third percentile) indicate a serious problem requiring immediate attention. In the case of infants, one should observe the infant feed, noting whether the child exhibits appropriate rooting and suck reflexes. The absence of these important reflexes may indicate neurologic deficiencies.

A complete head and neck examination should be performed. Craniofacial anomalies (e.g., cleft lip and/or cleft palate, retrognathia, macroglossia, and glossoptosis) should be noted, and the physician should maintain a high index of suspicion for genetic disorders and syndromes with characteristic facies.

Fiber-optic examination of the upper aerodigestive tract is an important tool in the evaluation of patients with dysphagia and is often the main reason for referral to an otolaryngologist. Examination should rule out nasal obstruction due to rhinitis, deviated nasal septum, choanal atresia, or adenoid hypertrophy. Evaluation of the hypopharynx may demonstrate the pooling of secretions or gross aspiration. Laryngeal abnormalities, both anatomical (e.g., laryngeal cleft, laryngomalacia) and functional (vocal fold paralysis), should be noted.

Finally, a neurologic examination should be performed. Obviously, special attention should be paid to the cranial nerves, although a peripheral examination is also important, and any abnormalities (e.g., hypotonia) documented.

69.6.3 Diagnostic Testing

Various radiologic studies are available to aid in the diagnosis. A chest X-ray can assess cardiac, tracheobronchial, and mediastinal abnormalities. Further evaluation with CT or MR imaging should be directed by the history and physical findings of a neck mass. Modified barium swallow uses fluoroscopy to visualize swallow function during the oral and pharyngeal phases. Information regarding aspiration can be obtained, and different consistencies of food used to determine the safety of oral feeding. Modified barium swallow is often combined with a barium esophagram to rule out structural or motility problems.

Functional endoscopic evaluation of swallowing can provide information on laryngopharyngeal sensation, laryngeal mobility, and aspiration. As with modified barium swallow, different consistencies of food can be used.

Twenty-four-hour pH probe studies are the gold standard for the diagnosis of reflux. Probes are positioned at the proximal and distal ends of the esophagus as well as the pharynx (in the case of a three-probe study). Esophageal manometry allows an assessment of esophageal motility. Endoscopy allows direct visualization of the esophagus and is indicated for both diagnosis and treatment (e.g., removal of a foreign body, dilation of a stricture).

69.6.4 Differential Diagnosis

In the evaluation of a patient with dysphagia, it is best to break down the myriad etiologies into a number of broad categories. It is important to recognize that multiple factors may be contributing to a patient's dysphagia.

69.6.5 Developmental Issues

Premature infants often require both ventilatory and feeding support. Such patients may have a weak suck reflex and difficulty coordinating feeding and respiration. They are maintained on alternate methods of feeding (gavage, gastrostomy). Fortunately, in the absence of neurologic injury, the majority of these patients will progress to normal oral intake.

69.6.6 Congenital Anatomical Defects

Defects involving the aerodigestive tract at any level from the nasal passage to the distal trachea and esophagus can interfere with normal swallowing. Obstruction of the nasal airway, as in piriform aperture stenosis, choanal atresia, or even severe septal deflections (as from birth trauma), can affect an infant's ability to coordinate feeding and respiration.

Craniofacial abnormalities can impair the feeding and swallowing mechanism in a number of ways. Children with cleft lip and palate are unable to generate an effective seal and must be fed with a special bottles and nipples. Patients with a cleft palate will also regurgitate feeds into the nasal cavity through direct communication via the cleft and defective velopharyngeal closure. Syndromes that include abnormalities in the growth, position, and proportions of the mandible and other facial bones can lead to feeding issues. Notable examples include Crouzon, Apert, Goldenhar, and Treacher Collins syndromes. When craniofacial disproportion is combined with a cleft palate and/or lip, the dysfunction becomes increasingly pronounced. Macroglossia, as seen in Down (trisomy 21) and Beckwith-Wiedemann syndromes, can interfere with the sucking mechanism, food bolus propulsion, and laryngeal protection. Finally, malposition of the tongue, due to macroglossia or retrognathia (as in Pierre Robin sequence), can cause airway obstruction and subsequent feeding problems.

Congenital laryngeal malformations such as laryngomalacia, laryngeal webs and clefts, and cysts cause dysphagia secondary to airway obstruction, aspiration, or both. Stridor and/or hoarseness should raise suspicion for a laryngeal cause of dysphagia.

Numerous tracheal and esophageal issues lead to dysphagia. Esophageal pathologies include atresia, duplication, tracheoesophageal fistula, webs, and strictures. Tracheoesophageal fistulas are often accompanied by other congenital defects, commonly involving the cardiac and genitourinary systems. Tracheoesophageal fistulas are seen in four typical configurations in association with esophageal atresia. Respiratory symptoms of choking, aspiration, and respiratory distress may be associated with the various types of tracheoesophageal fistula. The treatment of tracheoesophageal fistula involves surgical correction of the esophageal and tracheal abnormalities, typically soon after the condition is diagnosed in the infant.

Vascular rings can involve both the esophagus and the trachea, leading to stridor that worsens with feeding. Alternatively, dysphagia arising from such rings may not become apparent until the child begins eating solid food.

69.6.7 Acquired Anatomical Defects

Within this category, esophageal foreign body ingestion is likely the most common etiology encountered. The ingestion of caustic substances can cause dysphagia in the acute setting as well as later as a result of stricture of the esophagus. A good medical and surgical history should elucidate an iatrogenic cause of the patient's symptoms (intubation trauma, prior aerodigestive tract surgery). A history of tracheal or esophageal surgery, as well as any cardiac procedures, should raise suspicion for recurrent laryngeal nerve injury with vocal fold paralysis or superior laryngeal nerve injury resulting in alterations of laryngeal sensation.

69.6.8 Infectious and Inflammatory Disorders

Infections of the upper aerodigestive tract are common causes of odynophagia and dysphagia in children. Bacterial or viral pharyngitis is frequently seen in children and should be obvious on physical examination. Deep neck space infections (e.g., retropharyngeal and parapharyngeal abscesses) should be suspected in children with systemic signs of infection and complaints of odynophagia or refusal to eat. In immunocompromised patients, one should be alert to opportunistic infections of the esophagus with bacteria, *Candida* and other fungal agents, *Mycobacterium tuberculosis*, or viral pathogens such as cytomegalovirus and herpesvirus. Chagas disease, caused by the parasite *Trypanosoma cruzi*, is seen in Central and South America and leads to esophageal atonia (and ultimately megaesophagus).

Like adults, children may be affected by various connective tissue disorders that lead to dysphagia. Scleroderma affects smooth muscle and can limit esophageal motility, as well as lead to strictures due to severe reflux. Sjögren syndrome produces xerostomia. Juvenile rheumatoid arthritis (Still disease) can cause an arthritis of the cricoarytenoid joint, with pain on phonation and swallowing, as well as respiratory distress from fixation of the cricoarytenoid joint.

69.6.9 Neoplastic Conditions

Obviously, neoplasms within the upper aerodigestive tract can obstruct the passage of food, leading to the complaint of dysphagia. In addition, mediastinal tumors may extrinsically obstruct the esophagus. A history of progressive dysphagia, moving from problems with solids only to problems with both liquids and solids, is highly suggestive of obstruction due to neoplasm.

69.6.10 Neurologic Disorders

A neurologic cause of dysphagia should be considered when no other anatomical or functional cause can be found. Infants with central nervous system dysfunction may not demonstrate robust rooting and suck reflexes. They may have difficulty managing their secretions, with drooling and aspiration. Additional signs of neurologic impairment, including generalized hypotonia, may be present. Etiologies of the neurologic insult include hypoxia, trauma, infection, congenital defects (Chiari malformation), and genetic disorders (myasthenia gravis, muscular dystrophy).

69.6.11 Psychological/Behavioral Issues

Only after all organic causes of dysphagia have been ruled out should psychological reasons be considered. Clues in the history that may lead one to suspect the symptoms are behaviorally based are normal weight gain despite complaints and normal swallowing at meals, with symptoms occurring only between meals.

69.6.12 Other Gastrointestinal Disorders Affecting the Esophagus

Primary disorders of the gastrointestinal tract are relevant in the evaluation of dysphagia. Cricopharyngeal achalasia, or failure of the upper esophageal sphincter to relax with swallowing, causes the symptoms of gagging, regurgitation, and aspiration. Diffuse esophageal spasm, or "nutcracker esophagus," presents with odynophagia and chest pain and can be diagnosed via barium esophagram and esophageal manometry. Reflux of the gastric contents can cause symptoms of dysphagia and will be discussed in further detail in the following section.

69.6.13 Gastroesophageal Reflux

Gastroesophageal reflux occurs when relaxation of the lower esophageal sphincter allows reflux of the gastric contents into the esophagus. Gastroesophageal reflux disease (GERD) is the clinical manifestation of mucosal damage secondary to prolonged exposure to refluxed materials. Pathologic reflux is most often due to inappropriate so-called transient lower esophageal relaxations, but it may also be related to delayed gastric emptying and/or defective esophageal clearance.

History

Reflux in children may present with a variety of symptoms and signs but may be generally divided into two large categories: esophageal and extra-esophageal manifestations. Furthermore, within those groups, GERD presents differently in children of different age groups.

Esophageal Manifestations

Sporadic postprandial reflux, often accompanied by effortless regurgitation, is a normal occurrence in infants but typically disappears by 1 year of age. Infants with GERD may have more frequent regurgitation, choking, food avoidance, and back arching due to odynophagia and esophageal irritation; in the most serious cases, they may exhibit failure to thrive. Older children often complain of heartburn, dysphagia, and globus sensation.

Extra-esophageal Manifestations

GERD has been implicated in disorders involving the upper and lower airway, sinonasal system, and ears. Airway complaints in infants include stridor, cyanotic spells, and recurrent croup. In older children, one may see chronic cough, asthma, and recurrent pneumonia. Reflux has been implicated in the development of subglottic stenosis and must be a primary concern in any patient undergoing airway reconstruction. Reflux should be considered a contributing factor in patients with recurrent, chronic rhinosinusitis and otitis media.

Physical Examination

If the child has reflux beyond the upper esophageal sphincter into the pharynx, fiber-optic examination will reveal characteristic changes. Lymphoid hyperplasia secondary to chronic irritation can give the posterior pharyngeal wall a knobby, "cobblestone" appearance. Examination of the larynx may show erythema and edema of the postcricoid area and arytenoids. Other laryngeal findings include ulcerations, granulomas, and subglottic stenosis. Esophagoscopy may demonstrate mucosal erythema or ulceration.

Diagnostic Evaluation

In children with suggestive symptomatology and findings consistent with reflux on fiber-optic or rigid endoscopic examination, empiric antireflux therapy may be started with no further work-up. Indeed, studies have demonstrated similar sensitivities and specificities for endoscopic findings and other testing modalities. However, when the diagnosis is in doubt or the patient fails to respond to empiric therapy, additional testing may be required.

The 24-hour dual pH probe has long been considered the gold standard for the diagnosis of GERD. Two pH probes, one at the distal end of the esophagus and one at the proximal end of the esophagus or the pharynx, are used to record episodes of acid reflux. The standard criterion for GERD is a recorded esophageal pH of less than 4 for more than 5% of the recording time. This measure is inadequate for the diagnosis of extra-esophageal reflux disease. The pharynx and larynx lack the robust mucosal defenses of the esophagus and may be damaged by exposure to a much smaller amount of refluxate. Furthermore, there is strong evidence that much of the damage associated with reflux is caused not by acid but by pepsin, which has been shown to maintain some proteolytic activity at pH values up to 6.5.

Barium swallow and upper gastrointestinal series may show reflux but are unreliable; they are more useful for ruling out anatomical defects such as pyloric stenosis, which leads to feeding difficulties. Scintigraphy may demonstrate delayed gastric emptying or the aspiration of refluxed materials but is not sensitive for GERD. Esophageal biopsy may be indicated in recalcitrant cases to distinguish between GERD-related esophagitis and other entities, such as eosinophilic esophagitis. Findings at esophagoscopy that favor eosinophilic esophagitis include circular rings ("trachealization") of the esophagus, vertical linear furrows, and exudates. These disorders are differentiated via histologic examination.

Management

In less severe cases, management may begin simply with lifestyle changes, including upright feeding for infants, weight loss, avoidance of foods and drinks that induce reflux (spicy, acidic, or fatty foods; caffeine), and avoidance of meals 1 hour before sleep or exercise.

Medical therapy is indicated for patients with more severe symptoms, including airway involvement, and for those who do not respond to conservative management. Proton pump inhibitors (PPIs) are the mainstay of therapy. PPIs have been found to be metabolized faster in children than in adults, and as a result, higher doses and twice-daily administration are often necessary. Histamine$_2$ blockers may also be useful, either alone or in conjunction with PPIs. Promotility agents (metoclopramide, erythromycin, baclofen) may be of use in selected cases, especially if delayed gastric emptying is a concern.

Finally, in patients in whom severe symptoms remain despite maximal medical therapy, or in whom lifetime problems are anticipated (e.g. neurologic disorders), surgical therapy such as gastric fundoplication may be warranted.

69.7 Conclusion

The anatomy and physiology of the oral cavity and pharynx are complex, leading to a wide variety of disorders. Timely diagnosis and treatment are important because diseases in this region can have far-ranging effects on the growth and overall health of a child.

69.8 Roundsmanship

- Most disorders of the salivary glands in children are infectious or obstructive in nature; however, neoplasms are more likely to be malignant in children than in adults.
- Obstructive sleep apnea and recurrent tonsillitis or adenoiditis are common indications for adenotonsillectomy. Symptoms of obstructive sleep apnea in children differ significantly from those in adults.
- Obstructive sleep apnea can often be diagnosed based on the patient history. Polysomnography is the gold standard diagnostic tool for obstructive sleep apnea and may be helpful in children with comorbid conditions, or when the history is unclear.
- Gastroesophageal reflux disease has a wide array of extraesophageal manifestations in children. A definitive diagnosis is more difficult to obtain in children, and empiric trials of medication are often appropriate.

69.9 Recommended Reading

[1] Conner GH. Idiopathic conditions of the mouth and pharynx. In: Bluestone CD, Stool SE, Alper CM, et al, eds. Pediatric Otolaryngology. 4th ed. Philadelphia, PA: W. B. Saunders; 2003

[2] Derkay CS, Schechter GL. Dysphagia. In: Bluestone CD, Stool SE, Alper CM, et al, eds. Pediatric Otolaryngology. 4th ed. Philadelphia, PA: W. B. Saunders; 2003

[3] Gluckman JL, Righi PD. Inflammatory disease of the mouth and pharynx. In: Bluestone CD, Stool SE, Alper CM, et al, eds. Pediatric Otolaryngology. 4th ed. Philadelphia, PA: W. B. Saunders; 2003

[4] Miller CK, Willging JP. Advances in the evaluation and management of pediatric dysphagia. Curr Opin Otolaryngol Head Neck Surg 2003; 11: 442–446

[5] Sterni LM, Tunkel DE. Obstructive sleep apnea in children. In: Cummings C, Haughey B, Thomas JR, et al, eds. Otolaryngology: Head and Neck Surgery. 4th ed. Philadelphia, PA: Elsevier Mosby; 2005

[6] Zalzal GH, Tran LP. Pediatric gastroesophageal reflux and laryngopharyngeal reflux. Otolaryngol Clin North Am 2000; 33: 151–161

70 Pediatric Obstructive Sleep Apnea

Miguel Krishnan and Robin A. Dyleski

70.1 Introduction

Of the basic human needs, water, food, and sleep are essential for well-being. Sleep provides nourishment for both mind and body. It is a time of rest, recuperation, and regeneration from the day's demanding tasks. Pediatric obstructive sleep apnea (OSA) is one of the most commonly diagnosed ailments that may interfere with a child's ability to obtain good-quality sleep.

A child's struggle to breathe during sleep may manifest as a spectrum ranging from turbulent airflow that produces snoring to the extreme situation of complete airway obstruction and apnea. As apnea leads to hypoxia, the child is likely to change position, with a resultant fragmentation of sleep in order to maintain respiration. The outcome is that the child suffers more than just a loss of sleep; there are consequences that affect daytime development, as well.

Sir William Osler first described pediatric OSA in 1892. "Chronic enlargement of the tonsillar tissues is an affectation of great importance and may influence in an extraordinary way the mental and bodily development of children." At night, the child's sleep is greatly disturbed; the respirations are loud and snorting, and there are sometimes prolonged pauses, followed by deep, noisy respirations. The child may wake up in a paroxysm of shortness of breath.

Only in the past 20 years has the differentiation between adult and pediatric OSA become recognized as a topic of great importance. The prevalence, incidence, presentation, sequelae, and treatment of pediatric OSA vary greatly from those for the adult counterpart. Information about the differences between adult and pediatric OSA and new knowledge of pediatric OSA continue to be unveiled. Pediatric OSA has become a subject of great interest, especially with respect to its effect on children's behavior, psyche, and overall health.

70.2 Incidence

Pediatric OSA occurs in children between the neonatal period and adolescence. In neonates, it is usually due to craniofacial abnormalities, such as those associated with Down syndrome, Pierre Robin sequence, and choanal stenosis or atresia, as well as any chronic condition resulting in nasal obstruction or stenosis. In older children, OSA may be due to a multitude of factors.

The prevalence of pediatric OSA is 1 to 3%, with nearly 500,000 children affected in the United States. The cost to the health care system of children with OSA is increased by 226% compared with the cost of controls. After adenotonsillectomy is performed, this cost is noted to decrease by one-third.

Pediatric OSA shows no sex predilection in comparison with adult OSA. However, toward late adolescence, a slight male predominance is noted, as in adults. The incidence seems to be higher in African-Americans, which is felt to be due to their craniofacial structure. Although obesity does have some impact, most children who display symptoms of OSA are found to be underweight rather than overweight. However, as obesity continues to increase in the pediatric population, so does the incidence of pediatric OSA.

Snoring is nearly universally seen in pediatric OSA. Although snoring does not always suggest OSA, it is considered a hallmark of sleep-disordered breathing. Six to 27% of children snore on a regular basis, and 3% of children may have abnormalities of reduced gas exchange.

The incidence of pediatric OSA usually peaks in children between 2 and 8 years of age. This is the period during which the lymphoid tissue is largest in relation to the size of a child's pharyngeal airway space and head. The incidence of pediatric OSA is higher in children who have narrow pharyngeal airways, as well as in children who have craniofacial anomalies and syndromes associated with midface hypoplasia and pharyngeal disturbances.

70.3 Terminology and Classification

According to the American Thoracic Society, OSA of childhood is defined as a disorder of breathing during sleep characterized by prolonged partial upper airway obstruction and/or intermittent complete obstruction that disrupts normal ventilation during sleep and normal sleep patterns.

We have realized over the years that sleep disturbance can be attributed to a disturbance in breathing patterns during sleep. As in the classification of other ailments, categories of mild, moderate, and severe only scratch the surface of the true classification of cases of pediatric OSA.

Pediatric OSA is better defined as a point along a spectrum of sleep-disordered breathing. This spectrum commences with snoring, and as the condition intensifies in severity, it becomes sleep disordered breathing and finally frank pediatric OSA.

Primary snoring is snoring that is not associated with hypoxemia, hypercarbia, or apnea. Snoring is the first step toward the sleep apnea syndrome. It may occur every night or on an intermittent basis. It may be associated with a temporary condition of decreased nasal patency, such as that caused by allergic rhinitis, recurrent sinusitis, or chronic rhinorrhea.

The next entity along the spectrum is upper airway resistance syndrome. This is a combination of snoring with partial airway collapse during sleep. It is associated with restless sleep patterns and a reduction in airflow without hypoxemia, hypercarbia, or apnea.

Finally, the point on the spectrum at which the problem is most severe is OSA. This is characterized by snoring, upper airway resistance syndrome, hypercarbia, hypoxemia, hypoventilation, and frank apnea (▶ Fig. 70.1).

70.4 Etiology

The most common cause of pediatric OSA is chronic enlargement of the lymphoid tissues within the pharynx: in the nasopharynx, the nasopharyngeal tonsils (adenoids) and the

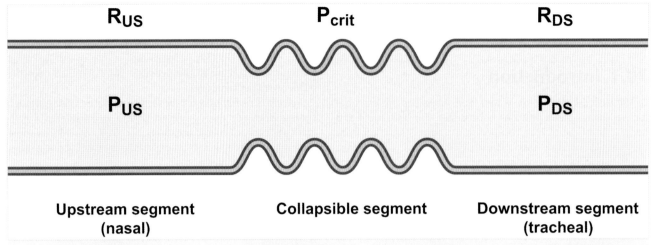

Fig. 70.1 Starling resistor model of the upper airway. R_{US}, upstream resistance; R_{DS}, downstream resistance; P_{US}, upstream intraluminal pressure; P_{DS}, downstream intraluminal pressure; P_{crit}, extraluminal pressure in collapsible segment. Airway obstruction occurs when P_{crit} exceeds intraluminal pressure in the collapsible segment.

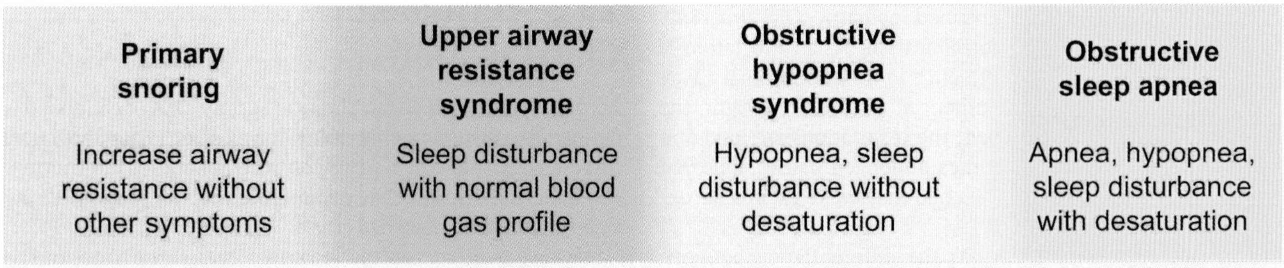

Primary snoring	Upper airway resistance syndrome	Obstructive hypopnea syndrome	Obstructive sleep apnea
Increase airway resistance without other symptoms	Sleep disturbance with normal blood gas profile	Hypopnea, sleep disturbance without desaturation	Apnea, hypopnea, sleep disturbance with desaturation

Fig. 70.2 The continuum of obstructive sleep-disordered breathing.

nearby tubal (Gerlach) tonsils; in the oropharynx, the pharyngeal tonsils; and at the base of tongue and vallecula, the lingual tonsils.

Although these four sets of tonsils are the most frequent culprits in the origin of pediatric OSA, pediatric OSA can realistically be caused by any of the structures that limit the size of the nasal and oral cavities, all the way to the glottis.

Other conditions within the nasal cavity that can cause OSA include nasal polyposis, nasal septal deviation, turbinate hypertrophy, allergic rhinitis, choanal stenosis/atresia, anterior piriform aperture, and midnasal stenosis.

The nasopharynx and the oropharynx contain more than 30 paired muscles, which maintain the intricate balance between airway patency and airway narrowing. According to the Starling resistor model and Bernoulli's principle, airway resistance is increased not only by relaxation but also by the dynamics of airflow (► Fig. 70.2).

These laws apply to the small airways associated with craniofacial syndromes and to the low level of muscle tonicity occurring in congenital neurologic conditions, further contributing to obstruction. Still, the most common areas involved in pediatric upper airway obstruction are the tonsils and adenoids, located in the nasopharynx and oropharynx (► Fig. 70.3 and ► Fig. 70.4).

A high incidence of OSA may associated with obesity, although OSA is more commonly noted in thin children. Obese children are more likely to present with snoring and sleep-dis-

ordered breathing than with frank OSA; however, it should be noted that some extremely obese children may have very severe OSA.

70.5 Sequelae

The consequences of pediatric OSA are diverse and can have lifelong, permanent effects upon a child's growth and development. As a child continues to mature anatomically, physiologically, and immunologically, his or her progress must be monitored with these effects kept in mind. The onset, duration, severity, and progression of OSA may increase a child's risk for developing long-term sequelae.

OSA can be difficult to diagnose in children (► Table 70.1). Their signs and symptoms do not always accurately reflect the severity of OSA disease, and not enough normative data are available to predict those who will have adverse outcomes.

Children may present with a variety of sequelae affecting multiple body systems, such as failure to thrive, neurocognitive deficits, and cardiopulmonary compromise. Somatic development can be affected; poor growth velocity despite adequate caloric intake and the absence of other chronic illness is a frequent pattern. Not only can adenotonsillar hypertrophy lead to decreased olfactory sensation and decreased taste, it also can cause dysphagia due to the direct impairment of oral and oropharyngeal swallowing.

The caloric expenditure of children who struggle to breathe during sleep may be increased by the effort needed to maintain adequate ventilation; the resultant hypercarbia can impair the physiologic release of insulin-like growth factor and lead to decreased linear growth. After adenotonsillectomy for obstructive apnea, children often exhibit significant weight gain and catch-up growth spurts.

The neurocognitive effects can lead to irritable behavior, lack of attention, and poor school performance. Contrary to popular belief, lack of sleep in the pediatric population leads to hyperactivity and an increase in aggressive behavior. Frequent snoring has also been associated with poor academic performance.

The cardiovascular sequelae can range from structural abnormalities to autonomic dysfunction. The consequences can include ventricular hypertrophy, pulmonary hypertension, systemic hypertension, cor pulmonale (right-sided heart failure),

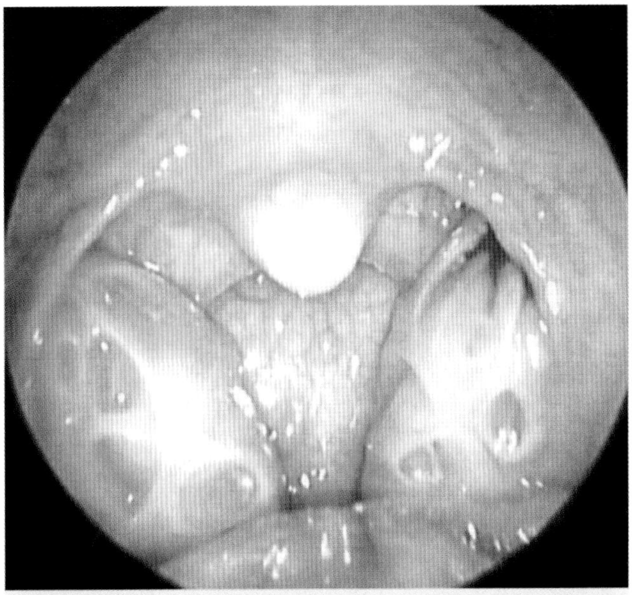

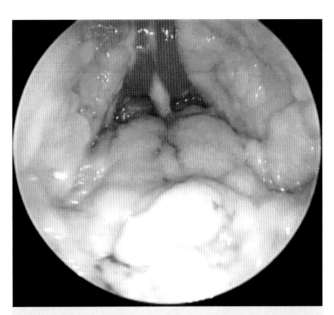

Fig. 70.4 Surgical view of adenoids with impairment of the posterior choanae and nasopharyngeal airway patency. The red rubber catheters at the top of image pass through the nasal cavity and are retracting the soft palate. The posterior ends of inferior turbinates are seen intranasally beyond the posterior choanae.

Fig. 70.3 Surgical view of tonsillar enlargement with limitation of the oropharyngeal airway.

Table 70.1 Childhood versus adult obstructive sleep apnea syndrome

	Child	Adult
Presentation		
Underweight/failure to thrive	Frequent	Rare
Daytime mouth breathing	Frequent	Rare
Adenotonsillar enlargement	Frequent	Rare
Daytime drowsiness	Rare	Frequent
Obesity	Common	Uncommon
Male-to-female ratio	1:1	2:1
Sleep pattern		
Obstructive	Obstructive apnea or hypoventilation	Obstructive apnea
Arousal with obstruction	Uncommon	Common
Disrupted	Uncommon	Common
Management		
Surgical	Definitive treatment in most patients	Minority of patients
Medical	Only in Selected Patients	Majority of Patients

Source: Adapted from Carroll JL, Loughlin GM. Diagnostic criteria for obstructive sleep apnea syndrome in children. Pediatr Pulmonol 1992;14(2):71–79.

and congestive heart failure. It is impossible to to predict which children are more likely to develop these serious sequelae, and all children with long-standing untreated obstructive sleep apnea are at risk for serious morbidity and mortality.

The pathophysiology of the cardiopulmonary problems is multifactorial. OSA results in increased levels of catecholamines, which may elevate the diastolic blood pressure; this process begins during sleep and persists into the awakening hours. Recurrent hypercapnia and hypoxia can elicit vasomotor recruitment of the pulmonary circulation, resulting in pulmonary hypertension. It is uncertain whether these sequelae reverse after the treatment of OSA.

70.6 Presentation

OSA may present in several different ways in children. These include loud snoring and restless sleep patterns, behavior problems in school, and cardiovascular manifestations leading to early mortality. The variety of possible presentations may lead to management by several independent specialists. Children may be brought to a developmental pediatrician because of failure to thrive; they may be referred to a neurologist for narcoleptic hypersomnolence or hyperactivity; they may be under the care of a psychologist for behavior issues or a pulmonologist for respiratory insufficiency; they may present to an otolaryngologist for snoring, mouth breathing, and enlarged tonsils. The presentation is complex, demonstrating that OSA may be the etiology of a variety of other problems. In many cases, the parents themselves may not even be aware that their child's snoring is abnormal.

Respiratory Disturbance Index (RDI) Formula

RDI= (# obstructive [apnea/hypopnea] cevents + # Central [apnea/hypopnea] events + # mixed [apnea/hypopnea]) x 60 / (# minutes of observed sleep)

The parental history and physical examination are ineffective for discerning the true severity of the disease. Although a child may present with snoring, it is difficult to distinguish primary snoring from frank OSA. Upon additional questioning, the parents may describe their child as a restless sleeper who moves all over the bed. The child may sleep in odd positions and use the accessory muscles of respiration (manifested as tracheal or sternal retractions) to relieve upper airway obstruction. The parents may observe choking or gagging respirations with periods of apnea, or they may describe "gasping" resuscitative breaths after apneic pauses. The parents often state that their child has very "frightening breathing."

70.7 Testing

During the history and physical screening process, the physician can determine if further testing is necessary. Family audio and video recordings can be reviewed for more information. These are useful when obtained during deep sleep, several hours after the child has gone to bed. The intensity of the noisy respirations and restlessness is often a better indicator of OSA than are the apneic episodes seen during sleep disturbance.

The physical finding of hypertrophic tonsils and adenoids does not always indicate the severity of OSA. It is the combination of enlarged lymphoid tissues and hypotonia during sleep that indicates the severity. However, if the findings on physical examination do not correlate with the history, further testing may be necessary.

A multitude of tests are available to ascertain the severity of sleep-disordered breathing. These vary from basic pulse oximetry to comprehensive polysomnography. Basic pulse oximetry is a good screening tool to identify patients with significant desaturations due to OSA; however, its negative predictive value is very poor, and further testing is required for clarification.

The 2-hour nap study, which is cost-effective, is performed during the daytime. Because of its brevity, it does not allow rapid eye movement (REM) sleep to be sustained. Therefore, a negative study may not rule out OSA.

Overnight polysomnography is the current gold standard for diagnosing and grading the severity of OSA. There are specific indications for polysomnography (see Box Indications for Polysomnography (p.559)). In addition to situations in which the history and physical examination are neither mutually suggestive nor exclusive, polysomnography is helpful in children who have craniofacial abnormalities, are obese or younger than 2 years of age, or have conditions such as mucopolysaccharidosis, neuromuscular disease, and sickle cell anemia.

Apnea–Hypopnea Index (AHI) Formula

AHI= (# obstructive [apnea/hypopnea] events) x 60 / (# minutes of observed sleep)

Polysomnography is a 6-hour overnight examination with multiple components for evaluating sleep disturbance, including electrocardiogram, electro-oculogram, electromyogram, electroencephalogram, pulse oximeter, end-tidal CO_2 monitor, snoring microphone, thoracic/abdominal piezo crystal, nasal thermistor, and videogram.

The following definitions are important in making the diagnosis of pediatric OSA.

1. Central apnea is the absence of chest wall motion with absence of airflow at the nose and mouth for at least 10 seconds.
2. Obstructive apnea is the presence of chest wall motion with absence of airflow at the nose and mouth for at least two respiratory cycles (a breath cycle defined as a cycle of inhalation and exhalation).
3. Hypopnea is a reduction in airflow of at least 50% or a 3 to 4% drop in oxygen saturation and/or arousal.
4. Mixed apnea is the combination of an obstructive component of any duration and a central component of at least 4 seconds' duration or twice the length of the respiratory cycle for that age group.

These components are used in calculating the indices for determining the severity of pediatric OSA. The respiratory disturbance index (RDI) is the sum of the obstructive apneas,

Table 70.2 Classification of pediatric obstructive sleep apnea based on the apnea index

Normal	AHI < 1.5
Mild OSA	1.5 < AHI < 5
Moderate OSA	5 < AHI < 15
Severe OSA	AHI > 15

Abbreviations: AHI, apnea–hypopnea index; OSA, obstructive sleep apnea.

hypopneas, central apneas, and mixed apneas per hour of sleep (see Box Respiratory Disturbance Index (RDI) Formula (p.558)). The apnea–hypopnea index (AHI) is the sum of all obstructive apneas and hypopneas per hour of sleep. The AHI is seen as a more sensitive indicator in pediatric OSA than in adult OSA (see Box Apnea–Hypopnea Index (AHI) Formula (p.558)). An AHI value below 1.5 (events per hour) is considered to be normal in pediatric patients (▶ Table 70.2). It is important to take into consideration the presence or absence of oxygen desaturation in conjunction with the AHI.

Indications for Polysomnography

- Differentiate between OSA and primary snoring
- Evaluate symptoms of excessive daytime sleepiness, growth delay, or failure to thrive
- Evaluate patients older than 6 years of age with enuresis refractory to treatment
- Evaluate patients with behavioral or attention disorders, especially when associated with intermittent hyperactivity
- Evaluate patients with unexplained cor pulmonale, pulmonary hypertension
- Confirm the diagnosis and assess the severity of OSA
- Assess the efficacy of adenotonsillectomy in a patient with documented severe OSA
- Determine the CPAP parameters to be used in treating OSA
- When performed with pH monitoring, provide information on the relationship of gastroesophageal reflux disease to respiratory events such as nocturnal asthma, nonproductive cough, and apnea or hypoxemia

Abbreviations: CPAP, continuous positive airway pressure; OSA, obstructive sleep apnea.

Source: Adapted with permission from Alkhalil M, Lockey R. Pediatric obstructive sleep apnea syndrome (OSAS) for the allergist: update on the assessment and management. Ann Allergy Asthma Immunol 2011;107(2):104–109.

An intermittent decrease in oxygenation below 90% or a sustained desaturation below 92% is considered hypoxemia. End-tidal CO_2 above 45 mm Hg for more than 60% of the total sleep time or end-tidal CO_2 above 53 mm Hg is considered hypercarbia. Airway events that result in hypercarbia cause blood gas chemistry changes that alert the body's homeostatic protective mechanisms to sustain adequate ventilation and oxygenation in distant tissues. This protective mechanism is known as an arousal. Arousals occur as a consequence of hypoxemia, hypercarbia, and upper airway resistance and are scored as

respiratory events resulting in arousal (RERAs). Arousals cause significant fragmentation in sleep and should be taken into consideration when the neurocognitive behavior of a child is being evaluated.

70.8 Treatment

Treatment protocols can be medical, nonsurgical, or surgical, depending on the symptoms, their severity, and parental preference. The site of obstruction is a key factor in determining which type of treatment may be used successfully in the management of pediatric OSA.

70.8.1 Medical Treatment Options

If the sleep apnea is mild and the nasal obstruction is caused by turbinate hypertrophy or enlarged adenoids, a trial of intranasal corticosteroids is a viable nonsurgical option. The use of a leukotriene inhibitor or intranasal corticosteroid has been shown to lessen the severity of pediatric OSA by relieving the nasal obstructive component. The effects are known to last for as long as 6 months after the termination of therapy.

Leukotrienes and their receptors are increased in adenotonsillar tissue, suggesting that topical intranasal corticosteroids may have additional beneficial effects in mild to moderate OSA.

In children with allergic rhinitis, montelukast in combination with an intranasal corticosteroid can result in adequate reduction of inflammation. This therapy has also been useful in the treatment of residual sleep-disordered breathing after adenotonsillectomy.

Some studies have shown that after the withdrawal of these medications, long-term effects continue. It is important to remember that a child's immunologic and anatomical status continually matures. Medical management can be used as a temporary treatment to help alleviate sleep apnea during the interim period of growth and development.

70.8.2 Nonsurgical Therapeutic Options

As the anatomical features of a child continue to grow, natural resolution is likely in many cases, given enough time. In mild to moderate OSA, short-term therapy may be all that is needed. In this situation, nonsurgical measures may be the best therapy.

A commonly used form of nonsurgical management is continuous positive airway pressure (CPAP). CPAP splints the airway open. Patient compliance, however, is usually very poor because of the inability to tolerate discomfort. The direct use of supplemental oxygen is not recommended for the treatment of pediatric OSA because it compromises the central respiratory oxygen drive mechanism and leads to further hypercarbia.

The association of OSA with morbid obesity is still unclear. Besides the direct adverse effect of obesity on the cardiovascular system, there is a direct effect of excess lipid deposits in the pharyngeal oral and neck tissues. Studies have not shown that morbid obesity has a direct correlation with the severity of pediatric OSA; however, weight loss is still a frequently recommended method to reduce the severity of pediatric OSA.

Other conservative measures that may resolve intermittent snoring due to inflammatory conditions include the avoidance of environmental allergens and irritants, such as tobacco smoke. Households with exposure to tobacco smoke have been shown to be strongly associated with snoring in children. Measures to reduce common allergens, such as dust and animal dander, are recommended. Avoidance of any food allergens is also helpful to increase nasal patency.

70.8.3 Surgical Options for Pediatric Obstructive Sleep Apnea

Adenoid, tonsil, and lymphoid hypertrophy is the primary source of upper airway obstruction in most children with OSA. Whether a child has complex medical problems or is otherwise normal, adenotonsillectomy is the initial treatment for alleviating pediatric OSA in the vast majority of patients.

Approximately 80% of children will require only an adenotonsillectomy to relieve their OSA. The remaining 20% will show improvement but may still need additional treatment.

Other recommendations may include the medical management of allergic rhinitis and allergen avoidance. The child with obstruction at other levels may need adjunctive surgeries. Relief of anatomical nasal obstruction may require septoplasty or inferior turbinate reduction. Uvulopharyngopalatoplasty, tongue base suspension, lingual tonsillectomy, or orthognathic surgery may be necessary in selected cases. The atypical child with complex medical problems, hypotonia, or uncorrectable obstruction may require tracheostomy for airway management.

Perioperative management must be individualized to each child's needs. The vast majority of children with mild OSA may successfully undergo adenotonsillectomy as an ambulatory surgery procedure. Children who have craniofacial anomalies, are younger than 3 years of age, have neuromuscular disorders, or have severe OSA should be admitted for postoperative monitoring for airway events and oral intake following surgery.

Contrary to the theoretical belief that edema may develop in the upper airway after surgery, objective polysomnographic measures have shown that surgical treatment for OSA in otherwise normal children significantly reduces obstruction as early as the first postoperative day. Although the airway is nearly always immediately improved, there may be residual abnormalities in the respiratory drive centers in children with severe OSA; these may take 24 to 48 hours to adjust to normal levels of carbon dioxide in the bloodstream. However, it is recommended to wait a minimum of 6 weeks before considering reevaluation with postoperative polysomnography.

70.9 Summary

Pediatric OSA is one of the most commonly diagnosed ailments and has multisystem effects on the development of a child. Previously grouped with adult OSA, pediatric OSA is now considered a separate entity, and its effects on behavior, cognition, and learning in children are well recognized. Accurate diagnosis and early intervention in cases of pediatric OSA are important in preventing long-term sequelae in growing children. Pediatric OSA comprises a broad spectrum ranging from snoring to sleep-disordered breathing to frank OSA. Although other areas may be involved, OSA is most commonly associated with adenotonsillar hypertrophy in children, and adenotonsillectomy is usually the recommended therapeutic intervention.

70.10 Roundsmanship

- Snoring and disturbed sleep patterns can be the harbinger of other long-term consequences, such as behavior problems, neurologic sequelae, and cardiovascular and pulmonary effects.
- Early diagnosis and treatment are necessary to promote the healthy development of a child.
- Adenotonsillectomy is generally the initial treatment and will cure or alleviate pediatric OSA in most healthy children.
- Postoperative monitoring should be performed on an individual basis for children who may have other risk factors.

70.11 Recommended Reading

[1] Alkhalil M, Lockey R. Pediatric obstructive sleep apnea syndrome (OSAS) for the allergist: update on the assessment and management. Ann Allergy Asthma Immunol 2011; 107: 104–109
[2] Au CT, Li AM. Obstructive sleep breathing disorders. Pediatr Clin North Am 2009; 56: 243–259, xii
[3] Carroll JL, Loughlin GM. Diagnostic criteria for obstructive sleep apnea syndrome in children. Pediatr Pulmonol 1992; 14: 71–74
[4] Church GD. The role of polysomnography in diagnosing and treating obstructive sleep apnea in pediatric patients. Curr Probl Pediatr Adolesc Health Care 2012; 42: 2–25
[5] Corbo GM, Forastiere F, Agabiti N et al. Snoring in 9- to 15-year-old children: risk factors and clinical relevance. Pediatrics 2001; 108: 1149–1154
[6] Helfaer MA, McColley SA, Pyzik PL et al. Polysomnography after adenotonsillectomy in mild pediatric obstructive sleep apnea. Crit Care Med 1996; 24: 1323–1327
[7] Katz ES, D'Ambrosio CM. Pediatric obstructive sleep apnea syndrome. Clin Chest Med 2010; 31: 221–234
[8] Kirk V, Kahn A, Brouillette RT. Diagnostic approach to obstructive sleep apnea in children. Sleep Med Rev 1998; 2: 255–269
[9] Loughlin GM, Brouillette RT, Brook LJ. American Thoracic Society Standards and indications for cardiopulmonary sleep studies in children. Am J Respir Crit Cure Med 1996; 156: 866–878
[10] Marcus CL, Keens TG, Ward SL. Comparison of nap and overnight polysomnography in children. Pediatr Pulmonol 1992; 13: 16–21
[11] Marcus CL, McColley SA, Carroll JL, Loughlin GM, Smith PL, Schwartz AR. Upper airway collapsibility in children with obstructive sleep apnea syndrome. J Appl Physiol 1994; 77: 918–924
[12] Montgomery-Downs HE, O'Brien LM, Holbrook CR, Gozal D. Snoring and sleep-disordered breathing in young children: subjective and objective correlates. Sleep 2004; 27: 87–94
[13] Shine NP, Coates HL, Lannigan FJ. Obstructive sleep apnea, morbid obesity, and adenotonsillar surgery: a review of the literature. Int J Pediatr Otorhinolaryngol 2005; 69: 1475–1482

71 Cleft Lip and Palate

Robin A. Dyleski and Kenneth M. Rosenstein

71.1 Introduction

Cleft lip and cleft palate are the most common birth defects seen in the head and neck in children. A cleft lip occurs when incomplete fusion of the maxillary and median nasal processes results in an opening of the upper lip. A cleft palate is an opening in the palate caused by failure of fusion of the lateral palatal shelves (▶ Fig. 71.1). Cleft lip and cleft palate occur together or individually, with or without other physical defects in the face or organs. Cleft lip and palate are immediately observed at birth, and in addition to the obvious deformity affecting the lip and palate, they may cause difficulties with respiration and feeding immediately following birth. In the emotional moments following a birth, the discovery of a cleft lip can be difficult for the parents. This chapter discusses the anatomical abnormality, genetics, and treatment of cleft lip and palate. Issues related to speech are also discussed, as well as management options. This chapter is not intended to supplant more comprehensive texts on this topic, but to provide an overview of the general care and management of children with cleft lip and palate.

71.2 Epidemiology and Genetics

Second in frequency only to clubfoot (talipes equinovarus), cleft lip and/or palate is the most commonly observed congenital malformation of the head and neck. In general, cleft lip with or without cleft palate is considered to be a distinct and separate condition from cleft palate without a cleft lip. The combined risk for cleft lip with or without cleft palate and cleft palate in the United States is about 1 in 600 live births. The risk for cleft lip with or without cleft palate is about 1 in 940 live births, whereas the risk for cleft palate without cleft lip is 1 in 1,500 live births, based upon the latest data (2006) from the National Institutes of Health Center for Dental and Craniofacial Research (▶ Table 71.1). Additionally, gender affects the prevalence of cleft lip with or without cleft palate, with boys twice as likely to be affected as girls. In the case of isolated cleft palate without cleft lip, girls are affected twice as frequently as boys. In the United States, ethnicity affects the rates of clefts; Native Americans have the highest rate of clefting, at 3.6 per 1,000 births, followed by persons of Asian descent, Caucasians, and African-Americans (▶ Table 71.2).

Both cleft lip with or without cleft palate and cleft palate may present as part of a syndrome or without any other identifiable malformations (nonsyndromic). Genetic counseling is highly recommended because of the high risk that the obvious cleft lip and palate are part of a recognized syndrome.

Specific genetic syndromes are inherited via single-gene transmission (autosomal-dominant, autosomal-recessive, X-linked) and via various chromosomal deletions, translocations, and additions, including trisomy. Many factors (both genetic and nongenetic) influence the development of cleft lip or palate. Well-known maternal risk factors include diabetes and gestational diabetes, folate deficiency, drug exposures (e.g., ethanol, phenytoin, thalidomide), and environmental exposures (e.g., to-

bacco smoke). The gene for transforming growth factor-α (TGF-αhas specifically been found to influence nonsyndromic cleft formation and is the focus of much research in cleft causation.

Syndromes that frequently include cleft lip with or without cleft palate are listed in ▶ Table 71.3. Increasingly, syndromes have become more often located to abnormalities at specific genetic loci. Knowledge of the presence of a syndrome benefits the child by allowing early access to programs that can assist parents in dealing with associated developmental problems the child may manifest.

71.3 Embryology

Cleft lip with or without cleft palate and isolated cleft palate are considered separate conditions not only because they seem to differ in epidemiologic expression but also because they occur at different times during embryologic development. Embryologic development of the lips and palate occurs very early in the fetus, in the first trimester. There are two related phases. The first begins in the fourth to fifth week of embryogenesis and involves formation of the lips, nose, and primary palate (the premaxilla, which is the bony palate consisting of the alveolus with the central four incisors anterior to the incisive foramen). The second phase, which begins around the eighth to ninth week, is closure of the secondary palate (the two lateral palatal shelves containing all the remaining teeth and the soft palate).

71.3.1 Embryology of the Cleft Lip

Around the fourth to fifth week, the ectoderm and mesoderm of the frontonasal and two lateral labial maxillary processes proliferate. The frontonasal process is destined to become three structures: (1) the philtrum (anterior labial segment), (2) the central alveolus containing the four upper incisors (anterior palatal segment), and (3) the hard palate anterior to the incisive foramen (posterior palatal segment). This process occurs and is completed by the end of the sixth week of development when the two lateral labial maxillary processes fuse with the central frontonasal process (▶ Fig. 71.2).

The frontonasal process forms with differentiation of the olfactory placode epithelium. Differential growth of the placode forms the curl of the nasal ala at the same time that the frontonasal process develops. Fusion begins at the nasal sill, forming the ovoid nostril shape, and continues down the upper lip to the free edge of the vermilion on the lip, while simultaneously the lateral palatal shelves fuse with the central premaxilla, closing the alveolus bilaterally. The current theory of labial and palatal formation involves epithelial contact of the edges of the processes with differential resorption of the surface epithelial cells, modulation and fusion of the mesodermal layer, and further differentiation of the germ layers into the bone, muscle, mucosa, and skin. The direction of the fusion of the three processes explains the great degree of variation in the severity of cleft lip and primary (alveolus) palate defects. Cleft lip can be unilateral or bilateral, complete (open all the way to the nose)

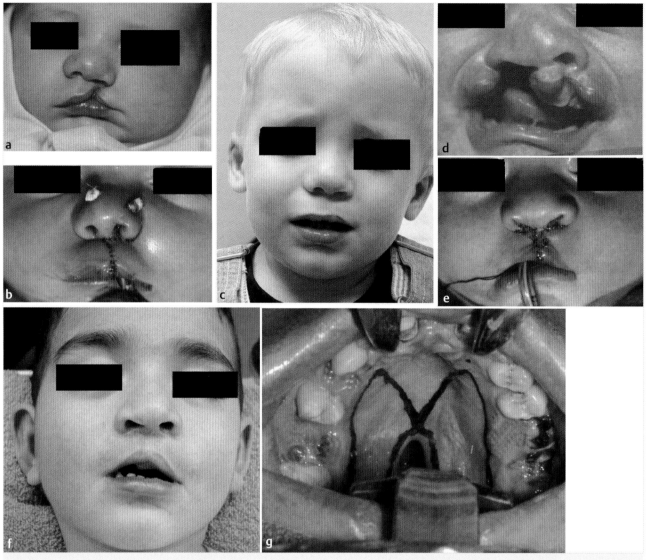

Fig. 71.1 (a) Child with unilateral cleft lip before repair. (b) Same child immediately after repair of cleft lip. (c) Same child, age 2 years. (d) Child with bilateral cleft lip before repair. (e) Same child immediately after repair of bilateral cleft lip. (f) Same child, age 3 years. (g) Unrepaired cleft palate.

Table 71.1 Average prevalence of cleft lip and palate and number of births affected by these defects each year in the United States, 2004 to 2006

	Prevalence[a]	Annual number of cases
Cleft palate only	6.35	2,651
Cleft lip with or without cleft palate	10.63	4,437

Source: Data from the U.S. Centers for Disease Control and Prevention (CDC) National Birth Defects Prevention Network (NBDPN). Cleft lip and palate data for 2004 to 2006 collected from 13 states (Arkansas, Arizona, California [eight-county Central Valley], Colorado, Georgia [five-county metropolitan Atlanta], Illinois, Iowa, Kentucky, Massachusetts, North Carolina, Oklahoma, Texas, and Utah) and Puerto Rico, representing 4,038,506 live births and adjusted for race-specific distribution.
[a]Prevalence per 10,000 live births.

Table 71.2 Rates of cleft lip with or without cleft palate within different ethnic groups in the United States

Ethnic group	Rate of cleft lip ± cleft palate (per 1,000 births)
Native Americans	3.6
Asians	2.1
Caucasians	1
African-Americans	0.5

or incomplete (extending partially from the free vermilion edge up to the nose). Also, the alveolus may be uninvolved (normal) or completely or incompletely cleft (▶ Fig. 71.3).

The second, or palatal, phase is complete by the 10th week. The lateral palatal shelves grow and protrude medially. Because the primary palate has fused (along with the lip) by the end of the sixth week, the secondary palate (the palate posterior and immediately lateral to the incisive foramen) is in position

Table 71.3 Common syndromes associated with cleft lip and palate

Syndrome	Cleft type	Inheritance Mode
Velocardiofacial	Cleft palate	Autosomal-dominant
Stickler	Cleft palate	Autosomal-dominant
Van der Woude	Cleft lip ± cleft palate	Autosomal-dominant
Orofacial digital I	Cleft lip ± cleft palate	X-linked
Orofacial digital II	Cleft lip ± cleft palate	Autosomal-recessive
Waardenburg	Cleft lip ± cleft palate	Autosomal-dominant
Ectodermal dysplasia	Cleft lip ± cleft palate	Autosomal-recessive

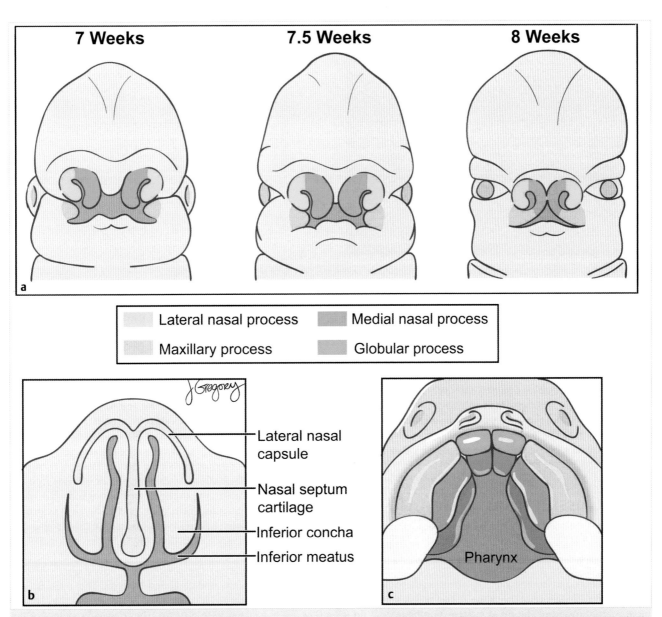

Fig. 71.2 (a) Embryology of the upper lip: three processes (7 weeks), partial fusion (7.5 weeks), and complete fusion (8 weeks). (b,c) Views of palatal fusion at 8 to 10 weeks.

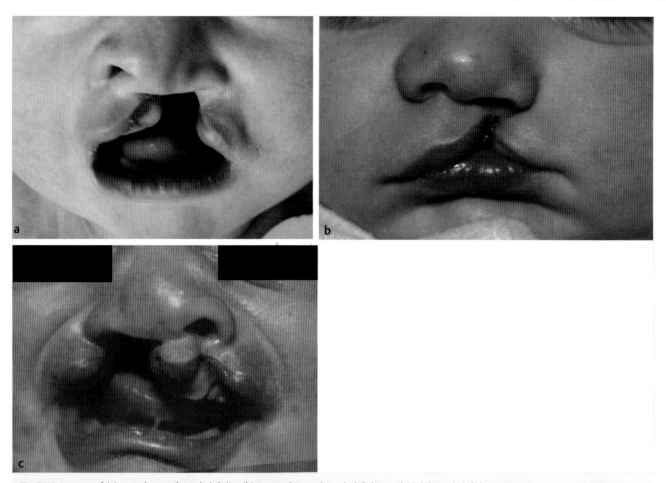

Fig. 71.3 Images of (a) complete unilateral cleft lip, (b) incomplete unilateral cleft lip, and (c) bilateral cleft lip.

to begin the process of making epithelial contact and undergoing epithelial resorption and mesodermal merging, with fusion at the midline. At the onset of this process, the forming tongue is located in the space between the lateral palatal shelves, causing a sloping cant to the lateral shelves. As the palate fuses from the incisive foramen anteriorly to the uvula posteriorly, the tongue position drops away. The process and direction of fusion explain the variety of cleft palates seen in our patients, with many degrees of incomplete closure ranging from cleft uvula to a complete cleft of the secondary palate (cleft extending to the incisive foramen; ▶ Fig. 71.4).

71.4 Classification of Cleft Lip and Palate

Understanding the embryology of cleft lip and palate has made it possible to devise a classification of cleft lip and palate for documentation and comparison. As mentioned earlier, clefts can be complete (failure of the entire fusion process) or incomplete (partial fusion of the lip or palate). Complete cleft lip is more commonly associated with complete cleft palate because the failure of closure of the lip and alveolus sets the secondary palate edges far enough apart to reduce the likelihood of contact and initiation of the fusion process.

In general, the most commonly used classification of clefts follows the scheme devised at the University of Iowa Department of Otolaryngology-Head and Neck Surgery (▶ Fig. 71.5). This classification divides clefts into four groups: group I, lip; group II, palate only; group III, alveolus and palate; and group IV, alveolus only. Group I (clefts of the lip) is subdivided into unilateral (right or left) and bilateral and further into complete and incomplete. Complete cleft lip (either unilateral or bilateral) extends completely into the nasal sill. An incomplete cleft lip extends a variable distance from the vermilion free edge.

In group II (palate-only clefts), the cleft is classified according to whether the cleft affects only the uvula or extends into the soft palate, and according to the degree of distance and shape of the hard palate component of the cleft. The cleft deformity seen in Pierre Robin sequence (an association of retrognathia/micrognathia, airway obstruction, and U-shaped cleft palate) is an example of group II-4, the U-shaped complete cleft palate.

Group III comprises the commonly seen variations of cleft lip with cleft palate, unilateral and bilateral. The alveolar (primary palate) clefts included in group IV are clefts of the alveolus that are associated with cleft lip. These alveolar clefts are not associated with a cleft of the secondary palate. The classification does not include the classic submucous cleft palate (diastasis of the soft palatal musculature, bifid uvula, and posterior V-shaped notching of the posterior midline hard palate), which is

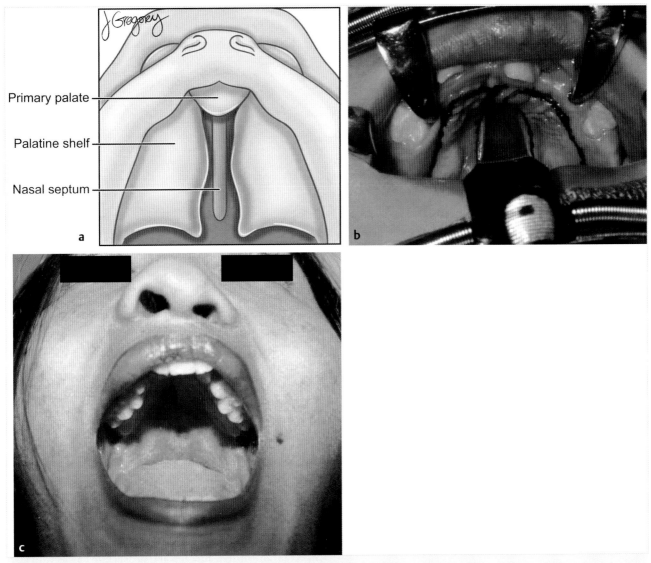

Fig. 71.4 (a) Palatal closure at 6.5 weeks. (b) Unrepaired complete cleft palate. (c) Submucous cleft palate.

a microform cleft palate. Submucous cleft palate is considered an incomplete cleft of the secondary palate.

71.5 Initial Evaluation and Care of the Infant with Cleft Lip or Cleft Lip and Palate

Babies born with cleft lip with or without cleft palate or cleft palate can have considerable difficulties in the newborn period. The first challenge these children face is respiration. The alteration in oral anatomy and the relationship of the tongue base to the pharynx and palate may result in airway obstruction requiring intervention. Most babies with cleft palate soon adapt to breathing with their cleft palate; however, various maneuvers can assist the child in accommodating, such as lateral positioning, placement of nasogastric tube (which moves the tongue

away from the posterior pharynx), and continuous positive airway pressure devices.

Feeding the baby with a cleft lip and palate can be difficult. After airway stability is established, maintaining oral feeding is essential. Children with cleft lip alone or with alveolar clefting only are usually able to use a standard nipple or be breastfed, but they may have some difficulty creating a seal around the nipple because of the lip defect. Babies with cleft palate have more special feeding needs. Because a cleft palate (except for incomplete alveolar clefts) prevents the infant from establishing oral suction, a child with a cleft palate usually needs a nipple that does not require sucking. Special nipples are available to facilitate feeding babies with cleft palate, such as the Pigeon and Haberman cleft palate nipples. These nipples contain one-way valves that allow milk to flow in only one direction: from the bottle into the nipple. The baby applies pressure from the alveolus to express the milk from the nipple. Most babies with cleft palate are able to feed and grow with these nipple systems.

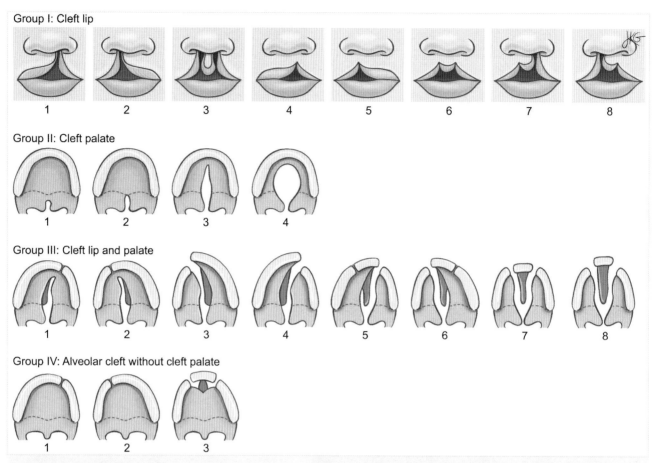

Fig. 71.5 Cleft classification used by the University of Iowa Department of Otolaryngology-Head and Neck Surgery.

71.6 Surgical Management of Cleft Lip and Palate

Cleft lip and palate repair is usually performed in the first year of life. In a child who is growing and gaining weight well, cleft lip and palate repair can proceed according to a general schedule used by most cleft surgeons.

71.6.1 Cleft Lip

Cleft lip repair helps the baby feed by improving its ability to seal its lips around the nipple. Most healthy children have gained sufficient weight by 8 to 12 weeks of age to undergo a safe cleft lip repair. In general, the "rule of tens" can be followed: cleft lip repair when the infant is about 10 weeks of age, weighs 10 lbs., and has a hemoglobin level of 10 g/dL. There are advantages to performing the cleft lip repair in the first few months of life in a child who is growing and thriving. The repaired cleft lip has a positive orthopedic effect on the width of the alveolar cleft in the patient with a complete cleft lip and palate, resulting in a significant narrowing of the alveolar and palatal cleft.

71.6.2 Cleft Palate

In the United States, repair of cleft palate is performed around 10 to 14 months of age in healthy children. Another "rule of tens" is generally used: age of 10 months, weight of 10 kg, and hemoglobin level of 10 g/dL. Other factors are considered in the timing of cleft palate repair, such as the width of the cleft palate (distance between the palatal shelves), degree of airway obstruction anticipated after repair (particular in babies with Robin sequence), and other medical comorbidities. The most commonly observed postoperative concern is airway obstruction resulting from the change in the baby's reconstructed oropharyngeal airway. This must be anticipated and monitored postoperatively. It is sometimes necessary to delay a palate repair for several months to allow the baby to grow and so avoid airway obstruction after repair.

71.6.3 Surgical Technique of Cleft Lip Repair

Many techniques for cleft lip repair have been developed, but the most commonly used repair follows the general design described by Dr. Ralph Millard in the 1950s: the rotation–advancement repair. This technique has been adapted over the years, but the general tenets remain constant: restoration of the natural Cupid's bow, camouflage of the scars in the philtral ridges, reconstruction of the orbicularis oris musculature, and correction of the nasal deformity seen in cleft lip. Bilateral cleft lip repair follows similar principles, but the surgeon must proceed without a "normal" side as a guide.

Unilateral Cleft Lip Repair

Although there are many techniques available for unilateral cleft lip repair, the Millard rotation–advancement technique will be described here. This technique is versatile and can be used in any unilateral cleft lip regardless of whether it is a microform cleft lip or a wide complete cleft. It is based upon the identification of key surgical landmarks (▶ Fig. 71.6a). The noncleft side is the rotation flap, and the cleft side–lateral lip is the advancement flap. An advantage of the rotation–advancement repair is the ability to modify the technique during the procedure as needed to fit the patient.

The landmarks 1 through 9 are marked with gentian violet or methylene blue as follows:
1. Nasal alar base on the noncleft side
2. Peak of Cupid's bow on the noncleft side
3. Midline of Cupid's bow (low point of the bow)
4. Peak of Cupid's bow on the cleft side (medial)
5. Peak of Cupid's bow on the cleft side (lateral, at the attenuation of the white roll and vermilion–cutaneous junction)
6. Point at the superior aspect of the advancement flap (lateral lip), which sets the "height" of the lip at the philtral ridge
7. Nasal alar base on the cleft side
8. Superior extent of the rotation incision, which should be about at the midline in the crease of the upper lip–nasal columella
9. Back cut incision length (if needed). This extra incision is used to lengthen the rotation incision and increase the degree of rotation of the rotation flap.

After these landmarks have been marked, the distances are measured for symmetry and then the proposed incisions are infiltrated with local anesthetic containing epinephrine. The rotation flap incisions are first incised and the rotation flap is checked for symmetry and a horizontal level at the Cupid's bow peaks. If the two Cupid's bow peaks are not in a horizontal plane, then the back cut (incision 8–9) is incised to make it horizontal (▶ Fig. 71.6b.)

The lateral lip segment (advancement flap) is incised along the cleft edge and a short distance from point 6 toward point 7. At this point, the nasal lower lateral alar cartilage is dissected free from its overlying skin (▶ Fig. 71.6c), if this is desired. The columella is reconstructed with rearrangement and closure of the back cut. The key tension-bearing stitch, which is the stitch that sets the uppermost aspect of the lip muscle, is placed (▶ Fig. 71.6d). If alar cartilage has been freed from the overlying nostril skin, it is positioned and held in place with nylon suture tied externally over bolsters (▶ Fig. 71.6e). The cleft incision is then closed in layers with absorbable suture in the orbicularis oris muscle, inner lip mucosa (not seen in figure), and then finally the lip skin and vermilion. Nonabsorbable sutures may be used, but some surgeons find that Dermabond (Ethicon, Somerville, NJ) leaves a more pleasing scar and requires less wound care on the part of the child's caregivers.

Bilateral Cleft Lip Repair

Bilateral cleft lip repair is more technically challenging than unilateral cleft lip repair. In bilateral cleft lip repair, it is necessary for the surgeon to create symmetry, particularly if the lip is not symmetric (one side is complete and the other side is incomplete). The general technique using specific anatomical landmarks is similar to that for the unilateral cleft. Millard introduced a technique in the 1950s that has remained popular to this time, with various modifications as needed to suit the patient's unique anatomical situation.

A recent innovation by Cutting and Grayson, nasoalveolar molding, has gained popularity because it permits treating the short columella along with narrowing the cleft width. Nasoalveolar molding requires the use of a prosthesis (▶ Fig. 71.7) that is constructed based on an impression of the patient's nasoalveolar cleft. Orthodontic taping and weekly adjustments to the prosthesis progressively elongate the columella. Surgical correction of the cleft lip is then performed at around 6 months of age. The innovation of nasoalveolar molding has improved the appearance of patients with bilateral cleft lip nasal deformities in a nonsurgical manner.

The repair begins with a determination of the surgical landmarks of the lip. The central lip element, the prolabium, is destined to be the future philtrum and is banked for future columella lengthening (if nasoalveolar molding is not performed). The height of the prolabium dictates the height of the repaired cleft lip. Children with a very small prolabium are problematic because there is no optimal way to lengthen a very short upper lip without creating a scar in an unnatural and unfavorable location.

The surgical landmarks are placed with gentian violet or methylene blue as follows (▶ Fig. 71.8):
1. Midpoint of the prolabium, the midpoint of the future Cupid's bow
2. and 3. Prolabium peaks of the future Cupid's bow, measured 2 to 3 mm lateral to point 1
4. and 5. Junction of the columella and the prolabium, future superior aspect of the philtrum ridges
6. and 7. The measured height of 2–4 marked at the white roll attenuation on the cleft edge
8. and 9. Similar to 6 and 7 on the opposite cleft edge
* Point at vermilion, measured distance of 1–2 plus 1 to 2 mm. This creates the hemivermilion flap under the Cupid's bow.

In bilateral cleft repair, the measurements are much more critical than in unilateral repair because symmetry is created in the design of the lip repair. After the landmarks and incisions have been marked (▶ Fig. 71.8a), local anesthetic containing epinephrine is injected. Prolabium incisions are made first, but the incisions at 1–2 and 1–3 are partial-thickness incisions because the mucosal "e" flap is pedicled upon the inferior aspect of the future philtrum at 1–2 and 1–3 (▶ Fig. 71.8b). Lateral flaps from the prolabium are raised if one wishes to "bank" them under the nostril for future columella lengthening or to use them in closing the nasal sill. Residual mucosa from the prolabium is used to line the anterior premaxilla (▶ Fig. 71.8c). Lateral incisions are made, with care taken to make sure that the "*" vermilion flaps are full-thickness flaps and contain sufficient mucosa to create the future labial tubercle at the middle of the lip under the philtrum. The lateral lip flap mucosa is closed with 5-0 chromic suture (▶ Fig. 71.8d). The orbicularis oris muscle in the lateral lip segments is approximated at the midline (▶ Fig. 71.8e). Then, the midline "*"flaps are sutured to each other to establish vermilion continuity with both deep

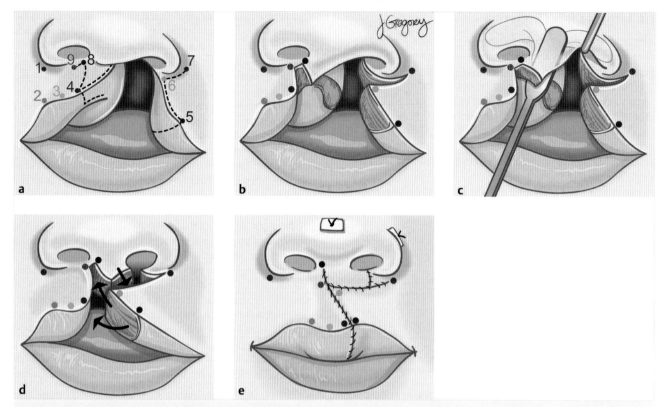

Fig. 71.6 Millard cleft lip repair. (a) Surgical marks for cleft lip repair. (b) Development of the advancement and rotation flaps. (c) Release of skin over the lower lateral cartilage on the cleft side. (d) Reconstruction of the columella and placement of tension-bearing sutures in the orbicularis oris muscle. (e) Final closure of the advancement and rotation flaps, with nasal bolsters in place.

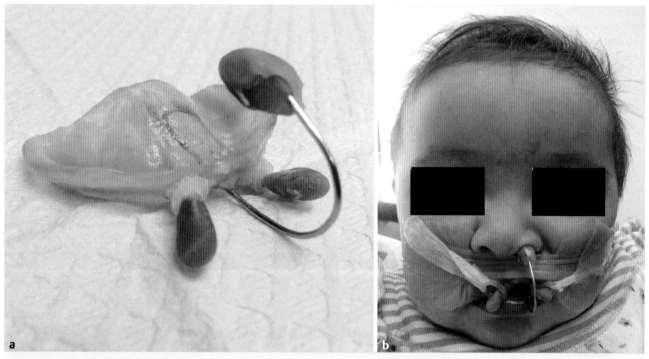

Fig. 71.7 (a) Nasoalveolar molding appliance. (b) Appearance of nasoalveolar molding in a patient with cleft.

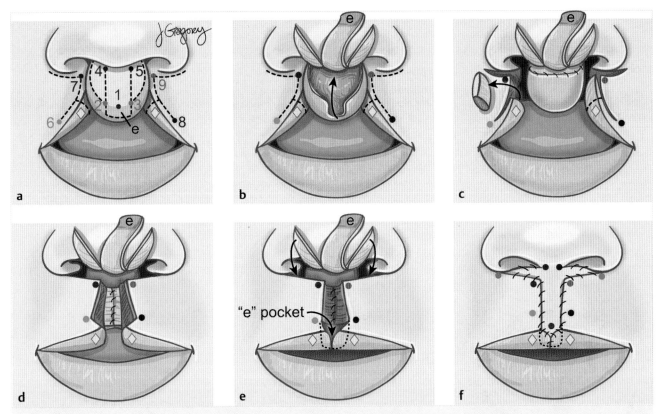

Fig. 71.8 Bilateral cleft lip repair technique. **(a)** Surgical markings. **(b)** Development of the "e" flap and lateral flaps pedicled on the superior prolabium. **(c)** Residual prolabial mucosa is used to line the anterior premaxilla, and full-thickness vermilion flaps are incised. **(d)** The mucosa of the lateral lip segments is closed with chromic sutures. **(e)** The fibers of the orbicularis oris muscle are aligned and approximated; the "*" vermilion flaps are sutured together. **(f)** The philtral flap is then sutured between the lateral lip segments, and the "e" flap is sutured behind the medial vermilion flaps; the lateral prolabial flaps are inset into the nasal sills and closed.

and mucosal sutures (▶ Fig. 71.8f). The philtrum with the attached "e" flap is then inserted between the lateral lip segments at the midline, with care taken to "tuck" the "e" flap into the space behind the "*" vermilion flaps, as depicted in panel 8G. The purpose of the "e" flap is to keep the philtrum from retracting superiorly, thus broadening the scar at the vermilion-cutaneous junction, and to provide bolstering and bulk to the vermilion tubercle. The two lateral prolabium flaps are sutured into position beneath the nasal sill (if needed or if future use is planned). The skin is closed with fine nonabsorbable suture, or Dermabond may be used when the edges are closely approximated (panel 8H).

71.6.4 Cleft Palate Repair

Historically, many techniques have been reported for cleft palate repair. The most commonly used palatoplasty procedures today are variations of the Wardill-Kilner-Peet repair (V to Y advancement), the Bardach two-flap repair, and the Furlow repair (double reverse Z-plasty). For many surgeons, the selection of the palatoplasty technique is related to the type of cleft present (complete vs incomplete) and the width of the cleft gap. All three procedures are good methods of repair. Palatoplasty includes treatment of the soft palate musculature with intravelar veloplasty (repair of the muscles within the soft palate with reorientation of the fibers), except when the Furlow technique is

performed on the soft palate. The Furlow palatoplasty technique can be used on the soft palate, with the Wardill-Kilner-Peet or the two-flap technique used for repair of the hard palate.

Bardach Two-Flap Palatoplasty

This procedure is often used for patients who have complete cleft palate. The procedure relies upon bilateral mucoperiosteal pedicled flaps based upon the descending palatine artery. It is performed by first infiltrating the palate with local anesthetic containing epinephrine. The cleft edges are incised, and lateral relaxation incisions are made along the alveolar ridge (▶ Fig. 71.9a). Subperiosteal flaps are elevated with preservation of the descending palatine artery, located as it exits its foramen at the lateral posterior hard palate border (▶ Fig. 71.9b). The vascular pedicles are carefully dissected to extend the range of rotation of the flaps. The soft palate muscles are then released from the posterior border of the hard palate. A vomer flap is elevated (▶ Fig. 71.9c) so that the nasal mucoperiosteal layer can be closed to seal the nose, with closure beginning anteriorly and proceeding posteriorly toward the uvula (▶ Fig. 71.9d). The soft palate muscle fibers are reoriented to lie horizontally in the soft palate and sutured together (the intravelar veloplasty). The soft palate mucosa and hard palate mucoperiosteal flaps are closed with absorbable suture (▶ Fig. 71.9e). The lateral relaxing incisions at the alveolus are

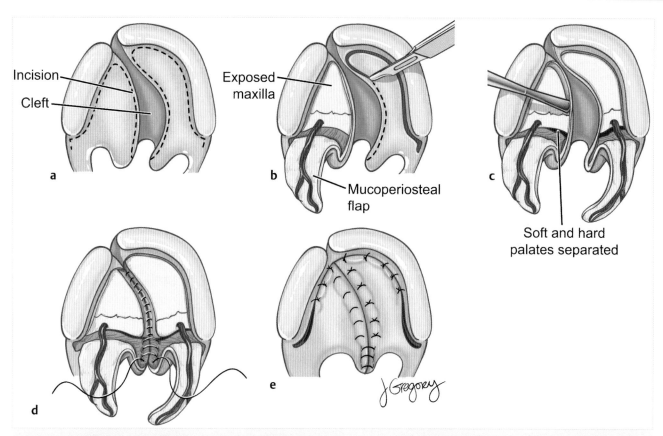

Fig. 71.9 Bardach two-flap palatoplasty. (**a**) Mucosal incisions. (**b**) Incisions are made along the cleft edge, allowing the development of nasal and palatal mucosal flaps. (**c**) The palatal flaps are raised and left pedicled posteriorly. (**d**) The soft tissues are released to allow full rotation about the vascular supply, the descending palatal artery; the vomer flap is elevated for use in nasal closure, and the nasal mucoperiosteum is closed. The soft palate muscles are reoriented and sutured together. (**e**) The palatal flaps are rotated and sutured.

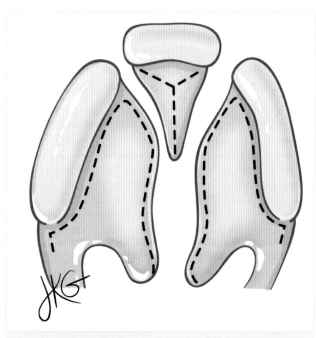

Fig. 71.10 Modification of the unilateral palate repair for bilateral cleft repair.

usually left open to close by secondary intention or are packed with microfibrillar collagen.

The benefits of this closure are that it is robust, with modifications easily made to close fairly wide cleft palate gaps (use more vomer flap), and that the Furlow palatoplasty (discussed later) may be used for closure of the soft palate. This procedure is also used with modification for bilateral cleft palate repair, with the midline vomer used to create flaps for closure of each side of the nasal floor (► Fig. 71.10).

Wardill-Kilner-Peet Palatoplasty (V to Y Advancement)

The V to Y advancement palatoplasty technique is often used to repair clefts of the secondary palate (those beginning at or posterior to the incisive foramen). It also can be combined with the Furlow palatoplasty (on the soft palate). The technique relies upon lateral palatal mucoperiosteal flaps, but they are "pushed back" toward the soft palate, providing some additional length to the palate (although this is somewhat limited). The flaps (► Fig. 71.11a) are designed such that the "point" of the flap is aimed toward the location of the canine teeth. The mucoperiosteal palate flaps and pedicles are raised (► Fig. 71.11b), as described for the Bardach two-flap repair. Similarly, nasal mucoperiosteal flaps are raised and closed to create the nasal floor. If the vomer is involved in the cleft, then the nasal floor should be closed on each side separately (► Fig. 71.11c). The procedure

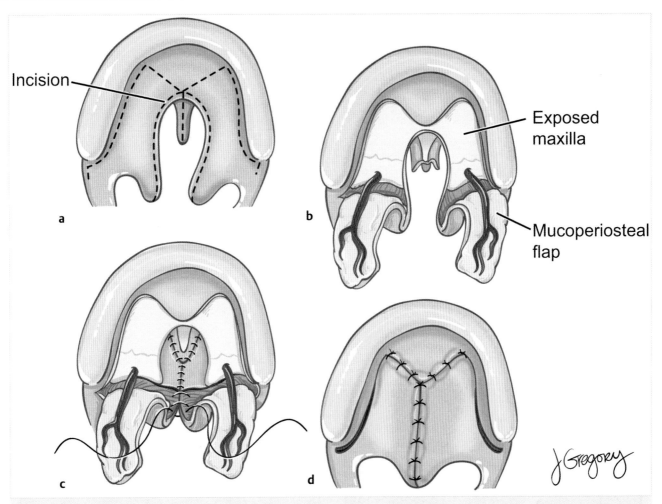

Fig. 71.11 Wardill-Kilner-Peet palatoplasty (V to Y advancement). (**a**) Incisions. (**b**) Nasal flaps and palatal flaps, based on the descending palatal artery, are raised. (**c**) The nasal flaps are repaired, and the soft palate muscles are reoriented and sutured together. (**d**) The mucosal flaps are rotated and closed, with lateral incisions allowed to heal by secondary intention.

continues with the intravelar veloplasty closure of the soft palate muscles. Finally, the mucoperiosteal flaps are closed at the midline and tacked to the anterior hard palate mucosa. The lateral relaxing incisions are filled with compressed microfibrillar collagen and allowed to close by secondary intention (▶ Fig. 71.11d).

Furlow Palatoplasty

The Furlow palatoplasty is radically different from the previously described techniques for repair of the cleft palate. In the previously described techniques, the soft palate is closed with a straight-line closure. In the Furlow technique, the soft palate is closed with Z-plasties on each side of the soft palate, one on the oral side and another on the opposite, nasopharyngeal side. The Furlow technique ("double opposing Z-plasty") can visibly lengthen the soft palate (because of the nature of the Z-plasty), with the entire soft palate moved closer to the posterior pharyngeal wall (making it easier to close the velopharyngeal space), and it also reorients the soft palate muscle fibers from a vertical to a horizontal direction. For these reasons, it has become a favored choice for cleft palate repair.

After the palate is injected with local anesthetic containing epinephrine, the cleft edges are incised. A Z-plasty is designed with the oral mucosa overlying the soft palate (▶ Fig. 71.12a,b). If the surgeon is right-handed, the soft palate muscles are elevated with the oral mucosal flap on the left hemipalate; the plane of dissection is between the soft palate muscles and the submucosa of the nasopharyngeal side of the soft palate (▶ Fig. 71.12c). Caution must be taken when this elevation is performed because the nasopharyngeal flap is very thin and easily perforated. The right oral hemipalatal flap is elevated between the submucosa and the soft palate muscle. The oral mucosal flap is much thicker than the corresponding submucosal flap on the nasopharyngeal side. The nasopharyngeal mucomuscular flap is then incised on the right hemipalate from the apex of the cleft toward the lateral pharyngeal wall (▶ Fig. 71.12d). The corresponding left nasopharyngeal mucosal flap is incised from the uvula anterolaterally toward the pharyngeal wall (see ▶ Fig. 71.12d). The nasopharyngeal flaps are interdigitated and sutured into position, followed by the oral flaps (▶ Fig. 71.12e,f).

When this technique is used for more extensive clefts involving the hard palate, one usually raises the hard palate flaps and inspects the vascular pedicles before committing to the Furlow

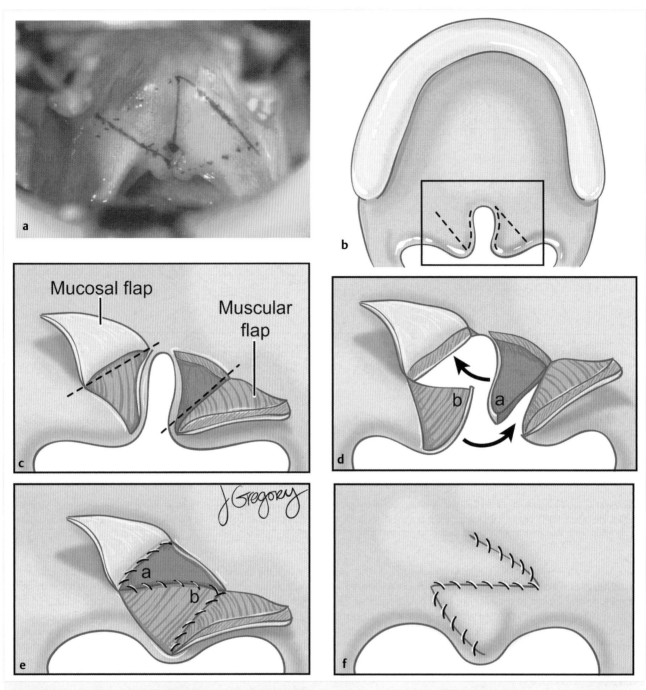

Fig. 71.12 Furlow palatoplasty technique. (**a**) Double opposing Z-plasties drawn on incomplete cleft palate. (**b**) The dotted lines represent incisions in the palatal mucosa. (**c**) The soft palate musculature is raised with the palatal mucosa on the left side, while the palatal flap on the right side is mucosa only; the nasal mucosa (with the musculature on the right side) is incised along the dotted line, and the soft palate musculature is left attached to the right nasopharyngeal mucosal flap, while the left side is mucosa only. (**d**) The nasopharyngeal mucosal flaps are transposed and (**e**) sutured together. (**f**) The nasal mucosal flaps are then transposed in the opposite direction and sutured together. The soft palate muscles are reoriented across the palate and moved posteriorly.

on the soft palate. Following successful dissection around the pedicle, the Furlow incisions and flaps are raised. The procedure is completed as described for each technique.

Complications in Palatoplasty

The most common immediate postoperative complication with all palatoplasty techniques is airway obstruction. This may be caused by postoperative tongue swelling (due to prolonged compression of the tongue with the mouth gag); thus, periodic inspection of the tongue with release of the gag is required. The most common reason for airway obstruction, however, is a direct effect of closure of the palate and the change in the oropharyngeal and palate shape after the repair. Most babies tolerate the changes following palatoplasty, but airway monitoring (with continuous pulse oximetry and a higher level of nursing

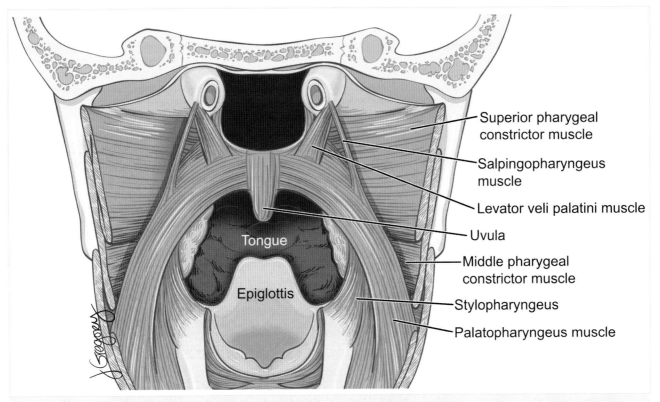

Fig. 71.13 Diagram of the oropharynx and soft palate musculature (posterior view), demonstrating the sphincteric structure of the velopharyngeal valve.

management) is mandatory after all but the most minor palato-plasty procedures. Intraoperative or postoperative hemorrhage is infrequent.

The most common complication after the immediate post-operative period is fistula. Dehiscence of the suture line may occur as a result of tension on the suture line, insufficient tissue, or thin mucoperiosteal tissue. The most likely site of fistula is at the junction of the hard and soft palate, where the mucoperiosteal tissue is thinnest. Fistulas should be allowed to heal for a minimum of 4 to 6 months before a repair attempt is made. Asymptomatic fistulas can be left until another surgical procedure is required.

71.7 Resonance and Speech Disorders

The velopharyngeal valve is a complex mechanism that plays an integral and unique role in human swallowing and speech function. Human evolution has combined the upper airway and digestive tract into a complex neuromuscular pathway with multiple functions. The primary role of the soft palate musculature is to allow positive pressure to build in the mouth for the propulsion of food during the initial phase of swallowing. Later, with the development of oral language, the same muscular valve was recruited to play an essential role in the articulation and resonance of human speech.

71.7.1 Anatomy and Function of the Velopharyngeal Valve

The velopharyngeal valve mechanism consists grossly of the soft palate and the lateral and posterior pharyngeal walls. In a simplified view, the mobile soft palate (velum) acts like a valve, rising and moving posteriorly to meet the pharyngeal walls; this effectively creates a seal and anatomically separates the nasopharynx from the oropharynx at the level of the soft palate (▶ Fig. 71.13).

Examination of the complex musculature and tissue properties of this region provides more detail. The most mobile portion of the valve mechanism is the muscle mass of the soft palate. Most of this mass and its mobility is provided by the levator veli palatini, a broad-based muscle that arises from the petrous areas of the temporal bone and cartilaginous portion of the eustachian tube and fans down to insert into its analogous partner at the soft palate midline, creating a sling. As these laterally oriented fibers contract, the mass of the soft palate is pulled both posteriorly and superiorly. This muscle's broad path is underscored by its complicated innervation; it receives fibers from the glossopharyngeal plexus, vagus nerve, and greater petrosal nerve of the facial nerve.

The tensor veli palatini is a smaller muscle arranged in a similar orientation that alone has limited mass to facilitate elevation of the velum. During swallowing, however, the tensor serves the unique purpose of opening the flexible cartilaginous portions of the eustachian tube, allowing the equilibration of middle ear pressure with atmospheric pressure via the nasopharynx. In conjunction with the musculus uvulae, the two lateral tensors help to stiffen the soft palate and create a more rigid surface against which food can be propelled during initiation of the pharyngeal swallow.

During swallowing, the oral tongue packages the food bolus to be swallowed and moves it posteriorly. The tongue rises against the hard palate and anterior velum to propel the bolus posteriorly. The passage of the bolus between the anterior tonsillar pillars initiates a reflex arc that terminates in stimulation of the pharyngeal plexus of the glossopharyngeal nerve. It is at this junction that the reflexive, nonvolitional swallow begins.

As the soft palate rises and separates the nasopharynx from the oral cavity, the base of the tongue is elevated by the palatoglossus, a slinglike muscle originating from the velum to the sides of the tongue. Tongue elevation also aids in stabilizing the soft palate and constricting the pharynx. The palatopharyngeus arises from the velum and inserts at the posterior border of the thyroid cartilage. As well as stabilizing the velum, the palatoglossus muscle is the first to reflexively elevate the larynx during swallowing to protect the upper airway.

Although the soft palate and its musculature provide most of the bulk and mobility of the velopharyngeal valve, the superior pharyngeal constrictor also has an integral role. During swallowing, the ringlike contraction of this muscle advances the posterior pharyngeal wall anteriorly and medializes the lateral pharyngeal walls. It is this muscle that is truly responsible for the sphincter-like nature of the velopharynx and makes it much more than a simple valve.

This sphincteric action increases oropharyngeal pressure and allows the targeted propulsion of food inferiorly. As a result, the sphincter prevents the nasopharyngeal regurgitation of food particles.

71.7.2 Role of the Aerodigestive Tract in Human Speech

The upper aerodigestive tract is designed for use in respiration and deglutition. As the human airway evolved, the larynx descended, and the pharynx and oral cavity became more suited to an incredible array of sound production. As the human larynx phonates, a buzzing fundamental frequency is created that has little resemblance to the tonality of speech. As the laryngeal sound passes through the oral cavity and nasopharynx, a full array of tones can be made with only slight modifications of the oral structures. These fully expired phonated tones comprise the vowels of all human language. For example, a high, anteriorly placed tongue and horizontal labial opening create a long "e" sound, while a rounded lip and posteriorly arched tongue create an extended "oo."

Spoken language, however, is not a series of vowels; it is characterized by a combination of resonant vowels and articulated phonemes. Phonemes are created in two ways, and the velum plays an important role in each. During the creation of most linguistic phonemes, the velum is closed, as in a swallow. This closure redirects all phonated expiration through the oral cavity. Through fine, targeted approximations of the tongue with the teeth, anterior hard palate, and soft palate, the consonants are articulated.

For example, to produce the word *teeth*, a person must close the velopharynx and expire through the mouth. The tongue is tapped against the hard palate directly behind the maxillary incisors to create a "t" sound. Instantaneously, phonation and an oral posture for "ee" create the vowel, and the tongue follows the vowel by inserting between the upper and lower incisors. Phonation ceases, yet expiration continues to create the "th" sound.

However, the production of a nasalized word like *man* requires initiation with phonation, an open velopharynx, and closed lips. Tightly closed lips allow the production of an "m" sound. The lips part briefly to produce the nasalized "a" vowel. The tongue tip then meets the alveolar ridge, stopping oral airflow again, and phonated air is redirected through the nasal airway, with the "n" sound produced.

It is through these articulated phonemes (nasal and oral) and vowels that the full array of all human speech, independently of language, is created. Because of the integral role of the velopharynx in both speech and swallowing, dysfunction of the velopharynx clearly has implications for an affected individual's health and ability to communicate.

71.7.3 Velopharyngeal Dysfunction

Dysfunction of the velopharyngeal mechanism is often separated into two major categories. Velopharyngeal insufficiency is characterized by an absence of sufficient anatomy for complete closure. In velopharyngeal incompetence, anatomical bulk and structure are sufficient for closure, but the neuromuscular mechanism is unable to provide adequate closure or correctly timed closure.

The most common cause of velopharyngeal insufficiency in a child is cleft palate. An unrepaired cleft palate causes significant nasal regurgitation and feeding problems in infancy. More subtle cases of submucosal cleft palate, in which the muscles are not joined at the midline, are often not recognized until later in life, when a child's developing speech is affected by resonance problems. Inadequate velar function predisposes a child to recurrent otitis media secondary to eustachian tube dysfunction.

After surgical reconstruction for cleft lip and palate, it is important to note that the arrangement of the velopharyngeal muscles is still deranged (even after intravelar veloplasty) because of the developmental absence of a midline raphe and decussation of the muscles of the soft palate. It is for this reason that velopharyngeal incompetence often persists despite adequate surgical repair.

Velopharyngeal incompetence is the neuromuscular dysfunction of an otherwise anatomically intact velopharyngeal mechanism. It is much less common than insufficiency. A new presentation of incompetence in an otherwise well child or adult is ominous for a progressive neurologic condition or skull base tumor affecting neurologic control. Resonance disorders of these types are characteristically seen in patients after significant head trauma or skull base surgery.

Two common yet nonpathologic forms of velopharyngeal dysfunction are also described. The first is the hypernasal speech that develops in a child after adenoidectomy. In children with large adenoids, the distance the velum must traverse to achieve adequate closure has been physiologically decreased by the physical presence of the adenoids. After surgery to remove the adenoids, the child's speech may sound hypernasal as the soft palate is initially unable to traverse the increased distance to the posterior pharyngeal wall (the increase due to the now-absent adenoid pad). These children are often monitored, and recovery of normal speech is typically gradual and complete over 3 to 6 months. Velopharyngeal dysfunction is considered pathologic only if it persists after this period.

Deaf speech is characterized by hypernasality and disrupted resonance patterns. Deaf persons learn speech through visualization and impersonation. Because the function of the velopharynx is visually hidden, it is a part of articulation that is nearly impossible for them to learn. Secondarily, it has been proposed that the increased vibratory conduction of nasal resonance provides important tactile feedback for speech production in deaf patients. These marked changes that characterize deaf speech stand as evidence of the important function of the velum. Because of this similarity, patients with abnormal resonance may be mistakenly presumed to have hearing impairment.

71.7.4 Diagnostics

Disorders of resonance are diagnosed primarily clinically. Severe anatomical deficits are apparent on a thorough clinical examination and rarely require additional work-up. Formal evaluation may include lateral neck radiography, nasometry, video nasopharyngeal endoscopy (nasopharyngoscope), and in some cases fluoroscopy.

Nasometry and fluoroscopy are the two modalities offering true functional information during speech. In nasometry, a receptor placed at the nasal aperture measures variations in air pressure during speech. Hypernasality is identified as relatively increased nasal airflow during the production of oral speech sounds in comparison with normative standards. Fluoroscopy is rarely used because of the risks of prolonged radiation exposure in children; however, motion of the soft palate is visualized well.

Video nasopharyngeal endoscopy is usually performed as an evaluation to determine the exact anatomical structure of the velopharynx during speech. A nasopharyngoscope is placed into the region of the choana under topical nasal anesthesia. With a speech pathologist directing the patient, the patient speaks test words and phrases that stress oral pressure consonants while the reviewer observes the closure of the velopharynx during the speech sample. The examination is recorded with both video and audio channels for the interpretation of velopharyngeal function. The patient's nasopharyngeal and velar movement is then graded for complete velopharyngeal closure or incomplete closure. Patients with complete closure are usually referred for speech therapy, whereas patients with incomplete closure who have exhausted speech therapy may be referred for physical management of their velopharyngeal insufficiency. Physical management may consist of surgical management or prosthetic management. The nasopharyngoscope is critical to planning the future surgical treatment of anatomical deficits.

In children with severe craniofacial deformities and syndromic findings accompanying velopharyngeal insufficiency, imaging studies are chosen accordingly. Intervention is planned based on the nature of the deficit.

71.7.5 Surgical Management of Velopharyngeal Insufficiency

In general, three surgical options are available for patients with cleft palate who have velopharyngeal insufficiency that is not correctable with speech therapy. There is usually a gap in the velopharyngeal valve that the patient cannot close despite maximal attempts. This gap represents the physical cross-sectional area that surgical management must fill for the velopharyngeal sphincter to be able to close. When the gap is due to a notch or groove in the posterior border of the soft palate, or there is a close but incomplete approximation of the soft palate to the posterior pharyngeal wall, a revision operation on the soft palate with a Furlow palatoplasty often is able to correct the velopharyngeal insufficiency. The increased length and closer approximation of the soft palate inherent in the Furlow palatoplasty make it an optimal choice in this situation. In addition, it is unlikely to cause airway obstruction and sleep apnea.

The other surgical procedures, pharyngeal flap and pharyngoplasty, are often used for the treatment of velopharyngeal insufficiency. These procedures can be used in patients who have velopharyngeal insufficiency without a cleft palate. They may be performed after or in combination with any of the previously described cleft palate procedures. Both of these procedures use pharyngeal tissues to create a narrowing of the velopharyngeal valve space.

The pharyngeal flap consists of a superiorly based rectangular flap of tissue harvested from the posterior pharyngeal wall (full thickness of mucosa and muscle; ▶ Fig. 71.14a). The flap of tissue is inset into the nasopharyngeal aspect of the soft palate (▶ Fig. 71.14b), with lateral openings (ports) remaining for nasal breathing and nasal resonance (▶ Fig. 71.14c). This procedure is best used when a large central gap is seen during the nasal endoscopy examination, usually in a patient with an adynamic palate. It relies upon lateral wall movement to close the two lateral ports during swallowing and speech. The drawback of this procedure is the risk for postoperative snoring and sleep apnea.

In the pharyngoplasty, the velopharyngeal sphincter is artificially made "tighter" by transposing tissue from the lateral pharyngeal walls up and behind the soft palate to narrow the inlet into the nasopharynx. Superiorly based flaps of tissue are harvested from the posterior tonsillar pillar (mucosa and muscle; ▶ Fig. 71.15a). They are rotated medially and inset into a site (previously determined during the nasopharyngoscope examination) on the posterior pharyngeal wall behind the soft palate (▶ Fig. 71.15b). These flaps narrow the lateral areas of the velopharyngeal sphincter and create a "speed bump" on the posterior pharyngeal wall against which the mobile palate can coapt during speech. The central opening is available for breathing and for air movement during speech. Although this procedure may induce postoperative snoring, the risk for chronic sleep apnea is less than with pharyngeal flap.

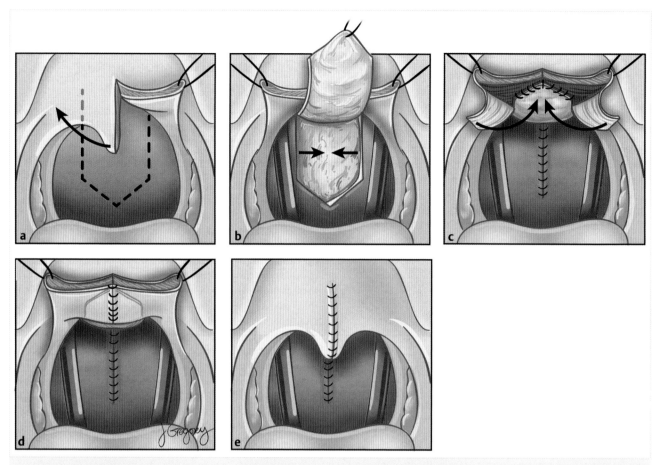

Fig. 71.14 Pharyngeal flap. (**a**) Superiorly based flap developed from the posterior pharyngeal wall, seen behind the split uvula. (**b**) The donor site on the posterior pharyngeal wall is closed primarily. (**c**) The flap is sutured to the nasopharyngeal side of the soft palate. (**d**) Nasopharyngeal flaps are sutured over the pharyngeal flap. (**e**) Uvular closure. Lateral ports in which red rubber catheters can fit are left for nasal respiration.

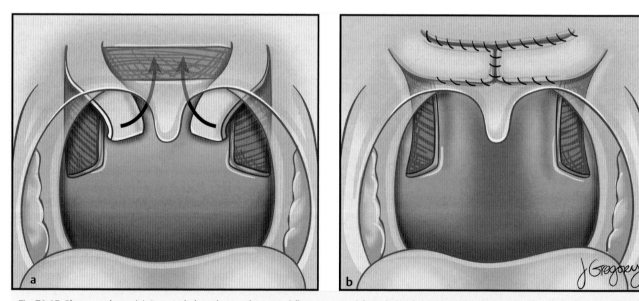

Fig. 71.15 Pharyngoplasty. (**a**) Superiorly based musculomucosal flaps are raised from behind the posterior pharyngeal pillars. The posterior pharyngeal wall between the base of these flaps is demucosalized. (**b**) The flaps are transposed and sutured to the denuded posterior pharyngeal wall to provide additional bulk and anterior projection and allow more complete closure of the velopharyngeal inlet.

71.8 Ear and Eustachian Tube Dysfunction

Children with cleft palate are at high risk for the development of middle ear effusion and conductive hearing loss. As described above, the tensor veli palatini muscle is a part of the soft palate musculature that is anatomically disrupted in cleft palate. As the only dilator of the eustachian tube, the tensor veli palatini is physically unable to dilate the eustachian tube until sometime after the cleft palate has been repaired. The development of middle ear effusion (typically mucoid) usually results in a conductive hearing loss. The placement of ventilating tubes (pressure equalization tubes) is required to correct the effusion and conductive hearing loss. Children with cleft palate often require several sets of pressure equalization tubes over a lifetime to prevent hearing loss and protect their ears against the effects of prolonged estachian tube dysfunction.

71.9 Cleft Palate Team Care

Children who are born with cleft lip and palate face many medical challenges. They usually have numerous needs and may have to see a number of different medical specialists and therapists early in life. Cleft palate and craniofacial teams are groups of specialists who are experienced in cleft and craniofacial care. The minimum team requirements are a reconstructive surgeon (who may be an otolaryngologist, plastic surgeon, or oral surgeon), a social worker, an orthodontist, and a speech pathologist, who meet face to face to discuss patient care coordination. Most teams have other specialists, including audiologists, nurses, ophthalmologists, pediatricians, geneticists, and dentists. The team approach allows a better coordination of care. Most children visit the specialists of the cleft and craniofacial team every 2 or 3 years (or more often if needed). Individual specialists see the patients independently as needed between team visits.

71.10 Roundsmanship

- Cleft lip and palate are the most common congenital malformation of the head and neck.
- Cleft lip and palate occur in approximately 1 in 600 live births in the United States. Native Americans and persons of Asian descent are at the highest risk.
- Cleft lip and palate may occur as an isolated malformation or as part of a syndrome.
- Cleft lip and palate are often a function of both genetics and environment, with some gene mutations now identified in patients with cleft lip and palate. Environmental etiologies have been identified that increase the risk for clefting.
- Lip embryogenesis begins at the fourth to fifth week and is complete by the end of the sixth week of gestation. Palate embryogenesis follows and is complete by the 10th week of gestation.
- Complete cleft lip and palate occur in 45% of all clefts; cleft lip with or without cleft alveolus occurs in 25%, and cleft palate only in 30%.
- "Rule of tens" for surgery. For cleft lip repair: 10 weeks, 10 lb, 10 g of hemoglobin. For cleft palate repair: 10 months, 10 kg, 10 g of hemoglobin.
- Most children who have cleft palate will develop a middle ear effusion with conductive hearing loss. The effusion is treated with the placement of pressure equalization tubes, and more than one set of tubes may be required.
- Team management allows coordinated care for the many problems that children with cleft lip and palate have to face.

71.11 Recommended Reading

[1] Cutting C, Grayson B, Brecht L, Santiago P, Wood R, Kwon S. Presurgical columellar elongation and primary retrograde nasal reconstruction in one-stage bilateral cleft lip and nose repair. Plast Reconstr Surg 1998; 101: 630–639

[2] Dionisopoulos T, Williams HB. Congenital anomalies of the mouth, palate, and pharynx. In: Tewfik TL, der Kaloustian VM, eds. Congenital Anomalies of the Ear, Nose, and Throat. New York, NY: Oxford University Press; 1997:243–262

[3] Furlow LT. Cleft palate repair by double opposing Z-plasty. Plast Reconstr Surg 1986; 78: 724–738

[4] Gorlin RJ, Cohen MM Jr, Hennekam RCM. Syndromes of the Head and Neck. 4th ed. New York, NY: Oxford University Press; 2001

[5] Johnston MC. Developmental biology of the mouth, plate, and pharynx. In: Tewfik TL, der Kaloustian VM, eds. Congenital Anomalies of the Ear, Nose, and Throat. New York, NY: Oxford University Press; 1997:229–242

[6] Lammer EJ, Shaw GM, Iovannisci DM, Van Waes J, Finnell RH. Maternal smoking and the risk of orofacial clefts: Susceptibility with NAT1 and NAT2 polymorphisms. Epidemiology 2004; 15: 150–156

[7] Millard DR Jr. Cleft Craft: The Evolution of Its Surgery. Vol I. The Unilateral Deformity. Boston, MA: Little Brown; 1976

[8] Millard DR Jr. Cleft Craft: The Evolution of Its Surgery. Vol II. Bilateral and Rare Deformities. Boston, MA: Little Brown; 1977

[9] Millard DR Jr. Cleft Craft: The Evolution of Its Surgery. Vol III. Alveolar and Palatal Deformities. Boston, MA: Little Brown; 1980

[10] Prescott NJ, Malcolm S. Folate and the face: evaluating the evidence for the influence of folate genes on craniofacial development. Cleft Palate Craniofac J 2002; 39: 327–331

[11] van Rooij IA, Vermeij-Keers C, Kluijtmans LA et al. Does the interaction between maternal folate intake and the methylenetetrahydrofolate reductase polymorphisms affect the risk of cleft lip with or without cleft palate? Am J Epidemiol 2003; 157: 583–591

[12] Vieira AR. Association between the transforming growth factor alpha gene and nonsyndromic oral clefts: a HuGE review. Am J Epidemiol 2006; 163: 790–810

72 Airway Disorders in Children

Robin A. Dyleski

72.1 Introduction

The airway of a child is susceptible to various congenital and acquired conditions because of intrinsic factors related to the size, position, and development of the airway. The pediatric airway is considered to begin at the nasal inlet at the nares and lips, and it extends to the main bronchi of the lungs; conditions affecting any of the areas between these sites can cause considerable respiratory difficulty in children. This chapter will address those conditions that affect the portion of the airway comprising the laryngeal and tracheal structures. Sometimes, several conditions may coexist within the same patient, and a careful history, examination, and diagnosis are necessary for adequate treatment and management of the breathing problem.

72.2 Developmental Anatomy

The formation of the aerodigestive tract begins early in fetal development. The fetal larynx, esophagus, trachea, and lungs have important functions in the fetus that change dramatically with the first breath at birth. Within the uterus, the larynx and trachea are essential to the growth and development of the lungs by modulating the "breathing" of amniotic fluid. Certain conditions that prevent the "breathing" of amniotic fluid frequently have significant effects upon the size and proper growth of the fetal lungs. With the newborn's first breath of air, the the larynx assumes three new roles: modulation of airflow into the trachea and lungs, protection of the lower airways (trachea and lungs) from the aspiration of secretions and swallowed food, and vocalization. Many congenital conditions can be understood more easily when the embryologic development of the airway is considered.

The anlagen of the larynx, trachea, and lungs originate from a ventromedial diverticulum in the developing pharynx (foregut) at about the 25th day of fetal development. This diverticulum, also known as the tracheobronchial groove, extends anterior to the developing esophagus as a solid tubelike structure, extending toward the thorax and developing chest. The caudal end of this structure will develop the trachea and the lung buds, the future lungs. By the fourth week, the esophagus can be distinctly identified.

The formation of the laryngeal anlage is affected by three tissue masses (anteriorly and laterally) at the fourth to fifth week that will become the future epiglottis, false and true vocal folds, arytenoids, and subglottis. By the sixth week of fetal development, the laryngeal structures and trachea are noted to have recanalized and are seen to have a distinct lumen. Later, after recanalization is completed, the fetus will "breathe" amniotic fluid into the lungs buds and subsequently into the developing lungs. The embryonic period of development sees the formation of the structural anatomy of the airway (▶ Fig. 72.1).

Because of the complex changes and modulations occurring in the embryologic development of the fetal larynx during the very early stages of gestation, there is a great potential for abnormalities in the structure and canalization of the airway lumen to arise. Congenital conditions such as laryngotracheal cleft, laryngeal webs, and certain cystic lesions are well-known examples of specific problems of developmental anatomy.

Congenital airway disorders usually manifest in the first days to weeks of life; however, they may not be discovered until much later, especially if mild. The discovery of a congenital lesion varies significantly depending upon the location of the lesion and its likelihood to cause symptoms in the child.

The fetal period of growth, starting at the third month of gestation, is marked by further growth of the larynx and trachea and the onset of lung development, along with the necessary muscular and neurologic development. The recanalization of the larynx and trachea is completed by the end of the third month, and the fetus then begins "breathing" amniotic fluid into the developing lungs.

Swallowing occurs in the fetus around the fourth month of gestation. Important neuromuscular reflexes develop in the

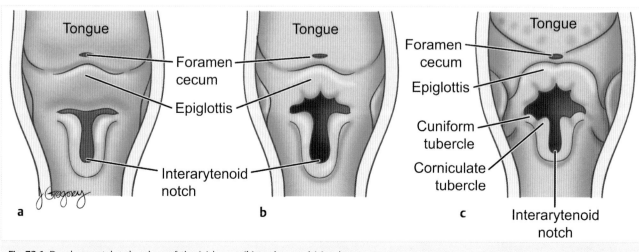

Fig. 72.1 Developmental embryology of the (a) larynx, (b) trachea, and (c) pulmonary tract.

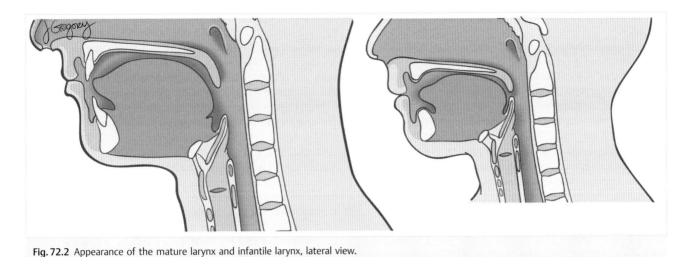

Fig. 72.2 Appearance of the mature larynx and infantile larynx, lateral view.

Table 72.1 Important components in the assessment of children in respiratory distress

History	Physical findings
History of intubation, instrumentation	Quality of stridor (inspiratory, expiratory, biphasic), constant or intermittent
Timing of the onset of respiratory distress (acute, gradual)	Use of accessory respiratory muscles (subcostal or sternal retraction, tracheal tug, flare of alae)
Qualities of the baby's cry	Oxygen saturation, respiratory rate
Presence of stridor	General appearance
Feeding problems, relationship of feeding to respiratory distress	Observation of feeding difficulties
What makes breathing better or worse	

successive months, with both esophageal swallowing and laryngeal breathing increased. The cellular linings of the larynx, trachea, and lower airway become populated with ciliated respiratory mucosa and squamous epithelium. The cartilages of the larynx and trachea develop enough strength to support a patent airway by the beginning of the third trimester. The onset of the third trimester marks the nearly complete development of the anatomical structures of the larynx and trachea. The larynx is fully capable at this point to complete its functions of respiration, protection, and phonation, even though the lungs and other body organs are often insufficiently developed.

72.2.1 Differences between the Infant and the Adult Larynx

Both the shape of the cartilage and the position of the larynx in the infant vary considerably from those in the mature adult. The thyroid cartilage in the infant is broader and shorter than the thyroid cartilage in the adult. The position of the true vocal folds is noted to be relatively higher within the infant thyroid cartilage, approximately one-half of the way rather than a third of the way from the inferior edge, as in the adult thyroid cartilage. In addition, the upper edge of the thyroid cartilage is usually tucked inside the hyoid bone in the infant, making the larynx higher within the infant's neck. The cricoid cartilage is typically found as high as the C4 vertebra in the infant neck,

compared with a much lower position, at the C6 vertebra, in the adult (▶ Fig. 72.2).

72.3 Clinical Evaluation of the Child with an Airway Problem

The evaluation of a child with an airway problem requires a careful and complete history, a perinatal and delivery history, and a thorough head and neck examination (▶ Table 72.1). An immediate assessment of the child is necessary to determine the urgency of the respiratory problem. The history includes a detailed assessment of the breathing difficulty, including the nature of the problem, the timing of the onset of the breathing difficulty, the presence of stridor (noisy breathing caused by laryngeal or tracheal disorders), the relationship of the respiratory distress to feeding, sleep and body position, and the presence or absence of cyanosis and apnea. It is imperative to learn whether anything eases or worsens the breathing problem. Sometimes, a video or audio tape made by the parents can help elucidate episodic concerns. Charting the patient's weight gains or losses on a standardized pediatric growth chart will provide information regarding the effect of the respiratory problem on the patient's ability to gain and maintain a normal weight.

Symptoms of stridor, apnea, cyanosis, and tracheal and/or subcostal retractions help not only to determine the severity of the problem but also to narrow the differential diagnosis. Information regarding prematurity and intubation or airway instrumentation at birth is an important facet of the child's history.

The physical examination includes a thorough head and neck examination and a general observation of the patient's respiration at rest, as well as the patient's voice or cry. For children with respiratory problems, this will include not only chest auscultation but also auscultation of the airway, with the stethoscope positioned over the patient's neck and in front of the mouth and nose to listen for stridor. Attention should be directed to determining if hoarseness or a weak cry is present, the nature of any stridor (including whether it is inspiratory, expiratory, or biphasic), and the presence of tracheal/chest retractions and apnea. Sometimes, feeding the child during the examination will demonstrate the symptoms of the airway problem (▶ Fig. 72.3).

The office or bedside examination will often require a flexible laryngoscopic examination, usually via the nostril or transorally for the smallest infants. Careful attention to both inspiratory and expiratory breathing is useful to determine vocal fold function and the effects of obstructive lesions and functional disorders. The flexible laryngoscope examination is usually the most important part of the evaluation of a patient with an airway problem because most pediatric problems can be visualized with this instrument. The flexible laryngoscopy examination,

however, is limited to the diagnosis of conditions affecting the supraglottis and glottis (▶ Fig. 72.4a). Typically, one is unable to definitively diagnose with a flexible laryngoscope lesions that are present in the subglottis or trachea (▶ Fig. 72.4b). Rarely, with use of the smallest-diameter flexible scopes, can a more distal lesion be visualized.

Radiologic evaluations, including plain X-ray films of the neck and chest, computed tomography (CT), and magnetic resonance (MR) imaging, are recommended for more distal lesions of the airways. These can delineate airway anatomy and the relationship of the airway to mediastinal structures (aortic arch, innominate artery) and identify congenital cardiac and mediastinal malformations. On occasion, ultrasonograpy or fluoroscopy may assist the diagnosis.

In selected cases, further evaluation with sleep/nap studies may determine the degree of apnea and oxygen desaturation. Pulmonary function assessment and pulmonary consultation are often helpful.

72.4 Stridor

Stridor is a symptom that is of concern to parents and physicians. Stridor is a respiratory noise created when airflow through the airway is turbulent. Airflow turbulence is most often caused by a partial airway obstruction, either anatomical or functional. Stridor is described according to when in the respiratory cycle it occurs. The quality of the stridor is important to note. Stridor may be described as fluttery, harsh, musical, or whistle-like. Stridor is described as *inspiratory* (commonly associated with supraglottic and glottic conditions), *expiratory* (commonly associated with tracheal problems), or *biphasic* (present during both inspiration and expiration, commonly associated with subglottic lesions). Various airway conditions are associated with different types of stridor, so that a description of the type of stridor helps to determine the type of airway lesion (▶ Table 72.2).

72.5 Airway Disorders

72.5.1 Laryngomalacia

Etiology

Laryngomalacia is the most common congenital airway disorder and the most common cause of stridor in infants and

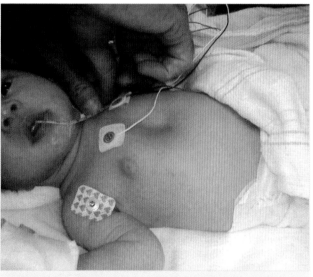

Fig. 72.3 Infant demonstrating severe sternal retractions.

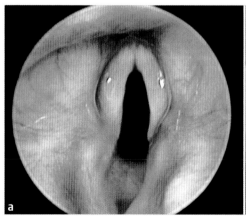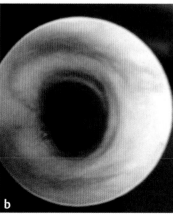

Fig. 72.4 (a) View of true vocal folds in a normal pediatric larynx. (b) Endoscopic view of normal subglottis.

Table 72.2 Types of stridor and airway conditions according to location of obstruction

Location	Voice	Stridor	Retraction	Feeding	Cough
Laryngeal: supraglottic	Muffled "hot potato"	Snoring, inspiratory and fluttering stridor	None until late	Difficult to impossible	Not noted
Laryngeal: subglottic	Normal, occasionally hoarse	Inspiratory and expiratory stridor, snoring	Intercostal early, then xiphoid	Normal	Barking (no other place in the airway)
Tracheal	Normal	Expiratory stridor and wheezing	None, except in severe obstruction	Normal	Brassy

Source: From Hartnick CJ, Cotton RT. Stridor and airway obstruction. In: Bluestone CD, Stool SE, Alper CM, et al, eds. Pediatric Otolaryngology. 4th ed. Philadelphia, PA: W. B. Saunders; 2003.

children. Laryngomalacia accounts for approximately 60% of all patients with stridor in this age group. The infant is usually born normally without any airway noise or stridor, but stridor begins variably between 1 and 4 weeks after birth.

Pathogenesis

Laryngomalacia is a specific supraglottic condition that manifests as stridor on inspiration. The stridor is caused by inward collapse of the epiglottis and aryepiglottic folds and by anterior prolapse of the redundant mucosa and cuneiform cartilages found over the arytenoids during inspiration. This collapse causes a variable obstruction of the glottic inlet and creates an intermittent, fluttery, inspiratory stridor. The supraglottic structures are pushed outward during expiration, allowing an unobstructed exhalation. This is to be differentiated from posterior disposition of the epiglottis due to an extremely posterior position of the tongue base, commonly seen in craniofacial disorders and mandibular growth conditions.

The exact cause of laryngomalacia is unknown, but a number of theories suggest that it is a neuromuscular developmental disorder of the larynx. One factor considered to be a contributory cause of laryngomalacia is laryngeal cartilage immaturity, or weakness of the laryngeal structural framework. Underdeveloped neuromuscular control of the pharyngeal and laryngeal supporting musculature is another component leading to laryngomalacia. This may occur in the absence of any other diagnosed neuromuscular conditions but manifest with airway issues, such as apnea and hypotonia.

Gastroesophageal reflux (GER) is strongly associated with laryngomalacia and is well described as a comorbid condition in children diagnosed with laryngomalacia. GER is often seen in the infant during diagnostic fiber-optic laryngoscopic examinations. GER is felt to worsen the symptoms of laryngomalacia, and also to be exacerbated by laryngomalacia. The airway obstruction caused by the inward collapse of the supraglottic structures in laryngomalacia results in an increased negative inspiratory pressure during breathing. This results in increased reflux of the gastric contents into the esophagus and up into the airway and pharynx. The effect of the acidic gastric contents on the laryngeal tissues frequently results in laryngeal edema, especially edema of the arytenoid mucosal region. GER-induced laryngeal edema worsens airway obstruction in children with laryngomalacia, thus exacerbating the general effects of laryngomalacia.

Natural History and Progression, Disease Complications, and Prognosis

Laryngomalacia varies in severity. It can be mild, with minimal symptoms other than intermittent mild stridor, or can be a life-threatening condition causing apnea and failure to thrive in the infant due to inability to feed. The variable severity is due to the variable degree of airway obstruction caused by inward collapse of the supraglottic structures.

In most infants, laryngomalacia responds well to medical treatment of the GER with H2 blockers or other anti-reflux medications, and improvement of the stridor is expected by the first birthday and resolution of symptoms by the age of 2 years. When infants have significant apnea, exhibit failure to thrive (fail to gain weight or fall off the normal growth curve), or are unable to tolerate GER medical regimens, surgical management is offered.

Presenting Symptoms

Babies who have laryngomalacia usually present within the first few weeks of life with the onset of intermittent, fluttery, or low-pitched stridor. The stridor is usually worsened by an increased respiratory rate, such as occurs during crying, feeding, or excitement; however, in some patients the stridor is loudest during sleep. Tracheal or sternal retractions are usually indications of more severe airway obstruction and are often associated with feeding problems. It is important to evaluate the amount of time that a baby with laryngomalacia needs to take a feeding; normal feedings usually require less than 30 minutes. Babies who need longer than 30 minutes are often at risk for failure to thrive because they expend more calories in feeding than they may be gaining from their formula.

The parents should also be questioned about the amount of "spitting up" or reflux symptoms they observe in the infant. Some infants have severe reflux symptoms and "spit up" after every feeding. Other symptoms that need to be assessed include potential apnea, cyanosis, episodes of complete airway obstruction, and resultant cardiac failure.

Medical Evaluation and Physical Examination

The infant with laryngomalacia is evaluated with a complete history (as described earlier in this section) and a general head and neck examination, with particular care taken to auscultate the baby's stridor over the chest and neck areas. The chest and

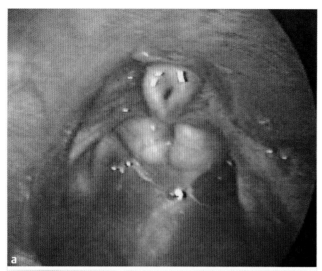

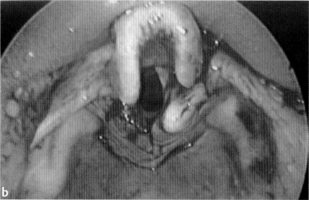

Fig. 72.5 (**a**) Laryngomalacia with severe inward collapse of the epiglottis and supraglottic structures on inspiration. (**b**) Laryngomalacia on inspiration following supraglottoplasty (with left cuneiform cartilage resection, right side present), demonstrating improvement in airway.

neck areas are observed for retractions, and a careful assessment of feeding is made in the history.

The main diagnostic examination for laryngomalacia is fiberoptic laryngoscopy. This can be safely performed in the ambulatory setting under topical nasal anesthesia, or via the unanesthetized oral cavity (in the youngest infants). With the fiber-optic laryngoscope in place, the baby is observed and the respiratory cycle is correlated with the laryngeal examination. This examination will usually reveal the following findings: (1) omega-shaped (tubular) epiglottis; (2) short aryepiglottic folds (that pull the epiglottis posteriorly and concomitantly pull the arytenoids anteriorly); (3) redundant arytenoid mucosa prolapsing anteriorly into the glottic opening; (4) prominent cuneiform laryngeal cartilages with prolapse into the glottic opening. These findings are diagnostic for laryngomalacia. There is a reported 15% incidence of concomitant aerodigestive tract anomalies when laryngomalacia is diagnosed (▶ Fig. 72.5a).

Treatment

Laryngomalacia is generally considered a medical condition of the airway because about 95% of patients in whom laryngoma-

lacia (plus concomitant GER) is diagnosed can be stabilized, with a decrease in symptoms of airway obstruction, stridor, and GER, through the use of anti-reflux medications until approximately 9 to 12 months of age. Responders have marked relief of their symptoms with normal growth and development.

Patients who have significant apnea, failure to thrive, or significant symptoms that do not respond to anti-reflux medications are usually considered for surgical treatment; they account for fewer than 5% of all patients in whom laryngomalacia is diagnosed. Surgical options require a careful assessment of the specific components of laryngomalacia that are causing airway obstruction in the patient. The usual procedure includes microlaryngoscopy (with the patient spontaneously breathing under general anesthesia), bronchoscopy, and supraglottoplasty (▶ Fig. 72.5b). The supraglottoplasty portion of the procedure frequently will include lysis of the aryepiglottic folds and excision of the cuneiform cartilage and redundant mucosa overlying the arytenoid cartilage. The patient is then observed via laryngoscopy upon emergence from anesthesia to confirm that the obstructing portions of the supraglottic larynx have been fully treated at the end of the procedure.

Complications of Medical and Surgical Options

The failure of medical treatment for laryngomalacia may delay definitive surgery. Unrecognized apnea and subsequent oxygen desaturation may occur in this setting. Fortunately, the vast majority of patients respond well to anti-reflux medications, and few patients with laryngomalacia who are initially medically managed proceed to surgical management.

Complications of surgical management are infrequent because of the intraoperative assessment of the efficacy of supraglottoplasty. When the supraglottoplasty is insufficient to relieve symptoms of airway obstruction, the patient may require an additional procedure to relieve airway obstruction, such as revision supraglottoplasty or tracheostomy.

72.5.2 Vocal Fold Paralysis

Etiology

Vocal fold paralysis (VFP) is a neurologic condition that may be congenital or acquired and unilateral or bilateral. VFP is the second most common cause of stridor in young children. There are many causes of acquired VFP, and specific etiologies may be more likely to cause unilateral or bilateral paralysis. In children, acquired VFP is often due to trauma, including birth-related injury, surgical trauma, and blunt or penetrating trauma. Other causes include infectious and inflammatory diseases, such as Lyme disease, Guillain-Barré syndrome, and other bacterial and viral diseases.

In cases of congenital VFP (unilateral and bilateral), the etiology is more frequently a central nervous system or cardiovascular system malformation than in acquired VFP. Congenital VFP may be found as a part of many syndromes.

Pathogenesis

True VFP can be caused by direct neuronal or central nervous system injury from trauma (including indirect trauma, such as stretch injury), inflammation, or infection or by a malformation of the central nervous system or the vagus nerve. Like all nerves, the vagus and recurrent laryngeal nerves are susceptible to injuries that result in various forms of dysfunction, in this case weakness (paresis) or complete absence (paralysis) of motor and sensory function. The recurrent laryngeal nerve is susceptible to various forms of injury, especially stretch-type injuries, because of its circuitous path (through the chest) to its target organ, the larynx.

In cases of congenital VFP, the pathogenesis is directly related to the underlying etiology of the VFP. In cases of central nervous system malformations, Arnold-Chiari malformation is the most often identified underlying deformity. Arnold-Chiari malformation is often associated with hydrocephalus with or without myelomeningocele and with inferior displacement of the medulla and cerebellum into the foramen magnum. This inferior herniation is felt to cause traction and pressure on the vagus nerves, resulting in impaired neuronal conduction, recurrent laryngeal nerve dysfunction, and VFP, particularly bilateral. Other central nervous system disorders and malformations can directly affect the vagus nerve, from its nucleus to the motor end plates of the nerve itself.

Mediastinal cardiac malformations, with abnormalities of the great vessels, can cause traction injuries to the vagus and recurrent laryngeal nerves. Patent ductus arteriosus is one of the most common causes of unilateral VFP, particularly left-sided VFP. Patent ductus arteriosus, which is treated surgically, is often seen in premature infants, and undiagnosed VFP may actually be present before patent ductus arteriosus is surgically managed.

In the case of infectious or inflammatory conditions, the brainstem itself or the vagus nerve is directly affected by the causative agent. These causes of VFP are in many cases transitory, and the VFP will resolve with time after resolution of the causative infection. In some cases, VFP may become permanent. Many cases of VFP are seen in which no causative agent, infection, or malformation is ever identified, and they remain classified as idiopathic.

Natural History, Disease Complications, and Prognosis

The causes of VFP, both unilateral and bilateral, are extensive (▶ Table 72.3). The natural history and prognosis of VFP depend on the cause. In cases of congenital, idiopathic VFP, either unilateral or bilateral, the severity of the symptoms will dictate the overall prognosis. The symptoms of airway obstruction and/or aspiration are the most important prognosticators of the patient's clinical course. In cases of bilateral VFP, the vocal folds are usually close together, with a more defined abduction paralysis resulting in more symptoms of airway obstruction. If this is not relieved, the patient will develop respiratory distress to a variable degree, with aspiration less likely. Unilateral VFP is more likely to result in aspiration problems unless the normally functioning vocal fold is able to compensate and hyperadduct to achieve glottic closure with the paralyzed side. When the VFP does not result in life-threatening airway obstruction or aspiration, especially when the condition is idiopathic, the expectation is that there will be partial or full recovery of nerve function. This may take several years to occur. At the time that unilateral or bilateral VFP is diagnosed, there is no test that can conclusively predict when recovery may occur, especially in very small children. Most clinicians will opt for observation in asymptomatic or mildly symptomatic children to allow for the possibility of spontaneous recovery of recurrent nerve function.

Presenting Symptoms

The most common presenting symptoms of unilateral VFP include a hoarse voice or cry, stridor, and aspiration or coughing with feedings. In cases of unilateral VFP, the degree of stridor is often mild (if present at all), and the most common symptom prompting consultation is a weak or hoarse cry. Any symptoms of cough or choking with feedings are usually the normal protective function of the larynx in response to actual aspiration during the feeding. These symptoms are found in both congenital and acquired forms of unilateral VFP.

The presenting symptoms of bilateral VFP contrast sharply with those of unilateral VFP; in bilateral VFP, there is usually a strong cry and frequently loud stridor with cry or agitation, in addition to other signs of airway obstruction, such as retractions, cyanosis, and oxygen desaturation. In bilateral VFP, the vocal folds are near the midline with a narrow glottic opening, maintaining their ability to coapt and produce a strong cry; however, because there is abductor muscle dysfunction, they are unable to lateralize properly, resulting in an insufficient glottic space and airway obstruction. The size of the glottic space will influence the degree of airway obstruction; the obstruction worsens with increases as respiratory rate. Aspiration is less common than in unilateral VFP because the narrow glottis inlet reduces inadvertent leakage into the airway during swallowing (▶ Fig. 72.6).

Table 72.3 Etiology of true vocal fold paralysis

Organ systems	Congenital	Acquired
Neurologic	*Arnold-Chiari malformation, hydrocephalus, peripheral nerve defects (myasthenia gravis), idiopathic*	*Multiple sclerosis, kernicterus, idiopathic*
Cardiovascular	Patent ductus arteriosus, cardiomegaly	Patent ductus arteriosus ligation, repair of coarctation of the aorta, acquired cardiomegaly
Infectious		Guillain-Barré syndrome, botulism, polyneuritis from viral etiology, syphilis, diphtheria
Trauma		*Birth canal trauma, postsurgical (thyroidectomy, tracheal reconstruction surgery), direct injury to neck or chest*
Other	Tracheo-esophageal fistula, mediastinal masses	

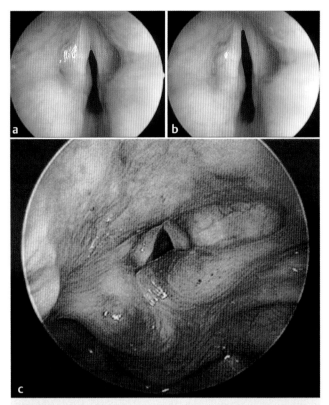

Fig. 72.6 Vocal fold paralysis. (**a**) Bilateral true vocal fold paralysis on inspiration (note medial position of the true vocal folds). (**b**) Bilateral true vocal fold paralysis with expiration (note that the true vocal folds are "pushed" apart by the airflow). (**c**) Unilateral true vocal fold paralysis (note the paramedian position of the the paralyzed right cord).

Medical Evaluation and Physical Examination

The diagnosis of VFP can be difficult in very small children. After a rapid assessment of the severity of the child's respiratory status, a detailed past and present medical history is obtained. The medical evaluation should detail any other known conditions afflicting the child, such as congenital cardiac or cerebral malformations or known syndromes, as well as any prior surgical interventions for these. Other areas of review must include significant precedent infectious or inflammatory conditions.

When the child is evaluated, an emphasis needs to be placed upon the presence of stridor, including all facets of its quality, its timing, the effect of positioning, and the degree of respiratory distress and airway obstruction. The relationship of feeding to the respiratory symptoms and weight gain is important information that can aid in establishing a correct diagnosis. This information may be directly observed or obtained from caregivers.

The physical examination remains similar to that for any child presenting with an airway problem—namely, a detailed head and neck examination with emphasis on the oral structures and neck. Auscultation of the chest and neck is usually performed to detect stridor; if stridor is heard, it should be characterized by its timing, quality, and frequency. Any heart murmurs are noted.

The diagnosis of VFP depends upon observation of the larynx and vocal folds with the patient spontaneously breathing. Flexible fiber-optic laryngoscopy, with topical anesthesia administered via the nostril or mouth, is usually performed at the bedside or in the office when VFP is suspected. The laryngeal examination notes the appearance of all laryngeal structures, with note taken of the shape and position of the epiglottis and other supraglottic structures, the false and true vocal folds, and the dynamics of laryngeal function during respiration and often swallowing. The vocal folds are observed for their appearance and surfaces, their position relative to each other and the midline, any swelling or mass effect, and movement with both inspiration (abduction) and expiration. The true cord movements may be enhanced with swallowing or cough (involuntary abduction of the true cords occurs following cough). In stable patients, observation with the flexible laryngoscope should be continued until the movement of the vocal folds is determined for both abduction and adduction.

In intubated or unstable patients who are unable to tolerate flexible fiber-optic laryngoscopy, the diagnosis is more difficult, and microlaryngoscopy and bronchoscopy in the operating room or neonatal intensive care unit (NICU) are advisable, when the patient is stable. Patients with severe stridor and airway obstruction may be intubated to secure a stable airway when severe airway obstruction, cyanosis, or desaturation occurs. If intubation is performed in the NICU, it is necessary to have oxygen, appropriate endotracheal tubes, and resuscitation equipment at the bedside. Microlaryngoscopy in the operating room is usually performed with light sedation that can be administered via intravenous or inhalational agents. Close communication between the surgeon and anesthesiologist is mandatory. Once the patient is anesthetized just enough to allow positioning of the laryngoscope, the larynx may be topically anesthetized with (2%) lidocaine solution to permit lessening of the general anesthetic, thus increasing the spontaneous respiratory effort of the patient. With a 0-degree rigid telescope, the larynx is observed under magnification for spontaneous vocal fold motion, and the movements of the true vocal folds are correlated with inspiration and expiration. This process is affected by the depth of general anesthesia, and it may take several minutes before vocal fold movement is clearly observed. Supplemental oxygen is administered via the suction port on the Parsons introducing laryngoscope or via a small, trimmed endotracheal tube placed in the hypopharynx.

Following the complete assessment of true vocal fold movement, the 0-degree telescope is passed distally, and the subglottis, trachea, and primary bronchi are examined to complete the airway assessment.

If the movement of one or both of the vocal folds is impaired, then it is necessary to palpate the arytenoids with a probe to confirm that the cricoarytenoid joint is freely mobile. Other conditions, such as fixation of the cricoarytenoid joint, can infrequently occur in children.

Radiographic studies may be useful in determining the etiology of VFP in children. Plain X-rays of the chest and neck in the anteroposterior and lateral projections can provide helpful information regarding associated malformations and conditions that result in unilateral or bilateral VFP. Plain film chest X-ray is especially helpful when there has been prior surgical management of patent ductus arteriosus, with the left mediastinal surgical clip plainly visible.

Modified barium swallow, performed in the radiology suite by the speech or occupational therapist, is a valuable video radiology study to evaluate the aspiration of liquids and pastes of various consistencies. The modified barium swallow can also provide specific information regarding aspiration reduction techniques and proper feeding options for children whose VFP results in aspiration. MR imaging and CT of the larynx do not provide specific information that will yield a diagnosis of VFP alone, but they can provide important information regarding associated medical conditions.

Treatment

In general, the treatment of VFP depends upon the etiology of the paralysis. When congenital VFP (either unilateral or bilateral) is diagnosed, the recommended treatment depends upon the severity of the symptoms. When the patient does not have signs and symptoms of airway obstruction, cyanosis, apnea, or aspiration, he or she is usually observed for possible spontaneous recovery. When the symptoms of respiratory distress are severe, operative microlaryngoscopy and bronchoscopy (if not already performed) are recommended to evaluate the airway for any other conditions for which intervention is warranted (e.g., a patient with both laryngomalacia and unilateral VFP from ductus arteriosus ligation). Subsequent tracheotomy is often necessary to maintain a satisfactory and consistent airway, especially in patients with bilateral VFP. Approximately 50% of patients with bilateral VFP have airway obstruction severe enough to require tracheotomy, whereas fewer than 10% of those with unilateral VFP require a tracheotomy for their airway demands. Approximately 50% of patients with Arnold-Chiari malformation have bilateral VFP, and they are in a special treatment category. Hydrocephalus in patients with Arnold-Chiari malformation can result in sufficient pressure on the vagus nerve rootlets to cause bilateral VFP. Often, immediate reduction of the hydrocephalus with a ventriculoperitoneal shunt is effective in reversing the bilateral VFP and restoring normal laryngeal function. In these patients with Arnold-Chiari malformation, the new onset of bilateral VFP is concerning for increased intracranial pressure, and treatment of that condition will often resolve the bilateral VFP.

Similar options exist for children with permanent acquired VFP or congenital VFP that does not resolve spontaneously. These options are used less frequently in pre-school-age children because of concerns about laryngeal growth and possible permanent effects on voice quality. Arytenoidectomy (partial or complete removal of the arytenoid cartilage and posterior portion of the vocal fold), arytenoid adduction (fixation of the medialized arytenoid to a more lateral position), injection of permanent and temporary filler agents (to medialize vocal folds that are too lateral), and thyroplasty procedures are all available surgical options for improvement of the airway and/or voice quality. These procedures are similar to their counterparts in the adult population, with some modifications made because they must be carried out under general anesthesia.

Complications of Medical and Surgical Options

Complications of the treatment of VFP are most commonly related to airway obstruction, apnea, cyanosis, and aspiration, which are found before the diagnosis in many patients with VFP, regardless of its cause. Tracheostomy placement may result in reactions to general anesthesia, tube dislodgement before tract healing, and pneumothorax. Fortunately, these complications are very rarely in properly staffed and equipped pediatric hospitals. Late complications from tracheotomy are also uncommon and include tracheotomy tube occlusion (from dried respiratory secretions), granulation tissue in the distal trachea (at the tip of the tube) and at the stoma, and accidental decannulation (dislodgement of the tracheotomy tube). Nursing care specialists commonly assist in identifying and avoiding such problems during home visits.

The need for a balance between adequate airway patency and vocal quality has made some of the decisions regarding the best treatment for children with VFP a dilemma. Discussions about procedures that may allow decannulation must always consider the effect on vocal quality. It is recommended that children participate in these decisions when they are old enough to comprehend the risks involved in balancing vocal quality with an adequate airway.

72.5.3 Masses and Tumors

Etiology

Masses and tumors of the larynx, trachea, and bronchi may be congenital or acquired. Although most congenital masses are diagnosed soon after birth, some may not become apparent until they enlarge and become symptomatic.

Recurrent respiratory papillomatosis is the most common tumor affecting the airway in young children, but a myriad of benign and malignant neoplasms of epithelial and connective tissue origin are also seen. Some tumors more commonly seen in children include hemangioma (especially in a subglottic location) and neurofibroma. Fortunately, tumors affecting the airways are rare, and it is even more rare for them to be malignant.

Recurrent Respiratory Papillomatosis

Pathogenesis

Recurrent respiratory papillomatosis (RRP) is known to be caused by infection with the human papillomavirus (HPV). More than 100 types of HPV are known, but RRP is most commonly associated with types 6 and 11. HPV infection is generally considered to be vertically acquired from an afflicted mother as a perinatal inoculaton during childbirth. Causative information is incomplete because the RRP infection rate is less than 1 per 500, whereas the maternal infection rate would predict an infection rate of 1 per 32 in infants (approximately 2,500 new cases are diagnosed annually). Transoral infection from vaginal and cervical secretions is the most commonly accepted transmission theory. It is believed that firstborn babies of susceptible young mothers have the highest infection rates of RRP. Interestingly, the siblings of RRP-afflicted children do not have increased rates of infection. The diagnosis is most commonly made around the age of 4 years.

Infection with HPV usually results in the growth of "papillomas," growths characterized by an irregular, exophytic surface and a nodular or pedunculated appearance. They can affect any part of the airway but tend to form in the glottic regions; the larynx is affected in nearly 100% of cases. Under magnification, the papillomas appear as projections of reddish to tannish tissue with sometimes visible vascular cores. On pathologic analysis, papillomas are covered by stratified squamous epithelium with fibrovascular cores and frequently show signs of dysplasia.

Natural History and Progression, Disease Complications, and Prognosis

Once papillomas form in a patient with RRP, continued growth of the lesions within the airway lumen, most often the larynx, is common. The unrelenting growth of laryngeal papillomas leads to progressive airway obstruction, hoarseness, and eventual death unless they are treated. Patients often have a significant papilloma load when they present.

RRP is a viral disease for which there is no known cure, and intermittent palliative procedures are required to maintain a patent airway. A number of clinical trials have attempted to develop an adjuvant medical regime to cure RRP or at least reduce the burden of multiple airway procedures required to clear the obstructing papillomas; mumps vaccine injection, interferon, 5-fluorouracil, acyclovir, and methotrexate have been tested. All trials showed a delay in disease progression in some patients, but none demonstrated the hoped-for cure for RRP. Ongoing trials of cidofovir show promise, but not all patients appear to respond.

The prognosis in RRP is mixed; spontaneous remission occurs in some patients, but many continue to live with disease. The spontaneous remissions rates seem to be higher at the time of school entry and around puberty, leading some investigators to consider that hormonal factors play a role in remission. It is likely that HPV infection in the laryngeal epithelium becomes dormant because some of the patients with spontaneous remissions experience recurrence as adults. It is hoped that the new vaccines against HPV will markedly reduce this disease by decreasing cervical infection in susceptible women.

Presenting Symptoms

RRP typically presents with hoarseness progressing to a whisper-like voice, stridor, wheezing, and increasing respiratory effort and distress. These symptoms are directly related to the location of papillomas in the larynx. Because the vocal folds are the most commonly affected regions of the larynx, vocal complaints are often the earliest symptoms. More subtle symptoms of progressive respiratory distress may be the presenting signs when the vocal folds are free of papilloma.

Medical Evaluation and Physical Examination

Patients with RRP present in either of two ways, depending upon the degree of airway obstruction. Patients with less severe disease often present to the doctor's office with chronic hoarseness, whereas patients with severe obstruction present to the

emergency department with symptoms of severe, progressive airway obstruction.

The medical evaluation of both types of patients includes a determination of the degree of respiratory distress, the duration of symptoms (especially hoarseness), and the presence or absence of stridor. Sometimes, small epithelial papillomas may be visualized in the oropharynx, particularly on the tonsils or uvula.

Flexible fiber-optic laryngoscopy is indicated for all but the most extremely symptomatic patients, whose symptoms may worsen significantly if they are upset or crying; they warrant evaluation in the operating room. The laryngeal examination characteristically reveals one or more visible papillomas in the glottic and supraglottic areas. The degree of airway obstruction should be estimated from this examination, to help determine the urgency of the need for surgical removal (▶ Fig. 72.7).

Treatment

Currently, the treatment of RRP is surgical palliation with removal of the airway papillomas. Patients who have RRP undergo suspension microlaryngoscopy with bronchoscopy on an intermittent schedule to maintain a patent airway. In severe cases, this interval may be as short as 2 to 3 weeks, which is typical in the youngest children. Often, the interval can be extended as the patients mature.

The surgical removal of papillomas in children may be performed as an ambulatory procedure. In many patients with RRP, general anesthesia is administered via an inhalation technique and maintained with an intravenous agent, which allows suspension microlaryngoscopy to be performed under spontaneous ventilation. After the laryngoscope is placed and lidocaine topically applied to the larynx, spontaneous ventilation allows all areas of the airway to be treated without the need for an endotracheal tube. Papillomas are removed most commonly with carbon dioxide laser, microforceps, or the laryngeal microdébrider. Pathologic inspection is routinely

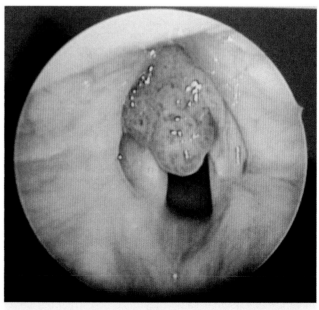

Fig. 72.7 Recurrent respiratory papilloma in the laryngeal glottis.

performed to monitor for rare malignant degeneration of a papilloma into squamous cell carcinoma.

When anesthesia cannot be maintained with spontaneous ventilation, other techniques, such as jet ventilation or apneic techniques, are used. In addition, children with severely obstructive papillomas may initially require intubation because of an inability to ventilate the partially obstructed airway. The endotracheal tube is gently twisted and pressed into the glottic area and slipped past the obstructing papilloma into the trachea. Generally, the endotracheal tube can be removed once the main obstruction is relieved.

Complications of Medical and Surgical Options

At this time, there is no consensus regarding the medical management of RRP, so the patients in each clinical trial are subject to possible complications of the medical treatment offered. All medical trials contain provisions for palliative surgical treatment of the airway with removal of obstructive papilloma.

In general, children with RRP tolerate the multiple operative procedures well. The main risk of repetitive papilloma removal is the formation of scar tissue on the vocal fold, particularly in the anterior commissure, resulting in poor vocal quality. This risk is diminished by keeping the intervals between procedures as long as possible yet safe for maintaining airway patency and recognizing that these procedures are aimed primarily at the maintenance of a patent airway, not the reduction of hoarseness.

The surgical complications of RRP treatment depend upon the instruments used to remove the papilloma. Although the carbon dioxide laser is commonly used because it removes papillomas with precision, it may rarely cause flash fires in the airway. Use of the laryngeal microdébrider "skimmer" is now common, but like all techniques, it may inadvertently remove normal tissue.

Subglottic Hemangioma

Etiology

Subglottic hemangioma is a congenital vascular tumor found in in the subglottis of infants. Subglottic hemangiomas are most commonly discovered in children between 3 and 6 weeks of age. Hemangiomas contain histologic tissue markers similar to those in placental tissue. Subglottic hemangiomas are more commonly found in children who have cutaneous hemangiomas, particularly those that affect the lower third of the face

and upper neck. A subglottic location may be noted up to 10% of the time in this subset of patients with hemangioma. Hemangiomas in the subglottic area result in variable degrees of airway obstruction.

Natural History and Progression

Subglottic hemangiomas, when located in the subglottic space, tend to become symptomatic. Hemangiomas are often sessile, flat lesions when first discovered, but within weeks to months they enter a proliferative phase during which they enlarge. The proliferative phase lasts for several months, with a change of texture and color beginning around the ninth month of life. This change, with softening and a whitish appearance noted on the hemangioma surface, marks the onset of the involution phase. Involution then proceeds for up to 5 to 7 years, with shrinkage of the hemangioma.

The prognosis for a patient with subglottic hemangioma is excellent because these lesions are expected eventually to involute and decrease in size. In addition to maturation and growth of the child's airway, regression leads to a decrease in symptoms, even when some hemangioma remains.

Presenting Symptoms

An infant with a subglottic hemangiomas usually will have an onset of stridor (usually inspiratory or biphasic) at around the age of 3 to 6 weeks, with a normal cry. The stridor may be associated with retractions in the pretracheal or sternal areas. The stridor progresses from intermittent to constant as the hemangioma enlarges during the proliferative phase. Some infants will develop feeding problems as the stridor worsens and the hemangioma becomes larger.

Cutaneous hemangiomas, present approximately in 50% of children with subglottic hemangiomas, will show similar signs of proliferation. About two-thirds of patients with hemangiomas of the lower third of the face are at risk and have airway hemangiomas. Subglottic hemangiomas are more common in girls.

Medical Evaluation and Physical Examination

A child with a cutaneous hemangioma presenting with inspiratory stridor should be suspected of having a subglottic hemangioma. Progressive worsening of stridor will be noted as the duration of the stridor lengthens. The evaluation includes flexible fiber-optic laryngoscopy (▶ Fig. 72.8). Hemangioma may be

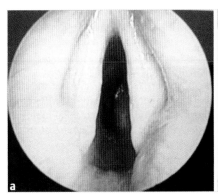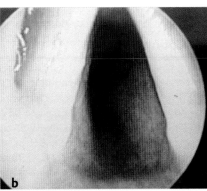

Fig. 72.8 (a) Image of subglottic hemangioma in the right posterior lateral subglottis. (b) Close-up view.

suspected by the observation of a reddish mass in the subglottis, particularly the posterolateral areas. Further evaluation requires microlaryngoscopy and bronchoscopy under general anesthesia. Findings include a smooth, dark red, mucosa-covered mass in the subglottis, sometimes with extension onto the edge of the true vocal fold. The mass is usually compressible and isolated to the subglottis. Tracheal involvement usually appears as a flat patch of reddish mucosa without encroachment into the airway lumen. Biopsy of the lesion is inadvisable because of the likelihood of significant bleeding.

Treatment

A subglottic hemangioma, if small, may be monitored and observed; however, the great majority of these are identified because of the significant symptoms they cause. A variety of treatment modalities are available for subglottic hemangioma, both medical and surgical.

Medical treatment is directed toward decreasing the symptoms of the hemangioma. Corticosteroids are the most commonly used agent for rapid airway symptom relief. Dexamethasone, in doses of up to 1 mg/kg/d initially, often will cause a marked decrease in stridor within 24 to 48 hours. Subsequent transition to prednisolone is sometimes used for up to several weeks once the stridor improves. Intralesional steroid use also has a desirable effect on hemangioma size and symptoms.

In the past, transition from systemic steroids to interferon alpha A was advocated for symptomatic hemangiomas. However this has fallen out of favor because of reports of spastic diplegia caused by myelination defects in the central nervous system.

Propranolol (3 mg/kg/d divided into three doses), a new treatment modality, has been observed to have a marked, rapid (within 24 to 48 hours) effect of decreasing the size and symptoms of airway hemangiomas in previously steroid-dependent children. The low dose of propranolol is well tolerated, and the low risk for systemic side effects (transient hypoglycemia and bronchospasm), combined with the dramatic decrease in symptoms, has made propranolol an agent of choice for many babies with subglottic and other airway hemangiomas.

Surgical management is offered in many situations to children with subglottic hemangioma. Excision of the hemangioma is effective in resolving symptoms in many patients. Excision may be performed with carbon dioxide laser, a microdébrider, or open surgical excision. Tracheotomy is an option for patients who cannot be treated medically (do not tolerate medical management) or who have a circumferential subglottic hemangioma. It is likely that medical therapy with propranolol will decrease the number of surgical procedures performed for subglottic hemangioma.

Complications of Medical and Surgical Options

The complications of medical therapy vary with the agent used. Systemic steroids are well-known to have severe systemic affects when used for a prolonged period of time. These include immune suppression, suppression of the adrenal hormonal axis, growth retardation, hyperglycemia, hypertension, and cushingoid appearance.

At this time, no severe side effects have been reported to occur with propranolol therapy. Patients are monitored for

hypotension, bronchospasm, and hypoglycemia; the risk for these decreases after the initiation of therapy, and most children are followed by a pediatric cardiologist while taking propranolol.

Surgical therapies risk the development of subglottic stenosis from scar formation at the site of the hemangioma. Additionally, incomplete resection of the hemangioma risks recurrence of the lesion in those sites where it remains.

72.5.4 Subglottic Stenosis

Etiology

Subglottic stenosis is characterized by a narrowing of the subglottic space, located just under the vocal folds and extending to the trachea. Stenosis can be congenital (absence of prior intubation and instrumentation of the airway, and abnormal size or shape of the cricoid cartilage lumen) or acquired (most commonly after intubation). Subglottic stenosis is the third most common cause of stridor in young children, although it can be found in all age groups. Inflammatory conditions may also cause subglottic stenosis in patients without a history of intubation.

Pathogenesis

The subglottic space in children is especially prone to the development of inflammation from trauma, including intubation injury. The subglottis is the narrowest portion of the pediatric larynx (as opposed to the glottis in adults) and is thus predisposed to injury from an endotracheal tube. The already small size of the neonatal airway, combined with any inflammation or scarring to the mucosal lining of the subglottis, makes it prone to luminal narrowing. It is well established that the placement of an endotracheal tube can cause pressure on the mucosal lining of the cricoid, resulting in decreased capillary refill and subsequent ischemic mucosal injury within hours of endotracheal tube placement. The ischemic damage to the mucosa can progress to edema and, if the pressure on the airway mucosa is unrelieved, ultimately to erosion and ulceration of the mucosa. In the most severe cases, there is the potential for a full-thickness mucosal injury, and even damage to the the the cricoid cartilage with destabilization of the lumen integrity.

Frequently, granulation tissue will be seen in the region of subglottic injury or at the vocal fold level, molded around the shape of the endotracheal tube on laryngoscopic examination. Healing takes about 3 weeks (once the endotracheal tube pressure is relieved), with ultimate re-epithelialization of the mucosal surface. The healing process results in the variable deposition of scar tissue with thickening of the submucosa in the subglottic space.

Other factors felt to play a role in the development of acquired subglottic stenosis in neonates include mucosal injury from endotracheal tube movement (shearing effect of the tube on the mucosa), injury from repetitive intubations, inflammation from bacterial contamination of the endotracheal tube, and the possibility of an underlying small airway (where even the smallest endotracheal tube is still too large).

The cross-sectional area of the subglottic lumen is related to the luminal radius: $A = \pi r^2$, where A is the cross-sectional

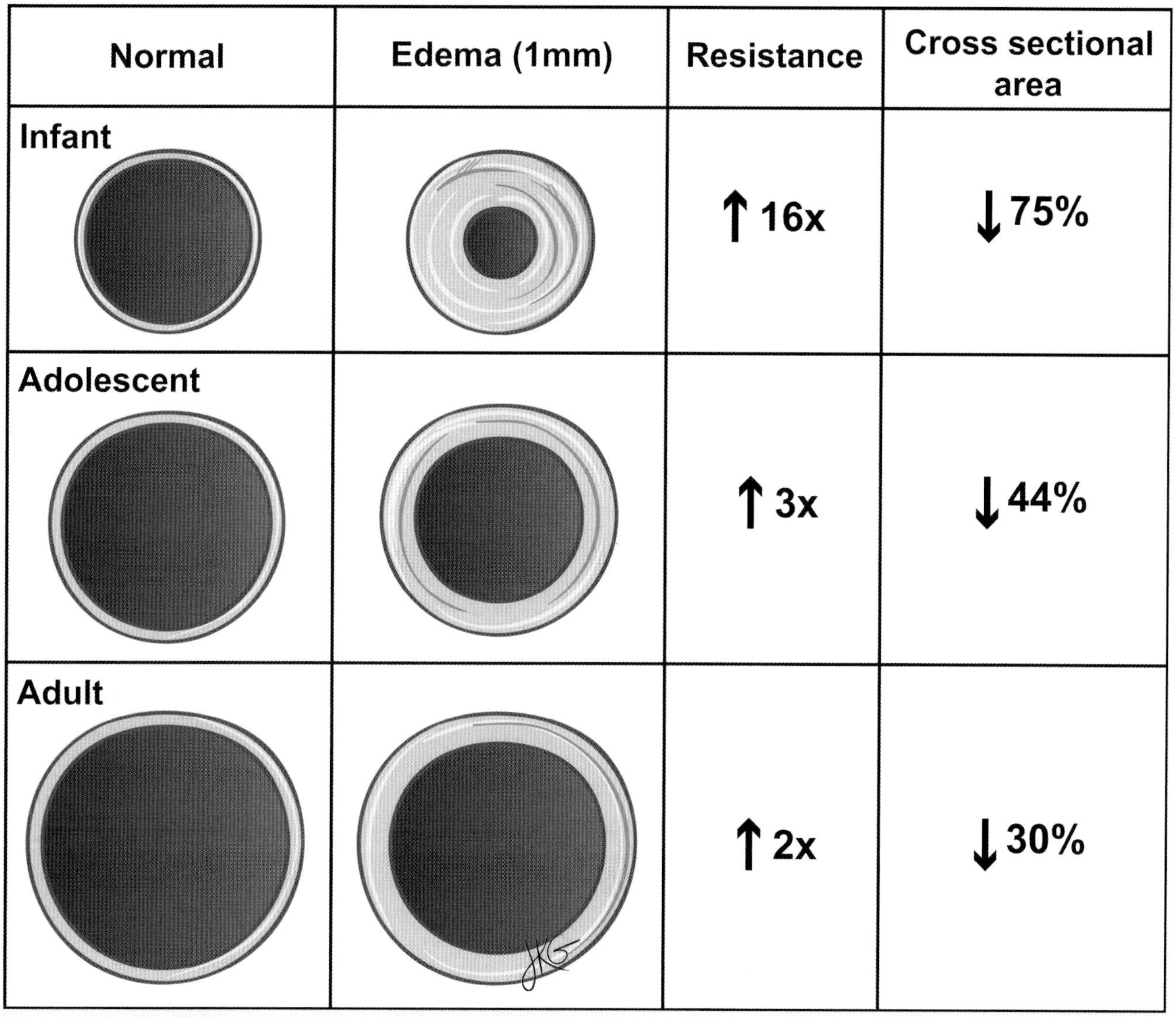

Normal	Edema (1mm)	Resistance	Cross sectional area
Infant		↑ 16x	↓ 75%
Adolescent		↑ 3x	↓ 44%
Adult		↑ 2x	↓ 30%

Fig. 72.9 The same degree of mucosal edema affects the smaller airways of children more severely than those of adults.

area and r is the radius of the subglottic lumen. Thus a very small decrease in the radius, for example from 4 to 3 mm, will decrease the cross-sectional area about 75%. This translates into a 16-fold increase in airflow resistance within the airway. Because of this effect on the luminal area, children are subject to significant respiratory disturbance from even minor respiratory conditions (▶ Fig. 72.9).

When the mucosal lining the airway is injured, it responds with an accumulation of inflammatory cells and mediators. The inflammatory response results in the development of edema within the mucosa. Depending upon the degree and severity of the inflammatory response and edema, tracheal intubation may be needed to maintain a patent airway despite the possibility of exacerbating the problem with the subglottic luminal size. Soon after the inciting event, increased fibroblast activity with collagen deposition will develop in the submucosa, and scar tissue will form in any areas of mucosal erosion. This process is stimulated and worsened by associated gastroesophageal reflux and acid contact with the mucosa. Once collagen and

scar tissue are deposited, the lumen remains narrowed. Direct (blunt or penetrating) trauma and endotracheal intubation are associated with the worst stenosis.

Congenital subglottic stenosis is present in babies at birth but may not be evident until an upper respiratory tract infection develops. The most common cause of congenital subglottic stenosis is an abnormally shaped cricoid cartilage or an abnormally formed cricoid with a smaller than normal lumen (▶ Fig. 72.10).

Natural History, Disease Complications, and Prognosis

The effects of subglottic stenosis vary greatly depending upon the severity. Subglottic stenosis can range from very mild, with minimal effect on the patient, to life-threatening. Perpetuation of the inciting cause of the stenosis can increase the degree of stenosis, so it is imperative to remove the causative agent as soon as possible. All care should be taken to use appropriately

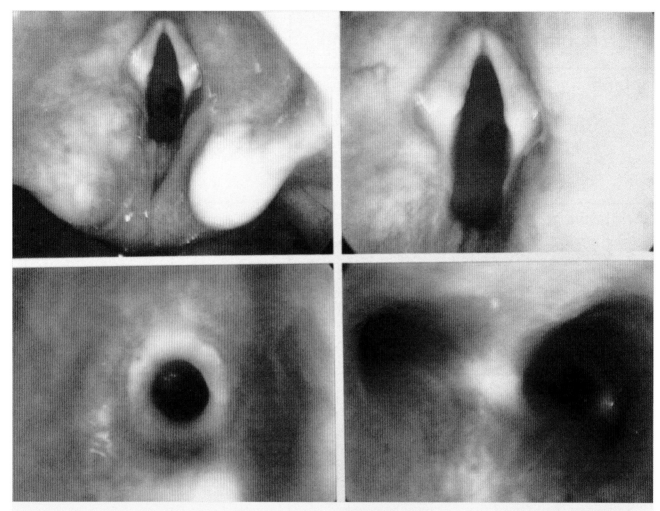

Fig. 72.10 Intraoperative images demonstrating grade II subglottic stenosis (*lower left panel*).

sized endotracheal tubes in children, and to ensure that the cuff of the endotracheal tube is located in the proper midtracheal position in order to protect the laryngeal subglottis.

In most cases, once subglottic stenosis has developed and the healing phase of subglottic injury has occurred, the stenosis is considered to have matured and stabilized. At this point, the narrowing becomes relatively fixed (barring any acute inflammation from upper respiratory infections, for example), and it is unlikely to resolve spontaneously. Some cases will continue to worsen because of continued trauma to the mucosa and submucosa from an unremedied inciting condition. Respiratory symptoms in these children may progress to severe distress and fatigue. At this point, it is necessary to secure the child's airway by intubation (if possible) or by tracheotomy (if the lumen will not permit passage of an endotracheal tube). High-potency steroids, such as dexamethasone, are frequently used in an effort to reduce inflammation, stabilize the mucosa, and prevent further edema. Death from airway obstruction may result if this process is delayed.

Subglottic stenosis is classified based upon the degree of narrowing in comparison with normal airway luminal size. The most commonly used grading scale is the Myer-Cotton system, which divides subglottic stenosis into four categories (▶ Ta-

Table 72.4 Myer-Cotton grading scale for subglottic stenosis

Grade	Percentage laryngeal luminal obstruction
I	0–50%
II	51–90%
III	91–99%
IV	No detectable lumen

ble 72.4). The categories are valuable in predicting the likelihood of success with the treatment options for subglottic stenosis. Grade I ranges from a normal luminal size to luminal obstruction of 50%, grade II indicates airway luminal obstruction of 51 to 90%, grade III is luminal obstruction of 91 to 99%, and grade IV indicates no detectable airway lumen.

In order to grade subglottic stenosis, the airway lumen must be examined and measured during laryngoscopy with the patient under general anesthesia. After inspection of the larynx, subglottis, and trachea, the airway is measured with a standard uncuffed endotracheal tube. The outer diameter of an uncuffed endotracheal tube is of uniform measured size and is used to assess the airway luminal size (although the "size" of a tube is

Table 72.5 Appropriate endotracheal tube size by patient age

Age	Endotracheal tube size (mm)
Premature	2.0–3.0
Birth–3 mo	3.0–3.5
3–12 mo	3.5–4.0
12 mo–2 y	4.0–4.5
2–4 y	4.5–5.0
4–6 y	5.0–5.5
6–8 y	6.0
8–10 y	6.5
10 y–adult	6.5 or larger

designated by its internal, not external, diameter). After placement of an uncuffed endotracheal tube, the airway is observed under magnification (typically a telescope is used) for air bubble escape as the anesthesiologist slowly increases the airway pressure. A normal leak is considered to be at a pressure of 18 to 24 cm H$_2$O. Lower pressures indicate excessive space around the tube, whereas higher pressures indicate that the tube is too large; the tube is exchanged for a larger or smaller one, and the leak pressure is measured again. The endotracheal tube size with which the pressure is closest to the normal leak pressure is deemed the airway size (▶ Table 72.5). Measurement of the airway size is a standard component of the endoscopic airway examination.

Presenting Symptoms

In either acquired or congenital subglottic stenosis, inspiratory or biphasic stridor is heard (biphasic stridor is noted in the most severe cases of luminal narrowing). The stridor may be constant, even during sleep and with quiet respiration. Feeding may be affected, and failure to thrive is frequent because the infant is unable to manage the increased respiratory effort needed to coordinate breathing and swallowing. In this situation, the child forgoes feeding and will lose weight because of the increased caloric energy needed for the work of breathing and the insufficient nutrients obtained from feeding.

Other symptoms of subglottic stenosis include chest and tracheal retractions, and a raspy or rattling sound may be heard during breathing when secretions are located at the stenosis site. Cyanosis and oxygen desaturation are late findings seen when respiratory failure is imminent.

Medical Evaluation and Physical Examination

The child with subglottic stenosis will typically present with stridor as the chief complaint. Because of the variable degree of luminal obstruction, it is imperative to determine the severity of airway compromise at the initial evaluation and take action immediately if there is severe respiratory distress.

In less severe cases, the medical evaluation should focus on any antecedent history of intubation, instrumentation in the airway, and conditions that may have led to airway trauma. The birth history and the need for airway support at birth are important. The history should reflect the effect of upper respiratory infections and any change in stridor/airway distress caused by those episodes. Feeding problems are important in determining the cause of airway distress.

The physical examination should focus on the airway and include both auscultation and inspection of the airway passages. Flexible laryngoscopy is integral in the diagnosis and should be performed in all but the most unstable children (in whom the airway often will need to be examined in the operating room, with ultimate treatment of the underlying condition). Despite the limitations of flexible laryngoscopy in visualizing the subglottis, it may reveal stenosis, and it is invaluable in excluding other causes of stridor. Ultimately, most children with subglottic stenosis require microlaryngoscopy with bronchoscopy under general anesthesia. Occasionally, imaging studies such as anteroposterior and lateral plain radiographs of the neck, CT fluoroscopy, and MR imaging are helpful in characterizing the stenosis. An evaluation of any coexistent gastroesophageal reflux is important because it is a known exacerbating factor.

Children who are intubated at the time of evaluation for subglottic stenosis present with a history of (often repetitively) failed extubation. The duration of intubation, reason for the initial intubation, and size of current and previous endotracheal tubes are important factors. The degree of prematurity and coexistent cardiac or pulmonary conditions all play a role in the evaluation. These children require evaluation of the airway under controlled conditions, usually in the operating room, with microlaryngoscopy and bronchoscopy. Granulation tissue, edema, and erosion in the subglottis and adjacent glottis are usually seen in patients with subglottic stenosis. The leak around the endotracheal tube is measured and compared with norms.

Treatment

The treatment of subglottic stenosis is tailored according to the degree of respiratory distress it induces. The vast majority of ambulatory children with mild (grade I) subglottic stenosis can be observed and managed expectantly. These children usually do not exhibit signs or symptoms of stridor or respiratory distress until an upper respiratory infection develops. The additional mucosal edema caused by the upper respiratory infection will often lead to the development of mild to moderate stridor, with a crouplike cough. Moderate retractions and distress often lead parents to bring these children for emergency treatment. In such cases, supportive management with corticosteroids for a few days and racemic epinephrine via nebulizer can provide substantial relief of their respiratory distress.

Children with higher grades of subglottic stenosis (grades II through III) frequently have symptoms of airway obstruction sufficient to require more aggressive management. Children with grade IV subglottic stenosis will always be tracheotomy-dependent because they have no discernible airway lumen. The airway obstruction of these children will have progressed from grade III to grade IV during the healing process. Children with grade IV stenosis will always require airway reconstructive surgery after decannulation. Children with grade II and grade III subglottic stenosis are often symptomatic and most often require intervention to improve their airway.

Neonatal Management

Babies with multiple failed attempted extubations who are found to have subglottic stenosis are usually managed based upon the findings at microlaryngoscopy and bronchoscopy. Infants with findings of mild edema, minimal to no mucosal ulceration, normal laryngeal function, and no other cause for the failed extubation attempts are frequently treated with the removal of any granulation tissue, polyp, or cyst found; reintubation with a smaller endotracheal tube (typically 0.5 mm to a full size smaller); the administration of dexamethasone; and observation for several days in anticipation of the reduction of any edema. The infant is then extubated following 48 to 72 hours of dexamethasone therapy (up to 1 mg/kg/d divided into two doses) and observed for the potential need for further airway support.

Anterior Cricoid Split

Some infants with isolated subglottic stenosis may benefit from an anterior cricoid split procedure. For infants who fail the above extubation protocol, or in whom an endotracheal tube of a smaller than usual size has been placed, an anterior cricoid split may be considered. Carefully selected candidates for anterior cricoid split are babies who weigh more than 1,500 g; have stable, controlled cardiac and pulmonary function; and have no other conditions preventing extubation (see Box Criteria for Anterior Cricoid Split).

Anterior cricoid split is performed through a horizontal midline neck incision. The cricoid cartilage is incised vertically to allow the subglottic lumen to expand. In this procedure, the only complete ring of the airway, the cricoid cartilage, is incised in one or more locations to allow the area of the subglottis to expand. An endotracheal tube one size larger than the tube previously used acts to distract the cricoid edges and stent the airway lumen during the healing period. The infant is then extubated after premedication with dexamethasone (up to 1 mg/kg/d) under controlled conditions, with a tracheostomy tray and intubation instruments immediately available, about 6 to 10 days after the procedure. In the event of respiratory distress or obstruction, the infant is intubated, or a tracheostomy is placed through the prior neck incision (▶ Fig. 72.11).

Criteria for Anterior Cricoid Split

1. Weight of more than 1,500 g
2. No assisted ventilation for > 10 days
3. Oxygen supplementation requirements < 35% FiO_2
4. Stable congestive heart failure for > 1 month
5. No hypertension medications required for > 14 days
6. Failed extubation two or more times with a laryngeal cause
7. Absence of pulmonary or airway infection

The anterior cricoid split procedure is useful in carefully selected patients and can avoid the need for more involved airway reconstructive surgery (laryngotracheal reconstruction procedures) and for tracheotomy. A current modification of the anterior cricoid split is to add a small piece of cartilage harvested from the conchal bowl or upper portion of the thyroid cartilage lamina as a stabilizing graft.

The complications of anterior cricoid split include failure of the procedure to relieve airway obstruction at the subglottis. Postoperatively, spontaneous ventilation is preferred over

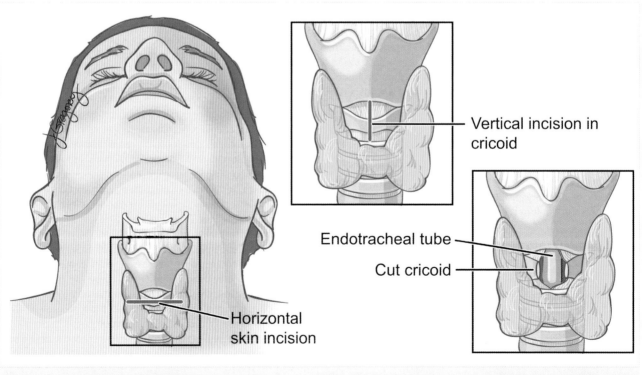

Fig. 72.11 Anterior cricoid split procedure.

mechanical ventilation because the former is associated with lower risk for pneumonia. Intubation must be secure, and the patient must not be accidentally extubated during the 6- to 10-day healing period. Signs of inadvertent dislodgement of the endotracheal tube include subcutaneous air with crepitus, pneumomediastinum, and pneumothorax. If the endotracheal tube becomes dislodged, it is best to reinsert it via the neck wound under direct vision in the emergency setting. Conversion to nasotracheal intubation either over a flexible bronchoscope or telescope allows the most accurate repositioning of the ETT.

Laryngotracheal Reconstruction

Laryngotracheal reconstruction involves expansion of the laryngotracheal structure to relieve an obstructed lumen. Successful laryngotracheal reconstruction requires a careful assessment of the length and exact location of the stenosis, and of the likelihood of continued or future need for prolonged intubation. Also required is optimization of the laryngeal obstruction, including treatment of the cause of the stenosis and the control of gastroesophageal reflux. Any child for whom laryngotracheal reconstruction is being considered must be a suitable candidate for the administration of general anesthesia.

Laryngotracheal reconstruction requires placement of a cartilage graft as well as stenting of the airway lumen. Various graft options are available, including costal cartilage (the most commonly used), auricular cartilage, and thyroid alar cartilage. The ribs are the preferred source of cartilage because of the large amount of donor material available and its excellent strength and robust qualities. Costal cartilage is usually harvested from the fifth or sixth anterior rib via a transverse incision placed under the breast. A generous graft is harvested, with care taken

to avoid injury to the perichondrium on the inner surface of the rib, which will cause pneumothorax.

Use of the thyroid ala cartilage is less frequent unless a small graft is necessary. The benefit of thyroid cartilage for grafting is that the donor site is within the surgical field. It is less useful when robust material is needed to distract the cricoid cartilage in higher-grade stenoses. Auricular cartilage has the least strength as a graft material because of its thinness in very young children. It often does not maintain the needed shape and has a tendency to buckle.

A stent is needed to maintain the airway lumen during the healing period after the procedure. Many patients who undergo laryngotracheal reconstruction require stenting for a prolonged period, extending from weeks to months in some cases. Stent materials vary, but many airways are stented with endotracheal tubes (when stenting is for 1 to 2 weeks) or with Teflon stents (Aboulker stent) for longer-term use. Different stents are used depending upon whether the patient has a preexisting tracheostomy at the time of the laryngotracheal reconstruction and on whether the laryngotracheal reconstruction is done as a single-stage or a double-stage procedure. It is important to note that the stent passes though the larynx, so it will prevent phonation and may increase aspiration while in place. The patient often will have a tracheotomy in place when a long-term stent is needed to maintain the airway. Stenting times increase with stenosis of a more advanced grade or the presence of significant scar tissue, and in previously reconstructed airways. Laryngotracheal reconstruction is performed after optimization of these factors.

The laryngotracheal reconstruction is performed through a horizontal neck incision (▶ Fig. 72.12). After the cartilage (usually costal) graft has been harvested, the larynx and trachea are exposed, and a vertical incision is made in the midline of

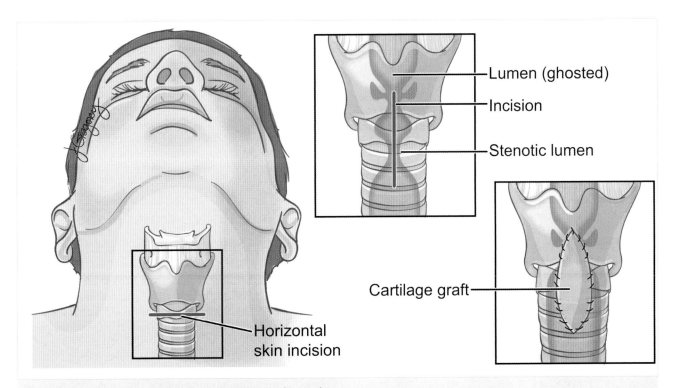

Fig. 72.12 Laryngotracheal reconstruction with cartilage graft procedure.

the cricoid cartilage with entry into the subglottic space. This incision is extended superiorly into the lower third of the thyroid cartilage, with care taken to avoid dividing the anterior commissure. The upper two tracheal rings are incised in continuity with the cricoid incision. At this point, either a stent is positioned into the airway (multiple-stage procedure with a tracheostomy in place) or the endotracheal tube is exchanged for another endotracheal tube that is 0.5 to 1.0 mm larger (single-stage procedure) and placed nasotracheally. The incision into the airway is then widened, and the cartilage graft is shaped to insert into the enlarged cricotracheal incision. The graft is sutured into position with 4–0 polypropylene sutures. A passive drain is placed over the reconstructed airway and the wound closed. If a stent is placed, it is secured with a transcricoid suture to avoid entry into the distal airway and resultant airway obstruction.

The patient is then monitored in a critical care unit (patients undergoing a single-stage procedure are monitored to prevent accidental premature extubation). The endotracheal tube is removed, and similar precautions are taken as for a patient undergoing anterior cricoid split (with a tracheostomy tray, intubation instrumentation, and laryngoscopy equipment at the bedside) following preparation with 24 to 48 hours of dexamethasone to reduce edema.

Patients who undergo double-stage laryngotracheal reconstruction are treated with a stent and a new or established tracheostomy. The stenting period will vary depending upon the patient's unique stenosis pattern. These stents require removal in the operating room, with a small neck incision to release the suture traversing the stent and endoscopic removal of the stent following premedication with dexamethasone. The tracheostomy is maintained until the reconstructed airway lumen is fully healed and adequate patency is ascertained.

In both types of laryngotracheal reconstruction, the endoscopic removal of granulation tissue and subsequent laser removal of residual scar tissue from the airway are often necessary. A carbon dioxide laser with a microscope and micromanipulator hand piece or fiber-optic contact delivery system is most commonly used.

Grade IV subglottic stenosis presents the most complicated situation in the relief of airway obstruction. In the past, four-quadrant laryngotracheal reconstruction was used, with anterior, posterior, and lateral cricoid incisions and prolonged stenting. More recently, cricotracheal resection has gained popularity. In this procedure, the entire airway obstruction is excised, along with the anterior and lateral aspects of the cricoid. Care is taken to avoid recurrent laryngeal nerve injury by maintaining the perichondrium and the posterior portion of the cricoid cartilage. The superior tracheal edge is then secured to the inferior edge of the thyroid cartilage with permanent suture. Stenting is with either an endotracheal tube (in a single-stage procedure) or a traditional Teflon stent and tracheostomy for a period of 7 to 21 days. A high rate of eventual decannulation can be achieved with this procedure.

Endoscopic Management of Subglottic Stenosis

In mild or limited cases of subglottic stenosis, and in postoperative patients following laryngotracheal reconstruction, endoscopic procedures are common. Scar and granulation tissue can be removed endoscopically with traditional forceps, microdébrider, or carbon dioxide laser. These techniques are very simple and may be repeated as needed to maintain and guide healing in the airway. The topical application of mitomycin C is a well-known treatment that is effective in reducing the development of scar tissue in the airway. Reported complications of mitomycin C application are infrequent. Laser is an acceptable treatment for stenotic lesions that are less than 10 mm in length, retain sufficient support of the cartilaginous structures, and are isolated in either the subglottis or upper trachea. The use of carbon dioxide laser outside these situations has an increased failure rate. Increasingly, high-pressure airway balloons are being applied in patients with airway stenosis. This dilation procedure is quite successful in breaking dense scar tissue and may have a long-lasting effect.

Complications

Complications of the surgical treatment of subglottic stenosis include those that occur during the procedure or in the early postoperative period and late complications. During the procedure, it is important to avoid lateral dissection around the trachea and inadvertent recurrent laryngeal nerve injury. Air leaking from the reconstructed airway into the surgical wound during emergence from anesthesia may result in subcutaneous emphysema with extension into the chest and the development of pneumomediastinum and pneumothorax. Proper passive drain placement helps to reduce this risk, which persists into the healing phase, especially the first few days following the procedure, until the reconstructed airway seals. It is imperative to avoid early drain removal.

Respiratory distress may follow stent migration or mucous plugging of the endotracheal tube or tracheotomy tube. This can be prevented by frequent suctioning and the use of humidified air. Problems associated with the graft itself include resorption and inward dislodgement. These graft issues may result in lumen intrusion and laryngotracheal reconstruction failure.

Late complications of laryngotracheal reconstruction include recurrence of stenosis with the need for revision surgery and endoscopic procedures. The voice may be poor because of the development of scar at the glottic level or true vocal fold paresis. If the graft protrudes into the lumen excessively, there can be continued airway obstruction. Attention to precise surgical technique and careful postoperative care is paramount for decreasing the occurrence of these problems.

72.5.5 Infectious Diseases of the Airway

Epiglottitis (Supraglottitis)

Epiglottitis is an infectious process affecting the epiglottis and supraglottic structures. In children, it is most often caused by *Haemophilus influenzae* type B (HIB), whereas adult epiglottitis is often caused by *Staphylococcus aureus*. Epiglottitis presents with a rapid onset of symptoms in children between the ages of 2 and 4 years. HIB causes a generalized infection of the epiglottis similar to cellulitis. The incidence of HIB epiglottitis has dramatically fallen in the United States in the last 20 years with the use of routine immunization against HIB, to the point that HIB epiglottitis has become rare.

Clinical Symptoms

The onset of epiglottitis is relatively rapid, with progression over just hours. The child will develop fever, airway distress, and later on stridor and drooling due to odynophagia. Patients often will lean forward and prop themselves up while sitting into a "tripod" position. These symptoms should make one consider epiglottitis as a diagnosis. The inspiratory stridor associated with epiglottitis is due to increasing edema of the supraglottis and impending obstruction.

Patient Examination and Evaluation

Supraglottitis and epiglottitis are serious medical emergencies with the potential to obstruct the airway. A patient suspected of having epiglottitis must be approached calmly and systematically. In order to reduce the child's anxiety, parts of the examination may even need to be omitted until epiglottitis has been excluded as a diagnosis. Although the gold standard is laryngoscopy, this may be deferred initially because of the possibility of making the child cry and subsequently obstruct the airway. In mild cases, a lateral neck X-ray may be obtained (as long as the child is accompanied by someone capable of providing emergency airway support). The typical diagnostic finding on lateral neck X-ray is a "thumb"-shaped density representing the swollen, edematous epiglottis. Older and calm children may tolerate fiber-optic flexible laryngoscopy, which visualizes the swollen epiglottis and supraglottis (▶ Fig. 72.13).

Children presenting with moderate to significant distress are taken immediately to the operating room for airway examination and management. The airway is inspected after the induction of anesthesia with inhalational agents, at which time the airway is secured, most frequently via intubation. (Alternatively, the patient can be ventilated through a rigid bronchoscope and then changed over to nasotracheal intubation.) The epiglottis is cultured. It is mandatory that a tracheotomy tray be open and ready in the event the airway becomes unstable.

Treatment

Epiglottitis is treated with parenteral antibiotics active against HIB. The culture is used to guide antibiotic therapy in refractory cases. Extubation success can be predicted by examining the supraglottic structures with a fiber-optic laryngoscope, and extubation is often possible after 48 to 72 hours of antibiotic therapy. Children with epiglottitis are expected to make a complete recovery and now rarely require a tracheotomy.

Complications

Epiglottitis is a well-known, potentially fatal infectious disease that is rarely seen today. Late diagnosis and misdiagnosis can result in worsening airway obstruction, hypoxemia, and the sequelae of hypoxia. Because of the rare occurrence of epiglottitis, it is necessary to maintain a high index of suspicion with this clinical presentation.

Croup (Laryngotracheobronchitis)

Croup (laryngotracheobronchitis) is an airway disorder affecting children from 6 months to 3–4 years of age. It is usually caused by a parainfluenza virus but may be caused by other respiratory viruses. Croup is more commonly seen in the cooler months and may affect babies and children repetitively, especially if there is an underlying airway anomaly.

Clinical Symptoms

The typical presentation of croup is a more gradual onset of the symptoms of an upper respiratory infection. The child may have rhinorrhea and a cough with a characteristic barky quality. As the infection progresses, a mild to moderate fever will develop. The child will not preferentially be in any position, nor will he or she appear "toxic" (like the child with epiglottitis); as the illness progresses, the voice will become slightly hoarse, and at this point inspiratory stridor (from narrowing at the subglottis and upper trachea) may become audible. The stridor may become biphasic as it worsens. The child may be symptomatic for 3 to 5 days while remaining infectious for up to 10 to 14 days.

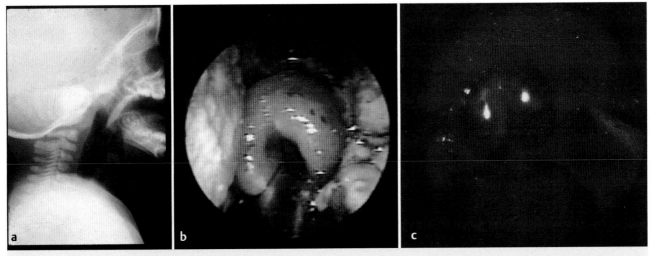

Fig. 72.13 Epiglottitis. (**a**) Lateral neck X-ray demonstrating thumb sign in dilated hypopharygeal air column. (**b**) Intraoperative view of acute epiglottitis; note the swollen epiglottis. (**c**) Laryngoscopic view of swollen, cherry red epiglottis in epiglottitis.

Patient Examination and Evaluation

The child with croup, despite having stridor, does not appear as ill as the child with epiglottitis. The findings of clear rhinorrhea, barky cough, and stridor all lead to the diagnosis of croup. The chest examination is usually normal. Diagnostic lateral and anteroposterior X-rays will often reveal the typical "steeple" sign indicating narrowing at the subglottic–tracheal junction (▶ Fig. 72.14).

Treatment

The treatment of croup (laryngotracheobronchitis) is aimed at decreasing airway edema. The home management of croup typically involves the use of humidification and cool air. Adequate hydration is essential. Most cases of croup are mild forms that can be managed at home.

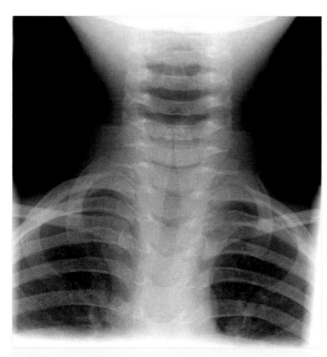

Fig. 72.14 Croup. Anteroposterior soft-tissue neck X-ray demonstrating the "steeple" sign typically seen in croup

Moderate to severe croup requires additional treatment at the clinic or emergency department. The administration of cool mist, along with nebulized racemic epinephrine, will help to reduce airway mucosal edema. Most children with croup at this stage will also benefit from systemic steroids. Steroids are well-known to reduce airway edema and have a prolonged effect. Most children are discharged home after a short stay at the emergency department. A small percentage of children do not respond well to this protocol and require hospitalization and possible intubation.

Complications

Although most children with croup have a complete resolution of their symptoms, a small number do not respond well to therapy. These children progress and often require endotracheal intubation, which entails a risk for subglottic stenosis because of the inflammation already present in the subglottis (▶ Table 72.6).

72.6 Pediatric Tracheotomy

Children who have airway obstruction that is not readily correctible may require tracheotomy to maintain a safe airway. Chronic respiratory failure, pulmonary conditions with ineffective cough, and other medical conditions require tracheotomy. Indications for pediatric tracheotomy are similar to those in adults, except for the duration of intubation. In general, children can remain intubated for up to several months (compared with several weeks for adults) because their more compliant airways are better able to tolerate the presence of an endotracheal tube than are those of adults.

Pediatric tracheotomy in children is routinely performed in the operating room. An anesthesiologist monitors the patient and assists by removing the tube when it is no longer needed. Endoscopic percutaneous tracheotomy is not recommended in children.

72.6.1 Technique

The patient is placed on a shoulder roll with the neck extended. The laryngeal cartilages are palpated, and the skin in the midline over the upper cervical trachea is infiltrated with a small

Table 72.6 Characteristics of epiglottitis and croup

Characteristic	Epiglottitis	Croup
Agent	Haemophilus influenzae type B	Parainfluenza virus
Age	2–5 y	6 mo–2 y
Cough	None	Barky
Drooling	Present	Absent
Stridor	Late, inspiratory	Inspiratory, then biphasic
Rate of onset	Rapid (hours)	Slow (days)
Position	Tripoding (leaning forward)	Any position
X-ray finding	Thumb sign	Steeple sign
Location affected	Supraglottis/epiglottis	Glottis to upper trachea

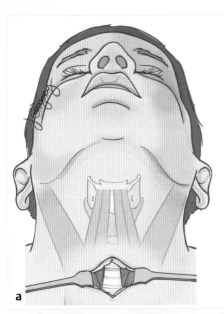
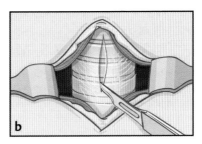
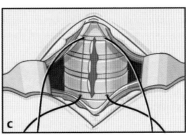
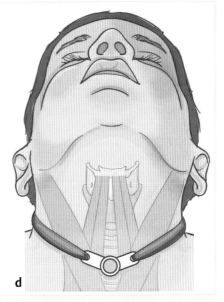

Fig. 72.15 Technique of pediatric tracheostomy. (a) Pediatric tracheostomy demonstrating vertical skin incision and retraction of the strap muscles laterally. (b) Vertical division of the pretracheal fascia exposing the cricoid cartilage and upper tracheal cartilage rings. (c) Placement of polypropylene stay sutures lateral to the vertical tracheotomy incision. (d) Tracheostomy tube in position with tracheostomy ties secured around the child's neck.

amount of local anesthetic (▶ Fig. 72.15). A vertical skin incision is made over the second to fourth tracheal cartilages. The immediate subcutaneous fat is dissected between the skin and cervical fascia and removed. The strap muscles are identified and separated at the midline raphe. The trachea and cricoid cartilage are visualized. Tracheal rings are palpated with a fingertip. Stay sutures are placed in the tracheal lateral to the incision and later marked "RIGHT" and "LEFT." After identification of the tracheal rings, a vertical incision is made through rings 2 to 4, between the two stay sutures. The endotracheal tube is directly visualized within the tracheal lumen. The skin may be sutured to the tracheal edges, maturing the stoma and reducing the risk for accidental false passage, with 5–0 chromic sutures.

At this point, the anesthesiologist slowly withdraws the endotracheal tube just until the tip of the tube is seen at the tracheal opening. A tracheostomy tube of the appropriate size is directly positioned into the trachea. The anesthesia circuit is attached to the tracheostomy tube, the chest is auscultated for bilateral breath sounds, and the end-tidal carbon dioxide values are observed on the anesthesia machine. Tracheotomy ties are secured around the patient's neck, and the tube may also be sutured to the neck skin if desired. A chest X-ray is taken to check the tube tip position relative to the carina and to check for pneumothorax.

72.6.2 Complications

Pediatric tracheotomy carries a low risk for intraoperative complications in trained individuals. The low risk is due to the superficial position of the trachea in the child. Tracheotomy in children with neck masses or tumors presents unique challenges, and adaptations are necessary in those cases. Improper tube selection is a potential complication leading to an early need to change the tracheotomy tube before an established tract is formed. This increases the risk for accidentally creating

a false passage and a malpositioned tube, with the potential complications of pneumomediastinum and pneumothorax. Potentially fatal mucous plugging occurs from a combination of two conditions, lack of adequate air humidification and insufficient suctioning.

Caregivers must learn the proper care and management of tracheostomy in children. This includes correct techniques for suctioning, cleaning the stoma, and changing the ties, as well as knowing how to change the tube. Visiting nurses can reinforce the proper techniques with caregivers and reduce complications in tracheotomy-dependent children.

72.7 Foreign Bodies in the Airway and Esophagus

72.7.1 Etiology

Children are prone to aspiration and the ingestion of foreign bodies because of their tendency to explore objects by placing them into the mouth. Children who are 3 years old and younger are at the greatest risk for choking on both small objects and small, hard foods. Each year, approximately 150 children die after ingesting or aspirating foreign bodies.

72.7.2 Pathogenesis

Foreign body ingestion and aspiration most commonly occur in children younger than 3 years of age, with far fewer foreign bodies found in the aerodigestive tract in older children. The combination of the oral exploration of objects, a high level of physical activity and running, the introduction of adult types of foods, and access to small objects and toy parts leads to increased risks in the toddler. Small, hard foods, such as popcorn kernels, nuts, and seeds, are the aspirated items most commonly found in young children. These foods present particular hazards to very young children until all 20 of their primary teeth have completely erupted (usually between 2 and 3 years of age) and they can sit and chew their foods thoroughly rather than hold them within the mouth (increasing the risk for aspiration).

Coins are the most common esophageal foreign body in children younger than 4 years of age, with pennies the most common foreign body extracted. Older children may ingest nickels, quarters, and other objects. The size of the esophagus and the coin diameter are the factors that determine esophageal passage or impaction.

72.7.3 Natural History

A foreign body within the aerodigestive tract usually will cause symptoms that require medical attention and subsequent removal of the foreign body. When foreign bodies are not detected, they may cause significant morbidity and possibly death from complications of their presence.

Foreign bodies within the tracheobronchial tree may present with intermittent symptoms of cough depending upon their location and whether they move around in the large airways. Impacted foreign bodies in the more distal bronchial airways will often cause the formation of a reactive granulation tissue (particularly if they consist of food matter), increased secretions, and subsequent distal pneumonia. Pneumonia that is refractory to appropriate treatment may be caused by an undetected foreign body. Long-standing foreign bodies may erode through the bronchus into the mediastinum or result in bronchiectasis.

Undetected foreign bodies in the esophagus create a risk for esophageal perforation. Long-standing or sharp-edged esophageal foreign bodies may create erosions of the mucosa and then the muscular layer of the esophagus, with ultimate perforation of the esophagus. Esophageal perforation can result in mediastinitis, with high rates of morbidity and mortality. Some children with esophageal foreign bodies may begin to "wheeze" if edema of the tracheo-esophageal wall develops, with resultant narrowing of the tracheal lumen.

72.7.4 Presenting Symptoms

Most children who have a foreign body in the aerodigestive tract present with an episode of choking or coughing after being observed to place an object or food substance in the mouth. These witnessed events require a careful evaluation to exclude an actual aspiration or ingestion of the object.

Airway foreign body aspiration may present with alteration of the voice, stridor, severe coughing, cyanosis, and wheezing, depending upon where the foreign body is located. Children who have bronchial foreign bodies may present with unilateral wheezing, a specific variety of stridor resulting from bronchial obstruction by the object. Oxygen saturation should be measured and hypoxemia immediately treated.

Children who have esophageal foreign bodies may initially not have many symptoms but will ultimately develop dysphagia or odynophagia, reduced oral intake, and drooling; older children will complain of chest pain. Some children who have long-standing esophageal foreign bodies may present with "wheezing" or the new onset of asthma due to swelling of the tracheo-esophageal wall. Disc battery ingestion may present with severe chest pain within hours of esophageal impaction as a consequence of the leakage of alkali from the battery.

72.7.5 Medical Examination

The examination of a child who has a foreign body in the airway or esophagus and in whom ingestion was witnessed or is suspected should immediately assess the severity of the problem. Airway foreign bodies may cause severe respiratory distress and hypoxemia, creating an urgent management situation. It is important to interview the caregivers/parents to determine the details of the ingestion, time since the incident, and any associated feeding or breathing problems before and after the incident.

Chest X-rays are the most useful imaging studies for both esophageal and airway foreign bodies. Most esophageal foreign bodies in this age group are radiopaque and will easily be seen on anteroposterior chest X-rays. Lateral chest X-rays are helpful in confirming an esophageal location and, in the case of disc-shaped objects, determining whether the object is a disc battery or a coin.

Airway foreign bodies also can be seen on anteroposterior and lateral chest X-rays, if radiopaque. With radiolucent objects, inspiratory and expiratory anteroposterior films may demonstrate air trapping on the affected side (▶ Fig. 72.16). In children too young for inspiration–expiration films to be obtained, a bilateral lateral decubitus chest series should be performed, again with observation for mediastinal shift and air trapping. Lung hyperinflation and atelectasis may also be seen when there is a foreign body in the airway.

72.7.6 Treatment

Documented esophageal and bronchial radiopaque and obvious foreign bodies are removed with rigid endoscopy under general anesthesia. Even when no foreign body is visible on radiographic examination, severe or prolonged symptoms often will lead to a diagnostic endoscopic examination under general anesthesia. In patients with severe symptoms of suspected foreign body aspiration, immediate endoscopy with general anesthesia is necessary (▶ Fig. 72.17).

Esophageal foreign bodies are usually removed via rigid esophagoscopy under general anesthesia, with protection of the airway. Methods such as Fogarty catheter extraction of a foreign body and flexible esophagoscopy without airway protection may compromise the airway in young children as the foreign body is extracted, and they are not advised. For children who have ingested smooth foreign bodies like coins, a brief period of observation for passage to the stomach, and proper NPO (nil per os) status, may be considered, with progression to rigid endoscopy if unsuccessful. Most coinlike foreign bodies will naturally pass from the gastrointestinal tract after they reach the stomach. If the object is suspected by history or X-ray to be a disc battery, endoscopic removal should proceed without delay in the hope of extracting the battery before leakage of the alkaline contents, which may occur within hours of the ingestion.

Removal of an esophageal foreign body is performed with endotracheal intubation and muscle relaxation, in order to prevent esophageal perforation by the esophagoscope during the procedure. After intubation, the patient is positioned and the

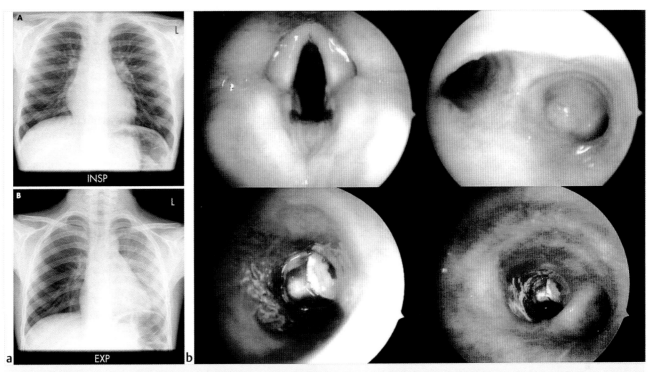

Fig. 72.16 Bronchial foreign body. (a) Upper panel: Inspiratory chest X-ray. Lower panel: Expiratory chest X-ray demonstrating air trapping in the right side of the chest caused by a right bronchial foreign body. (b) Endoscopic images of the removal of a right main bronchial foreign body.

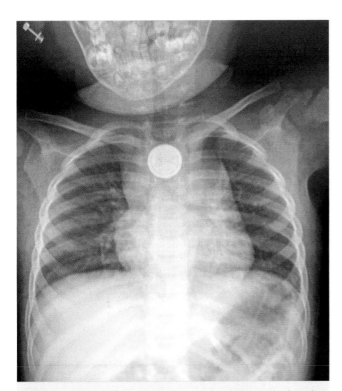

Fig. 72.17 Chest X-ray of a radiopaque esophageal foreign body at the level of the thoracic inlet, with the distinct rim appearance of a disc battery.

esophagoscope is carefully placed into the hypopharynx and then passed through the region of the cricopharyngeus muscle at the esophageal inlet. The scope is slowly and gently advanced, with the lumen always in view. The scope is advanced to the foreign body, the object is grasped with an appropriate forceps (most commonly the "coin-removing" forceps), and the object and scope are removed as a unit, with the foreign body trailing behind the scope. After the foreign body is removed, the esophagoscope is reinserted into the esophagus and the mucosa is inspected for injury from the foreign body. Long-term foreign bodies may have caused erosions of the mucosa or partial-thickness injuries of the muscle of the esophagus. Care must be taken to avoid converting a partial perforation into a full-thickness injury.

Bronchial foreign bodies require rigid endoscopic removal under general anesthesia, preferably with a pediatric anesthesiologist in attendance. Careful preparation of the instrumentation and joint management of the airway with the anesthesiologist are essential to success. The child is brought into the operating room, and general anesthesia is induced via either mask inhalation or a previously placed intravenous line. Careful laryngoscopy, with an inspection of all laryngeal surfaces and the application of a topical anesthetic to the larynx and trachea, is done after an adequate depth of anesthesia is established. Most commonly, the child remains spontaneously breathing throughout the procedure.

A telescope within the rigid bronchoscope is used to inspect the airway, and the patient is ventilated (spontaneously or with assistance) through the ventilating port of the rigid bronchoscope. The airway is examined, the normal bronchus first and then the bronchus with the foreign body. The normal side is initially studied to determine the presence of a single foreign body and a patent airway for ventilation if single-lung ventilation becomes necessary. Suitable optical forceps (containing a telescope) are selected depending upon the specifics of the foreign body, with the "peanut" forceps most commonly used. The foreign body is grasped and carefully removed, trailing behind the bronchoscope as the bronchoscope is withdrawn from the airway. Care is taken at the glottis because the object may become dislodged from the forceps. The bronchoscope is then reinserted to inspect for complete removal and for any trauma or injury to the impaction site. Granulation is frequently seen in cases of organic or long-standing foreign bodies, and postobstructive pneumonia with purulent secretions may be expected. Rarely, injuries to the bronchus may be noted and include perforation with bronchopleural fistula, pneumothorax, or pneumomediastinum. Children need to be observed following the procedure depending upon the antecedent symptoms and findings on bronchoscopy.

72.7.7 Prognosis

The vast majority of children with foreign body ingestion and aspiration make a complete recovery. In patients with a prompt diagnosis and removal of the foreign object, the postoperative course is usually uncomplicated. Patients with delayed or protracted symptoms of long-standing foreign bodies may require hospitalization for management of the underlying co-morbidities.

72.8 Roundsmanship

- The pediatric larynx is broader and higher in the neck than the adult larynx.
- A careful and complete history is critical in evaluating a child with a breathing problem. The evaluation includes an assessment for stridor and flexible laryngoscopy for a diagnosis.
- Laryngomalacia is the most common cause of stridor in infants. True vocal fold paralysis is the second most common cause of stridor in infants, followed by subglottic stenosis.
- Laryngomalacia is usually accompanied by gastroesophageal reflux. The medical management of laryngomalacia consists of treatment of the gastroesophageal reflux with histamine$_2$ blockers and proton pump inhibitors, with 95% of cases well controlled.
- Failure to thrive and obstructive apnea are the most common reasons for the surgical management of laryngomalacia. Supraglottoplasty is the procedure of choice.
- A patient with bilateral vocal fold paralysis has a good voice but commonly an inadequate airway due to the paramedian true vocal fold position.

- A patient with unilateral vocal fold paralysis often has a poor voice but a satisfactory airway.
- Left true vocal fold paralysis is more common that right true vocal fold paralysis. The left recurrent nerve has a longer course because it wraps around the ductus arteriosus and aortic arch and is at risk for injury when ductus arteriosus ligation is needed.
- Recurrent respiratory papillomatosis is a chronic condition requiring multiple periodic procedures to remove obstructive papillomas from the airway tract. Human papillomaviruses type 6 and type 11 are the main causative agents. Human papillomavirus vaccination may reduce the rate of recurrent respiratory papillomatosis in children.
- Hoarseness is the most common presenting symptom of recurrent respiratory papillomatosis.
- Hemangiomas are vascular tumors that may cause stridor. They are seen in the posterolateral aspect of the subglottis. The preferred treatment currently is oral propranolol. The hemangiomas usually also respond well to dexamethasone.
- Subglottis stenosis most frequently is acquired as a result of prolonged intubation in children. Treatment options vary depending upon the severity. Laser, balloon dilation, and subglottic expansion surgery for the stenosis are treatment options.

72.9 Recommended Reading

[1] Benjamin B, Inglis A. Minor congenital laryngeal clefts: diagnosis and classification. Ann Otol Rhinol Laryngol 1989; 98: 417–420

[2] Derkay CS, Wiatrak B. Recurrent respiratory papillomatosis: a review. Laryngoscope 2008; 118: 1236–1247

[3] Gallagher TQ, Hartnick CJ. Laryngotracheal reconstruction. Adv Otorhinolaryngol 2012; 73: 31–38

[4] Gustafson LM, Hartley BE, Liu JH et al. Single-stage laryngotracheal reconstruction in children: a review of 200 cases. Otolaryngol Head Neck Surg 2000; 123: 430–434

[5] Hartnick CJ, Cotton RT. Stridor and airway obstruction. In: Bluestone CD, Stool SE, Alper CM, et al, eds. Pediatric Otolaryngology. 4th ed. Philadelphia, PA: W. B. Saunders; 2003

[6] Horn DL, Maguire RC, Simons JP, Mehta DK. Endoscopic anterior cricoid split with balloon dilation in infants with failed extubation. Laryngoscope 2012; 122: 216–219

[7] Myer CM, O'Connor DM, Cotton RT. Proposed grading system for subglottic stenosis based on endotracheal tube sizes. Ann Otol Rhinol Laryngol 1994; 103: 319–323

[8] Myer CM, Cotton RT, Shott SR. The Pediatric Airway: An Interdisciplinary Approach. Philadelphia, PA: J. B. Lippincott; 1995

[9] Rosbe KW, Suh KY, Meyer AK, Maguiness SM, Frieden IJ. Propranolol in the management of airway infantile hemangiomas. Arch Otolaryngol Head Neck Surg 2010; 136: 658–665

[10] Williams H. Inhaled foreign bodies. Arch Dis Child Educ Pract Ed 2005; 90: ep31–ep33

73 Diseases and Disorders of the Pediatric Neck

James M. Pearson

73.1 Embryology and Anatomy

73.1.1 Embryology of the Larynx

The larynx, along with the rest of the respiratory system, is derived from the primitive pharynx. At 3 weeks gestation, the hypobranchial eminence forms. This will become the cartilaginous epiglottis. In the ventral foregut of the embryo, the laryngotracheal groove develops at 3 1/2 weeks. This groove is located posterior to the hypobranchial eminence, between the third and fourth branchial arches. The mesenchyme of the foregut grows in a lateral to medial direction, eventually bisecting this groove. Two separate tubes form that will ultimately become the esophagus and the laryngotracheal apparatus.

At 4 weeks, the cricothyroid and inferior pharyngeal constrictor muscles develop. These and other laryngeal muscles develop from the mesoderm of the fourth and fifth branchial arches and thus are innervated by cranial nerve X (vagus). At 5 weeks, the arytenoid masses appear; at this time, the thyroid and cricoid cartilages form, also derived from the fourth and fifth branchial arches, respectively. At 5 1/2 weeks, the interarytenoid and postcricoid muscles develop. In week 6, the lateral cricoarytenoid muscles appear. Between the weeks 5 and 7, the laryngeal lumen is obliterated, and by 7 weeks, chondrification of the thyroid and cricoid cartilages begins. Between weeks 8 and 10, the vocal folds are formed, while during week 9, the laryngeal lumen is reestablished. By 12 weeks, the arytenoids and corniculate cartilages, both derived from the fifth branchial arch, develop further and undergo chondrification; also at this time, the laryngeal ventricles appear. By 20 weeks, chondrification of the epiglottis takes place, and by 28 weeks, the cuneiform cartilage is seen, derived from the fourth branchial arch (▶ Fig. 73.1).

Congenital anomalies result from a failure of the normal sequence of embryonic development. The two arytenoid masses, which are seen by 5 weeks, are initially separated by a notch that is later obliterated. If this obliteration fails to occur, a pos-

terior laryngeal cleft may be seen. Such a cleft may open into the esophagus and cause severe aspiration in the newborn. Failure of the laryngeal lumen to recanalize by week 9 of development results in laryngeal atresia or stenosis.

73.1.2 Embryology of the Thyroid Gland

The thyroid gland derives from a diverticulum between embryologic tongue precursors at the site of the foramen cecum. Apparent at 4 weeks, this ventral (thyroid) diverticulum of endodermal origin is located between the first and second branchial arches. It then descends caudally in mesodermal tissues. By 6 weeks, the diverticulum is typically obliterated. Persistence of the tract of this descent may lead to the formation of a thyroglossal duct cyst later in life. The tract begins at the foramen caecum, passes either superficial to, through, or just deep to the hyoid bone, and continues caudally to the final location of the thyroid gland in the lower neck.

73.2 Anatomy of the Neck

The anatomical space of the neck is defined inferiorly by the clavicle and superiorly by the skull base posteriorly and the mandible anteriorly. The neck may be subdivided superficially by various triangular areas and in cross section by fascial planes.

Broadly, each side of the neck may be divided into two triangles, anterior and posterior, separated by the sternocleidomastoid muscle (▶ Fig. 73.2). The anterior cervical triangle is then subdivided into four smaller triangles: digastric, carotid, muscular, and submental. The posterior cervical triangle is subdivided into two smaller triangles: occipital and subclavian. These triangles are separated from one another by various bones, cartilages, and muscles. The contents of the triangles are clinically relevant in discerning structures that

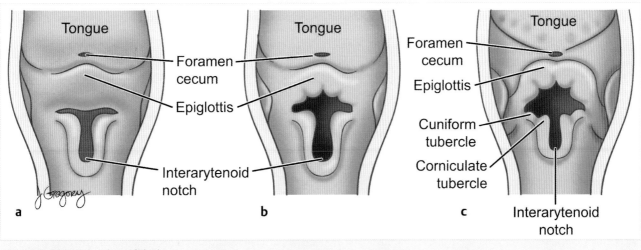

Fig. 73.1 (a–c) Embryology of the larynx.

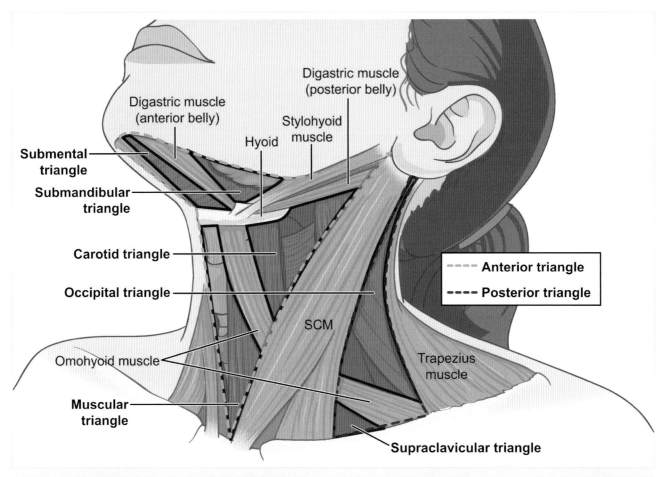

Fig. 73.2 Triangles of the neck. *SCM*, sternocleidomastoid.

may be involved in various pathologic conditions affecting the neck, ranging from cervical masses to penetrating trauma to infections.

When considered in cross section, the neck may be divided into spaces by anatomical fascial planes that separate the neck spaces and structures. Broadly, the fascial layers may be divided into the superficial and deep cervical fascia (▶ Fig. 73.3). The superficial cervical fascia envelops the platysma and the muscles of facial expression. The deep cervical fascia is subdivided into three layers: superficial, middle, and deep. The superficial layer of the deep cervical fascia envelops the trapezius, sternocleidomastoid, and strap muscles. The middle layer of the deep cervical fascia envelops the pharynx, larynx, trachea, esophagus, thyroid and parathyroid glands, buccinator and constrictor muscles of the pharynx, and strap muscles of the neck. The deep layer of the deep cervical fascia (also known as the prevertebral fascia) envelops the paraspinous muscles and the cervical vertebrae. Clinically, the fascial planes of the neck limit and direct the spread of infection and abscesses. Knowledge of the contents of these spaces can aid in differentiating the etiology, symptoms, and sequelae of various deep space neck infections.

Detailed descriptions of the borders and contents of each subtriangle and space are beyond the scope of this introductory chapter. The interested reader is directed to more detailed discussions of this topic.

73.3 Cervical Lymphadenopathy

By convention, the location of the cervical lymph nodes is described in terms of levels. The neck is subdivided into six levels. Level I denotes the neck inferior to the mandible, superior to the hyoid bone, and anterior to the sternocleidomastoid muscle. Levels II, III, and IV lymph nodes lie roughly along the sternocleidomastoid muscle; level II extends from the mastoid process superiorly to the level of the hyoid bone inferiorly, level III between the hyoid bone and the cricoid cartilage, and level IV from the cricoid cartilage to the clavicle. Level V lymph nodes are located posterior to the sternocleidomastoid muscle. Level VI lymph nodes are located in the lower anterior neck medial to the sternocleidomastoid muscle and inferior to the hyoid bone (▶ Fig. 73.4).

A thorough examination of the neck is an integral part of any pediatric otolaryngologic evaluation. The entire neck should be visually inspected and manually palpated. Often, lymph nodes will be palpable in the normal pediatric neck. Normal lymph nodes typically exhibit the following characteristics: nontender, mobile with regard to both the skin and deeper structures, spherical or ovoid in shape, and no larger than 10 mm in diameter. During or immediately following a head and neck infection or upper respiratory infection, it is not abnormal to find lymph nodes that are tender to palpation and/or larger than 10 mm. Isolated cervical lymphadenopathy should arouse suspicion in

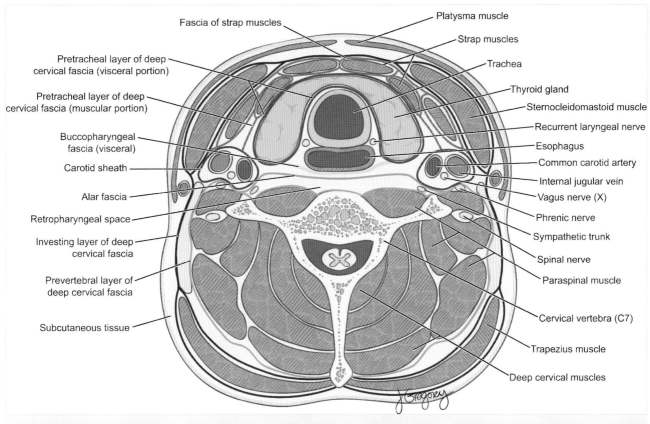

Fascia of strap muscles
Platysma muscle
Strap muscles
Pretracheal layer of deep cervical fascia (visceral portion)
Trachea
Pretracheal layer of deep cervical fascia (muscular portion)
Thyroid gland
Sternocleidomastoid muscle
Recurrent laryngeal nerve
Buccopharyngeal fascia (visceral)
Esophagus
Carotid sheath
Common carotid artery
Internal jugular vein
Alar fascia
Vagus nerve (X)
Retropharyngeal space
Phrenic nerve
Investing layer of deep cervical fascia
Sympathetic trunk
Spinal nerve
Prevertebral layer of deep cervical fascia
Paraspinal muscle
Cervical vertebra (C7)
Subcutaneous tissue
Trapezius muscle
Deep cervical muscles

Fig. 73.3 Fascial planes of the neck demonstrated in an axial section of the neck at the level of C7.

the clinician as to its cause. A detailed history and physical examination may uncover a subclinical infection. Cervical nodal characteristics that are suspicious include the following: nodes that are persistently enlarged to more than 10 mm and/or remain tender for more than 4 to 6 weeks after a precipitating infection has resolved, nodes fixed to skin or underlying structures, nodes larger than 20 mm even in the acute setting, and fluctuance, which may indicate abscess or necrosis within a node.

Physical examination alone may be adequate to evaluate cervical lymphadenopathy. In certain situations, imaging may be indicated. For example, nodes deep to the sternocleidomastoid muscle may not have palpable borders and may be indistinguishable from other masses of the neck. Similarly, when the entirety of a node cannot be palpated, the evaluation of nodal size may present a challenge. Finally, surgical planning and determining the relationship of a node of interest to adjacent structures and major blood vessels are greatly aided by the information provided by imaging. When indicated, radiographic imaging with contrast-enhanced computed tomography (CT) is the modality of choice. Consideration should be given to minimizing the exposure of patients in general, and especially children, to radiation so as to avoid the known serious sequelae of chromosomal damage and risk for future cancers.

The otolaryngologist is often called upon to evaluate cervical lymph nodes in children and to discern normal cervical nodes from pathologic ones. Using the information described above along with the rest of the clinical scenario, the clinician must make a decision to either observe or treat. Furthermore, the

clinician needs to be able to explain the rationale for that decision to the patient, family members, and the consulting pediatrician.

The treatment of cervical adenopathy in children depends on its etiology. Early on, the etiology may not be entirely clear, and the cervical nodes themselves are the focus of attention. When appropriate, a period of watchful waiting may be indicated—for example, during or immediately following a head and neck infection in an otherwise healthy and stable patient who has cervical adenopathy smaller than 20 mm and no suspicious characteristics. The family is reassured that the cervical adenopathy at hand does not demonstrate any suspicious findings and does not warrant any aggressive intervention at that time, and that the child will be closely followed for anticipated regression of the nodes in question. It is helpful if they are provided with a time frame within which to expect improvement or resolution, along with subsequent steps that may be taken if the nodes do not regress. Another option may be to treat with antibiotics cervical adenopathy that is suspected to be secondary to infection. A 10- to 14-day course of amoxicillin with potassium clavulanate, or clindamycin in the penicillin-allergic patient, may be employed. In more suspicious cases, fine-needle aspiration (FNA) biopsy performed in the clinic with cytopathologic interpretation, with or without culture of the aspirate, may be considered. Depending on the age, maturity, and cooperation of the child, this course of action may need to be performed under sedation or general anesthesia.

If there is a significant degree of clinical suspicion, when an FNA biopsy is insufficient or nondiagnostic, or when less

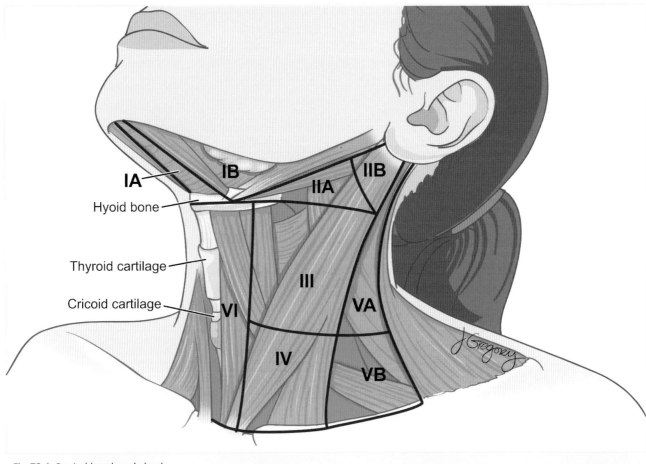

Fig. 73.4 Cervical lymph node levels.

invasive measures do not yield a diagnosis, excisional biopsy of an enlarged cervical node may be employed. This procedure typically requires general anesthesia and must be performed in the operating room. Once the specimen is removed, the surgeon may consider sending it fresh, along with cultures for bacteria (aerobic and anaerobic), fungi, and acid-fast bacilli. A fresh specimen, sent in saline, preserves the option of flow cytometry analysis should the pathologist's interpretation be suspicious for lymphoma.

73.4 Infections of the Deep Neck Spaces

Since their first detailed descriptions in the 1930s, the morbidity and mortality of deep space neck infections have decreased drastically. However, infections of the deep neck spaces are still seen with regularity, and the otolaryngologist is often called upon to diagnose the source or location of infection, differentiate infections from abscesses, and surgically treat appropriate cases. Earlier in this chapter, the fascial planes of the neck were introduced. Here, the cervical spaces defined by those fascial planes will be further explored, along with the etiology, spread, manifestations, and treatment of infections contained therein.

Deep space neck infections are typically polymicrobial infections caused by various oral aerobes and anaerobes, and occasional respiratory or skin pathogens. Common organisms include the following: *Staphylococcus* species (including methicillin-resistant *Staphylococcus aureus* [MRSA]), *Streptococcus* species (including *S. pneumoniae*), *Fusobacterium necrophorum*, *Bacteroides* species (including *B. fragilis*), *Haemophilus* species, *Klebsiella*, *Escherichia coli*, *Enterobacter*, *Enterococcus*, *Neisseria*, *Eikenella corrodens*, and *Prevotella* (*Bacteroides melaninogenicus*). The preferred empiric therapy is clindamycin, an augmented penicillin, or a third-generation cephalosporin. In children, the preferred alternative is vancomycin and metronidazole given together.

The well-known clinical fact that children have little physiologic reserve and may decompensate quickly must be acknowledged. In other words, children may appear only mildly sick upon presentation yet be gravely ill. However, their clinical condition can rapidly deteriorate to frank sepsis or airway compromise.

The descriptions below pertain to infections of specific cervical spaces, which may be suspected clinically based on their characteristic manifestations and/or radiographic appearance. The relevant anatomy is reviewed, and the common sources, routes of spread, characteristic manifestations, and complications of these infections are discussed, as well as their treatment.

Clinically, the infections often present with systemic symptoms of fever and leukocytosis. Head and neck findings that should arouse suspicion include odynophagia, dysphagia, trismus, "hot potato" voice, and asymmetry or fullness of the affected cervical region. In more advanced stages, intolerance of secretions (drooling) and difficulty breathing may be seen. Unlike adults, younger children may be unable to describe their symptoms; the clinician must then rely upon a history provided by the family and physical findings alone.

As a general rule, when a deep space neck abscess is suspected, radiographic imaging is often indicated to provide details regarding its size and location, and imaging is useful for surgical planning. If the abscess is not life-threatening and is superficial or limited to the peritonsillar area, treatment is often employed based on the history and clinical examination findings alone, without radiographic studies. When indicated, the preferred study is CT of the neck with intravenous (IV) contrast extending from the skull base to the clavicle.

Generally, the treatment of infections of the deep neck in children, as in adults, involves antibiotic therapy, protection of the airway, and surgical drainage when appropriate. If the airway is compromised, IV steroids may be considered; dexamethasone (up to 0.6 mg/kg/d administered IV and divided into doses given every 6 to 12 hours) is commonly used. If there is concern about impending loss of the airway, intubation may be undertaken prophylactically. In some cases, intubation is not possible, and urgent tracheostomy is the only means of obtaining an airway. In preparation for this, it is prudent to keep intubation and tracheostomy supplies readily available when caring for such patients. Antibiotic therapy is begun empirically with broad-spectrum antibiotics to cover the polymicrobial nature of such infections. If possible, culture is taken from the abscess cavity, and culture and sensitivity testing is performed by the microbiology laboratory. With a small or uncertain abscess, a trial of antibiotics may be appropriate. Clinical improvement is gauged over the following 24 to 36 hours based on symptoms, temperature curve, and other physical findings. For large or rapidly progressive abscesses, surgical drainage is often needed. The surgical approach depends on the site of infection, as detailed below.

73.4.1 Peritonsillar Space

Peritonsillar abscess (▶ Fig. 73.5) is the most frequently encountered deep space neck infection in practice. Suspected peritonsillar abscess is an extremely common source of consultation of the otolaryngologist by primary and urgent care physicians. Familiarity with the diagnosis and treatment of this condition and with differentiating abscess from tonsillitis or peritonsillar cellulitis is crucial.

The peritonsillar space is defined by the capsule of the palatine tonsil medially and the superior constrictor muscle laterally. Infections originate from the tonsils or pharynx. Clinical manifestations of a peritonsillar abscess include odynophagia, dysphagia, muffled voice, and trismus. Findings especially characteristic of peritonsillar abscess include contralateral deviation of the uvula across the midline and an inferomedially displaced and enlarged tonsil. Treatment entails perioral drainage by incision and drainage or needle aspiration; antibiotics against streptococci are given orally or IV. Patients with peritonsillar abscess must be able to tolerate adequate oral fluids before discharge. Complications include spread into the lateral pharyngeal space and reaccumulation of the abscess.

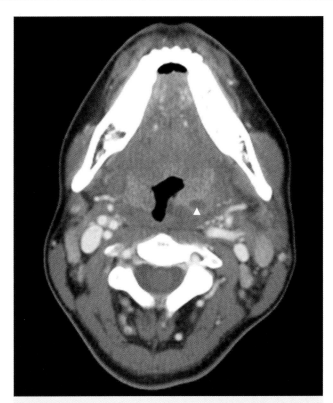

Fig. 73.5 Axial computed tomographic scan demonstrates a peritonsillar abscess medial to the left tonsil (*arrowhead*). (Courtesy of David Dascal, MD, and Mae Mae Chu, MD.)

73.4.2 Lateral Pharyngeal Space

The term *lateral pharyngeal space* is synonymous with *pharyngomaxillary space*. Conical in shape, the lateral pharyngeal space extends from the base of the skull superiorly to the hyoid bone inferiorly. This space is subdivided by the styloid process into prestyloid and poststyloid compartments. The prestyloid compartment (also known as the muscular compartment) is located anterior to the styloid process. It contains fat, lymph nodes, the internal maxillary artery, and several nerves (inferior alveolar, lingual, and auriculotemporal). The poststyloid compartment (also known as the neurovascular compartment) is located posterior to the styloid process. It contains the carotid artery, internal jugular vein, sympathetic chain, and cranial nerves IX, X, XI, and XII.

Infections of this space originate from various sources, including the tonsils, pharynx, teeth (especially the third molar), petrous portion of the temporal bone, parotid gland deep lobe, and lymph nodes draining the nose and pharynx. The spread of infection to this space occurs via direct extension from communicating spaces or extension from a peritonsillar abscess. Clinical manifestations include medial displacement of the lateral pharyngeal wall and tonsil, trismus, dysphagia, parotid edema, and fullness of the retromandibular neck. Treatment may involve tracheotomy (for establishment of a secure airway), along with external drainage through the submaxillary fossa. An intraoral approach should not be undertaken because in most cases, the great vessels (carotid artery and jugular vein) are medial to the abscess (between the pharynx and the vessels) and are at great risk for injury.

The complications of a lateral pharyngeal space infection may be quite serious. The most common complication is septic thrombosis of the internal jugular vein. The most common fatal complication is erosion of the carotid artery. Cranial nerve involvement can occur in the setting of involvement of the neural contents of the poststyloid compartment of this space. Mediastinitis may develop following spread along the carotid sheath.

73.4.3 Pterygopalatine Fossa

The pterygopalatine (pterygomaxillary) fossa communicates laterally with the infratemporal fossa via the sphenomaxillary fissure. It contains the maxillary nerve, sphenopalatine ganglion, and internal maxillary artery. Infections here may arise from maxillary molars (especially the third molar) and osteomyelitis of the maxilla in infants. Spread is through direct extension via the open communication, as noted above. Clinical manifestations include gingival pain and edema; cellulitis of the ipsilateral head (including the face, neck, and temporal region); orbital symptoms (lid edema, globe proptosis and fixation, abducens paralysis); severe trismus; and secondary infection of the maxillary sinus. Treatment requires external drainage through an intraoral approach (gingivobuccal sulcus) or a Caldwell-Luc incision.

73.4.4 Masticator Space

The masticator space is the subperiosteal space between the mandibular bone and the periosteum. It contains the mandibular bone, masseter and pterygoid muscles, temporalis muscle tendon, inferior alveolar nerve, and internal maxillary artery. Infections originate from the mandibular molars (especially the third molar). Clinical manifestations include trismus and painful swelling over the posterior ramus of the mandible. Treatment involves external drainage.

73.4.5 Parotid Space

The parotid space contains the parotid gland, cranial nerve VII (facial nerve), external carotid artery, and posterior facial vein. Infections originate from the parotid gland. Clinical manifestations include painful swelling near the angle of the mandible. Treatment involves external drainage via a parotidectomy incision. Complications include infectious spread into the lateral pharyngeal space with the potential for further spread to the mediastinum.

73.4.6 Submandibular Space

The submandibular space is subdivided by the mylohyoid muscle into the sublingual (supramylohyoid) space and the submaxillary (inframylohyoid) space. The sublingual space contains the sublingual gland. The submaxillary space contains the submandibular gland and lymph nodes (▶ Fig. 73.6). Infections here originate most often from the teeth, especially the third molars, but also from the salivary glands, pharynx, tonsils, and sinuses. Clinical manifestations include dysphagia and odynophagia. The treatment approach depends on the location. Sublingual space abscesses are approached intraorally, whereas a submaxillary space abscess is approached externally via a transverse incision below the mandible.

The complications of a submandibular space infection may be severe. Infection in the submandibular space, known as Ludwig angina, is a potentially life-threatening infection of the floor of the mouth and submental and submandibular spaces. Characteristic findings include a hard, "woody" induration of the anterior neck. Immediate attention must be given to airway maintenance because airway obstruction from posterior displacement of the tongue base is the most common cause of death with this condition. Tracheostomy is often indicated, along with external drainage; dental extraction of abscessed teeth is performed when necessary.

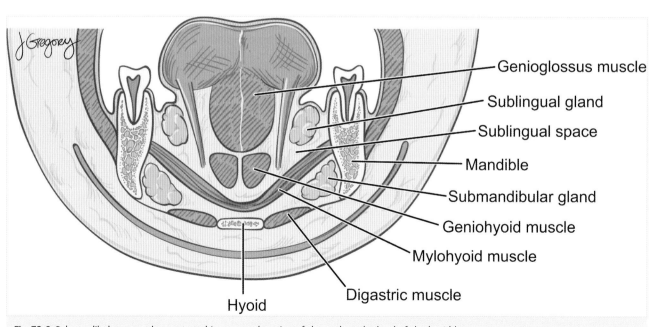

Genioglossus muscle
Sublingual gland
Sublingual space
Mandible
Submandibular gland
Geniohyoid muscle
Mylohyoid muscle
Digastric muscle
Hyoid

Fig. 73.6 Submandibular space demonstrated in a coronal section of the neck at the level of the hyoid bone.

73.4.7 Carotid Sheath Space

The carotid sheath space contains the carotid artery, internal jugular vein, and cranial nerve X (vagus). Infections here originate from other cervical spaces, including the lateral pharyngeal, submandibular, and visceral spaces. Clinical manifestations include pitting edema over the sternocleidomastoid muscle and torticollis. Treatment entails external drainage. Complications may be serious and include septic shock, carotid artery erosion, endocarditis, and cavernous sinus thrombosis.

73.4.8 Visceral Space

The visceral space contains the pharynx, esophagus, larynx, trachea, and thyroid gland. Infections in this space develop from the tonsils, esophageal perforation, laryngeal trauma with mucosal tear, or acute thyroiditis, or infection may spread from the chest. Clinical manifestations include dysphagia, odynophagia, hoarseness, and dyspnea. Treatment involves surgical drainage via transverse incision along the anterior border of the sternocleidomastoid muscle. Complications include extension into the adjacent mediastinum.

The retropharyngeal space, danger space, and prevertebral space lie adjacent to one another, oriented anteriorly to posteriorly, and are separated by three layers of fascia: the middle layer of the deep cervical fascia, also called the buccopharyng-eal fascia (the most anterior); the alar fascia; and the prevertebral fascia (most posterior; ▶ Fig. 73.7).

73.4.9 Retropharyngeal Space

Involvement of the retropharyngeal space is seen primarily in young children as a complication of upper respiratory infections. This is a consequence of the relatively larger number of lymph nodes in the retropharyngeal space found in children younger than 4 years of age. The retropharyngeal space extends from the skull base superiorly to the mediastinum inferiorly. The middle layer of the deep cervical fascia, which envelops the pharynx and esophagus, lies anteriorly, while the alar fascia is posterior. Infections in the retropharyngeal space arise from the nose, sinuses, adenoids, and nasopharynx. The clinical manifestations of retropharyngeal space infections include dysphagia, odynophagia, dyspnea, cervical rigidity, muffled voice, and unilateral bulging of the posterior pharyngeal wall. Surgical access may be via intraoral drainage (if caught early) or an external approach. Given the anatomy, mediastinitis is the most worrisome complication of retropharyngeal abscesses.

73.4.10 Danger Space

Just posterior to the retropharyngeal space lies the danger space, between the alar fascia anteriorly and the prevertebral

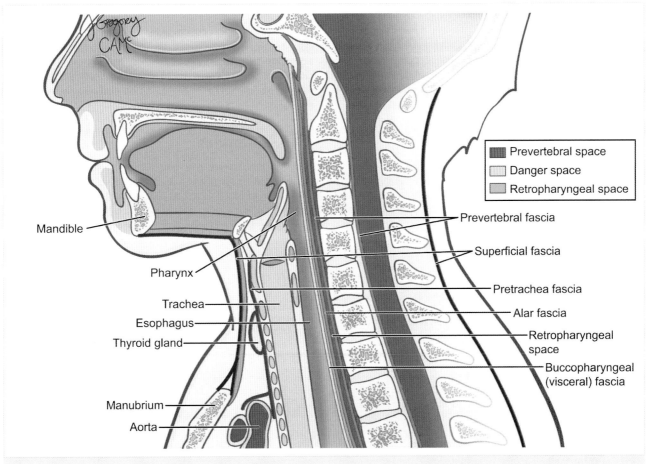

Fig. 73.7 Fascial planes of the neck demonstrated in a mid-sagittal section of the neck.

fascia posteriorly; this space contains only loose areolar tissue. Infections here are a result of spread from adjacent neck spaces. The danger space is so named because it extends from the base of the skull to the diaphragm and may channel the spread of infection along this course to the lower mediastinum.

73.4.11 Prevertebral Space

The prevertebral space lies just behind the prevertebral fascia and anterior to the vertebral bodies. It contains only areolar tissue. Infections here, which are uncommon in modern times, may result from the anterior spread of vertebral osteomyelitis.

73.5 Neck Masses: Diagnosis and Treatment

When a neck mass is being considered in the pediatric population, a complete differential diagnosis should be formulated based on the clinical scenario. The general categories of the differential to be considered include congenital, infectious and inflammatory, neoplastic, and traumatic etiologies.Congenital neck masses include hemangiomas, vascular malformations and tumors, dermoids, teratomas, thymic cysts, plunging ranulas, branchial remnants, and thyroglossal duct cysts.

73.5.1 Hemangiomas

Hemangiomas are the most common neoplasm of childhood. Epidemiologically, the head and neck are the most common sites of hemangioma (10% of cases in Caucasians), with a higher incidence in preterm infants and females; girls are three times more likely to be affected than boys. Typically, hemangiomas begin as small lesions that develop in the first few weeks of life and begin to enlarge several weeks later (proliferative phase); this phase lasts most of the first year of life. At 6 to 9 months of age, spontaneous regression (involutional phase) typically begins and lasts for several months. The diagnosis is usually made by the history and physical examination alone. With deeper lesions, imaging studies may be needed to delineate their size and extent. In the absence of significant symptoms, watchful waiting is often undertaken because of the expected natural course of involution. Symptoms of airway compromise, visual field involvement, and cosmetic deformity usually warrant consideration for more aggressive treatment. Treatment modalities include intralesional or systemic steroids, propranolol, laser therapy, and surgical excision.

73.5.2 Vascular Malformations

Vascular malformations and tumors can take several forms. They may be classified as purely venous, lymphatic, lymphaticovenous, or arteriovenous. Certain imaging modalities may aid in differentiating the various types from one another. CT, magnetic resonance (MR) imaging, and MR angiography are all employed as indicated. Treatment involves surgical resection. Arteriovenous malformations may be clinically discerned by findings related to their high rate of blood flow, including a palpable thrill, hyperthermia, an audible bruit, visible hypertrichosis, and hyperhidrosis. The treatment of arteriovenous

malformation entails preoperative embolization followed by surgical excision. Commonly employed adjuvant treatments include laser and sclerotherapy.

73.5.3 Dermoids

Dermoids by definition are derived from more than one embryonic layer and made up of a heterogeneous mixture of tissues, such as epithelium, bone, cartilage, and muscle. Clinically, they typically arise in the midline neck, usually in the submental region, are attached to the skin, and are asymptomatic. They may be differentiated from thyroglossal duct cysts, which also occur in the midline neck, by a lack of elevation upon swallowing. Surgical excision is the treatment of choice.

73.5.4 Teratomas

Teratomas are made of mature elements of ectoderm, mesoderm, and endoderm, in addition to immature embryonal tissue. Teratomas may present in newborns with respiratory symptoms due to tracheal compression. These masses are typically large, semicystic, and encapsulated. Ultrasound demonstrates mixed echogenicity and well-defined borders, which differentiate teratomas from lymphatic malformations; the latter are multiloculate with ill-defined borders on sonography. Treatment is by surgical excision.

73.5.5 Thymic Cysts

The third pharyngeal pouch gives rise to the thymus tissue during week 6 of development; by week 9, the thymus descends below the clavicles. Thymic cysts may derive from thymic remnants that persist along the course of embryologic thymic descent, from the angle of the mandible through the midline of the neck.

73.5.6 Ranulas

Plunging ranulas are pseudocysts of the floor of the mouth caused by blockage of a sublingual gland, which leads to the extravasation of mucus. Ranulas may present as a submental mass just off midline with or without an intraoral component in the floor of the mouth. Treatment is by surgical excision of the ranula in continuity with the affected sublingual gland.

73.6 Infectious and Inflammatory Diseases

Infectious and inflammatory conditions associated with pediatric neck masses involve cervical lymphadenitis from various causes, including cat-scratch disease, atypical mycobacterial infection, and Kawasaki disease.

73.6.1 Cat-Scratch Disease

Cat-scratch disease is caused by infection with the gram-negative bacillus *Bartonella henselae*. A history of exposure to cats is the basis for clinical suspicion. The patient will rarely provide this history unsolicited, so it should be explicitly sought in

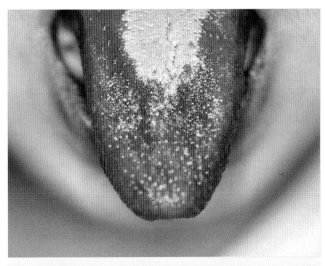

Fig. 73.8 Strawberry tongue.

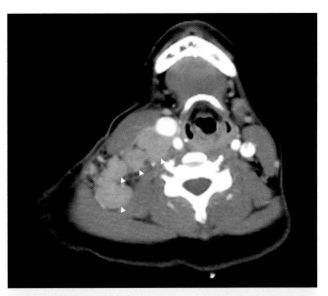

Fig. 73.9 Hodgkin lymphoma as seen on an axial computed tomographic scan of the neck. The bulky mass (*arrowheads*) is located on the right side of the neck medial and posterior to the sternocleidomastoid muscle. The mass displaces the internal jugular vein anteriorly on the right side. (Courtesy of David Dascal, MD, and Mae Mae Chu, MD.)

clinically appropriate circumstances. Aside from cervical lymphadenopathy, patients are typically asymptomatic. Treatment involves a course of azithromycin, which is usually curative. Surgery is reserved for abscesses requiring drainage.

73.6.2 Atypical Mycobacterial Infection

The atypical mycobacteria that are most often associated with cervical lymphadenitis are *Mycobacterium avium-intracellulare* and *Mycobacterium scrofulaceum*. Clinically, erythema of the overlying skin and spontaneous drainage of the affected nodes should arouse suspicion. The diagnosis is supported by the finding of caseating granuloma on a pathologic specimen. Confirmation of the diagnosis requires identification of the infecting organism. Because the culture of mycobacteria may require several weeks, polymerase chain reaction may be used to identify these organisms more expeditiously.

73.6.3 Kawasaki Disease

Kawasaki disease, also known as mucocutaneous lymph node syndrome, is a multisystem vasculitis. Its precise cause is not known, but an infectious etiology is suspected. Epidemiologically, it is seen most often in children younger than age 5. Clinical signs may include the following: nonsuppurative cervical adenopathy larger than 1.5 cm in diameter; mucosal findings of nonexudative conjunctivitis, fissured lips, or strawberry tongue (▶ Fig. 73.8); and skin signs including polymorphous truncal rash, palmar erythema, nonpitting edema of the extremities, and desquamation of the fingers and toes. The diagnosis requires fever lasting more than 5 days and at least four of the clinical signs listed. The most feared complication of Kawasaki disease is coronary aneurysm. Treatment is focused on the prevention of coronary complications and involves aspirin and IV immunoglobulin therapy.

73.6.4 Neoplasms

Neoplasms to be considered in children with a neck mass include rhabdomyosarcoma, lymphoma, and histiocytosis.

73.6.5 Rhabdomyosarcoma

Rhabdomyosarcoma is the most common soft-tissue tumor of childhood. Common sites in the head and neck include the orbit, nasopharynx, temporal bone (middle ear and mastoid), and sinonasal region. Biopsy is required for the diagnosis. Treatment depends on the stage of disease. Surgery should be considered for resectable lesions, because tumor staging is based on remaining disease after surgical biopsy and excision. Radiotherapy and chemotherapy are required for tumors that are not able to be completely resected during the biopsy procedure.

73.6.6 Lymphoma

Lymphoma typically presents with asymptomatic adenopathy. Lymphoma of all types is more common in males. The diagnosis is established by lymph node biopsy. The specimen must be sent fresh (not in formalin) to allow flow cytometry analysis. Treatment is nonsurgical. Early-stage disease is treated with radiation, whereas more advanced disease is treated with both radiation and chemotherapy.

Hodgkin lymphoma (▶ Fig. 73.9) is rare in children younger than age 5 and much more commonly seen in adolescents and young adults; it is twice as common in males. Cervical and supraclavicular lymph nodes are involved 90% of the time; the Waldeyer ring is rarely involved. Pathologically, the presence of Reed-Sternberg cells (multinucleated giant cells) is pathognomonic. Approximately 90% of patients have a good initial response to treatment. Survival in patients with early-stage disease is approximately 90% but decreases to 35% in those with advanced-stage disease.

Non-Hodgkin lymphoma is seen in children between 2 and 12 years old. Unlike in Hodgkin lymphoma, the Waldeyer ring may be involved. The incidence increases in immunosuppressed

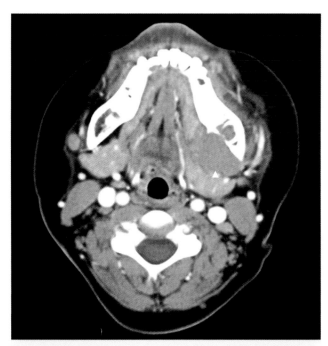

Fig. 73.10 Burkitt lymphoma as seen on an axial computed tomographic scan of the neck. The mass is located on the right side, adjacent to the inner cortex of the mandible (*white arrowhead*). (Courtesy of David Dascal, MD, and Mae Mae Chu, MD.)

patients. The prognosis is less favorable than for the Hodgkin type of lymphoma.

Burkitt lymphoma (▶ Fig. 73.10) is a type of non-Hodgkin lymphoma seen exclusively in children and is associated with Epstein-Barr virus (EBV) infection. Burkitt lymphoma is classified as of either the African type or the North American type of disease. African disease affects the maxilla or mandible. North American disease typically presents with an abdominal mass, with 25% of patients demonstrating head and neck involvement. Treatment involves chemotherapy. The 2-year survival is approximately 50%. Favorable prognostic indicators are age at presentation younger than 12 years and high anti-EBV titers in the North American type. Lymph node biopsy is usually necessary for diagnosis.

73.6.7 Histiocytosis

Histiocytosis is characterized by the abnormal non-neoplastic proliferation of the antigen-presenting Langerhans cell. This disease has a predilection for the anterior cervical lymph nodes. Males are more commonly affected. There are three clinical subtypes: eosinophilic granuloma (disease involving bone only); Hand-Schüller-Christian disease (characterized by fever, bone lesions, and diffuse scalp and ear canal eruptions; the Hand-Schüller-Christian triad is the constellation of diabetes insipidus, exophthalmos, and lytic bone lesions); and Letterer-Siwe disease (rapidly progressive proliferation of histiocytes, generally seen in patients younger than 2 years of age). The diagnosis is made following excisional lymph node biopsy. Treatment options include surgery for limited or focal lesions, radiotherapy for lesions not amenable to surgical excision, and adjuvant therapy for systemic disease. The prognosis is

excellent for patients with limited disease. Hand-Schüller-Christian disease may run a chronic course in more than half of patients. Patients with Letterer-Siwe disease have a 5-year mortality rate of 50% despite chemotherapy.

73.6.8 Fibromatosis Coli

Traumatic neck masses may be related to congenital torticollis (fibromatosis coli) or an arteriovenous fistula. Congenital torticollis presents within the first 6 weeks of life as an asymptomatic neck mass located within the sternocleidomastoid muscle. The diagnosis is based on the history and physical examination. A painless, firm, palpable mass is usually found within the belly of the sternocleidomastoid muscle. Spontaneous resolution is seen in most cases, but muscle shortening may occur. Treatment may involve observation, with physical therapy and range-of-motion neck exercises for infants if torticollis is seen clinically. Surgical release with sternocleidomastoid muscle lengthening is reserved for severe cases, when the child is older.

73.6.9 Laryngocele

Laryngoceles originate from the saccule of the laryngeal ventricle. Clinically, external laryngoceles may present laterally in the neck as a cystic mass located anterior to the sternocleidomastoid muscle. From the laryngeal ventricle, they extend through the thyrohyoid membrane to a position lateral to the thyroid cartilage. Internal laryngoceles are confined within the larynx and do not present as a neck mass. Symptoms associated with laryngoceles may include cough, hoarseness, and globus sensation. Surgery is indicated for symptomatic laryngoceles.

73.6.10 Thyroglossal Duct Cyst

Thyroglossal duct cysts (▶ Fig. 73.11) may arise anywhere along the course of the embryologic descent of the thyroid gland from the foramen caecum of the tongue to its final location in the lower neck. Clinically, they are midline and move with tongue protrusion. Movement with tongue protrusion differentiates thyroglossal duct cysts from other midline neck masses. Histologically, the cyst may contain ectopic thyroid tissue. In some cases, the body's only functioning thyroid tissue is contained within this cyst. Thus, ultrasound evaluation is indicated to confirm the presence of thyroid tissue in its typical position in the neck. Thyroid scanning or noncontrast CT of the neck may aid in determining the presence of normal, functioning thyroid tissue.

Surgical excision, the Sistrunk procedure, is the treatment of choice to prevent recurrence. This procedure removes not only the palpable cyst but also any remnants of the thyroglossal duct, which is followed up to the hyoid bone, and subsequently includes the middle third of the hyoid bone and a cone-shaped portion of the base of the tongue. A high recurrence rate is noted when the hyoid bone midsection and tongue base are not included in the thyroglossal duct cyst procedure. Infection of a thyroglossal duct cyst may be the presenting symptom and is usually treated with oral antibiotics active against streptococci and staphylococci. Incision and drainage may be necessary in refractory infections; if performed, the incision site must also

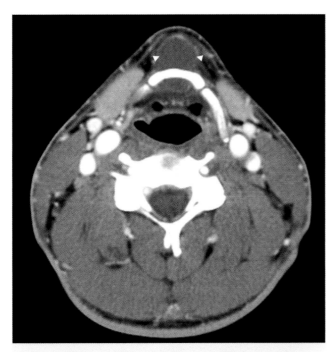

Fig. 73.11 Thyroglossal duct cyst as seen on an axial computed tomographic scan of the neck at the level of the hyoid bone. The cyst is located characteristically in the midline, anterior to and abutting the hyoid bone (*arrowheads*). (Courtesy of David Dascal, MD, and Mae Mae Chu, MD.)

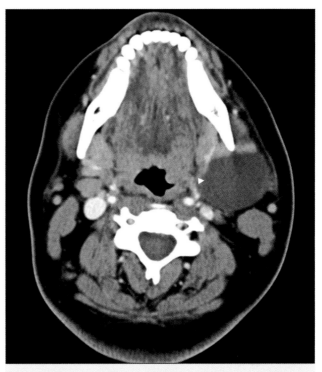

Fig. 73.12 Second branchial cleft cyst as seen on an axial computed tomographic scan of the neck. The cyst is located on the left side (*arrowhead*), characteristically anterior to the sternocleidomastoid muscle. (Courtesy of David Dascal, MD, and Mae Mae Chu, MD.)

be excised along with the lesion in the Sistrunk procedure to reduce the risk for recurrence.

73.6.11 Branchial Cleft Derivatives

Remnants of the embryologic branchial arches are a relatively common cause of pediatric neck masses, accounting for 17% of all such masses. Branchial anomalies may take the form of a fistula (having both an internal opening in the aerodigestive tract and an external opening in the skin), a sinus (having either an internal or external opening only), or a cyst. External openings may be found anywhere along the anterior border of the sternocleidomastoid muscle. Internal openings may be found in various locations within the aerodigestive tract, depending on the arch involved. Branchial anomalies may be classified as either first, second, third, or fourth arch anomalies. The tract of a given branchial anomaly courses caudal to the arch derivatives for which it is named and dorsal to the derivatives of the following arch. CT evaluation aids in the diagnosis. Treatment of each anomaly is by surgical excision. An understanding of the anticipated course of each anomaly aids in the safe and complete excision of each lesion.

First branchial arch anomalies appear on the face or are related to the auricle. They are divided into Work types I and II. Work type I anomalies contain only epidermoid elements, present as duplication anomalies of the external auditory canal, and may course near the facial nerve. Work type II anomalies are more frequently seen. They contain both ectoderm and mesoderm and present in the neck. Clinically, they become evident after infection, typically as an abscess below the angle of the mandible. They course through the parotid gland, either

medial or lateral to the facial nerve, and end inferior to or within the external auditory canal.

Second branchial arch anomalies are the most common type. The tract courses deep to second arch derivatives (external carotid artery, stylohyoid muscle, posterior belly of the digastric muscle) and superficial to third arch derivatives (internal carotid artery). Clinically, a second branchial arch anomaly presents as a painless, fluctuant mass in the lateral neck, anterior to the sternocleidomastoid muscle and below the angle of the mandible (▶ Fig. 73.12). The tract may open into the tonsillar fossa. Classically, the presentation follows an upper respiratory infection.

Third branchial arch anomalies are rare. The tract courses deep to third arch derivatives (internal carotid artery, glossopharyngeal nerve) and superficial to fourth arch derivatives (vagus nerve) to enter the pharynx at the piriform sinus or thyrohyoid membrane. Clinically, they present lower in the neck and anterior to the sternocleidomastoid muscle.

Fourth branch arch anomalies course from the apex of the piriform sinus inferior to the superior laryngeal nerve to the lower neck. They present clinically as recurrent thyroiditis or recurrent lower neck abscesses.

73.7 Thyroid Disorders

Thyroglossal duct cysts typically present as a midline neck mass anywhere along the embryologic pathway of descent of the thyroid gland. This condition has previously been discussed in greater detail.

73.7.1 Lingual Thyroid

Lingual thyroid tissue may be seen in children in the vicinity of the foramen caecum, located in the midline two-thirds of the way back on the dorsal tongue. Children with lingual thyroid may present with a globus sensation, chronic throat clearing, or asymptomatically with a visible mass in the posterior tongue on oral examination.

Like thyroglossal duct cyst, lingual thyroid may be the only functioning thyroid tissue in the body. Ultrasound or CT of the neck should be used to verify if there is thyroid tissue in its typical location in the neck. A thyroid scan may demonstrate the functional status of the lingual thyroid tissue or the thyroid gland. In most cases, a high level of suspicion, combined with the results of thyroid imaging and testing, will make the diagnosis, and biopsy is uncommonly required. Thyroid function testing should be performed because a hypothyroid state commonly accompanies lingual thyroid if it is the only functioning thyroid tissue in the patient. Symptomatic lingual thyroid tissue is treated with thyroid hormone suppression, and in refractory cases, surgical excision may be necessary when symptoms of a globus sensation are not relieved. Consultation with a pediatric endocrinologist is highly recommended.

Aside from thyroglossal duct cysts and lingual thyroid tissue, the incidence of thyroid pathology in the children seen by otolaryngologists in the United States is very low. It should be noted that thyroid nodules in persons younger than age 20 are more likely than those in older adults to harbor cancer, and the finding of a thyroid nodule in a child should be approached with a high index of suspicion.

73.8 Roundsmanship

- Cervical lymph nodes larger than 10 mm or tender for more than 6 weeks after a precipitating infection, fixed to skin, larger than 20 mm in an acute setting, or fluctuant should be considered suspicious.
- When a cervical lymph node biopsy is performed, the surgeon should consider sending the specimen in saline for aerobic and anaerobic bacterial, fungal, and acid-fast bacterial cultures and for flow cytometry, in addition to standard histopathology.
- Deep neck space infections can spread to specific adjacent areas, based on cervical fascial boundaries.
- Polymerase chain reaction testing can speed the identification of acid-fast bacilli infections.
- Kawasaki disease, a multisystem vasculitis, can lead to coronary artery aneurysms.
- Rhabdomyosarcoma is the most common soft-tissue tumor of childhood.
- Complete removal of a thyroglossal duct cyst requires excision of the cyst, the tract up to the hyoid bone, the midportion of the hyoid bone, and a conical section of the tongue base.

73.9 Recommended Reading

[1] Fairbanks DNF. Pocket Guide to Antimicrobial Therapy in Otolaryngology – Head and Neck Surgery. 13th ed. Alexandria, VA: American Academy of Otolaryngology – Head and Neck Surgery; 2007

[2] Janfaza P, Nadol J, Fabian R, Montgomery W. Surgical Anatomy of the Head and Neck. Philadelphia, PA: Lippincott Williams & Wilkins; 2000

[3] Pincus R. Congenital neck masses and cysts. In: Baily BJ, Johnson JT, Newlands SD, eds. Head and Neck Surgery–Otolaryngology. 3rd ed. Philadelphia, PA: Lippincott Williams & Wilkins; 2001

74 Laryngeal Anatomy

Michael J. Pitman

The structure of the mammalian larynx has developed in response to three important needs: protection of the lower airway from aspiration, sound making (phonation), and the generation and maintenance of positive intrathoracic air pressure to withstand compressive forces acting on the thorax. Although each category of demand has fostered its own special features of laryngeal anatomy, it is on the phonatory function and its anatomical adaptations that this section will focus. The phonatory function of humans is the most versatile, variable, and precise among those of the animals that use the larynx for sound making. It owes its capabilities to the evolution of special mechanisms of central nervous control and to special anatomical features, especially at the histologic level.

74.1 Regional Divisions of the Larynx

The interior space of the larynx is conventionally divided into three regions. The supraglottis includes the space that lies above the vocal folds, beginning at the lateral aspect of the ventricle. This region contains the epiglottis, ventricular folds, superior half of the ventricles, aryepiglottic folds, and arytenoid cartilages. The glottis is the space between the vocal folds. It extends from the lateral ventricle to the subglottis, which begins 10 mm inferior to the vocal fold edge anteriorly and 5 mm posteriorly. The subglottis extends to the bottom of the cricoid and is bounded superiorly by the conus elasticus.

Recognition of this vertical division of spaces is clinically important because of regional differences in the nature of the lymph drainage. Specifically, the supraglottic area has the highest density of lymphatic vessels and drains bilaterally into levels II and III. The lymphatic system of the subglottal area has bilateral drainage into the paratracheal and mediastinal lymph nodes. The glottal region is only sparsely supplied with lymphatic channels, and it drains unilaterally to levels II and III. The vocal folds serve as a barrier between the lymphatic systems of the supraglottal and subglottal regions.

74.2 Skeletal Elements

The skeleton of the larynx is cartilaginous and is illustrated somewhat schematically in ▶ Fig. 74.1 and ▶ Fig. 74.2. The cricoid cartilage, typically described as having the shape of a signet ring with a posterior flat lamina, joins the larynx to the trachea and is, in fact, the only complete ring of the trachea. The thyroid cartilage has approximately the form of an ancient war shield. The two flat alae of the thyroid cartilage meet at the anterior midline to form the angle of the thyroid cartilage, which ends superiorly at the thyroid notch. The human larynx is sexually dimorphic, with the male organ approximately 1 1/2 times the size of the female organ. The thyroid angle and thyroid notch are often prominent landmarks on the anterior neck surface, particularly in men. At the posterior–inferior edge of each thyroid ala, an inferior cornu articulates with the posterolateral region of the arch of the cricoid. The corresponding superior cornu and entire superior margin of the thyroid cartilage are suspended from the hyoid bone by the thyrohyoid membrane.

Articulating with the superior edge of the lamina of the cricoid cartilage are two roughly pyramidal arytenoid cartilages. At the triangular base of each arytenoid is the posterolateral muscular process, the point of attachment of the posterior and lateral cricoarytenoid muscles. The forward-projecting vocal process, at the anterior apex of the base of the arytenoid, is the point of attachment for the thyroarytenoid muscle and the connective tissue of the vocal fold. On top of each arytenoid sits the corniculate cartilage. The cuneiform cartilage is then slightly anterior to it and lies within the aryepiglottic fold. Finally, the triticeal cartilages, which are not always present, lie within the connective tissue between the superior horn of the thyroid cartilage and the hyoid bone. The corniculate, cuneiform, and triticeal cartilages are not of clinical significance.

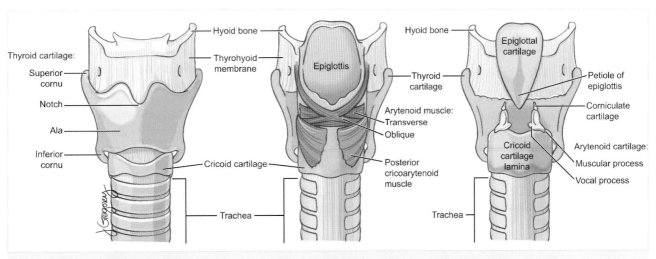

Fig. 74.1 Major structures of the larynx. (**a**) Anterior view. (**b**) Posterior view. (**c**) Posterior view of the cartilage.

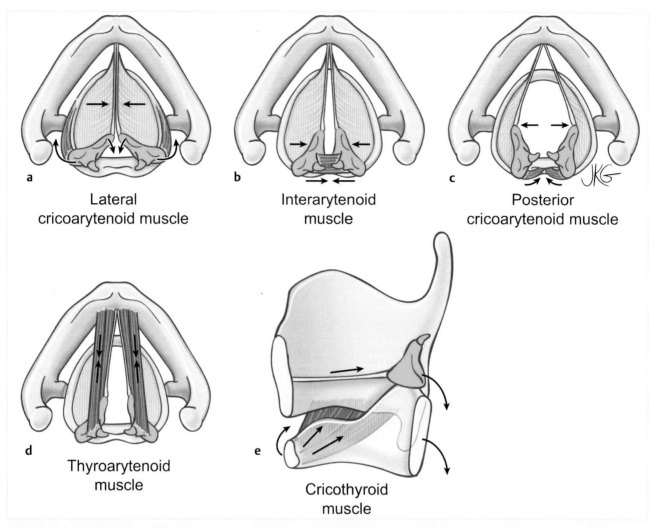

Fig. 74.2 (**a–e**) Gross anatomy of the intrinsic muscles of the larynx and their actions.

The thyroid, cricoid, and arytenoids are all hyaline cartilage—strong but relatively flexible. Beginning just after puberty, these cartilages begin to ossify, much more rapidly in men than in women. The process continues until most of the cartilaginous tissue has been converted, making the skeleton significantly more rigid.

The remaining significant cartilage is the epiglottis, a leaf-shaped elastic cartilage attached by its stem (the petiole) to the inner surface of the angle of the thyroid. It is curled somewhat along its vertical axis, so that it presents a concave shape to the airway. Because of the epiglottis and the walls formed by the alar portions of the thyroid cartilage, the opening to the intralaryngeal airway faces not upward but rather mostly posteriorly, toward the posterior pharyngeal wall. Sealing of the airway during deglutition is not accomplished by lowering of the epiglottis over the vocal folds, but rather primarily by motion of the entire larynx upward and posteriorly. As this occurs, the epiglottis is forced to retroflex against the pharyngeal wall. The epiglottis, which protrudes above the angle of the thyroid, then acts as a "prow," diverting ingested materials around the larynx and into the esophageal entrance.

74.3 Intrinsic Musculature and Displacement Forces

The intrinsic muscles of the larynx have small motor units and very rapid contraction times. The conventional approach to their gross anatomy is summarized in ▶ Fig. 74.2 and ▶ Table 74.1. All except the cricothyroid muscle are arranged as a quasi-sphincter around the glottis. In general, their combined gross actions serve to firmly seal the entrance to the airway against intrusion during swallowing, to close off the thorax and stabilize the chest wall during expulsive acts, and to withstand thrusting forces imposed by the arms.

Respiration and phonation require somewhat more subtle control of the glottal status and so a more finely individualized control of the intrinsic muscles. It is common to assign specific functions and highly individualized roles to each of the intrinsic muscles. It is important to realize that this approach is too simplistic. The muscles work in synergy, and the position and status of the vocal fold depend on the vector sum of the muscular and aerodynamic forces being generated at any given instant. Thus, in an important sense, the reality is that each muscle is an

Table 74.1 Intrinsic muscles of the larynx

Muscle	Attachments	Action	Innervation
Cricothyroid	Upper margin and exterior surface, anterior cricoid cartilage Lower margin and inferior horn, lateral thyroid ala	Approximate cricoid and thyroid cartilages (visor action) Increase thyroid-to-arytenoid (vocal fold) length	Superior laryngeal nerve
Posterior cricoarytenoid	Muscular process of arytenoid cartilage Cricoid cartilage lamina	Displace arytenoid posteriorly and move vocal process of arytenoid away from midline Open glottis	Recurrent laryngeal nerve
Lateral cricoarytenoid	Muscular process of arytenoid cartilage Superior margin of posterior cricoid ring	Displace arytenoid laterally and move vocal process of arytenoid toward midline Close glottis	Recurrent laryngeal nerve
Interarytenoid Transverse Oblique	Posterior facet of arytenoid cartilage Muscular process of one arytenoid cartilage to apex of the other; continues to lateral edge of epiglottis	Adduct arytenoids, close glottis Brace and stabilize arytenoids	Recurrent laryngeal nerve
Thyroarytenoid	Vocal process and nearby area of arytenoid cartilage to inner surface of thyroid angle	Decrease thyroid-to-arytenoid (vocal fold) length Increase vocal fold tension	Recurrent laryngeal nerve

auxiliary for all of the others. One important consideration is that the posterior cricoarytenoid muscles are the sole abductors of the vocal folds and so are responsible for establishing a glottal opening. There is a tendency in the literature to depict abduction as the result of rotation of the arytenoid cartilages about a vertical axis, but in fact significant rotary motion is prevented by the shape of the cricoarytenoid joint and its associated ligaments. Rather, the cricoarytenoid joint is a true diarthrodial joint; as such, the arytenoid slides along its articulatory facet, as well as rotates about an axis in the transverse plane. Together, these movements account for the posterior–superior displacement of the vocal process on abduction.

During phonation, the individual muscles are very finely controlled for positioning the vocal folds and adjusting their biomechanical properties. The lateral cricothyroid muscles generate the main adductor forces for glottal closure, along with the interarytenoid muscles, whose added adductor effect helps maintain glottal closure during episodes of high pulmonary air pressure.

The two remaining intrinsic muscle are largely responsible for the adjustment of the biomechanical properties of the vocal folds and so, in large measure, the control of important vocal qualities. Contraction of the cricothyroid muscle causes the vocal folds to lengthen by two different means. Contraction of the more posterior and oblique portion of the muscle pulls the thyroid cartilage forward or, equivalently, displaces the cricoid cartilage backward. This increases the distance between the posterior cricoid lamina and the thyroid angle. As the cricoid lamina moves relatively backward, it carries the arytenoid cartilages posteriorly, thus increasing the thyroid-to-arytenoid distance and lengthening the vocal fold. The second lengthening effect is somewhat less direct. Contraction of the vertical fibers of the cricothryoid muscle causes an approximation of the anterior portions of the thyroid and cricoid cartilages. This causes a rotation of the cartilages about the axis of their articulation at the inferior horn of the thyroid cartilage. The effect of this is to rotate the arytenoids, which ride on the upper edge of the cricoid, relatively backward and away from the thyroid angle, thus

lengthening the vocal fold. Increasing the vocal fold length increases the frequency of vocal fold vibration (see Chapter 75, Vocal Physiology).

The thyroarytenoid muscle forms the muscular body of the vocal fold. Its most medial portion is often referred to as the vocalis muscle. (This portion is not grossly separable from the rest of the muscle mass and is not strictly a muscle in its own right.) Isotonic contraction of the thyroarytenoid muscle shortens the vocal fold, which tends to lower vocal fundamental frequency, whereas isometric contraction increases vocal fold tension, thus raising vocal fundamental frequency. Finally, thyroarytenoid muscle contraction tends to rotate the arytenoid cartilage medially about its transverse plane rotational axis, which assists in closing the glottal space.

74.4 Membranous, Connective, and Secretory Tissues; Laryngeal Folds

Like the rest of the airway, the laryngeal region is lined with pseudostratified ciliated columnar respiratory epithelium, with the exception of one small but critical zone. The medial edges of the vocal folds are covered by stratified squamous epithelium, which is much better able to sustain the considerable collisional, frictional, and shear forces that are generated by phonatory oscillation. The membranous lining on each side is thrown into three anteroposterior folds.

The most superior of these, the aryepiglottic fold, extends from the apex of the arytenoid cartilage to the lateral margin of the epiglottis and plays a role in protecting the airway from intrusion. The ventricular folds and vocal folds are the main functional structures of the larynx. (The older term, *vocal cord*, still has some currency but has largely been abandoned in the scientific world in favor of the more accurately descriptive term, *vocal fold*. This is a literal translation of the earlier Latin name, *plica vocalis*. Similarly, the terms *true vocal cord* and *false vocal*

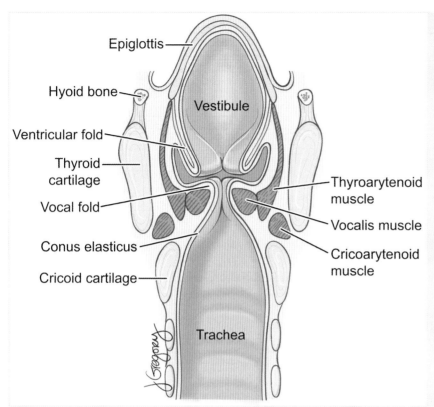

Fig. 74.3 Schematic coronal section illustrating the spatial relationship of the vocal folds and ventricular folds to one another and the entire larynx.

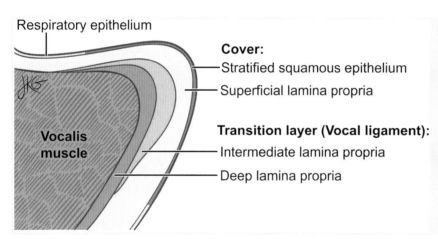

Fig. 74.4 Schematic organization of the five layers of the vocal fold.

cord have generally been replaced by the more accurate terms *vocal folds* and *ventricular folds*, respectively.) The main microscopic and gross anatomical features of these folds are shown in ▶ Fig. 74.3 and ▶ Fig. 74.4. Each is bulkier than the aryepiglottic folds, each has a distinct internal structure, and each plays a critical role in laryngeal function.

The ventricular folds are multilayered. Just deep to the covering respiratory epithelium is a zone of loosely organized connective tissue, the lamina propria. Deep to this zone is the stroma, a denser connective tissue region that forms the main structural support. Within the stroma is a dense assemblage of secretory glands that provide much of the protective and lubricating mucus of the active glottal region. The ventricular folds contain no intrinsic muscle fibers, although there are some deep muscle fibers that are an extension of the thyroarytenoid. Sphincteric closure of the glottal region can medialize the ventricular folds, and they may, in cases of disorder, be used to produce an abnormal phonation.

The quadrangular membranes arise from the lateral edges of the epiglottis and nearby inner surface of the thyroid cartilage. Each courses posteriorly downward to attach to the medial surface of the arytenoid cartilage. The inferior margin of the membrane is somewhat thickened and has often—but erroneously—been designated the ventricular ligament.

Much of the unique human ability to produce highly variable and exquisitely controlled phonation is due to the special anatomy of the vocal fold. Structurally, it is divisible into five layers, which are commonly lumped into three regions. In addition, a superficial membrane, referred to as the conus elasticus, lines the funnel-shaped subglottal region. This membrane joins the several periglottal cartilages to one another. It is divisible into a medial cricothyroid ligament and a lateral cricothyroid membrane and extends inferiorly to become continuous with the lining of the trachea.

The body of the vocal fold is the thyroarytenoid muscle, which lies deep within the fold. Contraction of this muscle can shorten the vocal fold or can increase its stiffness. Although the body of the vocal fold is not strongly involved in phonatory oscillation, it is important for helping to establish the biomechanical properties of the overlying, actively vibrating layers.

Medial to the body of the vocal fold is an organized zone of connective tissue referred to as the lamina propria. On the whole, the connective tissue of this region is not tightly packed, and the interfiber spaces are filled with a considerable amount of fluid-like material (proteoglycans, glycosaminoglycans). The lamina propria is divisible into three layers according to the amount and types of connective tissue fibers (elastin and collagen) and the way in which they are interwoven. Generally, the deeper the layer, the more collagen and the less elastin. The deep and intermediate layers are together referred to as the vocal ligament, while the combination of the superficial lamina propria and the squamous epithelium at the surface is called the vocal fold cover.

When the length of the vocal fold is changed, the physical properties, such as stiffness and thickness, of the vocal ligament and vocal fold cover are altered. This results in a change in the oscillatory response of the vocal fold to the driving air pressure. There is a change in the amplitude and frequency of vocal fold vibration. The rigidity of the body of the vocal fold also plays a role in controlling vocal fold vibration because the freedom of the cover tissues to vibrate is influenced by the freedom of the body to move. So, as vocal fold length increases, the tissues of the vocal fold become stiffer, but the relationship is highly nonlinear and includes significant hysteresis (i.e., the stretch–tension relationship differs depending on whether the folds are lengthening or shortening). Stiffer vocal folds oscillate at higher frequency, but the nonlinearity of the system ensures that the relationship is a complex one.

74.5 Innervation of the Larynx

The larynx is innervated by two branches of the vagus nerve (cranial nerve X), as summarized in ▶ Table 74.2. The origins of the vagus nerve lie mostly in the nucleus ambiguus of the brainstem, which also gives rise to glossopharyngeal (cranial nerve IX) and spinal accessory (cranial nerve XI) nerve fibers. Two enlargements of the nerve just outside the cranium, the nodose and jugular ganglia, contain the perikaryons of vagal afferent fibers. In the cervical region, the vagus nerve gives off several branches. The superior laryngeal nerve subdivides into an external and an internal branch (which is efferent and innervates the cricothyroid muscle). The internal branch provides sensory innervation to the membranes of the supraglottal region. The recurrent laryngeal nerve branches off the main trunk of the vagus nerve inferior to the level of the larynx. It provides sensory innervation to the glottal and subglottal membranes and motor innervation to all intrinsic muscles of the larynx (except the cricothyroid). It is of some clinical importance to note

Table 74.2 Summary of laryngeal innervation

Branch of vagus	Afferent	Efferent
Superior laryngeal nerve (internal branch and external branch)	Supraglottal mucosa	Cricothyroid muscle
Recurrent laryngeal nerve	Subglottal mucosa	Arytenoid, posterior cricoarytenoid, lateral cricoarytenoid, thyro-arytenoid muscles

that the right recurrent nerve loops around the junction of the common carotid and subclavian arteries before traveling superomedially to the larynx, whereas the left recurrent nerve descends into the upper thorax, where it loops around the aortic arch before ascending relatively vertically in the tracheo-esophageal groove back to the larynx. When a patient with a presumed injury of the left recurrent laryngeal nerve is evaluated, it is imperative that imaging extend into the thorax.

74.6 Roundsmanship

- The larynx is divided into the supraglottis, glottis, and subglottis. Each area has a distinct lymphatic drainage that affects both the treatment and prognosis of patients with neoplastic disease.
- The three main purposes of the larynx are protection of the lower airway from aspiration, phonation, and the generation and maintenance of positive intrathoracic air pressure to withstand compressive forces acting on the thorax.
- The cricoarytenoid joint is a true diarthrodial joint. This joint slides and rotates on an axis in the transverse plane.
- There are nine intrinsic muscles in the larynx.
- The medial edges of the vocal folds are covered by stratified squamous epithelium, which is better able than the surrounding respiratory epithelium to withstand the considerable collisional, frictional, and shear forces that are generated by phonatory oscillation.

74.7 Recommended Reading

[1] Hirano M. Phonosurgical anatomy of the larynx. In: Ford CN, Bless D M, eds. Phonosurgery: Assessment and Surgical Management of Voice Disorders. New York, NY: Raven Press; 1991:25–41

[2] Hirano M. Clinical Examination of Voice. New York, NY: Springer; 1981

[3] Jürgens U. The neural control of vocalization in mammals: a review. J Voice 2009; 23: 1–10

[4] Isshiki N. Phonosurgery. New York, NY: Springer; 1989

[5] Kirchner JA, ed. Vocal Fold Histopathology: A Symposium. San Diego, CA: College-Hill Press; 1986

[6] Sataloff RT, ed. Voice Science. San Diego, CA: Plural Publishing; 2005

[7] Sato K. Functional fine structures of the human vocal fold mucosa. In: Rubin JS, Sataloff RT, Korovin G, Gould WJ, eds. Diagnosis and Treatment of Voice Disorders. 2nd ed. New York, NY: Igaku-Shoin Medical Publishers; 1995:41–48

[8] Zemlin WR. Speech and Hearing Science: Anatomy and Physiology. Boston, MA: Allyn and Bacon; 1998

75 Vocal Physiology

Michael J. Pitman

75.1 Basic Conceptual Framework: The Source–Filter Model

The research of the past 70 years has validated the conceptualization of normal voice as the product of two active processes. The oscillation of the vocal folds results in periodic occlusion of the airway at the glottis, which divides the expiratory airstream into a series of airflow pulses. These glottal closures are the foundation for the generation of a nearly periodic acoustic wave train, referred to as the vocal source signal. This signal, in turn, is altered by the acoustic properties of the supraglottal airway, called the vocal tract. The acoustic characteristics of the vocal tract can be voluntarily modified by changing its shape. The upper airway, then, serves as a vocal tract filter. This source–filter model holds that the two aspects of voice production are essentially independent of each other. The assumption is not strictly true, but it is admissible for everyday clinical purposes.

Phonation is the generation of a periodic signal at the glottis: that is, the production of a source signal. Voice, on the other hand, is phonation that is acoustically modified, or filtered. Control of the vocal tract structures, which results in a modification of the filter's characteristics, is an articulatory, rather than a phonatory, function. Hence, some qualities commonly said to be vocal, including (most importantly) nasality, are really articulatory. These are outside the realm of vocal function strictly defined and will be not considered here.

The essential features of the source–filter model of voice production are summarized in ▶ Fig. 75.1, which will serve as a guide to the present brief exploration of vocal physiology.

75.2 The Power Supply: Air Pressure Generation

The acoustic power that is radiated as a voice or speech signal is drawn from the pressurized air that is provided to the vocal folds for phonation, and to the vocal tract directly for some speech sounds (consonant production). The source of pressurized air is, of course, the lungs. While the basic mechanisms of lung inflation and alveolar pressurization for speech are the same as for vegetative pulmonary ventilation, there are specific requirements, problems, and constraints that are imposed by the need for a stable phonatory product that can be easily and precisely modulated to meet the complex requirements of speech while, at the same time, satisfying the body's more general respiratory demands.

- Lung volumes for speech are typically greater than vegetative tidal volumes. The ventilatory tidal volume at rest is on the order of 0.5 L. However, speech breathing characteristically is initiated at an end-inspiratory lung volume of between 35% and 65% vital capacity (VC), and end-expiratory volume for speech is near (and often less than) REL, which is the rest position of the ventilatory system, at which expiratory and inspiratory recoil forces are equal and opposite. Loud speech is associated with larger lung volumes than soft speech.

- In tidal ventilation, the duration of inspiration is about 40% of the breathing cycle. Speech is normally produced only during expiration, so the interruption required for recharging the lungs must be minimized. Therefore, during speech, inspiration is typically shortened so as to occupy only about 10% of the cycle, with a corresponding increase in the magnitude of peak instantaneous inspiratory airflow.

- Tracheal air pressures during quiet tidal breathing are very modest, ranging between approximately -1 and $+1$ cm H_2O, of which the (positive) expiratory pressure is passively generated by recoil forces created during the preceding inspiratory phase. During speech, however, significantly higher inspiratory (negative) pressure is required in order to achieve rapid inspiration. More importantly, sound production calls for larger positive pressures, most commonly in the range of approximately $+4$ cm H_2O for soft phonation to about $+10$ cm H_2O for moderately loud phonation. Pressures in this range are higher than those usually produced by passive recoil and thus must be actively generated.

- Phonation and articulation for speech purposes require that the tracheal pressure be stable, and that it change only in response to the physiologic demands of the speech process and to the requirements of the linguistic features to be communicated. The mechanics of the lung and chest wall system therefore pose a problem. The recoil forces vary in a nonlinear manner as lung volume changes. Thus, at the end of a large inspiration, such as might occur in preparation for a long speech utterance, the tracheal pressure generated by recoil might well be more than is needed for phonation and speech. On the other hand, as the utterance comes to an end, the lung volume may be very low, in fact below the functional residual capacity (FRC). For this reason, passive pressure will probably be too low to drive phonation, or may be negative. Thus, for speech, active chest wall muscle activity is required to reduce (by delicately controlled inspiratory muscle action) excessively positive passive pressure, or to augment (by expiratory muscle activation) the inadequate or even negative passive tracheal pressure produced when lung volume has been depleted.

An additional problem, often overlooked, results from the fact that normal speech is characterized by large and sudden changes in airflow. As an example, when the word *she* is spoken, the peak airflow for "sh" is approximately 700 mL/s, but just a few tens of milliseconds later, airflow for the "e" is about 125 mL/s. Changes such as this can cause unwanted and sudden alterations of pressure. For speech purposes, therefore, the chest wall system is postured so as to optimize "load regulation." Compared with their positions during tidal breathing, the rib cage is typically somewhat expanded and the anterior abdominal wall somewhat more contracted, forcing the diaphragm upward a bit.

Unfortunately, the "rules" of breathing for speech are anything but clear. Different individuals appear to have very different ways of solving the biomechanical problems involved, and it is not uncommon for perfectly normal speakers to use ventilatory patterns that seem to fly in the face of the physiolo-

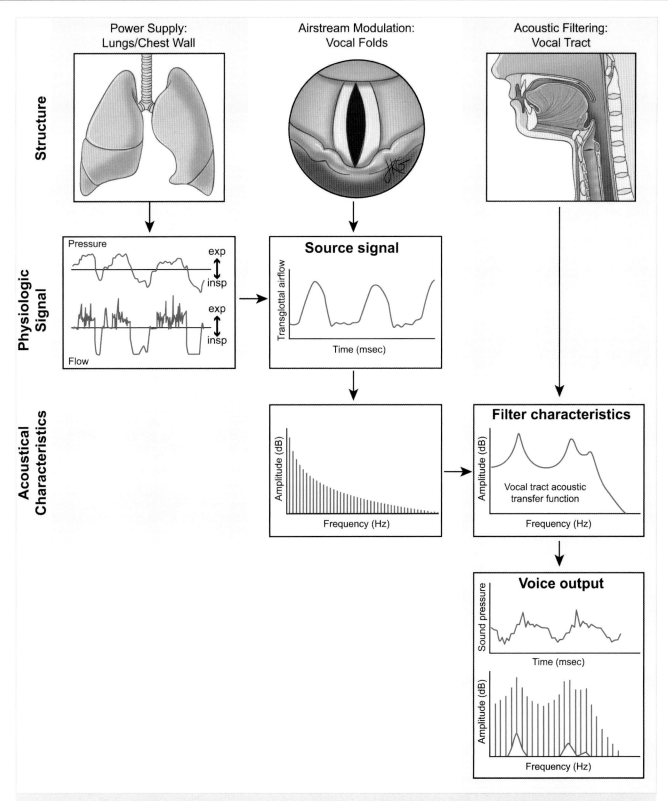

Fig. 75.1 Source–filter model of voice production. The pulmonary reservoir of air provides the power supply, while the airstream is modulated at the vocal fold level to produce a fundamental frequency and harmonics. These frequencies are modulated in the vocal tract.

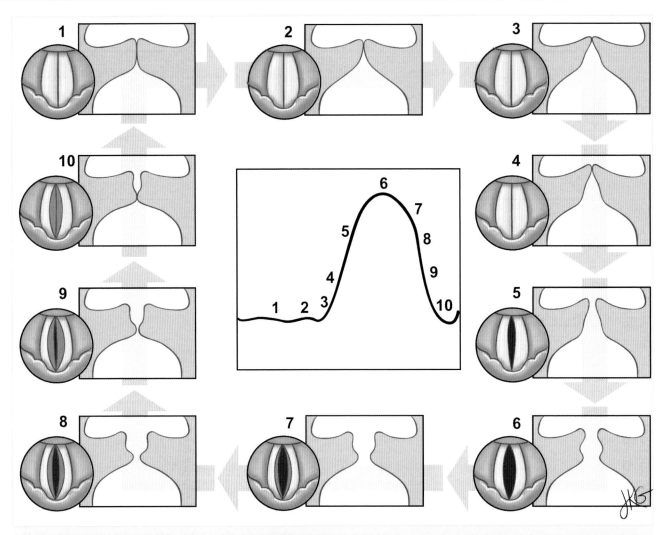

Fig. 75.2 The figures represent the position and contours of the vocal folds in coronal section and from above (*insets*) throughout the vocal fold vibratory cycle. The inner graph depicts airflow over time. (1) Complete glottis closure. (2) Opening of the lower border of the vocal folds. (3, 4) Progressive opening of the vocal folds. (5) Opening of the top and bottom of the vocal folds. (6) Complete opening of the glottis. (7–9) Closure of the lower border of the vocal folds. (10) Complete closure of the lower border and partial closure of the upper border of the vocal folds.

gists' expectations. Clinical pronouncements about "optimal" breathing patterns for speech, or about the role of ventilatory behavior in most instances of voice disorder, are almost always without empiric or even theoretical foundation and should be viewed with significant skepticism.

75.3 Phonation: Generating the Vocal Source Signal

The modern understanding of source signal production is referred to as the myoelastic–aerodynamic theory of phonation. It holds that the oscillation of the vocal folds is not due to the active rhythmic contraction of muscle fibers, as earlier models had posited, but is rather a passive result of the action of static and dynamic air pressures acting on the vocal folds, whose response is a function of their three-dimensional geometry and their biomechanical or rheologic properties. The aerostatic characteristics of the vocal system and the biomechanical properties of the vocal folds are, to a considerable extent, individu-

ally controllable, but they interact in complex and nonlinear ways and so are far from independent of each other. The regulation of phonation is largely a problem of controlling the trade-offs inherent in the aerodynamic–biomechanical interaction.

75.3.1 The Vocal Fold Vibratory Cycle and the Glottal Source Signal

▶ Fig. 75.2 provides a thumbnail sketch of the essentials of one cycle of vocal fold oscillation for the production of a transglottal airflow pulse, which is the basis of the vocal source signal. For more details, see Chapter 74. It is assumed that a tracheal pressure adequate to power the glottal cycle has been created through appropriate ventilatory muscle action.

Initially, the vocal folds have been adducted so as to make full contact at the midline, eliminating the glottal space. Tracheal air pressure acts perpendicularly against the underside of the folds. This pressure has the effect of pushing the lower margins of the vocal folds apart. As a result, a wave of separation begins to move superiorly as the pressure continues to act to "pry" the vocal folds away from each other. During this interval, vocal fold separation has not reached the upper surface, and so the glottis remains closed and there is no transglottal airflow. However, when the glottis opens as the upper edges of the vocal folds are finally blown apart, airflow through the glottis begins.

At this point, several features need to be considered. One is that almost all of the displacement of the vocal fold tissue is due to movement of the vocal fold cover, not the body (the thyroarytenoid muscle), which is almost always much stiffer than the combination of epithelial and connective tissue that constitutes the cover. Both structures, however, are essentially incompressible and elastic, so when they are displaced, they store energy that represents recoil forces that try to return the edges of the vocal folds to their original position. The greater the displacement from the rest position, the greater the restorative force that is generated. Hence, given the sequence of opening events, the lower edges of the vocal folds are farther from their original positions than the just recently opened upper edges, so the lower edges are subjected to significantly greater force pushing them back toward closure. Furthermore, with the release of air from the glottal space, the air pressure momentarily drops because of inertial effects. Thus, there is slightly less air pressure than previously to oppose the restorative forces.

With the opening of the glottis, another significant aerodynamic force is unleashed. The Bernoulli effect is the drop in pressure of a flowing fluid in a constriction. The vocal folds represent a narrowing in the airway, and when the glottis opens, a flow ensues. The pressure of the air in the space between the vocal folds will therefore be lower than the pressure in the trachea or in the supraglottal region. This means that the force acting to move or keep the vocal folds apart decreases when the open glottis permits airflow. In fact, it is possible for the intraglottal air pressure to be subatmospheric.

When the glottis is wide open and transglottal airflow is at a maximum, the lower margins begin to return to the midline while, thanks to momentum, the upper margins continue to separate, widening the glottis even more. This widening reduces the amount of constriction and so diminishes the Bernoulli effect. This fact, together with the greater displacement from their rest position that the upper margins have undergone, now puts the upper edges in the same situation that the lower edges were in just before, and the top part of the glottis begins to close. Of course, back in the lower glottal region, the nearing edges increase the amount of constriction in their neighborhood, thus increasing the relatively negative Bernoulli pressure, with the effect that there is now a tendency for the lower edges to be "sucked" together. Ultimately, the lower margins contact each other, the glottis closes, and flow is cut off. Without a flow, there is no Bernoulli pressure acting on the upper edges of the vocal folds, but there is also no tracheal pressure acting on them, so the tissue recoil forces are unopposed and the upper edges, too, are returned to the midline. This restores the glottis to the initial, completely closed position and sets up the conditions for the cycle to repeat.

What this vocal fold motion has accomplished is the release of a puff of air into the vocal tract. This is a physiologic signal whose characteristic shape is shown in ▶ Fig. 75.1 and in the center of ▶ Fig. 75.2. Under ordinary circumstances, the glottal movement pattern, and therefore the release of similar puffs of air, repeats at about 110 Hz (repetitions per second) in men and roughly twice as fast, at about 220 Hz, in women. This repetition rate is the fundamental frequency (F_0) of the glottal wave and is the primary determinant of the perceived musical pitch of the voice. On the whole, higher repetition rates are heard as higher pitches, and vice versa. A brief summary of vocal fundamental frequency and its control is provided in ▶ Table 75.1.

All other things being equal, the amplitude of the transglottal flow pulse is directly related to the tracheal pressure, referred to as the subglottal pressure by the voice physiologist. This amplitude in turn is largely, but not solely, responsible for the sound intensity of voice or speech. Sound intensity is the main determinant of perceived loudness.

Table 75.1 Actions that change vocal F_0

Factors	Action	Related changes and effects		ΔF_0
Static control factors	↑ VF rest length			↓ F_0
	↑ VF mass			↓ F_0
	↑ Baseline stiffness of VF			↑ F_0
	↑ Subglottic pressure			↑ F_0
Dynamic control factors	Cricothyroid muscle contraction	↑ VF length	↓ VF mass per unit of surface area	↑ F_0
			↑ Stretch of VF ↑ VF cover tension	↑ F_0
	Thyroarytenoid muscle contraction	↑ Stiffness of VF body		↑ F_0

Abbreviation: VF, vocal fold.

Table 75.1b Expected ranges of vocal F_0

Register	Female	Male
Modal	140–540 Hz	75–460 Hz
Loft ("falsetto")	500–1,100 Hz	275–640 Hz

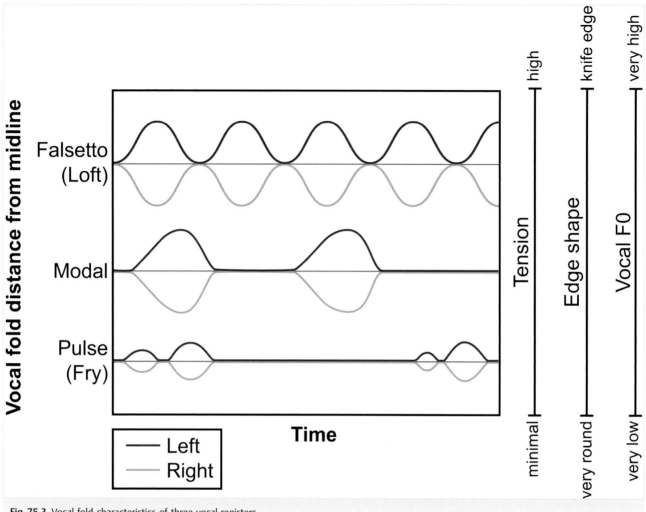

Fig. 75.3 Vocal fold characteristics of three vocal registers.

75.4 Acoustics of the Source Signal and Vocal Tract

The source signal produced by vocal fold oscillation is a nearly periodic wave train, meaning that it is a train of almost identical waves (see ▶ Fig. 75.1). Because it is periodic, the source signal is composed of a series of harmonics: sine waves at integer multiples of the fundamental frequency. The source signal can thus be represented, as it is in ▶ Fig. 75.1 under the heading "Airstream Modulation," either as a plot of airflow over time (upper plot) or as a series of sine waves of different amplitudes over frequency, which is referred to as a spectrum (lower graph). Thus, one can conceptualize the source signal not as a series of puffs of air but as a "bundle" of related frequencies injected into the bottom of the upper airway. An excellent and valid analogy is the way in which a trumpeter or other brass instrument player produces a series of air pulses by lip vibration into the instrument's mouthpiece. These air pulses, being nearly periodic, also inject a series of harmonic frequencies into the proximal end of the instrument's tube.

The vocal tract has acoustic properties determined by its length and shape, as does the tube of a trumpet. Some of the harmonic frequencies pass through the tract or tube relatively undiminished, while others are more or less attenuated. In short, the tract behaves as a complex acoustic filter. It is possible to plot the filter characteristics of the tract as a sort of "audiogram," showing the attenuation effect of the vocal tract as a function of harmonic frequency, as has been done in ▶ Fig. 75.1. This plot is formally said to show the "transfer function" of the vocal tract. When the spectrum that is the product of airstream modulation is introduced into the vocal tract filter, the extent to which any given frequency is transmitted to the filter's output at the lips is governed by the transfer function. The result, for the example of ▶ Fig. 75.1, is shown in the lower plot on the far right. The output spectrum now has peaks, harmonics that were transmitted with relatively little attenuation, and valleys, where harmonic frequencies were more strongly attenuated. The associated sound–pressure wave of the output spectrum is shown just above it. It is this pressure wave that reaches the listener's ear and that the listener perceives as the speaker's voice.

75.5 Registers

The model of phonation that has been considered thus far is valid for the most common pattern of vocal fold behavior—the mode that most speakers use most of the time. However, there are other ways in which the vocal folds may be adjusted to produce different vocal registers. Briefly, a register may be defined as a specific and reproducible mode of laryngeal action that is used over a range of contiguous frequencies to produce a consistent vocal quality. There is normally only a little overlap of register frequency ranges. (Musicians typically favor a much more complex—and less precise—definition of register that relies exclusively on perceived vocal quality. There is little agreement, and much acrimonious dispute, among different musical schools of thought about how many registers there are or what they should be called.) The physiologist recognizes three distinct vocal registers; they are schematized in ▶ Fig. 75.3, which emphasizes the differences, observable on endoscopic examination, in the displacement patterns of the vocal fold edges.

- *Modal register*, named for the statistical mode ("most common"), is the pattern of ordinary speech and is the one illustrated in ▶ Fig. 75.2. It employs moderate vocal fold tension, which results in somewhat rounded vocal fold edges. The glottal open phase is only somewhat longer than the closed phase. Moderate air pressure drives the system, producing vocal F_0 values in the mid frequency range (the mean F_0 of conversational speech is approximately 120 Hz for men and 210 Hz for women).
- *Falsetto* is an old musical term, still in common use, for the register at the highest vocal F_0 values. This register is also often referred to by the more modern term, *loft register*. High lung pressures are used to drive the vocal folds under very significant tension, such that the vocal folds have a knife edge configuration. The F_0 of phonation in this range is, on average, higher than approximately 275 Hz in men and approximately 500 Hz in women. The oscillatory pattern of the vocal folds is more sinusoidal in this register, and quite often no glottal closure occurs.
- *Pulse register*, also known, especially in the older literature, as *glottal fry*, occupies the F_0 range below approximately 30 Hz. It is not uncommon for individual glottal pulses to be separately perceptible. There may be a complete absence of tensioning; the vocal folds are floppy and blunt-edged, and the driving pressure is correspondingly low. Relatively brief glottal openings are followed by very long closed periods. Characteristically, vocal fold oscillation is only marginally periodic. A common but not essential feature of pulse register phonation is a "dichrotic" oscillatory pattern, in which a small, short opening is followed immediately by a larger and longer opening. Despite its rough perceptual quality, and notwithstanding its very poor periodicity, pulse register phonation is not inherently indicative of pathology, nor (long-standing clinical biases notwithstanding) is it injurious to the larynx.

75.6 Roundsmanship

- Both source and filter affect the human voice.
- During speech, inspiration as a percentage of the breathing cycle decreases from 40 to 10%.
- Tracheal air pressure during speech may increase by 10 times over that during quiet breathing.
- The myoelastic–aerodynamic model of phonation states that the oscillations of the vocal fold cover, under the influence of the intrinsic laryngeal muscles, create the fundamental frequency of vocalization and its harmonics. Signal modification in the vocal tract modifies the harmonic frequencies in a specific way.

75.7 Recommended Reading

[1] Hixon TJ, ed. Respiratory Function in Speech and Song. Boston, MA: College-Hill Press/Little Brown and Company; 1987

[2] Titze IR. Principles of Voice Production. Denver, CO: National Center for Voice and Speech; 2000

[3] Van Den Berg JW. Myoelastic-aerodynamic theory of voice production. J Speech Hear Res 1958; 1: 227–244

76 Pharyngeal Anatomy

Melin Tan

76.1 The Pharynx

The pharynx is a mucosa-lined musculomembranous tube that extends from the base of the skull to the lower border of the cricoid cartilage at the level of the sixth cervical vertebra, where it becomes contiguous with the esophagus (▸ Fig. 76.1). It is approximately 12 to 14 cm long and communicates with the nasal, oral, and laryngeal cavities, thus creating three distinct divisions: the nasopharynx, oropharynx, and hypopharynx (▸ Fig. 76.2). These three areas share the same general tubular structure of muscle and fascia lined superficially by mucosa.

The primary pharyngeal musculature is composed of three paired, overlapping constrictor muscles known as the superior, middle, and inferior pharyngeal constrictors. Together, the pharyngeal constrictors have a common insertion into the posterior pharyngeal raphe. However, their origins are complex. The superior constrictor muscle has four parts, which arise from four different areas: (1) the medial pterygoid plate and its hamulus; (2) the pterygomandibular raphe; (3) the alveolar process of the mandible; and (4) the lateral aspect of the tongue. The middle constrictor muscle arises from the hyoid bone and the stylohyoid ligament. The inferior constrictor muscle arises from the thyroid and cricoid cartilages. Superiorly, the superior constrictor muscle becomes replaced by the pharyngobasilar fascia, which attaches to the base of the skull at the pharyngeal tubercle. The gap between the superior constrictor muscle and the skull base is called the sinus of Morgagni.

The circular fibers of the constrictors surround the longitudinally running fibers of the palatopharyngeus, salpingopharyngeus, and stylopharyngeus muscles. These three muscles contribute to the movement of the pharyngeal wall. The palatopharyngeus muscle extends from the soft palate and pharyngeal wall to the thyroid cartilage, forming the substance of the posterior tonsillar pillar. It acts to elevate the pharynx and close off the nasopharynx during swallowing. The salpingopharyngeus muscle extends from the eustachian tube cartilage to interdigitate with the palatopharyngeus and acts to raise the pharynx and open the eustachian tube orifice during swallowing. The stylopharyngeus muscle originates at the styloid process, passes between the external and internal carotid arteries, and inserts on the superior posterior border of the thyroid cartilage; some fibers intermingle with the constrictor muscles. Like the salpingopharyngeus and the palatopharyngeus, it acts to elevate the pharynx, but it also minimally dilates the pharynx.

Two fascial layers envelope the muscular layers of the pharynx. The fibrous pharyngobasilar fascia begins at the pharyngeal tubercle of the skull base and extends inferiorly into the superior constrictor muscle. It sits between the skull base and the pharynx and helps to support the rigid structure of the nasopharynx. It thickens at the level of the tonsils and forms a fibrous tonsillar bed before becoming less recognizable at the lower part of the pharynx, where it eventually disappears. The buccopharyngeal (visceral) fascia is contiguous with the internal layer of the deep cervical fascia. Directly posterior to the buccopharyngeal fascia is the retropharyngeal space, which is contained by the alar fascia and communicates with the mediastinum. Posterior to this fascia is the prevertebral space; this extends to the sacrum and then the prevertebral fascia, which envelopes the prevertebral muscles. These layers are particularly important in the spread of infection and malignancy. Their separation also allows the free movement of the pharynx against the vertebral structures during swallowing.

The mucosal lining of the pharynx is a nonkeratinized stratified squamous epithelium. The posterior nasopharynx is distinct in that anteriorly, the mucosal lining is a ciliated, pseudostratified respiratory epithelium. This is consistent with the dominant respiratory epithelial lining of the nose. Posteriorly within the nasopharynx, the respiratory epithelium changes to nonkeratinized stratified squamous epithelium, which extends inferiorly to the rest of the pharynx.

The nerve supply to the pharynx is derived from the pharyngeal plexus, which is formed by the pharyngeal branches of the glossopharyngeal and vagus nerves, with lesser contributions from the superior cervical sympathetic ganglion. The vagus nerve supplies motor innervation. Additionally, through the auricular branch (Arnold nerve), the vagus may carry sensory information from the hypopharyngeal area that is perceived as originating in the external auditory canal and pinna. This explains the referred pain experienced by some patients with lesions in the hypopharynx. Sensory information otherwise travels along the glossopharyngeal nerve and the internal laryngeal branch of the superior laryngeal nerve.

The arterial blood supply of the pharynx comes from the major branches of the external carotid artery, including the ascending pharyngeal artery, tonsillar branches of the facial artery, and palatine branches of the maxillary artery. The primary venous drainage is via the pharyngeal veins, which then drain into the internal jugular vein. Lymphatic drainage of the pharynx is bilateral, which is important clinically in the spread and treatment of pharyngeal cancer.

76.2 Nasopharynx

The subsites of the nasopharynx are (1) the lateral walls, including the fossae of Rosenmüller and eustachian tube orifices; (2) the vault (roof); and (3) the posterior wall. The nasopharynx communicates with the nasal cavity via the choanae anteriorly. It is otherwise bound by the base of the skull superiorly and the upper surface of the soft palate inferiorly. The soft palate separates the nasopharynx from the oropharynx as it creates a narrowing in the pharynx known as the pharyngeal isthmus.

Each lateral wall is formed and supported by the margins of the superior constrictor muscle and the rigid pharyngobasilar fascia. The nasopharynx communicates with the middle ear cavity via the eustachian tube, located in the upper posterolateral wall. The torus tubarius is formed by the cartilaginous eustachian tube, the levator veli palatini muscle, and the overlying mucosa. The fossa of Rosenmüller lies just above the torus and is formed by the salpingopharyngeal fold, which extends from the torus to the posterior wall.

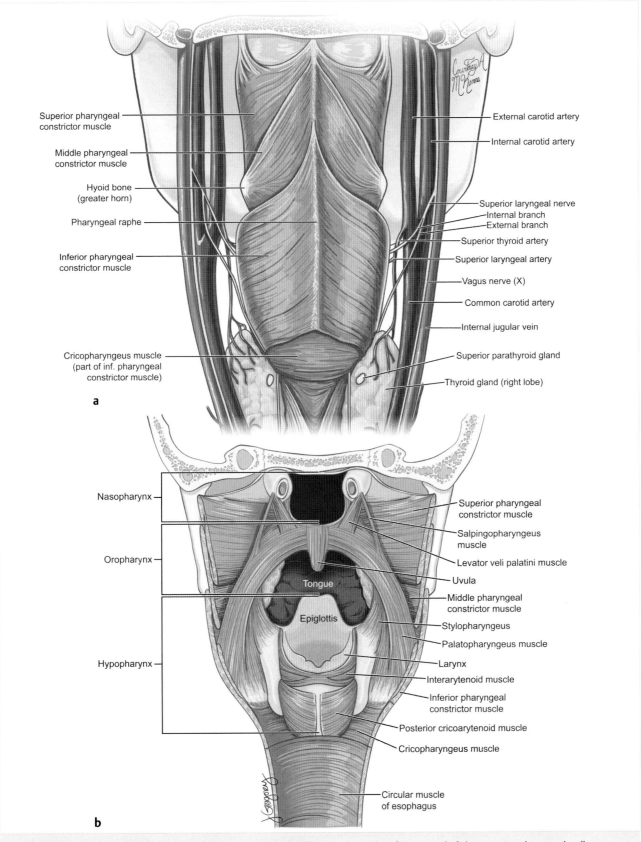

Fig. 76.1 (a) Posterior view of the pharynx. (b) Posterior view of the pharyngeal muscles after removal of the posterior pharyngeal wall.

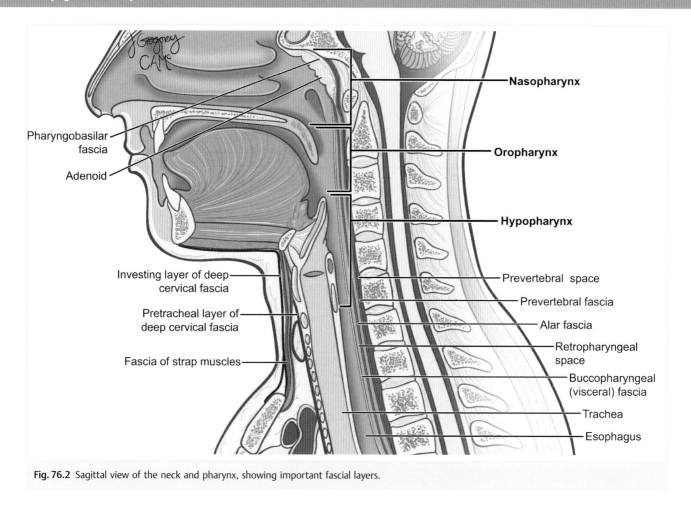

Fig. 76.2 Sagittal view of the neck and pharynx, showing important fascial layers.

The roof of the nasopharynx is created by the basisphenoid and the floor of the sphenoid sinus. Often, there is a depression in the midline of the bony roof, producing a concavity of the mucosa known as the pharyngeal bursa. Occasionally, a cystic mass, known as a Thornwaldt cyst, may be found in this area. Adenoids, or pharyngeal tonsils, are located in the midline roof of the nasopharynx, as well. They form the superior aspect of the Waldeyer ring, a loop of lymphoid tissue at the upper end of the pharynx that also includes the palatine tonsils and lingual tonsils.

Posteriorly, the buccopharyngeal fascia separates the nasopharynx from the deep fascial spaces and is thought to be a barrier to the deep spread of infection and early malignancy. The primary nodal drainage of the nasopharynx is via the retropharyngeal nodes; however, the lymphatic pathways are thought to become obliterated by adulthood as a result of the numerous pharyngeal infections that occur in childhood. Therefore, nasopharyngeal cancers often drain to second-order nodes in levels II, III, and occasionally IV.

76.3 Oropharynx

The oropharynx is the part of the pharynx that communicates with the oral cavity. It extends from the junction of the soft palate and hard palate superiorly to the vallecula inferiorly and the circumvallate papillae anteriorly. The subsites of the oropharynx are (1) the soft palate; (2) the base of the tongue; (3) the palatine tonsils; and (4) the lateral and posterior pharyngeal wall.

The soft palate plays an important role in separating the nasal cavity from the rest of the aerodigestive tract during speech and swallowing. It remains flaccid during respiration and elevates during deglutition to block communication between the nasal and oral cavities. The Passavant muscle is composed of fibers that arise laterally from the palatopharyngeus muscle and the posterolateral hard palate. When the fibers contract, they raise a ridge of soft tissue known as the Passavant ridge. This ridge opposes the elevated soft palate, thereby closing off the nasopharynx during swallowing. This function is also critical for preventing hypernasal speech.

The base of the tongue is the area of the tongue that is posterior to the circumvallate papillae. It plays a critical role in swallowing by propelling the food bolus into the hypopharynx.

The palatine tonsils are contained in the tonsillar fossa between the anterior and posterior faucial arches. The anterior arch, the glossopalatine fold, is formed by the palatoglossus muscle and its overlying mucosa. The posterior arch is formed by the palatopharyngeus muscle and its overlying mucosa. Deep to the tonsillar fossa are the superior pharyngeal constrictor muscles and the upper fibers of the middle constrictor muscles.

The primary lymphatic drainage of the oropharynx is to level II and level III nodes, the retropharyngeal nodes, and less commonly level V nodes. The palatine tonsils may also drain to the parotid nodes.

76.4 Hypopharynx

The hypopharynx extends from the tip of the epiglottis superiorly to the cricoid cartilage inferiorly, where it empties into the cervical esophagus. It abuts the larynx and is delineated from the oropharynx by the lateral glossoepiglottic folds, which, together with the medial glossoepiglottic folds, form the vallecula. The subsites of the hypopharynx are (1) the piriform sinuses; (2) the posterior pharyngeal wall; and (3) the postcricoid mucosa.

The piriform sinuses are mucosal recesses on either side of the laryngeal inlet. They are bounded by the inner surface of the thyrohyoid membrane, the thyroid cartilage, and the lateral surface of the aryepiglottic fold.

The posterior pharyngeal wall of the hypopharynx is the inferior continuation of the posterior wall of the oropharynx. The landmark between the two is the hyoid bone. The posterior cricoid region is the anterior wall of the hypopharynx from the arytenoid cartilages down to the inferior border of the cricoid cartilage.

The cricopharyngeus muscle sphincter is composed of horizontal fibers that extend from one side of the cricoid cartilage to the other, separating the hypopharynx from the cervical esophagus. It is tonically contracted and relaxes in response to the presence of a food bolus in the hypopharynx, allowing food to enter the esophagus. It then contracts again to close the esophagus and prevent reflux. When it does so, it increases the intrapharyngeal pressure, causing passive dilation of the pharynx (there is no major pharyngeal dilator muscle). Between the upper border of the cricopharyngeus and the lower border of the inferior pharyngeal constrictor muscle is a small, triangular, mucosa-covered space called the Killian dehiscence. It is through this area that a Zenker diverticulum most commonly arises.

The lymphatic drainage of the hypopharynx is directed to the jugulodigastric lymph nodes and spinal accessory chains. The piriform sinuses drain to level II and level III, and then secondarily to level V. The posterior wall of the hypopharynx drains to level II and level III nodes, as well as retropharyngeal nodes. The postcricoid lymphatics drain to levels III, IV, and VI nodes.

76.5 Roundsmanship

- The nasopharynx, oropharynx, and hypopharynx are divided into subsites for a consideration of function and oncologic factors.
- The layers of the posterior pharyngeal wall influence the spread of malignancy and infection.
- The pharyngeal constrictor muscles form a "sling" that surrounds the pharynx from the skull base to the cricopharyngeus muscle.

76.6 Recommended Reading

[1] Standring S, Borley NR, Collins P, et al, eds. Gray's Anatomy: The Anatomical Basis of Clinical Practice. Vol 1. 40th ed. London, England: Churchill Livingstone Elsevier; 2008
[2] Janfaza P, Nadol JB Jr, Galla RJ, Fabian PJR, Montgomery WW, eds. Surgical Anatomy of the Head and Neck. Vol 1. 1st ed. Philadelphia, PA: Lippincott Williams & Wilkins; 2001
[3] Mukherji SK. Head and Neck Imaging. Vol 2. St. Louis, MO: Mosby; 2003
[4] Netter F. Atlas of Human Anatomy. Vol 1.4th ed. Philadelphia, PA: Saunders Elsevier; 2006

77 Physiology of Swallowing

Amy L. Cooper

77.1 Introduction

The term *swallowing* refers to the entire act of deglutition, from the placement of food in the mouth through the oral and pharyngeal stages of the swallow until entry of the material into the esophagus through the cricopharyngeus and passage onward into the stomach.

77.2 Terminology

The highly complex process of swallowing can be divided into the following four phases: oral preparatory, oral, pharyngeal, and esophageal. These phases are interrelated, and the four phases must be appropriately timed and sequenced for the swallow to be achieved successfully. Approaching the act of swallowing from this perspective has implications for the management of swallowing disorders. As an example, the source of a swallowing difficulty may not be entirely obvious or easily understood; disruption in one phase may impact another phase. In addition, treatment aimed at one phase may enhance or alter the competency of another phase. Swallowing is best understood as a combination of preprogrammed events with neural circuitry that can adapt to change if needed. Therefore, swallowing can be thought of as a programmed response to stimuli rather than a true reflex. The duration and characteristics of each phase of swallowing depend on the type and volume of food being swallowed and on voluntary control. Swallowing occurs predictably based on the characteristics of the food swallowed and voluntary control.

77.3 Applied Anatomy

Clinicians involved in the diagnosis and treatment of swallowing disorders must be familiar with the basic anatomy of the upper aerodigestive system. Key structures include the jaw and lips anteriorly, the tongue (and its relationship to the velum and nasopharynx), the spinal column (and its relationship to the oropharynx anteriorly), the valleculae, the laryngeal inlet (and its relationship to the epiglottis and hypopharynx), the cricopharyngeus (and its relationship to the spinal column), and the closed esophagus (▶ Fig. 77.1). The key muscles of the head and neck used in swallowing are illustrated in ▶ Fig. 77.2.

77.4 Physiologic Phases of Swallowing

77.4.1 Oral Preparatory Phase

The sensory recognition of food approaching then entering the mouth is critical before oral preparatory movements can be initiated. The oral preparatory phase includes a transfer phase,

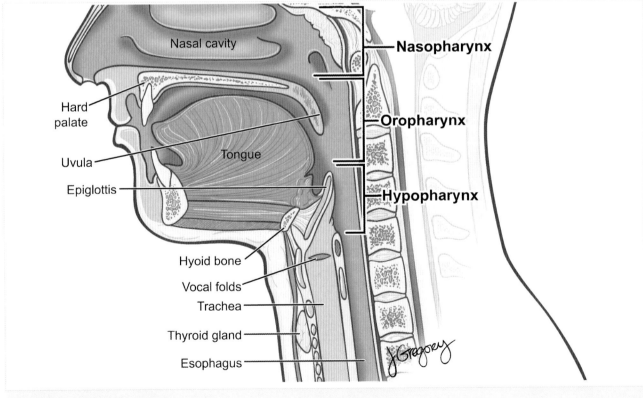

Fig. 77.1 Basic anatomy for swallowing.

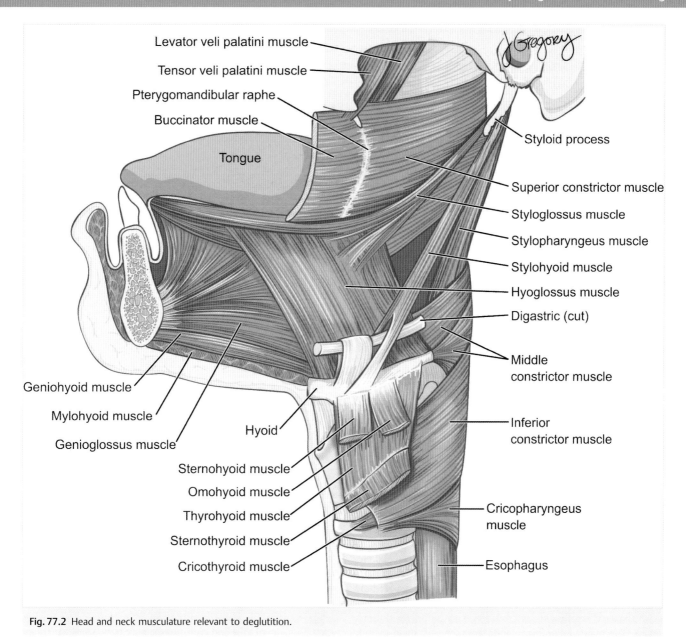

Fig. 77.2 Head and neck musculature relevant to deglutition.

during which the tongue arranges the bolus, a soft mass of food and/or liquid, and moves it posteriorly to an appropriate position for mastication (▶ Fig. 77.3a). Mastication involves a rotary lateral movement of the mandible and tongue. Food is chewed, ground, and mixed with saliva to form the bolus to be swallowed. The chewing activity stimulates the salivary glands, and the bolus is lubricated for swallowing ease. Although this activity is not required for a liquid bolus, momentary containment by the tongue is necessary so that the liquid bolus does not prematurely enter the oropharynx. Taste, temperature, viscosity, and bolus size are sensed (cranial nerves V, VII, and IX), and appropriate oral manipulations are carried out to prepare for the oral phase of swallowing.

77.4.2 Oral Phase

The oral phase of a swallow is basically a delivery system and is initiated when the tongue begins to move the bolus

posteriorly (▶ Fig. 77.3b). Before the swallow, the tongue (cranial nerve XII) cradles the bolus, pressing its edges against the hard palate as the swallow begins. This contact helps to prevent premature spillage into the oropharynx. When bolus preparation is complete, the bolus is positioned posteriorly on the tongue. The lips, buccal musculature, and velum work in tandem to build pressure and reduce the volume of the oral cavity, driving the bolus posteriorly. When contracted at the initiation of the swallow, the extrinsic tongue muscles (digastic, mylohyoid, and geniohyoid) enable this posterior movement. Any injury, neurologic disorder, or surgery affecting the muscles or nerves involved in the oral preparatory and oral phases of swallowing may negatively impact these phases. Decreased lip or buccal function may negatively impact the oral phase of swallowing with respect to oral containment of the bolus. Similarly, a decrease in tongue function is of concern because of reduced control and transport of the bolus.

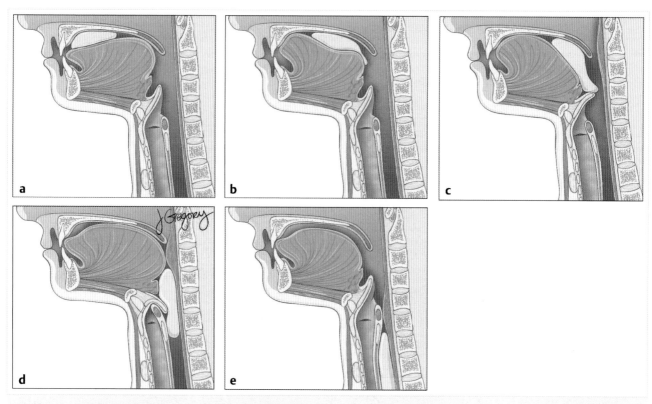

Fig. 77.3 (a–e) Phases of deglutition.

77.4.3 Pharyngeal Phase

The pharyngeal phase begins with triggering of the swallow, which should occur by the time the bolus head reaches the point where the mandible crosses the tongue base (▶ Fig. 77.3c). The pharyngeal trigger involves the complex action of tongue elevation, velopharyngeal closure, laryngeal elevation, and relaxation of the cricopharyngeus. All contribute to movement of the bolus through the pharyngeal area without penetration of and/or aspiration into the airway. The pharyngeal phase of swallowing is considered to be an involuntary phase. The major anatomical landmarks for this stage include the epiglottis, valleculae and piriform sinuses, thyroid and cricoid cartilages, larynx, cervical spine, and posterior pharyngeal wall. A number of physiologic activities occur as a result of pharyngeal triggering: (1) elevation and retraction of the velum with complete closure of the velopharyngeal port to prevent material from entering the nasal cavity; (2) tongue base retraction to contact the posterior pharyngeal wall; (3) progressive contraction of the pharyngeal constrictors; (4) elevation and anterior movement of the hyoid and larynx (which help to close off the airway and stretch/open the upper esophageal sphincter); (5) closure of the larynx at the laryngeal aditus (epiglottis and aryepiglottic folds), ventricular folds, and true vocal folds to prevent material from entering the airway; (6) cricopharyngeal sphincter relaxation to allow the upper esophageal sphincter to open and permit material to pass from the pharynx into the esophagus.

77.4.4 Esophageal Phase

Esophageal transit times can be measured from when the bolus enters the esophagus at the upper esophageal sphincter (▶ Fig. 77.3d) to when it passes into the stomach at the lower esophageal sphincter. This typically takes 8 to 9 seconds. The upper third of the esophagus is composed of striated and voluntary muscle tissue, the middle third is composed of a mixture of voluntary and involuntary muscle tissue, and the lower third is composed of smooth and involuntary muscle tissue. The peristaltic wave, which begins at the top of the esophagus, pushes the bolus ahead of it and continues sequentially until the lower esophageal sphincter opens to allow the bolus to enter the stomach. The opening or relaxing of the lower esophageal sphincter is referred to as descending inhibition. Primary peristalsis occurs when a swallow induces peristaltic activity, whereas in secondary peristalsis, a propogated contraction wave is initiated in the absence of a swallow. The initiation of secondary peristaltic contractions is involuntary and cannot be sensed. In the event that the bolus becomes trapped or moves more slowly than the primary peristaltic wave (as can happen when the bolus is poorly lubricated), stretch receptors in the esophageal lining are stimulated, and a local reflex response causes a secondary peristaltic wave to form around the bolus, forcing it farther down the esophagus. These secondary waves continue indefinitely until the bolus enters the stomach. Tertiary waves are often seen on barium swallow, manometry, and EGD (esophagogastroduodenoscopy) reports. They are defined

Table 77.1 Summary of cranial nerve participation in swallowing

Cranial nerve	Central nervous system	Autonomic nervous system
V: trigeminal	Sensory: touch, pressure in mouth Motor: muscles of mastication, tensor veli palatini, mylohyoid, anterior belly of digastric	None
VII: facial	Sensory: taste, anterior tongue Motor: orbicularis oris, posterior belly of digastric	Visceral motor: sublingual, submandibular glands
IX: glossopharyngeal	Sensory: taste, posterior tongue Motor: stylopharyngeus	Visceral motor: parotid gland
X: vagus	Sensory: sensation from larynx, pharynx, trachea, esophagus Motor: larynx, pharynx, esophagus	Visceral motor: smooth muscle of abdominal viscera
XI: accessory (cranial portion)	Motor: same contributions as cranial nerve X	
XII: hypoglossal	Motor: intrinsic and extrinsic tongue muscles, except for mylohyoid and anterior digastric muscles	

Source: Data from Crary M, Groher M. Introduction to Adult Swallowing Disorders. St. Louis, MO: Mosby Elsevier; 2003:22.

as contractions that occur simultaneously at different levels of the esophagus. These contractions are nonperistaltic, have no known physiologic role, and are observed with increased frequency in elderly people. This phenomenon has been called presbyesophagus in radiographic descriptions.

The esophageal phase of swallowing cannot be managed with therapeutic exercises. Patients with esophageal disorders should be referred to a gastroenterologist or otolaryngologist skilled in the evaluation and treatment of esophageal dysmotility.

77.5 Neural Control of Swallowing

The neural control of swallowing entails a very complex interaction of afferent sensory neurons, motor neurons, and interneurons that control the voluntary and involuntary/reflexive actions of swallowing. The somatic and autonomic components of cranial nerves V, VII, IX, X, XI (cranial portion), and XII are active in producing a normal swallow. Cranial nerve deficits cause changes in function that range from minor to life-threatening. ▶ Table 77.1 provides a summary of the cranial nerves directly involved in swallowing.

77.6 Summary

Swallowing is a highly coordinated series of events involving the entire act of deglutition, from the placement of food in the mouth through the oral and pharyngeal stages of the swallow until entry of the material into the esophagus through the cricopharyngeus and passage onward into the stomach. To effectively treat oropharyngeal swallowing disorders, the clinician must be able to define normal anatomy and physiology, as well as abnormal anatomical and physiologic features of the mechanism.

77.7 Roundsmanship

- Normal swallow consists of four distinct yet interrelated phases: oral preparatory, oral, pharyngeal, and esophageal.
- For swallow to be normal, the anatomical structures and their functions must be intact, and their actions must be appropriately timed and sequenced.

77.8 Recommended Reading

[1] Crary M, Groher M. Introduction to Adult Swallowing Disorders. St. Louis, MO: Mosby Elsevier; 2003:15–34
[2] Logemann J. Evaluation and Treatment of Swallowing Disorders. Austin, TX: PRO-ED; 1998:13–52
[3] Murray T, Carrau R. Clinical Manual for Swallowing Disorders. San Diego, CA: Singular Publishing Group; 2001:13–23

78 Voice Evaluation

Amy L. Cooper

78.1 Introduction

Abnormal voice is the product of inadequate or abnormal behavior of the vocal tract structures; an abnormal voice results from abnormal physiology. Because of structural, physiologic, acoustic, and perceptual factors, the evaluation of vocal function is a complex undertaking. In addition, the extraordinarily rapid development of both theory and technology in the past several decades has resulted in an explosive growth of evaluation techniques, many of which are as of yet unproven validity or utility in the assessment enterprise. A thorough review of the rationales, methods, and theoretical bases of vocal evaluation would require more resources than the present circumstances allow. The present purpose, therefore, is to provide a brief introduction to the rationale, methodology, and interpretation of the assessment of vocal function. A brief outline of the case history and the aerodynamic and acoustic factors pertinent to a patient's vocal function will be provided below. The physiologic significance of the phenomena discussed here was engaged in Chapter 75. Optimal diagnosis is essential in planning the therapeutic course.

78.2 Voice History

While the otolaryngologist focuses primarily on the structure of the larynx, the speech language pathologist (SLP) reports functional measures. The larynx is a dynamic structure, and a dynamic vocal assessment combining analyses of structure and function is required for the diagnosis and treatment of laryngeal disorders. The SLP begins by taking a case history incorporating aspects of the patient's medical and social history, which includes an assessment of the patient's vocal demands. The clinician provides a subjective impression of vocal quality (hoarse, breathy, harsh, aphonic, pitch breaks, tremor, diplo-

phonic, strained/strangled, glottal attack, glottal fry, vocal fatigue). These observations are used in conjunction with objective measures (acoustic, aerodynamic) that are discussed below. The behavioral assessment may also yield observations about breath patterns, including clavicular versus abdominal breathing, the presence or absence of stridor, and behaviors such as throat clearing. Additionally, rating scales, including the GRBAS Scale (see Box, below) and the CAPE-V Scale (see Box, below) can help quantify and qualify the degree of vocal aberrance. The Voice Handicap Index-10 (VHI-10; ▶ Table 78.1) is a questionnaire that can help define the patient's perceived disability in response to a voice disorder.

GRBAS Scale

Items are rated by the examiner on a scale of 0 (normal) to 3 (severe).
- Grade (overall severity)
- Roughness
- Breathiness
- Aesthenia (weakness)
- Strain

78.3 Acoustic Analysis

Acoustic analysis of the voice uses instrumentation to analyze the physiologically relevant properties of a sound wave. It provides measures of frequency, amplitude, disturbance (perturbation), harmonic content, noise, and other variables related to the function of the vocal tract and larynx. These measurements are intended to provide insight into the physiology, origins, and severity of dysphonia.

Table 78.1 Voice Handicap Index-10 (VHI-10)

Item	Grade
	Scale goes from 0 = never to 4 = always
My voice makes it difficult for people to hear me.	0 1 2 3 4
People have difficulty understanding me in a noisy room.	0 1 2 3 4
My voice difficulties restrict my personal and social life.	0 1 2 3 4
I feel left out of conversations because of my voice.	0 1 2 3 4
My voice problem causes me to lose income.	0 1 2 3 4
I feel as though I have to strain to produce my voice.	0 1 2 3 4
The clarity of my voice is unpredictable.	0 1 2 3 4
My voice problem upsets me.	0 1 2 3 4
My voice makes me feel handicapped.	0 1 2 3 4
People ask, "What's wrong with your voice?"	0 1 2 3 4

CAPE-V (Consensus Auditory-Perceptual Evaluation of Voice) Scale

Overall severity, roughness, breathiness, strain, pitch, and loudness are rated on a 100-mm visual analog scale. The rater places a vertical mark along each horizontal line; the far left end of the line represents least impaired status, and the far right end represents most impaired status.

Form:

Hospital #: _____ Date: _____

The following parameters of voice will be rated upon completion of the following tasks:

1. Sustained vowels /a/ and /i/ for 3 to 5 seconds' duration each.
2. Sentence production:

"The blue spot is on the key again."
"How hard did he hit him?"
"We were away a year ago."
"We eat eggs every Easter."
"My mama makes lemon muffins."
"Peter will keep at the peak."

1. Spontaneous speech. **Prompt as follows:**
   a) **New patient:** Tell me when your voice problem began, what you were noticing, and what you have done about it.
   b) **Return patients:** Tell me what's happened with your voice since last time you were here. What treatment have you had? Did it help?

Legend:

C, consistent
I, intermittent
MI, mildly deviant
MO, moderately deviant
SE, severely deviant

Overall Severity_____ /100
C I MI MO SE
Roughness_____ /100
C I MI MO SE
Breathiness_____ /100
C I MI MO SE
Strain _____ /100
C I MI MO SE
Pitch Loudness (Indicate the nature of the abnormality):
_____ /100
C I MI MO SE
Comments about resonance: Normal Other (Provide description): _____

_____

_____

Additional features (for example, diplophonia, fry, asthenia, aphonia, pitch instability, tremor, wet/gurgly, or other relevant terms):

G__R__B__A__S__ Clinician: _____

78.4 Aerodynamic Assessment

Measurements of airflow are of particular importance because they describe or quantify the power supply—that is, the subglottal pressure and transglottal airflow—for phonation. When available, spirometry is used to assess lung volume and lung capacity. Essential to insight into vocal efficiency are measurements of subglottal pressure and transglottal airflow. Vocal fold vibration is initiated and maintained by a pressure differential between the subglottal and supraglottal regions. An assessment of subglottal pressure and airflow permits inferences about what is happening at the level of the glottis. Abnormally high subglottic pressure and/or glottal resistance may be a sign of vocal hyperfunction or inflammation. Increased airflow may be a sign of vocal hypofunction or vocal fold paralysis/paresis. These measures are useful in treatment planning and can be used for comparisons before and after medical and surgical intervention. ▶ Table 78.2 summarizes the normative data for diagnostically significant vocal characteristics and their implications with regard to physiology.

78.5 Evaluation of the Vocal Fold Contact Pattern

The movements of the vocal folds are rapid and complex, and they unfold in three dimensions, as discussed in the chapter on vocal physiology. Endoscopic techniques, including videostroboscopy, videokymography, and high-speed video recording, make it relatively easy to assess the basic features of motion at the upper surface of the vocal folds and, during the glottal open phase, to get some sense of displacements of the glottal walls. However, the way in which the vocal folds contact each other, and the displacements or disruptions that may occur during the glottal closed phase, are hidden from visual inspection. A technique known as electroglottography (EGG) offers a way of visualizing these occult events.

EGG takes advantage of the fact that most tissues, having a high electrolyte content, are fairly good electrical conductors, whereas air is an extraordinarily poor electrical conductor. If electrodes are placed on the body surface over each thyroid ala, a weak high-frequency electric current can be passed between them through the tissues of the neck. During the open phase of the glottal cycle, the electrical resistance of this pathway will be comparatively high because the vocal folds are separated by an insulating volume of air. However, as the amount of vocal fold contact increases during glottal closure, the trans-neck resistance falls, reaching a minimum when the surface area of vocal fold contact is maximal; it then rises again to a maximum when the vocal folds fully separate. The magnitude of the current through the neck is thus a parameter of the vocal fold contact area.

In ▶ Fig. 78.1, the normal EGG of modal register phonation by a healthy male is compared with the EGG of a female patient who has vocal nodules. The abnormality of the latter pattern is clearly apparent and shows at least one way in which a clinically significant disruption of normal vocal fold contact may manifest. The interpretation of EGG records depends on both quantitative and qualitative methods that offer deeper insight into the bases of phonatory disorder.

Table 78.2 Expected values of diagnostically significant vocal characteristics

Variable	Test item	Expected values	Units	Implication of... Increase	Decrease
Power supply					
Subglottal (tracheal) pressure (P_s)	/pi/	5.4–9.7 ♀ 5.4–7.5 ♂	cm H_2O	Speech intensity ↑ Hyperkinetic disorder	Speech intensity ↓ Hypertonic chest wall Hypokinetic disorder
Phonation threshold pressure (PTP)	/pi/	≈ 3	cm H_2O	Hypertonic vocal folds Vocal fold tension/stiffness ↑ Vocal fold adduction ↑	————
Comfortable speech/ voice intensity	Sustained vowel /a/	≈ 75	dB	P_s ↑ Vocal fold hyperadduction	P_s ↓ Vocal fold hypoadduction Glottal gap
Maximum speech intensity	/a/		dB	————	Hypertonic chest wall Hypokinetic disorder
Glottal behavior					
Speaking fundamental frequency (SF_0)	/a/	180–250 ♀ 100–130 ♂ Hz 43–45 ♀ 33–38 ♂ ST (re 16.35 Hz)	Hz ST (re 16.35 Hz)	Vocal fold tension/stiffness ↑ P_s ↑ Hyperkinetic disorder	Vocal fold mass ↑ Vocal fold tension/stiffness ↓ P_s ↓
Maximum phonational frequency range (MPFR)	/a/	134–895 ♀ 77–576 ♂ Hz 36–85 ♀ 23–59 ♂ ST (re 16.35 Hz)	Hz ST (re 16.35 Hz)	Vocal fold tension/stiffness ↑	Vocal fold tension/stiffness ↓ Vocal fold paresis Cricothyroid paresis
Contact quotient (C_q) Closed quotient (C_q)	/a/	0.4–0.6		Vocal fold hyperadduction Vocal intensity ↑	Vocal fold hypoadduction Vocal intensity ↓
Speed quotient (S_q)	/A/	0.5		Vocal intensity ↑	Vocal intensity ↓
Harmonic-to-noise ratio (HNR)	/A/	>12	dB	————	Air stream turbulence Glottal gap Vocal fold hypoadduction Short-term F_0 instability Short-term intensity instability

Abbreviation: ST (re 16.35 Hz), semitones relative to 16.35 Hz.

78.6 Sound Spectrography

The ability to examine the acoustic content of the speech signal over time offers a means of assessing many features of the glottal source signal, of the vocal tract filter adjustment, and of the way in which these fundamental characteristics interact. The most common form of such an examination is the sound spectrogram, in which a gray scale is used to represent the evolution over time (horizontal axis) of the intensity of the speech signal as a function of frequency (vertical axis). It is possible to change the analytic parameters of the spectrogram to optimize frequency resolution, time relationships, vocal tract filter characteristics, noise elements, and so forth. This ability to optimize the spectrogram, and so derive the enormous amount of information that is contained in the resulting record, makes spectrography of enormous diagnostic value, especially in patients with complex disorders of the phonatory system.

▶ Fig. 78.2, which is the spectrographic analysis of a normal male saying "Joe took father's shoe bench out," gives some sense of the kinds of information that can be obtained. Each of the vertical lines seen during the vowels, for instance, is produced by a single glottal closure that pinches off the airflow (see Chapter 75), whereas the darker horizontal bands during the vowels result from peaks resonances in the vocal tract filter function or energy at nonharmonic frequencies. This can be seen during the "sh" of *shoe* and the "ch" of *bench*. The temporal relationships of laryngeal and vocal tract adjustments are relatively easily read by a professional experienced in spectrographic analysis.

78.7 Summary

The voice history and the results of acoustic and aerodynamic testing are critical parts of the diagnostic process. The evaluation of the dynamic physiology of phonatory and nonphonatory behavior is aided not only by visualization of the larynx but also by other forms of measurable documentation of laryngeal function. Of particular interest are the insights offered by inspection of the electroglottographic signal and sound spectrogram.

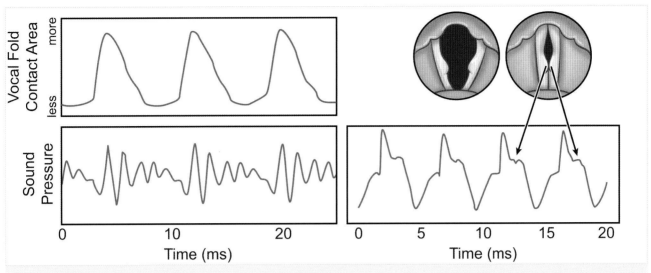

Fig. 78.1 Examples of electroglottographic (EGG) records. Left: The upper trace shows the changes in vocal fold contact area during three glottal cycles of a normal male voice. An increase in contact area (upward deflection) indicates more contact of one vocal fold to the other. It does *not* necessarily indicate greater glottal closure. The vocal signal generated by these glottal cycles is shown below the EGG. Right: Vocal fold contact pattern of a female speaker with vocal nodules. The protrusion of the relatively compliant masses causes the "shoulders" seen in the EGG record.

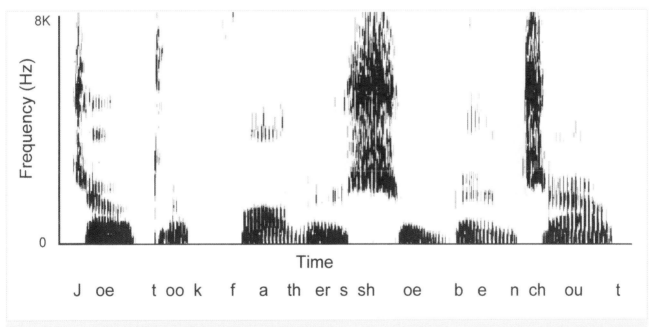

Fig. 78.2 Sound spectrographic analysis of a normal male saying "Joe took father's shoe bench out." It shows the intensity of the speech signal (the darker the marking, the more intense the sound) as a function of frequency (vertical axis) over time (horizontal axis). Glottal closures, noise elements, resonant frequencies of the vocal tract, and features of speech timing that are important in the assessment of complex speech and voice problems are demonstrated.

78.8 Roundsmanship

- An evaluation of laryngeal function is vital to treatment planning.
- The case history and the acoustic and aerodynamic data add vital information to laryngeal imaging.

78.9 Recommended Reading

[1] Baken RJ, Orlikoff RF. Clinical Measurement of Speech and Voice. 2nd ed. San Diego, CA: Singular Publishing Group; 2000

[2] Colton RH, Casper JK. Understanding Voice Problems: A Physiological Perspective for Diagnosis and Treatment. Baltimore, MD: Lippincott Williams & Wilkins; 1996

[3] Hirano M. Clinical Examination of Voice. New York, NY: Springer; 1981

[4] Isshiki N. Phonosurgery. New York, NY: Springer; 1989

[5] Jacobson B, Johnson A, Grywalski C et al. The voice handicap index (VHI): development and validation. Am J Speech Lang Pathol 1997; 6: 66–70

[6] Schwartz SK. The Source for Voice Disorders Adolescent & Adult. East Moline, IL: LinguiSystems; 2004:171–174

79 Laryngovideostroboscopy

Chandra M. Ivey

79.1 Introduction

Videostroboscopy is a technique for evaluating the vibration of the vocal folds. The human vocal folds vibrate too fast for the human eye to detect their motion. A flickered (strobed) light source directly over the vocal folds can effectively momentarily "freeze" this motion so that it can be perceived in pseudo-slow motion.

79.2 Incidence of Disease

Vocal fold irregularity can be seen in almost anyone, but videostroboscopy is used mainly as a tool for evaluating the dysphonic patient. Although visualization with still light via direct or indirect laryngoscopy allows lesions on the vocal cord to be detected, it does not provide a sufficient evaluation of the depth of an irregularity or the impact a lesion has on the vibration of the vocal fold. Videostroboscopy can assist in this evaluation, aid diagnosis and surgical planning, and improve the ability to predict outcomes after phonosurgery.

79.3 Applied Anatomy

Evaluation with videostroboscopy is based on the body–cover principle of vocal fold motion. For "normal" phonation, the vocal fold "cover" (the epithelium and superficial layers of the lamina propria) must move smoothly over the "body" (the thyroarytenoid muscle). The cover and body are attached to each other by the vocal ligament (the intermediate and deep layers of the lamina propria, which comprise the transitional layer;

▶ Fig. 79.1). The vocal body shortens and lengthens by relaxation or contraction of the thyroarytenoid and cricothyroid muscles in order to achieve a dynamic frequency range. These relative changes in the body result in tension changes in the cover. A short and relaxed body allows a lax cover to vibrate with large amplitude at lower frequency. A long and stiff body tenses the cover and results in smaller-amplitude vibrations at higher frequency. Any disease process that affects the ability of the cover to vibrate smoothly should cause predictable phonatory changes and be measurable.

According to Talbot's law, images persist on the human retina for 200 microseconds. Any stimuli presented faster than this are not perceptible as distinct images. When a series of still images are presented, each for less than 200 microseconds, an optical illusion of motion is created. This principle allows still images of multiple cycles of vocal fold vibration to be visually perceived as one cycle in pseudo-slow motion when the images are presented sequentially.

In order for videostroboscopy to work, vocal fold vibration needs to be fairly periodic in nature. The flashes of light can be entrained to a frequency slightly different from that of the vocal folds to give the perception of a moving wave. This is done by catching each cycle of vocal fold vibration in a slightly different position so that it appears to be slowly moving from closed to open. Although each frame captured is from an entirely different vibratory cycle of the vocal fold, the perception on the retina is that of a slowly vibrating vocal fold. ▶ Fig. 79.2a depicts the difference between stroboscopy and high-speed video imaging of vocal fold motion. ▶ Fig. 79.2b displays the averaged glottic cycle displayed during stroboscopy.

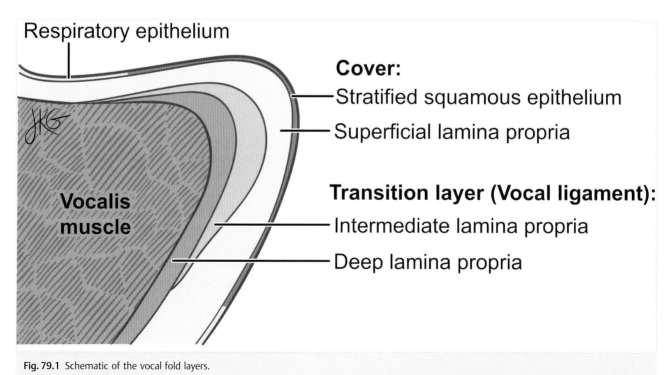

Fig. 79.1 Schematic of the vocal fold layers.

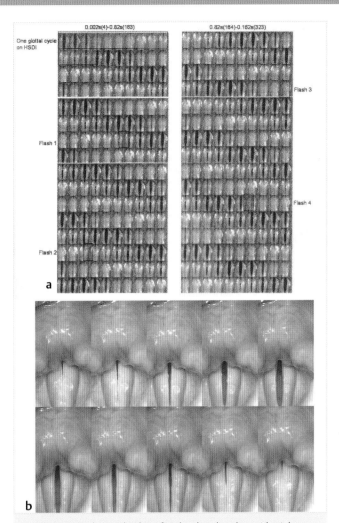

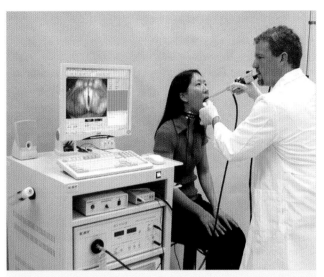

Fig. 79.3 Laryngovideostroboscopy equipment and examination. (Courtesy of Pentax of America, Montvale, NJ).

Fig. 79.2 (a) High-speed video of eight glottal cycles, with pink squares indicating the videostroboscopy light flash. Stacking of the pink frames results in a pseudo-slow motion vibration of the vocal folds. *HSDI*, high-speed digital imaging. (Reprinted with permission from Bless D, Patel RR, Connor N. Laryngeal imaging. In: Freid M, Ferlito A, eds. The Larynx. 3rd ed. San Diego, CA: Plural Publishing; 2009.) (b) Videomontage obtained with videostroboscopy.

79.4 Videostroboscopic Evaluation

79.4.1 Equipment

The basic equipment necessary for videostroboscopy includes the following:

1. Laryngoscope: Whether transnasal distal chip technology fiber-optic laryngoscopy or transoral rigid endoscopy is performed, consistent focused images of both vocal folds from the anterior commissure through the arytenoids are important for evaluation.
2. Video equipment: Recording capability allows multiple screenings of the vocal fold movement for a more complete evaluation. Some systems allow slowing the replay or playing the images in a frame-by-frame style, which can assist in a more accurate and consistent analysis.

3. Microphone: Voice recording allows measurement of the sound decibel (dB) level during videostroboscopy, as well as measurement of the voice fundamental frequency (F_0). These recordings serve as part of the medical record and document vocal changes over the course of treatment.
4. Entrainment system: For videostroboscopy to accurately depict a running image, the light must be triggered in a systematic fashion and relative to the phonatory frequency. The frequency is obtained either by using a laryngeal microphone or by electroglottography (EGG).
5. Strobed light source: This pulses bright light relative to the frequency of the vocal fold vibration to create the perceived slow motion vibration recorded in videostroboscopy.

79.4.2 Technique

Although each physician may have his or her own technique for videostroboscopy, the most important aspect of the evaluation is consistency. A typical examination is shown in ▶ Fig. 79.3.

Documentation at the patient's modal (or natural) pitch is standard, and the modal pitch should be the first pitch evaluated when data are recorded. The evaluation encompasses approximately 5 seconds of vocal fold vibration at this pitch and at a frequency of approximately 100 Hz higher. Observations are also made while the patient slowly raises his or her pitch to allow evaluation of the cricoarytenoid muscle contribution to phonation. These tasks are often recorded between 60 and 80 dB. Images taken at louder and softer voice ranges can add to the evaluation by changing the body–cover dynamics, which allows irregularities or lesions to be more easily identified. General laryngeal biomechanics are also noted.

Videostroboscopy is extremely useful for the identification and evaluation of irregular vocal fold vibration. Adjunct evaluation with voice recording and with acoustic and aerodynamic analysis can offer additional information for difficult cases or uncertain diagnoses.

79.4.3 Terminology

Many terms are used to describe abnormalities of vocal fold vibration in videostroboscopy:

- Vocal fold edge: The vocal fold should be straight from the anterior commissure to the vocal process. Any interruption in this is considered an irregularity.
- Glottal closure pattern: Description of the area between the vocal folds when they are fully adducted. Normal vocal folds are considered to have a complete closure pattern. Variations in this pattern that may indicate pathology are incomplete, spindle, hourglass, posterior chink, anterior chink, and irregular chink.
- Mucosal wave propagation: Description of the excursion of the moving wave over the body of the vocal fold. Typically, a wave that propagates across 50% of the superior surface of the vocal fold is considered normal. Propagation is typically greater with low-frequency vibration and smaller in high-frequency vibration. Similarly, the propagation increases with louder sounds. Areas of epithelial abnormality may show altered propagation, and in cases of severe scarring there may be absence of mucosal wave altogether.
- Vocal fold amplitude: The distance the vocal fold edge and thus the mass of the vocal fold are displaced from the midline during the glottic cycle. The typical amplitude is again 50% of the vocal fold width.
- Vibratory behavior: Description of the vibration of the vocal fold cover. In normal circumstances, the vibration of the cover is initiated on the infraglottic surface of the fold; it proceeds perpendicular to the vocal ligament and then across the superior surface of the vocal fold.
- Phase symmetry: Description of the cover vibration pattern of one vocal fold with respect to the other. Typically, each wave starts inferiorly and proceeds superiorly then laterally away from midline. When the vibration is in phase, the patterns mirror each other. When vocal fold pathology is present, the wave of one vocal fold may be altered in relation to the other so that they no longer mirror each other, and thus the vibratory patterns will be out of phase.
- Periodicity: In order to use videostroboscopy to evaluate the vocal folds, they must vibrate with predictable and measurable rhythm. If a lesion causes the vibration to vary too much from cycle to cycle, the strobe will not be able to sync with the frequency of vibration, and the vocal fold vibration will be perceived as "flickering" instead of moving in a wavelike fashion.

79.5 The Disease Process

79.5.1 Normal Stroboscopic Findings

Under normal conditions, each vocal fold has the same approximate tension and mass, allowing a precise, in-phase mucosal wave on each side. Each vocal fold edge should be straight, and the glottic configuration should show complete closure. The vocal folds tend to be closed for about 40 to 50% of the glottal cycle. The mucosal wave amplitude should be similar from side to side, and the vibration should proceed in an organized fashion from the infraglottic to the superior surface along the entire length of the vocal fold. The mucosal waves should be in phase, and the vocal folds should have the same periodicity.

79.5.2 Abnormal Stroboscopic Findings

Any epithelial or subepithelial lesion may disrupt the symmetry of the vocal fold edges. These lesions may also affect the glottic configuration because they may prevent full vocal fold closure and cause an hourglass or irregular closure pattern.

An increase in the mass of one vocal fold with respect to the other tends to increase the heaviness of that fold. If the change in mass is generalized, as in polypoid corditis of the vocal fold, it may cause an increased mucosal wave amplitude and propagation along the entire mucosal surface of the vocal fold, as well as an irregular periodicity. If the change in mass is due to the presence of a limited lesion—for example, a cyst or polyp—the area affected tends to move differently from the rest of the fold, causing a local change in mucosal wave and vibration, and likely a phase shift.

An increase in the stiffness of one vocal fold with respect to the other tends to create a reduced mucosal wave and vocal fold amplitude. This can create a phase asymmetry in which one vocal fold appears to be vibrating less. If a lesion affects both the cover and the ligament in a limited area of one vocal fold, videostroboscopy may reveal the absence of a mucosal wave, indicating loss of epithelium (as with scar), an inflamed subepithelial lesion (as with a cyst), or infiltration (as with invasive carcinoma) in that area.

The tension of each vocal fold may also affect the parameters measured with videostroboscopy. Because tension may affect both the mass and the stiffness of a vocal fold, it is important to evaluate whether the tension of each fold appears similar. At times, a vocal fold paresis may decrease the tension of one fold and cause changes in mucosal wave and vocal fold amplitude, resulting in phase asymmetry. Differential tension is often noted when there is a difference between the levels of the vocal folds.

It is important to remember that videostroboscopy is used to record vocal fold vibration in pseudo-slow motion, and then these videos are subjectively analyzed by the otolaryngologist. Consistent patterns of evaluation should be developed for reliable use.

79.6 Roundsmanship

- Videostroboscopy makes possible the evaluation of vocal fold vibration.
- As a consequence of Talbot's law, still images from multiple cycles of vocal fold vibration are visually perceived as one cycle in pseudo-slow motion when the images are presented sequentially.
- Many terms are used to describe vocal fold vibration in videostroboscopy, including the following: vocal fold edge, glottic closure pattern, mucosal wave propagation, vocal fold amplitude, vibratory behavior, phase symmetry, and periodicity.

- Changes in the mass, stiffness, and tension of the vocal folds are associated with predictable changes in the vibration characteristics displayed by videostroboscopy.

79.7 Recommended Reading

[1] Maunsell R, Ouaknine M, Giovanni A, Crespo A. Vibratory pattern of vocal folds under tension asymmetry. Otolaryngol Head Neck Surg 2006; 135: 438–444

[2] Titze IR. Vocal fold oscillation. In: Principles of Voice Production. Iowa City, IA: National Center for Voice and Speech; 2000: 87–122

[3] Verikas A, Uloza V, Bacauskiene M, Gelzinis A, Kelertas E. Advances in laryngeal imaging. Eur Arch Otorhinolaryngol 2009; 266: 1509–1520

[4] Woo P. Vocal fold vibration and phonatory physiology. In: Stroboscopy. San Diego, CA: Plural Publishing; 2010:39–52

[5] Woo P, Casper J, Colton R, Brewer D. Aerodynamic and stroboscopic findings before and after microlaryngeal phonosurgery. J Voice 1994; 8: 186–194

80 Laryngeal Electromyography

Rick M. Roark and Craig H. Zalvan

80.1 Introduction

Since the 1950s, laryngeal electromyography (EMG) has been a useful tool in the diagnosis of various neuromuscular disorders affecting the larynx. The percutaneous placement of needle electrodes within the laryngeal musculature allows the muscles to be studied at rest and during voluntary activation. The interpretation of electrical signals can be useful in determining the site of a lesion, degree of neuronal injury, and prognosis for reinnervation. It can also aid in differentiating between paralysis and mechanical fixation and can guide the injection of spasmodic laryngeal muscles with botulinum toxin.

80.2 Technical Information

Laryngeal EMG is routinely performed in the office setting. Most laryngeal electromyographers use a sensitive multichannel EMG system. A ground electrode is placed on the neck just lateral and inferior to the larynx. A reference electrode is placed away from the neck, typically overlying the angle of the mandible, the posterior triangle near the mastoid, or the clavicle. Both electrodes are amplified and the difference subtracted to generate a signal that best represents the electrical activity of the desired muscle and minimizes the background noise from other muscles, power sources, and other electromagnetic devices.

The sweep speed of the EMG display unit sets the rate at which the signal is horizontally traced to the display screen, with a setting of 10 ms/cm used for most purposes. Faster sweep settings (e.g., 1 ms/cm) facilitate a more detailed examination of signal shapes, whereas a slower sweep offers a more global view of the composite EMG signal. Gain, or sensitivity, of the EMG display adjusts the vertical extent to which the signal will be traced to the display screen and is typically set in the range of 50 to 200 mV/cm. When a general assessment of muscle activation is made, the sweep and gain settings are typically 100 ms/cm and 1,000 mV/cm, respectively. To examine the finer details of neuromuscular status (e.g., hierarchical recruitment of motor units during initial activation), settings of 1 ms/cm and 50 mV/cm are helpful. The indwelling electrode (either a bipolar concentric or a monopolar needle) is inserted at rest into the muscle of choice, followed by various voicing tasks to activate that muscle. Monopolar needles are thinner and cause less damage to tissue, as well as less pain. They record circumferentially at the site of interest and are less costly. Concentric needles do not require an external reference electrode because it is built into the needle itself; as such, a concentric needle results in less interference, which makes it optimal to evaluate the morphology of the laryngeal EMG results.

80.3 Technique

Laryngeal EMG is performed with the patient in a sitting or supine position (▶ Fig. 80.1). The head is slightly extended. Landmarks are first palpated: the cricothyroid membrane, the thyroid notch, and the trachea. Ground electrodes (and a reference

electrode, if a monopolar electrode is being used) are placed, and the area is prepared with alcohol. Once the needle is inserted into the skin and the EMG machine is turned on, sharp popping/crackling sounds are heard as the needle is advanced into muscle. The thyroarytenoid, posterior cricoarytenoid, and cricothyroid muscles are typically evaluated with diagnostic EMG.

80.3.1 Thyroarytenoid

To access the thyroarytenoid muscle, the needle is passed through the cricothyroid membrane just lateral to the midline on the side being tested. The needle is then advanced and angled 45 degrees upward and 20 to 30 degrees laterally (▶ Fig. 80.2). At times, the needle may penetrate the airway, which will result in a sinusoidal pattern on the screen and a loud monotone feedback from the speaker; it often will also elicit pain and cough from the patient. The needle is withdrawn slightly, repositioned, and advanced; when the needle is redirected, it should not be turned laterally while within the body, but rather withdrawn and turned in the desired direction to minimize tissue trauma. Advancing the needle forward will result in auditory evidence of muscle insertion. Testing of the thyroarytenoid muscle involves a period of rest to assess baseline activity followed by activation tasks; these include /i/ in short bursts, followed by a prolonged /i/ at both high and low pitch, a Valsalva maneuver, and a cough. These tasks adduct the vocal folds and activate the thyroarytenoid muscle. In addition, multiple repeated sniffing maneuvers test for synkinesis because the thyroarytenoid should be relatively quiet.

80.3.2 Posterior Cricoarytenoid Muscle

This muscle can be accessed in two ways. In young patients, the needle can be passed through the cricothyroid membrane and

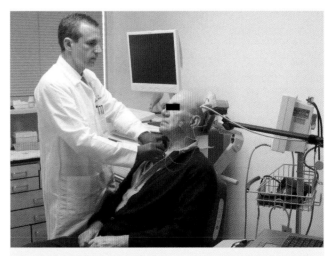

Fig. 80.1 Laryngeal electromyography is comfortably performed in an office setting.

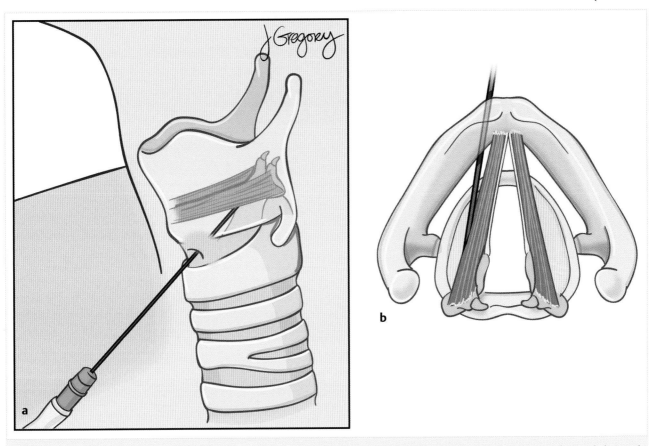

Fig. 80.2 (a) The needle is place through the cricothyroid membrane just lateral to the midline on the side of interest. (b) The needle is angled upward and laterally until the thyroarytenoid muscle is accessed.

directed into the airway, then slightly inferiorly and laterally into the posterior lamina of the cricothyroid cartilage. The needle is pushed through the cartilage until brisk pops are heard and motor unit action potentials are seen on the screen. The posterior cricoarytenoid is activated by a sniff maneuver. When the cartilage is ossified or the anterior approach is difficult, the posterior cricoarytenoid can be approached from the lateral neck. The larynx is grasped between the thumb on the lateral border and the pointer finger on the thyroid notch (for left posterior cricoarytenoid testing). The larynx is rotated away from the side being injected, and the EMG needle is advanced behind the lateral border of the thyroid cartilage at its lower border until the cricoid cartilage is encountered. At this point, the needle is retracted slightly, and a brisk signal will be heard when the patient sniffs if the posterior cricoarytenoid has been properly located (► Fig. 80.3).

80.3.3 Cricothyroid Muscle

The cricothyroid muscle is accessed by placing the needle through the skin overlying the cricoid slightly lateral to the cricoid itself. The needle is then advanced slightly medially and along the superior boarder of the cricoid until brisk potentials are heard and visualized. Absence of EMG activity during a head turn or chin raise will confirm that the needle is not within the strap muscles. To obtain activity of the cricothyroid muscle, the patient is asked to phonate a sustained /i/ at low pitch and then

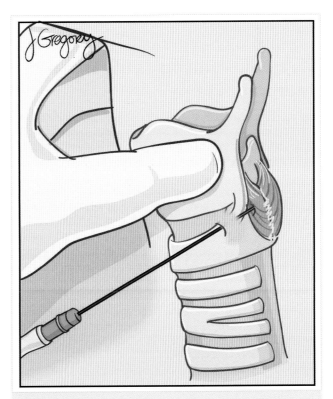

Fig. 80.3 Lateral approach to the posterior cricoarytenoid muscle.

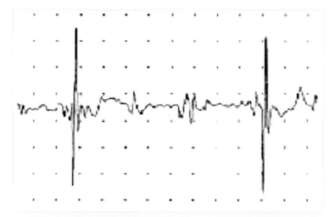

Fig. 80.4 Normal motor unit configuration (600 mV).

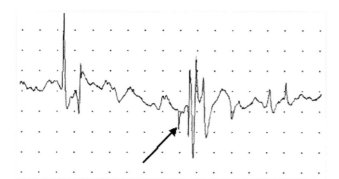

Fig. 80.6 Fibrillation potentials occurring with a polyphasic motor unit potential in a partially denervated thyroarytenoid muscle.

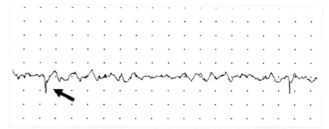

Fig. 80.5 Fibrillation potentials from partially denervated thyroarytenoid muscle.

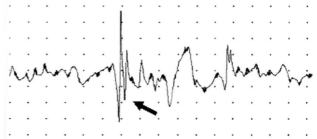

Fig. 80.7 Polyphasic motor unit action potential with increased amplitude (700 mV; *arrow*) from a thryoarytenoid muscle after recurrent laryngeal nerve injury during thyroidectomy.

at high pitch. Activation should increase substantially during high pitch phonation.

80.4 Electromyographic Signal Interpretation

Normal motor unit action potential (MUAP): The firing of each laryngeal motor unit creates a compound myoelectric potential called the MUAP. Individual MUAPs may be identified in the EMG signal during low-force activations (▶ Fig. 80.4) when few in number, but as additional motor units are recruited and firing rates are increased during greater force demands, the individual shapes become confounded. Normal MUAPs have a distinctive multiphasic wave shape indicating the four phases of compound muscle fiber depolarization. However, the specific MUAP morphology that is observed, with its distinguishing shape and timing characteristics, will depend greatly upon the size and geometry of the detector(s) and the recording setup (monopolar or bipolar). Although many of the important clinical impressions can be obtained when any recording scenario is used, more refined observations must often be paired with the specific electrodes used, the type of recordings, and the experience of the electromyographer.

Recruitment: As the volitional activity of a muscle persists or increases, adjacent motor units are recruited to activate more muscle fibers and increase or maintain the strength of contraction. When recruitment is normal, so many MUAPs are present

that individual MUAPs cannot be identified because they are obscured by one another. When this occurs, it is referred to as a full interference pattern. In cases of neural injury, fewer motor units are recruited, the interference pattern becomes thinned, and it is possible to identify individual units.

Insertional activity: When the needle enters the muscle, there may be brisk, sharp insertional activity due to brisk depolarization of the cell membranes. This typically lasts a few seconds. Prolonged insertional activity for longer than 300 ms may be indicative of muscle membrane instability from either a neuropathic or a myopathic process.

Fibrillation potentials/positive sharp waves: These are initial positive deflections of the MUAPs that are typically sharp, short, and repetitive (▶ Fig. 80.5). When present, they are indicative of denervated muscle fibers.

Polyphasic action potentials: A normal MUAP is biphasic or triphasic (phases indicate the number of times an MUAP crosses the baseline). Polyphasic (with four or more phases) action potentials are abnormal (▶ Fig. 80.6) and indicate active reinnervation by a damaged nerve. Polyphasic action potentials occur as nerve endings regrow to atrophied muscle fibers. The result of these immature synaptic transmissions is the appearance of MUAPs of lower amplitude and longer duration. The fibers eventually incorporate more muscle fiber units, resulting in increased MUAP amplitude but continued polyphasic morphology (▶ Fig. 80.7).

Giant waves: Muscle reinnervation following nerve injury will often be accompanied by one or more nonpolyphasic waves that have abnormally high amplitudes in the EMG signal. Giant waves (▶ Fig. 80.8) are formed as the axon branches in the newly reinnervated fibers of a motor unit begin to develop nodes of Ranvier and become myelinated, thus reducing the transport time of the action potential to the fiber end plate and

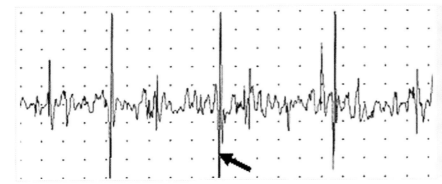

Fig. 80.8 Giant waves with amplitude of more than 900 mV (*arrow*).

so reducing the delay times of the fiber depolarization potentials to the recording electrode. Previously, the varied and prolonged delays that caused the depolarization potentials to sum into a polyphasic MUAP during early-stage reinnervation were reduced, causing the potentials now to sum supportively into an MUAP with a shorter duration and a greater amplitude. Although giant waves are consistent with muscle reinnervation physiologically, their presence is inconsistent with normal innervation anatomically because the bundling of fibers constituting the motor unit is closer than in a normal unit, in which fibers are more interspersed. Giant waves indicate a mature state of muscle reinnervation. An absence of vocal fold motion in the presence of giant waves suggests a poor prognosis.

The duration of the MUAP reflects the number of muscle fibers innervated by the axon being studied. Age tends to increase the duration as conduction velocity decreases. Temperature also affects duration, with hypothermia resulting in slower conduction and longer duration. In addition, chronic myopathic and neuropathic disease can increase the duration of the MUAP. The amplitude of the MUAP can similarly be affected by various myopathic and neuropathic conditions. The amplitude directly reflects the number of muscle fibers recorded per given axon. Thus, conditions that damage muscle or block neuromuscular transmission can result in decreased amplitude. Increased amplitude, conversely, is seen with reinnervation and inflammatory conditions.

80.5 Clinical Use

EMG can be a very useful tool in identifying neurologic and myopathic disorders of the laryngeal musculature. Common uses of laryngeal EMG include determination of the prognosis for recovery of a patient with vocal fold paralysis and EMG guidance for botulinum toxin injection. Other indications include testing for vocal fold paresis, myopathy, metabolic disorders, fixation of the cricoarytenoid joint, and other neuropathic conditions that are not covered in this chapter.

80.5.1 Vocal Fold Paralysis

EMG can be a useful tool to assess a patient presenting with vocal fold immobility. EMG does not predict the timing of return of function, nor does it guarantee a return of function. EMG is typically performed at least 3 weeks after an injury to allow wallerian degeneration to result in denervation and to allow fibrillation potentials to arise. Complete denervation is charac-

terized by an absence of recruitment and the presence of fibrillation potentials. In cases of neural recovery, polyphasic waves can be detected. EMG is relatively good at predicting the return of vocal fold function when performed between 2 and 6 months after injury, and a 60 to 90% correlation with clinical outcome has been observed in patients studied. Variability in these outcomes is likely due to timing of the study. Early after injury, the presence of polyphasics suggests an improved prognosis. Increasing recruitment on successive EMGs suggests an active reinnervation process and a higher likelihood of recovery. EMG is even better at predicting the lack of return of vocal fold motion. A lack of movement in the presence of giant waves portends a poor prognosis because maximal neuronal recovery has been achieved and the vocal fold is yet to move. Synkinetic reinnervation plays a large role in preventing vocal fold motion. If there is EMG evidence of significant synkinesis, then a return of motion is less likely. Data are lacking to define what should be considered significant synkinesis. Any synkinesis seen during recovery from a neural injury can lead to vocal fold immobility despite robust favorable EMG findings of return of function. Synkinesis is observed by EMG if there is recruitment in the thyroarytenoid during a "sniff" procedure, or in the posterior cricoarytenoid on phonation.

In addition to determining the prognosis of a patient with vocal fold paralysis, EMG can be useful for identifying the site of neural injury. A normal EMG of the cricothyroid muscle with an abnormal EMG of the thyroarytenoid muscle suggests a peripheral nerve injury below the branching of the superior laryngeal nerve at the nodose ganglion. If both the cricothyroid muscle and the thyroarytenoid muscle show evidence of neuronal injury, it is likely the injury occurred above this division and involves the vagus nerve along its course from the brainstem.

80.5.2 Vocal Fold Paresis

Based on the clinical history and physical examination, vocal fold paresis may be suspected as the etiology of a patient's dysphonia. It has been shown that this diagnosis is difficult to make based on history and physical examination alone because nearly 20% of patients in whom vocal fold paresis is suspected will have a normal EMG and no paresis. In addition, in the nearly 80% of those who do have paresis, identification of the paretic vocal fold based on physical examination alone is accurate only approximately 30% of the time. Hence, laryngeal EMG is very helpful in confirming vocal fold paresis and in identifying the side of weakness for possible surgical intervention.

80.5.3 Arytenoid Fixation

A normal EMG of the thyroarytenoid and cricothyroid muscles indicates no damage to the recurrent laryngeal nerve or superior laryngeal nerve and can suggest dislocation or fixation of the arytenoid joint. When used in this situation, EMG can be performed soon after injury because there is no need to wait for wallerian degeneration to occur. Causes of fixation include traumatic dislocation, arthritis, and posterior glottic scarring resulting in vocal fold immobility.

80.5.4 Spasmodic Dysphonia

EMG can be useful in diagnosing spasmodic dysphonia and other disorders of the basal ganglia. Intermittent breaks in voicing during connected speech associated with increased muscle firing is characteristic of spasmodic dysphonia. In addition, there is typically a delay between voicing and an increase in laryngeal muscle activity. The main use of EMG in this disorder is to guide injections of botulinum toxin into the thyroarytenoid and posterior cricoarytenoid muscles for therapeutic effect. Hollow needle electrodes can be attached to a syringe with appropriately diluted botulinum toxin, which is injected into the body of the appropriate muscle after electrical confirmation of proper needle placement into the muscle.

80.5.5 Lower Motor Neuron Disorders

Increased activity on needle insertion associated with findings of polyphasic innervation, positive sharp waves, and the presence of fibrillation potentials (▶ Fig. 80.8) are common findings in patients with diseases such as amyotrophic lateral sclerosis, degenerative diseases of the peripheral nerves, multisystem atrophy, post-polio syndrome, and Guillain-Barré syndrome. Often, there is also decreased recruitment as remaining nerve fibers cease functioning.

80.5.6 Myasthenia Gravis

Initial EMG of the larynx in patients with myasthenia gravis usually reveals normal insertional activity, amplitude, and duration of the MUAP. With repetitive stimulation, the amplitude and duration of the MUAP, as well as recruitment, decrease progressively over time.

80.6 Roundsmanship

- EMG is easy to perform in an ambulatory setting with minimal discomfort to the patient. It can be used to indicate the prognosis of a patient with injury, identify joint fixation, and guide the injection of botulinum toxin.
- EMG for vocal fold immobility in cases of iatrogenic trauma should be performed at least 3 weeks after the initial injury.
- EMG is useful in predicting a poor prognosis for functional return after vocal fold paralysis.
- EMG is a useful tool for guiding injections of botulinum toxin into the laryngeal musculature.
- Because EMG does require the use of a needle, insertional pain, bleeding, and rarely a hematoma can be encountered. Caution should be advised in patients with a history of anticoagulation or coagulopathy; however, significant morbidity from EMG is very rare.

80.7 Recommended Reading

[1] Basmajian JV, De Luca CJ. Muscles Alive: Their Functions Revealed by Electromyography. 5th ed. Baltimore, MD: Williams & Wilkins; 1985
[2] Hirano M. Electromyography of laryngeal muscles. In: Hirano M, ed. Clinical Examination of the Voice. New York, NY: Springer; 1981:11–24
[3] Munin MC, Murry T, Rosen CA. Laryngeal electromyography: diagnostic and prognostic applications. Otolaryngol Clin North Am 2000; 33: 759–770
[4] Sataloff RT, Mandel S, Heman-Ackah Y, Manon-Espaillat R, Abaza M. Laryngeal Electromyography. 2nd ed. San Diego, CA: Plural Publishing; 2006
[5] Sulica L, Blitzer A. Laryngeal electromyography: principles, applications, problems. In: Fried ML, Ferlito A. The Larynx. Vol 1. 3rd ed. San Diego, CA: Plural Publishing; 2009:211–225

81 Diagnostic Testing for Dysphagia

Craig H. Zalvan

81.1 Introduction

Like most diagnostic modalities, the history and physical examination are crucial in understanding the cause of dysphagia. A detailed history will point to the area causing the particular problem, which can then help guide the physician's choice of objective diagnostic testing. The field of dysphagia has experienced tremendous growth over the past few decades, and numerous diagnostic tests are available that can help pinpoint the etiology of dysphagia in many, although not all, cases.

In addition to a complete head and neck examination, including assessment of the cranial nerves, every examination for dysphagia must include visualization of the laryngopharynx (and possibly the trachea) with a flexible laryngoscope. Both anatomy and function are evaluated, including the following: mucosal lesions, velopharyngeal competence, epiglottic retroflexion with closure of the laryngeal vestibule, vocal fold mobility, pharyngeal squeeze, laryngeal elevation, and the presence of pooled secretions at baseline. Based on the history and results of this examination, objective testing is then ordered if deemed necessary. A battery of tests is available, each with advantages and disadvantages. An understanding of how each test is conducted and what information it may provide is necessary so that a prudent choice is made. If chosen correctly, these examinations may confirm a suspected etiology of the dysphagia, as well as its location and severity. Certain examinations can be used with real-time feedback to test the efficacy of swallowing maneuvers used in treatment.

81.2 Modified Barium Swallow

Modified barium swallow (MBS), or videofluorography, has long been the gold standard test for evaluating swallowing function. It is generally obtained to evaluate patients with suspected neurologic compromise, postoperative changes, upper esophageal sphincter dysfunction, or dysphagia to liquid boluses. This test is performed in the radiology suite with a radiologist and speech–language pathologist. The patient sits upright in the fluoroscopy suite and is fed a gradation of barium-coated boluses with consistencies ranging from thin liquid to solid, as well as varying sizes. This is an excellent test for identifying causes of dysphagia in the oral and pharyngeal phases of swallowing, as well as dysfunction of the upper esophageal sphincter. The esophageal phase can also be assessed. Premature bolus spillage, esophageal reflux, adynamic pharyngeal musculature, degenerative changes of the spine, and pooling of secretions are all assessed. Aspiration of material is easily detected, even when silent (absence of cough upon penetration or aspiration). In addition, the function of the cricopharyngeus and upper esophageal sphincter can be assessed, as well as the presence of a Zenker diverticulum. The MBS can be used to assess the success or failure of compensatory mechanisms and strategies taught to the patient; patients swallow while employing the compensatory maneuver, and its effect is observed in real time. The disadvantages of this test are the need for a radiology suite, a large team of health care workers, radiation exposure, and the inability to directly visualize the structures being assessed.

81.3 Flexible Endoscopic Evaluation of Swallowing and Sensory Testing

Flexible endoscopic evaluation of swallowing and sensory testing (FEESST) allows an evaluation of the oropharyngeal swallowing mechanism, as well as direct visualization of the oropharynx, hypopharynx, and larynx. It is generally employed in similar situations and as an alternative to MBS. This portable test is performed by passing a flexible laryngoscope through the nasal cavity into the pharynx to the level of the tip of the epiglottis. Baseline evaluation of secretions within the nasopharynx, vallecula, hypopharynx, posterior pharyngeal wall, and larynx is performed. The trachea can also be directly visualized. Vocal fold mobility is assessed, as is pharyngeal mobility, cough effectiveness, and pharyngeal squeeze (dynamic medial contraction of the pharyngeal walls during a high-pitched /i/). Sensory testing is then performed. A small puff of air is delivered to the arytenoid mucosa. When this is sensed, normal individuals respond with an abrupt closure of the larynx (laryngeal adductor reflex). The normal threshold is less than 4.0 mm Hg. If a response is not elicited, increasing pressure is used until a continuous pulse at 9 mm Hg is delivered. The absence of reflexive closure indicates the presence of a severe sensory deficit. Finally, foods of multiple consistencies mixed with food coloring are fed to the patient. The timing of the swallow, pooling of secretions, premature spillage, presence of residual food material, and penetration and aspiration before, during, and after the swallow, as well as the ability to clear the bolus, are all recorded.

The FEESST examination has many advantages. It is very easy to perform and highly portable. There is no radiation exposure. Direct visualization from the nasopharynx to laryngopharynx allows a direct evaluation of the anatomy. Neurologic information such as vocal fold mobility and sensation can be tested with FEESST. FEES can be used for biofeedback to help a patient learn swallow maneuvers and protective mechanisms.

The primary disadvantage is poor visualization during the actual swallow, with a brief period of "white out" during epiglottic inversion and pharyngeal contraction. The direct visualization of penetration or aspiration is not possible during the swallow; the presence of either can only be inferred by the appearance of food coloring in the structures of the larynx or subglottis after the swallow has finished. In addition, the cricopharyngeus, esophagus, and oral phase of swallow are not visualized during this procedure. The pooling of secretions in the hypopharynx may suggest cricopharyngeal abnormalities indicating the need for further investigation. Some patients may not be able to tolerate placement of the laryngoscope, either because of discomfort, which is very rare, or an inability to participate in the procedure because of neurologic compromise or mental status deficiencies.

81.4 Barium Swallow

A barium swallow (BS) allows an investigation of the anatomy and function of the hypopharynx, upper esophageal sphincter, esophagus, and cardia of the stomach. The patient swallows approximately 20 mL of thin barium liquid, which is evaluated with fluoroscopy. The barium distends the lumen of the aforementioned structures, so that they can be evaluated. It is ordered predominantly for patients experiencing dysphagia to solids. BS is helpful in the identification of mucosal irregularities, webs, rings, stricture, extrinsic compression, diverticula, foreign bodies, upper esophageal sphincter/lower esophageal sphincter/cricopharyngeal dysfunction, gastroesophageal reflux, airway aspiration, endoluminal masses, and esophageal dysmotility. The advantages of this examination include its noninvasive nature, low cost, and wide availability. The disadvantages include the need for radiation, relative anatomical imprecision, and lack of information about how foods and liquids of various consistencies are handled.

81.5 Transnasal Esophagoscopy

Transnasal esophagoscopy (TNE) has become a powerful tool in the diagnosis of dysphagia. Performed on unsedated patients in an office setting with the use of topical anesthesia, direct visualization from the nasopharynx to the stomach can be performed. Indications for this examination include dysphagia, laryngopharyngeal reflux disease (LPRD), chronic cough, globus, odynophagia, symptoms of gastroesophageal reflux disease (GERD), and suspected foreign body in the esophagus. It is also used as a screening tool for the evaluation of head and neck cancers and of Barrett disease. After the larynx is visualized for gross mobility, pharyngeal squeeze, and pooling of secretions, the patient is asked to swallow, and the endoscope is advanced through the cricopharyngeus. Cricopharyngeal opening and closure occur in less than 1 second, but the movement is captured digitally and can be reviewed. Cricopharyngeal relaxation is assessed. The scope is then passed toward the stomach with minimal insufflation of air. Mucosal irregularities and anatomical abnormalities, such as esophagitis, ulcers, webs, strictures, diverticula, varices, and masses, can be visualized as the scope is passed. Foreign bodies can also be identified and removed. The gastroesophageal junction is evaluated. Particular attention is paid to the Z-line, where the pale esophageal squamous epithelium transitions to the orange gastric columnar epithelium. It is assessed for continuity and regularity. Longitudinal blood vessels of the esophagus seen traversing the Z-line as well as Z-line irregularity may represent Barrett esophagus, which increases a patient's risk for esophageal carcinoma. A brush biopsy or four-quadrant cupped forceps biopsy of this area should be obtained. The lower esophageal sphincter is assessed for function, as well as for the presence of a hiatal hernia. The scope is then passed into the stomach and retroflexed, and the flap valve (closure of the gastroesophageal junction around the endoscope) is assessed from below. A patent flap valve occurs with a hiatal hernia and can predispose to reflux. Next, water and applesauce dyed with food coloring are swallowed. A normal swallow should allow pureed food to pass in less than 13 seconds. Clear water is then given to flush the esophagus and

allow an assessment of gross motility and peristalsis. The scope is withdrawn, and the mucosal surfaces are again visualized. The advantages of TNE include the office setting, topical rather than sedative anesthesia, minimal time lost from work, and lack of post- examination nausea or fatigue. In addition, this test can readily identify pathology along the entire upper gastrointestinal tract, providing quick diagnostic information. TNE is also less expensive when performed in the office setting. The disadvantages include occasional minor discomfort, the small caliber of the endoscope's operative port (which prevents the use of any equipment other than biopsy forceps), and the limited distal visualization to the stomach.

81.6 pH and Impedance Monitoring

In the past few decades, laryngopharyngeal reflux has been noted to be a significant cause of dysphagia in many patients. Reflux testing has evolved and can be an important tool in diagnosing reflux disease. To evaluate laryngopharyngeal reflux, pH testing is performed by placing a dual pH probe through the nose and into the esophagus. Ideally, this is accompanied by impedance testing, which detects the presence of liquid refluxate, either acidic or nonacidic. The upper probe is placed approximately 1 cm above the upper esophageal sphincter, either under direct vision or with the use of concurrent manometry. The level of acidity and presence of liquid refluxate are then recorded for a 24-hour period. Dietary intake and symptoms are recorded and compared with the pH and impedance tracing to isolate and correlate events with symptoms. A newer pH probe has recently been created that records pH of the nasopharynx only. This new system is more comfortable and provides information about the acidity of the naso-oropharynx for 24 hours. Placement is simple, via visualization of a guiding blinking light at the end of the probe, and a good position is confirmed with the sip of an acidic beverage. This new probe is helpful as a screening tool, but it does not provide the information on esophageal motility that is obtained with manometry (performed with the dual pH probe). pH tests can help guide treatment by quantifying the amount of reflux present, and patients can be evaluated while taking proton pump inhibitors to determine their response to this management. A patient can also be tested while off proton pump inhibitor therapy when it is expected that laryngopharyngeal reflux is not contributing the patient's disease and needs to be ruled out.

Impedance testing can be added to pH testing to evaluate for the presence of nonacidic reflux, which can be a cause of laryngeal symptoms but not respond to acid-suppressive medications. This can be performed at the same time as pH testing. An impedance catheter is placed within the esophagus. A series of electrodes detect changes in the electrical conductivity of the region of the esophagus in which the electrodes lie. Liquid and gas (refluxate) increase conductivity and thus change the impedance of an electrode, denoting the presence of refluxate.

The advantage of pH and impedance testing is that it provides objective information about the role of LPRD/GERD in patients' disorders. In addition, this type of testing has a very high degree of sensitivity. The disadvantages include the discomfort involved and the need to wear the equipment for 24 hours. The information obtained with this type of testing is subject to interpretation because a consensus on the interpretation of pH and impedance testing data has not been achieved.

81.7 Esophageal Manometry

This procedure involves placing a long catheter through the nose and into the esophagus as one would pass a nasogastric tube. The catheter has numerous pressure transducers along its length. The patient is instructed to swallow both dry and with liquids. The timing of pharyngeal and esophageal contractions, the strength of the contractions, and the sequencing of pressure events are recorded by this multichannel transducer. This test is useful for determining the strength of pharyngeal contraction, cricopharyngeal dysfunction (both patulous and nonrelaxing), esophageal motility disorders, and problems related to the discoordination of pharyngeal and esophageal contraction. Descriptions of absolute pressures and muscular coordination within the pharynx and esophagus are advantages of manometry. This information is easily obtained, is relatively inexpensive, and helps guide future therapy. The disadvantages include the discomfort sometimes involved during catheter placement and the lack of direct visualization of structures during the test.

81.8 Manofluorography

This technique simultaneously combines the fluoroscopic evaluation of swallowing with manometry. The advantage of this test is that it allows a precise temporal coordination of pressure information with the position of the bolus. Unfortunately, more equipment and significant expertise are required. Recent advances in technology are decreasing the level of expertise need to perform this test while increasing its accuracy, but the test is currently prohibitively expensive.

81.9 Scintigraphy

A bolus of food material coated with a short-lived isotope is administered orally to the patient. A gamma ray camera then measures the radioactivity as the bolus passes through the upper aerodigestive tract. Residue of material and aspiration can be detected. Transit of the bolus through the esophagus with timing and directionality can be assessed. The reflux of contents from the stomach and esophagus into the larynx can be assessed for hours after bolus ingestion. The food material is then monitored during its transit out of the stomach into the small intestine. This test is used primarily to study gastric emptying. It is easy to perform, causes no discomfort, and has minimal risk from low-dose radiation. It is sensitive for aspiration and reflux events. Quantitative analysis of the portion of the bolus aspirated can be done. The disadvantages are the need for low-dose radioactive material, the need for a gamma counter and experienced technicians, and the lack of direct visualization of the structures involved. In addition, multiple boluses are not used, and compensatory techniques cannot be assessed.

81.10 Ultrasonography

Ultrasonography is used primarily to evaluate the soft tissue of the oral cavity and oropharynx. Movement of the tongue and intrinsic musculature, the gross morphology, the presence of tumors, and the timing of swallow can be followed. In addition, multiple swallowing attempts can be assessed. Elevation of the hyoid can be tracked with ultrasonography. Endoluminal ultrasonography can be used to study the esophagus and cricopharyngeal region. Because of the lack of radiation, ultrasonography is a good technique to assess the oral and oropharyngeal phases of swallowing in children.

81.11 Computed Tomography and Magnetic Resonance Imaging

When a mass is suspected, the appropriate radiographic testing can be ordered. These techniques are covered elsewhere.

81.12 Conclusion

The history and physical examination should be used to guide the choice of diagnostic testing. In most cases, the cause of dysphagia can be pinpointed to a certain area of the upper aerodigestive tract. Testing is then ordered to confirm the area of dysfunction and/or elucidate the exact nature of the problem. If testing is chosen carefully, rarely does a patient need more than one test to confirm the diagnosis and initiate treatment. ▶ Table 81.1 outlines the preferred tests for particular problems.

81.13 Roundsmanship

- Dysphagia evaluation requires flexible fiber-optic nasopharyngolaryngoscopy for the examination of the involved anatomy and its function, including mucosal lesions, velopharyngeal competence, epiglottic retroflexion with closure of the laryngeal vestibule, vocal fold mobility, pharyngeal squeeze, laryngeal elevation, and the presence of pooled secretions at baseline.
- Modified barium swallow is generally used to evaluate patients with suspected neurologic compromise, postoperative changes, upper esophageal sphincter dysfunction, or dysphagia to liquid boluses. FEESST can also provide useful information in these situations.
- Barium swallow can aid in the diagnosis of mucosal irregularities, webs, rings, strictures, extrinsic compression, diverticula, foreign bodies, upper esophageal sphincter/lower esophageal sphincter/cricopharyngeal dysfunction, gastroesophageal reflux, airway aspiration, endoluminal masses, and esophageal dysmotility.
- Transnasal esophagoscopy can be used in patients with dysphagia, laryngopharyngeal reflux disease, chronic cough, globus, odynophagia, symptoms of GERD, and suspected foreign body of the esophagus. It is also useful as a screening tool for the evaluation of head and neck cancers and for Barrett disease.

Table 81.1 Comparison of diagnostic tests demonstrating which tests are better suited to detect particular symptoms and define location of etiology

	MBS	FEESST	TNE	US	Scintigraphy	BS	pH Testing	Manometry	Impedance
Oral dysphagia	++	–	–	+++	+	–	–	–	–
Oropharyngeal dysphagia	+++	+++	+	++	++	–	–	+++	–
Esophageal dysphagia	+	–	+++	+	+++	+++	–	+++	+++
Cricopharyngeal dysfunction	+++	+	++	++	++	++	–	+++	+
Aspiration	+++	+++	+	–	+++	++	–	–	–
Global swallow function	+++	++	++	+	+++	+	–	++	+
Muscular dysfunction	++	+	+	+	–	++	–	+++	–
Laryngopharyngeal reflux	+	+	+	–	+	+	+++	–	+++

Abbreviations: BS, barium swallow; FEESST, flexible endoscopic evaluation of swallowing and sensory testing; MBS, modified barium swallow; TNE, transnasal esophagoscopy; US, ultrasound.

- pH and impedence testing is highly sensitive can provide objective information in cases of suspected LPRD/GERD.
- Esophageal manometry can document the strength of pharyngeal contraction, hypo- and hyperfunctioning of the cricopharyngeus, disorders of esophageal motility, and problems related to discoordination of pharyngeal and esophageal contraction.

81.14 Recommended Reading

[1] Postma GN, Cohen JT, Belafsky PC et al. Transnasal esophagoscopy: revisited (over 700 consecutive cases). Laryngoscope 2005; 115: 321–323

[2] Weissman JL. The radiographic evaluation of dysphagia: the barium swallow (pharyngoesophagram) and the modified barium swallow. In: Carrau RL, Murry T, eds. Comprehensive Management of Swallowing Disorders. San Diego, CA: Singular Publishing Group; 1999:65–74

82 Evaluation and Management of the Hoarse Patient

Seth H. Dailey and Sunil P. Verma

82.1 Introduction

The ability to produce voice relies on three major components. The lungs serve as a generator to drive breath. The vocal folds serve as a vibrating source to make sound. The pharynx and oral cavity act as a filter to alter the sound into intelligible words.

The production of voice is integral for communication and enables an individual's personal and professional livelihood. As the ability to produce voice is an innate task, many take it for granted until an actual problem occurs. Hoarseness is a common problem, affecting approximately 20 million people in the United States at any one time.

82.2 Description of the Clinical Disorder

Hoarseness is a symptom of altered voice quality. Dysphonia is a disorder of voice production that impairs communication. Dysphonia may be a result of anatomical or functional components, and in some cases both. Causes range extensively from benign conditions such as muscle tension dysphonia to serious conditions such as a neurologic disease or malignancy. The keys to the diagnosis and management of dysphonia include a thorough history and physical examination that includes excellent visualization of the larynx.

82.3 Differential Diagnosis

- Infectious causes, such as viral, fungal, and bacterial infections. Fungal infections occur most commonly in patients who use inhaled steroids.
- Inflammatory causes, such as laryngopharyngeal reflux, post-nasal drip, allergies, and voice overuse.
- Phonotraumatic lesions, such as vocal fold cysts, polyps, nodules, and scar. These lesions most commonly occur in the mid-musculomembranous section of the vocal fold, where shear stress is the highest.
- Benign neoplasms, such as recurrent respiratory papillomatosis and granular cell tumors.
- Primary malignancies, including squamous cell cancer and minor salivary gland tumors. Secondary malignancies include invasive thyroid cancer and tracheal cancer.
- Neurologic conditions, such as spasmodic dysphonia, tremor, and Parkinson disease.
- Conditions of glottic insufficiency, including vocal fold paralysis, paresis, and presbylarynges. Affected individuals typically experience vocal fatigue and exhibit a diminished maximum phonation time.
- Vascular lesions, such as hemangiomas, varices, and ectasia. These may result in hemorrhage accumulating in the superficial layer of the lamina propria.
- Systemic conditions, including rheumatoid arthritis and amyloidosis. The former typically causes vocal fold immobility, and the latter is a multilobulated mass within the glottis.

- Traumatic lesions, including intubation injuries and external blunt or sharp trauma. Post-intubation hoarseness is a common phenomenon associated with vocal fold hypomobility due to cricoarytenoid joint fixation or recurrent laryngeal nerve neurapraxia. Blunt or sharp trauma is not as common.
- Insult to the vagus nerve or recurrent laryngeal nerve. This may be due to mass effect from lesions, iatrogenic injury, or pathology in the brainstem, neck, and chest.
- Iatrogenic injury to the recurrent laryngeal nerve is the most common cause of vocal fold paralysis. Surgeries with a risk for recurrent laryngeal nerve injury include intracranial surgery; neck procedures, such as surgery to the carotid artery, cervical spine, thyroid, and esophagus; and chest procedures, including pulmonary, cardiac, and vascular surgery.
- Functional voice disorders, such as muscle tension dysphonia.

82.4 Evaluation of the Disorder

82.4.1 History

An excellent is history is paramount in the evaluation of hoarseness. During the work-up, the patient should be questioned about the following:
1. Onset: gradual versus sudden. A gradual onset may be associated with neurologic conditions or malignancy. Causes of a sudden onset may include hemorrhage or even muscle tension dysphonia.
2. Duration of hoarseness.
3. Circumstances surrounding the onset.
4. Associated symptoms such as difficulty swallowing and shortness of breath often point to extensive laryngeal conditions.
5. Mitigating factors. Hoarseness that is constant often points to an anatomical lesion.
6. Social history, including tobacco or alcohol use.
7. Voice demands and use, both social and professional.

82.4.2 Physical Examination

All patients with hoarseness should undergo a complete head and neck examination. Special care should be taken with the cranial nerve examination, specifically examination of the palate and tongue for evidence of paresis, paralysis, or neurodegeneration. Neck palpation evaluates for the presence of neck masses, including lymphadenopathy and thyroid lesions.

Endoscopy of the larynx is critical to make a proper diagnosis. Endoscopy should assess for numerous items, including the following:
- Global evaluation of the laryngeal structures, including the epiglottis, arytenoid position, aryepiglottic folds, piriform sinuses, postcricoid area, false (vestibular) vocal folds, and true vocal folds.
- Vocal fold adduction and abduction. Limitations may point to a neurologic etiology, such as recurrent laryngeal nerve damage, or a mechanical etiology, such as joint fixation from rheumatoid arthritis or traumatic scarring.

- Vocal fold epithelium. Leukoplakia may be a result of hyperkeratosis and be associated with dysplasia or malignancy. Erythroplakia has a stronger association with malignancy than leukoplakia.
- Vocal fold vasculature. Normally, the vocal fold vasculature runs parallel to the vocal fold medial edge. Vasculature that travels perpendicular to this often "points" to phonotraumatic lesions. Tortuous vasculature may be associated with papilloma or malignancy. Ectasia and varices are typically results of trauma within the superficial layer of the lamina propria.
- Vocal fold symmetry, including epithelium, vasculature, and height. It is important to examine both vocal folds for abnormalities because phonotraumatic lesions are often bilateral. Specific attention should be paid to the vocal fold height because vocal fold paralysis may cause dysphonia when the two vocal folds differ in height.

An indirect examination of the larynx with a laryngeal mirror is important for many reasons. A mirror examination is a very quick procedure that provides a global view of the laryngopharynx. However, the examination is limited by a patient's gag reflex, provides only a transient view of the larynx, and does not allow the photodocumentation of findings.

Transoral rigid examination uses a 70-degree angled telescope for laryngeal visualization. Transoral laryngoscopy is best performed in patients with a limited gag reflex and may be carried out with halogen or stroboscopic light. Because of its large diameter, a rigid telescope provides abundant light to illuminate the larynx. A transoral telescope coupled with a camera permits the view to be magnified and recorded. Recording allows the surgeon to review an examination after it is performed and to compare it with later examinations during future visits.

Transnasal flexible endoscopy provides the advantage of being able to evaluate the larynx during connected speech. The examination is performed with the patient in a more "natural" position than during transoral endoscopy and is thought to provide a more accurate evaluation of laryngeal motion. Transnasal endoscopy can be performed with a flexible fiber-optic laryngoscope or a distal chip endoscope. The illumination and image quality are superb with the latter; however, its availability is limited by its expense. Transnasal flexible endoscopes may be coupled with halogen light, xenon light, or stroboscopic light.

The addition of stroboscopic light provides the physician with the ability to evaluate the membranous vocal fold in pseudo-slow motion. For this to occur, the frequency at which the stroboscopic light flashes is coupled to the frequency of the patient's voice, as measured by a microphone placed along the patient's neck external to a thyroid ala. The pseudo-slow motion image allows an evaluation of the mucosal wave, amplitude of vibration, any adynamic segments, phase closure, and periodicity. Laryngovideostroboscopy can be essential for the evaluation of a patient with hoarseness.

82.5 Testing

82.5.1 Radiography

Computed tomography (CT) of the larynx with intravenous contrast is helpful if an invasive process such as cancer is sus-

pected or if there has been laryngeal trauma. If vocal fold mobility is compromised, CT or magnetic resonance (MR) imaging is necessary to rule out pathology impinging upon the recurrent laryngeal nerve. The examination must include the vagus nerve from the skull base to the aortic arch.

82.5.2 Electromyography

Electromyography (EMG) is helpful in prognosticating the return of vocal fold motion in patients with 2 to 6 months of vocal fold immobility secondary to a neurogenic cause. It may also distinguish neurogenic from mechanical causes of vocal fold immobility, particularly after intubation trauma. EMG may be helpful in the diagnosis of vocal fold paresis as well.

82.5.3 Microbacterial Testing

Rarely, a culture of the larynx is performed if fungal or bacterial laryngitis is suspected but is atypical in presentation or unresponsive to empiric treatment.

82.5.4 Histopathology

A biopsy can be performed in the office or operating room for any suspected neoplasm.

82.6 Treatment

The etiology of dysphonia is often multifactorial, which is the reason for such a thorough investigation. Because of the numerous causes of dysphonia, it is difficult to describe thoroughly all possible treatment options. In general, the initial findings often dictate the first step in management and the need for further studies. For example, if a neurologic disorder is suspected, consultation with a neurologist specializing in movement disorders may be indicated.

If infection is suspected, then antivirals, antibiotics, or antifungals should be used appropriately. Swish and swallow antifungal medications should not be used because they are topical. Treatment with a systemic medication such as fluconazole is recommended.

Laryngopharyngeal reflux may contribute to voice disorders, causing symptoms of mild hoarseness, throat clearing, and globus sensation. Laryngopharyngeal reflux is managed with lifestyle changes; dietary changes are emphasized, including the avoidance of acidic foods and a decrease in meal sizes. Proton pump inhibitors may be initiated, with patients instructed to take their medication at least 30 minutes before meals.

Rhinitis with postnasal drip may be controlled with saline irrigation, nasal steroids, antihistamines, or anticholinergic nasal sprays. A through a work-up of allergic or chronic rhinosinusitis may be necessary.

Voice therapy is a key portion of the management of many voice disorders. Speech pathologists may work with patients regularly to improve voicing technique and efficiency. Voice therapy is an important tool for patients with functional voice disorders as well as those with lesions requiring surgery. Voice therapy should be used both before and after surgery to optimize results.

Phonomicrosurgery will benefit patients with benign lesions that are refractory to voice therapy.

Papillomatosis often requires multiple surgeries through a patient's lifetime. Adjunctive treatments include lasers and indole-3-carbinol. Cidofovir may benefit certain patients.

Patients who have spasmodic dysphonia and occasionally laryngeal tremor can be helped with botulinum toxin.

Patients with glottic insufficiency may benefit from voice therapy. In many cases, the vocal folds require augmentation, which may be performed with injection laryngoplasty or type I thyroplasty.

Unilateral type I thyroplasty with or without arytenoid adduction is a definitive treatment for patients who have unilateral vocal fold paralysis.

82.7 Roundsmanship

- Hoarseness is a symptom of altered voice quality. Dysphonia is a disorder of voice production.
- Although laryngopharyngeal reflux is present in many patients with hoarseness, a full work-up is warranted.
- The etiology of hoarseness is often multifactorial, and a proper diagnosis relies on an excellent history and physical examination, especially endoscopy.
- Laryngovideostroboscopy allows the evaluation of membranous vocal fold motion in pseudo-slow motion. Mucosal wave, amplitude of vibration, any adynamic segments, phase closure, and periodicity can be evaluated.
- A proper investigation for idiopathic vocal fold immobility includes CT or MR imaging along the course of the vagus nerve from the skull base to the aortic arch.

82.8 Recommended Reading

[1] Mau T. Diagnostic evaluation and management of hoarseness. Med Clin North Am 2010; 94: 945–960

[2] Sataloff RT. Professional Voice. The Science and Art of Clinical Care. 3rd ed. San Diego, CA: Plural Publishing; 2005

[3] Schwartz SR, Cohen SM, Dailey SH et al. Clinical practice guideline: hoarseness (dysphonia). Otolaryngol Head Neck Surg 2009; 141 Suppl 2: S1–S31

[4] Hoarseness , . . Arch Otolaryngol Head Neck Surg 2011; 137: 616–619

[5] Woo P, Casper J, Colton R, Brewer D. Diagnosis and treatment of persistent dysphonia after laryngeal surgery: a retrospective analysis of 62 patients. Laryngoscope 1994; 104: 1084–1091

83 Laryngitis

Craig H. Zalvan

83.1 Introduction

Laryngitis by definition refers only to inflammation of the larynx. The word *laryngitis* is commonly used erroneously by patients and physicians to describe symptoms such as change in voice, loss of voice, and/or discomfort in the throat. Laryngeal inflammation can be caused by a wide variety of conditions and associated with a myriad of other symptoms. This chapter will explore the causes of inflammation of the larynx that lead to symptoms referable to the larynx and pharynx. Noninflammatory conditions of the larynx leading to similar symptoms will be covered elsewhere.

83.2 Incidence

Although there are no data on "laryngitis" specifically, in 1996 there were 23.6 cases of the common cold and 36 cases of influenza per 100 people in the United States. Most patients with upper respiratory tract infections will have one symptom or another of laryngitis, and nearly everyone will experience laryngitis at some point in his or her life.

83.3 Classification

Acute laryngitis usually lasts up to 7 days and is typically self-limited. Subacute laryngitis lasts from 1 to 3 weeks. Laryngitis lasting for more than 3 weeks is considered chronic. In addition, patients can have recurrent bouts of laryngeal inflammation lasting for days to weeks. Laryngitis lasting longer than 3 weeks should be evaluated by an otolaryngologist, and direct visualization of the larynx should be performed.

83.4 Applied Anatomy

Laryngitis is confined principally to the mucosa of the larynx, which is covered by respiratory epithelium except for the true vocal folds, which are covered by squamous epithelium. The thin mucosa and superficial lamina propria vibrate together over the deeper layers of the lamina propria and the underlying vocalis muscle. This unique arrangement is easily compromised by edema, which leads to hoarseness.

83.5 The Disease Process

83.5.1 Etiology

Acute laryngitis: Most cases of acute laryngitis are temporary. The vast majority are virally mediated (▸ Fig. 83.1) and present as part of an upper respiratory infection with or without other symptoms, such as cough, rhinorrhea, nasal congestion, fever, headache, and malaise. Typically, as the respiratory symptoms improve, so do the voice and throat symptoms. Bacterial and fungal infection (▸ Fig. 83.2), although rare, must also be considered.

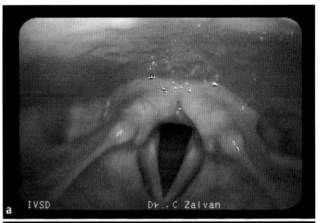
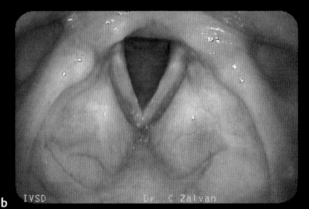

Fig. 83.1 (a) Normal laryngeal examination. Note the smooth mucosa, sharply defined borders of the arcuate line, smooth vocal fold edges, tan–pale coloration, and moist, glistening surfaces. (b) Viral laryngitis with mid-membranous vocal fold epithelial thickening as well erythema, edema, and hyperemia of the vocal folds.

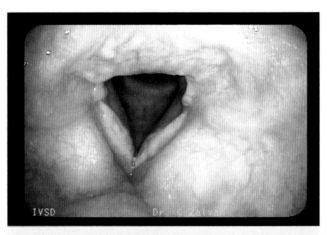

Fig. 83.2 Fungal laryngitis. Note the white fungal plaques covering the entire surface of both vocal folds. There are also incidental bilateral granulomas.

In addition to infection, acute vocal trauma from vocal overuse, misuse, or abuse is a common cause of acute laryngitis. Typically, patients will detail a vocal event that precipitated the acute change. Benign conditions such as vocal fold nodules, polyps, cysts, and muscle tension may predispose a patient to acute voice loss and discomfort. In severe instances, vocal trauma may result in vocal hemorrhage and lead to significant vocal fold inflammation and acute vocal changes.

Underlying laryngopharyngeal reflux may be exacerbated by stress, infection, medication, or dietary indiscretion. This can cause acute laryngeal inflammation and acute symptoms such as voice changes, throat clearing, globus pharyngeus, increased glottal mucus, and coughing.

Medications can secondarily lead to acute inflammatory changes by altering laryngeal hydration. Inhaled medication may directly cause inflammation from contact irritation as well as the initiation of a fungal infection. The increased use of inhaled steroids has led to an increase in the frequency of fungal laryngitis in immunocompetent individuals.

Allergies and environmental exposures can result in acute changes in breathing, respiration, mucosal hydration, and mucus production, all of which can lead to acute laryngitis.

Most cases of acute laryngitis are self-limited and improve over 1 to 3 weeks. Symptoms are often alleviated by conservative measures. Very rarely are antibiotics and steroids indicated for acute laryngitis.

However, some cases of acute laryngitis progress to chronic laryngitis after the initial acute phase has resolved. Chronic symptoms often prompt a visit to a medical doctor. Patients whose symptoms have lasted longer than 3 weeks should be evaluated by an otolaryngologist, who can visualize the larynx. This allows an accurate diagnosis to be made and treatment to be directed at the particular cause of the chronic symptoms.

83.5.2 Chronic Laryngitis

Laryngitis that persists more than 3 weeks is considered chronic. Systemic diseases (including collagen vascular disorders), insidious infectious disease, long-term environmental exposures, allergies, medications, and tumors are some of the more common causes of chronic laryngitis. Occasionally, acute laryngitis can cause secondary changes that result in chronic laryngitis. A careful history in a patient with symptoms of acute laryngitis often reveals chronic symptoms that have been present for weeks or months but were recently exacerbated. Laryngitis is often multifactorial. For example, viral laryngitis associated with a cough may cause a vocal hemorrhage, resulting in persistent hoarseness despite resolution of the viral component of the illness. Chronic laryngitis usually presents insidiously and progresses slowly over time. Any vocal changes, throat discomfort, or otalgia in a smoker requires evaluation by an otolaryngologist to rule out the possibility of laryngeal cancer.

83.5.3 Natural History

As stated above, most causes of acute laryngitis are virus-related and self-limited. Chronic laryngitis, if left untreated, can result in permanent changes in the vocal folds, such as thickening of the vocal fold mucosa, polypoid degeneration of the superficial lamina propria, and fibrosis or scarring.

83.5.4 Pathogenesis

Laryngitis is caused by acute or chronic changes to the larynx resulting from an inflammatory process. This involves a combination of humoral and cellular responses to mucosal irritation. The B-cell response to antibody–antigen activation leads to a cascade of inflammatory mediator release, cytokine release, complement activation, and cellular activation. Cell-mediated immunity results in the activation of macrophages, natural killer cells, and cytotoxic T cells. Acutely, tissue inflammation ensues, resulting in vasodilation with subsequent erythema, transudation of plasma with edema, inflammatory mediator release, and tissue destruction. Laryngeal edema, excess or insufficient mucus production, poor laryngeal closure, and mucosal stiffness result in the voice changes and discomfort associated with acute or chronic inflammation. Chronic inflammation can lead to localized fibrosis, scarring of the mucosa and superficial lamina propria, and a granulomatous reaction (▶ Fig. 83.3).

83.5.5 Potential Disease Complications

Acute laryngitis primarily causes discomfort of the laryngopharynx and dysphonia. This can lead to missed work, missed performances, and inconvenience for the patient. Rarely is there sufficient edema to cause airway compromise; however, this is may be a concern in a patient with an abnormally narrow glottis secondary to another disorder. Continued or excessive use of the voice during acute or chronic laryngitis can prolong and exacerbate symptoms, as well as lead to mucosal tears, acute hemorrhage, and muscle strain. Maladaptive phonatory behaviors secondary to acute or chronic inflammation can result in benign vocal fold lesions such as nodules, polyps, and cysts, as well as permanent fibrotic changes.

83.6 Medical Evaluation

83.6.1 Presenting Complaints

Dysphonia is defined as any change in voice: breathy, raspy, or rough voice; voice breaks or cracks; change in range; vocal

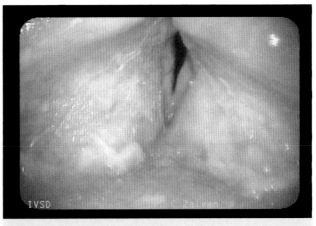

Fig. 83.3 Chronic laryngitis. Note the thickened mucosa of the entire supraglottis, with thick strands of white mucus; the smooth character of the mucosa is replaced with a rough, corrugated appearance.

fatigue or strain; loss of voice (aphonia) or whisper voice. Patients may describe a globus sensation (the feeling of having a lump in the throat) or discomfort in the throat; sharp pains or dull aches, either unilateral or bilateral, are often exacerbated by talking, swallowing, or eating. Occasionally, patients will have referred otalgia secondary to the shared vagal afferent innervation of the larynx and external auditory canal. In addition, the onset of laryngitis can often be accompanied by other respiratory tract symptoms, such as congestion, fever, headache, cough, and dysphagia. Airway symptoms such as stridor, dyspnea, croupy cough, and recurrent pneumonia should prompt immediate evaluation. Additionally, laryngitis in the setting of a preexisting airway abnormality, such as a tumor, laryngotracheal scarring, or vocal paralysis, can result in respiratory distress with airway compromise.

83.6.2 Evaluation

Most patients with acute laryngitis do not seek a medical evaluation. When symptoms are severe or long-lasting or cause functional difficulties for the patient, a medical evaluation is often obtained.

A thorough history is performed. A description of vocal changes and associated symptoms is obtained, including timing and severity. This is followed by questions about vocal hygiene, demands, use, and abuse, as well as the environment in which the voice is being employed, in order to obtain a sense of the patient's vocal behavior. In addition, information should be acquired about prior treatment, environmental exposures, laryngopharyngeal reflux symptoms, symptoms of allergy, medication use, history of systemic disease, and history of neurologic disorders or symptoms.

A thorough head and neck examination should be performed, followed by a laryngeal examination with a flexible laryngoscope. In cases of dysphonia, laryngovideostroboscopy should be performed as well, to assess vocal fold vibration and glottal function.

Acute laryngitis is often characterized by inflammation of the laryngeal structures with edema of the glottis and supraglottis. Hyperemia and surrounding erythema are more common in acute laryngitis. Excess mucus production is also common. Chronic laryngitis is often associated with excessive dryness of the larynx and mucosal thickening, with decreased mucosal wave on videostroboscopy. In some cases, granulation, keratosis, and fibrosis, as well as benign vocal fold changes such as a polyp, cyst, or nodule, may be seen. Of course, the presence of a malignant lesion must always be considered.

Typically, patients with acute laryngitis do not need further work-up unless the symptoms become chronic or worsen during treatment. Patients who present with recurrent episodes of acute laryngitis should not only be treated for the acute episode but also further evaluated to determine the underlying chronic disorder that predisposes them to these exacerbations.

Most cases of laryngitis, especially chronic cases, are multifactorial, and all the inciting and exacerbating factors need to be identified and addressed (▶ Fig. 83.4).

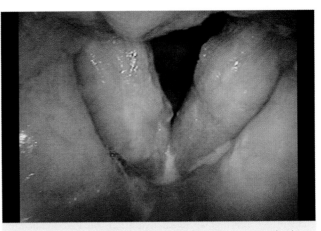

Fig. 83.4 Ulcerative laryngitis. Note the thickened mucosa with white coloration; anteriorly are bilateral tan–brown plaques that are completely stiff on stroboscopy. These areas can be confused with squamous cell carcinoma.

83.6.3 Testing

For patients with chronic laryngitis, further work-up is typically dictated by the response to medication, and a definitive diagnosis is determined by the history and physical examination (including laryngeal videostroboscopy) and failure to respond to treatment. This may include flexible endoscopic evaluation of swallowing and sensory testing (FEESST) for patients with dysphagia, pH testing for those with suspected refractory laryngopharyngeal reflux, modified barium swallow (MBS), allergy testing, and appropriate laboratory testing for suspected systemic disease: thyroid function tests; Lyme titers; erythrocyte sedimentation rate (ESR); C-reactive protein (CRP); angiotensin- converting enzyme (ACE); antinuclear antibody (ANA); rheumatoid factor (RhF); cytoplasmic and perinuclear antineutrophil cytoplasmic autoantibody (c-ANCA and p-ANCA). Electromyography (EMG) of the larynx can be performed for suspected neuromuscular disease. For any suspicious mass or lesion, an unsedated in-office biopsy or direct laryngoscopy with biopsy in the operating room should be performed.

83.6.4 Differential Diagnosis

- Laryngopharyngeal reflux
- Medications
  - Systemic effects
  - Local effects
- Infections
  - Viral
  - Bacterial
  - Fungal
  - Syphilis, leprosy, tuberculosis
- Environmental exposures
  - Smoking
  - Ethanol
  - Toxic inhalants
- Trauma, surgery
  - Vocal fold hemorrhage
  - Intubation
  - Postsurgical inflammation

- Bulimia, vomiting
- Caustic ingestion
- Hormones
  - Oral contraceptive pills
  - Hormone replacement therapy
  - Menopause
  - Menses
- Allergy
- Acute and chronic vocal fold misuse
- Dehydration
- Systemic disease
  - Amyloidosis, systemic lupus erythematosus, Wegener granulomatosis, rheumatoid arthritis
- Tumor
  - Benign
  - Malignant
  - Chemotherapy and radiation therapy

83.7 Treatment

83.7.1 Medical Treatment

The vast majority of patients with acute laryngitis need only treatment for symptomatic relief. Voice rest and modified voice use are instituted when voice changes are present. Hydration is extremely important and can be provided by having the patient drink at least eight glasses of water a day, inhale a cool mist via a personal or room humidifier, and use oral inhalation agents free of anesthetics and irritants (e.g., Entertainer's Secret Throat Relief Spray: www.entertainers-secret.com). Anti-inflammatory medications, antitussives, mucolytics, and nasal decongestants can be prescribed to alleviate acute symptoms. Patients should be counseled to avoid whispering to prevent long-term maladaptive compensatory behaviors. Rarely are antibiotics and antiviral medications warranted. For suspected laryngopharyngeal reflux, a reflux restricted diet is prescribed and proton pump inhibitors may be added, depending on the severity of symptoms and findings on examination. For patients who have severe dysphonia associated with severe laryngeal edema and need rapid resolution of their symptoms, oral or intramuscular steroids can be given. The larynx must be examined before steroids are prescribed to ensure the absence of vocal fold hemorrhage or mucosal abnormalities. The repeated use of steroids is not advised and is an indication of an underlying chronic condition that should be addressed. In cases of suspected fungal laryngitis, antifungal medications such as fluconazole are prescribed. Inhaled steroids should be discontinued; if this is not possible because of severe pulmonary disease, an aerosolized steroid should be prescribed and administered with a spacer at the minimal effective dose.

For patients with chronic laryngitis, an extensive otolaryngology evaluation should reveal the underlying disorder or disorders at which treatment will be directed. In all cases, the conservative treatment outlined above will be useful in alleviating some of the symptoms.

Although voice rest may be helpful in acute situations, it does not address underlying pathologic voice use patterns and is therefore beneficial only for acute treatment. Voice therapy may be helpful for patients with recurrent acute or chronic laryngitis. An evaluation by a speech–language pathologist will direct this aspect of a patient's treatment. Voice therapy helps identify poor vocal behaviors and targets treatment to address these behaviors via vocal retraining and exercise.

Careful follow-up should be arranged in cases of chronic laryngitis to optimize patient outcomes.

83.7.2 Surgical Treatment

Rarely is surgery indicated for cases of laryngitis, either acute or chronic. In acute laryngitis, airway intervention is rarely necessary but should be considered for patients with airway compromise. For patients with chronic laryngitis, biopsy of the larynx may be necessary to obtain a histopathologic diagnosis of an observed mass or lesion. This may be performed in the office with the patient unsedated or in the operating room via direct laryngoscopy with the patient under general anesthesia. Operative treatment may also be warranted in cases of laryngitis that have led to complications of benign vocal fold lesions, such as granulomas, fibrosis, nodules, polyps, or cysts.

83.8 Prognosis

The prognosis for full recovery in most cases of acute laryngitis is excellent, typically with complete resolution of the symptoms within 1 week. In cases of recurrent acute or chronic laryngitis, once the cause of the inflammation is diagnosed, the prognosis is generally excellent. In cases in which laryngitis is complicated by laryngeal fibrosis and scar formation involving the vocal folds, the prognosis for recovery is not as favorable. Chronic symptoms of dysphonia and discomfort may persist despite numerous and aggressive treatments or surgeries.

83.9 Roundsmanship

- Laryngitis by definition refers only to inflammation of the larynx. The word *laryngitis* is commonly used (incorrectly) by patients and physicians to describe symptoms such as change in voice, loss of voice, and/or discomfort in the throat.
- Most cases of acute laryngitis are virally mediated and require only conservative treatment to provide relief of symptoms in a few days or weeks.
- Recurrent acute laryngitis or the repeated use of steroids is an indication of an underlying chronic disorder.
- The etiology of chronic laryngitis is generally multifactorial.
- Once the multiple causes of chronic laryngitis are identified, the prognosis is excellent, except in cases complicated by vocal fold fibrosis and scarring due to severe or prolonged laryngitis.

83.10 Recommended Reading

[1] Dworkin JP. Laryngitis: types, causes, and treatments. Otolaryngol Clin North Am 2008; 41: 419–436

[2] Vital and Health Statistics. Current Estimates from the National Health Interview Survey, 1996. Series 10, No. 200. Atlanta, GA: Centers for Disease Control and Prevention, National Center for Health Statistics, 1999

[3] Woodson G. Laryngitis. In: Ossoff RH, Shapshay SM, Woodson GE, Netterville JL, eds. The Larynx. Philadelphia, PA: Lippincott Williams & Wilkins; 2003:151–158

84 Systemic Diseases of the Larynx

Melin Tan

84.1 Introduction

The larynx is a complex anatomical organ whose structure and function are influenced by its cartilaginous framework, muscles, mucosa, and cricoarytenoid joints. Many systemic diseases alter the function of the larynx or infiltrate the trachea, leading to a compromised airway and/or compromised phonation. This section will review the laryngeal manifestations of rheumatoid arthritis, systemic lupus erythematosus, relapsing polychondritis, sarcoidosis, Wegener granulomatosus, and amyloidosis. ▶ Table 84.1 summarizes the incidence of laryngeal findings in these disorders, in addition to their clinical manifestations, examination findings, diagnosis, and treatment.

84.2 Rheumatoid Arthritis

Rheumatoid arthritis is an autoimmune chronic inflammatory disease that affects synovial membranes, leading to bone and joint destruction. It is a systemic disorder with numerous extra-articular manifestations, including serositis, nodule formation, and vasculitis. Laryngeal manifestations of rheumatoid arthritis include cricoarytenoid joint arthritis, node formation on the true vocal folds, and rarely, amyloid deposition.

84.2.1 Incidence

Laryngeal involvement is common in RA; however, the true incidence is unknown.

84.2.2 Clinical Manifestations

Inflammation may occur in the cricoarytenoid joint, which is a true diarthrodial articulation formed by the cricoid and arytenoid cartilages. The symptoms of cricoarytenoid joint involvement are vague and nonspecific. They include globus (a sensation of fullness or tension in the throat), hoarseness, odynophagia, and pain during speaking or coughing. Hoarseness and stridor with exertion are mainly symptoms of chronic disease, as joint ankylosis may develop and cause airway obstruction. Alternatively, acute and chronic disease may be completely asymptomatic.

In addition to affecting the joint, rheumatoid arthritis may affect the membranous vocal fold. Cystic yellow nodes may develop in the submucosal space at the junction of the anterior and middle thirds of the vocal folds. They were first described in 1993 by Hosacko, who called them "bamboo nodes" because of their resemblance to bamboo joints (▶ Fig. 84.1 and ▶ Fig. 84.2). Since that time, bamboo nodes have been identified in several autoimmune diseases. Patients who have bamboo nodes generally present with dysphonia. The nodes are found mainly in patients with seropositive rheumatoid arthritis and tend to recur, in contrast to other laryngeal nodular or cystic lesions. Amyloid deposits are rare but have been found in the larynx of patients with rheumatoid arthritis and other autoimmune diseases.

84.2.3 Examination Findings

In the acute setting, direct laryngoscopy demonstrates inflamed and erythematous cricoarytenoid joints. The true vocal folds may appear normal or slightly edematous. Bamboo nodes are rarely present. Findings in the chronic phase include thickened mucosa over the arytenoids, a narrowed glottic chink, bowing of the vocal folds during phonation, and a variable degree of restricted mobility. The diagnosis is made by the clinical findings and confirmed by serology that shows an elevated erythrocyte sedimentation rate, elevated rheumatoid factor level, decreased complement levels, and an abnormal lupus panel.

84.2.4 Treatment

Medical management includes steroids or other anti-inflammatory medications. Surgical interventions include local injection of steroids into the cricoarytenoid joint or membranous vocal fold. Tracheostomy or cordotomy is performed for a compromised airway. The microsurgical excision of bamboo nodes is controversial because the results are inconsistent, and surgery in the face of such inflammation may lead to severe vocal fold scarring and increased dysphonia.

84.3 Systemic Lupus Erythematosus

Systemic lupus erythematosus is a common autoimmune disease in which circulating immune complexes cause damage to blood vessels, connective tissues, and mucosal surfaces, most often in the skin, joints, kidneys, and lungs. The most frequent otolaryngologic manifestation is the formation of ulcerative lesions of the oral cavity. The larynx is rarely involved, but the mucosa and submucosa of the laryngeal structures may be affected. When the larynx is involved, the glottis and cricoarytenoid joints are the most commonly affected areas.

84.3.1 Incidence

Laryngeal involvement is variable, appearing in from 1 to 30% of affected patients.

84.3.2 Clinical Manifestations

In the acute phase of systemic lupus erythematosus, mucosal ulceration and edema and submucosal hematomas may cause hoarseness, dyspnea, and throat pain. Late effects of the disease include corditis, mucosal thickening, laryngeal scarring with stenosis, and laryngitis sicca with dry, thickened vocal cords. The disease process may also lead to vocal fold fixation, perichondritis, and cricoarytenoid arthritis.

Table 84.1 Systemic diseases affecting the larynx

	Rheumatoid arthritis	Systemic lupus erythematosus	Relapsing polychondritis	Sarcoidosis	Wegener granulomatosus	Amyloidosis
Incidence of laryngeal involvement	Unknown	1–30% of affected patients	21–50% of affected patients	1–5% of affected patients	15–55% of affected patients	Unknown
Clinical manifestations	Cricoarytenoid joint inflammation and/or ankylosis Bamboo nodes	Ulcerative lesions of mucosal and submucosal surfaces Glottis and cricoarytenoid joints most commonly affected	Inflammation and loss of integrity of cartilaginous structures with resultant airway obstruction	Noncaseating granulomatous inflammation Supraglottis most commonly affected	Necrotizing granulomas and necrotizing vasculitis Subglottis most commonly affected	Amyloid deposition True and false vocal folds most commonly affected
Examination findings	Inflamed and edematous cricoarytenoid joints Bamboo nodes at the junction of the anterior and middle thirds of the vocal folds (▲ Fig. 84.1 and ▲ Fig. 84.2)	Can be normal Frank ulcerations of mucosa Erythematous and edematous larynx ± limited mobility of vocal folds	Glottic and supraglottic edema, laryngomalacia, tracheomalacia, and subglottic stenosis	Pale submucosal nodules in glottis and supraglottic structures (▲ Fig. 84.3) Thickened and inflamed laryngeal mucosa (▲ Fig. 84.4)	Edema, laceration, hemorrhage, stenosis, and necrosis	Smooth, pinkish gray or waxy yellow submucosal mass without ulceration of overlying mucosa (▲ Fig. 84.5)
Diagnosis	Clinical findings of multiple joint involvement ↑ESR and RF ↓Complement on serology	Clinical findings ↑ANA titer on serology	Clinical findings Biopsy of involved cartilage when clinical findings are equivocal	Chest X-ray Biopsy showing noncaseating granulomas Exclusion of other granulomatous disease	Clinical findings + c-ANCA on serology Biopsy showing granulomas and vasculitis	Biopsy showing apple green birefringence on polarized light after Congo red stain
Treatment	Systemic and/or intralesional steroids Anti-inflammatory medications Tracheostomy or cordotomy for airway obstruction	Systemic steroids Anti-inflammatory medications Antimalarials Tracheostomy or cordotomy for airway obstruction	Systemic steroids Immune suppressants Tracheostomy Intubation Airway stenting	Systemic, inhaled, and/or intralesional steroids Tracheostomy or cordotomy for airway obstruction	Systemic and/or intralesional steroids Cytotoxic agents Immune modulators Airway débridement or dilation, or stent insertion Laryngotracheoplasty, tracheal resection, and/or tracheostomy	For laryngeal amyloidosis endoscopic microsurgical removal of deposits For systemic amyloidosis systemic steroids and antimetabolites

Abbreviations: ANA, antinuclear antibody; c-ANCA, cytoplasmic antineutrophil cytoplasmic autoantibody; ESR, erythrocyte sedimentation rate; RF, rheumatoid factor.

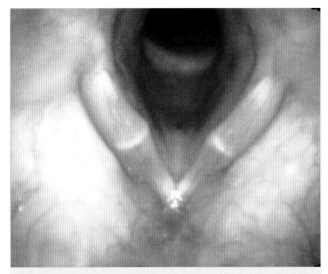

Fig. 84.1 "Joints" seen in "bamboo nodules" in the true vocal folds of a patient with rheumatoid arthritis.

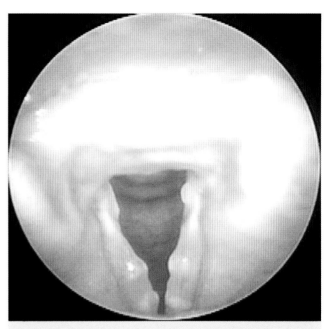

Fig. 84.2 Distinct nodes in rheumatoid arthritis.

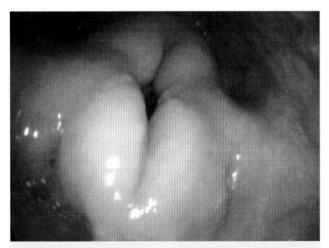

Fig. 84.3 Supraglottic edema in sarcoidosis.

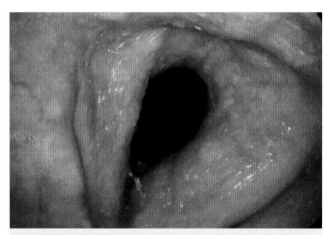

Fig. 84.4 Thickened and inflamed laryngeal mucosa in sarcoidosis.

84.3.3 Examination Findings

The diagnosis of systemic lupus erythematosus is based on clinical manifestations of disease involving two or more organ systems. Increased antinuclear antibody (ANA) titers are also sensitive for the disease. Anti-dsDNA (double-stranded DNA) antibody, a subtype of ANA, is highly specific for systemic lupus erythematosus and present in 70% of cases. In patients with an established diagnosis of systemic lupus erythematosus, the laryngeal examination may be completely normal; alternatively, the larynx may be erythematous and edematous, frank ulcerations may be present, and there may be abnormal vocal fold motion.

84.3.4 Treatment

Medical therapy for systemic lupus erythematosus includes high-dose steroids, nonsteroidal anti-inflammatory drugs, and antimalarial drugs. Tracheostomy or cordotomy may be performed for a compromised airway.

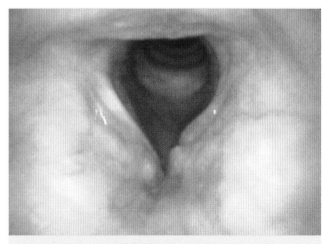

Fig. 84.5 Submucosal supraglottic accumulation of amyloid.

84.4 Relapsing Polychondritis

Relapsing polychondritis is a rare disorder characterized by recurrent episodes of inflammation of the cartilaginous and connective tissue. Auricular chondritis is the most common initial presentation, but episodes of inflammation can occur in any cartilaginous area. Laryngotracheal involvement is well recognized and is considered ominous because loss of the supportive cartilaginous scaffolding of the upper respiratory airways may lead to significant morbidity and mortality.

84.4.1 Incidence

From 21 to 50% of patients with relapsing polychondritis have symptomatic airway involvement, with a female predominance of 73:1.

84.4.2 Clinical Manifestations

Symptoms of airway involvement include cough, hoarseness, aphonia, choking sensation, and dyspnea. Patients may also demonstrate tenderness over the thyroid cartilage and anterior cervical trachea if these cartilages are affected. Airway obstruction can occur by several mechanisms: (1) airway encroachment by structures with inflammatory swelling in the active stage of the disease; (2) the formation of a mass of fibrous tissue with cicatricial contraction during the later stages of the disease; (3) dissolution of the tracheobronchial cartilage, with subsequent collapse of the airway during respiration.

84.4.3 Examination Findings

Laryngoscopy and bronchoscopy demonstrate variable findings, including glottic and supraglottic edema, laryngomalacia, tracheomalacia, bronchomalacia, and subglottic stenosis. The diagnosis of relapsing polychondritis is based on the clinical involvement of at least three cartilaginous areas. No serologic tests are sensitive or specific for relapsing polychondritis.

84.4.4 Treatment

The medical treatment for relapsing polychondritis includes steroids and immunosuppressive medications. Intubation in the patient with relapsing polychondritis may be difficult, depending on the degree of cartilaginous destruction in the upper airway. Dynamic obstruction from airway collapse may require continuous positive airway pressure (CPAP) or stenting. Tracheostomy is helpful only for proximal airway disease. Distal airway involvement may lead to death from obstructive respiratory failure if stenting is unsuccessful.

84.5 Sarcoidosis

Sarcoidosis is a chronic granulomatous disease characterized by noncaseating granulomatous inflammation. Although it may involve any organ system, it most commonly affects the lymph nodes, lungs, spleen, and liver. In the larynx, sarcoidosis generally affects the supraglottis, but it can affect any subsite of the larynx and also cause vocal fold paralysis via involvement of the recurrent laryngeal nerve. Chronic inflammation and granuloma formation distort the involved laryngeal tissues.

84.5.1 Incidence

Laryngeal involvement is estimated to occur in 1 to 5% of cases.

84.5.2 Clinical Manifestations

Initially, the laryngeal involvement may be relatively benign, appearing as pale submucosal nodules. These nodules eventually coalesce to produce pale, edematous tissue affecting mostly the epiglottis and other supraglottic structures (▶ Fig. 84.3). Lesions are rarely painful, and the symptoms depend on the site of involvement. The typical presentation is partial airway obstruction from distortion of the involved tissues, as well as dysphonia when the glottis is involved. The clinical course varies from spontaneous resolution to relentless progression and death.

84.5.3 Examination Findings

Laryngoscopy demonstrates edema of the epiglottis and supraglottic structures, or thickening and inflammation of the glottic and subglottic mucosa (▶ Fig. 84.4). Chest X-rays demonstrate hilar adenopathy. The diagnosis is confirmed by the microscopic appearance of noncaseating granulomas, epithelioid cells, macrophages, and giant cells with inclusion bodies on biopsy. Alternative granulomatous diseases, such as Wegener granulomatosis, tuberculosis, and fungal infection, must be ruled out. Serologic testing is notoriously insensitive and nonspecific, although angiotensin-converting enzyme levels can be used to track the activity of the disease.

84.5.4 Treatment

Medical therapy includes systemic steroids. Small lesions may benefit from intralesional steroid injection, and large lesions may require surgical debulking. Although the benefit is unclear, inhaled steroids may be effective in laryngeal disease. Tracheostomy or cordotomy is performed for airway obstruction.

84.6 Wegener Granulomatosis

Wegener granulomatosis is a well-defined syndrome of necrotizing granulomatous vasculitis of the upper airway, lower airway, and kidneys. Almost all patients with Wegener granulomatosis present with upper airway symptoms, and more than 90% have involvement of the nose or sinuses.

84.6.1 Incidence

Airway involvement affects 15 to 55% of patients with Wegener granulomatosis, and airway involvement tends to develop in patients younger than 30 years of age.

84.6.2 Clinical Manifestations

Wegener granulomatosis results in the development of necrotizing granulomas and necrotizing vasculitis. In the upper airway, it manifests as mucosal abnormalities, subglottic stenosis, tracheobronchial stenosis, and malacia. Symptoms therefore range from hoarseness and sore throat to cough, hemoptysis, wheezing, dyspnea, and stridor. Patients often have bloody nasal discharge. Stridor can be the first manifestation of airway involvement, and the onset may be sudden or progressive. Subglottic stenosis is the most common cause of stridor in Wegener granulomatosis, and the differential diagnosis in any patient with stridor should include this disease.

84.6.3 Examination Findings

Laryngoscopy and bronchoscopy demonstrate a wide range of mucosal abnormalities, including edema, ulceration, hemorrhage, stenosis, granulomas, and necrosis. Additionally, there may be cartilaginous deformities. The diagnosis is suggested by the clinical findings and by positivity for cytoplasmic antineutrophil cytoplasmic autoantibodies (c-ANCA) on serology. The diagnosis may be supported by biopsy of a site of active disease. Upper respiratory tract biopsy demonstrates acute and chronic inflammation, with granulomatous features and vasculitis of the small and medium-size vessels.

84.6.4 Treatment

Medical therapy for Wegener granulomatosis includes steroids, cytotoxic agents, antibiotics, and immune modulators. Surgical management of the airway includes intralesional steroid injection, airway débridement and dilation, stent insertion, laryngotracheoplasty, tracheal resection, and tracheostomy. Surgical manipulation of the airway should be minimized during active disease because the inflammation will often respond dramatically to medical management, and surgical intervention may result in the exacerbation of inflammation and stenosis.

84.7 Amyloidosis

Amyloidosis is an idiopathic disease characterized by the deposition of fibrillar proteins into tissues. Primary amyloidosis involves the spontaneous deposition of protein, whereas secondary amyloidosis occurs in conjunction with another systemic disease, such as rheumatoid arthritis or multiple myeloma.

84.7.1 Incidence

Amyloidosis accounts for 0.2 to 1.2% of all benign tumors of the larynx.

84.7.2 Clinical Manifestations

Laryngeal amyloidosis is usually a primary disease but it may be secondary with laryngeal localization. Pathologically, it is a deposition of amorphous fibrillar protein that defines amyloid. Laryngeal deposition may be secondary to systemic processes including Immunoglobulin light chain amyloidosis, monoclonal gammopathies or reactive processes related to chronic inflammatory conditions such as arthritis or Crohns disease. Alternatively, it may be an isolated process in the larynx or laryngotracheal complex. It is important to distinguish between primary and secondary amyloidosis because the distinction alters management. In the secondary form, systemic work up is warranted and the primary disease process is treated, controlling the formation of serum amyloid which then gets deposited into extracellular tissue. In the larynx, amyloidosis is more commonly a localized process; the true and false folds are the most common sites of involvement, followed by the aryepiglottic folds and subglottis (▶ Fig. 84.5). Unlike the amyloid in secondary amyloidosis, amyloid here is a proliferation of monoclonal cells with immunoglobulin light chains deposited into tissues. Four patterns of deposition have been described in the larynx: amorphous masses, deposits in vessel walls, deposits in the basement membranes of seromucous glands, and hyalinized rings in adipose tissue. Management generally involves conservative surgery aimed at maintaining airway patency and improving voice.

84.7.3 Examination Findings

Patients typically present with long-standing hoarseness or dyspnea. The typical appearance is a smooth, pinkish gray or waxy yellow submucosal mass without ulceration of the overlying mucosa. There may also be significant obstruction in the subglottic region. Computed tomography shows thickening of the involved tissues. The diagnosis is made by laryngoscopy and biopsy. Light microscopy demonstrates acellular, amorphous, homogeneous, eosinophilic material. Classic Congo red histologic stains demonstrate apple green birefringence under polarized light. Additional diagnostic tests, including complete blood cell count, electrocardiography, renal function studies, and urinalysis, are indicated in consideration of potentially devastating cardiac and renal involvement. Amyloid associated with multiple myeloma must be considered in patients with bone pain and proteinuria. A rectal or abdominal fat pad biopsy will aid in the evaluation for systemic disease.

84.7.4 Treatment

Systemic work up is warranted including laboratory tests of liver and kidney function, electrocardiography, chest x-ray and ultrasound examination of the abdomen. If systemic disease is revealed, the systemic disease process is treated and the larynx can be clinical monitored for resolution and airway maintenance. For primary laryngeal amyloidosis, steroids and antimetabolites have not been found to be helpful. The treatment for localized laryngeal amyloidosis is endoscpic microsurgical removal of deposits that interfere with phonation or the airway. Radiotherapy has also been noted to be successful in addition to surgery for airway maintenance. Bronchoscopy is warranted to evaluate for possible extent of disease into the trachea.

84.8 Roundsmanship

- Surgical intervention is based on restoring or preserving function in diseases that often respond to medical management.
- Surgical intervention in an acutely inflamed larynx or trachea may result in an exacerbation of the inflammation and stenosis.

- In the worst case scenario, a tracheotomy may be necessary to secure the airway.
- A high index of suspicion is needed to diagnose systemic disorders presenting with laryngotracheal or esophageal symptoms and signs.

84.9 Recommended Reading

[1] Bandi V, Munnur U, Braman SS. Airway problems in patients with rheumatologic disorders. Crit Care Clin 2002; 18: 749–765

[2] Bartels H, Dikkers FG, van der Wal JE, Lokhorst HM, Hazenberg BP. Laryngeal amyloidosis: localized versus systemic disease and update on diagnosis and therapy. Ann Otol Rhinol Laryngol 2004; 113: 741–748

[3] Ernst A, Rafeq S, Boiselle P et al. Relapsing polychondritis and airway involvement. Chest 2009; 135: 1024–1030

[4] Loehrl TA, Smith TL. Inflammatory and granulomatous lesions of the larynx and pharynx. Am J Med 2001; 111 Suppl 8A: 113S–117S

[5] Polychronopoulos VS, Prakash UB, Golbin JM, Edell ES, Specks U. Airway involvement in Wegener's granulomatosis. Rheum Dis Clin North Am 2007; 33: 755–775

[6] Staats BA, Utz JP, Michet CJ. Relapsing polychondritis. Semin Respir Crit Care Med 2002; 23: 145–154

[7] Voulgari PV, Papazisi D, Bai M, Zagorianakou P, Assimakopoulos D, Drosos AA. Laryngeal involvement in rheumatoid arthritis. Rheumatol Int 2005; 25: 321–325

85 Unilateral Vocal Fold Immobility

Jamie A. Koufman

85.1 Introduction

Unilateral vocal fold immobility may be due to laryngeal paralysis or fixation. Paralysis is much more common than cricoarytenoid joint fixation or other structural problems that may affect mobility. For phonation, normal vocal folds come together along their lengths like two hands clapping on a hinge; for swallowing, they close tightly, like a sphincter. The symptoms of unilateral vocal fold immobility depend to a great extent on the position on the vocal fold and the degree to which glottal closure is affected. Voice change, aphonia (absence of voice), dysphonia, and diplophonia (double tone) are the usual symptoms. Aspiration due to uncomplicated (peripheral neuropathic) unilateral vocal fold paralysis is uncommon; aspiration is seen more frequently with a central nervous system problem or concomitantly with superior laryngeal or vagal neuropathy.

85.2 Incidence of Disease

Among patients with laryngeal and voice disorders seen at a voice treatment center, unilateral vocal fold immobility accounts for 1 to 5% of cases, depending to some degree on the referral patterns of the center. At centers performing significant numbers of skull base surgeries and head and neck cancer surgeries, for example, the rates of iatrogenic vocal fold paralysis are relatively high. In addition, unilateral vocal fold paralysis is seen in as many as 1% of patients with endotracheal intubation.

85.3 Terminology and Classification of Process

Unilateral vocal fold paralysis is usually described by the position of the immobile vocal fold: *median* (in the midline), *paramedian* (near the midline), *intermediate* (partly open), or *cadaveric* (wide open). The latter position is also sometimes called *lateralized*. When the immobility is caused by a cricoarytenoid joint problem, it may be due to fibrosis, ankylosis, or even dislocation, although posttraumatic cricoarytenoid joint dislocation is uncommon.

85.4 Applied Anatomy

The innervation of the vocal folds is via the superior laryngeal nerve (SLN) and recurrent laryngeal nerve (RLN). The SLN is primarily a sensory nerve, and the RLN is principally motor. The RLN is so named because of its unusual course from the skull base down through the neck within the vagus nerve (in the carotid sheath) and then into the chest; on the left side, it dips under the aorta, and on the right it courses around the innominate artery. Finally, after sweeping around their respective arteries, the right and left RLNs ascend back into the neck in the tracheo-esophageal groove to enter the larynx posteriorly. It is important for the clinician to understand the anatomy of the

RLNs because they may be affected by occult disease anywhere along their lengths, including within the chest.

In addition to the innervation of the vocal folds, it is important to understand the anatomy of the cricoarytenoid complex. The arytenoids articulate with the posterior cricoid by facets on the superior surface. These are synovial joints. The movement of the arytenoids on the cricoarytenoid facets is three-dimensional. Not only do the arytenoids rotate and glide; they also tip and slide anteriorly, almost off the facets. The antagonistic pull of the opposing intrinsic and extrinsic muscles of phonation confer this remarkable degree of mobility on the arytenoids, the functions of which are involved in both phonation and airway protection. The height of the vocal processes of the two arytenoids must match so that the membranous vocals folds are at the same height. If the heights of the vocal processes (and so the membranous vocal folds) are asymmetric, dysphonia will result. Height mismatch of the vocal folds is an important indication for surgical intervention in unilateral vocal fold paralysis.

85.5 The Disease Process

85.5.1 Etiology

Paralytic dysphonia (unilateral vocal fold paralysis) is much more common than cricoarytenoid joint fixation. Fixation may be due to blunt trauma, endotracheal intubation, inflammation secondary to reflux disease, and/or rheumatologic diseases, especially rheumatoid arthritis. In addition, cartilage tumors such as cricoid chondrosarcoma can lead to unilateral vocal fold immobility due to fixation.

Unilateral vocal fold paralysis is most commonly idiopathic, although many patients date the onset of symptoms to an acute upper respiratory infection. After idiopathic vocal fold paralysis, the most common etiologies of unilateral vocal fold immobility are, in decreasing order of frequency, neck and chest surgery (iatrogenic), neurologic diseases, tumors of the neck and chest, endotracheal intubation, and neck and chest trauma (▶ Table 85.1).

Among iatrogenic cases, the rank order of occurrence has changed slightly in the last decade, with carotid endarterectomy (38%) now surpassing thyroidectomy (30%) as a cause. Skull base and head/neck cancer surgery accounts for 14% of cases, endotracheal intubation for 10%, and cardiac surgery and miscellaneous causes for 8%. The most common tumors associated with laryngeal nerve paralysis are apical lung cancer, thyroid cancer, esophageal cancer, and hypopharyngeal cancer.

85.5.2 Natural History and Progression

The most common symptom of unilateral vocal fold paralysis or fixation is dysphonia (hoarseness), although swallowing problems, cough, and aspiration can occur. In the patient's history, the onset of symptoms is important, in particular whether the onset was sudden or progressive. In general, a progressive onset of symptoms is more likely than a sudden onset to be associated

Table 85.1 Differential diagnosis of unilateral vocal fold immobility: paralysis and fixation

Etiology	Percentage of cases
Paralysis	
Sudden onset	95%
Neck/chest surgery	31%
Idiopathic	23%
Viral neuropathy	16%
Neurologic disorder	9%
Neck/chest neoplasm	8%
Endotracheal intubation	8%
Neck/chest trauma	4%
Gradual onset	5%
Central neurologic disease	50%
Multiple sclerosis	40%
Lyme disease	35%
Brain tumor	10%
Amyotrophic lateral sclerosis	10%
Shy-Drager syndrome	2%
Peripheral neurologic disease	50%
Benign and malignant tumors of head/neck/chest (e.g., thyroid tumors)	50%
Diseases of peripheral nerves (e.g., Lyme disease)	30%
Nerve tumors (e.g., vagus, glomus tumors)	10%
Chest tumors (e.g, apical lung cancer)	5%
Ortner syndrome (paralysis secondary to congestive heart failure)	2%
Fixation	
Sudden onset	
Blunt or penetrating laryngeal trauma with arytenoid dislocation	
Iatrogenic (e.g., endotracheal intubation, esophagoscopy)	
Gradual onset	
Rheumatoid diseases (e.g., arthritis)	
Cricoid cartilage disease/tumors (e.g., chondrosarcoma)	
Granulomatous diseases that affect the larynx (e.g., tuberculosis)	
Laryngopharyngeal reflux (interarytenoid or cricoarytenoid pericapsular fibrosis)	

with tumors affecting one or more of the laryngeal nerves or with a progressive neurologic disease.

When the paralysis is due to a known cause, such as surgery or trauma, almost half of patients regain normal or nearly normal voice within 1 year, even without any treatment, whether or not the paralyzed vocal fold regains movement. In this scenario, the vocal fold may be synkinetically reinnervated. Although this does not result in vocal fold motion, it may provide enough muscle tone to medialize the vocal fold with significant mass. This, and normal function of the opposite vocal fold, result in closure of the glottal gap, with the production of an adequate or even normal voice. In cases in which the RLN was left intact, complete spontaneous recovery with normal vocal fold motion may occur.

85.5.3 Potential Disease Complications

In addition to the dysphonia that results from vocal fold immobility, when the vocal folds are incapable of closing completely, secondary vocal fold pathologic lesions can develop in the striking zones (where they impact) as a result of the hyperkinetic compensatory processes of speaking. In other words, effortful vocal fold closure can lead to the development of vocal fold polyps, polypoid corditis, nodules, cysts, pseudocysts, and even

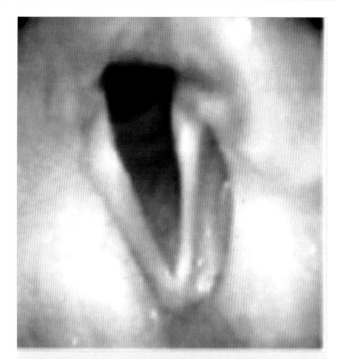

Fig. 85.1 Left vocal fold paralysis, with bowing and atrophy.

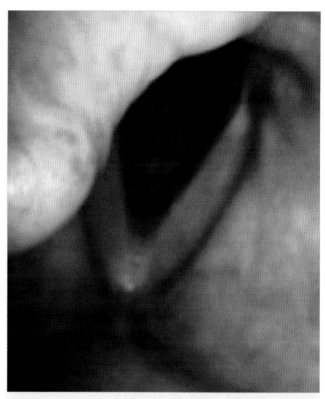

Fig. 85.2 Right vocal fold paralysis, with forward-tipped arytenoid and foreshortened vocal fold. The atrophy is less than that seen in ▶ Fig. 85.1.

vocal process granulomas. In addition, if the larynx cannot close during swallowing, aspiration (even aspiration pneumonia) can result.

85.6 Medical Evaluation

85.6.1 Presenting Complaints

Hoarseness (raspiness), diplophonia (double tone), effortful phonation (speaking), odynophonia (painful speaking), air hunger, vocal fatigue, aspiration, and chronic cough are the most common symptoms associated with unilateral vocal fold paralysis. In most patients, the glottal closure symptoms of consequence are hoarseness, vocal fatigue, and effortful phonation.

85.6.2 Clinical Findings, Physical Examination

As noted above, the duration of the onset of the symptoms is important. To determine the etiology, it is also prudent to note any synchronous events, such as an upper respiratory infection or head/neck or cardiothoracic surgery. To understand how urgent the need for vocal rehabilitation may be, it is imperative to inquire about the presence of aspiration, the patient's vocal needs, and how much the dysphonia is impacting his or her life.

Before performing laryngeal endoscopy, one should listen to the voice and note its character and severity. Is it a "wet" voice, suggesting decreased laryngeal sensation? Is there enough projection for conversation in a quiet room or over background noise? What is the quality of the cough? While a full head and neck examination is performed, special attention should be paid to an evaluation of cranial nerve function and a search for the presence of neck masses, especially in the thyroid, to detect secondary causes of the paralysis.

Ultimately, the diagnosis of unilateral vocal fold immobility requires a laryngeal examination. In the past, a mirror examination was performed, but this type of screening technique has become obsolete. Today, the laryngeal examination is most commonly performed with a flexible endoscope that allows an assessment of glottal function. Before the examination, it is worth teaching the patient the /i/sniff maneuver. Pronouncing a vowel like "eeeee" (/i/) brings the vocal folds together in adduction, and sniffing causes brisk vocal fold opening (abduction). The /i/sniff maneuver is an excellent vocal task for evaluating vocal fold mobility. In addition to vocal fold motion, the position of the folds, evidence of atrophy or bowing, and height of the vocal processes should be noted (▶ Fig. 85.1 and ▶ Fig. 85.2).

The most common findings in unilateral paralysis are hypomobility and bowing of the involved vocal fold, as well as hyperkinetic laryngeal biomechanics with supraglottic and pharyngeal squeezing (▶ Fig. 85.3). During high-pitched phonation, axial tilt and/or laryngeal rotation is common in patients with unilateral paralysis and/or bilateral paresis when there is significant asymmetric tension between opposing intrinsic laryngeal muscles, especially if one of the cricothyroid muscles is weak. Axial tilt and rotation are due to unbalanced closure of the right and left sides when one SLN is affected. (These findings are most common in patients with bilateral vocal fold paresis.)

With unilateral paralysis, stroboscopy will show increased amplitude on the paralyzed side, indicating decreased vocal fold tone. Stroboscopy also allows evaluation of the glottal chink, its size, and whether it is predominantly anterior or both anterior and posterior. The clinician should look for the vocal

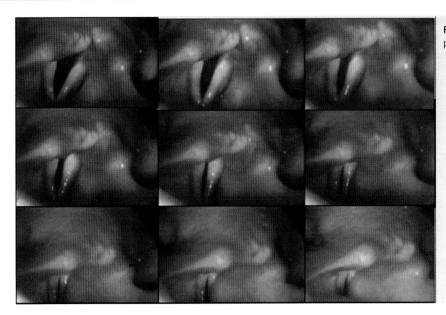

Fig. 85.3 Left vocal fold paralysis showing compensatory biomechanics.

process-to-vocal process contact point before compensatory biomechanics take over.

Finally, the presence of excessive secretions should be noted, whether there is pooling in the piriform or postcricoid area, or if there is penetration into the glottis or trachea. Gross sensation can be tested by palpating the supraglottis with the tip of the endoscope in an attempt to elicit an adductor reflex. Pharyngeal dysfunction is identified by the absence of a medial squeeze of the pharyngeal walls on a high pitched /i/ or the presence of a dilated piriform sinus. A combination of decreased sensation, pharyngeal dysfunction, and pooling secretions should serve as an alert to an increased risk for aspiration (even in a patient with a negative history because the patient could be experiencing silent aspiration).

85.6.3 Testing

The most important test that differentiates vocal fold paralysis from vocal fold fixation is laryngeal electromyography (EMG), which is an electrical neurodiagnostic test performed by placing a fine-needle electrode in the laryngeal muscles. Laryngeal EMG not only determines which muscles and nerves are affected but also indicates the prognosis for recovery. When the patient's prognosis is poor (between 2 and 6 months), one may proceed to a permanent rehabilitation procedure rather than wait a full 12 months, as was done historically. Other aerodynamic and acoustic tests and electroglottography can also be used to assess the severity of glottal closure problems.

When the etiology of the paralysis is unclear, most clinicians recommend a work-up for peripheral neuropathy, including blood tests to rule out vector-borne neurologic disease (e.g., Lyme disease, West Nile virus infection), as well as computed tomography (CT) of the neck to rule out a neoplasm affecting the laryngeal branches of the vagus nerve. At a minimum, a patient with a left vocal fold paralysis requires a chest X-ray to evaluate the thoracic component of the left RLN. CT of the chest may be the preferred examination because it is more sensitive for masses in the aortopulmonary window. If other neurologic symptoms suggest a demyelinating disease, then magnetic resonance (MR) imaging of the head and a neurologic consultation may be ordered.

In cases of idiopathic laryngeal paralysis, the author begins with laryngeal EMG, which can help determine the cause of the paralysis/paresis and whether it is "new" (of recent onset) or "old" (of remote onset). The presence of spontaneous activity implies ongoing denervation (i.e., "new"). Indeed, the radiologic work-up is EMG-guided. If the SLN (tested in the ipsilateral cricothyroid muscle) is not involved, CT of the neck (skull base through superior mediastinum) is obtained. If the SLN is involved (abnormal), then MR imaging of the brain and skull base is ordered, as well.

If, on the other hand, laryngeal EMG shows an "old" neuropathic pattern (characterized by large polyphasic motor units with no evidence of spontaneous activity), radiographic evaluations may be unnecessary. However, in case of doubt, imaging studies are the safe choice to be certain that the cause of the neuropathy is not neoplastic or a pernicious neurogenic pathologic process (e.g., multiple sclerosis).

85.7 Treatment

85.7.1 Medical Treatment

Many patients who have unilateral vocal fold immobility are able to compensate for their glottal closure problem with or without voice therapy. In these cases, the contralateral vocal fold becomes stronger and can be seen on laryngeal examination to cross the midline to achieve closure. In addition, the immobile vocal fold may have adequate tone and a good midline position secondary to nonfunctional synkinetic reinnervation. As many as 30 to 50% of patients with unilateral paralysis will not require surgical treatment. In addition, voice therapy can be very helpful in allowing patients to find adaptive compensatory laryngeal behaviors.

85.7.2 Surgical Treatment

The two basic surgical approaches, injection augmentation and medialization laryngoplasty ("Isshiki thyroplasty") with or without arytenoid adduction, have different advantages and disadvantages. Injection augmentation, which can be done in the office setting or in the operating room, involves the injection of an alloplastic material or autologous adipose tissue into the vocal fold itself. Although it requires a skin incision, medialization laryngoplasty provides permanent voice rehabilitation in the majority of cases. Unfortunately, today not many surgeons are skilled in this technique.

Arytenoid fixation from blunt and penetrating trauma is uncommon. It may also be due to traumatic endotracheal intubation and inflammatory joint diseases such as rheumatoid arthritis. The diagnosis of fixation can be confused with that of paralysis until a definitive diagnosis is made by laryngeal EMG and examination under anesthesia with passive mobility testing. Although some laryngologists believe that the arytenoid may be dislocated and then surgically reduced (i.e., "undislocated"), the author has never seen such a case and does not believe that "dislocation" is possible based upon the cricoarytenoid anatomy. On the other hand, damage to the joint can certainly occur, and endoscopic arytenoid repositioning is possible, assuming that the affected arytenoid can be mobilized.

85.7.3 Timing of Surgery and Choice of Procedure for Unilateral Vocal Fold Paralysis

Surgical treatment is reserved for patients with relatively severe glottal closure symptoms and/or aspiration. In the case of paralytic dysphonia, the term *relatively* is important. The need for surgery in each case is tempered by not only the severity of the dysphonia and/or aspiration but also the patient-specific consequences of failure to intervene surgically.

Patients who have glottal incompetence and obvious clinical and radiographic aspiration, with a risk for the development of life-threatening pneumonia, should undergo some type of glottal closure procedure. Which procedure(s) depend(s) on the symptom severity, prognosis for recovery, and overall medical status of the patient. Although it can be life-threatening, aspiration is a significant problem following unilateral vocal fold paralysis in fewer than 10% of cases.

The prognosis for patients who have aspiration associated with laryngeal paralysis is worst when (1) they have undergone skull base surgery for tumors with sacrifice of multiple cranial nerves (especially nerves IX through XII); (2) they have profound degenerative neurologic diseases such as amyotrophic lateral sclerosis; and (3) they have a history of cerebral vascular accident. For such patients, the surgical procedures may include total laryngectomy, tracheotomy with some type of feeding tube, injection augmentation, or laryngoplasty. For patients with moderate aspiration, even after skull base surgery, ipsilateral medialization with arytenoid adduction and possible cricopharyngeal myotomy will usually suffice to allow normal oral feeding. Such a procedure can usually be performed within 1 to 2 weeks of the skull base surgery. Patients with severe recalcitrant aspiration may require even more radical procedures, including tracheotomy, laryngotracheal separation, or laryngectomy.

The most common concern of the laryngeal surgeon is determining the method and timing for the treatment of patients with different levels of dysphonia, vocal demands, and progno-

ses. Obviously, for patients who have mild to moderate dysphonia and a good prognosis for recovery, no surgery may be appropriate. But what about a 75-year-old clergyman with vocal fold paralysis who is dysphonic? Such a patient will demand that something be done sooner rather than later. In such a case, knowing the prognosis may help answer the question. If the laryngeal nerve has little or no chance of recovery—such as after RLN sacrifice in thyroid cancer surgery—then medialization laryngoplasty with arytenoid adduction (if the posterior commissure is open or if the vocal folds are at different levels) may be an ideal solution to achieve excellent vocal rehabilitation in a timely fashion.

When the prognosis is not evident, laryngeal EMG may be very helpful. When performed between 2 and 6 months after the onset of paralysis, laryngeal EMG can predict the lack of return of vocal fold function with an accuracy of more than 95%. If such a result is found on EMG, a permanent procedure can be performed at that time. "Watching and waiting" or performing additional procedures to temporarily rehabilitate the voice would be unwarranted. If the result of laryngeal EMG is equivocal, a temporizing measure is often helpful in establishing a competent glottis while the result of reinnervation is awaited. Laryngologists now have several injection augmentation techniques and materials with different durability characteristics: temporary, semipermanent/durable, and permanent. Durable injectables will last from 6 months to 2 years. There is controversy as to whether any injectable is reliably permanent. Regardless, the availability of temporary and durable injections allows physicians to employ a practical strategy of achieving early surgical glottal closure with injection augmentation when the prognosis of a patient with vocal fold paralysis is unknown. Watching and waiting is not an appropriate plan unless the patient and surgeon have opted for this after considering temporary alternatives.

There are five techniques for performing injection augmentation and as many different materials. Injection augmentation can be done in the office or clinic setting with an awake patient, or it can be performed in the operating room while the patient is under general anesthesia, with the benefits of a motionless patient and magnification through an operating microscope. In truth, fewer than 25% of injection augmentation procedures are done in the operating room.

Performing procedures under general anesthesia is recommended for patients who are unwilling or unlikely to be cooperative when an awake technique is used (e.g., excessive gag reflex, difficult anatomy). General anesthesia usually allows more precise injection augmentation. If autologous adipose tissue (lipo-injection) is the implant/graft of choice, then general anesthesia is recommended.

For most patients with severe dysphonia and an uncertain prognosis after unilateral vocal fold paralysis, injection augmentation in the office is recommended with temporary or durable substances such as the following: Radiesse Voice Gel (Merz Aesthetics, San Mateo, CA); Cymetra (LifeCell, Branchburg, NJ); or even Radiesse Voice (Merz Aesthetics). In addition, if the paralysis is permanent but it is unclear whether the patient will benefit from vocal fold augmentation, a temporary injection can be used as a trial. The advantage of temporary materials is that they last only a few to several months; of course, this short duration is also a potential disadvantage. Neverthe-

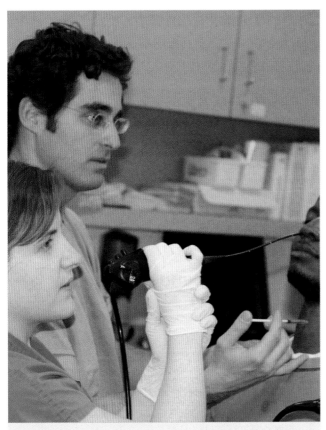

Fig. 85.4 Typical setup for in-office injection with transnasal endoscopic visualization.

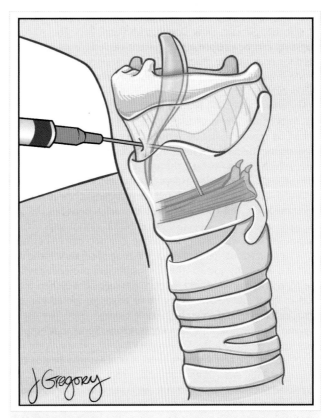

Fig. 85.5 Schematic of the thyrohyoid approach to injection for vocal fold augmentation.

less, repeated injections can help a patient over the initial period of relative vocal disability.

There are four different office-based techniques for performing injection augmentation in the awake patient: (1) percutaneous, from below, through the cricothyroid membrane; (2) percutaneous, directly through the thyroid cartilage (suitable only for relatively young patients without significant calcification of the thyroid cartilage); (3) percutaneous, from above, through the thyroid notch; and (4) peroral. All of these methods are done with simultaneous endoscopic (transnasal or peroral) laryngeal visualization (▶ Fig. 85.4 and ▶ Fig. 85.5).

Although some surgeons are proficient in many or all of the above approaches, the most popular technique for office-based vocal fold injection among contemporary laryngologists is the thyrohyoid approach with simultaneous transnasal flexible laryngoscopy. This technique has four advantages:
1. Minimal anesthesia is required.
2. It allows direct visualization of needle insertion.
3. It is well tolerated by patients.
4. There is a relatively easy learning curve for the surgeon.

For patients in whom vocal fold recovery is unlikely (e.g., malignant invasion of the RLN, transection or resection of the RLN, poor laryngeal EMG prognosis, paralysis for 9 to 12 months), a permanent treatment can be offered. If the glottal gap is very small or the patient's life expectancy is short, a "permanent injectable" may be used. Alternatively, a type I laryngoplasty with or without arytenoid adduction or an RLN–ansa cervicalis

reinnervation procedure (ANSA-RLN) may be performed. ANSA-RLN has a reported successful reinnervation rate of over 95%; it provides vocal fold bulk and tone, but not physiologic vocal fold movement. It takes 3 to 6 months for the innervation to begin to take effect, so a temporary injection must be performed to rehabilitate the voice and bridge this time gap. In reality, ANSA-RLN is the least commonly performed procedure for permanent vocal fold paralysis because of the excellent results and physician familiarity with laryngoplasty techniques, as well as the 3- to 6-month waiting period. Alternatively, ANSA-RLN is an excellent surgical option for pediatric patients because the procedure is performed with the patient under general anesthesia; laryngoplasty is performed with the patient under intravenous sedation, which is unlikely to be tolerated by a pediatric patient. ANSA-RLN is also optimal for immediate reinnervation at the time of RLN resection or transection. A successful ANSA-RLN in this scenario will spare the patient from future surgery for vocal rehabilitation.

Type I laryngoplasty with or without arytenoid adduction is the treatment of choice for the majority of patients with a permanent vocal fold paralysis; this surgery has a 96% success rate with minimal morbidity. The 4% revision rate is usually due to placing an implant too high and interrupting the mucosal wave. Laryngoplasty is performed under intravenous sedation to allow the patient to speak and provide the surgeon with vocal feedback when the implant is sized. Generally, a concomitant flexible laryngoscopy is performed to allow visualization of the vocal folds during the procedure, providing further feedback. Implants are generally made of e-PTFE (expanded polytetrafluoroethylene [Gore-Tex]; W. L. Gore Associates, Flagstaff, AZ) or silicone (Silastic; Dow Corning, Midland, MI). The silicone implants can be preformed or custom-carved. Aside from the need for revision, the other significant complication is infection of the implant. Although rare, implant removal is necessary if this occurs.

Arytenoid adduction is an adjunct to type I laryngoplasty. In this procedure, the muscular process of the arytenoid is accessed by removing the posterior aspect of the thyroid ala and medializing the piriform sinus. The process is lassoed with a suture, which is then passed through the paraglottic space and out through the anterior aspect of the larynx. Tension on the suture rotates the arytenoid and corresponding vocal process inferomedially. This corrects height mismatch between the vocal folds and closes a persistent posterior glottal gap, which cannot be done with an implant alone. The decision to perform an arytenoid adduction is made at the time of surgery. If the patient has a breathy voice or there is insufficient projection while the membranous vocal fold is optimally medialized, then most likely a vocal fold height mismatch or posterior glottal gap exists. This can be confirmed by flexible laryngoscopy. The use of arytenoid adduction varies among surgeons. Some may employ it as much as 30 to 40% of the time, whereas others rarely use it. The reason for this disparity is unclear, but it may be due to a lack of training and comfort with the procedure, as well as the increased operative time and risk. An arytenoid adduction adds approximately 30 minutes to the procedure and carries a very small risk for pharyngeal perforation as the piriform is medialized. The patient also experiences more discomfort when swallowing in the immediate postoperative period. In those patients who speak a significant amount, either socially or in business, the vocal improvement provided by an arytenoid adduction is likely worth the minimal risk and discomfort.

85.8 Roundsmanship

- The most common cause of unilateral vocal fold immobility is idiopathic vocal fold paralysis. Some of these cases may actually be due to a viral neuropathy.
- Unilateral vocal fold immobility presenting with progressive (gradual onset) hoarseness is associated with a relatively ominous differential diagnosis, including degenerative neurologic diseases and malignant tumors of the head, neck, and chest.
- Laryngeal electromyography is the most useful diagnostic test to determine the presence of neuropathy and the prognosis of vocal fold immobility.
- The voice symptoms of paralytic dysphonia can usually be surgically corrected by voice therapy, injection augmentation, or medialization ("Isshiki" type I) laryngoplasty with or without arytenoid adduction.

85.9 Recommended Reading

[1] Dursun G, Boynukalin S, Ozgursoy OB, Coruh I. Long-term results of different treatment modalities for glottic insufficiency. Am J Otolaryngol 2008; 29: 7–12

[2] Koufman JA, Postma GN, Whang CS et al. Diagnostic laryngeal electromyography: The Wake Forest experience 1995–1999. Otolaryngol Head Neck Surg 2001; 124: 603–606

[3] Koufman JA. Laryngoplasty for vocal cord medialization: an alternative to Teflon. Laryngoscope 1986; 96: 726–731

[4] McCulloch TM, Hoffman HT. Medialization laryngoplasty with expanded polytetrafluoroethylene. Surgical technique and preliminary results. Ann Otol Rhinol Laryngol 1998; 107: 427–432

[5] Miller FR, Bryant GL, Netterville JL. Arytenoid adduction in vocal fold paralysis. Oper Tech Otolaryngol Head Neck Surg 1999; 10: 36–41

[6] O'Leary MA, Grillone GA. Injection laryngoplasty. Otolaryngol Clin North Am 2006; 39: 43–54

[7] Rubin AD, Sataloff RT. Vocal fold paresis and paralysis. Otolaryngol Clin North Am 2007; 40: 1109–1131

86 Bilateral Vocal Fold Paralysis

Craig H. Zalvan

86.1 Introduction

Bilateral vocal fold paralysis is part of a spectrum of vocal fold immobility potentially resulting in airway compromise. Although there are many causes, only a few are relatively common. The work-up and treatment are coordinated to rule out potentially devastating disorders and ensure airway safety. Most causes of vocal fold paralysis are neurologic in nature, either direct neural trauma or a centrally mediated mechanism. Contrary to popular belief, patients with bilateral vocal fold immobility tend to have normal vocal quality, and most patients present with symptoms of airway obstruction: dyspnea on exertion, exercise intolerance, dysphagia, and stridor. Examination of the larynx demonstrates bilaterally immobile vocal folds with a resultant small glottic or interarytenoid gap. As the gap decreases in size, respiratory distress increases.

86.2 Incidence

Bilateral vocal fold paralysis is a very uncommon finding. Surgical trauma to both recurrent laryngeal nerves (RLNs) occurs in far fewer than 1% of thyroidectomies and other surgeries of the head and neck. Metastatic or direct invasion of the larynx resulting in bilateral RLN involvement is also a rare event. In children, approximately 2 to 5% of cases of bilateral vocal fold paralysis are congenitally acquired. Arnold-Chiari malformation is one of the more common causes of bilateral vocal fold paralysis in children. This malformation occurs in approximately 1 in 1,000 live births. The type II malformation most commonly causes bilateral vocal fold paralysis. Approximately one-third of children born with the type II malformation will have brainstem involvement by the age of 5 years. Of these, one-third will die, most commonly of respiratory complications.

86.3 Classification

Paralysis of the vocal folds is classified as unilateral or bilateral. In bilateral vocal fold paralysis, the position of the vocal folds determines the severity of symptoms. The position of the vocal folds can be described as medial, paramedian, or lateral. The more medial the vocal folds, the greater the degree respiratory compromise; the more lateral the vocal folds, the greater the degree of dysphonia and dysphagia.

86.4 Anatomy

Key anatomical relationships of the RLN along its entire course are important in determining the cause of bilateral vocal fold paralysis. The RLN, a branch of the vagus nerve, exits the brainstem from the medulla and courses through the jugular foramen to enter the neck. At the inferior (nodose) ganglion, the superior laryngeal nerve branches off from the main trunk to course adjacent to the pharynx and medial to the sheath of the carotid artery, further dividing into the internal and external branches. The left RLN/vagus nerve courses anterior to the carotid over the arch of the aorta, where the two components divide. The left RLN then courses posteromedial to the ligamentum arteriosum, ascends in the tracheo-esophageal groove, and enters posterior to the cricothyroid joint to innervate all motor components of the laryngeal musculature except the cricothyroid muscle. The right RLN branches off from the vagus nerve in the neck anterior to the right subclavian artery and then wraps around the artery to ascend in the right tracheo-esophageal groove before entering posterior to the cricothyroid joint. Familiarity with these anatomical relationships is important in understanding the causes of bilateral vocal paralysis. Any centrally mediated process (e.g., stroke, tumor, or hydrocephalus) can affect both RLNs at the level of the medulla. In all other cases of bilateral vocal paralysis, the cause must affect both nerves along their course if bilateral paralysis is to occur.

A detailed knowledge of the glottic space and arytenoid complex is also important in understanding airflow and vocal dynamics. The posterior glottis, or respiratory glottis, creates most of the space for airflow to occur. This region is the space posterior to the tip of the vocal processes and is bordered by both arytenoids, the interarytenoid muscle, and the mucosa (▶ Fig. 86.1). The posterior cricoarytenoid is solely responsible for abduction of the vocal folds. A distance of less than 4 mm between the arytenoid vocal processes is typically required to create stridor at rest (▶ Fig. 86.2). Increased airflow during increased activity may result in passive adduction of the vocal folds as a consequence of the Bernoulli phenomenon, leading to stridor in a compromised airway that has a diameter slightly larger than 4 mm.

86.5 The Disease Process

86.5.1 Etiology

The vast majority of cases of bilateral vocal fold paralysis are due to surgical trauma of both RLNs, typically during thyroidectomy (most often completion thyroidectomy in the setting of a preexisting unilateral vocal fold paralysis). In one series of 72

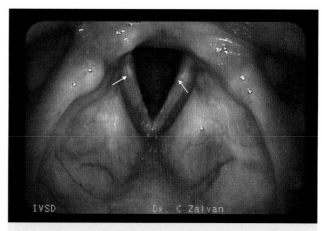

Fig. 86.1 Normal larynx with interarytenoid distance of approximately 2 cm. Arrows highlight the tips of the vocal processes.

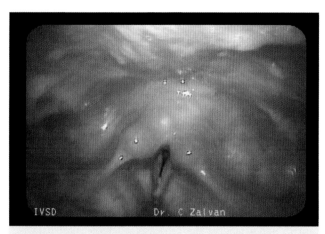

Fig. 86.2 Bilateral vocal fold paralysis in a patient with audible stridor. Note the posterior glottic gap of less than 4 mm.

adults with bilateral vocal fold immobility, surgical trauma (37%), malignancies (14%), endotracheal intubation (13%), neurologic disease (11%), and idiopathic immobility (11%) were the most common findings. Vocal fold paralysis is the second most common congenital anomaly of the pediatric airway, constituting 5 to 10% of congenital laryngeal lesions; bilateral paralysis occurs in 30 to 62% of this subgroup of patients. Airway intervention is required in over half of these children, often in the form of a tracheotomy. Arnold-Chiari malformation, hydrocephalus, and myelomeningocele are the most common causes of bilateral vocal fold paralysis in children. The majority of other cases are due to other neurologic diseases or are of idiopathic, iatrogenic, or traumatic origin.

86.5.2 Pathogenesis

Bilateral immobility of the vocal folds is due to systemic neuropathy, direct injury to both RLNs or the nucleus ambiguus, or mechanical fixation of both arytenoids. Airflow is then determined by the final resting position of the vocal folds, which evolves over time. When both vocal folds are immobile in the midline or a paramedian position, airway obstruction is more likely. When both are in the lateral position, breathy dysphonia and aspiration are common. Fixation of both arytenoids is rarely encountered but must be considered after laryngeal trauma or prolonged intubation, or in rheumatoid arthritis. Pressure necrosis, chronic inflammation with immune complex deposition, and fibrosis can result in immobility of the larynx if both arytenoids are affected. Neural integrity is intact, but effectively there is no mobility secondary to the failure of arytenoid rotation. The Box Causes of Bilateral Vocal Fold Paralysis in Adults (p.670) and the Box Causes of Bilateral Vocal Fold Paralysis in Children (p.671) summarize the differential diagnosis for bilateral vocal fold paralysis in adults and children, respectively.

Causes of Bilateral Vocal Fold Paralysis in Adults

- Iatrogenic
  - Thyroid and parathyroid surgery
    - Complete thyroidectomy
  - Tracheal resection
  - Cervical esophagectomy
  - Neurosurgery
    - Brainstem, skull base surgery
    - Anterior spinal approach surgery (with preexisting unilateral vocal fold paralysis)
  - Birth trauma
  - Contralateral carotid endarterectomy
  - Endoscopic laryngeal surgery (usually laser)
  - Radiation-induced fibrosis or chondronecrosis
- Malignancy
  - Laryngeal
  - Metastatic disease to the neck, brainstem, or mediastinum
  - Extension of pulmonary neoplasm
  - Lymphoproliferative disorders
- Central nervous system disease
  - Arnold-Chiari malformation
  - Neuromuscular disease
    - Amyotrophic lateral sclerosis, Shy-Drager syndrome, myasthenia gravis, Guillain-Barré syndrome, multiple sclerosis, Charcot-Marie-Tooth disease
  - Hydrocephalus
  - Cerebral vascular accident
- Systemic
  - Infectious
    - Lyme disease
    - Syphilis
    - Tuberculosis
    - Invasive fungal infection
  - Rheumatologic
    - Systemic lupus erythematosus, rheumatoid arthritis, relapsing polychondritis
  - Sarcoidosis
  - Wegener granulomatosis
  - Amyloidosis
- Metabolic
  - Hypocalcemia, hypokalemia, diabetes mellitus
- Local factors
  - Bilateral arytenoid dislocation
  - Bilateral arytenoid ankylosis
  - Blunt and penetrating trauma
  - Laryngospasm
  - Intubation injury
- Idiopathic

Causes of Bilateral Vocal Fold Paralysis in Children

- Neurologic
  - Arnold-Chiari malformation
  - Myelomeningocele
  - Hydrocephalus
- Iatrogenic
  - Cardiac surgery
  - Tracheo-esophageal fistula repair
- Systemic
- Traumatic
  - Intubation
  - Birth trauma
- Idiopathic

86.5.3 Natural History

Spontaneous recovery from bilateral vocal fold immobility occurred in 13% of adult cases in one retrospective case series, with most patients requiring tracheotomy for initial management. Of these cases, 15% were due to intubation injury, and of these, 44% recovered mobility in one or both vocal folds. In contrast, 48 to 60% of children recover.

Tracheotomy is required in fewer than 50% of adult patients with bilateral vocal fold paralysis. The rate of children requiring tracheotomy varies; study results range from 19 to 68%.

86.5.4 Potential Disease Complications

The most feared complication is airway obstruction and death from asphyxiation. Dysphonia, ineffective cough, chronic aspiration, aspiration pneumonia, and dysphagia are also common complications. Some patients experience chronic systemic fatigue due to the effort expended on respiration.

86.6 Medical Evaluation

86.6.1 Presenting Complaints

Contrary to popular belief, patients with bilateral vocal fold immobility tend to have a relatively normal vocal quality. Complaints are often of diplophonia, decreased vocal projection, vocal fatigue, vocal strain, and compensatory muscle tension. Breathy dysphonia occurs when there is lateral displacement of one or both immobile vocal folds with increased, unregulated airflow. Patients may also present with dysphagia, weak cough, and pneumonia secondary to loss of the laryngeal closure protective mechanism. The presentation of bilateral vocal fold paralysis is highly variable. At one extreme, a person may be completely asymptomatic, with normal voicing and respiration and no distress. This patient may describe intermittent episodes of feeling short of breath and mild stridor or "wheezing," typically during an upper respiratory illness; often, asthma is diagnosed. At the other end of the spectrum, the most typical presentation includes the onset of respiratory distress, shortness of breath, labored breathing, and stridor. Patients will complain of a "wheeze" during inspiration that represents stridor, which tends to be inspiratory early in the onset of bilat-

eral vocal fold paralysis but may become biphasic as the obstruction becomes more pronounced (depending on the resting position of the vocal folds). Following surgical trauma to both RLNs, patients may become acutely symptomatic after extubation in the operating room or recovery room, with stridor and distress. The symptoms may develop more insidiously over time as the vocal folds slowly medialize. These patients tend to adjust to the slow compromise of the larynx and may not have symptoms of obstruction until there is an abrupt change in the larynx. Any cause of laryngeal inflammation (e.g., laryngopharyngeal reflux, upper respiratory infection with laryngitis, weight gain) can exacerbate an already compromised larynx and lead to an acute exacerbation of symptoms.

86.6.2 Physical Examination

The examination of a patient with bilateral vocal fold paralysis begins with observation of the patient. Again, the degree of airway compromise dictates the degree and severity of the physical findings. A patient may be completely comfortable and appear calm or may present with extreme anxiety and a sense of impending doom. The vocal quality may be completely normal or characterized by breathiness, raspiness, and diplophonia. In addition, the patient may exhibit respiratory distress with labored breathing, stridor, the use of accessory muscles, supraclavicular retraction, and cyanosis. Flexible laryngoscopy is performed in the office setting, recovery room, or operating room if RLN damage is suspected. Laryngeal endoscopy on the operating room table after thyroidectomy or completion thyroidectomy in patients with preexisting unilateral vocal fold paralysis is helpful in identifying a bilateral paralysis and allowing rapid reintubation before the patient decompensates. The position of the vocal folds, size of the glottic airway, and presence of interarytenoid scarring or any other mechanically obstructive lesion are all noted. Videostroboscopy helps to ascertain vocal fold vibration and glottic closure on phonation.

86.6.3 Testing

Diagnostic laryngeal electromyography (EMG) can aid in developing a prognosis for recovery in cases of surgical trauma or neuropathy. Immediately after surgery, EMG can differentiate between vocal fold fixation (which is a very rare event) and traumatic RLN neuropathy. EMG performed 2 to 6 months after injury will help define the prognosis. If there are multiple polyphasic potentials and significant recruitment, the prognosis is favorable. Giant waves with no vocal fold motion, fibrillation potentials, poor recruitment, and synkinesis all portend a poor prognosis. In addition to aiding in the prognosis, EMG can help diagnose certain neurologic, metabolic, or myopathic causes of bilateral immobility. For more details, the reader is referred to Chapter 80 (Laryngeal Electromyography).

Imaging is necessary in cases of noniatrogenic bilateral vocal fold paralysis.. A chest X-ray is typically adequate to assess most tumors of the chest and mediastinum, although it is not as sensitive as computed tomography (CT) or magnetic resonance (MR) imaging in identifying masses in the cardiopulmonary window. MR imaging and/or CT from the vertex of the brain to the inferior aspect of the aortic arch should be performed to look for a lesion along the course of both RLNs, Arnold-Chiari malformation, brainstem lesions (tumors, metastatic disease, cerebrovascular anomaly), and other lesions of the brain.

The diagnostic laboratory work-up is usually limited but may include measurements of Lyme titer, fluorescent treponemal antibody absorbed (FTA-ABS), cytoplasmic antineutrophil cytoplasmic autoantibody (cANCA), purified protein derivative (PPD), rheumatoid factor (RF), antinuclear antibody (ANA), angiotensin-converting enzyme (ACE), erythrocyte sedimentation rate (ESR), and C-reactive protein (CRP) during investigations for a systemic cause of bilateral immobility in patients with a suggestive medical history.

Pulmonary function testing may be ordered to assess the degree of upper airway obstruction. The results can be highly variable, and pulmonary function testing should not be used as the primary diagnostic tool. Typically, blunting of the inspiratory curve is seen during forced inspiration, as well as flattening of the expiratory curve. Most studies show no correlation between pulmonary function testing results and glottic airway size; however, pulmonary function testing can be useful for the evaluation of airflow after intervention to demonstrate increased airflow.

An endoscopic evaluation should be performed in the operating room in cases of suspected interarytenoid scar formation or ankylosis of the cricoarytenoid joint. The latter does not occur often, but both should be suspected in patients with long-term intubation or a history of trauma to the neck or larynx. Palpation of the joint, independent motion of the arytenoids, and range of motion of the arytenoids are assessed. In addition, the subglottis and trachea should be inspected for signs of trauma, narrowing, or granulation.

86.6.4 Differential Diagnosis

There are multiple causes of bilateral vocal fold paralysis, and the frequencies of each differ between adults (see Box Causes of Bilateral Vocal Fold Paralysis in Adults (p.670)) and children (see Box Causes of Bilateral Vocal Fold Paralysis in Children (p.671)).

86.7 Treatment

86.7.1 Medical Treatment

Airway safety is the primary concern in patients with bilateral vocal fold paralysis. Postoperative patients may develop stridor and respiratory distress immediately upon extubation or, more commonly, during the few hours after extubation. Measures such as therapy with intravenous steroids, heliox, racemic epinephrine, and humidified oxygen may achieve a short-term resolution of respiratory distress. If respiratory distress continues or oxygen desaturation develops, emergent reintubation is performed. In rare cases, an emergent tracheotomy must be performed if the airway cannot be secured by intubation. A second attempt at extubation is made after the administration of intravenous steroids, typically 24 hours later. If a second attempt fails, tracheotomy is then performed to secure a safe airway. A tracheotomy provides the most stable and safe airway, as well as the best possible vocal result.

Patients with borderline toleration of their bilateral vocal fold paralysis may be candidates for botulinum toxin injection of both thyroarytenoid muscles. This results in immediate vocal fold bowing and long-term atrophy after serial injections, so that the glottic airway enlarges slightly. Although the change in the airway is minimal, it may be sufficient to provide a safe airway and obviate the need for a tracheotomy in these borderline patients. The injections generally need to be repeated every 6 to 12 months.

Patients who do not present with airway distress, significant dysphonia, or dysphagia can be monitored without intervention. Many patients will recover function of at least one vocal fold. Others with persistent bilateral paralysis remain stable and never require further intervention. These patients should be cautioned about acute respiratory compromise in the setting of laryngeal edema. They should be instructed to contact their physician or go the nearest emergency room immediately upon having any symptoms of airway distress. In these cases, conservative management with humidification, oral steroids, and mucolytics is often sufficient.

86.7.2 Surgical Treatment

As noted above, a tracheotomy provides the most stable and safest airway, as well as the best possible vocal result. Unfortunately, tracheotomy remains a very difficult social and physical burden for the patient. In addition, a long-term tracheotomy is associated with the potential complications of granulation formation, tracheal stenosis, dysphagia, aspiration, cellulitis, and skin breakdown.

For those patients who fail extubation, or have chronic symptoms of shortness of breath, stridor, exercise intolerance, or recurrent acute airway episodes necessitating hospitalization, procedures exist to create a more patent airway. The same procedures are available to patients who already have a tracheotomy but desire decannulation. Before performing a destructive procedure, the surgeon should be certain that recovery will not occur. To that end, the procedure should be delayed until either 1 year after the inciting injury or EMG evidence of a poor prognosis has been obtained.

The most conservative surgery involves a carbon dioxide laser posterior transverse cordotomy, which is performed endoscopically. An incision is made that separates the vocal process from the membranous vocal fold. This generally done unilaterally but may be done bilaterally if a unilateral procedure fails to create an adequate airway (▶ Fig. 86.3).

Alternatively, an endoscopic medial arytenoidectomy can be performed with a carbon dioxide laser (▶ Fig. 86.4). The medial wall of the arytenoid is removed, with or without a partial cordotomy. Traditionally, a complete arytenoidectomy was performed endoscopically by ablating the entire arytenoid or transcervically via laryngofissure. Because of the increased morbidity of these procedures, they have mostly been abandoned.

Laterofixation of one vocal fold can be performed via transcervical placement of a suture that wraps around the vocal process and posterior membranous vocal fold. Traction on the suture lateralizes the vocal fold. It is then tied in place over the strap muscles. In order to avoid a tracheotomy, laterofixation can be used as a temporary procedure in cases of surgical trauma to the RLN in a patient with a known intact RLN whose prognosis for recovery is good. The suture can be removed once

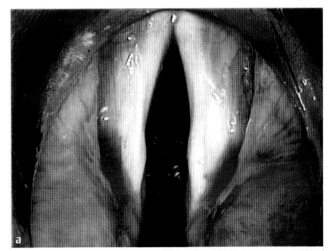

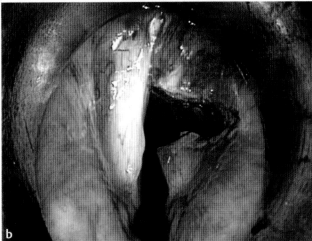

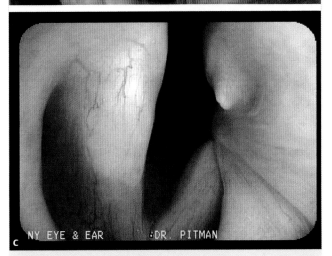

Fig. 86.3 Bilateral vocal fold paralysis (**a**) before posterior transverse cordotomy, (**b**) immediately after cordotomy, and (**c**) after healing is complete.

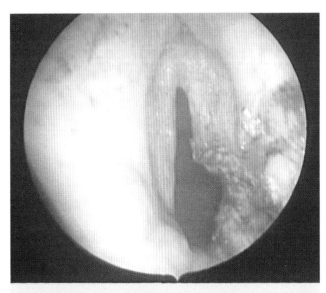

Fig. 86.4 Intraoperative view of medial arytenoidectomy.

A newly described technique is the abductor suture technique. This technique is truly reversible. It is a modification of the arytenoid adduction suture technique, which is often used in unilateral vocal fold paralysis. In the abductor technique, a permanent suture is placed through the muscular process of the arytenoid and then directed posteroinferiorly and tied to the inferior cornu of the thyroid cartilage. This procedure abducts the vocal process, thus enlarging the airway. It also allows adduction to occur if it is present. In the small series performed, all six patients had an improved airway; five were decannulated. Four patients had no vocal change, and two had increased breathiness.

These procedures can all be performed without a tracheotomy. The patients need to be selected carefully, with the full understanding of possible airway compromise from edema caused by the procedures. The procedures are also performed in patients with a tracheotomy so that they can be decannulated after intervention.

Overall, the success of these surgical procedures ranges from 80 to 100% when decannulation is used as the means of comparison. However, the literature lacks standardization of the success rates, and the results are varied with regard to complication rates. When performing these procedures, one must balance the benefit of an enlarged airway against the potential complications, which include aspiration resulting from an enlarged unprotected glottis, weak and breathy dysphonia, the urgent need for postoperative tracheotomy, surgical failure with the need for revision, or inability to decannulate the patient. The voice is always weaker after these procedures, excluding the arytenoid abduction procedure. The larger the airway, the better the breathing but the weaker the voice. This tradeoff must be well communicated to the patient. The patient must understand and accept it. The surgeon must negotiate this tentative balance when performing the surgery. The management of each case is based on the patient's clinical needs and physical findings, and the treatment is selected is based on the expertise and experience of the surgeon.

function has been restored. This suture technique can also be used as a permanent treatment. Although the technique is generally seen as nondestructive, the suture can saw through the membranous vocal fold with an irreversible outcome similar to that of a posterior transverse cordotomy.

Because destructive procedures are irreversible, a conservative approach should be taken during surgery. A 20% revision rate is to be expected. A second or even a third procedure with further resection of the arytenoid or vocal fold or surgery of the opposite side is preferable to excessive resection resulting in dysphonia or aspiration.

Laryngeal pacing and laryngeal reinnervation are potential treatment options in the near future. They are both in the experimental phase and aim to rehabilitate a larynx dynamically and restore vocal fold motion. Currently, a handful of patients have undergone these procedures, with mixed results. The standard of care still remains a tracheotomy for acute airway compromise. Secondarily, and often preferred, is a destructive procedure of the glottis to establish a larger airway caliber in patients unlikely to experience spontaneous recovery of laryngeal function and in those wishing to undergo decannulation.

86.8 Prognosis

Depending on the etiology, many patients with bilateral immobility will recover at least one functioning vocal fold. Patients with iatrogenic injury to a nerve or malignant involvement of a nerve are far less likely to show recovery. For those patients with little or no airway compromise, the prognosis is good for a normal quality of life. With even minor recovery of vocal fold abduction, airway intervention is typically not required. Intermittent respiratory distress associated with laryngeal edema is typically treated medically and resolves. Overall, approximately 50% of patients with permanent bilateral vocal fold paralysis will need surgical intervention. Spontaneous recovery of function in at least one vocal fold will occur in 20 to 60%, depending on the etiology.

86.9 Roundsmanship

- Many patients with bilateral vocal fold paralysis present with a normal voice.

- Airway compromise is the chief concern.
- Early electromyography can help identify patients with a poor prognosis for return of function and thus allow earlier surgical intervention.
- Tracheotomy is necessary in approximately 50% of patients with bilateral vocal fold paralysis.
- Bilateral thyroarytenoid botulinum toxin injection can result in a stable airway and avoid the need for tracheotomy or other permanent surgical procedures in selected cases.
- Surgical intervention can result in a safe airway, decannulation, and the preservation of adequate voice and swallow function.
- In destructive surgery to restore the glottic airway, one must balance the size of the airway against the ensuing dysphonia. Initial conservative surgery is ideal.

86.10 Recommended Reading

[1] Benninger MS, Gillen JB, Altman JS. Changing etiology of vocal fold immobility. Laryngoscope 1998; 108: 1346–1350

[2] Bosley B, Rosen CA, Simpson CB, McMullin BT, Gartner-Schmidt JL. Medial arytenoidectomy versus transverse cordotomy as a treatment for bilateral vocal fold paralysis. Ann Otol Rhinol Laryngol 2005; 114: 922–926

[3] Chen EY, Inglis AF. Bilateral vocal cord paralysis in children. Otolaryngol Clin North Am 2008; 41: 889–901

[4] Damrose EJ. Suture laterofixation of the vocal fold for bilateral vocal fold immobility. Curr Opin Otolaryngol Head Neck Surg 2011; 19: 416–421

[5] Dennis DP, Kashima H. Carbon dioxide laser posterior cordectomy for treatment of bilateral vocal cord paralysis. Ann Otol Rhinol Laryngol 1989; 98: 930–934

[6] Hillel AD, Benninger M, Blitzer A et al. Evaluation and management of bilateral vocal cord immobility. Otolaryngol Head Neck Surg 1999; 121: 760–765

[7] Rosenthal LH, Benninger MS, Deeb RH. Vocal fold immobility: a longitudinal analysis of etiology over 20 years. Laryngoscope 2007; 117: 1864–1870

[8] Woodson G, Weiss T. Arytenoid abduction for dynamic rehabilitation of bilateral laryngeal paralysis. Ann Otol Rhinol Laryngol 2007; 116: 483–490

87 Laryngopharyngeal (Airway) Reflux

Jamie A. Koufman

87.1 Introduction

Reflux is an expensive, high-prevalence disease, and it remains somewhat controversial because neither standardized diagnostic tests nor standard treatments exist. In addition, divisions between the medical specialties (otolaryngology, pulmonology, gastroenterology), each focusing on its own anatomical subdivision, has led to academic turf wars and further fragmentation of the medical care of patients with diverse manifestations of reflux. Nevertheless, reflux (particularly laryngopharyngeal reflux) affects almost half of patients with laryngeal and voice disorders, globus, and dysphagia, so the management of reflux is very important in the field of otolaryngology.

87.2 Prevalence of Reflux in America

Today, physicians and their patients are more attentive to esophageal and, to a lesser extent, airway reflux, particularly when its symptoms are "silent." This term has captured the public's awareness because people with silent reflux do not have heartburn and indigestion, the symptoms most commonly associated with esophageal reflux. Indeed, it is more common to underdiagnose or misdiagnose airway reflux because patients with laryngopharyngeal reflux usually do not have typical digestive symptoms.

The increased awareness of reflux diseases among physicians is not just a matter of experience and education; it is also a consequence of the fact that the prevalence of esophageal and airway reflux has skyrocketed since the 1970s. A comprehensive review of 20 prevalence studies reported the following: (1) The prevalence of reflux in America has increased by 4% per year since 1976. (2) Today, 40% of the American population has reflux, 22% has gastroesophageal reflux, and another 18% has airway (laryngopharyngeal) reflux. (3) Reflux-caused esophageal cancer has increased more than 650% in the last two generations, and esophageal adenocarcinoma is the fastest-growing cancer in America. (4) Barrett esophagus (a precancerous esophageal condition) is equally common (8%) among patients with esophageal reflux and those with airway reflux. These trends have been attributed primarily to the obesity epidemic and the use of food additives; however, it now appears that there may be more to the story. The American diet may be responsible for the reflux epidemic.

87.3 Terminology: Classification of Reflux Disease

Patients call it simply "acid reflux," but medical specialists have many different names and designations for diseases and disorders related to the backward flow of gastric contents into the esophagus and airway. In fact, different specialists use different terms that reflect their viewpoints (▶ Table 87.1). For example, when describing reflux, gastroenterologists generally refer to *gastroesophageal reflux disease*, which describes their focus, the esophagus and esophagitis. However, when the airway is involved, gastroenterologists use terms like *atypical, silent,* or *extra-esophageal reflux*. Airway specialists, such as otolaryngologists, generally use the term *laryngopharyngeal reflux* because the larynx and pharynx are the primary target organs when reflux escapes above the esophagus. The term *silent reflux* can be erroneous because most patients with reflux, particularly airway reflux, do have symptoms. Symptoms by definition cannot be silent, and the disease is not "silent" simply because the symptoms do not include heartburn or abdominal discomfort. It is worth noting that some people with reflux actually have no symptoms. Two groups of patients who warrant esophageal screening, even if they are completely asymptomatic, are those who have had heartburn that has abated and those older than 40 years of age with a family history of esophageal cancer or Barrett esophagus. In these two groups, reflux can be truly silent (no symptoms) and still associated with significant clinical disease.

Why are there so many different terms? Besides otolaryngologists and gastroenterologists, many other specialists, including allergists, pulmonologists, pediatricians, internists, family practitioners, anesthesiologists, and critical care specialists, regularly encounter the diverse manifestations of reflux. Because this chapter on reflux has been written for otolaryngologists, it makes sense to divide the aerodigestive tract into two basic components: the airway and the esophagus. These overarching designations make great sense; this chapter is entitled "Laryngopharyngeal (Airway) Reflux," but justifiably the title could have been "Airway Reflux" because the term *airway reflux* is more encompassing and descriptive than *laryngopharyngeal reflux*. In this chapter, the terms *airway reflux* and *laryngopharyngeal reflux* are used interchangeably, as are *esophageal reflux* and *gastroesophageal reflux disease*. As expected, the most popular terms across the medical literature are *laryngopharyngeal reflux* and *gastroesophageal reflux disease*.

Table 87.1 Most Common Medical Terms for *Acid Reflux*

Gastric reflux	Gastroesophageal reflux disease	Laryngopharyngeal reflux
Extraesophageal reflux disease	Supraesophageal reflux disease	Esophagopharyngeal reflux
Gastropharyngeal reflux	Atypical reflux disease	Esophageal erosions
Barrett esophagus	Reflux esophagitis	Silent reflux
Esophageal reflux	Airway reflux	

87.4 Applied Anatomy

The esophagus, airway, and lungs make up the aerodigestive tract (▶ Table 87.2). It is important to recognize that these structures and their functions are closely interrelated. The normal swallow represents a series of highly coordinated neuromuscular activities. After food is chewed and a bolus is formed, the tongue pushes it back to the oropharynx; the swallow is then initiated. After this, the swallow is an unconscious, brainstem-directed sequence. The tongue acts as a piston, forcing the bolus into the pharynx. Next, pharyngeal contraction propels the bolus downward. Meanwhile, there is reflex inhibition of respiration, and the larynx closes tightly to prevent aspiration. The bolus then travels the length of the esophagus, propelled by peristalsis, until it reaches the lower esophageal sphincter, which, like the upper esophageal sphincter, should open, allowing the bolus to pass, and then close behind it. Once inside the stomach, the bolus should remain there, where the process of digestion proceeds because of the presence of acid-activated pepsin.

Gastric reflux occurs when one or more flaws in the anatomical structures and/or their functions are present. Gastroesophageal reflux disease (GERD) is usually associated with (1) low pressure in the lower esophageal sphincter (LES), (2) transient LES relaxations (with or without increased intragastric pressure), and/or (3) esophageal dysmotility. In laryngopharyngeal reflux (LPR), the mechanisms of reflux are related to transient LES relaxations and poor upper esophageal sphincter (UES) function. Indeed, in many patients with reflux-related globus (the sensation of a lump in the throat), the UES pressure may be too low, too high, and/or poorly coordinated with pharyngeal and upper esophageal function.

One last anatomical consideration: the thresholds for acid- or pepsin-related tissue injury are vastly different for the esophagus and for the larynx. Just looking at normative pH monitoring data, 50 episodes of esophageal reflux per day are considered normal; by contrast, as few as three episodes of reflux into the laryngopharynx per week can lead to severe disease. Additionally, laboratory experiments have shown that the threshold for peptic injury in the esophagus is a pH below 4, compared with a pH below 5 for the larynx.

87.5 The Disease Process

87.5.1 Etiology: Risk Factors

Until 1980, the prevalence of obesity in America was stable, at approximately 15%. Since then, its rise has been astonishing. Today, more than 30% of Americans are obese, with a body mass index (BMI) above 30. Not surprisingly, the obesity trend in the United States parallels the rise of prepackaged and fast food, and especially the increased use of saturated fats and high-fructose corn syrup. Interestingly, patients with airway reflux (LPR) tend not to be obese. Furthermore, the prevalence of reflux in the 20- to 29-year-old age group is almost as high (37%) as it is in older people.

For more than two decades, otolaryngologists have recognized that the excessive consumption of carbonated beverages, especially caffeinated colas, is associated with LPR. In 2010, the American Beverage Association reported that the average 12- to 29-year-old consumes 160 gallons of soft drinks annually, or almost a half-gallon of soft drinks a day. The main problem is the acidity. Most beverages in bottles and cans have a pH of less than 4 and are just as acidic as stomach acid itself. However, soft drink consumption is only part of the picture.

Only in the past few years has the root cause of the American "acidity epidemic" become known and linked with the reflux epidemic. In 1973, following an outbreak of food poisoning (botulism), Congress enacted Code of Federal Regulations Title 21, Part 110, "Current Good Manufacturing Practice in Manufacturing, Packing, or Holding Human Food," mandating that the FDA ensure the safety of processed food crossing state lines. This was accomplished through the acidification of bottled and canned foods, which was intended to prevent bacterial growth and prolong shelf life. Today, almost everything in a bottle or a can has a pH of less than 4, and it appears that the acidity in food is a major risk factor for reflux disease. We also believe that the restriction of dietary acidity can have dramatic therapeutic benefits and should be a routine part of any antireflux therapy program. Identified causes and risk factors for reflux are summarized in ▶ Table 87.3.

87.5.2 Pathophysiology

Esophageal reflux may occur during the night or day, but typically GERD results from nighttime reflux, whereas LPR occurs during the daytime.

Table 87.2 Components of the Aerodigestive Tract

Nose, nasopharynx, and sinuses	Oral cavity, oropharynx, and pharynx
Hypopharynx and larynx	Trachea and lungs
Esophagus	Upper esophageal sphincter
Esophageal body	Lower esophageal sphincter
Stomach and small intestines	

Table 87.3 Most Commonly Reported Causes and Risk Factors for Reflux

Ethanol	Chocolate	Tobacco, smoking
Overeating, obesity	Tight clothing, belts	Carbonated beverages
Lying down after eating	Esophageal dysmotility	High-fat and fried foods
Xerostomia (e.g., after irradiation)[a]	Late-night eating (within 3 hours before bedtime)	Low pressure in lower esophageal sphincter

[a]The risk for reflux is extremely high in patients with irradiation-induced xerostomia, and reflux-related esophageal cancer is the most common subsequent cancer in patients who have been treated with irradiation.

The most common mechanism of reflux is transient LES relaxation. Unfortunately, the actual causes of this are so obtuse and numerous that the phenomenon remains rather mysterious. Clearly, increased intragastric and intra-abdominal pressure resulting from overeating, carbonation, certain medications, and too-tight clothing is a factor.

The typical patient with esophageal reflux has heartburn and indigestion, is obese, and experiences supine nocturnal reflux, esophageal dysmotility and LES dysfunction. Conversely, the typical patient with airway reflux/LPR has no gastrointestinal symptoms, is not overweight, has normal esophageal motility, but has UES dysfunction.

The UES is supposed to act as a second barrier (in addition to the LES), and under normal circumstances it prevents esophageal refluxate from entering the throat. The overlap of patients who have both LPR and GERD is approximately 25%. Despite this, it is felt that the pathophysiologic mechanisms in these two populations of patients with reflux are different, for reasons that are unknown.

The acid (pH) thresholds for cell damage of the larynx and esophagus are different. In general, esophageal damage occurs at a pH below 4 and laryngeal damage at a pH below 5. (Because the pH scale is logarithmic, a pH of 4 is 10 times more acidic than a pH of 5.) This variable pH threshold for laryngeal and esophageal tissue damage has important implications for both the diagnosis and treatment of LPR and GERD. Contrary to traditional belief, recent data indicate that it is not acid but pepsin that produces tissue injury. The confusion comes from the fact that the activation of pepsin, the primary and powerful proteolytic enzyme of the stomach, requires acid. As such, previous focus had been on acid, which actually is just the facilitator of pepsin activity. Without pepsin, acid itself is not nearly as damaging.

87.5.3 Cell Biology of Reflux and Carcinogenesis

The relationship between GERD and its progression from esophagitis through gastric metaplasia (Barrett esophagus) to dysplasia and finally adenocarcinoma has been well established. More controversial is the relationship between LPR and laryngeal cancer. It has been shown in humans with LPR, laboratory animals, and cell cultures that activated pepsin becomes tissue-bound, enters cells by endocytosis, and then adversely alters protective cell proteins, including E-cadherin (the mortar between squamous epithelial cells), carbonic anhydrase (responsible for maintaining adequate intracellular acid–base balance), and stress proteins (responsible for cell survival following stress).

Notably, laryngeal epithelial damage (e.g., the protein changes outlined above) occur with activated pepsin at pH 5. Recent studies have demonstrated that pepsin in laryngeal epithelial cell cultures upregulates all of the genetic markers associated with squamous cell carcinoma of the larynx. Clearly, the relationship between laryngeal cancer and reflux remains to be proved. However, considering these findings, the author strongly recommends pH testing and treating patients with laryngeal cancer as if they had severe LPR

87.6 Medical Evaluation

87.6.1 Symptoms and Manifestations of Airway Reflux

Of the many reported symptoms and manifestations of airway reflux, the most common are hoarseness, sore throat, chronic throat clearing, excessive throat mucus, chronic cough, choking episodes, shortness of breath, a sensation of a "lump in the throat" (globus), difficulty swallowing (dysphagia), and asthma (▶ Table 87.4).

87.6.2 Diagnosis

The symptoms and manifestations of airway reflux go beyond those typically associated with esophageal reflux, and there are red flags that make airway reflux highly likely. Awakening in the middle of the night from a sound sleep coughing and even gasping for air "like a fish out of water" (i.e., laryngospasm), chronic cough for more than 2 months (with a normal pulmonary evaluation), a chronic sensation of a lump in the throat other than during an actual meal (globus), morning hoarseness, chronic intermittent hoarseness, and difficulty swallowing (dysphagia), among others, can all be symptoms of LPR (▶ Table 87.5).

At present, there are many different ways to diagnose LPR. Unfortunately, there is still no single "gold standard" diagnostic test. The available methods are the following: (1) symptoms (reflux symptom index) and findings (reflux finding score); (2) conventional (sedated) and transnasal esophagoscopy; (3) reflux testing (pH monitoring and impedance); (4) biopsy (pepsin detection, histology, and other markers); and (4) a "diagnostic" therapeutic trial of antireflux treatment. Importantly, esophagoscopy cannot diagnose reflux; it only reveals the presence or absence of complications of reflux, such as Barrett esophagus and esophageal erosions, allowing the conclusion that pathologic reflux is present. However, the absence of complications does not allow one to conclude that pathologic reflux is not present; rather, it can only be concluded that if pathologic reflux is present, it has not resulted in visible complications.

Table 87.4 Symptoms of Airway Reflux

Regurgitation	Dysphagia (difficulty swallowing)
Chest pain	
	Dyspnea (shortness of breath, difficulty breathing)
Choking episodes	
Vocal fatigue	Globus (sensation of a "lump in the throat")
Voice breaks	Food becoming stuck
Chronic throat clearing	Airway obstruction
Excessive throat mucus	Wheezing
Postnasal drip	Chronic cough

Presently, there is no one diagnostic reflux test that provides more accurate information than the combination of pharyngeal, UES, and esophageal manometry with ambulatory 24-hour dual pH probe (simultaneous pharyngeal and esophageal) monitoring. Impedance monitoring is, in the author's experience, a much inferior choice for diagnosing airway reflux, although it is a good supplement to pH testing because it may identify injurious nonacid reflux. Under development are new diagnostic tests that are specific for airway reflux and use pepsin as a marker.

87.6.3 Differential Diagnosis

Many conditions can be misdiagnosed as reflux; likewise, reflux in many cases can be mistaken for something else (▶ Table 87.6).

Reflux should be considered in the differential diagnosis of almost all inflammatory and neoplastic conditions of the airway, but other etiologies must be considered, as well.

87.7 Treatment

Airway reflux (LPR) can be associated with minor symptoms (e.g., throat clearing) or with life-threatening disease (e.g.,

Table 87.5 Common Presentations of Airway Reflux

Dental caries and erosions	Posterior glottis stenosis
Esophageal spasm	Arytenoid fixation
Esophageal stricture	Paroxysmal laryngospasm
Esophageal cancer	Globus pharyngeus
	Laryngeal cancer
Endotracheal intubation injury	
Contact ulcers and granulomas	Paradoxical vocal fold movement
Vocal nodules and polyps	Recurrent leukoplakia
Pachydermia laryngitis	Polypoid degeneration
Laryngomalacia	Laryngospasm
Vocal cord dysfunction	Sudden infant death syndrome
Sinusitis and allergic symptoms	Sleep apnea
Asthma	

laryngeal stenosis, cancer, airway obstruction). It stands to reason that there cannot be any "one-size-fits-all" therapeutic regimen. Meanwhile, lifestyle, dietary, medical, and surgical treatment options are available.

87.7.1 Lifestyle and Dietary Treatment

Obesity and reflux go together, especially when the patient overeats; consumes a lot of fried and fatty foods, chocolate, and carbonated beverages; and eats late at night. Those are among the high-risk behaviors for reflux disease. Interestingly, smoking also causes reflux. The recommendations for lifestyle and dietary modifications are summarized in ▶ Table 87.7.

87.7.2 Medical Treatment

There are several different approaches to medical treatment: antacids, acid suppressants, mucosal protection, and promotility agents. These may be used alone or in combination, depending on the patient's reflux pattern and disease severity.

Antacids, once the cornerstone of antireflux treatment, are now reserved for patients with mild and intermittent symptoms or are used as adjunctive therapy to alleviate primarily heartburn in patients with recalcitrant disease. Today, proton pump inhibitors (PPIs) are the most commonly used antireflux drugs, followed by histamine$_2$ antagonists. Many different PPIs are available on the market today, and they account for $15 billion in annual sales in the United States alone.

PPIs provide the best acid suppression of any antireflux medication. However, their use has become more controversial in recent years because of concerns about rebound hyperacidity following drug cessation and side effects, as well as short- and long-term complications. When PPIs are used for airway reflux, they should be taken in twice-daily doses (before breakfast and before the evening meal). Patients with nocturnal reflux are also usually given a histamine$_2$ antagonist at bedtime because histamine$_2$ antagonists work better than PPIs during sleep.

Prokinetic agents (including baclofen, metoclopramide, erythromycin, and domperidone) can help improve gastric emptying, esophageal function (peristalsis), and sphincter function. They should be reserved for patients who demonstrate poor esophageal motility and/or sphincter function. Metoclopramide and domperidone should be used with caution because they can cause significant and permanent side effects. The numerous side effects of metoclopramide include irreversible tardive dyskinesia, and domperidone is not approved by the FDA for use in the United States.

Table 87.6 Differential Diagnosis of Airway/Laryngopharyngeal Reflux

Paradoxical vocal fold movement	Laryngospasm	"Vocal cord dysfunction"
"Irritable larynx"	Allergic rhinitis	Postnasal drip
Sinusitis	Vasomotor rhinitis	Asthma
Vocal cord granulomas	Muscle tension dysphonia	Vocal nodules and polyps
Infectious diseases: viral, bacterial, and fungal	Neoplasms	

Table 87.7 Recommended lifestyle and dietary modifications for reflux

General lifestyle recommendations	Top ten foods and beverages to avoid	Ten best foods for a patient with reflux
Stop smoking. Smoking causes reflux.	Onions (may not affect all patients)	Bananas (rich, low-acid fruit, although they are also a trigger food for 5% of people)
Avoid wearing clothing that is too tight, especially trousers, corsets, bras, and belts.	Peppers, hot sauce (including bell and black pepper)	Melons (best fruits for most patients with reflux: watermelon, cantaloupe, honeydew)
Avoid exercising right after eating (especially weight lifting, jogging, and yoga).	Citrus fruit and juice (naturally acidic, and more is added)	Aloe vera (great thickener and good for digestion)
Do not lie down right after eating, and do not eat anything within 3 hours before bedtime.	Deep-fried food (different from sautéed)	Rice and whole grains (brown rice, bulgur wheat, and whole-grain bread are best)
Elevate the head of the bed if there is nighttime reflux, with symptoms of hoarseness, sore throat, and/or cough in the morning.	Fatty meats (bacon, pork, lamb, some fatty steak cuts like rib eye)	Salads and vegetables (excluding onions, tomatoes, garlic, and peppers)
An overweight patient should start a low-acid, pH-balanced diet.	Alcoholic beverages	Oatmeal (one of the best breakfast foods)
	Chocolate (one of the most common foods that trigger reflux)	Ginger (spicy, zesty flavor and good for reflux)
	Almost all bottled and canned beverages (almost all are acidified)	Poultry (baked or grilled, not fried)
	Carbonated beverages (Coca-Cola, Pepsi-Cola, and all other "soft drinks")	Tofu (coagulated soy milk is a vegetarian staple protein)
	Anything eaten before bedtime is a "worst for reflux" food	Fish (all seafood—raw, grilled, baked, boiled, or broiled—is good for reflux)

Many patients with airway reflux need long-term medical treatment, but many also can discontinue their medications after the acute phase improves as long as they remain compliant with a reasonable maintenance antireflux diet.

87.7.3 Surgical Treatment

The primary surgical option for the treatment of reflux is a Nissen fundoplication, in which the dome of the stomach is wrapped around the esophagus and then sewn in place to produce a tight angle where the esophagus enters the stomach. The procedure is generally performed laparoscopically and is by far the single most effective treatment for both esophageal and airway reflux. There is controversy surrounding which patients with LPR are the best candidates for a fundoplication. Surgical treatment is often recommended for patients with lung disease related to reflux and for patients who cannot tolerate or fail medical treatment. When chosen correctly, the procedure is extremely effective, although the benefit can decrease over time if the wrap loosens; this may occur in as many as 10 to 30% of patients. A Nissen fundoplication can be associated with dysphagia, a gas bloat syndrome, dumping syndrome, and vagus nerve injury.

87.8 Roundsmanship

- LPR (laryngopharyngeal reflux)/airway reflux and GERD (gastroesophageal reflux disease) are both on the rise and presently affect as many as 40% of the American population.

- The increase in acid reflux may be due to the acidification of canned and packaged foods.
- The action of pepsin, facilitated by an acidic environment, may be the primary cause of tissue damage in LPR.
- Fragmentation between specialties (otolaryngology, gastroenterology, and pulmonology) has resulted in controversy and confusion about how to diagnose and treat reflux disease optimally.
- Only pharyngeal pH monitoring can positively confirm the diagnosis of LPR.
- When combined with a healthy antireflux diet, medical treatment with antacids, acid-suppressive medications, and/or prokinetic agents is effective in managing the vast majority of patients with reflux disease. Surgery (Nissen fundoplication) should be reserved for those who have complications of reflux disease and those shown to be suboptimally managed with medical treatment.

87.9 Recommended Reading

[1] Amin MR, Postma GN, Setzen M, Koufman JA. Transnasal esophagoscopy: a position statement from the American Bronchoesophagological Association (ABEA). Otolaryngol Head Neck Surg 2008; 138: 411–414

[2] Belafsky PC, Postma GN, Koufman JA. Validity and reliability of the reflux symptom index (RSI). J Voice 2002; 16: 274–277

[3] Belafsky PC, Postma GN, Koufman JA. The validity and reliability of the reflux finding score (RFS). Laryngoscope 2001; 111: 1313–1317

[4] El-Serag HB. Time trends of gastroesophageal reflux disease: a systematic review. Clin Gastroenterol Hepatol 2007; 5: 17–26

[5] Halum SL, Postma GN, Johnston C, Belafsky PC, Koufman JA. Patients with isolated laryngopharyngeal reflux are not obese. Laryngoscope 2005; 115: 1042–1045

[6] Johnston N, Bulmer D, Gill GA et al. Cell biology of laryngeal epithelial defenses in health and disease: further studies. Ann Otol Rhinol Laryngol 2003; 112: 481–491

[7] Johnston N, Dettmar PW, Bishwokarma B, Lively MO, Koufman JA. Activity/stability of human pepsin: implications for reflux attributed laryngeal disease. Laryngoscope 2007; 117: 1036–1039

[8] Koufman JA, Belafsky PC, Bach KK, Daniel E, Postma GN. Prevalence of esophagitis in patients with pH-documented laryngopharyngeal reflux. Laryngoscope 2002; 112: 1606–1609

[9] Koufman JA, Stern JC, Bauer MM. Dropping Acid: The Reflux Diet Cookbook & Cure. Minneapolis, MN: Reflux Cookbooks LLC (Brio Books); 2010

[10] Koufman JA. The otolaryngologic manifestations of gastroesophageal reflux disease (GERD): a clinical investigation of 225 patients using ambulatory 24-hour pH monitoring and an experimental investigation of the role of acid and pepsin in the development of laryngeal injury. Laryngoscope 1991; 101 Suppl 53: 1–78

[11] Reavis KM, Morris CD, Gopal DV, Hunter JG, Jobe BA. Laryngopharyngeal reflux symptoms better predict the presence of esophageal adenocarcinoma than typical gastroesophageal reflux symptoms. Ann Surg 2004; 239: 849–856, discussion 856–858

[12] Westcott CJ, Hopkins MB, Bach KK, Postma GN, Belafsky PC, Koufman JA. Fundoplication for laryngopharyngeal reflux disease. J Am Coll Surg 2004; 199: 23–30

88 Neurologic Disorders of the Larynx

Jihad Achkar and Phillip C. Song

88.1 Introduction

Neurolaryngology is the study and management of laryngeal dysfunction secondary to problems of neural control and coordination. Common neurolaryngologic disorders include entities that are specific to the larynx (e.g., spasmodic dysphonia, vocal fold paralysis and paresis), as well as others associated with more global neurologic problems (e.g., stroke, amyotrophic lateral sclerosis, basal ganglia pathology). The laryngopharynx depends on complex coordination between the central and peripheral neural pathways for the proper functioning of its multiple tasks. Neurologic disorders affecting either of these two pathways, or both, may have a significant impact on breathing, airway protection, swallowing, and phonation. Sensory deficits, motor weakness, or both compromise the function of the laryngopharynx, and the resultant dysphagia, aspiration, and dysphonia are frequently presenting symptoms in patients with neurologic disease. These problems are best addressed in a multidisciplinary manner, with coordination among an otolaryngologist, a neurologist, and a speech–language pathologist.

In this chapter, we attempt to highlight specific characteristics in the head and neck examination and laryngeal testing that are germane to recognizing neurologic disorders of the larynx. We also describe the presentation and approach to the treatment of several neurologic disorders that have a major impact on the laryngopharynx. Spasmodic dysphonia is discussed in Chapter 89, and vocal fold paralysis is covered in Chapter 85 and Chapter 86 .

88.2 Classification of the Disease Process

In general, neurologic diseases that affect the larynx can be categorized according to three broad themes of dysfunction: *dyscoordination*, *hypofunction*, and/or *hyperfunction*. Dyscoordination is a problem in the timing and sequence of motor events. Swallowing problems are often due to dyscoordination because a very tight and precise series of motor events (sequential contraction and elevation of the pharynx and larynx coordinated with relaxation of the cricopharyngeus and opening of the upper esophageal sphincter) occurs after a sensory trigger (oropharyngeal and pharyngeal sensory innervation). Often, there is a mixture of sensory and motor issues, but the problem is generally not purely within the peripheral nervous system. The classic example of a hypofunctional laryngeal disorder is vocal fold paralysis/paresis, which can occur in a purely motor form (recurrent laryngeal nerve paralysis), in a mixed motor and sensory form (high vagal injury), or as a manifestation of central nervous system (CNS) dysfunction (stroke, multiple sclerosis, amyotrophic lateral sclerosis). Hyperfunctional laryngeal disorders are generally central in origin. The classic hyperfunctional disorder is spasmodic dysphonia, which results in spasm of the intrinsic laryngeal muscles during vocalization.

88.3 Anatomy

Understanding the innervation of the larynx is key to evaluating patients with throat symptoms related to neurologic disorders. The recurrent laryngeal nerve (RLN) and superior laryngeal nerve (SLN) are the two branches of the vagus (10th cranial) nerve responsible for proper functioning of the laryngopharynx. They provide motor and sensory innervation to laryngeal and hypopharyngeal structures that allow breathing, airway protection, swallowing, and phonation.

88.3.1 Recurrent Laryngeal Nerve

The RLN nuclei lie within the nucleus ambiguus of the medulla oblongata. Axons exit with the vagus nerve through the jugular foramen and descend within the carotid sheath to branch off the vagus low in the neck. The right RLN loops around the anterior aspect of the right subclavian artery, whereas the left RLN loops around the aortic arch in the same manner. Each ascends in the tracheo-esophageal groove and enters the larynx just posterior and medial to the cricothyroid joint to innervate the intrinsic laryngeal muscles. A well-described anomaly of the right RLN has been found to occur in approximately 5 in 1,000 persons, in which the right RLN branches off the vagus at the level of the cricoid cartilage and enters the larynx directly without looping around the subclavian artery (nonrecurrent). This occurs in conjunction with an anomalous right retroesophageal subclavian artery. The RLN supplies motor innervation to the intrinsic muscles of the larynx, including the thyroarytenoid, lateral cricoarytenoid, posterior cricoarytenoid, and interarytenoid muscles. The posterior cricoarytenoid is the only muscle with the function of abducting the vocal folds. Although topographic distribution of the adductor and abductor fibers is seen in the brainstem and the distal portions of the RLN, in the main trunk of the nerve, the adductor and abductor fibers are mixed. The intrinsic laryngeal muscles are unilaterally innervated with the possible exception of the interarytenoids, which have crossing muscle fibers and may share a bilateral nerve supply. Neurologic disorders with resultant RLN palsies have the potential to affect all the major functions of the laryngopharynx.

88.3.2 Superior Laryngeal Nerve

The superior laryngeal nerve (SLN) branches off from the main trunk of the vagus high in the neck. Its sensory cell bodies lie in the nodose ganglion just superior to its branching point. It descends in the neck lateral to the pharynx and medial to the carotid sheath, and it divides into internal and external branches approximately 2 to 3 cm superior to the superior pole of the thyroid gland at the level of the hyoid bone. The internal branch enters the larynx, along with the superior laryngeal artery, through the thyrohyoid membrane. It supplies sensory innervation to the supraglottis. The external branch descends inferomedially on the pharyngeal constrictors to supply motor innervation to the cricothyroid muscle. The cricothyroid muscle is the tensor of the vocal folds and regulates the frequency of phonation.

Palsies of the SLN cause supraglottic sensory dysfunction, leading to a significant increase in the risk for aspiration. They may also lead to pitch alteration that can be detrimental to the function of professional voice users.

88.4 The Disease Process

88.4.1 Etiology and Pathogenesis

Neurologic disorders affecting the larynx have different etiologies, and the symptoms depend on the region of the nervous system affected.

Parkinson Disease

Parkinson disease is a disease of the basal ganglia and one of the most common neurologic disorders to affect the laryngopharynx. Parkinson disease is the result of progressive degeneration of the basal ganglia, mainly dopaminergic neurons of the substantia nigra pars compacta. Recent research suggests a genetic etiology, and ongoing investigation is under way to identify specific genes and pathways.

Stroke

Stroke is caused by the sudden interruption of blood supply to a brain region. The resultant corresponding neurologic deficits may vary in degree and distribution.

Multiple Sclerosis

Multiple sclerosis is an immune-mediated inflammatory disease of the CNS that results in the demyelination of axons. The subsequent neurologic deficits correspond to the affected regions of the brain.

Amyotrophic Lateral Sclerosis

Amyotrophic lateral sclerosis is an idiopathic neurodegenerative disease of upper and lower motor neurons. It leads to muscle weakness, atrophy, and spasticity.

Tremor

Essential tremor is a common movement disorder. It usually occurs with voluntary movement (action tremor), and to a lesser extent with posture holding. The tremors generally have a characteristic frequency of 4 to 10 Hz and mostly affect the upper extremities, neck muscles, and throat. Essential voice tremor is believed to be the phonatory manifestation of essential tremor.

Myasthenia Gravis

Myasthenia gravis is an autoimmune disorder affecting the neuromuscular junction. Autoantibodies target acetylcholine receptors, leading to a decrease in the number of receptors at motor end plates, with resultant weakness and fatigue of voluntary muscles.

88.4.2 Natural History and Progression

The severity of the symptoms of Parkinson disease vary greatly among individuals. It is not possible to predict how quickly the disorder will progress. The disease itself is not fatal, although secondary complications, such as pneumonia, fall-related injuries, and choking, may be.

Stroke is the third most common cause of death in the United States, and almost 5% of the population past the age of 65 years is affected. Dysphagia occurs in 27 to 50% of patients with stroke. The presence of dysphagia after a stroke significantly increases morbidity and mortality rates.

The course of multiple sclerosis varies among patients, and the disease may be remitting–relapsing, primary progressive, or secondary progressive in presentation. Multiple sclerosis, like other immune-mediated diseases, is more common in women and is estimated to have a female-to-male ratio of 3:2. Multiple sclerosis has been found to affect an estimated 400,000 individuals in the United States, but the highly variable disease course and presentation pose difficulties in diagnosis, and thus the actual numbers may be higher.

Respiratory muscle affliction is the symptom most detrimental to patients with disease progression of amyotrophic lateral sclerosis; dependence on mechanical ventilation ensues, and eventual death follows, usually at about 3 years after the establishment of a diagnosis.

Essential tremor is not life-threatening, although it can make communication difficult. Most individuals with myasthenia gravis lead a normal or nearly normal life with treatment. Occasionally, a myasthenic gravis crisis can result in respiratory failure, which requires immediate emergency medical care.

88.5 Medical Evaluation

The history of the present illness in suspected cases of neurologic dysfunction of the larynx needs to encompass a wide range of systems that may be beyond the head and neck. The neurologic history, an assessment of risk factors for stroke (e.g., hypertension, atrial fibrillation, hypercholesterolemia, smoking, patent foramen ovale), and the family history are important aspects of the history that may be relevant. Establishing the clinical course in the history is important because many neurologic diagnoses are based on the patient's symptoms and presentation, and specific diagnostic tests are not available. For laryngologic disorders, the presentation, symptoms, and examination characteristics may be subtle, especially at the onset, and a high degree of specificity needs to be established in order to recognize pathology. Specific questions about vocal strain, breathiness, vocal fatigue, and tremors may reveal important pathology. For instance, vocal fatigue, a common symptom of functional voice disorders, may be a manifestation of myasthenia gravis when it rapidly follows mild to moderate voice use. Vocal tremor is common in the elderly and is occasionally subtle enough to go unnoticed by physicians if they do not suspect the diagnosis. The findings associated with these disorders may not be the ones that are the most distressing to the patient and may have to be elicited through close questioning.

Dysphagia along with hoarseness should raise suspicion of a deeper neurologic condition. As previously mentioned, patients with vagus nerve injury experience motor and sensory consequences. Motor deficits can manifest as hypotonicity of the pharyngeal constrictor muscles, dilatation of the piriform sinuses, and vocal fold immobility. This affects the pharyngeal phase of swallowing and causes food material to pool in the dilated piriform sinuses. The loss of sensation and inability to protect the airway from the pooled material puts the patient at a serious risk for aspiration.

Among the rare manifestations of neurologic diseases affecting the larynx are stridor and breathing difficulties. Bilateral vocal fold paralysis, laryngospasm, and adductor laryngeal breathing dystonia may present primarily with stridor and difficulty breathing.

An accurate and thorough history helps direct the remainder of the evaluation toward the probable cause of the patient's complaints. After the history, a thorough head and neck examination and laryngoscopy are the next steps.

88.5.1 Clinical Features

The hallmark symptoms of Parkinson disease include bradykinesia, resting "pill-rolling" tremor, loss of postural reflexes, and rigidity. Voice and speech dysfunction can be subtle presenting symptoms in the early stages. Vocal symptoms include a monotonous, soft, and breathy voice that is typically perceived by patients to be of normal volume. There is often a flat affect to the voice, as well as to the facial features. Parkinson disease results in a loss of the "emotional" conveyance of the voice. Other symptoms may include difficulty initiating speech, vocal tremor, and sluggish articulation. Swallowing is not particularly a problem in patients with early parkinsonism. However, altered voluntary swallow may lead to drooling in some patients later in the course of the disease.

Manifestations can vary widely and depend on the region of the CNS affected. Patients often present with a mixture of motor and sensory deficits, with or without cognitive impairments. Generally, patients who have had a cerebrovascular accident may be globally debilitated, with cognitive deficits in addition to specific problems encountered within the larynx. When the insult involves the sensory and/or motor nuclei of the vagus nerve, laryngopharyngeal dysfunction ensues. As previously mentioned, the RLN and SLN branch out from the vagus to innervate the laryngopharynx and allow normal functioning. Therefore, multiple tasks, including swallowing, voicing, and breathing, are affected. If a patient with stroke presents with a weak, breathy voice, vocal fold paresis is generally suspected. Dysphagia can result from sensory and/or motor deficits leading to poor coordination during swallowing. The insensate supraglottis (SLN, internal branch) also predisposes patients to life-threatening aspiration. Typical symptoms of multiple sclerosis include limb weakness, eye symptoms (visual acuity and field defects), vertigo, and dermatomal sensory dysfunction. Dysphonia from glottal insufficiency can occur as a consequence of vocal fold immobility. Dysphagia and dysarthria are common presenting symptoms, as well.

In amyotrophic lateral sclerosis, lower motor neuron degeneration causes muscle weakness and atrophy, whereas degeneration of upper motor neurons presents with spasticity and abnormal reflexes. Patients can present with laryngopharyngeal dysfunction affecting any of the tasks of swallowing, phonation, articulation, and breathing. Oropharyngeal symptoms are present in as many as 25% of patients with amyotrophic lateral sclerosis. Involvement of the tongue, palate, and pharyngeal wall musculature can cause velopharyngeal insufficiency, dysarthria, and dysphagia. Pharyngeal muscular dyscoordination leads to frequent episodes of aspiration pneumonia that often have fatal consequences. The mixed dysarthria pattern of amyotrophic lateral sclerosis includes effortful, slow, short phrases with inappropriate pauses, imprecise consonants, and a strained or strangled voice, as well as decreased frequencies and volume.

It was formerly believed that essential voice tremor does not present as an isolated entity without other signs of tremor. In fact, Sulica et al have recently shown that half of vocal tremors occur with very subtle upper extremity symptoms that are no more severe than those seen in normal persons of similar age. In addition, patients with spasmodic dysphonia frequently present with a superimposed tremor component, causing an erroneous labeling of essential tremor as spasmodic dysphonia. Sulica et al also reported that one-third of the patients they reviewed had been given a diagnosis of spasmodic dysphonia. Vocal symptoms include voice instability that is very rhythmic in nature, increased phonatory effort, and decreased intelligibility. Voicing worsens with stress and during public speaking or telephone use. Alcohol will often relieve patients' tremors, adding further to the risks for misdiagnosis. The diagnosis is based on the clinical features and laryngoscopic findings. Endoscopy usually reveals involvement of the entire laryngopharynx with rhythmic tremors, albeit variably among individuals.

In myasthenia gravis, the most common presentation includes ptosis and diplopia. Otolaryngologic manifestations include dysphonia, dysphagia, and weakness of the muscles of mastication. Around 27% of patients report speech and swallowing difficulties as early symptoms. Voice symptoms include vocal fatigue, difficulty sustaining pitch, hypernasality, intermittent aphonia, and rarely stridor. A review of 40 cases of myasthenia gravis manifesting primarily in the larynx has recently been published. It details the presenting symptoms, examination findings, and treatment options. Dysphonia may result in subtle changes of voice (difficulty with high frequencies or inability to project or sustain volume or pitch).

88.5.2 Physical Examination

The neurolaryngologic assessment should focus primarily on function. Most throat conditions that are related to neurologic impairment have subtle, functional findings that unless actively elicited are easily missed.

The face and neck muscles should be evaluated for spasticity or asymmetry. Function of the vagus and glossopharyngeal nerves can be inferred by testing the gag reflex and observing for palatal deviation. Articulation difficulties almost always indicate a neurologic disorder.

Critical listening to the quality of the vocal signal is an invaluable skill in the evaluation of vocal complaints. An air leak during coughing signifies glottic incompetence. Severe vocal fold bowing and thinning in Parkinson disease may very well present with breathiness and hypophonia. Glottic incompetence may also reflect vocal fold weakness. A rhythmically tremulous voice quality during sustained /i/ phonation is highly suggestive of vocal tremor. A singer's inability to reach the high notes he previously hit easily during a *glissando* may represent SLN palsy, and this should be included in the differential diagnosis.

88.5.3 Testing

Laryngoscopy

Laryngoscopy is the critical component in the physical examination of patients with voice and swallowing difficulties. Flexible nasolaryngoscopy provides a general overview of the larynx in a physiologic position and allows the larynx to be examined during a variety of tasks. The examination should include tasks that are cortical (speaking and singing), volitional (simple /i/ or /a/), nonvolitional (spasms), vegetative (coughing, throat clearing, swallowing, and breathing), and emotional (laughing). Repetitive phonatory tasks may induce vocal fatigue and elicit evidence of subtle paresis and weakness. Video recording and archiving the examination allows a serial review of motion and function.

Weak adduction, vocal fold bowing, and a persistent chink in the mid-musculomembranous region are the most common findings in patients with Parkinson disease. During videolaryngoscopy in patients with stroke, the larynx is observed for gross asymmetries in configuration or movement. Unilateral vocal fold paralysis (RLN) generally manifests as an immobile vocal fold lying in the paramedian position. Hypotonicity of the lateral pharyngeal wall muscles and the resultant dilatation of the ipsilateral piriform sinus are commonly noted. The hallmark finding in myasthenia gravis on videostroboscopy is fluctuating impairment of vocal fold motion, bilateral or unilateral, and glottic incompetence in the absence of other structural abnormalities. Laryngeal electromyography (EMG) should be performed to confirm myasthenia gravis. Tensilon testing involves the administration of edrophonium (Tensilon), an anticholinesterase, to patients with suspected cases. The test result is considered positive if EMG demonstrates improved strength.

Laryngeal Electromyography

Laryngeal EMG evaluates electrical activity in the intrinsic laryngeal muscles and is a tool to differentiate neurologic vocal fold immobility from immobility with mechanical causes. Laryngeal muscle dyscoordination from synkinesis following nerve injury can cause vocal fold immobility and airway compromise and is accurately inferred by laryngeal EMG. Laryngeal EMG also offers the potential to predict the return of nerve function after a neurologic insult, and a patient may be directed toward early intervention when signs of a poor prognosis are elicited on laryngeal EMG.

Flexible Endoscopic Evaluation of Swallowing

Dysphagia may be evaluated via flexible endoscopic evaluation of swallowing (FEES). While the examiner keeps the flexible scope hovering at the level of the nasopharynx and looks down, different food consistencies are presented to the patient to observe bolus clearance. Pooling of secretions in the hypopharynx, penetration (entry of food into the larynx), or aspiration (passage beyond the vocal folds) may be observed. The treatment plan is determined accordingly.

Modified Barium Swallow

Different food consistencies are presented to the patient to test food bolus clearance. Swallowing maneuvers such as chin tuck–head turn and improvements in pre-swallow sensory input have shown benefit in decreasing the risk for aspiration and improving swallowing.

88.5.4 Differential Diagnosis

The full differential diagnosis of neurologic disorders that affect the larynx is extensive. ▶ Table 88.1 summarizes the differential diagnosis of neurologic disorders causing dysphagia, and ▶ Table 88.2 lists those causing vocal fold paresis and paralysis with dysphonia.

88.6 Treatment

The treatment of the laryngeal manifestations of a *stroke* is tailored according to the nature of the neurologic impairment. From least invasive to most invasive, interventions may include the following: dietary modifications, swallowing maneuvers, gastrostomy tube placement, vocal fold augmentation/medialization, and pharyngoplasty (open neck surgery to address a dilated piriform sinus). Pharyngoplasty results in a shallower pouch that collects less material and decreases the risk for aspiration. The treatment of glottic insufficiency in patients with stroke should aim for airway protection and voice improvement. Treatment options range from awake in-office injection medialization to open type I thyroplasty procedures. Medialization laryngoplasty increases airway protection by improving the valve effect and producing a stronger cough. Physical and occupational therapy should be a routine component of the recovery plan after a cerebrovascular accident.

Standard L-dopa treatment has not shown significant benefit for laryngeal symptoms related to *Parkinson disease.* Injection augmentation of the vocal folds has demonstrated temporary vocal improvement but requires repeated procedures and has limited benefit in severe cases. Bringing two nonpliable vocal folds together in the setting of poor lung effort and weak power supply can sometimes result in poorer voice quality. Behavioral therapy shows consistent beneficial results. Lee Silverman Voice Treatment (LSVT), an intensive voice therapy program that emphasizes the production of a loud voice with maximum effort, has shown excellent results in patients with bradykinetic speech. It allows patients to overcome the false perception that their usual-volume voicing is normal and leads to volume gain that is very beneficial. Swallowing function appears to improve after the treatment, as well. It has been shown that oral phase swallowing abnormalities are reduced by 51% after LSVT.

Steroids have been shown to be beneficial in the acute setting and are the mainstay for the treatment of *multiple sclerosis.* Plasmapheresis in severe attacks that are unresponsive to steroids has shown good results. Rehabilitation of speech and swallow dysfunction, as well as targeted treatment for specific deficits at the glottic level, is usually recommended for patients with multiple sclerosis.

The treatment of *amyotrophic lateral sclerosis* is generally supportive, with the goals of maximizing the strength and reserve of the tongue and pharyngeal muscles and reducing the

Table 88.1 Differential diagnosis of neurologic disorders causing dysphagia

Central nervous system disorders causing dysphagia	Peripheral nervous system disorders causing dysphagia
Delirium	Vocal fold paresis/paralysis
Dementia	Myasthenia gravis
Traumatic brain injury	Amyotrophic lateral sclerosis
Stroke/cerebrovascular accident	Progressive supranuclear palsy
Wallenberg syndrome	Post-polio syndrome
Cerebral palsy	Guillain-Barré syndrome
Neurodegenerative diseases	Neuropathy: diabetic, HIV infection
Parkinson disease	Myopathy
Huntington disease	Oculopharyngeal muscular dystrophy
Multiple system atrophy	Muscular dystrophy
Arnold-Chiari malformation	Dermatomyositis
Wilson disease	Polymyositis
Multiple sclerosis	Cricopharyngeal achalasia
	Botulism
	Lyme disease

Source: Adapted with permission from Blitzer A, Brin M, Ramig LO. Neurologic Disorders of the Larynx. 2nd ed. New York, NY: Thieme Medical Publishers; 2009.

Table 88.2 Differential diagnosis of neurologic disorders causing vocal fold paresis and paralysis with dysphonia

Central nervous system disorders causing vocal fold paralysis and paresis	Peripheral nervous system disorders causing vocal fold paralysis and paresis	
Stroke/cerebrovascular accident	Trauma	May be surgical, compressive, stretch, penetrating, or blunt
Brain or brainstem neoplasm	Idiopathic	
Arnold-Chiari malformation	Neoplasm	Neck, chest, or skull base tumors
Brainstem compression	Infection	Lyme, botulism, syphilis
Neurosarcoidosis	Neuropathy	HIV infection, diabetes, viral infection, medications, hypothyroidism, Guillain-Barré syndrome
Neurodegenerative disease	Myopathy	Myositis, myasthenia gravis

Source: Adapted with permission from Blitzer A, Brin M, Ramig LO. Neurologic Disorders of the Larynx. 2nd ed. New York, NY: Thieme Medical Publishers; 2009.

risk for aspiration. Symptom-based approaches are adapted to target affected organ systems. Velopharyngeal insufficiency and hypofunction of the tongue can be treated with the placement of a palatal prosthesis. Close collaboration with a speech–language pathologist is vital for voice rehabilitation, articulation, and swallowing.

The first-line treatment of *essential tremor* is pharmacologic. Propranolol and primidone have become the mainstays of treatment. Propranolol affects peripheral β-adrenergic receptors in skeletal muscle, resulting in symptomatic relief in up to 50% of patients. Primidone has approximately equal efficacy via a centrally acting mechanism of action. Unfortunately, neither of them has shown a consistent benefit in improving vocal tremor. Methazolamide, a carbonic anhydrase inhibitor, was recently shown to be promising in patients with vocal tremors; however, the results have not been supported by a subsequent blinded investigation. Botulinum toxin treatment has been tried for the treatment of vocal tremors with variable results. Botulinum toxin can be useful for reducing the amplitude and velocity of tremors.

The treatment of *myasthenia gravis* is usually pharmacologic, typically with anticholinesterase medication. When necessary, immunosuppressive agents, such as corticosteroids, azathioprine, cyclosporine, and intravenous immune globulin, may be included. Plasmapheresis and thymectomy may also be employed as immunomodulating therapies.

88.7 Conclusion

Neurologic disorders of the larynx comprise a diverse group of problems that affect swallowing, voice, and respiration. The key to a correct diagnosis is to look comprehensively beyond the anatomy of the larynx and to evaluate function, physiology, and motion with various laryngeal tasks. The neurologic manifestations may be subtle and intermittent, and thus awareness of the different possibilities enables the correct diagnosis. Testing for neurolaryngologic disorders should include perceptual auditory analysis, laryngeal examination, neurologic testing, FEES and/or modified barium swallow, and EMG. Multidisciplinary approaches are best suited for the diagnosis and treatment of these complex entities.

88.8 Roundsmanship

- The laryngopharynx depends on complex coordination between the central and peripheral neurologic pathways for proper functioning, and neurologic disorders affecting either, or both, may have a significant impact on breathing, airway protection, swallowing, and phonation, with resultant dysphagia, aspiration, and dysphonia.
- The key to a correct diagnosis is to look comprehensively beyond the anatomy of the larynx and to evaluate function, physiology, and motion with various laryngeal tasks.
- An accurate and thorough history helps to direct the remainder of the evaluation toward the probable cause of the patient's complaints.
- Critical listening to the quality of the vocal signal is an invaluable skill in the evaluation of vocal complaints, along with perceptual auditory analysis, laryngeal examination, neurologic testing, FEES and/or modified barium swallow, and EMG.

- These entities are best addressed in a multidisciplinary manner, with coordination among an otolaryngologist, a neurologist, and a speech–language pathologist.

88.9 Recommended Reading

[1] Alonso A, Hernán MA. Temporal trends in the incidence of multiple sclerosis: a systematic review. Neurology 2008; 71: 129–135

[2] Berke GS, Gerratt B, Kreiman J, Jackson K. Treatment of Parkinson hypophonia with percutaneous collagen augmentation. Laryngoscope 1999; 109: 1295–1299

[3] Duffy J. Motor Speech Disorders: Substrates. Differential Diagnosis, and Management. St. Louis, MO: Mosby; 1995

[4] Hollinshead WH. Anatomy for Surgeons: The Head and Neck. 3rd ed. Philadlephia, PA: Harper & Row; 1982

[5] Koller W, Graner D, Mlcoch A. Essential voice tremor: treatment with propranolol. Neurology 1985; 35: 106–108

[6] Logemann JA. Treatment of oral and pharyngeal dysphagia. Phys Med Rehabil Clin N Am 2008; 19: 803–816

[7] Louis ED, Ford B, Barnes LF. Clinical subtypes of essential tremor. Arch Neurol 2000; 57: 1194–1198

[8] Mao VH, Abaza M, Spiegel JR et al. Laryngeal myasthenia gravis: report of 40 cases. J Voice 2001; 15: 122–130

[9] Merati AL, Heman-Ackah YD, Abaza M, Altman KW, Sulica L, Belamowicz S. Common movement disorders affecting the larynx: a report from the neurolaryngology committee of the AAO-HNS. Otolaryngol Head Neck Surg 2005; 133: 654–665

[10] Muenter MD, Daube JR, Caviness JN, Miller PM. Treatment of essential tremor with methazolamide. Mayo Clin Proc 1991; 66: 991–997

[11] Osserman KE, Genkins G. Studies in myasthenia gravis: review of a twenty-year experience in over 1200 patients. Mt Sinai J Med 1971; 38: 497–537

[12] El Sharkawi A, Ramig LO, Logemann JA et al. Swallowing and voice effects of Lee Silverman Voice Treatment (LSVT): a pilot study. J Neurol Neurosurg Psychiatry 2002; 72: 31–36

[13] Sulica L, Louis ED. Clinical characteristics of essential voice tremor: a study of 34 cases. Laryngoscope 2010; 120: 516–528

89 Spasmodic Dysphonia

Michael J. Pitman

89.1 Introduction

Spasmodic dysphonia (SD) is a neurologic disorder of unknown origin that causes vocal fold spasms during speech. The spasms result in either excessive glottal closure or prolonged lateralization of the vocal folds, causing vocal breaks. The disease was first described by Traube in 1871 but was not accurately characterized as SD until 1968 by Aronson. Originally thought to be due to abnormalities of the basal ganglia, recent evidence suggests that the etiology is not so simple or localized.

89.2 Incidence of Disease

Although the exact prevalence of SD is unknown, there are thought to be 50,000 to 100,000 patients with this disorder in the United States. Of these, 62% are female. The typical age at onset is 39 to 45 years, but the condition has been known to begin anywhere between the second and ninth decades of life. Adductor SD occurs in 82% of patients, whereas 17% have abductor SD. Patients with adductor breathing dystonia or singer's dystonia comprise the remaining 1%.

89.3 Classification of the Disease Process

89.3.1 Adductor Spasmodic Dysphonia

In adductor SD, voice breaks are due to spasmodic hyperadduction of the vocal folds that interrupt phonation. As a result of the spasms, which generally occur with voiced vowels, vocal fold closure interrupts phonation, causing a strained or strangled vocal quality with intermittent vocal breaks.

89.3.2 Abductor Spasmodic Dysphonia

In abductor SD, voice breaks are due to spasmodic hyperabduction of the vocal folds that interrupt phonation. Patients have prolonged breathy voiceless breaks because of difficulties with voice onset following voiceless consonants such as /h/, /s/, /f/, /p/, /t/, and /k/. In addition, pitch changes and uncontrolled rises in vowel fundamental frequency may make them sound as if they are on the verge of crying.

89.3.3 Tremor

SD, like other neuromotor disorders, is frequently associated with tremor. In SD, the tremor is often localized to the larynx and pharynx. If tremor is present, then the SD is classified as the predominant type "with tremor" (e.g., adductor SD with tremor). This is clinically significant because the tremor aspect of the disorder does not respond as well as the spasms to treatment with botulinum toxin.

89.3.4 Adductor Breathing Dystonia and Singer's Dystonia

Because of the infrequency of these disorders, they will not be covered in depth here beyond being defined. Adductor breathing dystonia presents as persistent inspiratory stridor with normal voice and cough. Examination reveals paradoxical movement of the vocal folds on inspiration. Singer's dystonia has the symptoms of adductor SD, but the symptoms occur only during singing.

89.4 Applied Anatomy

All laryngeal muscles are involved in SD. In fact, in these patients, the findings of SD can be seen on an electromyographic (EMG) evaluation of the palatal muscles. It is the balance of the SD effect on the laryngeal muscles that determines whether a patient will have predominantly abductor SD, adductor SD, or occasionally mixed symptoms. In adductor SD, the thyroarytenoid and lateral cricoarytenoid muscles predominate. In abductor SD, the posterior cricoarytenoid muscles predominate. Occasionally, the interarytenoid or cricothyroid can play an influential role. Determination of which muscles are causing a patient's symptoms helps guide treatment with botulinum toxin injections.

89.5 The Disease Process

89.5.1 Etiology

SD is a focal dystonia that affects laryngeal muscle control during speech. The term *dystonia* refers to a syndrome of sustained muscle contraction. Focal dystonias involve abnormal activity in only a few localized muscles. The etiology of SD is currently unknown. Idiopathic dystonias, such as SD, are thought to be due to abnormalities of neurotransmitters in the basal ganglia (putamen, head of caudate, and upper brainstem). Despite this, it is clear the etiology of SD is more complex. It may be the phenotype of multiple abnormalities. Although a genetic basis of SD has not been established, 12% of patients will have a relative with some type of dystonia.

89.5.2 Pathogenesis

A study by Simonyan et al suggests that the pathophysiology of SD may be related to specific brain abnormalities in the corticobulbar and corticospinal tracts. Both diffusion tensor imaging and neuropathologic data show specific white matter changes along these tracts and in the brain regions contributing to them. Specifically, the genu of the internal capsule was found to have a decreased quality and density of axonal tracts. These changes suggest a deficiency in the connection between the cortical and subcortical regions, which is essential for voluntary voice production.

Ali et al used $H_2^{15}O$ positron emission tomography (PET) to examine speech-related changes in regional cerebral blood flow before and after botulinum toxin injection. Their data demonstrated differences between patterns of cerebral activity in patients with adductor SD and patterns in neurologically normal controls. Decreased activity was observed in sensory areas known to play a crucial role in coordinating oral–laryngeal movements. Three to four weeks after botulinum toxin therapy, the hypoactivity in the sensory areas normalized, with motor and premotor regions exhibiting an increase in cerebral blood flow. These changes may result in the more efficient processing of sensory signals and a return of normal inhibition. The findings of this study suggest that the pathophysiology of SD is related to abnormalities in sensory cortical areas as well as motor areas, and they may explain the efficacy of botulinum toxin beyond a simple weakening of the muscles injected.

89.5.3 Natural History and Progression

Patients with SD can associate the onset of their symptoms with either an upper respiratory infection (33%), parturition or pregnancy (10%), or a major life stressor such as divorce or a death (42%), whereas the remainder cannot identify an inciting event. The symptoms are generally progressive over the first few months to years and then stabilize. They do not spontaneously resolve. Approximately 15% of patients will develop dystonia elsewhere, most commonly cervical torticollis or writer's cramp.

89.5.4 Potential Disease Complications

Complications of the disease are mostly psychosocial and economic, caused by the impact of the dysphonia on patients' psyche and ability to communicate.

89.6 Medical Evaluation

89.6.1 Presenting Complaints

Patients present with dysphonia similar to that described in the section on classification of the disease process. Their symptoms are usually worse when they speak on the phone, publicly, or during periods of stress. There may be improvement with sedatives such as alcohol and benzodiazepines. Most can whisper normally, and some can sing or yell without difficulty. As stated, SD will often begin after an upper respiratory infection or in association with a major life stressor. Because of this and the presence of normal-sounding speech between vocal breaks or during certain phonatory tasks, the symptoms are often regarded as "psychological." Often, a patient will have visited many physicians and mental health professionals over years looking for a diagnosis and cure.

89.6.2 Clinical Findings, Physical Examination

Often, the diagnosis of SD is clear once the patient begins to speak. Nonetheless, it is vital that a complete history be taken and a physical examination performed, including a review of

systems. The physician should inquire about the events surrounding the onset of the disorder, its duration, and its severity. One should ask about the presence of other neurologic disorders or symptoms, as well as other areas of the body that may be affected by dystonia. A patient may have discomfort due to other focal dystonias that he or she is unaware of until directly questioned. The presence of other neurologic symptoms not associated with dystonia or tremor suggests that the SD may be secondary to another disease process.

A full head and neck and neurologic examination should be performed, with the examiner looking for signs of other neurologic diseases that may cause SD or be misconstrued as SD.

The most pertinent aspect of the physical examination is a subjective evaluation of the voice. This is performed by listening closely for phonatory breaks during the entire evaluation. In addition, the patient can be asked to count from 70 to 90 or to repeat sentences created to stimulate the phonatory breaks characteristic of SD (see Box Sentences Constructed to Stimulate the Phonatory Breaks of Spasmodic Dysphonia (p.688)). The patient is often asked to repeat the sentences in a whisper to see if the breaks subside, as would be expected in SD. Although this is less reliable, patients may also be asked to sing a familiar song to see if it can be done without phonatory breaks.

Sentences Constructed to Stimulate the Phonatory Breaks of Spasmodic Dysphonia

- Sentences that elicit adductor breaks when spoken include the following:
  - "I eat apples and eggs."
  - "The dog dug a new bone."
  - "We mow our lawn all year."
  - "Early one morning, a man and a woman were ambling along a 1-mile lane, running near Rainy Island Avenue."
- Sentences that elicit abductor breaks when spoken include the following:
  - "How high is Harry's hat?"
  - "Did he go to the right or to the left?"
  - "When he comes home, we'll feed him."
  - "He saw half a shape mystically cross a simple path, at least 50 or 60 steps in front of his sister Kathy's house."

89.6.3 Testing

Laryngoscopy or laryngovideostroboscopy with a transnasal endoscope is the primary test performed. The examination should be normal except for vocal fold spasms coordinated with vocal breaks. Having the patient read the sentences listed in the Box (see Box Sentences Constructed to Stimulate the Phonatory Breaks of Spasmodic Dysphonia (p.688)) with the endoscope in place often stimulates breaks. Laryngopharyngeal tremor may also be evidenced on examination if it is part of the disorder.

EMG is not typically used for the diagnosis of SD, although a typical burst of activity may be seen before a spasm.

When the diagnosis of SD is unclear, a trial injection of botulinum toxin may be used. The injection will mitigate SD but will not relieve or may even worsen muscle tension dysphonia (MTD), helping the clinician to distinguish between the two. In similar fashion, a trial of voice therapy will mitigate the symptoms of a patient with MTD but provide minimal relief to a patient with SD.

A neurologic consultation, brain magnetic resonance imaging, or computed tomography is reserved for patients with neurologic symptoms inconsistent with SD.

89.6.4 Differential Diagnosis

The main differential of SD is MTD. MTD is a disorder in which muscle tension and inefficient phonation result in dysphonia. The symptoms of MTD should persist during whispering, and the dysphonia should be consistent. This is in contrast to SD, in which normal fluent speech often occurs between phonatory breaks and the breaks are not present during whispering. The presentations of MTD and SD are not always typical, so it may be difficult to distinguish between the two disorders, especially when a consistent vocal strain is present. As previously discussed, a trial of botulinum toxin or voice therapy may help distinguish between SD and MTD.

89.7 Treatment

89.7.1 Medical Treatment: Botulinum Toxin

The oral medications used for dystonia, such as anticholinergics, benzodiazepines, and baclofen, provide minimal relief and have poor side effect profiles at the doses needed to affect the voice. Botulinum toxin injections are the current treatment of choice. Unfortunately, their effect is temporary, and injections must be repeated approximately every 3 months. Botulinum toxin is contraindicated in a small subset of patients (see Box Contraindications to Botulinum Toxin Injections (p. 689)).

Contraindications to Botulinum Toxin Injections

- Pregnancy: The use of botulinum toxin by women who are pregnant or lactating is not recommended.
- Aminoglycosides: The recent use of aminoglycosides interferes with neuromuscular transmission and may increase the effect of botulinum toxin therapy.
- Preexisting neurologic disorders (e.g., myasthenia gravis, Eaton-Lambert syndrome, motor neuron disease affecting the neuromuscular junction): Caution should be used when botulinum toxin is administered to patients with these disorders, especially if large doses are required. Although the amount of toxin that enters the systemic circulation after injection is minute, hyperkinetic symptoms can theoretically occur.

Botulinum toxin is produced by *Clostridium botulinum*. It causes a chemical denervation by splicing fusion proteins (SNAP [soluble NSF attachment protein]-25, syntaxin, synaptobrevin) and blocking the release of acetylcholine at the synaptic junction (▶ Fig. 89.1). Botulinum toxin A and botulinum toxin B are used in humans, A much more often. The clinical effect of botulinum toxin in SD is classically thought to result from the inhibition of acetylcholine release at the neuromuscular junction, weakening the laryngeal muscle and its spasms. Recent evidence shows that the toxin is found to directly affect not only extrafusal muscle fibers but also afferent muscle spindle output. It may also alter cerebral function, although this likely a secondary effect. These alternative pathways of botulinum toxin function are more likely to be responsible for its therapeutic effects than is weakening of the involved muscles.

To be effective, the botulinum toxin must be injected directly into the muscle, the thyroarytenoid for adductor SD and the posterior cricoarytenoid for abductor SD. A dosing protocol must be established for each patient individually because each person has a unique sensitivity. As such, each patient is started with a standard low dose. This is then increased or decreased based on the patient's side effects, symptom response, and individual needs. The onset of the botulinum toxin effect is usually within 48 to 72 hours, and the effect lasts 3 months until another injection is desired. Once an optimal dose is established for a patient, it will usually remain constant for years.

Dosage

The dosing protocols of individual practitioners may vary slightly; the one presented herein is the author's. Botulinum toxin is reconstituted with 4 mL of preservative-free 0.9% sodium chloride to create a concentration of 2.5 units/0.1 mL. The units needed for injection are drawn into a 1-mL syringe. If necessary, additional saline is drawn up so that the injection volume is 0.1 mL to allow optimal dispersion of the medication through the muscle. Traditionally, the botulinum toxin is injected within 24 hours of reconstitution, but recent studies show that if the toxin is frozen, the potency is stable for 4 to 8 weeks.

For the treatment of adductor SD, percutaneous injection of botulinum toxin into each thyroarytenoid muscle is performed at a starting dose of 0.75 units per muscle.

For the initial treatment of a patient with abductor SD, 5 units are injected unilaterally into the posterior cricoarytenoid muscle. The patient returns 2 weeks later for a contralateral injection if the results are not optimal. Before injection, flexible laryngoscopy is performed to confirm that the injected vocal fold is weakened and that adequate abduction is present so that airway compromise will not occur after a contralateral injection. If this is the case, then 1.25 units is injected into the contralateral posterior cricoarytenoid muscle. Once the optimal dosing is established, both sides can be safely injected at the same visit.

Patients are given a diary so that they can rate their voice and toxin side effects before the injection, then every day for 2 weeks after the injection, and then weekly until the next injection. This diary aids in the assessment of botulinum toxin dosing effectiveness and helps determine the optimal timing and dose for the next injection.

Technique

A Teflon-coated 27-gauge needle attached to an EMG unit is used to inject the botulinum toxin. EMG helps to localize the tip of the needle within an active area of the muscle for an optimal injection of toxin. When the needle is thought to be within the muscle, the patient is asked to perform a task to fire the muscle

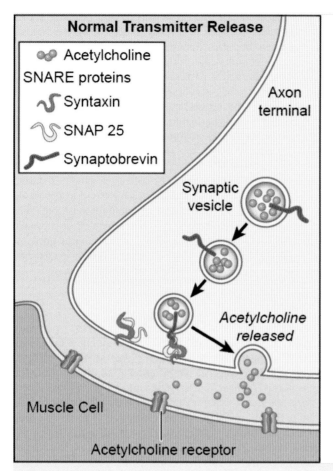

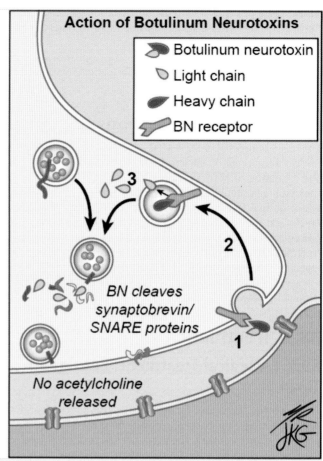

Fig. 89.1 Biochemistry of botulinum toxin A. *BN*, botulinum neurotoxin; *SNAP*, soluble NSF attachment protein; *SNARE*, SNAP receptor.

in question: sniff for the posterior cricoarytenoid; /i/ for the thyroarytenoid, lateral cricoarytenoid, or interarytenoid; glissando or high-pitched /i/ for the cricothyroid. If the needle tip is within the correct muscle, the EMG should be activated accordingly. Once crisp action potentials are obtained, the toxin should be slowly injected.

Thyroarytenoid injection: The needle is passed through the skin over the superior edge of the cricoid, just lateral to midline. The needle is advanced through the cricothyroid membrane and then as superiorly and laterally as possible into the right or left thyroarytenoid muscle. An attempt should be made to perform this maneuver completely submucosally so that airway stimulation and coughing are avoided (▶ Fig. 89.2).

Posterior cricoarytenoid injection: Either of two approaches can be used, transcricoid or lateral. The lateral approach is more often used. For the lateral approach, the larynx is grasped and rotated away from the site of the injection. The needle is passed through the skin just anterior to the sternocleidomastoid muscle at the height of superior aspect of the anterior cricoid ring. It is advanced to the posterior border of thyroid ala. The needle is then stepped posterior to the ala and advanced toward the posterior aspect of the cricoid. To confirm position, the needle tip can be balloted on the cricoid by applying pressure on the anterior aspect of the cricoid. The needle tip is then pulled slightly retrograde, and the position is confirmed with EMG (▶ Fig. 89.3). For the transcricoid approach, 2% lidocaine is

injected into the trachea for anesthesia via a cricothyroid membrane puncture. The needle with the toxin is then passed over the top of the cricoid just lateral to midline, through the airway, toward and through the lateral aspect of the posterior plate of the cricoid (▶ Fig. 89.4). This is done under laryngoscopic guidance. After the needle has passed through the cricoid, the position of the needle tip is confirmed on EMG (see ▶ Fig. 89.4).

Interarytenoid injection: After the trachea has been anesthetized as above, the needle is passed through the midline of the cricothyroid membrane and then upward at 45 to 60 degrees into the muscle, which sits above the posterior plate of the cricoid. The needle is passed under laryngoscopic guidance, and the intramuscular position is confirmed with EMG (▶ Fig. 89.5).

Cricothyroid injection: The needle is passed 1 cm lateral to midline over the superior boarder of the cricoid. It is passed straight posteriorly so that it is directed toward the medial border of the thyroid ala. Once the muscle is entered, a glissando or high-pitched /i/ is performed to confirm position (▶ Fig. 89.6).

Complications

In all cases, if a patient is underdosed, the mitigation of symptoms will be suboptimal. After injection for adductor SD, a patient who is overdosed may have a raspy or a weak and breathy voice, and may occasionally aspirate liquids. If this problem is

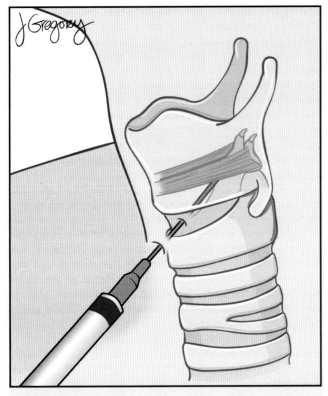

Fig. 89.2 Technique for botulinum toxin injection into the thyroarytenoid muscle.

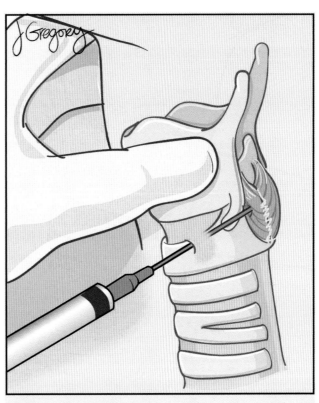

Fig. 89.3 Lateral approach for botulinum toxin injection into the posterior cricoarytenoid muscle.

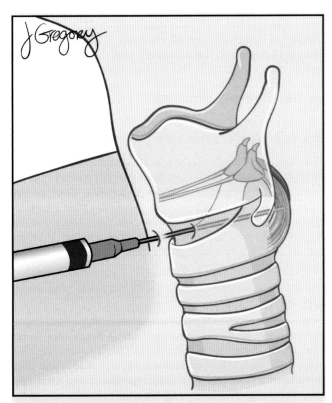

Fig. 89.4 Transcricoid approach for botulinum toxin injection into the posterior cricoarytenoid muscle.

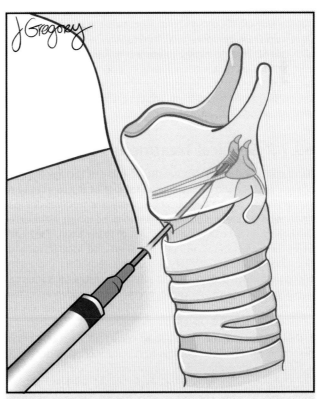

Fig. 89.5 Botulinum toxin injection into the interarytenoid muscle.

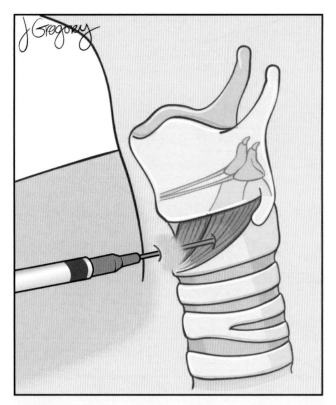

Fig. 89.6 Cricothyroid muscle injection.

severe, the patient can be instructed to perform a supraglottic swallow until the symptoms resolve. It may take days to weeks, but the side effects always resolve because the effects of botulinum toxin are temporary. Complications after injection for abductor SD include airway compromise. A patient may experience stridor or dyspnea on exertion, and airway obstruction can occur. Careful dosing at the beginning of treatment with staged injections to evaluate botulinum toxin sensitivity will help avoid such a disastrous consequence.

89.7.2 Surgical Treatment

Botulinum toxin injections are the first line of therapy because of their efficacy and minimal risk. Because of the morbidity of surgery and risk for complications, they are reserved for patients who fail botulinum toxin injections, no longer want to receive them, or have developed resistance to the toxin. The benefit of these operations, in both the short and long term, is in question. As a result, surgery for SD is a secondary procedure and is performed consistently at only a few institutions internationally. Before these procedures become more widely accepted, long-term follow-up data and reproduction of the results by other surgeons will be needed.

Dedo proposed and popularized recurrent laryngeal nerve resection for SD. This was the first and only procedure that achieved widespread use. Unfortunately, over the long term, the majority of patients experienced a return of their phonatory spasms. For this reason, the procedure was abandoned.

Isshiki proposed the type II laryngoplasty for adductor SD. This procedure relaxes and lateralizes the vocal folds. The anatomical alteration prevents the vocal fold spasm from forcefully obstructing airflow and causing a vocal break. If the surgery is overdone, a patient's speaking voice can be excessively raspy and breathy. In Isshiki's series of 41 patients, excellent results were reported in 70% after 6 months. Conflicting results have been presented by surgeons who could not replicate Isshiki's success.

Recurrent laryngeal nerve denervation and reinnervation was first described in 1999. In this procedure, the adductor branch of the recurrent laryngeal nerve is transected bilaterally. The distal branch is then reinnervated with the ansa cervicalis, and a lateral cricoarytenoid myectomy is performed. The ansa cervicalis reinnervation results in tone of the thyroarytenoid and lateral cricoarytenoid muscles and prevents reinnervation by the laryngeal nerves affected by SD. A retrospective study by Chhetri et al showed long-term (mean of 49 months) improvement in both patient subjective voice evaluation and expert perceptual voice evaluation. Of the patients, 26% had continued voice breaks, 30% had significant postoperative breathiness, 6% resumed botulinum toxin injections, and another 6% were undecided whether or not they should return to injections. Despite these results, 83% of patients said they would recommend the surgery. A Canadian group was able to reproduce these results in six patients who were treated without complications. One patient required continued botulinum toxin therapy.

A final surgical option for adductor SD is a bilateral thyroarytenoid and lateral cricoarytenoid myectomy. This procedure weakens the vocal folds bilaterally to prevent spasms. It is staged and performed under local anesthesia, and the breathiness is titrated to decrease the risk for overresection. Short-term results in five patients revealed improved fluency in all. Long-term studies are needed, especially in light of the failed history of myectomy for other dystonias, such as blepharospasm. After myectomy for blepharospasm, not only did symptoms usually recur, but the muscle often became dysfunctional secondary to fibrosis and scarring.

89.7.3 Voice Therapy

Voice therapy is of minimal benefit for the symptoms of SD. It is helpful in resolving the poor compensatory behaviors that patients have developed in attempts to decrease their spasms. Often, these behaviors spontaneously resolve after injections are begun, but that is not always the case. Voice therapy is also helpful when the clinician is unsure about whether a patient has SD or MTD. As noted, MTD should respond well to voice therapy, whereas SD does not.

89.8 Prognosis

Although the prognosis of surgery for SD is unclear, the results of botulinum toxin injections are well known. Patients report 90% and 71% of normal voice function after injection for adductor and abductor SD, respectively. Unfortunately, the effects are temporary, and the injections are somewhat painful. They also need to be repeated approximately every 3 months. It is evident the optimal treatment for SD has yet to be discovered.

89.9 Roundsmanship

- SD was originally thought to be due to abnormalities of the basal ganglia, but recent evidence suggests that the etiology is not so simple or localized.
- Alternative pathways of botulinum toxin function are more likely to be responsible for its therapeutic effects than is weakening of the involved muscles.
- Of patients with SD, 62% are female. The typical age at onset is 39 to 45 ears, and 82% of patients have adductor SD, whereas 17% have abductor SD.
- The most pertinent aspect of the physical examination is a subjective evaluation of the voice.
- Botulinum toxin dosing must be individualized for each patient to optimize the benefit and minimized the morbidity of treatment. It will often take multiple injection cycles to identify the optimal dose.
- Occasionally, traditional injections of the thyroarytenoid muscle and posterior cricoarytenoid muscle are not effective, and the injection of alternative muscles must be contemplated.
- Surgical alternatives have shown promise as secondary treatments but must be viewed skeptically without long-term follow-up or reproducibility by multiple surgeons.

89.10 Recommended Reading

[1] Ali SO, Thomassen M, Schulz GM et al. Alterations in CNS activity induced by botulinum toxin treatment in spasmodic dysphonia: an H215O PET study. J Speech Lang Hear Res 2006; 49: 1127–1146

[2] Blitzer A, Brin MF, Stewart C, Aviv JE, Fahn S. Abductor laryngeal dystonia: a series treated with botulinum toxin. Laryngoscope 1992; 102: 163–167

[3] Blitzer A, Brin MF, Stewart CF. Botulinum toxin management of spasmodic dysphonia (laryngeal dystonia): a 12-year experience in more than 900 patients. Laryngoscope 1998; 108: 1435–1441

[4] Chhetri DK, Mendelsohn AH, Blumin JH, Berke GS. Long-term follow-up results of selective laryngeal adductor denervation-reinnervation surgery for adductor spasmodic dysphonia. Laryngoscope 2006; 116: 635–642

[5] Childs L, Rickert S, Murry T, Blitzer A, Sulica L. Patient perceptions of factors leading to spasmodic dysphonia: a combined clinical experience of 350 patients. Laryngoscope 2011; 121: 2195–2198

[6] Hallett M. How does botulinum toxin work? Ann Neurol 2000; 48: 7–8

[7] Koufman JA, Rees CJ, Halum SL, Blalock D. Treatment of adductor-type spasmodic dysphonia by surgical myectomy: a preliminary report. Ann Otol Rhinol Laryngol 2006; 115: 97–102

[8] Sanuki T, Isshiki N. Overall evaluation of effectiveness of type II thyroplasty for adductor spasmodic dysphonia. Laryngoscope 2007; 117: 2255–2259

[9] Simonyan K, Tovar-Moll F, Ostuni J et al. Focal white matter changes in spasmodic dysphonia: a combined diffusion tensor imaging and neuropathological study. Brain 2008; 131: 447–459

[10] Stong BC, DelGaudio JM, Hapner ER, Johns MM. Safety of simultaneous bilateral botulinum toxin injections for abductor spasmodic dysphonia. Arch Otolaryngol Head Neck Surg 2005; 131: 793–795

90 Benign Lesions of the Larynx

Ted Mau

90.1 Introduction

Benign laryngeal lesions encompass a broad range of abnormalities with disparate pathophysiologic characteristics. They include lesions caused by vocal trauma, congenital or acquired structural aberrations, benign epithelial proliferations caused by human papillomavirus (HPV), and others. Although these lesions are often grouped together in the classification of head and neck diseases because of their common location and benign nature, each must be understood as a distinct entity with regard to pathogenesis, prognosis, and treatment.

90.2 Incidence of Disease

With the exception of papillomas, the incidence of benign laryngeal lesions is not precisely known. It would be reasonable to infer that lesions of the vocal folds occur in a subset of people with a self-reported voice disorder, and it has been estimated that 6% of the general public have a voice disorder at any given time. Of patients who seek treatment for their voice problems, 15 to 30% have been found to have benign vocal fold lesions in large series. The incidence of lesions caused by vocal trauma is likely highest in individuals whose occupations require heavy voice use: foremost in teachers, followed by counselors, attorneys, clergy, singers, call center workers, and others. Among nodules, polyps, and cysts, the incidence of nodules is the highest.

The incidence of laryngeal papilloma is likely close to the incidence of all forms of recurrent respiratory papillomatosis, estimated at 1.8 per 100,000 in U.S. adults.

90.3 Applied Anatomy

Most benign laryngeal lesions develop on the vocal folds. The fine structure of the vocal fold mucosa is crucial to an understanding of benign vocal fold lesions and their surgical management. The human vocal fold has a layered structure not found in other vocalizing mammals, and it is this unique composition that makes it possible for this seemingly simple pair of tissue folds to produce the acoustic range heard in speaking and sing-

ing. The vocal fold mucosa is made up of the epithelium and the lamina propria (▶ Fig. 90.1).

Histologically, the lamina propria consists of three layers: a superficial layer containing loosely organized elastin fibers in an extracellular matrix, an intermediate layer rich in longitudinally oriented elastin fibers, and a deep layer made up of predominantly collagen fibers. The superficial layer of the lamina propria (SLP), also called the Reinke space, is the most relevant for vocal fold surgeons. This layer imparts to the vocal fold mucosa its unique properties of self-sustained oscillation. Once lost through disease or trauma, it does not regenerate. Recognition of the importance of the SLP in phonatory function has led to the abandonment of the vocal cord stripping procedure in the treatment of benign vocal fold lesions. Deep to the three layers of the lamina propria lies the thyroarytenoid muscle, which tenses and relaxes to adjust the tension within the lamina propria and so modulate the frequency of vibration.

90.4 The Disease Process

90.4.1 Vocal Fold Nodules, Polyps, and Cysts

Terminology, Etiology, and Pathogenesis

There is no universally agreed-upon terminology for lesions caused by vocal trauma, commonly referred to as nodules, polyps, and cysts. There is some overlap in terminology, and even in the histologic appearance of these entities. What follow are commonly, though perhaps not universally, accepted definitions.

Nodules are bilateral, symmetric, or nearly symmetric lesions at the mid-membranous vocal folds (▶ Fig. 90.2). Nodules tend to be white to opaque and firm. After reaching a certain size, they can produce the classically described "hourglass" glottic closure pattern during phonation. Nodules are produced by vocal trauma but can also result from severe chronic cough. The repeated stress of mechanical impact between the two vocal folds is maximized at the point of largest vibratory amplitude during phonation, which is at the midpoint of the membra-

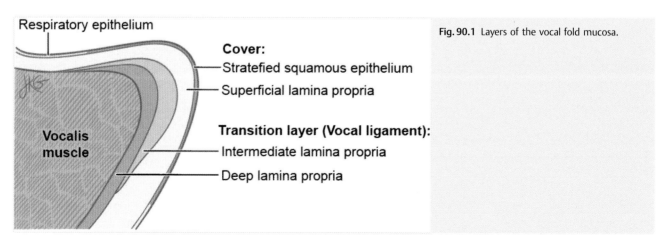

Fig. 90.1 Layers of the vocal fold mucosa.

Respiratory epithelium

Cover:
Stratefied squamous epithelium
Superficial lamina propria

Vocalis muscle

Transition layer (Vocal ligament):
Intermediate lamina propria
Deep lamina propria

nous vocal folds. Nodules form as a tissue response to injury and consist of thickened epithelium over a dense fibrous stroma rich in collagen. Epithelial keratosis accounts for the white appearance, and the dense fibrous stroma accounts for the firmness on palpation.

Polyps are also caused by vocal trauma, so they also tend to occur at the midpoint of the membranous vocal folds. They are more frequently unilateral but can occur bilaterally. They can be broad-based, pedunculated, or attached by a narrow mucosal stalk to the vocal fold, and they can vary in size from submillim-

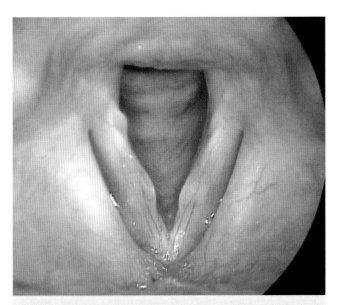

Fig. 90.2 Nodules at the junction of the anterior and middle thirds of the vocal folds.

eter lesions to lesions spanning almost the entire length of the membranous vocal fold. Polyps have been variably classified based on their gross appearance, as well as their composition. They can be translucent, vascular/hemorrhagic, fibrotic, or a combination thereof (▶ Fig. 90.3). Like nodules, polyps form as a tissue response to injury. In this case, the initiating event may be leakage from traumatized microvasculature that results in focal edema and eventual organization into a hyalinized stroma. Hemorrhagic or vascular polyps contain vascular telangiectasia and organized thrombus, suggesting the key role of vascular injury, deranged repair, and proliferation in the persistence of these types of polyps.

Cysts are entirely subepithelial and reside within the SLP. Two types are commonly acknowledged (▶ Fig. 90.4). A mucous retention cyst presumably results from an obstructed mucous gland duct. An epidermoid inclusion cyst can be congenital, iatrogenic, or possibly induced by vocal trauma. The cyst cavity is lined by squamous epithelium and has a keratin-rich and cholesterol-like filling. Finally, a superficial, translucent, broad-based polyp is referred to by some as a pseudocyst. It is "pseudo" in that it does not have a squamous epithelial lining.

Natural History and Progression

Because nodules, polyps, and some cysts are caused by vocal trauma, their fate is intimately tied to the patient's vocal behavior. If vocal trauma remains unabated, the lesions may enlarge and plateau at a certain size. On the other hand, most nodules will improve with voice rest and resolve with the cessation of traumatic vocal use. Some may not reverse completely, leaving smaller nodules that may be functionally acceptable. Polyps and cysts are more variable in their response to a reduction in vocal trauma. Small, hyaline polyps are more likely to regress,

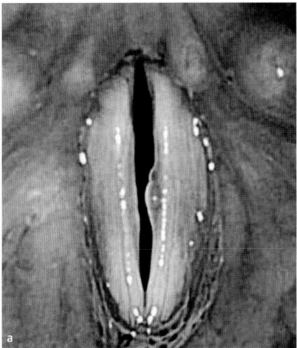
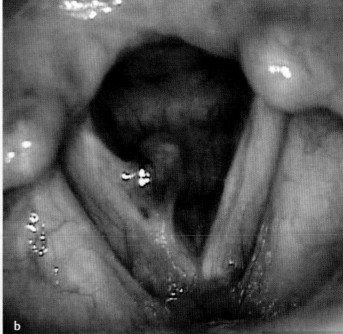

Fig. 90.3 Vocal fold polyps. (a) Translucent. (b) Hemorrhagic.

whereas translucent, hemorrhagic, and fibrotic/hyaline polyps may persist despite favorable modifications in vocal behavior. Cysts will not resolve with behavior modification, but the associated edema will improve along with vocal function. In the case of a cyst, excision is generally required to restore an acceptable voice.

Potential Disease Complications

Left untreated, nodules, polyps, and cysts will continue to interfere with vocal function. Over time, nodules and polyps that may have been amenable purely to voice therapy may progress so that behavior modification alone is no longer sufficient for resolution of these lesions and the patient's dysphonia.

90.4.2 Reinke Edema/Polypoid Corditis

Terminology, Etiology, and Pathogenesis

Reinke edema, also known as polypoid corditis or polypoid degeneration, is found almost exclusively in smokers and is much more prevalent in females (▶ Fig. 90.5). Unlike polyps, which are discrete masses, Reinke edema entails polypoid transformation of the vibratory mucosa along the entire length of the membranous vocal fold. This reflects chronic exposure of the vocal fold mucosa to smoke, as opposed to the localized mechanical or vascular trauma that gives rise to polyps. Although Reinke edema is sometimes mislabeled as simply a vocal fold polyp, the distinction between the two is important because they differ in etiology, anatomy, and surgical management. The term *edema* is descriptive of the gross appearance of the lesion but a misnomer at the histologic level. The SLP is not simply edematous but is transformed into a myxomatous stroma with unfavorable vibratory properties.

Natural History and Progression

Many smokers may have varying degrees of Reinke edema. They may remain asymptomatic aside from a gradual lowering of the pitch of their speaking voice and an increase in roughness, two hallmarks of the smoker's voice. As smoke exposure continues, the size and degree of the Reinke edema may increase, creating pedunculated lesions that function like a ball

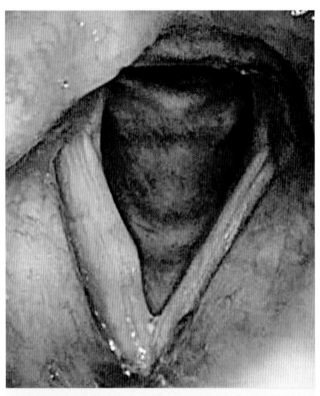

Fig. 90.4 Vocal fold cyst.

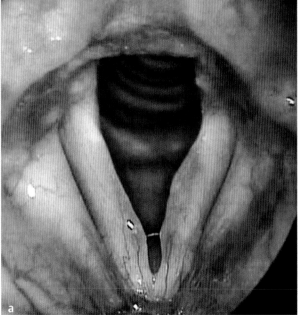
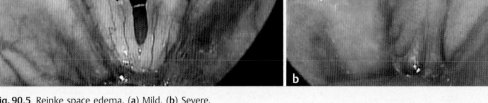

Fig. 90.5 Reinke space edema. (a) Mild. (b) Severe.

valve at the glottis. Because Reinke edema tends to be bilateral (but not necessarily symmetric), the ball valve component may cause mild to moderate airway obstruction. Some patients may seek medical attention after their voice or breathing has gradually deteriorated to an unacceptable point, or after a discrete episode of vocal trauma leads to an acute increase in the size of the lesion and symptom severity. Keratosis may also develop on the overlying epithelium and sometimes leads to concern for malignancy and biopsy. This keratosis, as well as Reinke edema, has not been associated with an increased risk for vocal fold malignancy. In fact, persons with Reinke edema are at a lower risk for developing laryngeal squamous cell carcinoma. Smoking cessation does not reverse the tissue change or reduce the lesion size, but it does prevent progression.

Potential Disease Complications

The deleterious effects of Reinke edema on the voice are self-evident in the rough quality and low frequency of the typical "smoker's voice." The effect of chronic airway obstruction from significant Reinke edema on cardiopulmonary health is unknown. Acute airway obstruction from sudden enlargement of Reinke edema due to mechanical trauma is possible.

90.4.3 Granulomas

Terminology, Etiology, and Pathogenesis

Granulomas in the larynx are not the immunologically mediated granulomas referred to elsewhere in medicine. They are akin to masses of granulation tissue and are found most often at the vocal processes (▶ Fig. 90.6). Occasionally, they are observed on the medial surface of the arytenoid body. They occur as the result of mechanical injury followed by an exuberant and aberrant reparative response. Mechanical injury can result from intubation (intubation granuloma) or vocal trauma (contact granuloma). Certain types of vocal behavior involve more forceful contact between the arytenoids and may be more likely to cause contact granulomas than other hyperfunctional vocal behaviors. Chronic cough and throat clearing fall into this category. The vocal hyperfunction that leads to granuloma formation can be a compensatory response to vocal fold paresis, atrophy, or other forms of glottic insufficiency. In the face of normal laryngeal anatomy, granulomas may form secondary to phonatory inefficiency and hard glottal onsets. Laryngopharyngeal reflux (LPR) is a commonly accepted etiologic factor for granulomas, although there is an obvious incongruence between the high estimated prevalence of LPR and the relatively rare finding of granulomas. It is likely that LPR is a major contributor to the development and persistence of granulomas once a mechanical injury has occurred, such that the injured mucosa is susceptible to a level of LPR that is ordinarily insufficient to cause symptoms on its own.

Natural History and Progression

It is likely that many granulomas develop and resolve on their own after the initial traumatic event. It is difficult to surmise what percentage of those brought to medical attention would regress on their own because intervention, chiefly in the form of acid suppression therapy and behavioral management, is in-

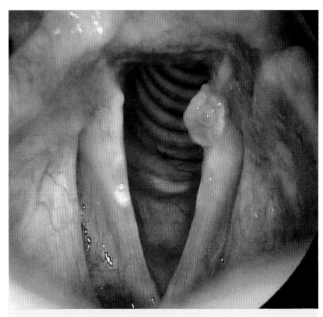

Fig. 90.6 Left vocal process granuloma.

variably implemented. Surgical excision alone carries a recurrence rate of more than 50%.

Potential Disease Complications

When large enough, granulomas will result in dysphonia. Acute enlargement of granulomas causing acute airway obstruction has been reported in isolated cases.

90.4.4 Papillomas

Terminology, Etiology, and Pathogenesis

Laryngeal papillomas, like their better-known counterpart in the genital tract, are "warts" caused by HPV. Unlike other entities described in this chapter, papillomas are neoplasms and have the potential (albeit a low one) for malignant transformation. They tend to develop at the transition between squamous epithelium and respiratory epithelium. Because the true vocal folds are lined with squamous epithelium while the surrounding structures are lined with respiratory epithelium, laryngeal papillomas are most often found on the true vocal folds. Papillomas have a distinct, warty appearance, with vascular stippling due to the fibrovascular stalks that project to the surface (▶ Fig. 90.7). More than 70 types of HPV have been identified. Some are associated with malignancy in the genital tract and are considered high-risk types. The low-risk HPV types 6 and 11 account for the vast majority of laryngeal papillomas.

Natural History and Progression

Untreated, laryngeal papillomas grow and produce progressively larger lesions locally. In the population with an adult onset, the rate of growth is highly variable among individuals and even within individuals when the lesions are followed for several years. Papillomas can also develop in noncontiguous sites in the proximal or distal airway; the likelihood is estimated to

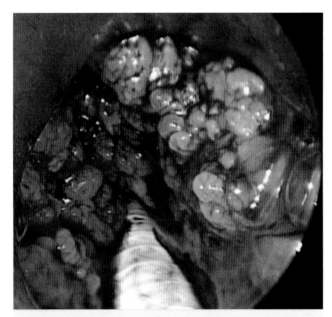

Fig. 90.7 Massive laryngeal papilloma obstructing the airway around an endotracheal tube.

be 10%. The soft palate, another structure with a squamous–respiratory epithelial transition, is a potential secondary site. More commonly, poorly controlled laryngeal papillomas lead to tracheal and even bronchial disease, presumably via a combination of airborne and iatrogenic seeding. Papillomas secondary to HPV type 11 are known to be more aggressive; these patients have a more severe laryngeal papillomatosis and a higher rate of development of tracheal and bronchial disease.

Potential Disease Complications

The most serious consequence of laryngeal papillomas is malignant conversion leading to squamous cell carcinoma of the larynx or tracheobronchial tree. The risk for conversion is 3 to 7%. Airway obstruction due to poorly controlled disease can be life-threatening. This is particularly a problem with tracheal papillomas, which are sometimes overlooked, less accessible surgically than laryngeal disease, and so less amenable to complete eradication.

90.4.5 Sulcus Vocalis

Terminology, Etiology, and Pathogenesis

A sulcus is a linear indentation, groove, or furrow. *Sulcus vocalis* is variably defined, and the term has been used to describe several entities that share the gross feature of a linear depression along the medial surface of the vocal fold. This can range from a focal deficiency of the SLP to invagination of the epithelium into the vocal ligament (▶ Fig. 90.8a). Sulci may be physiologic in that they do not affect vocal fold vibration. They can be congenital, in which case they are often bilateral. A sulcus can also be acquired (e.g., following excision of a vocal fold lesion that leaves a focal defect of the SLP). Theoretically, a sulcus may also be acquired after the rupture of a vocal fold cyst. Sulcus deformities have been categorized into three types by Ford. Type I is

physiologic and includes congenital sulcus with little voice impact and sulcus due to vocal fold atrophy. The mucosal wave is normal or minimally altered. Type II, or sulcus vergeture, consists of a contracted band along the medial vocal fold edge with adherence of the epithelium to the intermediate and deep layers of the lamina propria and a markedly reduced or absent mucosal wave. In type III, or sulcus vocalis, a pit-shaped, focal stiffness involves the vocal ligament, and the condition is associated with severe dysphonia (▶ Fig. 90.8b). The voice is typically thin with an elevated pitch, and patients complain of vocal fatigue and lack of projection.

Natural History and Progression

Sulcus vocalis will not change once formed. Patients may develop poor compensatory phonatory behaviors as they try to optimize their voice in the face of a sulcus.

Potential Disease Complications

No consequence beyond vocal impairment has been reported.

90.4.6 Saccular Cysts and Laryngoceles

Terminology, Etiology, and Pathogenesis

The laryngeal saccule is a blind pouch that extends superiorly from the anterior roof of the ventricle. A saccular cyst is a mucus-filled saccule sealed off from the laryngeal lumen and may be congenital or acquired. An anterior saccular cyst is localized and usually overhangs the anterior glottis. A lateral saccular cyst tends to be large and bulges the mucosa of the false vocal fold and aryepiglottic fold. This is sometimes called a congenital saccular cyst when noted in newborns with airway obstruction. A laryngocele is an air-filled dilatation of the saccule. It is believed to form after prolonged exposure to elevated intralaryngeal pressure in the setting of congenital weakness of the saccule lining. A laryngocele can be thought of as a large saccule that has become symptomatic. An internal laryngocele is confined within the cartilaginous laryngeal framework and appears as a submucosal swelling of the aryepiglottic fold. A mixed laryngocele is one that extends through the thyrohyoid membrane, lies lateral or external to the thyroid lamina, and can manifest as a lateral neck mass. A mixed laryngocele has both internal and external components.

Natural History and Progression

Saccular cysts and laryngoceles may enlarge over time. They may also remain relatively stable for long periods of time but suddenly enlarge in response to mucosal inflammation.

Potential Disease Complications

Saccular cysts and laryngoceles may cause voice change, dysphagia, and airway obstruction. They also may be secondary to a malignant neoplasm in the ventricle obstructing the introitus of the saccule. In this case, the mass would be the etiology of the saccular cyst or laryngocele. Isolated cases of sudden death due to rapid expansion of a saccular cyst causing airway distress have been reported.

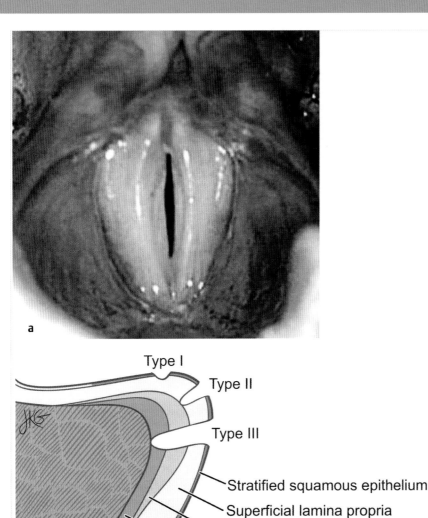

Type I

Type II

Type III

Stratified squamous epithelium

Superficial lamina propria

Intermediate lamina propria

Deep lamina propria

Fig. 90.8 Sulcus vocalis. (**a**) Bilateral sulci can be seen. (**b**) Sulcus vocalis classification. The schematic is only intended to illustrate the depth of involvement and not the size or shape of the defect.

90.5 Medical Evaluation

90.5.1 Presenting Complaints

The most common presenting complaints of benign laryngeal lesions relate to voice. The patient may describe a decline in voice quality—for example, an increase in roughness or raspiness. Sometimes, the complaint can be less tangible, such as the development of vocal fatigue or the lack of ability to raise vocal volume. The onset, duration, and progression of vocal symptoms are useful elements of the history. For example, lifelong dysphonia suggests a congenital lesion, such as a sulcus vocalis, whereas a steady progression of dysphonia may be due to a neoplastic process. Patients with a benign vocal fold lesion are unlikely to have any periods of normal voice, unlike patients with functional voice disorders.

Certain lesions have the potential to enlarge sufficiently to cause airway obstruction. Most of the time, however, progression is gradual, and patients present for their dysphonia before the development of dyspnea. Large saccular cysts or laryngoceles may cause swallowing discomfort or frank dysphagia if they impede epiglottic inversion during the swallow cycle.

90.5.2 Physical Examination and Testing

A dysphonic voice quality should be noted. The relative severity of the overall dysphonic quality can be recorded as mild, moderate, or severe and serves as a basis for comparison during follow-up examinations or after interventions. Subjective scales such as the GRBAS scale may be used to evaluate the voice. Patients' voices are evaluated on a scale of 0 to 3, with 0 normal and 3 severe. The overall grade, roughness, breathiness, asthenia, and strain are scored according to this scale. Objective voice measures such as acoustic parameters can be obtained. Any stridor should be noted. The key part of the evaluation consists of laryngoscopy, which can be considered an extension of the physical examination.

90.5.3 Laryngoscopy

Laryngoscopy can be carried out by indirect visualization with a mirror, transorally with a rigid angled endoscope, or transnasally with a flexible laryngoscope. Under most circumstances, this should suffice to identify Reinke edema, granuloma, papilloma, and submucosal bulges from saccular cysts and laryngoceles. Reinke edema involves distortion of the entire normal straight edge of the membranous vocal fold and may be bulky enough to produce a pedunculated mass with a smooth mucosa. Granulomas are distinguished mainly based on their location at the vocal processes or on the medial arytenoid bodies. Papillomas have a wartlike appearance with a distinct vascular stippling that may be discernible if the image quality is good. Some sulcus vocalis lesions, as well as some nodules, polyps, and cysts, may be sufficiently pronounced to be clearly visualized on routine laryngoscopy. Unilateral hemorrhagic polyps, for example, are easily identifiable. It may be difficult to discern smaller, bilateral vocal fold lesions as nodules versus polyps, or a smooth unilateral lesion as a polyp versus a cyst. For these situations, as well as to identify finer sulcus vocalis lesions and their effect on vocal fold vibration, videostroboscopy is recommended.

90.5.4 Videostroboscopy

The vocal folds are visualized under stroboscopy to produce a pseudo-slow motion video of vocal fold vibration (see Chapter 79 for more details on videostroboscopy). This allows the lesions to be seen at slightly different angles as they rock along the medial surface of the vocal fold if they are so located. This procedure also provides an assessment of the impact of the lesions on mucosal wave propagation, vibratory amplitude, glottal closure, and vibratory phase symmetry. Alterations in these parameters help differentiate lesions, as well as prognosticate potential surgical complexity and voice outcome. Nodules may cause a small to moderate decrease in the vibrational amplitude. Polyps, depending on their size, cause variable alterations in vocal fold amplitude and the mucosal wave simply by mass effect. The mucosal wave, although altered, is generally present or somewhat reduced. In contrast, cysts are distinguished by a significant reduction in the mucosal wave. This stroboscopic difference stems from the depth of the lesion and its adherence to the vocal ligament. As such, the pliability of the vocal fold cover is decreased, and mucosal wave propagation is severely retarded by the presence of the cyst. Although a polyp may be as large as or larger than a cyst, it involves the SLP and is not coupled to the vocal ligament. It therefore impacts the wave less. Videostroboscopy is also crucial in the assessment of sulcus vocalis. It reveals the impact of the lesion on mucosal wave propagation and estimates the depth of the sulcus.

90.5.5 Radiographic Imaging

Imaging has little role in the work-up of most benign laryngeal lesions except in the case of saccular cysts and laryngoceles. In these cases, computed tomography or magnetic resonance imaging of the neck is used to determine their anatomical extent and aid in surgical planning.

90.5.6 Differential Diagnosis

Laryngeal malignancies can mimic benign lesions. The most common laryngeal malignancy is squamous cell carcinoma and its variants. Much less common are salivary or mucous gland

tumors, cartilaginous tumors, sarcomas, and neuroendocrine tumors. Lymphomas have also been reported.

Various autoimmune and connective tissue disorders can manifest in the larynx. Bamboo nodules or rheumatoid nodules are submucosal masses found at the mid-membranous vocal folds. Because of their location, they can be mistaken as nodules caused by vocal trauma. Bamboo nodules have been described in isolated case reports of rheumatoid arthritis, systemic lupus erythematosus, progressive systemic sclerosis, Hashimoto thyroiditis, Sjögren syndrome, relapsing polychondritis, and mixed connective tissue disease. Sarcoidosis causes a pale, pink swelling of the supraglottic mucosa primarily. Amyloidosis is a disease of abnormal protein deposition and can be localized to the larynx. Amyloid deposits in the false vocal folds, ventricular floor, and true vocal folds can have a mass effect on the airway and cause dysphonia. The typical lesion is a multilobulated, irregular, smooth submucosal mass with an orange–yellow discoloration.

A history of prior vocal fold injection in the setting of a vocal fold abnormality should raise the possibility of a Teflon granuloma or superficial injectate in the SLP. These may not present as discrete lesions. Part or all of the membranous vocal fold may appear stiff, with a convex contour.

90.6 Treatment

90.6.1 Medical Treatment

With the exception of papillomas, most benign laryngeal lesions may not require treatment simply by virtue of their presence. Treatment is often implemented with the goal of symptom reduction, rather than lesion elimination. Most often, the treatment is surgical in nature.

Voice therapy plays several roles in the management of selected benign laryngeal lesions. Voice therapy is the first-line treatment for nodules and certain types of polyps that may reverse with the cessation of phonotraumatic vocal behavior. Voice therapy may be adjunctive in the treatment of laryngeal granulomas. For lesions that require excision, perioperative voice therapy may decrease the likelihood of persistence of the hyperfunctional vocal mechanism that contributed to lesion formation. Finally, if excision is expected to lead to a decline in voice quality because of necessary sacrifice of the vibratory mucosa, postoperative voice therapy serves to extract the best possible voice from a deficient sound source.

Acid suppression therapy with proton pump inhibitors is commonly used in the management of benign laryngeal lesions if LPR is thought to be a contributing factor. LPR is certainly not a factor in the development and propagation of all benign vocal fold lesions, and it is likely that it is currently being overdiagnosed. It is widely accepted that acid suppression therapy is central to the treatment of laryngeal granulomas. Acid suppression therapy is commonly employed postoperatively to minimize the likelihood of exposure of the surgical site in the larynx to acid.

Several adjunctive therapies have been used in addition to the surgical removal of papillomas. They are indicated when disease is extensive or a rapid return of papillomas requires frequent surgical extirpation. Generally, more than four surgical treatments per year will prompt a discussion of the use of adjuvant therapies. Oral indole-3-carbinol is a nutritional supplement found in high concentrations in cruciferous vegetables such as broccoli, cabbage, brussels sprouts, and cauliflower. Indole-3-carbinol is thought to modulate the proliferation of epithelial cells indirectly by altering estrogen metabolism. Although its benefit in controlling recurrent respiratory papillomatosis has only been suggested in a relatively small study, indole-3-carbinol has virtually no side effects. A cyclooxygenase-2 (COX-2) inhibitor, celecoxib, is currently being investigated for its effectiveness against recurrent respiratory papillomatosis in a Phase II multicenter randomized controlled trial. COX-2 is overexpressed in papillomas, and celecoxib has been shown to reduce papilloma cell proliferation in cell lines. Preliminary data seem to support the efficacy of celecoxib in achieving disease regression in a small group of patients. Results from the Phase II trial are pending. Cidofovir is a selective inhibitor of the herpesvirus DNA polymerase. It is commonly used off label as a surgical adjunct in an intralesional manner. Data on efficacy show an overall trend suggestive of benefit, although a large-scale randomized controlled trial is lacking. Cidofovir has also been administered intravenously in severe cases with lower airway involvement. Interferon alfa modulates the host immune response to increase antiviral activity. Its use in treating recurrent respiratory papillomatosis has been limited by a significant side effect profile. Finally, an angiogenesis inhibitor (bevacizumab) has shown some promise as a surgical adjunct when applied intralesionally.

Inhaled corticosteroids have been used in combination with proton pump inhibitors to treat laryngeal granulomas, although their efficacy as a single agent is unknown. Injection of botulinum toxin type A into the vocal fold adductors has also been used as a treatment for granulomas resistant to conventional management. In addition, patients who have granulomas secondary to laryngeal hyperfunction used to compensate for vocal fold atrophy may benefit from bilateral vocal fold injection augmentation to decrease the need for such hyperfunction.

90.6.2 Surgical Treatment

All techniques are carried out under general anesthesia via direct laryngoscopy with an operating microscope unless otherwise noted.

Cold Knife Excision

Polyps and cysts that fail to resolve after adequate voice therapy and remain symptomatic are typically excised with micro instruments in a microflap technique, described in Chapter 93 (Instrumentation and Techniques of Phonomicrosurgery). Cold knife excision can also be used to reduce the size of Reinke edema by debulking the diseased stroma in a similar microflap fashion. Complications with the cold knife technique relate mainly to excessive removal of the normal vocal fold lamina propria or epithelium, leading to vocal fold stiffness and permanent dysphonia.

Powered Laryngeal Microdébrider

The chief advantage of the microdébrider is rapid debulking of lesions in cases in which mucosal preservation is not war-

ranted. The main application is in papilloma removal, in which the toothed Tricut version of the débrider blade allows rapid debulking (Medtronic, Minneapolis, MN). The flat Skimmer version of the blade (Medtronic, Minneapolis, MN) minimizes the destruction of normal vocal fold mucosa and the underlying SLP. The microdébrider can also be used to debulk large granulomas. As with the cold knife technique, the main complication of microdébrider use is the loss of normal vocal fold lamina propria and epithelium, leading to permanent dysphonia.

Coblator

The Coblator (ArthroCare ENT, Austin, TX) is also excellent for debulking large amounts of papilloma. Compared with the microdébrider, it has the advantage that coblation minimizes bleeding. In contrast, it cannot be used near the epithelial basement membrane of the vocal fold because it does not provide enough control to precisely remove papilloma without excessive damage to the SLP or surrounding normal epithelium.

Carbon Dioxide Laser

The carbon dioxide laser can be used in an ablative fashion to remove papilloma. It can also be used in an excisional manner, akin to a hot knife, to remove large amounts of papilloma or a laryngocele. Both the internal and external parts of a laryngocele can be excised transorally with a carbon dioxide laser. Although the technique is rare, some authors use the laser at a low-power setting to assist in the dissection of vocal fold polyps or cysts. In all cases, the laser settings and technique used should be optimized to minimize irreversible thermal damage to the tissue adjacent to the target lesion. The most feared complication of laser use is an airway fire. Safety precautions include the avoidance of flammable inhalational anesthetic agents, the avoidance of flammable endotracheal tubes, protection of the endotracheal tube balloon with a saline-soaked pledget, the use of an FiO_2 (fraction of inspired oxygen) below 30%, and the application of moist towels to cover the patient's head and face.

Angioselective Lasers

The pulsed dye laser (PDL) and the pulsed potassium titanyl phosphate (KTP) laser have found increasing use in the treatment of benign vocal fold lesions. Both have wavelengths that coincide with the absorption peaks of oxyhemoglobin. Because of their angioselectivity, there is a theoretical advantage in their use for the treatment of lesions associated with rich vasculature, such as papillomas. Their use has been extended to the treatment of Reinke edema, granulomas, some polyps, dysplasias, and limited malignancies. The main advantage of these lasers is that they are delivered via a fiber that can be placed in the working channel of a flexible laryngoscope, allowing treatment to be carried out in an unsedated fashion in the office setting and avoiding the need for general anesthesia. In addition, their selective absorption by oxyhemoglobin decreases collateral damage to surrounding nonvascular tissue, such as the SLP. During direct laryngoscopy, these lasers can be used for the selective photoablation of vessels feeding hemorrhagic polyps, minimizing bleeding and optimizing the surgical field. They can also be used to treat the residual papilloma that is not excised at the anterior aspect of one of the vocal folds in order to prevent a glottic web when papilloma has been excised anteriorly from the other vocal fold. The papilloma treated with the photoangiolytic laser will slowly involute from ischemia without risk for the formation of an anterior glottic web. Like all lasers, photoangiolytic lasers are associated with a risk for airway fire when used in conjunction with an endotracheal tube, and all safety precautions must be applied.

90.7 Prognosis

Because the lesions discussed in this chapter are of a benign nature, the overall prognosis is excellent. The likelihood that vocal fold nodules, polyps, and cysts will resolve with a combination of behavioral and surgical intervention is excellent. Reinke edema can be surgically reduced to achieve an acceptable vocal outcome. Granulomas almost always resolve, although the time and intervention required may vary considerably. Focal, early laryngeal papillomas may be eradicated, but patients who have diffuse disease may require long-term, episodic maintenance with surgical procedures. Vaccination against HPV should lead to a greatly reduced incidence of disease in the decades to come. Sulcus vocalis has been a challenging entity to correct surgically. Advances in the treatment of sulcus vocalis may require novel techniques and materials to restore lamina propria defects. Finally, saccular cysts and laryngoceles can be managed successfully with surgery.

90.8 Roundsmanship

- The superficial layer of the vocal fold lamina propria is critical in normal vibratory function and must be maximally preserved in the surgical treatment of benign lesions. It does not regenerate once lost through disease or trauma. Vocal cord stripping is no longer an acceptable surgical procedure.
- Videostroboscopy should be performed in the assessment of vocal fold polyps, cysts, and sulcus vocalis to assess their impact on the mucosal wave, estimate the depth of their involvement, and enhance diagnostic accuracy.
- Benign-appearing laryngeal lesions with an atypical appearance should raise the possibilities of malignancy and of autoimmune, infectious, or connective tissue disorders.
- Voice therapy is the first-line treatment for patients with vocal fold nodules and some polyps. For patients whose lesions require excision, voice therapy still has a role in addressing the hyperfunctional vocal behavior that resulted in the development of such lesions in the first place.
- Acid suppression therapy and behavioral management, not excision, should be the first-line treatment for laryngeal granulomas.

90.9 Recommended Reading

[1] Gray SD, Hammond E, Hanson DF. Benign pathologic responses of the larynx. Ann Otol Rhinol Laryngol 1995; 104: 13–18

[2] DeSanto LW. Laryngocele, laryngeal mucocele, large saccules, and laryngeal saccular cysts: a developmental spectrum. Laryngoscope 1974; 84: 1291–1296

[3] Courey MS, Garrett CG, Ossoff RH. Medial microflap for excision of benign vocal fold lesions. Laryngoscope 1997; 107: 340–344

[4] Derkay CS, Wiatrak B. Recurrent respiratory papillomatosis: a review. Laryngoscope 2008; 118: 1236–1247

[5] Zeitels SM, Hillman RE, Bunting GW, Vaughn T. Reinke's edema: phonatory mechanisms and management strategies. Ann Otol Rhinol Laryngol 1997; 106: 533–543

[6] Ford CN, Inagi K, Khidr A, Bless DM, Gilchrist KW. Sulcus vocalis: a rational analytical approach to diagnosis and management. Ann Otol Rhinol Laryngol 1996; 105: 189–200

[7] Cohen SM, Garrett CG. Utility of voice therapy in the management of vocal fold polyps and cysts. Otolaryngol Head Neck Surg 2007; 136: 742–746

91 Adult Laryngotracheal Stenosis

Amanda Hu and Tanya K. Meyer

91.1 Introduction

Adult laryngotracheal stenosis is one of the more challenging disease entities faced by the airway surgeon. There is no treatment strategy that can be uniformly applied to all patients to guarantee excellent results. The larynx and trachea are both semirigid tubular structures. When injury occurs and wound healing progresses, circumferential scar contracture can cause narrowing of the airway. Furthermore, the larynx functions as a sphincter, opening to allow airflow and closing to allow phonation and facilitate swallowing. Scarring of the larynx may cause fixation of the vocal folds with airway compromise. Surgical attempts to open the airway statically may subsequently compromise phonation and swallowing. The plethora of surgical techniques available attests to the complexity of this problem.

91.2 Incidence of Disease

The true incidence of adult laryngotracheal stenosis is difficult to estimate. Prolonged intubation constitutes the most common cause of adult laryngotracheal stenosis in the modern era (▶ Fig. 91.1). The population incidence of laryngotracheal stenosis as a result of prolonged intubation is estimated at 1 in 200,000 adults per year. In the 1970s, Whited estimated that approximately 12% of patients intubated for more than 12 days would develop significant posterior glottic injury. This landmark article has led to changes by which many preventative measures are used in intubated patients to prevent laryngotracheal injury and has contributed to the practice of recommending a tracheostomy after 7 to 10 days of intubation.

91.3 Classification

There are several classification systems for laryngotracheal stenosis. These staging systems categorize the severity of disease to improve communication, help prognosticate the outcomes of surgery, and compare different methods of treatment. One commonly used classification system is the Cotton-Myer system (▶ Fig. 91.2), in which stenosis is graded on a scale from I to IV based on the degree of subglottic luminal obstruction. This is the simplest system; it is used more often in the pediatric population and only for subglottic stenosis. A system for grading the extent of posterior glottic stenosis was created by Bogdasarian and Olson in 1980 (▶ Fig. 91.3). There are four types, based on the degree of injury and arytenoid mobility and on the prognosis. A third clinical staging system is the McCaffrey system (▶ Table 91.1 and ▶ Fig. 91.4). This system is based on the location and length of the stenosis; the higher the stage number, the worse the prognosis for decannulation.

91.4 Applied Anatomy

The adult trachea is approximately 10 to 13 cm in length and 2.0 to 2.5 cm in diameter. It starts at the inferior border of the cricoid cartilage and extends to the bifurcation of the carina.

The fibromuscular tube of the trachea is supported by cartilaginous rings. These rings occupy the anterior two-thirds of the tracheal circumference and are incomplete posteriorly. There are approximately 14 to 20 tracheal rings.

The blood supply of the trachea is the same as that of the esophagus. The upper trachea is supplied by the inferior thyroid artery and tracheo-esophageal branches of the subclavian artery. The lower trachea is supplied by branches from the intercostal and internal mammary arteries. Because the blood supply approaches the tracheo-esophageal groove laterally, circumferential dissection of the trachea should be avoided to prevent devascularization.

The larynx is divided into the supraglottis, glottis, and subglottis. The supraglottis is defined as the area above the vocal cords and includes the ventricular folds, epiglottis, and arytenoids. The glottis includes the true vocal cords and the anterior and posterior commissures. It extends inferiorly from the true vocal fold edge 1 cm anteriorly and 5 mm posteriorly. The subglottis extends from the lower border of glottis to the inferior border of the cricoid. The glottis is the narrowest part of the adult airway, whereas the subglottis is the narrowest part of the pediatric airway.

91.5 The Disease Process

91.5.1 Etiology and Pathogenesis

Before the advent of prolonged intubation, most cases of laryngeal stenosis resulted from an infectious disease such as syphilis, diphtheria, tuberculosis, or typhoid fever. After World War II, with the advent of modern antibiotics and vaccinations, this etiology waned and was replaced by blunt trauma to the neck through motor vehicle accidents. Since the 1950s and the poliomyelitis epidemic, there has been a dramatic increase in the use of endotracheal tube intubation and mechanical ventilation with prolonged intubation. Correspondingly, prolonged intubation became and remains the predominant cause of laryngotracheal stenosis. Other etiologies are less commonly encountered and include iatrogenic injury, autoimmune and inflammatory conditions, and following radiotherapy. Some cases of laryngotracheal stenosis are idiopathic. Common etiologies of adult laryngotracheal stenosis are listed in ▶ Table 91.2. Some etiologies of interest are highlighted below.

Trauma

The most common cause of laryngotracheal stenosis is mechanical trauma from endotracheal intubation. This usually results in posterior glottic stenosis because the tube rests in the posterior commissure, applying pressure to the interarytenoid area, vocal processes of the arytenoids, and posterior cricoid plate. This pressure causes ischemic necrosis of the mucosa, leading to mucosal ulceration, bacterial infection, perichondritis and chondritis, and cartilage resorption (see ▶ Fig. 91.1). As the phases of wound healing progress, submucosal fibrosis occurs with scar contracture. Because the larynx and trachea are semi-

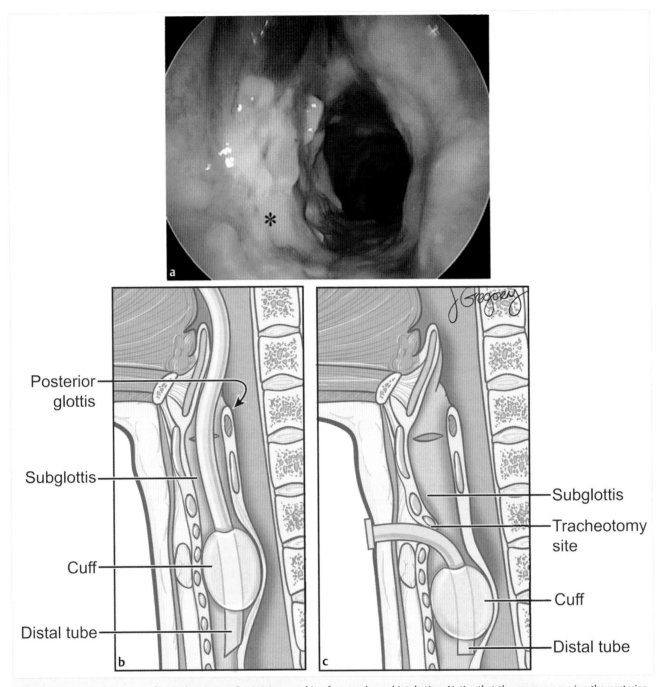

Fig. 91.1 (a) Endoscopic view of typical posterior glottic injury resulting from prolonged intubation. Notice that the mucosa covering the posterior glottis is absent, with cricoid cartilage exposure (*asterisk*), granulation at the cricoarytenoid joint, and irritation and granulation at the site of endotracheal tube pressure on the distal anterior tracheal wall. (b) Schematic of areas of injury due to intubation: posterior glottis, subglottis, cuff, and distal endotracheal tube tip. (c) Schematic of areas of injury due to tracheotomy: subglottis (if a high tracheotomy), tracheotomy site, cuff, and distal endotracheal tube tip.

rigid tubes, this causes stenosis of the airway. Factors related to the risk for stenosis include the following: tube size and composition, number of intubations, length of intubation, elective versus urgent intubation, concomitant nasogastric tube placement, laryngeal motion during intubation, and concomitant laryngopharyngeal reflux disease. High-pressure cuffs can also contribute to laryngotracheal stenosis. Modern practices use low-pressure cuffs, and cuff pressures are routinely monitored in patients who are chronically intubated or tracheotomized.

Tracheostomy can contribute to multiple airway abnormalities. A tracheostomy placed too high may cause cricoid erosion and subglottic narrowing. Excessive tracheal cartilage removal during fenestration at the time of tracheotomy can cause destabilization of the anterior tracheal wall. As healing occurs after decannulation, an "A-frame" stenosis can develop, often with associated malacia (▶ Fig. 91.5). Finally, stomal granulation tissue can develop and mature into cicatrix, and cuff and distal tube tip injury can occur.

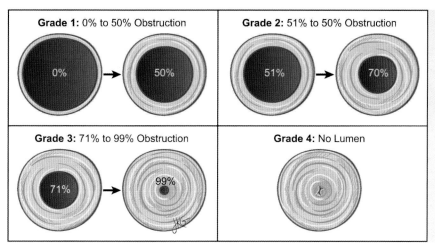

Grade 1: 0% to 50% Obstruction

0% → 50%

Grade 2: 51% to 50% Obstruction

51% → 70%

Grade 3: 71% to 99% Obstruction

71% → 99%

Grade 4: No Lumen

Fig. 91.2 Cotton-Myer classification of subglottic stenosis in the pediatric population.

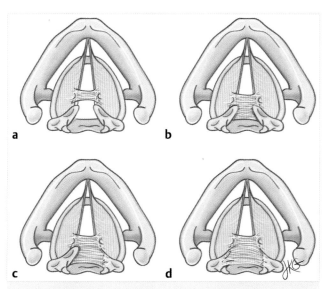

Fig. 91.3 Bogdasarian and Olson classification of adult posterior glottic stenosis. (a) Type I, vocal process adhesion or interarytenoid synechia. (b) Type II, posterior commissure stenosis with scarring in the interarytenoid plane and internal surface of the posterior cricoid lamina. (c) Type III, posterior commissure stenosis with unilateral cricoarytenoid joint ankylosis. (d) Type IV, posterior commissure stenosis with bilateral cricoarytenoid joint ankylosis.

Systemic Disease

Among the systemic diseases that can cause laryngotracheal stenosis, granulomatosis with polyangiitis, traditionally knows as Wegener granulomatosis, is the most common. Granulomatosis with polyangiitis is a multisystem autoimmune disease of unknown etiology. Its hallmark features include necrotizing granulomatous inflammation and pauci-immune vasculitis in small and medium-size blood vessels. Commonly involved organs include the upper and lower airways, lungs, and kidneys. Specific otolaryngologic findings include serous otitis media, ocular inflammation, epistaxis, sinusitis, nasal inflammation, saddle nose deformity, septal perforation, oral ulceration, palpable purpura, and skin ulceration. About one-fifth of patients will have subglottic stenosis.

Granulomatosis with polyangiitis is usually associated with the presence of diffusely staining cytoplasmic antineutrophil cytoplasmic autoantibodies (c-ANCA) directed against the serine proteinase 3 antigen (PR3-ANCA). Serum testing for c-ANCA and perinuclear antineutrophil cytoplasmic autoantibodies (p-ANCA) should be considered for patients with idiopathic subglottic stenosis. c-ANCA is 90% specific for granulomatosis with polyangiitis and varies with disease activity. p-ANCA is less specific. A negative c-ANCA does not eliminate the diagnosis of granulomatosis with polyangiitis. Limited granulomatosis with polyangiitis is often more difficult to diagnose than generalized forms, and serologic markers and biopsy may not be diagnostic. The medical treatment of granulomatosis with polyangiitis involves cyclophosphamide, prednisone, and trimethoprim/sulfamethoxazole. Surgical treatment should ideally be pursued after medical management has led to disease remission.

Relapsing polychondritis is another autoimmune disease with airway involvement. It generally presents with multiple areas of cartilage involvement, such as auricular and nasal cartilage inflammation. This results in a seronegative, nonerosive inflammatory polychondritis. Serum testing shows an increase in the erythrocyte sedimentation rate, and a cartilage biopsy should be performed. Treatment options include corticosteroids, nonsteroidal anti-inflammatory drugs (NSAIDs), colchicine, dapsone, methotrexate, and azathioprine.

Sarcoidosis is an idiopathic systemic disease characterized by the formation of noncaseating granulomas. It is more common in African-American women. Sarcoidosis may cause epiglottic swelling and subglottic stenosis. Other otolaryngologic manifestations include cervical lymphadenopathy, Heerfordt syndrome (uveoparotid fever), septal perforation, pulmonary hilar lymphadenopathy, and cranial neuropathies (e.g., facial paralysis and sudden sensorineural hearing loss). Diagnostic investigations include measurement of angiotensin-converting enzyme (ACE) and calcium levels, chest radiography, and purified protein derivative (PPD) testing (negative result). Medical treatment includes corticosteroids for acute exacerbations and conservative surgery.

Idiopathic Subglottic Stenosis

Idiopathic subglottic stenosis is a rare, nonspecific, progressive inflammatory disorder that causes subglottic and proximal

Table 91.1 McCaffrey classification of laryngotracheal stenosis

Stage	Description	Prognosis for decannulation
1	Lesions are confined to the subglottis or trachea and are less than 1 cm long.	90%
2	Lesions are subglottic stenoses longer than 1 cm within the cricoid ring without extension into the glottis or trachea.	90%
3	Lesions extend into the upper trachea but do not involve the glottis.	70%
4	Lesions involve the glottis with fixation or paralysis of one or both vocal folds.	40%

Source: Adapted from McCaffrey TV. Classification of laryngotracheal stenosis. Laryngoscope 1992;102:1335 and McCaffrey TV. Management of laryngotracheal stenosis on the basis of site and severity. Otolaryngol Head Neck Surg 1993;109:468.

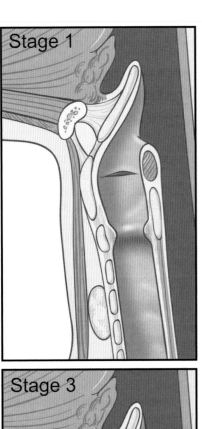
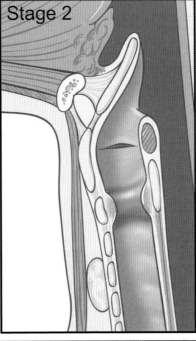
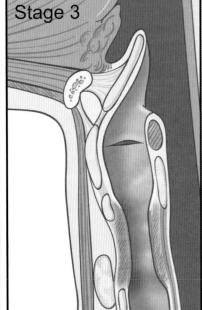
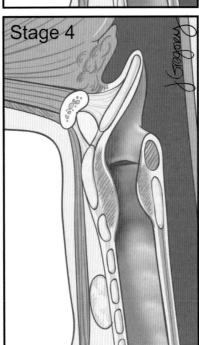

Fig. 91.4 McCaffrey classification of laryngotracheal stenosis. Stage 1: Lesions are confined to the subglottis or trachea and are less than 1 cm long. Stage 2: Subglottic stenoses longer than 1 cm are within the cricoid ring without extension into the glottis or trachea. Stage 3: Lesions extend into the upper trachea but do not involve the glottis. Stage 4: Lesions involve the glottis with fixation or paralysis of one or both vocal folds.

Table 91.2 Etiologies of adulty laryngotracheal stenosis

Trauma	Infection	Neoplastic lesions	Idiopathic
Endotracheal intubation	Syphilis	Benign	Laryngopharyngeal reflux
Tracheotomy	Diphteria	Malignant	
External laryngotracheal injury	Tuberculosis		
Iatrogenic injury	Typhoid fever		
Following radiotherapy	Systemic disease, granulomatosis with polyangiitis (Wegener granulomatosis)		
	Relapsing polychondritis		
	Sarcoidosis		

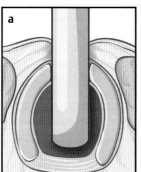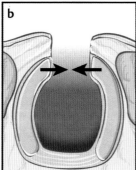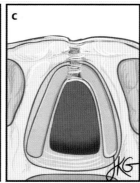

Fig. 91.5 (a–c) Evolution of an "A-frame" stenosis. Cross-sectional diagrams of the trachea at the stoma site. After the tracheotomy tube is removed, the anterior tracheal wall is destabilized (*arrows*), causing an A-frame stenosis, often with associated malacia.

tracheal stenosis. This disease affects middle-aged women (30 to 50 years of age) and is a diagnosis of exclusion made after other etiologies have been ruled out. It has been speculated, although not proved, that laryngopharyngeal reflux disease may contribute to idiopathic subglottic stenosis.

91.6 Medical Evaluation

91.6.1 Presenting Complaints

Symptoms often develop gradually and patients compensate, so airway narrowing can be quite advanced at the time of presentation. Presenting complaints include dyspnea (on exertion or at rest), exercise intolerance, inability to lie supine, and cough. Hoarseness may indicate glottic involvement. A misdiagnosis of refractory asthma may be made. A past medical history of intubation, tracheostomy, neck surgery, neck trauma, laryngopharyngeal reflux disease, or autoimmune disease is important. Previous operative reports of dilations or reconstructions should be obtained.

91.6.2 Clinical Findings, Physical Examination

Initially, stridor, patient discomfort or fatigue, use of accessory muscles, supraclavicular contractions, and vocal quality should be noted to assess the acuity of the airway and severity of the dyspnea, as well as the urgency or emergency of the situation.

The secondary goal of the clinical examination for a patient with suspected laryngotracheal stenosis is to determine the nature of airway dysfunction at all levels. The surgeon's choice of intervention is significantly affected by the ability to safely manipulate the patient's airway during general anesthesia and in the perioperative period. The physical examination should specifically include factors that affect ease of intubation and airway exposure, including mouth opening, Mallampati score, neck size, cervical mobility, laryngeal position, and cervical scars.

Because intubation can cause airway injury at multiple levels and is the most common cause of airway stenosis, it is essential to survey the entire airway for structural and functional deficits. Flexible laryngoscopy and bronchoscopy are critical in the assessment of dynamic airway function. The upper airway is evaluated for signs of sleep apnea, the larynx is inspected for appropriate neurologic function (sensation and vocal fold movement) and evidence of cicatrix, and the subglottis and trachea are examined for stenosis and malacia. It is important to evaluate the airway while the patient is awake and spontaneously ventilating because malacia is often elicited only when the patient is asked to cough volitionally. Most patients can tolerate bronchoscopy in the clinic with topical lidocaine, but this can also be performed in the operating room under light sedation.

Direct laryngoscopy and tracheobronchoscopy are performed under general anesthesia. The larynx is palpated to differentiate cricoarytenoid joint ankylosis from paralysis, and also to measure any areas of stenosis or abnormality. With a Hopkins rod-lens telescope, the distance of the stenosis from the superior surface of the vocal cords and the length of the stenosis can be determined. A small needle can be inserted into the airway through the cricothyroid space and at the sternal notch to determine the relation of the stenosis to these structures.

91.6.3 Testing

Testing includes serologic studies for autoimmune disorders, pulmonary function tests, chest radiography, and tissue biopsy. Fine-cut computed tomography from the hyoid to the carina will show subglottic or tracheal narrowing but will not give any information regarding glottic function or dynamic airway collapse.

91.6.4 Differential Diagnosis

The differential diagnosis of adult laryngotracheal stenosis is listed in ▶ Table 91.3.

Table 91.3 Differential diagnosis of laryngotracheal stenosis

Etiology of stenosis	Differential diagnosis
Congenital	Tracheomalacia, laryngomalacia, laryngeal cleft, congenital cysts
Infection	Laryngotracheobronchitis (croup), bacterial tracheitis
Trauma	Vocal cord paralysis, foreign body, external compression
Neoplasm	Benign: recurrent respiratory papillomatosis, subglottic hemangioma Malignant: squamous cell carcinoma of the larynx, chondrosarcoma
Systemic disease	Asthma, paradoxical vocal fold motion

91.7 Treatment

91.7.1 Medical Treatment

Comorbidities such as obstructive sleep apnea, diabetes, laryngopharyngeal reflux, and obesity should be optimized before any surgical intervention. Systemic inflammatory disease should be managed by an appropriate specialist. Inhaled, topical, and oral corticosteroids can be used. The prolonged use of oral steroids can have significant side effects, including cushingoid body habitus, hyperglycemic reaction, exacerbation of anxiety or depression, acne, increased intraocular pressure, gastrointestinal irritation, and avascular necrosis of the hip. Racemic epinephrine and heliox may be helpful in temporarily stabilizing the patient in situations of acute exacerbation of airway compromise. Voice and breathing retraining therapy administered by a knowledgeable speech–language pathologist can significantly help patients cope with their airway and voice limitations.

91.7.2 Surgical Treatment

When a surgical option is chosen, several factors must be considered: the location, length, and quality (soft vs fibrous) of the stenosis; dynamic malacia; associated impairment of vocal fold motion; extent of functional impairment; and medical comorbidities of the patient.

Endoscopic surgery is the method most commonly used to treat all levels of laryngotracheal stenosis. The major disadvantage is that laser incision or ablation of scar necessarily leaves a raw operative bed, potentially allowing the re-formation of cicatrix and a need for repeated procedures. About three-quarters of patients treated with endoscopic dilation as primary therapy will have recurrent stenosis and require subsequent treatment. Patients who are good candidates for endoscopic treatment include those with supraglottic or glottic stenoses, Cotton-Myer grade 1 or 2 subglottic stenoses, and soft or immature tracheal

Table 91.4 Surgical approaches to the treatment of laryngotracheal stenosis

Location of stenosis	Surgical approach	
Supraglottic		a) Endoscopic b) Open
Glottic	Anterior	a) Endoscopic b) Open: laryngofissure
	Posterior	a) Endoscopic • Carbon dioxide laser lysis of the interarytenoid synechia • Advancement of a posteriorly based mucosal flap • Posterior cordotomy/cordectomy • Arytenoidectomy b) Open posterior cricoid split with graft
Subglottic		a. Endoscopic (radial incision and dilation) b. Anterior cricoid split c. Anterior–posterior laryngotracheoplasty d. Cricotracheal resection
Tracheal		a) Endoscopic (radial incision and dilation) b) T-tube and stents c) Segmental resection d) Augmentation e) Slide tracheoplasty

stenoses of minimal thickness (< 1 cm). An endoscopic approach is often used initially, followed by an open procedure after recurrence.

Open surgical procedures can be broadly divided into two categories: laryngotracheal resection and laryngotracheal expansion. Laryngotracheal resection removes the area of stenosis, whereas laryngotracheal expansion enlarges the area of stenosis by splitting the airway and inserting a graft—often autologous rib cartilage.

Supraglottic Stenosis

Supraglottic stenosis is rare and can be caused by trauma, caustic injury, or infection. Endoscopic laser ablation of abnormal tissue is occasionally successful. If restenosis occurs, an external open approach is used, either via a transhyoid pharyngotomy or laryngofissure. Efforts are made to remove scar and preserve mucosa to cover denuded areas with mucosal flaps. If necessary, a buccal graft can be harvested for further coverage. A laryngeal stent is used during the healing process. Alternatively, a supraglottic laryngectomy can be performed.

Glottic Stenosis

Anterior Glottic Stenosis/Web

An anterior glottic web can be congenital or traumatic. In adults, it is most often iatrogenic, resulting from bilateral vocal fold surgery causing scarring at the anterior commissure. This disease can be managed by an endoscopic or an open approach. If the anterior glottic web extends less than 5 mm infraglottally, then endoscopic lysis of the web can be performed with a laser

or cold steel instrumentation. Lysis alone is rarely successful. Adjunctive procedures include injection of corticosteroids into the area of lysis, topical application of mitomycin C, and endoscopic placement of a Silastic keel with removal at 2 to 4 weeks.

If there is significant infraglottic extension of cicatrix, an anterior laryngofissure with resection of scar tissue, resurfacing with mucosal grafts, and placement of a soft, molded laryngeal stent should be performed.

Posterior Glottic Stenosis

Posterior glottic stenosis may also be managed endoscopically or by open surgery. The surgical choice is guided by the extent of posterior glottic involvement, as described in the classification of Bogdasarian and Olson. Type I is managed with endoscopic lysis of the interarytenoid synechia (▶ Fig. 91.6). Patients with type I posterior glottic stenosis have an excellent prognosis for decannulation, and many regain normal vocal fold motion. Types II and III can be managed with endoscopic laser resection of posterior scar tissue and advancement of a posteriorly based mucosal flap from the posterior cricoid mucosa. Type IV stenosis is the most severe, defined by bilateral cricoarytenoid joint ankylosis with scarring and contracture of the interarytenoid space. An endoscopic laser posterior cordotomy can statically enlarge the posterior respiratory glottis (▶ Fig. 91.7) while maintaining some phonatory function of the anterior glottis. An open or endoscopic arytenoidectomy can remove additional tissue, although patients may have postoperative dysphagia after resection of the lateral lamina of the arytenoid. It is important to counsel patients considering these procedures that they will be trading some voice and swallowing function

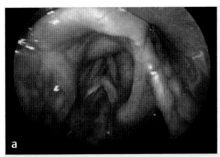
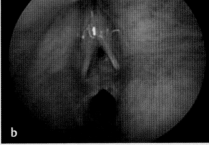
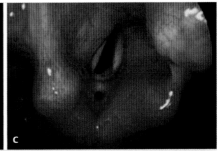

Fig. 91.6 Development of posterior glottic stenosis type I: interarytenoid synechia. (**a**) Endotracheal tube in place showing the development of florid posterior glottic granulation tissue and subglottic edema. (**b**) When the tube is removed, the granulation tissue prolapses into the airway. (**c**) If the granulation fronds fuse together, an interarytenoid synechia can develop.

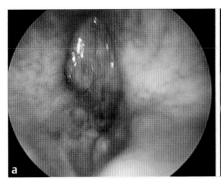
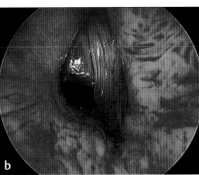

Fig. 91.7 (**a**) Preoperative and (**b**) postoperative views of a posterior cordotomy/cordectomy.

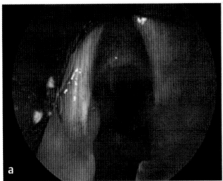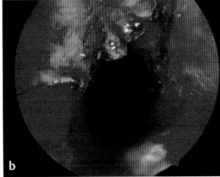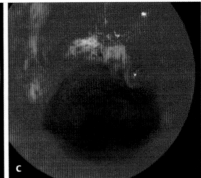

Fig. 91.8 (a–c) Radial incision and dilation of idiopathic subglottic stenosis.

for airway improvement. Open approaches include a posterior cricoid split with insertion of a rib cartilage expansion graft to separate the interarytenoid space. Alternatively, if the transcervical approach allows the restoration of arytenoid motion after scar resection, then the posterior glottis can be covered with a buccal graft or an advanced pharyngeal flap to prevent restenosis and restore glottal competence without a permanent deterioration of voice or swallowing function.

Subglottic Stenosis

Endoscopic Management

Endoscopic radial incision and dilation is the procedure most commonly used for subglottic stenosis (▶ Fig. 91.8). The stenotic area is incised with either sharp instrumentation or a laser. Dilation can be performed pneumatically or with rigid instrumentation. Theoretically, the radial incisions allow the preservation of intervening areas of mucosa, which will then epithelialize the dilated area and retard the re-formation of scar.

Adjunctive procedures include the topical application of mitomycin C to the dilated area. Mitomycin C is an antineoplastic antibiotic derived from *Streptomyces caespitosus* that preferentially inhibits fibroblast proliferation. One study showed a statistically significant increase in the success rate of endoscopic treatment of acquired upper airway stenosis from less than 20% to 75% when topical mitomycin C was added to the treatment regimen. Unfortunately, the efficacy of mitomycin C has been questioned in other studies, and possible complications include eschar formation (which can acutely obstruct the airway) and risk for malignancy. Other adjuncts that have been used include intralesional and systemic corticosteroids, perioperative antibiotics, and antireflux medications. Despite these measures, restenosis unfortunately commonly occurs.

Anterior Cricoid Split

Anterior cricoid split is a type of laryngotracheal expansion. It was first used in premature infants as an alternative to tracheotomy in the management of acquired subglottic stenosis. The anterior cricoid cartilage is divided in the midline, and the upper first and second tracheal rings are also split. This procedure allows the cricoid ring to expand. The patient may need to remain intubated for up to 10 days after the procedure, but a tracheostomy is ideally avoided.

Anterior and Posterior Laryngotracheoplasty

Anterior laryngotracheoplasty and posterior laryngotracheoplasty are laryngotracheal expansion procedures used in type III or IV subglottic stenosis or when an endoscopic procedure has failed. A laryngofissure is used to gain exposure, the anterior and/or posterior cricoid ring is divided in the midline, and cartilage grafts are placed to maintain expansion of the laryngotracheal framework. Cartilage grafts can be harvested from rib or nasal septum. This procedure requires a tracheostomy and usually placement of an endoluminal stent to support the grafts.

Cricotracheal Resection

When the stenosis involves the subglottic area but spares the vocal folds and leaves a small "antrum" of normal subglottis, the patient is a candidate for a cricotracheal resection (▶ Fig. 91.9). In this procedure, the stenotic tissue associated with the anterior cricoid ring can be resected and normal trachea inset into the demucosalized posterior cricoid plate. Some surgeons choose to place a "Grillo suture" from the chin to the presternal skin to encourage patients to remain in cervical flexion and prevent unnecessary tension on the anastomosis. In properly selected patients, the success rate can be over 90%. Most of these patients will develop some postsurgical voice change that may be permanent.

Tracheal Stenosis

Endoscopic Management

The endoscopic management of tracheal stenosis is very similar to that of subglottic stenosis. Laser or sharp instrumentation can be used for the incision or resection of cicatrix. Dilation can be performed with rigid or pneumatic instrumentation. Adjunctive measures include mitomycin C, intralesional and systemic corticosteroids, perioperative antibiotics, and antireflux medications.

T-Tube and Stents

In patients who have isolated tracheal or subglottic stenosis and normal laryngeal function, airway stenting can be judiciously considered. The role of airway stents is controversial in benign tracheal stenosis. Although the stent will provide imme-

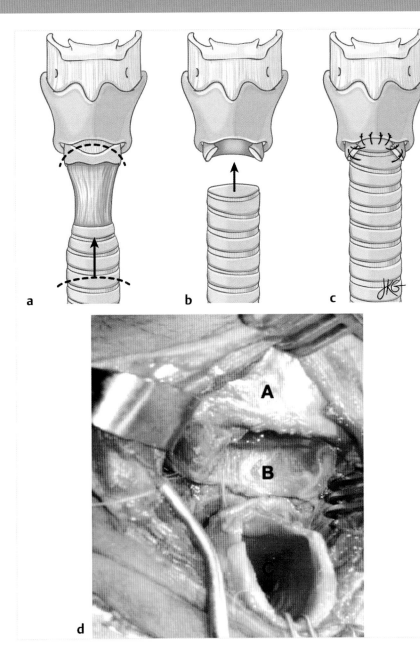

Fig. 91.9 Cricotracheal resection. (a–c) The stenotic tissue and anterior cricoid ring are resected, and normal trachea is advanced and inset into the demucosalized posterior cricoid plate. (d) Intraoperative view. *A*, thyroid cartilage. *B*, posterior cricoid plate with mucosa removed. The anterior arch of the cricoid has been resected. *C*, normal trachea, to be inset into the cricoid bed.

diate relief of the airway narrowing, the risks for the development of mucous plugs or granulation, stent migration, and long-term propagation of the damaged tracheal segment are serious considerations. Stents are most often selected for use in patients with malignant airway obstruction or inoperable lesions, and occasionally for the temporary support of a surgical repair.

For properly selected patients who require an airway appliance but cannot speak around a tracheotomy tube or whose tracheotomy tube cannot be capped because of suprastomal or subglottic stenosis, a T-tube can be used for airway support both inferior and superior to the stoma. This appliance is placed through an existing tracheal stoma and extends over the length of the stenotic or malacic segment. The external limb of the T-tube anchors the appliance in the proper position within the trachea to prevent migration, and it also allows access to the lumen for suction and the instillation of saline or medications. The external limb is *not* to be used as an airway but rather is kept capped to allow the patient to breathe and phonate through the glottis. This appliance does not have an inner cannula and is prone to mucous plug occlusion, especially if the external limb is left open and the natural process of humidification of inspired air in the upper airway is bypassed.

Segmental Resection

If the stenosis or malacic segment is isolated to the trachea, then a simple resection with an end-to-end anastomosis can be performed with a better than 90% success rate (▶ Fig. 91.10). Grillo et al reported on a series of 503 patients who underwent surgical treatment for post-intubation tracheal stenosis. A total of 471 patients reported good (87.5%) or satisfactory (6.2%) results. Complications included granulation, dehiscence, laryngeal nerve injury, airway obstruction, mediastinitis, hemorrhage, infection, myocardial infarction, tracheo-esophageal fistula, pneumothorax, deep venous thrombosis, recurrent stenosis, and death.

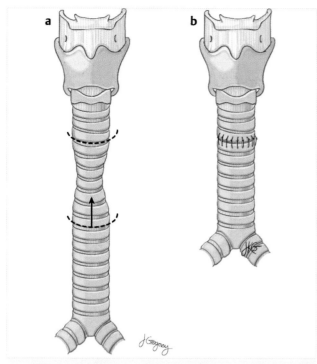

Fig. 91.10 (a) Segmental resection and **(b)** primary anastomosis of segments for isolated tracheal stenosis.

Augmentation

Augmentation tracheoplasty can be performed with autologous material such as rib cartilage, periosteum, pericardium, pedicled muscle flaps, composite grafts, esophagus, omentum, or solvent-preserved dura. Cartilage is commonly used as graft material for several reasons. It is a rigid autologous tissue. It derives its nutrition through diffusion and as a result can survive without a direct vascular supply. The surgical procedure follows the same principles as those used for other laryngotracheal expansion procedures.

Slide Tracheoplasty

A slide tracheoplasty can be used when segmental resection is not possible because of the length of abnormal trachea. This procedure is usually used for congenital stenosis in children and is not routinely applied in cases of traumatic stenosis (▶ Fig. 91.11).

91.8 Conclusion

This chapter has briefly reviewed key aspects in the evaluation and management of laryngotracheal stenosis. Treatment options are based on the severity and position of the stenosis. This is a challenging disease to manage, and patients need to be appropriately counseled regarding the risks and expectations of intervention.

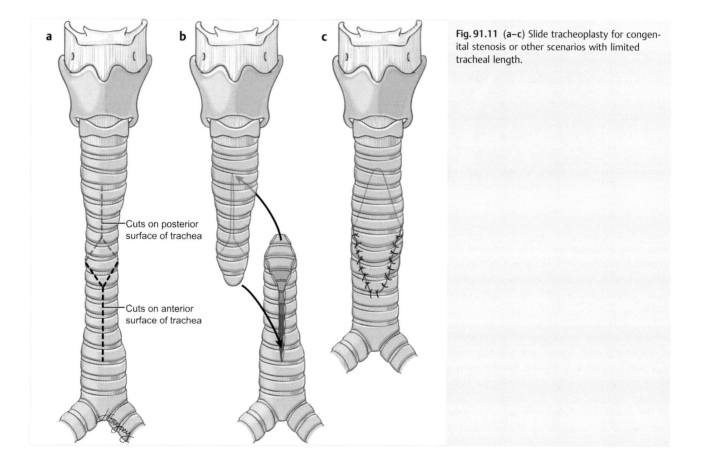

Cuts on posterior surface of trachea

Cuts on anterior surface of trachea

Fig. 91.11 (a–c) Slide tracheoplasty for congenital stenosis or other scenarios with limited tracheal length.

91.9 Roundsmanship

- The most common cause of laryngotracheal stenosis is prolonged endotracheal intubation; other causes include systemic inflammatory disease, infection, and neoplasm. Idiopathic subglottic stenosis is a diagnosis of exclusion.
- Airway obstruction may initially be misdiagnosed as asthma refractory to conventional treatment.
- Three important classifications for laryngotracheal stenosis are the Myer-Cotton, Bogdasarian and Olson, and McCaffrey systems.
- The surgeon's choice of intervention is significantly affected by the patient's underlying medical conditions, the ability to safely access the airway, and the nature of the airway deficits.
- Endoscopic incision and dilation can be used successfully to treat subglottic and tracheal stenosis. The main disadvantages are the risk for restenosis and the need for repeated procedures.
- Stents and T-tubes should be used judiciously in carefully selected patients. They both carry a significant risk for mucous plug formation and fatal airway obstruction.
- Open surgical procedures can be broadly divided into two categories: laryngotracheal resection and laryngotracheal expansion. Laryngotracheal resection removes the area of stenosis, whereas laryngotracheal expansion enlarges the area of stenosis by splitting the airway and inserting a graft.
- Placement of a tracheotomy tube is a time-honored option for patients with significant medical comorbidities or complicated multilevel stenosis.

91.10 Recommended Reading

[1] Bogdasarian RS, Olson NR. Posterior glottic laryngeal stenosis. Otolaryngol Head Neck Surg (1979) 1980; 88: 765–772

[2] Cotton RT, Myer CM. Contemporary surgical management of laryngeal stenosis in children. Am J Otolaryngol 1984; 5: 360–368

[3] Duncavage JA, Koriwchak MJ. Open surgical techniques for laryngotracheal stenosis. Otolaryngol Clin North Am 1995; 28: 785–795

[4] George M, Lang F, Pasche P, Monnier P. Surgical management of laryngotracheal stenosis in adults. Eur Arch Otorhinolaryngol 2005; 262: 609–615

[5] Grillo HC, Donahue DM, Mathisen DJ, Wain JC, Wright CD. Postintubation tracheal stenosis. Treatment and results. J Thorac Cardiovasc Surg 1995; 109: 486–492, discussion 492–493

[6] Lorenz RR. Adult laryngotracheal stenosis: etiology and surgical management. Curr Opin Otolaryngol Head Neck Surg 2003; 11: 467–472

[7] McCaffrey TV. Classification of laryngotracheal stenosis. Laryngoscope 1992; 102: 1335–1340

[8] McCaffrey TV. Management of laryngotracheal stenosis on the basis of site and severity. Otolaryngol Head Neck Surg 1993; 109: 468–473

[9] Meyer TK, Wolf J. Lysis of interarytenoid synechia (Type I Posterior Glottic Stenosis): vocal fold mobility and airway results. Laryngoscope 2011; 121: 2165–2171

[10] Perepelitsyn I, Shapshay SM. Endoscopic treatment of laryngeal and tracheal stenosis-has mitomycin C improved the outcome? Otolaryngol Head Neck Surg 2004; 131: 16–20

[11] Nouraei SA, Ma E, Patel A, Howard DJ, Sandhu GS. Estimating the population incidence of adult post-intubation laryngotracheal stenosis. Clin Otolaryngol 2007; 32: 411–412

[12] Whited RE. A prospective study of laryngotracheal sequelae in long-term intubation. Laryngoscope 1984; 94: 367–377

92 Laryngeal Trauma

Steven David Schaefer

92.1 Introduction

External laryngeal injuries are rare, accounting for only 1 in 30,000 emergency room visits. Early and careful management of these injuries has a profound consequence on the immediate probability of the patient's survival and long-term quality-of-life. Our approach to these injuries has been to apply the basic principles of laryngeal mechanics to repeated observation and to the refinement of medical and surgical treatment over the past 25 years.

92.2 Applied Anatomy and Physiology

The human larynx is a highly evolved respiratory sphincter. The laryngeal skeleton, which is a derivative of the second through sixth branchial arches, consists of the hyoid bone, three single cartilages (the thyroid, cricoid, and epiglottic cartilages), and three paired cartilages (the arytenoid, corniculate, and cuneiform cartilages). The cartilages are suspended together by fibrous ligaments and membranes. Phonation is the product of chest compression of subglottic air overcoming the elastic and muscular forces of vocal fold closure. Acting as a sound source, the larynx cycles between these two forces to produce a tone that is modulated by the vocal tract (broadly, the vocal tract can be defined as extending from the diaphragm to the lips). The complex interaction between vocal fold tension, mass, length, and mucosal covering and subglottic air pressure is best described by the myoelastic–aerodynamic theory. as we seek to repair the traumatized larynx, we must employ an understanding of laryngeal anatomy and physiology to guide us in deciding between medical and surgical management, and the extent of surgical treatment (see Chapter 74 for a detailed discussion of laryngeal anatomy and physiology).

92.3 The Disease Process

92.3.1 Etiology and Pathogenesis

External laryngeal injuries are now uncommonly seen in most emergency departments for several reasons. First, the overall incidence of neck trauma adjusted for the population has declined in comparison with the incidence in the early 1990s, reflecting safer designs in automobiles and decreasing violent crime in the United States. Second, the most severely injured patients die at the seen of the accident or assault and are not counted in estimates of laryngeal trauma. Third, the larynx is afforded partial protection by its position in the neck. Anteriorly, the inferior projection of the mandible partially shields the larynx from direct trauma; posteriorly, the rigid cervical spine protects the larynx. Nonetheless, injuries occur, and the resultant damage to the larynx is usually characteristic of the mechanism of injury. The mechanisms of external laryngeal injury can be divided into blunt trauma (including clothes-line, crushing, and strangulation injuries) and penetrating trauma.

Anterior blunt injuries are most commonly the result of motor vehicle accidents. If no seat belt is worn or if only a lap belt is used, the driver is thrust forward during rapid deceleration with the neck hyperextended. This position removes the bony protection of the mandible, exposing the larynx to anterior crushing forces. If the larynx then strikes the steering wheel or dashboard, it may be compressed between these objects and the cervical spine.

Clothesline injuries occur when the rider of a vehicle, such as a motorcycle or snowmobile, encounters a fixed horizontal object, such as a clothesline at neck level. This type of injury imparts the full momentum of the rider and the vehicle over the relatively small anterior neck, resulting in massive trauma. Many of these injuries lead to immediate death from a crushed larynx or separation of the cricoid from the thyroid or tracheal cartilage. The latter injuries are frequently accompanied by disruption of one or both recurrent laryngeal nerves. Strangulation injuries occur from manual compression, from assaults with strangulation by a soft object, or from attempted suicides by hanging. Typically, the initial finding may be hoarseness or abrasions on the overlying skin of the neck. However, these injuries may later (in 12 to 24 hours) be associated with marked edema of the larynx and resultant loss of airway. The magnitude of the force sustained to the anterior neck should be considered in the management of such patients to avoid subsequent potential loss of the airway. Overall, in blunt trauma to the anterior neck, fractures of the thyroid cartilage occur more frequently than of all other airway cartilages combined.

Injury from gunshot wounds depends on the type of weapon used, the effective range of the weapon, and the ammunition. Gunshots at close range impart intense energy to the soft tissues and are usually fatal. Low-velocity handguns (commonly used in domestic assaults) generally have only a moderate blast effect on surrounding tissue. These injuries may be misleading on initial examination because of the bullet's erratic course in soft tissues. High-velocity weapons, such as hunting rifles and military assault weapons, impart a significant amount of kinetic energy to the tissues. In these injuries, tissue viability is widely compromised, and initial impressions as to the extent of wounding are frequently inadequate. Knife injuries do not destroy tissue distant to the path of injury, and their course may be accurately estimated from the entrance and exit wounds.

The pediatric larynx is injured less often than the adult larynx. Situated higher in the neck than the adult larynx, the child's larynx is afforded greater protection by the caudal projection of the mandible. However, the pattern of injury reflects a dynamic between the loose attachments of the overlying mucous membranes and ligaments and the increased elasticity of the cartilaginous framework. Furthermore, the cross-sectional area of the pediatric larynx compared with that of the adult larynx is decreased. The combination of potentially increased soft-tissue injury and edema with decreased cross-sectional area makes the pediatric airway especially vulnerable to embarrassment. These injuries may be difficult to recognize because of the lack of obvious cartilaginous fractures.

92.4 Medical Evaluation

92.4.1 Acute Medical Evaluation and Management

When a patient with a neck injury presents to the emergency department, the first priority is to establish an airway. This may be very difficult and often requires emergent tracheotomy or cricothyroidotomy. Care should be taken to avoid manipulation of the neck. Until a cervical spine injury has been excluded, no extension of the neck should be allowed during either orotracheal intubation or tracheotomy. After the airway is secured, venous access should be obtained with at least two large-bore cannulas. Isotonic fluids are administered as needed to maintain circulation. The patient is then disrobed and examined for other injuries. If the patient is unstable after these measures, immediate surgery is needed. However, if the patient is relatively stable after these measures, diagnostic assessment may proceed. The minimum radiographic evaluation consists of a cervical spine series and a chest radiograph. After full assessment of all injuries, the various physicians involved should determine the order of management and proceed accordingly.

92.4.2 Secondary Medical Evaluation

The presentations of external laryngeal trauma vary from obvious open fractures to subtle aberrations of laryngeal function.

History

Understanding the mechanism of wounding is important to deciding on the immediate course of treatment and predicting the potential injuries. A patient arriving in the emergency department after striking the steering wheel with the anterior neck may appear stable within the first minutes after the accident. Within the next several hours, the initially normal findings of the examination, including laryngoscopy, may evolve into life-threatening endolaryngeal edema and hematomas. In such an example, the history of significant energy being imparted to the neck should alert the physician to the potential for an evolving catastrophic event. In contrast, a low-energy accidental blow of the fist or other less intense blow to the larynx can result in a displaced thyroid cartilage fracture. In penetrating trauma, the type of weapon and ammunition used, the range at which the injury occurred, and the anatomical site of the wound must all be considered. Having seen all of these events, we advocate that any patient with a history of trauma to the central compartment of the neck be considered to have a potential airway injury until proved otherwise.

Physical Examination

In our experience, only respiratory distress seems to correlate with the severity of blunt injury (▶ Table 92.1). Visual examination of the neck may reveal an open fracture or laryngocutaneous fistula, or more often nothing in the case of blunt trauma. The larynx should be palpated for crepitus. Tenderness to palpation, although not specific, is often present in significant injury. The skin of the neck may reveal contusions or abrasions from blunt trauma or a line pattern indicative of a strangulation injury. Penetrating injuries are examined for an entrance and an exit wound, and the most likely path of travel of the projectile should be determined. Open wounds are not explored with instruments, nor are they probed to avoid dislodging a hematoma and initiating further bleeding. The cervical spine should be palpated for any bony step-off fractures, dislocations, or tenderness. Hemoptysis may reveal an injury to the upper aerodigestive system, but it is often difficult to differentiate from bleeding caused by associated facial trauma.

External laryngeal injuries are often associated with a change in voice. A patient with severe trauma may be entirely aphonic. More commonly, a dysphonic voice is present secondary to alterations in the larynx, or the voice is muffled secondary to supraglottic or upper vocal tract injury. Hematomas of the true vocal folds add mass to these vibratory units and lower the fundamental frequency of vibration. Paresis of the vocal fold from damage to the recurrent laryngeal nerve or from mechanical dislocation of the cricoarytenoid joint may cause a weak, breathy voice. Finally, any injury to the larynx that changes the airflow patterns has the potential to alter the voice.

Among the most serious alterations of laryngeal function is the abnormal flow of air through the upper airway. In instances of cricotracheal separation, the partially transected airway may

Table 92.1 Presenting symptoms of 68 patients with laryngeal trauma

Presenting symptoms								Type of injury		
Group	Hoarseness	Pain/tenderness	Hemoptysis	Dysphagia	Subcutaneous emphysema	Impaired respiration	Hematoma	MVA	Blunt	Penetrating
I	8	7	1	1	1	1	0	7	3	1
II	10	2	2	2	5	18	3	7	9	19
III	4	1	1	1	5	8	1	2	2	8
IV	3	0	0	1	2	6	0	2	2	6

Abbreviation: MVA, motor vehicle accident.
Source: From Schaefer SD, Close LG. Acute management of laryngeal trauma. Update. Ann Otol Rhinol Laryngol 1989;98(2):98–104.
Note: Groups I through IV refer to the form of management and are discussed in ▶ Table 92.2. In group IV (patients with the most severe injuries), the severity of injury did not correlate with the presenting symptoms.

be maintained solely by a bridge of mucous membrane between the cricoid and trachea. In gunshot wounds, the path of the missile serves as a laryngocutaneous fistula and allows respiration despite obstruction at the glottic or supraglottic level. In this instance, airflow from the wound will be obvious, and no attempt should be made to cover, compress, or otherwise manipulate such a wound until the surgeon is ready to secure the airway. Stridor may be caused by bilateral vocal fold paresis or disruption or may result from any combination of unilateral immobility and subglottic, glottic, or supraglottic edema or hematoma. If severe enough, edema alone with healthy vocal fold movement may cause stridor. As discussed above, in some patients the edema or hematoma can evolve over a few hours, which may permit a recognition of subglottic, glottic, or supraglottic airway compromise. In many other patients, the airway comprise is too rapid to permit a distinction among inspiratory, expiratory, and mixed stridor. A third, more subtle form of laryngeal dysfunction is aspiration, which is usually caused by immobility of one or both vocal folds. Although not immediately clinically apparent after injury, aspiration may present later as pneumonia.

After the initial examination and securing of the airway, examination of the endolaryngeal anatomy is attempted. Since the 1980s, flexible fiber-optic laryngoscopic examination has made possible an improved nonoperative evaluation of the injured larynx. After careful insertion of the laryngoscope through the nares, the oropharynx and hypopharynx are examined for injury. The larynx is examined for hematomas and lacerations, and their size and location are noted. The arytenoids are evaluated for full range of motion during phonation and respiration. Partial limitation of range of motion indicates a structural deformity or dislocation of the arytenoids, whereas complete immobility is more suggestive of recurrent laryngeal nerve injury. Failure of the true vocal folds to meet in the same horizontal plane may indicate a structural change in the laryngeal framework or superior laryngeal nerve injury. In minor injuries with sufficient glottic closure to trigger a strobe, videostroboscopic laryngoscopy is helpful to reveal small alterations secondary to either muscle or mucosal injuries. Finally, exposed cartilage is recorded, along with the integrity of the surrounding mucous membrane.

92.4.3 Testing

Laryngeal Imaging

Plain films may identify gross fractures but are limited to a two-dimensional image of the relevant anatomy. Magnetic resonance imaging offers superior soft-tissue definition but does not permit visualization of the laryngeal hard tissue. In contrast, computed tomography (CT) permits an evaluation of the laryngeal skeletal and soft tissue in a noninvasive manner. We recommend reserving CT for patients in whom laryngeal trauma is suspected by history but in whom the extent of injury is not obvious on physical examination. Such patients are those who have only one sign or symptom of laryngeal trauma, such as hoarseness, and minimal physical findings suggestive of laryngeal injury. In this instance, CT may allow the surgeon to confirm the lack of injury in a noninvasive manner without direct, operative laryngoscopy and the concomitant need for

general anesthesia. CT may also be used to identify the patient with minimally displaced midline or lateral thyroid cartilage fractures that are otherwise unremarkable and minimally symptomatic. Such unrepaired lateral displacement of the thyroid cartilage impairs phonation by disrupting complete vocal fold closure or laryngeal valving. In a relatively small number of patients with massive edema or hematomas without lacerations, direct laryngoscopy has been insufficient to visualize the laryngeal framework. In these patients, CT is employed to search for laryngeal fractures. If none are detected, the patient undergoes a tracheotomy to preserve the airway and is observed, so that open exploration is avoided.

The management of injuries to the larynx is based on the mechanism and extent of injury found during the initial assessment. The first priority is always securing the airway. The long-term priority is the restoration of normal laryngeal function. To meet these goals, the initial management can be encompassed in four questions. First, does the patient have a tenuous airway? Given the propensity for central compartment neck trauma to compromise the laryngeal skeleton, this question should be cautiously answered. Second, how can the extent of injury best be evaluated? These options can include fiber-optic laryngoscopy, CT, or direct laryngoscopy. Third, after the first two questions have been satisfied, is the injury likely to heal spontaneously with a result equal to or better than that of surgical intervention? Forth, if the outcome of the injury is in doubt or so severe as to require surgical treatment, which procedures are indicated? The answers to the last two questions require a thorough knowledge of laryngeal mechanics and experience (▶ Fig. 92.1). The latter is increasingly difficult to acquire, given the rarity of these injuries.

92.5 Treatment

92.5.1 Medical Management

Medical management assumes that the patient does not require a tracheotomy and has an otherwise stable airway. If the patient has only the following injuries, we recommend close observation within the first 24 hours after injury and head-of-bed elevation. These injuries include (1) minor endolaryngeal mucosal lacerations without involvement of the anterior commissure or free margin of the true vocal fold; (2) single, nondisplaced, nonangulated fractures of the thyroid cartilage without overlying mucosal lacerations or exposed cartilage; (3) nonobstructing endolaryngeal edema; and (4) small, stable hematomas that are not causing respiratory embarrassment. Corticosteroids may be useful if given early after injury.

92.5.2 Surgical Management

Surgical treatment is indicated in injuries that will not spontaneously recover and therefore require surgical restoration of the traumatized larynx. These injuries are those (1) involving the anterior commissure or free margin of the true vocal fold, (2) resulting in exposed cartilage, (3) leading to multiple or displaced fractures of the thyroid cartilage or any fracture of the cricoid cartilage, (4) causing vocal fold paralysis or sufficient airway compromise to require intubation or tracheotomy, (5)

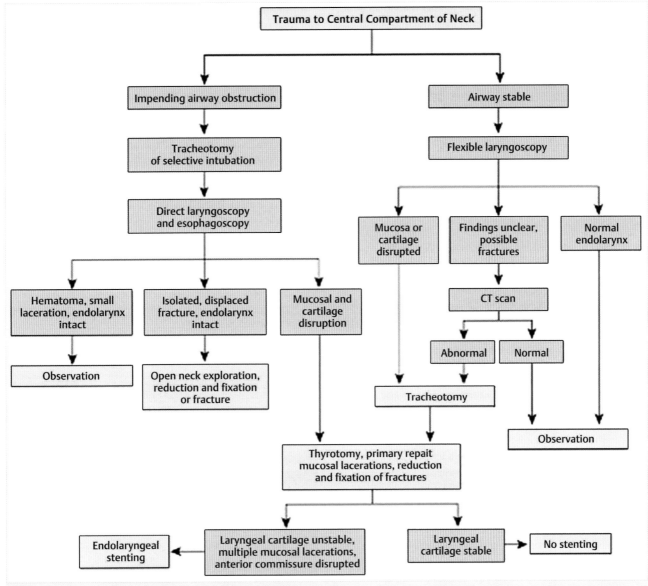

Fig. 92.1 Management protocol for the acutely injured larynx. CT, computed tomography. (Source: Adapted from Schaefer SD. The treatment of acute external laryngeal injuries. Arch Otolaryngol 1991;117:35.)

resulting in glottic or transglottic lacerations, and (6) associated with trauma to another area of the neck that requires surgical intervention. Repair of the larynx should be coordinated with all surgical teams involved and with the anesthesiologist. The person responsible for the airway at each stage of the procedure should be designated before the patient is brought to the operating room. Plans for emergently obtaining an airway and the instruments required for surgery should also be established.

The most conservative, reliable method of securing an airway in a patient with laryngeal injury is local tracheotomy while the patient is awake. Endotracheal intubation may further damage the larynx, be exceedingly difficult, interfere with subsequent examination and repair of the larynx, and convert an urgent procedure to an emergent one. Endotracheal intubation is acceptable when (1) the endolaryngeal mucous membrane is in-

tact, (2) the laryngeal skeleton is minimally displaced, and (3) the intubation is performed by one highly skilled in such procedures.

After local tracheotomy or the selective use of intubation, general anesthesia is induced followed by operative, direct laryngoscopy. The larynx is examined for exposed cartilage, hematomas, lacerations, and range of motion of the true vocal folds. The subglottis is evaluated for injury to the cricoid and trachea. Rigid esophagoscopy is performed to rule out injury to the esophagus.

Management of the traumatized pediatric airway presents special problems. Endotracheal intubation in the injured pediatric larynx has all of the same risks outlined above for the adult. The option of local tracheotomy is not feasible in a frightened, injured child. The time margin of error is also less because the arterial oxygen saturation drops more rapidly than in an adult. In this instance, rigid bronchoscopy is performed to secure the airway under direct visualization. A tracheotomy may then be performed over the bronchoscope.

After an airway has been obtained and endoscopy performed, and following review of the CT findings, the need for open exploration and repair is reevaluated. In patients with edema, hematomas, nondisplaced fractures of the thyroid cartilage, healthy true vocal fold motion, and no injury to the anterior commissure or free margin of the true vocal fold, no further surgery is usually indicated. Anesthesia is discontinued, the head of the bed is elevated, and the patient is observed carefully. Serial flexible fiber-optic laryngoscopic examinations are performed to ensure proper healing, and the tracheotomy tube is removed as soon as removal can be tolerated.

In patients with more severe injuries, surgical exploration is performed. In the past, controversy existed as to the optimal time for repair. Some authors had advocated delay of repair for 3 to 5 days to allow edema to subside, making it easier to identify mucosal lacerations. We believe that the best results are obtained with early repair, avoiding the morbidity of leaving open wounds in a contaminated field. Following exposure of the endolarynx via a thyrotomy, mucosal lacerations are meticulously repaired with 5–0 or 6–0 absorbable sutures. Dislocated arytenoids are reduced. In most injuries, wounds can be closed with adjacent mucosa. In cases involving military weapons or other instances in which the loss of tissue is large, regional mucosal flaps or skin grafts may be used to complete the lining of the larynx. After repair of the injured mucous membrane and muscle, the anterior commissure is reconstituted by suturing the anterior margin of the true vocal fold to the outer perichondrium. Regardless of the need for stenting, as is discussed below, reconstituting the anterior commissure is essential to maintain the scaphoid shape of this site and to preserve a normal voice. The thyrotomy is closed with permanent sutures, wire, or fixation plates.

The advantages of using a stent should be weighed against the risk for additional damage to the mucosa. Stents are recommended for injuries involving the anterior commissure, massive lacerations, comminuted fractures of the thyroid cartilage, and cases in which the architecture of the larynx is not maintained by open fixation of the fractures. The advantages of stenting in these instances are decreased web formation at the anterior commissure, decreased synechiae from extensive lacerations, and better support of the laryngeal architecture during healing. The placement of an endolaryngeal stent without open reduction and internal fixation of fractures and without closure of lacerations is unsatisfactory because both the injuries and the larynx are too complex to benefit from the placement of a lumen keeper. The choice of stents ranges from finger cots filled with foam rubber to commercially manufactured polymeric silicone stents. If preformed stents are not available, a finger cot stent can be made by packing it with gauze, or a silicone stent can be made from an endotracheal tube. This endotracheal tube stent is created by clapping the tube and then placing it in the autoclave for heating and reshaping (▶ Fig. 92.2).

All should be roughly in the shape of the larynx and made of soft material to avoid further mucosal damage. The stent should extend from the false vocal fold to the first tracheal ring to add stability and prevent endolaryngeal adhesions. Ideally, the stent should be secured in such a manner as to be easily removed with endoscopic techniques. Following repair of the laryngeal wounds, the strap muscles are reapproximated, and the wound is closed over a drain.

Various other injuries may also be encountered during surgery. As much as one-third of the anterior cricoid or trachea can be repaired by using the sternohyoid muscle and its overlying fascia. Loss of the anterior third of the thyroid cartilage or hemiglottis can be repaired by the closure of mucosal lacerations over a stent. If open reduction and internal fixation with stenting are unsuccessful in restoring the laryngeal architecture because of massive tissue loss, partial or total laryngectomy may be necessary. The decision for partial or total laryngectomy should be based on the defect, according to the same guidelines used in oncologic reconstruction. However, total laryngectomy has not been necessary in large series of cases of laryngeal trauma and is more likely to be considered acceptable management for military wounds.

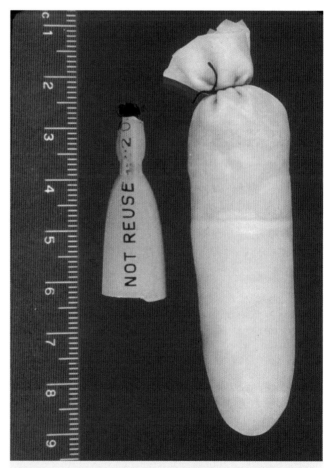

Fig. 92.2 Examples of a finger cot and a shaped endotracheal tube. These can be used as laryngeal stents if preformed stents are not available.

Table 92.2 Voice and airway results in evaluable patients by treatment group

Group	Voice			Airway			Total (N = 115)
	Good	Fair	Poor	Good	Fair	Poor	
I	20	0	0	20	0	0	20
II	38	3	0	40	1	0	41
III	18	3	0	21	0	0	21
IV	22	10	0	31	0	2	33

Source: From Schaefer SD. The acute management of external laryngeal trauma. A 27-year experience. Arch Otolaryngol Head Neck Surg 1992;118 (6):598–604.

Note: Group I patients had no airway compromise and were judged to have reversible injuries. They were managed by observation only. Group II patients had airway compromise and were considered to have reversible injuries. They were managed by tracheotomy, direct laryngoscopy, esophagoscopy, and observation. Group III patients were judged to have irreversible laryngeal fractures and/or lacerations that required management by open reduction and fixation of disrupted cartilage and/or mucous membrane. Group IV patients had more severe injuries, as discussed, and management differed from group III in that endolaryngeal stents were used.

92.5.3 Postoperative Care

We prescribe postoperative antibiotics for 5 to 7 days in an effort to reduce infection and the formation of granulation tissue. However, we are unaware of published verification of this practice. The head of the bed should be elevated, as tolerated, to minimize edema. The patient should be encouraged to ambulate as soon as ambulation can be tolerated. If a tracheotomy is present, routine care is provided. Stents placed at the time of surgery should be removed as soon as possible to prevent further mucosal damage, usually 10 to 14 days after surgery. Decannulation may be performed as soon as the stent is removed. Follow-up examinations should be scheduled for at least 1 year to assess the return of true vocal fold function and to monitor the development of subglottic stenosis. Proton pump inhibitors should be routinely used to prevent reflux, which may cause increased scarring of laryngeal tissues. When possible, nasogastric tubes are avoided to reduce reflux and prevent the posterior cricoid mucosal erosion associated with their use.

92.6 Complications

Complications after the repair of external laryngeal trauma include impaired vocalization, respiration, and deglutition. Postoperative granulation tissue may be seen after removal of the stent. This is best managed by prevention with meticulous closure of all mucosal lacerations at the time of surgery. Postoperative antibiotics and early removal of the stent may reduce the amount of granulation tissue. Profuse granulation tissue that persists may be debulked with the use of endoscopy.

Vocal fold immobility may cause a weak voice if unilateral; bilateral vocal fold involvement may result in aphonia and respiratory compromise. Unless the recurrent laryngeal nerve was known to be severed at the time of surgery, medialization procedures should be delayed for at least 6 months to permit delayed recovery. If after 6 months no mobility is present, electromyography is recommended. This permits differentiation between laryngeal denervation and arytenoid fixation, as well prognostication of the return of vocal fold function. At 6 to 12 months in the patient with a unilaterally denervated larynx, a medialization procedure may be performed to strengthen the voice or prevent aspiration. Further treatment of the denervated larynx and of laryngeal and/or tracheal stenosis is discussed elsewhere.

92.7 Prognosis

The outcome after laryngeal trauma depends on the extent of the original injury and the quality of subsequent repairs. For patients who do not require operative intervention, the prognosis for a full return of function is excellent. Patients requiring surgical intervention have an excellent chance of eventual decannulation with an adequate to good voice. Long-term complications after repair are uncommon. In our series of 139 patients with acute laryngeal trauma managed as presented in this chapter, only 2 patients were left with a poor airway, as defined by the inability to be decannulated (▶ Table 92.2). Time to decannulation in the patients undergoing tracheotomy along with exploration ranged from 14 to 35 days, whereas those with stents (usually reserved for more severe injuries) needed 35 to 100 days to decannulation. All but 13 of the 115 evaluable patients achieved a good voice; those 13 were classified as having a fair voice. In conclusion, the goal of the acute treatment of laryngeal injuries is preservation of the airway and the maintenance of laryngeal function.

92.8 Roundsmanship

- The early diagnosis and management of acute external laryngeal trauma are essential to optimal preservation of the airway and voice.
- Any individual with significant trauma to the anterior neck should be considered to have a laryngeal injury until proved otherwise.
- Flexible fiber-optic laryngoscopy is the cornerstone of the diagnosis of laryngeal injuries. Injuries may evolve over hours after the initial examination of the larynx and neck, and their potential airway complications may not fully manifest at first.
- Computed tomography should be employed when the findings can best direct the course of treatment, rather than routinely.
- Surgery is reserved for patients with thyroid and cricoid cartilage fractures and with mucosal lacerations. Laryngeal stenting is useful for unstable thyroid and cricoid fractures, large endolaryngeal lacerations, and disruption of the anterior commissure.

92.9 Recommended Reading

[1] Khokhlov VD. Knitted fractures of the laryngopharynx framework as a medico-legal matter. Forensic Sci Int 1999; 104: 147–162

[2] Kleinsasser NH, Priemer FG, Schulze W, Kleinsasser OF. External trauma to the larynx: classification, diagnosis, therapy. Eur Arch Otorhinolaryngol 2000; 257: 439–444

[3] Krekorian EA. Laryngopharyngeal injuries. Laryngoscope 1975; 85: 2069–2086

[4] Mancuso AA, Hanafee WN. Computed tomography of the injured larynx. Radiology 1979; 133: 139–144

[5] Nahum AM, Siegel AW. Biodynamics of injury to the larynx in automobile collisions. Ann Otol Rhinol Laryngol 1967; 76: 781–785

[6] Pennington CL. External trauma of the larynx and trachea. Immediate treatment and management. Ann Otol Rhinol Laryngol 1972; 81: 546–554

[7] Schaefer SD, Brown OE. Selective application of CT in the management of laryngeal trauma. Laryngoscope 1983; 93: 1473–1475

[8] Schaefer SD. The acute management of external laryngeal trauma. A 27-year experience. Arch Otolaryngol Head Neck Surg 1992; 118: 598–604

[9] Schaefer SD. Primary management of laryngeal trauma. Ann Otol Rhinol Laryngol 1982; 91: 399–402

[10] Stanley RB, Cooper DS, Florman SH. Phonatory effects of thyroid cartilage fractures. Ann Otol Rhinol Laryngol 1987; 96: 493–496

[11] Stanley RB, Hanson DG. Manual strangulation injuries of the larynx. Arch Otolaryngol 1983; 109: 344–347

[12] Van Den Berg J. Myoelastic-aerodynamic theory of voice production. J Speech Hear Res 1958; 1: 227–244

93 Instrumentation and Techniques of Phonomicrosurgery

Corbin D. Sullivan and Jonathan M. Bock

93.1 Introduction

Phonomicrosurgery is a highly specialized microsurgical technique designed to restore a patient's normal voice. Improved understanding of vocal fold histology, the innovation of microflap surgery, and the development of micro instruments has allowed surgeons to successfully restore vocal fold function after the surgical treatment of most benign vocal fold lesions.

93.2 Pertinent Anatomy

Successful surgery depends on a thorough understanding of vocal fold surgical anatomy. Hirano described the histology of the vocal fold as a complex layered structure with an outer epithelium, three layers of lamina propria, and the underlying vocalis muscle (▶ Fig. 93.1). The superficial layer of the lamina propria (SLP) is critical to maintaining normal vocal fold vibratory mechanics. Before Hirano's description, vocal fold stripping was commonly performed, essentially removing all layers of the lamina propria and epithelium above the muscle. The technique was imprecise and required healing of the entire vocal fold mucosa by secondary intent. After such an injury, epithelium regenerates, but the SLP does not have this capacity. This disordered and incomplete healing results in scarring and vocal fold stiffness. The more nuanced understanding of vocal fold histology introduced by Hirano led to the discovery that preservation of as much of the original architecture of the vocal fold as possible resulted in improved voice outcomes. This led directly to the central tenet of the microflap procedure: restoring normal vocal fold vibratory mechanics while preserving as much normal tissue architecture as possible. Most benign lesions involve only the epithelium and the SLP, just deep to the vocal fold epithelium, and are therefore amenable to microflap excision. The microflap limits the incision to the epithelium, and the benign lesion is then dissected free of the SLP with maximal tissue preservation and subsequent excellent voice outcomes.

93.3 Indications for Phonomicrosurgery

Successful phonomicrosurgery begins with proper patient selection. This includes a complete work-up and careful decision making regarding medical versus surgical management. Videostroboscopy is crucial to evaluate the effect of the lesion on vocal fold mucosal wave propagation, to diagnose the type of lesion, and to identify areas of possible scarring or sulcus. Conservative management may be warranted initially because many phonotraumatic lesions resolve without surgery. Such management will likely include voice therapy as well as the treatment of any underlying disorders contributing to the patient's pathology. Occasionally, a trial of strict vocal rest and steroids may be indicated. Indications for phonomicrosurgery of benign phonotraumatic lesions include failure of conservative measures to resolve the dysphonia to a point at which the voice returns to normal or has improved enough that the patient's morbidity is minimal. Other indications may include biopsy of surgical diseases such as papilloma and suspected carcinoma. When surgery is recommended, a thorough discussion of the operative indications, risks (oral and dental injury, tongue numbness and pain, taste changes, permanent hoarseness and airway compromise, need for further surgeries, inability to achieve exposure), benefits (diagnosis, improved voice), and alternatives (observation, medical treatment, possible in-office biopsy or laser procedure) is completed with the patient to ensure proper patient education regarding the planned procedure. Patients should be counseled to discuss stopping any blood thinners with their primary care physician before surgery if at all possible.

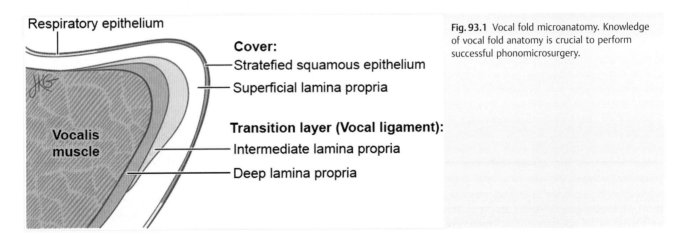

Fig. 93.1 Vocal fold microanatomy. Knowledge of vocal fold anatomy is crucial to perform successful phonomicrosurgery.

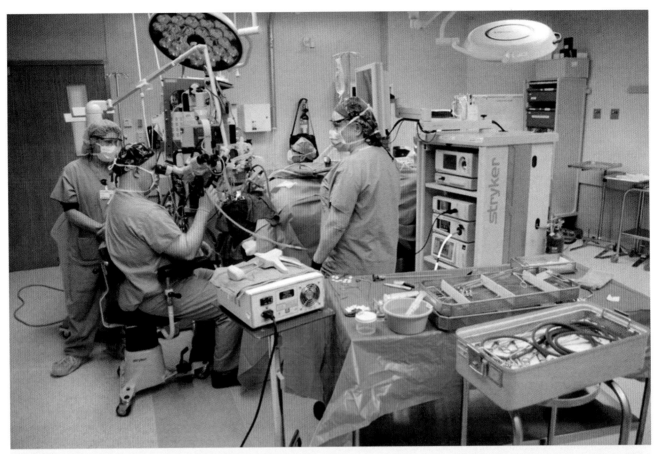

Fig. 93.2 Intraoperative room arrangement for phonomicrosurgery. The operating room table is generally turned 90 degrees away from anesthesia to allow room for the microscope, laser, surgeon's chair, and endoscopic towers.

93.4 Phonomicrosurgery Technique

93.4.1 Anesthesia and Perioperative Considerations

Appropriate communication with the anesthesiologist is essential throughout the process of microlaryngoscopy. Short-acting paralytic agents are generally used to allow easier laryngeal exposure. The anesthesiologist is asked to use the smallest allowable endotracheal tube, typically a 5.0- or 5.5-mm tube. Jet ventilation with 100% oxygen is used when adequate surgical exposure is not possible with an endotracheal tube or when surgery within the trachea or bronchus is anticipated. When laser use is a possibility, the endotracheal tube should be laser-safe, the FiO_2 should be kept below 30% to avoid airway fire, the patient's eyes should be protected with wet gauze, and wet towels should be placed over the patient's face. The patient's bed is generally turned 90 degrees away from anesthesia to allow easy interaction between the operating surgeon and the anesthesia team while affording complete access to the airway, with room for placement of operating room equipment (▶ Fig. 93.2). Universal precautions should also be observed by all operating room personnel, including wearing protective glasses, and appropriate warning signs should be posted for those who may enter during the laser portion of the procedure. A rigid bronchoscopy set should be immediately available to secure the airway if necessary, and a tracheotomy set should also be available for the possible emergent airway.

93.4.2 Instrumentation

Excellent surgical exposure of the larynx is crucial for successful phonomicrosurgery, and numerous laryngoscopes are available to facilitate success (▶ Fig. 93.3). The laryngoscopes used in phonomicrosurgery allow wide endolaryngeal exposure with binocular vision and bimanual instrumentation; often, a suction port is built into the laryngoscope for the clearance of smoke plume during laser procedures or for directing jet anesthesia. The authors prefer to start with either a regular Dedo (Pilling, Teleflex Medical, Research Triangle Park, NC; ▶ Fig. 93.3a) or laser Dedo laryngoscope (▶ Fig. 93.3b) for most patients because the wider posterior aperture and square corners provide excellent working space and instrument support during phonomicrosurgery. The Ossoff-Pilling laryngoscope (▶ Fig. 93.3c) is useful because it has a smaller endolaryngeal profile and often allows exposure of an anterior larynx while still permitting binocular vision and binocular instrumentation. The larynx of nearly every patient can be exposed with one of these two laryngoscopes with experience. The Ossoff-Karlan laryngoscope (Pilling) has a triangular back port, suction apparatus, and wide endolaryngeal posterior opening, which allows facile surgical exposure and laser use in the posterior larynx

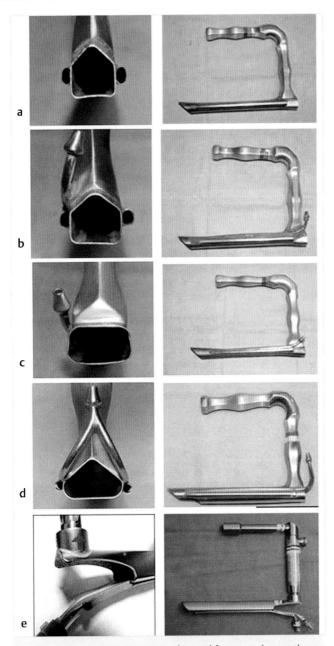

Fig. 93.3 Various laryngoscopes can be used for proper laryngeal exposure. (**a**) Dedo laryngoscope. (**b**) Laser Dedo laryngoscope. (**c**) Ossoff-Pilling laryngoscope. (**d**) Ossoff-Karlan laryngoscope. (**e**) Zeitels Universal Modular Glottiscope.

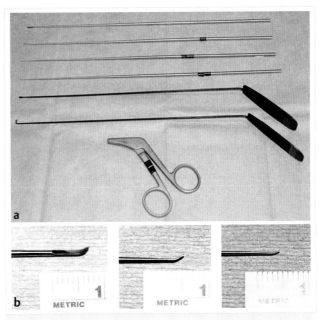

Fig. 93.4 Laryngeal microsurgical instrumentation. (**a**) From top to bottom: sickle knife; flap elevators (large, medium, small); ebonized straight blunt probe; ebonized 5-mm, 90-degree blunt probe; interchangeable handle for micro instruments. (**b**) Close-up view of instruments: sickle knife, medium 60-degree flap elevator, and small 30-degree flap elevator.

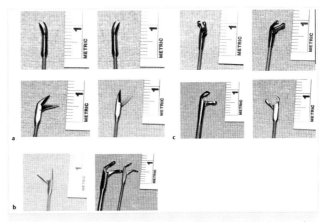

Fig. 93.5 Microlaryngeal instrumentation (Pilling). (**a**) Microlaryngeal scissors: left curved (top left), right curved (top right), up-angled (bottom left), and straight (bottom right) blades. (**b**) Microlaryngeal grasping forceps: straight "alligator" grasping (left) and medium and small up-angled grasping (right) forceps. (**c**) Microlaryngeal cup forceps: left (top left), right (top right), up-angled (bottom left), and straight (bottom right).

(▶ Fig. 93.3d). The Zeitels Universal Modular Glottiscope (Endo-craft, Providence, RI) is also widely used and offers a true gallows suspension exposure of the larynx (▶ Fig. 93.3e). A wide range of other laryngoscopes is available depending on surgeon experience and preference.

Microsurgical instruments are also critical to the success of a phonosurgical procedure. A variety of instruments are needed, including 0- and 90-degree blunt probes for laryngeal palpation, a sickle knife to make mucosal incisions, flap elevators of various sizes to elevate mucosal flaps (▶ Fig. 93.4), micro cup forceps (▶ Fig. 93.5), basket graspers, and microsuctions (▶ Fig. 93.6). A variety of laryngeal injection devices are also

available, including a butterfly needle, a Xomed injector (Medtronic Xomed, Jacksonville, FL), and a Zeitels injector for the subepithelial infusion of saline or epinephrine into the Reinke space or the injection of steroids or cidofovir. Steiner laryngeal suction cautery devices are also available if larger amounts of hemorrhage are anticipated. Photo documentation is essential in laryngology, and modern technology allows exceedingly high-quality imaging. Both 0- and 70-degree operating tele-

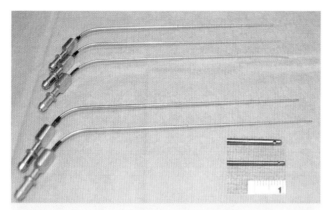

Fig. 93.6 Microlaryngeal suctions. From top to bottom: 7F, 5F, and 3F open-tip suctions; 5F and 3F velvet-eye (blunt tip, side port) suctions. Inset: close-up view of 5F and 3F velvet-eye suctions.

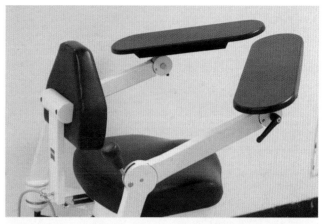

Fig. 93.7 Carl Zeiss Meditec (Dublin, CA) microsurgical chair with individual full arm supports and powered vertical height refinement, allowing total arm support and neutral ergonomic surgeon positioning during prolonged microsurgical cases.

scopes assist in the physical examination of the endolarynx, anterior commissure, and subglottis.

Proper surgical positioning starts with the precise support and positioning of the operating surgeon. Adequate support of the surgeon's arms is crucial for successful surgery because any mild tremor in movement is hugely magnified under the surgical microscope. In addition, proper surgeon positioning with a neutral shoulder and neck position allows comfortable working during prolonged surgical procedures and decreases the long-term incidence of neck and shoulder injuries. Chairs with finely adjustable arm supports are much preferred over the use of a Mayo stand, and many excellent versions are available (▶ Fig. 93.7).

93.4.3 Patient Positioning

The patient is placed in the prone position on the operating table, often with the table rotated 180 degrees to allow more room for the surgeon's legs under the head of the table. The operating room table is then turned 90 degrees from anesthesia to allow the laryngologist the most freedom of access and movement around the patient's head (see ▶ Fig. 93.2). An upper tooth guard must be used unless the patient is edentulous, in which case dentures should be removed, and wet gauze should be used to protect the upper alveolus. If the patient is partially edentulous, the remaining teeth are at particular risk during suspension laryngoscopy because of the uneven pressure that is applied over their surface during suspension. Unrolled moist gauze can be used to pack the open spaces between the teeth to disperse this pressure and add stability to the maxillary teeth during suspension laryngoscopy.

93.4.4 Operative Exposure

The approach to the initial exposure should be relatively consistent. The endotracheal tube is secured to the one side of the mouth, and the teeth or gums are protected. The patient is placed in the sniffing position with flexion of the lower cervical vertebrae and extension of the head at the atlanto-occipital joint. The laryngoscope is advanced down the side of the pharynx opposite the endotracheal tube. The laryngoscope is carefully placed underneath the epiglottis and advanced down to

the level of the true vocal cords under direct visualization. Before suspension, the oral cavity is inspected to ensure that the scope is adequately supported and that the lips are not being pinched. The posterior glottis can be examined by placing the laryngoscope behind the endotracheal tube and lifting forward, or by switching to jet anesthesia if indicated. Once the laryngoscope is properly positioned, the suspension apparatus is employed to expose the larynx and provide hands-free support of the patient's tissues for surgery. The suspension apparatus should be directly attached to the operating room table, not to a Mayo stand on the floor, because this allows easy adjustment of table angle during surgery and prevents inadvertent patient injury due to movement of the suspension gallows independently of the patient. Photo documentation with 0- and 70-degree operating telescopes can then be accomplished, and further refinement of the laryngoscope position can be completed based on endoscopic imaging of the larynx.

The surgeon can often anticipate difficulty with exposure based on the patient's examination and history. A patient with a Mallampati score of III or IV, poor mouth opening, a retrusive mandible, trismus, significant obesity, prominent incisors, previous cervical spine fusion, poor head extension/chest flexion, or radiation edema may pose a challenge for exposure. There are many adjustments in exposure technique than can be employed when laryngeal exposure is difficult. A shoulder roll induces neck extension and is counterproductive to obtaining the optimal neck flexion angle for laryngeal exposure. Elevating the head with folded blankets or clicking the table head up can assist in exposing the anterior larynx by increasing neck flexion. To enhance laryngeal exposure, anterior laryngeal counterpressure can also be applied with an assistant's hand, or with tape carefully placed from one side of the operating room table to the other across the patient's neck over a gauze pad to protect the skin (▶ Fig. 93.8). If the epiglottis is retroflexed or "floppy," gauze can be wrapped around the tongue to protrude the tongue and pull the epiglottis upward and out of the field while the laryngoscope is introduced. A perforating towel clamp can also accomplish this same purpose. Alternatively, the epiglottis can be directly grasped and elevated with a large alligator as the laryngoscope is passed beneath. At times, a smaller tooth

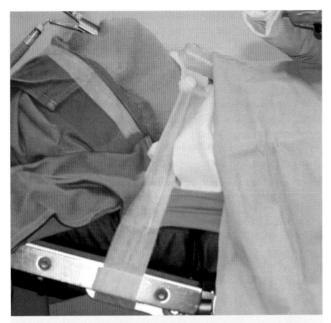

Fig. 93.8 Optimal patient positioning for microlaryngoscopy requires flexion at the neck and extension of the head to allow the best possible exposure. To assist with exposure, anterior laryngeal counterpressure can be applied with tape carefully placed from one side of the operating table to the other across the patient's neck over a gauze pad to protect the skin.

guard can also be useful, especially if the patient has prominent incisors. This may increase the risk for dental injury unless the guard has been made specifically for the patient. The best or most efficient method to attain exposure ultimately depends on the skill level and experience of the surgeon, but excellent exposure is necessary before the operation is continued..

93.4.5 The Microflap Surgical Procedure

Evaluation of the vocal fold lesion is begun by palpating the vocal fold with a straight or right-angle probe and noting the pliability of the lesion and its intracordal depth, any associated sulcus deformity, glottic webs, feeding vasculature, and possible extension into the subglottis or laryngeal ventricle. Vasoconstrictive agents are an essential component of phonomicrosurgery because they allow a dry operative field and obviate the use of electrocautery for hemostasis. Three commonly used vasoconstrictive agents, in order of decreasing potency, are cocaine, diluted epinephrine (generally 1:10,000 concentration), and oxymetazoline. Each is considered adequate for most procedures, and the choice is largely based on surgeon preference. Cocaine is the most potent vasoconstrictor and has the added advantage of conferring a topical anesthetic effect, but it does have some systemic absorption and can also trigger positive urine drug testing postoperatively. Both cocaine and epinephrine can have powerful cardiovascular effects, including hypertension and tachycardia. Oxymetazoline has the least systemic toxicity but is also the least effective vasoconstrictor. The agent of choice is applied via pledget for at least 1 to 2 minutes before incision to ensure adequate tissue penetration and vasoconstriction. If epinephrine is used, it may also be applied via subepithelial infusion, which has the dual benefits of vasocon-

striction and augmentation of the subepithelial or Reinke space. Augmentation increases the distance between the epithelium and vocal ligament, decreasing the risk for injuring the vocal ligament during incision. It may also clearly define a sulcus deformity or invasive lesion where the epithelium is adherent to the underlying vocal ligament. If laser use is anticipated, a saline-soaked pledget is placed into the subglottis to protect the endotracheal tube cuff before surgery.

The position of the incision for the microflap is recommended based on the nature and position of the surgical lesion. Generally, a medial incision is made for vocal fold polyps and striking zone lesions such as nodules; a lateral incision is made for intracordal cysts that are more adherent to the vocal ligament or for the excision of diffuse polypoid corditis (Reinke edema). Before incision, if the vasoconstrictive agents were topically applied, a subepithelial infusion with saline may be performed to augment the Reinke space. Incision into the vocal fold is made under microscopic guidance with a sickle knife, with care taken to incise only the vocal fold epithelium (see ▶ Fig. 93.4). The knife is often stabilized with both hands during incision. Any bleeding is then stopped by using a a large or micro pledget to repeat the application of vasoconstrictor. These agents are reapplied throughout the case as needed. Anterior or posterior extension of the incision can be easily accomplished with an up-biting scissor (see ▶ Fig. 93.5).

The flap elevator is then used in the ipsilateral hand with a laryngeal microsuction in the opposite hand to define the surgical plane under the epithelium. The flap elevator is angled to allow the atraumatic "heel" of the elevator to ride on the vocal ligament, thereby stabilizing the instrument, avoiding injury to the ligament, and ensuring maximal SLP preservation. Meticulous blunt and sharp dissection is often necessary to separate fibrosis surrounding the lesion from the epithelium and vocal ligament. This is often the case in chronic inflammatory conditions or a vocal fold cyst. Retraction of the epithelium with the velvet-eye microsuction allows the evacuation of any bleeding or serous fluid that may obstruct the field while keeping the vocal fold tissues on light tension. Using this instrument is more difficult than grasping the flap, but it is advantageous because of the constant fluid evacuation and the decreased risk for flap tearing as the suction will fall out of the surgical field if too much retraction is applied. Flap elevation proceeds in a lateral to medial direction until the entire lesion is freed from any scarring to the deeper vocal fold structures. Firmly adherent or particularly dense scarring may need to be incised or trimmed with a laryngeal microscissor.

When the lesion has been fully mobilized, it is grasped with a micro cup or basket grasper. The grasper is placed in the contralateral hand, and the surgical assistant guides the flap elevator or appropriate scissors—up, left, or right cutting—into the laryngoscope in the ipsilateral hand. The lesion is delivered as the final dissection is performed. It is removed in one piece if possible. If the epithelium will be clearly redundant, as is often the case with a polyp, the lesion does not need to be completely dissected out because it can be removed while still adherent to the redundant component of the epithelium. The remaining vocal fold epithelium is then redraped, and if there is remaining redundant epithelium, it is excised to allow the closest possible approximation of the epithelial edges for a "straight line" closure. At the completion of the resection, the surgical site is again inspected with 0- and 70 degree endoscopes to evaluate the surgical outcome. Postoperative photo documentation is then performed. Topical lidocaine (4%) is often applied at the end of the case to decrease the incidence of laryngospasm on emergence, and the laryngoscope is then carefully removed from the oral cavity. The teeth and lips are inspected for injury.

93.4.6 Postoperative Care and Voice Rest

Postoperative care following phonomicrosurgery involves pain management and vocal rest, both to varying degrees depending on the indications for and extent of surgery. Postoperative pain is usually minimal, and acetaminophen alone is often sufficient. The use of vocal rest after surgery varies markedly between practitioners, and some do not use it at all. Most laryngologists recommend roughly 1 week of strict voice rest following phonomicrosurgery. After the first postoperative visit on approximately day 5 to 7, the patient is placed on "modified voice use," meaning that the patient should not speak in a voice louder than can be heard at arm's length (the "arm's-length rule"). As a general guideline, the patient is allowed to speak for 10 minutes that day, then the allowance is doubled each day thereafter. The patient should refrain from significant phone use during the first few weeks, continue to use voice rest in noisy situations (bars, restaurants, concerts), and avoid singing, shouting, or screaming. Professional vocalists are often restricted from singing for at least 3 to 4 weeks postoperatively and are encouraged not to return to full performance for 2 to 3 months after surgery. Postoperative voice therapy and a measured return to performance or work requirements are critical for patients. Patients are generally examined with repeated videostroboscopy before a full return to work is allowed. The utility of these postoperative examinations lies in the careful inspection for the return of the mucosal wave, any untoward complications, or the return of signs of vocally abusive behavior. They can help guide the laryngologist in counseling the patient on a vocal behavior as well as postponing the return to work should healing be slow.

93.5 Risks and Adverse Effects of Phonomicrosurgery

Severe complications during phonomicrosurgery are rare. Many practitioners place their patients on perioperative proton pump inhibitor therapy to prevent laryngeal inflammation if they are concerned about laryngopharyngeal reflux. Most of the discomfort following phonomicrosurgery often involves tongue swelling and tenderness due to prolonged pressure from suspension laryngoscopy. Many patients will note some lingual paresthesia and dysgeusia following surgery that generally resolve within several weeks. Rarely, erosions along the lingual surface of the mandible and tooth pain can present postoperatively and war-

rant careful clinical follow-up. Dental injuries are a rare but predictably unfortunate consequence of the laryngeal exposure process despite the use of tooth guards, and all patients should be counseled about this before surgery. Edentulous patients may also have erosions of the maxilla from direct pressure of the laryngoscope. Oral and pharyngeal lacerations can also occur during exposure and are usually mild in nature. Postoperative stridor and airway compromise due to laryngospasm or redundant laryngeal tissue (from the excision of large polyps or stenosis surgery) can result in a requirement for emergency airway management, and all patients are counseled on this risk before surgery. Lastly, in some patients, it is simple not possible to achieve proper direct laryngoscopic exposure because of anatomy, cervical spine fixation, poor mouth opening, or other confounding factors. For these patients, in-office flexible laryngoscopic surgical techniques may be more appropriate.

93.6 Roundsmanship

- Phonomicrosurgery is predicated on the anatomical structure of the vocal fold. Mucosal dissection and resection can be performed under microscopic guidance while the important underlying tissues of the vocal fold are carefully preserved.
- Proper instrumentation is essential for successful phonomicrosurgery, including laryngoscopes that provide binocular microscopic vision and bimanual instrumentation, operating telescopes that allow a thorough and exact laryngeal examination, and microsurgical instruments that facilitate vocal fold incision, dissection, and lesion excision.
- Laryngeal exposure can be challenging, and the surgeon needs to be prepared to try different laryngoscopes and patient positioning strategies to facilitate an adequate surgical view.
- Meticulous dissection of the epithelium away from the underlying vocal ligament is paramount in microflap elevation, maximally preserving the superficial lamina propria while removing the epithelial or intracordal lesion that is interfering with vocal fold vibratory mechanics.

93.7 Recommended Reading

[1] Bastien RW. Benign vocal fold mucosal disorders. In: Flint PW, Haughey BH, Lund VJ, et al, eds. Cummings Otolaryngology. 5th ed. St. Louis, MO: Mosby Elsevier; 2010:chap 62

[2] Courey MS, Garrett CG, Ossoff RH. Medial microflap for excision of benign vocal fold lesions. Laryngoscope 1997; 107: 340–344

[3] Courey MS, Gardner GM, Stone RE, Ossoff RH. Endoscopic vocal fold microflap: a three-year experience. Ann Otol Rhinol Laryngol 1995; 104: 267–273

[4] Hirano M. Structure of the vocal fold in normal and disease states: anatomical and physical studies. In: Proceedings of the Conference on the Assessment of Vocal Pathology (ASHA Report II). Rockville, MD: The American Speech-Language-Hearing Association; 1981

[5] Sulica L. Microlaryngoscopy and endolaryngeal microsurgery. In: Fried MP, Ferlito A. The Larynx. Vol 2. 3rd ed. San Diego, CA: Plural Publishing; 2007: chap 13

94 Voice Therapy

Amy L. Cooper

94.1 Introduction

Voice therapy is an approach to treating voice disorders that involves vocal and physical exercises coupled with behavioral changes. The purpose of voice therapy is to help patients attain the best possible voice and the most relief from the vocal symptoms that are bothersome. Patients are referred to voice therapy when they have a voice disorder that does not warrant surgical intervention, when behavioral modification may decrease the likelihood of the need for surgical intervention, or when they require postoperative rehabilitation. The therapy is almost always initiated by referral from an otolaryngologist. It is extremely important for the otolaryngologist to strongly encourage voice therapy candidates to follow through with the recommended treatment; patients are sometimes put off by the time commitment therapy may entail (weekly sessions for up to 2 months). In a retrospective review of 294 charts at two voice institutions in Atlanta, 38% of patients did not adhere to the physician's recommendation to attend voice therapy. Of those who initiated follow-through, 47% did not return after the initial speech–language pathology evaluation session. Not unlike other therapies intended to change health behavior, voice therapy involves structured treatment sessions and follow-up work to be completed outside the therapy sessions to reinforce the behavior change. Also, not unlike other health care professionals, voice therapists must deal with the problems of resistance to change and lack of patient follow-through outside the therapy sessions.

94.2 Indications for Voice Therapy

The goal of voice therapy is to restore the best voice possible. The therapy program will vary from patient to patient, but in all cases the goal is a voice that is functional for employment and social communication. Voice therapy is conducted to address one of three types of disorders: hyperfunctional, hypofunctional, or dysfunctional. In each of these cases, a vocal fold lesion and/or neurologic abnormality may contribute to the voice disorder.

The most commonly observed voice problems are related to vocal hyperfunction. Hyperfunctional voice disorders are characterized by increased perilaryngeal and/or supralaryngeal tension. A decrease in these types of tension is targeted during voice therapy in order to improve glottal efficiency. Benign lesions, including nodules and polyps, are often present in conjunction with vocal hyperfunction. In these cases, therapy is geared not only at improving vocal efficiency but also at facilitating the healing of benign lesions.

Hypofunctional voice disorders result from incomplete or inconsistent glottal closure. Common diagnoses associated with vocal hypofunction include vocal fold paralysis or paresis and Parkinson-related dysphonia. Therapy techniques will typically consist of exercises to improve glottal closure, or to maximize resonance for improved vocal quality.

Patients who do not fit into either of the above categories are characterized as having a dysfunctional voice disorder. In these cases, the vocal mechanism is intact, but the patient is incapable of using the mechanism in an appropriate manner to attain adequate voice. Relevant diagnoses include puberphonia, paradoxical vocal fold movement, psychogenic dysphonia, and/or conversion disorders. In general, these diagnoses are well managed with voice therapy, although some patients may require psychological counseling, as well.

94.3 Evaluation

Voice therapy should be recommended only after a thorough examination of the vocal folds, preferably via videostroboscopy, as well as an analysis of vocal function. Videostroboscopy is a technique that allows a detailed visualization of not only the patient's laryngeal anatomy but also the patient's phonatory biomechanics. During laryngovideostroboscopy, the extremely rapid vibration of the vocal folds appears as a pseudo-slow motion event (see Chapter 79 for a more in-depth discussion of laryngovideostroboscopy). An evaluation of vocal function includes a detailed history and perceptual evaluation of the voice, as well as the collection of aerodynamic and acoustic data (see Chapter 78 for more information on voice evaluation). Pertinent information to be collected includes the medical history, any vocal misuse, and signs and symptoms of laryngopharyngeal reflux.

94.4 Treatment

A particular therapy regimen is individually developed based on each patient's (1) vocal fold pathology, (2) vocal demands, (3) baseline vocal behavior, and (4) compliance. Therefore, a voice therapy program for an 80-year-old retiree is likely to vary significantly from the voice therapy program for a 20-year-old college student. Uniformly, the individualized voice therapy program will incorporate the following:
- Application of the principles of vocal hygiene to the daily use of the voice
- A series of therapeutic vocal exercises aimed at altering vocal fold vibration and increasing the efficiency of the system through a balancing of the four subsystems of voice: respiration, phonation, resonation, and articulation

Both vocal hygiene and vocal exercise are important for success in voice therapy. Vocal hygiene consists of reducing environmental and behavioral factors that may cause damage to the vocal folds, including inadequate hydration, smoking, excessive alcohol intake, exposure to chemicals/fumes, excessive talking at loud volumes, and laryngopharyngeal reflux.

Management strategies differ among voice patients depending on whether their problems are related to vocal fold hyperfunction or hypofunction. The most commonly observed voice problems are related to vocal fold hyperfunction. Numerous exercises are geared at reducing the amount of "work" required for speaking. A voice therapy program for an individual with vocal hyperfunction would be selected from a variety of approaches, depending on the individual's causative and sustaining influences. For example, a trial lawyer who uses frequent glottal attacks may benefit from learning to reduce her rate of speech, adopting a smoother or more legato vocal style, opening her mouth more widely, and varying her intonation. The voice therapist is expected to select those therapy approaches that facilitate an easy, smooth style of voicing.

In the case of a patient with vocal fold hypofunction, treatment may be geared at increasing loudness or improving articulatory precision. A common neurologic voice disorder is Parkinson-related dysphonia. The Lee Silverman Voice Treatment has been demonstrated to be effective for treating this kind of dysphonia. The purpose of the treatment is to increase loudness, but it often results in improved respiratory output, decreased glottal incompetence, and overall improved intelligibility.

The vocal exercise regimen is developed on an individual basis to address specific biomechanical problems associated with particular voice disorders. ▶ Table 94.1 provides examples of 25 voice therapy facilitators and the vocal parameters affected. Selected therapy techniques facilitate a "target," or a more optimal vocal response by the patient. A part of voice therapy is searching with patients to find the selected therapy technique that seems to help them produce the desired vocal response. In the case of patients with degenerative organic pathology, voice therapy may be conducted to maintain the current level of function as long as possible and reduce ineffective compensatory behaviors. Therapy may be performed preoperatively or postoperatively. Preoperative voice therapy may be undertaken in an effort to eliminate vocally abusive behaviors and begin modeling postoperative voice production. Postoperative voice therapy is designed to help patients adjust to structural changes and to optimize healing in the postoperative period. It is of paramount importance that patients be made aware that restoring the voice to a previous or idealized level may not be possible.

Table 94.1 Voice therapy facilitators

Voice therapy approach	Pitch/frequency	Loudness/intensity	Quality
Auditory feedback		*	*
Varied loudness/intensity	*	*	*
Chanting		*	*
Chewing	*	*	*
Confidential voice		*	*
Counseling/explaining problem	*	*	
Digital manipulation	*		*
Elimination of vocally abusive behaviors		*	*
Establishing new conversational pitch	*		*
Tonal focus	*	*	*
Elimination of glottal fry	*	*	*
Posture	*		*
Hierarchy analysis	*	*	*
Inhalation phonation	*	*	
Laryngeal massage	*		*
Masking	*	*	
Nasal/glide stimulation			*
Open-mouth approach		*	*
Varied intonation	*		
Redirected phonation/imagery	*	*	*
Tension reduction exercises	*	*	*
Respiration training		*	*
Tongue protrusion during vowel production	*		*
Visual feedback	*	*	*
Yawn, sigh	*	*	*

There are cases in which the voice may never return to its previous state. An important component of voice therapy is counseling patients during this dramatic realization and managing their expectations.

The optimal voice for a particular patient should be reliably achieved in the clinical setting; otherwise, it is almost certain that the patient will fall short of the target voice in the real world. Carryover into everyday speech is essential. Skill drills should remind the patient of what he or she should be doing with his or her voice throughout the day. The clinician will focus on rebalancing respiration, phonation, and resonance; this is more important than individual skill drills. The clinician will also explicitly describe the need, purpose, and function of each therapeutic activity. It may be necessary to help a patient find a good voice despite the presence of pathology. This may involve developing the safest voice possible before the completion of medical or surgical treatment.

94.5 Special Considerations

There are some differences in the overall management of voice disorders in children versus those in adults. The age of the person, physical size of the laryngeal structures, and cognitive ability to understand the goals of therapy will dictate what can be done. As in all patients, heavy emphasis is placed on the evaluation in young children because certain pathologies, such as polyps, cysts, and recurrent respiratory papilloma, may be better managed surgically. Voice therapy for school-age children is usually geared at reducing hyperfunctional behaviors. The clinician will identify the situations in which the child is doing things that are vocally abusive and will work with teachers and family members to identify triggers and sustaining factors. A heavy burden is placed on family members to track vocally abusive behaviors outside the clinic setting. Children are often willing to reduce target behaviors when motivated by rewards and attention from caregivers. Obviously, a child must know that he or she has a voice problem before anything can be done about it. This is a major challenge because the child may remain unaware that there is a problem despite the best attempts of the physician, clinician, and parents. Therapy attempts are often deferred until the child matures enough to understand the problem more fully and to be an active participant in the therapy process.

A person of particular interest is the "professional voice user." This term can be used to describe any individual with heavy vocal demands, but in this case it is used to refer specifically to a performer. To achieve a better understanding of the demands that a performer makes on the vocal mechanism, it is useful to know something about the music or type of theater with which the performer is familiar. The goals of therapy are slightly different from those for a nonperformer. With a performer, there are no degrees of freedom with respect to the desired outcome, whereas with other voice patients, there is much more latitude in the range of vocal behaviors that constitute an acceptable outcome. Speech pathologists are always concerned about environmental contributors to voice disorders, but conditions in the performer's world may be somewhat unfamiliar. Studios, concert halls, rehearsal spaces, and practice rooms may be filled with dust, fumes, and ambient noise, and the temperatures may be variable. Additionally, stage direction, set design, and costume design must be considered. Another major source of pressure is that the professional voice user is constantly being judged by audiences, critics, conductors, managers, agents, coaches, and teachers. Rehabilitation professionals working with a performer need to be prepared for intense emotional reactions with regard to voice difficulties. The ongoing education and counseling, both a part of a voice therapy program for any patient, must be handled with special thoroughness and exquisite sensitivity in the case of the professional voice user.

Voice therapy should be performed only by a licensed speech–language pathologist who has training in voice disorders. Referring a patient to a clinician with little experience or interest in voice is not advisable because the odds of success decrease dramatically. In summation, voice therapy is individualized and is an essential component of treatment for many patients with voice disorders.

94.6 Roundsmanship

- Voice therapy is an approach to treating voice disorders that involves vocal and physical exercises coupled with behavioral changes.
- Voice disorders are hyperfunctional, hypofunctional, or dysfunctional.
- Voice therapy may be conducted as part of a conservative treatment plan, or it may be undertaken pre- and postoperatively when surgical management is deemed necessary.
- Voice therapy is best administered by a licensed speech–language pathologist who has a particular expertise in the area of voice disorders.

94.7 Recommended Reading

[1] Boone DR, McFarlane SC, Von Berg SL. The Voice and Voice Therapy. Boston, MA: Pearson Education; 2005
[2] Branski RC, Murry T. Voice therapy. Medscape. Otolaryngology and Facial Plastic Surgery. . Updated November 30, 2011. Accessed November 12, 2013
[3] Colton RH, Casper JK, Leonard R. Understanding Voice Problems: A Physiological Perspective for Diagnosis and Treatment. 3rd ed. Baltimore, MD: Williams & Wilkins; 1996
[4] Portone C, Johns MM, Hapner ER. A review of patient adherence to the recommendation for voice therapy. J Voice 2008; 22: 192–196
[5] Ramig LO, Pawlas AA, Countryman S. The Lee Silverman Voice Treatment: A Practical Guide for Treating the Voice and Speech Disorders in Parkinson Disease. Iowa City, IA: National Center for Voice and Speech; 1995
[6] Wider CN. Speech-language pathology and the professional voice user: an overview. In: Sataloff RT, ed. Treatment of Voice Disorders. San Diego, CA: Plural Publishing; 2005:11–15

95 Lasers in Laryngology

Philip A. Weissbrod

95.1 Introduction

Lasers have been used in laryngeal surgery since the 1970s. Originally used only in the operating room, they have become a mainstay in both office- and operating room–based laryngologic surgery. The original surgical laser, the carbon dioxide laser, is coupled to an operating microscope by way of an articulated arm and directed with a micromanipulator. More recently, with improved laser and fiber technology, a variety of lasers have been developed that deliver energy via fibers passed through the operating channel of a flexible laryngoscope. This has revolutionized the use of lasers in laryngology by making it possible to apply them in the awake office patient as well as in an operating room setting.

Lasers used in the operating room have great precision because of the stable surgical field provided by a patient under general anesthesia. However, as a consequence of the aforementioned advances, an increasing number of procedures can be effectively done in the office. The benefits of office-based procedures include avoidance of general anesthesia, decreased cost to the patient and the medical system, decreased procedure time, and few complications. For patients with disease processes that require multiple procedures, office-based surgery provides a safe and effective alternative to multiple trips to the operating room.

Despite improvements in technology, there are still instances where an operating room based approach is advantageous, especially in oncologic resections, situations where bleeding is expected, and where bulky or diffuse disease will make awake treatment difficult to complete in the office secondary to limitations in anesthesia.

95.2 Laser Terminology, Principles, and Mechanism of Action

The term *laser* is an acronym that stands for *l*ight *a*mplification by *s*timulated *e*mission of *r*adiation. There are some fundamental physics principles and terminology that must be understood to fully appreciate how lasers work and how lasers differ from one another. Photons, the basic unit of light and radiation, are integral to laser function. Photons have no mass, can act as a wave or a particle, and can be either absorbed or emitted by an atom. The basic unit of emission from a laser is a photon; therefore, we can discuss lasers as having certain characteristics of a wave, such as frequency, amplitude, and wavelength. Frequency is the number of times a wave repeats in a second and is measured in hertz (Hz). Amplitude is the height of a wave. Wavelength is the distance between waves and determines the color of a laser (▶ Fig. 95.1).

Lasers use the excitability of atoms or more specifically electrons to create photons. When an atom absorbs energy, its electrons enter into an excited state. When the electrons return to their ground state, energy is released in the form of a photon, a process called spontaneous emission. When an excited electron interacts with a photon equal to the energy difference between the electron's ground state and excited state, the photon will encourage the electron to release a photon, returning the electron to its ground state. The released photon will be identical to the original photon in wavelength, frequency, and phase. Because the original photon is not absorbed by the atom, there are now two identical photons. This process is called stimulated emission. Lasers take advantage of this principle to produce multiple photons with the same characteristics.

During the operation of a laser, absorption, spontaneous emission, and stimulated emission are all taking place. Initially, atoms are energized from the ground state to the excited state by a process called pumping. These atoms decay via spontaneous emission and emit photons, which are reflected back into the laser medium. Some of the photons are absorbed by atoms in the ground state, and others collide with atoms in the excited state. When photons collide with atoms in the excited state, this results in stimulated emission and increases the total number of photons. Optical amplification occurs when the number of photons being emitted is greater than the number of photons being absorbed, resulting in a continuously increasing number of photons. In order for optical amplification to occur, it is necessary to have more atoms in an excited than in a ground state so that emitted photons will not simply be absorbed by another atom in its ground state. This critical mass concept is called population inversion.

The external energy source that initially excites the atoms from the ground state is called the pump source. The source of the atoms that are pumped is termed the gain medium. The gain medium determines the laser's wavelength, or color. Gain mediums are housed in a space called the optical cavity and can be a gas, solid, or semiconductor depending on the type of laser.

Initially, when photons are produced, they are traveling in a multitude of directions. In order to encourage them to travel in a unified direction, they are reflected off mirrors (optical resonators) placed on either side of the optical cavity. One mirror has the capability to allow photons to leave the optical cavity in the form of a laser beam, or electromagnetic radiation, when triggered. The output can be in the form of a continuous wave of radiated energy or in a pulsed form (▶ Fig. 95.2).

The settings for most types of medical lasers include power, on–off interval, pulse width, and laser spot size or shape. Power

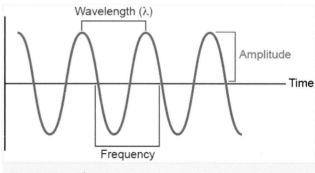

Fig. 95.1 Wave characteristics.

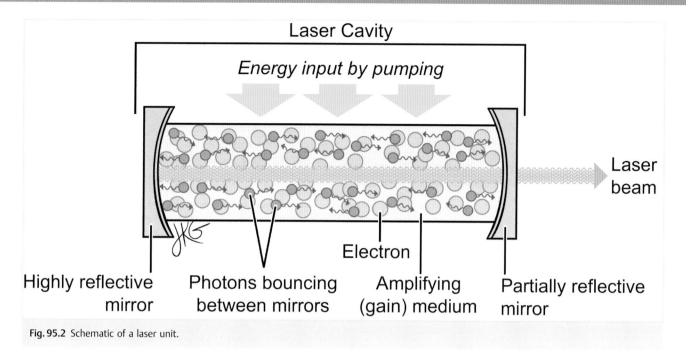

Fig. 95.2 Schematic of a laser unit.

Table 95.1 Correlation of tissue temperature with cellular injury

Tissue temperature (°C)	Cellular injury and tissue response
42–25	Beginning of hyperthermia, conformational changes, shrinkage of collagen
50	Reduction of enzymatic activity
60	Denaturation of proteins, coagulation of collagens
100	Tissue drying and formation of vacuoles
>100	Beginning of vaporization and tissue carbonization
300–1,000	Thermal ablation, photoablation, and disruption

is the amount of energy that a device emits and is measured in watts (W). The measure of emitted or received energy is called radiant energy. It is measured in joules (J) and accounts for power delivered over time.

•

When energy delivered to tissue is considered, the area over which the energy is delivered, or spot size, is of relevance. The spot size of a carbon dioxide laser can be adjusted by manipulating the depth of focus of the microscope or by altering the laser spot size directly. With a fiber-based laser, moving the fiber closer to the field can decrease the spot size. Irridance is power divided by area. Similarly, fluence, the total energy absorbed by a cross-sectional area, accounts for the distribution of energy over area.

•

In the case of a circular spot, the equation would be the following:

•

Therefore, as the fiber moves closer to the tissue, the radius decreases, and the irridance and fluence increase significantly. Ul-

timately, the reason why these concepts are important at the tissue level is that light energy is transformed into heat, which alters cellular structures. The degree to which tissue is heated determines the extent of damage (▶ Table 95.1).

Aside from adjustments to the power and spot size, the pulse width, or length of time in which a single burst of power is delivered, can alter the way in which tissue responds to a laser. Running a laser in continuous mode means that the energy at any given point in the "on" mode is constant. Alternatively, energy can be delivered in discrete pulses to minimize the transference of heat to surrounding tissue. The pulse duration should be less than the time necessary for heat to be conducted away from a laser-heated region. The time required for heat to dissipate is known as the thermal relaxation time. Thermal diffusion time, or the time that it takes for heat to flow into the tissue, is determined by characteristics specific to certain tissues, such as density, water content, and specific heat. If the pulse width is less than the diffusion time or relaxation time, thermal confinement exists. By keeping the pulse width shorter than the thermal diffusion or relaxation time, the zone of necrosis (▶ Fig. 95.3), or extraneous tissue injury, can be minimized.

95.3 Laser Applications in Laryngology

The clinical culmination of the above equations and terms is represented by the concept of selective photothermolysis. When lasers of different wavelengths are used (▶ Fig. 95.4), specific tissues will absorb energy selectively according to the concentration of water or the presence of pigment, as in blood or melanocytes. Therefore, the selection of a suitable laser relates to the inherent qualities of the laser and the characteristics of the tissue being treated. Although many lasers have been used over the past 20 years, a few have come to the forefront

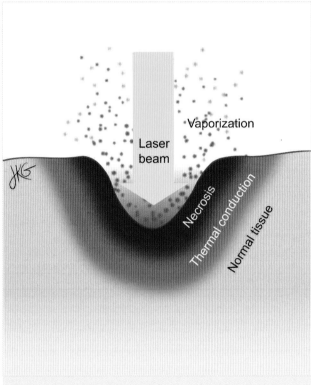

Fig. 95.3 Tissue alterations as a distance from incident laser.

for application in treating diseases of the larynx. In general, they can be separated into lasers that target the wavelength of oxyhemoglobin and those that target water (▶ Table 95.2).

The 585-nm pulsed dye laser and the 532-nm pulsed potassium titanyl phosphate (KTP) laser are two examples of lasers that target oxyhemoglobin and embody the concept of selective photothermolysis. The absorbance peaks of oxyhemeglobin are 541 and 571 nm. When this chromophore is targeted, energy can be directed specifically to the subepethelial microvasculature that supplies a lesion, where it will cause involution. Combining this directed therapy with pulsed energy delivery reduces collateral damage to surrounding tissues by respecting the thermal relaxation time of laryngeal tissue. Inadvertent lasering of healthy tissue during procedures has minimal voice implications, and studies have shown no long-term fibrotic injury from the use of these lasers. In the case of the true vocal folds, this is of vital importance because preservation of the superficial lamina propria and mucosa, the vibratory elements of the vocal fold, is maximized. Both the pulsed dye laser and the KTP laser are used to treat laryngeal papillomas, granulomas, Reinke edema, vocal fold polyps, leukoplakia, vascular lesions, ectasia, varices, dysplasia, and early glottic carcinoma. Given that these are fiber-delivered lasers, they are suitable for use in the operating room or office setting when directed through the operating port of a flexible laryngoscope.

As mentioned previously, office-based procedures have a number of benefits for patients; avoidance of anesthesia risk is the most substantial, especially for those who have medical comorbidities such as cardiopulmonary disease. Other benefits include a shorter recovery from anesthesia, shorter procedure times, and reduced cost to the medical system. Disadvantages of office-based procedures include patient discomfort, increased difficulty in treating the vocal fold because of movement, decreased reliance on biopsy for operative decision making, a potential increase in the total number of procedures for a given patient as a consequence of the ease of procedure administration, and perhaps decreased efficacy in comparison with operating room–based procedures.

The lasers in the other broad class used in laryngology are those that target water, such as the carbon dioxide laser and the thulium laser. These are better cutting instruments and have better hemostatic properties. They tend to generate more heat,

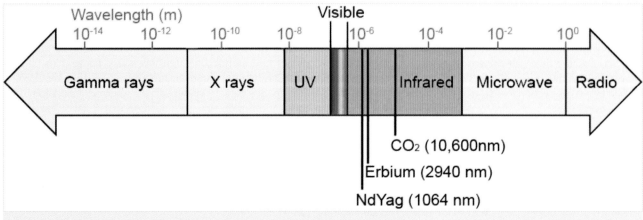

Fig. 95.4 Wavelengths of common laryngeal lasers. *Nd:YAG,* neodymium:yttrium-aluminum garnet; *UV,* ultraviolet.

Table 95.2 Common laryngeal lasers

Laser	Wavelength (nm)	Target chromophore	Delivery system
Potassium titanyl phosphate (KTP)	532	Oxyhemoglobin	Fiber-optic
Pulsed dye	585	Oxyhemoglobin	Fiber-optic
Neodymium:yttrium-aluminum garnet (Nd:YAG)	1,064	Oxyhemoglobin	Fiber-optic
Thulium (Tm)	2,013	Water	Fiber-optic
Holmium (Ho)	2,150	Water	Fiber-optic
Carbon dioxide (CO_2)	10,600	Water	Mechanical arm or photonic mirrored fiber

which causes tissue ablation instead of involution. Although at times desirable, this feature can lead to greater heat transference and an increased thermal effect on surrounding tissues, with the potential for increased scarring and fibrosis after treatment in comparison with the pulsed 500-nm lasers discussed previously.

The lasers that target water serve as excellent tools for the treatment of diseases such as recurrent respiratory papillomatosis and stenosis of the larynx or trachea, and for the resection of benign and malignant neoplasms. The most widely used laser in this class is the carbon dioxide laser. It is still used primarily in the operating room and delivered via a mechanical arm with articulating mirrors. Because it is in the invisible spectrum, a second coaxial helium-neon laser is used as an aiming beam. The beam is aimed with a micromanipulator hand piece attached to the microscope. This allows the precise delivery of carbon dioxide laser energy to a given lesion. The carbon dioxide laser is an excellent tool for laryngeal surgery but is limited in that it must be delivered in the direct line of sight. Recently, a new mirrored fiber delivery system has been developed that allows "fiber"-based delivery of the carbon dioxide laser.

Another recent advancement in carbon dioxide technology has come in the form of the AcuBlade (Lumenis, Yokneam, Israel), a robotic delivery system for carbon dioxide laser microsurgery. The device enables the surgeon to create an incision of varying length, shape, and depth, so that energy can be delivered in a uniform distribution along the length of an incision and a user is prevented from inadvertently incising too deeply. Proponents cite reduced surgical times, improved precision, less collateral tissue damage, and patient safety as benefits of the AcuBlade.

The thulium laser has effects on tissue similar to those of the carbon dioxide laser, but there is some experiential evidence that hemostasis is improved because of a greater thermal effect on tissue adjacent to ablated regions. The thulium laser is an extremely effective device for tissue ablation and cutting. Because it is delivered via a fiber, it can be used in the office as well as in the operating room.

95.3.1 Laser Safety, Risks, and Adverse Events

The use of lasers in both the office and the operating room requires that protective measures be taken for patients, physicians, and staff. All lasers require that staff and patients protect their eyes with glasses or goggles that are specific to the wavelength. For patients undergoing general anesthesia, all exposed skin in the perioral and facial region should be covered with moist towels, and eye protection should include the placement of moistened eye pads, ideally covered by paper tape.

Lasers have the potential to ignite combustible gas and plastic polymers. For this reason, to prevent fires, a laser-safe endotracheal tube should be used that consists of a metal-guarded tube or a polymer tube wrapped in metallic foil. The endotracheal tube balloon should be protected by placing a saline-soaked pledget in the subglottis, and the FiO_2 should be kept below 30% during laser applications. Should a fire occur, surgeons must be familiar with appropriate airway fire management. The procedure should be halted, gases shut off, and the endotracheal tube removed. If possible, direct visualization of the region allows the removal of remaining burning debris and flammable material. Saline should be flushed into the airway, and rigid bronchoscopy, reintubation, or tracheotomy should be considered to secure the airway.

95.4 Roundsmanship

- Lasers rely on photons to deliver energy to tissue.
- Optical amplification is necessary to achieve stimulated emission of radiation.
- Relevant chromophores in laryngology include oxyhemoglobin and water.
- The concept of selective photothermolysis is key in choosing lasers for laryngology procedures.
- Initial management of an airway fire includes turning off the gas and removing the endotracheal tube.

95.5 Recommended Reading

[1] Anderson RR, Parrish JA. Selective photothermolysis: precise microsurgery by selective absorption of pulsed radiation. Science 1983; 220: 524–527

[2] Franco RA. In-office laryngeal surgery with the 585-nm pulsed dye laser. Curr Opin Otolaryngol Head Neck Surg 2007; 15: 387–393

[3] Koufman JA, Rees CJ, Frazier WD et al. Office-based laryngeal laser surgery: a review of 443 cases using three wavelengths. Otolaryngol Head Neck Surg 2007; 137: 146–151

[4] Lin DS, Cheng SC, Su WF. Potassium titanyl phosphate laser treatment of intubation vocal granuloma. Eur Arch Otorhinolaryngol 2008; 265: 1233–1238

[5] Mallur PS, Branski RC, Amin MR. 532-nanometer potassium titanyl phosphate (KTP) laser-induced expression of selective matrix metalloproteinases (MMP) in the rat larynx. Laryngoscope 2011; 121: 320–324

[6] Raulin C, Karsai S. Laser and IPL Technology in Dermatology and Aesthetic Medicine. New York, NY: Springer; 2011

[7] Zeitels SM, Burns JA, Akst LM, Hillman RE, Broadhurst MS, Anderson RR. Office-based and microlaryngeal applications of a fiber-based thulium laser. Ann Otol Rhinol Laryngol 2006; 115: 891–896

[8] Zeitels SM, Burns JA, Lopez-Guerra G, Anderson RR, Hillman RE. Photoangiolytic laser treatment of early glottis cancer: a new management strategy. Ann Otol Rhinol Laryngo Supp l 2008; 117: 1: 99:3–24

[9] Zeitels SM, Burns JA. Laser applications in laryngology: past, present, and future. Otolaryngol Clin North Am 2006; 39: 159–172

[10] Zeitels SM, Burns JA. Office-based laryngeal laser surgery with the 532-nm pulsed-potassium-titanyl-phosphate laser. Curr Opin Otolaryngol Head Neck Surg 2007; 15: 394–400

96 Tracheo-Esophageal Puncture

Melda Kunduk and Andrew J. McWhorter

96.1 Rationale and Goals

Total laryngectomy is the definitive operation for malignancy of the larynx. It has evolved since its introduction by Billroth in 1873 but remains challenged by the functional deficits that it entails. Loss of oral communication is the greatest and most isolating of these deficits. Restoration of voice requires re-creation of a system with a generator, vibrator, and resonator. The three commonly used systems today are esophageal speech, artificial laryngeal speech, and tracheo-esophageal speech. In all three approaches, the pharyngoesophageal segment is used as the vibratory tissue to replace the vocal folds, and the resonator remains the pharynx, mouth, and nose. Esophageal speech requires regurgitation of air as the generator. It is a difficult technique to master and often requires extensive rehabilitation. The artificial larynx uses an external vibratory source such as an electrolarynx. It is limited by its mechanical sound quality with poor pitch modulation. Tracheo-esophageal speech has the advantage of restoring lung-driven speech that follows the normal cadence of respiration. There is typically greater volume and more voice modulation with tracheo-esophageal speech than with the other two methods.

Multiple procedures were originally developed by Conley and many others to create a mucosal shunt from the tracheostoma into the esophagus, but none was reliable enough to become widely used. Similarly, early attempts to deliver air into the esophagus with a diverse array of prostheses met with limited success. Drawing on an original description by Guttman, who reported a butcher who had fistulized himself with an ice pick and maintained a tracheo-esophageal fistula directly through the parting wall, Singer and Blom developed a technique as well as a prosthesis to create a safe fistula that restored voice in 90% of their patients. This technique was further enhanced by the development of more technologically advanced prostheses that provided a well-tolerated pathway and protected the airway from esophageal contents. Many developments have expanded on the original description of Singer and Blom, but all are based on the same principle in regard to both the procedure and the prosthesis.

96.2 Technique

The posterior membranous tracheal wall is visible through the stoma and lies below the level of the cricopharyngeus in the proximal cervical esophagus. The tracheo-esophageal puncture is a controlled fistula through this parting wall. It can be performed at the time of laryngectomy (primary) or at a later date (secondary). The primary puncture is performed following removal of the larynx and before closure of the pharynx. A fine, right-angle clamp is placed into the proximal cervical esophagus through the open pharynx from the laryngectomy defect. An incision is made over the clamp 1 to 1.5 cm below the superior border of the posterior tracheal wall in the stoma. A 14F to 16F red rubber catheter is then inserted, passed inferiorly, and secured (▶ Fig. 96.1). Alternatively, kits are available with which a measurement is made and the prosthesis is placed.

The original technique described by Singer and Blom was a secondary puncture. As originally described, rigid esophagoscopy is performed, and ballottement of the posterior membranous wall of the trachea is performed at the planned site for puncture within the stoma. After the position has been confirmed by visualization through the scope, the scope is turned 180 degrees so that the more distal lip sits posteriorly and protects the posterior esophageal wall. A needle is placed through the membranous tracheal wall into the esophagoscope. This

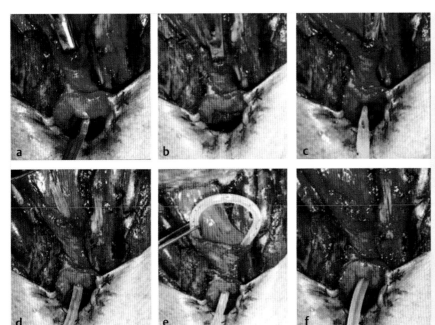

Fig. 96.1 Primary tracheo-esophageal puncture. (a) Incision over right angle passed through pharynx into proximal cervical esophagus. (b) Right-angle tips visible 1.5 cm below superior margin of the posterior tracheal wall. (c) Passing the catheter into the esophagus. (d) Advancement of the catheter into the pharynx. (e) Redirection of the catheter inferiorly into the distal esophagus. (f) Completed puncture with the catheter in position. (Courtesy of A. M. Pou and R. C. Hamaker.)

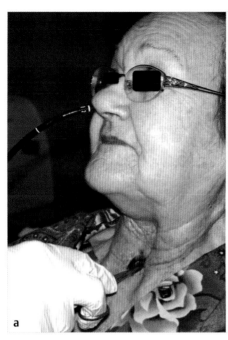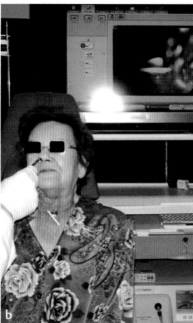

Fig. 96.2 Secondary tracheo-esophageal puncture with transnasal esophagoscope. (**a**) Patient is seated with the esophagoscope in position and the hemostat dilating the fistula puncture. (**b**) Patient with the prosthesis in place after sizing, visible at the stoma and in the esophagus on video monitor.

tract is then enlarged, and a catheter or prosthesis is placed. In a patient who has been irradiated or a patient with difficult access, rigid esophagoscopy can be difficult to perform. Flexible esophagoscopy can be used in a similar manner, with care taken to avoid injury to the posterior esophageal wall as the scope is not protecting it. Koch described using a Seldinger technique with a peel-away catheter, like those used in vascular access procedures. This facilitates placement of the catheter inferiorly, and it is rapid and easy to perform.

Alternatively, a secondary puncture can be performed in the office in an awake patient. Some instruments have been developed to facilitate this, but none has had a greater impact than the transnasal esophagoscope. The procedure was originally described in 2003 by Bach et al. It has the advantage of visualization similar to that of the operating room approaches, but with the added benefit of the patient being awake and upright. This prevents gravity from collapsing the esophagus, and air insufflation and patient swallowing open the esophagus for improved visualization. The patient is seated upright in the examination chair, and the posterior membranous trachea is injected with local anesthetic at the planned puncture site within the stoma. Typically, 1 to 2 mL of 1% lidocaine with 1:100,000 epinephrine is used. The technique is otherwise the same as the secondary puncture in the operating room, with either a needle or a stab incision performed following ballottement and confirmation of position with the transnasal esophagoscope in the proximal esophagus. Again, either a catheter or a prosthesis can be placed at this time (▶ Fig. 96.2). This technique has proved to be a successful and reliable way to create a tracheo-esophageal puncture. It is even applicable in patients with complex pharyngoesophageal defects repaired with free flap and gastric pull-up reconstructions. ▶ Fig. 96.3 demonstrates the step-by-step performance of the procedure as seen from the esophageal lumen.

Successful tracheo-esophageal voice creation does not depend only upon the puncture; it can be enhanced with other recommended preparatory steps for alaryngeal voicing. The performance of a unilateral pharyngeal plexus neurectomy or an inferior constrictor–cricopharyngeal myotomy at the time of laryngectomy has been popularized by Hamaker and repeatedly demonstrated to be very beneficial in the acquisition of good tracheo-esophageal voice. Both of these procedures allow the patient to have better reflux of air with less resistance for voicing. A neurectomy should not be performed bilaterally because it will result in an adynamic pharynx with increased dysphagia and a hollow voice. If a myotomy and a neurectomy are both performed, they should be ipsilateral. Similarly, the creation of an accessible stoma enhances the acquisition of hands-free speech by facilitating the use of an appliance for hands-free speech as well as finger occlusion. Suspending the trachea to the sternal or clavicular periosteum helps by reducing downward pull on the stoma. Release of the sternal heads of the sternocleidomastoid muscle flattens the anterior neck, effectively bringing the stoma forward. Addressing the pharynx and the stoma with these important steps is the key to the successful acquisition of tracheo-esophageal speech; they are more important than the puncture itself.

96.3 Risks and Adverse Effects

The only contraindication to performing the procedure as a primary puncture is separation of the parting wall. Separation can be suture-bolstered but carries an unwarranted increased risk for leak and infection. There are no contraindications to secondary puncture as long as the stoma and esophagus are accessible and patent. Microstomia and esophageal stricture should be addressed before puncture. There are, however, patients who are poor candidates for tracheo-esophageal speech. Lack of dexterity or visual acuity may limit the patient's ability to care for the prosthesis. Similarly, poor cognition or unfavorable social circumstances may prevent the patient from managing the continued care required for prosthesis and voice maintenance.

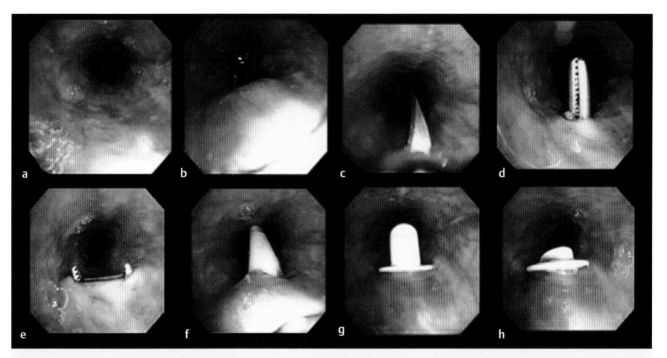

Fig. 96.3 Secondary tracheo-esophageal puncture with transnasal esophagoscopic view. (**a**) Proximal cervical esophagus. (**b**) Confirmation of position, with indentation visible. (**c**) No. 11 blade incision. (**d**) Placement of hemostat through incision. (**e**) Dilation of tract with spread of hemostat. (**f**) Placement of dilator through fistula. (**g**) Measurement of length of fistula tract with sizer. (**h**) Prosthesis in position.

Controversy initially existed as to the timing of the puncture. It was generally accepted that primary puncture had a better voice outcome, but other authors have demonstrated that when planned for properly, secondary puncture is equivalent to primary puncture. There are pros and cons to both approaches. Primary puncture can provide access for a feeding tube without the need for a nasogastric or gastric tube. It does require additional procedures aside from prosthesis placement. The prosthesis length is more likely to change with primary than with secondary puncture as the tissues mature in the healing process. Alternatively, secondary puncture allows exact placement of the fistula following healing and maturation of the stoma, especially in the setting of postoperative radiation. Some studies have suggested that after chemoradiation and salvage total laryngectomy, tracheo-esophageal puncture should be performed secondarily because of the potentially increased risk for pharyngocutaneous fistula with primary puncture.

In the perioperative period, the risks of the procedure are low. The most dangerous, although thankfully rare, risk is mediastinitis. Infection at the puncture site with parting wall abscess has been described, but the most common complication is dislodgement of the prosthesis or catheter with loss of the fistula.

More significant are the problems associated with voice acquisition and maintenance of the fistula on a long-term basis. Close teamwork with the speech–language pathologist is essential in assisting patients with both voice and prosthesis management. Pharyngoesophageal spasm is the greatest barrier to the acquisition of fluent speech. This should be a rare occurrence and is typically avoidable with the performance of a primary pharyngeal plexus neurectomy or cricopharyngeal my-

otomy. The spasm is clinically suspected but can be confirmed through fluoroscopy or endoscopy while the patient is voicing. Secondary neurectomies and myotomies can be performed. A less invasive alternative is botulinum toxin A injection into the pharyngoesophageal segment. This is highly effective, and the result may be permanent. Most common are problems with the prosthesis, such as dislodgement, potential foreign body aspiration, and prosthesis failure, which is usually secondary to fungal overgrowth. The patient should be trained to manage dislodgement with replacement of a prosthesis or a catheter into the fistula. A foreign body is easily managed through the immediately accessible stoma. Fungal overgrowth is the most common cause of prosthesis failure and leak due to loss of the valve competence (▶ Fig. 96.4).

Most troublesome are the problems associated with the fistula itself, especially thinning of the parting wall or enlargement of the fistula tract, creating peri-prosthesis leakage and aspiration. Close teamwork with the speech pathologist is invaluable. Downsizing the tract with a smaller catheter or a prosthesis with a larger posterior flange is the least invasive management alternative. Suture tightening of the fistula tract can be successful, as can the injection of collagen around the prosthesis. These problems can be difficult to manage and may require closure of the fistula with repuncture after healing.

Tracheo-esophageal puncture provides a safe and reliable method for voice restoration following total laryngectomy. Although multiple adjustments are necessary for the patient without a larynx, effective communication is most important to quality of life. Rehabilitation with the speech–language pathologist eases this transition and should be initiated in the preoperative period. Primary versus secondary puncture is less important in voice acquisition than are pharyngoesophageal segment

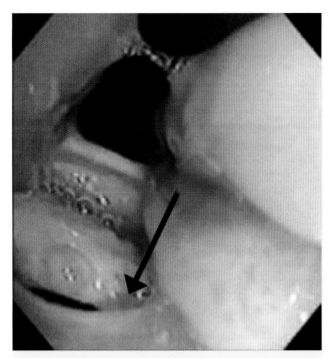

Fig. 96.4 Fungal overgrowth (*arrow*) on a tracheo-esophageal prosthesis causing valve failure from incomplete closure, as seen on transnasal endoscopy.

preparation with myotomy or neurectomy and appropriate stoma creation.

96.4 Roundsmanship

- Tracheo-esophageal puncture can be performed as a primary or secondary procedure with equal success.

- Primary puncture has the advantage of providing alternative access for feeding, but the prosthesis length is likely to change.
- The only contraindication to primary puncture is separation of the parting wall at the time of surgery.
- Secondary tracheo-esophageal puncture can be performed easily in the office under local anesthesia with transnasal esophagoscopy.
- The key to successful tracheo-esophageal voice acquisition is appropriate patient preparation with pharyngoesophageal myotomy or pharyngeal plexus neurectomy and appropriate stoma creation.

96.5 Recommended Reading

[1] Bach KK, Postma GN, Koufman JA. In-office tracheoesophageal puncture using transnasal esophagoscopy. Laryngoscope 2003; 113: 173–176
[2] Blom ED, Pauloski BR, Hamaker RC. Functional outcome after surgery for prevention of pharyngospasms in tracheoesophageal speakers. Part I: Speech characteristics. Laryngoscope 1995; 105: 1093–1103
[3] Brown DH, Hilgers FJ, Irish JC, Balm AJ. Postlaryngectomy voice rehabilitation: state of the art at the millennium. World J Surg 2003; 27: 824–831
[4] Emerick KS, Tomycz L, Bradford CR et al. Primary versus secondary tracheoesophageal puncture in salvage total laryngectomy following chemoradiation. Otolaryngol Head Neck Surg 2009; 140: 386–390
[5] Guttman MR. Rehabilitation of the voice in laryngectomized patients. Arch Otolaryngol 1932; 15: 478–479
[6] Izdebski K, Reed CG, Ross JC, Hilsinger RL. Problems with tracheoesophageal fistula voice restoration in totally laryngectomized patients. A review of 95 cases. Arch Otolaryngol Head Neck Surg 1994; 120: 840–845
[7] Koch WM. A failsafe technique for endoscopic tracheoesophageal puncture. Laryngoscope 2001; 111: 1663–1665
[8] LeBert B, McWhorter AJ, Kunduk M et al. Secondary tracheoesophageal puncture with in-office transnasal esophagoscopy. Arch Otolaryngol Head Neck Surg 2009; 135: 1190–1194
[9] Singer MI, Blom ED. An endoscopic technique for restoration of voice after laryngectomy. Ann Otol Rhinol Laryngol 1980; 89: 529–533
[10] Singer MI, Blom ED, Hamaker RC. Pharyngeal plexus neurectomy for alaryngeal speech rehabilitation. Laryngoscope 1986; 96: 50–54

97 Evaluation and Management of Esophageal Disorders

Catherine Rees Lintzenich and Kristin K. Marcum

97.1 Introduction

Esophageal disorders are common in the general population, and patients with associated symptoms frequently present to the otolaryngologist. Symptoms may include dysphagia, throat pain, globus sensation, heartburn, and regurgitation. Esophageal disorders account for the majority of swallowing complaints in young adults and a large proportion of swallowing complaints in older adults.

97.2 Esophageal Anatomy

The esophagus is a muscular conduit connecting the pharynx to the stomach for the transport of food. The normal esophagus is approximately 26 cm in length. It begins at the lower border of the cricoid cartilage opposite the transverse process of C6 and ends at the level of T10. At an early period in fetal development, the stomach is separated from the pharynx by the esophagus, which begins as a foregut structure. The future esophagus extends from the pharyngeal tube as far caudally as the liver outgrowth. By the end of the third week of development, the primitive foregut develops a ventral diverticulum from which the tracheobronchial tree develops. As a result of ingrowth by two lateral septa, the tracheo-esophageal septum gradually partitions this diverticulum, resulting in the formation of an anterior respiratory primordium and a posterior esophagus. During the fourth and fifth weeks of development, growth of the heart and liver allows the esophagus to stretch. As the esophagus elongates, its lumen is nearly completely obliterated, and recanalization occurs by week 8 to 10.

The mature esophagus is a collapsed tube beginning at the upper esophageal sphincter (UES) and coursing through the diaphragmatic hiatus at the lower esophageal sphincter (LES). The UES is more aptly described as the pharyngoesophageal segment because it is made up of the cricopharyngeus muscle, part of the inferior pharyngeal constrictor, and the most superior portion of the longitudinal esophageal muscular fibers. The cricopharyngeus muscle is a sling-shaped muscle arising from the posterior cricoid cartilage; it is tonically contracted, opening for swallowing and belching. The LES has a normal resting tone of 10 to 40 mm Hg and is normally positioned at or just below the diaphragm. The LES is not a true anatomical sphincter and is reinforced by the crura of the diaphragm. The esophagus comprises four layers: the mucosa, including stratified squamous epithelium, the lamina propria, and the muscularis mucosae; the submucosa; the muscularis propria; and the adventitia. The muscularis propria consists of proximal skeletal muscle and distal smooth muscle, which are arranged as inner circular muscle and outer longitudinal muscle. The cervical esophagus is composed primarily of striated muscle, and the distal two-thirds of the esophagus is composed of smooth muscle. A section consisting of mixed striated and smooth muscle between these areas is known as the transition zone. The innermost mucosal layer changes from nonkeratinized stratified squamous epithelium to columnar epithelium at the squamocolumnar

junction. The squamocolumnar junction can be recognized from the irregular Z-line separating the light pink esophageal squamous mucosa and the darker pink columnar gastric mucosa (▶ Fig. 97.1). The gastroesophageal junction is defined by the proximal margin of the gastric folds and the termination of the esophageal linear blood vessels. The squamocolumnar junction and gastroesophageal junction are normally located at the same level; however, the two are not one and the same. In patients with Barrett esophagus, the squamocolumnar junction is more proximal in the esophagus than the gastroesophageal junction, and in patients with a hiatal hernia, the gastroesophageal junction is more proximal than the diaphragmatic indentation.

The esophagus is innervated by both sympathetic and parasympathetic chains. There is also intrinsic innervation of the esophagus via nerve plexus. The Auerbach (myenteric) plexus is found between the circular and longitudinal muscles and functions to mediate intrinsic motor control of the esophagus. The Meissner plexus is within the submucosa and innervates the muscularis mucosae and secretory glands.

Swallowing begins when a food bolus is propelled into the pharynx from the mouth. The initiation of the swallow is voluntary, but the pharyngeal and esophageal phases that follow are involuntary. During ingestion of a meal, the pharyngeal constrictors contract, the UES relaxes, and distention of the proximal striated muscle initiates primary peristalsis. A rapidly progressing pharyngeal contraction then transfers the bolus through the relaxed UES into the esophagus, coordinated by the medullary swallowing center. As the UES closes, a progressive circular contraction begins in the upper esophagus and proceeds distally along the esophageal body to propel the bolus through the relaxed LES. Peristaltic pressures normally ranging from 30 to 180 mm Hg are generated. The LES subsequently closes with a prolonged contraction, preventing movement back into the esophagus. The mechanical effect of peristalsis is a stripping wave, so called because it strips the esophagus clean from its proximal to its distal end. Esophageal distention signals

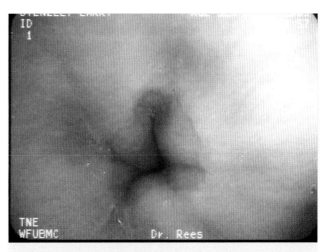

Fig. 97.1 Normal squamocolumnar junction.

secondary peristalsis to clear any remaining food. Finally, tertiary peristalsis consists of nonperistaltic contractions that may occur spontaneously or after swallowing.

Both the UES and LES are tonically contracted at rest. The closed state of the UES is primarily the result of continuous neural excitation. The resting state of contraction of the UES assists in preventing regurgitation and aspiration. It is believed that the tonic contraction of the LES is a function of the muscle itself and not dependent on neural effects. The stimulation of inhibitory fibers results in LES relaxation. The resting tone of the LES is typically between 15 and 45 mm Hg and is affected by a wide array of events, foods, drugs, and hormones. LES relaxation occurs not only in response to swallowing but also in response to esophageal distention.

97.3 Diverticula

Esophageal diverticula are small pouches or sacs in areas of weakness created by herniation of the lining of the esophagus through the muscular wall. True diverticula include all three layers of the esophagus, whereas in false diverticula, the mucosa and submucosa herniate through the muscular wall. The most common type of diverticulum is a Zenker diverticulum, which is a (false) pharyngoesophageal pulsion diverticulum typically associated with an underlying motility disorder and/or cricopharyngeal dysfunction. A Zenker diverticulum occurs proximal to the UES in the hypopharynx and involves the Killian triangle between the cricopharyngeus muscle and the raphe of the inferior pharyngeal constrictor muscles. A Killian-Jamieson diverticulum protrudes through a muscular gap (Killian-Jamieson triangle) in the anterolateral wall of the cervical esophagus inferior to the cricopharyngeus, superior to the circular muscle of the esophagus, and lateral to the longitudinal muscle of the esophagus. Killian-Jamieson diverticulum also has been called lateral cervical esophageal diverticulum. Zenker diverticulum is felt to be associated with chronic cricopharyngeal dysfunction and/or reflux. Symptoms include dysphagia, regurgitation, malodorous breath, cough, and aspiration. Zenker diverticulum is most readily diagnosed on fluoroscopic esophagram (▶ Fig. 97.2), although it may be seen on esophagoscopy at times. For symptomatic diverticula, endoscopic or open treatment can be performed, including a complete cricopharyngeal myotomy. For endoscopic diverticulotomy, the cricopharyngeal muscle is divided completely with a laser or surgical stapler device, effectively marsupializing the pouch so that it no longer collects food or saliva. In an open diverticulectomy, complete excision of the pouch is performed along with a cricopharyngeal myotomy (see Chapter 98 for further discussion of Zenker diverticulum).

97.4 Embryologic Disorders

Several esophageal disorders are a direct result of embryologic development disorders. The most common congenital anomalies are esophageal atresia and tracheo-esophageal fistula, which often present together as a result of failure of recanalization of the embryonic esophagus. The most common scenario is a distal tracheo-esophageal fistula and proximal atresia. Other, less common congenital abnormalities include esophageal

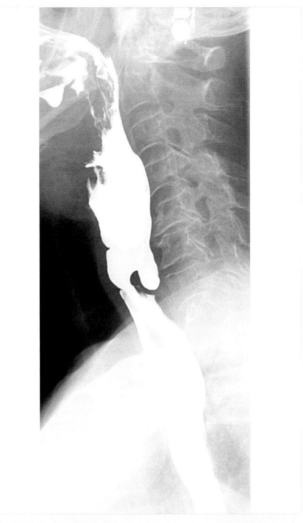

Fig. 97.2 Zenker diverticulum esophagram.

duplication cyst, which may present as a neck mass, and dysphagia lusoria, which is caused by compression of the esophagus by an anomalous retroesophageal right subclavian artery. Dysphagia lusoria is often associated with a nonrecurrent laryngeal nerve, and it may not present until middle age, when vessel elasticity is compromised. Children with tracheo-esophageal fistula may present very early in life with feeding difficulties, drooling, or respiratory distress. These children need to be evaluated for comorbidities because as many as 50% of them may have a cardiac or other abnormality. Radiographs may demonstrate a large amount of air in the stomach and proximal intestine. There may be inability to pass a nasogastric tube past 9 to 13 cm from the nares. Treatment for tracheo-esophageal fistula or atresia is urgent surgical repair in the newborn child. Dysphagia lusoria may be diagnosed by esophagram revealing a pulsatile horizontal bar at the obstruction site.

97.5 Cricopharyngeal Dysfunction

Cricopharyngeal dysfunction results from abnormal relaxation of the cricopharyngeus muscle and/or abnormal coordination between the pharynx and cricopharyngeus. Laryngopharyngeal

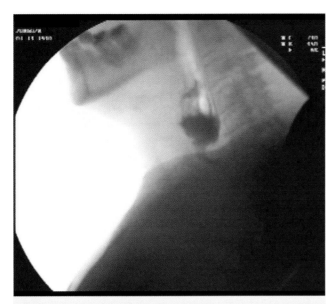

Fig. 97.3 Cricopharyngeal bar.

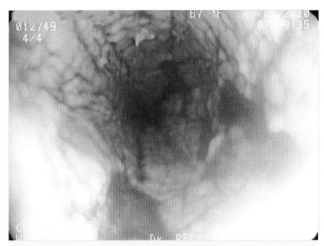

Fig. 97.4 *Candida* esophagitis.

reflux may contribute to cricopharyngeal dysfunction when chronic acid irritation triggers a neural reflex to increase UES pressure. The symptoms can be hard for patients to localize but are typically at the level of the cricoid cartilage or the suprasternal notch. Globus sensation and the sensation of effortful swallow or food sticking in the throat are common. Patients may describe a "choking" sensation, as well. It is very important to rule out distal esophageal problems in the presence of cricopharyngeal abnormalities because the cricopharyngeal dysfunction may be the result of compensation for a more distal esophageal problem. On fluoroscopic studies, the cricopharyngeus may appear prominent, looking like a "bar" during deglutition (▶ Fig. 97.3). Cricopharyngeal manometry is the best test for confirming cricopharyngeal dysfunction. The treatment of this region includes swallowing therapy, dilation, botulinum toxin injection, or cricopharyngeal myotomy (see Chapter 98 for further discussion of cricopharyngeal dysfunction).

97.6 Infectious and Inflammatory Disorders

There are many causes of nonspecific esophagitis that may present as heartburn or odynophagia. The most common infectious cause of esophagitis is *Candida albicans*. Patients often present with pain and dysphagia and are at increased risk if immunocompromised or on long-term antibiotics. Examining the oral cavity is not sufficient because esophageal candidiasis can present without findings of fungus in the oral cavity or pharynx. The fungal infection is suspected when white plaques with an erythematous base are seen on esophagoscopy (▶ Fig. 97.4). Treatment includes topical or systemic antifungals. Topical treatment may begin with nystatin swish and swallow (400,000 to 600,000 units four times daily or clotrimazole troches (one 10-mg troche dissolved slowly five times daily). With topical agents, successful therapy depends on adequate contact time between the agent and the oral mucosa. If the

patient does not respond to these local measures, the preferred therapy is oral fluconazole, A minimal starting dose is a 200-mg loading dose, then 100 to 200 mg daily for 14 to 21 days. When this treatment fails, biopsy with fungal culture should be performed.

Pill-induced esophagitis can cause punctate ulcerations that form as a result of prolonged contact of the esophageal mucosa with medications. The mechanism of pill-induced esophagitis is felt to involve delayed transit of the medication through the esophagus and local chemical irritation. Some of the more common offenders include tetracyclines, potassium chloride, doxycycline, aspirin, and bisphosphonates. Risk factors for pill-induced esophagitis include improper administration of medications (e.g., ingestion of the pill with inadequate volumes of fluid and/or taking medications just before lying down). The extent of injury caused by pill-induced esophagitis can range from superficial inflammation to deep ulceration and stricture formation. In general, pill-induced esophageal injuries heal without intervention within a few days, but avoiding the injurious drug is paramount. All medications should be converted to a liquid form, if possible, while the esophagus is healing. Acid suppression may be a useful adjunct treatment. A suspension of sucralfate may serve to layer a protective coating on the esophageal mucosa and promote healing. Patients should be instructed to remain upright and to drink copious amounts of water after taking the medication. For the patient who is unable to eat or drink because of severe odynophagia, a temporary period of parenteral hydration or alimentation may be required.

Eosinophilic esophagitis is an uncommon disorder of esophageal inflammation. According to an American Gastroenterological Association (AGA) consensus panel, eosinophilic esophagitis is a clinicopathologic disease characterized by the following: (1) symptoms including but not restricted to food impaction and dysphagia in adults; (2) feeding intolerance and symptoms of gastroesophageal reflux disease (GERD) in children; and (3) the presence of 15 or more eosinophils per high-power field on esophageal mucosal biopsy. The cause of the disorder is unknown, but it is increasingly diagnosed and has been linked to allergies. Two main hypotheses have been proposed to explain the pathogenesis of eosinophilic esophagitis. The first holds that

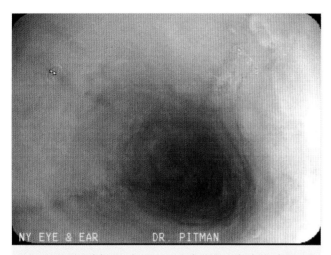

Fig. 97.5 Eosinophilic esophagitis. Note the mucosal edema, longitudinal furrows, "crepe paper mucosa," and white exudate.

a response to a food or an allergen triggers cytokine production. Recent studies exploring elemental diets in children have found that these diets can lead to a complete resolution of esophageal eosinophilia, confirming that food allergies are related to eosinophilic esophagitis in at least some patients. The second theory holds that GERD causes peptic damage to the epithelial tight junctions, which leads to increased permeability and subsequent recruitment of inflammatory cells, especially eosinophils. One of the consensus diagnostic criteria is the presence of 15 or more eosinophils per high-power field on biopsy. The esophageal mucosa is unique in the gut because it is normally devoid of any resident eosinophils. However, eosinophils accumulate in disease states such as GERD, Crohn disease, collagen vascular disease, connective tissue diseases, and drug-associated esophagitis. Therefore, a careful work-up to rule out existing conditions must be made before eosinophilic esophagitis can be diagnosed. The differential diagnosis in these cases must take into consideration the patient's history, clinical presentation, endoscopic features, and precise enumeration of eosinophils per high-power field. Adults with eosinophilic esophagitis usually do not have elevated eosinophil or immunoglobulin E levels in peripheral blood smears. Adults classically present with dysphagia to solids, food impaction, or strictures. Endoscopy may reveal trachealization of the esophagus with a ringed appearance; however, the esophagus may look normal, and therefore a high index of suspicion is warranted. The endoscopic features of eosinophilic esophagitis include longitudinal furrowing, friability, edema, longitudinal shearing, raised white lesions, whitish exudates, "crepe paper mucosa," a narrow esophagus, and transient or fixed rings (▶ Fig. 97.5). In the review by the AGA panel, 86% of patients were found to have rings, strictures, or a narrow esophagus. Although none of these features can be classified as pathognomonic, in the appropriate clinical context, the presence of more than one of these findings is strongly suggestive of the diagnosis. After endoscopy and biopsy, the treatment options include ingested or topical steroids, allergy evaluation, and elimination trials. Caution is advised during esophagoscopy because patients with eosinophilic esophagitis are prone to superficial lacerations and are at higher risk for esophageal perforation.

Polymyositis is a type of muscle weakness due to inflammation and degenerative changes in striated muscle. Proximal muscle weakness in the shoulder and hips is the most common presenting symptom. When associated with skin rashes, the disorder is termed dermatomyositis. Peristalsis is diminished and poorly coordinated, and the esophagus may be dilated. Manometry reveals decreased UES pressure and reduced peristaltic waves. The goals of treatment are to improve muscle strength and to avoid the development of extramuscular complications. In patients with dermatomyositis, resolution of the cutaneous manifestations is an additional goal. Patients with polymyositis are generally referred to rheumatology for an immunologic work-up and treatment. Treatment generally consists of glucocorticoids; other treatment options can include azathioprine or methotrexate. Patients may be on systemic steroid therapy for as long as a year.

GERD is the backward flow of gastric contents into the esophagus and overall the most common cause of inflammatory esophagitis. Further backward flow into the pharynx is known as laryngopharyngeal reflux (LPR), or extraesophageal reflux. Typical symptoms of GERD include regurgitation, heartburn, and chest pain. Symptoms of LPR include dysphagia, intermittent dysphonia, throat clearing, globus sensation, and cough. The mechanism of GERD is related to transient inappropriate LES relaxations and gastric distention. The mechanism of LPR is less well understood but may involve inappropriate UES relaxation, as well. Refluxate may consist of food, gas, stomach acid, bile acids (bile reflux), or esophageal contents (esophagopharyngeal reflux). Esophageal injury from reflux may manifest as erosive esophagitis (▶ Fig. 97.6) or peptic stricture. Endoscopic changes in the mucosa of the esophagus are not required for the diagnosis of reflux (nonerosive reflux disease). Reflux is frequently seen in the setting of a hiatal hernia. Prolonged GERD predisposes to Barrett esophagus and adenocarcinoma. However, the "spectrum of disease" approach has been challenged by the view that GERD may be a disease with "categories," such as nonerosive disease, erosive esophagitis, and Barrett esophagus, and that conversion from one disease state to another is distinctly unusual. Data suggest that although GERD may progress in severity, the reported rates of progression are relatively low over a 20-year period. GERD is often evaluated with ambulatory pH monitoring and manometry. Manometry may confirm that the pH probe is in the correct location, as well as evaluate for motility disorders. All proton pump inhibitors should be held before the ambulatory pH monitoring. The AGA recommends that endoscopy with biopsy be performed for patients with GERD and dysphagia who have not responded to an empiric trial of twice-daily proton pump inhibitor therapy. The treatment of reflux includes lifestyle modifications and acid-reducing medications, such as proton pump inhibitors. Proton pump inhibitors do not physically stop reflux; instead, they reduce the acidity of the refluxate (increase the pH). Unfortunately, weakly acidic refluxate or even refluxate with a neutral pH may be injurious to the esophageal lining and cause reflux symptoms.

Barrett esophagus is a potentially serious complication of long-standing GERD. It occurs when the normal stratified squamous epithelium of the distal esophagus has been replaced by intestinal columnar epithelium (metaplasia). Barrett esophagus is the most significant outcome of chronic GERD and a risk factor for esophageal adenocarcinoma. Thus, it is recommended

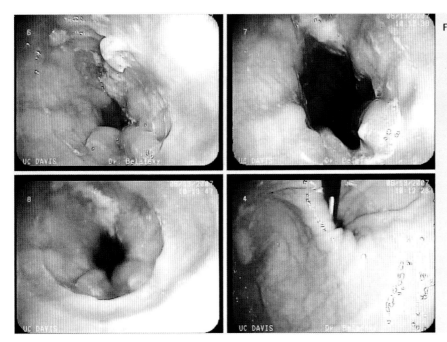

Fig. 97.6 Erosive esophagitis.

that patients with prolonged GERD symptoms, especially middle-aged white men, undergo endoscopic screening for Barrett esophagus. If Barrett esophagus is confirmed, these patients require continued endoscopic surveillance to detect the development of dysplasia and adenocarcinoma. The risk for esophageal adenocarcinoma in Barrett esophagus is approximately 0.5% annually, but the risk increases substantially in patients with longer (> 3 cm) affected esophageal segments and with high-grade dysplasia. The goal of surveillance is to detect cancer at an earlier and potentially curable stage. Endoscopic surveillance guidelines suggest four-quadrant biopsies at 2-cm intervals along the entire affected length of the esophagus at varying time periods depending on the presence or severity of dysplasia.

97.7 Trauma

Esophageal injuries may be iatrogenic or induced. Mallory-Weiss tear is an incomplete tear of the esophageal mucosa and laceration of submucosal arteries resulting from increased abdominal pressure. It is commonly associated with retching in alcoholics and may present as upper gastrointestinal bleeding. In Boerhaave syndrome, increased abdominal pressure causes all three layers of the esophagus to rupture; patients have severe symptoms of hematemesis, chest pain, and hypovolemic shock. Esophageal perforations, whether due to trauma or instrumentation, including endoscopy and nasogastric tube placement, should all be considered otolaryngologic emergencies. In patients at risk for esophageal perforation, tachycardia, chest pain, dysphagia, or dyspnea should be immediately evaluated.

97.8 Foreign Body Ingestion

Foreign body ingestion is most common in children. Foreign bodies tend to lodge at three areas of natural constriction in the esophagus: the level of the cricopharyngeus, the aortic arch, and the LES. Patients who have esophageal foreign bodies present with drooling, dysphagia, or dyspnea from compression of the adjacent membranous posterior tracheal wall. Common esophageal foreign bodies include coins, food, toys, and disc batteries. Upon the patient's presentation to the emergency department, both lateral and anteroposterior films should be obtained. If there is a concern for foreign body ingestion by history, physical examination, or imaging findings, the patient should undergo endoscopy. Disc batteries can often be differentiated from coins by the appearance of a small double ring on an anteroposterior film or a slight "step-off" on a lateral film (▶ Fig. 97.7). Disc battery damage is predominantly from an external current that causes electrolysis of tissue fluids, generating hydroxide. Any patient who has ingested a disc battery should be taken urgently to the operating room. Airway compromise from esophageal edema has been reported as early as 3 hours after ingestion, and esophageal injury has occurred in patients with a battery lodged for less than 2 hours. The longer the battery has been in the esophagus, the more edematous the mucosa becomes and the more tightly the battery adheres to the mucosa, making extraction more difficult and dangerous. If the battery remains in place, ulceration and perforation can occur. Treatment depends on the extent of injury and parallels that for ingested caustic materials, discussed below. In the case of any suspected esophageal foreign body, general anesthesia with endotracheal intubation is recommended to protect the airway. The otolaryngology team should perform the intubation in the case of a second foreign body in the oropharynx or hypopharynx. After removal of the foreign body, the esophagus should be assessed for underlying pathology, such as stricture. Complications from the removal of foreign bodies are uncommon but may include esophageal perforation and delayed stricture formation.

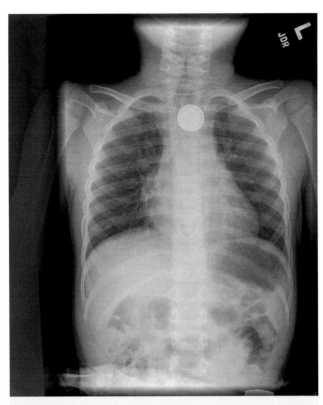

Fig. 97.7 Note the double ring of a disc battery on anteroposterior view.

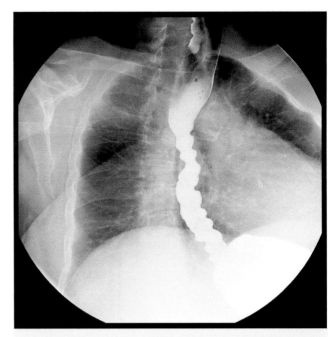

Fig. 97.8 Corkscrew esophagram.

97.9 Ingestion of Caustic Materials

Ingestion of caustic materials generally occurs in children but may occasionally also occur in adults, most commonly in psychotic persons, the elderly, or prisoners. Alkaline ingestion causes liquefaction necrosis and more severe damage than acidic ingestion, which causes coagulation necrosis. The coagulum that forms in acid ingestion may help to limit the depth of penetration of the caustic substance. The severity of oropharyngeal and external injury does not always correlate with the severity of esophageal injury. Symptoms include drooling, mouth pain, stridor, chest pain, and abdominal pain. The oral cavity may appear normal, and a normal appearance does not rule out esophageal injury. Injury occurs in stages; within the first 24 hours, a dusky edema develops and ulceration may appear; then, submucosal inflammation occurs over the next few days, followed by a sloughing of the superficial layer at 5 to 7 days. Fibrosis of the deep layers with scar and stricture may develop in 1 to 4 weeks. The general consensus recommends endoscopy within the first 24 to 48 hours of presentation. Delayed evaluation may increase the risk for perforation on endoscopy. Esophageal injury is graded at the time of endoscopy. Grade 1 injury consists of edema and erythema, and patients with grade 1 injury can usually be fed normally and discharged home. Grade 2 esophageal injury consists of linear ulcerations and necrotic tissue with whitish plaques of necrosis. These lesions rarely progress to esophageal stenosis, although some patients may require esophageal dilation. Grade 3 esophageal injury is characterized by circumferential injury, which may be transmural with mucosal sloughing. Patients with grade 3 injury require

placement of a feeding tube under direct vision or intravenous nutrition. Grade 3 injuries carry a higher risk for stricture in the future. The feeding tube not only provides a method for nutrition but also serves as a stent to maintain a lumen during stricture formation. Patients with evidence of grade 4 injury (perforation seen on radiology or endoscopy) have a very poor prognosis and a high fatality rate due to systemic complications. Some grade 3 and most grade 4 injuries will require temporary diversion or esophagectomy. Long esophageal strictures have been reported in up to 40% or more of pediatric patients who have grade 2 or grade 3 injury following an alkali ingestion. In 80% of the patients in whom strictures ultimately develop, the strictures develop within 8 weeks after the ingestion. Corticosteroids are controversial; some authors report benefit for grade 2 or 3 injuries, but most authors opine that steroids do not decrease the rate of stricture. Charcoal, gastric lavage, and emetics are contraindicated. The induction of vomiting is contraindicated because vomiting may lead to additional esophageal injury if the gastric contents come in contact with the esophageal mucosa. Diluting or neutralizing agents are not effective in preventing esophageal injury and may lead to vomiting.

97.10 Esophageal Motility Disorders

Motility disorders may be classified as hypo- or hyperkinetic disorders. Hyperkinetic motility disorders include nutcracker esophagus and distal esophageal spasm, both of which usually present with noncardiac chest pain. The diagnostic work-up includes manometry with an assessment of esophageal pressures along the pharynx and esophagus. Manometry reveals normal peristalsis with high-amplitude esophageal contractions in nutcracker esophagus versus nonperistaltic contractions (with normal or elevated pressure) in esophageal smooth muscle in distal esophageal spasm. Newer testing includes impedance, which examines bolus transit along the esophagus. In distal esophageal spasm, the esophagram may show a "corkscrew" appearance, but it is more commonly normal (▶ Fig. 97.8). Treatment consists of nitrates, calcium channel blockers, anticholinergics, and possibly dilation or botulinum toxin injections in advanced cases. Nutcracker esophagus is treated with antireflux therapy, calcium channel blockers, and/or nitrates to decrease the amplitude of the contractions.

Hypokinetic motility disorders include achalasia and progressive systemic sclerosis. In achalasia, degeneration of the Auerbach plexus results in aperistalsis and a poorly relaxing LES. Symptoms may include progressive dysphagia, vomiting, malodorous breath, chest pain, and weight loss. Progressive systemic sclerosis is an autoimmune disease that causes small-vessel vasculitis, widespread collagen deposition, and fibrosis of smooth muscle in the lower two-thirds (smooth-muscle portion) of the esophagus. Symptoms include severe GERD, dysphagia, and tight sclerotic skin. The work-up includes manometry and barium swallow. In achalasia, manometry most often reveals an esophageal amplitude of less than 30 mm Hg and an increased LES pressure with poor relaxation. Diagnosis by barium swallow may reveal a pointed "bird's beak" appearance at the LES, air–fluid levels, and/or aperistalsis (▶ Fig. 97.9). Progressive systemic sclerosis is also diagnosed by barium swallow. The flaccid, dilated esophagus is similar to that seen in achalasia; however, the LES is patent. Manometry will show normal UES pressure, loss of tone of the LES, and aperistalsis because only smooth muscle is affected. The treatment of achalasia can include serial dilation; a Heller myotomy of the esophagus, LES, and cardia; botulinum toxin A injections to the LES; and calcium channel blockers to decrease LES pressure. Progressive systemic sclerosis has a higher risk for reflux because the LES is incompetent. Treatment includes antireflux medication, calcium channel blockers, and systemic steroids.

97.11 Esophageal Stenosis

Esophageal stenosis may be due to a multitude of conditions, including stricture, esophageal rings, and uncommonly Plummer-Vinson syndrome. Esophageal strictures may develop from a multitude of causes, including reflux, radiation injury, and caustic ingestion, among others. The proximal esophagus is particularly susceptible to radiation-induced stricture after treatment for head and neck cancer because of its more tenuous blood supply. An esophageal lumen narrowed to less than 13 mm generally will cause symptoms of dysphagia. Esophageal rings include both type A and type B rings. Type A rings uncommonly develop from muscular hypertrophy at the proximal LES. Type B rings, or Schatzki rings, occur at the squamocolumnar junction and are associated with reflux and hiatal hernias (▶ Fig. 97.10). Plummer-Vinson syndrome may occur in patients with a long history of iron deficiency and is more common in middle-aged women of Scandinavian descent. Patients may present with microcytic anemia, cheilitis, splenomegaly, and dysphagia due to a degeneration of esophageal muscle that leads to the formation of cervical pharyngoesophageal webs. Because of an increased risk for esophageal carcinoma, patients

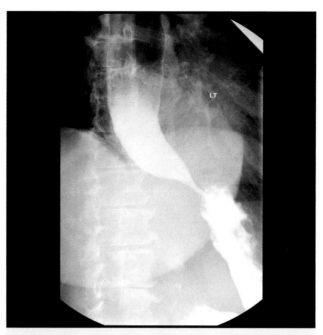

Fig. 97.9 Achalasia "bird's beak" esophagus.

warrant close follow-up. Other treatments include cautious dilation and iron supplementation. Esophageal stricture is usually treated by serial dilation with balloons, bougies, or Savory dilators. Type A esophageal rings are often treated with botulinum toxin A injection, whereas type B Schatzki rings can be treated with dilation. Antireflux therapy is advisable to prevent recurrence.

97.12 Esophageal Neoplasms

Neoplasia in the esophagus is relatively uncommon but when present is typically malignant. In 2012, there were 17,460 new cases of esophageal carcinoma in the United States and 15,070 deaths. The two main pathologies are squamous cell carcinoma and adenocarcinoma. For most of the 20th century, the vast majority of esophageal cancers were squamous cell carcinomas. In the 1960s, squamous cell carcinoma accounted for more than 90% of all esophageal tumors in the United States, whereas esophageal adenocarcinomas were considered so uncommon that some authorities questioned their existence. For the past three decades, however, the frequency of adenocarcinoma of the esophagus, esophagogastric junction, and gastric cardia has increased dramatically in Western countries, so that adenocarcinoma now occurs with greater frequency than squamous cell carcinoma. Risk factors for squamous cell carcinoma of the esophagus include alcohol and tobacco abuse, and it is usually found in the thoracic esophagus. The incidence rates for esophageal squamous cell carcinoma were highest in blacks (8.8 per 100,000 per year) and Asians (3.9 per 100,000 per year). In contrast, adenocarcinoma presents in the distal esophagus at the gastroesophageal junction and is associated with GERD and Barrett esophagus. Adenocarcinoma is largely a disease of Caucasians and males, with the incidence in males outnumbering that in females by as much as 6:1. Barrett esophagus is usually

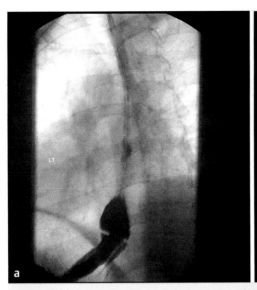
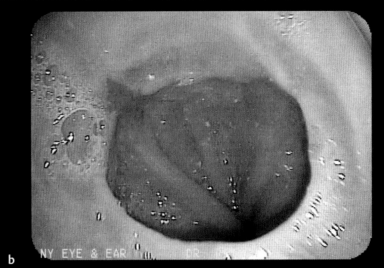

Fig. 97.10 Schatzki ring. (**a**) Radiograph. (**b**) Esophagoscopic appearance.

discovered during endoscopic examinations of middle-aged and older adults, whose mean age at the time of diagnosis is approximately 55 years. Patients who have an esophageal malignancy typically present with dysphagia and weight loss due to mechanical obstruction. Under most circumstances, esophageal cancer is identified at a late, incurable stage. Endoscopic resection is considered appropriate therapy for neoplastic lesions limited to the superficial mucosal layers because these tumors have low rates of lymph node metastasis (< 3%). There is less consensus, however, with regard to lesions that extend to the muscularis mucosae. Most centers consider endoscopic treatment for this early neoplasia acceptable, although others disagree. Esophagectomy is preferred for lesions that invade the submucosa, given the significantly higher rates of lymph node metastasis associated with these lesions. There is some hope that with increased screening and surveillance for Barrett esophagus in patients who have GERD, adenocarcinoma will be detected at an earlier and potentially curable stage. However, at this time, palliative care remains a high priority for patients with advanced disease.

97.13 Roundsmanship

- Esophagitis due to infectious, caustic, medical, or irritant causes should be evaluated in patients with throat pain.
- Reflux may cause esophagitis, with sequelae of strictures, motility disorders, and intestinal metaplasia.
- Eosinophilic esophagitis should be considered in adults with a history of food impaction, persistent dysphagia, or gastroesophageal reflux disease (GERD) that fails to respond to medical therapy. In children, symptoms that may be associated with eosinophilic esophagitis vary by age and include feeding disorders, vomiting, abdominal pain, dysphagia, and food impaction.
- Esophageal foreign bodies should be imaged with two views; disc batteries lodged in the esophagus must be emergently removed by endoscopy.

- Esophageal masses are predominantly malignant. Adenocarcinoma is increasing in frequency to become the most common esophageal neoplasm in the United States.

97.14 Recommended Reading

[1] Amin MR, Belafsky PC. Cough and swallowing dysfunction. Otolaryngol Clin North Am 2010; 43: 35–42

[2] Castell DO, Richter JE. The Esophagus. 4th ed. Philiadelphia, PA: Lippincott Williams & Wilkins; 2004

[3] Elliott EJ, Thomas D, Markowitz JE. Non-surgical interventions for eosinophilic esophagitis. Cochrane Database Syst Rev 2010: CD004065

[4] Francis DL, Katzka DA. Achalasia: update on the disease and its treatment. Gastroenterology 2010; 139: 369–374

[5] Gaudreault P, Parent M, McGuigan MA, Chicoine L, Lovejoy FH. Predictability of esophageal injury from signs and symptoms: a study of caustic ingestion in 378 children. Pediatrics 1983; 71: 767–770

[6] Hirano I, Richter JE Practice Parameters Committee of the American College of Gastroenterology. ACG practice guidelines: esophageal reflux testing. Am J Gastroenterol 2007; 102: 668–685

[7] Joffe MM, Love LA, Leff RL et al. Drug therapy of the idiopathic inflammatory myopathies: predictors of response to prednisone, azathioprine, and methotrexate and a comparison of their efficacy. Am J Med 1993; 94: 379–387

[8] Kahrilas PJ, Smout AJ. Esophageal disorders. Am J Gastroenterol 2010; 105: 747–756

[9] Kay M, Wyllie R. Caustic ingestions in children. Curr Opin Pediatr 2009; 21: 651–654

[10] Liacouras CA, Furuta GT, Hirano I et al. Eosinophilic esophagitis: updated consensus recommendations for children and adults. J Allergy Clin Immunol 2011; 128: 3–20, e6, quiz 21–22

[11] Marcum KK, Mott RT, Rees CJ. Eosinophilic esophagitis. Ear Nose Throat J 2009; 88: 1258–1259

[12] Pappas PG, Kauffman CA, Andes D et alInfectious Diseases Society of America. Clinical practice guidelines for the management of candidiasis: 2009 update by the Infectious Diseases Society of America. Clin Infect Dis 2009; 48: 503–535

[13] R, Castell DO. Esophageal motility disorders (distal esophageal spasm, nutcracker esophagus, and hypertensive lower esophageal sphincter): modern management. Curr Treat Options Gastroenterol 2006; 9: 283–294

98 Management of Oropharyngeal Dysphagia

Neel Bhatt and Stacey L. Halum

98.1 Introduction

There are many diverse and frequently occurring pathologies that lead to oropharyngeal dysphagia. Although the presentations of dysphagia may often appear similar, careful investigation, including a thorough clinical history and selective imaging methods, can help identify the underlying pathology. In this chapter, important causes of oropharyngeal dysphagia are outlined, with particular emphasis placed on the evaluation and treatment of each disorder. Topics discussed in this chapter include the management of aspiration, cricopharyngeal dysfunction, Zenker diverticula, neurogenic dysphagia, and dysphagia following therapy for head and neck cancer.

98.2 Evaluation and Management of Aspiration

98.2.1 Description of Dysphagia with Aspiration

Aspiration is characterized by the improper passage of oropharyngeal or hypopharyngeal contents into the larynx and lower respiratory tract, beyond the level of the true vocal folds. Aspiration may occur throughout any age group, but its frequency appears to be greatest among the elderly because of the increasing incidence of dysphagia with aging. Aspiration occurring with deglutition or secondary to laryngopharyngeal reflux events is often related to a multitude of reasons, such as a weak cough reflex, lack of motor coordination/function, or impaired laryngeal sensation. Many of the causes are discussed in greater detail throughout this chapter.

The risk for developing aspiration pneumonia from inhaled oral contents necessitates the proper and effective prevention of recurrent aspiration. The oropharyngeal bacteria within the aspirated contents are believed to be the nidus for infection in the development of aspiration-related pneumonia. The chief pathogens responsible for pneumonia are *Streptococcus pneumoniae* and *Haemophilus influenzae*, which normally colonize the nasopharynx and oropharynx. Chemical pneumonitis, which may occur acutely or chronically, is irritation and damage of the lung parenchyma after the aspiration or inhalation of noninfectious agents. Many studies suggest that approximately half of healthy adults aspirate small quantities of oropharyngeal contents. However, as a consequence of low bacterial counts in the oropharyngeal contents, a vigorous coughing reflex, epithelial ciliary transport, and both cellular and humoral immunity, the aspirated contents typically do not lead to the development of pneumonia in healthy individuals.

98.2.2 Differential Diagnosis of Dysphagia with Aspiration

The differential diagnosis of dysphagia with aspiration is important to consider because populations at high risk for aspiration tend to have a multitude of cardiac and pulmonary comorbidities. Pulmonary edema, often seen among individuals with decompensated heart failure or fluid overload, may present similarly to aspiration pneumonia with shortness of breath, dyspnea on exertion, and tachypnea. Unlike aspiration pneumonia, pulmonary edema tends to present with crackles on pulmonary auscultation. A chest radiograph will generally show bilateral opacities, compared with dependent lobe opacification in aspiration pneumonia. Leukocytosis tends to be absent in pulmonary edema. A beta-natriuretic peptide (BNP) test and echocardiography can further clarify the etiology of a patient's complaint.

In the diagnosis of aspiration pneumonia, the possibility hospital-acquired or community-acquired pneumonia must be considered. Atypical organisms, not normally observed in aspiration pneumonia, may be detected with appropriate antigen testing, serology, or culture. Finally, fluoroscopic or endoscopic evaluation can help in determining whether aspiration is the likely causative means for the development of pneumonia.

98.2.3 Evaluation of Dysphagia with Aspiration

The clinical features of aspiration pneumonia vary considerably based on its severity. Generally, patients who have aspiration pneumonia present with a cough productive of purulent sputum, fever, chills, pleuritic chest pain, and shortness of breath. The aspiration event or events leading to pneumonia are typically not observed, a situation often described as "silent aspiration." Therefore, the diagnosis is usually made based upon the clinical presentation, suspicion of aspiration risk, and radiographic evidence demonstrating infiltrates in the dependent pulmonary lobes. In patients at high risk for the development of silent aspiration pneumonia, early antibiotic therapy may be warranted based on symptoms alone (fever, dyspnea and cough) because plain radiographs can miss approximately one-third of developing pneumonias. Although CT is highly sensitive for the detection of pneumonia, its time-consuming nature and high cost make it impractical for the diagnosis of aspiration pneumonia, which generally requires expedient recognition and the initiation of treatment to avoid associated symptom progression and respiratory decompensation.

Speech Pathology Evaluation

Patients presenting with aspiration pneumonia should undergo a videofluoroscopic evaluation of swallow (modified barium swallow [MBS]) or a flexible endoscopic evaluation of swallow (FEES) with a speech–language pathologist. Although there is ongoing debate about which swallowing assessment tool is the most sensitive for detecting aspiration and predicting future risk for aspiration pneumonia, both MBS and FEES are overall highly sensitive (>85%) in detecting aspiration (▶ Fig. 98.1). Bedside swallowing evaluations may be considered, but their sensitivity for detecting aspiration is significantly lower than

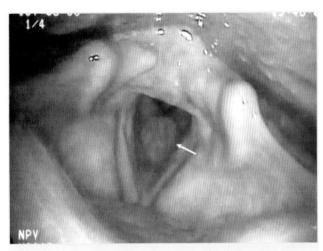

Fig. 98.1 A patient with impaired sensation demonstrates no cough reflex upon aspiration of a thick nectar bolus during flexible endoscopic evaluation of swallow (FEES). The material in the subglottic airway (*arrow*) was effectively cleared when the patient was cued to voluntarily cough and swallow.

that of MBS and FEES, especially in patients with silent aspiration (absence of spontaneous cough reflex).

98.2.4 Treatment of Dysphagia with Aspiration

Antibiotic Therapy

Antibiotics are always indicated for acute or chronic aspiration pneumonia. For nontoxic patients, early and aggressive antibiotic therapy is essential to prevent the progression of symptoms and avoid the need for parenteral antibiotics and hospitalization. Such cases typically can be managed with broad-spectrum antibiotics, such as ceftriaxone with azithromycin, levofloxacin, or moxifloxacin. In the inpatient setting, the goal remains to provide broad coverage that includes gram-negative bacteria, so that third-generation cephalosporins, fluoroquinolones, and piperacillin are appropriate antibiotic choices. If the patient has been recently hospitalized, antibiotics may be required that cover specific pathogens, including methicillin-resistant *Staphylococcus aureus* (MRSA), *Klebsiella pneumoniae*, and *Pseudomonas aeruginosa*. Sputum cultures with the early initiation of culture-directed antibiotic therapy are important in management.

Positioning Maneuvers and Swallowing Exercises

During the MBS or FEES, the speech–language pathologist can determine whether compensatory swallowing techniques can be employed to minimize the aspiration of food contents. Swallowing techniques are widely recommended as compensatory strategies for individuals with oropharyngeal dysphagia, although the efficacy of some techniques remains controversial. The benefits of the following techniques are highly dependent on the mechanism of the swallowing dysfunction. They must be tailored to fit the patient's specific swallowing deficits and

must be feasible based on the patient's comorbidities, cognitive abilities, and motivation. The most basic recommendations are postural techniques, which include chin tuck, head turn, and head tilt. The chin tuck maneuver brings the patient's chin closer to the chest, thereby decreasing the size of the laryngeal opening by moving the base of the tongue and epiglottis posteriorly. In the head turn technique, the patient turns the head toward the weaker, less sensate, or damaged side (e.g., a patient following a stroke or peripheral paresis). With this technique, twisting the neck toward the injured side prevents a food bolus from traveling down the weaker side of the pharynx, allowing it to be more efficiently propelled along the stronger side. In the head tilt maneuver, the patient tilts the head toward the stronger side, encouraging bolus transmission down this side. Other swallowing maneuvers include the supraglottic swallow, super-supraglottic swallow, effortful swallow, and Mendelsohn maneuver. Each technique requires more deliberate action with each swallow. In the Mendelsohn maneuver, the patient physically holds up the larynx to keep it elevated immediately after swallowing. This technique is usually indicated for individuals with limited laryngeal excursion and a reduced cricopharyngeal opening. The supraglottic swallow is helpful for patients with aspiration during the swallow, especially patients with reduced laryngeal sensation. Patients are instructed to hold their breath throughout the entire swallow, then cough immediately thereafter to prevent aspiration. Finally, the super-supraglottic swallow is a slightly modified version of the supraglottic swallow, in which patients perform a Valsalva maneuver while holding their breath to maximize posterior glottic closure during the swallow.

Exercises can also be prescribed to help strengthen the muscles of deglutition. The patient can practice forceful swallowing, which helps to generate more pressure during actual swallowing. In the falsetto exercise, the patient practices phonation while sliding up a scale to the highest pitch possible. This particular exercise results in a level of laryngeal elevation similar to that in swallowing. The breath-hold exercise, in which the patient inhales and holds the breath for a few seconds, helps strengthen the airway closure at the level of the vocal folds. Additional exercises are used to strengthen the tongue and increase the range of motion of the jaw, lips, and tongue. For pharyngeal constrictor and strap muscle strengthening, Shaker exercises are often prescribed, in which the patient performs repetitive, gentle cervical flexion against gravity while in a supine position.

Surgical Management

The surgical management of chronic aspiration is often warranted when improvement is not observed with medical management or speech–language therapy. The type of surgery depends on the mechanism of aspiration.

A wide variety of surgical options are available, including vocal fold medialization with or without arytenoid adduction, vocal fold injection augmentation, chemical or surgical cricopharyngeal muscle (CPM) myotomy, pharyngoplasty procedures, supraglottoplasty procedures, and various forms of laryngeal suspension. Vocal fold medialization or injection augmentation, for example, may be indicated in patients who have persistent and incomplete glottic closure due to unilateral vocal fold motion impairment, vocal fold scarring, or a decrease in vocal fold tissue. In patients with cricopharyngeal achalasia, chemodenervation with botulinum toxin and CPM myotomy via a transcervical or an endoscopic approach are appropriate options. Temporary injection with botulinum toxin may precede definitive surgical treatment because it can be useful in predicting candidates who are likely to improve with a surgical CPM myotomy.

Beyond individualized surgeries to minimize aspiration, a gastrointestinal procedure such as a feeding gastrostomy may be required if the patient's swallowing function is not capable of supporting adequate nutrition. In patients who are already dependent on a gastric feeding tube and continue to have problems due to reflux-related aspiration, the tube can often be advanced into the jejunum to help prevent reflux. When oropharyngeal secretions lead to chronic aspiration (as seen in cerebral palsy), these can be controlled with the surgical excision or botulinum toxin injection of salivary glands or the ligation of salivary ducts. In extreme cases, separation of the airway and digestive tract is necessary. These approaches render patients aphonic, and they must rely on alternative communication devices or on esophageal or tracheo-esophageal prosthetic speech. There are numerous long-term surgical options. Two that are potentially reversible include laryngotracheal separation and tracheo-esophageal diversion. In both, a tracheostoma is created. In the separation, the proximal end of the trachea is closed upon itself in a blind pouch, whereas in the diversion it is anastomosed to an esophagotomy to divert aspirate into the esophagus. The gold standard and the most definitive option for preventing aspiration is a total laryngectomy. This should be reserved for patients whose swallowing dysfunction is not expected to improve with time.

98.3 Evaluation and Management of Cricopharyngeal Muscle Dysfunction

98.3.1 Description of Cricopharyngeal Muscle Dysfunction

The CPM, a major contributor to the upper esophageal sphincter (UES), is an essential muscle in the mechanism of swallowing. The CPM is tonically contracted at baseline, then relaxes and dilates during swallow to permit bolus advancement through the UES into the esophagus. Normal UES function relies not only on the neuromuscular integrity of the CPM but also on the function of the surrounding muscles of deglutition. Thus, UES dysfunction can be either primary or secondary in nature; primary dysfunction occurs when the CPM itself is responsible for dysphagia, whereas secondary dysfunction typically occurs as a result of more global problems with dyscoordination or neuromuscular swallowing dysfunction (e.g., decreased laryngeal elevation or weak pharyngeal propulsion). Primary UES dysfunction is often idiopathic but may result from peripheral neurogenic injury or from disease processes like polymyositis. In primary UES dysfunction, the CPM exhibits chronic hypertonicity and spasm, failing to relax/dilate to allow bolus to advance through the UES. Because laryngeal elevation in an anterosupe-

rior direction and pharyngeal propulsion are necessary to draw open the UES and advance bolus through the UES, respectively, secondary UES dysfunction occurs when the CPM fails to open normally because of poor anterosuperior elevation of the larynx and/or decreased pharyngeal bolus pressure during swallowing. Patients who have poor laryngeal elevation and pharyngeal function, such as those who have had a stroke or have undergone extensive irradiation of the neck (strap muscles), may have such secondary UES dysfunction on videofluoroscopic swallowing examinations. The thyrohyoid muscle is particularly important in anterosuperior elevation of the larynx during swallow, which results in secondary mechanical opening and stretching of the CPM to allow bolus advancement. Experimental therapies such as implantable electrical stimulation and magnetic devices to promote bolus advancement through the UES have typically targeted methods to pull the larynx or cricoid in an anterosuperior direction to mechanically open the CPM. Patients with lack of laryngeal elevation during swallow and weak pharyngeal propulsion subsequent to stroke, irradiation, or other etiologies often fail to respond well to CPM myotomy or CPM chemodenervation because of insufficient opening of the UES for bolus transport despite the absence of underlying primary CPM resistance. In contrast, patients with isolated primary UES dysfunction have a much better response to CPM surgical and chemodenervation treatments.

98.3.2 Differential Diagnosis of Cricopharyngeal Dysfunction

There are a multitude of pathologies that are important to consider in the evaluation of CPM dysfunction. A thorough work-up, including endoscopy, can help eliminate other conditions that may be easily mistaken for CPM dysfunction. Diffuse or focal esophageal spasm and esophageal motility disorders typically present with dysphagia, regurgitation, and the sensation of a food bolus sticking to the throat. Individuals with esophageal spasm and motility disorders often will describe noncardiac chest pain, an important distinguishing characteristic of CPM dysfunction. Generalized pharyngeal or base of tongue weakness can also mimic CPM dysfunction, although patients often demonstrate pooling of bolus in the piriform sinuses and vallecula after swallowing. In cases of isolated pharyngeal weakness, the pharyngeal constrictors will fail to effectively propel bolus through the CPM, thus resulting in piriform pooling and the appearance of poor CPM dilation/opening on videofluoroscopic study. If such a situation is suspected, CPM dilation with botulinum toxin injection can be helpful in distinguishing CPM dysfunction from isolated pharyngeal weakness. If the procedure fails to relieve the swallowing dysfunction, aggressive pharyngeal constrictor strengthening exercises should be initiated.

Esophageal strictures also present with symptoms similar to those previously discussed. Strictures may develop in a primary process, such as fibrosis or neoplasm, or secondarily, such as in patients who have chronic acid reflux or are taking certain medications. A thorough clinical history can help elucidate potential causes of secondary esophageal stricture. When a primary process leading to stricture is suspected, endoscopy with biopsy can effectively differentiate it from other etiologies.

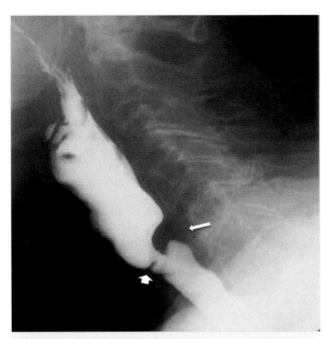

Fig. 98.2 Cricopharyngeal muscle (CPM) dysfunction. A prominent CPM bar is seen on radiographic modified barium swallow (*arrow*). This patient ultimately underwent endoscopic CPM myotomy with excellent response. There is also an incidental cervical esophageal web seen anteriorly (*arrowhead*).

98.3.3 Evaluation of Cricopharyngeal Muscle Dysfunction

The presentations of individuals experiencing CPM achalasia are varied. Patients often experience the sensation of solid food becoming stuck at the level of the cricoid during swallowing; they also experience choking or coughing. Although the diagnosis of CPM achalasia may be suggested by a thorough history and physical examination, endoscopic and radiographic evaluations are necessary steps in the evaluation. Endoscopic examination will rule out another cause of dysphagia, such as vocal fold dysfunction or laryngopharyngeal carcinoma. Radiographic studies can determine if a cricopharyngeal bar, dyscoordination, or pharyngeal diverticula are present (▶ Fig. 98.2).

The presence of a CPM bar alone is neither highly sensitive nor specific for CPM dysfunction, and manometry assessment should be considered in equivocal cases. Manometry of the UES is sensitive and specific in detecting CPM hypertonicity in experienced hands, although the reliability and accuracy of the results can be suboptimal in institutions without special expertise in UES assessment.

98.3.4 Treatment of Crichopharyngeal Muscle Dysfunction

CPM achalasia is typically unresponsive to medical intervention, such as therapy with systemic muscle relaxants. Botulinum toxin injection is a nonsurgical treatment option for relaxing the UES. Botulinum toxin promotes muscle relaxation by inhibiting the release of acetylcholine at the neuromuscu-

lar junction. Periodic injections of botulinum toxin into the CPM can provide temporary muscle relaxation and relieve dysphagia. The duration of action of botulinum toxin typically ranges from 3 to 9 months in most patients. The use of botulinum toxin is not a permanent solution for individuals with CPM achalasia and best serves as a trial of therapy when it is unclear if a myotomy will be effective. If the patient's symptoms improve upon administration of the botulinum toxin, then CPM achalasia is likely the correct diagnosis. In-office injection with electromyographic guidance can be effective in the treatment of elderly patients who have significant comorbidities and cannot undergo general anesthesia. If patients can tolerate general anesthesia, botulinum toxin injection is often performed simultaneously with dilation of the UES because it is believed that fibrosis of the CPM may coexist with CPM neurogenic changes in many patients who have primary UES dysfunction.

The risks of botulinum toxin are generally related to inaccurate injections or diffusion of the toxin, which can lead to paralysis of the adjacent muscles (posterior cricoarytenoid, inferior pharyngeal constrictor, upper esophageal musculature), temporarily worsening dysphagia or impairing vocal fold motion. This is much more common after in-office injections. Unfortunately, as described above, these are often performed in sicker patients and can result in severe morbidity or even mortality secondary to increased dysphagia. Therefore, many practitioners have abandoned in-office injections for this set of patients.

After conservative management (e.g., swallowing exercises, head-positioning maneuvers) has failed, surgical intervention for CPM achalasia is warranted provided that previous clinical evidence, videofluoroscopy, and in some cases manometry support the diagnosis. There are several approaches for the treatment of CPM achalasia. The most widely used technique is transcervical cricopharyngeal myotomy. This surgery is typically performed under general anesthesia, often with placement of an esophageal bougie or orogastric tube to improve visualization of the CPM fibers and prevent esophageal mucosal violation during the myotomy. The CPM fibers, which extend in horizontal bands originating from the posterior lateral border of the cricoid cartilage, are carefully incised, and a segment of muscle may be removed to prevent recurrent fibrosis of the muscle edges.

The CPM may also be readily exposed via an endoscopic technique. Endoscopically, the submucosal prominence of the CPM is exposed in the postcricoid region with either a Weerda (Karl Storz, Tuttlingen, Germany) or Slimline (Karl Storz) diverticuloscope. After the scope is suspended, the prominence should be examined and palpated under microscopy to ensure correct positioning. With carbon dioxide laser, the mucosa is incised in the midline to reveal the underlying transverse running muscle fibers (▶ Fig. 98.3).

These are carefully and completely transected until the underlying buccopharyngeal fascia is identified. Leaving the fascia intact is a crucial step. It provides a protective barrier preventing leakage into the danger space with resultant infection (mediastinitis). If there is any question about the integrity of the underlying fascia, closure with fibrin glue and/or endoscopic suture reapproximation of the mucosa should be performed.

98.4 Evaluation and Management of Zenker Diverticulum

98.4.1 Description of Zenker Diverticulum

Zenker diverticulum is a false diverticulum consisting of an outpouching of hypopharynx mucosa and submucosa. The diverticulum typically occurs in an area of muscle weakness in a region between the inferior constrictor and the CPM known as the Killian triangle. Although the exact mechanism for the development of a Zenker diverticulum is not known, it is believed to be secondary to high intrabolus pressures generated by failure of the CPM to adequately relax during swallowing.

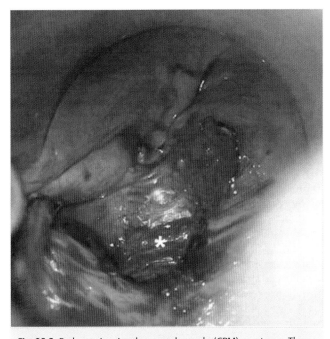

Fig. 98.3 Endoscopic cricopharyngeal muscle (CPM) myotomy. The CPM fibers retract laterally under the mucosa as they are transected with the carbon dioxide laser. The horizontal fibers of the CPM (*asterisk*) can be appreciated during the carbon dioxide laser dissection. A defocused laser beam can be appreciated at the superior edge of the defect (bottom of figure).

Zenker diverticula typically occur in older adults beginning after the sixth decade of life; however, they have been described in much younger individuals, including children. Early in the development of a diverticulum, oropharyngeal dysphagia to solids is the most common presenting feature. Over time, the size of the diverticulum increases, leading to the retention of food and secretions in the pouch. Particularly when a diverticulum is large, patients may have halitosis, dysphagia, cough, weight loss, regurgitation, aspiration, and even recurrent pneumonia. The prevalence of Zenker diverticula among the general population is low (0.01 to 0.11%).

98.4.2 Differential Diagnosis of Zenker Diverticulum

The evaluation of a Zenker diverticulum requires consideration of other, similarly presenting pathologies. Diverticula can occur anywhere along the esophageal lining, although they occur more frequently in the middle and distal portions of the esophagus. If a diverticulum protrudes through the anterolateral wall of the cervical esophagus just inferior to the CPM and lateral to the longitudinal muscle of the esophagus (the Killian-Jamieson space), it is called a Killian-Jamieson diverticulum. Esophageal diverticula most typically present with dysphagia, regurgitation, achalasia, and aspiration. As previously discussed, esophageal spasms and strictures may present with clinical features similar to those of Zenker divercticula. For each differential diagnosis, fluoroscopic evaluation with barium contrast can identify the specific location of the diverticulum.

98.4.3 Evaluation of Zenker Diverticulum

The diagnosis of Zenker diverticulum is determined by a barium swallow study (▶ Fig. 98.4). Manometry is not typically performed; however, it may prove helpful in determining the etiology of the diverticulum. Endoscopy may be indicated if the barium contrast study or history suggests the possibility of neoplasm. Although FEES is generally not a very sensitive test for detecting a Zenker diverticulum, patients with a Zenker diverticulum can occasionally be noted to have the classic finding of delayed regurgitation of bolus back into the hypopharynx several seconds after swallowing. FEES can also be important in excluding causes of secondary dysphagia, such as vocal fold paresis and base of tongue weakness.

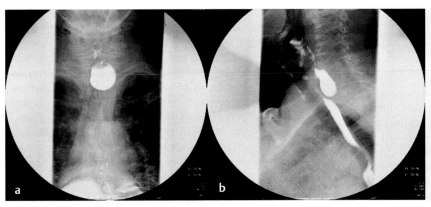

Fig. 98.4 Zenker diverticulum on barium esophagram. (**a**) Posteroanterior view demonstrates a large, circular sac just to the left of midline that measures just over 3 cm in maximal diameter. (**b**) On lateral view, the barium-filled sac can be appreciated posteriorly, with the cricopharyngeal muscle–containing party wall visible between the sac and the esophageal lumen.

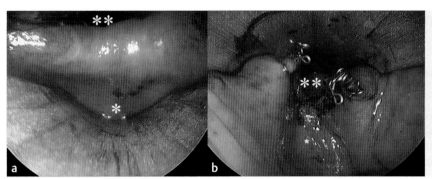

Fig. 98.5 Endoscopic Zenker diverticulum. (**a**) A small Zenker sac is exposed, with the sac posterior (*asterisk*) and the esophagus anterior (*double asterisk*) to the parting septum; the septum contains the cricopharyngeal muscle. (**b**) After stapling, most of the septum has been divided, but the base of the septum remains, which can be further transected with a laser if desired. The esophageal lumen is visible (*double asterisk*) as well as the residual posterior sac (*asterisk*).

98.4.4 Treatment of Zenker Diverticulum

The treatment modality for symptomatic Zenker diverticula is predominantly surgical. Several surgical methods are used. In the choice of a method, the many factors to be considered include the health and physiologic age of the patient. As discussed previously, CPM dysfunction is believed to be a major mediator in the development of Zenker diverticula. Therefore, cricopharyngeal myotomy must be performed alone or in conjunction with a procedure that addresses the diverticulum. In patients who cannot tolerate a surgical procedure, botulinum toxin injection into the CPM alone often results in dramatic symptom relief.

Similar to CPM myotomy, the surgical management of a Zenker diverticulum can be performed via an external or an endoscopic approach. Several endoscopic procedures are routinely used in which the party wall is transected in the midline to create a common cavity encompassing the diverticulum and the esophagus. Regardless of the technique, transoral surgery requires direct visualization of the septum, esophageal lumen, and diverticular pouch (▶ Fig. 98.5a). When an endostapler is used, the septum between the esophageal lumen and the diverticulum is divided and the edges are sealed by the staples (▶ Fig. 98.5b).

Alternatively, a laser can be used to incise the septum between the esophagus and the Zenker sac. Because the septum contains the CPM, the procedure involves a CPM myotomy; simultaneously, a common cavity and continuity between the sac and proximal esophagus are created. One reason for the failure of stapler diverticulotomy in small sacs is an incomplete CPM myotomy when the CPM extends beyond the base of the sac. For patients who cannot tolerate general anesthesia, flexible endoscopic procedures may be used. In general, endoscopic procedures cause fewer complications, require a shorter hospital stay, and allow a more rapid resumption of an oral diet.

In some cases, severe kyphosis, osteophytes, and/or a limited oral opening prevent adequate exposure of the Zenker diverticulum via a transoral approach, and an external approach is required. In conjunction with a cricopharyngeal myotomy, a diverticulectomy or diverticulopexy may be performed. Diverticulectomy consists of suturing or stapling the neck of the diverticulum and excising the pouch. Because of the risk for postoperative leak at the base of the diverticulum, this procedure carries a higher risk for mediastinitis. In addition, care needs to be taken to avoid excessive excision of the esophageal wall, which can result in postoperative esophageal stenosis. There-

fore, the excision is often performed with a bougie in place to prevent excessive resection. Diverticulopexy is performed by inverting the diverticulum and anchoring the pouch to the posterior pharyngeal wall. This procedure is typically recommended for patients with extensive comorbidities because there is no excision or division of the esophagus or pharynx, thereby decreasing operative and recovery time and the risk for posteroperative mediastinitis.

98.5 Evaluation and Management of Neurogenic Dysphagia

98.5.1 Description of Neurogenic Dysphagia

Dysphagia is a common manifestation of a disease or disorder of the central or peripheral nervous system. For functional swallowing to occur, a multitude of neural pathways and muscles must coordinate properly. Lesions in the cerebral cortex, basal ganglia, brainstem, or cerebellum may prevent normal swallowing function. Examples of such neurogenic pathology include stroke, traumatic brain injury, benign or malignant neoplasms, cerebral palsy, myasthenia gravis, and multiple sclerosis. Degenerative diseases such as Alzheimer disease, Parkinson disease, Huntington disease, Wilson disease, amyotrophic lateral sclerosis, dementias (frontotemporal, Lewy body, vascular), olivopontocerebellar atrophy, and progressive supranuclear palsy may also cause neurogenic dysphagia. Finally, iatrogenic injury to the territories of cranial nerves IX, X, and XII can result in significant neurogenic dysphagia.

Acute stroke causing a lesion in the cerebral cortex is by far the most common cause of central neurogenic dysphagia. Dysphagia from stroke usually occurs with hemiplegia. However, as seen in patients with small lacunar infarcts or specific brainstem lesions, dysphagia may occasionally be the only clinical neurologic sign. Dysphagia following stroke is often transient if direct brainstem injury is not involved. The vast majority of patients who have had a stroke recover their swallowing function. Those with persistent dysphagia have significantly higher rates of morbidity and mortality from their stroke. Therefore, it is important that patients with stroke be screened for dysphagia, and stroke needs to be considered in the differential diagnosis for patients with isolated dysphagia.

The most common causes of peripheral neurogenic dysphagia are injuries affecting cranial nerve IX, X, or XII. Of these, iatrogenic injuries to cranial nerve X are the most common, often occurring at the time of skull base surgery, cervical surgery, or carotid endarterectomy. Distal injuries affecting the recurrent laryngeal nerve in isolation result in unilateral vocal fold paralysis, often with coexistent UES dysfunction. With high cranial nerve X injury, patients are more likely to have dysphagia because the paralyzed vocal fold often remains in a lateral position, impairing glottic closure during swallowing. More significantly, superior laryngeal nerve involvement results in impaired laryngopharyngeal sensation, exacerbating the risk for aspiration.

98.5.2 Differential Diagnosis of Neurogenic Dysphagia

In most of the aforementioned neurologic disorders, dysphagia is a very common feature. This association necessitates a thorough evaluation for other etiologies of dysphagia often obscured by the neurologic disorder. In patients with neurodegenerative diseases, the course of dysphagia tends to worsen progressively. Therefore, the sudden development of worsening dysphagia should prompt investigation into additional causes, such as neoplasms, strictures, and diverticula, as discussed throughout this chapter.

98.5.3 Evaluation of Neurogenic Dysphagia

In all patients with dysphagia, signs of coexisting neurologic deficits, such as dysarthria, blunted affect, velopharyngeal insufficiency, and vision changes, warrant further evaluation by a neurologist to assess for a systemic neurologic disorder. Although many patients may present with a well- established diagnosis of stroke, traumatic brain injury, or iatrogenic neurogenic injury, other neurologic diseases can manifest with more subtle changes, and dysphagia can be an initial complaint. For example, patients who have myasthenia gravis, which affects the neuromuscular junctions, present with variable difficulty swallowing that worsens throughout a meal or the day. Often, the laryngeal, oral, and velopharyngeal muscles are all affected, while CPM function remains normal. Because of the velopharyngeal involvement, patients often experience nasal regurgitation of bolus during swallowing and may have problems with hypernasal speech. Videofluoroscopy shows dysfunction in the oral preparatory phase and the pharyngeal phase. Although myasthenia gravis is caused by antibodies to nicotinic acetylcholine receptors, acetylcholine antibody receptor testing has poor sensitivity (60%), so a therapeutic trial of pyridostigmine is often the most reasonable initial step when myasthenia gravis is strongly suspected. If further diagnostic testing is needed, the diagnosis can usually be confirmed with single-fiber electromyography. As another example, amyotrophic lateral sclerosis can present with progressive motor neuron death leading to bulbar weakness. During progression of the disease, patients tend to have increasing difficulty with solids as a consequence of inadequate generation of muscle force in both the oral and pharyngeal phases of swallowing. The insufficient force and failure of the CPM to relax decrease UES opening and increase dysphagia. Clinically, many patients with amyotrophic lateral sclerosis will present with dysphagia, weight loss, and recurrent episodes of aspiration pneumonia, and often with coexisting dysarthria (slow, slurred speech).

In individuals suspected to have neurogenic dysphagia, FEES is a reasonable screening approach because it is highly sensitive in the detection of aspiration. However, videofluoroscopic swallow study is still considered the gold standard for evaluating patients with neurogenic dysphagia because the test allows direct visualization of the oral preparatory phase, reflex initiation, and pharyngeal transit more clearly than does FEES alone.

98.5.4 Treatment of Neurogenic Dysphagia

With many specific neurologic diseases, either peripheral or central in origin, the management of dysphagia varies considerably, depending on the disease process. The overall goal of managing neurogenic dysphagia is to prevent aspiration while maintaining adequate nutrition. For individuals who are unable to meet their nutritional requirements by mouth because of severe dysphagia, gastrostomy can help to supplement nutrition. The incorporation of postural and swallowing techniques, as discussed earlier in this chapter, should also be emphasized to further limit aspiration. Based on the cause of the disease, food consistency should be optimized to facilitate ingestion. For most patients with neurogenic causes of dysphagia, liquids pose a greater challenge than solids. Therefore, attempts should be made to increase the viscosity of fluids when beneficial.

Patients with isolated cranial nerve X injury (recurrent laryngeal nerve and/or superior laryngeal nerve) often experience significant improvement in swallowing after surgical treatment to improve glottic closure (injection laryngoplasty or medialization laryngoplasty with arytenoid adduction) and CPM myotomy to minimize resistance at the UES. In such cases, pharyngoplasty to minimize pooling in the piriform sinus on the paralyzed side can also be considered. In patients with systemic neurologic diseases and more diffuse neuropathy, cricopharyngeal myotomy or botulinum toxin injection can be performed as a treatment if there are signs of CPM dysfunction with retention of an adequate oral phase, pharyngeal peristalsis, and reflex mechanisms. Many individuals with neurogenic dysphagia have severe deficits in these aforementioned phases of swallowing, making cricopharyngeal myotomy or relaxation an ineffective intervention.

98.6 Evaluation and Management of Dysphagia following Head and Neck Cancer Therapy

98.6.1 Description of Dysphagia following Head and Neck Cancer Therapy

The standard treatment modalities for patients with locally advanced head and neck cancer involve surgical resection, chemotherapy, and radiation therapy. These options, although often curative in eliminating the cancer, can be extremely disfiguring and disruptive of normal anatomy and neuromuscular function,

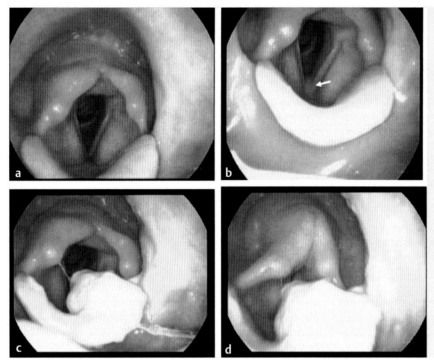

Fig. 98.6 Multifactorial dysphagia in a patient with head and neck cancer. Flexible endoscopic evaluation of swallow (FEES) images of a patient with previous irradiation for a base of tongue malignancy, impaired sensation, and deficient laryngeal elevation during swallowing. (**a**) Intact vocal fold mobility noted. (**b**) Pooling in the vallecula and silent aspiration noted (*arrow*) with diluted applesauce. (**c**) Graham cracker bolus with severe laryngeal penetration. (**d**) Upon instruction, the patient could adduct the vocal folds and then repetitively complete forceful swallows and chin tuck to advance the bolus without aspiration.

leading to dysphagia. The extent and type of dysphagia following treatment for head and neck cancer varies considerably depending on the location of the cancer, tissues removed, methods used for reconstruction, and type of rehabilitation therapy. For instance, it has been well established that irradiation to the base of the tongue can lead to swallowing dysfunction secondary to prolonged oral preparatory times, slowed bolus transit times, and increased oropharyngeal residues (▶ Fig. 98.6). Patients with laryngeal or hypopharyngeal malignancies who undergo irradiation or chemoradiation protocols are more likely to have problems of impaired laryngeal sensation, weak laryngeal elevation, and impaired UES opening.

98.6.2 Differential Diagnosis of Dysphagia following Head and Neck Cancer Therapy

Because therapies for head and neck cancer are inherently associated with a high rate of dysphagia, dysphagia or aspiration secondary to other causes may be unsuspected or missed in patients with head and neck cancer. In the clinical management of a patient following therapy for head and neck cancer, it is important to identify the expected level of dysphagia following treatment. If the patient experiences symptoms that are unexpected or far more severe than anticipated, a thorough work-up should be conducted to assess for other causes, such as stroke, esophageal neoplasms, diverticula, strictures, and achalasia.

98.6.3 Evaluation of Dysphagia following Head and Neck Cancer Therapy

Radiation therapy leads to the fibrosis and necrosis of tissue, which are particularly difficult to treat because there are no

beneficial long-term management options for reversing the damage. The tissue damage leads to oropharyngeal complications, including xerostomia, mucositis, and strictures. Therapeutic doses of radiation have the capacity to significantly damage salivary glands, causing a permanent decrease in salivary flow. Patients will often complain that boluses of dry foods such as crackers and breads become stuck, and water is required to advance the bolus, compensating for the decline in saliva production. Mucositis, which is characterized by irritation and ulceration of the oral mucosa, is also a common manifestation of radiation therapy. Clinicians will often recommend that a patient maintain proper oral care while avoiding spicy or irritating foods. Although xerostomia and mucositis are common in patients with dysphagia after irradiation for head and neck cancers, neither of them alone has been shown to alter bolus transit times; typically, the patients who have been treated with irradiation and have the greatest swallowing impairment are those with a combination of mucositis, xerostomia, and severe alterations in anatomy and neuromuscular function. One possible alteration in anatomy is the development of a stricture that physically impedes bolus passage at the level of the pharynx or esophagus. Typically, strictures respond well to esophageal dilation, which can be done as standard blind bougie dilation or, in tight cases, dilation over a wire. In cases of complete stenosis, a dual endoscopy approach or "rendezvous procedure" (retrograde flexible esophagoscopy via the patient's gastrostomy site with anterograde esophagoscopy and dilation) can be performed under fluoroscopic guidance with recanalization of the esophagus.

In the most severe cases of dysphagia, there is often impaired neuromuscular function that attenuates the laryngeal protective mechanisms present in a normal swallow. For example, laryngeal elevation anterosuperiorly is a critical movement for triggering UES opening and protecting the laryngeal inlet from aspiration. In many patients who have undergone irradiation, severe fibrosis of the strap muscles, such as the thyrohyoid muscles, develops and causes them to be dysfunctional, with absence of laryngeal elevation during swallow, aspiration, and piriform sinus pooling. Although neuromuscular stimulators, magnetic devices, and laryngeal repositioning surgeries are currently being explored for the "frozen larynx" syndrome, to date there is no actual cure for this problem. Aggressive swallowing therapy with a speech–language pathologist remains the standard of care. There may be some benefit to initiating swallowing therapy early in the course of irradiation, before fibrosis and dysphagia have developed, although this remains controversial. Finally, in addition to functional motor impairments, many patients have severe impairment of sensory function, resulting in loss of cough reflex and silent aspiration. Therapy with supraglottic/super-supraglottic swallow may help reduce aspiration and facilitate modest dietary intake, but generally these patients are at extremely high risk for aspiration pneumonia and pneumonitis because they do not have a reactive cough during secretion-related or reflux-related aspiration events. In severe cases of chronic aspiration, tracheo-esophageal diversion, laryngotracheal separation, or total laryngectomy must be considered.

The management of dysphagia following treatment for head and neck cancer requires proper imaging studies, including MBS or FEES. MBS can more accurately determine the presence of deficits with each stage of the swallow. FEES permits direct visualization of the neuromuscular function and anatomical deficits contributing to the dysphagia, which can be beneficial if some type of augmentation or surgical treatment is anticipated.

98.6.4 Treatment of Dysphagia following Head and Neck Cancer Therapy

Therapy with swallowing maneuvers, postural techniques, and swallowing exercises, as discussed previously, is critically important to help prevent and manage dysphagia following head and neck cancer therapy. In patients at high risk for dysphagia after therapy, a pretreatment assessment of swallowing should be considered. This formal evaluation by a speech–language pathologist before oncologic intervention allows time to develop specific compensatory maneuvers and plan rehabilitation. In addition, a pretreatment assessment can determine the baseline oropharyngeal function, which may assist in developing the most appropriate surgical plan for preserving swallow function. If patients undergoing radiation therapy or chemoradiation therapy develop dysphagia during or after their treatments, they should meet with a speech–language pathologist early in the course of their dysphagia so that they can work on techniques to curb the development of tissue fibrosis and maintain muscular strength and coordination.

In addition to the surgical options already outlined in this chapter, patients with head and neck cancer may benefit from augmentation procedure(s) to help minimize the underlying anatomical defects that are impairing swallow function. For example, patients with oropharyngeal malignancy in whom severe velopharyngeal insufficiency develops after therapy may benefit from a palatal augmentation/pharyngoplasty procedure. Those with large base of tongue defects after cancer resections (with resultant pooling in the defect) may benefit from lipoinjection augmentation of the tongue defect to help minimize pooling. Patients with unilateral vocal fold paralysis or loss of vocal fold tissue may benefit from some type of vocal fold augmentation, with lipoinjection a reasonable option for mild glottic closure impairment and muscular flap reconstruction an option for larger defects. Because of the high risk for poor wound healing, extrusion, and/or laryngocutaneous fistula after irradiation, standard medialization laryngoplasty with synthetic implants should be performed with great caution in cancer patients who have previously been treated with irradiation to the neck.

Depending on the sites involved with head and neck cancer, a variety of deficits may be demonstrated. Thus, treatments need to be tailored to the individual. Ideally, the physician team and speech–language pathologists will work closely together to optimize each patient's swallowing function and provide him or her with realistic expectations for the future.

98.7 Roundsmanship

- Although bedside swallowing evaluations may be considered for detecting aspiration, their sensitivity is significantly lower than that of modified barium swallow (MBS) and functional endoscopic evaluation of swallow (FEES), especially in patients with silent aspiration (absence of a spontaneous cough reflex).
- Botulinum toxin injection is a nonsurgical treatment option for relaxing the UES and generally results in significantly improved swallowing function in patients with primary UES dysfunction.
- Because cricopharyngeal muscle dysfunction is believed to be a major mediator in the development of Zenker diverticulum, cricopharyngeal myotomy should be included with any procedure done to address the diverticulum.
- In individuals suspected to have neurogenic dysphagia, flexible endoscopic evaluation of swallow (FEES) is a reasonable screening approach to detect aspiration; however, videofluoroscopic swallow study is the gold standard because it allows assessment of the oral preparatory phase, reflex initiation, and pharyngeal transit.
- In patients at high risk for dysphagia following therapy for head and neck cancer, a pretreatment swallowing assessment should be considered. A formal evaluation by a speech–language pathologist before oncologic intervention allows time to develop specific compensatory maneuvers and plan rehabilitation.

98.8 Recommended Reading

[1] Al-Kadi AS, Maghrabi AA, Thomson D, Gillman LM, Dhalla S. Endoscopic treatment of Zenker diverticulum: results of a 7-year experience J Am Coll Surg 2010; 211: 239–243
[2] Bakheit AMO. Management of neurogenic dysphagia Postgrad Med J 2001; 77: 694–699

[3] Basi SK, Marrie TJ, Huang JQ, Majumdar SR. Patients admitted to hospital with suspected pneumonia and normal chest radiographs: epidemiology, microbiology, and outcomes Am J Med 2004; 117: 305–311

[4] Dantas RO, Cook IJ, Dodds WJ, Kern MK, Lang IM, Brasseur JG. Biomechanics of cricopharyngeal bars Gastroenterology 1990; 99: 1269–1274

[5] Langmore SE, Schatz K, Olson N. Endoscopic and videofluoroscopic evaluations of swallowing and aspiration Ann Otol Rhinol Laryngol 1991; 100: 678–681

[6] Marik PE. Aspiration pneumonitis and aspiration pneumonia N Engl J Med 2001; 344: 665–671

[7] Marik PE, Kaplan D. Aspiration pneumonia and dysphagia in the elderly Chest 2003; 124: 328–336

[8] Pauloski BR. Rehabilitation of dysphagia following head and neck cancer Phys Med Rehabil Clin N Am 2008; 19: 889–928

[9] Ramsey DJC, Smithard DG, Kalra L. Early assessments of dysphagia and aspiration risk in acute stroke patients Stroke 2003; 34: 1252–1257

[10] Repici A, Pagano N, Fumagalli U et al. Transoral treatment of Zenker diverticulum: flexible endoscopy versus endoscopic stapling. A retrospective comparison of outcomes Dis Esophagus 2011: 235–239

99 Evaluation and Management of Tracheobronchial Infections and Masses

Christopher R. Gilbert, Lonny Yarmus, and Lee M. Akst

99.1 Introduction

Tracheobronchial masses and infections are rather uncommon within the general population. Unfortunately, few symptoms are specific for these diseases; most present with some combination of cough, dyspnea, wheezing, respiratory failure, and hemoptysis. Because their presentation can be quite similar to those of many other diseases, they are often considered relatively late in the differential diagnosis, which can lead to a delay in diagnosis and treatment. This chapter will focus on the most common etiologies of tracheal masses and infections seen in clinical practice. It will also concentrate on common tracheobronchial infections and tracheal masses that generally require endoscopic evaluation. A more in-depth review of covered topics is available within our reading list at the end of this chapter.

99.2 Tracheal Infections

99.2.1 Etiology, Pathogenesis, and Natural History

Upper respiratory tract infections are quite common and often caused by viruses. They typically present with viral-type prodromes and are frequently self-limited. However, certain tracheal infections, albeit rare, are very important to recognize because they have the potential to be fatal if left untreated.

Bacterial tracheitis (also known as exudative tracheitis) is believed to occur as a complication of viral croup or laryngotracheitis, and therefore its incidence is highest in the fall and winter months. Bacterial tracheitis can present in the adult or pediatric population; however, the adult form is often self-limited, so many people may not seek medical attention. Adults will often present with productive cough and fevers, but because of the larger size of the adult trachea, obstruction is quite rare. Most children will present acutely ill and within a few hours to days experience the onset of an acute "barking" cough, fever, hoarseness, and stridor. Unfortunately, because of the rapidly progressive nature of the disease, many children can develop respiratory distress within hours. There is usually no drooling or dysphagia, which is more common in patients with supraglottitis. The two most common pathogens identified appear to be *Staphylococcus aureus* and *Moraxella catarrhalis*.

99.2.2 Diagnostic Testing

Endoscopic examination remains the mainstay of both the diagnosis and treatment of suspected tracheobronchial infection. We review the role of biopsy versus tracheal aspiration in the situations presented below.

Endoscopic examination will confirm the diagnosis of bacterial tracheitis, revealing marked edema, purulent exudate, mucosal ulceration, pseudo-membrane formation, and mucosal sloughing within the tracheal lumen, all of which can contribute to airway obstruction. Blood cultures are frequently negative, but tracheal cultures will often identify the pathogen. Examination of the airway is best accomplished within the controlled confines of the operating room and often requires the use of rigid bronchoscopy for the adequate suctioning and removal of pseudo-membranes. The majority of affected children will need mechanical ventilation during the acute phase of the illness, mainly for airway protection, but once the mucosal inflammation has subsided, most are safely extubated and do well.

Radiographic imaging may be helpful in formulating a diagnosis of endobronchial tuberculosis, but 20% of patients with isolated endobronchial tuberculosis have normal findings on chest imaging. It therefore remains important that bronchoscopy and subsequent microbiological analysis be performed for the diagnosis. Varying mucosal or submucosal pathologic changes, including ulcer, granuloma, infiltration, fibroplasia, and stenosis, have been described. Patients with suspected isolated endobronchial tuberculosis require direct biopsy sampling of the endotracheal lesions because noninvasive respiratory sampling tends to be nondiagnostic.

For those patients in whom tracheobronchial fungal infections develop, endoscopic examination is warranted to obtain a diagnosis as well as examine the extent of disease. The limited data available regarding fungal tracheobronchitis provide an incomplete description of the endoscopic presentations; however, a number of case reports are available. There appear to be two common descriptions: (1) intraluminal involvement with circumferential growth and invasion and (2) diffuse plaquelike involvement of the trachea.

99.2.3 Differential Diagnosis

Because of the nonspecific symptoms of cough, fever, and dyspnea, the differential often remains relatively broad. However, the development of stridor and/or hoarseness, especially over a short period of time, should raise concern for bacterial laryngotracheitis. The possibility of tuberculosis exposure in a patient's history raises concern for endobronchial tuberculosis, although some patients have no clear exposure history identified. Endobronchial tuberculosis often has a biphasic age distribution, commonly presenting in young females as well as in the elderly. Immunosuppressed patients will be at increased risk for the development of fungal infection, including laryngotracheitis.

99.2.4 Treatment

The antibiotic selected should provide empiric gram-positive and gram-negative coverage until the Gram stain returns. With the continued rise of methicillin-resistant *S. aureus* (MRSA), most suggest vancomycin until pathogen identification. The duration of antibiotic therapy often ranges from 10 to 14 days.

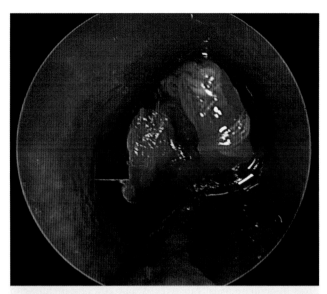

Fig. 99.1 Endotracheal *Aspergillus* infection. A large fungating mass is seen emanating from the right main stem; culture of this mass grew *Asperigillus*.

The treatment for endobronchial tuberculosis includes the use of standard anti-tuberculosis therapy. Some advocate corticosteroids to decrease tracheobronchial stenosis; however, the data remain largely from case series and retrospective studies. One needs to consider the risk for the systemic advancement of tuberculosis secondary to the use of steroids. In cases of severe tracheobronchial stenosis, more invasive therapeutic interventions are often indicated, including the use of balloon dilation and stent placement. Focal stenosis may be amenable to surgical resection once infection control is achieved.

The long-term sequelae of fungal tracheobronchitis are not well-known because most of the patients appear to die of their underlying illness. Aspergillosis is the most common fungal infection reported (▶ Fig. 99.1). Treatment also appears highly individualized; however, antifungal use is reported in most series. Descriptions of survivors have ranged from asymptomatic to severely stenotic.

99.3 Tracheal Masses

99.3.1 Etiology, Pathogenesis, and Natural History

The incidence of tracheal masses in the general population is relatively rare, with some estimates of two cases per every million persons. Presenting symptoms can range from cough and dyspnea to respiratory failure from central airway obstruction. It is quite common for patients with less severe symptoms to be given a misdiagnosis of asthma, bronchitis, or chronic cough before the correct diagnosis. This delay in accurate diagnosis appears most likely related to the nonspecific presentation and rarity of tracheal masses.

99.3.2 Diagnostic Testing

Endoscopic airway evaluation is invaluable for establishing the diagnosis of an endotracheal mass. It is performed via flexible or rigid bronchoscopy, as well as direct laryngoscopy, depending on the location of the lesion and the preference of the physician. Lesions are inspected, and biopsies can be obtained.

Endobronchial Masses Related to Systemic Diseases

Wegener Granulomatosis

Patients with Wegener granulomatosis (WG) generally test positive for cytoplasmic antineutrophil cytoplasmic autoantibody (c-ANCA); however, up 20% of patients with airway involvement may be negative for c-ANCA. The results of further diagnostic testing, such as biopsy demonstrating necrotizing vasculitis of small vessels, can help confirm the diagnosis.

Amyloidosis

The diagnosis of amyloidosis requires a tissue biopsy in which characteristic amyloid fibrils stain pink with hematoxylin–eosin as well as demonstrate green birefrigence under polarized light microscopy after being stained with Congo red.

Sarcoidosis

Endoscopy in patients with sarcoidosis will often reveal diffuse hyperemia, edema, and less commonly ulceration. Nodules and mass lesions have also been well described. Supraglottic structures may be involved, with subglottic disease much less common. A classic "turban-like thickening" of the larynx can be seen, and most believe this is related to diffuse infiltration and swelling of the supraglottis. A diagnosis of sarcoidosis requires biopsies of affected areas as well as a negative work-up for tuberculosis. These biopsies should identify well-defined noncaseating granulomas without evidence of vasculitis, necrosis, or infection. Pulmonary nodules on chest X-ray or computed tomography (CT) and an elevated angiotensin-converting enzyme (ACE) level may also help in the diagnosis, although these results can be normal in approximately 10% of cases.

Tracheobronchopathia Osteochondroplastica

Endoscopy for tracheobronchopathia osteochondroplastica (TO) is diagnostic with the visualization of innumerable small, hard nodules extending from the subglottic space to the carina. The nodules can cause tracheal narrowing and rigidity if sufficiently large and numerous. One of the distinguishing features of TO is the absence of involvement of the posterior membranous wall.

Nonmalignant and Malignant Tracheal Tumors

Recurrent Respiratory Papillomatosis

The diagnosis of recurrent respiratory papillomatosis (RRP) is suspected with the endoscopic visualization of characteristic hypervascular papillary lesions (▶ Fig. 99.2), but the diagnosis is confirmed by pathologic analysis.

Suspected neoplasms within the tracheobronchial tree should be confirmed pathologically. This can be performed via flexible or rigid bronchoscopy, as well as direct laryngoscopy, depending on the location of the lesion and the preference of the physician. Once a diagnosis is obtained and the endoluminal extent of disease has been assessed, further treatment options can be discussed. Endobronchial ultrasound is a minimally invasive tool that helps identify the degree of airway invasion. A number of studies have identified a strong correlation between endobronchial ultrasound definition of airway invasion and histologic invasion. The 20-MHz radial probe is able to identify distinct layers of the airway wall (▸ Fig. 99.3, ▸ Fig. 99.4, ▸ Fig. 99.5). The depth of invasion and the delineation between

normal and abnormal tissue are easily identified invasively with the endobronchial ultrasound probe.

Pulmonary function testing can be helpful in identifying central airway obstruction. The typical flat truncation of inspiratory and expiratory limbs is suggestive of a fixed airway obstruction (see ▸ Fig. 99.4). CT of the chest and neck may also be helpful in identifying tracheal pathology. However, an

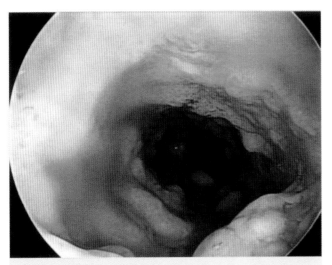

Fig. 99.2 Endotracheal papilloma seen in the distal trachea of a 25-year-old man with HIV infection and recurrent respiratory papillomatosis, first diagnosed at the age of 18 years.

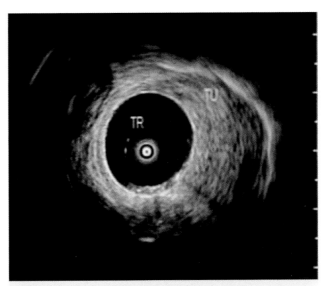

Fig. 99.3 Radial endobronchial ultrasound image of trachea. TR, radial probe ultrasound balloon; TU, tumor invasion of the tracheal wall.

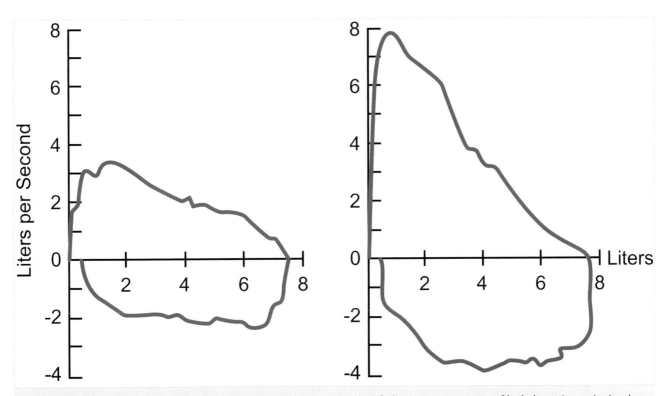

Fig. 99.4 Flow–volume loop of a patient with tracheal stenosis. The curve on the left demonstrates truncation of both the expiratory (top) and inspiratory (bottom) limbs. This is suggestive of a fixed airway obstruction. The curve on the right demonstrates the flow–volume loop obtained after endoscopic dilation of the stenosis.

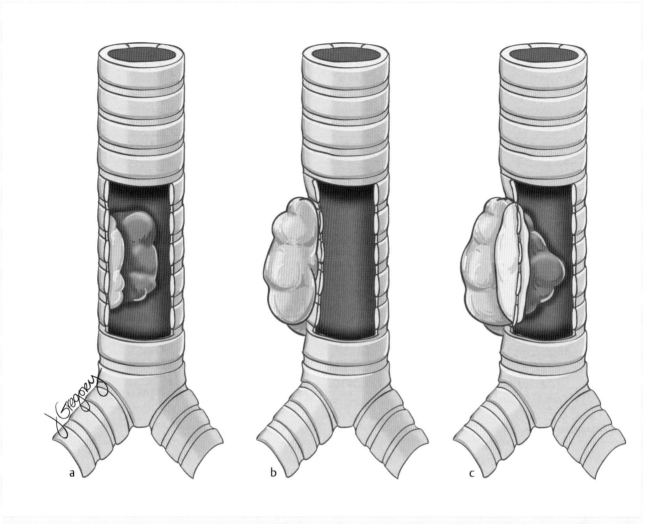

Fig. 99.5 Airway tumor classification. (**a**) Intrinsic disease, (**b**) extrinsic disease, and (**c**) mixed intrinsic/extrinsic disease.

endoscopic evaluation during each patient's work-up remains essential.

99.3.3 Differential Diagnosis

The differential diagnosis for tracheobronchial masses is rather broad, although most of the etiologies are quite rare. The most common masses in adults are related to malignant disease, whereas in children the most common masses are nonmalignant in nature (▶ Table 99.1 and ▶ Table 99.2). There are also a number of systemic diseases that can initially present with tracheobronchial masses, or new evidence of tracheobronchial involvement may appear further along in the disease course. We briefly review the more common tracheobronchial masses seen with their initial presentations.

Endobronchial Masses Related to Systemic Diseases

Wegener Granulomatosis

WG is a multisystem disease often affecting adults in the fourth and fifth decades of life. It is pathologically defined by necrotiz-

ing granulomatous vasculitis involving the small vessels, but well-defined granulomas can also be located within the tracheobronchial tree. WG commonly involves three distinct areas: the upper respiratory tract, lower respiratory tract, and kidneys. WG involves the tracheobronchial tree in only 10 to 20% of cases but can present with symptoms such as hoarseness, dyspnea, stridor, and progressive central airway obstruction. However, because central airway obstruction can be a presenting feature, an aggressive evaluation of hoarseness or unexplained dyspnea in patients with known or suspected WG is necessary.

Amyloidosis

Amyloidosis is a multisystem disorder characterized by the deposition of insoluble fibrillar proteins in tissues. It may be idiopathic and primary, or secondary to a systemic disease such as multiple myeloma. Both upper and lower respiratory tract disease can occur. Tracheal and lower respiratory tract amyloidosis is especially common in patients with primary amyloidosis.

The most commonly described pattern in amyloidosis is the presence of multifocal plaques within the tracheal and bron-

Table 99.1 Tracheal tumors occurring in the adult population

Nonmalignant (10%)	Malignant (90%)	
	Primary	Metastatic
Squamous papilloma	Squamous cell carcinoma	Thyroid cancer
Granular cell tumor	Adenoid cystic carcinoma	Lung (squamous cell and non–squamous cell carcinoma)
Chondroma	Carcinoid	Esophageal carcinoma
Adenoma	Mucoepidermoid carcinoma	Melanoma
Leiomyoma	Adenocarcinoma	Sarcoma
Myoepithelial cell tumor	Small cell carcinoma	Renal cell carcinoma
Lipoma	Leiomyosarcoma	Breast carcinoma
Fibroma	Chondrosarcoma	
Schwannoma	Spindle cell sarcoma	
Hemangioma		
Paraganglioma		
Fibrous histiocytoma		
Neurofibroma		
Chondroblastoma		
Benign mucoepidermoid tumor		
Angiofibroma		
Xanthoma		
Myoblastoma		
Hamartoma		
Glomus tumor		
Intratracheal goiter		

chial submucosa without extension beyond the airway wall. More localized disease in the form of masslike tumors may also appear in the trachea or bronchi.

Sarcoidosis

Sarcoidosis is a chronic granulomatous disorder of unknown etiology with the potential to involve virtually any organ system. Although otolaryngologic manifestations may occur in up to 40% of patients with sarcoidosis, primary involvement of the trachea or esophagus occurs in fewer than 1% of cases. The true pathogenesis of sarcoidosis is not well defined, but the primary hypothesis suggests that exaggerated cellular immune responses lead to the injury, disruption, and destruction of affected organs. The disease is often self-limited and relatively benign, except when it causes damage to vital organs such as the heart and lungs.

Tracheobronchopathia Osteochondroplastica

TO remains a rare disease characterized by the presence of nodules of cartilage, bone, or both within the submucosa of the

trachea. It was first described in 1855, and as of 1992, only 350 cases had been reported in the literature.

Nonmalignant Tracheal Tumors

Nonmalignant tracheal tumors are oftentimes small (< 2 cm), round, and soft. The term *nonmalignant* is preferred to *benign* given that although these tumors may not have metastatic potential, their anatomical location is not benign, and they can cause critical airway obstruction.

Recurrent Respiratory Papillomatosis

The most common nonmalignant tumor of the trachea is squamous cell papilloma, also referred to as recurrent respiratory papillomatosis (RRP). This disease has a bimodal onset with both pediatric and adult forms; the pediatric form is typically more aggressive and more likely to involve the tracheobronchial tree than the adult form, which shows a predilection for isolated laryngeal involvement. The true incidence is unknown, but most believe it ranges between 1.5 and 4.5 per 100,000. It appears to occur most often in patients who are immunocom-

Table 99.2 Tracheal tumors occurring in the pediatric population

Nonmalignant (80%)	Malignant (20%)	
	Primary	Metastatic
Squamous papilloma	Carcinoid	Melanoma
Granular cell tumor	Mucoepidermoid	Sarcoma
Pleomorphic adenoma	Leiomyosarcoma	
Myoepithelial cell tumor	Spindle cell sarcoma	
Lipoma	Paraganglioma	
Fibroma	Lymphoma	
Schwannoma	Rhabdomyosarcoma	
Hemangioma	Melanoma	
Paraganglioma		
Fibrous histiocytoma		
Neurofibroma		
Chondroblastoma		
Angiofibroma		
Myoblastoma		
Hamartoma		
Glomus tumor		

promised, with HIV infection/AIDS the most common primary illness.

RRP is a disease of viral etiology, linked to human papillomavirus types 6 and 11. Morbidity and mortality are not related to the viral infection itself, but rather to the small risk for malignant transformation, the impact of mass lesions on laryngeal function, and airway obstruction. Presenting symptoms of papillomatosis may include cough and hoarseness, but it may also present with stridor and central airway obstruction. The duration of symptoms before diagnosis may vary because a misdiagnosis of asthma or allergies is common.

Granular Cell Tumors

Granular cell tumors were first described in 1926 and thought to be myogenic in origin, but they have more recently been attributed to a neurogenic origin. These lesions are mainly intraluminal in nature but can also invade locally. Malignant transformation has been reported in up to 2% of cases, with tumors larger than 8 mm carrying the highest risk for transformation.

Chondromas

Chondromas are mesenchymal tumors often described as hard, broad-based, and covered by mucosa. They are often found on the internal aspect of the posterior cricoid lamina, but they have been reported throughout the trachea. Calcification commonly occurs but unfortunately does not help distinguish

benignity. Malignant chondrosarcomas may also calcify, and therefore this type of lesion requires further investigation.

Leiomyomas

Leiomyomas commonly occur in the membranous portion of the trachea and originate in smooth muscle within the tracheal wall. Endoscopically, most appear as smooth, polypoid-type masses.

Hemangiomas

Hemangiomas of the upper airway have been described in both the adult and pediatric populations. Endoscopically, they often appear as blue, smooth, broad-based lesions emanating from the posterolateral aspect of the subglottic area. These lesions are covered by normal respiratory epithelium and may simply regress over a period of observation.

Malignant Tracheal Tumors

The most common tracheal tumors are malignant in nature and may contribute to mortality in either of two distinct manners: asphyxiation from central airway obstruction or locoregional invasion with progression of disease. Unfortunately, most patients remain without a diagnosis and present late. The importance of early diagnosis cannot be overstated because patients presenting with early-stage disease and undergoing surgical resection fare better than those presenting later with more advanced disease. Surgical resection rates for tracheal tumors remain low, with most series in the 10% range. Many patients who have potentially resectable tracheal tumors appear to be treated initially with modalities other than curative surgery for unclear reasons.

Squamous cell carcinoma and adenoid cystic carcinoma appear to be the most common primary malignancies of the trachea, together accounting for over three-quarters of all tracheal carcinomas. Other malignant tumors include mucoepidermoid carcinoma, carcinoid, non–squamous cell bronchogenic carcinoma, melanoma, sarcoma, and lymphoma.

Squamous Cell Carcinoma

Squamous cell carcinoma is the most common tracheal tumor. Unfortunately, it presents with a rather rapid progression and is often not amenable to surgical resection. Men are twice as likely to develop squamous cell carcinoma, with 90% of all cases related to tobacco abuse. Squamous cell carcinomas often demonstrate exophytic growth with ulceration and bleeding. The lateral tracheal wall is often involved. In patients with posterior wall involvement, invasion from an esophageal primary should always be considered.

Adenoid Cystic Carcinoma

Adenoid cystic carcinoma is reported as the second most common malignant tracheal tumor. There appears to be no sex predilection, and the age of patients in reported cases ranges from 30 to 90 years, with the average age in the middle forties. Adenoid cystic carcinoma has been described as a relatively low-grade malignancy originating from the epithelium of mucosal glands lining the respiratory tract. Microscopically, it appears as small, uniform cells that are arranged in a tubular, sheetlike pattern. Adenoid cystic carcinoma will often arise from the posterolateral distal two-thirds of the trachea.

Lymphoma

The incidence of lymphoma has been increasing. The increase is thought to be related to the population with HIV infection; 75,000 new cases occurred in the year 2008. Approximately 75% of lymphomas presenting in the neck region will have nodal involvement, with the remaining 25% being extranodal.

Metastatic Malignant Tumors

Metastatic implants to the trachea fortunately remain uncommon; however, they have been well reported. The most common tumors reported to metastasize to the trachea include thyroid, esophageal, laryngeal, and lung tumors.

99.3.4 Treatment

The etiology of the mass will dictate the overall management, but patients with large obstructing masses will require relief of central airway obstruction through the use of endoscopic methods or the placement of a tracheostomy. One of the particularly challenging aspects surrounding the management of central airway obstruction is that patients typically present late in their course with a critical airway. The first step in the management of central airway obstruction is to secure a stable airway. Because of the complexity of many of these cases, a multidisciplinary approach to further treatment is recommended.

Although the complete management of central airway obstruction is beyond the scope of this chapter, a brief overview of the authors' general approach is provided. Rigid bronchoscopy remains the procedure of choice because of the ability to achieve immediate airway stabilization while providing oxygenation, ventilation, and diagnostic and therapeutic intervention.

The optimal endobronchial therapy depends on the characteristics of the mass. Three types of airway obstruction have often been described, which are illustrated in ▶ Fig. 99.5. Extrinsic obstruction and mixed obstruction respond well to endobronchial balloon dilation and stenting, whereas intrinsic disease may respond favorably to direct tumor destruction and excision (laser vaporization, cryotherapy, and/or mechanical débridement). The presence of purely extrinsic disease remains a contraindication to the use of the destructive therapies such as laser and cryotherapy because these damage the airway wall.

Because many patients with obstruction will present late in the disease course (and therefore may not be eligible for tracheal resection), tracheal stents remain a good option. Stents palliate the dyspnea resulting from central airway obstruction and may help liberate patients from the ventilator. The most common types of stents available in the United States are silicone and self-expanding metal stents. Silicone stents come in various sizes and are easy to modify. They are also easy to remove or reposition, but placement can be more difficult and requires the use of rigid bronchoscopy. Metal stents can be placed via flexible bronchoscopy but are more expensive; in addition, granulation tissue is more likely to develop, which limits removal or repositioning.

Endobronchial Masses Related to Systemic Diseases

Wegener Granulomatosis

The management of tracheobronchial WG can be difficult, and a multidisciplinary approach should be used. Systemic symptoms are often treated with steroids, but more potent immunomodulators may be required. Airway disease may not respond in the same fashion as systemic disease and therefore may need to be treated independently. Endoscopic and/or surgical therapy is indicated in those with central airway obstruction. Direct intralesional treatment with corticosteroids or mitomycin has been reported. Other potential interventions include balloon dilation, stent placement, and resection. Because of high rates of restenosis in the face of active disease, surgical resection should be reserved for cases in which WG has resolved.

Amyloidosis

A diagnosis of amyloidosis should prompt referral to a medical oncologist for systemic evaluation; however, no medical therapy available at this time appears to modify its overall course. For patients with secondary amyloidosis, treatment of the underlying disease appears to delay amyloid deposition and disease progression. Surgical treatment should focus on maintaining airway patency, preserving laryngeal function, and improving voice quality. Complete resection at the cost of function is discouraged because recurrence is common regardless of the extent of excision. Localized laser and microdébrider resection are the modalities most commonly used.

Sarcoidosis

The treatment of sarcoidosis commonly involves the use of systemic corticosteroids, which has been associated with improvement in more than 80% of cases of laryngeal sarcoid. Systemic steroids remain the first-line treatment in all patients, except those with central airway obstruction. If central airway obstruction is severe, airway interventions may be required; these include balloon dilation, endoscopic excision or destruction, and/or stent placement. Urgent tracheostomy may be required for patients with critical airway disease. Direct intralesional treatment with corticosteroids or mitomycin has been reported but will not have an immediate effect.

Nonmalignant Tracheal Tumors

Recurrent Respiratory Papillomatosis

Although current medical and vaccine therapies are the subjects of active investigation, current clinical care is directed at removing the lesions. The treatment of RRP focuses on the surgical débridement of lesions in order to control symptoms. Most advocate early and aggressive intervention for patients presenting with any form of progressive airway obstruction. Laser therapy and débridement for papilloma destruction are the most commonly performed procedures. Other therapeutic options include photodynamic therapy, with one study showing a small but statistically significant decline in papilloma recurrence. Nonsurgical approaches include the use of antiviral agents such as acyclovir, cidofovir, interferon, and ribavirin. More recent work has demonstrated a significant decrease in papilloma recurrence after the initiation of antireflux therapy, most notably ranitidine, which may have an immune-modulating effect.

Chondromas

Definitive treatment requires surgical resection because of a high incidence of recurrence with endoscopic resection.

Leiomyomas

Tracheal resection is recommended because recurrence and death related to hemorrhage after endoscopic excision have been reported. Although the data are limited, some experts recommend bronchoscopic excision only when a lesion is clearly pedunculated because of the previously mentioned risk for hemorrhage.

Hemangiomas

In patients with symptomatic hemangiomas, surgical resection has traditionally been the treatment of choice. However, recent work suggests that propranolol may replace surgery as a first-line treatment. The data remain retrospective and are derived from small case series, but because of the significant improvements noted and the minimal side effect profile of propranolol, this treatment continues to hold promise. Other options include steroids, interferon, or laser therapy.

Malignant Tracheal Tumors

Treatment for a patient with tracheal cancer remains highly individualized, with little literature available to help guide one's decisions during planning. Unfortunately, there is currently no universally accepted, data-driven staging system for tracheal carcinoma. The prognostic implications of local lymph node involvement also remain unclear. In contrast, evidence of metastatic disease does appear to correlate with worse outcomes. The most important prognostic factors related to survival appear to be the histology of malignancy, along with the ability to achieve a histologically complete resection. Patients with adenoid cystic carcinoma or mucoepidermoid carcinoma appear to do better than those with other malignancies.

Patients undergoing resection appear to do better, and those undergoing complete resection seem to do the best. This is the case not only in patients with local disease but also in those patients with advanced disease who undergo a local resection. Surgical resection remains the procedure of choice for malignant tracheal tumors. Despite this, large series from Europe show that only 10% of patients with tracheal cancer undergo resection, whereas another 40% could have been offered resection. Experts in tracheal resection believe that up to 50% of the trachea can safely be resected without causing significant stress or anastomotic compromise. Thanks to the pioneering research of Hermes Grillo and his colleagues, tracheal resection techni-

ques continue to improve, and the larger centers quote operative mortality rates of around 3%.

Patients with obvious widespread metastatic disease and a large tumor burden should be offered palliative interventions, whereas resection should be considered for those with local disease and no comorbidities. When patients present with locoregional disease, a multidisciplinary approach to their disease and therapeutic options should be used. It is important that these patients undergo evaluation and treatment at large tertiary centers with extensive experience in complex airway management and tracheal resection. This type of centralized care will not only improve patient care but also provide large databases to help promote research within this disease.

Endoscopy is often used as a treatment for patients with central airway obstruction and as a palliative measure for those with unresectable disease. It is also used to evaluate and treat hemoptysis, and to aid in surgical planning. Similarly, radiotherapy can be utilized either as a primary mode of treatment or as adjuvant therapy after resection. High-dose radiation to the chest remains is relatively contraindicated because it results in changes and scarring when generally surgical excision would be a viable alternative. Adjuvant radiotherapy appears to increase survival times; this is thought to be related mainly to improved local control of disease. Few data exist regarding systemic chemotherapy in the treatment of tracheal malignancies. Because of the paucity of data, we recommend chemotherapy only for patients in clinical trials who have primary tracheal malignancies.

The outcomes of patients with tracheal malignancies remain poor, with 5-year survival rates in the 10 to 15% range. However, as noted above, observational data sets have found that those undergoing surgical resection of their malignancy appear to have improved outcomes, with some studies quoting 5-year survival rates higher than 50%.

Lymphoma

One obvious exception to the above treatment paradigm is lymphoma within the tracheobronchial tree. Options for both diagnosis and treatment may vary among institutions. There still remains significant debate regarding the proper method of obtaining tissue. Most pathologists prefer excisional biopsies to help diagnose lymphoma and define the particular subtype. Fine-needle aspiration can often provide a diagnosis, but the lack of architecture sometimes makes subtype definition difficult. Lymphoma is generally treated with chemotherapy and radiation; surgery rarely if ever plays a role in the disease. However, the presence of central airway obstruction will often be an indication for airway stabilization until a response to chemotherapy and radiotherapy has begun.

Metastatic Malignant Tumors

Metastatic disease should always be confirmed pathologically if the confirmation will influence future treatment or if there is a question regarding the diagnosis. No specific treatments are available to individualize care; rather, it is recommended to proceed with a general approach to airway obstruction and palliation.

99.4 Roundsmanship

- Cases of bacterial and fungal tracheobronchitis remain relatively rare; however, they can be life-threatening if misdiagnosed.
- Endobronchial tuberculosis remains a worldwide infectious disease problem with the potential to cause recalcitrant tracheobronchial stenosis.
- Nonmalignant tracheal tumors are more common in the pediatric population and are often best treated with surgical resection.
- Surgical resection with curative intent remains the goal in patients who have localized primary tracheal malignancies
- Endoscopic methods remain a mainstay for the treatment of malignant disease during attempts to palliate central airway obstruction.

99.5 Recommended Reading

[1] Denlinger C, Patterson GA. Diagnosis and management of tracheal neoplasms. In: Flint PW, Haughey BH, Lund J, et al. Cummings Otolaryngology: Head and Neck Surgery. 5th ed. Philadelphia, PA: Mosby Elsevier; 2010:1611–1624

[2] Duncan N. Infections of the airway in children. In: Flint PW, Haughey BH, Lund J, et al. Cummings Otolaryngology: Head and Neck Surgery. 5th ed. Philadelphia, PA: Mosby Elsevier; 2010:2803–281

[3] Gaissert HA, Grillo HC, Shadmehr MB et al. Uncommon primary tracheal tumors. Ann Thorac Surg 2006; 82: 268–27–3

[4] Gorden JA, Ernst A. Endoscopic management of central airway obstruction. Semin Thorac Cardiovasc Surg 2009; 21: 263–273

[5] Leahy K. Laryngeal and tracheal manifestations of systemic disease. In: Flint PW, Haughey BH, Lund J, et al. Cummings Otolaryngology: Head and Neck Surgery. 5th ed. Philadelphia, PA: Mosby Elsevier; 2010: 889–893

[6] McCarthy MJ, Rosado-de-Christenson ML. Tumors of the trachea. J Thorac Imaging 1995; 10: 180–198

100 Tracheobronchoscopy and Esophagoscopy

Thomas L. Carroll

100.1 Introduction

Tracheobronchoscopy and esophagoscopy are essential, fundamental tools for the otolaryngologist. They afford the evaluation, management, and surveillance of subglottic, tracheal, bronchial, and esophageal disease and injury. Familiarity with the anatomy of the larynx, hypopharynx, esophagus, and lower airway is paramount for those performing these interventions. A thorough understanding of the available instrumentation, the techniques of use, and the advantages and disadvantages of both rigid and flexible endoscopy are required for the operating surgeon.

100.2 Tracheobronchoscopy

100.2.1 Anatomy

The subglottis begins approximately 5 mm below the upper lip of the true vocal folds. It extends to the inferior border of the cricoid cartilage, where the trachea begins. The cricoid is the only complete ring in the airway. The trachea, with its membranous posterior wall, extends approximately 10 cm (in adults) to the carina, where the right and left main bronchi begin. The main bronchi further divide into lobar bronchi (three on the right, two on the left), and yet again into lobar segmental bronchi (18 in all). The trachea, bronchi, and further diminishing levels of the lower airway are also referred to as generations; the trachea is the zero generation, the main bronchi are the first generation, and so forth. Each of the lobar and lobar segmental bronchi has a specific, anatomically appropriate name (▶ Fig. 100.1).

100.2.2 Indications

Indications for tracheobronchoscopy are categorized as either diagnostic or therapeutic. Evaluations for secondary malignancy in head and neck cancer and for stridor with concern for airway stenosis or foreign body aspiration are the most common reasons for an otolaryngologist to perform tracheobronchoscopy. Other reasons to perform this intervention include unexplained hemoptysis, chronic cough, unexplained wheezing or dyspnea, infectious concerns, and imaging findings requiring direct evaluation. These indications often lead to interventions that include bronchoalveolar lavage, transbronchial or intraluminal biopsy, removal of a foreign body, assistance in intubation (endotracheal tube positioned over a flexible bronchoscope), assistance in the placement of a percutaneous tracheotomy tube, and suctioning of inspissated secretions or blood clots.

100.2.3 Equipment

Tracheobronchoscopy can be performed with either rigid or flexible endoscopes; both types have unique roles in the management of tracheobronchial pathology. Although they are used to evaluate the subglottis, trachea, and bronchi, these pieces of equipment are typically referred to as bronchoscopes. Their inherent advantages and disadvantages in both the operative and office settings must be understood by the operating surgeon to obtain the best possible visualization and most facile completion of the indicated intervention.

Rigid Bronchoscopy

Rigid bronchoscopes are specialized metal tubes available in a variety of lengths and diameters. They are often divided arbitrarily into pediatric and adult sets. They typically range from 3 to 8.5 mm in diameter and increase in length to proportionally accommodate the size of the patient's larynx and trachea (▶ Fig. 100.2). The tip of a rigid bronchoscope is beveled to facilitate passage through the oral cavity, larynx, and carina. The wall of the distal end of the scope is perforated to allow ventilation during rigid tracheobronchoscopy (▶ Fig. 100.3). Although pediatric and adult models can vary, the proximal end has an adapter for a light source and an anesthesia ventilation circuit. The proximal end also allows the placement of a rigid Hopkins rod telescope of exact length, as well as flexible suction tubing and working instrumentation through an airtight rubber gasket (▶ Fig. 100.4). The working instruments are of a precise length so that their tips to exit just beyond the distal end of the bronchoscope. Visualization through the rigid scope occurs when the examiner looks either directly through a glass window at the proximal end or through the eyepiece of an inserted Hopkins rod telescope (with or without a camera/video system attached). The direct view can be somewhat limiting; therefore, a Hopkins rod telescope with a straight or angled lens is used to place the point of visualization at the distal end of the scope, nearest the pathology of interest. Most surgeons attach a video camera to the eyepiece of the Hopkins rod telescope to project the picture of the airway onto a monitor in front of them. Video technology also provides a means to photo document a procedure and work in a more ergonomically comfortable position.

Rigid bronchoscopy is performed exclusively in the operating room and almost exclusively under general anesthesia. The primary advantages of a rigid bronchoscope include a large lumen and the ability to ventilate the patient directly through the scope during an intervention. These two advantages make it possible to remove large foreign bodies, control brisk bleeding for which the passage of a larger-diameter suction is required, debulk airway tumors, and discharge airway stents. Pediatric otolaryngologists and surgeons who remove foreign bodies from the trachea and proximal bronchi almost exclusively use rigid bronchoscopy as a first-line intervention for the aforementioned reasons and have various sizes available as needed. Rigid bronchoscopes have the primary disadvantage of being too stiff, short, and wide to allow access to most second-generation (lobar) and third-generation (lobar segmental) bronchi.

Flexible Tracheobronchoscopy

Flexible bronchoscopes, transnasal esophagoscopes, and flexible laryngoscopes can all be used to evaluate the lower airway.

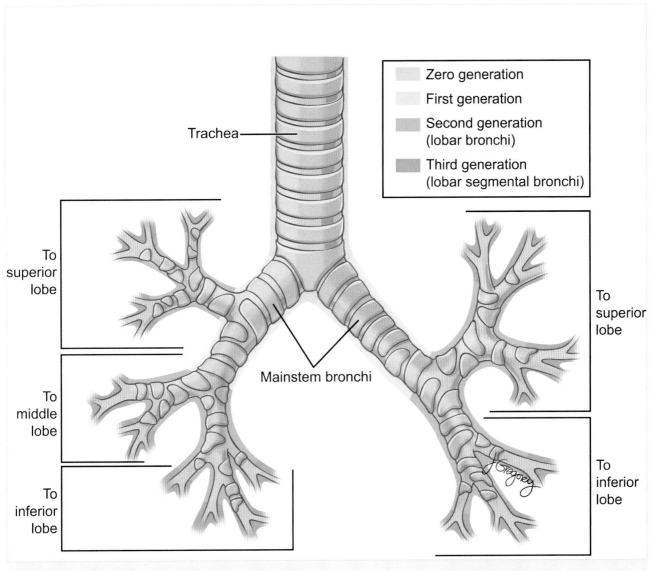

Trachea

Zero generation
First generation
Second generation (lobar bronchi)
Third generation (lobar segmental bronchi)

To superior lobe

To middle lobe

To inferior lobe

Mainstem bronchi

To superior lobe

To inferior lobe

Fig. 100.1 Tracheobronchial tree.

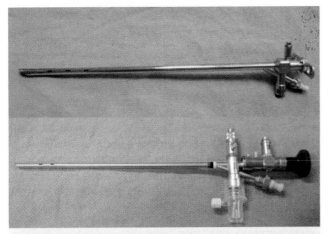

Fig. 100.2 Adult (*top*) and pediatric (*bottom*) rigid bronchoscopes.

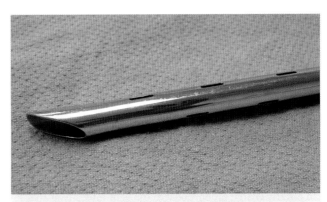

Fig. 100.3 Ventilation ports at the distal end of a rigid bronchoscope.

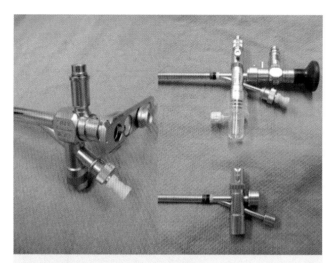

Fig. 100.4 Proximal ends of rigid bronchoscopes, with rigid endoscope inserted (*top right*).

Each has its advantages and limitations; the flexible broncho- scopes and transnasal esophagoscopes are similar. The scopes can vary in length and diameter, but are all comparable in terms of their features. A typical adult flexible laryngoscope is ap- proximately 30 cm in length and 4.1 mm in diameter. The aver- age adult bronchoscope is 60 cm in length and 6 mm in outer diameter, and the average transnasal esophagoscope is 60 cm in length and 5.1 mm in diameter. These lengths and sizes vary among manufacturers, and the scopes for the pediatric popula- tion can be as small as 2.2 mm in diameter. The anatomical area being evaluated and the patient's age and ability to tolerate an office-based procedure will typically dictate the length and di- ameter of the flexible endoscope used, the type and level of anesthesia required, and the location of the procedure. The en- doscopes are available with and without working channels that allow suctioning and the passage of small (usually less than 2 mm in diameter) instruments for endoscopic procedures. Commonly used channel instruments include cup forceps, laser fibers, balloons, injection/biopsy needles, and foreign body re- trieval tools, such as baskets and graspers.

Flexible endoscopes are available in two forms: fiber-optic and distal chip. Although distal chip technology is becoming more accessible and popular, flexible fiber-optic scopes contin- ue to be commonplace. Fiber-optic bronchoscopes are flexible plastic and metal tubes composed of bundles of glass fibers that transmit light to the scope's distal end and an image directly to a proximal eyepiece. The glass fibers are delicate; if the scope is mishandled, fiber breakage can lead to a patchy image. Alterna- tively, chip tip digital endoscopes use a charge-coupled device to capture an image. As the image is projected through a lens onto the capacitor array (a two-dimensional photoactive re- gion) of the charge-coupled device, each capacitor accumulates an electric charge proportional to the light intensity at that lo- cation. A control circuit ultimately converts the charges of the entire array into a sequence of voltages. In the chip tip scope, these voltages are then sampled, digitized, and projected as a digital video image that can be displayed and recorded. Chip tip digital endoscopes are less delicate than their fiber-optic equiv- alents. They create clear, crisp images without the pixilation

seen in the images of even the most pristine fiber-optic scopes. Some of the digital processors have the added ability to simu- late light filters to more clearly define vascular and neoplastic lesions. Chip tip digital endoscopes are more expensive and re- quire specialized processing devices for visualization of the image (there is no way to directly visualize through a chip tip scope); therefore, they are not as appealing to some clinicians. Both fiber-optic and chip tip endoscopes can be attached to vid- eo recording devices with monitors for documentation pur- poses.

The primary advantage of flexible bronchoscopy is the ability to visualize and intervene in smaller, more distal second- and third-generation bronchi. A flexible scope also provides angles of visualization and larger visual fields that are impossible with a fixed, rigid Hopkins rod. The scope can often be passed, diam- eter permitting, through the lumen of an endotracheal or tra- cheotomy tube. The disadvantages of flexible bronchoscopes in- clude the inability to suction at high volume, pass large instru- ments for intervention, and ventilate through the instrument.

100.2.4 Technique

Rigid Tracheobronchoscopy

In the adult patient, general anesthesia is typically induced, and ventilation proceeds via a face mask. As an alternative, sponta- neous ventilation techniques can be used and are often pre- ferred in pediatric cases. The adult patient is placed with the neck flexed and the head extended (sniffing position) to allow better visualization of the larynx. This position may be changed to facilitate access to the trachea and distal bronchi as the case proceeds. The table is turned toward the operating surgeon who takes over mask ventilation temporarily while positioning himself or herself at the head of the bed. The surgeon places an upper dentition mouth guard or protects the upper gingiva with gauze. The dominant hand introduces the rigid broncho- scope into the oral cavity while the nondominant hand opens the mouth and stabilizes the scope. The bevel of the distal bron- choscope should be in the anterior (neutral) position to allow elevation of the base of the tongue and epiglottis as the larynx is visualized directly (▶ Fig. 100.5). The bronchoscope should be passed through the vocal folds with the beveled edge rotated 90 degrees from neutral to avoid unnecessary trauma. Locating the glottis can be difficult when this direct method is used. An al- ternative technique is to use an anesthesiologist's straight or curved blade laryngoscope in the nondominant hand to better expose the endolarynx while placing the bronchoscope be- tween the vocal folds with the dominant hand. Once the bron- choscope is in place, the surgeon removes the laryngoscope blade while visualizing through the bronchoscope to ensure that its position is maintained. It is common to use either meth- od with a Hopkins rod telescope already inserted into the rigid scope for visualization on a video monitor.

After the rigid bronchoscope is safely in the trachea, the anes- thesia team can attach the ventilation circuit to its proximal ventilation port, and ventilation can safely proceed. Standard positive-pressure ventilation is not always possible if the bron- choscope must be frequently removed during the case or if the pathology is in the proximal trachea, resulting in a situation in which the ventilation ports on the bronchoscope are proximal

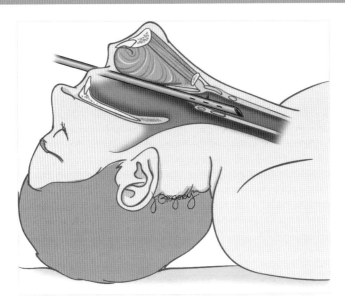

Fig. 100.5 Rigid bronchoscopy is performed by aligning the axis of the oral cavity, glottis, and trachea with head extension and neck flexion.

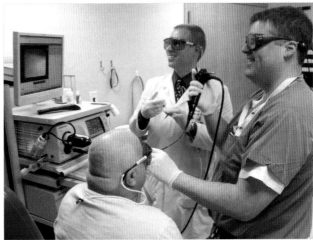

Fig. 100.6 Flexible tracheobronchoscopy can be performed comfortably under topical anesthesia.

to the vocal folds. In these instances, a jet ventilation technique can be used via the bronchoscope or, alternatively, via a catheter placed into the airway outside the bronchoscope.

When the main bronchi are evaluated, it is often necessary to manipulate the neck to obtain a better angle for access to the more distal airway. In such a scenario, the head is tilted so that the ear is brought closer to the contralateral shoulder. The rigid bronchoscope has been mostly supplanted by the flexible bronchoscope, but it is still preferred for the retrieval of foreign bodies, especially if the objects are sharp. Because of the hollow lumen and steel structure of the endoscope, a sharp object can be delivered into it, after which both can be removed together so that the sharp object cannot injure tissue or become snagged as it is withdrawn.

Flexible Tracheobronchoscopy

Flexible tracheobronchoscopy can be performed in multiple settings under various levels of anesthesia. It can be successfully accomplished without sedation but with topical local anesthesia in the office setting, under conscious sedation with topical anesthesia in an endoscopy suite, or under general anesthesia via an existing endotracheal tube. A flexible endoscope passed through the nose is easily manipulated during an evaluation of the subglottis, trachea, and main bronchi in the office setting. Office tracheobronchoscopy without sedation is performed with the patient seated upright (▶ Fig. 100.6). If the subject does not have a tracheotomy, nebulized 4% plain lidocaine is administered orally. At the same time, the nasal passages are topically decongested and anesthetized. With the surgeon facing the patient, a flexible endoscope is placed through the more patent nasal passage. The larynx is visualized and evaluated for pathology, abnormalities of vocal fold motion, and glottic stenosis. If the larynx remains too sensate for the procedure to proceed, additional 4% lidocaine is applied to the vocal folds through the working channel of the endoscope. For the tracheotomized patient, lidocaine applied via the working channel and

the tracheostoma can also be used to anesthetize the larynx and lower airway. In addition, the distal examination can be performed via the tracheotomy. If it is not possible to offer nebulized treatments in the office setting or a scope with a working channel is not available, lidocaine can alternatively be applied by injecting it into the airway percutaneously. This produces a cough, which distributes the medicine. Lidocaine can also be applied transorally with an Abraham cannula. Taking the time to slowly and comfortably topically anesthetize a patient is invaluable for the patient's experience. It also allows the surgeon to survey the anatomy methodically and perform any procedures deemed necessary.

When it is necessary to evaluate the lower airway beyond the main bronchi, sedation is often needed, so the procedure is performed in a monitored endoscopy suite with the patient in the supine position. In addition to the intravenous sedatives given, topical local anesthesia is routinely administered directly to the larynx and trachea to decrease the need for excessive sedation and allow the patient to maintain satisfactory respiration. With the endoscopist at the head of the bed for orientation, the flexible bronchoscopy proceeds. It is imperative to remain aware of the anteroposterior and lateral orientation during flexible tracheobronchoscopy in the awake/office or sedated/endoscopy suite setting. General anesthesia can be administered for flexible bronchoscopy if the patient cannot tolerate the procedure because of anxiety or a severe gag reflex, or if the delicate nature of the procedure requires respiration to be held temporarily.

100.2.5 Risks and Adverse Effects

The most severe complication of rigid tracheobronchoscopy is pneumothorax or pneumomediastinum. If this is suspected, a chest X-ray is obtained after the procedure. Depending on the severity of the intervention, a chest X-ray may also be obtained after flexible bronchoscopy. An unsedated transnasal bronchoscopic procedure may have to be aborted approximately 3% of the time because of a narrow nasal vault, epistaxis, or patient intolerance. Loss of the airway requiring surgical intervention is possible during rigid bronchoscopy, as is the case in any procedure in which general anesthesia is administered and an endotracheal tube is not placed. This possibility should be considered preoperatively for any patient with potentially obstructing lesions of the oral cavity, larynx, or pharynx or any patient with limited neck mobility. The surgeon should have appropriate instrumentation available for emergent tracheotomy during all airway cases.

100.3 Esophagoscopy

100.3.1 Anatomy

The esophagus is a muscular tube that extends from the hypopharynx to the stomach. It is composed of only four layers, lacking a serosa outside the adventitial layer. The muscular layer, deep to the mucosa and submucosa, is composed of skeletal muscle in the proximal third and smooth muscle in the lower third of the esophagus (the muscular layer of the middle third is mixed). The upper esophageal sphincter (UES) is the tonically contracted proximal margin of the esophagus located approximately 16 cm from the incisors at the level of the sixth cervical vertebra. For all landmarks, an additional 3 cm can be added when they are measured from the nasal sill. The UES is 2 to 4 cm in length and is a functional unit that is composed of the cricopharyngeus muscle as well part of the inferior constrictor, upper esophagus, and the cricoid and arytenoid cartilages. The esophagus length ranges from 20 to 24 cm, extending to the lower esophageal sphincter (LES). The LES is not a true sphincter but a 2- to 4-cm area composed of tonically contracted smooth muscle from both the esophagus and diaphragm; it is both a physiologic and an anatomical entity located approximately 39 cm from the incisors at the level of the 11th thoracic vertebra adjacent to the cardia of the stomach. The rugae of the stomach meet the smooth wall of the esophagus at the gastroesophageal junction. A location of the gastroesophageal junction more than 2 cm above the diaphragmatic pinch is considered a hiatal hernia. The squamous epithelium of the esophagus meets the gastric columnar epithelium of the stomach at the squamocolumnar junction, also known as the Z-line. This is approximately 40 cm from the incisors and should correlate with the termination of the longitudinal submucosal vessels of the esophagus and gastroesophageal junction. Irregularities of the Z-line can be indicative of esophagitis or possibly Barrett esophagus (squamous metaplasia). Barrett esophagus should be suspected when tongues of what appear to be gastric mucosa migrate proximal to the gastroesophageal junction, infringing on the area of the longitudinal esophageal vessels. The squamocolumnar junction and the gastroesophageal junction, when normal, are found at the same level but are, by definition, different.

Other anatomical areas of interest are the external compressors of the esophageal lumen. Moving distally through the esophagus, they are the aorta (pulsatile, approximately 23 cm from the incisors); the left main bronchus (approximately 27 cm from the incisors); and the diaphragmatic pinch (approximately 38 cm from the incisors; ▶ Fig. 100.7).

100.3.2 Indications and Patient Selection

Rigid esophagoscopy and flexible esophagoscopy are typically performed for both diagnostic and therapeutic purposes. Esophagoscopy can be used to inspect the lumen of the esophagus

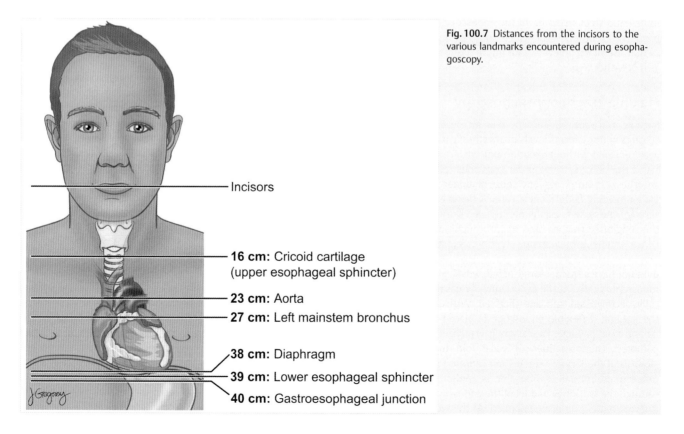

Fig. 100.7 Distances from the incisors to the various landmarks encountered during esophagoscopy.

Incisors

16 cm: Cricoid cartilage (upper esophageal sphincter)

23 cm: Aorta

27 cm: Left mainstem bronchus

38 cm: Diaphragm

39 cm: Lower esophageal sphincter

40 cm: Gastroesophageal junction

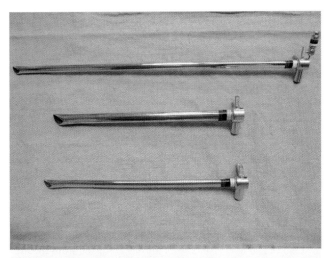

Fig. 100.8 Rigid esophagoscopes.

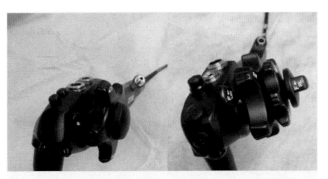

Fig. 100.9 (a) Transnasal endoscope and (b) flexible gastroscope.

Rigid Esophagoscopy

A rigid esophagoscope is a hollow, oval metal tube with a flared, blunt tip and a proximal "keel" for easier manipulation and orientation. It is available in many lengths and diameters (▶ Fig. 100.8). Unlike rigid bronchoscopes, rigid esophagoscopes typically do not have a separate port for a telescope and do not have a proximal adapter for instrumentation. Light is delivered via a long light carrier that is inserted through a separate, smaller port and emerges near the distal tip. The proximal opening is the only place through which both visualization (with or without a Hopkins rod telescope) and instrumentation occur. Rigid esophagoscopy is superior for evaluating the cervical esophagus because of difficulties of insufflation and visualization in the area of the UES. It is also preferred when larger biopsies or higher-volume suction is needed.

Flexible Esophagoscopy

Flexible esophagoscopes are available in two varieties. Transnasal esophagoscopes are intended for use in an awake, office setting, whereas flexible gastroscopes are used for sedated, transoral esophagoscopy in the operating room or monitored endoscopy suite. Both types of flexible esophagoscope routinely incorporate chip tip digital technology, deliver air and water for visualization, have at least a 2-mm working channel for suction and the insertion of smaller biopsy forceps and intervention devices, and are available in various diameters and lengths. A typical transnasal esophagoscope is 4.5 mm in diameter, whereas a gastroscope ranges from 9 to 12 mm in diameter and can deliver larger working instrumentation compared with a transnasal esophagoscope. Transnasal esophagoscopes have only one control wheel that flexes and extends the scope in one plane, whereas gastroscopes have two control wheels that allow flexion and extension of the tip in two planes perpendicular to each other (▶ Fig. 100.9).

Flexible esophagoscopy can be performed without general anesthesia and is not challenged by cervical spine anatomy/limitations. It provides better visualization of the squamocolumnar junction and gastroesophageal junction, and the examiner can visualize the gastroesophageal junction from within the stomach by retroflexing the endoscope. Unsedated office-based transnasal esophagoscopy can avoid the need for sedation and its attendant risks. The patient is also free to return to unrestricted activity after the procedure is complete. It is well

for pathology including tumor, strictures, foreign bodies, and changes to the mucosal surface caused by infectious or inflammatory conditions. Diagnostic biopsies can be performed as necessary. Esophagoscopy is not an effective tool to evaluate peristalsis because the presence of the scope in the esophagus alters its function. Esophagoscopy is often used to deliver instruments for therapeutic interventions, including balloons for dilation, graspers, laser fibers, and devices for cutting and radio-frequency ablation. Esophagoscopy also aids in the placement of tracheo-esophageal puncture devices after laryngectomy.

Patients are chosen for esophagoscopy based on their history, their response or lack of response to medical therapies, or the results of other diagnostic tests. Radiographic studies such as chest X-ray and barium esophogography may reveal foreign bodies; anatomical abnormalities such as webs, strictures, and diverticula; or evidence of achalasia that warrants visualization or intervention. The indications for esophagoscopy in patients with laryngopharyngeal reflux are ill defined. Recent findings suggest that patients presenting with symptoms of laryngopharyngeal reflux without symptoms of gastroesophageal reflux disease (GERD) may be at an elevated risk for esophageal adenocarcinoma. Thus, the presence of laryngopharyngeal reflux in and of itself may warrant esophagoscopy to rule out Barrett esophagus, erosive esophagitis, or adenocarcinoma. Unexplained esophageal dysphagia, weight loss, hemoptysis, hematemesis, odynophagia, and regurgitation are also indications for esophagoscopy. Patients who have head and neck cancer with esophageal symptoms require esophageal screening to rule out secondary malignancy or alternative pathology.

100.3.3 Equipment

Both rigid and flexible esophagoscopes are available and have inherent advantages and limitations. Rigid esophagoscopes are employed exclusively in the operating room, whereas flexible esophagoscopes can be used both in the operating room and in the office with an unsedated patient.

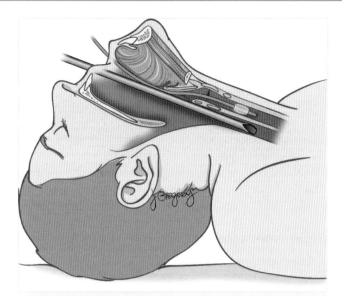

Fig. 100.10 Rigid esophagoscopy is performed with the middle finger of the nondominant hand on the patient's hard palate and the esophagoscope resting on and advanced by the thumb.

tolerated with the application of only topical nasal decongestant and anesthetic. The procedure, not including the time needed for topical anesthesia to take effect, lasts approximately 5 to 10 minutes. Sedated flexible esophagoscopy is usually preferred if numerous biopsies are indicated with a resulting increase in the duration of the procedure. If evaluation of the stomach or upper duodenum is indicated by a patient's history of abdominal pain, nausea, or vomiting, a sedated procedure with the appropriate scope is indicated.

100.3.4 Technique

Rigid Esophagoscopy

Rigid esophagoscopy is performed in the operating room under general endotracheal anesthesia (although monitored anesthesia care and local anesthesia are possible) with the patient supine. One should avoid using a shoulder roll or any other positioning that causes extension of the neck. The patient's upper teeth are protected with a tooth guard. The surgeon stands at the head of the bed and uses the nondominant hand to simultaneously open the mouth, stabilize the scope off the teeth, and advance the scope. The instrument is inserted under direct visualization through the oral cavity in a perpendicular trajectory toward the pharynx. The dominant hand serves only to support the length of the rigid scope and alter the angle of insertion. At the base of the tongue, the contour of the posterior pharyngeal wall is followed, and the esophagoscope is eventually aligned parallel with the esophagus. When the postcricoid area is reached, the larynx is lifted anteriorly to expose the esophageal introitus, which is usually slightly to the left of midline (▶ Fig. 100.10). The rigid scope is then advanced to the gastroesophageal junction if there is no obstructing pathology. The mucosal lining is visualized and instrumented as needed as the scope is slowly retracted. A Hopkins rod telescope can be inserted once the scope is in the esophagus for photo documentation and superior visualization.

Flexible Esophagoscopy

Transnasal esophagoscopy is performed with the patient seated in the office examination chair in a comfortable position. Cotton soaked in oxymetazoline and 4% lidocaine is placed in both nares for 10 minutes. If needed, benzocaine spray is applied to the oropharynx, or 2% viscous lidocaine is ingested. The scope is inserted through the more patent nasal passage and the larynx is visualized. While the tip of the scope is positioned just above the postcricoid area on the left, the patient is asked to swallow, and the scope is inserted into the esophagus while simultaneously engaging a small puff of air. With the use of a combination of insufflation, water, and suction, the scope is passed into the stomach and the stomach is insufflated. Retroflexion is performed to visualize the gastroesophageal junction from below. The scope is then pulled back into the esophagus, where the Z-line is visualized. Biopsies are taken from the area of the squamocolumnar junction and gastroesophageal junction if abnormalities are visualized. The mucosa of the entire esophagus is then carefully inspected as the scope is withdrawn. This procedure can be recorded through still images or video.

Sedated esophagoscopy with a flexible scope is performed with the patient in the lateral decubitus position. An oral appliance is inserted between the teeth to direct the flexible endoscope to the midline of the oropharynx. Under direct visualization, the endoscope is inserted past the tongue base and via the piriform sinuses into the esophagus. The examination proceeds as above for the transnasal esophagoscope once the instrument is in the esophagus. If a sedated or general anesthesia esophagoscopy procedure is performed without incident, the patient can be started on clear liquids in the postanesthesia care unit, and eating can proceed later in the day if the patient is otherwise asymptomatic.

100.3.5 Risks and Adverse Effects

Approximately 3% of the time, unsedated transnasal esophagoscopy is aborted because of a narrow nasal vault, patient discomfort, or epistaxis. Esophageal perforation is the most significant complication of esophagoscopy. If the patient has symptoms of chest pain, odynophagia, dyspnea, or tachycardia after the procedure, this must be ruled out. If it is suspected during the procedure, a nasogastric tube can be placed under direct visualization and intravenous antibiotics started. If perforation is suspected in the postanesthesia care unit, a chest X-ray is indicated to evaluate for free air or pneumothorax, and esophogography with a water-soluble contrast material should be performed when the patient is stable. Esophageal perforation can be avoided by never forcing an esophagoscope when it meets resistance and always having clear visualization of the esophageal lumen before advancing the scope.

100.4 Roundsmanship

- Tracheobronchoscopy and esophagoscopy are invaluable tools for the otolaryngologist, serving both diagnostic and therapeutic purposes.
- Patient positioning is the key to successfully completing rigid tracheobronchoscopy and esophagoscopy.

- Instrumentation for both rigid and flexible tracheobronchoscopy and esophagoscopy is available in multiple lengths and diameters, and the appropriate size must be chosen. This is especially important in pediatric and smaller adult patients. Having alternate sizes of rigid bronchoscopes available and ready if need be is paramount in the setting of obstructing airway cases.
- In-office, nonsedated options exist for both tracheobronchoscopy and esophagoscopy, and these techniques are often preferred by both patient and provider.
- Taking the time to topically anesthetize patients so that they are comfortable is invaluable during the performance of unsedated in office procedures.
- Complications from tracheobronchoscopy and esophagoscopy typically present immediately postoperatively, and the operating surgeon should always be ready to care for a perforation of the trachea or esophageal lumen. The surgeon should have a low threshold for obtaining a postoperative chest X-ray when performing these procedures.

100.5 Recommended Reading

[1] Belafsky PC, Postma GN, Daniel E, Koufman JA. Transnasal esophagoscopy. Otolaryngol Head Neck Surg 2001; 125: 588–589

[2] Garner J, Schweinfurth J, May W, Faust J. The transnasal esophagoscopy documentation dilemma. Laryngoscope 2007; 117: 1143–1145

[3] Lee KH, Rutter MJ. Role of balloon dilation in the management of adult idiopathic subglottic stenosis. Ann Otol Rhinol Laryngol 2008; 117: 81–84

[4] Postma GN, Belafsky PC, Aviv JE. Atlas of Transnasal Esophagoscopy. Philadelphia, PA: Lippincott Williams & Wilkins; 2007

[5] Rosen CA, Amin MR, Sulica L et al. Advances in office-based diagnosis and treatment in laryngology. Laryngoscope 2009; 119 Suppl 2: S185–S212

[6] Tsao GJ, Damrose EJ. Complications of esophagoscopy in an academic training program. Otolaryngol Head Neck Surg 2010; 142: 500–504

[7] Young VN, Smith LJ, Sulica L, Krishna P, Rosen CA. Patient tolerance of awake, in-office laryngeal procedures: a multi-institutional perspective. Laryngoscope 2012; 122: 315–321

101 Evaluation of the Rhinosinusitis Patient and Surgical Considerations

Steven David Schaefer

101.1 Introduction

The time-honored rhinologic history and physical examination are the mainstay of the evaluation of a patient presenting for the medical or surgical treatment of sinonasal disease. A third diagnostic element, computed tomography (CT), has emerged as an essential part of furthering our understanding of the extent of sinonasal disease and of surgical planning.

101.2 History

Common clinical complaints are summarized in the Box Clinical Complaints Associated with Rhinosinusitis (p. 774), below. Today, our understanding of sinusitis extends beyond an identification of the classic triad of headache, nasal obstruction, and mucopurulent rhinorrhea. We now recognize that shared respiratory epithelium and the anatomical proximity of the sinuses and nasal passages predispose to an inflammatory process incompletely described by the term *sinusitis*. A more inclusive term is *rhinosinusitis*. (The two terms are used interchangeably in this text.)

Clinical Complaints Associated with Rhinosinusitis

Major complaints
- Facial pain, pressure
- Facial congestion, fullness
- Nasal obstruction, blockage
- Nasal discharge, purulence; discolored postnasal discharge
- Hyposmia, anosmia
- Purulence in nasal cavity

Minor complaints
- Headache
- Halitosis
- Fatigue
- Dental pain
- Cough
- Ear pain, pressure, fullness

Source: Modified from Lanza DC, Kennedy DW. Adult rhinosinusitis defined. Otolaryngol Head Neck Surg 1997;117(3 Pt 2):S1–S7.

In communicating the clinical diagnosis of sinusitis, the temporal aspect of the process is essential to planning treatment. Historically, no good consensus exists for differentiating acute from chronic sinusitis. The American Academy of Otolaryngology-Head and Neck Surgery Task Force resolved these issues by defining acute sinusitis as sinusitis with a duration of less than 4 weeks, subacute sinusitis as that with a duration of 4 to 12 weeks, and chronic sinusitis as that with a duration of longer than 12 weeks (▶ Table 101.1). Common symptoms are headache, facial pain and pressure, and mucopurulent rhinorrhea.

Headache is a common symptom of rhinosinusitis as well as of various intracranial and extracranial pathologic processes. The location of the headache, in addition to its character, response to prior treatment, timing, and associated symptoms, should be documented. Headache due to sinus disease is usually localized to the involved sinus and contiguous structures; for example, maxillary sinusitis leads to pain in the upper jaw. Disease within the sphenoid sinus presents more of a diagnostic challenge because the pain is typically referred to the vertex region. In contrast, headache or pain in the occipital region suggests a neuromuscular or intracranial vascular origin. Headache accompanied by cranial nerve findings, such as vertex symptoms with cranial nerve II, III, IV, or V findings, suggests a medical emergency such as cavernous sinus thrombosis. The character of the headache may offer a useful diagnostic clue because sinus pain tends to be more focal, whereas neurovascular headache is associated with other symptoms, such as the "sick headache" of migraine, or may be related to the menstrual cycle. This picture can be particularly confusing if the sinus disease triggers a migraine. A response to decongestants or antibiotics suggesting rhinosinusitis versus a response to specific medications for neurovascular disease should be elicited to help differentiate between these two common conditions. Finally, the history should include the time of day when headache occurs and its relationship to events in the day and accompanying symptoms, such as the visual aura of neurovascular headache.

Facial pain and pressure: The patient usually uses the term *facial pain* to describe various levels of discomfort over a specific region of the face. This symptom, particularly if accompanied by tenderness, is more specific for rhinosinusitis than is headache. Pressure or a sense of fullness within the sinuses or adjacent region of the nose is a complaint probably reflecting the inability of the obstructed sinus ostium to permit equilibration with the ambient atmosphere.

Mucopurulent rhinorrhea: The presence of anterior or posterior mucopurulent rhinorrhea correlates well with sinonasal disease. As a generalization, this complaint is more often seen in association with other symptoms of sinus disease in acute infections, whereas it may be the sole manifestation of chronic rhinosinusitis. Care should be taken in the history to distinguish between actual infectious rhinorrhea and the clear or white secretions suggestive of allergic rhinitis.

Previous surgical treatment: A knowledge of any previous surgical treatment is very useful in understanding the pathogenesis of current disease and identifying potential pitfalls in revision surgery. This is important because patients have been found to fail surgery for the following reasons: (1) failure of the previous surgery to address the site of disease (e.g., only a Caldwell-Luc procedure performed for combined maxillary and ethmoid sinusitis; (2) incomplete ventilation of a diseased sinus, particularly retention of infected ethmoid cells; (3) inadequate

Table 101.1 Clinical categories of rhinosinusitis (from the 1996 American Academy of Otolaryngology-Head and Neck Surgery Task Force)

	Duration	Strong history	Include in differential	Special notes
Acute	Up to 4 wk	2 major factors OR 1 major factor, 2 minor factors OR Nasal purulence on examination	1 major factor, 2 minor factors	Fever or facial pain does not constitute suggestive history in absence of other nasal symptoms or signs
Subacute	4–12 wk	Same as chronic	Same as chronic	Complete resolution after effective medical therapy
Chronic	12 wk	2 major factors OR 1 major factor, 2 minor factors OR Symptoms or nasal purulence on examination	1 major factor, 2 minor factors	Facial pain does not constitute suggestive history in absence of other nasal symptoms or signs
Recurrent acute	Four episodes per year, each episode last 7–10 days; absence of intervening signs of chronic rhinosinusitis	Same as acute rhinosinusitis		
Acute exacerbations of chronic	Sudden worsening of chronic rhinosinusitis, return to baseline after treatment			

Modified from Lanza DC, Kennedy DW. Adult rhinosinusitis defined. Otolaryngol Head Neck Surg 1997;117(3 Pt 2):S1–S7.

postoperative care; (4) lack of identification of confounding disease processes, such as allergic fungal sinusitis with polyps or AERD (*a*spirin-*e*xacerbated *r*espiratory *d*isease); (5) iatrogenic sinusitis induced by obstruction of a preoperatively normal sinus resulting from postoperative alterations of the outflow tract of the sinus; and (6) idiopathic disease. Knowledge of the previous surgery is also useful in identifying potential pitfalls of revision surgery because the earlier operations may have resulted in dehiscence of the lamina papyracea or skull base with subsequent herniation of orbital or cranial contents into the sinuses. In such patients, the history may range from rather vague indications, such as "some polyps were removed from my nose 10 years ago," to the rather obvious indication of skull base penetration from a history of "clear fluid drains from my nose since sinus surgery." The more information the history conveys to the surgeon, the more likely it will be that the surgeon can preoperatively obtain the appropriate tests and consultations to manage these pitfalls (▶ Fig. 101.1).

101.2.1 Surgical Considerations

The essential questions to be resolved in considering surgery for a patient are these: Has medical therapy proved inadequate or unlikely to manage the sinonasal disease? Is surgery appropriate and likely to significantly improve the patient's state of health? Surgery should be reserved for those patients whose disease is refractory to repeated courses of prolonged appropriate antibiotic therapy: one or more broad-spectrum antibiotics for 3 weeks or longer. Surgical indications are further strengthened by increases in the duration, morbidity, severity, or frequency of infection despite good medical treatment. Other considerations are the actual measures being employed to diagnose a sinus infection. Many of the measures or symptoms used to diagnose rhinosinusitis are rather vague or nonspecific, such as

headache. Others—for example, mucopurulent rhinorrhea—are more consistent with acute or chronic sinusitis. A history of polyps does not necessarily indicate the need for surgical treatment. However, polyps refractory to allergic management that are associated with nasal obstruction, with or without exacerbation of asthma, are properly treated by surgery. On the other hand, surgical treatment of asthma and nasal polyposis without consideration of aspirin sensitivity is a missed opportunity to manage aspirin-exacerbated respiratory disease. Finally, the history should be correlated with a physical or radiographic finding before surgery is considered. Significantly, an opacified sinus on imaging without a history of sinusitis or evidence of neoplasm is not alone an indication for surgery.

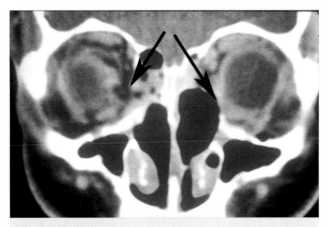

Fig. 101.1 Postoperative coronal computed tomographic scan of a patient with iatrogenic blindness. Note the bilateral loss of the lamina papyracea and air within both orbits (*arrows*).

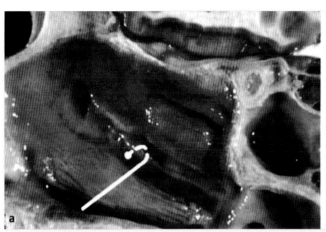 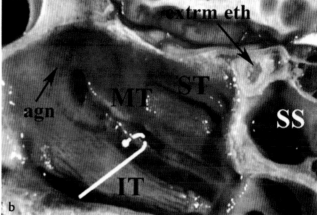

Fig. 101.2 (a) Sagittal cadaver section showing the right lateral nasal wall. Probe in middle meatus or ostiomeatal complex. (b) Same view as in (a) *agn*, agger nasi; *extrm eth*, extramural ethmoid cell; *IT*, inferior turbinate; *MT*, middle turbinate; *SS*, sphenoid sinus; *ST*, superior turbinate.

101.3 Physical Examination

101.3.1 Nasal Endoscopy

The second element of an evaluation for the medical or surgical treatment of sinus disease is careful endoscopic examination of the nose. The concept of using an optical telescope to examine the nose is not new; however, advances in the last three decades in optics and illumination have led to significant supplementation of conventional anterior rhinoscopy with nasal endoscopy. Endoscopy is directed toward confirming the history and documenting evidence of sinonasal disease—in particular, obstruction of the ostia of the sinuses. The office examination should begin with vasoconstriction and, if needed, anesthesia to permit maximal visualization of the nose. The nose should be examined with a rigid 0-degree and/or a 30- or 45-degree telescope. A flexible endoscope is an alternative instrument, but the optics are inferior to those of the rigid endoscope. The first passage of the endoscope should be along the floor of the nose (▶ Fig. 101.2).

This first phase of endoscopy permits visualization of the orifice of the nasolacrimal duct (in the inferior meatus), inferolateral nasal wall, eustachian tube orifice, and nasopharynx. The second passage of the endoscope is immediately inferior to the middle turbinate and provides a view of the sphenoethmoid recess, middle meatus, and sphenoid ostium. Each of these sites may be variably difficult to examine because of the presence of polyps, degenerated mucous membrane, or pneumatization of the middle turbinate. The last passage of the telescope should be directed toward the frontal recess, thus crossing adjacent to the junction of the middle turbinate and the agger nasi. Coupled with a good history, nasal endoscopy should be regarded as a highly sensitive and specific measure of sinonasal disease. Potential findings include the following.

Polyps

The identification of massive polyposis is not difficult, nor is it solely in the realm of the skilled nasal endoscopist. In contrast, recurrent ethmoiditis due to a small polyp obstructing the ostiomeatal complex can be difficult to diagnose and often goes unrecognized during anterior rhinoscopic examinations.

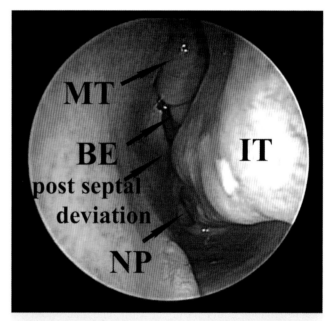

Fig. 101.3 Zero-degree endoscopic view of the left side of the nose. The inferior turbinate, middle turbinate, inferior aspect of the bulla ethmoidalis, nasopharynx, and a posterior septal deviation are well visualized. *BE*, inferior aspect of the bulla ethmoidalis; *IT*, inferior turbinate; *MT*, middle turbinate; *NP*, nasopharynx.

Mucopurulent Secretions

When the history is used to direct the examination, the endoscopic documentation of mucopurulent secretions draining from the ostium of the involved sinus is "the gold standard" in making the diagnosis of sinusitis.

Deviated Nasal Septum

The relationship of a partially deviated nasal septum to sinusitis or otitis media has been and remains the subject of much discussion in otolaryngology (▶ Fig. 101.3). Less controversial is lateral compression of the middle turbinate by the deviated septum as a cause of recurrent sinusitis. In the absence of sinus disease, this form of airway obstruction is corrected by septoplasty. In contrast, impaction of the middle turbinate into the lateral nasal wall with sinusitis is treated by septoplasty and surgery of the involved sinus.

Concha Bullosa

Pneumatization of the anterior aspect of the middle turbinate is referred to as a concha bullosa. Many such conchae have little clinical significance. A concha bullosa is significant when such enlargement of the turbinate obstructs the ostiomeatal complex or is the actual site of infection.

Fungal Sinusitis

Two forms of fungal sinusitis may be recognizable on nasal endoscopy: invasive and noninvasive. Probably less frequent in incidence but better known to physicians is invasive fungal sinusitis, which comprises acute fulminant, chronic, and granulomatous forms. Mucormycosis is an acute fulminant invasive fungal sinusitis that is typically seen in compromised patients. This entity is characterized by various degrees of bone and soft-tissue destruction on both endoscopic and CT examination; it is treated with aggressive surgery and systemic antifungal agents. Less known is noninvasive fungal sinusitis, which includes fungal balls and allergic fungal sinusitis. Allergic fungal sinusitis presents with nasal polyps, a green "slimelike" fungal debris within the sinus lumen, and areas of increased density within opacified sinuses on CT and variable bone resorption on scanning. This entity is a localized, extramural immune response to noninvasive dematiacious fungi (e.g., *Bipolaris*) and is managed by removal of the polyps and fungus, continual aeration and cleaning of the involved sinus, and corticosteroids as needed (▶ Fig. 101.4).

Tumors

The diagnosis of benign and malignant tumors of the sinonasal region has been greatly enhanced by the ability of the endo-

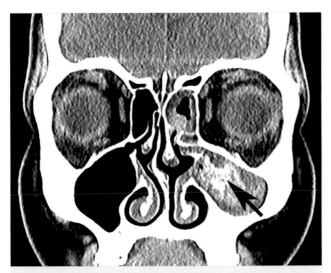

Fig. 101.4 Coronal computed tomographic scan of a patient with allergic fungal sinusitis involving the left maxillary sinus. Note area of hyperdensity (*arrow*) within the maxillary sinus.

scope to magnify, illuminate, and view sites at various angles from the optical axis of the instrument. Often, a history of epistaxis with accompanying evidence of soft- or hard-tissue invasion and the endoscopic identification of a friable, irregular mass within the nose lead to a histopathologic confirmation of carcinoma. More challenging is the diagnosis of a unilateral sinonasal polyp versus inverting papilloma in the patient with a history of multiple "polyp surgeries" and the endoscopic picture of a rather unimpressive mass in the nose. In the case of a sinonasal tumor, the diagnosis can be confirmed by biopsy in the office, whereas for some inverting papillomas, formal surgery is required to obtain sufficient tissue for pathologic examination (▶ Fig. 101.5).

Epistaxis

Bleeding from the nose is often due to the erosion of blood vessels supplying the anterior nasal septum. Other common sites of bleeding are along the anterior aspect of the inferior or middle turbinates. Less common is bleeding in the posterior region of the nose or the nasopharynx. All patients with either prolonged or frequently recurrent epistaxis should undergo a complete endoscopic examination to rule out occult neoplasms or vascular malformations. In the postpubertal male, epistaxis may be associated with a benign tumor known as a juvenile nasopharyngeal angiofibroma. This tumor, which most often presents with nasal obstruction and subsequent epistaxis, arises between the basiocciput and basisphenoid. Bleeding from a sinus cavity into the nose should alert the physician to a possible tumor within the sinus and necessitates CT.

101.3.2 General Otolarygologic Examination

Other aspects of the physical examination include evaluation of the following.

Olfaction

Various methods exist to roughly quantify olfaction, but many of these suffer from a lack of standardization and degradation of the substances causing the odor over time. An excellent alternative a commercially available smell identification test, which is based on the University of Pennsylvania Smell Identification Test (UPSIT). This test, which uses a normalized "scratch and sniff" measurement of olfaction, is administered within 15 minutes by the patient (Sensonics, Haddon Heights, NJ). Contrary to popular opinion, impaired olfaction is complicated and is often not due to simple obstruction of the nose by a deviated septum or nasal polyps. Many a surgeon and patient have been disappointed after surgery performed to restore olfaction.

Vision

The evaluation of vision is guided by the history. For example, chronic ethmoid or sphenoid sinusitis may first present as alterations in visual acuity or visual fields. Any infectious, inflammatory, or benign or malignant process may first present with compromise of vision and/or an abnormal appearance of the eyes. Although Graves disease or thyroid eye disease is often

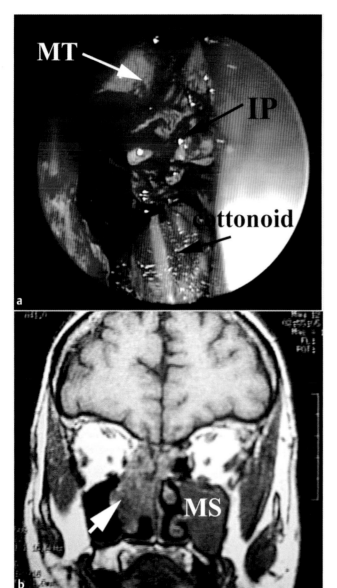

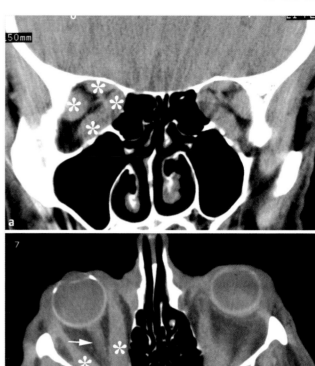

Fig. 101.6 (a) Coronal computed tomographic (CT) scan of a patient with bilateral thyroid eye disease. Note typical hypertrophic extraocular muscles (*asterisks*), which compress the optic nerve. (b) Axial CT scan of another patient with bilateral thyroid eye disease. The optic nerve (*arrow*) is compressed by extraocular muscles (*asterisks*).

Fig. 101.5 (a) Endoscopic intraoperative photograph of inverting papilloma of the right side of the nose. Neurosurgical cottonoid appears in the inferior region of the nose. *IP*, inverting papilloma; *MT*, middle turbinate. (b) Coronal magnetic resonance image showing inverting papilloma (*arrow*) in the same patient as in (a). The contralateral maxillary sinus is opacified because of sinusitis, not tumor. The maxillary sinus on the same side as the tumor is not opacified. *MS*, maxillary sinus.

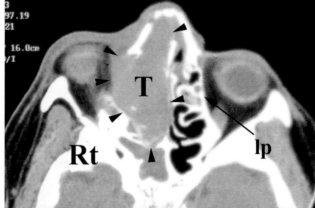

Fig. 101.7 Axial computed tomographic scan of a malignant tumor (*arrowheads*) of the right side of the nose invading the ipsilateral orbit. In contrast, the contralateral lamina papyracea is intact. *lp*, lamina papyracea; *T*, tumor.

considered the most likely cause of unilateral exophthalmos, any mass-occupying process that extends into the orbit may present with this finding (▶ Fig. 101.6 and ▶ Fig. 101.7).

Infections of the face or sinuses (viscerocranium) may spread to the eye and brain (neurocranium). Early infections of the eye limited anteriorly to the periosteum of the orbit or septumorbitale present with edema and erythema of the eyelids. As the infection spreads into the orbit, proptosis develops and extraocular movement declines. Further involvement of the superior

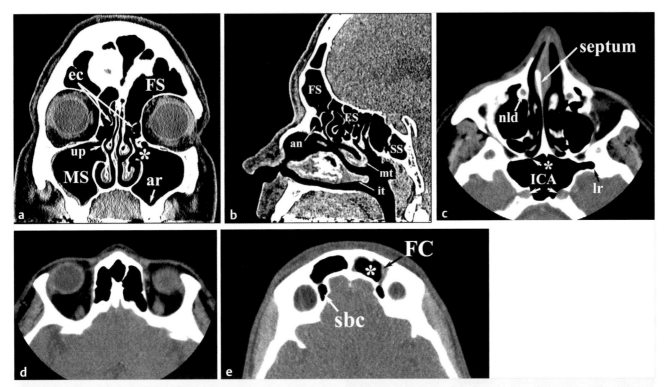

Fig. 101.8 (**a**) Coronal computed tomographic (CT) scan of a patient after antibiotic treatment for acute sinusitis showing only mild residual thickening of the mucous membrane lining the right maxillary sinus. The uncinate process, ostium of the maxillary sinus (*asterisk*), anterior ethmoid cells, alveolar recess of the maxillary sinus, and frontal sinus are all normal. *ar*, alveolar recess of the maxillary sinus; *ec*, anterior ethmoid cells; *FS*, frontal sinus; *MS*, maxillary sinus; *up*, uncinate process. (**b**) Sagittal CT scan through the plane of the right frontal recess. An agger nasi cell is extending into the frontal recess of the frontal sinus and slightly narrowing the outflow tract of this sinus. Other structures noted are the sphenoid sinus, ethmoid sinus, middle turbinate, and inferior turbinate. *an*, agger nasi cell; *ES*, ethmoid sinus; *FS*, frontal sinus; *it*, inferior turbinate; *mt*, middle turbinate; *SS*, sphenoid sinus. (**c**) Axial CT scan through the mid plane of the sphenoid sinus showing the internal carotid arteries, sphenoid sinus ostium (*asterisk*), nasolacrimal duct, lateral recess of the sphenoid sinus, and deviated nasal septum. *ICA*, internal carotid arteries; *nld*, nasolacrimal duct; *lr*, lateral recess of the sphenoid sinus. (**d**) Axial CT scan of the same patient as in (a–c) showing normal outflow tract of the frontal sinus. (**e**) Axial CT scan through the mid body of the left frontal sinus in another patient. This patient has a frontal cell arising within the frontal sinus, which partly contains air (*asterisk*); the drainage pathway distal to the cell is obstructed. Posteriorly, a suprabullar ethmoid cell extends into the frontal recess. *FC*, frontal cell; *sbc*, suprabullar ethmoid cell.

orbital fissure leads to a loss of extraocular movement. Infection or any other process that compromises the optic nerve between the retina and the optic chiasm leads to a Marcus Gunn pupil or afferent pupillary defect. Such a process is detected by moving a flashlight from one eye to the other. Normally, there is both a direct and consensual constriction of the two pupils. In the presence of an afferent pupillary defect, the involved eye minimally constricts during direct illumination with the flashlight, giving the impression of pupillary dilation, while the uninvolved eye constricts. Shining a light in the normal eye causes both pupils to constrict because of an intact pupillary afferent pathway. Another name for such an abnormal finding is *positive swinging flashlight test*. Visual impairment of the contralateral eye indicates extension of the disease process into the cavernous sinus. As is true in any patient with ophthalmologic symptoms, joint management with an ophthalmologist is required.

Neuropathy

Additional dysfunction of cranial nerves III through VI further localizes potential benign and malignant processes to within the sinuses with or without extension to the cavernous sinus.

101.4 Computed Tomography and Magnetic Resonance Imaging

CT is the third element of the evaluation of a patient with sinusitis and the radiographic sinus examination of choice. From a practical standpoint, coronal CT of the paranasal sinuses may be far more cost-effective than repeated plain films and is far more likely to aid in the patient's treatment. As both computer and X-ray detection technologies evolve, modern CT scanners capture multiple images in an axial plane and reformat the images in axial, coronal, and sagittal projections. With the knowledge that a patient who has a simple upper respiratory infection may have abnormal findings on a CT scan of the sinuses, the timing of imaging has been further refined. The "best practice" today is to perform CT several weeks after the completion of prolonged antibiotic therapy unless the patient's condition warrants immediate intervention (▶ Fig. 101.8). Magnetic resonance (MR) imaging is selectively employed to discern the contents of an opacified sinus with or without CT cisternography (▶ Fig. 101.9a), which aids in imaging the extension of sinus disease into adjacent structures such as the eye and brain (▶ Fig. 101.9b).

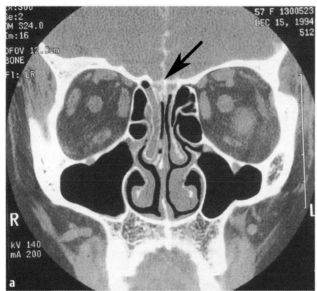

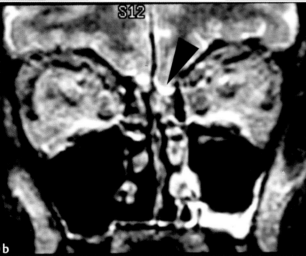

Fig. 101.9 (a) Contrast computed tomographic cisternogram showing cerebrospinal fluid (CSF) fistula (*arrow*) in the roof of the right ethmoid sinus. (b) Magnetic resonance image with a small polyp-like structure in the superior region of the left side of the nose in a patient with intermittent CSF rhinorrhea is found to be an encephalocele (*arrowhead*).

Reading any form of imaging of the sinus should begin with what is obvious, and sometimes overlooked: first verify that the scans are from the patient of interest, the date of the examination, and the quality of the images. CT is employed in the following situations.

101.4.1 Extension of Disease beyond Sinuses

Infections of the eye or brain may result from either hematogenous or direct extension of sinusitis. CT is important in both evaluating the involvement of other organs and planning treatment, such as drainage of a subperiosteal orbital abscess into the ethmoid cavity via an endoscopic ethmoidectomy. MR imaging may be complementary to better discern the disease process and the extent of disease beyond the sinuses (▶ Fig. 101.10).

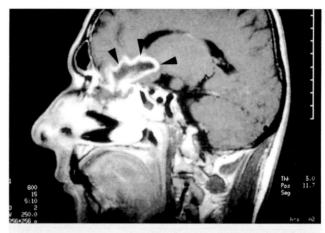

Fig. 101.10 Iatrogenic brain abscess following sinus surgery (*arrowheads*), best demonstrated on sagittal magnetic resonance image.

101.4.2 Problem Diagnosis

Some patients present with a sole complaint indicative of either sinusitis or another disease process. In the absence of physical findings (see Box Physical Findings in Rhinosinusitis (p. 780)), CT is helpful in such cases to rule out chronic sinus infection before proceeding with other forms of treatment (e.g., migraine headache or migraine exacerbated by sinusitis). Another problem diagnosis is the so-called silent sinus syndrome. This disorder is characterized by an inward displacement of the roof and the posterior walls of the maxillary sinus. The uncinate process uniformly approximates the medial inferior orbit. The maxillary sinus is opacified on CT scans even though frequently the patient is unaware of any sinus disease. However, as the walls of the sinus collapse inward, the floor of the orbit continues to implode into the sinus, leading to inferior displacement of the globe and subsequent diplopia (▶ Fig. 101.11). Double vision may be the first symptoms of this atypical form of sinusitis.

Physical Findings in Rhinosinusitis

- External physical findings
  - Swelling and erythema: maxillary, orbital, and frontal regions
- Findings on anterior rhinoscopy
  - Hyperemia
  - Edema
  - Crusts
  - Purulence
  - Polyps
- Findings on nasal endoscopy
  - Bluish discoloration of turbinates
  - Purulence at sinus ostia
  - Polyps, note size and location
  - Septal deflection: note compromise of sinus ostia
  - Concha bullosa
  - Paradoxical turbinates
- Other abnormalities

Modified from Hadley JA, Schaefer SD. Clinical evaluation of rhinosinusitis: history and physical examination. Otolaryngol Head Neck Surg 1997;117(3 Pt 2):S8–S11.

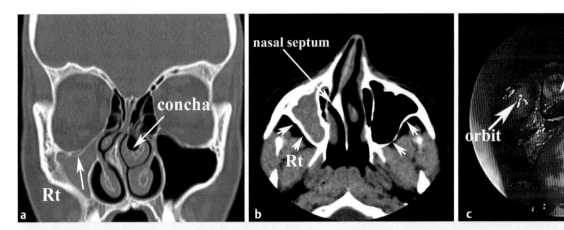

Fig. 101.11 (a) Coronal and (b) axial computed tomographic scans from a patient with silent sinus syndrome. The floor of the right orbit (*arrow*) is displaced or contracted inferiorly, causing a more inferior location of the globe compared with the normal left orbit. The uncinate process completely approximates the inferior medial right orbit. The coronal image also shows a nasal septum deviated to the right and excessive pneumatization of the anterior aspect of the left middle turbinate, known as a concha bullosa (*concha*). The axial image shows the loss of the *S* appearance of the posterior maxillary wall (*short arrows*), which follows from the inward collapse of the roof and posterior walls of this sinus. (c) The surgical findings in this patient. *ES*, ethmoid sinus; *MT*, middle turbinate; *orbit*, inferomedial wall of orbit.

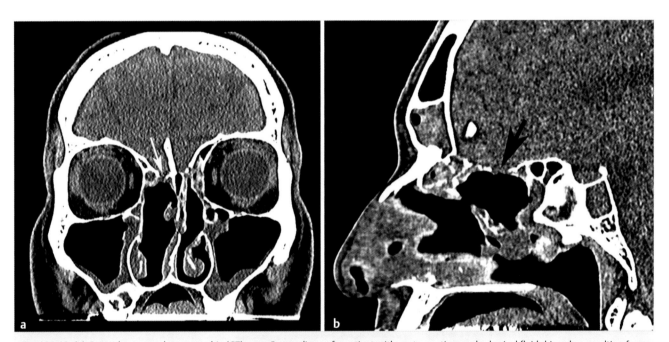

Fig. 101.12 (a) Coronal computed tomographic (CT) scan, 2-mm slices, of a patient with postoperative cerebral spinal fluid rhinorrhea resulting from injury to the roof of the right ethmoid sinus (*arrow*). (b) Sagittal CT scan of patient in (a) showing the skull base defect. The site of the injury is typical; instruments can be directed through the skull base as the surgeon progresses to the posterior ethmoid cells.

101.4.3 Recurrent Sinusitis

Because plain films of the sinuses are neither sensitive nor specific for many of the disease processes affecting the paranasal sinuses, CT is employed in patients with multiple episodes of sinusitis and/or nasal polyps. This examination clearly delineates the extent and severity of disease. In contrast, isolated anterior ethmoiditis can easily be unrecognized on a Caldwell radiograph because this film reflects the sum of all the bone and soft-tissue densities within the sinus. In cases of allergic fungal sinusitis, MR imaging is a useful supplement to CT because fungal concretions appear as low signal intensity or signal voids on T2-weighted images.

101.4.4 Recurrent Disease after Surgery

Patients with recurrent sinusitis or polyps after surgery are difficult to evaluate by any modality because of a loss of normal sinonasal architecture and fibrosis. CT is strongly recommended for any such patient in whom postoperative medical therapy fails after a trial of 2 to 3 months or for whom revision surgery is contemplated. If the history or physical examination suggests that the prior procedures may have injured the floor of the anterior cranial fossa or orbit, 1- to 2-mm coronal slices are recommended (▶ Fig. 101.12). MR imaging is particularly useful for identifying encephaloceles and mucoceles, which may not be apparent on CT scans (▶ Fig. 101.13).

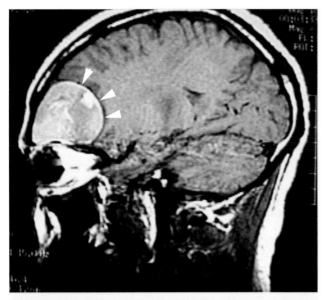

Fig. 101.13 Sagittal T1-weighted magnetic resonance (MR) image showing epidural mucopyocele (*arrowheads*) arising from the frontal sinus. MR image reveals heterogeneous contents of the mucocele, which would not be discernible on computed tomography.

101.4.5 Surgical Planning

The CT scan provides an essential road map in both planning and performing endoscopic sinus surgery. In the operating room, particular attention should be given to the following: (1) angle or plane of the lateral lamella of the cribriform plate relative to the cribriform plate and the roof of the ethmoid sinus, which may predispose to penetration of the anterior cranial fossa; (2) proximity of the maxillary ostium to the orbital floor; (3) extent of pneumatization of the ethmoid sinus, which can be minimal anteriorly, thereby increasing the risk for penetration of the orbit, or extensive posteriorly, with cells surrounding the optic nerve; (4) number and location of septa relative to the midline of the sinus; (5) location and any dehiscence of the optic nerve or carotid artery within the lateral wall of the sphenoid sinus; (6) anterior–posterior pneumatization of the frontal sinus, which influences access to the sinus through the frontal recess; and (7) extent of residual sinus architecture to aid in the identification of surgical landmarks.

101.4.6 Staging Rhinosinusitis

CT provides an objective measure of the extent of rhinosinusitis. Staging benign sinus disease, much like the staging of neoplasms, has evolved as a means to convey the extent of the

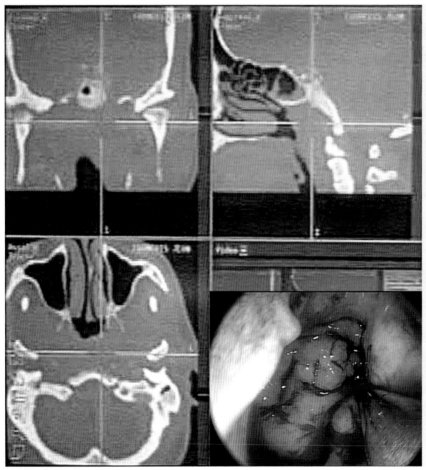

Fig. 101.14 Intraoperative computer-assisted image guidance. Lower right quadrant shows biopsy site of left clival mass. The other three quadrants show localization of the tumor in three projections during surgical removal.

disease process and audit therapeutic outcome. Of the various proposed staging systems, the modified Lund-Mackay system has proved both simple to use and sufficiently precise to satisfy these goals. After appropriate medical treatment, CT scans of all four sinuses are evaluated. Each sinus is assigned a numeric value: 0, no abnormality, 1, partial opacification; or 2, total opacification. The anterior and posterior ethmoid sinuses are separately evaluated and graded. Each ostiomeatal complex is included in the staging and is given a value of 0 for no obstruction and 2 for obstruction. A total score of 0 to 12 for each side is possible, with the higher number reflecting more severe rhinosinusitis.

Regarding intraoperative computer-assisted image guidance, as CT and stand-alone work station computing power increased in the 1990s, digital data from imaging studies were reprocessed and coupled to electromagnetic and infrared detectors to guide surgery within the brain and face, in a process much like that of a GPS (ground-positioning satellite) system (▶ Fig. 101.14).

101.5 Roundsmanship

- A complete history and a carefully performed physical examination (including nasal endoscopy) are critical for treating patients presenting with sinus or nasal problems.
- Mucopurulent rhinorrhea is the most consistent symptom of bacterial sinusitis.
- The majority of patients with sinusitis spontaneously improve with minimal physician management. A minority of these patients require antibiotics. When surgery is being considered, the physician should taken into account the length of treatment and the antibiotics previously used. Too frequently, patients are treated for a week or so with one antibiotic, followed by another trial of one or more antibiotics. Once medi-

cal management has failed, the decision to perform surgery should also be based on the imaging findings of refractory sinusitis and the physical findings.
- The preoperative CT scan is a road map to surgery. In those patients who have had prior surgery, imaging should delineate why it failed and forewarn the surgeon of potential pitfalls, such as prior injury or vulnerability to injury of the eye or brain.

101.6 Recommended Reading

[1] Anon , ymous. . Report of the rhinosinusitis task force committee meeting. Alexandria, Virginia, August 17, 1996.. Otolaryngol Head Neck Surg 1997; 117: S1–S68

[2] Berges-Gimeno MP, Simon RA, Stevenson DD. The natural history and clinical characteristics of aspirin-exacerbated respiratory disease. Ann Allergy Asthma Immunol 2002; 89: 474–478

[3] Doty RL, Shaman P, Dann MS. Development of the University of Pennsylvania Smell Identification Test: a standardized microencapsulated test of olfactory function. Physiol Behav 1984; 32: 489–502

[4] Hadley JA, Schaefer SD. Clinical evaluation of rhinosinusitis: history and physical examination. Otolaryngol Head Neck Surg 1997; 117: S8–S11

[5] Lanza DC, Kennedy DW. Adult rhinosinusitis defined. Otolaryngol Head Neck Surg 1997; 117; (3 Pt 2): 1–7

[6] Lund VJ, Mackay IS. Staging in rhinosinusitis. Rhinology 1993; 31: 183–184

[7] Manning SC, Schaefer SD, Close LG, Vuitch F. Culture-positive allergic fungal sinusitis. Arch Otolaryngol Head Neck Surg 1991; 117: 174–178

[8] McClay JE, Marple B, Kapadia L et al. Clinical presentation of allergic fungal sinusitis in children. Laryngoscope 2002; 112: 565–569

[9] Som PM, Lawson W, Biller HF, Lanzieri CF. Ethmoid sinus disease: CT evaluation in 400 cases. Part I. Nonsurgical patients. Radiology 1986a; 159: 591–597

[10] Som PM, Lawson W, Biller HF, Lanzieri CF, Sachdev VP, Rigamonti D. Ethmoid sinus disease: CT evaluation in 400 cases. Part III. Craniofacial resection. Radiology 1986b; 159: 605–609

[11] Zinreich SJ. Rhinosinusitis: radiologic diagnosis. Otolaryngol Head Neck Surg 1997; 117: S27–S34

102 Anatomy and Physiology of the Nose and Paranasal Sinuses

Steven David Schaefer and Ameet R. Kamat

102.1 Introduction

An understanding of the anatomy and physiology of the nose and paranasal sinuses is essential to optimize the diagnosis and treatment of diseases of these organs. The evolution of computed tomography (CT) and magnetic resonance (MR) imaging, coupled with advances in our understanding of the pathogenesis of upper respiratory tract disease and its treatment, has reawakened otolarygologists' interest in this heretofore underappreciated organ system. The advent of improved surgical optics and endoscopes requires that the otolaryngologist–head and neck surgeon be thoroughly familiar with the anatomy of the upper respiratory tract. This requirement is reflected in the detailed anatomical citations in this chapter.

102.2 Applied Anatomy

102.2.1 Anatomy of the Nose

As the most prominent facial feature, the nose has been the subject of both Western and Eastern art for millennia. In ancient India, the practice of amputating the nose as a punishment for adultery led to a practical understanding of the external nasal anatomy as surgeons developed forehead and arm flaps to reconstruct the skin and nasal skeleton. The nasal skeleton is a pyramid consisting (superiorly) of paired bones and (inferiorly) of paired upper and lower lateral cartilages. The nasal bones overlap the upper lateral cartilages, which are attached to the internal surface of the bones. The inferior third of the external nose is supported by the semilunar or archlike lower lateral or alar cartilages. The medial crura join together to form the columella, which is connected to the caudal septal cartilage by the membranous septum. The lateral crura provide the structural support to the nasal introitus and abut the upper lateral cartilages to form the limen nasi. The narrowest part of the nasal airway is the internal nasal valve, which is roughly bounded medially by the septum, inferiorly by the nasal floor, laterally by the inferior turbinate, and superiorly the limen nasi. The regulation of inspiratory nasal airflow begins with dilation of the nostrils by the facial muscles; airflow is constricted by the nasal valve and modified by the turbinates and the cartilaginous–bony septum. The inferior, middle, superior, and rarely supreme turbinates are the most prominent appendages of the lateral nasal wall. The inferior, middle, and superior turbinates, or bony conchae, are medial to the outflow tract of the nasolacrimal duct, the outflow tract of the ethmoid, maxillary, and frontal sinuses, and the outflow tract of the posterior ethmoid sinus, respectively (▶ Fig. 102.1). The midline septum consists of the anterior quadrilateral cartilage and four bones: the perpendicular plate of the ethmoid posterosuperiorly, the vomer posteriorly, and the crests of the maxilla and palatine bones inferiorly. Posteriorly, the nasal cavity communicates with the nasopharynx via the choanae (▶ Fig. 102.2).

The external and internal blood supply to the nose is the carotid artery. The internal carotid artery gives rise via the ophthalmic artery to the anterior and posterior ethmoidal arteries (▶ Fig. 102.3). These vessels provide blood to the superior lateral nasal wall and superior septum. The external carotid artery vascularizes the remaining nose. The greater palatine and facial arteries supply the anteroinferior nasal septum and lateral nasal wall. The inferoposterior septum and nasal wall receive their primary blood supply from the sphenopalatine artery, which is one of the five branches of the internal maxillary artery. A confluence of the anterior branches of the internal and external carotid arteries at the anterior nasal septum forms the Kiesselbach plexus or Little area. Given the turbulent airflow across the anterior septum, particularly in the presence of a deviation of the caudal septum, and the abundant blood supply, the Kiesselbach plexus is the principal site of epistaxis. Venous drainage of the nose is primarily via the facial, sphenopalatine, and ophthalmic veins. This rich venous plexus may drain to the intracranial veins, forming the so-called danger triangle, from which infection can ascend from the skin and soft tissue bounded by the nasal root and oral commissures and the nasal cavity to the brain.

102.2.2 Anatomy of the Paranasal Sinuses

The investigation of paranasal sinus anatomy may have begun with the anatomist Galen in the second century AD, although

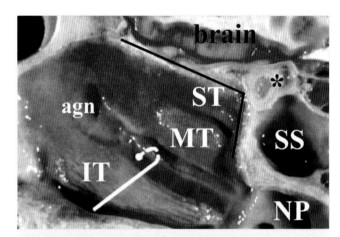

Fig. 102.1 Sagittal cadaver section showing left lateral nasal wall. The black line parallel to the floor of the anterior cranial fossa and the second line parallel to the anterior wall of the sphenoid sinus emphasize the posterior–inferior 15-degree slope of the skull base. During intranasal sinus surgery, the surgeon must adjust the dissection of the ethmoid sinus inferiorly during advancement into the posterior region of the nose. *agn,* agger nasi; *asterisk,* extramural ethmoid cell; *IT,* inferior turbinate; *MT,* middle turbinate; *NP,* nasopharynx; *SS,* sphenoid sinus; *ST,* superior turbinate.

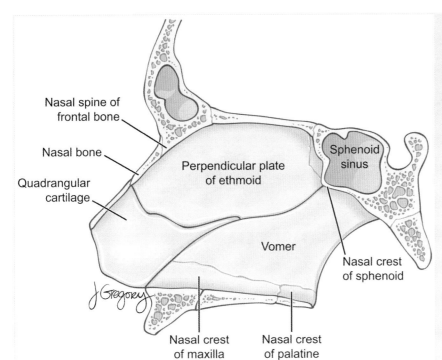

Fig. 102.2 The nasal septum comprises the quadrangular cartilage and the nasal crest of the palatine bone, maxillary crest, vomer, nasal crest of the sphenoid, and perpendicular plate of the ethmoid. The blood supply consists of the anterior and posterior ethmoidal arteries, which are branches of the internal carotid artery via the ophthalmic artery, and the sphenopalatine, sublabial, and greater palatine arteries, which are branches of the external carotid artery.

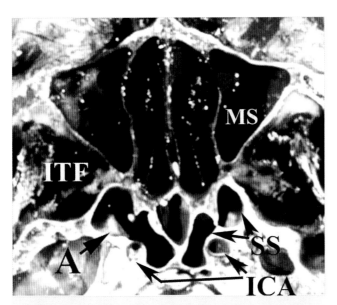

Fig. 102.3 Axial cadaver section through the sphenoid and maxillary sinuses. In some individuals, posterior ethmoid cells expand into the sphenoid bone. Less commonly, these extramural ethmoid cells (i.e., pneumatizing beyond the ethmoid bone) expose the optic nerve. The extramural cells are referred to as Onodi cells. *A*, optic nerve; *ICA*, internal carotid artery; *ITF*, infratemporal fossa; *MS*, maxillary sinus; *SS*, sphenoid sinus.

themselves. Most of these works, however, were by individuals concerned not with detailed, precise anatomy but with more theoretical questions addressing functional explanations for the existence of these "hollow" spaces in the cranium. Anatomical observations by such individuals were not usually performed for a systematic assessment of structure; rather, they appear to have been used to buttress their particular functional theories. In the late 19th century, the Austrian anatomist Emil Zuckerkandl published the first detailed and systematic anatomical and pathologic description of the paranasal sinuses.

During the preantibiotic era of the early part of the 20th century, anatomical studies focused upon descriptions that could improve procedures for the cannulation or drainage of pathologic sinuses. After treatment, sinus infections were observed often to recur in the same treated sinus, and to spread and infect the other, untreated sinuses. These secondary infections were explained by the close and intimate relationships seen in the anatomy of the paranasal sinuses. The importance of understanding prenatal development as a vehicle to understanding sinus surgery became more fully appreciated. Later, technologic advances saw the development of external and endonasal (intranasal) microscopic and endoscopic sinus procedures. The advent of endoscopes, CT, and other technologies has lead to a renaissance in our understanding of the anatomy and physiology of the sinuses.

Ethmoid Sinus

The ethmoid and other paranasal sinuses originate from the primordia of the cartilaginous nasal capsule, and their pneumatization follows from epithelial budding into the bony elements of the cranium, thus establishing a communication network with the nasal cavity throughout life. The prenatal development of the paranasal sinuses begins as an evagination of respiratory mucosal epithelium from the nasal capsule invading two bony

his writings do not mention the sinuses by name. The depth and nature of descriptions of the sinuses have varied considerably throughout history, usually mentioned within larger works. Notable in this regard were da Vinci's discussions of the maxillary sinus and Berengario da Carpi's initial descriptions of the sphenoid sinus (in the 16th and 17th centuries). In the 17th and 18th centuries, studies began to focus upon the sinuses

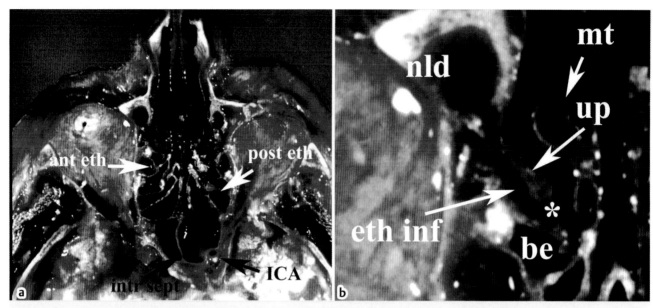

Fig. 102.4 (a) Axial cadaver section through the ethmoid sinus, orbit, and sphenoid sinus. The ethmoid sinus is anatomically divided into an anterior and a posterior ethmoid sinus. The sphenoid sinus is vertically separated into a right and left sinus by the intrasinus septum. In this specimen, the right internal carotid artery is seen as it passes through the cavernous sinus. *ant eth*, anterior ethmoid sinus; *ICA*, internal carotid artery; *intr sept*, intrasinus septum; *post eth*, posterior ethmoid sinus. (b) Enlargement of (a) showing from above left the ostiomeatal complex. *asterisk*, hiatus semilunaris; *be*, anterior aspect of bulla ethmoidalis; *eth inf*, ethmoid infundibulum; *mt*, middle turbinate; *nld*, nasolacrimal duct; *up*, uncinate process.

elements of the splanchnocranium (i.e., maxillary and ethmoid bones). Once mesenchymal differentiation in the area of the inferior nasal conchae ensues, it has the effect of producing a more prominent fold of the conchae and aids in accentuating the depth of these grooves, or furrows. The developing folds are considered the primitive step for conchal formation, whereas the furrows constitute the future inferior and middle meatus. By the 63rd to 70th day of prenatal development, six major furrows develop along with their corresponding ridges or folds, called the ethmoturbinals (i.e., turbinates arising from the ethmoid). The number of these folds and furrows that persist during fetal development varies. For example, from the seventh month to term, one can find three to five ethmoidal conchae with a corresponding number of intervening meatus, but after birth, because of either fusion or obliteration, only two or three ethmoidal conchae may persist (i.e., middle, superior, or supreme ethmoidal conchae).

The first primary furrow of the lateral nasal wall is located between the first and second ethmoturbinals, sometimes referred to as the first interturbinal furrow. The appearance of the first furrow is also an important developmental stage because its descending anterior region will become the ethmoid infundibulum, while the superiorly ascending region will become the frontal recess (▶ Fig. 102.4). The former is an important region into and through which a number of the paranasal sinuses will eventually drain to the nasal cavity. The frontal recess, on the other hand, undergoes further development with the appearance of additional furrows, what Kasper termed *pits*, which are outgrowths of epithelium that appear as spherically shaped excavations in this region. Pneumatic invasion of the frontal bone originating from one of these pits in the frontal recess results in the development of the frontal sinus.

At birth, the ethmoid sinus consists of anterior and posterior divisions. The ethmoid labyrinth may be visualized consistently by plain film radiography only after the first year post partum and only if the air-filled divisions of the ethmoid sinus are well developed. At the ages of 4 to 8 years, the ethmoid sinus system is 18 to 24 mm in length, 10 to 15 mm in height, and 9 to 13 mm in width. By the 12th year, the ethmoids have reached nearly adult size, with expansion during puberty involving primarily the bones outside the ethmoid capsule.

In the adult, the ethmoid sinus viewed in a transverse section forms a pyramid, with a blunted apex located anteriorly and a wider base located posteriorly. The entire sinus measures 4 to 5 cm anteroposteriorly, 2.5 cm inferosuperiorly, 0.5 cm wide anteriorly, and 1.5 cm posteriorly. Various descriptions of the ethmoid roof, such as fovea and foveolae ethmoidales, have caused considerable confusion over the years. Lateral to the lamina cribrosa of the cribriform plate, the insertion of the middle turbinate, and the lateral lamella of the cribiform plate, numerous ethmoid air cells open superiorly and are closed by the frontal bone. Because the indentations or foveolae (from the Latin, *foveolae ethmoidales ossis frontalis*, "ethmoid pits of the frontal bone") are invaginations into the frontal bone, this bone and a portion of the fovea form the roof of the ethmoid sinus (▶ Fig. 102.5). The roof of the ethmoid articulates with the lateral lamella of the cribriform plate. The length and orientation of the lateral lamella, the thinnest bone in the entire skull base, determines the depth of the olfactory fossa and relates to the vulnerability to intracranial penetration. The lateral wall of the ethmoid bone is the lamina papyracea (orbital plate), which forms the most constant component.

The actual size of the sinus and the number of cells present vary in each reported series. The ethmoid cells are divided into

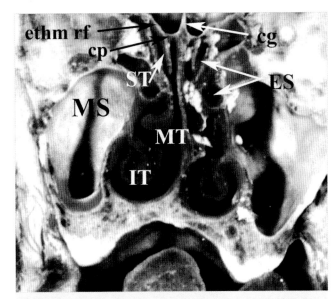

Fig. 102.5 Coronal cadaver section through the mid plane of the maxillary sinuses. The superior, middle, and inferior turbinates are well seen, along with the attachment of the middle turbinate to the cribriform plate and roof of the ethmoid sinus. The section also passes through the anterior ethmoid sinus and crista galli. *cg*, crista galli; *cp*, cribriform plate; *ES*, ethmoid sinus; *ethm rf*, roof of the ethmoid sinus; *IT*, inferior turbinate; *MS*, maxillary sinuses; *MT*, middle turbinate; *ST*, superior turbinate.

those that are within the ethmoid bone, or intramural, and those that are outside the ethmoid bone, or extramural. The anterior ethmoid cells can be further subdivided based on their location or that of their ostia. However, cells of a given origin frequently invade the territory usually occupied by cells of another origin, and at least some authors favor classification by the location of their ostia.

During development, the attachments of the various bony structures arising from the ethmoid (i.e., conchae, uncinate process) to the lateral wall are formed by one of several ground plates, or basal lamellae. While the lateral attachments of these lamellae end abruptly, their medial aspects project beyond the labyrinth and form prominences that extend into the nasal cavity. The most anterior of the lamellae is the lateral extension of the uncinate process. The second lamella is referred to as the anterior plate of the bulla because its extension into the nasal cavity forms the bulla ethmoidalis, while the third lamella serves as the attachment of the middle turbinate. The third lamella is an important anatomical structure, demarcating the division between the anterior ethmoid cells and the posterior cells and so essentially dictating the drainage patterns of these air cells into the middle and superior meatus, respectively. The third lamella is also clinically significant because it is considered a natural boundary to the spread of infection into the posterior ethmoid, and it is the posterior landmark in anterior ethmoidectomy. The fourth lamella is at the attachment of the superior turbinate, and when a supreme turbinate is also present, a fifth lamella arises lateral to this turbinate.

Among the various classifications proposed, the Ritter nomenclature system conveys most clearly the origin and drainage of the ethmoid cells. In the Ritter classification, the most

anterior cells are the frontal recess cells (range, 0 to 4 cells), which arise from the anterosuperior growth of the ethmoid cells into the frontal bone. These cells may come to rest within the frontal bone by forming the frontal sinus, giving rise to the frontal bullae, bulging into the frontal sinus floor, or forming the supraorbital ethmoid cells as they pneumatize the orbit.

The bullar cells drain into the middle meatus via crescentic ostia that lie superiorly, posteriorly, and parallel to the much larger semilunar cleft in the lateral nasal wall, the entrance of which Zuckerkandl described as the hiatus semilunaris (see ▶ Fig. 102.4b). The hiatus semilunaris forms the curved groove between the bulla ethmoidalis, which borders it posteriorly, and the uncinate process, a ridge of bone formed by the ramus descendens of the first ethmoturbinal, which borders it anteriorly. The anteroinferior boundary of the hiatus semilunaris is the uncinate (from the Latin *uncinia*, "hook") process, also a semilunar structure, which has an anterosuperior to posteroinferior sagittal orientation. This structure attaches to the lamina perpendicularis of the palatine bone and the ethmoid processes of the inferior turbinate. The anterior aspect of this attachment to the lateral nasal wall has been called the maxillary line.

Conchal cells are ethmoid air cells that invade the middle conchae, and when these cells are located in the anterior aspect of the conchae, the condition is referred to as a concha bullosa. The concha bullosa cells are clinically important because they can be an isolated source of recurrent ethmoiditis or may obstruct the middle meatus. The middle turbinate, being a medial appendage of the lateral nasal wall, overhangs the bulla ethmoidalis, the hiatus semilunaris, and the uncinate process. On occasion, both the uncinate process and the hiatus semilunaris are not covered by the downward expansion of this 3.5- to 4-cm-long important bony structure. Anteriorly, the middle turbinate is attached superiorly to the cribriform plate, with a 15-degree slope posteroinferiorly so that the posterior tip lies at, or immediately inferior to, the sphenopalatine foramen.

The posterior ethmoid cells (range, 1 to 7 cells), which invade the posterior ethmoid capsule, may also involve the middle turbinate, sphenoid, palatine, and maxillary bones. The posterior cells drain into the superior and, to a lesser degree, the supreme meatus. An important form of extramural extension of the posterior ethmoid cells is the migration of these cells to the medial aspect of the optic nerve within the sphenoid bone. Collectively, these cells are known by various names, including postrema cells. When the cells are superior and inferior to the optic nerve, they are known as Onodi cells. Such cells are clinically important because the optic nerve may be covered by relatively thin bone and vulnerable to injury during dissection posterior to the anterior face of the sphenoid bone. The anterior ethmoidal canal containing the artery and nerve of the same name runs between 2 mm inferior and 4 mm superior to the cribriform plate. The anterior ethmoidal artery originates from the ophthalmic artery to course through the orbital region and passes through the anterior ethmoidal canal onto the anterior cranial fossa to finally enter the nasal cavity. The posterior ethmoidal canal traverses the ethmoid bone at a plane approximately 1.5 mm (range, 0 to 3.1 mm) above the cribriform plate, and it may, like the anterior canal, be partially dehiscent of bone (▶ Fig. 102.6).

Maxillary Sinus

The maxillary sinus has been referred to as the antrum of Highmore in honor of the English anatomist Nathanial Highmore, whose 1651 treatise *Corporis Humani Disquisitio Anatomica* describes and illustrates this sinus. However, the person recognized as the earliest known discoverer of the maxillary sinus is Leonardo da Vinci, who both illustrated and described this sinus in 1489.

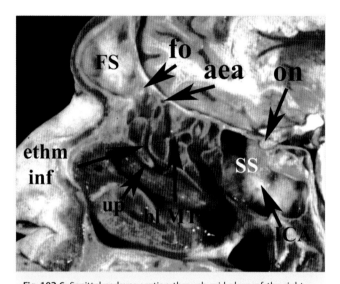

Fig. 102.6 Sagittal cadaver section through mid plane of the right ethmoid sinus. Beginning anteriorly, the frontal sinus communicates with the nose through its ostium. Defining the posterior aspect of the frontal recess is the anterior ethmoidal artery. Inferior to this vessel is the bulla ethmoidalis, and approximately 10 mm posterior to the anterior ethmoidal artery is the posterior ethmoidal artery. The anterior ethmoid sinus is separated by the basal lamella of the middle turbinate from the posterior ethmoid sinus, and posterior to this sinus is the sphenoid sinus. The optic nerve passes through the superior aspect of the lateral wall of the sinus. Within the lateral wall of the sphenoid is the bony prominence surrounding the internal carotid artery. Other important structures are the ethmoid infundibulum and uncinate process. *aea*, anterior ethmoidal artery; *bl MT*, basal lamella of the middle turbinate; *ethm inf*, ethmoid infundibulum; *fo*, frontal sinus ostium; *FS*, frontal sinus; *ICA*, internal carotid artery; *on*, optic nerve; *SS*, sphenoid sinus; *up*, uncinate process.

The maxillary sinus, lying within the body of the maxillary bone, is the largest and most constant of all four paranasal sinuses. The maxillary sinus is generally described as shaped like a pyramid. Its anterior wall is the facial surface of the maxilla, where the facial vein and artery run, while the posterior wall is the infratemporal fossa, where the maxillary artery and vein are located. The medial wall constitutes the lateral wall of the nasal cavity, where a number of vascular structures are situated (e.g., branches of the sphenopalatine, the septal branch of the superior labial, and the ethmoidal arteries). The superior wall or roof of this sinus is the floor of the orbit, and the floor of the maxillary sinus is the alveolar process of the maxilla. It becomes evident from its topographic relationship to contiguous structures that infections and tumors of the maxillary sinus can spread in multiple directions, especially to the dentition (see ▶ Fig. 102.5).

Development of the maxillary sinus begins by the 65th day of gestation, so that it is the first sinus to develop in utero. At birth, the sinus has an average volume of 6 to 8 mL but is fluid-filled, making the interpretation of plain film radiographs difficult. The maxillary sinus then undergoes two periods of rapid growth: one between birth and 3 years, and the other between the ages of 7 and 12 years. Between these two growth periods, at around 4 years of age, the sinus extends laterally past the infraorbital canal. After the second period of rapid growth (▶ Table 102.1), subsequent expansion involves pneumatization of the alveolar process of the maxilla. Before growth is completed, the maxillary sinus descends from 4 mm above the floor of the nasal cavity at birth to the same level as the nasal floor at the age of 8 to 9 years, and then a final drop of 4 to 5 mm below this level occurs by adulthood.

In the adult, the maxillary sinus can be roughly described as triangular in shape, measuring 25 mm along the anterior limb of its base, 34 mm in depth, and 33 mm in height. The primary or natural ostium of the maxillary sinus is located in the superior aspect of the medial wall of the sinus, and the sinus drains via its infundibulum into the ethmoid infundibulum and thus the hiatus semilunaris. The natural ostium tends to be elliptical, measuring from 1 to 20 mm in length. In addition, accessory maxillary sinus ostia have been found in 15 to 40% of subjects examined by various authors. These ostia may be located in the ethmoid infundibulum or the membranous region of the medial sinus wall (known as the membranous meatus or fontanel),

Table 102.1 Embryologic patterns of sinus development

Paranasal sinus	Embryologic appearance	Postnatal appearance	Growth spurt interval
Ethmoid sinus	Development begins in third fetal month.	Present at birth	First growth spurt occurs between first and fourth years, second growth spurt between fourth and eighth years.
Maxillary sinus	Development beings by 65th day of gestation.	Present at birth	First growth spurt occurs between birth and 3 years, second growth spurt between 7 and 12 years.
Frontal sinus	Development begins in fourth fetal month.	Detected at 7 to 12 years of age	Adult size is attained by 20 years.
Sphenoid sinus	Development begins in third fetal month.	Detected at 3 to 4 years of age	By seventh year, sinus begins to extend posteriorly toward the sella turcica.

Source: Data from Rice D, Schaefer S. Endoscopic Paranasal Sinus Surgery. 3rd ed. Philadelphia, PA: Lippincott Williams & Wilkins; 2004.

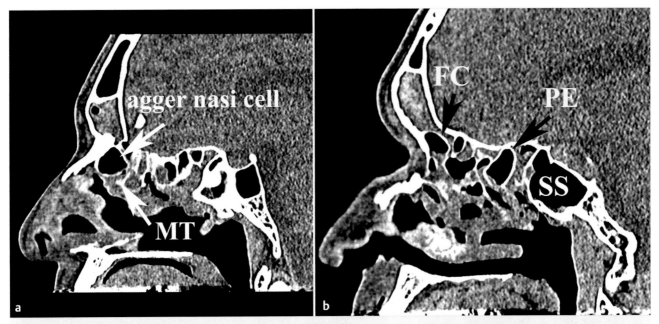

Fig. 102.7 Sagittal computed tomographic (CT) scans through the ethmoid and frontal sinuses. (a) An ethmoid cell is pneumatizing the agger nasi and forming an agger nasi cell, which is one of several cells that populate the frontal recess in this patient. The anterior aspect of the middle turbinate is posterior to this cell and confirms the origin of the cell within the agger and not within more posterior cells, such as lacrimal cells. Note the obstruction of the frontal sinus outflow tract into the nose by the cell. *MT*, middle turbinate. (b) Sagittal CT scan through the ethmoid sinus, frontal sinus, and sphenoid sinus (*SS*). The outflow tract of the frontal sinus is occluded by a frontoethmoid or frontal cell. Posterior to this cell is another frontal cell, which is superior to the bulla ethmoidalis; therefore, this cell is referred to as a suprabullar cell. Posterior to the anterior ethmoid cells, there is one large posterior ethmoid cell. Between this cell and the anterior wall of the sphenoid sinus is the sphenoethmoid recess. *FC*, frontal cell; *PE*, posterior ethmoid cell; *SS*, sphenoid sinus.

which is inferior to the uncinate process and superior to the insertion of the inferior turbinate.

Frontal Sinus

Volcher Coiter of Holland, a pupil of Fallopius and Eustachius, is said to have been the first to describe the frontal sinus. Interestingly, Berengario da Carpi described the frontal bone region as having "two tables within which there is a notable vacuity so as to not weigh down the body," but da Vinci, in 1489, may have been the first to recognize its existence and illustrate its morphology.

The development of the frontal sinus is initiated in the fourth fetal month, when the entire nasofrontal area is represented by the frontal recess, and it is the last paranasal sinus to develop. The usually paired frontal sinuses have several possible origins, each of which influences the relationship of this sinus to the lateral nasal wall and its drainage pattern within the middle meatus. In a study of 100 adult specimens and 15 late-term fetuses, Kasper found the most common origin of the frontal sinus to be pits or furrows within the frontal recess, which are considered rudimentary anterior ethmoid cells. *The anatomy of this region is challenging because there is neither a clear developmental pattern nor any constancy in the differentiation of the frontal pits.* One can have as many as four pits, or there can be a total absence of pit formation. When there is no pit formation, the frontal recess remains a simple blind outgrowth from the middle meatus without configuration of its lateral wall. Which of these pits is variably present and which goes on to become the frontal sinus determine the specific pattern of sinus

drainage. If the most anterior pit (i.e., pit 1) migrates in a ventral direction, it may pneumatize the agger nasi bone, becoming an agger nasi cell, whereas the second most anterior pit (i.e., pit 2) may migrate anterosuperiorly to become the frontal sinus (see ▶ Fig. 102.6). Thus, the terms *agger nasi* (referring to the mound of bone anterior to the insertion of the middle turbinate) and *agger nasi cell* (referring to the cell that pneumatizes the agger nasi) are not interchangeable because each represents a distinct anatomical entity (▶ Fig. 102.7). Moreover, a markedly pneumatized agger nasi cell can have pathophysiologic consequences in frontal sinus drainage. Another variant of frontal sinus formation can occur if no anterior ethmoid air cells develop in the frontal recess; ethmoid air cell extension from the ethmoid infundibulum then can create a frontal sinus.

At birth, the sinus has little clinical relevance, and it is often indistinguishable from the anterior ethmoid cells. At 3 years of age, the frontal sinus is observed 3.8 mm above the nasion (a craniometric point defined as the junction between the nasal and frontal bones at the midline), and it continues its vertical growth trajectory at an average annual rate of 1.5 mm until the 15th year. Final growth is completed before the 20th year.

The adult frontal sinus, when viewed in a transverse section, has been classically described as pyramidal in shape by Mosher. The base or inferior floor of the pyramid is the orbital nasal portion of the splanchnocranium, the apex extends outward a variable distance over the orbit, the anterior wall is subcutaneous, and the posterior wall is cerebral. The dimensions of the adult frontal sinus have been reported as measuring 28 mm in height, 27 mm in width, and 17 mm in length. This ideal sinus is a representative average, with the actual size and configuration

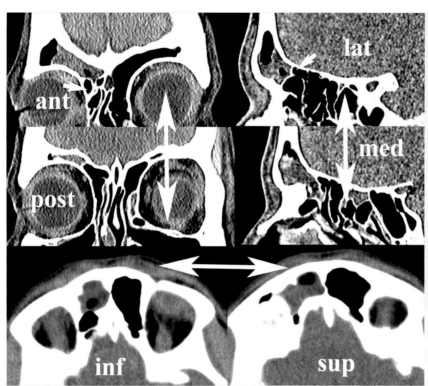

Fig. 102.8 Composite of computed tomographic scans through the frontal sinus outflow tract. Coronal (*upper left*), sagittal (*upper right*), and axial (*lower*) images are paired—that is, anterior to posterior, medial to lateral, and inferior to superior. When the images are viewed collectively, the obstruction to the right frontal outflow tract is seen to be due to frontal cells, noted best in the upper right sagittal lateral image (*arrow*). *ant*, anterior; *inf*, interior; *lat*, lateral; *med*, medial; *post*, posterior; *sup*, superior.

reflecting the origin of the cavity and the superior development into the squama of the frontal bone. At the inferior aspect in the midsagittal plane, the anterior or outer table of the frontal sinus is approximately twice as thick as the posterior or inner table. Historically, the communication of this sinus with the nasal cavity has been described as a distinct nasofrontal duct, although others prefer the term *frontal recess*. The term *nasofrontal duct*, which is used to describe the communication of the frontal sinus through the middle meatus with the nasal cavity, is anatomically and developmentally incorrect. To confuse the issue even further, the terms *frontal recess*, *frontal infundibulum*, and *nasofrontal duct* have also been used interchangeably when in reality they represent different anatomical structures. Conceptually, the frontonasal outflow tract has been likened to an hourglass, with the upper portion being the body of the frontal sinus, the neck being the ostium (varying 2 to 10 mm in diameter), and the lower portion beneath the neck being the frontal recess. However, the term *frontal recess*, introduced by Killian, is based on the prenatal observation of a space that is the continuation of the ascending branch of the first primary interturbinal furrow, with the descending branch becoming the ethmoid infundibulum. The frontal infundibulum was defined by Killian as the superior opening of the frontal sinus drainage tract. A more recent interpretation of this anatomy defines the frontal infundibulum as viewed from within the frontal sinus as the funnel-shaped narrowing toward the frontal ostium. Finally, the nasofrontal duct as defined by Lang is any mucosa-lined bony passage longer than 3 mm. We would question this definition because the outflow tract of the frontal sinus is potentially narrowed by the ethmoid bulla, or the lamella of the bulla, posteriorly and by agger nasi cells anteriorly rather than forming a true duct. In 1939, Van Alyea described the outflow tract of the frontal sinus as the *frontal recess*, and despite its earlier mean-

ing, this term best describes the area. The developmental variability of the frontal sinus leads to the observed multiple drainage patterns, which can be further complicated by the highly variable pneumatization of the adjacent ethmoid air cells and by the position of the uncinate process (▶ Fig. 102.8).

Sphenoid Sinus

In 1521, Giacomo Berengario da Carpi was the first to describe the sphenoid sinuses, but it was Tillaux who suggested that this sinus is part of the other paranasal sinus complex. According to Dixon, the sphenoid sinus is the most variable cuboidally shaped sinus of all the paranasal sinuses. The average adult sinus has six surfaces: the anterior, posterior, superior, inferior, medial, and lateral walls (▶ Fig. 102.9). In addition, the sphenoid bone, where this sinus resides, is strategically located in one of the most complex regions in all of human anatomy. The endocranial surface of this bone serves as a seat for endocrine activity; as a conduit for the cranial nerves responsible for vision, ocular movements, nasal mucosal gland stimulation, and nasal sympathetic innervation; and as a conduit for the major vascular supply of the nasal cavity.

Growth of the usually paired sphenoid sinuses is initiated during the third month of intrauterine development. The two sinuses generally develop asymmetrically because usually one sinus encroaches upon and limits the other's growth to a rudimentary size. The vertical bony partition between the two sinuses has been incorrectly termed *median septum*. Congdon suggested the more appropriate term *intersinus septum* because the partition is frequently more lateral than medial, and this is the accepted term today. Both complete and partial septation of the sinuses is frequent because no clear pattern has emerged from a number of studies. When the sinus is viewed

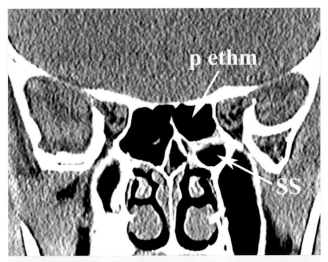

Fig. 102.9 Coronal computed tomographic scan through the sphenoid bone. The left sphenoid bone is pneumatized superiorly by an extramural posterior ethmoid cell and inferiorly by the sphenoid sinus. Because the sphenoid sinus does not have a horizontal septum, the appearance of such a structure implies an extension of the ethmoid sinus into the sphenoid bone. *p ethm*, posterior ethmoid cell; *SS*, sphenoid sinus.

in a coronal plane, a horizontal partition may be present. In reality, the extramural posterior ethmoid cells have pneumatized the superior aspect of the sphenoid bone, and the sphenoid sinus lies inferior to the "horizontal septation."

Around the time of birth, the sphenoid sinus is primarily an evagination of the sphenoethmoid recess, with essentially no growth until the age of 3 years. It is not until the third year of life that the sphenoid conchae become attached to the presphenoid and the cavity develops into the definitive sphenoid sinus. In the most common developmental type, the postsellar type, the sinus extends posteriorly toward the sella turcica by the age of 7 years. Development may continue into adulthood and involve the basisphenoid, with arrest in pneumatization accounting for the tremendous variations in the sinus size.

The average adult sinus measures 20 mm in height, 23 mm in length, and 17 mm in width. The volume varies from 0.1 to 30 mL, with the average ranging from 5 to 7.5 mL. As the sinus expands, vessels and nerves in the lateral aspect of the body of the sphenoid bone come to lie as indentations in the wall of the sinus. The sphenoid sinus drains by a single ostium into the sphenoethmoid recess. This ostium, in the clinical setting, is 2 to 3 mm in diameter and may be either round or elliptical. The sinus depends on mucociliary flow for drainage because the ostium is located typically 10 to 15 mm superior to the floor of the sinus, or 8 mm from the cribriform plate (range, 1 to 15 mm) and 5 mm lateral to the nasal septum. Our own experience suggests that in most cases the ostium is observed inferior rather than superior to the average location and generally lies at a 30-degree angle from the floor of the nose and at the inferior plane of the superior turbinate. The pneumatization of the posterior aspect of the middle turbinate may make visualization of this ostium difficult. Because of the importance of such identification in surgery, various measurements have been reported. Mosher found that the anterior face of the sphenoid sinus averaged 7 cm from the nasal spine at an angle of 30 degrees.

102.3 Physiology

The lining of the nasal vestibule is essentially a continuation of the adjacent facial skin and consists of squamous epithelium with sebaceous and sweat glands and course hairs known as vibrissae. Within the nasal cavity, the epithelium transitions from squamous and transitional to respiratory, pseudostratified columnar epithelium (posteriorly) consisting of ciliated (columnar) cells, nonciliated (columnar) cells, goblet cells, and basal cells. This epithelium lies on a basement membrane and a lamina propria. All of the glands, as well as the neural and vascular structures, are found within the lamina propria. The nose and sinuses are cleansed by mucus produced by the goblet cells. Mucociliary clearance is accomplished by cilia that beat at a rate of approximately 1,000 strokes per minute and direct the mucus within the sinuses and nose in a specific pattern (▶ Fig. 102.10).

Olfactory epithelium forms the third type of lining in the nose and covers the superior turbinate and adjacent nasal septum. This pseudostratified epithelium contains bipolar neurons that have specific receptors for odorants, so that they are the first-order neurons in a complex pathway for smell via the limbic system, reticular formation, hippocampus, thalamus, hypothalamus, and frontal lobe. Although olfaction is relatively "insensitive" in humans compared with that in many animals, it remains an important sense and an essential requirement for complex taste.

Nasal airflow is regulated by the autonomic nervous system via parasympathetic innervation of the nasal glands through the sphenopalatine ganglion and by vasodilation. The nasal mucous membrane covering the inferior and middle turbinates becomes engorged with blood secondary to vascular control by the sympathetic nervous system. The relative inputs of the two elements of the autonomic nervous system alternate from side to side approximately every 2 to 4 hours. This nasal cycle results in maximal patency or obstruction of one airway. Patients may perceive this normal nasal physiology as an indication of an airway problem. In persons who have other mechanical obstructions of the nose, such as a deviated septum or polyps, cycling of the airway may compound the nasal obstruction. Furthermore, the turbinates will become engorged with blood as an individual turns the head from side to side while sleeping. Pregnant women are particularly sensitive to nasal obstruction due to hormone-induced engorgement of the mucous membranes, with some prone to rhinitis or sinusitis, a condition known as rhinitis of pregnancy.

102.4 Roundsmanship

- The discrete anatomy of the paranasal sinuses is extremely variable. Each sinus develops within certain parameters and shares physical features and relationships with the other sinuses and the nose.
- The ethmoid is the key sinus both anatomically and functionally. The proximity of this sinus to the frontal and maxillary sinuses accounts for the spread of disease from former to the latter, and for obstruction of the outflow tracts of the frontal and maxillary sinuses from ethmoid sinusitis, polyps, or tumors.

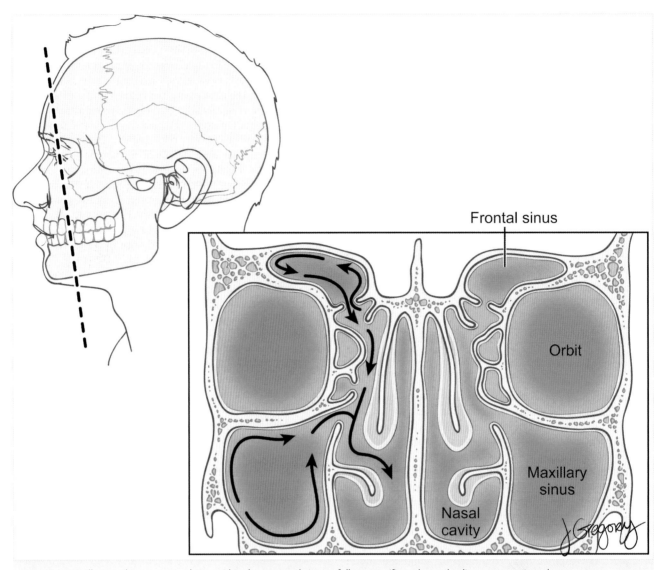

Fig. 102.10 As illustrated, mucous circulation within the paranasal sinuses follows specific pathways leading to egress into the nose.

- The complex embryologic origins of the frontal sinus determine the structure of its outflow tracts and the likelihood of frontal sinusitis.
- The maxillary and ethmoid sinuses are both present at birth, with develoment of the former beginning in the first trimester and development of the latter in the third trimester.
- Nasal airway patency is regulated by the autonomic nervous system, with airway resistance varying between the sides every 2 to 4 hours. Therefore, patients may complain of nasal airway problems that are simply reflections of normal airway physiology.

102.5 Recommended Reading

[1] Mosher HP. The applied anatomy of the frontal sinuses. Laryngoscope 1904; 14: 830–855

[2] Mosher HP. The surgical anatomy of the ethmoidal labyrinth. Ann Otol Rhinol Laryngol 1929; 38: 869–901

[3] Negus V. The Comparative Anatomy and Physiology of the Nose and Paranasal Sinuses. London, England: E & S Livingstone; 1958

[4] Ritter FN. The middle turbinate and its relationship to the ethmoidal labyrinth and the orbit. Laryngoscope 1982; 92: 479–482

[5] Zinreich SJ. Rhinosinusitis: radiologic diagnosis. Otolaryngol Head Neck Surg 1997; 117: S27–S34

[6] Schaeffer JP. The sinus maxillaris and its relations in the embryo, child, and adult man. Am J Anat 1910; 10: 313–367

[7] Schaeffer JP. The genesis, development, and adult anatomy of the nasofrontal region in man. Am J Anat 1916; 20: 125–143

[8] Stammberger HR, Kennedy DW Anatomic Terminology Group. Paranasal sinuses: anatomic terminology and nomenclature. Ann Otol Rhinol Laryngol Suppl 1995; 167: 7–16

[9] Stoney P, MacKay A, Hawke M. The antrum of Highmore or of da Vinci? J Otolaryngol 1991; 20: 456–458

[10] Van Alyea OE. Ethmoid labyrinth. Anatomic study, with consideration of the clinical significance of its structural characteristics. Arch Otolaryngol 1939; 29: 881–902

[11] Van Alyea OE. Frontal cells. An anatomic study of these cells with consideration of their clinical significance. Arch Otolaryngol 1941; 34: 11–23

103 Nasal Immunity

William R. Reisacher and Emily Z. Stucken

103.1 Introduction

Strategically positioned at the entry point of the respiratory tract, the nasal cavity constantly processes stimuli from the environment. These include particles, such as microbes, chemicals, and proteins, as well as factors related to air quality, such as temperature and humidity. The nasal cavity is forced to decide whether or not a particular stimulus is dangerous to the body, and then take the necessary steps to either neutralize or tolerate it. To perform this function, the nasal cavity possesses an elaborate system of both innate and adaptive immune mechanisms. The innate immune system is the first line of defense and uses both specific and nonspecific mechanisms, whereas the adaptive immune system demonstrates both specificity and memory through the clonal proliferation of T and B lymphocytes. Any errors in these systems, through either a deficient or a hypersensitive response, may produce damage to the respiratory tract and subsequent disease.

103.2 Histology of the Nasal Cavity

The vestibule of the nasal cavity is lined with keratinized, stratified squamous epithelium that is contiguous with the skin of the external nose. At the limen nasi, this squamous epithelium changes first to nonciliated cuboidal or columnar epithelium before transitioning to the respiratory epithelium that lines the remainder of the nasal cavity and paranasal sinuses. This respiratory mucosa is a pseudostratified, ciliated, columnar epithelium made up of three cell types: ciliated cells, goblet cells, and basal cells (▶ Fig. 103.1). Ciliated cells are the most prevalent cell type lining the surface epithelium. Each cilium has nine microtubule doublets surrounding two central singlet microtu-

bules, in a configuration similar to that of cilia found elsewhere in the body, with dynein arms articulating between the outer microtubules (▶ Fig. 103.2). Each ciliated cell contains over 200 cilia, which beat at 10 to 20 cycles per second to power mucociliary clearance. Goblet cells rest on the basement membrane and produce mucus that is expelled from the apical surface. The third cell type that makes up the respiratory epithelium, the basal cell, sits on the basement membrane and serves as a source of regenerating ciliated and goblet cells.

Other cell types found in the nasal cavity include melanocytes and intraepithelial lymphocytes, as well as scattered plasma cells, mast cells, and eosinophils. The intraepithelial lymphocyte population within the nasal cavity is composed strictly of T cells with few, if any, B cells. This likely explains the finding that the majority of lymphomas of the nasal cavity are NK/T-cell lymphomas. Lymphomas of the paranasal sinuses, in contrast, tend to be of B-cell origin.

103.3 Innate Immune System

The most basic features of the innate immune system are the barrier of the nasal respiratory mucosa and mucociliary clearance. Mucus, which is primarily composed of high-molecular-weight, heavily glycosylated macromolecules, sits on a less dense layer of serous fluid produced from seromucinous glands in the underlying lamina propria. The viscous mucinous layer traps inhaled particulate matter, while the serous layer allows the underlying cilia to beat freely and direct mucus-trapped foreign matter toward the nasopharynx to prevent damage to the respiratory tract (▶ Fig. 103.3). The efficiency of this system is regulated by the physical properties of mucus, as well as the frequency of the ciliary beat.

In primary ciliary dyskinesia, the microstructure of the cilia are altered because of defects in the dynein arms. As a result,

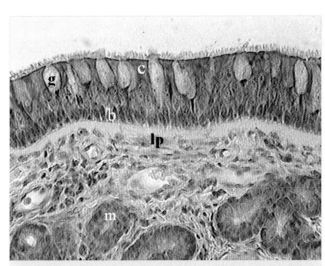

Fig. 103.1 Photomicrograph of the nasal respiratory epithelium. *b*, basal cell; *c*, ciliated cell; *g*, goblet cell; *lp*, lamina propria; *m*, seromucinous gland.

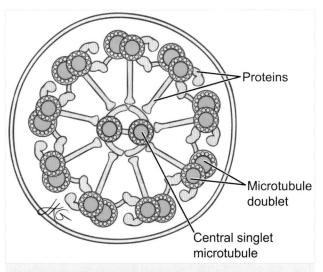

Fig. 103.2 Cross section of a cilium, demonstrating the arrangement of microtubules and cross-linking proteins.

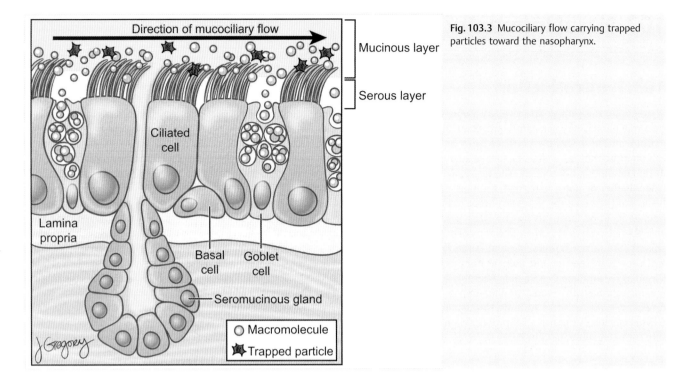

Fig. 103.3 Mucociliary flow carrying trapped particles toward the nasopharynx.

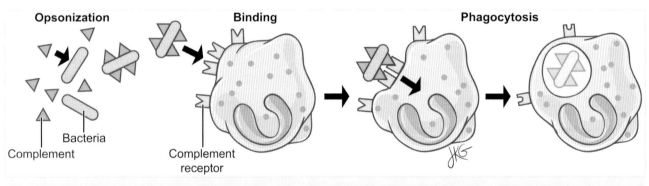

Fig. 103.4 The opsonization of pathogens and foreign debris allows more efficient binding and phagocytosis by activated cells.

mucociliary clearance is impaired. Patients with primary ciliary dyskinesia are susceptible to recurrent episodes of sinusitis, bronchitis, and bronchiectasis as a result of mucociliary stasis. These patients often present with respiratory distress in the neonatal period. They go on to develop chronic cough and rhinitis in early childhood, with recurrent episodes of rhinosinusitis, otitis media, bronchitis, and pneumonia. Male infertility is also common. The triad of recurrent rhinosinusitis, bronchiectasis, and situs inversus is known as Kartagener syndrome. A brush biopsy of the nasal mucosa for ultrastructural analysis can establish the diagnosis of primary ciliary dyskinesia.

Particles on the mucosal surface of the nose are also detected by the surface receptors of macrophages and dendritic cells, which then engulf and internalize them. This function is enhanced by a process known as opsonization, in which the particles are coated with antibodies or complement (▶ Fig. 103.4). Opsonization also attracts and activates other inflammatory cells located in the lamina propria, such as lymphocytes, neutrophils, eosinophils, basophils, mast cells, and plasma cells.

Although this is largely a nonspecific process, the structure of certain opsonins allows some specificity, as well. Serum amyloid A is an opsonin secreted by respiratory epithelial cells that binds directly to gram-positive bacteria, and surfactant proteins (SP-A and SP-D) have the ability to bind and agglutinate bacteria, fungi, and allergens, as well as inorganic particles.

Respiratory epithelial cells secrete small, extracellular peptides, such as β-defensin, as well as larger proteins, such as cathelicidin, lysozyme, and lactoferrin; these can inhibit the growth of microbes, have immediate microbicidal activity, or even possess immunomodulatory capabilities. Lysozyme, an enzyme that is also secreted by monocytes and macrophages, is directed against the peptidoglycan cell wall of certain bacteria, such as *Streptococcus* and *Pseudomonas*. The destruction of gram-negative bacteria by lysozyme requires the presence of certain cofactors, such as ascorbic acid, antibody–complement complexes, and lactoferrin, which is an iron-binding protein found in neutrophil granules. The protein psoriasin increases the cell wall permeability of bacteria such as *Escherichia coli*, and calprotectin has both antibacterial and antifungal activity.

The human body is exposed to viruses on a regular basis, and the respiratory tract is their primary target. The first lines of defense against viruses are nasal air filtration, the mucous barrier, and the secretion of immunostimulatory cytokines and chemokines from epithelial cells, macrophages, and neutrophils. The most important of these chemical messengers are the interferons IFN-α and IFN-β, which upregulate genes that protect cells against viral replication. Current efforts are under way to identify pharmacologic agents that could activate this gene pathway and produce a rapid but nonspecific defense against viruses during epidemics when vaccines are not effective.

Nasal defense against parasitic infections occur primarily through complement proteins involved in opsonization, chemoattraction, cellular activation, and the direct killing of parasites. Other proteins that perform similar functions include collectin and petraxins (C-reactive protein and serum amylase proteins), which may be either secreted or membrane-bound. Another line of defense is the chitinase family—specifically, acid mammalian chitinase (AMCase)—which is a class of genes that are regulated by interleukin-13 (IL-13), a major Th2 cytokine. The products of these genes act upon chitin, which is abundant in parasites, nematodes, insects, and fungi. It is theorized that allergic disease, also dominated by Th2 inflammation, represents an over activation of the evolutionarily beneficial ability to defend against these previously common invaders. Current evidence suggests that AMCase expression is highly associated with recalcitrant chronic rhinosinusitis (CRS).

Another protein of the innate immune system that may cause problems when overactivated is B-cell activating factor (BAFF), a member of the tumor necrosis factor (TNF) family. BAFF is produced in epithelial as well as submucosal cells of the sinonasal tract and regulates B-cell survival, proliferation, and antibody production. Evidence suggests that increased BAFF expression, which is seen in patients who have chronic rhinosinusitis with nasal polyposis (CRSwNP), may enhance immunuglobulin A (IgA) synthesis and eosinophilic inflammation. In addition to BAFF, other cytokines that modulate the B-cell response in patients with CRSwNP include B-cell attracting chemokine-1 (BCA-1) and stromal cell-derived factor-1α (SDF-1α).

Toll-like receptors (TLRs) are specific pattern recognition receptor proteins that are present in soluble, transmembrane, or cytosolic forms on macrophages, dendritic cells, or epithelial cells in the respiratory tract. These genetically ancient receptors are able to recognize certain pathogen-associated molecular patterns (PAMPs), such as bacterial lipopeptide, endotoxin, flagellin, double-stranded RNA, and bacterial DNA. By unknown mechanisms, TLRs are able to tolerate normal bacterial flora, but when activated by pathogens, they initiate both innate and adaptive processes. TLR9, one of the 11 known mammalian TLRs, has been studied for its ability to stimulate a Th1 immune response while inhibiting a Th2 response. CpG, a bacterial DNA sequence and TLR9 agonist, has been investigated for use as an adjuvant for hepatitis and cancer vaccines, as well as an immunostimulatory agent for the treatment of allergy, asthma, and CRS.

103.4 Adaptive Immune System

The adaptive immune system in humans is a mechanism by which the body mounts an antigen-specific response to a particular insult. The main components of the adaptive immune system are B and T lymphocytes and the family of immunoglobulins. B cells originate in the bone marrow and are initially coated with surface IgM and IgD. After leaving the bone marrow, they migrate to secondary lymphoid organs and proliferate in response to antigen stimulation and T-cell interactions. When stimulated, B cells mature into immunoglobulin-secreting plasma cells that are antigen-specific. These plasma cells undergo class switching to elude other immunoglobulin classes, including IgA, IgG, and IgE, each of which has a specific immune role. Two immunoglobulin classes, IgA and IgE, perform important functions within the nasal cavity and paranasal sinus environment and deserve special attention.

IgA is the most prevalent immunoglobulin in the nasal cavity. It exists in monomeric and dimeric forms, but the IgA in the nasal cavity and paranasal sinuses is largely in the dimeric form of secretory IgA (SIgA). SIgA is a 390-kDa dimer linked by a J chain and containing a secretory component that allows active passage across the nasal epithelium. The SIgA found in nasal mucus coats bacterial and other antigenic material and prevents it from breaching the nasal mucosa.

The importance of IgA in protecting the nasal mucosa from foreign invaders is demonstrated in patients who lack this immunoglobulin. Selective IgA deficiency is the most common isolated immunoglobulin deficiency, with incidence rates ranging from 1 per 223 to 1 per 1,000 individuals in the United States. In this patient population, IgA-laden B cells lack the capacity to differentiate into IgA-secreting plasma cells. Patients with selective IgA deficiency often have a commensurate increase in IgM levels. Their clinical presentation ranges from asymptomatic to prone to the development of recurrent sinonasal, pulmonary, and gastrointestinal infections. Sinus infections are mainly bacterial in origin. Allergic disease and autoimmune disorders are also more prevalent in this patient population. The management of patients with selective IgA deficiency includes the treatment of acute bacterial infections or the daily administration of prophylactic antibiotics, depending on the severity of symptoms.

The second immunoglobulin that plays a pivotal role in the local immunity of the nasal cavity is IgE. IgE is the main immunoglobulin involved in the allergic response and is important in the pathophysiology of allergic rhinitis. Although IgE-producing plasma cells are not a normal component of the nasal mucosa, an increase in allergen-specific IgE has been found in the nasal turbinate tissue of allergic patients. There is evidence that the IgE permeating the nasal tissues of allergic individuals may be produced locally rather than migrate from distant sources. Several studies have shown that immunoglobulin class switching can occur in the local environment of the nose, and ex vivo studies have demonstrated that allergen-induced class switching occurs in isolated nasal turbinate tissues. Investigators have also demonstrated an increase in antigen-specific IgE in patients who have rhinitis with negative results on serum allergy testing. It has been suggested that a local allergic response may be the inciting factor in these patients, who have previously been categorized as having nonallergic rhinitis based on the results of systemic testing. Further discoveries in this field may lead to an improved understanding and treatment of this patient population.

T cells are the second class of lymphocytes that make up the adaptive immune system. T cells originate in the thymus, where they mature and undergo differentiation. Autoreactive cells are selected for apoptosis before leaving the thymus. Once T cells exit the thymus, they are attracted to lymphoid organs by cellular signaling. When an antigen is encountered, a T cell becomes activated and undergoes clonal expansion with specificity to that antigen. T cells differentiate into one of two lineages: helper T cells, which are positive for CD4, and cytotoxic T cells, which are positive for CD8. CD4 + T helper cells further differentiate into either Th1 cells or Th2 cells, which can be distinguished by differences in their cytokine profiles and functionality. Th1 cells produce IL-2 and IFN-γ, which are involved in cytotoxic inflammatory reactions in response to intracellular pathogens. They participate in delayed-type hypersensitivity reactions, act primarily through cell-mediated interactions and communication through cytokines. Th2 cells produce IL-1, IL-4, IL-5, IL-9, and IL-10, favoring IgE-mediated allergic inflammation and eosinophil production (▶ Fig. 103.5). The cytokines produced by each cell type inhibit the activation of the other cell type, thus preventing the activation of conflicting inflammatory pathways.

Differential activation of Th1 and Th2 pathways within the nasal cavity promotes differential expression of rhinologic disease. In chronic rhinosinusitis with nasal polyps (CRSwNP), the local inflammatory environment exhibits a predominance of Th2 cells and the Th2-related cytokines IL-4 and IL-5. This is significantly different from chronic rhinosinusitis without nasal polyps (CRSsNP), which is generally a Th1-driven process. Activation of the Th2 cytokine profile is associated with the influx of eosinophils, which comprise 60 to 90% of the cell population in nasal polyps. The inflammatory products of eosinophils have the capacity to inflict local tissue damage, which has been proposed to account for the inflammatory reactions that occurs in nasal polyposis. The predominance of a Th2- and eosinophilia-mediated reaction also accounts for the association of nasal polyps with allergy and asthma, which are also Th2-driven processes.

103.5 Roundsmanship

- Nasal immunity relies on both innate and adaptive mechanisms.
- Deficiencies, as well as hypersensitivities, of nasal immunity can produce disease.
- Mucociliary clearance moves pathogens and foreign particles toward the nasopharynx.
- Innate defense mechanisms may be antigen-specific, as well as nonspecific.
- Opsonization both attracts and activates other inflammatory cells.
- Chemical messengers are able to activate genes that assist in the body's defense against pathogens.
- B-cell differentiation and IgE production may occur on the local level.

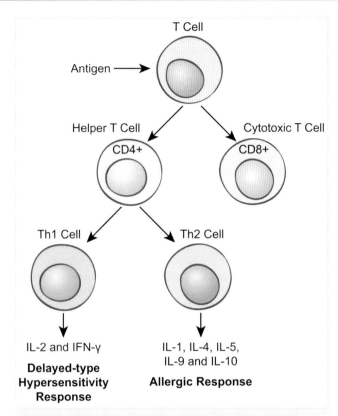

Fig. 103.5 T-cell lineage and pathways of differentiation into Th1 and Th2 helper cells. *IFN*, interferon; *IL*, interleukin.

- The balance of Th1 and Th2 cytokines may play a role in certain disease processes, such as nasal polyposis.

103.6 Recommended Reading

[1] Balogh K, Pantanowitz L. Mouth, nose, and paranasal Sinuses. In: Mills SE, ed. Histology for Pathologists. 3rd ed. Philadelphia, PA: Lippincott Williams & Wilkins; 2007:403–430

[2] Cheng G, Wang LCS, Fridlender ZG et al. Pharmacologic activation of the innate immune system to prevent respiratory viral infections. Am J Respir Cell Mol Biol 2011; 45: 480–488

[3] DeMarcantonio MA, Han JK. Nasal polyps: pathogenesis and treatment implications. Otolaryngol Clin North Am 2011; 44: 685–695, ix

[4] Knowles MR, Boucher RC. Mucus clearance as a primary innate defense mechanism for mammalian airways. J Clin Invest 2002; 109: 571–577

[5] Michalek M, Gelhaus C, Hecht O et al. The human antimicrobial protein psoriasin acts by permeabilization of bacterial membranes. Dev Comp Immunol 2009; 33: 740–746

[6] Patadia M, Dixon J, Conley D et al. Evaluation of the presence of B-cell attractant chemokines in chronic rhinosinusitis. Am J Rhinol Allergy 2010; 24: 11–16

[7] Ramanathan M, Lee WK, Lane AP. Increased expression of acidic mammalian chitinase in chronic rhinosinusitis with nasal polyps. Am J Rhinol 2006; 20: 330–335

[8] Ramanathan M, Lane AP. Innate immunity of the sinonasal cavity and its role in chronic rhinosinusitis. Otolaryngol Head Neck Surg 2007; 136: 348–356

[9] Wise SK, Ahn CN, Schlosser RJ. Localized immunoglobulin E expression in allergic rhinitis and nasal polyposis. Curr Opin Otolaryngol Head Neck Surg 2009; 17: 216–222

104 Olfaction and Taste Disorders

William R. Reisacher and Saral Mehra

104.1 Introduction

The ability to smell and taste plays an important role in our enjoyment of life, as well as our survival in the world. These senses help us identify which foods to eat, as well as alert us about potentially dangerous substances in the environment. The sense of smell is linked to sexual attraction, and certain odors and tastes can evoke powerful emotions and bring back vivid memories many years after the initial experience. For the otolaryngologist, disorders of olfaction and taste are amongst the most difficult to diagnose and treat. Because the perception of flavor represents a complex integration of olfactory and gustatory signals in the orbitofrontal and other areas of the cerebral cortex, disorders of taste and smell are often analyzed together. However, the two systems are quite different in terms of anatomy, physiology, and pathology, and separate discussions are warranted.

104.2 Olfaction Disorders

104.2.1 Applied Anatomy

The pathway for the sensation of smell begins when odorant molecules access the olfactory epithelium via airflow. The olfactory epithelium is composed of a 1- to 2-cm^2 patch of pseudostratified columnar epithelium on the cribriform plates, segments of the superior and middle turbinates, and superior nasal septum. The olfactory epithelium contains nerve endings of the olfactory sensory neurons of cranial nerve I (and some endings of cranial nerve V, which sense compounds such as menthol, mustard, and capsaicin). Olfactory cells are bipolar sensory neurons within the nasal epithelium that have nonmotile cilia (▶ Fig. 104.1). These neurons extend their unmyelinated axons in bundles through the cribriform plates to synapse with cells in the olfactory bulbs. Axons from cells in each bulb coalesce to form the olfactory tract on each side. These tracts then send their signals to a wide number of brain areas, which together are called the primary olfactory cortex. The pattern of receptor stimulation is unique for each particular odorant, and this pattern is reassembled centrally for processing.

A multigene family has recently been identified in humans that encode approximately 500 G-protein–coupled odorant receptors (GPCRs), which are expressed only on the dendrites and axons of olfactory sensory neurons. Although the neurons expressing a particular receptor are randomly distributed in the olfactory epithelium, each projects to a topographic region in the olfactory bulb that is specific to that receptor.

104.2.2 Terminology

A smell disorder can be described as either a quantitative or a qualitative problem. A diminished sense of smell is *hyposmia*, and a total absence of smell is *anosmia*. Qualitative disorders, which can collectively be called *dysosmias*, include *parosmia* (an altered perception of smell that is usually foul), *phantosmia* (perception of smell in the absence of a physical stimulus), and *agnosmia* (the inability to verbally differentiate a smell despite being able to distinguish between odorants).

An etiologic classification system also exists, and clinical olfactory disorders can be transport (conductive), sensory, or neural. Transport loss is a decreased access of odorant molecules to the olfactory epithelium, sensory loss involves damage

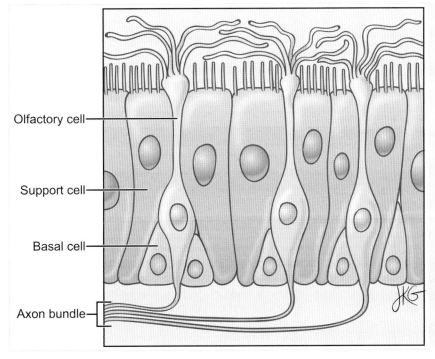

Fig. 104.1 Structure and cellular population of the olfactory epithelium.

Olfactory cell

Support cell

Basal cell

Axon bundle

to the neuroepithelium, and neural disorders reflect injury to the olfactory bulb and central olfactory pathways.

104.2.3 The Disease Process

Etiology

Loss of smell is usually caused by nasal or sinus disease, upper respiratory tract infection, head trauma, or side effects from a large variety of medications. A comprehensive differential diagnosis for olfaction disturbances is shown in ▶ Fig. 104.1.

Pathogenesis

The pathogenesis of disorders involving olfaction depends on the etiology. The mechanism of chronic rhinosinusitis (CRS) is likely a mixed transport and sensory problem consisting of obstruction and direct injury to the neuroepithelium, resulting in baseline olfactory sensory neuron death. This mixed loss theory is supported by the finding that a number of patients who have adequate medical or surgical treatment for other sinonasal complaints have persistent osmias. The pathogenesis of olfactory disorders following viral infection is postulated to involve the olfactory receptor cells; however, a central mechanism cannot be completely ruled out. There is also a strong association between olfaction disorders and neurodegenerative diseases such as Parkinson disease and Alzheimer disease. Finally, malingering must be included in the differential diagnosis of smell disorders, and a number of objective tests are designed to detect malingerers.

104.2.4 Medical Evaluation

Presenting Complaints

A thorough patient history will include the timing of the olfactory problem (sudden, gradual, fluctuating); previous incidents of the problem; antecedent events (head trauma, upper respiratory infection); associated symptoms (nasal obstruction, rhinorrhea); the presence of other neurologic deficits, such as memory impairment and motor findings; and a history of nasal surgery.

Physical Examination

The physical examination should include a thorough otologic, upper respiratory, and head and neck evaluation. The nasal examination should include endoscopy evaluating the middle meatus, sphenoethmoid recess, nasopharynx, and olfactory cleft; any anatomical obstructions to airflow, such as polyps, masses, or edematous mucosa, should be noted. In addition, a comprehensive neurologic examination should be conducted that emphasizes the cranial nerves and general sensorimotor function.

Testing

Tests of olfaction disorders are useful in confirming patient complaints, documenting the level of impairment, and evaluating improvement over time. Qualitative olfactory impairment can be tested with a forced-choice verbal identification of odors

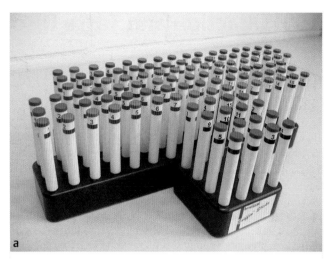

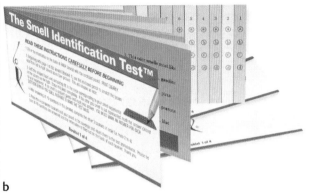

Fig. 104.2 Some commonly available tests to assess olfactory function. (a) Sniffin' Sticks. (Courtesy of Burghart Messtechnik, Wedel, Germany). (b) University of Pennsylvania Smell Identification Test (UPSIT). (Courtesy of Sensonics, Haddon Heights, NJ).

such as in the University of Pennsylvania Smell Identification Test (UPSIT), "Sniffin' Sticks," and the Connecticut Chemosensory Clinical Research Center Test (▶ Fig. 104.2). The UPSIT uses 40 scratch-and-sniff odors; the patient must choose from one of four and identify the odor. This test can also be helpful in identifying malingering. Threshold tests, discrimination tests, and objective tests (e.g., chemosensory event-related potentials, odor-induced changes on electroencephalogram and electro-olfactogram) can also be conducted as indicated. Serum testing for systemic diseases should include blood glucose, thyroid function, erythrocyte sedimentation rate, and liver function. Finally, skull base and/or brain imaging with computed tomography (CT) or magnetic resonance (MR) imaging is indicated as guided by the medical evaluation.

104.2.5 Treatment

Treatment should focus on the etiology and may involve a multidisciplinary team. For patients with a transport smell disorder, medical management of allergies, infections, and inflammation is frequently effective. Surgery may be indicated when polyposis, nasal septal deviation, or CRS results in a transport disorder. However, it is important to remember that CRS may cause direct toxicity to the olfactory nerve, which may result in persistent olfactory loss even after polyp removal and sinus reventilation.

104.2.6 Prognosis

Although there is no proven effective treatment for a sensorineural olfactory loss, spontaneous recovery and regeneration are common in postviral olfactory disorders and may occur up to 2 years after viral exposure. Similarly, in olfactory dysfunction following head trauma, improvement may occur without intervention because of the regenerative capacity of the olfactory system. One study that tested olfactory function in 66 patients with olfactory dysfunction following head injury found that 36% improved, 45% showed no change, and 18% worsened. Treatment is warranted because patients risk injury from their inability to detect gas leaks, smoke, spoiled foods, and other warning signs of impending danger. Also, quality of life is significantly affected in patients whose enjoyment from tasting foods is diminished, leading to weight loss, malnutrition, impaired immunity, and worsening of medical illness, particularly in the elderly.

104.3 Taste Disorders

104.3.1 Applied Anatomy

The sense of taste occurs when chemicals bind to taste receptors, which are polarized neuroepithelial cells that form columnar, pseudostratified "islands" in the surrounding oral cavity epithelium. Clusters of approximately 50 to 100 taste receptors, known as taste buds, are located at various places within the oral cavity, including the edges of the tongue, anterior and dorsal surfaces of the tongue, soft palate, pharynx, and larynx. On the tongue, taste buds are located within fungiform, foliate, and circumvallate papillae. Fungiform papillae are on the anterior two-thirds of the tongue and can contain up to 15 taste buds. Foliate papillae are located on the posterior and lateral edges of the tongue and typically contain many more taste buds than fungiform papillae. The approximately nine circumvallate papillae are located on the posterior tongue, separating the anterior tongue from the base of the tongue.

Taste receptor cells share almost all of the properties of neural cells except that they have no axons (▶ Fig. 104.3). Sensory information is transmitted to afferent nerve fibers located within the taste buds, which have cell bodies in the sensory ganglia of cranial nerves VII, IX, and X. Fibers from these ganglia project into the central nervous system at the level of the rostral solitary nucleus of the brainstem. Signals then travel via thalamic pathways to the primary opercular and insular taste cortex, as well as the orbitofrontal cortex, cingulate gyrus, and other integrative projection areas. Cranial nerve VII, whose cell bodies are within the geniculate ganglion, transmits taste information through two branches, the chorda tympani and the greater superficial petrosal nerve. Cranial nerve IX, whose cell bodies are in the petrosal ganglion, innervates most of the foliate and circumvallate papillae. Cranial nerve X, whose cell bodies are in the nodose ganglion, innervates taste buds in the pharynx and larynx via the superior laryngeal nerve.

The five basic tastes in humans are sweet, sour, bitter, salty, and umami. Sweet taste encourages the consumption of carbohydrates, which are required for energy. Sour taste is associated with acids, which increase as foods begin to spoil. Likewise, many substances that are poisonous to humans have a bitter taste. Salt intake is necessary for maintaining water balance and blood circulation, and umami, which is the taste of L-glutamate, signals the presence of proteins in food. Certain visual and textural cues can also have an impact on the perception of how food tastes, and many genetic, cultural, and developmental factors contribute to an individual's attraction to certain foods.

104.3.2 Terminology

A quantitative reduction in gustatory sensitivity is referred to as *hypogeusia*, whereas the absence of this sense is called *ageusia*. Certain central nervous system diseases, such as multiple sclerosis, are capable of producing a taste disturbance on half of the tongue, called *hemiageusia*. A qualitative reduction in gustatory sensitivity is referred to as *dysgeusia*. An altered perception

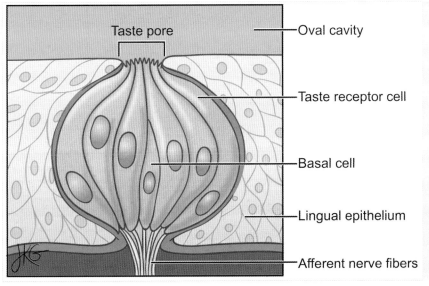

Fig. 104.3 Organization of taste receptor cells within a taste bud.

Taste pore

Oval cavity

Taste receptor cell

Basal cell

Lingual epithelium

Afferent nerve fibers

Table 104.1 Differential diagnosis of olfactory and taste disorders

Etiology of olfactory disorders	Etiology of taste disorders
Nasal and sinus disease	**Oral and perioral infections**
Allergic or vasomotor rhinitis	
Chronic sinusitis	**Aging**
Nasal polyps	
Adenoid hypertrophy	**Iatrogenic causes**
Following viral upper respiratory infection	Oral appliances
	Dental procedures
Head trauma	Middle ear surgery
Direct injury	Oncologic surgery
Nerve injury	Procedures with lingual compression
Brain injury	Tonsillectomy, oropharyngeal surgery
	Microlaryngoscopy
Neurodegenerative disease	Endotracheal intubation
Alzheimer disease	
Parkinson disease	**Trauma**
Multiple sclerosis	Fractures of the skull base or midface
Aging	**Neurologic conditions**
	Idiopathic mononeuropathy, polyneuropathy (e.g., Bell palsy)
Exposures and nutritional factors	Cerebrovascular disorders, accidents
Medications	Gustatory aura with epilepsy or migraine
Cigarette smoking	Multiple sclerosis
Cocaine abuse (intranasal)	
Toxic chemicals	**Systemic disease**
Industrial agents	Sjögren syndrome
Vitamin and trace metal deficiency	
Radiation treatment of head and neck	**Endocrine disorders**
	Adrenocortical insufficiency
Congenital conditions	Diabetes mellitus
Congenital anosmia	Hypothyroidism
Turner syndrome	
Kallmann syndrome	**Congenital conditions**
	Kallmann syndrome
Neurologic conditions	Turner syndrome
Neoplasm or brain tumor	
Epilepsy (olfactory aura)	**Exposures and nutritional factors**
Migraine headache (olfactory aura)	Medications
Cerebrovascular accident	Vitamin and trace metal deficiency
Parkinson disease	Malnutrition

Table 104.1 *continued*

Etiology of olfactory disorders	Etiology of taste disorders
Parkinsonian syndromes	Toxic chemicals and industrial agents
Alzheimer disease	Radiation treatment for head and neck cancer
Motor neuron disease	
Tremor	
Huntington disease	
Inherited ataxia	
Psychiatric conditions	
Malingering	
Schizophrenia	
Depression	
Olfactory reference syndrome	
Endocrine disorders	
Adrenocortical insufficiency	
Diabetes mellitus	
Thyroid disorder	
Primary amenorrhea	
Pseudohypoparathyroidism	
Systemic conditions	
Sjögren syndrome	
Systemic lupus erythematosus	
Pregnancy	

of taste without any stimulation is known as *parageusia*. Dysgeusia and parageusia can be further described depending on the type of taste that is present. The perception of a foul taste may be referred to as *cacogeusia*, and that of a metallic taste may be called *metallogeusia*.

104.3.3 Medical Evaluation

Presenting Complaints

The diagnosis of taste disorders begins with a detailed history, starting with a description of the problem. The physician should ask when the problem first was noted and about events that occurred around that time, such as illnesses, radiation treatments, or new medications. The history should also elicit information about recent trauma or surgical procedures, particularly those occurring in the oral cavity or oropharynx.

Physical Examination

During the physical examination, the otolaryngologist should perform a complete head and neck examination, including a thorough assessment of the sinonasal tract with nasal endoscopy. It is important to remember that many complaints of taste disturbance actually stem from olfactory deficits. A careful examination of the oral cavity should be done to assess for oral and perioral infections, as well as for dental carries and gingival disease. Middle ear function should be evaluated with otomicroscopy along with audiography and tympanometry. A full cranial nerve examination should be performed, and any positive findings should prompt a consultation by a neurologist. Because many causes of taste disturbance may be systemic in nature, such as chronic renal failure and liver disease, it is recommended that each patient also have a complete evaluation by his or her primary care physician.

Testing

Testing should focus on identifying the etiology, assessing the patient's function, and determining the impact on the patient's quality of life. Blood testing may be useful to diagnose nutritional deficiencies, such as vitamin D and zinc deficiencies, which can lead to taste disturbance. CT or MR imaging may be obtained to rule out CRS, temporal bone disease, or brain abnormalities. There are a limited number of objective tests to assess taste function, but one of the most common is electrogustometry (EGM), in which stimulation of the taste buds in various parts of the tongue, either with an electric stimulus or with flavored paper discs, is followed by a measurement of threshold. In general, increased thresholds on both sides of the tongue are associated with peripheral damage to the receptor systems and the tongue by physical or chemical trauma, whereas asymmetric abnormalities are usually associated with peripheral nerve damage or central nervous system causes. Instruments to help assess the impact of disease on quality of life include the Short Form 36 Health Survey (SF-36) and the Beck Depression Inventory.

Differential Diagnosis

Some common medications that may lead to taste disturbances include angiotensin-converting enzyme (ACE) inhibitors, calcium channel blockers, diuretics, chemotherapeutic agents, and topical antihistamines. Approximately one-third of adults undergoing tonsillectomy experience taste disturbances 2 weeks after surgery, decreasing to fewer than 10% after 6 months. A comprehensive differential diagnosis for taste disorders appears in ▶ Table 104.1.

104.3.4 Treatment

The treatment for taste disturbance focuses primarily on identifying the underlying cause. The physician must also keep in mind that the perceived intensity of taste generally diminishes with age, as well as with psychological problems. Oral hygiene must also be discussed, along with the importance of smoking cessation. Acute disturbances in taste are typically transient in nature and require no specific treatment. In 2009, there was a sharp rise in reports of metallogeusia after the consumption of pine nuts, which was believed to have occurred after a type of pine nut containing a toxin had entered the human food supply. The condition became known as "pine mouth" and produced symptoms lasting for up to 2 weeks after the ingestion of breads or sweet foods. It has recently been discovered that certain genes control the temperature dependence of sweet taste

receptors, and studies are under way evaluating the utility of hot and cold stimulation in the treatment of sweet dysgeusia.

104.4 Roundsmanship

- The perception of flavor is a complex integration of olfactory and taste stimuli in the cerebral cortex.
- Disorders of smell can be classified as quantitative (hyposmia or anosmia), qualitative (dysosmia), or based on the site of pathology (transport, sensory, or neural).
- The five basic tastes in humans are sweet, sour, bitter, salty, and umami, each of which has a proposed survival or homeostatic function.
- A quantitative reduction in gustatory sensitivity is referred to as hypogeusia or ageusia; a qualitative reduction in gustatory sensitivity is referred to as dysgeusia.
- The possible etiologies of taste and smell disorders are large and varied, and the clinical evaluation must focus on identifying the most likely cause.
- Disorders of smell and taste can be dangerous because they may lead to weight loss, malnutrition, and the inability to sense danger, particularly in the elderly.

104.5 Recommended Reading

[1] Axel R. Scents and sensibility: a molecular logic of olfactory perception (Nobel lecture). Angew Chem Int Ed Engl 2005; 44: 6110–6127
[2] Berling K, Knutsson J, Rosenblad A, von Unge M.. Evaluation of electrogustometry and the filter paper disc method for taste assessment. Acta Oto l aryngol; 131: 488–493
[3] Chaudhari N, Roper SD.. The cell biology of taste. JCell Biol; 190: 285–296
[4] Chester AC, Antisdel JL, Sindwani R. Symptom-specific outcomes of endoscopic sinus surgery: a systematic review. Otolaryngol Head Neck Surg 2009; 140: 633–639
[5] Doty R L, Mishra A.. Olfaction and its alteration by nasal obstruction, rhinitis, and rhinosinusitis. Laryngoscope; 111: 409–423
[6] Doty R L, Yousem DM, Pham LT, Kreshak AA, Geckle R, Lee WW.. Olfactory dysfunction in patients with head trauma. Arch Neurol; 54: 1131–1140
[7] Duncan HJ, Seiden AM. Long-term follow-up of olfactory loss secondary to head trauma and upper respiratory tract infection. Arch Otolaryngol Head Neck Surg 1995; 121: 1183–1187
[8] Flesch F, Rigaux-Barry F, Saviuc P et al. Dysgeusia following consumption of pine nuts: more than 3000 cases in France. Clin Toxicol (Phila) 2011; 49: 668–670
[9] Fujiyama R, Ishitobi S, Honda K, Okada Y, Oi K, Toda K.. Ice cube stimulation helps to improve dysgeusia. Odontology; 98: 82–84
[10] Heiser C, Landis B N, Giger R et al.. Taste disturbance following tonsillectomy—a prospective study. Laryngoscope; 120: 2119–2124
[11] Snow JB. Causes of olfactory and gustatory disorders. In: Getchell TV, Bartoshuk LM, Doty RL, Snow J. Smell and Taste in Health and Disease. New York, NY: Raven Press; 1991:445–449

105 Benign Nasal Obstruction

Anthony P. Sclafani and Anthony M. Sclafani

105.1 Introduction

Nasal obstruction is a common complaint frequently experienced during a number of normal and pathologic conditions. When chronic, however, nasal obstruction can cause significant morbidity and reduction in quality of life. The physician must determine the specific etiology and direct treatment toward it; however, the etiology may often be multifactorial, and treatment plans should be created that most effectively address these factors.

105.2 Incidence and Prevalence of Disease

All patients have experienced nasal congestion at some point in their lives, but persistent nasal obstruction for more than a month should be evaluated. Symptomatic and persistent nasal obstruction is estimated to affect 20% of the population. Eighty percent or more of individuals in the population have a septal deviation of some degree, and approximately 5% of people have symptomatic nasal obstruction associated with a deviated septum.

105.3 Terminology

The diagnosis and management of nasal obstruction are greatly facilitated by a consideration of structural versus functional nasal obstruction. Nasal obstruction from a fixed, structural cause such as a deviated septum is typically constant and usually of long duration. Obstructive symptoms that are of recent development or that vary over time suggest a pathophysiologic cause and may be more amenable to medical treatment. The term *nasal cycle* refers to the cyclical alternation of vasocongestion and decongestion naturally occurring in the nose. This cycle is coordinated between the two sides of the nose; the vasoerectile tissue on one side undergoes engorgement while the opposite side shrinks because of diminished blood flow. In most persons, the pattern reverses every 4 to 6 hours. The term *laminar airflow* refers to the smooth, nonturbulent flow of air through the nasal cavity.

105.4 Applied Anatomy

The nasal cavities are bounded bilaterally by three sets of turbinate bones, the nasal sidewalls, and the alae, and medially by the nasal septum and columella. The caudal end of the nasal bones is termed the *piriform aperture*. The posterior choanae are the junctions of the two nasal cavities with the nasopharynx. The internal nasal valve is a physiologic area bounded by the inferior turbinate (anterior head), the junction of the upper lateral cartilage (ULC) and lower lateral cartilage (LLC) (the "scroll"), the nasal septum, and the nasal floor. The attachment of the ULC and septum should form an angle of about 10 to 15 degrees (▶ Fig. 105.1). The external nasal valve is the rim of the

ala. The inferior turbinate, a separate bone (inferior concha) forming the lower part of the lateral nasal sidewall, is covered by vasoerectile mucosa that responds to both environmental and physiologic stimuli. More superiorly, portions of the ethmoid bone, including the middle turbinate, complete the lateral and superior nasal walls. Medially, the nasal septum is composed of the quadrangular cartilage, which rests upon the maxillary crest, a ridge of bone rising up from the palate. Dorsally, the nasal septum fuses with the ULCs to make up the lower nasal dorsum. Posteriorly, the quadrangular cartilage articulates with the vomer (inferiorly) and perpendicular plate of the ethmoid bone (superiorly). Submucosal blood vessels running in the perichondrium supply nutrients to the septal cartilage. Small areas of the septum are contributed by the palatine and sphenoid bones (▶ Fig. 105.2).

105.5 The Disease Process
105.5.1 Etiology

Given the multiple potential causes of nasal obstruction, it is impractical to discuss each in detail here; most are covered more comprehensively elsewhere in this book. Deviated nasal septum may occur congenitally, as a result of birth trauma, or as a result of nasal trauma later in life, but most often it is developmental, becoming evident in adolescence or after puberty. Minor deflections of either the bony or cartilaginous septum are very common, even in relatively asymptomatic patients, but some patients with minor deviations may complain significantly of obstructive symptoms. Likewise, turbinate enlargement can be congenital/developmental, with bulky turbinate bone. More common is mucosal hypertrophy (secondary to chronic rhinitis or sinusitis) with or without bony enlargement. Internal nasal valve dysfunction can be idiopathic or can be related to prior nasal surgery; intercartilaginous incisions and removal of portions of the lateral crura during rhinoplasty can

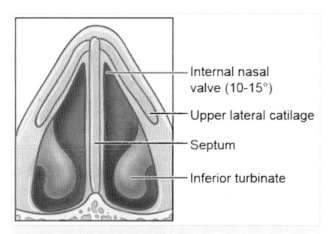

Fig. 105.1 The internal nasal valve is defined by the nasal septum, nasal floor, anterior end of the inferior turbinate, and lateral nasal sidewall. The internal nasal valve angle is roughly 10 to 15 degrees.

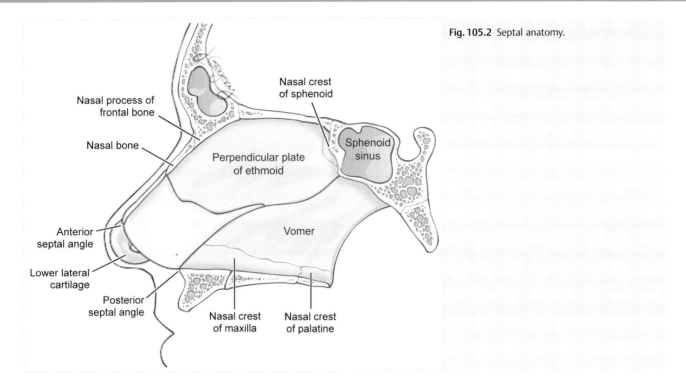

Fig. 105.2 Septal anatomy.

Nasal process of
frontal bone

Nasal bone

Nasal crest
of sphenoid

Perpendicular plate
of ethmoid

Sphenoid
sinus

Anterior
septal angle

Vomer

Lower lateral
cartilage

Posterior
septal angle

Nasal crest
of maxilla

Nasal crest
of palatine

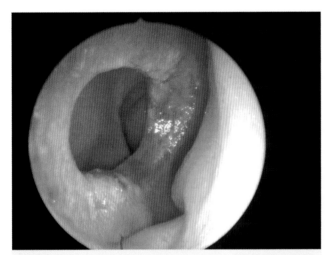

Fig. 105.3 Septal perforation viewed from the patient's left nasal cavity. The anterior end of the left inferior turbinate is seen on the right side of the photo, while the right and middle turbinates can be seen through the septal perforation.

105.5.2 Pathogenesis

Inspired air is directed posteriorly after entering the nasal cavity, passing the area of the internal nasal valve about 15 to 20 mm from the alar margin and then continuing to the nasopharynx. Fifty percent of total airway resistance occurs during the passage of air through the nose. Quiet inspiration is generally laminar in nature, whereas expiration may be more turbulent. Turbulent airflow facilitates air distribution within the nasal cavity, but requires more energy and may lead to a sensation of nasal obstruction. Turbulent airflow occurs in the setting of higher transnasal pressures and faster air speeds; hence, narrow nasal passages will require faster air flow to deliver the same volume of air to the nasopharynx, leading to more turbulent airflow. By Poiseuille's law of the flow of a fluid through a tube,

where in this case P equals the transnasal pressure drop, μ represents the fluid viscosity, L stands for the length of the nasal cavity, Q is the volume flow rate, and r is the radius of the nasal cavity. As the radius decreases, the pressure change across the nasal length increases by the fourth power; therefore, even a moderate reduction of the nasal cavity radius can cause a significant increase in transnasal pressure unless it is compensated for by a large reduction in the rate of airflow. As can be seen, a deviated nasal septum, enlargement of the turbinate, partial inward collapse of the internal nasal valve, significant nasal polyposis, or masses will reduce the nasal airway radius and greatly increase the transnasal pressure differential. This pressure gradient may also cause dynamic inspiratory collapse at the semicollapsible internal nasal valve. Furthermore, airflow velocity necessarily increases as the airway radius decreases in order for the same air volume to be delivered to the nasopharynx. As noted earlier, an increase in flow rate increases the turbulent aspects of airflow, and turbulent airflow further contributes to the sensation of nasal obstruction.

weaken the lateral support of the nasal valve and lead to medial collapse of the valve. Similarly, the ULC can become flail and prone to collapse after dorsal nasal reduction because the fusion of the ULC with the septum may be removed when a cartilaginous dorsal hump is removed, and injudicious rasping of a bony hump may disarticulate the ULC from its attachment to the undersurface of the caudal end of the nasal bone. Septal perforation (▶ Fig. 105.3) or excessive removal of the inferior turbinate ("empty nose syndrome") can also cause subjective symptoms of nasal obstruction associated with turbulent nasal airflow, crusting, and dryness. Prior septal surgery is the most common cause of nasal septal perforation; intranasal use of illicit drugs (e.g., cocaine) is also quite common.

105.5.3 Natural History and Progression

Nasal obstruction, in and of itself, represents an impairment of quality of life. It may lead to chronic mouth breathing, dry mouth, and snoring, but alone it will not cause obstructive sleep apnea. The treatment of other symptoms associated with nasal obstruction, such as epistaxis, chronic rhinorrhea, and sinus infection, is best directed at the underlying cause. Nasal obstruction from a fixed cause, such as a deviated septum, will not progress, but obstruction from a physiologic cause may progressively worsen until the obstruction is chronic and complete unless the root cause is treated. Not uncommonly, the development and progression of a functional cause of nasal obstruction may be associated with a previously tolerated or compensated structural cause: again, the treatment of both causes is reasonable in symptomatic patients.

105.5.4 Potential Disease Complications

Nasal obstruction, if it affects areas of sinus outflow, can increase the likelihood of sinus infection. A severely deviated septum can compromise the nasal cavity in the area of the middle turbinate, causing the latter to remain fairly lateral during development, obstructing the middle meatus and infundibulum. Areas of a severely or sharply angulated deviated septum can become dessicated and therefore points of epistaxis, as can chronically inflamed and hyperemic septal or turbinate mucosa. Nasal obstruction can be associated with chronic mouth breathing and fatigue (especially during strenuous activity), although dry mouth and snoring may be the most prominent symptoms noted by patients; however, as noted above, they will not cause obstructive sleep apnea. Hyposmia may result from severe nasal obstruction because airflow to the olfactory nerve endings in the superior nasal cavity can be compromised by severe nasal obstruction; anosmia, however, is typically not caused by nasal obstruction alone, and other causes of anosmia must be sought.

105.6 Medical Evaluation

The central piece of the medical evaluation for nasal obstruction is the physical examination. Anterior rhinoscopy with a nasal speculum and head mirror/light should be performed both before and after the topical application of a nasal decongestant. The color and degree of congestion of the mucosa, as well as the response to the decongestant, should be noted. Once decongested, the posterior nares are more viewable. However, rigid nasal endoscopy is invaluable in inspecting the posterior nares, middle meatus, and posterior choanae. Flexible endoscopy may be necessary when a severe caudal septal deflection prevents an adequate posterior inspection. Nasal polyps, debris, mucopurulence, and cobblestoning of the mucosa should be noted; any localized or atypical soft-tissue mass should be noted and biopsy considered. The integrity of the entire septum should be ascertained. Crusts of dried mucus or blood should be removed with forceps or suction so that all mucosal surfaces can be inspected; small septal perforations or masses may lurk beneath this debris.

105.6.1 Presenting Complaints

In addition to simple nasal obstruction, patients may also report intermittent headaches, nasal discharge, and/or facial pain and pressure; these symptoms may suggest sinusitis, and radiographic imaging is often necessary to eliminate the possibility of sinusitis. Other symptoms may include chronic mouth breathing, dry throat, snoring, decreased sense of smell, and, in the case of nasal obstruction caused by allergic rhinitis, postnasal drip and rhinorrhea.

105.6.2 Clinical Findings, Physical Examination

The diagnosis of a deviated septum is relatively straightforward; a portion of the septum deviates significantly from the midline (▶ Fig. 105.4). An enlarged turbinate likewise fills a disproportionate amount of the airway and narrows the functional lumen of the nose. Collapse of the internal nasal valve may be suggested by narrowing (especially at the dorsal junction of the ULC and septum), but the diagnosis is made when there is visible and symptomatic inward collapse on inspiration, with a reduction or elimination of symptomatic obstruction when this area is stabilized (not splayed laterally) with a small curet or forceps. The Cottle maneuver manually stabilizes the cheek lateral to the ala (without distracting the ala laterally) in order to prevent internal nasal valve collapse on inspiration; patients with internal nasal valve collapse will note improvement in breathing during the Cottle maneuver. Among the more common causes of nasal obstruction, allergic rhinitis and sinusitis are discussed elsewhere in this book.

A septal disorder, such as perforation or hematoma, can also cause nasal obstruction. A perforation can cause symptoms of nasal obstruction, either by serving as a nidus for mucous crusting or by causing turbulent airflow; it may be obvious on physical examination or may be seen only endoscopically after débridement of the nose. Nasal polyps, although common, cause nasal obstruction only when massive. More commonly, physiologic causes of nasal obstruction include rhinitis of pregnancy (secondary to elevated estrogen levels and generally seen in the

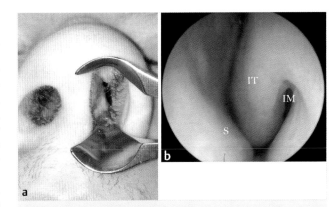

Fig. 105.4 (a) Severe caudal septal deviation seen by anterior rhinoscopy. (b) Low septal deviation encroaching on left inferior turbinate and obstructing the airway. The inferior meatus is seen. *IM*, inferior meatus; *IT*, inferior turbinate; *S*, septum.

third trimester of pregnancy and in the first 6 months post partum); classic rhinitis medicamentosa (rhinitis secondary to the administration of α-adrenergic topical agents); and drug-induced rhinitis (particularly β-blockers, angiotensin-converting enzyme [ACE] inhibitors, and oral contraceptives). Rhinitis of pregnancy and rhinitis medicamentosa generally have a pale, swollen, and "boggy" mucosa (especially the inferior turbinate). Especially in the case of rhinitis medicamentosa, an unusually rapid decongestion may be seen after the application of a decongestant spray.

More uncommonly, inflammatory conditions such as sarcoidosis, systemic lupus erythematosus, and Wegener granulomatosis may cause mucosal edema and nasal obstruction; sarcoidosis, in particular, may present with a pale, "cobblestone" mucosa. Tumors of the nasal cavity are relatively rare, with inverting papilloma the most significant. Arising from the lateral nasal sidewall, inverting papilloma may vary in appearance from polypoid to wartlike and may degenerate to a squamous cell carcinoma. Finally, masses of the nasopharynx or stenosis/atresia of the posterior choanae can cause nasal obstruction, so a complete evaluation of the nose and nasopharynx is mandatory.

105.6.3 Testing

Physical examination of the nose, including nasal and nasopharyngeal endoscopy, is the first step in the evaluation of nasal obstruction. Computed tomography (CT; ▶ Fig. 105.5) is indicated in the presence of any bony or soft-tissue erosion or mass, or if sinusitis is suspected; contrast-enhanced CT or magnetic resonance imaging is indicated if a malignancy is considered.

Functional testing may include rhinomanometry, acoustic rhinometry, or peak nasal inspiratory flow. Rhinomanometry simultaneously measures air pressure in the nasopharynx and anterior nares, but it is cumbersome and generally limited to research applications. Acoustic rhinometry determines the internal cross-sectional area of the nose by measuring the reflectance of sound waves and can be performed easily in the office setting; it can be useful in evaluating changes in the internal nasal structure, but its accuracy decreases posteriorly in the setting of significant anterior obstruction. Peak nasal inspiratory flow measures the maximal airflow through the nose, but normative data are lacking, hindering its clinical use. If an inflammatory process is suspected, biopsy and serologic testing are performed as indicated.

105.6.4 Differential Diagnosis

The differential diagnosis of nasal obstruction is broad, including common as well as uncommon causes. Principal primary causes of nasal obstruction include deviated nasal septum (congenital, developmental, or traumatic; ▶ Fig. 105.6), inferior turbinate hypertrophy, and internal nasal valve collapse. Common secondary causes of nasal obstruction include upper respiratory tract infections; sinusitis; rhinitis (allergic or nonallergic); rhinitis medicamentosa; rhinitis of pregnancy; and medications (especially β-blockers, ACE inhibitors, oral contraceptives, and many psychotropic medications). More uncommon causes include septal hematoma or perforation; nasal polyps; choanal atresia/stenosis; nasal foreign bodies; nasopharyngeal masses;

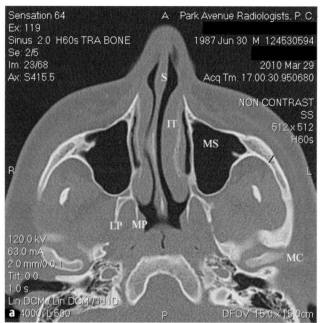

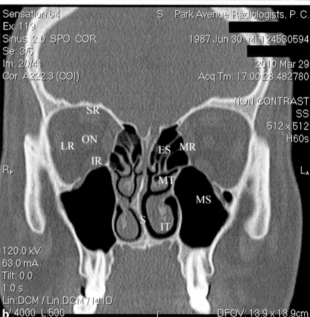

Fig. 105.5 (**a**) Axial computed tomographic (CT) scan demonstrates deviation of the septum from the midline. The left inferior turbinate fills in much of the void created by the deviation. The maxillary sinus is well aerated and has no evidence of mucosal disease. The zygoma, mandibular condyle, and medial pterygoid and lateral pterygoid processes are also seen in this projection. *IT*, inferior turbinate; *LP*, lateral pterygoid; *MC*, mandibular condyle; *MP*, medial pterygoid; *MS*, maxillary sinus; *S*, septum; *Z*, zygoma. (**b**) Coronal CT scan of the same patient further demonstrates the severity of the septal deviation. The inferior turbinate fills much of the space voided by the septal deviation. The middle turbinate is seen, and the ethmoid sinuses and maxillary sinuses are free of disease. The orbital muscles are seen: the superior rectus, lateral rectus, and inferior rectus; the medial rectus is seen just below the superior oblique muscle (not marked). The optic nerve is clearly seen. *ES*, ethmoid sinuses; *IR*, inferior rectus; *IT*, inferior turbinate; *LR*, lateral rectus; *MR*, medial rectus; *MS*, maxillary sinuses; *MT*, middle turbinate; *ON*, optic nerve; *S*, septum; *SR*, superior rectus.

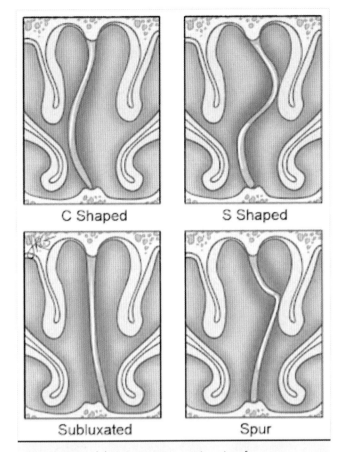

C Shaped S Shaped

Subluxated Spur

Fig. 105.6 Septal deviations can present in various forms.

inflammatory disorders (Wegener granulomatosis, sarcoidosis, systemic lupus erythematosus); nasal tumors (inverting papilloma, carcinoma); and hypothyroidism.

105.7 Treatment

105.7.1 Medical Treatment

The medical management of nasal obstruction is directed at the underlying cause. In general, nasal obstruction from noninfectious, noninflammatory disorders is treated symptomatically. Nasal saline sprays and rinses, along with topical emollients, may help relieve or reduce symptoms, as well as assist the natural cleansing mechanism of the nose by facilitating the débridement of dried mucus. Topical nasal corticosteroids, in most cases and unless contraindicated, may help relieve primary or reactive mucosal edema, thereby providing a more patent airway. Topically applied nasal steroids typically begin to demonstrate an effect in 7 to 10 days. The most common side effects of intranasal steroids include headache, postnasal drip, and nasal dryness. Patients should be advised to avoid spraying the medication directly toward the septum to avoid chemical irritation of the mucosa and the possibility of a septal perforation. Patients should be counseled to administer the spray with the contralateral hand, aiming toward the ipsilateral medial canthus.

Nasal decongestants may provide some mild temporary relief by reducing the vascular engorgement of (primarily) the inferior turbinates, but this is generally acceptable to patients only for short-term relief, as in an upper respiratory tract infection or seasonal allergic rhinitis. Directly applied topical decongestants cause a more potent decongestion of the nasal mucosa, but routine use for more than 3 to 4 days may induce a relative resistance to normal, physiologic adrenergic stimuli—hence, the severe rebound congestion associated with rhinitis medicamentosa.

In the case of nasal obstruction caused by septal perforations, most symptoms can be relieved with saline sprays, nasal rinses, and topical emollients. A septal button can be placed through the perforation to reduce symptomatic whistling. Made of soft silicone, this two-piece device is inserted bilaterally and snapped together through the perforation, limiting or eliminating airflow across the perforation.

105.7.2 Surgical Treatment

The four most common reasons for surgical treatment of nasal obstruction are correction of nasal septal deviation, treatment of turbinate hypertrophy, internal nasal valve repair, and repair of septal perforation.

Correction of Deviation of the Nasal Septum

Modern corrective septal surgery can be divided into two basic categories: subtotal septectomy, popularized by Killian, and septoplasty, described by Cottle. The Killian approach is more direct, removing deviated septal cartilage and bone, whereas the Cottle philosophy is predicated upon managing the natural tendency of the cartilage to warp while maximally preserving cartilage. Ultimately, all septal manipulations are performed in a submucoperichondrial and submucoperiosteal plane in order to preserve septal blood supply.

The Killian incision is made parallel and 10 mm posterior to the caudal septum. Before elevating a mucosal flap, it is essential to perform proper hydrodissection of the mucoperichondrium by injecting local anesthetic into both sides of the septum. Correct injection is evidenced by blanching and elevation of the mucosa and represents separation of the mucoperichondrium from the cartilage. The plane is further developed, the ipsilateral mucosal flap is raised over both the cartilaginous and the bony septum, and an incision through the cartilage is made parallel to the mucosal cut; this provides access to the contralateral submucoperichondrial plane, which is similarly elevated. Once both mucosal flaps are elevated, a cartilage cut is made and continued to the bony septum, parallel to (but at least 10 mm below) the dorsal septal edge. The cartilage is freed from its posterior bony attachments to the perpendicular plate of the ethmoid and vomer, and then cut from its attachment to the maxillary crest. Once this outlined segment of cartilage is removed, only a caudal/dorsal L-shaped strut of cartilage remains. It is essential that this L-strut be located at least 10 mm caudally and dorsally to avoid a tip collapse and a saddle nose deformity, respectively. Any deviated portions of posterior septal bone or maxillary crest are then removed with rongeurs or an osteotome, as described in the section on septoplasty (▶ Fig. 105.7).

The Killian submucous resection offers simple and quick access to the mid and posterior septum. However, exposure of the caudal portion of the L-strut is very limited, and the elevation

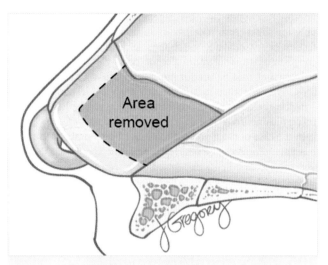

Fig. 105.7 Killian submucous resection of the septum removes maximal amounts (*shaded area*) of septal cartilage.

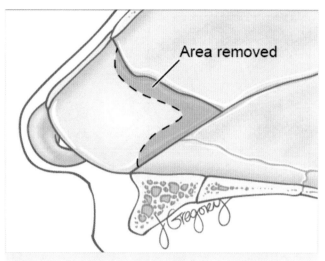

Fig. 105.8 Cottle septoplasty preferentially removes minimal amounts of cartilage to allow the creation of a "swinging door" of quadrangular cartilage.

of bilateral complete septal flaps is necessary. A large potential space for fluid collection (septal hematoma or seroma) is created, and a significant portion of the remaining quadrangular cartilage has been separated from its blood supply, the mucoperichondrium. Deviated portions of cartilage are removed, rather than remodeled, and so deviations of the remaining L-strut are not addressed by the classic submucous resection.

Septoplasty is classically performed through a Cottle hemitransfixion incision, placed at the margin of the caudal septum. An ipsilateral mucosal flap is elevated along the length of the septum, including the maxillary crest. Decussating fibers of periosteum and perichondrium often make this elevation more difficult, and a two-tunnel (one along the inferior septum, one along the medial nasal floor) approach is used, enabling sharp division of the decussating fibers if needed. A "swinging door" of cartilage is created by first removing an inferior strip of cartilage along the length of the maxillary crest, incising cartilage, and dissecting this strip from the contralateral mucoperichondrium. Next, the quadrangular cartilage is disarticulated from the bony septum, allowing elevation of the contralateral mucoperichondrium from the bony septum. A Takahashi forceps is used to remove small fragments of bone to allow free movement of the septal cartilage. Significant bony septal deviations are more carefully removed by first incising the bone superior to the deviation sharply with bone scissors; it should be remembered that the perpendicular plate inserts into the anterior cranial fossa floor, and rough handling of this bone can lead to a cerebrospinal fluid leak. If the remaining quadrangular cartilage (pedicled on its dorsal attachments and on one unelevated mucoperichondrium) can be moved to the midline easily, no further intervention is needed (▶ Fig. 105.8). However, in most cases there are still substantial deviations remaining. Along concave areas, a series of partial-thickness cartilage incisions can be made, parallel to the axis around which cartilage warping is desired (▶ Fig. 105.9). Significant deviations that still remain may be incised and dissected off the contralateral mucosal flap. Finally, the caudal septum can be dissected from the anterior nasal spine (anterior-most portion of the maxillary crest)

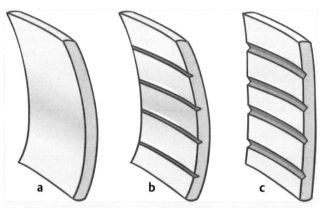

Fig. 105.9 (a–c) Partial-thickness cartilage incisions promote warping away from the cuts around an axis parallel to the cuts and can be used to promote septal cartilage remodeling.

and sutured as necessary to the nasal floor periosteum or through a hole drilled into the maxillary crest.

The main advantage of the Cottle septoplasty is the greater amount of structure preserved and the avoidance of bilateral mucoperichondrial elevation. This makes septal cartilage resorption, saddle nose deformity, and septal hematoma formation less likely. However, cartilage warping can be unpredictable and may leave residual deviations.

Regardless of the specific technique used, once the deviation has been corrected, the mucosal flaps are quilted together with a transseptal 4–0 plain gut running suture and the incision closed with interrupted 4–0 chromic sutures. It is good practice to close mucosal tears with 4–0 plain sutures, and these should always be closed if a tear is located nearby on the contralateral flap. In these cases, or if there is excoriation of the mucosa, soft silicone splints should be placed bilaterally and sutured together with transseptal 2–0 silk sutures. Septal perforations, although uncommon, are most frequently seen after septal surgery. Hemostasis should be excellent at the conclusion of the surgery, and nasal packing is almost always unnecessary because epistaxis after septal surgery is uncommon (1%). It should be noted that because the growth centers of the nose are located in the inferior quadrangular cartilage, driving the growth of the nose during puberty, septal surgery is generally deferred until age 15 years in girls and 16 years in boys; premature disturbance or destruction of the nasal growth centers can stunt full growth of the nose to adult size.

Treatment of Turbinate Hypertrophy

Multiple treatments of turbinate hypertrophy have been described, but these can be categorized loosely as those that reposition, those that remove bone, and those that treat cartilage. Long-term control of mucosal hypertrophy with depo injections of corticosteroids has been described, but the potential for retrograde injection into orbital vessels, causing blindness, has led to the abandonment of this practice. Mucosal and submucosal cauterization of the turbinates will induce some fibrosis after tissue death, leading to some contracture of the mucosal surfaces. However, with all turbinate therapies, untreated mucosa will undergo additional enlargement if the underlying cause of the hypertrophy is not addressed. Fracturing the turbinate (outfracture) laterally alone can relieve nasal obstruction, but only briefly (3 to 6 months). Total removal of the inferior turbinate, addressing both bone and mucosa, was similarly advocated but subsequently abandoned. Total removal frequently injured the sphenopalatine artery at the posterior end of the turbinate, causing massive epistaxis; in the long term, these patients frequently developed atrophic rhinitis. Patient complaints of nasal obstruction after total turbinectomy are believed to be the result of a lack of mucosal surface area for air humidification and the production of mucus, and this is difficult to treat adequately. Partial turbinectomy, removing the anterior one-third of the turbinate, is highly effective in relieving nasal obstruction caused by turbinate enlargement because this area is the narrowest portion of the nasal airway. After the mucosa in this area has been crushed with a curved hemostat to reduce bleeding, the turbinate bone and mucosa are cut with turbinate scissors along the line of crushed tissue, and the anterior turbinate is removed with Takahashi forceps; the stump of the turbinate is cauterized and the remaining turbinate outfractured. A submucous resection of the turbinate is similar, except that the mucosa is first incised along the free turbinate margin, and a flap of mucosa is elevated from the medial side of the turbinate bone. The turbinate bone, along with the mucosa on the lateral side of the turbinate, is crushed and excised. Following cauterization of the stump, the mucosa flap is redraped over the raw surface. Submucous resection of the turbinate generally is associated with less postoperative crusting than partial turbinectomy. Newer technologies, such as radio-frequency ablation and submucosal powered débridement, also lead to less bleeding, but only submucosal powered débridement has been shown to be associated with lasting results similar to those of partial or submucous resection of the turbinates.

Because the inferior turbinates are covered with vasoerectile tissue, bleeding is the most common complication (5%) of turbinate surgery. Adequate hemostasis should be ensured by the conclusion of surgery, and consideration given to the placement of resorbable gelatin hemostatic sponge material over the cut surfaces of the turbinate; however, as with septal surgery, nasal packing is rarely needed. Patients should be started early on saline nasal sprays to diminish crusting and promote rapid mucosal healing. In general, after this and most other nasal surgeries, it is good practice to advise patients against nose blowing, head hanging, and strenuous activities for 10 days after surgery to avoid postoperative epistaxis.

Internal Nasal Valve Surgery

As mentioned earlier, the internal nasal valve is formed by the caudal end of the ULC, inferior turbinate, septum, and nasal floor. Narrowing of the cross-sectional area of the airway will increase air speed and the transnasal pressure gradient. Weakness of any wall of the valve area will lead to inward inspiratory collapse. In addition to correcting any septal deformities and/or turbinate enlargement, increasing the nasal valve angle (between the ULC and the septum, normally approximately 10 to 15 degrees) or strengthening the lateral wall of the valve (the ULC, LLC, and their articulation at the "scroll"; see Chapter 53) can reduce or correct impaired inspiratory airflow.

The two main surgical maneuvers in valve repair are spreader and alar batten grafts. Both can be placed through either closed or open rhinoplasty approaches. To create a spreader graft, cartilage is harvested (ideally from the nasal septum or the conchal bowl) and shaped into a rectangular block 2 to 3 mm wide, 12 to 15 mm long, and 3 to 4 mm thick. It is then sutured in a submucosal pocket after the ULC has been divided from the dorsal septum. This will widen the nasal valve cross-sectional area by maintaining the ULC more laterally (▶ Fig. 105.10). The alar batten graft is used for more flail caudal ULC and LLCs, including their attachment to each other at the scroll. This area may be weak congenitally because of malposition of the lateral crus or (most commonly) because of lateral crus resection during reduction rhinoplasty. An alar batten graft is tucked into a soft-tissue pocket laterally over the piriform aperture while the medial end is sutured to the dorsal septum (▶ Fig. 105.11). The caudal ULC and lateral crus can then be "suspended" by sutures from this more rigid structure, raising the lateral sidewall of the internal valve. Care should be taken to position both grafts precisely so they do not add bulk without adding support. There is generally an excellent "take" of these grafts, and when the procedure is performed properly, they function quite well. However, if not secured properly at its ends, an alar batten graft may add bulk to the valve and cause further inward collapse.

Septal Perforation Repair

The repair of septal perforations uses existing nasal mucosa; therefore, as the size of a perforation increases, the amount of available mucosa is reduced, and ultimately the complete closure rate decreases. A perforation of the septum lacks underlying cartilage as well as mucosa; as a result of both the underlying cause of the perforation and chronic crusting and bleeding at the edge of the perforation, the repair of a septal perforation generally requires the removal of 2 to 3 mm of the rim of the perforation to provide a reasonably healthy tissue edge with which to work.

Perforations smaller than 5 mm in diameter can usually be repaired through an intranasal approach, whereas larger perforations are best repaired through an external rhinoplasty

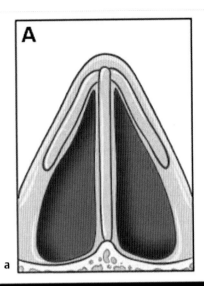
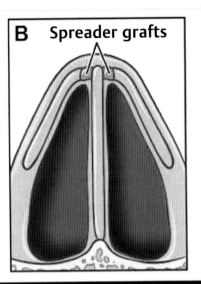
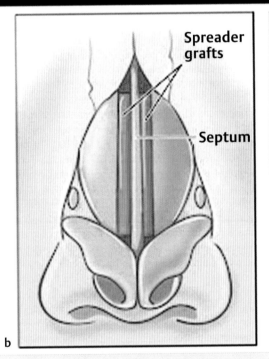
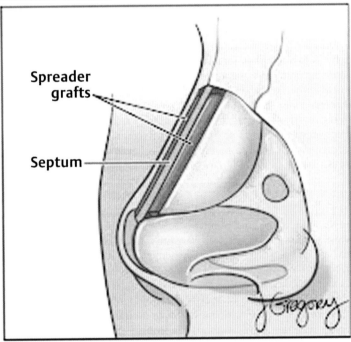

Fig. 105.10 A spreader graft is placed between the upper lateral cartilage and dorsal septum to (a) widen the nasal valve and (b) support the medial upper lateral cartilages.

approach. Regardless of its size, the repair of a septal perforation requires bilateral mucosal flap elevation, advancement/rotation of the mucosal flap edges with suture repair, and placement of an interposition graft of cartilage or soft tissue (temporalis fascia or acellular dermis) between the repaired flaps to serve as a scaffold for full healing. Repaired mucosal flaps are protected with soft silicone splints for 2 to 6 weeks. Perforations smaller than 5 mm can be repaired by first widely elevating the mucosal flaps. Relaxing incisions are made in the flaps in areas where the contralateral flap is intact: superior to the perforation and parallel to the dorsum on one side, posterior to the perforation and perpendicular to the dorsum on the other side. The flaps are then closed in a horizontal fashion on the first side and vertically on the other side, limiting the overlap of the repairs. The relaxing incisions, with cartilage nourished by intact mucosa on the opposite side, will heal by secondary intention. These repairs are generally (> 85%) successful.

Perforations 5 to 25 mm in size can require more extensive surgery. A large, posteriorly based mucosal flap can be elevated from the septum, nasal floor, and lateral sidewall on each side of the nose. A releasing incision is made along the underside of the turbinate origin from the lateral sidewall, allowing free transposition of the flap onto the septum to close the perforation. Denuded bone at the nasal sill occasionally requires coverage with a skin graft. Once the flaps have been used for bilateral perforation repair, the interposition graft is placed, and the mucosal flaps are quilted together with a running plain gut suture.

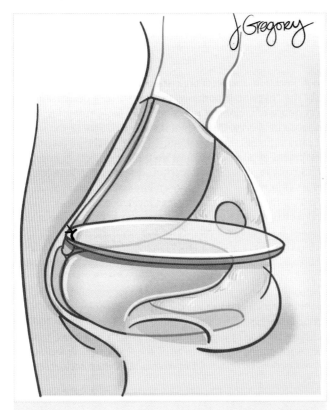

Fig. 105.11 An alar batten graft spans the space between the caudal upper lateral cartilage and cephalic lower lateral cartilage and between the piriform aperture and the dorsal septum to strengthen the internal nasal valve.

Silicone splints are then placed over both sides of the septum, sutured together through the septum, and left in place for 6 weeks. With this technique, perforations of 25 mm or more can be closed successfully in up to 80% of cases.

Caudal septal perforations present a unique problem because it may be impossible to rotate a nasal mucosal flap sufficiently for complete perforation repair. In these cases, a buccal mucosal flap can be raised from the gingivobuccal sulcus and left pedicled near the midline. A temporary fistula is created through the sulcus into the nasal sill medially, and the flap is brought through into the nose. The flap is then sutured to the edges of the perforation. Two to three weeks later, the pedicle can be divided and the fistula closed, but often the pedicle is auto-amputated and the fistula closes spontaneously.

The most likely adverse outcome after septal perforation repair is incomplete closure of the perforation. In general, the success rate for this surgery decreases as the diameter of the perforation increases. Small perforations can be closed in 85 to 90% of cases, whereas the closure of medium to large perforations may be successful in only 75 to 80% of cases. Care should be taken to avoid destabilization of the caudal and (especially) the dorsal cartilage struts, to avoid the development of a saddle nose deformity. Epistaxis from raw mucosal turbinate edges is generally mild and self-limited.

105.8 Roundsmanship

- Nasal obstruction is a sensation of poor nasal inflow that may or may not directly correlate with the physical examination findings.
- Symptoms of nasal obstruction are increased in situations of turbulent nasal airflow.
- Even small changes of nasal diameter in the areas of airway narrowing can have significant effects on nasal airflow.
- Unless otherwise contraindicated, nonsurgical treatment of nasal obstruction should always be tried before surgery is considered.
- Nasal obstruction may be associated with chronic mouth breathing, dry mouth, and snoring; however, it is not a proximate cause of obstructive sleep apnea.
- The success of septal perforation repair is related to the size of the defect; small perforations are usually closed in 85% of cases, whereas medium to large perforations may be closed in only 75 to 80% of cases.
- Killian submucous resection of the septum classically removes maximal amounts of septal cartilage, leaving only the dorsal and caudal struts; conversely, septoplasty preserves maximal amounts of cartilage and relies in part on the natural tendency of the cartilage to warp away from the side of partial-thickness cartilage incisions.

105.9 Recommended Reading

[1] Canady JW. Evaluation of nasal obstruction in rhinoplasty. Plast Reconstr Surg 1994; 94: 555–559
[2] Jessen M, Janzon L. Prevalence of non-allergic nasal complaints in an urban and a rural population in Sweden. Allergy 1989; 44: 582–587
[3] Jessen M, Malm L. Definition, prevalence and development of nasal obstruction. Allergy 1997; 52 Suppl: 3–6
[4] Mladina R. The role of maxillar morphology in the development of pathological septal deformities. Rhinology 1987; 25: 199–205
[5] Teichgraeber JF, Wainwright DJ. The treatment of nasal valve obstruction. Plast Reconstr Surg 1994; 93: 1174–1182, discussion 1183–1184
[6] Constantian MB, Clardy RB. The relative importance of septal and nasal valvular surgery in correcting airway obstruction in primary and secondary rhinoplasty. Plast Reconstr Surg 1996; 98: 38–54, discussion 55–58

106 Allergic and Nonallergic Rhinitis

Jennifer S. Collins

106.1 Introduction

Rhinitis has both allergic and nonallergic causes. It is a complex of symptoms characterized by sneezing, runny nose (rhinorrhea), nasal congestion, and nasal itching. Associated symptoms of itchy and watery eyes, itchy ears, sinus pressure, and sleep disturbance may be present. Frequent comorbidities of rhinitis include sinusitis, asthma, eczema, and recurrent otitis media. Mucus in the nose has protective, barrier, and antimicrobial properties; however, too much mucus causes a major disturbance in daily life. The impact and importance of rhinitis are often diminished by practitioners and patients alike, and the symptoms affect almost every aspect of daily activities. Interference with learning, absenteeism from school and work, and disordered sleep create enormous costs to society. A multimodal approach in treatment is often required, including behavioral modifications, antihistamines, topical corticosteroids, and immunotherapy.

106.2 Incidence of Disease

Rhinitis is an exceedingly common global health problem, affecting a quarter of the world's population (approximately 1.6 billion people). Numbers are similar in the United States; approximately 25% of the population suffers from rhinitis. Allergic rhinitis is the most common type; however, cases of nonallergic rhinitis and cases of mixed allergic and nonallergic rhinitis account for approximately 10%–40% of all adult cases. An estimated 17 million individuals are affected by nonallergic rhinitis.

Rhinitis in all forms represents a terrific cost to society. It is one of the top 10 reasons for consultation in primary care clinics in the United States. In the mid 1990s, $1.8 billion was spent annually on physician visits and medication. Indirect costs to society are equally as great, and in the 1990s there were 811,000 lost work days, 842,000 lost school days, and 4.23 million days of decreased activity.

The incidence of allergic rhinitis varies by sex, age, socioeconomic class, and region. Interestingly, allergic rhinitis was case-reportable in the 19th century. However, over the next 100 years, the incidence of allergic rhinitis rose sharply, and it continues to rise for unknown reasons. Forty percent of children have allergic rhinitis. Boys have the disease more commonly than girls. As we age, for unknown reasons these sexual discrepancies disappear. All races are affected equally. Higher socioeconomic classes often have a higher incidence of disease. The prevalence increases from west to east in Europe. Additionally, English-speaking and industrialized countries have a higher prevalence.

In contrast, nonallergic rhinitis typically presents after the age of 20 years and affects women more than men. We do not see the same differences in prevalence between socioeconomic classes that are seen in allergic rhinitis.

The epidemiology of allergic rhinitis has been the focus of many studies. Factors considered include incidence of childhood infection, socioeconomic status, family size, and birth order. The "hygiene hypothesis" proposes that a decrease in the occurrence of childhood infections may be contributing to the increase in allergy. Other studies show evidence of the impact of early antibiotic and acetaminophen use on the increasing development of allergy. Evidence from birth cohorts in Europe is conflicting regarding the impact of socioeconomic status on allergic rhinitis. When Swedish children were followed in the 1950s, a three- to fourfold higher incidence of allergic rhinitis was noted in those with a higher socioeconomic status. Other studies have shown evidence to the contrary. Furthermore, a protective effect of (1) a large family size, (2) being a middle child, (3) maternal exposure to farm work during pregnancy, and (4) rural upbringing has been shown.

Finally, several risk factors for developing allergic rhinitis were identified and include the following: family history of allergic disease, serum immunoglobulin (IgE) level above 100 kU/L before the age of 6 years, being first-born, male sex, tobacco exposure during the first year of life, early use of antibiotics, positive skin testing to allergens, and higher socioeconomic class.

106.3 Classification of Disease

Rhinitis is classified as allergic, nonallergic inflammatory, or nonallergic noninflammatory. Classification is not exclusive, and approximately 34% of individuals have mixed allergic and nonallergic cases (see Box Types of Rhinitis (p.812)).

Traditionally, allergic rhinitis was classified as seasonal, most commonly caused by aeroallergens and pollens, or perennial, most commonly caused by environmental allergens such as dust mite and cat. This classification posed problems for a number of reasons. Certain allergens vary from year to year, and pollens can last upward of 10 months. Traditional perennial allergens may be in an environment where exposure is intermittent. For example, a patient may be exposed to an animal only at a relative's home.

Types of Rhinitis

- Allergic
  - Seasonal or perennial (chronic), mild intermittent, mild persistent, moderate/severe intermittent, moderate/severe persistent
- Nonallergic inflammatory
  - Occupational, drug-induced, infective, aspirin-sensitive, nonallergic rhinitis with eosinophilia syndrome (NARES), cerebrospinal fluid leak
- Nonallergic noninflammatory
  - Atrophic, emotional, idiopathic, gustatory, hormonal, rhinitis medicamentosa, vasomotor

To account for these issues, the classification of allergic rhinitis was changed to mild intermittent, mild persistent, moderate/

Mild Normal sleep No impairment of daily activities	**Mild** Normal sleep No impairment of daily activities	**Moderate/Severe** Abnormal sleep Impairment of daily activities Troublesome symptoms	**Moderate/Severe** Abnormal sleep Impairment of daily activities Troublesome symptoms
Intermittent < 4 days per week < 4 weeks	**Persistent** > 4 days per week > 4 weeks	**Intermittent** < 4 days per week < 4 weeks	**Persistent** > 4 days per week > 4 weeks

Fig. 106.1 Classification of rhinitis.

severe intermittent, and moderate/severe persistent, depending on the severity (mild or severe) and duration(intermittent or persistent) of symptoms (▶ Fig. 106.1). For symptoms to be mild, there must be normal sleep and no impairment of daily activities.

Nonallergic disease can be either inflammatory or noninflammatory. Inflammatory disease is further divided based on the presence or absence of eosinophilic infiltration as nonallergic rhinitis eosinophilic syndrome (NARES) or occupational/ irritant rhinitis. Noninflammatory disease includes atrophic disease, gustatory rhinitis, hormonal rhinitis, rhinitis medicamentosa, and vasomotor rhinitis.

106.4 The Disease Process

106.4.1 Allergic Rhinitis

The etiology of allergic rhinitis is complex, involving genetic and environmental interactions. The expression of allergic disease is autosomal-dominant with incomplete penetrance. Genes located in the major histocompatibility complex (MHC) on chromosome 6 dictate the production of high levels of IgE by B lymphocytes after allergen challenge. The production of IgE facilitates the allergic reaction. The stimulus for turning on the MHC complex is unknown.

The allergic reaction is a complicated chain of events involving the interaction of many cells, chemical mediators, and cellular products. Our knowledge of events comes from in vitro studies and studies in which humans are exposed to various allergens, after which nasal washes, nasal biopsies, and analysis for cellular infiltrate are performed.

In general, it begins with antigen processing, including dendritic cells, B lymphocytes, and macrophages. Antigen presentation occurs in the lymph node to type 2 CD4 + T helper (CD4 + Th2) lymphocytes. Next, B lymphocytes produce allergen-specific IgM and are signaled by the CD4 + Th2 lymphocytes to isotype switch to IgE. Allergen-specific IgE binds to its high-affinity IgE receptor, Fc epsilon (FcεR), on mast cells and basophils. A complex of allergen-specific IgE bound to FcεR cross-links the receptors, resulting in the subsequent degranulation of basophilic cells (mast cells and basophils). The degranulation products of mast cells and basophils act in cellular recruitment and the inflammatory stimulation seen in individuals with allergic rhinitis. This intricate and forever-evolving process is discussed in further detail below (▶ Fig. 106.2). For complete details, the reader is referred to a textbook of immunology.

Antigen Processing and Presentation

Uptake and allergen processing by the B lymphocytes in the respiratory epithelium begins the process. Specific allergens are loaded into MHC class II and transported to the cell membrane, where they are presented to the CD4 + Th2 lymphocytes. Two signals are required to stimulate the B lymphocytes to produce IgM. The first is recognition of the allergen–MHC complex by CD4 + Th2 lymphocytes via the T-cell receptor. The second is interaction of the CD40 ligand on the CD4 + Th2 lymphocytes and the CD40 receptor on the B lymphocytes. Interaction delivers a critical second signal to the B lymphocytes, triggering the production of allergen-specific IgM. Activation of the CD4 + Th2 lymphocyte results in interleukin-4 (IL-4) cytokine secretion. IL-4 has many actions; however, it is critical in inducing isotype switch from IgM to IgE in B lymphocytes. B lymphocytes mature into long-lived plasma cells dedicated to the production of allergen-specific IgE.

Stimulation of basophilic cells: Preformed, circulating, allergen-specific IgE binds to the high-affinity FcεR on basophilic cells, mast cells, and basophils. When free allergen binds to the allergen-specific IgE–FcεR on the cell membrane, crossing-linking of these receptors occurs. Cross-linking results in (1) the immediate degranulation of preformed mediators, primarily histamine, within the mast cell or basophil; and (2) activation of phospholipase A2 in the cell membrane (▶ Fig. 106.2).

Basophilic cells release multiple chemicals, including exoglycosidases, tumor necrosis factor-α (TNF- α), and the granule-associated products tryptase (only in the mast cells), chymase, peroxidase, and arylsulfatase B, into the epithelium. These chemicals result in increased vascular permeability, vasodilation of the nasal mucosa, and direct stimulation of sensory nerve fibers, causing the acute symptoms of rhinitis: itch, sneeze, rhinorrhea, and nasal congestion. Histamine is the primary mediator of these events, which are referred to as the early-phase response.

Cross-linking of the FcεR also results in the transcription of cytokines and the initiation of arachidonic acid metabolism. Secretion of these cytokines and chemokines amplifies the allergic reaction. The production of vasoactive agents and cytokines, including IL-1, IL-2, IL-3, IL-4, IL-5, IL-6, granulocyte–monocyte colony-stimulating factor (GM-CSF), and TNF- α, promotes chemotaxis, proliferation, IgE production, and activation of a cellular infiltrate in the nasal mucosa, further contributing to the allergic response (see Box Cytokines and Effects in an Allergic Reaction (p.814)). Cellular mixture is a combination of eosinophils, T and B lymphocytes, and mast cells. In particular, IL-5 is

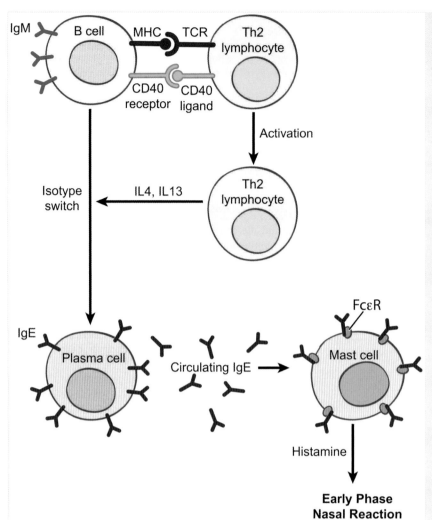

Fig. 106.2 The pathophysiology of allergic rhinitis. *FcεR*, Fc epsilon receptor; *Ig*, immunoglobulin; *IL*, interleukin; *MHC*, major histocompatibility complex; *TCR*, T-cell receptor; *Th2*, type 2 CD4 + T helper lymphocyte.

fundamental to eosinophil proliferation, survival, and chemotaxis in the nasal mucosa. The degranulation of eosinophils releases highly toxic oxygen radicals and proteins that damage the nasal epithelium.

Cytokines and Effects in an Allergic Reaction

- Interleukin-2: activation of T and B cells
- Interleukin-4: autoproliferation of T cells, activation of B cells, and recruitment of inflammatory cells
- Interleukin-5: recruitment and proliferation of eosinophils
- Interleukin-13: recruitment and proliferation of eosinophils

Arachidonic acid metabolites are potent mediators of the allergic reaction. Cross-linking of FcεR activates phospholipase A2, releasing arachidonic acid from the cell membrane. Arachidonic acid is metabolized via two separate pathways: (1) the cyclooxygenase pathway to form prostaglandin A2 and (2) the thromboxane or the lipoxygenase pathway to form leukotrienes (see ▶ Fig. 106.3). Products of this cascade are responsible for nasal congestion, neutrophilic infiltrate, vasodilation, and cellular chemotaxis.

Fifty percent of individuals with allergic rhinitis will experience a second-phase reaction 2 to 6 hours later, called the late-phase response. We believe that basophils are responsible for the late-phase response because nasal washes from these patients reveal increases in the same mediators involved in the early-phase response, with the exception of prostaglandin D2, given that basophils do not produce prostaglandin D2 while they are present in the nasal mucosa after allergen challenge.

Two other important factors contributing to the symptoms of allergic rhinitis are nasal priming and nasal hyperreactivity. Nasal priming occurs with chronic exposure to allergen, resulting in chronic inflammatory changes. Lower and lower thresholds of allergen are required to stimulate rhinitis in these individuals. Additionally, the chronic inflammatory changes result in nasal hyperreactivity, whereby nonspecific irritants, such as strong odors, pollution, and smoke, cause symptoms of rhinitis.

Environmental influences are additional important considerations in the development of allergic rhinitis. Of particular interest is the activation of protease-activated receptors. There are four types of protease-activated receptors; types 2 and 4 are important in allergic disease. These receptors are seven transmembrane G protein coupled receptors widely expressed on many types of cells, including those of the respiratory mucosa. Stimulation of these receptors is irreversible and is accom-

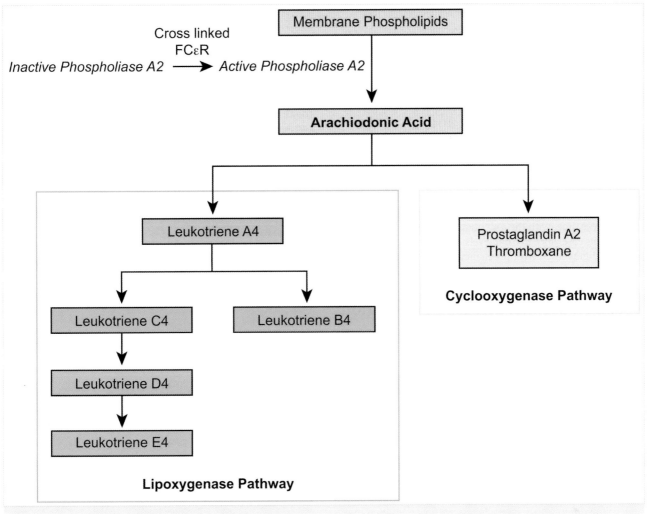

Fig. 106.3 The arachidonic acid cascade. *FcεR*, Fc epsilon receptor.

plished by endogenous and exogenous serine proteases. Endogenous proteases include tryptase, a degranulation product of mast cells and eosinophils; exogenous proteases include dust mite, *Alternaria*, *Aspergillus*, and cockroach. Stimulation of these receptors results in increased IgE production, angiogenesis, scarring, leukocyte infiltration, and airway hyperresponsiveness. The overall effect of stimulation of these receptors is that environmental allergens are able to penetrate into the mucosal layer. Exposure to exogenous proteases early on may be a risk factor for the development of allergic disease.

106.4.2 Nonallergic Rhinitis

The causes of nonallergic rhinitis are varied and depend on the cause. In general, we know little about its development and/or causes.

Autonomic dysregulation is common to all types of nonallergic rhinitis. Autonomic dysregulation is characterized by an exaggerated or diminished neural response to typical triggers. In normal anatomy, parasympathetic neurons contain acetylcholine, peptide histidine, and vasoactive intestinal peptide. Secretion of these neuropeptides into the nasal epithelium causes vasodilation of capillaries and tissue, resulting in rhinorrhea. In contrast, sympathetic neurons contain norepinephrine and neuropeptide Y. Secretion of these neuropeptides leads to vasoconstriction, resulting in congestion.

In noninflammatory forms of rhinitis, abnormality of the autonomic nervous system leads to increased rhinorrhea (parasympathetic stimulation) and/or congestion (sympathetic stimulation). Additionally, there is a heightened response to nonspecific triggers (environmental irritants), histamine, and cold stimulation of the extremities and nasal mucosa, as well as a decreased response to vasoconstrictive stimuli. For example, patients with gustatory rhinitis have symptoms when they ingest spicy foods. These events result in increased concentrations of intranasal neuropeptides and symptomatology.

Local intranasal allergen-specific IgE was recently identified as playing a potential role in the pathophysiology of nonallergic rhinitis. Despite normal levels of total IgE and negative results of skin prick testing and serum testing for allergic sensitization in some patients with nonallergic rhinitis, intranasal washes from these patients revealed local allergen-specific IgE. Additionally, increased levels of high-affinity FcεR were found in some patients with nonallergic rhinitis. Finally, 50% of these individuals experienced an increase in rhinitis symptoms with dust mite allergen challenge. This suggests that a local allergic reaction may be causing symptoms not detected by traditional testing methods.

In pregnancy-induced rhinitis, a history of smoking and IgE sensitization to dust mite may play a role, although this is unclear. Some studies suggest that nonallergic rhinitis may precede the development of allergic rhinitis.

106.4.3 Natural History and Progression

The key events that cause rhinitis to start and stop are elusive. Studies that followed college students with allergic rhinitis over 23 years showed a trend decreasing symptoms and disease over time. In contrast, the symptoms of nonallergic rhinitis tend to worsen over time, with the exception of hormone-induced rhinitis. In this case, once thyroid levels are normalized or delivery is induced in women with pregnancy-induced rhinitis, the rhinitis symptoms resolve.

106.4.4 Potential Disease Complications

Psychosocial and medical complications are associated with rhinitis. Embarrassment, social isolation, sleep disturbance, poor school and work performance, and interference with daily activities are significant complications of disease and should be addressed thoroughly. Medical complications include chronic serous otitis media, eustachian tube dysfunction, perforated tympanic membrane, and rhinosinusitis (both acute and chronic).

Importantly, allergic rhinitis is commonly associated with other disease processes, such as asthma, sinusitis, eczema, and recurrent otitis media. Both nonallergic rhinitis and allergic rhinitis of childhood are associated with a two- to fourfold increase in the risk for the development of asthma in children and young adults. Early intervention with immunotherapy in children may prevent the development of asthma.

Nonallergic rhinitis with eosinophilia syndrome (NARES) may be a risk factor for the development of aspirin-exacerbated respiratory disease; however, this relationship is unclear.

Allergic rhinitis and nonallergic rhinitis are associated risk factors for chronic rhinosinusitis. However, we do not know if there is a risk that untreated disease will progress to chronic rhinosinusitis (see Chapter 107 for more details).

106.5 Medical Evaluation

A thorough history is the key to differentiating allergic from nonallergic rhinitis (see Box Highlights of an Allergy History (p.816)). Allergy is the most common cause of rhinitis, and allergic rhinitis should be ruled out before rhinitis with other causes is considered and treated. Important clues in the history that suggest allergic causes are seasonal exacerbations, triggers on exposure to certain substances, and resolution when the exacerbating substance is removed. The onset of nonallergic disease is at a later age, and nasal congestion and postnasal drainage are more prominent in nonallergic rhinitis. Exacerbating factors suggesting autonomic dysregulation are often noted in nonallergic disease, including temperature changes, food, and nonspecific irritants like strong odors and smoke. Hormonal conditions, including hypothyroidism and the changes associated with pregnancy, may cause nonallergic rhinitis. Pregnancy-induced rhinitis occurs in the second to third trimester, was not present before pregnancy, and resolves within 2 weeks after delivery. Finally, the development of symptoms in association with a new medication may provide an important clue in the history and suggest medication-induced rhinitis (see Box Medications That May Cause Nonallergic Rhinitis (p.816)). Treatment-resistant disease and unilateral symptoms of congestion, pain, and pressure are red flags for a more severe disease process such as cerebrospinal fluid leak or malignancy. The presence of these signs warrants further work-up.

Highlights of an Allergy History

- Establish the main complaint: nasal congestion, pruritus, rhinorrhea, sneezing, decreased sense of smell.
- Establish the duration: Did the symptoms start gradually or acutely? Is there a history of symptoms during childhood? Is there a history of head trauma?
- Establish the frequency of symptoms: intermittent, chronic, seasonal, with known exposures (e.g., at work, school).
- Are the symptoms unilateral or bilateral?
- Are there alleviating or aggravating factors?
- What symptoms are associated? Sleep disturbance, postnasal drip, fever, cough, sinus pressure, tooth pain, loss of smell or hearing?
- How severe are the symptoms? Do they affect daily life, sleep, work, or school activities?
- Is there a history of eczema, asthma, food allergy, or oral allergy?
- Is there a family history of allergic disease?
- Are there exposures in the environment that might be contributing to symptoms (e.g., animals, feathers, mold, leaks, job exposures, tobacco)?
- Which medications have been tried in the past? Have they been tried in combination? Were they being used correctly?

Medications That May Cause Nonallergic Rhinitis

- Analgesics: nonsteroidals, aspirin
- Antihypertensives: angiotensin-converting enzyme inhibitors, amiloride, β-blockers
- Psychotropics: risperidone, chlorpromazine, amitriptyline
- Phosphodiesterase type 5 inhibitors: sildenafil, tadalafil, vardenafil
- Others: cocaine, gabapentin, catecholamines, imidazoles

106.5.1 Presenting Complaints, Clinical Findings, Physical Examination, Testing

Regardless of the cause, patients who have rhinitis present with a symptom complex of nasal congestion, rhinorrhea, nasal pruritus, and/or sneezing. There are many associated symptoms, including sleep disturbance, itchy and watery eyes, ear pain or pressure, diminished or lost sense of smell, postnasal drip, and cough, that are important to describe. Diminished quality of life is a major factor as symptoms of fatigue, depression, and embarrassment are common.

A general head and neck examination should be performed in all patients with rhinitis. Observe for the presence of allergic stigmata: "allergic shiners" (dark circles under the eyes), the "allergic salute" (a transverse supratip crease caused by habitual upward nose wiping), boggy or edematous turbinates and nasal mucosa, nasal polyps, deviated septum, internal nasal valve collapse, and cobblestoning. Nasal endoscopy provides a detailed and complete examination of the nasal cavity. A rigid or flexible endoscope allows the examiner to visualize the middle meatus, eustachian tube, nasal polyps, sphenoethmoid recess, and posterior choanae, which cannot be visualized during direct observation with a nasal speculum. This is particularly important in the identification of polyps, masses, and adenoid hypertrophy.

Skin prick testing is helpful in providing clues of allergic sensitization. The total serum IgE and allergen-specific IgE levels in the blood provides supportive data for the cause of rhinitis and aid in determining appropriate treatment. The results of these tests may guide treatment toward avoidance and immunotherapy.

Treatment-resistant disease may require radiographic imaging, including sinus X-rays and noncontrast computed tomography (CT) of the sinuses. X-rays are inadequate to quantify sinus disease, and CT is the gold standard.

106.5.2 Differential Diagnosis

The differential diagnosis of rhinitis includes allergic rhinitis, nonallergic rhinitis, rhinitis caused by mechanical factors, granulomatous diseases, defects in cilia, neoplastic diseases, and cerebrospinal fluid rhinorrhea (see Box Differential Diagnosis of Rhinitis (p.817)).

106.6 Treatment

The treatment of allergic rhinitis involves the avoidance of triggers, pharmacotherapy, and immunotherapy. The treatment of nonallergic rhinitis involves avoidance, pharmacotherapy, and surgery (▶ Table 106.1 and ▶ Fig. 106.4; see Box Treatment of Nonallergic Rhinitis (p.817)).

Differential Diagnosis of Rhinitis

- Allergic: intermittent and chronic
- Nonallergic, inflammatory: atrophic, emotional, idiopathic, gustatory, hormonal, rhinitis medicamentosa, vasomotor
- Nonallergic, noninflammatory: occupational, drug-induced (cocaine), aspirin-sensitive, nonallergic rhinitis eosinophilic syndrome (NARES)
- Nasal polyposis
- Mechanical factors: septal deviation, foreign body, choanal atresia, adenoidal hypertrophy, external valve collapse.
- Granulomatous diseases: sarcoidosis, Wegener granulomatosis, malignant midline granuloma
- Defect in ciliary function: primary ciliary dyskinesia
- Neoplastic diseases: malignant or benign
- Cerebrospinal fluid rhinorrhea: traumatic or spontaneous
- Infective: viral, bacterial, fungal, parasitic

Treatment of Nonallergic Rhinitis

- Inflammatory
  - NARES: topical intranasal corticosteroids, decongestants, and antihistamines
  - Irritant/occupational: exposure avoidance, topical intranasal corticosteroids, decongestants, antihistamines
- Drug-induced: exposure avoidance
- Noninflammatory
  - Atrophic: débridement, nasal lavage, topical antibiotic creams
  - Vasomotor: ipratroprium bromide, intranasal corticosteroids
  - Hormonal: chromones
  - Rhinitis medicamentosa: weaning regimen overlapped with intranasal corticosteroids

Table 106.1 Medications for the treatment of rhinitis

	Sneezing	Rhinorrhea	Nasal obstruction	Nasal pruritus	Ocular symptoms
H₁ antihistamines					
Oral	2+	2+	1+	3+	2+
Intranasal	2+	2+	1+	2+	-
Intraocular	-	-	-	-	3+
Corticosteroids	3+	3+	3+	2+	2+
Cromoglycates					
Intranasal	1+	1+	1+	1+	-
Intraocular	-	-	-	-	2+
Anticholinergics	-	2+	-	-	-
Antileukotrienes	-	1+	2+	-	2+

Source: Adapted from Al Sayyad JJ, Fedorowicz Z, Alhashimi D, Jamal A. Topical nasal steroids for intermittent and persistent allergic rhinitis in children. Cochrane Database Syst Rev 2007;(1):CD003163.

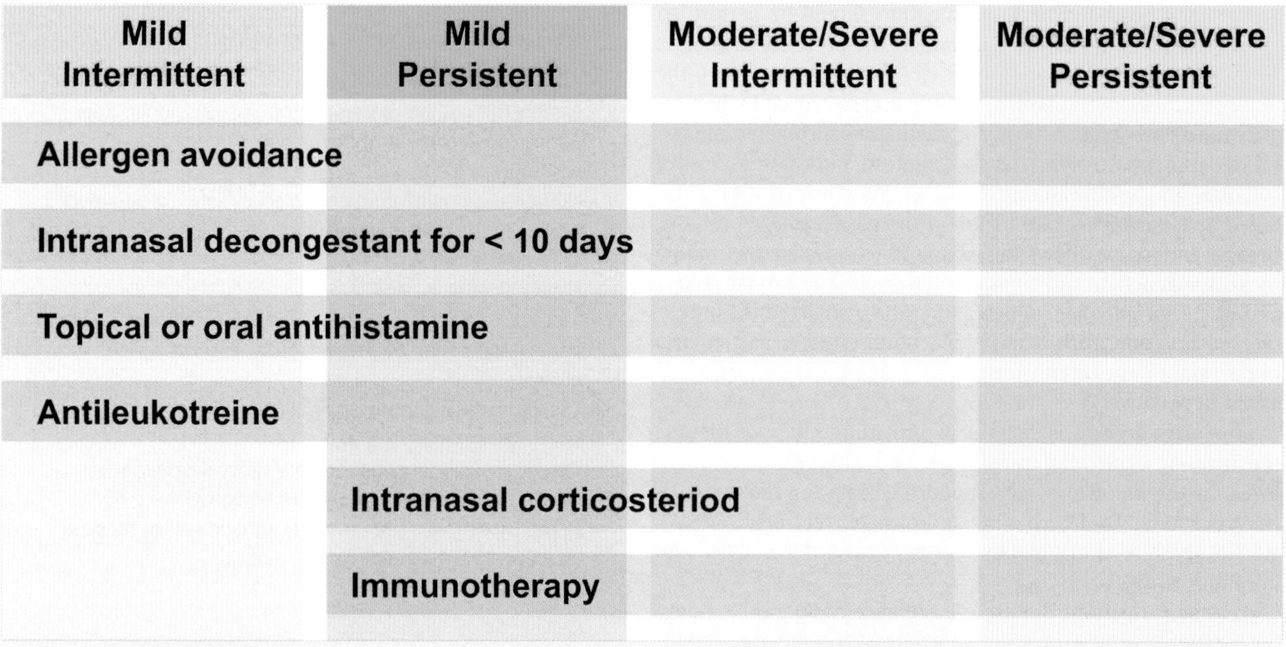

Mild Intermittent	Mild Persistent	Moderate/Severe Intermittent	Moderate/Severe Persistent
Allergen avoidance			
Intranasal decongestant for < 10 days			
Topical or oral antihistamine			
Antileukotreine			
	Intranasal corticosteriod		
	Immunotherapy		

Fig. 106.4 Treatment of allergic rhinitis. (Source: Data from Orban N, Saleh H, Durham S. Allergic and non-allergic rhinitis. In: Adkinson NF Jr, Bochner BS, Busse WW, Holgate ST, Lemanske RF Jr, Simons FER, eds. Middleton's Allergy: Principles & Practice. 7th ed. Philadelphia, PA: Mosby Elsevier; 2009:973–990.)

The first-line treatment for both allergic and nonallergic rhinitis should focus on the avoidance of any identified triggers. All patients should be counseled on appropriate avoidance techniques. This can be done best by an allergist/immunologist.

In most individuals, pharmacotherapy is required and should be tailored based on symptomatology. Individuals with mild intermittent disease will most likely be managed effectively with one therapy. Others, with more severe disease, will require a multimodal approach. Treatment during pregnancy and nursing requires special attention. Most antihistamines and topical intranasal corticosteroids are pregnancy class C. Of note, diphenhydramine, montelukast, and budesonide for inhalation are pregnancy class B. All medications used in the treatment of rhinitis are secreted into the breast milk, and caution should be used.

Immunotherapy is an important aspect in the treatment of allergic rhinitis. Consideration for the initiation of immunotherapy requires the presence of both symptoms on allergen exposure and allergen-specific IgE. Important factors to be noted before the initiation of therapy include inadequate symptom control with medications, compliance with the medical regimen, cost of the medications, and exposure. Immunotherapy reduces symptoms in approximately 80 to 85% of individuals and has the potential to alter the immune response in a semipermanent way. In general, patients experience symptom relief after 6 months of therapy. Published guidelines on adequate dosing should be followed. The duration of treatment affects efficacy, and studies suggest that a minimum of 3 to 5 years is required to achieve a lasting effect. Individuals on immunotherapy should be monitored yearly for symptom improvement. Importantly, some studies suggest that immunotherapy in children may prevent the progression of airway disease to asthma. Finally, cautious use in certain groups of patients is warranted,

including persons with preexisting autoimmune disease or HIV infection, those on β-blocker therapy, and pregnant women.

Uncontrolled case series have reported on the role of surgical interventions in the treatment of nonallergic rhinitis. Patients who have symptoms that are difficult to treat and who are unresponsive to a multimodal approach of 6 to 12 months of pharmacotherapy should be considered candidates for surgical intervention. Turbinectomy is beneficial when severe nasal congestion is present. In the past, vidian nerve resection, electrocoagulation of the anterior ethmoidal nerve, and sphenopalatine ganglion block were used; however, none of these techniques has been shown to have long-term benefits. Additionally, some patients experienced persistent pain, which outweighed any benefit of the procedure.

106.7 Roundsmanship

- Rhinitis is a symptom complex characterized by rhinorrhea, sneezing, congestion, and nasal pruritus.
- There are allergic, nonallergic, and mixed causes of rhinitis; rhinitis with nonallergic causes is a diagnosis of exclusion.
- Risk factors for the development of allergic rhinitis are family history of allergic disease, serum IgE level above 100 kU/L before the age of 6 years, being first-born, male sex, tobacco exposure during the first year of life, early use of antibiotics, positive result of skin testing with allergens, and higher socioeconomic class.
- Comorbidities are asthma, eczema, sinusitis, and otitis media.
- Allergic rhinitis is caused by a classic type I IgE-mediated response; nonallergic rhinitis is caused by autonomic dysregulation.
- Treatment is multimodal and includes corticosteroids, antihistamines, and immunotherapy.

106.8 Recommended Reading

[1] Jacobsen L, Niggemann B, Dreborg S et al. Specific immunotherapy has long-term preventive effect of seasonal and perennial asthma: 10-year follow-up on the PAT study. Allergy 2007; 62: 943–948

[2] Linna O, Kokkonen J, Lukin M. A 10-year prognosis for childhood allergic rhinitis. Acta Paediatr 1992; 81: 100–102

[3] Orban N, Saleh H, Durham S. Allergic and non-allergic rhinitis. In: Adkinson NF Jr, Bochner BS, Busse WW, Holgate ST, Lemanske RF Jr, Simons FER, eds. Middleton's Allergy: Principles & Practice. 7th ed.Philadelphia, PA: Mosby Elevier; 2009:973–990

[4] Rondon C, Romero JJ, Lopez S et al. Local IgE production and positive nasal provocation test in patients with persistent nonallergic rhinitis. J Allergy Clin Immunol 2007; 119: 899–905

[5] U.S. Department of Health and Human Services. Agency for Healthcare Research and Quality. Management of Allergic and Nonallergic Rhinitis. May 2002. AHQR publication 02:E023. Summary, Evidence Report/Technology Assessment: No 54

[6] Wallace DV, Dykewicz MS, Bernstein DI et alJoint Task Force on PracticeAmerican Academy of Allerg,Asthma and ImmunologyAmerican Costhma and ImmunologyJoint Council of Alhma and Immunology. The diagnosis and management of rhinitis: an updated practice parameter. J Allergy Clin Immunol 2008; 122 Suppl: S1–S84

107 Medical Management of Acute and Chronic Sinusitis

Jennifer S. Collins

107.1 Introduction

Acute rhinosinusitis (ARS) and chronic rhinosinusitis (CRS) are distinct entities. ARS is an acute infection lasting anywhere up to 12 weeks. In contrast, CRS comprises a spectrum of disease and complex pathophysiology resulting in more than 12 weeks of inflammation of the paranasal passages and nasal mucosa despite medical management. Previously, the treatment of CRS varied depending on the specialty; however, multidisciplinary expert panels put forth guidelines to direct diagnosis and management. The term *sinusitis* was changed to *rhinosinusitis* to reflect the involvement of the nasal and paranasal passages. The causes of CRS are varied and often elusive. Differences in allergic sensitization, cellular infiltrates, cytokine expression, and the host response account for the spectrum of disease seen in CRS. The approach to treatment is multidisciplinary and involves medical and surgical modalities.

107.2 Incidence

ARS is the most common health care complaint in the United States, affecting over 1 billion people annually. The cost to society, however, is difficult to estimate because the costs of ARS are often grouped with the costs of CRS. ARS is associated with a significantly decreased quality of life, absence from school and/or work, and increased medication use.

CRS is one of the three most common health care complaints and accounts for 22 million office visits and 500,000 emergency department visits per year in the United States. CRS affects approximately 15 to 30% of the U.S. population, and over $3.5 bil-

lion is spent annually in its treatment. CRS is subdivided into CRS with nasal polyposis, CRS without nasal polyposis, and allergic fungal sinusitis (AFS). CRS without nasal polyposis is the most common form of the disease, accounting for 60 to 65% of all cases. Cases of CRS without polyposis develop in males and females in equal numbers.

CRS with nasal polyposis accounts for 20 to 35% of all cases. The prevalence of CRS with nasal polyposis is higher in patients who have certain comorbidities, including allergic rhinitis, asthma, aspirin sensitivity, and cystic fibrosis. Aspirin sensitivity is present in 15% of patients with nasal polyps. The late onset of asthma frequently coincides with the development of polyposis in adults. Approximately 40% of patients with cystic fibrosis will have nasal polyps, and any child or adolescent with nasal polyps should be screened for cystic fibrosis. More males are affected than females, and the incidence of polyps increases after the age of 40 years.

AFS accounts for 8 to 12% of all cases of CRS. AFS typically develops in young adults. The mean age of patients at diagnosis is 22 years, and males and females are equally affected. Atopy is a risk factor for disease, and elevated levels of total immunoglobulin E (IgE) are common. There appears to be a geographic distribution of disease, with a higher incidence in more temperate climates.

107.3 Classification of Disease

The classification of rhinosinusitis is based on the duration of illness and the presence or absence of nasal polyps (▶ Fig. 107.1). Rhinosinusitis can be acute, recurrent acute, or

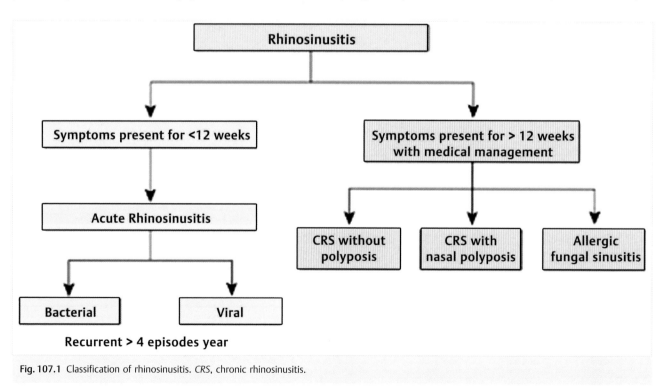

Fig. 107.1 Classification of rhinosinusitis. *CRS*, chronic rhinosinusitis.

chronic, or it can be an acute exacerbation of chronic disease. Acute sinusitis is sudden in onset, and symptoms can last for up to 12 weeks. Typically, if the symptoms worsen over 5 days or last longer than 10 days, bacterial causes should be suspected. In children, viral infections are more common than bacterial infections. Recurrent rhinosinusitis is characterized by the occurrence of more than four separate episodes in a single year. Individuals are symptom-free between episodes.

CRS is characterized by symptoms lasting longer than 12 weeks despite adequate medical treatment. CRS is further classified by the presence or absence of nasal polyps and by whether criteria consistent with AFS have been met (allergic mucin, fungal hyphae, and IgE-mediated fungal allergy). Patients with AFS are immunocompetent and tend to have allergic rhinitis.

107.4 Applied Anatomy

The exact function of the paranasal sinuses is unknown; however, it is probable that they function to humidify and warm inspired air, lighten the skull, improve vocal resonance, absorb shock to the face or skull, and secrete mucus to assist with air filtration. The paranasal sinuses develop as outpouchings of the nasal mucosa. Narrow ostia connect the sinuses to the nasal cavity. The sinuses are lined with ciliated pseudostratified columnar epithelium with goblet cells. The ostia of the frontal, maxillary, and anterior ethmoid sinuses open into the ostiomeatal complex. The ostiomeatal complex includes the area lateral to the middle meatus and middle turbinate. This unit is important because all sinuses except the sphenoid and posterior ethmoid sinuses drain through it. The posterior ethmoid and sphenoid sinuses open into the superior meatus and sphenoethmoid recess. Anything that obstructs this unit causes symptoms of facial pain/pressure, congestion and disturbance of normal airflow.

The sinus epithelium is important because it is thinner and less richly supplied with blood vessels and glands than the mucosa of the nasal cavity. Overlying the mucosal layer is a thin layer of mucus infiltrated with cilia, comprising a mucociliary clearance system. The mucociliary clearance system enables the mucosa to remove particulate matter and debris. Particular matter is trapped in this bilayered system and mobilized by beating cilia that sweep mucus toward the ostia clearing debris. Hair cells in the nasal cavity actively catch particles larger than 15 μm in size. These particles are trapped within the mucosal layer.

107.5 Etiology and Pathophysiology

107.5.1 Acute Rhinosinusitis

The most common cause of acute sinusitis is viral infection. Only 0.2 to 5% of these episodes are further complicated by bacterial infections. The most common viruses causing acute sinusitis are rhinovirus, influenza virus, and parainfluenza virus.

Direct inoculation of the nasal mucosa with virus results in ARS. Viral replication begins immediately, and detectable levels are present within nasal secretions in less than 10 hours.

Symptoms begin approximately 12 hours after inoculation. Virus spreads via direct and systemic methods throughout the paranasal sinuses, causing inflammation. Neutrophils infiltrate the mucosal layer in response to infection, resulting in hypersecretion of glands, increased vascular permeability, and transudation of fluid into the nasal cavity and sinuses. Direct toxic effects of some viruses and/or bacteria on the nasal cilia can disrupt the mucociliary clearance system. Mucosal edema, distortion of the composition of normal mucous secretions, and ciliary dyskinesia result in sinus obstruction.

The most common cause of damaged epithelium is viral infection, which allows the normal respiratory flora to infect the nasal epithelium. This typically occurs 2 to 4 days after the initial viral infection. Normal respiratory flora are typical responsible for infection and include coagulase-negative staphylococci, *Corynebacterium*, and *Staphylococcus aureus*. The most commonly associated bacteria are *Streptococcus pneumoniae, Haemophilus influenzae*, and *Moraxella catarrhalis*. Seventy-five percent of cases of bacterial sinusitis are caused by *S. pneumoniae* and *H. influenzae*. Microaerophilic and anaerobic bacteria should be considered in the setting of dental root infection with extension into the maxillary sinus cavity. Importantly, viral infections are not the only cause of damaged epithelium. Allergic disease, mechanical obstruction (e.g., obstruction of the ostiomeatal complex, septal deviation), swimming, odontogenic infections, intranasal cocaine use, impaired mucociliary clearance (e.g., cystic fibrosis, cilia dysfunction), and immunodeficiency should be considered in appropriate patient groups.

107.5.2 Chronic Rhinosinusitis

The etiology of chronic rhinosinusitis remains elusive despite intensive research efforts. In the past, a lack of clear terminology and varied approaches to treatment and study designs contributed to our lack of understanding of these disorders.

We do know that CRS is a heterogeneous group of disorders with different etiologies and pathophysiologies. Complex inflammatory changes occur within the nasal and paranasal mucosa of individuals with CRS. Differences in inflammatory cell infiltrate, type of T-lymphocyte response, and remodeling patterns result in the assorted disease patterns observed. In general, the role of bacterial infection is controversial in CRS both with and without nasal polyposis. Immunodeficiency should be ruled out in patients who have CRS without nasal polyposis. Aspirin intolerance is seen only in CRS with nasal polyposis. IgE and IgG sensitization to fungus and allergic mucin must be present in AFS.

Risk factors for CRS include allergic rhinitis, active tobacco use, immunodeficiency, defects in mucociliary clearance, recurrent viral upper respiratory tract infections, systemic diseases (including Churg-Strauss vasculitis, sarcoidosis, and Wegener granulomatosis), and anatomical abnormalities (▶ Table 107.1). Allergic sensitization to dust mites, cockroach, and molds is common in all diseases. This may be in part due to the activation of protease-activated receptors (see Chapter 106 for a full discussion). Importantly, any cause of obstruction (e.g., nasal polyps, granulomatous disease, allergies, mucosal edema) of the ostiomeatal complex can create the sensation of facial pain/pressure, nasal congestion, or disturbance of airflow.

Table 107.1 Risk factors for the development of chronic rhinosinusitis

CRS risk factor	CRS with polyps	CRS without polyps	AFS
Atopy	Common	Common	Common
Immunodeficiency	Rare	Immunodeficiency in 12%	Rare
Environmental irritants	Common	Common	Common
Aspirin intolerance	Common	Rare	Rare

Abbreviations: AFS, acute fungal sinusitis; CRS, chronic rhinosinusitis.

Each disease entity has a distinctive pathophysiology and response to treatment and management, and each is discussed separately below.

Chronic Rhinosinusitis without Nasal Polyposis

CRS without nasal polyposis is the most common form of CRS. Various processes, including allergic, nonallergic, immunologic, and structural abnormalities, contribute to the chronic changes observed in the mucosal layer. Analysis of sinus fluid reveals a neutrophilic infiltrate, as well as low numbers of eosinophils, mast cells, and basophils. Histologic changes within the mucosal lining include thickening of the basement membrane, edema, and hyperplasia of goblet cells, in addition to a submucosal monocytic infiltrate of neutrophils and macrophages.

The cytokine profile in CRS without nasal polyposis is unique. There are elevations in CD4+T helper type 1 (CD4+Th1) lymphocytes and in the lymphocyte-associated cytokines interleukin-1β (IL-1β), interferon-γ (IFN- γ), tumor necrosis factor-α (TNF-α), and TGF-β. Elevations in TGF-β result in the characteristic fibrosis seen in CRS without nasal polyposis. This cytokine is noticeably absent in CRS with nasal polyposis.

The role of chronic bacterial infections in CRS without nasal polyposis is debatable. Studies are flawed based on patient selection, culture techniques, and prior use of antibiotics. Recurrent and/or chronic bacterial infections can cause permanent anatomical changes. Additionally, biofilms, which are complex aggregations of bacteria embedded within an extracellular polymeric substance on chronically inflamed surfaces, may be present. These microcommunities of bacteria are difficult to eradicate and may represent a hidden source of chronic infection impenetrable to antibiotics.

Chronic Rhinosinusitis with Nasal Polyposis

CRS with nasal polyposis is the second most common form of CRS. By definition, polyps must be present. Polyps are edematous, semitranslucent masses in the nasal and paranasal cavities that have no pain fibers. There are two types of polyps: ethmoidal and antrochoanal. Ethmoidal polyps are more common, emerge from the ethmoid sinus via the ostiomeatal complex, and are bilateral. In contrast, antrochoanal polyps arise from the maxillary sinus via the middle meatus and are unilateral. Antrochoanal polyps are less likely to be associated with allergic disease. The presence of unilateral polyps is uncommon and should prompt consideration of more severe diseases, including inverted papilloma and nasal tumors.

Epithelial damage with a thickened basement membrane is shown on histologic analysis of polyp tissue. There is an eosinophilic infiltrate, and stromal tissue exhibits fibrosis or edematous changes, decreased blood supply and glands, and the absence of neural tissue. Mature polyps may form pseudocysts with surrounding fibroblasts and inflammatory cells.

The inflammatory infiltrate in the nasal polyps associated with cystic fibrosis and primary ciliary dyskinesia shows important differences. Unlike the eosinophilic infiltrate typically seen in CRS with nasal polyposis, a characteristic lymphocytic and neutrophilic infiltrate is revealed by histology. The presence of this cellular infiltrate in children warrants further screening for disease.

The cellular and cytokine profile of CRS with nasal polyps is in contrast to that of CRS without polyps. It is characterized by activated CD4+Th2 lymphocytes, increased amounts of IL-5, IL-13, and histamine, and the absence of TGF-β. IL-5 and Il-13 are key cytokines in the proliferation and survival of eosinophils. The cellular and cytokine profile suggests an allergic role in the development of nasal polyps.

Although the cause of nasal polyposis remains elusive, it probably represents a heterogeneous disease with varied causes, including allergic and infectious conditions and aspirin sensitivity. Allergic disease most likely plays a role, and up to 60% of patients with polyposis will have atopy. Additionally, IgE is increased locally within polyp tissue. Local IgE production and a type I mediated allergic reaction may have a role in the etiology of polyposis.

A unique subset of adult patients with nasal polyposis will also have aspirin hypersensitivity with aspirin-induced bronchial asthma and/or aspirin- induced rhinitis (aspirin-exacerbated respiratory disease, or Samter triad). In this group of patients, defective inhibition of the cyclo-oxygenase enzyme 1 in the arachidonic acid pathway (see Chapter 106 for full details) leads to the excessive production of leukotrienes. The ingestion of aspirin leads to symptoms of bronchospasm and/or rhinitis 30 minutes to 4 hours later. Symptoms of worsening asthma, nasal polyposis, and rhinitis develop slowly over years despite avoidance of the drug. It is important to recognize and treat this sensitivity because these patients are 10 times more likely to require repeated surgical interventions for polyp management. The diagnosis is made through challenge testing with lysine-aspirin by an allergist/immunologist. Desensitization and long-term aspirin therapy can be effective in treating up to 60% of these patients.

The role of bacterial infections and superantigen activation of T lymphocytes remains controversial. Studies reveal an increased colonization of *S. aureus* in patients with nasal polyps or aspirin-sensitive asthma versus controls. *S. aureus* produces enterotoxins that act as superantigens, directly activating T lymphocytes, as in atopic dermatitis. Additionally, patients with nasal polyposis have an increased local presence of *S. aureus* enterotoxin–specific IgE. This IgE is not found in the serum, suggesting that a type I mediated allergic reaction to the enterotoxin may occur within the paranasal sinuses, resulting in the formation of nasal polyps.

Allergic Fungal Sinusitis

The pathophysiology of AFS is poorly defined, but it is most likely an infectious and/or allergic process. Presumably, a complex reaction involving both an immediate type I IgE-mediated response and a type III immune complex deposition (fungus-specific IgG and fungus) results in mucosal edema, eosinophilic infiltration, and allergic mucin formation. Supporting evidence includes the presence of fungus-specific IgE and IgG locally and in the serum. Total levels of quantitative IgE are elevated in these patients. Histology of the nasal mucosa reveals eosinophilic infiltrates.

Allergic mucin, present within the sinuses, varies in color and can be anywhere from light tan to dark green, with a thick, peanut butter–like consistency. The function is unknown. Allergic mucin contains degranulated eosinophils, Charcot-Leyden crystals (a by-product of degranulated eosinophils), and fungal hyphae. The identification of fungal hyphae in allergic mucin is problematic, and these are not always identified.

The fungi associated with AFS are ubiquitous in the environment and are in the dematiaceous family. Because of their omnipresence in the environment, exposure does not equate with disease. In children and adults, *Bipolaris* and *Curvularia* are most commonly isolated from the mucin. In adults, *Alternaria* and *Aspergillus* species also play an important role.

107.6 Medical Evaluation

107.6.1 Presenting Complaints

A thorough history is important in the diagnosis of ARS and CRS. Information regarding the nature and duration of symptoms, triggers, alleviating factors, and comorbid conditions (including allergy, asthma, recurrent infections, intranasal drug use, and aspirin sensitivity), as well as previous treatment, imaging, and surgical interventions, should be documented.

Disease is classified based on symptom duration and the presence or absence of nasal polyps and/or allergic mucin. The symptoms of ARS and CRS are similar and divided into major and minor symptoms (▶ Table 107.2). Any patient reporting changes in vision, diplopia, severe headache, proptosis, or focal neurologic or meningeal signs requires immediate attention and imaging. Patients with ARS report the acute onset of nasal congestion and obstruction, purulent nasal discharge, maxillary tooth discomfort, and facial pain or pressure that is worse when they bend forward. Symptoms start acutely and can last anywhere up to 12 weeks.

CRS commonly starts with an indolent infection or upper respiratory infection that never resolves. Two of the four hallmark signs of CRS (mucopurulent drainage, nasal obstruction, facial pain/pressure, and decreased sense of smell) must be present in

Table 107.2 Symptoms associated with rhinosinusitis

Major symptoms	Minor symptoms
Facial pain/pressure	Headache
Facial congestion/fullness	Fever
Nasal obstruction/blockage	Halitosis
Nasal discharge/purulence; postnasal drip	Fatigue
Hyposmia/anosmia	Dental pain
	Cough
	Ear pain/pressure/fullness

Source: Adapted from Lanza DC, Kennedy DW. Adult rhinosinusitis defined. Otolaryngol Head Neck Surg 1997;117(3 Pt 2):S1–S7.

conjunction with mucosal inflammation for CRS to be considered. Each type of CRS can present characteristically in its own way (see Box Typical Presenting Symptoms of Chronic Rhinosinusitis (p.823)).

Typical Presenting Symptoms of Chronic Rhinosinusitis

- Chronic rhinosinusitis with nasal polyposis: gradual worsening of nasal congestion and facial fullness/pressure; diminished sense of smell
- Chronic rhinosinusitis without nasal polyposis: facial pressure/pain and mucopurulent drainage in association with fatigue and low-grade fever
- Allergic fungal sinusitis: dramatic or progressive presentation of severe nasal congestion, facial asymmetry, and vision changes; thick, "peanut butter–like" discharge from the nose

107.6.2 Physical Examination and Evaluation

An algorithm for the diagnosis and work-up of ARS and CRS is presented in ▶ Fig. 107.2. In general, a head and neck examination should be done for all patients presenting with these complaints. Observe for signs of facial asymmetry, proptosis, inflamed nasal mucosa, visible polyps, septal deviation, mucupulent drainage, and lymphadenopathy. Rigid or flexible endoscopy is useful in both ARS and CRS and should be performed if available. The observation of obstruction of the ostiomeatal complex is important.

No radiologic imaging is necessary for ARS. If symptoms persist despite treatment, multiplanar noncontrast sinus computed topography (CT) is the imaging modality of choice to document CRS. Sinus mucosal thickening, sinus ostial obstruction, polyps, and radiographic evidence of sinus opacification are commonly documented in CRS.

The presence of certain diseases warrants further work-up. All children with nasal polyposis should be screened for cystic fibrosis. Patients with recurrent ARS and symptoms of allergic disease and all patients with CRS should undergo an allergy work-up that includes an evaluation for sensitivity to perennial and seasonal allergens and measurement of total IgE. Desensitization should be considered for patients who have CRS with

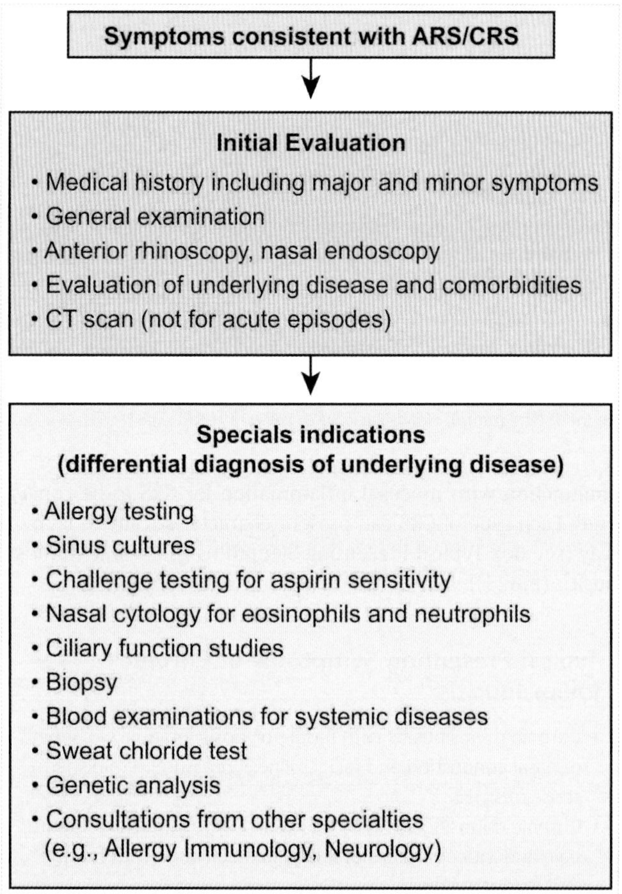

Symptoms consistent with ARS/CRS

Initial Evaluation

- Medical history including major and minor symptoms
- General examination
- Anterior rhinoscopy, nasal endoscopy
- Evaluation of underlying disease and comorbidities
- CT scan (not for acute episodes)

Specials indications
(differential diagnosis of underlying disease)

- Allergy testing
- Sinus cultures
- Challenge testing for aspirin sensitivity
- Nasal cytology for eosinophils and neutrophils
- Ciliary function studies
- Biopsy
- Blood examinations for systemic diseases
- Sweat chloride test
- Genetic analysis
- Consultations from other specialties
  (e.g., Allergy Immunology, Neurology)

Fig. 107.2 Algorithm for the diagnosis of rhinosinusitis. *ARS*, acute rhinosinusitis; *CRS*, chronic rhinosinusitis; *CT*, computed tomography. Source: Data from Bachert C, Gevaert P, van Cauwengerge P. Nasal polyps and rhinosinusitis. In: Adkinson NF Jr, Bochner BS, Busse WW, Holgate ST, Lemanske RF Jr, Simons FER, eds. Middleton's Allergy: Principles & Practice. 7th ed. Philadelphia, PA: Mosby Elsevier; 2009:991–1003.

nasal polyposis and a history of aspirin sensitivity. Finally, patients who have recurrent ARS and CRS without nasal polyposis should be evaluated for possible acquired immunodeficiency (isolated and total hypogammaglobulinemia, selective IgA deficiency, HIV). As advancements are made regarding our knowledge and treatment options for innate immunodeficiencies, including toll-like receptor defects and disorders of complement, defects in these pathways should also be considered. Referral to a specialist in allergy/immunology is indicated for laboratory evaluation, including screening for HIV infection, quantitative immunoglobulins, IgG subclasses, and evidence of immune titers to vaccines.

Nasal swabs provide little or no useful information regarding culprit bacteria and should not be performed. Bacterial cultures via direct sinus puncture or middle meatal endoscopy in patients with CRS can be helpful.

107.6.3 Differential Diagnosis

The differential diagnosis of rhinosinusitis includes allergic and nonallergic rhinitis, atypical migraine headaches, disorders of

olfaction, gastroesophageal reflux, laryngeal reflux, and head and neck tumors.

107.7 Medical Treatment

The goal of medical and surgical treatment is to reduce symptoms and eradicate bacterial and/or fungal infections. Symptom reduction can be achieved with supportive measures of humidified air, saline nasal rinses, and oral decongestants. Monotherapy with intranasal corticosteroids may provide beneficial symptom reduction in ARS and is indicated in combination with other medications in CRS. Maximal treatment of allergic disease should be instituted in appropriate patients (▶ Table 107.3).

107.7.1 Acute Rhinosinusitis

The benefits of antibiotic therapy in ARS are controversial, and it should be initiated with care. Cochrane Reviews report a limited role for antibiotics in ARS. In patients who have symptoms for less than 7 days, antibiotic treatment shows a small benefit. When antibiotic therapy is initiated, the first-line treatment against normal respiratory flora should guide the choice. Patients who have fever above 101°F, moderate to severe facial pain, progression of symptoms, or symptoms for longer than 14 days should be treated with antibiotics. Typically, amoxicillin, cephalosporins, and sulfa-based antibiotics are adequate. Macrolide antibiotics may also be used as an alternative.

107.7.2 Chronic Rhinosinusitis

In contrast to ARS, combination therapy with oral or topical corticosteroids and oral antibiotics is recommended for the treatment of CRS with and without nasal polyposis. Treatment with oral corticosteroids is often required. The optimal dosing regimen and treatment duration vary among practitioners.

All patients with CRS should be treated maximally for allergic disease, and immunotherapy should be considered. Identified immunodeficiencies and systemic illnesses contributing to the disease process should be addressed.

Antibiotic choice is guided by drug allergy status, prior use of antibiotics, and culture results. Amoxicillin/clavulanate is the first-line choice in patients without penicillin allergy; in allergic patients, a quinolone antibiotic may be used safely. Clindamycin is an alternative antibiotic for penicillin-allergic patients or for those in whom methicillin-resistant *S. aureus* infection is suspected. Treatment typically is continued for at least 3 weeks to induce remission of symptoms. Multiple courses in combination with surgical intervention are often required.

Patients who have aspirin-sensitive CRS with nasal polyposis may benefit from aspirin desensitization, leukotriene synthesis inhibitors (zileuton), and/or leukotriene antagonists (montelukast), although these are off-label uses. Patients on zileuton should be monitored for evidence of hepatic impairment. Aspirin challenge should be considered in patients with a history of allergy and/or asthma. Other systemic causes of nasal polyposis should be considered and treated.

The treatment of AFS begins with surgery, and medical management follows. Oral corticosteroids are the backbone of

Table 107.3 Medical treatment of acute and chronic sinusitis

Condition	Treatment	
ARS	Antibiotics for 10–14 days	First line: amoxicillin, cephalosporins, trimethoprim/sulfamethoxazole, macrolides Second line: amoxicillin/clavulanate, levofloxacin
	Supportive therapy	Intranasal corticosteroids, nasal decongestants, saline rinses
	Antibiotics for 3 weeks	Amoxicillin/clavulanate, clindamycin
CRS without nasal polyposis	Corticosteroids	Intranasal corticosteroid sprays ± systemic corticosteroids
	Allergy treatment	Maximize medical therapy for allergies Consider immunotherapy
	Supportive therapy	Saline rinses and nasal sprays
	Antibiotics for 3 weeks	Amoxicillin/clavulanate, clindamycin
CRS with nasal polyposis	Corticosteroids	Intranasal corticosteroid sprays Prednisone 40 mg/d for 5 days, then 20 mg for 5 days, then 10 mg for 5 days, then 5 mg for 5 days
	Allergy treatment	Maximize medical therapy for allergies Consider immunotherapy
	Supportive therapy	Saline rinses and nasal sprays
	Leukotriene synthesis inhibitor/leukotriene antagonist	Monteleukast and zileuton
	Allergy treatment	Allergy evaluation and maximal therapy Aspirin challenge and desensitization
	Surgery	Disease-directed sinus surgery
AFS	Corticosteroids	Prednisone 0.5 mg/kg for several weeks, tapered to 10 mg/d; continue taper to lowest dose that maintains remission Intranasal corticosteroid sprays
	Allergy treatment	Immunotherapy
	Antifungals	Oral and topical nasal rinses controversial

Abbreviations: AFS, acute fungal sinusitis; ARS, acute rhinosinusitis; CRS, chronic rhinosinusitis.

maintaining remission in the postsurgical patient. Immunomodulation and suppression of the inflammatory response by the corticosteroids reduces relapses. Dosing guidelines and duration of treatment are unknown and should be based on patient symptom scores.

Immunotherapy may be a powerful treatment tool in AFS. Previously, it was felt that immunotherapy with the inciting fungus might exacerbate disease and should be removed from the treatment regimen. However, three small studies showed that patients receiving immunotherapy for fungus for 3 to 5 years had a reduction in symptom scores, were able to stop oral and topical corticosteroid use, and had decreased relapse rates up to 3 years later. A promising treatment option may be recombinant IgE (omalizumab) therapy. Limited case reports/series suggest decreases in symptom scores and relapse rates.

In the past, oral antifungal therapies for AFS were proposed; however, they have serious side effects, and there is little evidence to support their use. Topical antifungal therapy may add some benefit in reducing symptoms of AFS, but studies are lacking.

107.8 Prognosis

ARS typically responds well to first-line antibiotics. Progression of symptoms or lack of improvement after 7 days of therapy should be considered treatment failure. In these cases, the empiric use of second-line antibiotics (levofloxacin or amoxicillin/clavulanate) is indicated.

Patients should be counseled that CRS is a chronic illness requiring lifelong treatment. The rates of lifelong exacerbations and recurrences of CRS despite maximal therapy are high, particularly in patients with AFS, 10 to 100% of whom experience recurrence.

107.9 Complications

All patients with ARS or CRS may develop complications secondary to a delay in diagnosis, recurrence of disease, or treatment failure. Transient hyposmia or anosmia is typically reversible in cases of virally induced ARS. In rare cases of bacterial ARS,

Table 107.4 Orbital complications of sinusitis

Group	Complication	Description
I	Preseptal cellulitis	Inflammatory edema limited to area anterior to orbital septum, caused by restricted venous drainage; eyelids swollen but not tender, extraocular muscle movement unaffected, no chemosis; proptosis, if present, mild
II	Orbital cellulitis	Pronounced edema of orbital (retroseptal) contents without abscess; chemosis and proptosis, but vision loss rare
III	Subperiosteal abscess	Abscess between bone and periosteum of orbital bone; orbital contents displaced inferolaterally by accumulating pus; chemosis and proptosis; decreased vision or ocular mobility rare
IV	Orbital abscess	Intraorbital collection of pus; severe proptosis, ophthalmoplegia, and vision loss common
V	Cavernous sinus thrombosis	Bilateral ocular signs, fever, headache, photophobia, proptosis, ophthalmoplegia, rapid vision loss, and involvement of cranial nerves III, IV, V_1, V_2, and VI

abscesses involving the eye, meninges, or brain may ensue. The most common complication of ARS is progression to CRS.

The most worrisome complication of CRS is extension to and/or involvement of the brain via the orbit (▶ Table 107.4). Signs of extension into the orbit include proptosis (forward displacement of the eye), gaze restriction, decreased visual acuity, color vision defects, and an afferent pupillary defect. These symptoms in the setting of fever, headache, and cranial nerve palsy suggest the most troublesome complication, the development of cavernous sinus thrombosis.

Alternative complications and concerns of therapy are medication side effects, the emergence of antibiotic resistance, and the development of antibiotic allergy.

107.10 Roundsmanship

- ARS and CRS differ in the duration of illness but have similar symptoms.
- Most cases of ARS are virally induced; patients with symptoms lasting less than 2 weeks do not require antibiotics.
- CRS represents a spectrum of disease depending on the immunologic reaction to environmental allergens and infection.
- CRS is a chronic relapsing and remitting disease.
- CRS is strongly associated with allergic disease.
- The four cardinal signs of CRS are mucopurlent drainage, nasal obstruction, hyposmia/anosmia, and facial pain/pressure; two must be present along with evidence of mucosal inflammation to consider CRS.

- Treatment of ARS rarely requires antibiotics; treatment of CRS requires a multi-modal approach including medical and surgery.
- Signs of proptosis, gaze restriction, decreased visual acuity, color vision defects, and an afferent papillary defect should alert you the possibility of orbital extension and immediate work up should ensue.

107.11 Recommended Reading

[1] Ahovuo-Saloranta A, Borisenko OV, Kovanen N et al. Antibiotics for acute maxillary sinusitis. Cochrane Database Syst Rev 2008; 16: CD000243

[2] Bachert C, Gevaert P, van Cauwengerge P. Nasal polyps and rhinosinusitis. In: Adkinson NF Jr, Bochner BS, Busse WW, Holgate ST, Lemanske RF Jr, Simons FER, eds. Middleton's Allergy: Principles & Practice. 7th ed. Philadelphia, PA: Mosby Elsevier; 2009:991–1003

[3] Dykewicz MS, Hamilos DL. Rhinitis and sinusitis. J Allergy Clin Immunol 2010; 125 Suppl 2: S103–S115

[4] Lanza DC, Kennedy DW. Adult rhinosinusitis defined. Otolaryngol Head Neck Surg 1997; 117: S1–S7

[5] Sweet JM, Stevenson DD, Simon RA, Mathison DA. Long-term effects of aspirin desensitization—treatment for aspirin-sensitive rhinosinusitis-asthma. J Allergy Clin Immunol 1990; 85: 59–65

[6] Slavin RG, Spector SL, Bernstein IL et alAmerican Academy of Allergy, Asthma and ImmunologyAmerican College of Allergy, Asthma and ImmunologyJoint Council of Allergy, Asthma and Immunology. The diagnosis and management of sinusitis: a practice parameter update. J Allergy Clin Immunol 2005; 116 Suppl: S13–S47

[7] Rosenfeld RM, Andes D, Bhattacharyya N et al. Clinical practice guidelines: adult sinusitis. Otolaryngol Head Neck Surg 2007; 137: 1–31

[8] J Allergy Clin Immunol 1998; 102; (6 Pt 2): S107–S144

108 Surgical Treatment of Sinusitis

Steven David Schaefer

108.1 Introduction

Over the past century or more, surgical procedures to treat sinusitis and related diseases evolved. The various procedures can be roughly divided into those that entered the affected sinus through face and those that approached the paranasal sinuses through the nose. The former (open) techniques progressed over a century to become well standardized by the 1950s, and although less often employed today, they remain useful in selected patients. The latter (*intranasal*, referred to as *endonasal* in Europe) techniques were more problematic in their early development and required modern optical telescopes or endoscopes to visualize and operate on all four sinuses through the nose. The popularization of these less invasive techniques awaited not only the development of surgical endoscopes, but also a convergence of our understanding of sinus anatomy, pathophysiology, and function.

108.2 Open Surgical Techniques

108.2.1 Maxillary Sinus

Before the popularization of endoscopic intranasal sinus surgery, the Caldwell-Luc operation was the most common procedure for the treatment of maxillary sinus disease. This procedure was indicated to treat chronic infection refractory to medical treatment, cysts or polyps within the maxillary sinus, dental fistulas, and fractures of the maxilla; it was also used for decompression or removal of the floor of the orbit in the treatment of thyroid eye disease and biopsy of neoplasm. The procedure consists of two elements: fenestration of the canine fossa and creation of the nasal antral window (antrostomy). The procedure begins with an incision beneath the upper lip in the gingivobuccal sulcus above the roots of the teeth. The soft tissue over the maxilla is elevated in the subperiosteal plane to expose and preserve the infraorbital nerve. The anterior wall of the maxillary sinus is opened (fenestrated) with various types of

surgical burs, bone-cutting forceps, or osteotomes (▶ Fig. 108.1). Cysts, polyps, tumors, or diseased mucous membrane is then removed through the fenestration. Next, an approximately 1 x 2-cm rectangle of bone beneath the inferior turbinate is removed to create a nasoantral window. The procedure is completed with reapproximation of the soft tissue over the anterior maxillary sinus wall with suture.

108.2.2 Frontal Sinus

Chronic frontal sinusitis and polyps, mucoceles, and tumors within the frontal sinus have been addressed with multiple approaches to the frontal sinus (▶ Fig. 108.2). Perhaps the first form of frontal sinus surgery was trephination, a fenestration of the anterior wall of the sinus through a skin incision over the brow. Because in the preantibiotic era the treatment of osteomyelitis often required the débridement of infected bone, the next procedure in the evolution of the treatment of infections within the frontal sinus was the Riedel operation. In 1898, Riedel described ablation of the frontal sinus by removal of its anterior wall and floor (▶ Fig. 108.3). This permitted wide access through the forehead skin but left a significant cosmetic deformity. Killian modified the Riedel procedure in 1904 by preserving a 10-mm-wide bridge of bone at the supraorbital rim, which resulted in less disfiguration than the Riedel operation. In the same year, Hoffman described opening the anterior wall of the frontal sinus while preserving its blood supply via the periosteum of the frontal bone, a procedure later termed *osteoplastic frontal sinusotomy*. In 1914, Lothrop described a combined intranasal and external procedure that resulted in removal of the floor of the entire frontal sinus, as well as removal of the adjacent nasal septum and intra-frontal sinus septum. This procedure would await the advent of the surgical microscope and endoscopes to be repopularized as an intranasal frontal sinus drainage procedure. Using an external approach to remove the cells of the ethmoid sinus and the middle turbinate, Lynch in 1920 described removal of the floor of the frontal sinus. Over

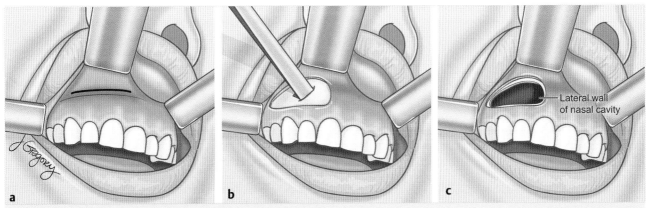

Fig. 108.1 Caldwell-Luc procedure. (**a**) Buccal–gingival incision to expose the anterior face of the maxilla. (**b**) The anterior face of the maxillary sinus is exposed, and a surgical chisel is used to create an opening into the maxillary sinus. (**c**) A generous fenestration allows adequate exposure for the removal of mucosa of the right maxillary sinus.

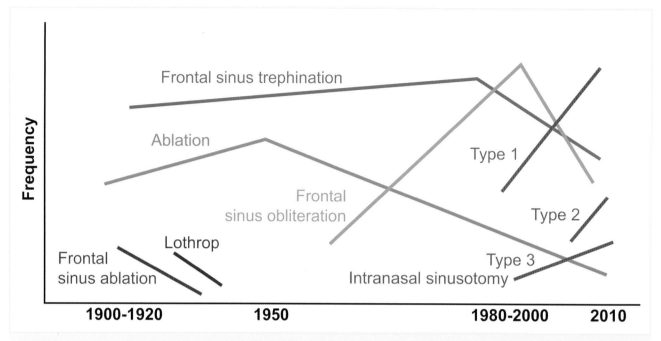

Fig. 108.2 Progression of frontal sinus surgical procedures during the past century. In the early 1900s, ablation, or removal of the anterior, the posterior, or both walls of the frontal sinus, was the most common procedure for the treatment of chronic frontal sinusitis. Trephination was a common form of surgical treatment since the time of the ancient Egyptians. In 1904, Hoffman introduced the osteoplastic frontal sinusotomy, which consisted of opening and replacing the anterior wall of the frontal sinus as a means to access this sinus for treatment. The procedure would later be reintroduced in the 1950s, and for many years it served as the most frequent form of frontal sinusotomy. In 1914, Howard Lothrop proposed draining the frontal sinus into the nose by removing the entire floor of this sinus and the adjacent nasal septum. Beginning in the 1980s, a series of intranasal microscopic and endoscopic frontal sinusotomies was popularized in Europe and later in the United States.

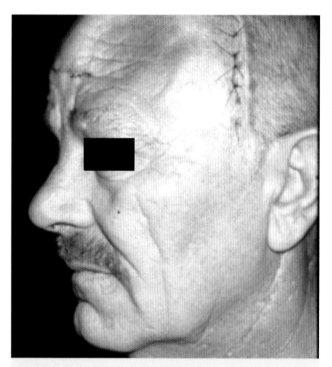

Fig. 108.3 Patient several days after removal of the anterior wall of frontal sinus, or ablation procedure of Riedel, for osteomyelitis of the frontal bone.

the next 60 years, several unsuccessful modifications to the procedure were made in order to avoid collapse of the soft tissue of the adjacent orbit into the drainage pathway into the nose. Although variations of the above procedures are still occasionally used, the next major advance in frontal sinus surgery was to combine the osteoplastic frontal sinusotomy with obliteration of the frontal sinus with fat, as described by Goodale and Montgomery in the 1950s. The procedure uses Hoffman's exposure of the frontal sinus via a vascularized anterior frontal sinus bone–periosteal flap to carefully remove all normal and diseased mucous membrane within the sinus, repair fractures, or remove tumors (▶ Fig. 108.4). The sinus is then obliterated with abdominal fat, which remains partially viable for many years. When performed correctly, this operation has consistently yielded the best long-term results and has been referred to as the gold standard in frontal sinus surgery. However, the advent of optical endoscopes and various intranasal frontal sinus procedures has significantly reduced the use of the osteoplastic frontal sinusotomy.

108.3 Intranasal (Endonasal) Techniques

In the United States, Harris Mosher was an early proponent of intranasal sinus surgery. His anatomical studies of the ethmoid and sphenoid sinuses formed the basis for intranasal ethmoidectomy and sphenoidotomy. Others, such as Howard Lothrop, reported draining the frontal sinus into the nose via

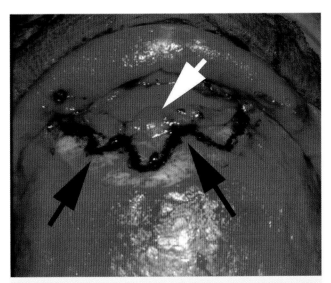

Fig. 108.4 Osteoplastic frontal sinusotomy via a coronal forehead skin incision, as viewed by the surgeon at the head of the table. The outer periosteum (*white arrow*), or pericranium, of the frontal bone remains intact, with the anterior wall of the frontal sinus serving as its blood supply. Thus, the procedure is referred to as an osteoplastic frontal sinusotomy. The osteotomy, or incision into the anterior wall of the frontal sinus, is outlined (*black arrows*), and the anterior wall is incised with fine-cutting burs or saws.

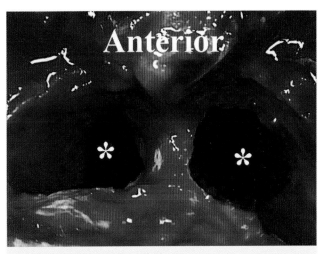

Fig. 108.5 Transfrontal drainage via an osteoplastic frontal sinusotomy into the nose. This so-called marsupialization of the frontal sinus into the nose shares the elements essential to the Lothrop or type III frontal sinusotomy. That is, the floor of the frontal sinus, the intrasinus septum, and the adjacent nasal septum are removed to create a maximal sinusotomy (*asterisks*).

the combination of intranasal removal of the floor of this sinus and an external opening through the brow, or sinusotomy (▶ Fig. 108.5). Because these are difficult procedures to perform with only a headlight and potentially more dangerous than the open approaches, early proponents would later question the wisdom of such surgery. By 1929, Mosher described intranasal ethmoidectomy as "one of the easiest operations with which to kill a patient." Over the next 40 years, relatively few surgeons used intranasal approaches to the sinuses. However, by the early 1980s, Wigand in Germany and Messerklinger in Austria had modified existing intranasal sinus procedures so that they could be performed safely, although not necessarily easily, with the use of endoscopes. Wigand used a headlight and an endoscope to begin his surgery with resection of the middle turbinate to gain exposure to the posterior ethmoid cells and face of the sphenoid sinus. Next, he cannulated the sphenoid sinus ostium, removed the anterior wall of the sphenoid sinus, and performed a total ethmoidectomy. This approach permitted surgery to be performed with the illumination and magnification of endoscopes while the ethmoidectomy was begun posteriorly and the retrograde dissection of the ethmoid cells was directed away from the skull base. Given the statements of Mosher and others, surgeons were well aware of the risk for intracranial injuries during intranasal sinus surgery.

In contrast to this procedure, Messerklinger and Stammberger used their studies of the physiology of the sinuses to apply the optical telescope to modify the anterior ethmoidectomy of Halle. This procedure has the advantage of selectively limiting surgery to the pathologic sinuses. In an anterior-to-posterior approach, the surgery begins with anterior ethmoidectomy and is extended posteriorly depending on the diseased sinuses. The

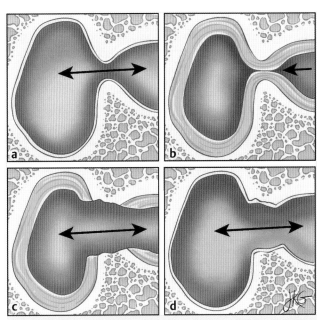

Fig. 108.6 Normal sinus function can be restored following surgical removal of an obstruction to normal ventilation of the sinuses. (**a**) Normal egress of mucus and ventilation of air into a sinus. (**b**) With obstruction of this pathway, the mucous membrane becomes hypertrophic, and sinusitis then develops as a result of stasis of secretions within the sinus. (**c**) The selective removal of the obstructing site by enlarging the ostium of a sinus restores normal ventilation and mucociliary flow. (**d**) Resolution of the mucous membrane hypertrophy and return of normal sinus function.

disadvantage of such a technique is the anterograde dissection of the ethmoid cells and potential penetration of the skull base.

Building upon the concepts of Messerklinger, Wigand, and Stammberger, Kennedy offered the concept of "functional endoscopic surgery" (▶ Fig. 108.6). Such surgery recognizes the

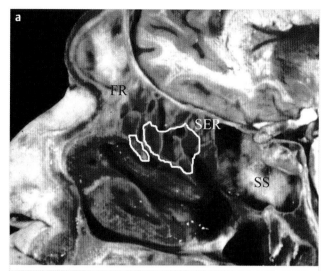

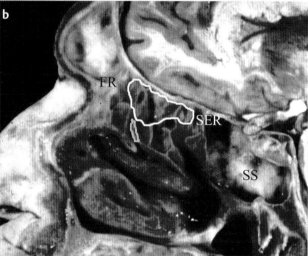

Fig. 108.7 (a) Cadaver section showing removal of the inferior two-thirds of the ethmoid cells and uncinate process (outlined by *white lines*) in the anterior-to-posterior approach during a combined approach to endoscopic intranasal ethmoidectomy. *FR*, frontal recess; *SER*, sphenoethmoid recess; *SS*, sphenoid sinus. **(b)** Sagittal cadaver section shows the retrograde, or posterior-to-anterior, approach to complete the removal of the remaining superior ethmoid cells. Removal of the superior uncinate process is shown in blue. *FR*, frontal recess; *SER*, sphenoethmoid recess; *SS*, sphenoid sinus.

principle of the "potential for reestablishing sinus drainage and mucosal recovery" through correction of the obstructing sinus ostium or isthmus, and removal of devitalized mucous membrane or bone. The goals of the aforementioned surgeons for the treatment of *extensive* sinusitis or polyposis over time became the same, and differed only in regard to such elements as preservation of the middle turbinate and dissection of the ethmoid labyrinth. The combination of these approaches seeks to bring together the salient features of the anterior-to-posterior and posterior-to-anterior approaches, while observing the concept of functional endoscopic sinus surgery (FESS; ▶ Fig. 108.7).

The basic elements of modern intranasal sinus surgery incorporate a *disease- and anatomy-oriented* surgical approach, preserving sinus anatomy and using anatomical relationships to conform to fundamental surgical principles. A disease-oriented, or functional, approach to sinus surgery assumes that in many patients, chronic sinusitis develops from medically irreversible obstruction of the outflow tract of the sinuses. Such obstruction occurs at the narrowest point of communication of a sinus with the nasal cavity, often the infundibulum or ostium of the involved sinus. Surgery is directed toward removing such restrictions to reestablish normal mucociliary flow.

The first step is exposure of the contents of the lateral nasal wall—that is, the maxillary and ethmoid sinuses. A 0-degree endoscope is use to identify and remove the uncinate process (▶ Fig. 108.8). Complete uncinectomy is necessary to begin the anterior-to-posterior exenteration of the inferior ethmoid cells. This permits visualization of the more lateral ethmoid cells and the lamina papyracea. The lamina papyracea should be regarded as a landmark and is exposed through exenteration of the ethmoid cells. The complete removal of the uncinate process should expose the natural ostium of the maxillary sinus (▶ Fig. 108.9). If the ostium cannot be discerned, the uncinate process or polyps are obstructing visualization and should be removed. If the ostium appears normal and there is no intrinsic maxillary sinus disease, it is left intact. If the ostium is small or stenotic, it is inferiorly or posteriorly enlarged with either a débrider or forceps. Disease within the sinus is removed with angulated double-spoon or giraffe forceps.

Next, the inferoanterior wall of the bulla ethmoidalis, or second basal lamella, is removed with microcuret, forceps, or more recently surgical débrider. If disease is limited to the anterior ethmoid sinus, individual cells are exenterated to the basal lamella of the middle turbinate (▶ Fig. 108.10). The superior–anterior ethmoid cells are then removed in retrograde fashion with microcuret, débrider, or forceps under 30- or 45-degree endoscope visualization. *If disease involves the entire ethmoid sinus*, the exenteration continues posteriorly to the face of the sphenoid sinus. *When indicated by disease, the anterior wall of the sphenoid is removed*. Although the sphenoid sinus can be entered medial or lateral to the middle turbinate, we prefer identifying the ostium just inferior to the superior turbinate. The sinusotomy is enlarged with bone-cutting forceps. With the use of a 30- or 45-degree endoscope to visualize the skull base, the residual superior ethmoid cells are exenterated in a posterior-to-anterior or retrograde dissection. Superior cells are removed by grasping or curetting in a pulling motion rather than by directing instruments toward the skull base (▶ Fig. 108.11). This motion, as previously noted, reflects translation of the wisdom of Mosher into modern surgical technique to permit safe intranasal sinus surgery. In the absence of frontal sinusitis, the anterior boundary of the procedure is the ethmoid infundibulum.

In the presence of frontal sinusitis, the location of the obstruction to the outflow tract of the frontal sinus and the presence of intrinsic disease or anatomical variations determine the type of opening or sinusotomy performed. These variations in intranasal frontal sinus surgery are classified as types I, IIa, IIb, and III frontal sinusotomy (Draf types I through III) procedures. The complexity of these procedures results from the developmental competition of the uncinate process and ethmoid cells extending into frontal recess to form the outflow tract of the sinus. A type I sinusotomy removes the anterior ethmoid cells obstructing the outflow tract of the frontal sinus within the frontal recess. The frontal recess is defined as a space bounded

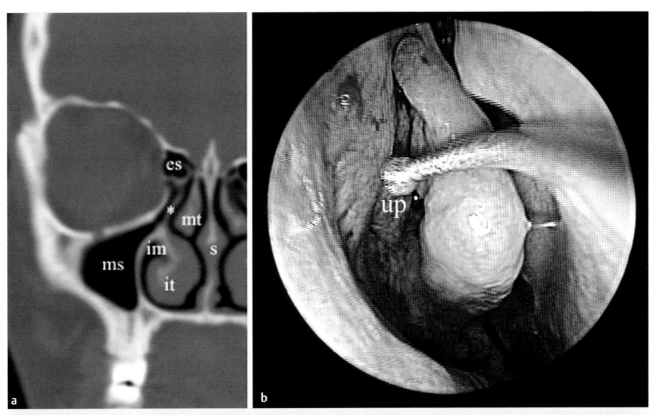

Fig. 108.8 (a) Coronal computed tomographic scan shows relevant landmarks near the right ostiomeatal complex. *asterisk*, uncinate process; *es*, ethmoid air cell; *im*, inferior meatus; *it*, inferior turbinate; *ms*, maxillary sinus; *mt*, middle turbinate; *s*, septum. (b) Intraoperative view of the right middle turbinate (held medially by the curved probe, exposing the uncinate process). The uncinate process forms the anterior and medial boundaries of the ostiomeatal complex and must be completely removed to fully visualize the natural ostium of the maxillary sinus, the lateral ethmoid cells, and the frontal recess cells. *up*, uncinate process.

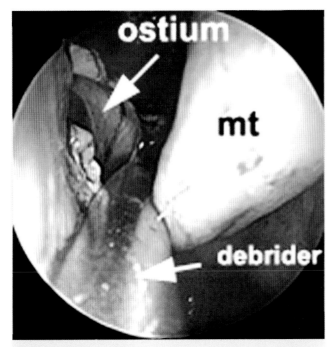

Fig. 108.9 Endoscopic exposure of the right natural ostium of the maxillary sinus after removal of the uncinate process with a débrider. *mt*, middle turbinate.

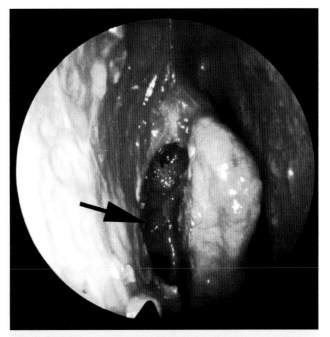

Fig. 108.10 Exposure of the basal lamella (*arrow*) of the middle turbinate after completion of anterior ethmoidectomy.

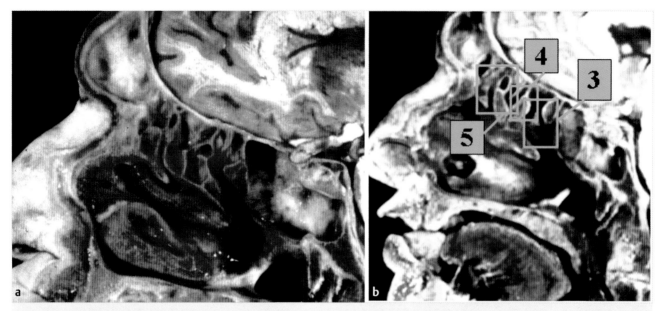

Fig. 108.11 (a,b) Retrograde dissection of the superior ethmoid cells is illustrated in steps 3 through 5.

anteriorly by the pneumatization of the lacrimal bone, posteriorly by the anterior ethmoidal artery, medially by the middle turbinate, and laterally by the lateral nasal wall. A type IIa frontal sinusotomy includes removal of the frontal recess cells and the floor of the frontal sinus bordered by the middle turbinate and lateral nasal wall. The type IIb sinusotomy differs from the type IIa procedure in that it involves total removal of the floor of the sinus. The type III sinusotomy is the most extensive procedure and has three elements: removal of the adjacent superior nasal septum, removal of the entire floor of the frontal sinus, and removal of the intra-frontal sinus septum (▶ Fig. 108.12). The resulting sinusotomy permits maximal drainage of this sinus into the nose. This procedure is also known as the modified Lothrop procedure because it encompasses the elements of the original surgery described in 1914. In recent years, the type III sinusotomy has been increasingly employed for the removal of benign frontal sinus tumors and as a portal to the anterior cranial fossa for the resection of skull base tumors.

108.4 Complications

The most serious complications in sinus surgery involve the orbit and cranium. Both types of complications may be minimized, but not necessarily completely avoided, by careful preoperative evaluation of the patient and the patient's imaging, and by meticulous surgical technique. The preoperative evaluation should include any history of prior sinus surgeries. In such cases, one should inquire about the postoperative course. Surprisingly, patients may not volunteer that after surgery they developed a fever and stiff neck and were admitted to the hospital for intravenous antibiotics, or they may wonder why they had clear fluid dripping from their nose. In both examples, the integrity of the anterior cranial fossa floor was breached. The following should be identified on preoperative imaging: (1) The depth of the olfactory fossa and the plane of the lateral lamella of the cribriform plate. The lateral boundary of the olfactory

fossa is the lateral lamella of the cribriform plate. The deeper the olfactory fossa, the more vertical the lateral lamella becomes. As the lateral lamella becomes more vertical, the likelihood of bony dehiscence of the lamella increases, as does the risk for intracranial injury. (2) The vertical height of the maxillary sinus relative to the vertical height of the ethmoid sinus (▶ Fig. 108.13). In most individuals, the ratio of the vertical height of the ethmoid to the vertical height of the maxillary sinus is 1:2. As that ratio declines to less than 1:2, the "vertically shorter" ethmoid sinus results in less vertical volume or space. Consequently, the working distance within the ethmoid sinus between the floor and the roof is reduced, and the incidence of intracranial injury increases. (3) Bony dehiscence of the carotid artery and optic nerve within the sphenoid sinus. As the sphenoid sinus pneumatizes into the sphenoid bone, there may be little or no bone surrounding the medial borders of both the internal carotid artery and the optic nerve. (4) Expansion of the posterior ethmoid cells into the sphenoid bone. As extramural ethmoid cells pneumatize the sphenoid bone, they present significant surgical hazards. First, these cells may expose the medial surface of the optic nerve, forming what is referred to as an Onodi cell. When this variation is present, the optic nerve will appear as a tubular structure coursing through the lateral wall of the Onodi cell and therefore should be avoided. Extramural ethmoid cells may also expand into the central portion of the sphenoid bone, giving the appearance on coronal computed tomographic (CT) scans of a horizontal septum dividing the sphenoid into a superior and an inferior sinus. At sphenoidotomy, surgeons may erroneously believe that they are within the sphenoid sinus, which is inferior to the extramural ethmoid cell. (5) The posterior–inferior slope of the anterior cranial fossa floor. As a generalization, the anterior cranial fossa floor slopes 15 degrees posteroinferiorly. However, sagittal CT scans reveal that some individuals have either a nearly horizontal floor or an inferior expansion into the roof of the ethmoid sinus. (6) The position and presence of bony dehiscence of the anterior and

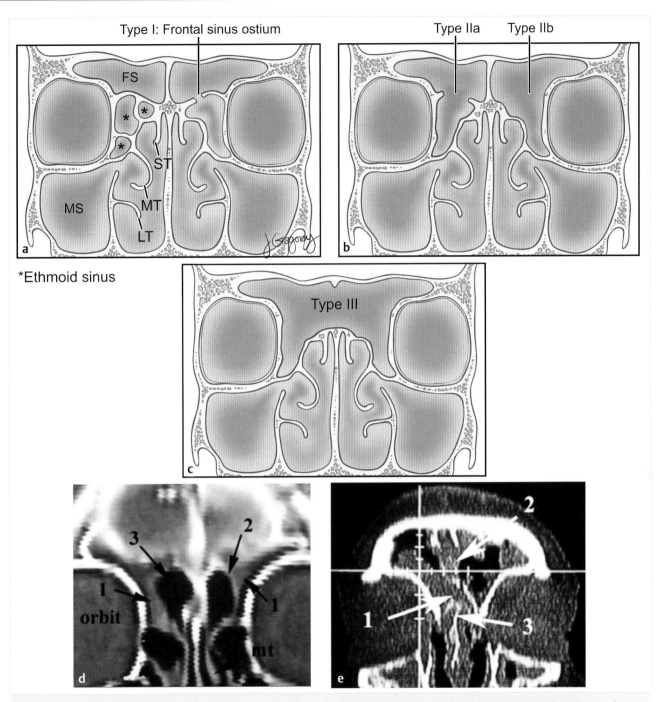

Fig. 108.12 (a) Type I intranasal frontal sinusotomy. This procedure consists of removing the anterior ethmoid cells within the frontal recess that are obstructing the outflow tract of the frontal sinus. Note that the floor of the frontal sinus is not altered in this procedure. *asterisks*, ethmoid sinus; *FS*, frontal sinus; *LT*, lower turbinate; *MT*, middle turbinate; *MS*, maxillary sinus; *ST*, superior turbinate. (b) Type IIa frontal sinusotomy. Unlike in a type I frontal sinusotomy, the floor of the frontal sinus between the lamina papyracea and the middle turbinate is removed. (c) The elements of a type III frontal sinusotomy are removal of the entire floor of both frontal sinuses; the intrasinus septum, which divides the frontal sinus into a left and a right cavity; and the upper nasal septum. (d) Coronal computed tomographic (CT) scan of patient with bilateral frontal sinusitis (*1*) secondary to extension of ethmoid cells (*2*), also described previously as frontal cells, into the floor of the frontal sinus. These ethmoid cells literally balloon into the floor of the frontal sinus and are visible because of the contrast between the mucus in the frontal and ethmoid sinuses (*1*) and the air within the ethmoid or frontal cells (*3*). (e) Intraoperative CT reconstruction using computer-assisted image-guided surgery. In this image, the end of a probe placed within the right frontal sinus is identified at the convergence of the vertical and horizontal lines. To restore drainage of the frontal sinus, the floor of the sinus (*1*) is removed, as are the intrasinus septum (*2*) and the upper nasal septum (*3*).

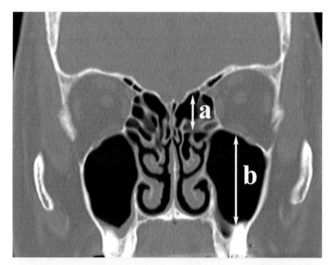

Fig. 108.13 Coronal computed tomographic scan illustrating the vertical relationship of the ethmoid and maxillary sinuses to each other. The potential for intracranial injury increases in those individuals with a relatively "short" vertical height of the ethmoid sinus (*a*) compared with the height of the maxillary sinus (*b*).

posterior ethmoidal arteries. As the ethmoid cells expand into the ethmoid bone during fetal and early postnatal development, these vessels are skeletonized, becoming more vulnerable to injury during surgery. (7) Bony dehiscence of the lamina papyracea. The bony integrity of the lamina varies between individuals, and the lack of an intact lamina makes the orbit more vulnerable to surgical injury. Such injuries are even more likely when surgical débriders are used because the periorbita, orbital fat, and muscles can be aspirated into the débrider.

At surgery, several routine precautions or practices should be employed, including the following: (1) Minimizing intraoperative hemorrhage. Increased intraoperative bleeding increases the risk for complications. Reducing hemorrhage begins several minutes before the actual surgery with the appropriate use of vasoconstrictive agents and the infiltration of all surgical sites with a combination vasoconstrictive–anesthetic agent, such as 1% lidocaine with 1:100,000 epinephrine. (2) Avoiding myopic surgery. In using endoscopes, the novice surgeon tends to place the optic too close to site of surgery and in doing so loses perspective and anatomical awareness of important landmarks. The endoscope is best kept at a slight distance from the point of surgery and brought closer to the site of interest as more magnification is required. (3) Avoiding directing instruments into the skull base. As discussed previously in the section on intranasal ethmoidectomy, as surgery proceeds anteriorly to posteriorly within the nose, instruments must be rotated inferiorly rather than advanced superiorly. This observation is the basis for combining an anterior-to-posterior approach for removal of the majority of the ethmoid cells with a posterior-to-anterior (retrograde) dissection of the remaining superior ethmoid labyrinth. In the latter element of the procedure, instruments are directed away from rather than into the skull base. (4) Controlling bleeding to maintain visualization. Too often, the surgeon may attempt to continue surgery when bleeding obscures the surgical field. In such cases, the nose should be packed with cottonoids and the sites of bleeding cauterized. If bleeding is still problematic, pack that side of the nose and work on the

other side. If this fails, discontinuing surgery is the wisest course.

Intracranial injury is uncommon and variable, and it requires immediate attention. Because the roof of the ethmoid sinus is the floor of the anterior cranial fossa, a violation of this bone is likely to cause cerebrospinal fluid rhinorrhea. Although many methods of repairing such defects have been described, we strongly recommend the placement of fat through the defect and into the subarachnoid space. One continuous piece of fat should be used, with approximately three-quarters of the fat placed intracranially and one-quarter within the nose. This "dumbbell"-shaped fat graft should immediately stop the rhinorrhea. A second graft of either mucous membrane or an alloplastic material may be placed intranasally to approximate roof of the ethmoid and held in place with tissue glue and/or absorbable packing. Postoperatively, the patient should be instructed to avoid for several weeks nose blowing and any other activity that increases intracranial pressure. Perioperative antibiotics at the time of injury are appropriate, whereas the sustained postoperative use of antibiotics should be based on the likelihood of overt wound contamination and the virulence of the sinusitis. Following such injuries, most patients do well provided there is no residual intracranial communication. In contrast, the worst outcomes follow vascular injuries; subarachnoid hemorrhage causes intense vasoconstriction of the cerebral vasculature, and even when the site of hemorrhage is controlled, the patient may have a poor outcome.

Orbital injuries vary from hemorrhage to direct trauma to the eye, extraocular muscles, or optic nerve. Hemorrhage may result from a transected ethmoidal artery bleeding into the orbit or injury to the orbital vasculature. Because the orbit is a closed space bounded anteriorly by its periosteum (septum orbitale) and the condensations of this fibrous tissue (the medial and lateral canthal tendons) that fix the septum to the bony orbit, hemorrhage rapidly compromises vision. Increasing pressure within the orbit and eye requires immediate attention and consultation with ophthalmology. As a first step, all packing within the nose should be removed. If ophthalmologic help is not immediately available, a lateral canthotomy and transection of the lateral canthal tendon at its insertion on the orbital rim should be performed. This procedure permits the eyeball to be displaced anteriorly, resulting in additional volume within the orbit and lower pressure. If intraorbital bleeding continues, then the orbit should be explored. Injuries to the extraocular muscles, eye, or optic nerve should all be treated in consultation with an ophthalmologist.

108.5 Roundsmanship

- Frontal sinus surgery has evolved over the past century along two different approaches: drainage of the sinus into the nose and obliteration or ablation of the sinus. In the past 20 years, intranasal endoscopic approaches to the frontal sinus have reduced, but not eliminated, the need for external procedures.
- Intranasal sinus surgery is common today, but historically it was uncommonly used in the United States because of the potentially high complication rate. With the advent of surgical endoscopes to enhance illumination and visualization of the nose and sinuses, and improved techniques.

- FESS (*functional endoscopic sinus surgery*) is a concept, not a procedure, such as ethmoidectomy. The concept is based on the potential recovery of hypertrophic or chronically infected sinus mucous membrane following the restoration of normal sinus aeration and mucociliary transport.

108.6 Recommended Reading

[1] Halle M. Die intranasalen operationen bei eitrigen erkrankungen der nebenhohlen der nase. Arch Laryngol Rhinol 1915; 29: 73–112

[2] Kennedy D, Zinreich SJ, Rosenbaum AE, Johns ME. Functional endoscopic sinus surgery. Theory and diagnostic evaluation. Arch Otolaryngol 1985; 111; (9): 576–582

[3] Lawson W. The intranasal ethmoidectomy: an experience with 1,077 procedures. Laryngoscope 1991; 101: 367–371

[4] Messerklinger W. Endosckopiche diagnose und chirugie der rezidivierenden sinusitis. In: Krajina Z, ed. Advances in Nose and Sinus Surgery. Zagreb, Yugoslavia: Zagreb University; 1985

[5] Mosher HP. The surgical anatomy of the ethmoidal labyrinth. Ann Otolaryngol 1929; 38: 869–901

[6] Schaefer SD. An anatomic approach to endoscopic intranasal ethmoidectomy. Laryngoscope 1998; 108: 1628–1634

[7] Stammberger H. Endoscopic endonasal surgery—concepts in treatment of recurring rhinosinusitis. Part II. Surgical technique. Otolaryngol Head Neck Surg 1986; 94: 147–156

[8] Weber R, Draf W, Kratzsch B, Hosemann W, Schaefer SD. Modern concepts of frontal sinus surgery. Laryngoscope 2001; 111: 137–146

[9] Wigand ME, Steiner W, Jaumann MP. Endonasal sinus surgery with endoscopical control: from radical operation to rehabilitation of the mucosa. Endoscopy 1978; 10: 255–260

109 Tumors of the Nose and Paranasal Sinuses

Ameet R. Kamat and Steven David Schaefer

109.1 Introduction

Benign and malignant tumors of the nose and sinuses arise from the uniquely ectoderm-derived epithelium known as schneiderian epithelium, in recognition of the contributions of Victor Conrad Schneider to our understanding of this organ system. Schneiderian epithelium arises from the primitive nasal sacs that invaginate to form the nasal placodes and, subsequently, the nose and sinuses. In contrast, the laryngobronchial tree forms from endoderm or foregut-derived epithelium. Within the lining the nose and sinuses, mucoserous glands form by an interaction between the ectoderm and mesoderm. This complex embryogenesis gives rise to two types of neoplasia: that resulting from metaplastic epithelium, forming squamous cell tumors, and that originating from mucoserous epithelium.

109.2 Incidence of Disease

A recent Danish review of the various sinus and nasal cavity tumors detailed their frequency (▶ Table 109.1).

109.3 The Disease Process

109.3.1 Etiology and Pathogenesis

Generally, benign and malignant tumors of the sinus and nasal cavities share many initial symptoms, depending on their origin, anatomical site, and rate of growth. Tumors arising within the nose or involving its lateral wall can present early with epistaxis or nasal airway obstruction. Aside from the benign, much more common inflammatory nasal polyps, papillomas arise from the nasal and rarely from the sinus mucous membrane. Because these neoplastic growths develop from the schneiderian mucous membrane, arising nearly uniformly from either the lateral nasal wall or septum, appear either fungiform or sessile, and have a variable behavior, they are also designated schneiderian papillomas. Histologically, the papillomas appear

either papillary and exophytic, or exhibit an inverting epithelial growth into the underlying stroma. This variant of schneiderian papillomas, also commonly referred to as an inverting papilloma, is more frequently associated with the lateral nasal wall and sinuses. On nasal endoscopy, papillomas are significantly more solid than inflammatory polyps and have irregular surfaces.

109.3.2 Natural History and Progression

Relatively few schneiderian papillomas arise directly from the sinus cavities; rather, they extend into the sinuses. Patients may develop proptosis or diplopia as the papilloma continues to grow, expands into the bony orbit, and compresses, without infiltrating, the orbital periosteum or periorbita. Fewer than 5% of schneiderian papillomas are associated with squamous cell carcinomas. It remains unclear if such carcinomas arise within anaplastic changes in existing papillomas, occupy a cavity that had preexisting papillomas, or begin within foci of carcinoma in existing papillomas. Whatever the origin of these epithelial carcinomas, their clinical course rapidly departs from that of a mass obstructing the sinus or nasal cavities; they have the potential to cause epistaxis and directly extend into adjacent structures, invading the orbit, brain, facial soft tissues, muscles, and nerves.

Progressive invasion leads to impaired vision, trigeminal nerve sensory and motor changes, and potentially altered mentation as the tumors invade the brain; regional and distant metastasis may also occur.

109.4 Medical Evaluation

109.4.1 Imaging

Computed tomography (CT) and magnetic resonance (MR) imaging are complementary examinations to evaluate both benign and malignant tumors of the nasal and sinus cavities (▶ Fig. 109.1 and ▶ Fig. 109.2). CT remains the diagnostic test of choice for defining changes within the facial skeleton as tumors erode or invade bone. The rate of growth of a tumor may be inferred from the radiographic findings. As slowly growing tumors compress bone, the bone is remodeled and forms a thin shell around the tumor. Although this finding may suggest benign disease, a slowly growing malignant tumor may have a similar radiographic appearance. More typically, malignant tumors grow rapidly and destroy bone as they invade the facial skeleton. MR imaging better delineates tumors and dramatically reveals differences within the density of soft tissue. CT may show only an opacified sinus, whereas MR imaging reveals the whole range of possible reasons for the opacification. During tumor evaluation, the outflow tract of the sinus may be obstructed by the neoplasm and the sinus cavity filled with mucus. MR imaging can define the extent of disease and allow treatment planning. At the skull base, CT and MR imaging are

Table 109.1 Distribution of sinus and nasal cavity tumors

Tumor type	Percentage of cases
Squamous cell carcinoma	55%
Adenocarcinoma	28.5%
Adenoid cystic carcinoma	5%
Undifferentiated carcinoma	4.5%
Mucoepidermoid carcinoma	2.5%
Transitional cell carcinoma	1.7%
Small cell carcinoma	1.2%
Carcinoma, not otherwise specified	0.8%

Source: Data from Throup C, Sebbesen L, Danø H, et al. Carcinoma of the nasal cavity and sinuses in Denmark 1995–2004. Acta Oncol 2010;49 (3):389–394.

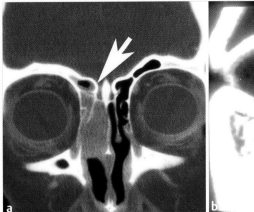

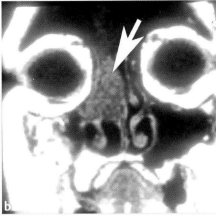

Fig. 109.1 (a) Coronal computed tomographic (CT) scan of a patient with esthesioneuroblastoma of the right ethmoid sinus (*arrow*). (b) Coronal magnetic resonance image. Superior to the arrow, the image shows the intracranial extent of tumor, which is much less obvious on the CT scan.

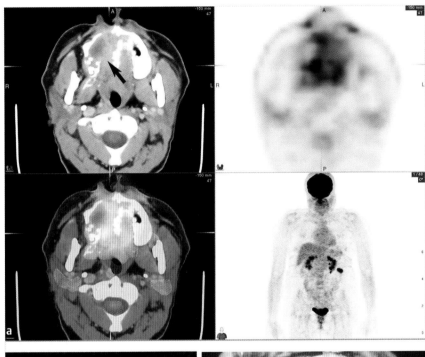

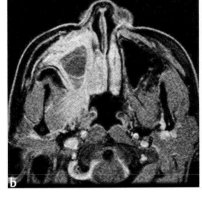

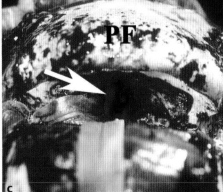

Fig. 109.2 (a) Positron emission tomography (PET)–computed tomography (CT) of a 55-year-old woman with adenoid cystic carcinoma arising in the right maxillary sinus and extending through the ipsilateral orbit to the dura of the right middle fossa. On the left, axial CT scans through the mid plane of the tumor (*arrow*) show excessive erosion of bone. At the upper right, PET–CT shows moderate uptake of the glucose tagged isotope, known as avidity and quantified by the standard uptake value (SUV), reflecting metabolic activity of the tumor. At the lower right, PET–CT shows tumor only at the primary site. (b) Axial contrast-enhanced fat-suppressed T1 magnetic resonance (MR) image of the same patient at the mid plane of the right maxillary sinus emphasizes the soft-tissue elements of the tumor and its invasion of surrounding structures. With this MR imaging protocol, the tumor signal is best separated from the surrounding tissue, permitting maximal identification of neoplasia. (c) Intraoperative photograph of patient showing craniofacial resection of tumor. Arrow indicates resection of the roof of the right ethmoid sinus, which forms part of the floor of the right anterior cranial fossa. A pericranial flap, which is derived from the superficial periosteum of the frontal bone and adjacent soft tissue, is routinely used to reconstruct the floor of the anterior cranial fossa. *PF*, pericranial flap.

complementary, showing bone, dural, and brain involvement. Recently, positron emission tomography (PET) has been combined with CT to investigate unknown primary neoplasms, differentiate infection from benign or malignant disease, stage known tumors by searching for regional and distant metastasis, and monitor patients after treatment for potential residual or recurrent disease.

109.4.2 Differential Diagnosis

A second group of nonepidermoid epithelial neoplasms arise from either the surface epithelium or any structure within its ducts. These tumors comprise salivary and nonsalivary histologic types. Examples of the former are benign neoplasms such as pleomorphic adenomas and oncocytomas and malignant tumors such as adenoid cystic, mucoepidermoid, acinic cell, and ductal carcinomas. Nonsalivary neoplasms include various types of adenocarcinomas, olfactory neuroblastomas, and adenosquamous carcinomas. Another malignant neoplasm originates within the melanocytes normally present within the mucosa and submucosa of the nasal and sinus cavities. The development of these mucosal melanomas is often heralded by epistaxis; they appear as black–brown pigmented lesions and may initially seem to be confined to an isolated site. However, distant metastasis is frequently later evident, and 5-year survival is rare. Olfactory neuroblastomas, also known as esthesioneuroblastomas, are derived from olfactory epithelium. These malignant tumors often present with epistaxis and nasal obstruction, and they may be confined to the nose or involve the anterior or middle cranial fossa (see ► Fig. 109.1).

109.5 Disease Staging

Sinus tumors are staged with the TNM (tumor node metastasis) classification and are grouped into maxillary sinus tumors and tumors involving the ethmoid sinuses and nasal cavity.

A T1 lesion of the maxillary sinus is limited to the mucosa of the sinus itself, with no bony involvement. T2 lesions include those with bony involvement of the hard palate and/or middle meatus, without extension to the posterior wall of the sinus or pterygoid plates. A tumor that involves the posterior wall of the sinus, subcutaneous tissues, floor or medial wall of the orbit, pterygoid fossa, or ethmoid sinuses is considered a T3 lesion. A tumor with any invasion of the anterior orbit, skin of the cheek, pterygoid plates, infratemporal fossa, cribriform plate, or sphenoid or frontal sinuses is classified as a T4a tumor. T4b lesions may invade the orbital apex, dura, brain, or middle fossa; involve any cranial nerve other than cranial nerve V$_2$; or extend to the nasopharynx or clivus.

Ethmoid sinus and nasal cavity cancers are graded similarly, with some differences based on anatomy. T1 lesions are restricted to one subsite (nasal cavity: vestibule, floor, lateral wall, septum; ethmoid sinus: left or right), with or without bony invasion. T2 tumors involve two subsites in a single region or extend into an adjacent region within the nasoethmoid complex, regardless of bony invasion. T3 cancers extend to the medial wall or floor of the orbit, maxillary sinus, palate, or cribriform plate. T4a tumors can invade the anterior orbital compartment, skin of the nose or cheek, pterygoid plates, or sphenoid or frontal sinuses or can have minimal extension into the anterior fossa. T4b lesions, similar to T4b lesions of the maxillary sinus, may invade the orbital apex, dura, brain, middle fossa, cranial nerves other than the maxillary division of the trigeminal nerve, or the nasopharynx or clivus.

The grading of nodal involvement is the same for both areas. Involvement of a single, ipsilateral node smaller than 3 cm is considered N1 disease. N2a nodal disease indicates involvement of a single, ipsilateral node 3 to 6 cm in size. N2b disease is involvement of bilateral or contralateral nodes smaller than 6 cm, while N2c disease is involvement of at least one lymph node larger than 6 cm.

Staging is done uniformly for both maxillary sinus and nasoethmoid malignancy. T1 lesions without nodal or distant metastasis are stage I, and similarly, T2 lesions without nodal involvement or metastasis are considered stage II disease. Stage III includes any T3 lesion without nodal or distant metastasis and any T1–T3 lesion with N1 neck disease. Stage IVa includes any T4a lesion or any T1–T3 lesion with N2 nodal involvement, and stage IVb indicates any T4b lesion. Any distant metastasis must be stage IVc disease.

109.6 Surgical Treatment

Given the greater prevalence of maxillary sinus carcinomas than of other paranasal sinus carcinomas, it is understandable that treatment for the past century or more has focused on this sinus. Early attempts to remove the maxilla surgically proved difficult, and surgery was later combined with (and in some cases replaced by) radiation therapy. Because of the propensity of ethmoid, frontal, and sphenoid carcinomas to involve the eyes and cranial cavity and the relative rarity of these tumors, the concept of craniofacial surgery and multidisciplinary therapy has been developed. More recently, the experience gained from endoscopic intranasal sinus surgery has made it possible to perform less invasive surgery in carefully selected patients. Radiation and chemotherapy are often now applied pre- or postoperatively to permit the possibility of preserving important organs, such as the eyes, and improving patient survival. In this chapter, a range of oncologic procedures are presented.

109.6.1 Maxillectomy

This procedure, an en bloc resection of the maxilla, is used primarily for the surgical treatment of malignant tumors arising within or substantially involving the maxillary sinus. In its classic form, a lateral facial skin–muscle flap is developed immediately superficial to the maxilla and adjacent facial skeleton. The most common flap uses a Weber-Fergusson incision, which begins lateral to the orbit, runs horizontally immediately beneath the ipsilateral eyelid, and then progresses inferiorly in the nasofacial crease and around the nasal ala to the upper lip philtrum (► Fig. 109.3). The upper lip is then divided by the incision, which is further carried into the labial and gingival–buccal sulcus. After exposure of the maxilla, osteotomies are made through the malar eminence to transect the zygoma and frontal bone. The orbital floor and its rim are incised and form the superior aspect of the resection unless the eye or skull is compromised by tumor. The hard palate is divided in the midline (with preservation of the soft palate), and the ethmoid sinus is separated from the maxilla. The final osteotomy is transection of the pterygoid plates, which are included in the surgical resection.

Medial Maxillectomy

As the next step in the evolution of surgery for maxillary sinus neoplasm, medial maxillectomy has advanced significantly in the past 40 years. As initially described, a Weber-Fergusson incision was used to expose the maxilla, and the medial maxillary sinus and lateral nasal wall were removed for low-grade malignancies and benign neoplasms of this site (► Fig. 109.4). The next modification of maxillectomy was exposure of the maxilla in selected tumors via midface degloving, which involves separating the facial soft tissue overlying the maxilla through circum-malar, gingivolabial, and gingivobuccal incisions. The soft

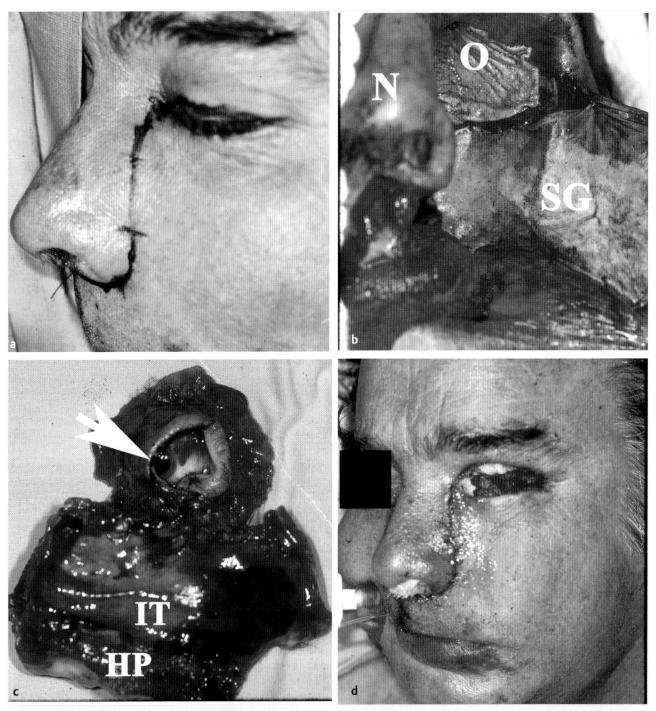

Fig. 109.3 (a) A Weber-Fergusson incision is outlined on this patient, who is undergoing radical maxillectomy with orbital exenteration for squamous cell carcinoma of the left maxillary sinus involving the orbit. The eyelid incision in this patient is on the upper lid for oncologic reasons; typically, the incision runs just below the lashes of the lower eyelid. (b) Intraoperative photograph of the patient in (a) showing exposure of the maxillary and orbital cavities after removal of the sinus tumor and left eye. *N*, nose; *O*, orbital cavity with split-thickness skin graft lining the cavity; *SG*, skin graft surfacing facial flap used to expose the maxilla via the Weber-Fergusson incision. (c) Surgical specimen from patient consisting of the maxillary sinus and contents of the orbit. *arrow*, left eye; *HP*, hard palate; *IT*, inferior turbinate;). (d) Intraoperative photo showing closure of wound and packing in left orbit supporting the skin graft lining the cavity.

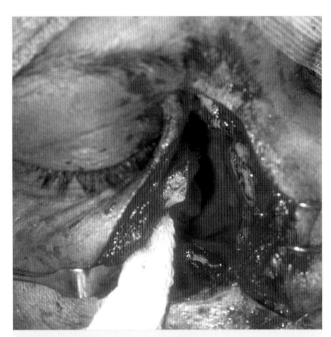

Fig. 109.4 An external approach to a right medial maxillectomy through a nasofacial crease incision provides good exposure of the medial wall of the maxillary sinus.

tissues of the midface are elevated and the maxilla is accessed from a sublabial direction.

Endoscopic Medial Maxillectomy

This is the most recent procedure in the century-long evolution of maxillectomy. Like open approaches to the lateral nasal wall and medial maxillary sinus, this modification includes a complete resection of this site. Because the nasolacrimal duct is transected during the procedure, placing a stent in the duct into the nose or dacryorhinocystostomy is recommended to prevent epiphora. In general, endoscopic medical maxillectomy serves most patients well. However, the limitations of the procedure are poor exposure of the anterior wall of the maxillary sinus and a lack of sufficient experience by most surgeons.

109.6.2 Craniofacial Resection

Multiple surgical approaches are now available for the resection of benign and malignant tumors involving the face and neurocranium. Most paranasal sinus tumors are approached via some form of frontal craniotomy to expose the anterior cranial fossa floor. The standard bifrontal craniotomy provides the best exposure of the tumor but may involve the greatest degree of frontal lobe retraction and therefore the slowest postoperative recovery for the patient (see ▶ Fig. 109.2). Tumor removal depends on the degree of dural and frontal lobe infiltration, the health of the patient, and the ability to reconstruct the surgical defect. As a generalization, the floor of the anterior cranial fossa is reconstructed with a pericranial flap or free flaps, and forehead defects are repaired with various forms of bone grafts. Radiation therapy is used in most centers, with or without chemotherapy, depending on the type and extent of tumor.

Preoperative radiation and chemotherapy may permit organ-sparing surgery; some esthesioneuroblastomas or squamous cell carcinomas that approximate the optic nerve may be selectively managed by induction chemotherapy and radiation, allowing preservation of the nerve. In contrast, adenoid cystic carcinomas are resistant to chemotherapy and radiation and require aggressive surgical resection.

109.6.3 Endoscopic Skull Base Resection

Building upon the surgical skills acquired from extensive endoscopic sinus surgery, more surgeons are using intranasal endoscopic approaches to remove benign and relatively low-grade malignant neoplasms, such as esthesioneuroblastomas. The ability to successfully and oncologically remove such tumors depends on the following: (1) the surgeon's experience in endoscopic medial maxillectomy and the other approaches used for tumor removal; (2) the surgeon's experience in the repair of cerebrospinal fluid fistulas and encephaloceles, necessary to gain the skills needed for intranasal reconstruction of the skull base; (3) the surgeon's experience in orbital and optic nerve surgery; and (4) the extent of the tumor. When these conditions are met, the surgeon must seek to remove the entire tumor, but the means by which this is achieved may differ from those used in external surgery. For example, a large, bulky tumor with relatively little invasion of the anterior skull base over the nose and septum prevents easy exposure of the normal tissue margins. If the center of the tumor is removed, so that the mass collapses upon itself, then each margin can be identified and the tumor completely resected. The next obstacle the surgeon must overcome is "watertight" reconstruction of the dura. With small dural defects, such reconstruction with fascia or allografts is relatively easy. After complete removal of the skull base, reconstruction is problematic and remains a barrier to a more universal application of the endoscopic approach. However, there is little question that a properly performed and oncologically sound endoscopic resection is preferred by patients (▶ Fig. 109.5).

109.7 Prognosis

The object of tumor staging is to relate the clinical findings to the prognosis and to manage treatment based on that prognosis. Approximately 5% of all human neoplasms occur in the head and neck, and 5% of these are within the nose and sinuses. Neoplasms are more common in the maxillary than in the ethmoid sinuses, and frontal neoplasms and sphenoid neoplasms each constitute only 4 to 5% of sinus malignancies. The prognosis worsens as the neoplasm extends beyond the nasal or sinus cavity, invades vital structures, involves regional lymphatics, or metastasizes to distant sites. In the maxillary sinus, the Öhngren line, an imaginary line drawn from the medial canthus to the angle of the mandible, is a useful means to predict prognosis and is significant in tumor staging; maxillary sinus cancers superior to this line (suprastructure neoplasms) can invade the orbit and spread posteriorly into the infratemporal and pterygopalatine fossae. Such neoplasms carry a much worse prognosis than do infrastructure malignancies (inferior to the Öhngren line; ▶ Fig. 109.6).

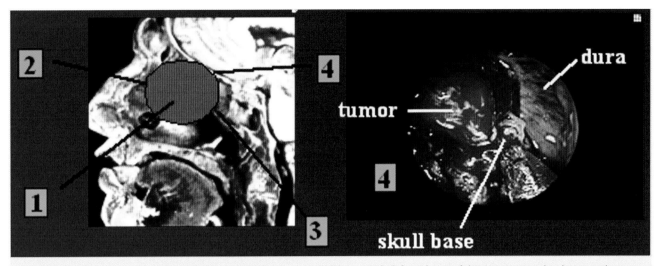

Fig. 109.5 Endoscopic resection of an inverting papilloma invading the skull base. On the left, each step of the resection is outlined. Step 1: The tumor is debulked to permit visualization of the margins. Step 2: The anterior margin of the resection is cleared of tumor and frozen section sent for pathologic examination. Step 3: The posterior or most distal margin is defined and resected. Step 4: Resection of the skull is performed. This is the most critical aspect of the surgery and requires maximal exposure. The endoscopic view of the resection and the dura is seen on the right.

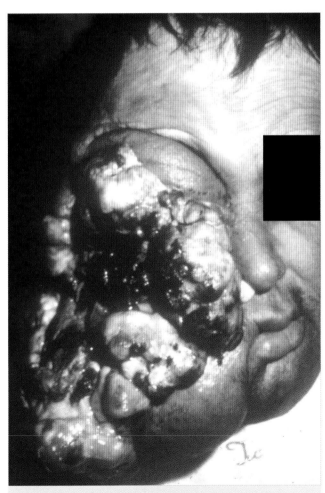

Fig. 109.6 An untreated squamous cell carcinoma of the right maxillary sinus illustrates the natural history of this disease.

109.8 Roundsmanship

- Tumors of the nose arise from the uniquely ectoderm-derived epithelium known as schneiderian epithelium.
- Inverting papillomas are a variant of schneiderian papillomas, arising from an inversion of epithelial growth into the underlying stroma. They most frequently are found within the lateral nasal wall and sinuses. Squamous cell carcinomas are associated with inverting papillomas, but their etiology is unclear.
- Epistaxis and nasal airway obstruction must be evaluated by nasal endoscopy. All patients with such symptoms of more than 4 weeks' duration should be assumed to have a nasal/sinus tumor until it is proven otherwise by nasal endoscopy.
- Computed tomography and magnetic resonance imaging are complementary modalities that should both be employed in evaluating nasal, sinus, and skull base tumors.
- The surgical treatment of sinus/nasal tumors has progressed over the past century toward intranasal endoscopic approaches. Whatever approach is used, complete resection of the tumor is mandatory, and all surgeons must have the ability to use intranasal and external approaches as indicated.

109.9 Recommended Reading

[1] Batsakis JG. The pathology of head and neck tumors: nasal cavity and paranasal sinuses, part 5. Head Neck Surg 1980; 2: 410–419

[2] Ketcham AS, Wilkins RH, Vanburen JM, Smith RR. A combined intracranial facial approach to the paranasal sinuses. Am J Surg 1963; 106: 698–703

[3] Ohngren LG. Malignant tumours of the maxillo-ethmoid region: a clinical study with special reference to the treatment with electrosurgery and irradiation. Acta Otolaryngol 1933; 19 Suppl: 1–276

[4] Sessions RB, Larson DL. En bloc ethmoidectomy and medial maxillectomy. Arch Otolaryngol 1977; 103: 195–202

[5] Thorup C, Sebbesen L, Danø H et al. Carcinoma of the nasal cavity and paranasal sinuses in Denmark 1995–2004. Acta Oncol 2010; 49: 389–394

110 Surgical Techniques for the Anterior Skull Base

David Henry Hiltzik and Homere Al Moutran

110.1 Comprehensive Anterior Skull Base Anatomy and Pathology

The subspecialty of cranial base surgery requires a large amount of resources, knowledge, training, and multispecialty collaboration. The anatomical, pathologic, and surgical complexity of the cranial base requires a multidisciplinary approach comprising a dedicated group of professionals. An understanding of neurosurgery, head and neck surgery, medical and radiation oncology, ophthalmology, anesthesia, and especially pathology is critical in the treatment of cranial base neoplasms and diseases. In this chapter, the pathology, surgical approaches, and complications of the anterior fossa will be described and discussed.

110.1.1 Pertinent Anatomy

The anterior cranial base provides support for the frontal lobes of the brain and the grooves for the olfactory nerve. The paranasal sinuses, specifically the frontal and ethmoid sinuses, along with the orbital roofs, are the focal points of the anterior skull base anatomy. The posterior wall of the frontal sinus is the anteriormost limit of the anterior skull base. The ethmoid bone and sinuses, including the cribriform plate, fovea ethmoidalis, and orbital roofs, comprise the floor, along with the planum sphenoidale (▶ Fig. 110.1).

Superiorly, the olfactory apparatus lies in the cribriform plate (i.e., the foramina of the anterior cranial base that allow sinus access to the central nervous system). The keel-like crista galli divides the cribriform plate in the midline and is the area where the dura is most adherent. Its position just posterior to the foramen caecum marks the origin of the sagittal sinus. This foramen can be a source of bleeding during anterior craniofacial surgery if not appropriately ligated during exposure. The fovea ethmoidalis makes the greatest contribution to the central anterior floor (see ▶ Fig. 110.1).

However, the dura is more adherent to the cribriform than to the fovea because of the penetration of the olfactory filaments through the cribriform plate into the superior nasal vault. Despite this fact, the fovea is still the area most susceptible to iatrogenic cerebrospinal fluid (CSF) leak, particularly during endoscopic sinus surgery. Both the anterior and posterior ethmoid arteries and their adjoining vessels help identify the floor of the anterior cranial base. The optic nerve lies in the optic canal approximately 5 mm posterior to the posterior ethmoid artery (▶ Fig. 110.2). It sits immediately lateral to the planum sphenoidale, which demarcates the posteriormost border of the anterior skull base. The lamina papyracea, a rather permeable structure that may allow penetration into the orbit, comprises the lateral edge of the ethmoid sinuses. While the periosteum is a barrier to tumor spread, the thin fascial layer that surrounds the orbital fat contributes greatly to orbital integrity, thereby allowing an additional level of resection.

The predominant blood supply of the ethmoids and anterior skull base is derived from both the internal and external carotid artery systems, through the internal maxillary artery and the anterior and posterior ethmoidal arteries, respectively. Similarly, the venous drainage is through the nasal veins, which drain into the jugular system, and the ethmoidal veins, which drain into the cavernous sinus. The sensory nerve supply is though the trigeminal nerve divisions V_1 and V_2.

110.1.2 Tumors of the Anterior Skull Base: Types, Incidence, and Progression

Cranial base tumors, as an aggregate, are relatively rare with varied pathologies. Anterior skull base tumors are largely epithelial, olfactory, or salivary in origin. There is also a large set of tumors that metastasize to the skull base. Sinonasal tumors that involve the anterior cranial base are those that extend superiorly through the skull at the ethmoid roof, cribriform plate, or

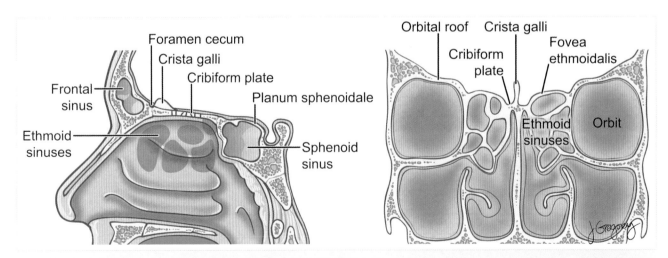

Fig. 110.1 Sagittal and coronal cuts that demonstrate the anterior skull base. Note the distinction between the fovea ethmoidalis and the cribriform plate.

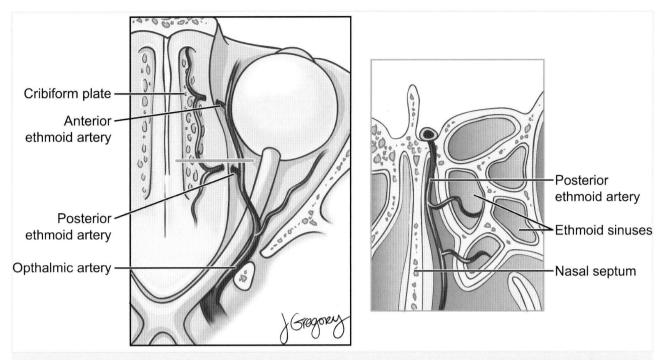

Fig. 110.2 The relationship of the anterior and posterior ethmoid arteries and the optic nerve is shown relative to the ethmoid and sphenoid sinuses.

planum sphenoidale, or posteriorly through the posterior wall of the frontal sinus. Benign processes, such as angiofibromas, inverted papillomas, chondromas, and encephaloceles/mucoceles, as well as malignant processes that are prevalent in these anatomical locations require surgical intervention.

Malignant tumors of sinonasal origin are of endodermal, mesodermal, and epidermal derivation; they include squamous cell carcinoma, esthesioneuroblastoma (olfactory neuroblastoma), sarcoma, adenoid cystic carcinoma, mucoepidermoid carcinoma, melanoma, lymphoma, hemangiopericytoma, malignant giant cell tumor, basal cell carcinoma, and metastatic malignancies. The most common tumor pathologies vary from study to study and from region to region in the world. Squamous cell carcinomas, sarcomas, esthesioneuroblastomas, adenoid cystic carcinomas, and adenocarcinomas are most prevalent in the Americas. In European studies, however, intestinal-type adenocarcinomas (rare in American studies) predominate, and in Brazil skin tumors top the list.

Paranasal tumors are generally locally invasive, with little involvement of the regional lymph nodes (8%) or metastases. Numerous classification systems have been attempted, including the Kadish stage, TNM (tumor node metastasis) system, and international system, but none has significant prognostic value. Overall, the 5-year disease-free survival rate is 50%; adenocarcinoma has a better prognosis than squamous cell carcinoma. Although much has been written about the technical details of the surgeries, few studies have made a great impact with regard to prognosis and long-term results. The international collaborative study group that included 1,307 patients collected from 17 institutions concluded that the histology of the primary tumor, the status of the surgical margins, and intracranial involvement are significant predictors of recurrence-free and disease-specific survival. Other significant factors found in

smaller studies include tumor grade, orbital involvement, and sphenoid sinus involvement. It is critical to recognize that tumor histology coupled with the potential for complete resection, rather than the TNM staging system, is by far the most important criterion affecting cure.

110.2 Preoperative Evaluation

110.2.1 Presentation, Signs, and Symptoms

A common or "standard" presentation for cranial base tumors does not exist because these lesions are asymptomatic until they compromise neighboring structures. Therefore, they are frequently found at advanced stages. The presenting symptoms usually depend on the size and location of the tumor in the skull base and on the related structures. Also, a percentage of tumors are identified incidentally on computed tomography (CT) or magnetic resonance (MR) imaging performed as a result of a generalized, nonfocal complaint of headache.

The anterior skull base and involved paranasal sinuses are closely related to the orbit and to the cribriform plate. If the tumor is predominantly in the nasal cavity, then nasal congestion, epistaxis, anosmia, and unilateral otitis media (effusion) are some of the possible initial symptoms. Tumors of the anterior skull base often produce orbital signs resulting from mass or destructive effects, such as visual disturbances in the form of diplopia or orbital displacement in the form of proptosis, as well as epiphora and visual loss. Because of the close vicinity of the cribriform plate, alterations of taste and smell are possible. Neurologic findings become apparent when tumors erode into the pterygomaxillary space, epidural space, or brain tissue itself

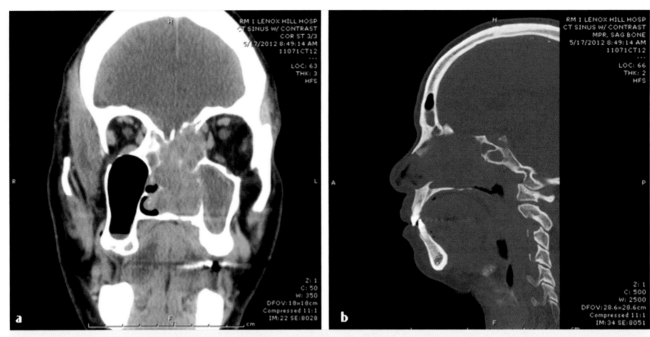

Fig. 110.3 (a) Coronal (soft-tissue window) and (b) sagittal (bone window) computed tomographic scans of a large sinonasal malignancy with mild erosion of the right skull base and invasion into both orbits.

and can manifest as headaches, cranial neuropathies, and even frontal lobe symptoms, such as alterations in personality. Visual changes demonstrate involvement of cranial nerves II, III, IV, or VI or of the orbit. Pain and a variety of dysesthesias result from involvement of trigeminal nerve divisions V_1 and V_2, especially the supratrochlear, supraorbital, and infraorbital nerves. This is particularly true of adenoid cystic cancers, which have the potential for substantial perineural spread with minimal tumor mass formation.

110.2.2 Radiology

CT, positron emission tomography (PET) coupled with CT (PET–CT), and MR imaging are the mainstays of the preoperative evaluation other than direct biopsy. All lesions of the cranial base require both CT and MR imaging for diagnosis and treatment. Usually PET–CT coupled with MR imaging is employed. CT provides an in-depth understanding of the craniofacial skeleton and its bony relationship to these lesions, whereas MR imaging provides a detailed soft-tissue description. Axial and coronal CT scans are required, along with both soft-tissue and bone algorithms (▶ Fig. 110.3). MR imaging generally includes axial, coronal, and sagittal images obtained from both T1 with and without contrast and T2 series (▶ Fig. 110.4).

These MR imaging techniques differentiate various tissue types on the basis of signal response. MR angiography can also be of valuable clinical use. A synthesis of both modalities allows a detailed characterization of the tumor with regard to differential diagnosis and of its extent and resectability with regard to preoperative planning. This information is extremely valuable considering the common deficiency in receiving a tissue diagnosis before surgery as a result of the locations of many skull base tumors. Because of the clarity of tumor location and tissue characteristics provided by CT and MR imaging, a narrow range of histologic types can be defined and treated accordingly.

PET has become increasingly valuable in the evaluation of cranial base tumors. It plays a significant role with regard to initial metastatic work-up as well as postoperative surveillance. Preoperatively, it contributes to the staging of cranial base lesions and the detection of metastases, which may result in a change of treatment plan. Postoperatively, these scans are important in differentiating between postoperative tissue fibrosis and previously undetected tumor. The development of fusion PET–CT allows the simultaneous acquisition of anatomical and metabolic data. This technology makes possible the early detection of tumor recurrence, guides endoscopic biopsies, and assists in the selection of an overall treatment plan.

110.3 Surgical Techniques

In 1954, Smith first described anterior craniofacial resection for a tumor arising in the frontal sinus. Ketcham subsequently published the first series of cases and established the first indications, morbidity issues, and outcomes of this type of surgery. Later on, Tessier and Derome improved the technique and introduced modifications to the first approach described.

Since then, anterior craniofacial surgery has been improved by multiple variations and refinements, especially with the revolution of endoscopic technology. Numerous variations and approaches have been described in the literature, as follows:
- Transcranial
  - Standard bifrontal craniotomy
  - Extended frontal craniotomy
  - Frontotemporal craniotomy
- Transfacial/transnasal
  - Endonasal (endoscopic, microscopic)
  - Midfacial degloving
  - Lateral rhinotomy (Lynch approach)

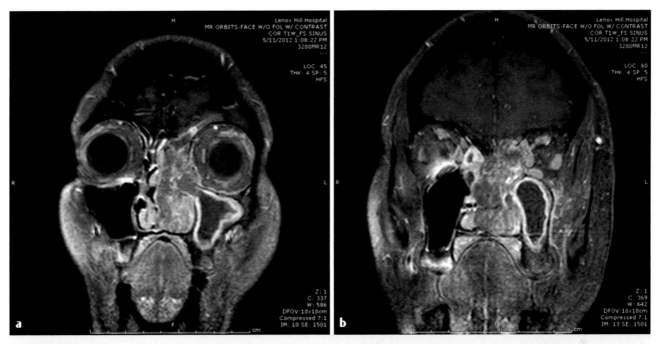

Fig. 110.4 Magnetic resonance (MR) image of the same patient depicted in the computed tomographic scan in ▶ Fig. 110.3. These **(a)** anterior and **(b)** more posterior coronal MR imaging sections demonstrate the dura and orbital contents more clearly, along with the postobstructive sinusitis in the maxillary sinus on the left.

Of note, transcranial and transfacial approaches are often integrated to resect a single tumor.

110.3.1 Open Approach to the Anterior Skull Base

For most anterior craniofacial approaches, the patient should be placed in a supine position. The head usually is rested on a horseshoe-shaped holder but can be fixed with a Mayfield-type pinning system.

The transcranial approach is preferred in most cases in light of its excellent visualization and its ability to provide broad access to the entire anterior skull base laterally from orbit to orbit and anteriorly to posteriorly from the fovea and cribriform to the planum sphenoidale (▶ Fig. 110.5). This approach allows a complete, often en bloc resection with minimal aesthetic and functional deficit. The transfacial approaches often leave scarring on the face and offer little added access to the sinonasal cavity and anterior fossa. With the transcranial subfrontal approach, the transfacial approaches are largely used if there is lateral extension of the tumor into the orbit, lateral maxillary sinus, and infratemporal fossa.

Mobilizing soft tissues from the coronal (frontoparietal) suture to the superior orbital rims anteriorly and all the way to the zygomatic arch laterally usually necessitates a bicoronal incision regardless of the tumor location. The scalp elevation can be done in the subperiosteal or subgaleal plane, depending on the surgeon's preference, where a pericranial flap can still be harvested from the cutaneous flap at the end of the surgery (▶ Fig. 110.6).

Dissection is done deep to the temporoparietal fascia flap to the level of the temporalis fat pad, where the deep temporalis fascia is duplicated. At this point, the fat pad is entered and the superficial layer of the deep temporalis fascia is elevated with the skin flap protecting the forehead branches of the facial nerve.

The traditional bifrontal craniotomy begins a few centimeters above the supraorbital rims (see ▶ Fig. 110.6). Stopping at this level can result in retraction of the frontal lobes to access the planum sphenoidale and more posterior structures. For an improved visualization of the tumor, facilitating its total removal and decreasing, although not eliminating, the morbidity due to brain retraction, the frontal bar (also called sub-basal or extended frontal) approach is favored. Various other craniotomies are also described to accomplish the goal of minimal brain retraction. They involve additional osteotomies that enable removal of the supraorbital rims and nasion en bloc.

This approach exposes the whole area from the rhinion anteriorly to the sella posteriorly and the orbits on the sides. The size of the frontal bone and the amount of the orbital rims included in the flap are determined by the amount of exposure that will be needed.

The supraorbital neurovascular structures are dissected carefully out of the bony foramina, thereby preserving sensation to the forehead and blood supply to an eventually needed pericranial flap. Following craniotomy, dural elevation can extend posteriorly to the tuberculum sellae, falciform ligaments over the optic nerves, and lesser wings of the sphenoid bone.

For unilateral tumors that extend into an adjacent orbit or the cavernous sinus, a frontotemporal craniotomy with orbito-zygomatic osteotomy allows a better access to the superior orbital fissure. The open approaches can also be used in conjunction with the transfacial approaches, including midfacial degloving and lateral rhinotomy. For reasons of cosmesis and functional preservation, the subfrontal approach is preferred when an "open approach" is needed.

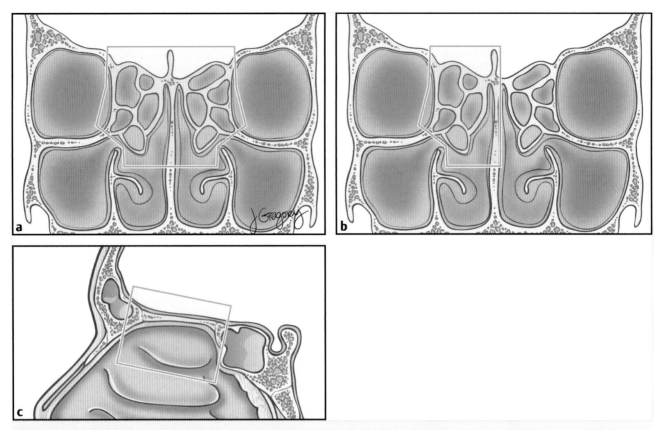

Fig. 110.5 Schematic depicting the desired extent of resection for (a) bilateral and (b) unilateral anterior (c) craniofacial resection.

The approaches from above allow the resection of larger tumors involving dura or brain with complete vascular control and the ability to achieve an en bloc resection with negative margins. The entire sinonasal cavity can be well visualized and accessed, allowing complete exenteration of the ethmoid, maxillary, frontal, and sphenoid sinuses, if necessary, as well as the nasal floor with minimal morbidity.

Once the resection is performed, the skull base must be reconstructed to prevent communication between the sinus and intracranial cavity. If a CSF leak is created, then a watertight seal must be achieved. The pericranial flap is the mainstay of anterior fossa reconstruction in the open approaches. A temporoparietal flap or temporalis muscle flap, as well as fascia lata or a variety of biomaterials, can also be used. Exenteration of the frontal sinus and obliteration of the frontal recess are important components in the closure of these cases to prevent pneumocephalus in the short term and mucocele formation in the long term. The nasal cavity is often packed, and nasal trumpets are placed to avoid pneumocephalus, as well.

110.3.2 Endoscopic Endonasal Approach to the Anterior Skull Base

Technologic advancements in the form of intraoperative navigation and instrumentation plus the acquisition of endoscopic skills and expertise through a better understanding of the anatomy of the skull base "from below" over the last 15 years have brought a true paradigm shift in skull base surgery.

Endoscopic skull base surgery comprises a series of approaches or "corridors" through the sinonasal passages, with the maximum of lateral extension obtained between the two medial orbital walls at the middle of the cribriform plate (mean distance, 25 to 33 mm), while the mean distance between the anterior and posterior ethmoidal arteries at the level of the lamina papyracea is 16 mm. Therefore, the endoscopic endonasal route can be considered a minimally invasive technique for approaching an area limited by the sella posteriorly, orbits laterally, and frontal recess at the junction of the crista galli anteriorly.

The endoscopic approach to the anterior skull base is performed with a "four-handed" technique in which two surgeons use a transethmoid and a transcribriform approach. This dissection extends from the posterior wall of the frontal sinus to the planum sphenoidale. At the beginning of the case, the patient is positioned with the navigation apparatus and thoroughly decongested. The approach is initiated by resecting the attachment of the anterior portion of the nasal septum to the cranial base after the middle turbinates have been removed. A total ethmoidectomy along with an endoscopic modified Lothrop procedure (wide opening of the frontal recesses with a drilling out of the frontal sinus floor and intersinus septum) is then performed. After wide exposure and visualization of the floor of the entire anterior fossa have been attained, the fovea ethmoidalis and cribriform plate are removed bilaterally. The limits of this module are both laminae papyraceae laterally, the frontal sinus anteriorly, and the transition with the planum sphenoidale posteriorly. Although the cribriform exposure damages olfaction, it is likely that olfaction has already been compro-

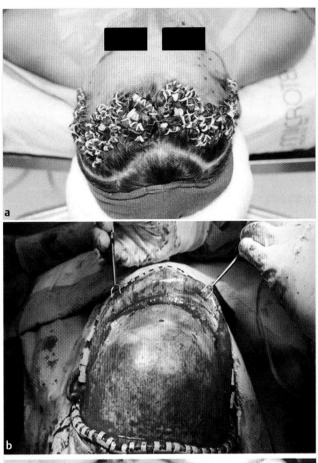

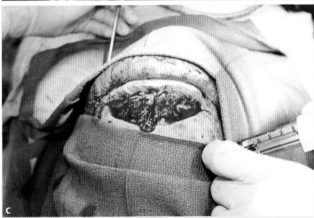

Fig. 110.6 (a) The bicoronal incision is marked. The hair is not shaved and is completely preserved after the surgery. (b) The scalp flap is elevated, with the pericranium preserved in the scalp for later use in reconstruction of the skull base. (c) The frontal bone flap is removed.

110.4 Complications of Cranial Base Surgery

Cranial base surgery poses serious surgical challenges that are reflected in the relatively high rate of postoperative complications. These tumors involve critical structures, so that wide and extensive access is required in both open and endoscopic approaches, often leaving extensive and challenging defects. Because of an average complication rate of 30 to 50%, proper preoperative planning with regard to approach and reconstruction must be performed. Potential risk factors for complications must also be assessed, including patient demographics and comorbidities, prior surgical and radiation treatment, the extent of anatomical involvement of the lesion, and the biology of the tumor type. Although the surgical mortality of these procedures is less than 4%, central nervous system, wound, and systemic medical complications occur in up to 40% of patients. The majority of complications are related to CSF leak, meningitis, and wound infection. Postoperative emergencies specific to any intracranial procedure include cerebral edema, thrombosis, pseudoaneurysm, air embolism, and postoperative seizures.

In most large studies of the complications of skull base surgery for malignant tumors, postoperative wound infections have been reported to occur in up to 20% of cases. These include superficial wound infections, osteomyelitis, intracranial abscess, and bone flap failures. Medical comorbidities and prior radiation therapy have been shown to be predictive factors.

Cranial nerve and orbital complications are of concern in both the intraoperative and the postoperative period and are therefore often predicted based on tumor location and type of approach. Neurophysiologic monitoring understandably plays a crucial role in cranial base surgery. Any orbital involvement or resection of the surrounding structures can produce diplopia and visual disturbances. Epiphora can occur secondary to lacrimal duct complications and an insufficient dacryocystorhinostomy. Deficits of cranial nerves III, IV, and VI are most common in resections involving the cavernous sinus; combined paralysis is therefore called cavernous sinus syndrome. Total ophthalmoplegia and diplopia can be expected in these circumstances, along with conjunctival injection and edema.

CSF leaks, along with wound infections, account for over half of all postoperative complications after cranial base surgery. They occur in 2 to 20% of cases and can often be predicted by radiology showing tumor involvement of the dura, brain, middle ear, and eustachian tube. Prior radiation therapy, dural invasion, and brain involvement are significant predisposing factors. CSF leaks can be categorized as low-flow or high-flow leaks. They are detected by the history and the clinical and radiologic examination. Depending on the surgical site, patients may present with clear rhinorrhea or otorrhea at rest or on exertion, which is often associated with a salty taste and a halo sign (a dark ring surrounding a more lightly stained center) on the patient's dressings or sheets. A collected fluid sample can be assayed for β_2-transferrin, a protein found only in CSF, perilymph, and vitreous humor. If this is not feasible and the location of the leak cannot be determined, MR imaging or, more commonly, CT cisternogragraphy can be performed; CT before and after an intrathecal injection of a radiopaque dye can identify the leak location. Patients can also present with pneumocephalus and, in

mised by the disease in question. Once the entire bony floor of the anterior fossa is removed, the dural and intracranial portion of the tumor can be resected with negative margins. Reconstruction of the skull base is performed, preferably with local vascularized tissue. If vascular tissue is unavailable, avascular dermal grafts are employed. In simple terms, the "endoscopic approach" can accomplish the same resection as the "open approach," except that is done from below the skull base instead of above it and with fewer incisions.

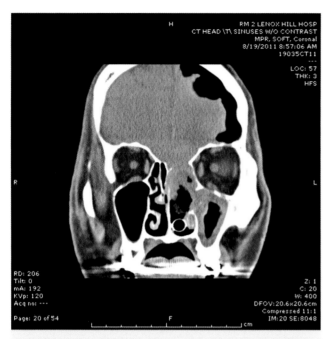

Fig. 110.7 Computed tomographic scan of a large pneumocephalus secondary to a postoperative communication between the nasal cavity and intracranial space.

the worst case, a life-threatening tension pneumocephalus (► Fig. 110.7).

High-flow leaks are most often treated urgently by direct surgical closure with nonvascularized tissue such as fat or fascia, alloplastic materials, or a combination of both along with a tissue sealant. These leaks can be addressed by either open or endoscopic approaches. Low-flow leaks can often be resolved by lumbar drain or, if necessary, ventricular or lumbar shunt placement in intractable situations. Excessive drainage must be avoided to prevent pneumocephalus.

Meningitis is the most undesirable complication of cranial base surgery. The risk for meningitis increases in the presence of a CSF leak, especially in anterior skull base surgery, when the intradural space is directly exposed to the paranasal sinuses.

Meningitis usually presents with fever, headache, nausea, vomiting, and mental status changes. There should be a low threshold for initiating a work-up in the clinical setting of any of these symptoms. CT of the head is performed to rule out increased intracranial pressure and dilated ventricles. A lumbar puncture then allows analysis of the CSF for color, protein, glucose, red blood cells, and white blood cells, and a Gram stain is performed. Postoperatively, meningitis is usually aseptic or of bacterial origin; a viral origin is unlikely. Aseptic meningitis usually results from meningeal irritation by surgical intervention, blood, or breakdown products. Bacterial meningitis, which is more common, is devastating and often the result of large defects that are at risk for CSF leaks. Once meningitis is diagnosed,

treatment with intravenous antibiotics and close monitoring of the CSF leak is initiated.

Cranial base surgery is a complicated and demanding subspecialty with a high risk for complications as well as the potential for great rewards. Patients requiring an anterior craniofacial resection must undergo a thorough work-up with a detailed history, physical examination, and radiologic studies, including CT, MR imaging, and PET. Presurgical planning is crucial and necessitates a multidisciplinary team. The surgical approach depends on a multitude of factors, and close postoperative follow-up is essential to avoid serious complications.

110.5 Roundsmanship

- Skull base surgery requires a multidisciplinary approach across a broad range of subspecialties, with the participation of a head and neck surgeon, neurosurgeon, oncologist, radiologist, and pathologist.
- CT, MR imaging, and PET–CT are all necessary in the evaluation of anterior fossa tumors.
- The surgical approach to the anterior fossa depends on the pathologic type and stage of the tumor, the patient's anatomy, and the surgeon's skill set.
- The complications of skull base surgery can be devastating and must be avoided with the exercise of surgical judgment and close postoperative monitoring.

110.6 Recommended Reading

[1] Cantù G, Riccio S, Bimbi G et al. Craniofacial resection for malignant tumours involving the anterior skull base. Eur Arch Otorhinolaryngol 2006; 263: 647–652

[2] Cantú G, Solero CL, Mariani L, Mattavelli F, Pizzi N, Licitra L. A new classification for malignant tumors involving the anterior skull base. Arch Otolaryngol Head Neck Surg 1999; 125: 1252–1257

[3] Danks RA, Kaye AH. Carcinoma of the paranasal sinuses. In: Kaye A, Laws ER Jr, eds. Brain Tumours: An Encyclopedic Approach. New York, NY: Churchill Livingstone; 1995:809–824

[4] Donald PJ. Complications in skull base surgery for malignancy. Laryngoscope 1999; 109: 1959–1966

[5] Gil Z, Even-Sapir E, Margalit N, Fliss DM. Integrated PET/CT system for staging and surveillance of skull base tumors. Head Neck 2007; 29: 537–545

[6] Irish JC, Gullane PJ, Gentili F et al. Tumors of the skull base: outcome and survival analysis of 77 cases. Head Neck 1994; 16: 3–10

[7] Kaplan MJ, Fischbein NJ, Harsh GR. Anterior skull base surgery. Otolaryngol Clin North Am 2005; 38: 107–131

[8] Ketcham AS, Wilkins RH, Vanburen JM, Smith RR. A combined intracranial facial approach to the paranasal sinuses. Am J Surg 1963; 106: 698–703

[9] Kraus DH, Shah JP, Arbit E, Galicich JH, Strong EW. Complications of craniofacial resection for tumors involving the anterior skull base. Head Neck 1994; 16: 307–312

[10] Kryzanski JT, Annino DJ, Heilman CB. Complication avoidance in the treatment of malignant tumors of the skull base. Neurosurg Focus 2002; 12: e11

[11] Patel SG, Singh B, Polluri A et al. Craniofacial surgery for malignant skull base tumors: report of an international collaborative study. Cancer 2003; 98: 1179–1187

[12] Vrionis FD, Kienstra MA, Rivera M, Padhya TA. Malignant tumors of the anterior skull base. Cancer Contr 2004; 11: 144–151

111 Anatomy and Embryology of the Ear

Christopher J. Linstrom

111.1 Introduction

An understanding of any pathologic process is based upon a thorough knowledge of the normal, including normal development. This is especially true for all structures of the head and neck, and most importantly for the ear. It is impossible to completely understand the basis for much otologic and neurotologic disease without a firm grounding in the embryology and anatomy of the ear.

111.2 Ear Development: The Short of It

Humans are vertebrates, and the auditory system in all vertebrates has the following similar structures (▶ Fig. 111.1):
1. A sound-directing appendage, the auricle.
2. A connection between the external sound source and the outer surface of a sound-conducting membrane. Sound pressure (force per unit area) is slightly diminished as sound travels through this junction and must be reamplified.
3. A sound reamplification system. Most, but not all, vertebrates have three ossicles: two long levers (malleus and incus) articulating with a small receiver (stapes).
4. An air pressure–to–fluid compression sound wave transformation system (cochlea). Reamplified sound passing through the stapes sets up a series of waveforms that are carried through a closed fluid space (perilymph). Shearing forces change the resting volume and shape of the endolymph.

5. A fluid wave–to–electrical depolarization transformation system (cochlea). Fluid waves deforming the resting position of the inner and outer hair cells depolarize them, thus transforming the envelope of analogue sound into an electrical representation of sound that is carried along cranial nerve VIII to the brainstem, midbrain, and cortex, where sound is recognized centrally (Broca speech area).

The human ear develops from three tissue sources:
1. The otocyst (▶ Fig. 111.2) will form the membranous (cochlear and vestibular) labyrinth. Mesenchyme around the otocyst forms cartilaginous rests, which then ossify to become the endochondral bone of the otic capsule, the densest of the human bones. The petrous portion of the temporal bone is so named because of the dense otic capsule within it.
2. Branchial arches 1 and 2, together with the first pharyngeal pouch, will form all of the structures of the external auditory canal and middle ear except the footplate of the stapes (▶ Fig. 111.3). The first pharyngeal pouch develops into the pharyngotympanic (eustachian) tube and middle ear cavity. The middle ear cleft develops around the cartilage of the first and second branchial arches to give rise to the ossicles (▶ Fig. 111.4).
3. The six mesodermal hillocks from branchial arches 1 and 2 develop to form the auricle. The superficial mesoderm of branchial arches 1 and 2 gives rise to six preauricular cartilaginous hillocks arranged around the dorsal part of the first branchial cleft. These auricular hillocks (▶ Fig. 111.5, ▶ Fig. 111.6, ▶ Fig. 111.2) grow and mature to give rise to the

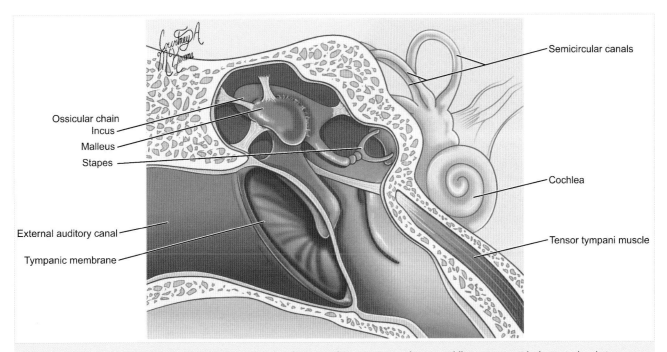

Fig. 111.1 Coronal view of a right ear showing the external auditory canal, tympanic membrane, middle ear space with the ossicular chain, tensor tympani muscle, and structures of the inner ear.

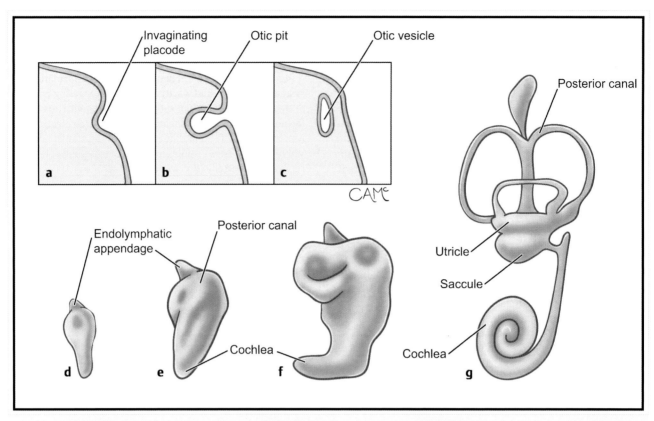

Fig. 111.2 (a–g) Schematic showing development of the membranous vestibular and cochlear labyrinths from the otic pit/vesicle.

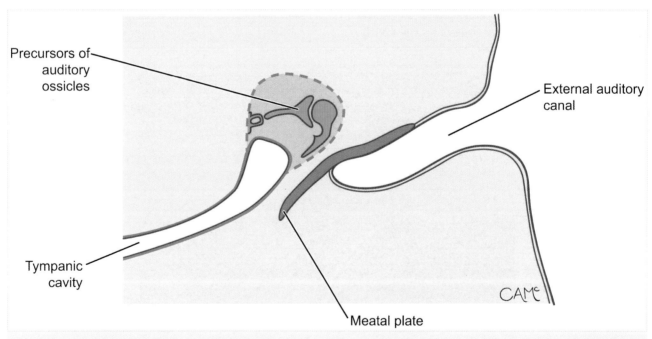

Fig. 111.3 Coronal view of a left ear. Branchial arches 1 and 2 give rise to the first branchial cleft, which invaginates and meets the first pharyngeal pouch to form the external auditory canal, tympanic membrane, and middle ear cleft.

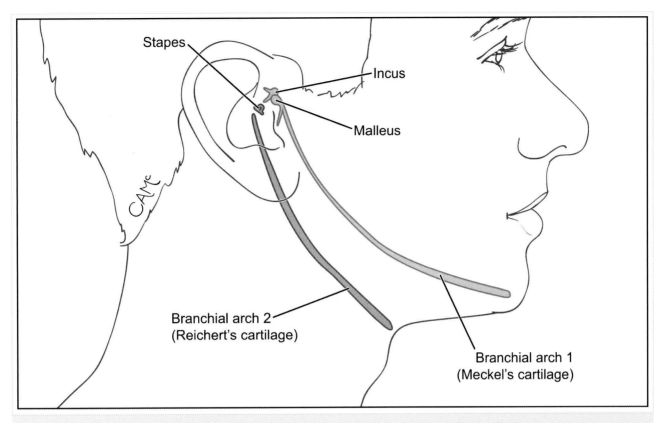

Fig. 111.4 Derivatives of the cartilage of branchial arch 1 (Meckel cartilage) and branchial arch 2 (Reichert cartilage).

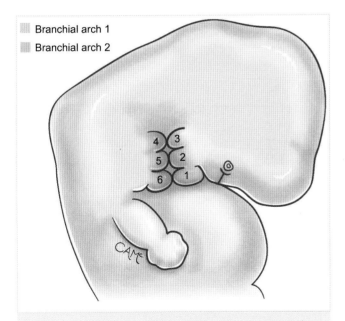

Fig. 111.5 Branchial arches 1 and 2 give rise to the six preauricular cartilaginous hillocks that will form the auricle.

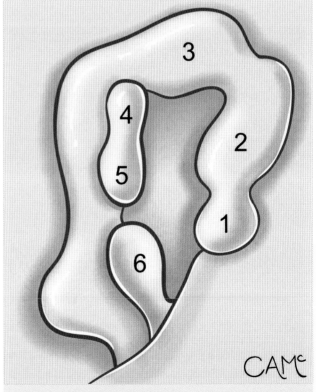

Fig. 111.6 Further development of the six preauricular hillocks into the cartilaginous skeleton of the auricle.

851

tragus (hillock 1), anterior helix (hillock 2), remainder of the helix (hillock 3), superior part of the antihelix (hillock 4), inferior part of the antihelix (hillock 5), and the antitragus and lobule (hillock 6). The outer and middle ear should be thought of as one developmental "unit." The inner ear develops simultaneously, but as a separate entity.

111.2.1 Early Embryonic and Fetal Life

The primordium of the inner ear appears in early embryonic life as a collection of plaquelike ectodermal cells on the cephalic end of the embryo next to the open neural tube of the rhombencephalon. This plaque, the otic placode (see ▶ Fig. 111.2), migrates medially into the surrounding mesenchyme and pinches off to form a pit, the otic vesicle. The otic vesicle continues to migrate medially toward the acoustic ganglion of the developing brain, from which it will derive its innervation. It migrates to lie near the first and second branchial arches. The five branchial arches in the human embryo (1, 2, 3, 4, and 6; 5 is rudimentary) are separated from one another by clefts (outside) and pouches (inside). Each arch has a mesodermal core, is covered with surface ectoderm, and is in close proximity to a pharyngeal pouch with its endodermal lining. Each branchial arch thus has all three structural subunits of development. The mesodermal center develops into the cartilage of the arch: the Meckel cartilage in branchial arch 1 and the Reichert cartilage in branchial arch 2. Each arch will have an arterial supply that involutes and is replaced by a named artery, a corresponding vein, and a nerve. The artery and nerve of branchial arch 1 are the external maxillary artery and the mandibular division of

the trigeminal nerve (V_3); the arterial supply and nervous supply of branchial arch 2 are the facial artery and nerve, respectively.

As the tubotympanic recess of pharyngeal pouch 1 migrates laterally through mesenchyme, it forms the eustachian tube and middle ear cleft. Its endodermal lining envelops the ossicles and will ultimately invest them with respiratory epithelium (pseudostratified columnar epithelium containing supporting cells and mucus-producing goblet cells). Meanwhile, the cleft between branchial arches 1 and 2 (first arch cleft) migrates medially to meet pharyngeal pouch 1. A "sandwich" of these three tissue layer derivatives will form the tympanic membrane: ectoderm (squamous epithelium) laterally, mesenchyme (fibrous middle layer of the tympanic membrane) centrally, and endoderm (respiratory epithelium) medially.

111.3 Ear Development: The Long of It

111.3.1 The Inner Ear

By the first month after conception, the otic placode (ectoderm; see ▶ Fig. 111.2) has formed in the region of the rhombencephalon. This deepens and migrates medially to form the otic pit, subsequently separating from the surface and becoming the otic vesicle. This is lined by ectoderm (and will be innervated by neural crest cells derived from the neural crest of the rhombencephalon, the acousticofacial ganglion) and is termed the otocyst. Two regions of each otocyst soon become recognizable: a dorsal or utricular portion (▶ Fig. 111.8), from which the endolymphatic duct arises, and a ventral or saccular portion. The otic vesicle then begins to divide into three basic subunits (see ▶ Fig. 111.2 and ▶ Fig. 111.8; ▶ Fig. 111.9, ▶ Fig. 111.10, ▶ Fig. 111.11).

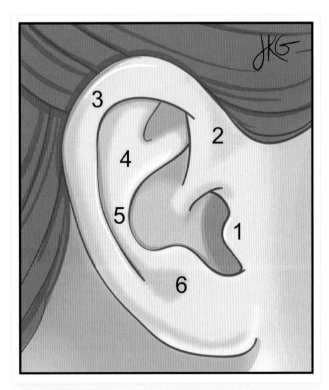

Fig. 111.7 Derivatives of the six preauricular hillocks in the normal human auricle.

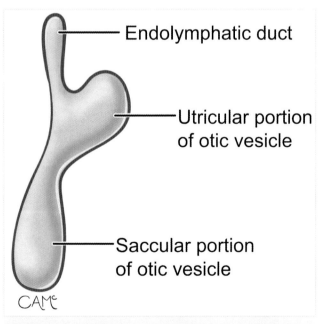

Fig. 111.8 The otocyst differentiates into a dorsal (utricular) portion, which also gives rise to the endolymphatic duct, and a ventral (saccular) portion.

1. First fold → endolymphatic sac.
2. Second fold → pars superior or vestibular section (phylogenetically older) → semicircular canals and utricle.
3. Third fold → pars inferior or cochlear section (phylogenetically newer) → cochlea, including the footplate of the stapes and saccule.

The second and third folds are connected by a constricted area called the utriculosaccular duct, leading from the pars superior (vestibular) to the pars inferior (cochlear) to the endolymphatic duct and sac. The saccule is separated from the cochlea by a deep constriction, termed the ductus reuniens. The membranous labyrinth is formed by the end of the seventh embryonic week.

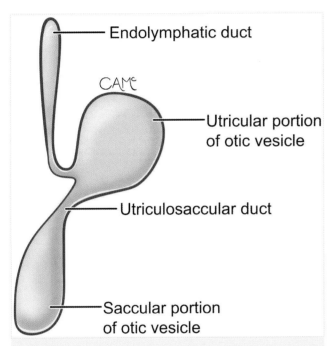

Fig. 111.9 Derivatives of the pars superior are the vestibular labyrinth, utricle, and endolymphatic sac. Derivatives of the pars inferior are the saccule, cochlea, and medial portion of the stapes footplate.

111.3.2 The Semicircular Canals, Utricle, and Saccule

Three flat, disclike diverticula grow out from the utricular portion (from the pars superior), and soon the central portions of the walls of these diverticula fuse and then disappear (see ▶ Fig. 111.2, ▶ Fig. 111.8, ▶ Fig. 111.9, ▶ Fig. 111.10, ▶ Fig. 111.11). The peripheral, unfused portions of the diverticula become the semicircular ducts, which are attached to the utricle and enclosed within the semicircular canals of the labyrinth. The three semicircular canals develop ampullated ends, all of which will eventually lie near the facial nerve, oriented roughly in the x, y, and z planes; each ampullated end contains a cupula comprising a gelatinous layer with both supporting and neuroepithelial cells, stereocilia, and kinocilia. The semicircular canals detect angular acceleration when the endolymph moves toward or away from the kinocilia, which serve as a reference. The saccule and utricle develop into gravity-sensing organs with a gelatinous otolithic membrane, upon which microscopic calcium carbonate crystals (otoconia) lie. These have mass and are affected by gravity. The innervation is from below the supporting and neuroepithelial cells. The superior portion of the vestibular ganglion innervates the cristae ampullares of the lateral and superior semicircular canals and the macula of the utricle. The inferior portion of the vestibular ganglion innervates the crista ampullaris of the posterior semicircular ampulla and the macula of the saccule.

111.3.3 The Cochlea

From the ventral (saccular) portion of the otocyst, a tubular diverticulum, the cochlear duct, grows and coils like a snail in two and three-quarter turns to form the cochlea. As the membranous labyrinth enlarges, vacuoles appear in the cartilaginous otic capsule and soon coalesce to form the perilymphatic space. The membranous labyrinth is now suspended in a fluid, the perilymph, within the perilymphatic space. The perilymphatic space related to the cochlear duct develops into two divisions: the scala tympani and the scala vestibuli. The cochlear duct is seen in the adult as the scala media. The scala tympani and scala vestibuli communicate at the helicotrema; the scala media is

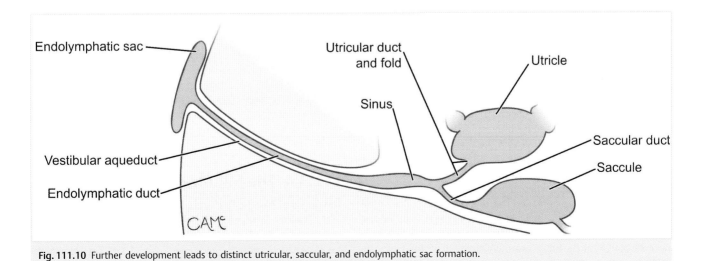

Fig. 111.10 Further development leads to distinct utricular, saccular, and endolymphatic sac formation.

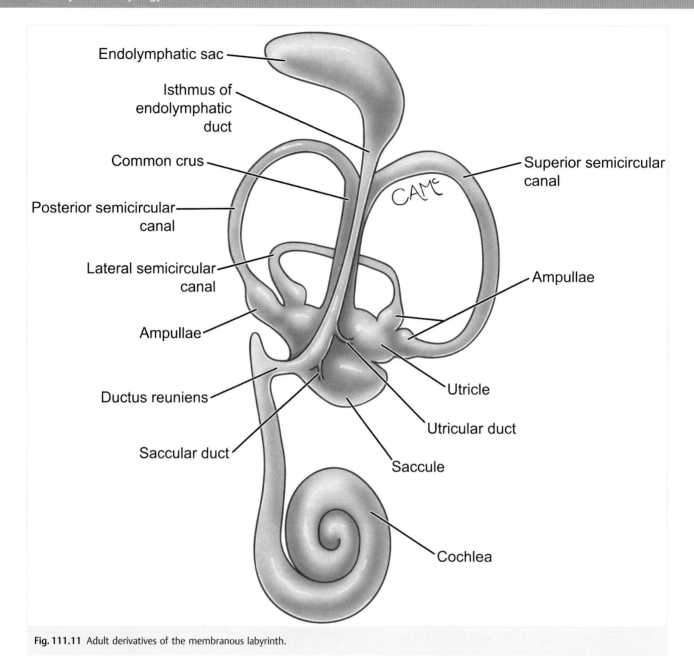

Fig. 111.11 Adult derivatives of the membranous labyrinth.

always separate. Within the cochlear duct (scala media), the connection of the cochlea with the saccule (pars inferior) becomes constricted to form the narrow ductus reuniens (see ▶ Fig. 111.11).

The organ of Corti differentiates from cells in the wall of the cochlear duct. Ganglion cells of cranial nerve VIII migrate along the turns of the cochlea and form the spiral ganglion, which innervates the organ of Corti. Within the organ of Corti, the epithelial cells differentiate into two columnar ridges, the inner ridge and the outer ridge, which elaborate the tectorial membrane. The inner ridge, called the spiral lamina, becomes the anatomical anchoring point for the organ of Corti. The spiral lamina, together with the helical bony nerve canal, is called the modiolus. The cartilaginous otic capsule ossifies from cartilaginous rests to form the bony (osseous) labyrinth of the inner ear.

The membranous labyrinth attains its adult size in the fetus. The surrounding otic capsule mesenchyme first chondrifies, then ossifies from approximately 14 to 16 ossification centers. Enchondral ossification takes place in all areas of the petromastoid temporal bone except in those areas with endosteal or periosteal surfaces (e.g., fissula ante fenestram). Therefore, three bony layers are histologically present within the temporal bones: the endosteal, enchondral, and periosteal layers.

111.3.4 The Middle Ear and Ossicles

The dorsal end of the first branchial arch cartilage (pars dorsalis of the Meckel cartilage) is closely related to the developing ear and becomes ossified to form the first two bones of the middle ear, the malleus and the incus (see ▶ Fig. 111.4). The intermedi-

Table 111.1 Auricular derivatives of the hillocks of His

Hillock No.	Derivative
1	Tragus
2	Anterior helix
3	Majority of the helix
4	Antihelix (superior part)
5	Antihelix (inferior part)
6	Antitragus and lobule

ate portion of the cartilage regresses and forms the anterior malleolar ligament. The trigeminal nerve (cranial nerve V) is the nerve of the first arch. Its derived and innervated muscles include the tensor tympani and the tensor veli palatini, and the anterior belly of the digastric muscle.

The dorsal end of the second arch cartilage (pars dorsalis of the Reichert cartilage) ossifies to form the stapes (all except the footplate) and the styloid process of the temporal bone. The facial nerve (cranial nerve VII) is the nerve of the second branchial arch, and its derived and innervated muscles include the muscles of facial expression, stapedius muscle, and posterior belly of the digastric muscle.

The primitive pharynx is wide cranially and narrows caudally as it joins the esophagus. Pairs of pharyngeal pouches lined by endoderm develop in a craniocaudal sequence between the branchial arches. The first pharyngeal pouch thus lies between the first and second branchial arches. The first pharyngeal pouch expands into an elongated tubotympanic recess and envelopes the structures of the middle ear cleft, creating an investiture of respiratory epithelium over all of the structures within the middle ear. The expanded distal portion of this recess contacts the first branchial groove (primordium of the external acoustic meatus) and later contributes to the formation of the tympanic membrane. During the late fetal period, the tympanic cavity gives rise to the mastoid antrum. The tubotympanic recess invaginates and pneumatizes the mesenchyme posterior to the ossicles, forming the aditus ad antrum and the antrum. Even in very poorly pneumatized temporal bones, the antral air cells are almost always found because their formation is an early developmental event. Further mastoid pneumatization occurs during childhood and depends upon normal eustachian tube function. The epithelial lining of the middle ear induces erosion of the surrounding mastoid bone; this is at least in part due to the fact that the partial pressure of air within the middle ear, aditus ad antrum, and antrum is greater than the resting pressure of bone marrow.

111.3.5 The External Ear

The external acoustic meatus develops from the dorsal end of the first branchial groove. The ectodermal cells at the bottom of this funnel-shaped tube proliferate and extend inward as a solid epithelial plate, the meatal plug. By the early part of month 7 of gestation, the central cells of this plug degenerate, thereby forming a cavity that becomes the inner part of the external acoustic meatus. The early tympanic membrane is composed of the ectoderm of the first branchial membrane, which separates the first branchial groove and the first pharyngeal pouch. The middle layer of mesenchyme of the first and second branchial arches persists between these two as the fibrous layer of the tympanic membrane.

The auricle develops from the superficial mesoderm of branchial arches 1 and 2, which give rise to the six preauricular cartilaginous hillocks arranged around the dorsal part of the first branchial cleft. The preauricular hillocks grow and mature to form the auricle (▶ Table 111.1; see ▶ Fig. 111.5, ▶ Fig. 111.6, ▶ Fig. 111.7).

The parts of the auricle derived from the first branchial arch are supplied by the mandibular branch of the trigeminal nerve; those derived from the second branchial arch are supplied by cutaneous branches of the cervical plexus, especially the lesser occipital and great auricular nerves. The facial nerve has few cutaneous branches, but some fibers contribute to the sensory innervation of the skin in the mastoid region and auricle.

111.4 Roundsmanship

- The external and middle ear clefts should be thought of as linked developmental entities.
- Any end organ innervated by the central nervous system develops from ectoderm. The development of the inner ear should be thought of as an event that occurs simultaneously with but separately from the development of the external and middle ear clefts.
- The external auditory canal develops from the first branchial cleft.
- The cartilaginous anlage of the first branchial arch is the Meckel cartilage, which gives rise to the malleus and incus.
- The middle ear, the eustachian tube, and its adnexa develop from the first pharyngeal pouch.
- The cartilaginous anlage of the second branchial arch is the Reichert cartilage, which gives rise to the stapes (except the footplate) and the styloid process.
- The auricle (pinna) develops from six auricular hillocks of cartilage, three each from branchial arches 1 and 2.

111.5 Recommended Reading

[1] Anson BJ, Donaldson JA. Surgical Anatomy of the Temporal Bone. 3rd ed. Philadelphia, PA: W. B. Saunders; 1981

[2] Gulya AJ. Developmental anatomy of the temporal bone and skull base. In: Gulya AJ, Minor LB, Poe DS, eds. Glasscock-Shambaugh's Surgery of the Ear. 6th ed. Shelton, CT: People's Medical Publishing House-USA; 2010:3–27

[3] Gulya AJ. Schuknect HF. Anatomy of the Temporal Bone with Surgical Implications. 3rd ed. New York, NY: Informa Healthcare; 2007

[4] Moore KL, Persaud V. The Developing Human. Philadelphia, PA: W. B. Saunders; 2003

112 Auditory Function and Dysfunction

Mila Quinn, Miriam I. Redleaf, and Christopher J. Linstrom

112.1 Introduction

The auditory system has several major distinctions from the vestibular system. The auditory system depends upon a physical interface with the environment: that is, sound vibrations must have open access to entry points into the primary receptive organ, the cochlea. Unlike in the vestibular system, there is no central compensation for unilateral auditory loss. Unlike vestibular sensations, auditory sensations are usually forefront in the conscious mind and are extensively manipulated for the pleasure they bring. The effects of untreated bilateral loss of auditory function are devastating, interrupting the acquisition of information, social contact, and personal growth.

112.2 Transmission of Sound Waves

The anatomical structure that allows the propagation of sound waves is in theory simple. The external auditory canal must have an air-filled lumen—an unobstructed air passage—to allow sound to arrive at the tympanic membrane. Additionally, each external canal has a resonant frequency that amplifies sound in the range of 3 to 4 kHz, much like a narrow-mouthed bottle. Structurally, the external auditory canal is lined with skin containing normal appendages as well as ceruminous glands. The medial portion of the canal is bony, whereas the lateral portion is cartilaginous. The physiologic purpose of the external auditory canal is to direct sound toward the tympanic membrane. However, many factors, both congenital and acquired, can cause canal occlusion.

The most common adult otologic complaint is cerumen impaction associated with secondary conductive hearing loss. Other causes of canal occlusion in adults include chronic ear canal dermatitis (i.e., chronic otitis externa), chronic infection, trauma, osteomata, and exostoses. In children, canal occlusion is most often caused by cerumen. Clearing the external ear of cerumen and/or other debris in most cases immediately improves hearing, usually to the level of the preoccluded state.

112.3 Congenital Auricular Atresia/Microtia

Congenital auricular atresia with microtia occurs rarely (approximately 1 in 1,000 live births), and the incidence varies by race. Congenital canal atresia typically presents very early in life. Despite the desire of parents and referring physicians for early intervention, only otoacoustic emissions testing of the normal ear is appropriate at this time. If the results of otoacoustic emissions testing are normal in the unaffected ear, it is highly likely that this ear will hear well and that the child will develop speech normally; however, if the results are abnormal or unobtainable, an auditory brainstem reflex test (ABR), either with sedation or under general anesthesia, is required to document the level of audition. In cases of bilateral congenital auricular atresia,

otoacoustic emissions testing is not possible, and an ABR with bone stimuli is required. Imaging studies, such as computed tomography (CT) of the temporal bones, add nothing to the immediate diagnostic needs of the child, expose the patient to approximately 50 times the radiation dose of a chest X-ray, and should be performed only before a surgical intervention. The banded bone-anchored hearing aid (BAHA) or baby BAHA is FDA-approved in the United States for children ages 6 months and older. Thus, there is time for both adequate diagnostic testing and therapeutic intervention, even in a child who has bilateral congenital auricular atresia with microtia.

The rare indication for CT before planned surgical correction of congenital auricular atresia (usually no sooner than the end of the child's sixth or seventh year) is to rule out cholesteatoma. This may hasten the time course of intervention but is usually not the only deciding factor. Surgery is generally not performed until the child is old enough to cooperate with postoperative care of the ear.

An older child without amplification may have speech delay or speech inaccuracies as a consequence of bilateral auricular conductive hearing loss. Again, emphasis should be placed on thorough audiometric testing of each ear and age-appropriate audiometric intervention, either with an air-level hearing aid, if possible, or with a vibrotactile hearing aid such as the banded BAHA. The insertion of the flange fixture for the BAHA is FDA-approved in the United States after the fifth birthday. If the child is very small, surgical intervention may be delayed until the skull is large and thick enough to accommodate a 3- or 4-mm flange fixture, usually after the sixth or seventh year. Unlike in adults, the insertion of a BAHA in children should be staged, with a 6-month period allowed for osseointegration of the flange fixture before the abutment is attached and the surrounding soft tissue is thinned.

Adult patients with partial stenosis of the external auditory canal may complain vigorously about itching in and drainage from the canal, and they may present with a history of recurrent ear infections accompanied by hearing loss. Physical examination of an adult will reveal the stenotic canal, and the skin may be visibly inflamed. If indicated, CT of the temporal bones demonstrates the extent of bony narrowing of the external ear, anatomy of the middle ear, integrity of the ossicular chain, anatomy of the otic capsule, and intratemporal course of the facial nerve.

Both medical treatment and surgery of the stenotic or atretic canal are difficult but not impossible. Inflamed and thickened canal skin can occasionally be treated successfully with topical steroids, antifungals, and antibiotics. Definitive treatment often involves excision of the occluding skin, canalplasty (widening of the bony canal), and placement of a thin split-thickness free skin graft to resurface the bony canal. The external auditory canal must be carefully packed to support the new grafts and treated with meticulous care during the healing period (approximately 6 weeks).

In pediatric cases of canal atresia, the treatment is more problematic. The atretic soft tissue and the calvaria adjacent to the external auditory canal, the atretic plate, span the site where the external canal would normally be located. The ossicles are often malformed; the malleus and incus are typically fused and attached to the bone of the tympanic ring, and there is no tympanic membrane. The facial nerve may run through the middle ear space in an expectedly abnormal course. Because of the lack of height of the tympanic ring, the distance from the glenoid fossa to the middle cranial fossa may be too small to accommodate a neocanal with an adequate lumen. The lack of adequate height forces the neocanal to be located more posterosuperiorly, and the canal may not line up perfectly with the reconstructed tympanic membrane. Reconstruction of an atretic external auditory canal in children is successful only with perfect surgical technique and meticulous postoperative care. This is not an operation for the occasional or inexperienced otologist. The parents must be told that at least some form of postoperative stenosis is likely to occur, even if the initial meatus is widely patent, and that revisions are commonly necessary. A molded ear plug taken at the time of the initial surgery or revision and used during sleep may help to keep the reconstructed canal patent. Meticulous and frequent care is always required. Even if the conductive hearing loss is not improved to the level of soft speech (30 dB), the presence of a patent external auditory canal may allow placement of an air-level hearing aid.

Another successful option for hearing rehabilitation may be the placement of a bone conduction hearing aid. This can be a bone-anchored hearing aid (BAHA) in adults 18 years of age or older or in children older than 5 years, a dentally fixed conduction device in adults 18 years of age or older (SoundBite; Sonitus Medical, San Mateo, CA), or a traditional head-banded bone conduction hearing aid in children (e.g., the banded BAHA). Each device is a vibrotactile stimulator of the cranium and cochlea. The flange fixture (screw) of the BAHA undergoes osseointegration with the cranium behind the stenotic canal. The dental appliance is attached to the subjacent maxillary molars, and the traditional bone conduction aid vibrates against the adjacent cranium via the scalp. The vibratory signal propagates through the entire cranium, stimulating the ipsilateral cochlea. These devices usually eliminate a significant portion of the conductive hearing loss (i.e., only the neurosensory reserve of the cochlea is important in the preoperative evaluation). Because the BAHA is a percutaneous device, the skin over and adjacent to the flange fixture must be pierced and thinned.

112.4 Ossicular Amplification of Sound Vibrations

The next physiologic step in the auditory system is amplification of the sound waves. Transmission of sound waves to the inner ear is accomplished by the tympanic membrane, ossicles, and oval window footplate. The auricle helps to locate sound in the vertical plane. The external canal has its own resonance, which amplifies the 3- to 4-kHz range. Physiologically, the major factors that amplify incoming sound waves are the ratio of the area of the tympanic membrane to the area of the oval window footplate, and the lever action of the ossicles (▶ Fig. 112.1).

The sound pressure (pressure = force/area) at ear level is naturally amplified 20-fold by the ratio of the tympanic membrane area to the footplate area, and the lever action of the native unobstructed ossicles increases the sound pressure by 1.3. Together, these increase the signal of the sound vibrations by

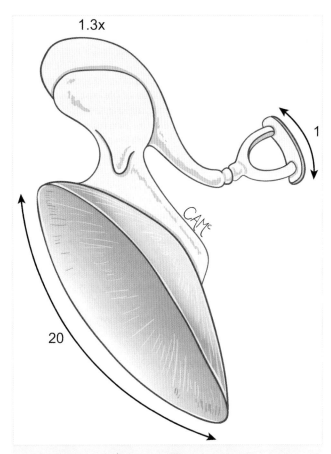

Fig. 112.1 Schematic of the ratio of tympanic membrane size to oval window size (power = force/area = 20), and the lever action of the ossicles (1.3). The sum of these two actions increases the power (power = force/area) of footplate displacement 26 times, which is a net gain of 28 dB in amplitude.

28 dB from the lateral surface of the tympanic membrane to the undersurface of the stapes footplate.

Any pathology that interrupts sound wave amplification to the tympanic membrane and/or ossicles, or impedes ossicular vibration, may cause a mechanical (conductive) hearing loss; middle ear fluid, tympanic membrane perforation, tympanosclerosis, tympanic membrane retraction, ossicular erosion, malleus fixation, and otosclerosis are common middle ear pathologies. This set of problems represents reversible otologic disease. Common problems of the tympanic membrane and/or ossicles can be treated surgically.

Within the middle ear, the most common pathology that impedes ossicular vibration is fluid from otitis media, either the purulence of acute otitis media or the serous effusion of chronic otitis media. Children may not notice or care about their hearing loss, but adults are more apt to notice the change in hearing and will seek medical attention. In addition to the physical and audiometric examinations, CT of the temporal bone may reveal chronic mastoiditis, dehiscence of the tegmen, and/or encephalocele formation. Eustachian tube dysfunction may lead to chronic middle ear and mastoid hypoventilation, and chronic infection may develop. Attempts have been made to correct eustachian tube dysfunction with medical or surgical intervention. These techniques include nasal steroids and other medications, almost all of which are ineffective. Surgical approaches include partial resection of the cartilaginous meatus in the nasopharyngeal fossa of Rosenmüller and balloon tuboplasty. These are technically difficult to perform with insufficient proof of universal benefit, and they are not part of standard practice. The discipline of surgical manipulation of the eustachian tube is developing. For adults and children, the standard treatment for middle ear fluid is the pressure equalization tube.

Problems of the tympanic membrane and ossicular chain tend to be acquired rather than congenital in both adults and children. In children, congenital ossicular malformations are usually found in combination with canal atresia and tend to consist of misshapen or fused ossicles that are fixed laterally to the atretic plate. Correcting any ossicular problem is secondary to the atresia repair.

If the external auditory canal is patent, the otoscopic examination will help determine the size and location of a tympanic membrane perforation, but an intact tympanic membrane is a natural barrier to full visualization of the middle ear. An audiogram is absolutely required and should demonstrate a conductive or mixed hearing loss in the setting of tympanic membrane or middle ear pathology. A well-performed CT of the temporal bones with thin cuts (1-mm slices) and edge enhancement will usually reveal fenestral otosclerosis or ossicular discontinuity

when these are present. Chronic inflammation may obscure the ossicular chain. It is important that the CT be performed and the results reviewed by an experienced radiologist. CT is the imaging modality of choice when superior canal dehiscence, malleus fixation, or wide cochlear aqueduct is suspected to be the cause of conductive hearing loss (▶ Fig. 112.2). It is important to bear in mind that tympanosclerosis is hyalinized scar tissue and not ordinarily calcified. Its characteristic signal on CT is that of a dense shadow, not of calcified tissue.

Conductive hearing loss can be treated medically with a hearing aid in patients of any age, or with a bone conduction aid, as previously described. Surgical interventions for tympanic membrane and ossicular pathology should be well-known to otolaryngologists. Tympanic membrane perforations may be grafted, the ossicular chain may be reconstructed, a stapes prosthesis may be placed, or a BAHA may be inserted.

112.5 Fluid-Filled Spaces of the Cochlea

At the stapes footplate, sound waves are transformed from vibration of the ossicles to undulation of the perilymph in the scala vestibuli. The neuroepithelium of the cochlea is located in

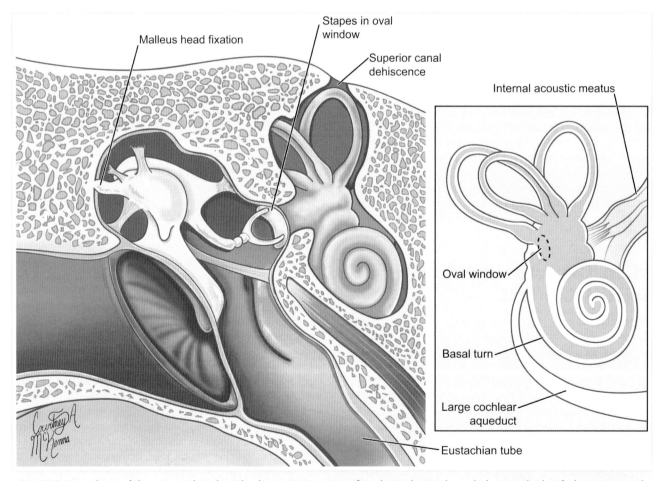

Fig. 112.2 Coronal view of the otic capsule and ossicles demonstrating causes of conductive hearing loss, which are easily identified on a computed tomographic scan: superior canal dehiscence, malleus fixation, and large cochlear aqueduct. The large cochlear aqueduct is in a different coronal plane and is superimposed upon this image.

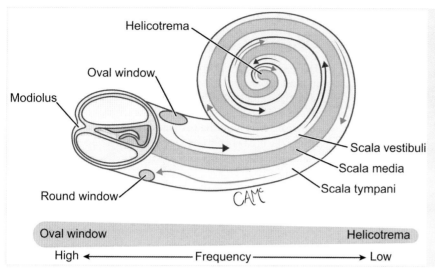

Fig. 112.3 The cochlea as an uncoiled tube. Oval window vibration causes the perilymph of the scala vestibuli to vibrate, propagating sound waves in fluid around the helicotrema to the scala tympani and round window. The neuroepithelium in the scala media (cochlear duct) is tonotopically arranged, with the highest frequencies represented near the oval window and the lowest frequencies at the helicotrema.

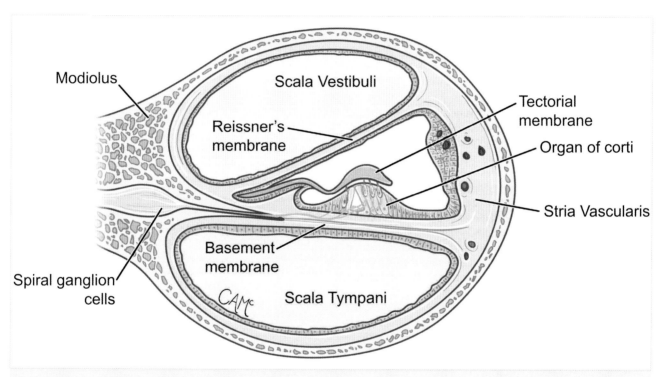

Fig. 112.4 Displacement of the scala media basement membrane by the perilymph of the scala tympani occurs tonotopically and changes the rate of firing of hair cells in the organ of Corti. Afferent signals are transmitted by the nerve fibers of the spiral ganglion cells.

the endolymph of the scala media, a closed tube surrounded by a continuous cushion of perilymph (▶ Fig. 112.3). At the same temperature, fluid is neither compressible nor distensible. Sound pressure at the medial surface of the stapes footplate is transmitted throughout the entirety of the perilymphatic space via the helicotrema. Vibration of the stapes footplate at the scala vestibuli is propagated to the tip of the cochlea, the helicotrema, and travels back down the length of the cochlea in the scala tympani to be "relieved" at the round window membrane. Anatomically, the neuroepithelium near the oval window—the base of the cochlea—is most stimulated by high-frequency sounds, whereas the area near the helicotrema is most stimulated by low-frequency sounds.

Neuroepithelial afferent signals depend on two broad conditions: the endolymphatic potential and the undulating displacement of the scala media basement membrane by the perilymph. The differential ion concentrations of the perilymph (low K^+, high Na^+) and endolymph (high K^+, low Na^+) are maintained by sodium–potassium pumps in the stria vascularis (▶ Fig. 112.4). The net outcome is an 80-mV positive charge in the endolymphatic spaces, which is necessary for neuroepithelial function. Physiologically, two mechanisms appear to focus the undulations of the perilymph to narrow the area of stimulation of the neuroepithelium. The lumen shape and tissue dynamics of the perilymph of the scala tympani displace the basement membrane of the scala media at frequency-specific locations. And, as will be seen later, there is modulation of the afferent neural signal via efferents and via the outer hair cells.

Pathologic conditions are those that interfere with the composition of the endolymph and the undulation of the perilymph. These conditions are for the most part acquired, not congenital. Otosclerosis of the cochlear otic capsule causes atrophy of the subjacent stria vascularis, disrupts the endolymphatic potential, and causes a concomitant sensorineural hearing loss. The undulating perilymphatic wave is disrupted by many disease processes. Labyrinthitis or meningitis can cause the scalae to fill with new bone (labyrinthitis ossificans). Formation of a "third window"—an opening into the cochlea in addition to the oval and round windows—may cause a conductive hearing loss. This is seen in superior or posterior canal dehiscence. Meniere disease, or endolymphatic hydrops, classically causes *unprovoked* episodes of aural fullness and pressure, tinnitus, and acute hearing loss, followed by minutes to hours of vertigo. With repeated attacks, there may be slowly progressive hearing loss, which may be related to the distortion and dilation of the scala media.

The primary complaint in all of these conditions is hearing loss. The otologic examination is usually normal. On tuning fork examination, the Weber test may be abnormal; the Rinne test is usually normal. A standard audiogram is required to assess the side and type of hearing loss. Asymmetries of sensorineural hearing are never normal, regardless of the putative diagnosis, and must be further evaluated with an appropriate retrocochlear test: contrast-enhanced magnetic resonance (MR) imaging or CT with contrast. Vestibular evoked myographic potential (VEMP) testing, described extensively in Chapter 113, may help diagnose superior canal dehiscence syndrome. CT can be helpful because it can demonstrate fenestral and/or cochlear otosclerosis, and it usually is quite helpful in identifying ossification of the scalae and canal dehiscence. If superior canal dehiscence syndrome is suspected, then CT should be performed in an orientation orthogonal to the superior semicircular canal.

Treatment for these conditions includes hearing aids. It is important to note that in Meniere disease, the patient's narrowed dynamic range may result in hyperacusis and/or recruitment, causing the amplified signal to become painful and/or distorted; amplification clipping essential, so that the amplified signal from the hearing aid will not cause discomfort. Similarly, in semicircular canal dehiscence syndrome, amplification may cause dizziness (Tullio phenomenon). These potential problems must be considered by the dispensing audiologist.

Sensorineural hearing loss due to scala tympani ossification and far-advanced otosclerosis can be compensated by cochlear implantation. The conductive hearing loss of superior canal dehiscence can be arrested or sometimes improved with canal occlusion via a middle cranial fossa approach, but this is a technically difficult operation. The hearing loss of Meniere disease may be arrested or sometimes improved by endolymphatic sac decompression and/or shunting, an operation whose efficacy remains controversial because the perceived improvements may be due to the natural unpredictable fluctuations of Meniere disease or a placebo effect.

112.6 Neuroepithelium of the Organ of Corti

The cochlea, seen schematically in ▶ Fig. 112.5, is 35 mm long in most people and is coiled in two and one-half turns. The scala media contains the primary auditory organ, the organ of Corti (see ▶ Fig. 112.5), whose function is to transduce the mechanical displacement of the perilymph wave into neurotransmitter firing. The organ of Corti is a complex collection of neuroepithelium consisting of inner and outer hair cells, as well as essential supporting cells (▶ Fig. 112.6).

The inner hair cells synapse with afferent fibers of the auditory nerve, while the outer hair cells synapse with efferent fibers from the same nerve. The organ is elongated, running the entire length of the scala media. The composition of the endolymph creates a positive potential relative to the perilymph. Within the tunnel of Corti (the space between the inner and outer hair cells), a different electrolyte composition creates yet another functionally distinct space. The tips of the inner and outer hair cells have stereocilia, which extend into the tectorial membrane. When the basement membrane undulates, these stereocilia are sheared one direction, then another, altering the firing rates of the hair cells.

The sensory information from the hair cells travels medially into the osseous spiral lamina toward the neurologic center of the cochlea, the modiolus (see ▶ Fig. 112.5). Type 1 and type 2 spiral ganglion cells are the primary sensory afferent cell bodies for the auditory nerve.

Many pathologic conditions affect the function of the organ of Corti. The congenital disorders that cause organ of Corti malformations and dysfunction are numerous. The types of congenital malformations of the otic capsule associated with varying degrees of membranous labyrinth dysgenesis and organ of Corti malformation are shown in ▶ Fig. 112.7. Most of these malformations are visible with the resolution available on fine-cut CT. However, in most congenital forms of hearing loss, the CT scan appears normal, and in recent years evaluation has relied more heavily on genetic studies. The current classification system for congenital hearing loss is the dfna/dfnb/dfnx and mito system. In this classification, *dfn* denotes nonsyndromic hereditary deafness, *a* indicates an autosomal-dominant mode of inheritance, *b* indicates autosomal-recessive inheritance, *x* denotes X-linked inheritance, and *mito* indicates mitochondrial inheritance. The most common form of nonsyndromic sensorineural hearing loss identified at present is malformation of the connexin genes, which encode gap junction proteins between cell membranes and may be responsible for maintaining the sodium–potassium gradients essential for neuroepithelial function.

The types of congenital hearing losses that are associated with other disorders or syndromes are diverse. For example, a widened vestibular aqueduct and enlarged endolymphatic sac can be associated with Pendred syndrome (thyroid goiter/hypothyroidism and bilateral congenital sensorineural hearing loss). Many of the craniofacial syndromes, such as Apert syndrome (acrocephalosyndactyly), Crouzon syndrome (craniosynostosis, low-set ears, exophthalmos, hypertelorism, hypoplastic mandible, often with patent ductus arteriosus and coarctation of the

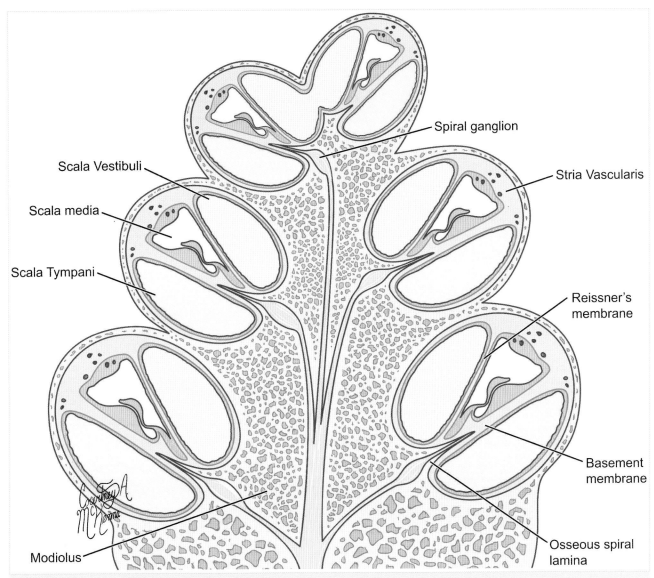

Fig. 112.5 The scalae of the cochlea, coiled 2.5 times in successively smaller turns. The scala media (cochlear duct) with the organ of Corti is seen, along with the scala vestibuli and scala tympani, osseous spiral lamina, stria vascularis, modiolus with spiral ganglion cells, and auditory nerve.

aorta), and Waardenburg syndrome (iris pigment abnormality, white forelock or white hair on other areas of the body, hypertelorism), are apparent on first examination. It is standard to look for disorders of thyroid and kidney function during the routine laboratory testing of children with sensorineural hearing loss, and to check for Usher syndrome (retinitis pigmentosa) by referral to an ophthalmologist for an examination of the retina and possibly an electroretinogram. An electrocardiogram is required to rule out Jervell syndrome and Lange-Nielsen syndrome, in which a mutation of genes coding for potassium channels may cause prolongation of the QTinterval, in addition to sensorineural hearing loss. It remains unclear how these congenital structural malformations and gene defects impair hair cell signaling at the cellular level. Repair at the cellular level is not possible at this time.

The infant is often identified because he or she has failed a newborn hearing screening examination and is referred for further testing. An older child will be given the benefit of the doubt for about 12 months. If the child does not say "mama" or "dada" by then, patience and denial of the problem are exhausted, and parents want a swift diagnosis. The hearing screen can be performed with otoacoustic emissions testing, which measures cochlear events, or with an ABR, which is a more involved test of both the peripheral and central auditory system. The ABR is an early-latency evoked response in that the waveforms elicited occur within a few milliseconds of the stimulus. In most cases, the child will eventually be referred for otologic evaluation, which involves a gestational and family history, physical examination, age-appropriate audiometric confirmatory testing, imaging, laboratory testing, and genetic counsel-

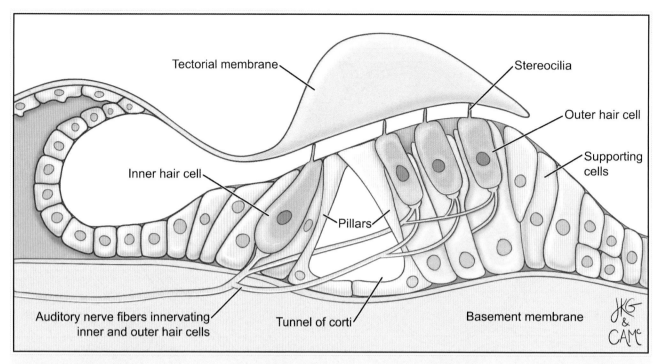

Fig. 112.6 Structure of the organ of Corti, showing the inner and outer hair cells, tunnel of Corti, and supporting cells. Shearing of the hair cell stereocilia modulates firing rates.

Malformation	Description	CT Findings
Scheibe	Cochleosacular membranous aplasia	Normal
Scheibe-Bing-Siebenmann	Complete labyrinthine membranous aplasia	Normal
Mondini	Incomplete interscalar septal formation, reduced number of cochlea turns	Fig. 7
Michel's Aplasia	No inner ear formation	No structures on CT
Large Vestibular Aqueduct	Large vestibular aqueduct	Fig. 7

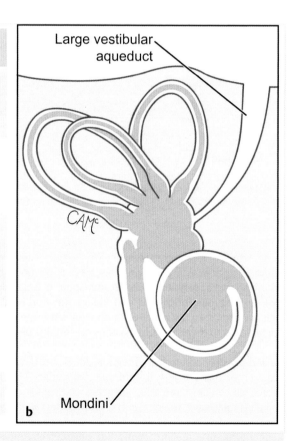

a

b

Fig. 112.7 (a) Congenital malformations of the otic capsule. (b) Corresponding computed tomographic profiles. *CT*, computed tomography.

ing. It is important not to jump to diagnostic or therapeutic conclusions on the first visit. Even if severe or profound hearing loss is suspected, it is initially very difficult for parents to understand and accept this in their child. In many cases, a brief trial of amplification and repeated testing may be performed to help parents to understand the severity of the problem. Above all, the physician must be empathetic and absolutely sure that the audiometric evaluation has been performed thoroughly and properly before making any significant recommendations, such as cochlear implantation.

Acquired hearing loss in adults is quite common. The most common type is presbycusis, which is the down-sloping high-frequency hearing loss of aging. The actual mechanism remains unclear, as does prevention. Noise exposure and exposure to ototoxic medications have long been known to cause sensorineural hearing loss. Otosclerosis may cause conductive or mixed hearing loss. Autoimmune hearing loss, or autoimmune inner ear disease, ordinarily follows a pattern of a downward fluctuation and inexorable diminution of hearing. It is usually bilateral, but the hearing loss may be sequential (i.e., one ear may lose hearing and then the other after a delay of 6 to 12 months). The pattern of fluctuation is very important in making the diagnosis. Many batteries of serologic testing are available, much as for any rheumatologic disease. These should be done to help support or refute the diagnosis of autoimmune inner ear disease.

The causation of hearing loss in adults often remains uncertain. The audiogram describes the pattern of loss, not the reason for the loss. Otoacoustic emissions, which reflect outer hair cell function, are usually absent. CT of the temporal bone is usually normal. MR imaging of the brain with contrast, with particular attention to the internal auditory canal, is usually normal. The patient is often left with the diagnosis of "sensorineural hearing loss" but not a reason for the loss. It should be a comfort for the patient that a thorough diagnostic evaluation will definitively exclude a retrocochlear tumor as a cause of the hearing loss.

By far the most frustrating form of acquired hearing loss is "sudden deafness," or sudden idiopathic sensorineural hearing loss, which occurs unilaterally over a period of minutes or hours (by definition, a 30-dB interaural difference in three adjacent frequencies over a period of no more than 3 days) and for which no real etiology is identified. Sudden idiopathic sensorineural hearing loss is thought to be a cochlear event. Because nobody dies of this condition, there is no event-related histopathology to define the cause. Oral or intratympanic steroids are currently the treatment of choice and may reverse the hearing loss if given in a timely fashion and in large enough quantities. There is no place for antiviral medication in the treatment of sudden idiopathic sensorineural hearing loss.

The treatment of sensorineural hearing loss in children and adults is amplification. Hearing aids are tried first, even in children with profound sensorineural loss. Parents are instructed on how to watch for any benefit from hearing aid use, such as startling to noises, recognizing and mimicking environmental sounds, and beginning to phonate. Adults who start using hearing aids can be tested behaviorally and can describe for themselves how amplification may be helping. If the hearing aids are of limited benefit, evaluation for cochlear implantation can be initiated.

112.7 Auditory Nerve and Central Pathways

The cell bodies for the auditory nerve are the spiral ganglion cells in the modiolus of the cochlea. These become the auditory nerve and travel in the internal auditory canal to synapse in the ipsilateral cochlear nucleus. From there, ipsilateral and contralateral projections travel to higher centers, merging with input from the contralateral auditory nerve (▶ Fig. 112.8).

Rarely, there is congenital absence of the auditory nerve. This is suspected during newborn auditory screening and is usually accompanied by a malformation of the otic capsule on CT. The internal auditory canal can be narrow. MR imaging can help in identifying how many nerves are present in the internal auditory canal. If only one nerve is identified, and if the face has normal function, the nerve is assumed to be the facial nerve. An electrical ABR, in which an electrode is placed transtympanically into the promontory to stimulate the spiral ganglion cells, can help determine if there is a functioning cochlear nerve. The presence of a wave v on an electrical ABR indicates function of the auditory nerve and would support cochlear implantation, if the bilateral hearing level is appropriately diminished.

Another pediatric diagnosis in hearing loss is central auditory neuropathy; the best-understood example of this is the presence of central hemosiderin deposits (kernicterus) in newborns with high postpartum bilirubin levels. Central auditory neuropathy is also diagnosed functionally in patients with auditory neuropathy (auditory dyssynchrony). These patients have poor sensorineural function. Although otoacoustic emissions may be present, the ABR is abnormal and often absent, indicating a disconnect between the cochlea and the eighth cranial nerve. Although these patients may not be the very best candidates, cochlear implantation is indicated because amplification is of very little benefit, if any.

Pathologic conditions of the auditory nerve in adults cause sensorineural hearing loss that is characterized by disproportionately low speech discrimination scores. The most common acquired benign pathology of the auditory nerve is a vestibular schwannoma (or acoustic neuroma), which grows from either the superior or inferior vestibular nerve and impairs auditory function by direct compression of the auditory nerve. The auditory nerve also may be implicated in presbycusis.

Any neurologic condition that occurs spatially in areas of central auditory pathways can affect hearing. Multiple sclerosis can cause sensorineural hearing loss, as can other central autoimmune diseases, such as polyarteritis nodosa. Central auditory processing testing can identify central presbycusis. Any intracranial space-occupying lesion can affect hearing.

The diagnosis of hearing loss is properly made by an audiogram. An unexpectedly low speech discrimination score and normal otoacoustic emissions, a test of outer hair cell function, suggest problems in the auditory nerve or centrally. Central auditory processing tests, such as auditory discrimination tests, temporal processing and pattern discrimination tests, and dichotic speech tests, can help distinguish peripheral dysfunction from central dysfunction. After these functional tests are

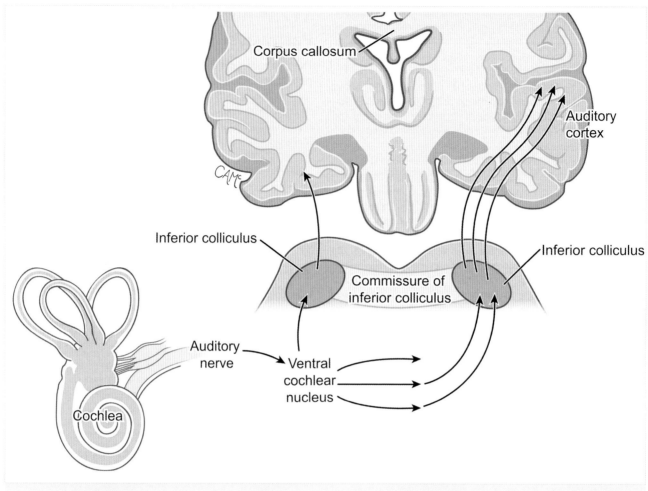

Fig. 112.8 Central projections of the auditory nerve.

obtained, MR imaging of the brain and internal auditory canals with and without gadolinium is imperative. When a neurologic disease is suspected, a neurology consult is appropriate. Any disease process that may be identified should be treated appropriately.

The treatment of sensorineural hearing loss, whether of cochlear or retrocochlear etiology, is amplification. Cochlear implantation is an appropriate treatment modality for those people who cannot be helped with hearing aids. At one time, the replacement of cochlear function with a cochlear implant was considered inappropriate treatment for central sensorineural hearing loss, but opinion on this has changed. These patients comprehend speech better with a cochlear implant than with a hearing aid. The patients must be instructed, however, that the possible improvement after cochlear implantation will be limited by the underlying pathology. Specifically, their speech understanding (especially in noise) may not be as good as that of traditional users of cochlear implants. Hearing retraining programs are now available for adults with decreased central auditory processing, although improvements in central auditory processing disorder tests after retraining have not been established. Perhaps the appropriate metric to quantify improvement has not yet been found.

112.8 Disease-Specific Diagnostic Testing

It is sometimes helpful to reconsider mechanisms of hearing loss and to survey the tests that help clarify each situation. The most common cause of hearing loss is middle ear fluid. This is diagnosed by visualization of the tympanic membrane and insufflation with a pneumatic otoscope. The tympanogram in the setting of middle ear fluid is usually, but not always, flat. Myringotomy may reveal middle ear fluid even in patients with normal otoscopy and peaked tympanogram tracings. Finally, CT can identify fluid in the middle ear and mastoid, especially in the case of chronic mastoiditis.

Conductive hearing loss is diagnosed by tuning fork testing and audiography. The Weber and Rinne tests show characteristic findings, with the Weber test lateralizing to the affected ear. Air conduction may be less than bone conduction in the affected ear, while air conduction is greater than bone conduction in the normal ear. The audiogram usually shows an air–bone gap. However, bone thresholds may be unreliable, especially if there are bilaterally reduced thresholds and if there is difficulty in masking out one side. Very rarely, what is interpreted by the audiologist as a sensorineural loss may in fact be a conductive loss. Because crucial hearing-related advice and decisions are based upon audiometric testing, the audiologist must be well trained and experienced. Self-administered hearing tests are notoriously unreliable and should not be used. CT at thin slice intervals and with edge enhancement may be helpful in defining the cause of conductive hearing loss. It can show soft tissue in the middle ear space, ossicular erosion, otosclerosis, malleus fixation, a large cochlear aqueduct, and dehiscence of the superior or posterior semicircular canal.

Sensorineural hearing loss should be suspected in anyone with nonpulsatile tinnitus, whether or not the individual is aware of any hearing loss. The Weber and Rinne tests can identify asymmetric hearing loss because air conduction will exceed bone conduction bilaterally, and the Weber test will lateralize to the unaffected side. These tests yield information about the physics of audition but not about the level of audition. Professionally performed audiography is required to demonstrate sensorineural loss. Speech discrimination scores that are lower than pure tone thresholds may indicate dysfunction of the auditory nerve or central hearing loss. The presence of recruitment with tuning fork testing is diagnostic of cochlear losses. Normal otoacoustic emissions, which reflect outer hair cell integrity and function, suggest retrocochlear rather than cochlear losses. In cases of asymmetric sensorineural hearing loss, MR imaging of the internal auditory canals with gadolinium contrast should be obtained to rule out a cerebellopontine angle or an internal auditory canal mass.

The presence of a "third window" should be suspected in adults with no history of otitis who have unilateral conductive hearing loss documented on an audiogram. Vestibular evoked myographic potential (VEMP) testing shows a lower threshold in the affected ear. CT may identify the site of otic capsule dehiscence.

112.9 Roundsmanship

- Physiologically, the major factors that amplify incoming sound waves are the ratio of the area of the tympanic membrane to that of the oval window footplate, and the lever action of the ossicles.
- The neuroepithelium near the oval window (basal turn of the cochlea) is most stimulated by high-frequency sounds, whereas the area near the helicotrema is most stimulated by low-frequency sounds.

- Neuroepithelial afferent signals from the cochlea depend on two broad conditions: the endolymphatic potential and the undulating displacement of the scala media basement membrane by the perilymph.
- Type 1 and type 2 spiral ganglion cells are the primary sensory afferent cell bodies for the auditory nerve.
- From the cochlear nucleus, ipsilateral and contralateral projections travel to higher centers of the brain and merge with input from the contralateral auditory nerve.
- The most common cause of hearing loss is middle ear fluid. This is diagnosed by visualization of the tympanic membrane and insufflation with a pneumatic otoscope.
- The most common cause of acquired hearing loss in adults is presbycusis.
- Sensorineural hearing loss should be suspected in anyone with nonpulsatile tinnitus, whether or not the individual is aware of any hearing loss.
- Pathologic conditions of the auditory nerve in adults cause sensorineural hearing loss, which is characterized by disproportionately low speech discrimination scores.
- The treatment of sensorineural hearing loss, whether of cochlear or retrocochlear etiology, is amplification.

112.10 Recommended Reading

[1] Guinan JJ, Salt A, Cheatham MA. Progress in cochlear physiology after Békésy. Hear Res 2012

[2] Heman-Ackah SE, Roland JT, Haynes DS, Waltzman SB. Pediatric cochlear implantation: candidacy evaluation, medical and surgical considerations, and expanding criteria. Otolaryngol Clin North Am 2012; 45: 41–67

[3] Joshi VM, Navlekar SK, Kishore GR, Reddy KJ, Kumar EC. CT and MR imaging of the inner ear and brain in children with congenital sensorineural hearing loss. Radiographics 2012; 32: 683–698

[4] Merchant SN, Rosowski JJ. Conductive hearing loss caused by third-window lesions of the inner ear. Otol Neurotol 2008; 29: 282–289

[5] Schow RL, Seikel JA, Chermak GD, Berent M. Central auditory processes and test measures: ASHA 1996 revisited. Am J Audiol 2000; 9: 63–68

[6] Schwander M, Kachar B, Müller U. Review series: The cell biology of hearing. J Cell Biol 2010; 190: 9–20

[7] Shearer AE, Hildebrand MS, Sloan CM, Smith RJ. Deafness in the genomics era. Hear Res 2011; 282: 1–9

[8] Ulfendahl M, Flock Å . Outer hair cells provide active tuning in the organ of corti. News Physiol Sci 1998; 13: 107–111

[9] Willi UB. Middle-ear mechanics: the dynamic behavior of the incudo-malleolar joint and its role during the transmission of sound [dissertation]. Zurich, Switzerland: University Hospital; 2003:1–26

113 Equilibrium Function and Dysfunction

Mila Quinn, Miriam I. Redleaf, and Christopher J. Linstrom

113.1 Introduction

A normally functioning vestibular system calls no attention to itself. When everything is working well, individuals are unaware of balance, much as they are unaware of a normally functioning heart. A normally functioning system can be manipulated to bring casual pleasure, such as rolling down a snow-covered hill, going on "fun rides," or watching a large-screen IMAX movie. Other than these entertainments, most people rarely think about spinning or balance. In contrast, any dysfunction of the vestibular system is acutely noted by most individuals, who are unable to ignore their symptoms. They usually cannot tell which side is malfunctioning, or what activities elicit their unsteadiness; however, they are usually intensely bothered by their imbalance and demand comfort and relief. It only complicates the picture that any medication or illness can be associated with imbalance and that imbalance occurs in 100% of the population. The goal of this chapter is to guide the general otolaryngologist toward a diagnosis and treatment plan for patients with vestibular complaints. It is unreasonable to expect that the otolaryngologist will cure every patient. The role of the medical professional is to diagnose the end organ that is the likely cause of the problem and to offer reasonable treatment.

This chapter provides an outline of the functional components of the vestibular system. For each functional component, the anatomy, physiology, dysfunction, diagnostic tests, and treatment options are surveyed.

113.2 Orientation of the Peripheral and Central Vestibular Systems

The peripheral vestibular system consists of a bony capsule surrounding membranous canals that are floating in perilymph and filled with endolymph. This fluid in turn bathes the five functional neuroepithelium end organs: the three ampullae of the semicircular canals and the two maculae of the utricle and saccule (▶ Fig. 113.1). The electrolyte composition of the endolymph and perilymph differs because of the actions of sodium–potassium pumps. Stimulation of the neuroepithelium causes changes in the discharge rates of the type 1 and type 2 hair cells that make up the maculae and ampullae. These vestibular hair cells synapse with the bipolar neuronal cells of the Scarpa ganglion, the cell bodies of the two vestibular nerves. Impulses

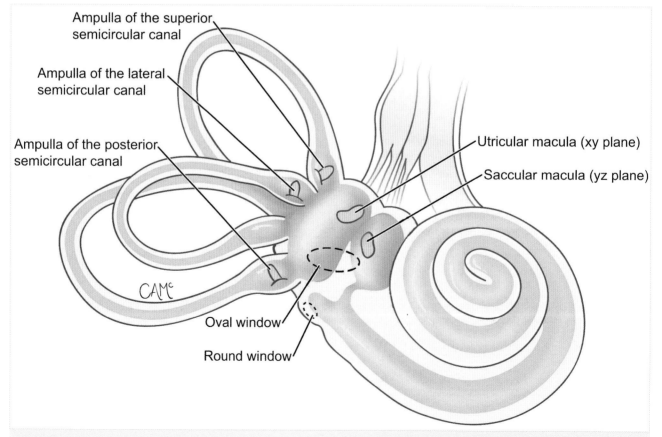

Fig. 113.1 Drawing of the peripheral vestibular system, illustrating the otic capsule, ampullae of the semicircular canals, maculae of the utricle and saccule, and inferior and superior vestibular nerves.

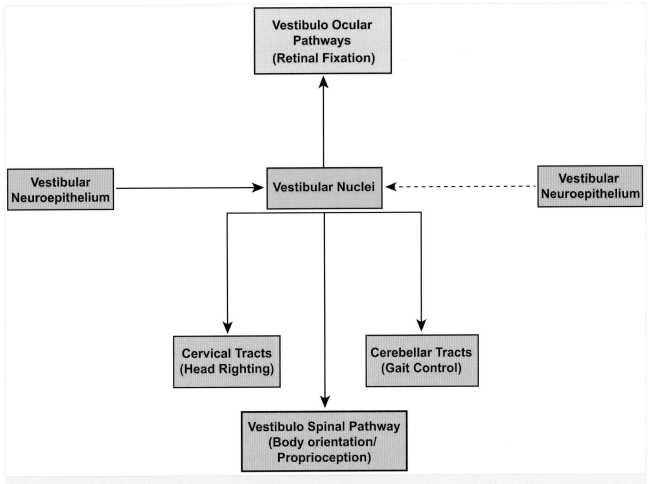

Fig. 113.2 Schematic of the vestibular nerves and their central connections to the cerebellar, ocular, cervical, and proprioceptive systems.

from the five loci of neuroepithelium continue centrally to form elaborate connections to the ocular nuclei, cerebellum, proprioceptive tracts, and cervical nuclei (▶ Fig. 113.2). The peripheral vestibular system is enclosed in a continuous bony capsule that has only one opening—the vestibular aqueduct connecting the vestibule to the posterior cranial fossa. Only two structures adjacent to a nonpathologic vestibular capsule can affect equilibrium: (1) The air of the middle ear space is adjacent to the lateral semicircular canal, and changes in air temperature can cause the sensation of motion, and (2) motion at the stapes footplate can also cause the sensation of motion. Some individuals are so sensitive to alterations in footplate dynamics that any dysfunction of the eustachian tube ventilation causes dizziness.

113.3 Bony Anatomy and Physiology of the Peripheral Vestibular System

The bony otic capsule encloses the semicircular canals and the vestibule. The resulting capsule is the only endochondral bone in the body, and it cannot repair itself if fractured. Instead, fibrous tissue forms in the fracture line, but this repair usually cannot preserve function. By the time of birth, the otic capsule has attained adult size and is completely formed of endochodral bone.

Any of the three perpendicular semicircular canals can undergo erosion, which uncovers the perilymph and exposes the endolymph within the membranous canal to pressure changes, causing disequilibrium (▶ Fig. 113.3). This is termed *semicircular canal dehiscence*. Erosion of the lateral semicircular canal by cholesteatoma causes imbalance with Valsalva maneuver, with finger pressure in the ear canal, or with loud noises. The superior semicircular canal can be uncovered by middle cranial fossa erosion, resulting in the array of symptoms seen in this dehiscence syndrome: general unsteadiness, autophonia, unsteadiness caused by loud noises (Tullio phenomenon), conductive hearing loss, and occasional hyperacusis. Less commonly, the posterior semicircular canal can become dehiscent as a consequence of cholesteatoma, a prominent jugular bulb, or a cerebellar plate in a hypoaerated temporal bone.

The diagnosis of dehiscence in any of the semicircular canals can be established with fine-cut computed tomography (CT) of the temporal bone. Dehiscence of the lateral semicircular canal can be seen on axial or coronal CT. Dehiscence of the posterior semicircular canal is well seen on the Poschl projection, which consists of sections parallel to the superior semicircular canal.

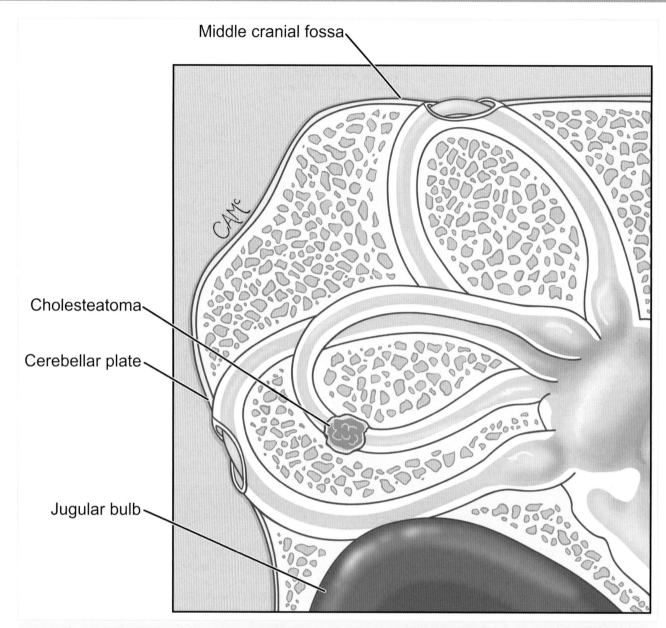

Fig. 113.3 Erosion of the superior, lateral, and posterior semicircular canals. Superior canal dehiscence from erosion of the middle cranial fossa dura, lateral canal dehiscence from cholesteatoma, and posterior canal dehiscence from the jugular bulb or cerebellar plate.

Erosion of the lateral semicircular canal can be established with a fistula test, in which a reliable seal is made between an insufflating ear canal speculum and the skin of the external canal. Positive pressure is applied without a leak, so that the tympanic membrane is compressed toward the promontory. This in turn compresses the exposed lateral semicircular canal periosteum. In lateral canal dehiscence, any positive pressure will cause the eyes to deviate away from the insufflated ear (Hennebert sign).

Vestibular evoked myogenic potentials (VEMPs), also called balance evoked myogenic potentials (BEMPs), are illustrated in ▶ Fig. 113.4. The physiology of the response is based on a primitive pathway in which the saccule, normally a vestibular organ, functions as a mixed auditory and vestibular organ. When noise is introduced into the ear canal, and ultimately to the stapes footplate, the auditory impulse stimulates central pathways for proprioception and spatial orientation. The VEMP response

therefore is the involuntary motion of the extraocular muscles or involuntary relaxation of a tensed sternocleidomastoid muscle when noise is introduced unilaterally into an ear canal. The decibel threshold for the causing this muscular response is usually roughly equivalent in each ear. However, in the superior canal dehiscence syndrome, the decibel threshold in the affected ear is reduced relative to that in the unaffected ear.

The treatment for canal dehiscence is surgical. Cholesteatomas that erode the lateral or posterior semicircular canals put hearing at risk and will deafen the patient if left untreated. These must be meticulously removed under microscopic magnification and the canal immediately patched with appropriate materials, such as fascia or periosteum. In a large dehiscence, the lumen of the canal can be obliterated with bone paste or bone cement, with every effort made not to tear the membranous canal. Superior canal dehiscence from erosion of the middle cranial

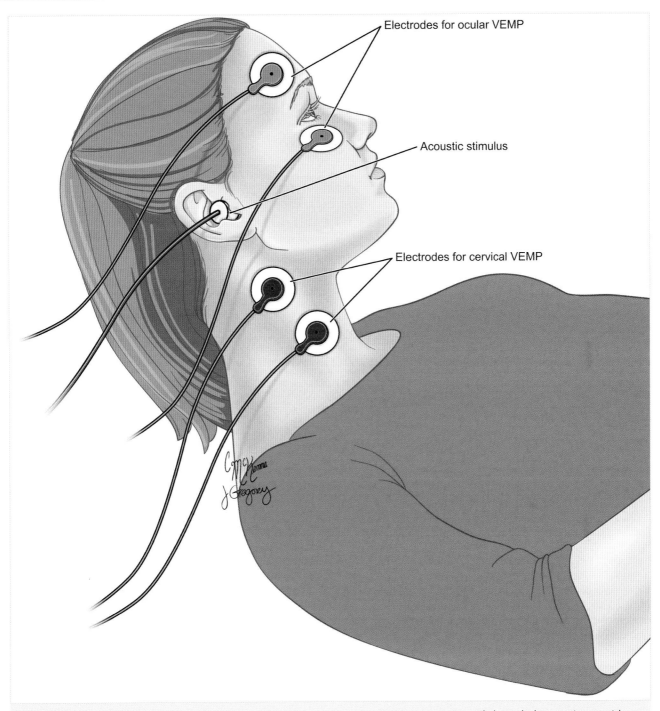

Fig. 113.4 Positioning of electrodes, of acoustic stimulation, and of the patient for VEMP testing. *VEMP*, vestibular evoked myogenic potential.

fossa dura carries less risk for inner ear fistula and sensorineural hearing loss. Instead, the discomfort from conductive hearing loss and dizziness must be weighed against the morbidity of a middle cranial fossa approach to canal plugging.

113.4 Membranous Endolymphatic Canals

The membranous vestibular labyrinth is enclosed by the bony vestibular capsule (▶ Fig. 113.5). The membranous labyrinth is filled with endolymph, in which the ratio of potassium to sodium is higher than in perilymph. Because of the difference between the ratios of K^+ to Na^+ in the two fluids, endolymph has a net positive charge of 89 mV compared with perilymph. The membranous canals are continuous with the scala media of the cochlea via the ductus reuniens, and continuous with the endolymphatic sac on the cerebellar plate via the vestibular aqueduct. The connection between the vestibular aqueduct and the posterior cranial fossa, although porous, is not directly open. Any breach of the membranous labyrinth causes marked

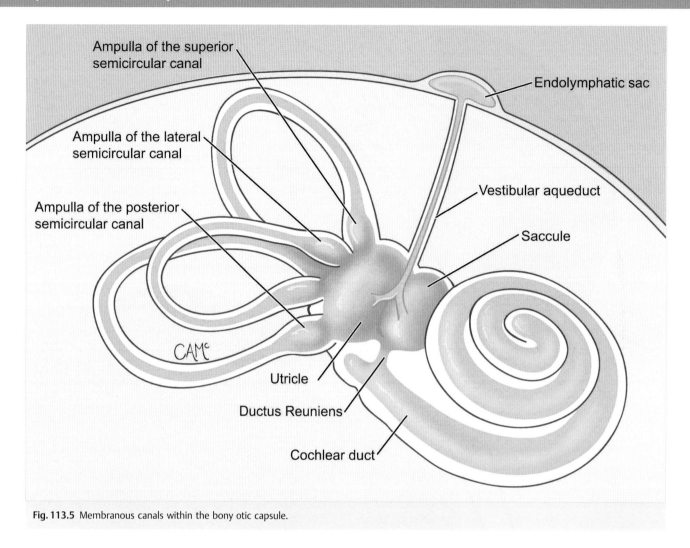

Fig. 113.5 Membranous canals within the bony otic capsule.

vestibular symptoms and may be the basis for the disabling vertiginous episodes that occur in Meniere disease.

Most balance disturbances related to the endolymphatic canals are not caused by actual rupture of the membranous canal. Instead, exposure of the perilymph to direct pressure or leakage of perilymph usually causes imbalance. As previously mentioned, dehiscence of the semicircular canals causes imbalance when pressure changes are introduced to the exposed periosteum of the canal. Additionally, imbalance can be caused by leakage of perilymphatic fluid. Leakage is usually from the vestibule via the oval window, fissula ante fenestram, or fossula post fenestram, but sometimes from the scala tympani of the cochlea via the round window niche, or from the ampullated end of the posterior semicircular canal via the Hyrtl fissure (▶ Fig. 113.6). The fissula, fossula, and Hyrtl fissure are congenital fissures filled with soft tissue that are present in all temporal bones, but they usually are not porous.

Diagnostic tools to distinguish perilymph exposure, perilymph leak, and Meniere disease are varied. The eyes deviate away from the affected ear with positive pressure and toward the affected ear with negative pressure. This is the Hennebert sign.

When this maneuver seems unambiguous, leak can be confirmed by direct observation of the round and oval window niches. Rarely, a sample of clear fluid from these sites can confirm the presence of β₂-transferrin. Semicircular canal dehiscence has previously been described and can be identified with VEMP testing and Poschl views on temporal bone CT.

Meniere disease has a typical and reliable set of symptoms, in which recurrent episodes of unilateral ear pressure, tinnitus, and hearing loss are accompanied by disabling vertigo. The episodes last for hours, but not days, and audiometric testing confirms a low-frequency sensorineural hearing loss that is worst during the acute spell and gradually returns to a new baseline afterward. The pathophysiology of the disease is thought to be increased fluid pressure in the endolymphatic canals, causing dilation of the membranous canals. The abnormal physiology of Meniere disease can be detected by electrocochleography, which shows the ratio of the summation and action potentials in response to an auditory stimulus to be abnormally large (SP/AP > 0.50; ▶ Fig. 113.7). It would be reassuring to assert that electrocochleography is the gold standard for establishing Meniere disease in a dizzy patient, but the changes seen on electrocochleography are unreliable, and the test is uncomfortable for most patients and difficult to organize.

Treatment for exposure of the membranous labyrinth or leakage of perilymph is surgical. Fistulas are approached via middle ear exploration with the placement of fat, fascia, or areolar tissue into the most likely sites of leak. Canal resurfacing with fascia or periosteum and canal plugging with bone paste

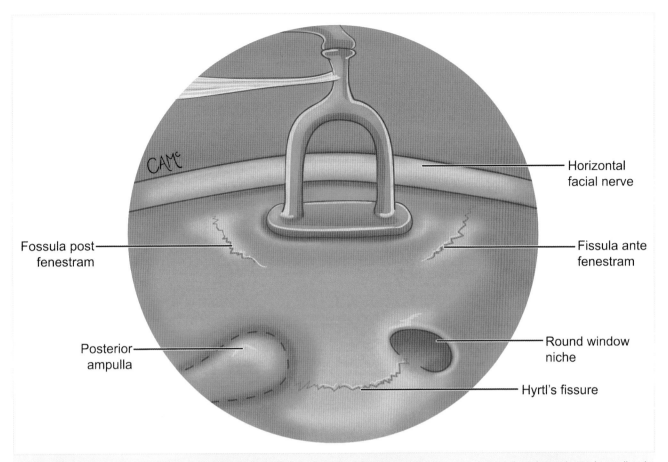

Fig. 113.6 Sites of perilymph leakage: the fissula ante fenestram, fossula post fenestram, scala tympani via the round window niche, and ampullated end of the posterior semicircular canal via the Hyrtl fissure.

as well as bone cement have previously been described. Treatments for Meniere disease range from stress reduction to craniotomy with vestibular nerve section. Because Meniere disease is very responsive to increases in psychological stress, simple information about the disease and what to expect, and referral for psychological techniques of stress reduction, are enough to manage the disease in some patients. The next tier of treatments involves salt restriction and daily diuretics. Some patients benefit from the placement of a pressure equalization tube in the affected ear, and some benefit from tube placement followed by the application of positive pressure for 5 minutes several times per day (the Meniett machine). Decompression of the endolymphatic sac can bring relief for some patients, although this may be a placebo effect. Destructive interventions are intratympanic instillations of gentamicin, sacculotomy, labyrinthectomy, and intracranial vestibular nerve section. Although gentamicin is considered a selective vestibulotoxin, it often causes incidental sensorineural hearing loss, and the patient must be cautioned of this risk.

113.5 Neuroepithelium

The peripheral sensory organs for balance are the ampullae of the lateral semicircular canals and the maculae of the utricle and saccule. The canals are perpendicular to one another, although they are all tilted up at an angle of 30 degrees from the horizontal. Therefore, the horizontal semicircular canal is 30 off the horizontal plane, and the two other canals are perpendicular to that plane. The semicircular canals detect angular motions and turns. When the head moves, the endolymph moves relative to the ampulla of the canal, and that deflection of the crista of the ampulla causes an increase or decrease in the baseline firing rate of the type 1 and type 2 vestibular hair cells (▶ Fig. 113.8). The presence of cold or warm water in the ear canal changes the temperature of the middle ear space, cooling or warming the endolymph of the lateral semicircular canal and causing that ampulla to deflect away from the vestibule or toward the vestibule.

The utricle is located on the ceiling of the vestibule, directly inferior and medial to the horizontal facial nerve as it courses over the oval window niche. The utricle is basically in the x-y plane. The saccule is located on the anterior medial wall of the vestibule, just anterior and medial to the anterior lip of the oval window. The saccule is basically in the y-z plane. These two organs detect linear acceleration and falling. The sensory neuroepithelium of the utricle and that of the saccule are the maculae, in which the type 1 and type 2 hair cells are oriented toward a central striola; their baseline firing rates are modified by acceleration.

Disorders of the neuroepithelium are twofold; those resulting from abnormal stimulation of the neuroepithelium or those caused by death or hypofunction of the neuroepithelium.

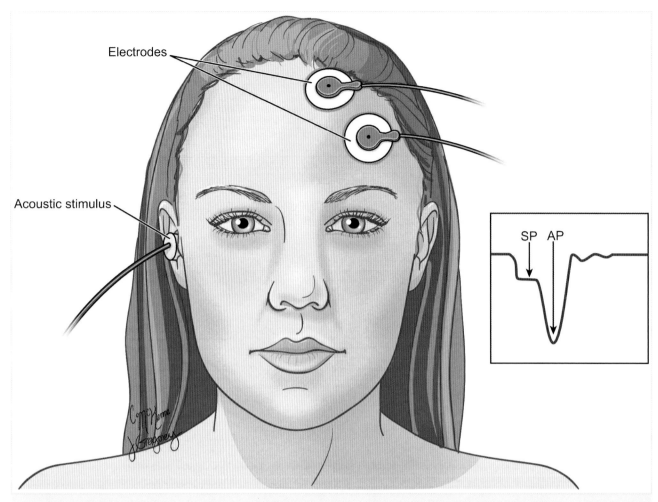

Fig. 113.7 Electrocochleography technique. Acoustic stimuli can be introduced via the canal or transtympanically. An electrical response within the first 2.0 milliseconds consists of the summation potential and action potential. *SP*, summation potential; *AP*, action potential.

Benign paroxysmal positional vertigo (BPPV) is caused by nonphysiologic stimulation of the ampullae by otoliths, which are loose neuroepithelial components composed of calcium carbonate around a matrix protein. In this disorder, which tends to occur most often in the posterior semicircular canal, normal head motions cause abnormal stimulation of the posterior canal neuroepithelium with an exaggerated central response that patients find unpleasant. BPPV is diagnosed by Dix-Hallpike testing (▶ Fig. 113.9), in which the patient is positioned with the head turned and hanging so that the aberrant otoliths of the posterior semicircular canal cause maximal stimulation and nystagmus. The characteristic result is a rotatory and lateral nystagmus that beats toward the ground when the subject's head is hanging backward with the problem ear down. The nystagmus begins a second or two after the provocative position is assumed, grows in intensity, and then abates. Sitting up reverses the direction of the nystagmus. Each subsequent cycle of stimulation is shorter and less intense. BPPV is by far the most common reason for referral to an otolaryngologist's office for imbalance.

Other disorders of the neuroepithelium result from death of the type 1 and type 2 hair cells. Ototoxins, usually intravenous antibiotics given for life-threatening infections, cause generalized nonresponsiveness of the ampullae and maculae to stimu-

lation. Caloric testing elicits reduced or no symptoms and nystagmus. The patient cannot fix any visual target on the retina while the head is moving (oscillopsia), resulting in an inability to read signs or recognize faces while walking.

Labyrinthitis (infection or inflammation of the perilymph or endolymph) causes hair cell death and nonfunction. This would be identified by a reduced response on caloric testing or by enhancement in one labyrinth on magnetic resonance (MR) imaging with and without gadolinium. A key feature of true labyrinthitis is that the intraotic inflammation and infection are devastating to vestibular and auditory function, and the patient becomes quite ill, with roaring tinnitus in the affected ear. In the long term, unilateral peripheral vestibular loss would be expected, with completely absent caloric responses and robust horizontal nystagmus toward the unaffected ear when vibration is applied to the mastoid of the affected side.

Loss of utricle function can be identified by the ocular countertorsion test, in which the subject sits with the head upright. The examiner picks a landmark on the subject's iris and then tilts one ear up, looking for physiologic righting of the iris—an ocular countertorsion. If this does not occur, if the iris tilts with the head without compensation, hypofunction of the superior utricle is indicated.

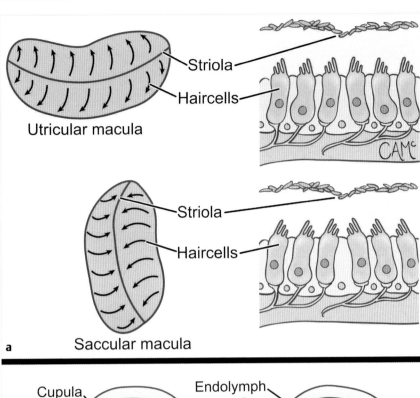

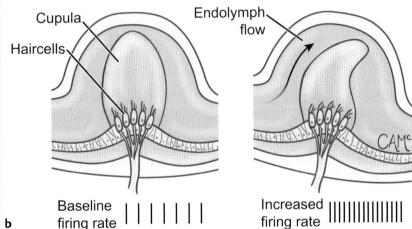

Fig. 113.8 (a) Maculae and (b) ampullae: orientation of type 1 and type 2 hair cells and the response of firing rates to hair cell deflection.

A common and perhaps more serious malfunction of the neuroepithelium is alcohol intoxication. As ingested alcohol diffuses into the endolymph, the endolymph rises, giving the subject a sensation of motion. A characteristic nystagmus follows. Although this condition requires no treatment except time, it is probably responsible for more deaths, in motor vehicle accidents, than any other form of dizziness.

The treatment for loss of neuroepithelial function consists of supportive care in the short term and physical therapy in the long term. There is no method of restoring the lost function, and in the acute phase of unequal vestibular inputs from the two ears, a vestibular suppressant and medical leave are the best that can be offered. In the long term, when vertigo has given way to general unsteadiness, physical therapy can help the patient regain some balance, independence, and confidence.

The treatment for BPPV, on the other hand, can intervene at the site of the problem and show good results. The treatments for BPPV range from interventions during a single office visit to surgical obliteration of the malfunctioning semicircular canal.

The particle repositioning (Epley) maneuver can allow the loose otoliths to fall into the vestibule, where they become asymptomatic. Habituation exercises can retrain the central vestibular system to ignore the aberrant information from the affected ear. In patients with long-term BPPV, the posterior semicircular canal can be obliterated, or the cingulate nerve can be sectioned in an infracochlear approach.

113.6 Vestibular Nerves

The five islands of vestibular neuroepithelium transmit their varying discharge information to the superior and inferior vestibular nerves, which are afferent (sensory) nerves. The macula of the utricle and ampullae of the superior and lateral semicircular canals synapse with the superior vestibular nerve, while the macula of the saccule and ampulla of the posterior semicircular canal synapse with the inferior vestibular nerve. The portion of the inferior vestibular nerve that travels from the

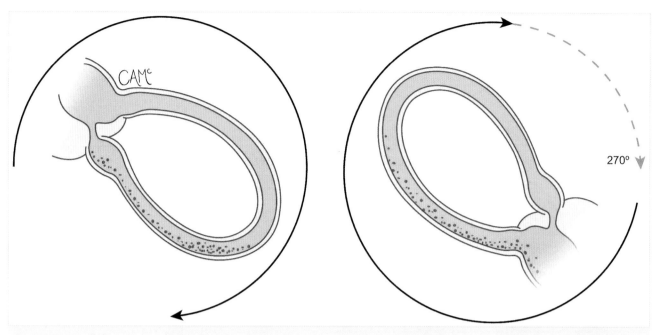

Fig. 113.9 Dix-Hallpike testing: position of the left posterior semicircular canal in the left head-hanging position. The canal is positioned to cause maximal stimulation and pooling of the otoconia away from the ampulla. In the Epley maneuver, the canal is then rotated 270 degrees to allow the otoconia to pour into the vestibule. The canal is pictured in mid rotation as the otoconia begin to fall into the vestibule.

ampulla of the posterior semicircular canal is called the cingulate nerve. The nerve cell bodies for the bipolar primary axons of the vestibular nerves are located in the internal auditory canal, forming the Scarpa ganglion. From the internal auditory canal, the nerves progress across the cerebellopontine angle to enter the brainstem.

Isolated dysfunction of any of these nerves can occur. The reasons are usually hard to identify. Isolated neuronitis occurs secondary to autoimmune disease, presumed viral infection, idiopathic inflammation, and neoplasms along the nerve route. The symptoms are nonspecific and usually consist of generalized unsteadiness and spinning without ear symptoms or position sensitivity. A coordination of tests can help identify which vestibular nerve is hypofunctioning; absent caloric responses identify superior vestibular nerve malfunction because lateral canal stimulation is ineffective. Increased VEMP thresholds identify inferior vestibular nerve malfunction because the saccule requires more auditory stimulation to elicit the primitive auditory–vestibular response. Normal hearing (by an audiogram and/or otoacoustic emission testing) helps to exclude labyrinthitis as a possible cause of dizziness because the hearing in the putative ear should be affected as well as balance in labyrinthitis.

If the hearing is symmetrical and unchanged, the diagnosis of vestibular neuritis (aka vestibular neuronitis) may be supported by a reduced bithermal caloric response on one side or abnormal results of symmetry, phase and gain testing on the Harmonic Rotation Chair test. Of these examinations, the bithermal caloric test on the Visual Electronystagmogram (VNG) done with infrared goggles or on the Electronystagmogram (ENG) performed with transdermal electrodes is both localizing (what place within the inner ear?) and lateralizing (which side?).

Like the treatment for neuroepithelial loss, previously described, the treatment for vestibular nerve hypofunction consists of supportive care in the acute phase and physical therapy in the long term.

113.7 Central Pathways

The many and complex central connections for the afferent vestibular impulses are diagrammed in ▶ Fig. 113.3. The central downstream cross-connections for the afferent vestibular information appear to coordinate two major systems. The information from the two peripheral vestibular organs is coordinated so that a stimulus of the canals of one ear is interpreted along with an equal and opposite counterstimulus of the canals of the contralateral ear. Far more complex than this coordination, however, is the constant repositioning and reassessment of the orientation of the ocular globe, the head on the neck, and the entire body along its vertical axis. The central connections for the vestibular system therefore interpret the differing afferent information from each ear and instruct the rest of the body—eyes, neck, and posture—to adjust.

Any central disease can cause malfunction of the coordination of the vestibular input and therefore can cause imbalance. Multiple sclerosis, cerebral vascular events, cerebral inflammatory diseases, and migraine can all cause vestibular dysfunction. On testing in these cases, the audiogram tends to be symmetric and uninformative. Simple cerebellar testing—finger to nose, repetitive motions, Romberg test—may identify problems in cerebellar function. The caloric responses are normal in each ear. However, the head thrust test, in which the clinician rotates the subject's head quickly to the side, may reveal that the eyes do not stay fixed on their target but instead show a compensatory saccade after the thrust is complete. Similarly, oculokinetic tests may find that the eyes do not track normally. Many other findings on electronystagmography (ENG) are indicative of

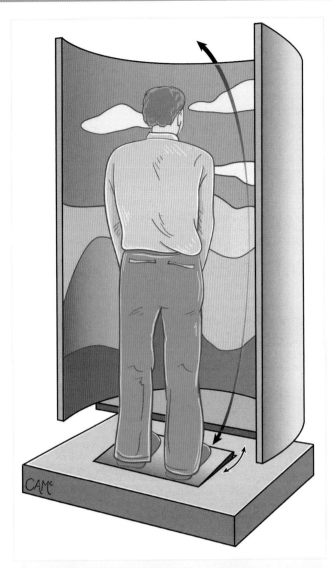

Fig. 113.10 Posturography measures the subject's maintenance of vertical body orientation in progressively more difficult conditions. The visual background is fixed or sways. The platform on which the subject stands is flat or wobbles. The subject's eyes may be open or closed.

nonspecific central disease: nystagmus, which does not depend upon position and which is not suppressed; the inability to track a sinusoidal motion; and the inability to perform saccades.

Posturography (▸ Fig. 113.10) tests the input and integration of the peripheral vestibular system, eyes, and proprioceptive tracts. These may be quite abnormal in central disease. Posturography is also a good tool for identifying malingerers, who tend to sway and almost fall during the easiest conditions but will manage to keep their balance during the more challenging conditions to avoid hurting themselves.

If central disease is suspected, MR imaging of the brain and internal auditory canals with and without gadolinium can be performed.

Migraine-equivalent vertigo may be the diagnosis for many patients who simply defy classification. Pathognomonic symptoms are the conversion of migraine headaches into vertiginous episodes that have the same temporal patterns and the same triggers. For example, a 40-year-old woman has experienced migraines at the same time as her menstrual cycle for years. Then suddenly the migraines stop, and she instead experiences vertiginous episodes at the same time of the month and for the same number of days. These patients respond well to preventive measures and to topiramate or verapamil. However, many patients who most likely have this syndrome do not fit easily into this pattern of symptoms. Patients who experience episodes of imbalance with no audiologic findings, and with normal ENG and normal MR imaging findings, may warrant a closely monitored trial of verapamil.

113.8 Directed Diagnostic Inquiries

The diagnosis and treatment of patients with dizziness is not a science derived from first principles. Instead, it is a struggle through inexact histories, contradictory tests, the patient's despair, and the clinician's frustration at not being able to help. A further complicating feature is that people who report several episodes or days or years of dizziness often have additional episodes of dizziness resulting from a new cause. For example, people with Meniere disease may have recurrent episodes of BPPV. The key to managing the stresses of the clinic visit and subsequently to devise a reasonable treatment plan is to try to keep the many diagnostic possibilities in mind.

The history can give significant clues. Effort should be made to obtain a concise and specific answer to one key question: Did this dizziness start one day and has it continued since then, or does it come in episodes? The answer to this question is usually very difficult to elicit because most people cannot verbally distinguish between a constant symptom of varying intensity, like BPPV or an ototoxic effect, and a symptom that started years ago but is episodic. Patients prefer to describe how uncomfortable they are and will have to be redirected until this key question is answered. Although most referrals to the otolaryngologist's office office for imbalance are ultimately for BPPV, the majority of patients with pathognomonic nystagmus on Dix-Hallpike testing do not give a history of vertigo after position change.

Because most dizziness is BPPV, the most important feature of the physical examination is the extent to which the dizzy patient unconsciously guards against head motion during the interview. A look at the tympanic membrane usually does not add any information. A special feature of the physical examination is insufflation with a pneumatic speculum to look for eye deviation toward the contralateral ear in cases of perilymphatic fistula.

An audiogram must be performed to look for unilateral otologic loss and for Meniere disease. Patients with unilateral losses often are unaware of them. Otoacoustic emissions establish cochlear function and can help distinguish labyrinthitis from neuronitis.

Office tests for vestibular function include the Dix-Hallpike test, ocular countertorsion test, head thrust, and vibration test, These maneuvers look for BPPV, utricular failure, central dysfunction, and unilateral peripheral vestibular loss, respectively.

VEMP testing can help identify superior canal dehiscence if the threshold is lower in the affected ear, or unilateral inferior vestibular nerve dysfunction if the threshold is higher. ENG can distinguish central from peripheral dysfunction, and caloric testing can help identify superior vestibular nerve hypofunction. Electrocochleography is not helpful practically, but theoretically it can help identify Meniere disease. Rotatory chair testing can help identify unilateral vestibular loss.

Posturography gives an overall view of visual and proprioceptive balance integration. CT identifies canal dehiscence, and MR imaging looks for inflammation of the vestibular labyrinth and nerves and for central disease.

113.9 Roundsmanship

- When the head moves, the endolymph moves relative to the ampulla of the canal, deflecting the crista of the ampulla and causing an increase or decrease of the baseline firing rate of the type 1 and type 2 vestibular hair cells.
- The macula of the utricle and the ampullae of the superior and lateral semicircular canals synapse with the superior vestibular nerve, while the macula of the saccule and the ampulla of the posterior semicircular canal synapse with the inferior vestibular nerve.
- Leakage or exposure of the perilymph to direct pressure, or any breach of the membranous labyrinth, causes marked vestibular symptoms.
- It is very helpful to obtain from the patient a specific answer to the question, Did this dizziness start one day and has it continued since then, or does in come in episodes?
- The most important feature of the physical examination is the extent to which the dizzy patient unconsciously guards against head motion during the interview because most dizziness is benign paroxysmal positional vertigo.
- In lateral canal dehiscence, any positive pressure will cause the eyes to deviate away from the insufflated ear (Hennebert sign).
- Any of the three mutually perpendicular semicircular canals can undergo erosion, which uncovers the perilymph, exposes the endolymph within the membranous canal to pressure changes, and can cause disequilibrium.
- The diagnosis of canal dehiscence in any of the semicircular canals can be established with fine-cut CT of the temporal bone.
- Benign paroxysmal positional vertigo is caused by nonphysiologic stimulation of the ampullae by loose neuroepithelial components termed *otoliths*.

- The abnormal physiology of Meniere disease can be detected by electrocochleography, in which the summation and action potentials in response to an auditory stimulus show an abnormally large ratio ($SP/AP > 0.50$).
- Electroneurography can distinguish central from peripheral dysfunction, and caloric testing can help identify superior vestibular nerve hypofunction.
- Posturography tests the input and integration of the peripheral vestibular system, eyes, and proprioceptive tracts.
- The treatments for benign paroxysmal positional vertigo range from interventions during a single office visit to surgical obliteration of the malfunctioning semicircular canal.
- The treatment for loss of neuroepithelial or vestibular nerve function consists of supportive care in the short term and physical therapy in the long term.

113.10 Recommended Reading

[1] Brantberg K. Vestibular evoked myogenic potentials (VEMPs): usefulness in clinical neurotology. Semin Neurol 2009; 29: 541–547

[2] Buchholz D. Heal Your Headache. 1st ed. New York, NY: Workman Publishing; 2002

[3] Chien WW, Carey JP, Minor LB. Canal dehiscence. Curr Opin Neurol 2011; 24: 25–31

[4] Cianfrone G, Pentangelo D, Cianfrone E et al. Pharmacological drugs inducing ototoxicity, vestibular symptoms and tinnitus: a reasoned and updated guide. Eur Rev Med Pharmacol Sci 2011; 15: 601–636

[5] Ferraro JA. Electrocochleography: a review of recording approaches, clinical applications, and new findings in adults and children. J Am Acad Audiol 2010; 21: 145–152

[6] Fife TD, Tusa RJ, Furman JM et al. Assessment: vestibular testing techniques in adults and children: report of the Therapeutics and Technology Assessment Subcommittee of the American Academy of Neurology. Neurology 2000; 55: 1431–1441

[7] Helminski JO, Hain TC. Evaluation and treatment of benign paroxysmal positional vertigo. Ann Long-Term Care 2007; 15: 33–39

[8] Konrad-Martin D, Gordon JS, Reavis KM, Wilmington DJ, Helt WJ, Fausti SA. Audiological monitoring of patients receiving ototoxic drugs. Persp ect 2005; 9; (1): 17–22

[9] Markley BA. Introduction to electronystagmography for END technologists. Am J Electroneurodiagn Technol 2007; 47: 178–189

[10] Minor LB, Schessel DA, Carey JP. Ménière's disease. Curr Opin Neurol 2004; 17: 9–16

[11] Nashner LM. Computerized dynamic posturography. In: Jacobson GP, Newman CW, Kartush JM, eds. Handbook of Balance Function Testing. San Diego, CA: Singular Publishing Group;1997:280

[12] Neuhauser H, Lempert T. Vertigo and dizziness related to migraine: a diagnostic challenge. Cephalalgia 2004; 24: 83–91

[13] Whitney SL, Sparto PJ. Principles of vestibular physical therapy rehabilitation. NeuroRehabilitation 2011; 29: 157–166

114 Diagnostic Audiology

Shlomo Silman and Carol A. Silverman

114.1 Introduction

This chapter provides an overview of tuning fork tests; behavioral hearing tests, including pure-tone threshold tests, masking, and speech audiometry; physiologic measures of auditory function, including tympanometry, acoustic reflex threshold and acoustic reflex adaptation testing, and otoacoustic emissions testing; auditory evoked potentials testing, including electrocochleography, auditory brainstem response testing, and auditory steady-state testing; testing for the identification of functional hearing loss; hearing screening; pediatric audiologic assessment; and vestibular testing, including electronystagmography, videonystagmography, sinusoidal harmonic acceleration, computerized dynamic platform posturography, and vestibular evoked myogenic potential testing. Understanding the interpretations of these audiologic tests will assist the otolaryngologist in the diagnosis and management of hearing and vestibular disorders.

114.2 Tuning Fork Tests

Tuning forks have two tines that, when struck against an object, produce a tone close to a pure tone at a specific frequency (with some lower-intensity overtones [harmonics]). The most commonly employed tuning fork is the 512-Hz tuning fork. The 1024- and 2048-Hz tuning forks generally provide supplemental information. The 256-Hz tuning fork can produce vibrotactile sensations that the patient may mistake for sound, so this tuning fork is infrequently used. The most useful tuning fork tests are the Weber and Rinne tests.

With the Weber tuning fork test, the tuning fork base is placed on the midline of the forehead, and the patient is asked on which side the sound is louder. If the sound is equally loud in both ears or heard in the center of the head, the absence of lateralization is consistent with symmetric hearing loss or symmetric, normal hearing sensitivity. Lateralization indicates: (1) conductive hearing loss in the ear to which the sound lateralized; (2) sensorineural hearing loss in the ear opposite the ear to which the sound lateralized; or (3) asymmetric sensorineural hearing loss that is worse in the ear opposite the ear to which the tone is lateralized. Sound will lateralize to the ear with conductive hearing loss because of one of the following: (1) an occlusion effect that traps sound pressure generated in the external ear canal with vibration of the ear canal walls; (2) a reduced middle ear resonant frequency with a mass-loaded ear (as in ossicular discontinuity or some cases of middle ear effusion with more viscous fluid); or (3) a phase advance with a stiffening pathology (e.g., ossicular fixation or some cases of middle ear effusion with less viscous fluid) that creates a tight coupling between the footplate and oval window, resulting in a more direct path to the inner ear.

In the Rinne tuning fork test, bone-conduction (BC) hearing is compared with air-conduction (AC) hearing. The base of a vibrating tuning fork is held firmly against the mastoid process for about 2 seconds; the tuning fork then is held vertically with the tips of the tines located at about 1 to 2 cm lateral to the entrance of the ear canal. If hearing by AC produces a louder sensation than hearing by BC, the result is consistent with normal hearing sensitivity or sensorineural hearing loss; this result is termed a positive Rinne (AC > BC). If hearing by BC produces a louder sensation than hearing by AC, then the result is consistent with conductive hearing impairment; this result is termed a negative Rinne (BC > AC). If the loudness sensation by BC is equal to that by AC, the result is classified as an equivalent Rinne (AC = BC), consistent with normal hearing sensitivity or a mild conductive hearing loss. A study of the accuracy of the Rinne test on 100 ears with various conductive pathologies (with masking of the contralateral, nontest ear) revealed that the minimum air–bone gap for the Rinne tuning fork test to meet a 75% correct detection criterion is 55 to 60 dB at 512 Hz and larger at 1024 Hz; trial performance of the Rinne test with the 2048-Hz tuning fork fails to meet even a 50% (chance) correct detection criterion even for the largest air–bone gaps. Thus, the Rinne tuning fork test is not useful in the detection of minimal air–bone gaps or conductive pathologies producing high-frequency hearing losses.

114.3 Behavioral Hearing Tests

114.3.1 Classification of Type and Magnitude of Hearing Loss Based on the Pure-Tone Audiogram

Hearing sensitivity conventionally is assessed at the pure-tone octave frequencies of 250, 500, 1000, 2000, 4000, and 8000 Hz. Pure-tone AC threshold testing is done with earphones placed over the pinnae of the outer ears or with insert earphones worn in the ear canals. BC threshold testing is performed with a bone vibrator/oscillator placed on the mastoid process of the temporal bone. The outcome of threshold testing is recorded on an audiogram (▶ Fig. 114.1), which displays test frequency along the x-axis and intensity along the y-axis. A threshold that is better than 0 dB HL (decibels hearing level; e.g., –5 dB HL) indicates hearing sensitivity that is better by 5 dB than the hearing sensitivity of a young adult without hearing or ear problems.

When BC testing is performed, the threshold results furnish information about the sensorineural mechanism. Auditory signals delivered through an earphone worn over the pinna or an insert receiver in the ear canal pass through the ear canal into the middle ear and cochlea, where the sound is transduced into a neural impulse that then travels through the auditory nerve and cochlear nuclei (and through the rest of the auditory brainstem to the auditory cortex). Thus, an AC threshold reflects integrity of both the sensorineural and conductive mechanisms. An elevated AC threshold therefore indicates a hearing problem in the conductive and/or sensorineural mechanism. The difference in decibels between the AC and the BC thresholds is referred to as the *air–bone gap* (ABG), which yields information on the status of the conductive mechanism.

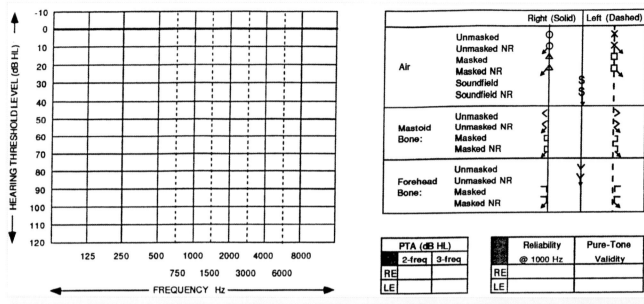

Fig. 114.1 Audiogram template. Intensity is shown on the ordinate, and frequency is shown on the abscissa. Thresholds are reported based on the use of a 5-dB-intensity step size. The legend shows the symbol used for recording pure-tone air conduction and bone conduction thresholds for each ear, and in the sound field. *LE*, left ear; *NR*, no response; *PTA*, pure-tone average; *RE*, right ear.

The upper limit of the normal range of BC thresholds is 15 dB HL, although some clinicians consider 25 dB HL to be the upper limit. The upper limit of the normal range of AC thresholds is 25 dB HL in adults. With conductive hearing impairment, the BC threshold is within normal limits but the AC threshold is elevated beyond the normal limit, yielding a significant (> 10 dB) ABG. With sensorineural hearing impairment, the AC and BC thresholds both are elevated beyond the normal limits and are approximately equal, without significant ABGs. Mixed hearing impairment (hearing impairment affecting both the conductive and sensorineural mechanisms) is characterized by AC and BC thresholds that are elevated beyond the upper limit of normal and AC thresholds worse than BC thresholds, yielding significant ABGs. A medically significant conductive mechanism problem can be present without a hearing impairment per se, as significant ABGs can be present although neither the AC nor BC threshold exceeds the upper limit of normal (normal hearing sensitivity with significant ABGs). A mixed hearing loss is present only when elevated AC and BC thresholds and a significant ABG are present at the same frequency. Various types of hearing loss are shown in ▶ Fig. 114.2. Common causes of conductive and sensorineural hearing loss are shown in ▶ Table 114.1.

The magnitude of the hearing impairment is specified based on the pure-tone average (PTA), which usually is a 3-frequency average of the AC thresholds for 500 Hz, 1000 Hz, and 2000 Hz, but also can be a 4-frequency average (e.g., 500, 1000, 2000, and 3000 Hz or 500, 1000, 2000, and 4000 Hz). The Committee on Hearing and Equilibrium of the American Academy of Otolaryngology—Head and Neck Surgery has adopted the use of a 4-frequency PTA (based on 500, 1000, 2000, and 3000 Hz) for the evaluation of Meniere disease, vestibular schwannoma, and conductive hearing loss. In their guidelines for the evaluation of conductive hearing loss, they also specify the use of this 4-frequency average for reporting ABGs.

▶ Table 114.2 shows a classification of the degree of hearing loss based on the PTAs over the so-called speech frequencies (500, 1000, and 2000 Hz); the classification ranges from normal to profound. Note that the classification of the degree of hearing loss is similar for children and adults except that the upper limit of normal hearing sensitivity is 15 dB HL for children and 25 dB HL for adults; consequently, the range from 16 to 25 dB HL is classified as slight hearing loss in children. This table also shows the impact of the various degrees of hearing loss on speech understanding without amplification, given that soft conversational speech is approximately 35 dB HL, conversational speech is approximately 45 to 50 dB HL, and loud conversational speech is approximately 65 dB HL. ▶ Table 114.2 also shows the predicted impact of various degrees of hearing loss on speech and language when early intervention is not provided. Persons with a normal PTA but with hearing impairment in the high frequencies may experience difficulty hearing conversations in noisy, group, or reverberant situations, even when the high-frequency impairment is mild. The effect of a unilateral hearing loss is less adverse than that of a bilateral hearing loss, but it becomes more pronounced in more competitive listening situations.

Frequency-specific threshold data based on a behavioral audiologic evaluation often can be obtained from infants having a cognitive age as young as 6 months. In an infant with a cognitive age younger than 6 months, behavioral observation audiometry is limited as it can help rule out only moderate or worse hearing impairment in at least one ear.

Pure-Tone Configuration

The pure-tone audiogram can be classified not only in terms of the type and degree of hearing loss, but also in terms of its audiometric configuration. ▶ Fig. 114.3 illustrates some common audiometric configurations, such as flat, sloping, rising,

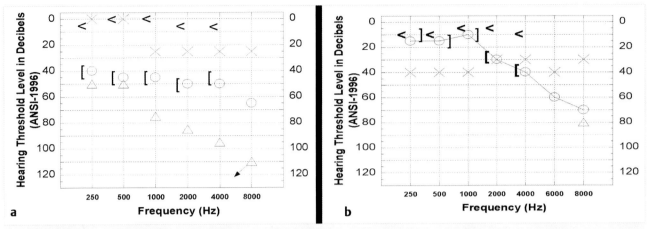

Fig. 114.2 (a) In the right ear at the low frequencies, the masked (true) right bone conduction (BC) thresholds are beyond the normal limits and the masked (true) air conduction (AC) thresholds are also beyond the normal limits without significant air–bone gaps (ABGs), consistent with the presence of sensorineural hearing loss at these frequencies; in the right ear at the higher frequencies above 500 Hz, the masked (true) right BC thresholds beyond the normal limits and the masked (true) right AC thresholds beyond the normal limits, with significant ABGs (30 to 50 dB), are consistent with the presence of a mixed hearing loss at these frequencies. In the left ear at the low frequencies, the unmasked BC thresholds represent the cochlear reserve of the left ear (although the symbol indicates BC vibrator placement on the right mastoid); the masked (true) BC thresholds for the right ear are elevated, so the unmasked BC thresholds must represent the BC hearing for the left ear. The unmasked BC thresholds (representing left BC hearing) and the left AC thresholds both are within normal limits without significant ABGs, so they are consistent with normal hearing sensitivity at these low frequencies. In the left ear at frequencies above 500 Hz, the unmasked BC thresholds (representing left BC hearing) and left AC thresholds remain with normal limits, but significant ABGs are present (20 to 25 dB), consistent with normal hearing sensitivity with significant ABGs at these frequencies. (b) In the left ear at the low–mid frequencies through 1000 Hz, the left masked (true) BC thresholds are within normal limits but the left AC thresholds are elevated beyond the normal limits with significant ABGs (30 to 35 dB), consistent with conductive hearing impairment at those frequencies; at frequencies above 1000 Hz, the unmasked BC thresholds (representing left BC hearing) remain within normal limits and the left AC thresholds remain beyond the normal limits with significant ABGs (20 to 25 dB), also consistent with conductive hearing impairment at these frequencies in the left ear. In the right ear at low–mid frequencies through 1000 Hz, the unmasked BC thresholds, representing right BC hearing, and the AC thresholds are within normal limits, consistent with normal hearing sensitivity at those frequencies; above 1000 Hz, the right masked (true) BC thresholds and right AC thresholds are elevated beyond normal limits without significant ABGs, consistent with a sensorineural hearing loss at those frequencies. *ANSI*, American National Standards Institute.

trough, high-frequency, low-frequency, inverted scoop or trough, fragmentary or corner, notched, and peak. The audiometric configuration may be suggestive of an etiology but usually is not pathognomonic. A flat audiometric configuration is seen, for example, with late-stage Meniere disease. Sloping audiometric configurations are commonly seen in presbycusis. Ears with relatively early-stage Meniere disease often show a rising audiometric configuration. Some individuals with congenital hearing loss have a trough audiometric configuration, whereas individuals with an inverted scoop or inverted trough audiometric configuration have a hereditary hearing loss. Some cases of hereditary hearing loss produce a fragmentary or corner audiogram. Occupational hearing loss often initially produces a hearing loss with a notch centered at frequencies within 3000 to 6000 Hz. Some patients with Meniere disease display a 2000-Hz peak audiogram whereby the pure-tone thresholds are within normal limits at 2000 Hz but then increase as frequency increases above and decreases below the peak frequency.

Audiometric configuration also is affected by the type of conductive hearing impairment. An audiogram with a stiffness tilt refers to an audiometric configuration for a stiffening conductive lesion in which the conductive hearing loss preferentially affects low frequencies, whereas one with a mass tilt refers to an audiometric configuration for a mass conductive lesion (e.g., ossicular discontinuity) in which the conductive hearing loss affects the high frequencies more than the low frequencies. A Carhart notch refers to an audiometric configuration often seen in patients with otosclerosis whereby the BC threshold is poorer at 2000 Hz than at the adjacent frequencies because of loss of ossicular resonance. Some cases of middle ear effusion and chronic ear disease show a peak audiogram whereby the AC threshold peaks at 2000 Hz; this finding suggests the presence of a stiffness effect at the low frequencies that disappears at 2000 Hz, together with a mass effect that begins to be observed above 2000 Hz.

Ototoxic Monitoring with Standard Pure-Tone Audiometry

Ototoxic (cochleotoxic and/or vestibulotoxic) effects may be observed in patients receiving aminoglycoside antibiotics (e.g., kanamycin and amikacin), loop diuretics (e.g., ethacrynic acid and furosemide), cancer agents (e.g., cisplatin and carboplatin), or high doses of aspirin and antimalarials (e.g., quinine). Often, these effects are permanent, although they may be temporary and reversible. Patients receiving ototoxic drugs should have audiologic monitoring. A commonly employed protocol established by the American Speech-Language-Hearing Association (ASHA) is to obtain a baseline audiogram before or within 72 hours after the first dose of an aminoglycoside, and within 1 week before or within 24 hours after the first dose of a chemo-

Table 114.1 Common causes of conductive and sensorineural hearing loss

Conductive	Sensorineural: cochlear	Sensorineural: eighth nerve or cochlear nuclei
Aural atresia	Noise-induced hearing loss	Vestibular schwannoma
Eustachian tube dysfunction	Ototoxicity	Auditory neuropathy spectrum disorder
Otitis media	Meniere disease (endolymphatic hydrops)	Some cases of vascular loop syndrome
Cholesteatoma	Presbycusis	Presbycusis
Temporal bone trauma/fracture affecting the outer ear and/or middle ear	Temporal bone trauma/fracture affecting the cochlea	Temporal bone trauma/fracture affecting the auditory nerve and/or cochlear nuclei
Otosclerosis	Otosyphilis	Otosyphilis
Glomus tumor within the middle ear space (occasionally mixed hearing loss when the tumor invades the cochlea)	Meningitis	Meningitis
Exostoses and osteomas that are large enough to close off the ear canal	HIV/AIDS	HIV/AIDS
External otitis with swelling of the ear canal sufficient to close off the ear canal	Other infections affecting newborns (Rh incompatibility, cytomegalovirus infection, rubella, toxoplasmosis)	Other infections affecting newborns (Rh incompatibility, cytomegalovirus infection, rubella, toxoplasmosis)
Hereditary (genetic)	Hereditary (genetic)	Hereditary (genetic)
Tympanosclerosis	Perilymph fistula (can also be mixed hearing loss)	
Ossicular chain discontinuity	Idiopathic sudden sensorineural hearing loss	
Larger tympanic membrane perforations	Diabetes mellitus	
	Autoimmune inner ear disease	
	Superior semicircular canal dehiscence syndrome (air–bone gaps are considered to be artifactual)	

therapeutic agent. In responsive patients, the AC thresholds should be done over the range of 250 through 8000 Hz. The ASHA protocol specifies weekly monitoring for aminoglycoside antibiotics and monitoring within 24 hours of each dose of a platinum derivative. A change in hearing sensitivity, calculated with reference to the baseline results, is a worsening of threshold by at least 20 dB at any one frequency or by at least 10 dB at any two frequencies, or a loss of response at three consecutive test frequencies at which responses previously could be recorded. Any change needs to be confirmed at a retest within 24 hours. If any change is significant, then acoustic admittance and BC threshold testing needs to be done to rule out changes due to a conductive component. With unresponsive patients, physiologic measures such as otoacoustic emissions testing and auditory brainstem response testing should be used for audiologic monitoring of patients receiving ototoxic drugs.

Extended High-Frequency Audiometry

Extended high-frequency pure-tone AC testing involves obtaining thresholds above 8000 Hz—that is, at 9000, 10,000, 11,200, 12,500, 14,000, 16,000, 18,000, and 20,000 Hz. Ultra-high-frequency audiometry has been used to monitor ototoxic hearing changes because many ototoxic drugs (e.g., cisplatin) may affect the ultra-high frequencies before affecting the traditional audiometric frequency range (250 through 8000 Hz). Various rapid protocol threshold test procedures involving extended

high-frequency audiometry frequently have been employed to identify the so-called sensitive range of ototoxicity (SRO). A significant limitation of extended high-frequency audiometry is that the threshold increases with frequency, and also with age. Thus, a baseline threshold may be beyond the output limits of the audiometer, precluding the possibility of seeing ototoxic changes at that frequency, particularly in older adults.

114.3.2 Speech Audiometry

The procedure for measuring the speech recognition threshold (SRT) involves having the patient repeat spondaic words spoken with equal stress on each of the two syllables. The SRT is the lowest intensity at which the patient can correctly repeat the speech stimuli with 50% accuracy. Agreement between the SRT and PTA is determined by measuring the decibel difference between these measures. When the audiometric configuration is flat within the speech frequencies (i.e., not more than a 5-dB difference between two adjacent octave frequencies in the 500- through 2000-Hz range), the comparison is made between the SRT and 3-frequency PTA. Similarly, with sloping or rising audiometric configurations, whereby more than a 5-dB difference exists between two adjacent octave frequencies in the 500 through 2000 Hz range, the comparison is made between the SRT and the 2-frequency PTA based on the best two AC thresholds among 500, 1000, and 2000 Hz. Agreement, as indicated by a small decibel difference between the SRT and PTA, substanti-

Table 114.2 Pure-tone average, degree of hearing loss, impact of hearing loss on speech, and impact of hearing loss on speech and language

Pure-tone average (dB HL)	Degree of hearing loss	Impact on hearing and speech (without amplification)	Impact on speech and language without intervention
0–15	Normal	None	None
16–25 (children)	Slight	May have hearing difficulty in the classroom	May have slight articulation, language, and educational problems
16–25 (adults)	Normal	None or minimal when listening to conversation in competitive situations	None
26–40	Mild	May have difficulty understanding faint speech, speech at a distance, or speech in competitive situations	Adults: none Children: more likely to show some articulation, language, and educational problems
41–55	Moderate	Difficulty generally experienced hearing conversational speech at 3 to 6 feet, as well as difficulty hearing faint or distant speech or speech in competitive situations	Adults: usually none Children: effects of hearing loss on articulation, voice quality, language, and educational achievement more pronounced than for mild hearing loss
56–70	Moderate to severe/severe	Usually difficulty hearing loud as well as conversational speech, faint or distant speech, or speech in competitive situations	Adults: deterioration in speech may occur Children: increasingly adverse effects of hearing loss on articulation, voice quality, and educational achievement
71–90	Severe	May hear some loud sounds near the ear; difficulty hearing loud and conversational speech as well as faint or distant speech, or speech in competitive situations	Adults: usually deterioration in articulation and voice quality Children: in addition to adverse effects on articulation, voice quality, language, and educational achievement, speech and language generally do not develop spontaneously
91 +	Profound	Will not hear faint or distant speech, conversation in quiet surroundings at 3 to 6 feet, loud speech, or speech at 1 foot from the ear	Adults: more pronounced adverse effects on articulation and voice quality Children: increasingly adverse effects on articulation, voice quality, language, and educational achievement; speech and language generally do not develop spontaneously; benefit substantially more limited for hearing aids than for cochlear implants

Abbreviation: dB HL, decibels hearing level.

ates the validity of the AC thresholds for a given ear. If technical factors can be ruled out, an SRT significantly better (> 12 dB) than the PTA may indicate the presence of functional (nonorganic) hearing impairment. If the SRT is significantly worse (> 12 dB) than the PTA, the difference is usually attributable to language factors.

Supra-threshold speech recognition performance (speech discrimination) is obtained for each ear under the earphones to determine how well a person can understand speech at an intensity that is well beyond the SRT. The material used for suprathreshold speech recognition testing ranges from nonsense syllables to words to sentences, but most commonly involves monosyllabic words. The speech recognition score for a given ear generally is reported as the percentage of items correctly repeated by the patient when the speech is presented at

a level that is at about 25 to 40 decibels sensation level (SL: dB above the SRT). A high speech recognition score in a person with a hearing loss suggests that a patient will obtain significant benefit from amplification. Frequently, a patient who is fitted with a hearing aid also receives speech recognition testing in noise in sound field (stimuli delivered through a loud speaker rather than through an earphone) to determine how well a patient will function with a hearing aid in noisy situations.

A statistical approach has been applied to analysis of the speech recognition scores as the 95% confidence limits have been established for each percentage word recognition score. These 95% critical differences limits can be used to compare word recognition performance between ears, assuming most importantly that the pure-tone thresholds are essentially equivalent for the two ears and that recorded materials are used. If

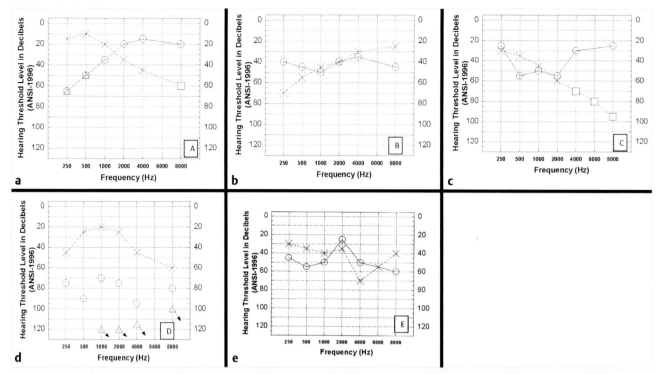

Fig. 114.3 Various audiometric configurations. (**a**) A high-frequency hearing loss audiometric configuration refers to a hearing loss present only at high frequencies (left ear). A low-frequency hearing loss audiometric configuration refers to a hearing loss present only at low frequencies (right ear). (**b**) With a flat audiometric configuration, the pure-tone thresholds generally are roughly equivalent (within about ± 20 dB) across the frequency range (right ear). With a rising configuration, the pure-tone thresholds improve as the frequency increases (left ear). (**c**) With a sloping audiometric configuration, the pure-tone thresholds worsen as the frequency increases (left ear). With a trough (also called saucer) audiometric configuration, the pure-tone thresholds are worse in the mid frequencies than in the low or high frequencies (right ear). (**d**) An inverted scoop or inverted trough audiogram has a configuration that is the opposite of that for the trough or saucer audiogram, with pure-tone thresholds worse in the low and high frequencies than in the mid frequencies (left ear). A fragmentary or corner audiogram refers to an audiogram with hearing thresholds present only for the low frequencies near the output of the audiometer (right ear). (**e**) A notched audiometric configuration is indicative of hearing loss within a restricted frequency range that recovers above and below the notch frequencies (left ear). A peak audiogram refers to an audiogram with pure-tone thresholds that are normal at a single or restricted range of frequencies but are consistent with hearing loss at frequencies above or below the peak frequency (right ear). *ANSI*, American National Standards Institute.

the score for one ear falls significantly outside this range, it can be concluded that word recognition performance is significantly poorer for one ear than for the other ear. Such a finding may suggest a retrocochlear pathology, but the utility of such a finding is somewhat limited, given that vestibular schwannomas are likely to be associated with asymmetric audiometric configurations. The 95% confidence limits may be more useful for comparing speech recognition performance in a given ear at a past test session with performance at a current test session, provided that the pure-tone results have remained stable over time.

The sizes of the 95% confidence intervals are narrower for scores at the extreme ends of the range (i.e., close to 0% or 100%) and for longer word lists, and are wider for scores in the middle of the range and for shorter word lists. These 95% confidence intervals have been widely employed in audiology. For example, they have been used to determine which hearing aid or hearing-aid electroacoustic characteristic produces a significant improvement in the word recognition score or to determine whether aural rehabilitation produces a significant benefit in communicative efficiency.

An individual with normal hearing sensitivity who presents with deficits in auditory processing, such as diffi-

culty understanding speech in background noise, distractibility or difficulty attending to speech, auditory memory problems, or difficulty in auditory discrimination, may have a central auditory disorder. A battery of sensitized speech tests (e.g., filtered speech, speech in noise, rapid speech) and electrophysiologic measures has been employed to detect central auditory disorder in individuals with normal hearing sensitivity and auditory-processing deficits.

114.3.3 Masking

Clinical masking of the nontest ear (NTE) during audiologic assessment often is necessary to prevent the NTE from participating in the assessment of the test ear (TE). In some situations, sound presented to the test ear is heard by the nontest ear, yielding a false impression of the hearing sensitivity of the test ear.

An understanding of the concepts of interaural attenuation, crossover, and cross-hearing is required to understand when masking is required to block out participation of the NTE. Interaural attenuation refers to the loss in intensity of a sound as it travels from the TE to the NTE by BC. A sound presented by AC loses approximately 40 dB as it travels from the TE to the NTE.

Hence, the interaural attenuation for AC sounds is approximately 40 dB. The interaural attenuation largely reflects the difference in impedance between air and the skull, resulting in rejection of energy when AC sound penetrates and sets the skull bones and the cochleae into vibration; little loss of intensity then occurs as the sound travels by BC through the skull bones to the cochleae of both ears. If a tone is presented to the right ear at 70 dB HL by AC (through the earphone), then it is estimated to arrive at the cochlea of the left ear at 30 dB HL. Thus, the crossover level of that 70-dB HL tone presented to the TE is 30 dB HL. Cross-hearing occurs if the BC threshold of the NTE is sufficient to hear the crossover level (i.e., is 30 dB HL or better in this example). If cross-hearing occurs, then the unmasked AC threshold for the TE represents the hearing sensitivity of the NTE rather than that of the TE; masking of the NTE is required to establish the true AC threshold of the TE. A general rule for AC masking, based on this interaural attenuation for AC, is to mask whenever the threshold of the TE minus 40 dB equals or exceeds the BC threshold (or AC threshold since the AC threshold sometimes is slightly better than the BC threshold). The need to obtain a masked AC threshold should be based on comparison of the AC threshold for the TE with the AC threshold for the NTE. For example, if the right ear AC threshold is 20 dB HL and the left ear AC threshold is 70 dB HL, then the masked left ear AC threshold needs to be obtained with masking noise in the right ear. The masked AC threshold can be equivalent to the unmasked AC threshold or up to about 60 or 65 dB poorer than the BC threshold of the TE because the largest possible ABG is approximately 60 to 65 dB.

The results of several studies suggest that the interaural attenuation for insert earphones is significantly greater than that for traditional supra-aural earphones. Thus, we suggest the following rule when insert earphones are used: If the depth of the insert earphone insertion is deep, then consider the interaural attenuation to be 65 dB at 250 and 500 Hz, and 55 dB at the higher frequencies; if the depth of the insert earphone insertion is shallow, then use interaural attenuation values that are 5 dB lower than those for deep insertion.

The interaural attenuation for BC sounds is essentially 0 dB, which means that sounds delivered through the bone oscillator travel by BC to the cochleae of both ears, essentially with no loss in intensity. If a tone is presented to the right ear at 70 dB HL by BC (through the bone oscillator), then it is estimated to arrive at the cochlea of the left ear at 70 dB HL (70 dB HL – 0 dB interaural attenuation). Because the interaural attenuation for BC is approximately 0 dB, the unmasked BC threshold represents the better cochlea, regardless of whether the bone vibrator is placed on the right or left mastoid process of the temporal bone. Thus, the unmasked BC threshold is needed for only one ear, and the obtained BC threshold represents the cochlear integrity of the better ear. The ABG should be examined in each ear to determine the need for obtaining a masked BC threshold whereby the true BC threshold for the TE is obtained by using a bone vibrator on the mastoid process of the TE while masking noise is presented by AC through an earphone on the NTE. If the ABG in a given ear exceeds 10 dB, then the masked BC threshold should be obtained.

Consider an example in which the unmasked BC threshold is 30 dB HL, the right AC is 30 dB HL, and the left ear is 40 dB HL. In this example, the left BC threshold must be 30 dB HL (it cannot be any better than the unmasked BC threshold, and it cannot be poorer than the AC threshold of that ear). In the left ear, the best the BC threshold can be is 30 dB HL, and the worst it can be is 40 dB HL (equivalent to the right AC threshold). Thus, masking is unnecessary in this situation as we can consider the BC threshold to be 30 dB HL, bilaterally. Consider another example in which the unmasked BC threshold is 30 dB HL, but the right and left AC thresholds are 50 dB HL. In this example, the ABG is 20 dB, bilaterally, so masked BC thresholds need to be obtained for both ears. The clinician obtains the masked BC threshold first for the right ear, putting masking noise in the left ear, and obtains a right masked BC threshold of 45 dB HL. This shift would obviate the need for obtaining the masked BC threshold for the left ear, which can be assumed to be 30 dB HL (the unmasked BC threshold), which has to represent the BC threshold for at least one ear. If, however, the right masked BC threshold did not change significantly from 30 dB HL, then the left masked BC threshold would need to be obtained because it could be 30, 35, 40, 45, or 50 dB HL.

The situation for masking during speech audiometry is similar to the situation for pure-tone testing except that the speech level in the TE is compared against each BC threshold (and AC threshold to be conservative) at all frequencies. Masking should be employed whenever the speech level in the TE exceeds any AC or BC of the NTE by 40 dB or more.

Masking cannot always be achieved because in some situations the masking noise in the NTE will cross over and reach the BC threshold of the TE, thereby resulting in cross-hearing of the noise by the TE. In such a situation, the masking noise in the NTE has confounded threshold measurement in the TE. This is termed a masking dilemma. The audiometric configuration that is most likely to be associated with a masking dilemma is maximal bilateral ABGs. For example, let us consider the situation in which the unmasked BC threshold is 10 dB HL and the unmasked AC threshold is 60 dB HL. In this example, when a masked BC threshold is obtained for one of the ears, say the right ear, a relatively high starting level of masking noise needs to be introduced into the left ear because the AC threshold is relatively high there. It is possible that the noise crosses from the NTE to the TE with an interaural attenuation of 40 dB (the noise is presented by AC) and may reach the BC threshold of 10 dB in the TE, thereby elevating the BC threshold in the TE.

▶ Fig. 114.4 shows the unmasked and masked pure-tone and speech results in a patient with an asymmetric hearing loss.

114.4 Physiologic Measures of Auditory Function

114.4.1 Acoustic Admittance Testing

A tympanogram is a graph of the admittance (Y) of the middle ear as a function of the air pressure introduced into the ear canal through a probe inserted into the ear canal. The variation in air pressure generally is in the range of about +200 to –300 decapascals (daPa) A probe tone is introduced through a speaker in the probe assembly; some of the energy is admitted into the middle ear through the tympanic membrane, and some of the energy is rejected at the tympanic membrane. The microphone in the probe assembly picks up the

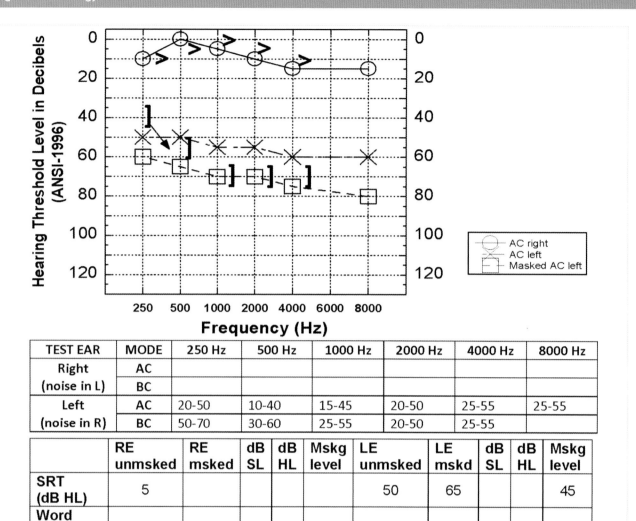

TEST EAR	MODE	250 Hz	500 Hz	1000 Hz	2000 Hz	4000 Hz	8000 Hz
Right	AC						
(noise in L)	BC						
Left	AC	20-50	10-40	15-45	20-50	25-55	25-55
(noise in R)	BC	50-70	30-60	25-55	20-50	25-55	

	RE unmsked	RE msked	dB SL	dB HL	Mskg level	LE unmsked	LE mskd	dB SL	dB HL	Mskg level
SRT (dB HL)	5					50	65			45
Word Recog. Score (%)	100		35	40			76	30	95	75

Fig. 114.4 The unmasked and masked pure-tone and speech results in a patient with an asymmetric hearing loss. Note that the unmasked air conduction (AC) thresholds for the right ear range between 0 and 15 dB HL, consistent with normal hearing sensitivity. The unmasked AC thresholds for the left ear, ranging between 50 and 60 dB HL, are 40 to 50 dB poorer than the AC thresholds for the right ear; because the interaural attenuation for AC is 40 dB, subtracting 40 dB from the unmasked AC thresholds of the left ear indicates that the right ear may be cross-hearing the tones presented to the left ear; therefore, masking noise was presented to the right ear while the AC thresholds were reestablished in the left ear to obtain the true masked AC thresholds for the left ear. The levels of masking noise are shown in the table below (test ear left, noise in R), mode AC, and the masked left AC thresholds (see box symbols) are shown at levels between 60 and 80 dB HL. Note that the unmasked bone conduction (BC) thresholds were obtained with the bone vibrator placed on the left ear; these thresholds, between 0 and 15 dB HL, reflect the integrity of the cochlea on the right side because the interaural attenuation of BC is 0 dB, and the ear with the better cochlea is the right ear. To determine the masked true left ear BC thresholds, masking noise was presented to the right ear while the BC thresholds were reestablished in the left ear. The levels of masking noise are shown in the table below (test ear left, noise in R), mode BC, and the masked left BC thresholds (see bracket symbols) are shown at levels that are between more than 40 dB HL at 250 Hz (output limit for BC is 40 dB at that frequency) and 70 dB HL at 4000 Hz. Thus, this patient has a flat sensorineural hearing loss in the left ear of moderately severe degree. The speech table shows that the speech recognition threshold (SRT) is 5 dB HL in the right ear, consistent with the normal-hearing pure-tone threshold levels in that ear; the unmasked SRT in the left ear is 50 dB HL. Because the interaural attenuation for speech AC stimuli is about 40 dB, and because some of the right AC and BC thresholds are 10 dB HL or better, the right ear may be cross-hearing the speech stimuli presented to the left ear, so the left masked, true SRT needs to be reestablished while masking noise is presented in the right ear. The masked left SRT is 65 dB HL, consistent with the masked left pure-tone AC thresholds. As the speech table shows, word recognition testing was done at 35 dB SL re: SRT in the right ear (so the presentation level was the SRT level of 5 plus 35 dB, which equals 40 dB HL) and at 30 dB SL re: SRT in the left ear (so the presentation level was the SRT level of 65 plus 30 dB, which equals 95 dB HL). With a word-presentation level of 40 dB in the right ear, the crossover level into the left ear is 0 dB HL, so cross-hearing by the left ear is not possible, and masking noise in the left ear was not needed while the word recognition score was obtained for the right ear, which was 100%. But with a word-presentation level of 95 dB HL in the left ear, the crossover level is 95 dB – 40 dB = 55 dB HL, resulting in cross-hearing in the right ear. Thus, masking noise was needed in the right ear (75 dB HL of masking was used) while the word recognition score was obtained for the left ear, which was 76%. *ANSI,* American National Standards Institute; *dB HL,* decibels hearing level; *dB SL,* decibels sensation level; *LE,* left ear; *RE,* right ear.

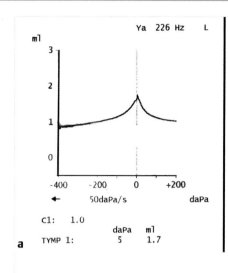

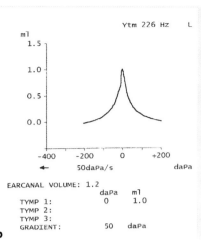

Fig. 114.5 (**a**) A tympanogram obtained in the baseline-off mode. (**b**) A tympanogram obtained in the baseline-on mode. The tympanometric peak pressure (TPP) is 5 daPa in (**a**) and is 0 daPa in (**b**). Note that in the tympanogram in (**a**), the ear canal volume (Vec) can be read by looking at the ordinate value associated with an air pressure of +200 daPa and also by reading the C1 value (1.0) below the tympanogram. The value of 1.7 ml represents the combined admittance of the outer and middle ear, so the peak-compensated static-acoustic admittance is obtained by subtracting the C1 value (1.0) from the ml value at the TPP (1.7) to yield 0.7 mmho. In the tympanogram in (**b**), the Vec cannot be read from the tympanogram curve; the value is displayed below the tympanogram as 1.2 cc. The peak-compensated static-acoustic admittance is the value (1.0 mmho) on the ordinate associated with the TPP; it also is displayed below the tympanogram.

rejected energy and transmits it to a device that measures its admittance in millimhos (mmho). The admittance of the middle ear provides information regarding the presence of any stiffening (e.g., otosclerosis) or loosening (e.g., mass lesion such as ossicular discontinuity) in the middle ear.

Tympanometric Peak Pressure

The peak of the tympanogram occurs when the ear canal air pressure against the lateral side of the tympanic membrane from the probe assembly inserted in the ear canal equals the air pressure exerted laterally from the middle ear against the medial side of the tympanic membrane. The air pressure at which this occurs is referred to as the tympanometric peak pressure (TPP), measured in decapascals. The TPP also represents the ear canal air pressure at which the admittance of acoustic energy into the middle ear from the ear canal is maximal (▶ Fig. 114.5). Although it correlates closely with middle ear pressure, the TPP is not an exact measurement of the pressure in the middle ear. In patients older than 12 years of age, the TPP is considered to be within normal limits if it is greater than –50 daPa. A TPP that is equal to or more negative than this cutoff reflects eustachian tube dysfunction in that ear, with or without middle ear effusion; the TPP is obliterated (beyond the negative limit of the air pressure range employed by the device) when the fluid level in the middle ear in cases of middle ear effusion is sufficient to reach the ossicles.

Peak-Compensated Static-Acoustic Admittance and Equivalent Ear Canal Volume

The peak-compensated static-acoustic admittance (in millimhos) is obtained from the tympanogram. When the tympanogram is run at "baseline on" (▶ Fig. 114.5b), the device will exclude the admittance from an extreme ear canal air pressure such as +200 or –300 daPa, which grossly represents the admittance of the ear canal (termed the equivalent ear canal volume in cubic centimeters), from the tympanogram. So, the tails of the tympanogram generally will be at about 0 mmho, and the

peak-compensated static-acoustic admittance, in mmho, which can be read from the ordinate at the peak height of the tympanogram, essentially is the admittance of the middle ear. For the 226-Hz probe tone, 1 mmho = 1 cm^3. If the tympanogram is run at "baseline off" (▶ Fig. 114.5a), then the admittance at the TPP represents the combined admittance of the outer ear and middle ear, and the clinician must subtract the displayed equivalent ear canal volume from this combined admittance of the outer ear and middle ear to derive the peak-compensated static-acoustic admittance.

A normal range for peak-compensated static-acoustic admittance is approximately 0.35 to 1.30 mmho. A peak-compensated static-acoustic admittance that is significantly reduced (< 0.35 mmho) is consistent with the presence of a stiffening middle ear disorder. A peak-compensated static-acoustic admittance that is significantly increased (> 1.30 mmho) is consistent with the presence of ossicular discontinuity or a stiffening middle ear pathology in conjunction with a flaccid tympanic membrane (or healed tympanic membrane perforation) when significant ABGs are present. Because of the considerable overlap in peak-compensated static-acoustic admittance between normal and pathologic ears, this parameter should be interpreted in conjunction with the audiometric and other acoustic admittance findings. An abnormally large value of the equivalent ear canal volume (Vec), above 2.5 cm^3 in adults or above 2.0 cm^3 in children, is consistent with the presence of tympanic membrane perforation or a patent tympanostomy tube. In such cases, the tympanogram will appear to be flat because the TPP will be absent. If the Vec in a patient with a known tympanostomy tube is significantly below 2.5 cm^3 in an adult or significantly below 2.0 cm^3 in a child, then the finding may be suggestive of a blocked tympanostomy tube; in such cases, if the blockage is limited to the tympanostomy tube, a TPP will be seen, probably within normal limits.

The shape of the tympanogram traditionally has been classified as type A, type A$_D$, type A$_s$, or type B (▶ Fig. 114.6). Type A, with a normal TPP and normal peak amplitude, is interpreted as consistent with normal middle ear function. Type A$_D$, with a greater than normal peak amplitude or a peak in which the

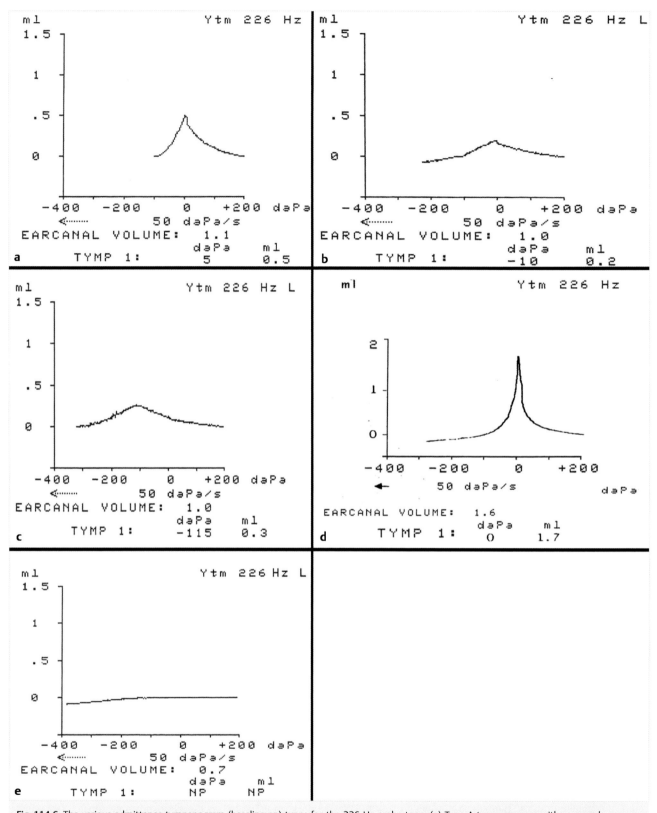

Fig. 114.6 The various admittance tympanogram (baseline on) types for the 226-Hz probe tone. (**a**) Type A tympanogram with a normal tympanometric peak pressure (TPP) of 5 daPa and a normal peak-compensated static-acoustic admittance of 0.5 mmho. (**b**) Type A$_S$ tympanogram with a normal TPP (−10 daPa) but a reduced peak-compensated static-acoustic admittance (0.2 mmho). (**c**) Type C tympanogram with a significantly negative TPP (−115 daPa). (**d**) Type A$_D$ tympanogram with an abnormally increased peak-compensated static-acoustic admittance (1.7 mmho). (**e**) Type B tympanogram is flat, with an absent TPP.

right and left slopes do not meet, is consistent with increased admittance of sound energy in the middle ear, which can occur with ossicular discontinuity. Type A$_s$, characterized by a peak amplitude that is reduced and a normal TPP, has been interpreted as consistent with a stiffening middle ear pathology, such as ossicular fixation. Type C, with a significantly negative TPP, has been interpreted as consistent with eustachian tube dysfunction. Type B is consistent with an associated pathology that produces greatly increased stiffness, such as middle ear effusion, or a condition such as tympanic membrane perforation, in which the admittance in the middle ear does not vary with air pressure. However, we believe it is more useful to interpret TPP and peak-compensated static-acoustic admittance first separately and then together, rather than to interpret just the shape of the tympanogram. If these tympanogram classifications are used, then the peak amplitude should be considered normal if the peak-compensated static-acoustic admittance is within the normal range; similarly, the peak amplitude should be considered reduced if the peak-compensated static-acoustic admittance is below the normal range, and it should be considered increased if the peak-compensated static-acoustic admittance is beyond the normal range. Type C should not be interpreted as consistent with the absence of middle ear effusion. Also, because many stiffening and mass lesions may have peak-compensated static-acoustic admittance values within the normal range, many of these stiffening and mass lesions yield a normal type A tympanogram.

High-Frequency Tympanometry in Older Children and Adults

As mentioned in the previous section, significantly high peak-compensated static-acoustic admittance values can be seen in ears with ossicular discontinuity and in ears with otosclerosis in conjunction with either a flaccid tympanic membrane or a healed tympanic membrane perforation. However, these pathologies also can yield peak-compensated static-acoustic admittance values within the normal range. When peak-compensated static-acoustic admittance exceeds 0.75 mmho and the audiogram shows significant ABGs, consistent with the presence of middle ear pathology, high-frequency tympanometry performed with the 678-Hz probe tone may help differentiate between ossicular discontinuity and ossicular fixation with either a flaccid tympanic membrane or a healed tympanic membrane perforation.

In order to perform high-frequency tympanometry with the 678-Hz probe tone, the major components of admittance—susceptance and conductance—have to be examined. Acoustic susceptance comprises stiffness susceptance and mass susceptance. The former represents the acceptance of sound energy into stiffness; the latter represents the acceptance of sound energy into mass. Conductance represents the acceptance of sound energy into resistance. With the 226-Hz probe tone, the admittance (Y) tympanogram is obtained. With the 678-Hz probe tone, tympanograms for the susceptance component of admittance (symbol is B) and for the conductance component of admittance (symbol is G) are obtained. The susceptance and conductance tympanograms for this probe tone frequency have certain characteristics for ears with ossicular discontinuity that differ from the characteristics for ears with ossicular fixation in

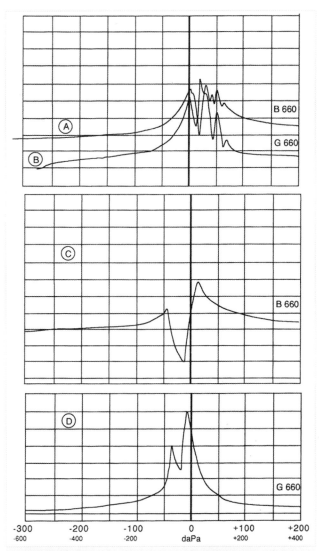

Fig. 114.7 High-frequency tympanometry (660-Hz probe tone) for an ear with ossicular discontinuity and for an ear with otosclerosis in conjunction with a flaccid tympanic membrane or a healed tympanic membrane. The susceptance (B) and conductance (G) tympanograms are shown for each ear. Both of these ears had abnormally large peak-compensated static-acoustic admittance values on the admittance tympanogram for the low-frequency probe tone (not shown here). (A) and (B) show the B and G tympanograms for the ear with ossicular discontinuity. The findings are consistent with ossicular discontinuity as more than 3 extrema (positive and negative peaks) are seen for G and more than 5 extrema are seen for B. (C) and (D) show the B and G tympanograms, respectively, for an ear with otosclerosis and a flaccid tympanic membrane. This ear shows 3 extrema for the B tympanogram and 3 extrema for the G tympanogram, and the number of extrema does not exceed normal limits, so ossicular discontinuity is not present. (Used with permission from Silman S, Silverman CA. Auditory Diagnosis: Principles and Applications. San Diego, CA: Singular Publishing; 1997.)

conjunction with either a flaccid tympanic membrane or a healed tympanic membrane perforation.

▶ Fig. 114.7 illustrates high-frequency tympanograms (678-Hz probe tone) for an ear with ossicular discontinuity and for an ear with otosclerosis in conjunction with a flaccid tympanic membrane or a healed tympanic membrane. Note the multiple positive and negative peaks (called extrema) for both the B and G tympanograms in the case of the ear with ossicular discontinuity. More than 5 peaks are present for both the B and G tympanograms, consistent with the presence of a mass-loaded middle ear system, which has shifted the resonance frequency of the middle ear downward from the normal of around 900 Hz. In contrast, note that only three extrema are seen in the B and G tympanograms in the ear with otosclerosis and a flaccid tympanic membrane or a healed tympanic membrane perforation. The criteria for abnormal high-frequency (678-Hz probe tone) tympanometric findings are as follows: (1) more than 5 extrema for the B tympanogram; or (2) more than 3 extrema for the G tympanogram; or (c) the air pressure interval between the outermost extremum for a tympanogram with 5 extrema (either B or G) exceeds 100 daPa, or the air pressure interval for the outermost extremum for a tympanogram with 3 extrema (either B or G) exceeds 75 daPa. The air pressure interval between the outermost extremum in the ear with ossicular discontinuity with a flaccid tympanic membrane or a healed tympanic membrane perforation is less than 75 daPa for both the G and B tympanograms; this finding, along with the number of extrema not exceeding 3 for both the B and G tympanograms, is consistent with the absence of ossicular discontinuity and points to ossicular fixation with a flaccid tympanic membrane or a healed tympanic membrane perforation.

114.4.2 Acoustic Reflex Threshold and Decay

The acoustic reflex primarily involves contraction of the stapedius muscle in response to a sufficiently intense sound. The stapedius muscle originates from the pyramidal eminence on the posterior wall of the tympanic cavity of the middle ear, and its tendon inserts onto the neck of the stapes. Activation of the acoustic reflex decreases the volume of the middle ear as contraction causes medial movement of the ossicles and tympanic membrane medially. The decreased volume leads to increased stiffness, resulting in the rejection of sound energy (decreased admittance of sound in the middle ear).

The acoustic reflex is bilateral, even for acoustic signals presented to only one ear. Therefore, the change in acoustic admittance elicited by a sound can be monitored either in the ear receiving the intense auditory signal (ipsilateral acoustic reflex threshold testing) or in the opposite ear (contralateral acoustic reflex threshold testing). Ipsilateral acoustic reflex threshold (ART) testing involves, like tympanometry, insertion of a probe assembly into one ear. An intense activator (e.g., at 500, 1000, and/or 2000 Hz) is presented through the speaker of the probe assembly into the ear canal. The clinician adjusts the air pressure to match the TPP through one of the tubes of the probe assembly. A constant probe tone (typically 226 Hz) at about 85 dB SPL also is introduced into the ear canal through the probe assembly. A microphone in the probe assembly measures the dB SPL in the ear canal, and the acoustic admittance device converts that reading into acoustic admittance. If the acoustic reflex does not occur, then no change in dB SPL or acoustic admittance occurs. If the acoustic reflex is elicited by a sufficiently intense activator, the dB SPL and acoustic admittance will increase because of the effect of the acoustic reflex on the middle ear volume and admittance. Contralateral ART testing is similar

to ipsilateral ART testing, except that the activator is presented through an insert in the ear canal opposite to the one that has the probe assembly. The intensity of the activator is increased in one ear until a deflection is observed in the contralateral ear with the probe assembly. The ARTs generally are reported for each ear for each activator (conventionally 500, 1000, and 2000 Hz) for the ipsilateral and/or contralateral mode of testing. The ART is labeled for the ear that receives the activator. Therefore, for contralateral ART testing, if the probe assembly is in the right ear, the activator is in the left ear, and the recorded ART is the left contralateral ART because the activating sound in the left ear triggered the acoustic reflex.

The ART represents the lowest sound intensity that yields a detectable decrease in acoustic admittance on the readout of the acoustic admittance device when the device is set to display the acoustic admittance as a function of time lapsing from presentation of the sound.

The ARTs are affected by conductive pathology, significant sensorineural hearing impairment attributed to cochlear causes, and disorders of the acoustic reflex arc, which affect cranial nerve VIII (cochleovestibular nerve), the cochlear nuclei of the auditory brainstem, the superior olivary complex of the auditory brainstem, the motor nucleus of cranial nerve VII (facial nerve), or cranial nerve VII, which innervates the stapedius muscle. The acoustic reflex pattern can be predicted by considering whether the pathology affects the afferent acoustic reflex arc and/or the efferent acoustic reflex arc. In the case of the acoustic reflex, the afferent (sensory) arc involves sound transmission through the outer ear, middle ear, cochlea, cochleovestibular nerve, cochlear nuclei, and superior olivary complex. The efferent (motor) arc involves the motor nucleus of the facial nerve, facial nerve, stapedius, and stapes.

A cochlear hearing loss of approximately 50 dB or more is sufficient to affect the ART by elevating it or making it absent. Cochlear hearing losses involve the afferent arc, so, for example, if the hearing loss is in the right ear, then the right contralateral ART and right ipsilateral ART will be affected because right contralateral and right ipsilateral acoustic reflex testing involve activator presentation to the right ear, which then carries the auditory information through the right cochleovestibular nerve to the superior olivary complex. The effect is frequency specific, so the ART is affected at activator frequencies with significant cochlear hearing loss. Vestibular schwannomas also involve the afferent arc in a similar manner to cochlear hearing losses, except that the effect on the ART is more pronounced than that of cochlear hearing losses and the frequency effect is unpredictable. The Silman and Gelfand 90th percentiles, when applied to the contralateral ARTs, can enable differentiation between cochlear and retrocochlear lesions and can enable the detection of retrocochlear pathology when the hearing sensitivity is normal and ABGs are not present. The 90th percentiles establish the cutoffs for the effect of cochlear pathologies of varying magnitudes and normal hearing sensitivity. Therefore, if the ART is elevated beyond the 90th percentile (and ABGs are absent), then the finding may be consistent with retrocochlear pathology. The 90th percentiles cannot be applied when the cochlear hearing loss reaches a magnitude of 80 dB HL or more.

A facial nerve lesion that is medial to the origin of the nerve to the stapedius muscle can affect the ART by affecting the efferent arc. Therefore, if the lesion affects the right facial nerve medial to the branch to the stapedius, then the left contralateral ART and right ipsilateral ART will be affected (elevated or absent) at one or more frequencies; left contralateral ART testing involves the affected efferent arc on the right side, and right ipsilateral ART testing involves the affected efferent (as well as afferent) arc on the right side.

A conductive pathology has dual effects. The afferent arc is affected because sound transmission through the middle ear is affected by the ABG. The efferent arc is affected because the pathology prevents acoustic reflex contraction in the ear with the conductive pathology at all activator frequencies. In the case of a right middle ear effusion, the right contralateral ART will be elevated or absent at a given activator frequency according to the magnitude of the ABG at that frequency, which affects the afferent arc; the activator is in the ear with the ABG (afferent arc), and the probe assembly is in the normal ear in which the acoustic reflex is monitored (efferent arc is intact). With left contralateral ART testing, the activator is in the normal left ear (afferent arc), but the probe is in the ear with the conductive pathology; the conductive pathology in the left ear prevents the acoustic reflex from contracting, so the efferent arc is affected and the left contralateral acoustic reflexes will be absent at all activating frequencies. The right ipsilateral ART will be absent for all activators because the efferent arc is impaired by the conductive pathology in that ear, which prevents the acoustic reflex from contracting. The left ipsilateral ART will be present at expected levels as both the activator and probe are in the normal ear. ARTs are more sensitive to conductive pathology than any other acoustic admittance measure. With bilateral conductive pathology, right and left contralateral and ipsilateral ARTs all will be absent at all activator frequencies because all ART testing will involve insertion of the probe in an ear with a conductive lesion that affects the efferent arc, so that acoustic reflex contraction cannot occur. Eustachian tube dysfunction without middle ear effusion generally is too mild to affect the ARTs unless the dysfunction is severe (extremely negative TPP). Recall that ART testing is done at TPP, which generally overcomes the effect of the negative TPP.

114.4.3 Acoustic Reflex Adaptation

Acoustic reflex adaptation (ARA) or decay represents the decrease in magnitude of the acoustic reflex over time during the presentation of an acoustic stimulus over a period of about 10 seconds. Like ART testing, ARA testing can be performed in the ipsilateral or contralateral mode with the probe tone frequency at 226 Hz and activating stimuli at 500 and 1000 Hz. The activating stimuli are presented at 10 dB SL re: ART. Thus, ARA may not be accomplished if the ART is absent or elevated near the output of the acoustic admittance device. If the magnitude of the acoustic reflex decays by 50% or more over a period of 10 seconds, then the ARA is recorded as positive, possibly consistent with retrocochlear pathology. Differentiation between a retrocochlear lesion affecting the afferent arc and a facial nerve lesion (medial to the branch to the stapedius) affecting the efferent arc can be made based on the comparison of ipsilateral and contralateral ARA findings for each ear, similar to the comparisons between the ipsilateral and contralateral ARTs.

The sensitivity and false-positive rate for the differential diagnosis of retrocochlear pathology based on combined contrala-

teral ART testing using the Silman and Gelfand 90th percentiles and ARA testing are 83% and 10%, respectively.

114.4.4 Otoacoustic Emissions

Otoacoustic emissions (OAEs), low-level sounds generated in the cochlea of the inner ear, can be detected with a sensitive, low-noise microphone placed within the external auditory meatus. They represent a by-product of normal auditory physiologic processes involving the interaction between the outer hair cells and the traveling wave along the basal membrane. Spontaneous otoacoustic emissions (SOAEs) occur in the absence of sound stimulation. They are generated at specific sites along the basal membrane of the cochlea and produce two waves traveling in opposite directions. The wave traveling toward the apical end of the basal membrane dissipates; however, the wave traveling backward in the basal direction stimulates the ossicles of the middle ear and tympanic membrane, generating sound in the external ear canal. SOAEs have little clinical applicability because they are absent in approximately 30% of individuals with normal hearing.

Transient otoacoustic emissions (TOAEs) and distortion product otoacoustic emissions (DPOAEs) are *evoked* otoacoustic emissions because sound stimulation is necessary for their generation. With TOAEs, a cochlear echo is generated by an outgoing wave; this represents a reflection of the traveling wave along the basal membrane that is produced at a point of irregularity along the basal membrane. The outer hair cells enhance the reflected wave in a nonlinear manner, so damage to these hair cells adversely affects the OAEs. The latency of the so-called cochlear echo is roughly 3 to 10 milliseconds, representing the travel time through the ear to the point on the basal membrane where the reflected wave is generated and then the travel time for the wave to be propagated back outward. This mechanism involving irregularities of the basal membrane and the reflected traveling wave also underlies DPOAEs. With DPOAEs, two short-duration pure-tone signals of different frequencies are simultaneously presented into the ear canal. Because of outer hair cell nonlinearities, intermodulation distortion products are produced, resulting in emissions at frequencies that represent certain sums and differences of the stimulating frequencies. The intermodulation distortion product occurring at the frequency representing $2f_1 - f_2$ usually is the one measured and reported in DPOAE testing because this intermodulation distortion product is the largest of the intermodulation distortion products.

Transient Otoacoustic Emissions

▶ Fig. 114.8 shows a tracing for TOAEs in an adult ear with normal hearing sensitivity and normal middle ear function. Suggested criteria for a pass result on TOAEs are as follows: (1) signal-to-noise ratio of at least 6 dB for at least four of the following frequencies (1000 Hz, 2000 Hz, 3000 Hz, 4000 Hz, and 6000 Hz); (2) 70% or greater stability of the stimulus peak dB SPL; and (3) overall waveform reproducibility of at least 70%. Studies show that when the average pure-tone thresholds across the entire audiometric frequency range do not exceed 20 dB HL, the probability of passing TOAE testing exceeds 90%. For average pure-tone thresholds between 20 and 40 dB HL, the

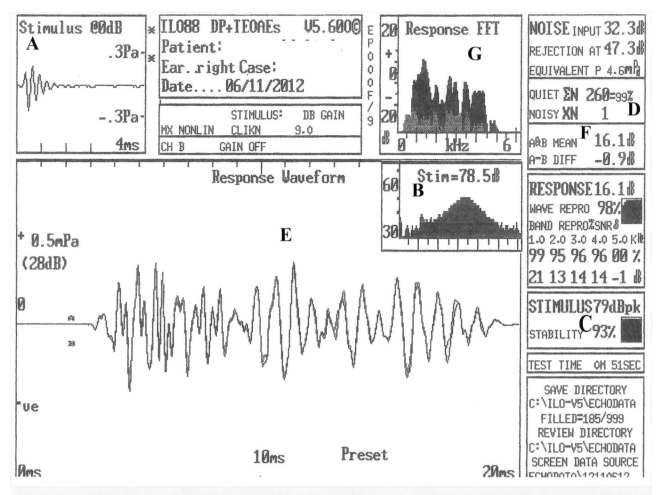

Fig. 114.8 A transient otoacoustic emissions (TOAEs) recording in a normal ear. Section A represents the waveform (intensity over time) of the click stimulus. Section B shows the frequency spectrum (intensity as a function of frequency) for the click stimulus, which has a peak sound pressure level (SPL) of 78.5 dB in this example. Section C shows a 93% stability of the stimulus peak dB SPL during this recording. Section D shows a 32.3-dB SPL noise level measured in the ear canal during the recording; with a noise level for rejection of sweeps set to 47.3 dB, only one sweep was rejected (see *NOISY XN*), which is extremely low. The lower part of the figure (section E) shows the amplitudes of the section A and section B TOAE waveforms over a 20-ms period. The mean amplitude of the section A and section B averages of the response waveform (*A&B MEAN*) is 16.1 dB SPL (section F). The A-B difference (*A-B DIFF*) is −0.9 dB, indicating that the noise level in the ear canal is very low. The amplitude of the response (16.1 dB SPL) is shown below this, with a waveform reproducibility (*WAVE REPRO*) of 98%. Also shown are the reproducibility and signal-to-noise ratios for each of five frequency bands centered at 1000, 2000, 3000, 4000, and 5000 Hz. Here, the signal-to-noise ratios greatly exceed 6 dB at 1000, 2000, 3000, and 4000 Hz. Section G shows the frequency analysis of the noise (*light shaded area*) compared with the frequency analysis of the TOAEs (*dark shaded area*).

probability of passing TOAE testing declines as the hearing loss increases, from over 90% at 20 dB HL to approximately 50% at 30 dB HL and approximately 8% at 40 dB HL. Thus, a pass result of the TOAE may not rule out slight to mild hearing loss up to about 40 dB HL. TOAEs are obliterated with conductive pathology for ABGs of at least 20 to 25 dB. They also are obliterated with a substantially negative TPP less than or equal to −200 daPa, even when ABGs are not present. Approximately 80% of patients with retrocochlear pathologies fail OAEs testing; one reason for this, in the case of vestibular schwannomas, is involvement of the cochlear artery.

Distortion Product Otoacoustic Emissions

▶ Fig. 114.9 shows a tracing for DPOAEs in an adult ear with normal hearing sensitivity and normal middle ear function.

Various clinics employ different pass criteria for the DPOAEs. We suggest that the criterion for a pass result on the DPOAEs be a signal-to-noise ratio of at least 6 dB at 1000, 2000, 3000, and 4000 Hz; the presence of a signal-to-noise ratio of at least 6 dB at 1500, 5000, and 6000 Hz as well as at the other frequencies strengthens a pass finding.

Studies show that when the average pure-tone thresholds across the entire audiometric frequency range do not exceed 20 dB HL, the probability of passing DPOAE testing exceeds 90%, similar to the probability of passing TOAE testing. For average pure-tone thresholds between 20 and 25 dB HL, the probability of passing DPOAE testing declines to about 60% at 25 dB HL. For average pure-tone thresholds between 25 and 40 dB HL, the probability of passing DPOAE testing declines further to 12% at 40 dB HL (for traditional high-level-stimulus intensities). The probability of passing DPOAE testing with average pure-tone

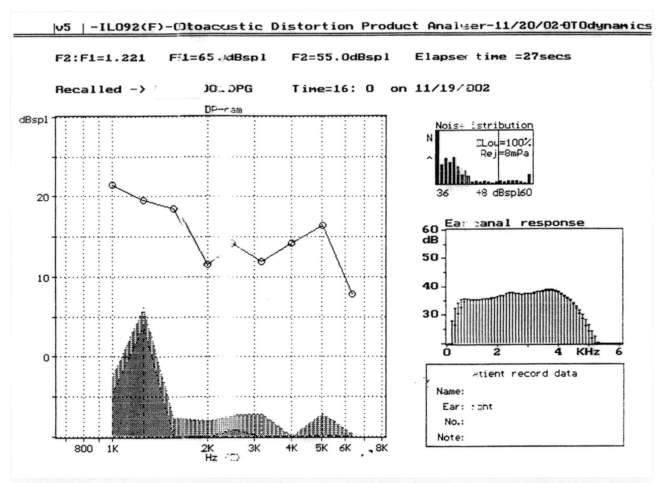

Fig. 114.9 A distortion product otoacoustic emissions (DPOAEs) recording. The f_2/f_1 ratio, shown at the top of the recording, is 1.221. The intensities for f_1 and f_2, also shown at the top of the recording, are 65 dB SPL and 55 dB SPL, respectively. The "Ear canal response" shows the frequency spectrum of the noise in the ear canal before testing is initiated. The DP-gram is a frequency spectrum. The light and dark shaded areas in the DP-gram show the frequency spectrum of the noise levels during testing. The open circles show the intensity of the emissions at each frequency, usually f_2, as shown here. The SPL values for the emissions should be compared against the SPL values of the noise to determine the signal-to-noise ratio. In this example, the SPL values for the emissions are substantially more than 6 dB greater than the noise levels across the frequency range. The graph labeled "noise distribution" shows the amplitude distribution of the noise floor.

thresholds equivalent to 50 dB HL is about 5%. Thus, a pass result on DPOAE testing may not rule out slight to borderline moderate hearing loss up to about 40 to 45 dB HL. Like TOAEs, DPOAEs are obliterated with conductive pathology for ABGs of at least 20 to 25 dB and with a substantially negative TPP less than or equal to –200 daPa (even when ABGs are not present).

114.5 Auditory Evoked Potentials

Auditory evoked potentials represent changes in the electroencephalogram (EEG) during auditory stimulation. Recording electrodes, usually placed on the scalp, detect the electrical activity from the brain. Recordings of auditory evoked potentials show the response waveform (amplitude of the electrical activity elicited by the sound stimulation over time [latency]). Because the voltage of the background EEG with electrophysiologic noise is much larger than the voltage of the potential elicited by sound stimulation, averaging of responses to numerous signal presentations, amplification of the response, response filtering, and other procedures are employed to enhance the

evoked potential and reduce the background EEG and noise. The auditory evoked potential tests that have the greatest application for otolaryngologists include electrocochleography (ECochG), auditory brainstem response (ABR) testing, and auditory steady-state response (ASSR) testing.

114.5.1 Electrocochleography

The evoked potentials that are typically recorded and interpreted in ECochG include the summating potential (SP) and the action potential (AP). The SP is a direct current potential that represents the extracellular activity of the hair cells within the organ of Corti of the cochlea. Its amplitude is on the scale of microvolts (μV), ranging from about a fraction of a microvolt up to about 1 μV in a normal ear, for extratympanic placement. Slightly larger amplitudes are obtained with transtympanic placement. The AP is an alternating-polarity potential that represents the synchronous firing of the thousands of fibers of the auditory nerve for a short-duration stimulus such as a click. Its amplitude also is on the scale of microvolts, typically about 2.0

ECOG-right ear

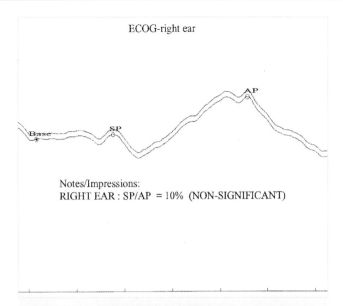

Notes/Impressions:
RIGHT EAR : SP/AP = 10% (NON-SIGNIFICANT)

Fig. 114.10 An electrocochleographic recording for a normal ear. The amplitude is 0.03 µV (measured from the base) for the summating potential and 0.25 µV (measured from the base) for the action potential. Thus, the amplitude ratio is 0.03 µV/0.25 µV, which equals 0.1 or 10%, which is non-significant for Meniere disease. *AP*, action potential; *SP*, summating potential.

µV, but can be as large as about 5 µV Its latency ranges from about 1.3 to 1.7 milliseconds (roughly around 2.0 milliseconds); the latency of the SP, which precedes the AP, is slightly less than that of the AP.

ECochG can be performed with the transtympanic or extratympanic placement of the active (noninverting) electrode. The former involves insertion of a needle electrode through the tympanic membrane onto the promontory of the cochlea and generally is done under local anesthesia. It is more invasive than ECochG recorded with extratympanic electrodes. Extratympanic placement can involve placement of an electrode at the tympanic membrane or more laterally in the ear canal. The TIPtrode (Etymotic Research, Elk Grove Village, IL) extratympanic electrode is a gold foil–wrapped inserted earphone with a foam tip that is placed near, but not at, the tympanic membrane. Regardless of the approach, a ground electrode is placed on the forehead, and the reference (inverting) electrode is usually placed on the contralateral earlobe. The amplitudes of the ECochG potentials decrease as the electrode placement becomes more lateral; thus, they are larger for transtympanic than for extratympanic electrode placement. The stimulus usually is a high-intensity click at approximately 80 to 95 dB nHL.

▶ Fig. 114.10 shows an ECochG recording. Note that the SP precedes the AP. ECochG typically has been employed in patients suspected of having endolymphatic hydrops. In such cases, the SP/AP amplitude ratio is calculated for each ear, and an elevated SP/AP ratio (due to elevation of the SP) is considered consistent with endolymphatic hydrops; an enlarged ratio also is seen in perilymphatic fistula and some cases of superior semicircular canal dehiscence. The specific SP/AP ratio that is the cutoff for normalcy should be determined by each clinic; generally, this ratio ranges from about 0.35 to 0.5. The results of several investigations reveal a lack of sensitivity of the SP/AP

ratio (25 to 55%) for Meniere disease, regardless of the disease classification as definite versus less than definite. Study findings also reveal that the sensitivity of this ratio is lower if ECochG is performed when no vertigo is present than if it is performed when vertigo is present. Some have suggested that the sensitivity of the SP/AP ratio is enhanced with transtympanic electrodes, but this is not universally accepted.

114.5.2 Auditory Brainstem Response Testing

Neurodiagnostic Auditory Brainstem Response

ABR (brainstem auditory evoked potentials [BAEPs] or brainstem auditory evoked responses [BAERs]) waveforms include a series of peaks (▶ Fig. 114.11) and generally occur within about 10 milliseconds after stimulus onset. Wave I is generated at the distal part of the auditory nerve and represents the status of the cochlea. Wave II is generated at the proximal part of the auditory nerve (junction of the auditory nerve with the auditory brainstem). Wave III is generated mainly by the ipsilateral cochlear nucleus and may receive a small contribution from the eighth nerve fibers entering the cochlear nuclei. Wave IV is probably generated mainly by the midline brainstem structures (e.g., superior olivary complex, trapezoid bodies, and acoustic stria). The origin of the positive component of wave V primarily is the contralateral lateral lemniscus (side opposite the side of stimulation). Although waves I and II have single generator sites, the later waves have multiple generator sites. The multiplicity of generator sites for the later waves makes it difficult to localize the lesion to a specific generator site. The major waves that are evaluated diagnostically are waves I, III, and V. The mean latencies in normal individuals at moderately high to high intensities are roughly 1.5 milliseconds for wave I, 3.5 milliseconds for wave III, and 5.5 milliseconds for wave V. The absolute peak latencies decline with maturation in infants. Wave I achieves adult latency values at about 3 months of age, and wave V achieves adult values at about 1.5 to 3 years of age. The interwave interval (IWI), also called the interpeak latency, represents the difference in absolute latency between two waves, such as the I to III IWI, III to V IWI, and I to V IWI. The I to III IWI, approximately a little more than 2.0 milliseconds, traditionally was thought to represent the travel time through the auditory nerve and caudal auditory brainstem; the III to V IWI, approximately a little less than 2.0 milliseconds, traditionally was thought to represent the travel time through the rostral auditory brainstem to the level of the lateral lemniscus; and the I to V IWI, approximately 4.0 milliseconds in normal individuals, traditionally was thought to reflect travel time from the distal auditory nerve to the lateral lemniscus. The I to V IWI also has been referred to as the central conduction time or brainstem transmission time, although peripheral pathology and stimulus parameters do slightly affect the interpeak latency. Because peak latencies shorten with maturation, the I to V IWI does not achieve adult values until about 3 years of age.

Another important measure for the evaluation of the neurodiagnostic ABR is the interaural latency difference of wave V (ILD V); this is the difference between the latencies of wave V in the two ears. The ILD in normal ears typically does not exceed

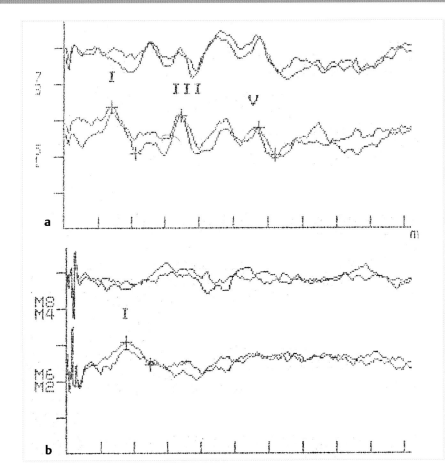

Fig. 114.11 Auditory brainstem response recordings in an individual with a right acoustic tumor. (**a**) Tracings from a normal ear and (**b**) tracings from an ear with a 3-cm acoustic tumor of the cerebellopontine angle. In both ears, the top tracings are the contralateral recordings (test and retest), and the bottom tracings are the ipsilateral recordings (test and retest). In (**a**), the absolute peak latencies are as follows: 1.40 milliseconds for wave I (amplitude of 0.37 μV), 3.48 milliseconds for wave III, and 5.72 milliseconds for wave V (amplitude of 0.21 μV). Thus, the I to III interwave interval (IWI) is 2.08 milliseconds, the III to V IWI is 2.24 milliseconds, and the I to V IWI is 4.32 milliseconds. All absolute peak latencies and IWIs are within normal limits for this ear. In (**b**), only wave I is present at 1.76 milliseconds (amplitude of 0.18 μV). Although wave I is within normal limits, the large tumor has obliterated the later waves. Such tumors do not affect wave I because wave I is generated on the auditory nerve distal to the auditory brainstem.

0.3 to 0.4 milliseconds. The peak amplitude, largest for wave V and smallest for wave I, generally does not exceed 1 μV. The amplitude parameter is not as sensitive to retrocochlear pathology as the IWI or ILD V. Wave V is the most robust wave, and it generally is the only wave seen at threshold. Wave I is the first wave to disappear with stimulus intensity reduction.

The electrode montage typically involves placement of the active (noninverting) electrode on the vertex of the skull or upper forehead, reference (inverting) electrode on the medial earlobe of the ear receiving auditory stimulation, and the ground (common) electrode. Stimuli typically include clicks for neurodiagnostic ABRs and tone bursts for the estimation of behavioral thresholds from the ABR. The transducer can be earphones or a bone vibrator.

The effect of cochlear pathology is to prolong the peak latencies. As the magnitude of the hearing loss increases, the probability of an absent wave I also increases, which in turn results in a decrease in the probability of obtaining the I to V IWI. Cochlear hearing loss is not associated with prolongation in the I to V IWI. Some clinicians obtain a latency–intensity function for wave V in which the wave V latency is shown on the ordinate and the stimulus intensity on the abscissa of a graph. In normal individuals, the slope of this function is downward because the wave V latency decreases as intensity increases. In persons with cochlear hearing loss, the slope becomes steeper than what is seen in individuals with normal hearing or in individuals with conductive hearing loss. Thus, at the lower intensities, the wave V latency is prolonged in comparison with that in individuals with normal hearing, but at the highest intensity levels, it

becomes equivalent to or nearly equivalent to that seen in individuals with normal hearing. Similar findings are obtained when the magnitude of a flat cochlear hearing loss reaches or exceeds about 60 dB HL, except that the wave V latency at the highest intensities does not approach that seen in individuals with normal hearing. With steeply sloping high-frequency cochlear hearing impairment, the function may be shifted significantly to the right of that of individuals with normal hearing, and the wave V latency value may plateau at a significantly prolonged value (i.e., not show further decline with continued increases in stimulus intensity).

With a conductive hearing impairment, the I to V IWI, if wave I is present, is not prolonged. The wave V latency–intensity function is shifted to the right of the function seen in individuals with normal hearing, and the degree of shift correlates with the magnitude of the ABG.

The effect of an eighth nerve retrocochlear pathology such as a vestibular schwannoma or meningioma is to prolong the I to V IWI, and especially the I to III IWI; the cutoff value depends on the clinic normative data, but this value usually approximates 2.3 to 2.4 milliseconds. The III to V IWI usually is unaffected by this kind of lesion unless the lesion is affecting the auditory brainstem because of its large size; the cutoff value depends on the clinic normative data, but this value usually approximates 2.1 milliseconds. The I to V IWI will be prolonged if either the I to III or the III to V IWI or both are prolonged. Although the cutoff value for the I to V IWI should depend on the clinic normative data, this value is approximately 4.3 to 4.4 milliseconds. The sensitivity and false-positive rate of the I to

III/I to V IWIs are approximately 90% and less than 10%, respectively. ABR testing is the audiologic measure within the audiologist's armamentarium that has the greatest sensitivity with respect to eighth nerve and auditory brainstem tumors. Nonetheless, the sensitivity of ABR to eighth nerve tumors is markedly reduced when tumor size is below 1 cm. If wave I is absent, then the interaural wave V is a useful diagnostic indicator of retrocochlear pathology, except if the pathology is bilateral. With bilateral prolongations of wave V latency, when the I to V IWI is absent because of an absent wave I, the wave V latency should be compared with the normative data, and the patient should be considered to be at risk for retrocochlear pathology if the latency is prolonged beyond 2 to 3 standard deviations above the mean. With some eighth nerve tumors that are large enough to displace the auditory brainstem, the ABR is obliterated in the affected ear, but a contralateral effect on the ABR latencies is seen in the unaffected ear. The III to V IWI traditionally has been considered as an indicator of pathology in the high auditory brainstem, but eighth nerve tumors also can affect the III to V IWI, and high auditory brainstem lesions can be associated with absence of the later waves, preventing measurement of an IWI. Correction factors that increase latency cutoff values for increasing hearing loss should not be employed because they lead to increased false-negative rates.

Although reported in one case study, the use of a high stimulus repetition rate should not be considered as a sensitized ABR measure for the detection of eighth nerve pathology.

Bone Auditory Brainstem Response

ABR threshold testing with BC stimulation, employing click or tone bursts, has been used to estimate the cochlear reserve, particularly in infants and children and individuals with aural atresia. Although peak latencies for BC ABRs are prolonged in comparison with those for AC ABRs in adults (the reverse is true in infants), the ABR thresholds are essentially similar for AC and BC in individuals with normal hearing. Careful calibration of the BC stimuli is essential. Because of output limitations with the BC transducer compared with the AC transducer, maximum BC presentation levels are at about 50 to 60 dB HL. Masking of the contralateral ear is always required when a BC ABR test is done because the BC stimulation is arriving at both ears at the same intensity. The ABG can be grossly estimated by comparing the BC ABR threshold with the AC ABR threshold.

114.5.3 Auditory Steady-State Response

The ASSR is the latest auditory evoked potential technology developed to estimate behavioral audiometric thresholds beyond the capability of the ABR, which is limited when individuals with hearing loss over 80 dB HL are tested. ASSR testing commonly employs amplitude-modulated stimuli because (1) the auditory nervous system is very responsive to amplitude modulation and (2) amplitude modulation greatly reduces the spectral splash of the stimulus so that high ASSR thresholds are valid estimates of the behavioral thresholds. The ASSR printout shows a threshold audiogram (▶ Fig. 114.12). The ASSR thresholds generally are within 5 to 10 dB of the behavioral thresholds.

In addition to the fact that ASSR testing can quantify hearing losses up to 120 dB HL (ABR testing is difficult with hearing loss

greater than 80 dB HL), a statistical algorithm is employed by ASSR devices for objective detection of the threshold in a standard manner, whereas threshold identification in ABR testing (with diagnostic devices) generally involves the subjective judgment of the clinician. Another advantage of ASSR testing is that multiple stimulus frequencies in both ears can be tested simultaneously. The major limitation of ASSR testing is its lack of sensitivity to mild hearing loss. However, OAEs and/or ABR is sensitive to mild hearing loss.

114.6 Testing for Functional Hearing Loss

The presence of discrepant findings within an audiologic evaluation or between audiologic evaluations that cannot be attributed to a known organic cause is referred to as functional hearing loss. Other terms, such as *nonorganic hearing loss* and *malingering*, have been used; the former term is inaccurate because a functional overlay often occurs in individuals with an organic hearing loss, and the latter term implies conscious deception by the patient. Functional hearing loss is more prevalent in workers in industrial settings who file compensation claims for hearing impairment caused by occupational noise exposure, veterans who file compensation for service-connected hearing loss, and children who are experiencing unexplained academic difficulties.

114.6.1 Functional Indicators within the Routine Audiologic Evaluation

Several measures within the basic audiologic examination can provide indications of the possible presence of functional hearing loss. Pure-tone AC threshold testing routinely involves a retest threshold at 1000 Hz in both ears. Such test–retest reliability normally is within ±5 dB. Test–retest reliability of ±15 dB or more is seen in approximately 10% of patients with functional hearing loss. Lack of test–retest reliability is not pathognomonic for functional hearing loss.

In individuals with an asymmetric hearing loss, the absence of a shadow curve in the AC configuration whereby the difference in unmasked AC thresholds exceeds 85 dB also is suggestive of functional hearing loss because interaural attenuation values for AC signals are not this large.

The presence of a significant discrepancy or disagreement between the SRT and the PTA, with the SRT significantly better than the PTA, can be indicative of functional hearing loss when other factors (e.g., instrumentation, lack of understanding of instructions, language familiarity) are ruled out. Speech stimuli are louder than pure-tone stimuli, so a patient using a mental yardstick to respond to stimuli will respond to speech stimuli at lower levels than pure-tone stimuli. The sensitivity of this measure for functional hearing loss is approximately 60 to 70% and may be higher in children because of their naïveté.

The pure-tone or speech Stenger can be performed when the interaural difference in unmasked AC thresholds (or SRTs in the case of a speech Stenger) is at least 40 dB. It is based on the Stenger principle: when two tones are presented bilaterally at the same frequency, the tone is heard only in the ear receiving

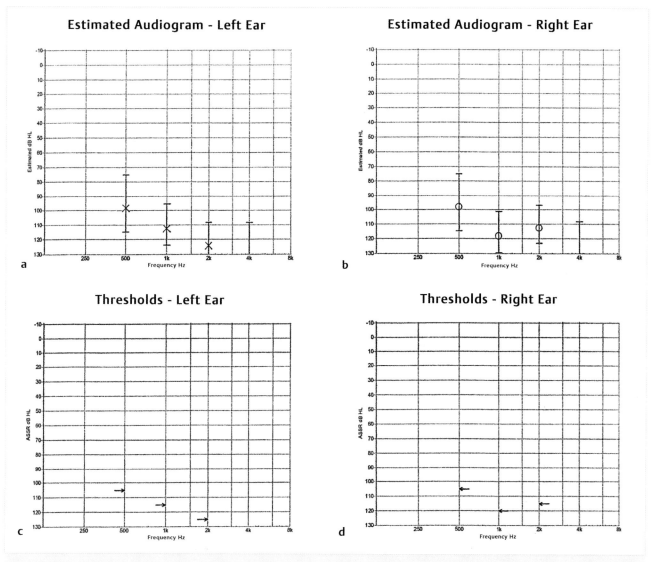

Fig. 114.12 Auditory steady-state response (ASSR) recording for a 15-month old girl. (**a,b**) ASSR thresholds are shown for both ears. (**c,d**) Estimated behavioral pure-tone thresholds are shown for both ears. At 500 Hz, the ASSR results suggest a severe hearing loss at best and a profound hearing loss at worst, bilaterally; at the higher frequencies, the results suggest a profound hearing loss bilaterally.

the tone at a higher threshold. For example, if the AC threshold is 20 dB HL in the right ear and is 60 dB HL in the left ear, then presentation of a tone at 30 dB HL to the right ear but at 85 dB HL in the left ear results in a sensation level of 10 dB in the right ear and 25 dB in the left ear; thus, the tone is heard only in the poorer, left ear. A patient with functional hearing loss, hearing the tone only in the poorer ear, may make the conscious decision not to respond to the tone in the poorer ear. By keeping the tone at a constant 10 dB SL re: threshold in the better ear and then raising the intensity of the tone in the poorer ear until the patient stops responding (or the admitted threshold is obtained), the threshold of the poorer ear can be estimated to be 15 dB better than the level at which the patient stopped responding. A similar procedure is followed for a speech Stenger, except that spondaic words rather than pure-tone stimuli are presented.

Some clinicians posit the presence of functional hearing loss based on subjective behavioral signs, such as intense lip

reading, exaggerated attempts to hear, and unfamiliarity with amplification if the patient wears amplification. These behavioral signs are not diagnostic of functional hearing loss because many persons with organic hearing loss demonstrate these behaviors. The presence of these behaviors should serve to alert the clinician to the possibility of a functional hearing loss on objective audiologic measures.

114.6.2 Physiologic and Electrophysiologic Measures

ARTs cannot occur at levels equivalent to, or below, the admitted behavior thresholds because acoustic reflexes are elicited by intense acoustic stimulation. In fact, functional hearing loss should be suspected even if the ARTs are elicited at 10 dB SL re: admitted pure-tone thresholds. Electrophysiologic threshold testing with ABR or ASSR can enable objective estimation of the pure-tone thresholds in each ear. Otoacoustic emissions testing can be helpful in supporting the auditory evoked potential findings, particularly when OAEs are present.

114.7 Hearing Screening

The US Preventive Services Task Force recommends hearing screening in all newborns. The task force has identified the following indicators of risk for permanent, bilateral, congenital hearing loss: stay in the neonatal intensive care unit for 2 or more days, family history of hereditary childhood sensorineural hearing loss, craniofacial abnormalities, and congenital syndromes and infections known to be associated with hearing loss. It recommends the use of a one- or two-step validated protocol, such as OAEs testing with ABR testing done if OAEs testing is failed. Newborns failing hearing screening should receive audiologic and medical follow-up after discharge and before 3 months of age so that early intervention services can be implemented.

The Committee on Practice and Ambulatory Medicine and the Section on Otolaryngology-Head and Neck Surgery upheld prior recommendations of the American Academy of Pediatrics for newborn hearing screening and periodic hearing screening throughout childhood until 21 years of age. The committee further recommended that any child with one or more risk factors for hearing loss should receive hearing screening appropriate for developmental age with at least one comprehensive audiologic evaluation by 2 to 2.5 years of age. All children with fail results on hearing screening should undergo comprehensive audiologic follow-up. Hearing screening should be performed upon parental expression of concern regarding the child's hearing status. The committee also recommends referral for follow-up by an otolaryngologist and pediatric audiologist when factors such as developmental and behavioral delay and problems may affect the validity of routine hearing screening. When hearing loss is documented, follow-up with the implementation of early intervention should involve the specialties of otolaryngology, audiology, speech–language pathology, and genetics.

The guidelines promulgated by the American Speech-Language-Hearing Association for pure-tone hearing screening in children between 3 years of age and third grade are as follows: pure-tone AC screening at 1000, 2000, and 4000 Hz if acoustic admittance testing is part of the identification protocol and also at 500 Hz (provided ambient noise levels do not exceed permissible levels) if acoustic admittance screening is not part of the identification protocol. The screening level is 20 dB HL at all frequencies. A child must pass all frequencies in both ears to pass the hearing screen; any other result is a fail result. All screening failures must be rescreened within 2 weeks, preferably within the same test session after removal and repositioning of the earphones and reinstruction. A child with pure-tone hearing screening failure should be referred for an audiologic evaluation.

A very diverse range of protocols has been used for hearing screening in the elderly, in whom the prevalence of sensorineural hearing loss is high. A commonly employed approach to hearing screening in the elderly involves the AudioScope (Welch Allyn, Skaneateles Falls, NY), a hand-held otoscope that also can be used for pure-tone AC hearing screening at 500, 1000, 2000, and/or 4000 Hz at the level of 20, 25, and/or 40 dB

HL. The highest sensitivity (over 90%), with good specificity (about 70 to 80%), is achieved with 2000 Hz at 40 dB HL. Some studies suggest that individuals who fail pure-tone hearing screening at this level are more likely to go for audiologic follow-up than individuals who fail at lower levels. Another approach to geriatric hearing screening is the 10-item screening version of the Hearing Handicap Inventory for the Elderly (HHIE), which is a self-administered questionnaire that was developed to examine the effects of hearing impairment on social and emotional adjustment. A score of at least 10 (scale of 0, associated with no handicap, to 40, associated with maximum handicap) suggests that the individual perceives that he or she has a hearing handicap and should be referred for audiologic rehabilitative follow-up. Some protocols for hearing screening in the elderly employ both approaches.

114.8 Behavioral Audiologic Testing in the Pediatric Population

Generally, by 6 months, infants begin to localize to sound by turning their head. The use of visual reinforcement audiometry (VRA) in children who are developmentally between 6 months and 2.5 years of age is based on the emergence of this auditory developmental milestone. With VRA, auditory stimuli are presented through a loudspeaker in a sound-treated audiometric booth. A toy that lights up (sometimes it also makes noise) on top of the speaker usually resides within a smoked plastic enclosure and does not become active (illuminated with or without noise) until the audiologist presses the control button. A limitation of VRA in sound field is that the thresholds represent the hearing sensitivity only for the better ear, so VRA usually fails to detect a unilateral hearing loss. Pure-tone AC testing through earphones (traditional or insert earphones) may be employed in VRA in many children within this range who are developmentally older (perhaps about 1 year of age or more). Conditioning would be accomplished in a manner similar to that for auditory stimulus presentation through a speaker. The use of traditional or insert earphones in VRA allows an ear-specific assessment.

Play audiometry generally is performed in children who are developmentally between 2.5 and 4 years of age. Traditional or insert earphones are used for AC testing, allowing ear-specific assessment, and the bone vibrator is used for BC testing. If only one audiologist is doing the hearing testing, a screening audiometer is used, the earphones are placed on the table, and a tone at a moderately intense level is presented; the audiologist then guides the child to perform a task such as throwing a block into a box. Any behavioral task can be employed, such as building a pyramid, stacking rings on a peg, or even clapping or slapping the audiologist's hand. SRT testing often can be accomplished by using a smaller set of spondaic words that are intended for young children or by using spondaic words for which there are picture or toy representations. Supra-threshold SRT may be accomplished by using word lists with vocabularies developed specifically for the assessment of young children.

Hearing testing in older children usually can be accomplished with conventional audiometry involving hand-raising responses to sound presentations.

114.9 Vestibular Testing

The basic vestibular test battery includes videonystagmography (VNG), which has largely replaced electronystagmography (based on recordings of the corneoretinal potential), sinusoidal harmonic acceleration (SHA) testing, computerized dynamic platform posturography (CDPP) testing, and vestibular evoked myogenic potential (VEMP) testing. Both VNG and SHA testing are based on the vestibulo-ocular reflex (VOR).

The cristae ampullares, the sensory receptors of the ampullae of the semicircular canals in the vestibular labyrinth, detect angular acceleration (head turns in the horizontal and/or vertical planes). The right and left horizontal semicircular canals detect angular acceleration in the horizontal plane. Detection of angular acceleration in the vertical planes is accomplished by pairing of the left posterior semicircular canal and right anterior semicircular canal, which are in parallel planes, and by pairing of the right posterior canal and left anterior semicircular canal. When an individual is standing so that the head is upright, the electrical activities generated by the cristae ampullares of the right and left horizontal (lateral) semicircular canals are equal. With head turn to the right (right angular acceleration), the endolymph within the membranous labyrinth of both horizontal canals lags the head turn because of inertia, and its movement is in the opposite direction (leftward). Because the location of the utricle is medial to each of the horizontal canals, the endolymph in the right horizontal canal moves toward the right utricle (utriculopetal) and the endolymph in the left horizontal canal moves away from the left utricle (utriculofugal). Utriculopetal stimulation will result in bending of the kinocilia of the hair cells in the crista ampullaris of the right horizontal semicircular canal toward the utricle in the right labyrinth, resulting in increased electrical discharge from that canal; additionally, the utriculofugal stimulation will result in bending of the kinocilia of the hair cells of the left horizontal semicircular canal away from the utricle in the left labyrinth, resulting in decreased electrical discharge from that canal. Therefore, the right vestibular nerve is excited, whereas the left vestibular nerve is inhibited. The increased electrical activity from the right vestibular nerve is transmitted to the right vestibular nuclei and then through several neurons to lateral rectus extraocular muscle of the left eyeball and to the medial rectus extraocular muscle of the right eyeball. The activation of these muscles moves the eyes slowly to the left. This slow eye movement to the left is facilitated by inhibition of the left vestibular nerve. This chain of events describes the VOR, the purpose of which is to maintain visual fixation on an object through compensatory eye movements when the head turns.

At the end of the VOR, when the slow eye movement deviates from the midline to a critical extent, a central process is triggered that moves the eyes quickly to the right to return the eyes to midline. This fast movement is a saccade. The combination of the slow-phase eye movement in one direction (away from the head movement) followed by a fast-phase saccade in the direction opposite that of the slow-phase eye movement is termed *nystagmus*, which is said to beat in the direction of the fast phase (saccade). Thus, head turn to the right yields slow eye movement to the left, which, if the deviation is great enough, triggers a saccade to the right, yielding right-beating nystagmus. The slow-phase velocity (SPV) is the physiologic component of eye movement, and the saccade is the corrective phase of the eye movement. In normal individuals, the amplitude of the VOR is greatest in a dark environment and least in a light environment.

Each of the three semicircular canals in each labyrinth responds best to head rotation in its plane. In this way, the semicircular canals translate head rotation direction in the three-dimensional space.

Nystagmus can be induced in a normal person when warm or cool water or air is injected into an ear canal. The injection of warm water into the right ear canal causes the endolymph in the right horizontal semicircular canal to expand and rise, thereby moving in a utriculopetal direction. Thus, the electrical discharge from the right horizontal semicircular canal is increased relative to the electrical discharge from the left horizontal semicircular canal. Ultimately, the left lateral rectus and right medial rectus muscles are activated, so the slow phase is to the left and the fast phase is to the right, consistent with right-beating nystagmus. The injection of cool water into the right ear canal causes the endolymph in the right horizontal semicircular canal to contract, become denser and falling, thereby moving in an utriculofugal direction. Thus, the electrical discharge from the right horizontal semicircular canal is decreased relative to the electrical discharge from the left horizontal semicircular canal. Because the asymmetry in electrical discharge from the right and left canals favors the left side, ultimately the right lateral rectus muscle and the left medial rectus muscle are activated, so both eyeballs are pulled slowly to the right. When the slow eye movement to the right exceeds a certain point, a central process is triggered that moves the eyes quickly to the left to return the eyes to midline. Thus, the injection of cool water in the right ear yields slow eye movement to the right, and then a fast phase to the left, yielding left-beating nystagmus.

Note that in the vestibular system, a peripheral disorder is one that affects the vestibular labyrinth and/or the vestibular nerve. The vestibular nuclei are considered to be part of the central vestibular system. A left peripheral vestibular lesion reduces the electrical activity generated by the crista ampullaris of the left horizontal canal, in comparison with the electrical activity generated by the crista ampullaris of the right horizontal canal. The asymmetry in electrical discharge between the right and left sides favors the right side, so the right vestibular nerve is excited, and the chain of events is similar to that described for warm water stimulation of the right ear canal. Thus, left-sided Meniere disease causes a slow-phase eye movement to the left and fast-phase eye movement to the right; this represents right-beating nystagmus.

114.9.1 Electronystagmography and Videonystagmography Standard Battery

In electronystagmography (ENG), electrodes are placed on the outer canthus of each eye and a ground electrode is placed on the middle of the forehead (electrodes are also placed above and below one eye if eye movements are recorded in the vertical plane). ENG is based on the corneoretinal potential. The eyes have an electrical potential (corneoretinal potential) whereby the cornea has a positive electrical charge and the retina has a negative electrical charge. The electrical potential difference between the cornea and retina makes the eye behave like a dipole. When horizontal eye movements are recorded, the noninverting electrode is placed on the outer canthus of the right eye and the inverting electrode is placed on the outer canthus of the left eye. When the eyes move to the right, the noninverting electrode detects a large positive charge; the positive cornea moves away from the inverting electrode, which therefore detects a smaller positive charge that is inverted to become a small negative charge. The resultant charge is positive. Thus, rightward eye movement is associated with a positive charge, and the pen of the device records an upward deflection. When the eyes move to the left, the noninverting electrode detects a small positive charge (because of dipole movement), and the inverting electrode detects a large positive charge that is inverted to become a large negative charge. The resultant charge is negative. Thus, leftward eye movement is associated with a negative charge, and the pen of the device records a downward deflection. ▶ Fig. 114.13 shows right-beating and left-beating nystagmus for an ENG recording.

Many vestibular clinics have adopted video recording techniques in place of the corneal retinal potential recording techniques in ENG devices. VNG devices substitute video eye tracking for measurement of the corneal retinal potential, so VNG testing is done without electrodes. The video eye tracking uses a video camera to measure pupil position and gaze angle. Generally, with VNG, the patient wears goggles within which a camera(s) is mounted. The goggle lens acts like a mirror to reflect the image of the pupil to the infrared camera, the output of which is fed to a computer (for analysis of the eye movements) and to a video monitor (for direct observation of the eye movements). Based on the reflection from the cornea, the x- and y-coordinates of the center of the pupil then are used to determine eye position and angle of gaze.

Clinics increasingly have adopted VNG testing in place of ENG testing because video eye tracking is more convenient than the use of electrodes. Additionally, VNG does not require time for light or dark adaptation, as does ENG. Other advantages of VNG over conventional ENG include increased accuracy of saccade velocity measurements, absence of muscle artifacts and electrical interference, and stability of the recording over time. VNG testing also can be performed in many blind individuals who lack or have an insufficient corneal retinal potential. Calibration must be accomplished at several points through the ENG test battery but is generally necessary only at the beginning of VNG. Regarding the magnitude of the SPV, the interpretation is very similar for ENG and VNG. ▶ Fig. 114.14 shows the results of a VNG test battery for a patient.

Saccade Test

Saccades originate from the frontal eye field of the cortex, which projects to the contralateral pontine paramedial reticular formation. Neural activity then is transmitted through neurons to the ipsilateral abducens nucleus (ultimately to the ipsilateral lateral rectus muscle) and to the contralateral oculomotor nuclei (and ultimately to the contralateral medial rectus muscle). Thus, a left saccade is controlled by the right frontal eye field, left pontine paramedial reticular formation, left abducens nucleus to the left lateral rectus muscle, and right oculomotor

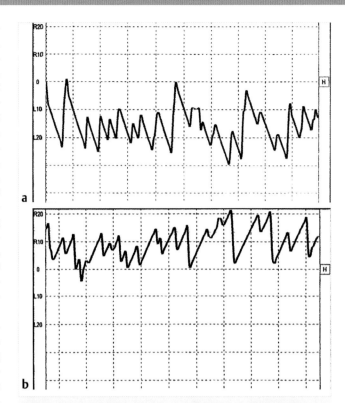

Fig. 114.13 Electronystagmography (ENG) recording (horizontal channel) showing (a) right-beating nystagmus and (b) left-beating nystagmus. (a) The diagonal line on the right side of any vertical line shows that the eye movement is slowly to the left (slow phase) because the pen deflection is downward from the top of the vertical line; the vertical line that follows, a rapid upward deflection, shows that the eye movement is quickly to the right (fast phase), bringing the eyes back to midline. Because the fast component is to the right, it is labeled as right-beating nystagmus. (b) The diagonal line on the left side of the vertical line shows that the eye movement is slowly to the right (slow phase). The steep downward vertical line that follows shows that the eye movement is then quickly to the left (fast phase), bringing the eyes back to midline. Because the fast component is to the left, it is labeled left-beating nystagmus. A quick method for determining beating direction is to look at a vertical line and a diagonal line beginning at the top of the vertical line; if that diagonal line is on the right side of the vertical line, then the nystagmus is right-beating; if the diagonal line is on the left side of the vertical line, the nystagmus is left-beating.

nuclei to the right medial rectus muscle. The saccade test usually involves a light bar. The patient is instructed to quickly look between two targets (without head turns) in the horizontal and vertical planes. The tracing of the saccade waveform can be obtained in VNG as well as ENG; it shows rectangular waves in normal individuals. The VNG printout for the saccade test shows (1) peak SPV as a function of degrees from the midline, (2) accuracy of the saccade (degree of overshoot or undershoot) as a function of degrees from midline, and (3) latency of the saccade (time from the onset of the target to the onset of the eye movement) as a function of degrees from midline. The latency parameter is more susceptible to aging effects. Saccade test results for a patient are shown in ▶ Fig. 114.14. Abnormalities on saccadic testing, such as saccadic dysmetria (overshoot or undershoot of saccades, primarily affecting

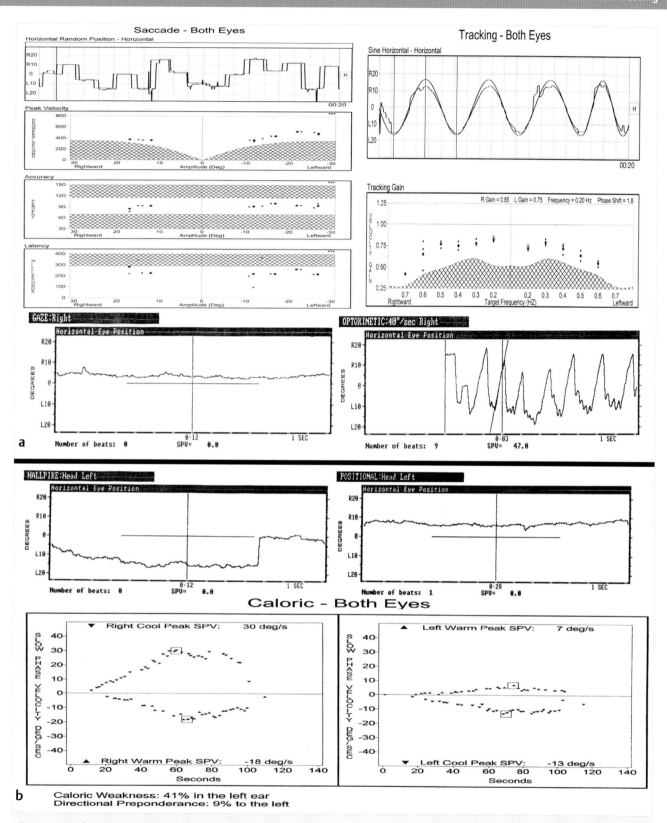

Fig. 114.14 Videonystagmography (VNG) test results. (**a**) Saccadic tracking (slow-phase velocity [SPV], accuracy, and latency) is within normal limits in this patient. Gaze testing (shown only for gaze right) reveals no nystagmus for gaze center, left, or right. Pendular tracking is within normal limits (see smooth sinusoidal curves and tracking gain within normal limits). (**b**) Hallpike maneuver produced no nystagmus with head right or left (only head left shown). Positional testing produced no nystagmus with head supine, right, left, or hanging (only head left is shown here). Bithermal calorics revealed a total right ear SPV of 48 degrees (30 minus −18) and a total left ear SPV of 20 (7 minus −13). Unilateral weakness (%) is calculated as [(48 − 20)/(48 + 20)] × 100 = 41% weakness in the left ear in this case. Directional preponderance (DP; %) reveals a total right-beating nystagmus of [− (−18) + −13] = 31 degrees per second and a total left-beating nystagmus of (30 + 7) = 37 degrees per second, so the DP is (31 − 37)/(31 + 37) × 100 = −9% (DP to the left, within normal limits). The caloric findings are consistent with left peripheral vestibular pathology. A left acoustic neuroma was confirmed at surgery.

accuracy), saccadic slowing (SPV abnormally reduced), and delayed saccades (abnormally increased latencies), may be consistent with central nervous system disorder. Fatigue, inattention, and drug effects need to be ruled out with saccadic slowing and delayed saccades.

Smooth Pursuit (Tracking) Test

The smooth pursuit system enables the tracking of a target moving slowly and smoothly in a sinusoidal manner. The smooth pursuit system maintains the image of the target on the fovea during the sinusoidal movement of the target. The origin of smooth pursuit eye movements is the parieto-occipital visual association area of the cerebral cortex ipsilateral to the direction of movement of a target. Thus, visual pursuit of a target slowly moving to the left is controlled by the left hemisphere. Neural activity from the parieto-occipital visual association area of the cerebral cortex is transmitted through neurons to the ipsilateral pontine paramedial reticular formation, and then to the ipsilateral abducens nucleus (and ultimately to the ipsilateral lateral rectus muscle) and contralateral abducens nucleus (and ultimately to the contralateral medial rectus muscle). The patient is instructed to visually follow a light target moving sinusoidally (back and forth), usually on a light bar. The tracing of the smooth pursuit waveform can be obtained with VNG as well as ENG; it shows a smooth, sinusoidal waveform in normal individuals. With VNG, the measures of interest are (1) velocity gain (peak eye velocity divided by peak target velocity) as a function of frequency for rightward and leftward target movement and (2) phase angle (degree to which eye movement lags or leads target movement) as a function of frequency in each direction. Smooth pursuit test results for a patient are shown in ► Fig. 114.14. Bilateral saccadic pursuit, manifested by reduced velocity gain (< 0.2), may be consistent with a central nervous system disorder; drug effects, inattention, and lack of understanding of the instructions must be ruled out. Unilateral saccadic pursuit, manifested by asymmetry in velocity gain, is a nonlocalizing finding. Unilateral saccadic pursuit may be consistent with acute spontaneous nystagmus associated with an acute peripheral vestibular lesion; in this case, the saccadic pursuit is impaired, with visual pursuit in the direction of the fast phase of the spontaneous nystagmus.

Optokinetic Test

In traditional ENG testing, the optokinetic eye movement system was presumed to be involved when an individual attempted to follow visual targets moving across the visual field, such as a display of vertical stripes moving with a constant velocity toward the right or toward the left. With a light bar, the stimuli are a series of lights (like pulses) moving to the right followed by a series of lights (like pulses) moving to the left. The patient is instructed to watch the images without head turns. The use of a monitor or projection system enables a much greater proportion of the visual field (ideally, at least 90%) to have repeated moving stimuli; this kind of stimulus is more effective than the light bar stimulus, which involves a limited visual field. Studies suggest that the nystagmus recorded on the optokinetic test includes a smooth pursuit as well as an optokinetic component. The smooth pursuit component is minimized

during the "optokinetic after nystagmus" component whereby recording continues in darkness after about 30 seconds of recording in the light condition. The instructions influence the nature of the response in optokinetic testing. If the patient is instructed to follow a single target in the optokinetic visual field, the smooth pursuit component is emphasized in the response; the response to this instruction is called "look nystagmus." If, however, the patient is instructed to stare at the center and attempt to count the number of targets passing by, the smooth pursuit component is minimized, and the optokinetic component is maximized in the response; the response to this instruction is called "stare nystagmus." The parameter of interest for optokinetic nystagmus (look or stare) is the velocity gain as a function of time for each stimulus (e.g., 40 degrees per second for the images moving left and 40 degrees per second for the images moving right). ► Fig. 114.14 shows the results of optokinetic testing for a patient. Bilaterally reduced optokinetic nystagmus, manifested by bilaterally reduced velocity gain, may be consistent with a central nervous system disorder; drug effects, visual impairment, and inattention must be ruled out. Unilaterally reduced optokinetic nystagmus, manifested by asymmetric velocity gain, may be consistent with a central nervous system disorder or may reflect the presence of spontaneous nystagmus. The clinical significance of abnormal optokinetic findings is strengthened when they are obtained in conjunction with other abnormal ENG/VNG findings. Aging also increases the likelihood of abnormal findings on optokinetic testing. These limitations reduce the clinical utility of this ENG/VNG optokinetic subtest.

Gaze Test

During the gaze test, the patient sits with the head erect and looks straight ahead at a light target on the light bar at different points, such as, midline, 25 to 30 degrees to the right of midline (horizontal right), 25 to 30 degrees to the left of midline (horizontal left), 25 to 30 degrees above midline (vertical up), and 25 to 30 degrees below midline (vertical down). The presence of spontaneous nystagmus is established by examining the recordings of the eyes midline with vision and also with vision occluded (by "shuttered" goggles in VNG or by eye closure in ENG). The VNG printouts show the SPV over time (waveform). ► Fig. 114.14 shows the results of gaze testing for a patient. In normal individuals, spontaneous nystagmus is absent or minimally present during the gaze midline (or with vision occluded). The presence of significant spontaneous nystagmus is a nonlocalizing finding. If spontaneous nystagmus is present and is unchanged in intensity and direction with eccentric gaze positions, then the gaze nystagmus reflects spontaneous nystagmus; if it changes in intensity or direction with gaze position, then gaze nystagmus also is present.

Bilateral gaze nystagmus that is right-beating for right gaze and left-beating for left gaze, and that has an intensity in the nonoccluded vision condition that is undiminished compared with that in the occluded vision condition, may be consistent with central nervous system pathology, usually brainstem pathology; drug effects, however, must be ruled out.

If significant spontaneous nystagmus is present and gaze nystagmus beats in the same direction as the spontaneous nystagmus in both eccentric gaze positions, then the possibility of a pattern reflecting Alexander's law should be considered, whereby the nystagmus intensity increases with gaze in the direction of the fast phase of the spontaneous nystagmus. For example, a patient demonstrates left-beating spontaneous nystagmus and left-beating nystagmus on right and left horizontal gaze that is strongest for the left horizontal gaze (because of the additive effects of combining spontaneous and gaze nystagmus when the direction of the gaze is in the direction of the spontaneous nystagmus) and weakest for the right horizontal gaze (because the gaze is in the direction opposite that of the spontaneous nystagmus). Such pattern is usually consistent with peripheral vestibular pathology (in this example, on the right side), although the possibility of central nervous system pathology cannot be ruled out. Horizontal unilateral gaze nystagmus refers to nystagmus for a single eccentric gaze direction; this finding may be consistent with a central nervous system disorder if its intensity in the normal visual condition is undiminished relative to that in the occluded vision condition (or the nystagmus is present in the normal visual condition but not in the vision occluded condition).

Vertical gaze nystagmus (down-beating or up-beating) may be consistent with a central nervous system disorder.

Dix-Hallpike Procedure

The Dix-Hallpike procedure usually is performed before static positional tests so that if benign paroxysmal positional vertigo (BPPV) is present, movement into the various positions during static positional testing does not fatigue the BPPV. Posterior semicircular canal BPPV can be identified with the Dix-Hallpike procedure. With the traditional maneuver, the patient sits with the head turned slowly 45 degrees to the right and with the eyes open. The clinician, who is behind the patient and has one hand at the top of the patient's head and the other hand on the patient's back, then rapidly pulls the patient back down, keeping the head in the turned position, until the patient is lying supine with the head hanging to the right over the end of the examining table. The patient is asked whether any dizziness is experienced. The nystagmus should be up-beating and torsional toward the ear that is underneath. The patient then is returned to the sitting position, and the procedure is repeated if nystagmus was present to determine if the response is fatigable. This entire procedure then is repeated with the head turned to the left (after the patient is brought back to the sitting position). The most useful parameters to examine are the SPV over time and the nystagmus waveforms. The Dix-Hallpike results for a patient are shown in ▶ Fig. 114.14. The classic response, consistent with posterior semicircular canal BPPV, is characterized by the following: (1) Latency of the nystagmus is less than 10 seconds; (2) the nystagmus, which develops in intensity and then declines in intensity, is transient and has a duration of less than 1 minute; (3) the nystagmus and symptoms of dizziness are fatigable on the repeated maneuver; and (4) the nystagmus is up-beating with a torsional component in the direction of the underneath ear when the patient is brought to the supine position. Thus, classic Dix-Hallpike findings are both localizing and lateralizing. The response is nonclassic if any of these features are not noted, and the results are nonlocalizing.

Static Positional Tests

With positional testing, recordings are made with the patient in various positions, including the following: (1) supine with head elevated 30 degrees, (2) supine with head turned 90 degrees to the right or right lateral (whole body right on the right side), (3) supine with the head turned to the left 90 degrees or left lateral (whole body left on the left side), and (4) head hanging (lying on the examination table with the head hanging over the end of the table). Lateral positions are preferred to the head-turned positions because the latter can elicit cervical vertigo in some individuals and neck rotation ability is restricted in some individuals. All positional testing is accomplished in the vision occluded condition (eyes closed in ENG). The patient performs mental tasking (e.g., count by twos, name animals) to prevent nystagmus suppression. If nystagmus is present in any position, then testing under visual fixation is performed to determine whether visual fixation can reduce the nystagmus; inability of visual fixation to reduce the nystagmus is suggestive of a central nervous system disorder. The parameters of interest are the SPV over time and any nystagmus waveforms. Static positional test results for a patient are shown in ▶ Fig. 114.14.

Positional nystagmus that is present in the eyes occluded condition (and is absent under the visual fixation condition) is considered to be abnormal if its SPV exceeds the normative cutoff value (e.g., 4 degrees per second for VNG, 6 degrees per second for ENG) for at least one position. It is a nonlocalizing (peripheral or central vestibular pathology) finding.

Horizontal positional nystagmus that is present in the eyes occluded condition and is direction-changing within a single head position in the eyes occluded condition may be consistent with a central nervous system disorder.

Positional nystagmus (any intensity) present in the eyes occluded condition and in the visual fixation condition is a pathologic, nonlocalizing finding if visual fixation significantly reduces the intensity; it is consistent with a central nervous system disorder if visual fixation fails to significantly reduce the intensity.

Vertical positional nystagmus in the eyes occluded condition is considered to be consistent with a central nervous system disorder if its magnitude exceeds the normative cutoff value (about 6 to 7 degrees per second) and visual fixation fails to reduce the intensity of the nystagmus.

Alcohol ingestion should be ruled out if (1) direction-changing geotropic nystagmus is obtained whereby the nystagmus is right-beating with the right ear down and left-beating with the left ear down (and absent in the sitting and supine positions) or if (2) direction-changing ageotropic nystagmus is obtained whereby the nystagmus is right-beating with the left ear down and left-beating with the right ear down.

Caloric Testing

Standard alternate binaural bithermal caloric testing involves the injection of cool or warm water or air directly into an ear canal with the patient supine and the head elevated about 30 degrees. Testing is done with vision occluded (eyes closed in ENG) and then in the normal visual condition (eyes open in ENG) to test for visual fixation suppression after peak SPV is obtained in the vision occluded condition. The patient does mental tasking during the vision occluded condition to prevent nystagmus suppression. Each ear is irrigated, one at a time, with a cool stimulus or a warm stimulus (or vice versa). With water irrigation, the cool temperature is set to about 30°C and the warm temperature is set to about 44°C. With air irrigation, the cool temperature is set to about 21°C and the warm temperature is set to about 51°C. In normal individuals, the SPV of the nystagmus is within normative limits and approximately equal for the two ears for each temperature, and it is right-beating for right warm and left cool irrigations and left-beating for left warm and right cool irrigations. The parameter of greatest interest is the SPV over time for each irrigation. Caloric test results for a patient are shown in ▶ Fig. 114.15

The presence of bilateral weakness is assessed by looking at (1) the sum of the peak SPV across the four irrigations, (2) the sum of the peak SPV for the right ear (across the warm and cool irrigations) and the sum of the peak SPV for the left ear (across the warm and cool irrigations), and (3) the peak SPV for each irrigation. If the total peak SPV across the four irrigations is assessed, bilateral weakness is thought to be present when it is less than approximately 20 to 22 degrees per second. If the individual ear SPV (across both temperature irrigations) is assessed, then bilateral weakness is thought to be present when the peak SPV for each ear is less than about 12 degrees per second. If the SPV for each irrigation is assessed, then bilateral weakness is through to be present when each peak SPV is less than approximately 8 degrees per second. Bilateral weakness is consistent with bilateral peripheral vestibular pathology or a central nervous system disorder. The peak SPV also is examined for the presence of hyperactive responses (> 60 to 150 degrees per second) in one or both ears; the normative cutoff value differs widely among investigators but more commonly ranges between about 140 and 150 degrees per second. It is a relatively rare finding, particular when it is unilateral, and may be consistent with cerebellar dysfunction when tympanic membrane perforation and technical factors are ruled out. Some clinics also perform ice water calorics when caloric responses are absent to determine if any residual response is present with ice water stimulation.

If bilateral weakness is absent, the presence of unilateral weakness (as a percentage) is calculated with the following formula: {[(right cool peak SPV – right warm peak SPV) minus (left warm peak SPV – left cool peak SPV)]/(right cool peak SPV + right warm peak SPV + left cool peak SPV + left warm peak SPV)} x 100. This formula essentially is equivalent to the total peak SPV for the right ear minus the total peak SPV for the left ear, with this difference then divided by sum of the total peak SPV across all four irrigations, times 100. Unilateral weakness is abnormal if its absolute value exceeds a criterion level (20 to 25%). A significantly positive unilateral weakness indicates left ear weakness, whereas a significantly negative unilateral weakness indicates right ear weakness (peripheral vestibular pathology). Any spontaneous nystagmus should be considered in the interpretation of caloric responses.

Typically, right warm and left cool irrigations yield right-beating nystagmus, and left warm and right cool irrigations yield left-beating nystagmus. In normal individuals, the right-beating nystagmus and left-beating nystagmus are similar in magnitude (although opposite in direction). An individual has directional preponderance (DP) if the magnitudes of the caloric responses beating in one direction are stronger than those beating in the other direction. Thus, the DP (%) = {[(–peak SPV right warm – peak SPV left cool) minus (peak SPV right cool + peak SPV left warm)]/(peak SPV right warm + peak SPV left cool + peak SPV left warm + peak SPV right cool)} x 100. The clinical significance of DP is controversial and neither lateralizing nor localizing; however, the presence of significant DP does indicate whether the nystagmus beats more strongly in one direction than another. DP is significant if it is greater or equal to 25 to 30%. A positive DP value indicates that responses obtained from the left cool and right warm irrigations (right-beating) are stronger than the responses from the right cool and left warm irrigations (left-beating); a negative DP value indicates that the left-beating responses are stronger than the right-beating responses.

Failure of fixation suppression (%) is calculated by dividing the SPV obtained just before the effect of visual fixation is determined by the peak SPV (normal visual condition after visual fixation). This generally is measured for at least two irrigations

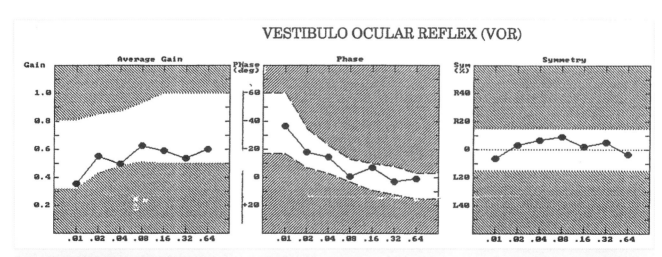

Fig. 114.15 Sinusoidal harmonic acceleration results in a normal patient. Note that the gain, phase, and symmetry are within the normal range at all chair oscillation frequencies.

(right and left warm or right and left cool). Complete suppression by fixation yields a fixation index near 0%, whereas complete lack of fixation yields a fixation index exceeding 100%. Abnormal failure of fixation suppression greater than approximately 50 to 60% is consistent with a central nervous system disorder.

A recent study of 77 patients with unilateral peripheral vestibular pathology and 80 control subjects revealed caloric test sensitivity and specificity values of 83% and 78%, respectively. The most important caloric parameter was unilateral weakness, followed by the SPV for warm irrigations, followed by SPV for cool irrigations. DP was of limited clinical importance in the differential diagnosis of unilateral peripheral vestibular pathology.

114.9.2 Sinusoidal Harmonic Acceleration

SHA testing involves measurement of the slow-phase velocity (SPV) of nystagmus induced by side-to-side sinusoidal rotations of a motorized chair in a dark room; the patient is tested (the head is tilted downward by about 30 degrees for perpendicular orientation of the horizontal semicircular canals relative to the rotational axis) with the eyes open (and performs mental arithmetic to prevent suppression of nystagmus), and recording electrodes are placed at the outer canthi of the eyes with a ground electrode on the forehead. With chair rotation in the clockwise direction, the SPV of the nystagmus is counterclockwise, and vice versa. Chair rotation typically is performed over at least five multiple sinusoidal oscillation frequencies (e.g., 0.01, 0.02, 0.04, 0.08, 0.16, 0.32, and 0.64 Hz) with peak angular velocities of 50 to 60 degrees per second. The instrumentation performs a fast Fourier transform analysis to remove the fast phase so that the eye SPVs can be reported in comparison with those of the head/chair. The parameters generally measured include phase, gain, and symmetry. Phase represents the temporal relation between SPV (degrees per second) of the eyes and SPV of the head/chair and is expressed in degrees. With a phase lead, the peak SPV of the eyes occurs before the peak SPV of the head/chair; with a phase lag, the peak SPV of the eyes occurs after the peak SPV of the head/chair. The gain parameter represents the SPV of the eyes divided by the SPV of the head/chair. Symmetry (%) refers to the difference between peak SPV of the eyes in the condition in which the chair moves clockwise (slow phase of the eye movement is in the opposite direction) and peak SPV of the eyes in the condition in which the chair moves counterclockwise (slow phase of the eye movement is in the opposite direction), referenced to the total of the maximum eye SPVs in both directions. The instrumentation printout of the rotary chair results generally displays each of these parameters as a function of chair oscillation frequency. ▶ Fig. 114.15 displays the SHA results from a normal individual.

Typical findings for a unilateral acute peripheral vestibular lesion such as vestibular neuritis or active Meniere disease include the following: abnormally increased phase leads, largely at the lower oscillation frequencies, and asymmetry, whereby the peak SPV in one direction (usually toward the side of the lesion) is greater than that in the opposite direction, particularly at the higher frequencies. In the case of a slowly developing peripheral vestibular lesion, such as a vestibular schwannoma, a vestibular compensation process occurs that often normalizes results for the symmetry parameter; thus, if vestibular compensation has occurred, then the sole abnormal finding may be increased phase leads that are greatest at the lower oscillation frequencies. When abnormal findings are obtained on the symmetry measure, they can be monitored over time to see if central compensation occurs, which is correlated with a diminution of the subjective feeling of dizziness. Symmetry results need to be adjusted when spontaneous nystagmus is present; for example, a left-beating spontaneous nystagmus augments the left-beating nystagmus that occurs with right rotations and decreases the right-beating nystagmus that occurs with left rotations. The results of a recent large sample study of patients with a variety of peripheral vestibular disorders and a control group revealed that the correct classification of individuals as normal or as having unilateral peripheral vestibular impairment is best for the 0.01-Hz frequency, second best for the 0.1-Hz frequency, and third best for the 0.05-Hz frequency (the oscillation frequencies evaluation included frequencies of 0.01, 0.02, 0.05, 0.1, and 0.2 Hz at the peak velocity of 50 degrees per second). The phase parameter had the greatest diagnostic utility. SHA test sensitivity and specificity at 0.01 Hz were 84% and 64%, respectively. The sensitivity and specificity of the unilateral weakness measure on caloric testing in this group were 83% and 79%, respectively.

Gain often is abnormally reduced in bilateral peripheral vestibular pathology. Abnormally reduced gain has sometimes been observed in unilateral acute peripheral vestibular lesions. Very low gain results limit the diagnostic utility of other SHA parameters.

The SHA test yields information about asymmetry in the peripheral vestibular system in response to low-frequency (slow) stimulation. A benefit of the SHA test is that it furnishes information about the presence of residual caloric responses in patients who have absent response to bithermal caloric stimulation, including ice testing. Also, similar to caloric vestibular testing, the SHA test is sensitive only to pathologies that affect the horizontal semicircular canal or superior vestibular nerve. The best application of SHA testing is for the detection of bilateral vestibular pathologies; it is more challenging to detect unilateral vestibular disorders with SHA testing, which involves the simultaneous stimulation of both ears. SHA testing also has value for monitoring central compensation over time in unilateral peripheral vestibular disorders.

114.9.3 Computerized Dynamic Platform Posturography

CDPP provides an evaluation of the patient's ability to use visual, vestibular, and somatosensory/proprioceptive input to remain standing upright without swaying or falling. This ability not only depends on the reception of appropriate sensory input by the brain but also requires coordination of the muscles such that the body mass is centered over an area spanned by the feet (center of gravity [COG]); the ability to stand upright involves both sensory and motor components. Sway refers to movement in the COG and is assessed in the anteroposterior and lateral planes. Pressure sensors on the force plate(s) of the platform detect pressure changes exerted on the platform associated with sway with feet and/or body movement.

Table 114.3 Conditions for each component of the sensory organization test in computerized dynamic platform posturography

Sensory organization test	Platform, visual surround, eyes open or closed	Sensory input to the brain: visual, vestibular, somatosensory
1	Eyes open Visual surround stable Platform fixed	Visual accurate Vestibular operational Somatosensory accurate
2	Eyes closed Platform fixed	Visual absent Vestibular operational Somatosensory accurate
3	Eyes open Visual surround changes Platform fixed	Visual conflict Vestibular operational Somatosensory accurate
4	Eyes open Visual surround stable Platform moves	Visual accurate Vestibular operational Somatosensory inaccurate
5	Eyes closed Platform moves	Visual absent Vestibular operational Somatosensory inaccurate
6	Eyes open Visual surround moves Platform moves	Visual inaccurate Vestibular operational Somatosensory inaccurate

The patient stands on a platform while wearing a harness to prevent falls. A visual surround is in front and to the sides of the patient. Both the visual surround and/or the platform can move under computer control. The test is performed in the eyes open and eyes closed condition; in the eyes open condition, the test is administered under normal vision and distorted vision (the visual surround sways so that visual cues are inaccurate).

The two components of the CDPP test are the sensory organization test (SOT) and the motor control test (MCT). The SOT has six subtests (▶ Table 114.3). The most difficult subtest is SOT 6 because both visual input and somatosensory input are distorted, creating sensory input conflict to the brain; balance in this subtest is dependent upon the vestibular system. Distorted input affects balance more than absence of input. The equilibrium score (%) is provided for each subtest based on the magnitude of sway. A composite equilibrium score across the subtests also is provided. The range in equilibrium scores is 0 to 100%, with 0% indicating a fall and 100% indicating no sway and good stability.

▶ Fig. 114.16 shows the CDPP test findings in a patient. The sensory analysis looks at the pattern of results across the SOT subtests and displays how well the patient uses somatosensory input to maintain postural control (based on a comparison of the results of SOT1 and SOT2), visual input to maintain postural control (based on a comparison of SOT1 and SOT4), and vestibular input to maintain postural control (based on SOT1 and SOT5), and the degree to which reliance on visual input is appropriate (based on SOT3 and SOT6). Higher scores indicate better performance. The COG alignment scatterplot shows the COG relative to the center of base support before each trial. In normal individuals, the COG is near the center of the base. The strategy analysis results indicate the extent to which a patient moves his or her COG around the ankle or hip to maintain postural control; the ankle strategy is dominant in normal individuals, and the less efficient hip strategy is dominant in many individuals with equilibrium problems. Unlike electromyography recordings, CDPP testing does not involve the placement

of transdermal electrodes on the body. Therefore, conclusions about ankle versus hip strategies based on CDPP findings are subject to the disadvantage of a lack of direct muscle information.

In the MCT, the platform makes sudden front-to-back or back-to-front jerk movements (translations) of small, medium, and large amplitudes. The muscle reaction latency of each foot to each of these two types of translations is reported. The MCT results also are shown in ▶ Fig. 114.16. Prolonged MCT latencies may be suggestive of a lesion within the long loop pathway involving the nonvestibular, spinal cord, brainstem, and/or subcortical components of the pathway. Examples of pathologies that may be associated with bilaterally prolonged MCT latencies include peripheral neuropathy and multiple sclerosis. Examples of localized brainstem lesions that may be associated with prolonged MCT latencies include stroke and cerebral palsy.

The major purpose of CDPP testing is to examine postural control in patients whose sole balance complaint is unsteadiness or unexplained falls and in patients with bilateral hypofunction, which puts them at increased risk for falls, particularly as age increases. Some have suggested such testing in all patients who experience unsteadiness or balance difficulty during periods when vertigo is absent. Thus, from the otologic perspective, CDPP essentially represents functional assessment for the purpose of planning and monitoring vestibular and balance rehabilitation to reduce the risk for and rate of falls.

114.9.4 Vestibular Evoked Myogenic Potential Testing

In the VEMP test, change in muscle tone is elicited by brief, intense acoustic stimulation and is recorded electromyographically with surface electrodes placed on the skin overlying the neck or spinal muscles. The VEMP is a vestibulocollic reflex originating in the saccule with neural transmission through the inferior vestibular nerve and descending vestibular spinal

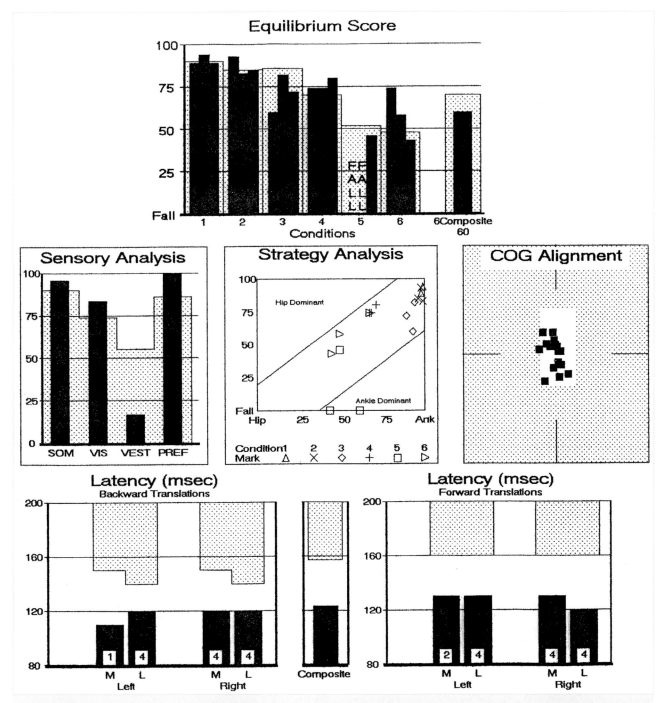

Fig. 114.16 The results of computerized dynamic platform posturography testing in a patient with a confirmed right acoustic neuroma. The results of sensory analysis are consistent with a significant abnormality in the vestibular modality. See text for more details. *COG*, center of gravity.

pathways that supply the neck and spinal muscles. The saccule is positioned in the labyrinth just below the anterior half of the stapes footplate, so intense sound may elicit responses from the hair cells of the maculae of the saccule, which ultimately result in muscle tone changes within a contracted muscle. The maculae of the saccule detect linear acceleration in the horizontal or vertical plane when the head and body move together as a single unit. The VEMP notably differs from an auditory evoked potential in that it can be elicited by nonacoustic (e.g., tactile) as well as acoustic stimulation and is myogenic rather than neurogenic.

Elicitation of VEMPs is optimized with tone bursts at the nominal frequency of 500 or 1000 Hz. As with auditory evoked potentials, averaging and filtering of the responses are employed. The most commonly employed electrode sites (ipsilateral to the ear receiving acoustic stimulation) involving the sternocleidomastoid muscle (cervical VEMP) are as follows: (1) noninverting (active) electrode on the upper belly of the sternocleidomastoid muscle, inverting electrode on the sternum, and ground over the sternocleidomastoid muscle; (2) noninverting electrode on the forehead, inverting electrode over the

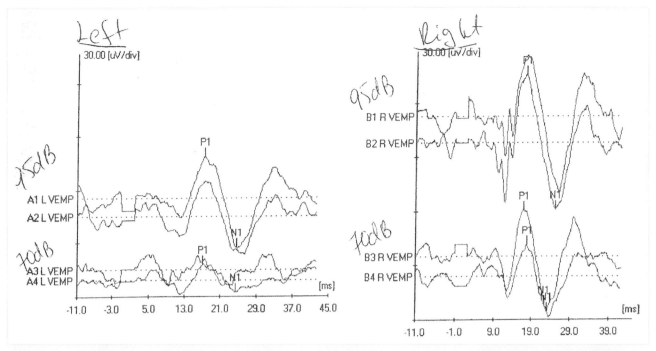

Fig. 114.17 Vestibular evoked myogenic potential recording from a normal individual.

belly of the sternocleidomastoid muscle, and ground over the middle of the sternocleidomastoid muscle. The former montage yields an initial positive deflection that is upward (P1) and then a negative deflection (N1); with the latter montage, deflections are in the reverse direction (i.e., downward for P1 and upward for N1). ► Fig. 114.17 shows a VEMP from a normal individual. The VEMP also can be recorded from the infraorbital region; the literature for cervical VEMPs is much larger than that for infraorbital VEMPs because the infraorbital VEMP is an emerging technology. The origins of infraorbital VEMPs currently are believed to be the utricle and superior vestibular nerve.

In a commonly employed approach to achieve sufficient tensing of the sternocleidomastoid muscle, the patient is lying down in a supine position (typically at a 30-degree angle, as for caloric vestibular testing) and in a semirecumbent position with the neck turned maximally to the side away from the ear receiving the acoustic stimulation; the patient then lifts his or her head just off the table. Often, the ongoing electromyographic activity is monitored to ensure that muscle tension during testing remains stable. The signal stimulation period needs to be short to reduce the adverse effects of muscle fatigue on the response and to minimize the possibility that the patient will recruit other muscles to maintain the head elevation. The VEMP parameters of interest include its threshold, P1 latency, N1 latency, and the P1–N1 (VEMP) amplitude in each ear. The interaural latency difference is measured based on P1 and N1. The asymmetry ratio (%) is calculated as follows: [VEMP amplitude (right – left)] divided by [VEMP amplitude (left + right)] x 100. For cervical VEMPs in a normal adult, the VEMP threshold occurs at about 70 to 90 dB HL, P1 latency is about 12 to 13 milliseconds, and N1 latency is about 22 to 23 milliseconds. Normative data based from the individual testing center are used to define the upper limits of normalcy for these parameters. Conductive hearing impairment generally abolishes an AC VEMP.

A major application of the VEMP has been to evaluate patients with superior semicircular canal dehiscence. The VEMP threshold may be significantly better (i.e., lower) in patients with superior semicircular canal dehiscence than in normal individuals because the dehiscence shunts sound energy away from the cochlea through the vestibular labyrinth.

The VEMP is absent or its amplitude is reduced in approximately 80% of patients with vestibular schwannoma, reflecting involvement of the inferior vestibular nerve, and it may be abnormal even when caloric findings are normal; low specificity rates around 50% have been reported.

Study findings suggest that absent VEMPs or VEMPS with decreased amplitude may occur in patients with vestibular neuritis when the inferior vestibular nerve is involved.

A limitation of the VEMP affecting test–retest reliability and intersubject comparisons is normalization of muscle tone. Obtaining a prestimulus, baseline electromyogram to normalize the electromyogram helps alleviate this limitation but does not overcome it because of muscle tone changes during acoustic stimulation. Maturation and aging affect the VEMP, so normative data for the various age groups need to be obtained. Given the sensitivity and specificity rates in the literature for the various disorders, and the great diversity in recording, stimulus, and instrumentation parameters, VEMPs should interpreted cautiously and in conjunction with other vestibular, otologic, and audiologic findings.

114.10 Internet Resources

- AudiologyOnline (http://www.audiologyonline.com)
- Audiology Educational Resources Online (http://www.worldaudiology.com/resource/audiology-educational-resources/)
- Audiogram Tutorials and Audiology Links (http://audsim.com/Business/linksbusiness.htm)

114.11 Recommended Reading

[1] American Speech-Language-Hearing Association (ASHA). Guidelines for the audiologic management of individuals receiving cochleotoxic drug therapy. ASHA 1994; 36 Suppl 12: 11–19

[2] American Speech-Language-Hearing Association. Guidelines for identification audiometry. ASHA 1985; 27: 49–52, 40

[3] Committee on Hearing and Equilibrium of the American Academy of Otolaryngology–Head and Neck Surgery. Committee on Hearing and Equilibrium guidelines for the diagnosis and evaluation of therapy in Meniere's disease. Otolaryngol Head Neck Surg 1995; 113: 181–185

[4] Committee on Hearing and Equilibrium of the American Academy of Otolaryngology–Head and Neck Surgery. Committee on Hearing and Equilibrium guidelines for the evaluation of hearing preservation in acoustic neuroma (vestibular schwannoma). American Academy of Otolaryngology-Head and Neck Surgery Foundation, INC. Otolaryngol Head Neck Surg 1995; 113: 179–180

[5] Committee on Hearing and Equilibrium of the American Academy of Otolaryngology–Head and Neck Surgery. Committee on Hearing and Equilibrium guidelines for the evaluation of results of treatment of conductive hearing loss. AmericanAcademy of Otolaryngology-Head and Neck Surgery Ffoundation, Inc. Otolaryngol Head Neck Surg 1995; 113: 186–187

[6] Harlor AD, Bower C Committee on Practice and Ambulatory MedicineSection on Otolaryngology-Head and Neck Surgery. Hearing assessment in infants and children: recommendations beyond neonatal screening. Pediatrics 2009; 124: 1252–1263

[7] Gelfand SA. Clinical precision of the Rinne test. Acta Otolaryngol 1977; 83: 480–487

[8] Kaplan H, Gladstone S, Lloyd LL. Audiometric Interpretation: A Manual of Basic Audiometry. 2nd ed. Boston, MA: Allyn & Bacon; 1993

[9] Maes L, Vinck BM, Wuyts F et al. Clinical usefulness of the rotatory, caloric, and vestibular evoked myogenic potential test in unilateral peripheral vestibular pathologies. Int J Audiol 2011; 50: 566–576

[10] Silman S, Gelfand SA. The relationship between magnitude of hearing loss and acoustic reflex threshold levels. J Speech Hear Disord 1981; 46: 312–316

[11] Silman S, Silverman CA. Auditory Diagnosis: Principles and Applications. San Diego, CA: Singular Publishing; 1997

[12] US Preventive Services Task Force. Universal screening for hearing loss in newborns: US Preventive Services Task Force recommendation statement. Pediatrics 2008; 122: 143–148

115 Radiology of the Temporal Bone

George Alexiades

115.1 Introduction

Temporal bone imaging is an important diagnostic tool for the otolaryngologist–head and neck surgeon. The two main imaging modalities used today are computed tomography (CT) and magnetic resonance (MR) imaging. The strength of CT lies in optimal viewing of the bony architecture of the temporal bone, whereas MR imaging is excellent at delineating soft-tissue structures. MR imaging does not image bone well at all.

115.2 Computed Tomography

CT is the process of using a computer to create an image from multiple "slices" of X-rays. The early CT machines were known as CAT (computed axial tomography) scans because they generated images only in the axial plane. Newer machines are able to gather the data and reformat the image in any plane, or even create a three-dimensional image.

In temporal bone imaging, CT is excellent for showing the bony architecture. (From this point forward, all references to CT scans will be with the assumption that they are weighted for bone—i.e., the contrast and brightness of the image were changed to reveal bony architecture while showing all soft-tissue densities as a medium gray.) This is in contrast to typical soft tissue–weighted CT scans, which can show different densities of soft tissues; however, they tend to overexpose bone and obscure its architecture. On the temporal bone scan, bone and highly calcified tissue will appear white, air will appear black, and soft tissue and fluid will appear gray (▶ Fig. 115.1).

The temporal bone is actually made up of five different bones: the squamous bone, petrous bone, mastoid, tympanic ring, and styloid process. The squamous bone is the lateral flat bone to which the temporalis muscle attaches. The petrous portion comprises the medial pyramidal bone, which houses the otic capsule and middle ear space. The mastoid comprises the lateral aerated portion of the temporal bone. The tympanic ring is a U-shaped bone that forms the anterior, inferior, and posterior walls of the external auditory canal. The tympanic ring articulates with the squamous bone anteriorly (forming the tympanosquamous suture) and with the mastoid bone posteriorly (forming the tympanomastoid suture). Finally, the styloid process arises out of the inferior aspect of the temporal bone and serves as an excellent landmark for the stylomastoid foramen, through which the facial nerve exits the temporal bone.

In assessing temporal bone CT scans, it is important to view the bone globally before focusing on the pathology. The lifelong history of the temporal bone can be deduced by its characteristics on the scan. The three main features of the temporal bone to assess on a CT scan are its development, pneumatization, and aeration.

Development refers to the presence, absence, or malformation of the labyrinthine structures: the cochlea, semicircular canals, vestibule, and internal auditory canal. In a well-developed bone, these structures will all appear normal, signifying normal development of the ear in utero (weeks 3 to 16 of gestation).

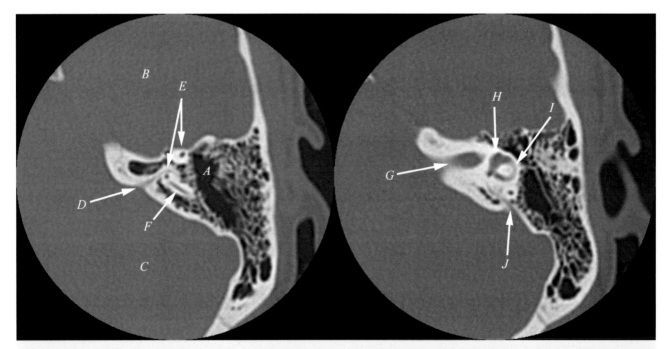

Fig. 115.1 Axial computed tomographic scans of the left temporal bone. The scan on the left is a more superior cut. *A*, antrum; *B*, middle cranial fossa; *C*, posterior cranial fossa; *D*, subarcuate artery; *E*, superior semicircular canal; *F*, posterior semicircular canal; *G*, internal auditory canal; *H*, vestibule; *I*, lateral semicircular canal; *J*, vestibular aqueduct.

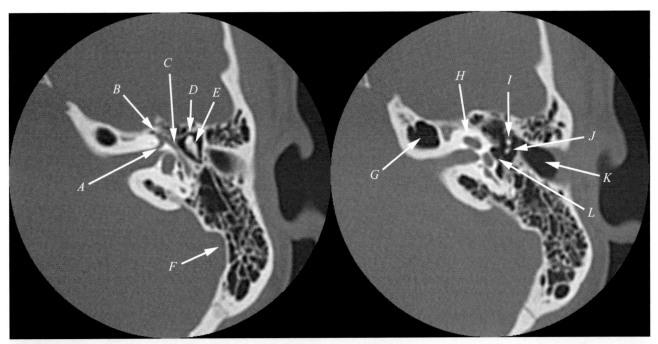

Fig. 115.2 Axial computed tomographic scans of the left temporal bone. The cuts are more inferior than the cut in ▶ Fig. 115.1, and again the scan on the left is a more superior cut. *A*, labyrinthine segment of facial nerve; *B*, geniculate ganglion; *C*, tympanic segment of facial nerve; *D*, head of malleus; *E*, body of incus; *F*, sigmoid sinus; *G*, petrous apex; *H*, cochlea; *I*, manubrium of malleus; *J*, long process of incus; *K*, external auditory canal; *L*, stapes suprastructure (very faint) and footplate.

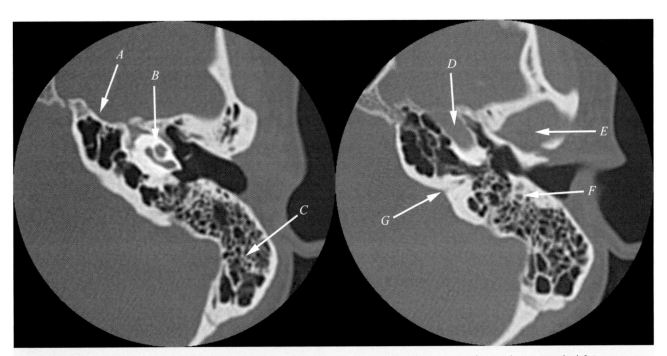

Fig. 115.3 Axial computed tomographic scans of the left temporal bone. These are more inferior cuts, and again the scan on the left is a more superior cut. *A*, foveate depression (gasserian ganglion lies within it); *B*, basal, middle, and apical turns of the cochlea; *C*, mastoid air cells; *D*, petrous carotid artery; *E*, temporomandibular joint; *F*, descending facial nerve; *G*, cochlear aqueduct.

Pneumatization refers to the presence or absence of air cells in the mastoid. A well-pneumatized bone will show extensive air cells in the mastoid and minimal bone marrow in the mastoid tip. Oftentimes, there is pneumatization of the petrous apex. Pneumatization occurs from birth until early adolescence and is inhibited by frequent episodes of otitis media or prolonged serous otitis media. However, inhibition can be reversed by ventilating the middle ear space with tubes. Finally, *aeration* refers to the status of the air cells present—whether they are filled with air or fluid. This refers to the short-term status of the ear.

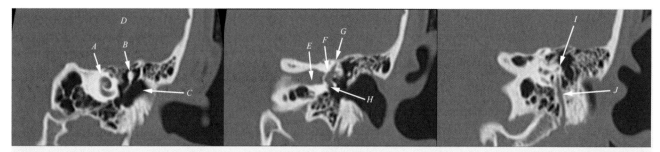

Fig. 115.4 Coronal computed tomographic scans of the left temporal bone, moving in an anterior to posterior direction (left to right). *A*, cochlea; *B*, malleus; *C*, external auditory canal; *D*, middle cranial fossa; *E*, internal auditory canal; *F*, vestibule; *G*, superior semicircular canal; *H*, round window niche; *I*, lateral semicircular canal; *J*, descending facial nerve.

An ear can have poor pneumatization and normal aeration, which would signify frequent ear infections during childhood that the patient is no longer experiencing. Conversely, a well-pneumatized temporal bone that is poorly aerated signifies a current problem in the ear, without necessarily a chronic history of infections.

▶ Fig. 115.1, ▶ Fig. 115.2, and ▶ Fig. 115.3 show all the major landmarks in the temporal bone through a series of axial images as one progresses in a superior to inferior direction. ▶ Fig. 115.4 shows coronal cuts through the temporal bone. It is important to note that a CT scan shows the bony anatomy of the ear and that these structures are identified as such. The membranous structures of the inner ear lie within these bony structures. The vestibule is the central bony chamber that houses the utricle and saccule and that the semicircular canals enter. The internal auditory canal is the bony canal through which the facial, cochlear, and superior and inferior vestibular nerves all course on their way from the brainstem to the otic capsule. The vestibular aqueduct is a bony channel that houses the endolymphatic duct as it courses to the endolymphatic sac. Finally, the cochlear aqueduct is a bony channel that lies parallel and inferior to the internal auditory canal and courses from the cerebellopontine angle to the basal turn of the cochlea at the round window. It does not house any structures but is often patent in younger persons and serves as a tract for inflammation in the cochlea and subsequent hearing loss in patients with meningitis, which explains why there is preferential ossification of the cochlea at the basal turn in these instances.

Cholesteatoma is one of the more common diagnoses for which a CT scan is obtained. The diagnosis of cholesteatoma is based on the physical examination, and the CT scan serves only to delineate its extent. Only in infrequent cases can a definitive diagnosis of cholesteatoma be made on a CT scan. ▶ Fig. 115.5 shows an axial and a coronal cut through a temporal bone with cholesteatoma. Here, scalloping of the bone is clearly evident, which is a hallmark of cholesteatoma. Erosion of the otic capsule is another sign of an erosive lesion. Ossicular erosion can be seen in chronic otitis media and cannot be used for the diagnosis of cholesteatoma.

In addition, a contrast agent can be used during CT to identify vascular lesions. Iodine is the contrast agent used, and care must be taken in individuals with an allergy to iodine, asthma, or renal insufficiency. MR imaging has largely replaced CT of the temporal bone with contrast because it offers much better contrast of the soft-tissue structures.

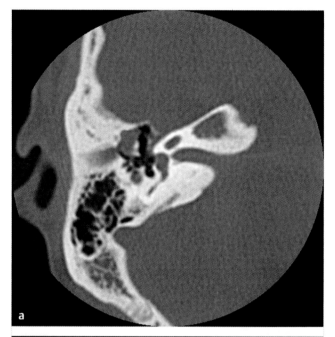

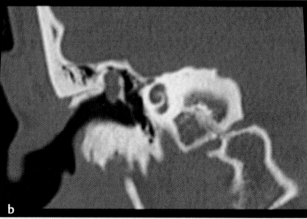

Fig. 115.5 (a) Axial and **(b)** coronal temporal bone computed tomographic scans demonstrating a cholesteatoma lateral to the incudomalleolar joint, with erosion of the scutum.

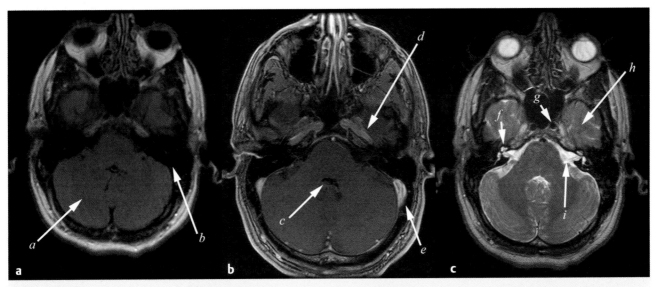

Fig. 115.6 Axial magnetic resonance images of normal internal auditory canals. (**a**) T1 before contrast. (**b**) T1 after gadolinium contrast (note enhancement of the sigmoid sinus and nasal mucosa). (**c**) T2 sequence (note that the cerebrospinal fluid spaces and globes are bright). *a*, cerebellum; *b*, mastoid; *c*, fourth ventricle; *d*, carotid artery; *e*, sigmoid sinus; *f*, cochlea; *g*, carotid artery; *h*, temporal lobe; *i*, cerebellopontine angle (note cochlear and inferior vestibular nerves traversing angle and entering the internal auditory canal).

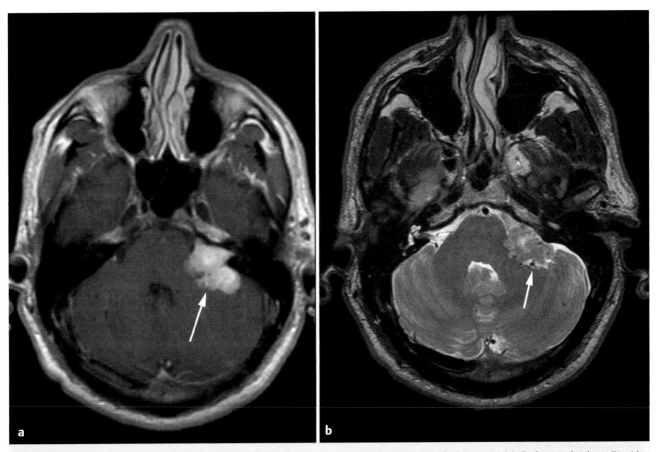

Fig. 115.7 Magnetic resonance images showing a large left vestibular schwannoma that is indenting the brainstem. (**a**) The lesion is bright on T1 with gadolinium (*arrow*). (**b**) It is darker on T2 (*arrow*).

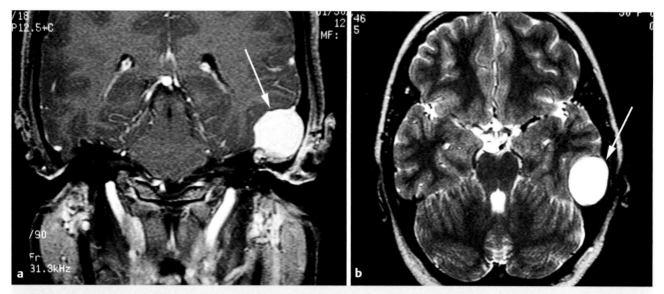

Fig. 115.8 (a) Coronal T1-weighted magnetic resonance (MR) image with gadolinium shows a cholesterol granuloma extending from the mastoid up into the temporal lobe (*arrow*). (b) Axial T2-weighted MR image of the same patient. Note that the lesion is bright on both T1 and T2 imaging (*arrow*).

115.3 Magnetic Resonance Imaging

MR imaging technology is relatively new; it was first used in humans in 1977. Unlike CT, which uses ionizing radiation, MR imaging uses powerful magnetic fields to align hydrogen atoms in the body. In temporal bone radiology, whereas CT is used to visualize the bony anatomy, MR imaging is excellent for delineating soft-tissue anatomy. Various pulse sequences can be used to increase the contrast between tissues. This depends on the time of excitation (TE) and the repetition rate (TR) of the magnetic field. Furthermore, contrast (gadolinium) can be used during MR imaging to help identify lesions with increased vascularity. MR imaging machines today typically use a 1.5-T (tesla) magnet, with 3.0-T magnets becoming more commonplace. With increased strength comes increased resolution.

The first sequence created for MR imaging was the T1-weighted sequence. This sequence has a relatively short TE and TR. In MR imaging of the brain, the cerebrospinal fluid (CSF) will appear dark, subcutaneous fat will have a higher density, and there will be good contrast between the gray and white matter. Intravenous gadolinium is often used with T1-weighted imaging to visualize neoplasms. T2-weighted imaging uses a relatively long TE and TR; as a result, CSF and other tissues with a high water content appear very bright. Fat-density tissues appear much darker on T2-weighted than on T1-weighted images; this weighting is very good for demonstrating edema in tissues. The FIESTA (*f*ast *i*maging *e*mploying *s*teady-*s*tate *a*cquisition) sequence is a high-resolution T2-weighted imaging sequence that is often used to visualize the internal auditory canals and cerebellopontine angles to identify neoplasms, even in the absence of contrast injections. A FLAIR (*f*luid-*a*ttenuated *i*nversion recovery) sequence is created to suppress the signal of CSF. This is often useful in visualizing lesions such as multiple sclerosis plaques or in assessing whether fluid in the mastoid is CSF in cases of suspected CSF leak. Many other sequences are available for MR imaging but fall outside the scope and depth of this chapter.

One of the most common indications for ordering MR imaging of the internal auditory canals is to rule out the presence of a cerebellopontine angle lesion in the evaluation of asymmetric sensorineural hearing loss (▶ Fig. 115.6). Of these lesions, vestibular schwannoma, also known as acoustic neuroma, is the most common. This is covered in depth in Chapter 134, Posterior Skull Base Diseases and Surgery. ▶ Fig. 115.7 shows the imaging characteristics of a typical vestibular schwannoma. The lesion is of medium density on T1 sequencing and enhances with gadolinium contrast. On T2, the lesion fades and is usually seen as a filling defect of the internal auditory canal. Similar imaging characteristics exist for meningiomas, which are also commonly found in the cerebellopontine angle, with the exception that meningiomas can be differentiated by "dural tails." Because meningiomas arise from the dura, enhancement of the dura often extends beyond the border of the tumor. Also, meningiomas are not always based in a pattern concentric to the internal auditory canal, but may arise in a fashion eccentric to the internal auditory canal.

Cholesterol granuloma is another common lesion of the temporal bone and often arises in the petrous apex of a well-pneumatized temporal bone. In this location, obstructed air cells subsequently bleed into themselves, creating a slowly expanding mass that can be quite destructive if left untreated. Because of the presence of blood breakdown products and a high water content, cholesterol granulomas tend to be bright on T1 and T2 sequences (▶ Fig. 115.8).

115.4 Roundsmanship

- CT of the temporal bone is excellent for delineating bony anatomy, whereas MR imaging is excellent for providing soft-tissue detail.
- MR imaging rule of thumb: as one goes from T1- to T2-weighted images, fat fades (becomes dark on T2) and inflammation enhances (becomes brighter on T2).

115.5 Recommended Reading

[1] Harnsberger R, Glastonbury CM, Michel MA, Koch BL. Diagnostic Imaging: Head and Neck. Diagnostic Imaging Series. Salt Lake City, UT: Amirsys Publishing; 2010

[2] Swartz JD, Loevner LA. Imaging of the Temporal Bone. New York, Ny: Thieme Medical Publishers; 2008

[3] Valtonen HJ, Dietz A, Qvarnberg YH, Nuutinen J. Development of mastoid air cell system in children treated with ventilation tubes for early-onset otitis media: a prospective radiographic 5-year follow-up study. Laryngoscope 2005; 115: 268–273

116 Diseases of the External Ear

Christopher J. Linstrom

116.1 Introduction

The typical otolaryngologist–head and neck surgeon sees many patients with infections of the external ear. The infections may be classified by location, cause, and time course as acute, subacute, or chronic. Before discussing the individual disease processes, we review the normal anatomy and physiology of the external ear.

116.2 Anatomy and Physiology

The external ear is composed of the auricle and external auditory canal (EAC). Both contain elastic cartilage derived from mesoderm and a small amount of subcutaneous tissue, covered by skin with its adnexal appendages. There is fat but no cartilage in the lobule. The auricle is derived from six hillocks, three each from branchial arches 1 and 2 (▶ Fig. 116.1). During normal gestation, the cartilaginous hillocks merge to form the auricle, and with selective growth of the mandible, the auricle rises from its original position near the lateral commissure of the mouth to the temporal area. The tragus and antitragus form a partial barrier to the entrance of macroscopic foreign bodies.

The EAC canal is derived from the first ectodermal branchial groove between the mandibular (1) and hyoid (2) arches. The epithelium lining this groove contacts the endoderm of the first pharyngeal pouch, thus forming the tympanic membrane, the

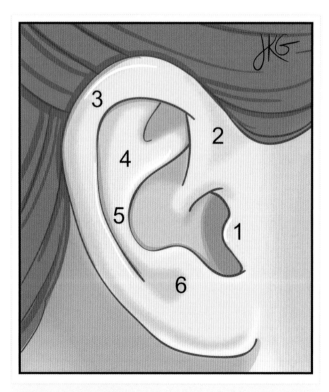

Fig. 116.1 The auricle is formed from six auricular hillocks, three each from branchial arches 1 and 2.

most medial extent of the EAC. Connective tissue of mesodermal origin is found between the ectoderm and endoderm and becomes the fibrous layer of the tympanic membrane. Because of its origin, the EAC, including the lateral surface of the tympanic membrane, is derived from ectoderm and is lined by squamous epithelium.

The process of canalization is complete by about week 12 of gestation, at which time the canal fills with epithelial tissue. The canal ordinarily recanalizes by about week 28 of fetal life.

The outer 40% of the EAC in its anterior and inferior aspect is cartilaginous and contains a thin layer of subcutaneous tissue between the skin and cartilage. The inner 60% is osseous, is formed primarily by the tympanic ring, and contains very scant soft tissue between the skin and periosteum. The average length of the adult external auditory canal is 2.5 cm. Because of the oblique position of the tympanic membrane, the posterosuperior part of the canal is about 6 mm shorter than the anteroinferior portion. The junction of the cartilaginous and bony portions of the canal is a narrowed section termed the *isthmus*.

Laterally to medially, the canal curves slightly superiorly and posteriorly in a gentle 'S' shape. Three macroscopic defense mechanisms protect the EAC and lateral surface of the tympanic membrane: the tragus and antitragus, the skin with its cerumen coat, and the isthmus of the canal.

The skin of the cartilaginous canal contains many hair cells and sebaceous and apocrine glands, such as cerumen glands. Together, these three adnexal structures provide a protective function and are termed the *apopilosebaceous unit*. Glandular secretions combine with sloughed squamous epithelium to form an acidic coat of cerumen, one of the primary barriers to infection of the canal. An invagination of the epidermis forms the outer wall of the hair follicle, and the hair shaft forms the inner wall. The follicular canal is the space between these two structures. The alveoli of the sebaceous and apocrine glands empty into short, straight excretory ducts, which drain into follicular canals. Obstruction of any part of the ductal system predisposes to infection.

The canal is normally a self-protecting and self-cleansing structure. The cerumen coat gradually works its way past the isthmus to the lateral part of the canal and sloughs externally. Instrumentation and excessive cleansing of the canal disturb this primary protective barrier and may lead to infection. Individual variations in the anatomy of the canal may predispose some people to wax accumulation.

The canal interfaces on all but its lateral surface. Medially, it is bound by the tympanic membrane, which when intact is a good barrier to the spread of infection. The horseshoe-shaped tympanic ring separates the canal from the middle cranial fossa. The posterior bony canal serves as the anterior boundary of the mastoid cavity. Several vessels penetrate the canal, especially along the tympanomastoid suture, which may be involved in the hematogenous extension of infection from the canal to the mastoid segment. Posterior to the cartilaginous canal, dense connective tissue overlies the mastoid, which may become secondarily infected.

Superiorly, the canal is bound by the middle cranial fossa and inferiorly by the infratemporal fossa and base of the skull. Infections extending through the roof of the canal may extend into these structures. Anteriorly, the canal is bordered by the temporomandibular joint and the parotid gland.

The lymphatic drainage of the canal is an important channel for the spread of infection. Anteriorly and superiorly, the canal drains to the preauricular lymphatics in the parotid gland and the superior deep cervical nodes. The inferior portion of the canal drains into the infra-auricular nodes near the angle of the mandible. Posteriorly, the lymphatics drain into the postauricular nodes and the superior deep cervical nodes. The auricle and EAC receive their arterial supply from the superficial temporal and posterior auricular branches of the external carotid artery. Venous drainage from the auricle and meatus is via the superficial temporal and posterior auricular veins. The former joins the retromandibular vein, which usually divides and joins both jugular veins; the latter joins the external jugular vein but may also drain to the sigmoid sinus through the mastoid emissary vein.

Sensation to the auricle and EAC is supplied by cutaneous and cranial nerves, with contributions from the auriculotemporal branches of the trigeminal (V), facial (VII), glossopharyngeal (IX), and vagus (X) nerves and the great auricular nerve from the cervical plexus (C2–C3). The vestigial extrinsic muscles of the ear—anterior, superior, and posterior auricular—are supplied by the facial nerve (VII).

116.3 Infectious and Inflammatory Diseases

116.3.1 Otitis Externa

Otitis externa is a spectrum of infection of the EAC. The appearance of the canal varies according to the time course of infection: acute, subacute, or chronic.

Acute otitis externa is a bacterial infection of the canal caused by a break in the normal skin/cerumen protective barrier in the milieu of elevated humidity and temperature. Acute otitis externa may be caused by anything that results in removal of the protective lipid film from the canal, allowing bacteria to enter the apopilosebaceous unit. It usually begins with itching in the canal, and scratching by the patient allows bacteria to proliferate in locally macerated skin and sets up an itch–scratch cycle. The moist environment of the canal is now a perfect medium for rapid bacterial growth. Later, pain ensues as the swollen soft tissues of the canal distract the periosteal lining of the bony canal. As the disease progresses, purulent discharge begins, and the auricle and periauricular soft tissues may become involved.

In patients in whom the disease does not resolve after treatment, a subacute or chronic form may occur. This condition represents a spectrum of disease ranging from mild drying and scaling to complete obliteration of the canal by chronically infected, hypertrophic skin.

Bacteriology

The usual pathogens responsible for acute otitis externa are *Pseudomonas aeruginosa*, *Proteus mirabilis*, staphylococci, streptococci, and various gram-negative bacilli. For a mild or uncomplicated infection, culture of the canal is ordinarily not taken because it will usually demonstrate a mixed pattern of growth. For recalcitrant infections, culture may identify a predominant organism and assist in the choice of antibiotic therapy.

Natural History

The natural history of untreated acute otitis externa is one of increasing pain, swelling, and discharge from the canal. The infection may spread to the adjacent periauricular soft tissues, face, and neck. In an immunocompromised patient, what began as an isolated superficial infection of the apopilosebaceous unit of the EAC may progress to perichondritis, chondritis, cellulitis, and erysipelas. Rich lymphatic and hematogenous drainage pathways favor the spread of infection to local and regional sites in the head and neck. Few patients progress to such an advanced stage before seeking medical attention.

The natural history of chronic otitis externa is far less dramatic than that of its acute counterpart. The chronic scaling and itching may lead to repeated episodes of acute otitis externa. With time, the canal skin may become lichenified, and ultimately the canal may become completely obliterated.

Medical Evaluation

The history and functional inquiry should include information regarding duration, number of occurrences, nature and severity of pain, antecedent otologic disease, previous auricular instrumentation or trauma (especially the use of cotton-tipped applicators), and predisposing factors, such as diabetes, radiotherapy, or any condition causing immunosuppression. Any previous otologic or head and neck surgery is noted.

Pain, fullness, itching, and hearing loss are the four major symptoms of external otitis, although not every patient has each symptom.

Physical Examination

On initial inspection, redness, swelling, lateral protrusion, discharge, and evidence of cellulitis involving the periauricular tissues should be noted. Pain with distraction of the auricle is typical in the setting of otitis externa.

The canal should be thoroughly débrided and examined. Topical and local anesthesia is usually of little effect in hyperemic, macerated tissue and no substitute for reassurance and patience. The canal may be cleaned with suction, a cerumen loop, or alligator forceps. Gentleness and thoroughness in cleaning the ear are very important.

Differential Diagnosis

The differential diagnosis of external otitis is large and includes conditions with similar features, such as necrotizing otitis externa, bullous external otitis, granular external otitis, perichondritis, chondritis, relapsing polychondritis, furunculosis, and carbunculosis, as well as many dermatoses, such as psoriasis and seborrheic dermatitis. All have features in common with acute and chronic external otitis yet enough dissimilarities to be considered distinct clinical entities.

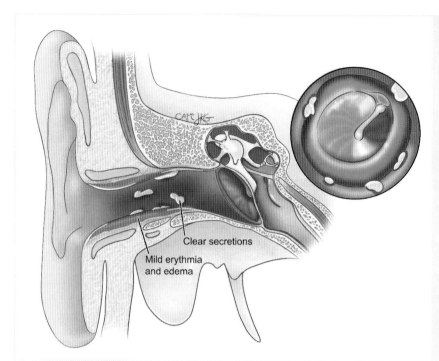

Clear secretions

Mild erythmia and edema

Fig. 116.2 Otitis externa, moderate acute inflammatory stage. The external auditory canal is more edematous than in the acute stage, with the lumen nearly obliterated and with a more profuse exudate.

Carcinoma involving the EAC may present as infection, and in its earliest stages it is often mistaken for infection and treated inappropriately. The most common malignant neoplasm of the external ear is squamous cell carcinoma, although other primary carcinomas have been described: basal cell carcinoma, malignant melanoma, ceruminous adenoma or adenocarcinoma, adenoid cystic carcinoma, and metastatic carcinomas to the temporal bone with extension to the EAC, such as breast, prostatic, small (oat) cell, and renal cell carcinomas.

Staging

The clinical course of external otitis may be divided into the following stages: preinflammatory; acute inflammatory (mild, moderate, or severe); and chronic inflammatory. Typically, the preinflammatory stage begins when the stratum corneum becomes edematous because of removal of the protective lipid layer and acid mantle from the canal, resulting in plugging of the apopilosebaceous unit. As obstruction continues, a sense of fullness and itching begins. The disruption of the epithelial layer allows the invasion of bacteria that either reside in the canal or are introduced on foreign objects inserted into the canal. This produces the acute inflammatory stage, which is accompanied by pain and tenderness of the auricle. In the earliest stage, the skin of the EAC shows mild erythema and minimal edema (▶ Fig. 116.2). A small amount of a clear or slightly cloudy secretion may be seen in the canal. As pain and itching increase, the disease progresses to the moderate stage, in which the canal shows more edema and a thicker, more profuse exudate (▶ Fig. 116.3). Further progression of the inflammation leads to the severe inflammatory stage, characterized by increased pain and obliteration of the lumen of the canal. A profuse, purulent exudate and edema of the canal skin may obscure the tympanic membrane. In addition, small white papules are often visible on the surface of the canal skin. *P. aeruginosa* or another gram-negative bacillus can almost always be cultured at this stage. In the severe stage, the physician often sees evidence of extension of the infection beyond the canal to involve the adjacent soft tissues and cervical lymph nodes.

In the chronic inflammatory stage, the patient experiences less pain but more profound itching. The skin of the external canal is thickened, and superficial flaking may be seen. This condition is likened to eczema and may range from mild drying and thickening of the canal to complete obliteration of the external canal by chronically infected, hypertrophic skin (▶ Table 116.1).

Medical Treatment

The four fundamental principles in the treatment of external otitis in all stages are: (1) frequent and thorough cleaning; (2) the judicious use of appropriate antibiotics; (3) the treatment of associated inflammation and pain; and (4) recommendations regarding the prevention of future infections. In any stage of infection, thorough cleaning is a priority. In the preinflammatory stage, a complete cleaning may be all that is required. In the absence of purulence, a brief course of an acidifying drop such as aluminum sulfate–calcium sulfate is effective in discouraging bacterial or fungal growth.

Treatment of the acute inflammatory stage varies with the extent of disease. In the mildest form, cleaning as above is indicated. An antibiotic otic drop is recommended to cover what is probably a *Pseudomonas* infection. At this stage, edema of the EAC should not be severe, and the patient should be able to instill drops into the ear by tilting the head to the side or by lying down with the involved ear upright. In the moderate stage of inflammation, edema of the canal may interfere with the instillation of drops. The physician should then insert a porous expandable wick into the canal and instill drops on it. Often, the canal may accommodate two or even three wicks. As the wick expands, it presses the soft tissues and periosteum centrifugally; this alone may relieve pain. The wick is removed by the

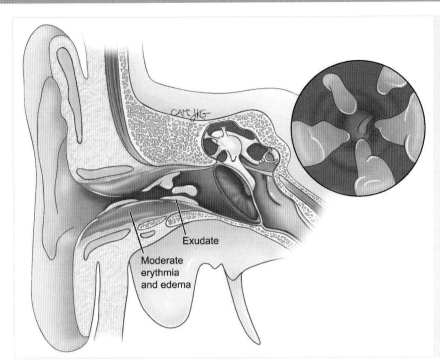

Fig. 116.3 Otitis externa, severe stage. Infection extends beyond the limits of the canal to involve adjacent soft tissues and cervical lymph nodes. Erythema of the conchal skin and scaliness are secondary to profuse drainage.

Exudate

Moderate erythmia and edema

Table 116.1 Diagnosis of otitis externa

History	Physical examination		Laboratory	
Pain	Preinflammatory	Mild erythema	Culture	*Pseudomonas aeruginosa*
Fullness		Edema		*Proteus mirabilis*
Itching	Acute inflammatory	Auricular tenderness		*Staphylococcus* species
Discharge		Erythema		*Streptococcus* species
		Edema	Radiology	Rarely indicated
		Discharge		
	Chronic inflammatory	Thickening, flaking of canal skin		
		Eczematization		
		Ulceration		

physician at the time of reexamination. If the edema has not been significantly reduced, repacking is indicated. Antibiotic drops should be continued for at least 2 to 3 days after the cessation of pain, itching, and drainage so that complete eradication of infection may be ensured. An oral analgesic is often prescribed for pronounced pain. The patient is cautioned to avoid manipulation of the canal. If the infection has not spread beyond the boundaries of the external canal, the use of oral antibiotics will be of little to no value.

In the severe stage, infection usually extends beyond the limits of the canal. In addition to the cleaning, packing, and use of antibiotic drops discussed previously, soft-tissue involvement is treated by administering an oral antibiotic with broad-spectrum coverage. In addition to antipseudomonal ear drops, common choices of oral antibiotics include antipseudomonal fluoroquinolones (e.g., ciprofloxacin or levofloxacin), antistaphylococcal penicillins, and cephalosporins. In children younger than 12 years of age, one should discuss the use of these medications with the patient's pediatrician before prescribing oral fluoroquinolones.

Warm soaks (normal saline or a mild aluminum sulfate–calcium acetate solution) are also useful for treating the crusting and edema involving the auricle and surrounding skin. Culture of the canal for aerobic bacteria and/or fungi is indicated only for patients in the severe stage or for patients who have previously been treated without resolution. Treatment is generally continued for 10 to 14 days if there is a good response. For the rare patients who do not respond to this regimen, hospitalization, vigorous daily local care, repeated culturing, and intravenous antibiotics are indicated.

The chronic stage of external otitis is manifested by marked thickening of the skin of the EAC due to long-standing infection. Examination reveals flakes of dry, scaly skin in the canal. Although removal of debris is recommended, this may be difficult because of narrowing of the lumen of the canal. Repeated cleaning and the instillation of antibiotics and steroids are indicated. Triamcinolone acetonide 0.25% cream or ointment, fluocinolone 0.01% oil, or dexamethasone sodium phosphate 0.1% ophthalmic drops may be used. A final office visit is important to ensure that the infection has completely resolved and the canal is back to its normal state.

All patients should be instructed to avoid future infections by not instrumenting the ear. Swimmers should be taught to towel dry the concha and lateral canal, to shake water out of the canal, or to instill an acidifying drop after swimming. Patients who have repeated infections are best advised to use an acidifying drop composed of equal measures of vinegar and water, or ethyl alcohol and water, when exposed to high humidity. One should suspect otomycosis if all other reasonable measures have failed and should treat with drying agents, especially powders. Custom-made ear molds are useful for these patients.

Recalcitrant Otitis Externa

The physician will be able to judge very quickly which patients are responding. The prolonged use of antibiotic drops may suppress the return of the normal flora of the external canal and lead to a fungal superinfection. This should be suspected, especially if a grayish matted discharge is found in the ear even when telltale hyphae are absent. If a fungus has been cultured, the infection should be treated with drying agents such as powders, an antifungal drop, or a systemic oral antifungal medication such as fluconazole. If no progress is made in the office, rare patients may have to be admitted as inpatients. Frequent and thorough examination and cleaning are essential. Subtle signs of chronic middle ear disease (e.g., granulation tissue or the opening of a tiny perforation) may be obscured by a swollen tympanic membrane, giving a "fish mouth" appearance to the perforation. A "sewer cap" of crust on the drum may reveal a cholesteatoma underneath. Signs of underlying chondritis or perichondritis, especially diffuse crusting or exudative weeping, may be present. Computed tomography (CT) of the temporal bones may give additional information.

The patient is placed on daily aural drops, preferably one covering *P. aeruginosa*, and intravenous antibiotics with gram-positive and gram-negative coverage. Ciprofloxacin is a reasonable initial treatment, but in very rare cases, a cephalosporin together with an aminoglycoside is a logical combination if monotherapy is unsuccessful. Therapy should be tapered according to culture and sensitivities. Severely swollen ears may calm down with required steroids.

Many recalcitrant infections occur because of noncompliance or chronic instrumentation of the canal skin. The patient should be counseled to amend bad habits. The rare patient will need to be admitted for intravenous antibiotics and daily aural toilet (see Box Treatment of Otitis Externa (p.918)).

Surgical Management of Hypertrophic Chronic Otitis Externa

When such local measures are insufficient to eradicate infection and reestablish the lumen of the canal, it is necessary to remove the involved canal skin and any adjacent involved cutaneous or cartilaginous tissue. This is very rarely required but is best done through a postauricular incision, which allows better visualization of the involved tissues. A generous amount of conchal cartilage is removed to effect a wide meatoplasty. The bony canal is enlarged with a drill; the intraoperative use of a facial nerve monitor facilitates protection of the vertical segment of the facial nerve. The canal is resurfaced with a split-thickness skin graft that is temporarily held in place with stents or packing.

Treatment of Otitis Externa

Medical
- Frequent, thorough cleaning
- Antibiotic coverage
  - Drops
  - Oral
  - Intravenous as needed
- Treatment of inflammation, pain
- Recommendations for prevention

Surgical
- Excision of involved canal skin
- Wide meatoplasty
- Resurfacing of the canal with a split-thickness skin graft

116.3.2 Skull Base Osteomyelitis (Necrotizing [Malignant] Otitis Externa)

This potentially life-threatening disease should be viewed within the larger context of osteomyelitis of the temporal bone and skull base. Thanks in large part to newer antipseudomonal antibiotics, the prevalence of skull base osteomyelitis (SBO) has decreased significantly, although the disease still may be seen, especially among diabetics, the immunocompromised, and the elderly. SBO remains within the differential diagnosis of a refractory external ear infection in the patient at risk.

Bacteriology

The causative organism is almost always *P. aeruginosa*, although other organisms, such as *P. mirabilis*, *Aspergillus fumigatus*, *Proteus* species, *Klebsiella* species, and *Staphylococcus* species, have been isolated.

Natural History

The natural history of SBO is one of relentless progression to involve the cranial nerves, especially the facial nerve. The pain is inexorable and deep-seated. Multiple cranial nerves may be affected, especially cranial nerves VII, IX, X, and XI.

Presenting Complaints

The diagnosis of SBO is made in a patient with the appropriate history, physical examination findings, and supporting laboratory findings. Four key features are seen: (1) persistent, deep-seated, severe otalgia for longer than 1 month; (2) persistent purulent otorrhea with granulation tissue for several weeks; (3) diabetes mellitus, another immunocompromised state, or advanced age; and (4) cranial nerve involvement.

SBO usually begins as an acute external otitis that does not resolve despite medical therapy, as described previously. The history is significant for a long-standing infection of the external canal accompanied by aural discharge and severe, deep-seated pain. The disease usually occurs in elderly patients with poorly controlled diabetes, although it may be found in any chronically ill, debilitated, or immunocompromised patient, and the HIV status should be assessed if unknown.

Physical Examination

Most patients with SBO have granulation tissue visible in the inferior aspect of the canal (or even extruding from it) that may obscure the tympanic membrane (a rare finding in routine cases of otitis externa). The skin of the canal is often erythematous, indurated, and sometimes macerated. Purulent secretions are common. Lower cranial nerve palsies may be seen.

Radiographic Findings

CT of the temporal bone with contrast will yield excellent bony detail, with less precise information about soft tissue. It may define subtle bony changes, such as erosion of the anterior canal wall with involvement of the temporomandibular joint and erosion of the tympanic ring and base of the skull. It may demonstrate soft-tissue thickening and mastoid clouding.

Magnetic resonance (MR) imaging without and with gadolinium enhancement may be advantageous in defining the medial extent of disease at the skull base. Dural enhancement and involvement of the medullary bone spaces are seen with central skull base invasion. Underlying cerebral involvement is easily visualized with gadolinium-enhanced MR imaging. MR imaging yields very imprecise information about bone. The patency of the dural sinuses and great vessels of the neck may be assessed in a noninvasive fashion with MR angiography or venography. Changes seen on MR imaging do not quickly resolve with clinical improvement, so although MR imaging is a useful diagnostic tool to assess the extent of disease, it is less useful to follow the clinical course of SBO.

Technetium 99 m bone scanning and gallium 67 scanning have been advocated in the evaluation of SBO. Their sensitivity for the presence of infection is far greater than their specificity for the cause. ^{99m}Tc scanning gives excellent information about bone function but poor information about bone structure. A positive scan is thought to represent osteoblastic activity as little as 10% above normal. The scan is positive in acute and chronic osteomyelitis and in areas of active bone repair without infection, as in trauma. Its use in the evaluation of SBO is complementary to that of ^{67}Ga scanning. ^{67}Ga is thought to be incorporated into proteins and polymorphonuclear leukocytes at sites of active infection as a ^{67}Ga–lactoferrin complex. It will highlight an acute infective focus but not the full extent of an osteomyelitic process. As treatment progresses, the ^{67}Ga scan will revert to normal (negative), while the ^{99m}Tc scan will lag behind for many months. Baseline studies with both are thus recommended, so that sequential imaging can be used to monitor the response to therapy. Planar scintigraphy with indium 111–labeled leukocytes has been demonstrated to yield better results for the detection of osteomyelitis than either planar scintigraphy or tomography with ^{67}Ga- and/or ^{99m}Tc-methylene diphosphonate and may replace the former two radionuclide modalities in the evaluation of patients suspected to have SBO (▶ Table 116.2).

Differential Diagnosis

Other diseases to be included in the differential diagnosis are severe acute otitis externa, squamous cell carcinoma, glomus jugulare tumor, cholesteatoma, nasopharyngeal carcinoma, Hand-Schüller-Christian disease, eosinophilic granuloma, Wegener granulomatosis, and clival chordoma. In the appropriate clinical setting, a high index of suspicion is appropriate.

Medical Treatment

Swab and/or tissue cultures of the EAC should be obtained. If present, granulations should be biopsied and sent to rule out carcinoma or other pathology. Because *Pseudomas* is so frequently the predominant organism, the patient is treated with antipseudomonal antibiotics for an extended period, often for 6 weeks or more. Monotherapy is discouraged in the treatment of

Table 116.2 Diagnosis of necrotizing external otitis

History	Physical examination	Laboratory	
Persistent otalgia	Granulation tissue in external canal	Culture	*Pseudomonas aeruginosa* (almost always)
Persistent purulent otorrhea			*Proteus mirabilis*
	Purulent discharge		*Aspergillus fumigatus*
Diabetes mellitus	Cranial neuropathy, especially in cranial nerve VII		*Klebsiella* species
Advanced age			*Staphylococcus* species
		Radiology	Computed tomography with contrast
Immunocompromise			Magnetic resonance imaging with contrast
			Technetium 99 m scan
			Gallium 67 scan

SBO. Two antipseudomonal antibiotics are ordinarily chosen from among several alternatives (including gentamicin or tobramycin with or without ticarcillin or piperacillin) to achieve synergy and to avoid the emergence of a resistant strain of bacteria. Alternative antibiotics include mezlocillin or azlocillin, ceftazidime, imipenem, aztreonam, amikacin, norfloxacin, and ciprofloxacin or any of the other appropriate antipseudomonal fluoroquinolones. If an aminoglycoside is chosen, peak and trough levels and hearing must be carefully monitored. It is wise to treat in concert with an infectious disease colleague to help select those medications that will be of greatest benefit with the least toxicity. If the ear remains purulent despite adequate intravenous antibiosis and local care, cultures should be repeated to look for the emergence of a resistant organism; ciprofloxacin resistance has been reported in 20% of patients undergoing long-term (6 weeks or more) therapy for osteomyelitis.

An early clinical feature of successful treatment is the cessation of pain, and patients may be tempted to discontinue therapy once this occurs. Regardless of the choice of medication or mode of delivery, patients must understand that they will require meticulous aural toilet and antibiotic treatment for at least 6 weeks and vigorous management of their serum glucose levels. Either in the hospital or in the office, the ear is débrided carefully under the microscope on a regular basis until granulations have subsided. The patient is placed on antipseudomonal otic drops and appropriate systemic antibiotics. Diabetes is aggressively managed and the diet carefully monitored.

Hyperbaric oxygen is thought to facilitate osteoneogenesis and to promote the repair of diseased bone and thus may be of value in the most severe cases. The cost and inconvenience of hyperbaric oxygen therapy have limited its availability. Its use is recommended for patients who have advanced disease with significant skull base or intracranial involvement, recurrent disease, or infections refractory to antibiotic treatment.

Patients with disease refractory to intravenously administered antibiotics may require surgical control of the infected site.

Surgical Treatment

Most patients can be managed medically, and the role of surgery in SBO remains controversial. Surgical débridement of tissue and osteomyelitic bone is usually reserved for patients who do not respond to conventional therapy. Additionally, surgery provides tissue for culture in these refractive cases to look for resistant organisms or for a new organism, such as an invasive fungus. The progression of pain despite aggressive medical therapy, the persistence of granulations, and the development of cranial nerve involvement are all ominous signs that call for more aggressive medical therapy and possibly surgical intervention.

With the onset of facial paralysis, early surgical removal of granulation and, when necessary, decompression of the descending facial nerve have provided excellent return of function. The primary surgical goal is to relieve the entrapped nerve and allow its natural return of function. Serial electroneuronography (ENOG) has been used to detect the electrical degeneration of cranial nerve VII in patients with clinically complete facial paralysis. Electroneuronography showing more than 90% electrical degeneration of the facial nerve may support surgical

Table 116.3 Treatment of necrotizing external otitis

Medical Treatment	Surgical Treatment
Hospital admission	Excision of granulation tissue
Intravenous antibiotics	± Middle ear exploration
Daily cleaning, débridement	± Mastoidectomy
	± Facial nerve decompression
	± Temporal bone resection if no response

decompression of the involved segment of the nerve. However, the entire concept of facial nerve decompression in the context of SBO remains controversial; the mainstay of therapy for SBO remains medical, not surgical.

Surgical treatment, including abscess drainage, débridement of sequestra, and more extensive resection of bone and soft tissue, should be individualized depending upon the patient's overall health status and response to more conservative measures (▶ Table 116.3).

Prognosis

Mortality remains significant, especially in the immunocompromised patient. The progression of disease results in severe, unremitting pain within the ear and at the base of the skull and extension of the infection to the mastoid, parotid, lower cranial nerves, and transverse and sigmoid sinuses. Osteomyelitis of the skull base may lead to meningitis, brain abscess, and death. Poor prognostic factors include facial paralysis, polyneuropathy and intracranial extension (see Box Complications of Necrotizing External Otitis (p.920)).

Complications of Necrotizing External Otitis

- Cranial neuropathy (cranial nerve VII and lower)
- Progression despite aggressive local care (to mastoid, parotid, lower cranial nerves, base of skull, dural venous sinuses, and brain)
- Meningitis
- Brain abscess
- Death

The diagnosis and management of SBO remains an otolaryngologic challenge. Perhaps the greatest advances in its treatment have resulted from the recognition of SBO as a distinct entity and a clear understanding of its pathophysiology. A team approach involving the cooperation of otolaryngology, endocrinology, and infectious disease may enhance the overall outcome. The advent of the fluoroquinolones and other antipseudomonal antibiotics has significantly lowered the morbidity and mortality associated with SBO.

116.3.3 Conditions Related to External Otitis

Several other infectious and inflammatory diseases are included in the differential diagnosis of otitis externa.

Radiation-Induced Otitis Externa

Another form of otitis externa occasionally occurs after radiotherapy of the region of the external ear. The predominant symptoms result from the inflammation and infection that result when radiotherapy weakens local defense mechanisms and resident bacteria flourish. When the otitis externa is limited to the skin of the EAC, treatment measures, with particular attention to water avoidance, are appropriate. In the worst form of osteoradionecrosis with purulent infection, sequestra of devitalized tissue should be removed and replaced with vascularized tissue.

Bullous External Otitis

Bullous external otitis is a very painful condition in which vesicles or bullae are noted in the bony portion of the external canal. The vesicles are commonly hemorrhagic and should not be ruptured because secondary infection may ensue. *Pseudomonas* may be one of the causative organisms, so appropriate otic drops are recommended. Packing and irrigation of the canal should be avoided because they tend to prolong the course of this disease.

Granular External Otitis

Granular external otitis often resembles the earliest stage of necrotizing external otitis in that there may be small granular plaques or pedunculated granulations in the external canal. This condition may occur in patients who have not been fully treated for a previous episode of external otitis; it may also occur as a result of contact dermatitis (e.g., exposure to hairspray). After the topical or local anesthesia, the removal of granulation tissue, placement of a wick in the canal, and instillation of antibiotic drops will usually resolve the problem. Oral antibiotics should be given if the infection extends beyond the canal. If the patient is diabetic or debilitated, the diagnosis of necrotizing external otitis is entertained and treated appropriately.

Perichondritis and Chondritis

Perichondritis (inflammation of the perichondrium) and chondritis (inflammation of the cartilage) may follow or complicate infections of the EAC or result from accidental or surgical trauma to the auricle. The condition is painful, and the patient often describes severe itching deep within the canal. With time, the skin over the affected area becomes crusted with squamous debris, and the involved cartilage begins to weep. The ear is indurated and erythematous; often, the canal swells shut. The surrounding soft tissues of the face and neck may become involved.

In the mildest stages, thorough débridement and treatment with topical and oral antibiotics are generally sufficient. If these measures do not succeed, the ear is débrided again, and cultures are taken. Appropriate treatment for common pathogens, especially *Pseudomonas*, is begun and tapered according to culture results. Ciprofloxacin is a logical choice for moderate stages, combined with an antipseudomonal drop such as gentamicin or a fluoroquinolone drop.

If the infection spreads to involve regional soft tissues and lymphatics, the patient should be hospitalized and parenteral treatment with adequate coverage for *Pseudomonas* begun. In difficult cases, the ear should be cultured before treatment is started. For patients with recalcitrant infections, infectious disease consultation is often helpful. At every stage of the disease, frequent and thorough débridement of the canal is essential. The metabolic requirements of cartilage are low, and its blood supply is appropriately diminished. Once infection has become established in the perichondrium or cartilage, it is extremely difficult to treat. If subacute or chronic infection, evidenced by inexorable weeping, continues, surgical intervention is indicated.

The affected area is cleansed and injected with local anesthetic containing epinephrine. Incisions are made, and the dissection is taken down to the affected cartilage. If it has lost its normal "pearly white" appearance, it is most likely necrotic and should be excised. Often, necrosis extends farther than can be grossly visualized. Small irrigation drains are placed beneath the flaps and sutured to the skin. The skin flaps are closed. The drainage ports are irrigated with an antibiotic (e.g., 50,000 U of bacitracin dissolved in 250 mL of normal saline). The drains are advanced as the condition resolves. Parenteral antibiotics, otic drops, and aggressive local care continue until the infection has resolved.

Furunculosis and Carbunculosis

Furunculosis and carbunculosis are conditions resulting from gram-positive infections, usually staphylococcal, of the hair follicles. The primary lesion is usually a small, well-circumscribed pustule that may enlarge to become a furuncle or merge with several similar lesions to form a carbuncle. The infection occurs most commonly at the junction of the concha and canal skin.

For treatment to be successful, any accumulated infectious material must be removed. Spontaneous drainage can often be encouraged with the use of warm soaks, supplemented by topical and oral antibiotics and wicks if necessary. If these measures fail to relieve obstruction of the canal, incision and drainage under local anesthesia are indicated.

Infectious Eczematoid Dermatitis

Infectious eczematoid dermatitis results from the drainage of contaminated or purulent material from the middle ear into the floor of the external ear and adjacent infra-auricular skin. This drainage causes a secondary infection or an autosensitization phenomenon manifested by crusted plaques in the canal. Treatment is directed at control of the underlying middle ear infection. Supportive treatment of the external canal reaction consists of the removal of accumulated debris, application of sterile saline soaks to the crusted areas, and application of an antibiotic cream or ointment.

Otomycosis

Otomycosis is a fungal infection of the skin of the external canal. Although fungi may be the primary pathogens, they are usually superimposed on a chronic bacterial infection of the external canal or middle ear. Secondary otomycosis tends to recur if the underlying primary infection is not controlled. All fungi have three basic growth requirements: moisture, warmth, and darkness. Altering moisture will discourage fungal growth. *Aspergillus* species are the most common, usually *A. niger*. If aural culture should grow *A. fumigatus* or *A. flavus*, one should consider a more invasive infection.

Pruritus is the primary clinical complaint. The otoscopic examination commonly reveals a white, black, or dotted gray membrane. Thorough cleaning under a microscope with the patient supine to remove any fungal debris is the first and absolutely most important step in therapy. Thorough aural toilet is supplemented by the topical application of an acidifying solution such as aluminum sulfate–calcium acetate or of a drying powder such as boric acid. Clotrimazole cream or solution may also be used. In the presence of a tympanic membrane perforation or a patent ventilation tube, the application of clotrimazole drops or lotion may be very painful. Thorough cleaning and drying therapies such as powders are best. Metacresyl acetate may be painted on the margin of a perforation or an infected ventilation tube. This is best done under the microscope. This medication should not enter the middle ear cleft because it is quite irritating. In recalcitrant infections, a foreign body such as a ventilation tube acts as the nidus for infection and should be removed. Tympanoplasty is best performed to close an intermittently draining perforation with a superimposed fungal infection.

Gentian violet is usually well tolerated in patients with mastoid cavities, although it is best left out of the middle ear cleft in the presence of a perforation. Because it will permanently stain skin and clothing, small amounts are used with adequate protection of the surrounding area.

Treating physicians should realize that all drops are formulated with moisture and do not persist indefinitely in a homogenized state. Eventually, the water component will separate from the precipitate of the active medical ingredient. Water is exactly what fungi need to grow. Adding drops indefinitely to an ear with otomycosis may prove counterproductive, and an acidifying powder such as boric acid or a compounded powder (as described below) will often help dry an ear with a refractory infection.

Many patients with refractory otomycotic infections may have had previous mastoid surgery, and often the canal wall has been taken down. Because of moderate to severe hearing loss, these patients may need to wear a hearing aid with a closed mold. Careful instruction to the patient, meticulous débridement of the ear, and the use a drying agent such as boric acid powder, chloromycetin–sulfanilamide–amphotericin B powder, or chloromycetin–sulfanilamide–tolnaftate powder will often help clean the cavity. The use of ointments in cavities with closed hearing aids may promote fungal growth due to the accumulation of moisture. In refractory cases, gentian violet or metacresyl acetate may be used topically.

Herpes Zoster and Herpes Simplex

Herpes zoster and herpes simplex are viral infections known to affect the EAC. The patient initially experiences a period of burning pain or localized headache, and vesicles usually appear within several days. When the vesicles coalesce and rupture, crusts are formed. Herpes zoster tends to appear unilaterally in a dermatomic distribution. Involvement of the facial nerve may produce paresis or paralysis (herpes zoster oticus or Ramsay Hunt syndrome). Treatment is supportive, with the topical application of a drying agent, such as hydrogen peroxide, for crusts. The status of the facial nerve is carefully followed; surgical decompression of the facial nerve may be a consideration if it is clinically paralyzed and electrical criteria are met by ENOG testing. Many patients excoriate the blisters, and bacitracin ointment or a suitable substitute should be applied to prevent superinfection. Acyclovir, famciclovir, and valacyclovir have been shown to ameliorate herpetic infections, especially herpes zoster oticus. The latter two have easier dosing schedules and are better absorbed orally than acyclovir. Also, famciclovir may reduce the duration of postherpetic neuralgia. However, it will cause a transitory rise in hepatic enzyme production and must be used with caution.

Dermatoses

Allergic and irritant contact dermatoses may mimic diffuse external otitis. Causative agents may be absolute (so noxious that a reaction occurs in everyone exposed, such as strong acids or alkali) or relative (noxious to susceptible individuals, usually after repeated exposures, such as various soaps or the plastic mold of a hearing aid). Allergic contact dermatitis refers to a delayed hypersensitivity reaction resulting from substances such as poison ivy, nickel compounds (found in some earrings), and rubber compounds (especially in headphones). The typical reaction presents as erythema, weeping, and vesiculation accompanied by itching. The patient may produce a secondary infection by scratching. Treatment consists of removal of the causative agent and the use of topical steroids and astringents. Topical or systemic antibiotics are indicated for the treatment of infection. Systemic steroids may be indicated for severe cases. In rare cases (e.g., a patient with a cochlear implant and hypersensitivity to plastic), the external, ear level receiver/stimulator may be painted with a different material or covered with a cloth casing to separate it from the skin.

External Ear Disease and HIV Infection

Among the external ear manifestations seen in HIV disease is Kaposi sarcoma, which presents with reddish blue lesions typically described as hemorrhagic nodules. The lesions may be discrete or confluent. Although chemotherapy, radiotherapy, and interferon alfa have been used for therapy, the treatment of auricular and canal lesions is rarely necessary. Infections of the external ear in HIV-infected patients are caused by both typical and atypical pathogens. Recurrent herpetic infections and *Pneumocystis carinii*–infected aural polyps have been reported in the EAC as a result of chronic otitis media.

Another external ear manifestation of HIV disease is seborrheic dermatitis, which tends to be more widespread and refractory to treatment than the same condition in HIV-negative patients. Necrotizing external otitis in the HIV-positive patient adds another level of concern regarding its treatment. An infectious disease consultant should be involved in the overall care of the HIV-positive patient. The use of the protease inhibitor medications has made these otologic manifestations exceedingly rare.

116.3.4 Relapsing Polychondritis

Relapsing polychondritis is an intermittently progressive disease marked by the inflammatory destruction of cartilage. Although it is thought to be an autoimmune disorder, the exact cause is unknown. Cartilage of the external ears, larynx, trachea, bronchi, and nose may be involved. The symptoms are episodic, with fever, anemia, erythema, swelling, and pain, and an elevated sedimentation rate is noted during acute episodes. Sparing of the earlobe is the rule and is useful in distinguishing this disease from a cellulitis. As the disease progresses, symptoms of increasing respiratory obstruction may become apparent if tracheal cartilage is involved. Labyrinthine disturbances are rarely present. The diagnosis is made on the basis of the history and physical examination, supported by an elevated sedimentation rate. Biopsy of the involved cartilage may show necrosis, inflammation, and fibrosis. Treatment is with oral corticosteroids, and rarely with intravenous steroids.

116.4 Traumatic Injuries of the External Ear

116.4.1 Blunt Injuries

Shearing forces to the auricle, commonly seen in sports such as boxing and wrestling, may disrupt the normal perichondrium of the auricular cartilaginous framework, causing seroma or hematoma formation. The lobule is composed primarily of fat covered with skin and is less susceptible to injury. Because it is malleable throughout life, auricular cartilage is more likely to be injured by shearing forces than by blunt trauma. It rarely fractures.

If uninfected, very small seromas of the auricle may be observed, and larger ones aspirated. If the seroma reaccumulates, it should be treated under sterile conditions with drainage; a bolster-type dressing with dental rolls and through-and-through, nonabsorbable sutures should be placed to obliterate the potential space for reaccumulation of the seroma. If the seroma is infected, there is a risk that the cartilage itself may become necrotic and lost. The ear should be incised and drained and the patient put on broad-spectrum antibiotic coverage; drains should be placed. The goal is to prevent loss of the cartilaginous frame.

The same principles apply to hematomas of the auricle, except that observation is rarely an option. Because the cartilaginous frame is at greater risk, the hematoma should be drained and a compressive dressing applied with dental rolls sutured on either side. If the hematoma reaccumulates or is very large, drains should be placed, and the ear should be treated until the skin flaps remain flat. Preservation of the cartilaginous framework with prevention of a "cauliflower" or "boxer's" ear is the goal. Once auricular cartilage has been lost and reparative scarring has begun, the auricle is doomed to reparative malformation. Intervention must be undertaken soon after any injury if it is to be effective.

116.4.2 Sharp Trauma to the Auricle

The result of sharp trauma to the auricle may range from a small injury, such as an earlobe torn during piercing, to complete avulsion of the auricle, usually after a motor vehicle accident. The auricle has a plentiful blood supply and as a general rule will heal if the cartilaginous and soft-tissue structures remain even partly attached, less so if complete avulsion has occurred. If remnants or the entire auricle can be salvaged, these should be cleansed and reimplantation attempted in the acute situation.

Torn lobes may be caused by gravity when a heavy earring works its way over time through the lobe or by acute injury when an earring tears through the lobe. Inflammation and infection should be treated. The torn lobe may be repaired in the office; the lobe may be repierced at a later stage.

Animal and human bites of the auricle are by definition contaminated. The edges of the wound must be decontaminated with local antisepsis. Tetanus toxoid should be given. Broad-spectrum antibiotic coverage for the most likely oral flora, including microaerophilic streptococci and anaerobes such as *Bacteroides*, is indicated. If remnants of the auricle have been salvaged, these may be thoroughly washed, decontaminated, and reattached with sutures. If only the auricular cartilage remains, it should be cleaned of soft-tissue attachments, decontaminated, and buried in a subcutaneous pocket (e.g., behind the auricle, in the forearm or abdomen) for later use.

Shearing avulsions are much more difficult to treat. The auricular remnant, if found, may be mangled, torn, or abraded. If a part or all of it appears viable, an attempt at surgical reattachment is worthwhile, with all rules of antisepsis obeyed. However, if it has been lost or is beyond retrieval, the edges of the EAC should be freshened and tacked away and the canal packed with Gelfoam (Pfizer, New York, NY) or another material to help prevent acquired stenosis of the EAC. The patient must then be counseled regarding the main steps of auricular reconstruction (costochondral cartilage harvest, sculpture, and subcutaneous implantation; lobular transposition; auricular lateralization) as required. A very good option in these severe cases is the insertion of osseointegrated titanium posts for anchoring an auricular prosthesis. A well-made auricular prosthetic device for the properly selected patient is an excellent option with very acceptable cosmetic results. As well, porous high-density polyethylene (Medpor; Porex Surgical, Newnan, GA), covered with a vascularized temporoparietal flap, can yield an excellent aesthetic result; however, in many cases, implant exposure or infection has occurred years after surgery with resultant stenosis of the EAC. This type of repair must be chosen carefully with regard to the age and usual activities of the recipient.

116.4.3 Thermal Injuries

Burns of the auricle are classified by their nature (thermal burns, ultra-cooling burns due to frostbite) and the degree of the injury to the skin: first-degree leading to erythema, second-degree (blistering), or third-degree (full-thickness) burns. In first- and second-degree burns, pain is present; in third-degree burns, the sensory nerve endings have been destroyed and the affected area is anesthetic. It is of great importance to elicit a detailed history of the nature and time course of the injury.

Upon inspection, the area may be erythematous and blistered (first- and second-degree burns), blackened with eschar (third-degree burns), or white, hard, and cold (frostbite) as a result of extreme vasoconstriction. It is important to suspect that the extent of the injury extends beyond what is apparent on inspection. This is especially true in electrical injuries. A thermal burn should be cooled quickly with cold/iced compresses to waste the built-up heat within the tissue in an attempt to prevent necrosis by cell expansion and disruption. Frostbite is rewarmed more slowly with warming compresses. If frostbite extends to larger areas of the body, the patient may be placed in a warming bath, or warming intravenous solutions may be used. The extremity should not be rubbed lest shearing forces cause further damage.

Broad-spectrum antibiotic coverage against expected organisms such as *Pseudomonas* species and common skin flora (streptococci and staphylococci) should be given. Topical ointments and creams such as 1% silver sulfadiazine creams may be used. Surgical débridement should be delayed until the wound "declares itself" and a line of demarcation between healthy and dead tissue becomes apparent. Once this has happened, the débridement of dead tissue and application of topical antiseptic ointments may encourage healing in first- and second-degree burns. More severe burns may require split- or full-thickness grafting. There is no reason to rush into repair until the full extent of the injury is obvious. A facial plastic surgeon experienced in the treatment of burns and in reconstructive surgery is an important colleague in the care of patients with thermal and frostbite injuries to the auricle and EAC.

116.4.4 Acid Burn of the External Auditory Canal and Auricle

This rare occurrence causes massive denaturation of the skin, surrounding soft tissue, and supporting cartilage and may result in partial or complete loss of the auricle and EAC. Acids of industrial concentration, such as sulfuric acid and other fortified acids (or alkalis), are the usual agents. The injury is almost never accidental but is part of a criminal assault. As with any chemical burn, the caustic agent must be removed with copious and prolonged irrigation.

If the auricle has been severely damaged, it may ultimately undergo partial or complete autoamputation. A hypertrophic scar and/or keloid will inevitably form and is treated with compressive dressings and/or steroid injections (triamcinolone 10 mg/mL or 40 mg/mL) as necessary. The injured auricle may be allowed to "declare itself," as with thermal and frostbite burns. It is important to inspect the EAC and tympanic membrane and to make every effort to flush any noxious agent from these areas and salvage as much normal tissue as possible. The EAC may be packed with medicated Gelfoam or another packing material.

These types of injuries are almost never isolated but are often part of a much larger picture, including inhalation injuries and trauma to vital internal organs and the extremities. It is important to think "beyond the ear," especially if there has been a history of smoke inhalation. These patients are properly assessed by the trauma and burn services, as well as otolaryngology.

116.4.5 Fractures of the External Auditory Canal

Foreign objects placed into the EAC may cause lacerations of the canal. These types of injuries are rare. Far more common are injuries to the EAC caused by trauma to adjacent structures. Because of its anatomical boundaries, the EAC is susceptible to injuries associated with trauma of the temporomandibular joint (e.g., a blow to the jaw) or fractures of the temporal bone, most commonly longitudinal fractures.

Inspection of the EAC reveals a "step" deformity of the canal. A flail piece of bone may be seen, with or without an accompanying laceration. Passive movement of the jaw may cause the bone fragment to move.

The patient should be inspected for additional areas of injury, both fractures of the jaw and other otologic injuries, such as traumatic perforation of the tympanic membrane, damage to the ossicular chain, facial nerve injury, and injury to the vestibular labyrinth. A tuning fork test should, at a minimum, be done; ideally, a screening audiogram should be performed. Radiographic studies (e.g., mandibular views, panorex, CT of the petrous temporal bones) should be obtained as indicated.

Treatment is of the underlying cause; if the mandible has been fractured, the fracture must be reduced and the patient usually placed in intermaxillary fixation. Temporal bone fractures, even those associated with cerebrospinal fluid (CSF) otorrhea, are ordinarily observed, with the patient placed in bed at about 45 degrees until the CSF otorrhea subsides. The ear should not be manipulated. If there is witnessed and progressive facial nerve dysfunction, in which case the likely site of injury is at the geniculate ganglion, the nerve is followed clinically and electrically with serial ENOG and/or needle electromyographic studies and may need to be decompressed.

If a flail piece of bone in the EAC, usually at the scutum or tympanomastoid suture line, becomes infected or otherwise bothersome, it may be removed. It is rarely necessary to repair soft-tissue lacerations. The EAC may be packed with Gelfoam moistened with otologic drops or another packing material.

116.5 Noninflammatory Lesions of the External Ear

116.5.1 Lesions of the Auricle

Congenital Lesions

Preauricular Skin Tags

These consist of redundant tissue, usually comprising skin and fat, found near or just anterior to the tragus. If the mass contains cartilage, it is a remnant of auricular tissue, left over from auricular development. It may be a duplication of one or several of the ectodermal hillocks of His. Preauricular skin tags or auricular remnants are nonfunctional, and most parents request that they be removed. However, they may carry with them cultural connotations, such as a child being "favored." If held on with only a soft-tissue stalk, the skin tag may be lassoed with a silk suture, tied at the base, and allowed to undergo necrosis and fall off. If cartilage is found within the lesion, excision should be done in the operating room, with the knowledge that the facial nerve may be very superficial in young children. The patient is seen as needed until the scar has healed. Electrocautery is rarely necessary in the excision of these lesions and should be used carefully.

Preauricular Pits

These are depressions or sinuses lined with squamous or columnar epithelium that are found in front of the anterior root of the helix. They are heritable and often bilateral; inheritance is thought to be in an autosomal-dominant fashion with variable expression. The pits may elaborate keratin and/or mucous and may become infected. If quiescent, they are observed. If filled with uninfected debris, they may be treated with warm compresses and the material expressed from outside the opening. If the pit or sinus becomes recurrently infected, it may require excision. It is important to remove the entire tract if it is excised.

First Branchial Cleft Cysts, Sinuses, and Fistulas

These result from anomalous duplication of the EAC and may occur between the EAC and structures anterior or inferior to the auricle, including the neck. They are classified according to the Work system. Work type I anomalies contain only ectodermal derivatives and may be thought of as a "parallel" duplication of the EAC. Work type II anomalies contain both ectodermal and mesodermal derivatives and may be found extending between the EAC and the parotid in any relationship to the extratemporal facial nerve, including bisecting the nerve. The treatment of first branchial cleft cysts, sinuses, and fistulas is by excision. These anomalies may contain keratin debris that can become infected. If infected, they may require incision and drainage, but this is not recommended if it can be avoided. The cyst, sinus, or fistula may be gently probed with a sterile, malleable lacrimal probe or another suitable instrument to map out its pathway. The opening may be gently filled with dye such as methylene blue before excision. A rim of tissue around the internal opening is resected with the specimen, and every attempt is made to excise the tract in toto, leaving none of it behind. If the tract is suspected to course in any relation to the extratemporal facial nerve, the excision should be done in a more formal way. A modified Blair incision is made and the parotid is exposed, as is the facial nerve at least from the stylomastoid foramen to the pes anserinus and distal branching points, with the use of intraoperative facial nerve monitoring. The cyst, sinus, or fistula must be carefully dissected from the intact and stimulated facial nerve. The first attempt at excision is usually the most thorough because the anatomy of the lesion is best preserved. With each incision and each subsequent surgical attempt at removal, the anatomy becomes more distorted and the chance of complete resection less.

Cutaneous Cysts

Cysts of ectodermal and sebaceous origin may be found in any relationship the auricle. If growing and painful, a cyst should be excised along with an ellipse of skin over the lesion to be used as a soft-tissue "handle," allowing excision of the cyst with its tract and surrounding soft tissue. It is important to make every attempt to identify and excise every bit of the cyst lining; there always is one. If the cyst has become acutely infected and is ready to burst, the patient is treated with oral antibiotics and warm soaks. The cyst may need to be incised and drained, but this is not optimal. Once the acute infection has subsided, the cyst should be excised.

Acquired Lesions

Chondrodermatitis Nodularis Chronica (Winker Nodule)

This is a benign lesion with the appearance of a "punched-out crater." It is found most commonly in older men at the rim of the helix, as well as in other areas of the auricle. It is thought to be caused by the breakdown of elastic fibers due to chronic sun exposure. The lesion may be painful to touch or pressure. This distinguishes it from other dermatologic lesions, such as senile keratosis, keratoacanthoma, cutaneous horn, and skin cancer (squamous or basal cell), which are usually painless.

Treatment is by full-thickness excision that includes the supporting cartilage. The defect is reconstructed with a full-thickness skin graft or local advancement flaps.

Gouty Tophi of the Auricle

These are deposits of uric acid in crystalline form in the auricle, often at the helix. The patient will have hyperuricemia and should have other markings of gout, such as arthropathy(ies) and involvement of the great toe(s). Serologic markers for uric acid will confirm the suspected underlying diagnosis. If quiescent, the nodule may be observed. If painful or inflamed, it is removed under local anesthesia. Histopathologic examination will reveal fusiform, washed-out casts of monosodium urate with an accompanying inflammatory surround: polymorphonuclear leukocytes, histiocytes, and foreign body giant cells.

The patient should be treated for gout with the daily administration of allopurinol. Colchicine and other anti-inflammatory medications are used for acute exacerbations.

Bacterial Perichondritis

This is distinguished from relapsing polychondritis, which is a nonbacterial autoimmune condition that is treated with steroids. Bacterial perichondritis is distinguished by crusting, weeping, and exudate from the auricle and by pus. If there are signs of bacterial infection, the ear must be treated with antibiotics.

Infection of the perichondrium of the auricle and supporting cartilage is an urgent problem. It may be a sequela of otologic surgery or trauma, or it may follow external otitis. Predisposing factors include diabetes and any cause of relative immunosuppression. The patient presents with a swollen, painful, erythematous auricle, usually crusting and weeping. Swabs are taken for Gram stain, culture, and sensitivity. The most common organism isolated is *P. aeruginosa*. Oral antibiotics with good gramnegative coverage, such as fluoroquinolones, should be started along with warm soaks. Treatment may begin at home, but the patient must be seen frequently, even daily, until the ear either improves or fails to. In the latter case, the patient should be hospitalized, broad-spectrum intravenous antibiotics started, and drains placed under the skin of the auricle and irrigated with an antibiotic solution such as bacitracin. Diabetes must be brought under strict control; patients often require a sliding scale of insulin. Necrotic cartilage should be excised and every effort taken to save as much of the cartilaginous auricular framework as possible.

Sebaceous Cysts

These true cystic collections occur as a result of sebaceous gland obstruction. They have a true lining and may occur anywhere in the head and neck. The scalp, nape of the neck, and auricle are favored sites. If small and nonpainful, they may be observed. The acutely infected sebaceous cyst is treated with a broad-spectrum oral antibiotic and may occasionally have to be drained. If it becomes larger and painful, the sebaceous cyst is excised, with care take to remove all of the cyst lining. This is best done when the cyst is distended and not infected. If any of the cyst lining is left behind, it will likely regrow.

Neoplasia of the Auricle and External Auditory Canal

The auricle and EAC may give rise to both benign and malignant neoplasia, based upon the cell of origin. Benign processes include actinic keratosis, papilloma, and other lesions. Cancers of the auricle and EAC include basal cell carcinoma, squamous cell carcinoma, and melanoma (melanotic and amelanotic). Rarer cancers of the auricle and EAC include Kaposi sarcoma (now much less frequent in HIV disease since the advent of protease inhibitors and other reverse transcriptase inhibitors) and ceruminous adenocarcinoma, seen either alone or in association with multiple cylindromas of the scalp, face, and EAC.

Malignancies with the potential for hematogenous metastasis to the temporal bone (but not necessarily to the auricle or EAC) include renal cell carcinoma, small (oat cell) adenocarcinoma of the lung, breast cancer, cancer of the prostate, and cutaneous melanoma.

In the majority of skin cancers, malignancy is an end-stage result of chronic sun (actinic) exposure. The amount and longevity of sun exposure are of the greatest importance. Tanning lotions with protection against the ultraviolet ways of the sun are of relative recent widespread use. A thorough history of sun exposure, the work history (indoor vs. outside work), and a history of the use of tight-fitting ear molds leading to chronic irritation of the EAC should be elicited.

Slowly growing malignancies such as basal cell cancer may persist for years before the patient seeks help. Far less frequently, advanced cancers of the auricle may occur as part of an aggressive picture of skin cancer, especially squamous cell carcinoma of high grade. In this small number of cases, the auricle and/or skin of the EAC must be partially or completely resected, possibly with a neck dissection and possibly with a lateral temporal bone resection, and the wound closed with local, pedicled, or free vascularized flaps. The extent of the disease, assessed by clinical examination, radiographic examination, and examination of the histopathologic margins, will determine the extent of the dissection. Surveillance and local control may help to avoid these more advanced cases.

116.5.2 Lesions of the External Auditory Canal

Keratosis Obdurans

This is an acute-upon-chronic condition of the external ear in which the EAC is plugged by an accumulation of dense, inspis-sated keratin debris. Acute infection, swelling, pain, and hearing loss follow. In very advanced cases, in response to chronic irritation and infection, the normally thin architecture of the squamous epithelium lining the canal may become lichenified, and the canal may be plugged by dense debris and secondarily stenotic.

The typical patient with this problem is elderly, often in a nursing home in which care of the ear is neglected. If and when the ear becomes acutely infected, the patient will be brought to the otologist. It is important to distinguish this entity, if possible, from acute otitis externa, osteomyelitis of the skull base, and other plausible conditions. The history usually yields the answer if it can be accurately obtained.

These ears are difficult to treat, in large measure because of pain, but will usually respond well to careful, thorough cleaning under microscopic vision in the office, rarely in the operating room, and very rarely under general anesthesia. The ears are exquisitely painful to clean, and thus pain must be eliminated before aural toilet. The patient may require a four-quadrant block of the EAC with local anesthesia. Most patients will allow the ear to be cleansed in the office. There is usually an "onion skin" appearance to the epithelial debris because it has been collecting for many months to years. Although the diagnosis is apparent with gross inspection, material should be sent for pathologic examination to ascertain that this is keratin debris and nothing else. The physician may not be able to clean the ear completely in one sitting; the patient may need to return for several sessions and the ear be medicated with an appropriate acidifying solution between visits.

The important difference between this and other, similar conditions, such as cholesteatoma of the EAC, is that once it is completely cleaned and topically medicated, the ear with keratosis obdurans will often slowly and gradually revert back toward a healthy appearance. The change toward health may be quite remarkable once aural toilet commences. The inciting event of dense packing of squamous debris and superinfection has been cured, and the ear can now resume a more normal appearance. This does not happen with external ear cholesteatoma. Prevention of recurrence is via appropriate ototopic therapy and routine office-based débridement.

External Auditory Canal Cholesteatoma

This is a cyst of squamous debris found in the EAC. It has many features in common with primary acquired cholesteatoma: it has an active matrix that elaborates keratin debris, and it may locally erode bone and soft tissue. Unlike keratosis obdurans, it does not revert toward a normal state once obstruction and local infection have been relieved and treated. There may be an antecedent history of trauma, otologic surgery, acquired stenosis, or chronic inflammation, but most patients have no identifiable cause. The tympanic ring, especially its anterior and inferior aspects, is a favored site for EAC cholesteatoma. The patient may initially present with otologic complaints due to blockage by keratin debris: hearing loss, fullness, symptoms of infection, rarely dizziness or vertigo, and most rarely involvement of the facial nerve.

An edge-enhanced CT of the temporal bones reveals features of cholesteatoma with bony erosion and scalloped edges. EAC cholesteatoma is usually a localized disease process, often unilateral, bilateral in fewer patients. Depending upon the site and size of the EACC, there may be normal hearing, hearing loss of a conductive or mixed nature, or, if the otic capsule has been violated, anacusis. Facial nerve involvement is rare.

The mainstay of treatment is routine office-based débridement, advice to the patient about water precautions, and the judicious use of acidifying drops and/or powders as needed. If the EAC cholesteatoma becomes obstructed, rendering the ear difficult to clean, limited localized surgery including meatoplasty may be indicated to facilitate aural toilet. Surgery to eradicate all foci of the cholesteatoma has proved of little value, and so EAC cholesteatoma, unlike primary and secondary cholesteatoma of the middle ear and mastoid, is managed medically, not surgically. There is really very little need for surgery in even the most advanced cases.

The surgeon must also have a precise mental road map of the problem with microscopic detail. This may be facilitated by CT, but there is no substitute for careful microscopic evaluation. In very advanced cases, the jugular bulb, tympanic facial nerve, and structures of the otic capsule may be exposed. Extreme caution must be used in dealing with these most delicate structures.

Having the patient soften the squamous debris at home for several days with an organic solvent (baby oil, olive oil, docusate) before scheduled office débridement will greatly facilitate cleaning. If inner ear structures of the vestibular labyrinth have been exposed, the patient may experience precipitous and violent vertigo due to the caloric effect of the suction. It is best to débride the ear manually under the microscope with small tools such as a cerumen loop, round knife, or alligator forceps while the patient is in the supine position, and to use a minimal amount of suction just at the end of the cleaning. Because cleaning may be needed as often as every 3 to 4 months, the physician and patient must work together to achieve the best system that will keep the erosive potential of EAC cholesteatoma in check and cause the least amount of discomfort to the patient.

It is important to be aware of developmental defects in the formation of the tympanic ring that may lead to chronic irritation, weeping, and the collection of keratin debris and so mimic cholesteatoma of the EAC and other entities. A persistent foramen tympanicum, or foramen of Huschke, is an anatomical variation of the tympanic portion of the temporal bone due to a defect in normal ossification of the tympanic ring during the first 5 years of life. It is not a true foramen because no neurovascular structures traverse it; rather, it is is a defect of tympanic bone ossification due to abnormal mechanical forces during early postnatal life or to genetic factors, thus far undefined. Its location is at the anteroinferior aspect of the EAC, posteromedial to the temporomandibular joint. Based on retrospective radiographic series, persistent foramen tympanicum has been estimated to occur in 4.6 to 9.1% of individuals, with an average dimension of 4.2 mm in the axial plane and 3.6 mm in the sagittal plane. CT of the temporal bone performed at thin intervals (0.6-mm section thickness, 0.3-mm section increment) with an ultra-high resolution filter will best image this entity if it is present.

Persistent foramen tympanicum, or foramen of Huschke, should be kept in the differential diagnosis in cases of refractory chronic otitis externa and especially of cholesteatoma of the EAC. It may predispose the patient to injury of the EAC, tympanic membrane, or middle ear cleft during temporomandibular joint arthroscopy and may facilitate the spread of infection or tumor from the EAC into the infratemporal fossa and vice versa.

Cerumen Impaction

The subject of wax impaction may seem banal, but few other conditions in our specialty can be remedied within a single office visit to the tremendous relief and satisfaction of the patient. Many patients with wax impaction will present with hearing loss, fullness, tinnitus, autophony, and rarely imbalance or vertigo. The history and physical examination, including tuning fork testing, will usually confirm the diagnosis and exclude other causes. Most patients will admit to using cotton squabs and other foreign bodies in the EAC. Patients wearing tightly fitting hearing aid molds or other ear pieces may be predisposed to wax impaction. The treatment and prevention of wax impaction, however nonglamorous, are fundamental to what we do, and one should develop a reliable method to care for this most common problem.

Realizing that the ear is exquisitely sensitive, especially an erstwhile normal EAC now impacted with wax, the physician must treat carefully, cautiously, slowly, and with reassurance. Patients can tolerate many manipulations of the ear if what will be done is explained to them and is done slowly. A few extra seconds of counsel and reassurance are well worth the effort. All reasonable attempts should be made to thoroughly clean wax impactions in *one* office visit.

There are a few important factors to remember: (1) Avoid blind, forceful irrigation. (2) The patient should assume a comfortable position, which may vary from sitting to lying recumbent. (3) The physician should anticipate a vasovagal response and be prepared to treat it immediately because it may occur with any instrumentation of the EAC. (4) A microscope provides better visualization than a hand-held otoscope, as well as the ability to work bimanually. (5) Reassure the patient; a relaxed patient will allow a more thorough procedure. (6) Use reasonable techniques for a reasonable length of time. (7) Have pressed gelatin foam and alligator forceps readily available, which can be applied focally if the canal skin is abraded during manipulation. (8) Inspect all parts of the tympanic membrane to look for other signs of disease, such as a perforation or attic retraction cholesteatoma, after the ears have been cleaned.

Patients should be counseled to avoid placing any foreign body into the ear to clean it. A weekly rinse of 3% hydrogen peroxide or an acidifying drop may help the ear to cleanse itself. However, some patients will require manual débridement at regular intervals to maintain canal patency.

Foreign Body

Foreign bodies in the EAC may be either organic or inorganic. Several broad principles must be observed in treating a patient with a suspected or known foreign body, all based upon common sense. (1) For young children, "if one foreign body, there may be two or three." Remember to check the nose in addition to the ears for foreign bodies. (2) Living foreign bodies (usually insects) must be killed first, then removed. The patient is usually quite bothered by the beating of an insect's wings or other movement. This is silenced with lidocaine or mineral oil. (3) Batteries and acid-eluting foreign bodies must be removed as soon as possible because they may cause extensive chemical burns to the EAC. This is a rather urgent otologic situation, and the patient should be treated in the office or operating room without delay. (4) Do not attempt to remove foreign objects, such as beans or bugs, with irrigation because they may swell and compound the problem. (5) The ear is exquisitely sensitive. A patient who cannot tolerate the pain may need to be immobilized to prevent tympanic membrane or middle ear injury during removal of the foreign body. For an uncooperative or hysterical patient, general anesthesia may be required. (6) Only an experienced physician with proper instruments and magnification and in the proper setting should attempt to remove any foreign body from the EAC. If these are not available, the patient should be taken to the operating room. (7) A reasonable attempt to establish audition in the ear in question with at least a tuning fork test should be made before the removal of a densely impacted foreign body.

Aural Polyp

Polyps are soft-tissue masses, usually circumscribed and glistening, that often obstruct the EAC. An aural polyp may be thought of as a flag—an indicator of an underlying disease such as chronic otitis media or a cholesteatoma with concomitant inflammation. The polyp usually arises from the middle ear mucosa (respiratory epithelium) but may arise directly from the tympanic membrane as a reaction to a foreign body, such as a ventilation tube.

An aural polyp is often a physical obstruction to local medical treatment of disease in the EAC. Polyps may be treated in several ways: locally with astringents (e.g., silver nitrate, trichloroacetic acid, 20% phenol) to reduce the mass of the polyp or by removal. Astringents tend to work well because of the myxedematous nature of polyps; they are inflammatory tissue and contain a lot of water. Reducing this fraction alone will shrink the mass and allow topical therapy to start working.

An aural polyp must be removed with caution. The surgeon should have a clear idea of the most likely site of origin: a perforation, a cholesteatoma, or a foreign body reaction to a tube. If there is any suspicion that the polyp is attached to a deeper structure, such as the facial nerve, the stapes footplate, or a dehiscence of the vestibular labyrinth, or if a herniation of the meninges and/or brain (meningoencephalocele, encephalocele) cannot be excluded, the polyp should not be manipulated until definitive radiologic studies (CT and/or MR imaging with and without +/- contrast) more precisely define the anatomical site of origin.

The polyp, once grasped with an appropriately sized instrument, should be "smeared" and never forcibly removed from the ear. An inflammatory polyp will easily yield to gentle manipulation. Another underlying disease process may be more resistant, and again, the polyp should never be removed with force.

All material removed from the body must be sent for pathologic examination, and an aural polyp is no exception. Once removed, the polyp should be examined histologically, even if the tissue removed has all of the gross features of a polyp, and definitely identified as an inflammatory polyp; other entities, such as glial tissue, brain, and neoplasm, must be excluded.

Dermatologic Conditions of the External Auditory Canal

The EAC may be thought of as a blind pouch lined with skin. There are several differences between the skin of the EAC and skin elsewhere in the body. Specialized systems, such as the apopilosebaceous unit and ceruminous glands, are present in the skin of the EAC, but not elsewhere. The EAC is thus susceptible to many of the dermatologic processes found elsewhere in the body. Much of what otologists treat may be generally classified as chronic otitis externa, but the EAC may also manifest purely local problems, such as contact dermatitis and neurodermatitis (lichen simplex chronicus). The EAC may also manifest systemic conditions such as psoriasis, eczema, atopic dermatitis, seborrheic dermatitis, acne vulgaris, and sarcoidosis.

The patient may present with an acute otitis externa and typical symptoms of itching, serous or mucous drainage, fullness, and hearing loss. The history is a key feature toward a correct diagnosis. Both ears must be given careful scrutiny under the microscope, and the physician will often see a similar state in the EAC for many dermatologic conditions. Very dry skin and signs of mechanical excoriation aid in determining the root cause; the baseline problem is that the skin is too dry, leading to pruritus, scratching, and violation of the skin and its lymphatics. The result is a perfect setup for acute otitis externa: a warm, moist, dark environment—just what bacteria and fungi need for growth. This set of otologic problems is cyclical. The baseline is "too dry," but acute exacerbations may cause the ear to become moist and acutely infected.

Drops do not remain drops forever; eventually, they become the residue of the drops and the liquid into which the active ingredient of the drops was dissolved. Therefore, drops add fluid and often water to the ear, again providing an enhanced environment for bacterial overgrowth. Desiccating powders are often a better choice in the acutely infected, moist ear. Once the ear has reached its "baseline," gentle moistening with steroid oils (e.g., fluocinolone 0.01% oil; prednisolone forte 1% ophthalmologic solution) or creams/ointments (triamcinolone 0.025%) once or twice a week may maintain the ear. The patient must be cautioned not to instrument the ear.

Unfortunately, chronic otitis externa is poorly understood by most general physicians and also by many otolaryngologists. The typical patient has been treated with several different drops in the hope that finding "the perfect drop" will solve the problem. Ultimately, there is no *cure* for many of these conditions, but the treatment of acute exacerbations and the judicious use of steroids will go a long way to help care for the patient.

Osteomas and Exostoses of the External Auditory Canal

Osteomas

Osteomas (▶ Fig. 116.4) of the external auditory canal are true neoplasms; they are often unilateral, solitary, and peduncu-

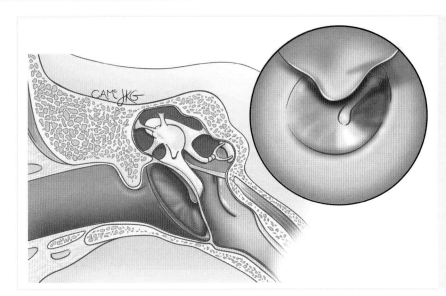

Fig. 116.4 (a) Coronal and **(b)** sagittal section of a right ear showing a single stalk of an osteoma.

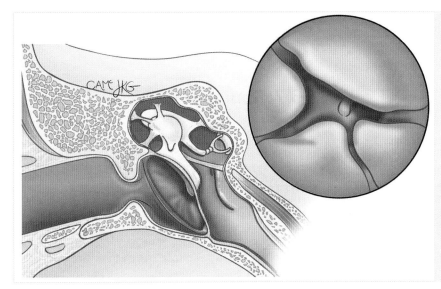

Fig. 116.5 (a) Coronal and **(b)** sagittal section of a right ear showing broad-based growth centers of exostoses.

lated, and they are not related to exposure to cold water or air. They usually occur at the tympanosquamous suture line in a more lateral location than exostoses. A solitary, large osteoma may fill a good portion of the EAC, causing all of the problems of advanced exostoses. On CT, an osteoma may be more heterogeneous, with areas of cancellous bone, and less dense than an exostosis. Usually, a stalk leading to the osteoma can be seen under the microscope or on CT.

Exostoses

Exostoses (▸ Fig. 116.5 and ▸ Fig. 116.6) of the EAC are acquired, benign, broad-based growths of bone occurring within the EAC, most often near the tympanomastoid or tympanosquamous suture line. They are often bilateral and more advanced in one ear than in the other. Exostoses are not true neoplasms. They are bony calluses or hyperostoses arising from the tympanic ring. They typically do not have a stalk. The presumed pathophysiology is refrigeration osteitis, the effect of chronic exposure of the bone of the EAC to cold water or air in activities such as swimming, surfing, skiing, and boating.

If the one or several bony lesions are small and most of the tympanic membrane is clearly visible, the ear is observed. There are several reasons to shave down an exostosis or to remove an osteoma:

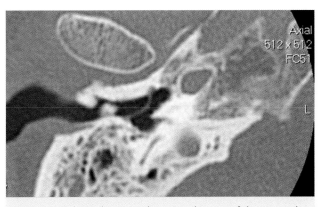

Fig. 116.6 Right axial computed tomographic scan of the temporal bone showing exostoses.

1. The patient has recurrent infections of the EAC. Trapped squamous debris and wax will become a nidus of recurrent EAC infections, and the obstruction should be removed.
2. The patient has conductive hearing loss due to wax/debris impaction. With severe obstruction(s), even a small amount of wax and debris will cause conductive hearing loss.
3. The usual bony and soft tissue landmarks are less distinct. It is not wise to wait this long because the surgeon must rely upon landmarks of the EAC to perform the surgery.
4. It will allow the patient to be properly fitted with a hearing aid.

Exostoses may occur along with other conditions (e.g., otosclerosis). If the exostoses are too large for the usual transcanal approach to be used, they should be removed from the ear with the greater hearing loss. The ear should be allowed to heal, the hearing retested, and then the stapedectomy performed.

All patients for whom surgery is being considered must have a formal hearing test and an edge-enhanced, noncontrast CT of the temporal bones to show landmarks around the bony lesion(s): the tympanic membrane, middle ear and ossicular chain, and tympanic and vertical course of the facial nerve. The surgeon should have a very good idea during the preoperative preparation not only of what the ear looks like under the microscope, but also of what radiologic landmarks will help to guide the dissection.

Surgery may be done through the EAC or through a postauricular approach. The important word is to "shave" the exostosis(es) carefully. Exostoses grow slowly, and by the time the patient requires surgery, these lesions have been present for many years; it is highly unlikely that they will grow back any more quickly. Therefore, there is no need to remove every millimeter of neo-ossification. A reasonable goal is to be able to see most of the perimeter of the tympanic membrane and to know that the EAC, after it heals, will be large enough to hold an ITC (in the canal) hearing aid mold. Because of the proximity of the vertical portion of the facial nerve and the tympanic membrane, nothing more than shaving the bone need be done. It is wise to perform this surgery under general anesthesia and to monitor the facial nerve electrophysiologically.

In the extremely rare cases in which all landmarks have been lost, it is best to dissect anteriorly and superiorly, where the facial nerve is unlikely to be found, until a known landmark (such as the tympanic membrane) is encountered. Approaching from behind while the vascular strip is retracted with a Penrose drain or another suitable retractor may also provide landmark clues.

The surgical technique for the removal of an osteoma is somewhat more straightforward and simpler than that for exostoses. The lesion is ordinarily removed via a transcanal approach, but a postauricular approach may be required for an extremely large osteoma. Because there is ordinarily a stalk leading to the osteoma, it can be tapped with a 2- to 4-mm nasal osteotome and the osteoma delivered. The remaining stalk can be shaved down with a diamond bur. The remainder of the care is the same as with exostoses.

Although the patient is ordinarily asked to give consent for a split-thickness skin graft, this is almost never necessary because of the redundancy of skin over the exostoses or osteoma.

The skin of the EAC is incised in a horizontal fashion around the midpoint of the lesion(s) with a round knife or similar instrument, and the skin is "window-shaded" fore and aft away from the bony growth, which is then shaved with an appropriately sized diamond bur or tapped out with an osteotome. Once the bony growths have been reduced and the tympanic membrane is easily seen, the remaining skin is placed back flat and trimmed if necessary, and the EAC is packed for about 3 to 4 weeks. The patient must be advised that the ear will take about 6 to 8 weeks to heal properly. It is extremely rare to have to revise this type of surgery if it is done carefully and conservatively.

116.6 Conclusion

With a thorough knowledge of the normal embryology, anatomy, and physiology of the external ear, in addition to an understanding of the natural history of the various common disease processes that occur in this location, the treatment of the patient with external ear disease becomes logical. However, it is not always easy. Most conditions can be managed with the recommendations outlined in this chapter. There is no substitute for patience and thoroughness.

116.7 Roundsmanship

- An understanding of the various disease entities occurring in the external ear is predicated on a knowledge of the embryology, anatomy, and physiology of the canal.
- Infection and blockage of the apopilosebaceous unit are the precursors of infectious otitis externa.
- Otitis externa presents as a spectrum of disease and may be classified into preinflammatory, acute inflammatory, and chronic inflammatory stages.
- Four principles form the basis of treatment for all stages of infection of the external ear: thorough cleaning, antibiotic therapy, control of inflammation and pain, and recommendations to prevent infection. Of these, the first is the cornerstone of therapy.
- Recalcitrant and recurrent otitis externa must be treated aggressively with daily local care and antibiotics, often in the hospital. Patience and thoroughness are needed for successful treatment.
- Necrotizing external otitis is a disease occurring in immunosuppressed patients. It must enter the differential diagnosis of any patient with nonresolving acute external otitis.
- There are four hallmarks of necrotizing external otitis: persistent otalgia; persistent otorrhea and granulation tissue; diabetes mellitus, advanced age, or immunocompromised state; and cranial nerve involvement.
- Necrotizing external otitis must be treated aggressively. Management includes proper radiographic imaging to map the extent of disease, meticulous local care, control of diabetes or immunodeficiency (when possible), and antibiotics. Surgery is rarely required. Mortality remains significant in patients with cranial nerve involvement.

116.8 Recommended Reading

[1] Carfrae MJ, Kesser BW. Malignant otitis externa. Otolaryngol Clin North Am 2008; 41: 537–549

[2] Chandler JR. Malignant external otitis and osteomyelitis of the base of the skull. Am J Otol 1989; 10: 108–110

[3] Chandler JR. Malignant external otitis. Laryngoscope 1968; 78: 1257–1294

[4] Damiani JM, Damiani KK, Kinney SE. Malignant external otitis with multiple cranial nerve involvement. Am J Otol 1979; 1: 115–120

[5] Darr EA, Linstrom CJ. Conservative management of advanced external auditory canal cholesteatoma. Otolaryngol Head Neck Surg 2010; 142: 278–280

[6] Gangadar SS, Kwartler JA. Skull base osteomyelitis secondary to malignant otitis externa. Curr Opin Otolaryngol Head Neck Surg. 2003; 11: 316–323

[7] Lacout A, Marsot-Dupuch K, Smoker WRK, Lasjaunias P. Foramen tympanicum, or foramen of Huschke: pathologic cases and anatomic CT study. AJNR Am J Neuroradiol 2005; 26: 1317–1323

[8] Okpala NC, Siraj QH, Nilssen E, Pringle M. Radiological and radionuclide investigation of malignant otitis externa. J Laryngol Otol 2005; 119: 71–75

[9] Raines JM, Schindler RA. The surgical management of recalcitrant malignant external otitis. Laryngoscope 1980; 90: 369–378

[10] Shupak A, Greenberg E, Hardoff R, Gordon C, Melamed Y, Meyer WS. Hyperbaric oxygenation for necrotizing (malignant) otitis externa. Arch Otolaryngol Head Neck Surg 1989; 115: 1470–1475

[11] Toulmouche MA. Observations d'otorrhée cérébrale suivis des réflexions. Gazette Medicale de Paris 1838; 6: 422–426

[12] Van Gilse PHG. Des observations ultérieures sur la genèse des exostoses du conduit externe par l'irrigations d'eau froide. Acta Otolaryngol 1938; 26: 343

[13] Weber PC, Seabold JE, Graham SM, Hoffmann HH, Simonson TM, Thompson BH. Evaluation of temporal and facial osteomyelitis by simultaneous In-WBC/Tc-99m-MDP bone SPECT scintigraphy and computed tomography scan. Otolaryngol Head Neck Surg 1995; 113: 36–41

[14] Work WP. Newer concepts of first branchial cleft defects. Laryngoscope 1972; 82: 1581–1593

117 Conditions of the Middle Ear and Mastoid

Ronald A. Hoffman

117.1 Introduction

Conditions of the middle ear and mastoid can be categorized as infectious/inflammatory, neoplastic, metabolic/genetic, and iatrogenic/traumatic. Because of anatomical and physiologic interdependency, diseases arising in the middle ear often affect the mastoid, and vice versa. Disease limited to the middle ear usually presents as hearing loss or otorrhea. Mastoid disease may be silent, unless there is an acute suppurative component or associated bone destruction. Facial nerve paresis or paralysis, vertigo, or central nervous system complications may implicate mastoid extension.

117.2 Infectious/Inflammatory Conditions

117.2.1 Otitis Media with Effusion

The most common disorders of the middle ear are infectious/inflammatory, in particular otitis media (OM) of childhood (▶ Fig. 117.1). Otitis media is the most common reason for childhood visits to the pediatrician, and it is estimated that 80% of children will have at least one episode by the age of 5 years. Otitis media can be subdivided into two general types: otitis media with effusion (previously and often still referred to as serous otitis media) and acute otitis media (previously called acute suppurative otitis media). Otitis media with effusion and acute otitis media result from poor eustachian tube function and the general immunologic immaturity of childhood. The

eustachian tube, lined with upper respiratory tract mucosa, is normally closed but is opened by the action of the muscles of chewing and swallowing. Normal eustachian tube function allows aeration of the middle ear space and contiguous mastoid air cell system, as well as egress of the secretions from the middle ear. The eustachian tube becomes obstructed in children in association with upper respiratory tract mucosal diseases, primary ciliary dyskinesia, enlarged adenoids, and adenoid infection, and in association with general anatomical and physiologic immaturity. Eustachian tube dysfunction in adults usually results from upper respiratory tract mucosal disease, an acquired disease such Wegener granulomatosis, or nasopharyngeal malignancy. A unilateral serous otitis media in an adult (particularly one of Chinese origin and especially one with ipsilateral cervical lymphadenopathy) without a history of preceding upper respiratory tract infection or barotrauma should alert the clinician to the possibility of nasopharyngeal carcinoma.

When the eustachian tube fails to function normally, middle ear gases are absorbed by the middle ear mucosa, creating negative middle ear pressure. Negative pressure and the activation of inflammatory mediators cause the egress of fluid into the middle ear, creating otitis media with effusion. Such fluid usually resolves spontaneously as the pathology affecting the eustachian tube resolves. The most common symptoms of otitis media with effusion are ear fullness and hearing loss. In many children, particularly younger children, otitis media with effusion may be asymptomatic. Physical findings include a dull and immobile tympanic membrane that does not move on pneumatic otoscopy. There may be a visible air–fluid level or air bubbles in the middle ear.

In otherwise healthy children who have no speech or language delays and no evolving pathologic changes to the tympanic membrane, the treatment of otitis media with effusion can be expectant observation, often for 6 to 9 months. If there is upper airway disease, treatment should be oriented toward improving upper airway health, with secondary improvement in eustachian tube function. Oral decongestants and steroid nasal sprays are often useful in the presence of active upper airway disease, but there is little evidence that these modalities are of value in the absence of such pathology. A course of oral antibiotics is reasonable, even though otitis media with effusion does not present with the signs or symptoms of the acute infection of otitis media (see below). Studies have shown that as many as 30% of fluid specimens from patients who have otitis media with effusion may be culture-positive. However, antibiotics are not recommended as prophylaxis to prevent otitis media with effusion, particularly with the increased incidence of antibiotic-resistant microbes.

Ultimately, if middle ear fluid does not resolve, a myringotomy with insertion of a ventilation tube is indicated. This surgical procedure is usually performed under light general anesthesia. A small incision is made in the tympanic membrane (myringotomy), and a ventilating tube is placed into the incision. Small ventilation tubes will usually remain in place and aerate the middle ear for 6 to 9 months. Longer-lasting tubes should be reserved for recurrent disease. Most authors agree

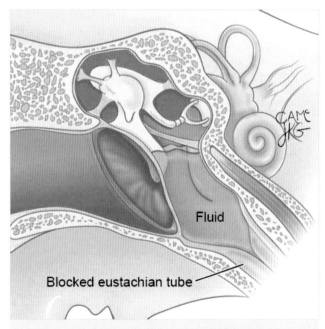

Fig. 117.1 Coronal schematic of the structures of the ear, demonstrating eustachean tube dysfunction and effusion in the middle ear.

that the adenoids should not be removed at initial myringotomy; removal should be reserved for recurrent cases. Eighty-five percent of children need tubes only once. The most common complication of myringotomy with tube insertion is otorrhea, which occurs in approximately 10% of cases. Other, less common complications include a persistent tympanic membrane perforation, cholesteatoma, or chronic otorrhea.

117.2.2 Acute Otitis Media

Acute otitis media is an acute infection of the middle ear space that may be viral or bacterial in origin. The most common bacterial pathogens are *Streptococcus pneumoniae, Haemophilus influenzae, Moraxella catarrhalis*, and group A streptococci. Acute otitis media can be an isolated occurrence or recurrent. In children, otitis media with effusion and acute otitis media often represent a continuum of disease. A middle ear effusion is repeatedly infected, and the effusion persists between acute exacerbations. The signs and symptoms of acute otitis media include fever, pain, and otorrhea if the tympanic membrane spontaneously ruptures. Young children will often be toxic, with a high fever, diarrhea, irritability, and general lethargy. Physical examination reveals pus in the external auditory canal if the tympanic membrane has ruptured. If the tympanic membrane is intact, the middle ear may appear white, or the tympanic membrane may be bulging and erythematous.

In May 2004, the American Academy of Pediatrics and the American Academy of Family Physicians jointly issued a clinical practice guideline for the treatment of children with acute otitis media, encouraging less use of antibiotics and greater use of analgesics. Children older than 2 years of age who are not febrile and are mildly symptomatic can be treated with expectant observation and oral analgesics. Children younger than 2 years of age should be treated with a 10-day course of oral antibiotics. Amoxicillin is the initial drug of choice, followed by amoxicillin/clavulanate or cefuroxime. Bacterial resistance has become an increasing problem. Accordingly, myringotomy with ventilating tube insertion has become more commonly used as a treatment of acute otitis media.

117.2.3 Bullous Myringitis

Bullous myringitis is characterized by the presence of one or more bullae on the tympanic membrane or, less commonly, on the wall of the external auditory canal. Bullous myringitis has historically been said to be caused by *Mycoplasma pneumoniae*. However, studies have failed to establish such a relationship. Rather, bullous myringitis appears to be a specific clinical manifestation of the same pathogens that are usually associated with acute otitis media. The clinical hallmark of bullous myringitis is disproportionate pain, relieved as the blisters rupture. There is often bloody drainage into the external auditory canal after rupture. Treatment is with oral antibiotics and analgesics.

117.2.4 Tuberculous Otitis Media/ Mastoiditis

Tuberculous otitis media usually involves both the middle ear and contiguous mastoid. Tuberculous otitis, caused primarily by

Mycobacterium tuberculosis (less often by atypical mycobacteria) is rare, accounting for 0.04% of cases of chronic suppurative otitis media. Tuberculous otitis media is usually diagnosed based on cultures obtained when infection has been resistant to standard oral antibiotic therapy, or on histopathology of biopsies obtained at surgery. No definitive signs or symptoms lead to the diagnosis of tuberculous otitis. Although tuberculous otitis has historically been said to cause multiple tympanic membrane perforations, it more often presents as a single perforation associated with conductive hearing loss and/or painless otorrhea. If a biopsy specimen is available, pathology will reveal noncaseating granulomas and acid-fast bacilli. Polymerase chain reaction testing may confirm the presence of acid-fast bacilli before cultures become positive. A past medical history of tuberculosis, as well as evidence of systemic disease, should be sought. Treatment is medical, usually 6 to 9 months of oral antituberculous drugs, often in combination. Infectious disease consultation is appropriate.

117.2.5 Sequelae of Otitis Media

The most common complication of untreated or persisting otitis media with effusion is chronic adhesive otitis, in which the tympanic membrane retracts and adheres to middle ear structures (► Fig. 117.2). The most common symptom is hearing loss. There is a characteristic "sunken" appearance on physical examination and a lack of tympanic membrane motion on

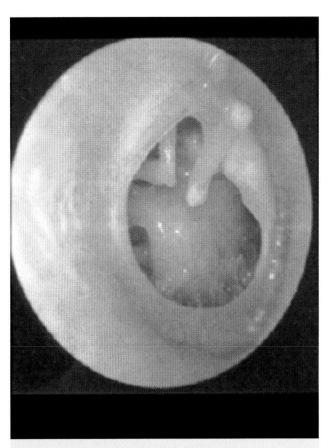

Fig. 117.2 Perforation of a right tympanic membrane.

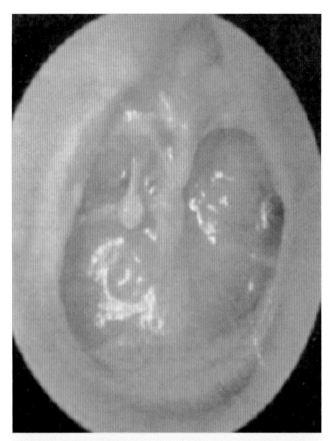

Fig. 117.3 Severely atelectatic right middle ear.

pneumatic otoscopy. Audiometric studies will usually reveal a conductive hearing loss. The treatment of adhesive otitis includes addressing the underlying eustachian tube dysfunction and the insertion of a myringotomy tube. Cartilage reinforcement tympanoplasty, in which cartilage is incorporated into the tympanic membrane, may successfully increase tympanic membrane rigidity and prevent recurrent retraction.

Adhesive otitis media or recurrent acute otitis media may predispose to chronic suppurative otitis. Chronic suppurative otitis media can result in or be associated with a perforation of the tympanic membrane (▶ Fig. 117.3) or chronic infection in the mastoid bone. Tympanic membrane perforations can be asymptomatic or can present with hearing loss or otorrhea. When they are acutely infected, there can be pain. The perforation should be visible on otoscopy. Acute rupture of the tympanic membrane usually heals spontaneously. Chronic perforations that do not heal on their own may necessitate surgical reconstruction.

All infectious or inflammatory processes that arise within the middle ear have a propensity to affect the mastoid. Computed tomography (CT) of the temporal bones performed in the presence of otitis media with effusion will virtually always show asymptomatic opacification of the mastoid. An acute suppurative component will lead to symptomatic mastoiditis, usually presenting as pain. In younger children, the presenting features may be fever and a postauricular, subperiosteal abscess that is secondary to rupture through a thin lateral mastoid cortex. Rarely, the presenting symptom is a secondary complication, such as facial nerve paresis or paralysis, vertigo secondary to a

labyrinthine fistula, or a central nervous system complication, such as an epidural or brain abscess. CT is the key to accurate diagnosis and may reveal coalescent mastoiditis or more aggressive bone destruction. Surgical exploration is often necessary, in addition to appropriate antibiotics, to make a definitive histopathologic diagnosis and effect a cure.

Cholesteatoma is an abnormal cystic mass of exfoliated keratin, shed from skin (▶ Fig. 117.4). There are many descriptors of cholesteatoma. Cholesteatoma can be acquired or congenital. Congenital cholesteatoma arises as a result of epithelial rests that fail to migrate from the middle ear to the external auditory canal during embryogenesis. Congenital cholesteatoma often presents as an asymptomatic white mass behind an intact tympanic membrane in a child without a prior history of ear surgery.

An acquired cholesteatoma resulting from untreated chronic otitis may be secondary to adhesive otitis media (retraction cholesteatoma) or to a tympanic membrane perforation (perforation cholesteatoma). The cholesteatoma can be further categorized anatomically as a pars flaccida, pars tensa, or combined cholesteatoma. A cholesteatoma can also be characterized as cystic, shed (a buildup of a mass of free keratin debris), or en plaque (as when skin migrates on the undersurface of the tympanic membrane and invades the adjacent mesotympanum and epitympanic recesses).

Adhesive otitis media can cause retraction pockets, which are deeply retracted areas of the tympanic membrane. Shed skin from the normal surface epithelium of the tympanic membrane can build up in these deep pockets and expand to form a "cystic" cholesteatoma, with a matrix surrounding the keratin debris. Alternatively, cholesteatomas occurring in the presence of a chronic tympanic membrane perforation may develop from external tympanic membrane skin that migrates through the perforation. Lacking a capsule, they may shed a mass of skin that builds up in the middle ear or, less commonly, the mastoid. The migrating skin may shed little or no keratin debris and simply be en plaque.

Finally, cholesteatomas can be classified as traumatic or iatrogenic. Traumatic cholesteatomas can be secondary to an implosive injury to the tympanic membrane, as may be caused by an inserted Q-tip or a water skiing fall, or secondary to a basilar skull fracture. Basilar skull fracture can cause a direct invagination of skin into the mastoid. Iatrogenic cholesteatoma can be secondary to any middle ear surgery.

On physical examination, cholesteatoma has a characteristic, white appearance. Laboratory testing includes audiometry and imaging studies, usually CT of the temporal bone. Untreated cholesteatoma usually results in chronic middle ear or mastoid infection. This most often presents as painless ear discharge and/or hearing loss. Local bone destruction can cause permanent conductive or sensorineural hearing loss, vertigo due to a labyrinthine fistula, or facial nerve paralysis. Untreated cholesteatoma can be associated with intracranial extension and present as an epidural abscess, brain abscess, or meningitis.

Cholesteatoma is treated surgically in the majority of cases. The three goals of cholesteatoma surgery are (1) eradication of disease, (2) reconstruction of the tympanic membrane and/or ossicular chain, and (3) prevention of residual/recurrent disease. Eradication of disease is a technical challenge because any

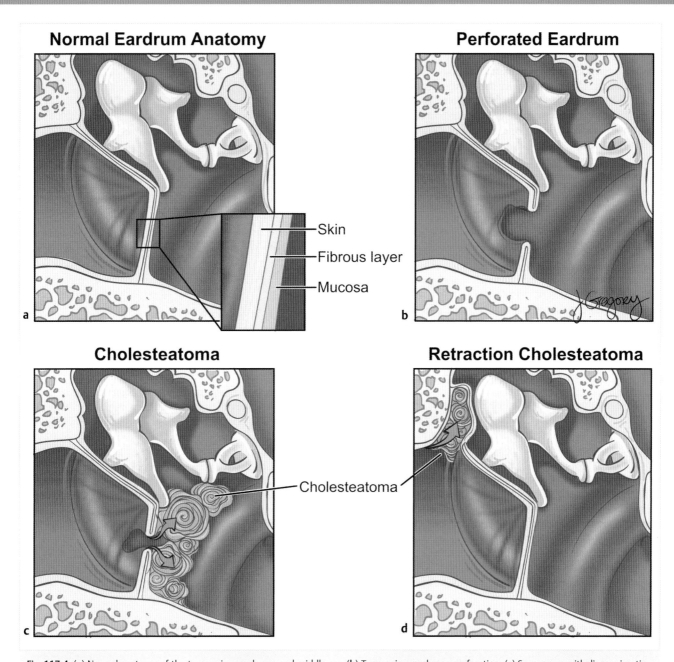

Fig. 117.4 (**a**) Normal anatomy of the tympanic membrane and middle ear. (**b**) Tympanic membrane perforation. (**c**) Squamous epithelium migrating through a tympanic membrane perforation into the middle ear to form a perforation cholesteatoma. (**d**) Development of a retraction cholesteatoma in an attic retraction pocket.

small residue of cholesteatoma matrix in the middle ear or mastoid can lead to residual disease, and the incidence of residual cholesteatoma is reported to be as high as 25%. Residual cholesteatoma occurs most often in the middle ear and epitympanum. It usually presents as a small "pearl" of cholesteatoma at the site of the abandoned matrix. Residual disease can be difficult to diagnose. Many surgeons advocate a planned second-look surgical procedure for residual disease 9 to 12 months after the initial surgery. CT may be useful in identifying residual disease, particularly if a baseline study demonstrates a well-pneumatized middle ear and mastoid. A small opacity that enlarges over time strongly suggests residual disease. There has been a recent trend toward using non-echo-planar diffusion-

weighted magnetic resonance (MR) imaging to detect residual disease. Dremmen et al reported a positive predictive value of 93% for the detection of cholesteatoma including lesions as small as 2 mm.

There are numerous technical approaches to reconstructing the tympanic membrane and ossicular chain, which are beyond the scope of this chapter. The critical factors for success include removing all disease, grafting the tympanic membrane with cartilage to prevent recurrent retraction disease, and adequately assessing the status of the ossicular chain in order to maximize reconstructive efficacy. Recurrent disease, which develops in about 25% of patients, is best prevented by cartilage reinforcement tympanoplasty.

There continues to be controversy regarding canal wall up versus canal wall down tympanomastoid procedures. Ears in which the normal anatomy is preserved with canal wall up mastoidectomy certainly heal faster, may have better postoperative hearing, and do not require the maintenance of a mastoid bowl, which is associated with complications. Taking the canal wall down can improve mastoid and attic exposure, particularly when the dura is low-lying or the sigmoid sinus is located far anteriorly. There is general agreement that the canal wall should be taken down if a patient is likely to be unreliable in follow-up because a canal wall down ear is generally safer. In other settings, the key issue should be the location of the disease. Taking the canal wall down does not improve exposure of the middle ear, facial recess, or sinus tympani. If disease is in the epitympanum, a transcanal or transmastoid atticotomy may suffice. Taking the canal wall down, with proper exteriorization of the epitympanum, nearly eliminates the possibility of recurrent retraction disease. Residual disease in the mastoid should be easily managed in the office setting with a canal wall down procedure. A middle ear that becomes adhesive following a Bondy modified radical mastoid procedure, in effect, autoconverts to Bondy radical.

117.3 Middle Ear Neoplasms

Middle ear tumors, other than cholesteatoma, are unusual. A glomus tumor is a benign nonchromaffin paraganglioma arising from paraganglia (glomus bodies) of the parasympathetic nervous system. Glomus bodies are small (0.25 to 0.50 mm) ovoid patches of paraganglionic cells that are dispersed throughout the body, mostly in association with autonomic nervous tissue. In the head and neck, glomus bodies are found at the carotid bifurcations, along the vagus nerve, and in the temporal bone arising along the Jacobson nerve (tympanic branch of the glossopharyngeal nerve, or cranial nerve IX). When functionally active, glomus bodies are chemoreceptive organs that detect changes in arterial partial pressures of oxygen and carbon dioxide and increase or decrease stimulation to the brainstem respiratory centers.

Glomus tumors, after cholesteatomas, are the most common tumors of the middle ear. Glomus jugulare tumors arise over the dome of the jugular bulb and extend into the middle ear and mastoid. Glomus tympanicum tumors arise on the promontory and are more often limited to the middle ear. Both present as a middle ear mass, often with a red hue (▶ Fig. 117.5). The average age at presentation is 52 years, and females are more commonly affected than males in a ratio of 5:1 to 6:1. Rarely, glomus tumors can metastasize to distant organs, even though they do not appear histologically malignant. One to three percent are endocrinologically active, secreting catecholamines or dopamine. Symptoms associated with endocrine activity include excessive sweating, hypertension, tachycardia, anxiety, and weight loss.

The most common symptoms are pulsatile tinnitus and hearing loss. The diagnosis is suspected upon otoscopic identification of a middle ear mass. CT of the temporal bones helps differentiate isolated glomus tympanicum tumors from larger, extensive glomus jugulare tumors. Of critical importance, CT rules out an ectopic carotid artery or a jugular bulb diverticulum, either of which can mimic a glomus tumor. MR imaging

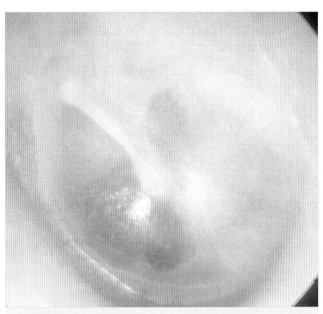

Fig. 117.5 Small, posteroinferior glomus tympanicum tumor of the right ear.

and angiography are helpful diagnostic adjuncts. The treatment of glomus tympanicum tumors is surgical removal. Glomus jugulare tumors can be embolized and surgically removed, or if large, they can be embolized and treated with radiation. Occasionally, what was thought to have been a glomus tumor will turn out postoperatively to have been a lower cranial nerve schwannoma, a meningioma, or a benign adenomatous tumor of the middle ear mucosa. Primary malignancies of the middle ear are extremely rare.

117.4 Metabolic Disorders of the Middle Ear

117.4.1 Otosclerosis

Otosclerosis is a disorder of bone remodeling that affects the bone of the otic capsule but no other bone in the human body. There are two phases to this process: a continuous resorption of the dense bone of the cochlear capsule and the simultaneous deposition of new, softer, more vascular bone. The etiology of otosclerosis is unknown. Approximately 50% of patients with otosclerosis have a positive family history, strongly suggesting a genetic factor that is yet to be identified. Other proposed etiologies include a metabolic disease of bone, an autoimmune disorder, a response to measles virus, and an abnormal response to hormonal factors. Otosclerosis usually begins in the late twenties or thirties, is more common in women than in men, and is bilateral in half of patients.

Otosclerosis occurs most often as a distinct focus of abnormal bone at the juncture of the anterior edge of the footplate of the stapes and the adjacent otic capsule. This focus of abnormal bone fixes the stapes and causes a conductive hearing loss, which is the most common presenting symptom of otosclerosis. Other associated symptoms include tinnitus, sometimes pulsatile, and ear fullness. The physical exanimation is normal, with the exception that tuning fork tests suggest a conductive hearing loss. On occasion, there is a red blush to the promontory of the middle ear due to the underlying hypervascular bone, the so-called Schwartze sign. Audiometric testing reveals a predominantly conductive hearing loss. Therapeutic options include expectant observation, hearing aids, and surgery. Expectant observation may be acceptable if the hearing loss is mild or unilateral. Amplification, in the form of a hearing aid, should restore hearing to normal or nearly normal and is risk-free. Stapedectomy, the surgical removal of the stapes and replacement with a stapes prosthesis, returns hearing to nearly normal in 97% of patients. The main risk of stapedectomy surgery is complete loss of hearing in the operated ear due to inner ear injury. This complication occurs in approximately 1% of surgeries. Other risks include the new onset of tinnitus, dizziness, facial nerve injury, and postoperative taste disturbance.

Occasionally, otosclerosis will diffusely invade the surrounding otic capsule and cause a severe to profound sensorineural hearing loss. This can happen with or without disease affecting the stapes. If there is no conductive component, such patients are not candidates for stapedectomy. They benefit from hearing aids until their hearing loss reaches a degree at which a cochlear implant is merited. Some data support the use of oral fluoride and calcium to stabilize the sensorineural component of otosclerosis.

117.4.2 Paget Disease

Paget disease is characterized by increased osteoclastic activity that causes extensive remodeling of bone. The skull and temporal bone are often involved. The most common otologic symptom is progressive hearing loss, which is usually a mixed loss. The hearing loss may be associated with tinnitus and dizziness. The diagnosis is made with imaging studies. Treatment is medical.

117.4.3 Osteogenesis Imperfecta

Osteogenesis Imperfecta is a genetic connective tissue disorder that affects collagen. The hallmarks of osteogenesis imperfecta are brittle bones that easily fracture, blue sclerae, and hearing loss. Osteogenesis imperfecta may be associated with a conductive hearing loss due to a discrete bony focus similar to that seen in otosclerosis or a sensorineural hearing loss due to cochlear involvement. The diagnosis is made by family history, genetic testing, and imaging studies. A stapedectomy is an option in patients with limited disease causing a conductive hearing loss.

117.5 Autoimmune Disorders Affecting the Middle Ear and Mastoid

Rarely, an autoimmune disorder can present as chronic, non-cholesteatomatous otitis. Wegener granulomatosis is a systemic disease characterized by necrotizing granulomatous vasculitis of the upper and lower respiratory tract and renal disease. The presenting ear symptoms may be serous otitis media secondary to nasopharyngeal obstruction of the eustachian tube, or chronic middle ear and mastoid granulomatous disease. The diagnosis is made on biopsy and serologic identification of cytoplasmic antineutrophil cytoplasmic autoantibiodies (c-ANCA) in peripheral blood. Recently, autoimmune disease related to immunoglobulin G4 (IgG4) has been reported to mimic recurrent, chronic otitis and mastoiditis. IgG4-related disease is characterized by an overabundance of IgG4-positive plasma cells in affected tissues and, frequently, elevated serum IgG4 levels. This clinical entity was first described in the context of autoimmune pancreatitis. The diagnosis is made by the identification of plasma cells immunohistochemically positive for IgG4 and an elevated peripheral serum level of IgG4. In both cases, the treatment in medical.

117.6 Traumatic Injuries to the Middle Ear

Traumatic injuries to the middle ear are often self-inflicted. Manipulation of the ear with a Q-tip, hair pin, or pen can result in a perforation of the tympanic membrane and disarticulation of the ossicular chain. If the trauma results in sensorineural hearing loss or vertigo, emergent surgical exploration may be necessary to seal a possible perilymphatic fistula of the inner ear. Blunt trauma to the head can cause a temporal bone fracture. Temporal bone fractures are classically categorized as longitudinal (along the axis of the external auditory canal) or transverse (perpendicular to and traversing the internal auditory canal). Many temporal bone fractures are a complex combination of the two. Temporal bone fractures, particularly longitudinal, can cause a tympanic membrane rupture and ossicular discontinuity. The diagnosis is confirmed on CT. If there is a sensorineural component to the hearing loss, a perilymphatic fistula should again be suspected. Occasionally, severe trauma can lead to cerebrospinal fluid otorrhea through a tympanic membrane perforation.

117.7 Roundsmanship

- The most common disorders of the middle ear are infectious/inflammatory, in particular otitis media of childhood.
- Unilateral serous otitis in an adult, particularly in association with ipsilateral cervical lymphadenopathy, suggests carcinoma of the nasopharynx.
- A red mass of the middle ear is most often a glomus tumor, but imaging is essential to rule out an ectopic carotid artery or a jugular bulb diverticulum.
- Adequate treatment of cholesteatoma is predicated on a thorough knowledge of the anatomy and location of the pathology.
- The most common cause of a unilateral conductive hearing loss, in the absence of a prior history of ear infection or surgery, is otosclerosis.

117.8 Recommended Reading

[1] Daly KA, Hoffman HJ, Kvaerner KJ, et al. Epidemiology, natural history and risk factors: Panel report from the Ninth International Research Conference on Otitis Media. Int J Pediatr Otorhinolaryngol 2010;74(3):231–240

[2] Campbell RG, Birman CS, Morgan L. Management of otitis media with effusion in children with primary ciliary dyskinesia: a literature review. Int J Pediatr Otorhinolaryngol 2009; 73: 1630–1638

[3] Griffin GH, Flynn C, Bailey RE, Schultz K. Antihistamine and/or decongestants for otitis media with effusion (OME) in children. Otolaryngol Head Neck Surg 2007; 136: 11–13

[4] Koopman L, Hoes AW, Glasziou PP et al. Antibiotic therapy to prevent the development of asymptomatic middle ear effusion in children with acute otitis media: a meta-analysis of individual patient data. Arch Otolaryngol Head Neck Surg 2008; 134: 128–132

[5] Vlastarakos PV, Nikolopoulos TP, Korres S, Tavoulari E, Tzagaroulakis A, Ferekidis E. Grommets in otitis media with effusion: the most frequent operation in children. But is it associated with significant complications? Eur J Pediatr 2007; 166: 385–391

[6] Kotikoski MJ, Kleemola M, Palmu AA. No evidence of Mycoplasma pneumoniae in acute myringitis. Pediatr Infect Dis J 2004; 23: 465–466

[7] Dale OT, Clarke AR, Drysdale AJ. Challenges encountered in the diagnosis of tuberculous otitis media: case report and literature review. J Laryngol Otol 2011; 125: 738–740

[8] Shin-Ichi J, Atsuko T, Ryuzaburo N, Hiroshi T. Residual cholesteatoma. Arch Oto laryngol H ead N eck S urg 2008; 134; (6): 652–657

[9] Dremmen MH, Hofman PA, Hof JR, Stokroos RJ, Postma AA. The diagnostic accuracy of non-echo-planar diffusion-weighted imaging in the detection of residual and/or recurrent cholesteatoma of the temporal bone. AJNR Am J Neuroradiol 2012; 33: 439–444

[10] Cruise AS, Singh A, Quiney RE. Sodium fluoride in otosclerosis treatment: review. J Laryngol Otol 2010; 124: 583–586

[11] Wierzbicka M, Szyfter W, Puszczewicz M, Borucki L, Bartochowska A. Otologic symptoms as initial manifestation of wegener granulomatosis: diagnostic dilemma. Otol Neurotol 2011; 32: 996–1000

[12] Schiffenbauer AI, Wahl C, Pittaluga S et al. IgG4-related disease presenting as recurrent mastoiditis. Laryngoscope 2012; 122: 681–684

118 Surgery for Chronic Ear Disease

John F. Kveton and Christopher J. Linstrom

118.1 Introduction

The successful management of chronic ear disease depends upon the surgical techniques employed to eradicate the disease within the temporal bone. The surgeon must possess a solid understanding of the basic surgical approaches to the temporal bone and, more importantly, must know when to adapt these particular approaches to the surgical situation at hand. This chapter will outline a systematic, step-by-step approach that should be employed by the surgeon to manage chronic ear disease. A disciplined surgical perspective is critical for the successful application of this approach to obtain deeper exposure within the temporal bone.

118.2 A Systematic Approach to the Temporal Bone

The easiest way to understand this approach to chronic ear disease is to remember how temporal bone dissection is learned in the temporal bone laboratory. One begins by first learning the surface anatomy of the temporal bone, followed by a cortical mastoidectomy. Deeper dissection progresses to expose the antrum and the ossicular heads in the epitympanum. One next proceeds with identification of the facial nerve and chorda tympani nerve, opening of the facial recess, and exposure of the stapes and long process of the incus within the middle ear. Finally, for a wider-field exposure of the middle ear and anterior epitympanum, the posterior canal wall is removed. This method of exposing the mastoid and middle ear regions can be adapted to deal with any disease encountered within the temporal bone and can be successfully employed if the surgeon develops a disciplined attitude to adhere to this method in all cases.

118.2.1 Incision

A postauricular incision is mandatory in the management of patients with chronic ear disease. Transcanal approaches should be reserved for noninfected middle ear procedures, such as tympanoplasty for a dry tympanic membrane perforation or ossiculoplasty. Endaural approaches to the mastoid are mainly of historical interest and will not be described in this chapter. The postauricular approach to the mastoid is safer and is the foundation for this systematic approach to mastoid surgery. Before the postauricular incision, vascular strip incisions are made in the ear canal (▶ Fig. 118.1).

The postauricular incision is made 5 to 10 mm behind the postauricular crease after the region has been infiltrated with local anesthetic with epinephrine. This incision should begin 10 mm above the crus of the helix and extend around to the mastoid tip. The incision should involve only the subcutaneous tissue, avoiding the temporalis muscle and musculoperiosteal layer over the mastoid bone. The subcutaneous layer over the temporalis muscle should be developed, and either the areolar tissue over the temporalis fascia or the temporalis fascia should

be harvested. After placement of a self-retaining retractor to expose the musculoperiosteum over the mastoid, the mastoid region should be palpated to identify the temporal line (which becomes the root of the zygoma in the anterior margin of the exposure). This is an important landmark in the initial exposure for mastoid surgery because the middle cranial fossa dura is almost never inferior to the temporal line. With electrocautery, an incision is now made through the temporalis muscle 5 to 10 mm superior and parallel to the temporal line, as far as the retraction allows. Electrocautery is now used to make another incision perpendicular to the temporal line down to the mastoid tip. The musculoperiosteal flaps are elevated to expose the whole mastoid bone, and the self-retaining retractor reflects the flaps to maintain exposure. The vascular strip elevates out of the ear canal with the anterior musculoperiosteal flap so that the ear canal and middle ear are accessible through this exposure. Middle ear disease can now be addressed and preparation for tympanoplasty accomplished. Disease around the oval window should be left in place at this time and the middle ear packed with epinephrine-soaked absorbable gelatin material.

118.2.2 Simple Mastoidectomy

All procedures for chronic ear disease begin in this manner. Under the operating microscope, the mastoid cortex is inspected, with note taken of the temporal line and its relationship to the spine of Henle and fossa mastoidea. This provides a rough indication of the proximity of the middle cranial fossa dura to the ear canal, and therefore of how difficult the mastoid procedure will be.

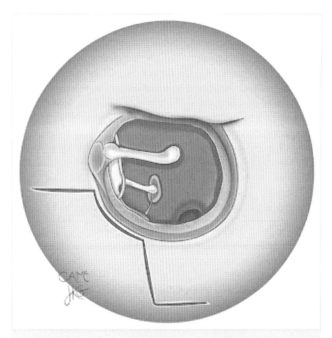

Fig. 118.1 Before the postauricular incision, a vascular strip is outlined with angles and straight Beaver blades.

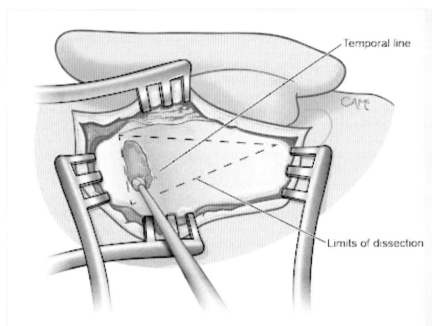

Temporal line

CArt

Limits of dissection

Fig. 118.2 Mastoidecotmy is begun by using a large cutting bur to identify the middle fossa dura along the temporal line.

With a cutting bur and continuous suction–irrigation, drilling is now begun about two drill diameters above the temporal line. Drilling should begin anteriorly above the external auditory canal and extend posteriorly to the incision in smooth continuous strokes until the dura is identified through a thin layer of bone (▶ Fig. 118.2). Once the dura has been identified, the mastoid cortex can be removed inferior to the dura, down to the mastoid tip and skeletonizing the posterior canal wall. The central mastoid air cells are now removed by following the sigmoid sinus medially and maintaining the dural plate over the tegmen superiorly. Following the tegmen, the Körner septum is encountered, and once it has been removed, the lateral semicircular canal is seen in the antrum. With the lateral semicircular canal in view, progressively smaller burs can be used to open the aditus ad antrum until the short process of the incus is identified. Further dissection anteriorly will expose the heads of the incus and malleus. The remaining central mastoid cells and mastoid tip are opened to remove residual mastoid disease. The vertical segment of the fallopian canal may be exposed if necessary at this time (▶ Fig. 118.3).

With this exposure, most chronic mastoid and middle ear inflammatory disease can be managed. All thickened granulation tissue can be removed in the mastoid and attic regions through the mastoid, and the middle ear disease can be managed through the ear canal. Successful disease removal can be measured by the free flow of irrigation fluid from the attic into the middle ear. Once this is accomplished, tympanoplasty can be performed.

118.2.3 Facial Recess Exposure

Exposure of the middle ear and ossicles via the facial recess is an indispensable tool for the otologic surgeon to effectively eradicate disease that is too extensive for a simple mastoidectomy exposure. The facial recess approach is mandatory in cholesteatoma surgery in which a staged approach is planned, and

in fact it should be used in any case of posterior–superior retraction pocket disease or attic cholesteatoma. This approach is also helpful in chronic inflammatory disease when the ossicular chain is encased in granulation tissue. Working through the facial recess allows complete removal of disease around the ossicular chain to correct the associated conductive hearing loss. In the event that ossicular erosion has occurred, the facial recess provides a better approach for measurement and placement of the ossicular prosthesis, whether it is an autograft or prosthesis.

Whether the decision to use the facial recess approach is made at the onset of the surgery (as in cholesteatoma cases) or during the simple mastoidectomy, the surgical technique should not vary. Once the attic has been widely opened, the vertical segment of the facial nerve is defined. The digastric ridge in the opened mastoid tip should be traced anteriorly, and the vertical segment of the facial nerve will be identified as it enters the stylomastoid foramen. With a thin a layer of bone kept over the fallopian canal, the nerve should be followed superiorly toward the lateral semicircular canal until the second genu has been uncovered. In this process, the chorda tympani nerve will be identified as it courses somewhat posterior to the plane of the vertical segment, so that as the vertical segment is being identified, care must be taken to avoid injury to the chorda tympani. The chorda tympani should be preserved at this time in the surgery to serve as the lateral limit of dissection. Drilling lateral to the chorda tympani nerve will result in entering the ear canal lateral to the anulus of the tympanic membrane. Once the vertical segment of the facial nerve has been identified, progressively smaller smooth diamond burs are used to remove all bone lateral to the vertical segment but medial to the chorda tympani to complete the facial recess approach (▶ Fig. 118.4).

In cases of chronic suppurative otitis media, granulation tissue can now be removed from the posterior tympanum and the ossicular chain assessed. In these cases, the posterior bony

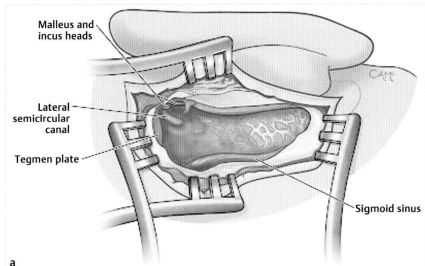

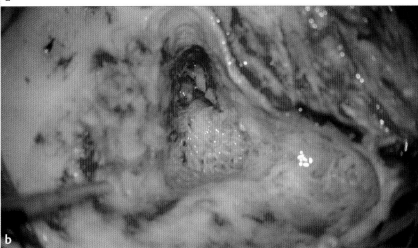

Fig. 118.3 (a) Upon completion of s simple mastoidectomy, the tegmen plate, sigmoid sinus, malleus and incus heads, and lateral semicircular canal are identifiable. (b) As seen intraoperatively in a left ear, the bluish shade indicates thin bone at the tegmen tympani and overlying the sigmoid sinus.

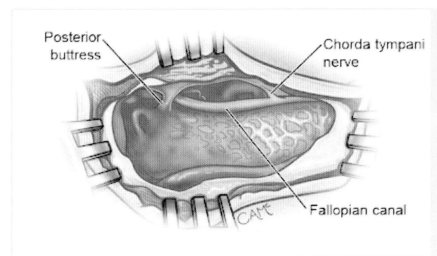

Fig. 118.4 The boundaries of the facial recess are the posterior buttress superiorly, the chorda tympani nerve laterally, and the fallopian canal medially.

buttress is maintained to stabilize the incus at the posterior incudal ligament.

The visualization of the posterior tympanum that is provided by the facial recess approach makes possible the resection of the vast majority of cholesteatomas encountered by the otologic surgeon, so that the need for a canal wall down procedure

is avoided. The number of canal wall down procedures would dramatically increase if the facial recess approach were not used because most cholesteatomas cannot be totally removed with the simple mastoidectomy approach.

Cholesteatoma management through the facial recess approach begins by viewing the cholesteatoma and its relationship

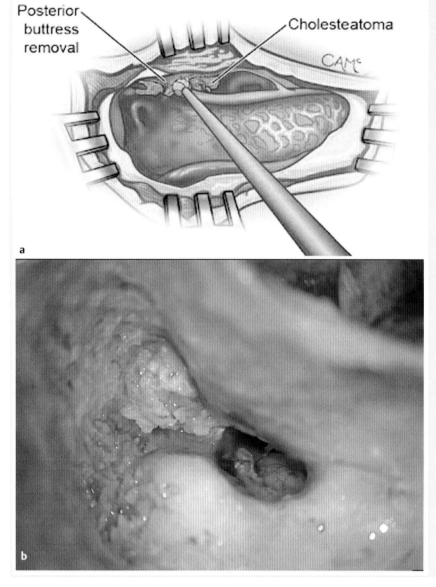

Posterior buttress removal

Cholesteatoma

a

b

Fig. 118.5 (a) Removal of the posterior buttress provides better access to the anterior epitympanum for (b) removal of the malleus head and cholesteatoma in the posterior tympanum and anterior epitympanum.

to the ossicular chain. If the cholesteatoma is medial to the incus or anterior to the malleus head with an intact ossicular chain, the ossicular chain must be disarticulated to remove the disease. If ossicular erosion is present, disarticulation of the remaining ossicles is necessary. Disarticulation of the intact ossicular chain is begun by first cutting the incudostapedial joint, then separating the incudomalleolar joint with a sickle knife and removing the incus from the surgical field. With a 2-mm smooth diamond bur, the posterior bony buttress is removed, and the internal portion of the second genu of the facial nerve is defined as it enters the horizontal segment of the facial nerve, so that the facial nerve can now be traced from the horizontal segment through the second genu to the vertical segment. With this enhanced exposure, cholesteatoma can be removed from the stapes, oval window, and most of the middle ear. If the chorda tympani nerve is involved in cholesteatoma, it should be cut and removed with the specimen. If cholesteatoma is entering the sinus tympani, a small diamond bur can often remove a bony overhang inferior to the pyramidal eminence and anterior to the vertical segment of the facial nerve to provide access for

removal of the disease. Extending the facial recess exposure by removing the chorda tympani to drill more inferiorly may be necessary (▶ Fig. 118.5).

The majority of attic cholesteatomas involve the malleus as well, and inadequate resection of the malleus and surrounding bone is a common reason for recurrence. Recurrence in the attic can be reduced by adhering to the surgical steps of facial recess cholesteatoma resection. After the cholesteatoma has been managed around the stapes and oval window region, a small diamond drill is used to expose the malleus head. The head of the malleus is amputated to expose the anterior epitympanum. A diamond drill is used to smooth out the tegmen plate and open the anterior epitympanum. The cog must be removed to obtain this exposure. Any cholesteatoma remnants can now be removed, and the horizontal segment of the facial nerve can be examined as it progresses superior to the cochleariform process on its way to the geniculate ganglion. This exposure also provides better visualization of the semicanal of the tensor tympani region toward the eustachian tube orifice. Finally, a small diamond bur should be used to drill the bony margins of

Posterior canal wall

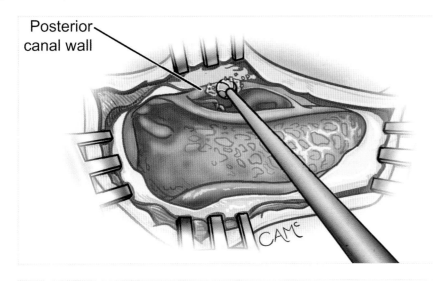

Fig. 118.6 Wider removal of the superior canal wall once the posterior canal wall has been removed allows better healing of the mastoid defect.

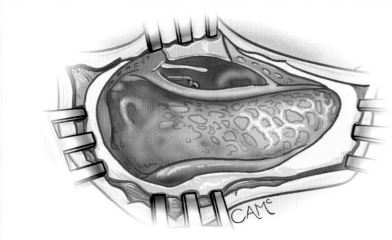

Fig. 118.7 Attention to the inferior bony transition into the mastoid tip results in a more rounded mastoid cavity that will reepithelialize more uniformly.

the attic defect (if present) to ensure complete removal of the disease before reconstruction.

118.2.4 Canal Wall Down Mastoidectomy

Removal of the posterior bony canal wall is the final step in this systematic approach to the surgical removal of middle ear and mastoid disease. Even if the surgeon identifies the need to take this step early in the procedure, he or she must follow the previous steps of the facial recess exposure to perform the procedure appropriately. The surgeon must identify the facial nerve and develop the facial recess before proceeding with the posterior canal removal. Disciplined adherence to this technique protocol will result in a more successful outcome because of the importance of a low-lying facial ridge for healing and later cleaning of the mastoid defect.

Once the facial nerve has been identified via the facial recess approach, the major portion of the posterior canal can be removed with several bites of a bone rongeur or a large cutting bur (▶ Fig. 118.6). The most critical stage of this procedure now occurs, which is the development of smooth bony transitions into the attic superiorly and into the inferior bony canal inferi-

orly. Progressively smaller diamond burs are used to remove residual bone covering any air cells within the anterior epitympanum, making the tegmen essentially continuous with the anterior–superior external canal. Removal of these anterior epitympanic cells usually uncovers cholesteatoma and also avoids mucoid drainage after healing. Inferiorly, varying amounts of bone are removed to widen access to the tympanic membrane and produce a smooth, wide transition into the mastoid tip. This technique prevents the accumulation of keratinous debris in the postoperative cavity. The wide exposure can be expanded to resect any residual cholesteatoma within the hypotympanum by drilling down the inferior anulus. Cholesteatoma in the sinus tympani can be reached by removing more bone anterior to the vertical segment of the facial nerve once the posterior canal wall has been removed (▶ Fig. 118.7).

As important as the bony dissection is for the removal of chronic disease, the development of an appropriately sized external meatus is critical for the long-term success of a canal wall down procedure. The conchomeatoplasty begins after all bone dissection has been completed. The medial surface of the conchal cartilage is exposed by sharply dissecting all soft tissue away with a curved iris scissors. A semilunar incision is then made as the cartilage turns laterally so that auricular protrusion is preserved while maximal expansion of the external auditory

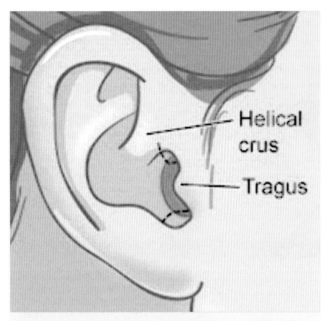

Fig. 118.8 Development of the superiorly based conchomeatal flap is key to successful healing of a canal wall down mastoidectomy.

meatus is obtained. Now, beginning in the ear canal, an incision is made in the inferior canal at 6 o'clock and carried straight out of the ear canal through the meatus to the new margin of the cartilage. The incision is then turned along the margin of the cartilage halfway up the distance of the conchal bowl. A second incision is begun at 12 o'clock in the ear canal and is carried out of the ear canal between the tragus and the root of the helical crus (▶ Fig. 118.8). Hemostasis should be quickly achieved, and any exposed cartilage at these incisions is sharply resected with a curved iris scissors or No. 15 blade. This superiorly based conchomeatal flap should line the posterior–superior aspect of the mastoid defect and serve as a source of reepithelialization of the mastoid bowl (▶ Fig. 118.9). Once this flap has been developed, closure of the middle ear can be performed with a large piece of temporalis fascia or pericranium. Gelfoam (Pfizer, New York, NY) should be placed into the Eustachean tube and the anterior mesotympanum, but the graft should be placed onto the promontory and span the oval window to lie directly on the facial nerve and lateral semicircular canal. If the stapes is absent, a bone strut or cartilage may be used for ossicular reconstruction, but the purpose of this procedure is the development of a dry ear with a sealed middle ear rather than hearing restoration. The auricle is then reflected into position, and the conchomeatal skin flap may be secured posteriorly by placing two absorbable sutures at the lateral margins of the flap and securing them posteriorly to the musculoperiosteal layer. The postauricular incision is then closed with a deep subcuticular stitch. The mastoid defect may be filled with ophthalmic antibiotic ointment or packed with surgical Nu-Gauze (Johnson & Johnson, New Brunswick, NJ) impregnated with antibiotic ointment.

118.3 Tympanoplasty

After disease in the middle ear and mastoid has been dissected and removed, in most cases the tympanic membrane will at least need to be reinforced if not reconstructed. A study of various techniques of tympanoplasty is therefore logical after a discussion of mastoidectomy; these may be performed with mastoidectomy or alone.

Other than traumatic perforations in an erstwhile *normal* drum, almost all perforations of the drum occur in the context of chronic otitis media or cholesteatoma and involve at least partial eustachian tube dysfunction. The surgeon must keep this in mind. It is not uncommon in the technique of tympanoplasty to account for poor eustachian tube function by placing a ventilation tube through the grafting material in order to ventilate the middle ear.

Tympanoplasty is the placement of soft tissue or cartilage without or with adnexal attachments in a favorable way to reconstruct a defect in the ear drum. Paper patching of an acute perforation involves many of the same principles as a Wullstein type I tympanoplasty, to be discussed, but it does not use soft tissue to repair the drum and therefore is not properly considered a tympanoplasty.

The basic mechanism of repair is that the freshened epithelial edge from the rim of the perforation or from the surrounding external auditory canal will migrate over the scaffold of soft tissue until it meets another area of squamous epithelium, when it will stop proliferating as a consequence of contact inhibition. It is essential that there be absolutely no entrapment of squamous epithelium beneath the soft-tissue scaffold. If it is trapped, it will almost always result in the formation of a keratoma or a cholesteatoma.

118.3.1 Classification

Tympanoplasty may be classified in several ways:
1. By the technique of soft-tissue placement used (overlay technique, underlay technique, combined technique)
2. By that part of the *native* ossicular chain before reconstruction to which any prosthetic or soft tissue is applied (Wullstein classification)
3. By combined techniques that use soft tissue and cartilage or another strengthening material (e.g., cartilage tympanoplasty)

118.3.2 Technique of Soft-Tissue Placement

Overlay Technique

The overlay technique is indicated for large, nearly total or total perforations; for previous tympanoplasty failures; for large perforations in which there is a severely blunted anterior angle of the external auditory canal; and for cases in which the primary goal is to achieve a grafted, safe, and dry ear, with hearing a secondary and minor consideration.

Approach

Although any tympanoplasty may be performed via a transcanal approach, the best view of the ear will be obtained via a postauricular approach. This is the recommended technique and allows not only the best view but also perfect placement of all grafting material. The auricle itself will hide a well-placed

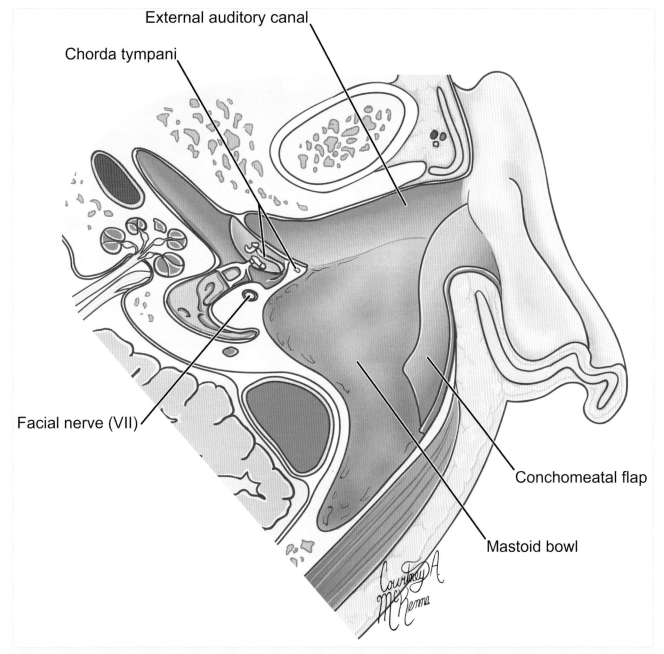

Chorda tympani

External auditory canal

Facial nerve (VII)

Conchomeatal flap

Mastoid bowl

Fig. 118.9 Reepithelialization of the mastoid bowl will occur from the conchomeatal flap in the sinodural angle and the anterior canal wall skin.

postauricular incision. The incision need not be long. If there is a bony excrescence, a prominent anterior overhang, or a pronounced tympanomastoid or tympanosquamous suture line, this will need to be drilled down, which is best done from behind, with the ear opened maximally. The vascular strip incisions (▶ Fig. 118.10) may be done through the canal or from behind, according to the preference of the surgeon, but the exposure should be as great as possible, with every millimeter of the drum remnant easily visible.

The overlay grafting technique requires that all of the squamous epithelium surrounding the perforation and the surrounding skin of the external auditory canal be removed and saved to graft the lateral surface of the new scaffold of fascia as a free graft of squamous epithelium (▶ Fig. 118.11). If there is a

prominent anterior bony overhang, the skin over it should be carefully "window-shaded" away from the middle ear cleft and held away while the bony external auditory canal is carefully drilled down and shaped so that every millimeter of the fibrous anulus can be seen (▶ Fig. 118.12). This is often a quick task, but it *must not* injure an intact, mobile ossicular chain. Acoustic trauma due to a rapidly rotating microdrill will be transmitted through the ossicles, causing a high-tone (usually > 6 kHz) acoustic trauma. To thin the anterior bony canal, diamond drills alone should be used because they are less likely to skip or jump. It is of the utmost importance that the ossicular chain be visible and indeed viewed at every moment of drilling. If the bone is too thin, the drill may approach the glenoid fossa, the capsule of which lies just anterior to the tympanic ring. If

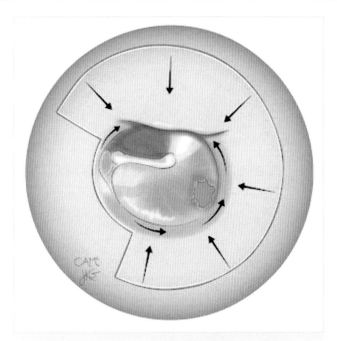

Fig. 118.10 Overlay technique of tympanoplasty begins with vascular strip incisions and elevation.

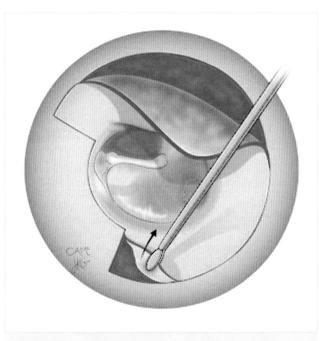

Fig. 118.11 The residual tympanic membrane and surrounding external canal skin are elevated and saved for later grafting.

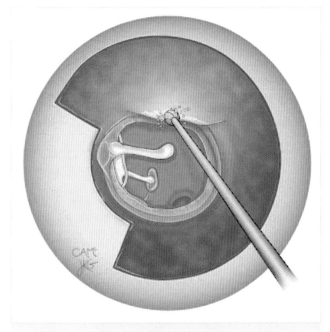

Fig. 118.12 Bony overhangs of the medial canal are removed to allow complete visualization of the anulus.

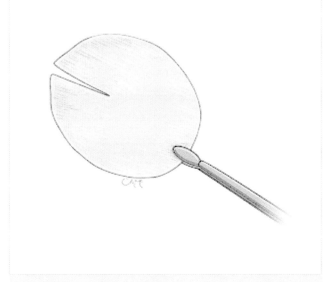

Fig. 118.13 Dried temporalis fascia is cut to size and split to allow passage below the handle of the malleus.

yellow fat is encountered, the dissection has proceeded too far anteriorly. The fat should be gently reduced with a bipolar cautery and otherwise left alone. The patient may have trismus postoperatively.

Once all portions of the tympanic membrane remnant have been visualized, the squamous epithelium over the drum and the anterior canal is removed and saved as a free graft. There is usually a remnant of the fibrous anulus left, but very little else of the native drum. Temporalis fascia that has been air-dried is

now cut in the shape of the new drum, and a slit is fashioned to allow the handle of the malleus to pass above (lateral) to the graft (▶ Fig. 118.13). The slit is cut in such a way that the redundant fascia will drape over the upper part of the malleus. The fascia is supported medially with absorbable gelatin sponge (Gelfoam) or another packing material. The fascia is now spread out to cover the entirety of the perforation and often resembles an intact, healed drum (▶ Fig. 118.14). The free graft of epithelium is spread out into the anterior angle between the edge of the fascia and the anterior tympanic ring (▶ Fig. 118.15). A folded piece of dry Gelfoam (the "dry roll") is tucked carefully

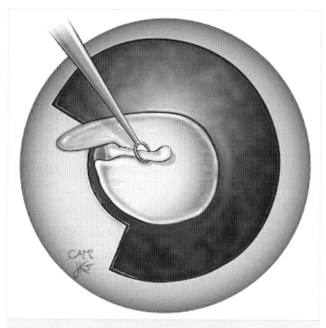

Fig. 118.14 The fascia is placed under the malleus.

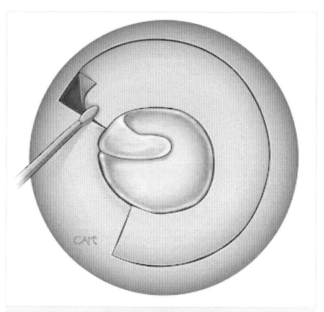

Fig. 118.15 The free graft is placed over the fascia.

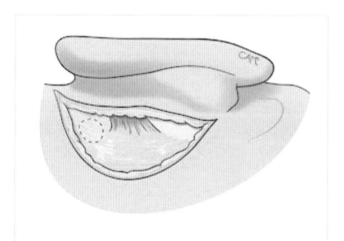

Fig. 118.16 Postauricular incision provides access to the external canal as well as to temporalis fascia.

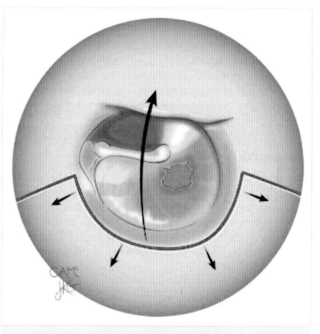

Fig. 118.17 Overlay tympanoplasty begins with vascular strip incisions and elevation of the tympanomeatal flap anteriorly.

into this anterior angle. This will help jump-start the epithelialization of the lateral surface of the drum. If other pieces of thin skin are available, they may be placed epithelial side up on the lateral surface of the fascia to encourage epithelialization. The lateral surface of the fascia and squamous epithelium "sandwich" is now supported with either dry or moist Gelfoam. It is helpful to place a leaf of moistened Gel*film* (Pfizer) immediately lateral to the fascia to help prevent fibroblast invasion of the fascia and Gelfoam. This will greatly facilitate cleaning the ear in the postoperative stage. The vascular strip is returned to its proper position, and the postauricular incision is closed in layers. As a final check, the vascular strip is carefully everted, then replaced to its proper position and held there by pieces of Gelfoam. Cotton or another packing material is placed into the meatus, and the ear is dressed with a dry mastoid or similar dressing.

Underlay Grafting Technique

This technique is ideal for smaller, discrete perforations with an intact, articulated, and mobile ossicular chain. A posterior approach is preferred (► Fig. 118.16). All steps of the approach to and the preparation of the perforation are the same as for the lateral grafting technique (► Fig. 118.17), except for the placement of the fascia. Once the perforation has been prepared, the fascia is placed underneath the perforation, as far anteriorly toward the eustachian tube orifice as possible. The fascia is supported on its medial surface with pieces of Gelfoam, either dry

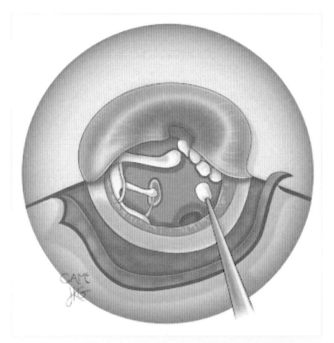

Fig. 118.18 Gelfoam is placed in the middle ear cleft to support the fascial graft.

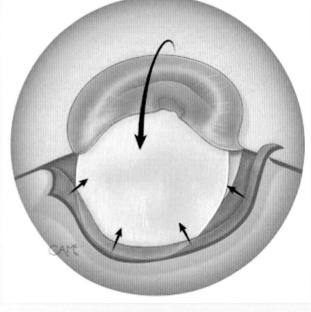

Fig. 118.19 The tympanomeatal flap is replaced over the temporalis fascia.

or moistened (▶ Fig. 118.18). The combined fascia and drum remnant are returned to their proper positions, with the edges of the squamous epithelium unfurled (▶ Fig. 118.20). The lateral surface of the reconstructed drum is packed with Gelfoam (▶ Fig. 118.20). The remainder of the technique is the same as with lateral grafting.

Combined Technique

All steps of this technique are the same as with the underlay grafting technique except that the drum remnant is taken off the long process of the malleus. The fascia is placed under the remnant of the drum but then over the handle of the malleus. The fascia is supported on its medial and lateral surfaces with Gelfoam. The remainder of the technique is the same as with underlay grafting.

118.3.3 Ossicular Reconstruction

The classification of tympanoplasty by the level of ossicular reconstruction was first described in the 1950s by Horst Wullstein. The five subdivisions describe increasingly more medial repairs. The recipient *native* ossicle defines the classification. Even if an ossicular reconstruction augments the native ossicle, or if a prosthesis (partial or total ossicular prosthesis) is to be used, the nomenclature is nonetheless derived from the native ossicle remaining before reconstruction. The actual technique of fascial grafting does not affect this classification.

1. Wullstein I: The drum is repaired to an intact *malleus* and mobile ossicular chain.
2. Wullstein II: The drum is repaired to an intact and mobile *incus*.
3. Wullstein III: The drum is repaired to an intact and mobile *stapes superstructure (columellar repair)*.

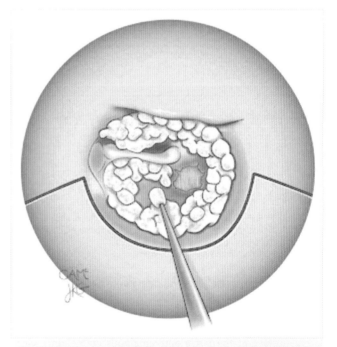

Fig. 118.20 The vascular strip is replaced and the canal packed with Gelfoam for lateral support.

4. Wullstein IV: The drum is repaired to an intact and mobile *stapes footplate*.
5. Wullstein V: The drum is repaired to a controlled fenestration into the *otic capsule* (generally to a fenestration of the horizontal or lateral semicircular canal or of an immobile stapes footplate).

118.3.4 Combined Technique

There is a growing awareness among otologists that fascia by itself is not strong enough to withstand the negative pressure of chronic eustachian tube dysfunction. In some cases of pronounced eustachian tube dysfunction, a pressure-equalizing tube is placed through the fascial graft before reconstruction. In other cases, stronger grafting material (e.g., a very thin piece of cartilage) is used either as a cantilever from the scutum or as a replacement of part or all of the drum.

118.4 Risks and Complications of Chronic Ear Surgery

Most complications associated with chronic ear surgery occur because of loss of surgical orientation and can be avoided by following this disciplined approach with precise dissection and meticulous hemostasis. Sensorineural hearing loss may occur by ossicular trauma or inadvertent fenestration of the otic capsule. Contact of the incus with the otologic drill during either the mastoidectomy or tympanoplasty, especially at the posterior buttress, produces high-frequency sensorineural hearing loss. Such loss can also be caused by the forceful manipulation of any ossicle, but especially the stapes, during the resection of disease in the oval window. Fenestration of the otic capsule can lead to partial and often total hearing loss, depending on the size of the fenestration and the length of time between the injury and recognition of the injury. The lateral semicircular canal is most vulnerable to injury with the otologic drill. This usually occurs in a contracted mastoid with low-lying dura or in a bloody surgical field when the surgeon has become disoriented. Fistulization of a semicircular canal or the cochlea can be found during removal of cholesteatoma. A small fistula (< 2 mm) may be uncovered and sealed with hydroxyapatite cement or bone wax, but cholesteatoma matrix must be maintained in larger fistulas. The most critical feature in the management of otic capsule fistula is prevention of the loss of perilymph. Avoidance of suctioning during manipulation of the fistula will prevent significant loss of perilymph with subsequent hearing loss. Avulsion of the stapes footplate during the removal of chronic granulation tissue or cholesteatoma is another cause of hearing loss. Fistulization of the otic capsule is also associated with vestibular injury. Permanent vestibular damage produces immediate severe vertigo with usual compensation of balance function over 6 to 12 weeks. Positional vertigo or mild disequilibrium may be permanent after severe injury.

Injury to the facial nerve is the most feared risk associated with chronic ear surgery. Continuous facial nerve monitoring is mandatory for these cases, but it should not be viewed as an assurance that facial nerve injury will not occur. The most common site of injury to the facial nerve is at the second genu as the nerve enters the vertical segment. The angle of the nerve at the second genu is highly variable, and often the nerve sheath can be mistaken for granulation tissue in a chronically infected mastoid. To avoid facial nerve injury in this area, the surgeon can positively identify the lateral semicircular canal by following the middle cranial fossa dura into the antrum, then dissect more inferior to the lateral semicircular canal along the vertical segment of the facial nerve before approaching the second genu

region. The horizontal segment of the facial nerve is the next most common site of injury; injury here is usually caused by the manipulation of disease in the presence of a dehiscent nerve. If disease is identified in the oval window region, a facial recess exposure is mandatory to ensure removal without facial nerve injury. In these cases, the second genu of the facial nerve should be clearly identified, and a small diamond drill should be used to follow the nerve into the horizontal segment. Any manipulation of disease should then be in a plane parallel to the facial nerve, with gentle palpation performed to assess dehiscence of the fallopian canal. Injury to the proximal portion of the horizontal segment of the facial nerve can be avoided by noting the cochleariform process and following the nerve superior to this bony landmark. Dysgeusia can occur after chronic ear surgery as a consequence of removal of the chorda tympani nerve. Taste disturbances are a recognized result of chronic ear disease and often predate surgical intervention. In the presence of cholesteatoma, the chorda tympani nerve should be resected with the disease. Dysgeusia is usually self-limiting over several months.

Dural injury, with or without cerebrospinal fluid (CSF) leak, can be avoided by immediate identification of the dura on beginning the mastoid procedure and skeletonization of the dural plate with a diamond drill during the procedure. At times, disease may erode through the dural plate, causing dural thinning and CSF leak. Dural exposure can be managed by gentle bipolar cauterization, which will remove any residual disease and contract the dura. In the presence of a CSF leak, reconstruction of the tegmen plate with hydroxyapatite cement is most effective. Inadvertent opening of the sigmoid sinus can be managed with bipolar cauterization in small tears, but a large tear of the sinus requires suture repair and possible extradural sinus obliteration. Unintentional fenestration of the posterior bony canal wall should be avoided by careful monitoring of the drill during the mastoid procedure. In the treatment of attic cholesteatomas, reconstruction of the canal wall defect is mandatory. This is best accomplished with tragal cartilage attached to perichondrium that spans the surrounding bone. Bone PATE should be used to repair small bone defects or reinforce thinning of the canal bone more laterally.

The greatest risk associated with tympanic membrane grafting techniques of any sort is graft failure. Tympanoplasty, in experienced hands, should succeed in more than 90% of cases, and the success rate should approach 95 to 97%.

Ossicular reconstruction with tympanoplasty carries a built-in risk for trauma to the oval window and thereafter to the inner ear, especially in the context of severe eustachian tube dysfunction. The tonic, progressive inward migration of a middle ear prosthesis may eventually penetrate the integrity of the oval window, leading to partial or complete neurosensory hearing loss, vertigo, and tinnitus. This must be anticipated and managed with a pressure-equalizing tube, a cartilage tympanoplasty, or staging. A postoperative dead ear is a devastating complication.

Failure of tympanic membrane repair, with or without conductive hearing loss, can occur after tympanomastoidectomy. This usually is a result of uncontrolled infection in the immediate postoperative period and is associated with persistent purulent discharge after surgery. Delayed or recurrent perforation is the result of poor eustachian tube function.

118.5 Roundsmanship

- A disciplined approach to mastoid dissection results in more efficient, complication-free surgery.
- Identification of the mastoid tegmen is the first step in a simple mastoidectomy.
- Following the dura into the antrum will prevent injury to the lateral semicircular canal.
- A facial recess approach is mandatory when cholesteatoma is identified during surgery for chronic ear disease.
- To remove the posterior bony canal, the facial recess approach should be performed first.
- Do not suction over an otic capsule fistula.
- Regardless of the technique used, success in tympanoplasty is directly proportional to the careful visualization and preparation of the perforation and the placement and stabilization of the soft-tissue graft.
- All soft-tissue grafts must be placed so that no squamous epithelium is trapped underneath it. Because skin has minimal growth requirements, trapped squamous epithelium will almost always result in keratoma or cholesteatoma formation.
- If superficial temporalis fascia has already been used and is in short supply, consider using pericranium.
- Severe and chronic Eustachian tube dysfunction is not affected by surgery on the tympanic membrane. The deleterious effect of Eustachian tube dysfunction on healing and aeration of the middle ear cleft must be anticipated, and the placement of a pressure-equalizing tube or a cartilage graft to support the drum may be of benefit in these cases.

118.6 Recommended Reading

[1] Copeland BJ, Buchman CA. Management of labyrinthine fistulae in chronic ear surgery. Am J Otolaryngol 2003; 24: 51–60

[2] Gacek RR. The surgical management of labyrinthine fistulae in chronic otitis media with cholesteatoma. Ann Otol Rhinol Laryngol 1974; 83 Suppl 10–1–19

[3] Glasscock ME. Tympanic membrane grafting with fascia: overlay vs. under-surface technique. Laryngoscope 1973; 83: 754–770

[4] Harner SG, Leonetti JP. Iatrogenic facial paralysis prevention. Ear Nose Throat J 1996; 75: 715–771, 718–719

[5] Ho SY, Kveton JF. The efficacy of the 2-staged procedure in the management of cholesteatoma. Arch Otolaryngol Head Neck Surg 2003;129(5):541–545

[6] Kveton JF. Revision mastoidectomy. In: Haberman RS, ed. Middle Ear and Mastoid Surgery. New York, NY: Thieme Medical Publishers; 2004:74–80

[7] Kveton JF, Goravalingappa R. Elimination of temporal bone cerebrospinal fluid otorrhea using hydroxyapatite cement. Laryngoscope 2000; 110: 1655–1659

[8] Kveton JF. The facial nerve in revision mastoid surgery: avoiding complications. Oper Tech Otolaryngol Head Neck Surg 1992; 3: 69–72

[9] Kveton JF. Open mastoid cavity operations. In: Gulya AJ, Minor LB, Poe DS, eds. Surgery of the Ear. 6th ed. Shelton, CT: People's Medical Publishing House-USA; 2010:515–528

[10] Magliulo G, Colicchio MG, Appiani MC. Facial nerve dehiscence and cholesteatoma. Ann Otol Rhinol Laryngol 2011; 120: 261–267

[11] McRackan TR, Abdellatif WM, Wanna GB et al. Evaluation of second look procedures for pediatric cholesteatomas. Otolaryngol Head Neck Surg 2011; 145: 154–160

[12] Neumann A, Kevenhoerster K, Gostian AO. Long-term results of palisade cartilage tympanoplasty. Otol Neurotol 2010; 31: 936–939

[13] Sheehy J. Mastoidectomy: the intact canal wall procedure. In: Brackmann D, ed. Otologic Surgery. 2nd ed. Philadephia, PA: W. B. Saunders; 2001:166–177

[14] Weber PC. Iatrogenic complications from chronic ear surgery. Otolaryngol Clin North Am 2005; 38: 711–722

[15] Wullstein H. Theory and practice of tympanoplasty. Laryngoscope 1956; 66: 1076–1093

119 Syndromic and Nonsyndromic Hearing Loss

Carol A. Silverman

119.1 Introduction

Universal newborn hearing screening programs in which the hearing of all newborns is screened (based on electrophysiologic techniques) before discharge from the newborn nursery have been legislated or voluntarily implemented throughout all states and territories of the United States. Although these programs have enabled the early identification of many children with hereditary hearing loss, they can never succeed in identifying all cases of genetic hearing loss because some forms of genetic hearing loss do not manifest until long after birth. The early identification of hearing loss, especially before 6 months of age, affords the opportunity for early intervention, such as speech–language therapy, hearing aid amplification, or cochlear implantation, which in turn promotes the acquisition of speech and language and maximizes favorable educational outcomes.

Hereditary hearing loss accounts for at least 60% of the occurrences of hearing loss in developed countries. More than 400 genes for hearing loss have been identified. Nonsyndromic hearing loss accounts for approximately 70 to 80% of cases of genetic hearing impairment; syndromic hearing loss accounts for the remainder of cases of genetic hearing impairment.

The term *congenital hearing loss* signifies the presence of hearing impairment at birth, such as that associated with cytomegalovirus infection. Hereditary hearing loss can manifest at birth or after birth, sometimes many years after birth. The nature of the hearing loss can be progressive or nonprogressive and unilateral or bilateral. The degree and configuration of the hearing loss are variable across various genetic disorders and can be variable even within a particular genetic disorder.

119.2 Mendelian and Nonmendelian Inheritance

119.2.1 Mendelian Inheritance

Mendelian patterns of inheritance include autosomal-dominant (AD), autosomal-recessive (AR), X-linked recessive, and X-linked dominant. With AD inheritance, the typical mating is between an affected parent who is heterozygous for the condition (one altered allele of the gene and one unaltered allele of the gene) and an unaffected parent who is homozygous (identical unaltered alleles). The so-called Punnett square (▸ Table 119.1) for this situation demonstrates that the probability of an offspring expressing the AD hearing loss trait is 50%. An offspring who does not inherit the *Dd* genotype will not be a carrier of the allele for hereditary hearing loss. A pedigree of the affected individuals in each generation of a family tree usually shows vertical transmission, in which the hearing loss trait appears in multiple, successive generations. With AD inheritance, there generally is no predilection for gender, so the hearing loss is transmitted equally by each parent. A mating between two affected parents, each with AD hearing loss, yields a Punnett square reflecting *Dd* by *Dd* mating, which is associated with a 25% probability of a homozygous affected offspring (*DD*), a 50% probability of a heterozygous affected offspring (*Dd*), and a 25% probability of an unaffected offspring (homozygous *dd* genotype). The phenotype of a homozygous affected offspring (*DD* genotype) typically is more severe than the phenotype of a heterozygous affected offspring (*Dd* genotype). An unaffected offspring (homozygous *dd* genotype) does not pass on the disorder to future offspring.

A genotype associated with a particular condition (e.g., *Dd*) in which the condition (e.g., hearing loss) is not expressed is said to be incompletely penetrant. The term *expressivity* describes variation in the phenotype associated with a specific genotype (e.g., *Dd*) such that two individuals with the same genotype may display different phenotypes.

With AR inheritance, the typical mating is between two carrier parents who both are heterozygous for the condition (one altered allele of the gene and one unaltered allele of the gene) and who do not exhibit hearing loss. For AR inheritance, the Punnett square (▸ Table 119.2) displays a 25% probability that an offspring will express an AR hearing loss trait and a 50% probability that an offspring will be a carrier. With AR inheritance, a pedigree showing the affected individuals in each generation of a family tree usually indicates horizontal transmission, in which the hearing loss trait appears within a single generation rather throughout multiple, successive generations. As

Table 119.1 Punnett square for autosomal-dominant inheritance

		Unaffected parent: genotype	
		d	*d*
Affected parent: genotype	*D*	*Dd* (hearing loss, heterozygous genotype)	*Dd* (hearing loss, heterozygous genotype)
	d	*dd* (no hearing loss, homozygous genotype)	*dd* (no hearing loss, homozygous genotype)

Table 119.2 Punnett square for autosomal-recessive inheritance

		Carrier parent: genotype	
		R	*r*
Carrier parent: genotype	*R*	*RR* (no hearing loss, homozygous genotype)	*Rr* (carrier, heterozygous genotype)
	r	*Rr* (carrier, heterozygous genotype)	*rr* (hearing loss, homozygous genotype)

Table 119.3 Punnett square for X-linked recessive inheritance

		Carrier female: genotype	
		x	*X*
Male parent: genotype	*X*	*xX* (carrier female, heterozygous genotype)	*XX* (girl without hearing loss, homozygous genotype)
	Y	*xY* (boy with hearing loss, hemizygous genotype)	*XY* (boy without hearing loss, hemizygous genotype)

Table 119.4 Punnett square for X-linked dominant inheritance from an affected mother (hemizygous)

		Affected female parent: genotype	
		X	*x*
Unaffected male parent: genotype	*X*	*XX* (female without hearing loss, homozygous genotype)	*xX* (female with hearing loss, heterozygous genotype)
	Y	*XY* (boy without hearing loss, hemizygous genotype)	*xY* (boy with hearing loss, hemizygous genotype)

Table 119.5 Punnett square for X-linked dominant inheritance from an affected mother

		Unaffected female parent: genotype	
		X	*X*
Affected male parent: genotype	*x*	*xX* (female with hearing loss, heterozygous genotype)	*xX* (female with hearing loss, heterozygous genotype)
	Y	*XY* (boy without hearing loss, hemizygous genotype)	*XY* (boy without hearing loss, hemizygous genotype)

with AD inheritance, there generally is no predilection for gender, and the hearing loss is transmitted equally by each of the parents. With a mating between two parents who have AR hearing loss, the Punnett square is *rr* by *rr*, which yields 100% of offspring with AR hearing loss.

For X-linked recessive inheritance, the phenotype is expressed in males having an altered allele on the X chromosome and in females having two copies of the altered allele. The most typical mating is between a carrier female and an unaffected male. For X-linked recessive inheritance, the Punnett square (▶ Table 119.3) indicates that the probability of a girl being a carrier is 50% and that the probability of a boy having a hearing loss is 50%. An affected man does not transmit the disorder to any son; a male offspring receives the unaffected Y chromosome from the father and the X chromosome from the mother. A carrier woman can transmit the altered allele to either her son or her daughter. A mating between an affected male and a carrier female represents *xY* by *xX*; for this mating, the probability that a male offspring will have X-linked recessive hearing loss is 50%, the probability that a female offspring will have X-linked recessive hearing loss (*xx* genotype) is 50%, and the probability that a female offspring will be a carrier is 50%.

X-linked dominant inheritance is much less common than X-linked recessive inheritance. For X-linked dominant inheritance, a mating between an affected female and an unaffected male represents the *xX* by *XY* genotype. The phenotype is expressed with the *xX* genotype, as in AD inheritance. With a mating between an affected female (who usually is heterozygous) and an unaffected male, the Punnett square displaying the probabilities of inheritance of particular genotypes (▶ Table 119.4) shows that the chance that a female offspring will have hearing loss (*xX* genotype) is 50% and that the chance that a male offspring will have hearing loss (*xY* genotype) is 50%. A mating between an unaffected female and an affected male represents

the *XX* by *xY* genotype. With this mating (▶ Table 119.5), 100% of all female offspring will have hearing loss because the altered *x* allele is inherited from the father, and none of the male offspring will have hearing loss because the unaltered *X* allele is inherited from the mother.

The severity of the phenotype in X-linked dominant inheritance is greater in males than in females. In women with the *xX* genotype, one allele is normal, whereas in men with the *xY* genotype, there is only one allele, that on the X chromosome, and that altered allele is producing an abnormal (or no) protein.

The existence of sign language and schools for the deaf has enabled deaf persons to form communities, and as a result, the frequency of matings between deaf individuals, known as *assortative mating*, has increased. Parents who both have the same form of AR deafness are homozygous for the same recessive allele. Consequently, 100% of their offspring will be deaf; such matings, which yield deafness in 100% of the offspring, are termed *noncomplementary matings*. The term *complementary mating* is used if all offspring from matings between individuals with different forms of genetic deafness (or between individuals with environmentally induced deafness or between an individual with environmentally induced deafness and an individual with recessive deafness) have normal hearing.

119.2.2 Mitochondrial Inheritance

DNA is found not only in the nuclei of cells, but also in the mitochondria within cell cytoplasm. Mitochondria supply energy to the cell in the form of adenosine triphosphate (ATP) and also are involved in other cellular processes, such as cell differentiation, cell death, and cell signaling. Each cell has hundreds of mitochondria. If a cell has both altered and normal mitochondrial DNA, the condition is termed *heteroplasmy of mitochondrial DNA*. If the cells have only altered mitochondrial DNA, the condition is termed *homoplasmy of mitochondrial DNA*. Homoplasmy is associated with more severe symptoms and an earlier onset of symptoms than heteroplasmy. Heteroplasmy is more common than homoplasmy; because the number of affected mitochondria inherited can vary, the phenotypic expression can be more variable with heteroplasy than with homoplasmy. Mitochondrial DNA inheritance is solely through the mother, and not the father, because mitochondrial DNA is found in oocytes but not in sperm cells. The prevalence of mitochondrial hearing loss has been estimated to be 1% in the population with prelingual hearing loss and 5 to 10% in the population with postlingual, nonsyndromic hearing loss.

119.3 Nonsyndromic Hearing Loss

The vast majority of cases of genetic hearing loss (70 to 80%) are nonsyndromic. Of individuals with nonsyndromic hearing loss, approximately 60 to 75% have AR inheritance of the hearing loss. The locus of each of the genes associated with nonsyndromic AR hearing loss is labeled DFNB with an Arabic numeral postscript.

119.3.1 Connexin Hearing Loss

The most common nonsyndromic AR hearing loss results from mutations in the connexin family of genes, particularly in the *GJB2* gene (gap junction protein β_2), which encodes connexin 26, and the *GJB6* gene (gap junction protein β_6), which encodes connexin 30. Mutations in the *GJB2* gene may account for up to 50% of cases of nonsyndromic AR severe to profound hearing loss in several populations. The genes of the connexin family are responsible for the formation of gap junction proteins that enable the recycling of potassium ions after sensory hair cell stimulation in the cochlea. The most common connexin gene mutation is the *GJB2* mutation, and the most common of the connexin 26 gene mutations is 35delG/30delG (most frequently observed in the European and American Caucasian populations). The 167delT mutation is most commonly observed in Ashkenazi Jews, the 235delC mutation is specific to Asian populations, the R143W mutation is most commonly observed in some African populations, and W24X mutation is seen primarily in Spanish/Slovak and Indian populations. Approximately 90 different *GJB2* mutations have been identified. Although the vast majority of *GJB2* mutations are associated with nonsyndromic AR deafness, some rare mutations have been associated with AD syndromic forms of deafness (e.g., Vohwinkel syndrome, ectodermal dysplasia keratitis–icthyosis deafness syndrome).

The hearing loss is of prelingual onset. In one study of 234 patients having *GJB2* mutations, approximately 82% demonstrated severe or profound sensorineural hearing loss, and the remaining 18% had mild to moderate sensorineural hearing loss. The audiometric configuration was a corner audiogram (with hearing present only at the lowest frequencies) in about 41%, downsloping in about 29%, flat in about 24%, and U-shaped in 5%. A rising (upsloping) audiometric configuration was not observed in any of the individuals. The audiometric configuration of the hearing impairment was more likely to be symmetric than nonsymmetric.

Some mutations in the connexin 32 gene have been associated with X-linked dominant Charcot-Marie-Tooth type I disease. This form, which affects 7 to 10% of individuals with Charcot-Marie-Tooth disease, is associated with a variable phenotype that sometimes shows mild-to-moderate sensorineural hearing loss but more commonly displays gait disturbances and Achilles contractures.

119.4 Syndromic Hearing Loss

119.4.1 Autosomal-Dominant (DFNA) Hearing Loss

Waardenburg Syndrome

The most common cause of AD syndromic hearing loss is Waardenburg syndrome, which has variable penetrance. Approximately 1 to 2% of cases of profound hearing loss result from Waardenburg syndrome. The most common forms of Waardenburg syndrome are type I and type II. Type I Waardenburg syndrome is more frequent and is associated with mutations in the *PAX3* gene, which encodes the paired box 3 transcription factor. Clinical features associated with Waardenburg syndrome type I include the highly penetrant dystopia canthorum (more laterally situated medial canthi of the eyes) and one or more of the following: sensorineural hearing loss that usually (but not always) is congenital, nonprogressive, bilateral, and symmetric (hearing loss penetrance is 36 to 58%); a broad and high nasal bridge; synophrys ("unibrow"); iris pigmentation abnormalities such as heterochromia iridis (different colors of the iris), intensely blue eyes, or bicolored eyes; hair that is prematurely gray or has a white forelock, or eyebrows or eyelashes that show whitening; hyperpigmentation and/or hypopigmentation of the skin (e.g., white or light skin patches); and vestibular symptoms (vertigo, dizziness, or imbalance) and abnormalities on various vestibular function tests.

Type II Waardenburg syndrome is distinguished by the general absence of dystopia canthorum, the presence of more highly penetrant hearing loss (less severe than in type I, but usually progressive), and the presence of heterochromia iridis. The most common gene mutation associated with type II Waardenburg syndrome is the *MITF* gene mutation; the *MITF* gene encodes the microphthalmia-associated transcription factor. Types III and IV Waardenburg syndrome are rare forms; the former is associated with the clinical features of type I in conjunction with upper limb contractures and hypoplastic muscles, and the latter is associated with the clinical features of type II in conjunction with Hirschsprung disease, manifested by obstructions and dilations of the colon resulting from dysfunction in colonic autonomic innervation.

Branchio-otorenal Syndrome

The inheritance pattern of branchio-otorenal syndrome usually is AD. The most commonly occurring clinical features of this syndrome include the following: (1) usually severe (but can be mild to profound) hearing loss (conductive, sensorineural, or most commonly mixed) that can be progressive and of delayed onset; (2) preauricular pits; (3) bilateral renal defects varying from hypoplasia or dysplasia to agenesis; and (4) branchial fistulas involving the lower neck. Less frequently occurring clinical features include malformed pinnae (e.g., cupped pinnae or lopped ears with malformation of the antihelix), external auditory canal stenosis, preauricular skin tags, and lacrimal duct aplasia. In addition to external auditory canal stenosis, temporal bone abnormalities can involve the ossicles, cochlea, vestibular aqueduct (e.g., enlarged vestibular aqueduct), and horizontal semicircular canal. The syndrome usually results from a mutation in the *EYA1* gene, which encodes transcription factors.

Treacher Collins Syndrome (Mandibulofacial Dysostosis or Franceschetti-Klein Syndrome)

Treacher Collins syndrome, an AD disorder of craniofacial morphogenesis resulting from impaired embryologic development of the first and second branchial arches, results from a de novo mutation in 60% of cases. Penetrance is high and expressivity is variable. The mutation generally is found in the *TCOF1* gene but also may be found in the *POLR1D* and *POLR1C* genes on chromosome 5q. The estimated incidence is 1 in 50,000 live births.

Clinical features involve the head and neck. The dysmorphologic facial features include the following: downward-sloping (antimongoloid) palpebral fissures; colobomas of the lower eyelids; depressed malar bones (cheek bones); colobomas (gaps or defects) of the lower eyelids, often with absent eyelashes on the lower lid medial to the colobomas; retrognathia; malformed auricles; broad mouth; and pointed nasal prominence. Some may have cleft lip and/or palate. The soft-tissue facial dysmorphology generally is bilaterally symmetric, whereas the bony facial features can be asymmetric. The facial bone hypoplasia often is associated with dental malocclusion and numerous dental caries.

The otologic clinical features include bilateral auricular malformations with microtia in up to 85% of patients, stenosis or atresia (often complete) in one-third of patients, fused malleus/incus remnant in 90%, and abnormal stapes in 73%. The radiologic findings often reveal failed pneumatization of the mastoid bone and a bony cleft on the lateral temporal bone that makes the facial nerve susceptible to surgically induced injury. The small middle ear space and the bony cleft on the lateral temporal bone limit the number of patients who have Treacher Collins syndrome with atresia who can be considered as candidates for surgery. Obstructive sleep apnea was present in 54% of children and 41% of adults in a recent cohort study of patients with Treacher Collins syndrome. The obstruction is multilevel but is most significant at the level of the oropharynx/hypopharynx.

Audiologic evaluation usually reveals a maximal, bilaterally symmetric conductive hearing loss with a rising audiometric configuration that may also slope at the high frequencies. In approximately 17%, the hearing loss is mixed. A recent study revealed that bone-anchored hearing aids (BAHAs) can be successfully implanted with greater functional gain than can be achieved with conventional bone conduction hearing aids. Because the thickness of the calvarial bone often is poor or irregular, additional holes need to be drilled or materials for bone augmentation need to be employed for sufficient placement of the fixture.

Because this syndrome can be identified by prenatal testing in embryos, prenatal diagnosis and genetic counseling should be recommended to parents. Additionally, a multidisciplinary approach to management should be employed, including otolaryngology, audiology, speech and language pathology, general dentistry, and orthodontics evaluations.

Neurofibromatosis

Neurofibromatosis type I (von Recklinghausen syndrome) accounts for the vast majority of cases of neurofibromatosis, and the prevalence of unilateral vestibular schwannoma is approximately 2 to 4%. The National Institutes of Health diagnostic features of neurofibromatosis type I (NF1) include at least two of more of the following: six café au lait spots, two or more neurofibromas of any form or at least one plexiform neurofibroma, optic pathway glioma, two or more Lisch nodules (iris hamartomas) that extend from the iris but do not impair vision, an osseous lesion (e.g., sphenoid dysplasia or tibial pseudoarthritis), axillary or inguinal freckling, and first-degree relative with NF1. Although the inheritance is AD in approximately half of cases, a de novo genetic mutation is involved in the other half of the cases.

Although bilateral vestibular schwannomas occur in approximately 95% of patients with neurofibromatosis type II (NF2), this type of neurofibromatosis accounts for only a small proportion (5 to 10%) of cases of neurofibromatosis. The estimated incidence of NF2 ranges from 1 in 33,000 live births to 1 in 87,410 live births. The *NF2* gene (tumor suppression protein) mutation is located on chromosome 22, whereas the *NF1* gene is located on chromosome 17. The Wishart form of NF2 (more severe form) is associated with early onset of the disease; numerous schwannomas and meningiomas develop, and death by 40 years of age may be the final outcome. The Gardner form (less severe form) is generally associated with later onset of the disease; the schwannomas remain relatively stable for years, and fewer schwannomas and meningiomas develop. Approximately one-third of individuals with NF2 are mosaic for the mutation; therefore, individuals with mosaicism may have tumors in a localized area of the body.

The vestibular schwannomas, which generally develop by 30 years of age, are associated with sensorineural hearing loss and other symptoms that can be found in persons with vestibular schwannomas (e.g., vertigo or other balance problems, tinnitus). Other cranial nerve schwannomas may also develop, particularly involving the trigeminal or oculomotor nerves bilaterally. Other tumors associated with NF2 most commonly include intracranial meningiomas, multiple cutaneous tumors (generally peripheral nerve schwannomas), and multiple spinal tumors. Cutaneous lesions are generally less prominent in individuals with NF2 than in those with NF1. Visual impairment and eventual blindness may result from cortical and posterior subcapsular cataracts; the visual impairment less frequently is associated with retinal hamartomas.

The modified National Institutes of Health diagnostic criteria for NF2 include any one or more of the following: (1) bilateral vestibular schwannomas; (2) first-degree relative with NF2 and either a unilateral vestibular schwannoma or at least two of the following: meningioma, schwannoma, glioma, neurofibroma, posterior subcapsular lenticular opacities; (3) unilateral vestibular schwannoma in conjunction with at least two of the following: meningioma, glioma, neurofibroma, posterior subcapsular lenticular opacities; (4) two or more meningiomas in conjunction with either a unilateral vestibular schwannoma or at least two or more of the following: schwannoma, glioma, neurofibroma, cataract.

Vestibular schwannomas may be managed by watchful waiting in patients with small tumors and good hearing, surgical tumor removal (hearing-conservative approaches vs hearing-ablative approaches), or stereotactic irradiation. The hearing loss can be managed with aural rehabilitation, hearing aids, sign language, or cochlear auditory brainstem implants. Patients with NF2 should have imaging studies of the entire central nervous system (intracranial and spinal) and neurologic, oto-logic, neuro-ophthalmologic, and audiologic examinations. Genetic testing and counseling should be recommended. Annual monitoring, from about 10 years of age until approximately the fourth decade of life, should include intracranial magnetic resonance (MR) imaging, brainstem auditory evoked potentials testing, and audiologic evaluation. Siblings also should be screened (MR imaging or genetic testing) for NF2.

Other

The inheritance mode of otosclerosis, discussed elsewhere in this book, is thought to be AD with reduced penetrance. The absence of a positive family history in up to half of the cases has led to the hypothesis of complex inheritance representing interactions between various genetic and environmental factors.

119.4.2 Autosomal-Recessive Hearing Loss

Usher Syndrome

Usher syndrome is a group of AR conditions associated with congenital, bilateral sensorineural hearing impairment and retinitis pigmentosa (a retinopathy affecting the rod photo-receptors); the retinitis pigmentosa is manifested initially by impaired night vision and later by tunnel vision, sometimes resulting in total blindness. Usher syndrome is phenotypically and genetically heterogeneous. The prevalence of Usher syndrome is 2 to 4% in the profoundly deaf population and is 50% in the deaf–blind population in the United States.

Usher syndrome is classified as follows: type I (30 to 40%), type II (60 to 70%), and type III (2 to 4%). Type I Usher syndrome is characterized by congenital, bilateral profound deafness; absence of vestibular function (which is associated with delayed motor developmental milestones); and progressive retinitis pigmentosa, the onset of which generally occurs before puberty. Type I Usher syndrome has been associated with mutation in any one of seven genes, with USH1B the most common genetic subtype. Management of the hearing loss with cochlear implantation generally is beneficial.

Type II Usher syndrome, which is less severe than type I, is characterized by congenital sloping, moderate to severe sensorineural hearing loss (management usually is with hearing aids), normal vestibular function, and retinitis pigmentosa, the onset of which typically is before the age of 20 years. The hearing loss may be slowly progressive. The vast majority of genetic mutations associated with type II Usher syndrome are attributed to the USH2A gene, which encodes usherin (a transmembrane protein).

Type III Usher syndrome is characterized by progressive sensorineural hearing loss of variable onset, retinitis pigmentosa of variable onset, and vestibular function that ranges in degree from normal to absent. Type III Usher syndrome is the most commonly occurring form of this syndrome in the Ashkenazi Jewish population. The predominant genetic subtype is USH3A, which encodes clarin-1 (a transmembrane protein). The retinal impairment associated with Usher syndrome can be detected by electroretinography before the development of visual signs and symptoms; thus, persons who are at risk for Usher syndrome should undergo electroretinography to allow maximal time for adapting to the visual impairment.

Pendred Syndrome

Pendred syndrome may account for approximately 7 to 10% of cases of hereditary prelingual deafness. It is largely characterized by sensorineural hearing loss (which typically is profound and prelingual) and goiter. The goiter, present in the majority of individuals with Pendred syndrome, usually appears after the first decade of life; affected patients are more frequently euthyroid than hypothyroid. The inclusion of goiter as a criterion for the diagnosis of Pendred syndrome results in substantial underassessment. Positive findings on the perchlorate discharge test are seen in the vast majority of individuals with Pendred syndrome.

In a report of 33 patients, nearly all demonstrated bilateral, symmetric, sloping, severe to profound hearing loss. The patients generally reported that the onset of hearing loss had been during early childhood or that it had been present at birth; 27% reported progressive hearing loss. Based on a difference of more than 8% on the duration parameter, unilateral weakness of 9 to 100% was observed in 41% of patients, bilateral weakness in 50% of patients, and a complete absence of caloric responses in one individual. In approximately 90% of those who underwent radiologic testing, computed tomography (CT) revealed an enlarged vestibular aqueduct (with enlarged contents), and in 18% of those with an enlarged vestibular aqueduct, a Mondini cochlear malformation also was present.

Mutations of the SLC2A4 (PDS) gene, which encodes pendrin, are largely responsible for Pendred syndrome. Pendrin, a transporter of chloride and iodide, is expressed in the inner ear, thyroid, and kidney.

An enlarged vestibular aqueduct in conjunction with sensorineural hearing loss also can occur in individuals who do not have Pendred or branchio-otorenal syndrome.

Jervell and Lange-Nielsen Syndrome

This syndrome is characterized by a markedly prolonged QT interval on the electrocardiogram, which indicates abnormal cardiac repolarization, in conjunction with sensorineural hearing loss. The cardiac abnormality can lead to recurrent syncope, ventricular arrhythmia, and sudden death in childhood. It is the more severe of the variants of the long-QT syndrome. Another variant of long-QT syndrome is Romano-Ward syndrome, which has cardiac features that are similar to those in Jervell and Lange-Nielsen syndrome but is not associated with sensorineural hearing loss. The Jervell and Lange-Nielsen syndrome, characterized by AR inheritance, is associated with mutations of the gene *KCNQ1* or *KCNE1*, which encodes proteins that conduct the I_{ks} current. It may be responsible for as much as 1% of the population with profound hearing loss.

A multinational study of 186 patients with Jervell and Lange-Nielsen syndrome revealed that cardiac arrest and sudden death occurred in 27%; the median age at death was 8.5 years. At least one cardiac event occurred in 86%; by the age of 3 years, 50% had experienced a cardiac event. In 93% of the life-threatening cases (cardiac arrest and sudden death), the triggers were exercise and emotions. In 90.5%, the mutation involved the *KCNQ1* gene, and in 9.5%, the mutation involved the *KCNE1* gene. A QT interval longer than 550 milliseconds in conjunction with syncope during the first year of life represented a significant risk factor for a life-threatening cardiac event. The severity of the cardiac events was substantially greater for boys than for girls. The efficacy of therapy with β-blockers was limited; a life-threatening event occurred in 27% of the patients while they were on such therapy. The authors proposed that defibrillator implantation be considered for those infants and children with Jervell and Lange-Nielsen syndrome who also have this risk factor (prolonged QT interval of > 550 milliseconds and syncope during the first year of life).

Sickle Cell Disease

Sickle cell disease, which affects 1 in 400 African Americans in the United States, is a hereditary disorder associated with abnormal protein in the erythrocytes, which leads to a change in their morphology. Sickle cell disease comprises a group of hemoglobinopathies associated with abnormal forms of hemoglobin: sickle cell anemia (hemoglobin SS), hemoglobin SC disease, hemoglobin D disease, β-thalassemia, and hemoglobin E disease Affected erythrocytes have difficulty traversing blood vessels because of their sickle shape, and they are also stickier than normal erythrocytes, even when their morphology is unsickled. As a result, blood flow is occluded. Characteristics of sickle cell disease include the following: hand–foot syndrome (swelling of the hands and feet because of obstructed blood flow); splenic sequestration (enlargement of the spleen resulting from insufficient blood flow through the spleen because of an excessive number of sickle cells); hemolytic anemia (premature breakdown of the blood cells); painful episodes or crises (which occur when sickle cells become trapped in the small blood vessels); stroke or brain damage; renal failure; pneumonia or acute chest syndrome similar to pneumonia; leg ulcers; and stroke. The estimated prevalence of sensorineural hearing impairment varies considerably from study' to study. The sensorineural hearing loss, hypothesized to result from sickling/stickiness of the erythrocytes in the stria vascularis, can be unilateral or bilateral and is variable in degree. One study indicated that 80% of patients with sickle cell disease and hearing impairment have the hemoglobin SS sickle cell variant. The percentage of patients with hearing impairment in addition to sickle cell disease was low, not exceeding 7%, for the other sickle cell disease variants.

119.4.3 X-Linked (DNF) Hearing Loss

Alport Syndrome

The mode of inheritance in Alport syndrome is X-linked dominant. Features of this syndrome include sensorineural hearing loss, progressive glomerulonephritis (inflammation of the glomeruli of the kidneys), and ocular abnormalities, most notably ocular flecks and lenticonus (bulging of the lens capsule and underlying cortex). The bilateral, high-frequency (generally > 3,000 Hz) sensorineural hearing loss results from lesions of the capillary basement membrane of the stria vascularis, analogous to the lesions in the glomerular capillary basement membrane. The onset of hearing loss generally is within the first two decades of life and is progressive during childhood, stabilizing in adulthood. Hearing loss penetrance is about 83% in males and 57% in females. The progressive kidney disease begins with hematuria; by about 25 years of age, 94% of males and 3% of females demonstrate renal insufficiency evidenced by abnormally elevated serum creatinine. The ocular flecks appear as yellow or white spots in the macular and midperipheral regions of the retina. The lenticonus usually is anterior and bilateral, resulting in refractive errors.

The results of a large genotype–phenotype correlational study (N = 681 from 175 families) of X-linked Alport syndrome in the United States revealed hearing loss in 89% and ocular abnormalities in 30%. Hematuria was present in microscopic form in 91% and in macroscopic form in 49%. Proteinuria followed the onset of hematuria in 85%. The average age at the onset of end-stage renal disease varied with the type of mutation; it was 25 years for those with truncating mutations and as late as 37 years for those with missense mutations. Renal failure progressed to end-stage renal disease in 60%, generally in conjunction with hypertension. Ocular abnormalities were less frequent in those with missense mutations (20%) than in those with other mutations (36 to 50%). Similarly, hearing loss, a predominant feature regardless of mutation type, was less frequent in those with missense mutations (84%) than in those with other mutations (94 to 100%).

Alport syndrome is genetically heterogeneous—X-linked dominant in 85% of cases and AR or AD in about 15% of cases. Various mutations in the *COL4A5* gene, which encodes type IV collagen, expressed in the basement membranes of the kidney, ear, and eye, are responsible for the X-linked form of Alport syndrome.

Congenital Fixation of the Stapes Footplate with Perilymphatic Gusher

A stapes gusher is a serious and unusual complication of stapes footplate surgery in males with X-linked recessive hearing loss (combined low-frequency conductive and high-frequency sensorineural hearing loss) in which opening of the stapes footplate leads to a profuse outflow of perilymphatic fluid, and consequently severe to profound hearing loss and dizziness. Radiographic imaging can reveal congenital malformations of the audiovestibular system (enlarged vestibule and dilation of the lateral end of the internal auditory canal along with deficiency/absence of bone between the lateral end of the internal auditory canal and basal end of the cochlea). The hearing loss and malformations generally are milder in female carriers.

Snik et al commented on the surprising finding of acoustic reflexes in these patients despite the presence of significant air–bone gaps. They hypothesized that the air–bone gaps reflect an asymmetry between the scala tympani and the scala vestibuli that increases the efficiency of the transduction of skull vibrations during bone conduction testing into cochlear fluid vibrations, and that ultimately yields better than expected bone conduction thresholds and artifactual air–bone gaps. Their audiologic investigations of a patient who had not undergone stapes surgery revealed normal tympanometric findings with present contralateral acoustic reflex. The latencies on auditory brainstem response testing were consistent with the presentation level rather than with the presentation level corrected for the air–bone gap (because conductive components are expected to decrease the effective stimulation level at the cochlea). They concluded that the third window (aqueducts and vascular and neural channels of the cochlea) is enlarged in patients who are stapes gushers, resulting in more efficient transduction of skull vibrations into cochlear fluid vibrations and ultimately better than expected bone conduction thresholds and significant, artifactual air–bone gaps. This condition is associated with mutations largely in the *POU3F4* gene, which encodes a POU homeodomain transcription factor.

119.4.4 Mitochondrial Hearing Loss

MERRF and MELAS

The sample sizes in studies of mitochondrial disorders in children generally have been small. A recent study of 26 children with established mitochondrial disorders and audiologic data revealed that 58% had hearing loss (38% sensorineural, 8% conductive, and 4% mixed; normal hearing sensitivity in the remainder). Approximately 47% were female. Of the 9 children who were followed over time, 44% had progressive hearing loss. Of the 15 children with hearing loss, MERRF (myoclonic epilepsy with ragged red fibers) had been diagnosed in 1 and MELAS (mitochondrial myopathy, encephalopathy, lactic acidosis, stroke-like episodes) had been diagnosed in 3. These two disorders are mitochondrial encephalopathies. The features of MERRF include mitochondrial myopathy and progressive myoclonus epilepsy. The features of MELAS include encephalomyopathy with strokelike episodes and lactic acidosis. In the children with MELAS, the hearing loss was symmetric and sensorineural, but the configuration and severity were variable; one child, with bilateral, symmetric, moderately rising to mild sensorineural hearing loss, appeared to have findings possibly consistent with auditory neuropathy spectrum disorder (as evidenced by sensorineural hearing loss with present otoacoustic emissions). The child with MERRF appeared to have a progressive disorder because the otoacoustic emissions amplitude decreased over time and the cochlear microphonic was absent; the sensorineural hearing loss was asymmetric (moderate in the right ear and mild in the left). All waves were absent bilaterally on auditory brainstem response testing. The findings were possibly suggestive of auditory neuropathy spectrum disorder. In light of the possible progression of hearing loss and possible occurrence of auditory neuropathy spectrum disorder, the authors recommend audiologic monitoring including auditory brainstem response and otoacoustic emissions testing.

MELAS and MERFF are genetically heterogeneous disorders. The variability in clinical features is consistent with heteroplasmy of the mitochondrial DNA.

Aminoglycoside Ototoxicity and Maternally Inherited Diabetes and Deafness

The mitochondrial A1555G mutation in the 12S rRNA gene confers susceptibility to bilateral sensorineural hearing loss from aminoglycoside antibiotics. This mutation also can be associated with nonsyndromic hearing loss. The frequency of the mitochondrial A1555G mutation in aminoglycoside ototoxicity appears to be greatest in Asian populations. In the United States, the mitochondrial A155G mutation is seen in approximately 15% of individuals with hearing loss from aminoglycoside antibiotics.

Maternally inherited diabetes and deafness (MIDD) is largely associated with a point mutation (A to G substitution) at position 3243 of the mitochondrial DNA that encodes the gene for transfer RNA. Characteristics of MIDD include diabetes, usually of insidious onset; sensorineural hearing loss; possibly abnormalities on brain scans (present in more than 50%); psychiatric disorders (e.g., recurrent depression, schizophrenia, various phobias); macular retinal dystrophy (present in 86%); myopathy observed as exercise-induced muscle cramps or weakness; cardiac abnormality (e.g., left ventricular hypertrophy without hypertension or cardiac autonomic neuropathy); renal disease; short stature resulting from a deficiency of hypothalamic growth-releasing hormone; and gastrointestinal complaints (e.g., constipation and pseudo-obstruction). The onset of the bilateral sensorineural hearing loss, which is of cochlear etiology, usually is in early adulthood and usually precedes the diagnosis of diabetes; the hearing loss is either slowly or rapidly progressive, initially high-frequency in configuration, then becomes more severe and affects all frequencies. The severity is worse and the rate of progression is faster in males than in females.

119.5 Genetic Aspects of Age-Related Hearing Loss

Susceptibility genes may underlie the variability in the configuration and degree of sensorineural hearing loss associated with aging. Heritability estimates range from 35 to 55%, suggesting that about 35 to 50% of the variability in hearing sensitivity in older adults is due to genetic factors, with the remaining proportion associated with environmental factors.

The apolipoprotein E (*APOE*) gene encodes apolipoprotein E, a component of very low-density lipoproteins, which play a role in keeping cholesterol levels within normal limits. This gene has been implicated in Alzheimer disease, generalized atherosclerosis, stroke, and macular degeneration. The *APOE* ε4 allele is the variant that most strongly predisposes to these disorders. A recent study has implicated the *APOE* genotype in age-related hearing loss. In this population-based study of elderly individuals (85 years of age or older), after adjustments for atherosclerosis and cognitive function, the degree of age-related hearing loss was most severe in those with the *APOE* ε4/*APOE* ε4 genotype, second most severe in those with only one copy of the *APOE* ε4 allele, and least severe in those without the *APOE* ε4 allele.

119.6 Genetic Testing and Counseling

The GTR: Genetic Testing Registry Web site (http://www.ncbi.nim.nih.gov/gtr) provides information on the specific genetic tests available on a research or diagnostic test basis. Genetic testing as part of newborn hearing screening programs is becoming more widespread. The results of genetic testing may yield information (e.g., possible progressive nature of hearing loss, association with other symptoms that need management) that can guide parents and families in the planning process, and that may obviate the need for other expensive and more invasive medical tests. Genetic testing can be (1) prenatal, based on samples collected from an embryo or fetus during amniocentesis or chorionic villus sampling; (2) diagnostic, to identify the genetic aspect of a medical condition; (3) part of the newborn screening process, to identify a particular hereditary form of deafness, such as that associated with abnormalities of connexin 26; or (4) carrier screening to identify disorders such as sickle cell disease. Parents must be afforded the opportunity to decline genetic testing. Usually, genetic testing is based on a blood sample.

Genetic testing can have significant implications for family relationships. Many individuals are concerned that employer or health/life insurer access to the results of genetic testing can lead to job discrimination or health/life insurance discrimination. Federal legislation, particularly the Genetic Information Nondiscrimination Act (GINA) of 2008, as well as legislation passed by many states, does exist to protect individuals from discrimination based on genetic information, but increased legislation is needed for more comprehensive protection from discrimination.

Medical professionals, including otolaryngologists, need to be sensitive to cultural issues related to deafness. Within the Deaf community, deafness often is not viewed as a disability to be prevented or cured. Rather, being Deaf (capitalization of the letter *D* to signify deaf culture with communication by American Sign Language) is valued by the Deaf community, so that genetic testing procedures employed by members of the Deaf community may be viewed as a means to ensure that the unborn child will be deaf.

Genetic counseling may have to be recommended to explain the implications of the results of genetic testing, including those regarding family planning and future pregnancies.

119.6.1 Comprehensive Evaluation Procedures

A comprehensive otolaryngologic evaluation should include a physical examination to identify features associated with syndromic hearing loss: craniofacial/cervical abnormalities or facial asymmetries; ear or cervical pits/tags; hypopigmentation or hyperpigmentation of the skin, or café au lait spots; prematurely gray hair or a white forelock; small or malformed pinnae; canal stenosis; tympanic membrane abnormalities; goiter; abnormal shape, slant, and color of the eyes and intercanthal distance; abnormal number of fingers or toes, or webbed fingers or toes. Balance and gait also should be assessed because abnormalities can be associated with syndromic or nonsyndromic hearing loss.

A family history should include questions about consanguinity in the family and whether any family member has one or more of the following features: hearing impairment or the need to use a hearing aid, particularly during childhood or early adulthood; premature graying of the hair or a white forelock; renal or urinary problems; cardiac problems; thyroid problems; widely spaced or multicolored or differently colored eyes, or visual problems including night blindness, tunnel vision, cataracts, and glaucoma; pits or tags on the ear or neck; ears that are abnormal in shape or size; bones that break easily or frequently; arthritis or problems with joints. A pedigree analysis based on the history contributes to the arousal of suspicion for particular inheritance patterns. The ethnicity and country of origin should be established for family members with hearing loss.

A complete audiologic evaluation should be done to establish the type and severity of the hearing loss and its configuration, and serial audiologic testing should be done to rule out the progression of hearing loss. A hereditary hearing impairment can be of delayed onset, occurring many years after birth, particularly some forms of AD hearing loss. If hereditary hearing loss is suspected, family members should be tested because individuals with hearing loss may be unaware of their hearing problem. Auditory brainstem response testing can be used to estimate behavioral thresholds in infants, including those who are difficult to test, and also to determine the site of a lesion (cochlear vs retrocochlear). Otoacoustic emissions testing helps to determine the presence of peripheral hearing loss. Audiologic management may include evaluation and fitting for a hearing aid or other sensory aid, such as a cochlear implant, and/or assistive listening device.

If balance or gait problems are present or suspected, a vestibular evaluation should be performed, which may include electronystagmography/videonystagmography, rotary chair testing, and posturography. Such testing can help differentiate between Usher type I and type II syndrome.

Patients with visual problems (e.g., Alport syndrome, Stickler syndrome, NF2, Norrie disease, Usher syndrome) should be referred to ophthalmology. Urinalysis and laboratory tests (for serum creatinine levels) should be performed, and referral to a nephrologist for renal follow-up should be considered when a syndrome with renal impairment (e.g., Alport syndrome, branchio-otorenal syndrome) is suspected. Referral to a cardiologist should be considered when cardiac problems are present that raise suspicion for syndromes associated with cardiac abnormalities (e.g., Jervell and Lange-Nielsen syndrome). Radiologic studies such as a high-resolution CT of the temporal bone should be considered to document inner ear malformations (e.g., branchio-otorenal syndrome, Pendred syndrome, Treacher Collins syndrome). MR imaging studies should be considered when (1) NF2 is suspected, (2) progressive hearing loss is present but CT scans are normal, or (3) the audiologic findings are consistent with a retrocochlear site of the lesion. Referral to endocrinologist should be considered when diabetes is suspected or for thyroid function testing (e.g., perchlorate discharge) when Pendred syndrome is suspected; a limitation of perchlorate discharge testing is that it is nonspecific.

When hereditary hearing loss is identified in children, referral for psychoeducational management should be made so that an individualized education plan can be developed. The pediatrician is an important member of the interdisciplinary team in children with hearing loss. Family members need to be fully informed of the various treatment/habilitation options.

The 2002 (reaffirmed in 2005) American College of Medical Genetics (ACMG) statement "Genetics Evaluation Guidelines for the Etiologic Diagnosis of Congenital Hearing Loss" presents triage/testing as follows:

1. Upon suspicion of syndromic hearing loss, gene-specific mutation testing often can be done.
2. Upon suspicion of nonsyndromic hearing loss when the hearing loss is an isolated case in the family, do cytomegalovirus testing and *GJB2* (connexin 26) mutation screening.
3. Upon suspicion of nonsyndromic hearing loss when two or more first-degree family members (including the patient) have hearing loss, do *GJB2* (connexin 26) mutation screening.
4. Upon suspicion of nonsyndromic hearing loss in conjunction with the presence of a pedigree suggestive of dominant inheritance, do mutation screening for connexin-related deafness and other genes.
5. Upon suspicion of nonsyndromic hearing loss in conjunction with a pedigree suggestive of mitochondrial inheritance, test for the A1555G mutation and the A7445G mutation.
6. Upon suspicion of nonsyndromic hearing loss when both parents have hearing loss, connexin-related deafness may be involved, and the mating may be between individuals who both have *GJB2* hearing loss. Genetic testing can reveal if the child has *GJB2* deafness. The ACMG Expert Panel cautions that a negative mutation screen does not rule out genetic hearing loss.

A recent study was performed on the diagnostic yield of various tests within a test battery ordered for 270 children referred to the otolaryngology department of two large city hospitals. The results revealed that the diagnostic yield of the entire battery (CT of the temporal bone, MR imaging of the brain and internal auditory canal with contrast, connexin 26 genetic testing, genetics consultation, ophthalmologic consultation, electrocardiography, renal ultrasound, and fluorescent treponemal antibody absorption [FTA-ABS] testing) was 43%. The diagnostic yield for the stepwise addition of each test/consultation was determined because uniform application of the entire test would have resulted in an inefficient use of health care resources and would have necessitated numerous health care visits. The first test, CT, was found to have a diagnostic yield of 14%. Addition of the second test, MR imaging, increased the diagnostic yield to 24%. Addition of the third test, connexin 26 testing, raised the diagnostic yield to 38%. Addition of the fourth test, genetics consultation, further increased the diagnostic yield to 42%. The fifth test, renal ultrasound, increased the diagnostic yield only slightly (to 43%). The diagnostic yield did not increase further with the addition of ophthalmology, electrocardiography, and FTA-ABS testing.

No overlap was found between the group of children who were positive on imaging testing and the group of children with connexin 26 mutations. The diagnostic yields of imaging and ophthalmologic consultation were greater when syndromic hearing loss was suspected than when nonsyndromic hearing loss was suspected. On the other hand, the diagnostic yield of connexin 26 testing was significantly greater when nonsyndromic hearing loss was suspected. MR imaging and CT had similar sensitivities in detecting inner ear abnormalities, although the latter was slightly more sensitive in the detection of enlarged vestibular aqueducts and the former had slightly higher sensitivity in the detection of hypoplastic or aplastic cochlear nerves. Additionally, MR imaging identified brain pathology associated with congenital cytomegalovirus infection.

119.7 Internet Resources

1. OMIM (http://www.ncbi.nlm.nih.gov/omim)

This Web site is a comprehensive compendium providing descriptions of the clinical features, inheritance, gene mapping, and clinical management for different genetic syndromes, with references.

1. Hereditary Hearing Loss Homepage (http://hereditaryhearingloss.org)

This Web site furnishes descriptions of genetic syndromes with links to OMIM. It is maintained by Guy Van Camp (University of Antwerp) and Richard Smith (University of Iowa).

1. GTR: Genetic Testing Registry (http://www.ncbi.nim.nih.gov/gtr)

This Web site furnishes extremely wide-ranging information on genetic diseases, including descriptions of the genetic tests for various genetic disorders; the locations of genetic clinics (evaluation and counseling); the National Society of Genetic Counselors directory; the American Board of Medical Genetics list of board-certified geneticists; access to *GeneReviews*, which provides summaries of various hereditary disorders (including disease characteristics, diagnosis/testing, and genetic counseling); a talking glossary of genetic terms; and access to the orphaned portal on rare diseases and orphan drugs.

1. Harvard Medical School Center for Hereditary Deafness (http://hearing.harvard.edu)

This Web site furnishes information on hereditary hearing loss and genetic tests, consumer resources, PowerPoint lectures on genetics, and research opportunities.

1. Interactives DNA (http://learner.org/interactives/dna/index.html)

This interactive Web site furnishes information on DNA; the history of the discovery of DNA; the Human Genome Project; genetic inheritance, including Mendelian inheritance and complex inheritance; Punnett squares; sex linkage; genetic engineering; and associated ethical and social issues.

119.8 Roundsmanship

- The vast majority of cases of genetic hearing loss (70 to 80%) are nonsyndromic. Inheritance of the hearing loss is AR in approximately 60 to 75% of individuals with nonsyndromic hearing loss.

- The most common nonsyndromic AR hearing loss results from mutations in the connexin family of genes, particularly the *GJB2* gene (gap junction protein β$_2$), which encodes connexin 26.
- Obtain audiologic evaluations of family members when genetic hearing loss is suspected.
- Mitochondrial inheritance plays an important role in maternally inherited diabetes and deafness (MIDD) and aminoglycoside ototoxicity.
- Genetic testing is possible for many genes. Mutations in the *GJB2* gene may account for up to 50% of cases of nonsyndromic, AR, severe to profound hearing loss in several populations.
- The diagnostic work-up of a patient with suspected hereditary hearing loss can follow the triage/testing approach recommended in the American College of Medical Genetics (ACMG) statement "Genetics Evaluation Guidelines for the Etiologic Diagnosis of Congenital Hearing Loss," or the stepwise diagnostic battery recommended by Lin et al.

119.9 Recommended Reading

[1] Bekheirnia MR, Reed B, Gregory MC et al. Genotype-phenotype correlation in X-linked Alport syndrome. J Am Soc Nephrol 2010; 21: 876–883

[2] Bindu LH, Reddy PP. Genetics of aminoglycoside-induced and prelingual non-syndromic mitochondrial hearing impairment: a review. Int J Audiol 2008; 47: 702–707

[3] Burch-Sims GP, Matlock VR. Hearing loss and auditory function in sickle cell disease. J Commun Disord 2005; 38: 321–329

[4] Chennupati SK, Levi J, Loftus P, Jornlin C, Morlet T, O'Reilly RC. Hearing loss in children with mitochondrial disorders. Int J Pediatr Otorhinolaryngol 2011; 75: 1519–1524

[5] Cremers CWRJ, Smith R, eds. Genetic Hearing Impairment: Its Clinical Presentations (Advances in Oto-Rhino-Laryngol Vol 61). Basel, Switzerland: Karger; 2002

[6] Ferner RE. The neurofibromatoses. Pract Neurol 2010; 10: 82–93

[7] Genetic Evaluation of Congenital Hearing Loss Expert Panel. ACMG statement. Genetics Evaluation Guidelines for the Etiologic Diagnosis of Congenital Hearing Loss. Genet Med 2002; 4: 162–171

[8] Lin JW, Chowdhury N, Mody A et al. Comprehensive diagnostic battery for evaluating sensorineural hearing loss in children. Otol Neurotol 2011; 32: 259–264

[9] Liu XZ, Pandya A, Angeli S et al. Audiological features of GJB2 (connexin 26) deafness. Ear Hear 2005; 26: 361–369

[10] Luxon LM, Cohen M, Coffey RA et al. Neuro-otological findings in Pendred syndrome. Int J Audiol 2003; 42: 82–88

[11] Marsella P, Scorpecci A, Pacifico C, Tieri L. Bone-anchored hearing aid (Baha) in patients with Treacher Collins syndrome: tips and pitfalls. Int J Pediatr Otorhinolaryngol 2011; 75: 1308–1312

[12] Schwartz PJ, Spazzolini C, Crotti L et al. The Jervell and Lange-Nielsen syndrome: natural history, molecular basis, and clinical outcome. Circulation 2006; 113: 783–790

[13] Snik AF, Hombergen GCH, Mylanus EA, Cremers CW. Air-bone gap in patients with X-linked stapes gusher syndrome. Am J Otol 1995; 16: 241–246

120 Noise-Induced Hearing Loss and Hearing Protection

Maurice Miller

120.1 Introduction

Exposure to noise in and out of the workplace accounts for more new cases of sensorineural hearing loss and accompanying tinnitus than all other causes combined. Presbycusis is believed by some to be the most common etiology of hearing loss in the adult American population. However, exposure to noise and aging typically occur simultaneously because while workers are employed for 40 years or longer in industries where they are exposed to high levels of noise, they simultaneously experience a four-decade-long aging of their auditory system. Current regulations to prevent hearing loss resulting from exposure to high levels of noise assume an *additive* effect of noise and age, but these factors may operate synergistically; exposure to high levels of noise may hasten premature aging of the auditory system.

Some reports indicate that acetylsalicylic acid, which typically has transient effects on hearing, may cause permanent, irreversible hearing loss in persons employed in noisy operations. Such interactive relationships need to be explored and reflected in updated criteria to provide more realistic methods of protecting workers' hearing.

Exposure to noise in recreational environments is a significant additional factor contributing to sensorineural hearing loss (SNHL) and tinnitus. Loud musical performances and the use of MP3 players for extended periods of time at high-intensity levels can affect the hearing of young persons who are not yet employed. More than 61 million Americans are exposed, on a regular basis, to various forms of nonoccupational hearing loss. Audio-protective agents to prevent or reverse noise-induced hearing loss are under active investigation and will be discussed later.

120.2 Legislative Background

It has been estimated that more than 10 million American workers are exposed to time-weighted levels of sound pressure of 85 dBA and greater. Among the industries in which such levels routinely occur are agriculture, mining, construction, manufacturing, utilities, transportation, and the military, although other industries and occupations may also expose workers to such high levels of noise.

Occupational noise and many other occupational hazards are not controlled by marketplace incentives alone, and government bodies have become involved in addressing, controlling, and regulating these hazards. Regulations to control the noise hazard in industry fall within the province of the federal government, specifically the Occupational Safety and Health Administration (OSHA), a branch of the U.S. Department of Labor. All industrial and occupational operations are within its jurisdiction, although "small business employers," usually defined as those with fewer than 25 employees, are exempt from OSHA regulations. The OSHA Hearing Conservation Amendment to the Occupational Noise Exposure Standard (29 CFR 1910.95) was passed in March 1983 and was implemented in April of that year, although a number of specific and important modifications have occurred since its passage.

Although it was preceded by various organizational consensus statements, the 1983 OSHA Occupational Noise Exposure Standard remains the national basis for most occupational hearing conservation programs. It is arguably the most important regulation designed to protect hearing since the beginning of the Industrial Revolution, yet it represents a *minimal* rather than an *optimal* effort to preserve worker hearing. The OSHA regulation is designed primarily to protect workers' hearing from exposure to noise in the workplace.

It is important to note the distinction between workers' compensation, which covers occupational hearing loss to varying degrees, and federal legislation. In the United States, state governments are responsible for promulgating compensation laws, whereas workplace health and safety standards fall under the jurisdiction of the U.S. Department of Labor. Coverage for occupational hearing loss varies from state to state, but federal regulations are uniform throughout the nation.

120.3 Pathophysiology of Noise Exposure

Noise can damage hearing when direct cochlear injury results from acoustic trauma during a single or a few exposures to extremely high levels of acoustic energy (e.g., an explosion). Isolated acoustic trauma can also damage the middle ear (e.g., ossicular chain discontinuity or tympanic membrane injury from sudden pressure changes). In acoustic trauma, the sound reaching the sensory structures in the cochlea exceeds the physical limits of these elements, and hair cells in the cochlea and supporting structures are damaged.

Far more frequent, and a major concern of occupational hearing conservation programs, are the effects of *long-term chronic* exposure to occupational noise. Chronic exposure to noise initially causes a temporary hearing loss, and the shift in hearing usually recovers within 14 hours. Repeated exposures may result in a permanent noise-induced hearing loss. The change to permanent loss is related to the intensity of the sound, duration of the exposure, frequency characteristics of the sound, and individual susceptibility, a risk criterion probably related to genetic factors.

Long-term exposure to moderate levels of noise usually causes edema and the distortion of sensory cells, a group of changes that have been termed *physiologic metabolic exhaustion*. Metabolic exhaustion is the point at which the threshold shift, usually in the range of 3,000 to 6,000 Hz and often bilateral, is a recoverable SNHL. Further exposure of unprotected and vulnerable ears has been shown to result in the complete absence of hair cells or their replacement by scar tissue, primarily in the basilar turns of the cochlea. When the degeneration of hair cells occurs, there is a permanent, usually irreversible, SNHL. Exposure to high levels of noise results in hair cell trauma. If the damage exceeds the ability of the hair cells to repair themselves, they die. Hair cells can die in different ways—either through apoptosis (an *active* mode of hair cell death requiring an energy supply) or through necrosis (a *passive* mode of cell death resulting in an early disintegration of cells).

120.4 Hearing Impairment and Tinnitus from Blast Trauma and Traumatic Brain Injury

The auditory system has been particularly at risk for damage during military deployment in Iraq and Afghanistan because most injuries are the result of blast explosions from improvised explosive devices: mortar, suicide bombs, and others. It has been estimated that 20% of the 1.6 million troops deployed in Iraq and Afghanistan have experienced traumatic brain injury. The most common residual long-term symptoms in military personnel with traumatic brain injury are intractable tinnitus and hearing loss, which were reported by 27% of veterans in 2007.

Head injury, by definition, can damage the central nervous system. The early and thorough identification and diagnosis of central auditory processing disorders in patients with head injury are crucial to improving and maintaining central auditory processing ability, as well as overall auditory function. Traumatic brain injury can also affect any part of the peripheral auditory system, and a complete evaluation of function from the outer and middle ear to the temporal cortex (early and later auditory evoked responses) is essential; disorders of both peripheral and central auditory function often coexist.

120.5 Occupational Hearing Conservation Program

The main components of an occupational hearing conservation program to protect worker hearing are the following:
1. Measurements of sound pressure levels in the work environment and levels of worker exposure to quantify the need for the program
2. Periodic audiometric testing of workers
3. Review of audiometry findings and case histories by a professional and appropriate referral
4. Personal hearing-protective devices and employee education program
5. Evaluation of the effectiveness of the program

Our discussion concentrates on the role of the hearing professional in the occupational hearing conservation program, particularly the audiologic and otologic aspects.

In many work environments, different departments assume responsibilities for the various aspects of the program: engineering or industrial hygiene departments for noise measurements, safety or industrial hygiene departments for hearing-protective devices, and nursing for audiometry. The hearing professional needs to have an ongoing relationship with each of the above departments or other departments that are involved in execution of the program. Although the hearing professional may not be directly involved in noise measurements or the personal hearing-protective aspects of the program, it is his or her responsibility to make sure that these critical aspects of the program are being covered and properly managed.

Sound level meters record noise *levels*, and *audio* or *noise dosimeters* measure noise *exposures*. The latter, which are worn on the worker's body, are preferred when noise exposure changes during the course of a workday. Dosimeters also record the varying noise levels and times of exposure, permitting the occupational hearing conservation team to identify and in many cases provide solutions to high-level exposures during a workday.

In the absence of data provided by use of the above instruments, a noisy area that needs attention to preserve worker hearing can be suspected when any of the following occur:
1. Workers must increase their voice levels to communicate with fellow employees.
2. Workers need to be within 1 to 2 inches of fellow workers to be heard.
3. Worker complaints of tinnitus and muffled hearing are reported after exposure to the work environment.

OSHA requires that all employees whose noise exposure reaches or exceeds the "action level" (85 dBA) for a time-weighted average of 8 hours undergo pure-tone air conduction audiography. Baseline and annual audiograms are required. The required audiometric test for noise-exposed workers consists of air conduction threshold measurements at 500, 1,000, 2,000, 3,000, 4,000, and 6,000 Hz in each ear. The addition of 8,000 Hz can aid in distinguishing noise-induced hearing loss from presbycusis. The majority of these tests are performed by occupational hearing conservationists, and microprocessor audiometers are used for such tests. In a review of the audiometric and case history data, the specialist should be familiar with the worker's specific occupation, the degree and level of occupational noise exposure, the ambient noise level in the audiometric test environment, the date of the most recent audiometer calibration, and relevant case history data.

It is appropriate for the professional to recommend otologic and/or audiologic evaluation, as indicated, including specific procedures, such as auditory brainstem response (ABR) testing, otoacoustic emissions (OAEs) testing, and vestibular evaluation. Employees requiring middle ear surgery, surgical relief of Meniere disease, or management for acoustic tumors should be referred to experienced otologic surgeons in the area where the employee lives or works.

120.5.1 Data Collection and Analysis

Shortly after the initiation of the program, companies with a significant number of noise-exposed employees will be generating a significant amount of audiometric and audiologic data. The employees' noise exposure, use of personal hearing protection, and air conduction thresholds are recorded, along with the results of a baseline test noting the presence or absence of a standard threshold shift (STS) at 2,000, 3,000, and 4,000 Hz for each ear. The results of the otoscopic screening examination are collected and can be managed with analyzed with dedicated software.

The audiometric data can be used to assess the effectiveness of the overall program, alert workers to impending hearing loss, and reveal potential employer liabilities for compensable hearing loss. The incidence of occupational noise-induced hearing loss, evidenced by the STS (an average change of 10 dB or greater at 2,000, 3,000 and 4,000 Hz in either ear compared with the baseline, with age adjustments allowed), is one indicator of the effectiveness of the occupational hearing conservation program. Incidence rates of 5% or less, decreasing with each year, provide such evidence.

120.5.2 Protection of Residual Hearing and Prevention of Further Hearing Loss

Among the most significant components of the occupational hearing conservation program is protection of the workers' hearing. Engineering controls that reduce noise exposure at the source represent the ultimate solution for noise control. Rotating or administrative controls that move employees to quieter areas of the industrial operation, so that total exposure during the workday is kept to a "safe" level, have limited applications and are impractical in many operations. Until noise can be and is controlled at the source, personal hearing-protective devices, properly fitted and consistently used, will remain the major method for protecting and preserving workers' hearing. The occupational hearing conservation team is faced with a general unwillingness of workers to use hearing protection, who offer a variety of reasons for noncompliance. Although protection of the eyes is generally widely accepted, hearing protection is not because the onset of chronic noise-induced hearing loss is a gradual, subtle, painless, and bloodless process. Although the issuance and monitored use of hearing-protective devices often falls within the province of a company's safety department, the hearing professional must be assured that appropriate hearing protection is being issued and its use monitored. And just as ineffective hearing protection must be avoided, overprotection is similarly to be avoided because it encourages nonuse, may unnecessarily interfere with interpersonal communication, and may prevent the detection of important warning signals.

Personal hearing-protective devices provide a barrier between the noise source and the cochlea. The basic types are ear plugs, ear muffs, and semiaurals. Ear plugs are the predominant form of protection and used in about 80% of industrial applications. The most widely used type is the user-molded or formable plug made of a soft polymer. Ear muffs consist of a plastic cup attached to an adjustable headband. The cups are made to fit snugly against the head with foam or liquid-filled cushions. Ear plugs are subject to variations from the manufacturer's stated noise reduction ratio (NRR) when a worker inserts the device into his or her external auditory canal. Ear muffs are less subject to such variations, although they too can be "sabotaged" in a number of ways. Ear plugs should be used with caution, if at all, by any workers with insulin-dependent diabetes, particularly those working in areas where fresh running water is not available.

The hearing professional should be aware of the procedures implemented to determine the degree of use and effectiveness of noise protectors, as defined by the National Institute of Occupational Safety and Health (NIOSH).

Experts in the field of hearing protection recently reached a consensus on a revised American National Standards Institute (ANSI) standard for measuring the real-ear attenuation (REAT) of hearing-protective devices. The REAT measures the *change* in the sound level entering the ears of a subject wearing a hearing-protective device in an occupational hearing conservation program after placement of the device either by a thoroughly trained user (method A) or by an inexperienced, novice user (method B).

Critical to the success of the hearing-protective device program is the employee education program. Attendance at the annual employee education program is required (unlike audiometric testing, which is nonmandatory but must be made available to the employee). The employee education program explains the effects of noise on hearing, the purpose and use of various personal hearing-protective devices, and the audiometric procedures that will be offered. The hearing professional is strongly advised to be an integral part of the employee education program and should be personally present to answer questions from employees in attendance. In many respects, the employee education program is the most critical component of the occupational hearing conservation program.

Although the majority of ear plugs in use are *passive*, there is also a role, albeit a limited one, for *active* hearing protectors. Active devices can increase the attenuation of low-frequency noise by about 15 to 20 dB in comparison with the attenuation provided by the widely used passive protectors. The active type provides low-frequency protection when the worker is exposed to repetitive or continuous noises that are relatively constant in their frequency spectrum and level. They incorporate microphones and amplifiers that transmit external sounds to earphones mounted inside the hearing-protective device.

120.5.3 Otoprotective Agents for Noise-Induced Hearing Loss

Many agents have and are being tested in animals to determine if they can prevent or lessen the effects of temporary or permanent noise-induced SNHL. Some agents are administered to prevent these losses and are designed to be used before noise exposure. A few, referred to as *rescue agents*, are taken within hours or a few days after the noise exposure to prevent permanent hearing loss and are designed to act before cochlear damage becomes permanent.

No otoprotective agents are currently approved by the FDA. ACEmg (β-carotene, vitamin C, vitamin E, and magnesium) and D-met (D-methionine) appear to be the most promising otoprotective agents, although NAC (N-acetylcysteine) and ebselen are also contenders. These agents, based on studies in rodents, appear to provide protection from aminoglycoside- and cisplatinum-induced damage to hair cells. An oxidative mechanism may explain their action against these toxicities.

120.6 Roundsmanship

- Noise-induced hearing loss is a ubiquitous threat to hearing in the modern, noisy world.
- Groups of patients especially at risk include teenagers and young adults, especially those individuals who frequent rock concerts and other venues where music in electronically amplified to aphysiologic levels.

- Any period of exposure to noise loud enough to cause tinnitus has probably caused a temporary threshold shift in hearing. This should be understood as a severe warning sign—the ear will not tolerate this level of noise exposure repeatedly.
- Individuals who must be or choose to be exposed to noise should wear hearing protection. It is not possible to protect the ear completely from unwanted noise exposure. Hearing protection may significantly help decrease noise-induced hearing loss in these individuals.
- For any patient at risk for noise-induced hearing loss, an annual hearing test is the minimum requirement for hearing safety.

120.7 Recommended Reading

[1] ANSI. American National Standard: Methods for Measuring the Real-Ear Attenuation of Hearing Protectors. New York, NY: American National Standards Institute; 1997

[2] Berger EH. Hearing protection devices. In: Berger EH, Ward WD, Morrill JC, Royster LH, eds. Noise and Hearing Conservation Manual. 5th ed. Akron, OH: American Industrial Hygiene Association; 1986

[3] Bohne BA, Harding GW, Lee SC. Death pathways in noise-damaged outer hair cells. Hear Res 2007; 223: 61–70

[4] Dobie RA. Medical-Legal Evaluation of Hearing Loss. New York, NY: Van Nostrand Reinhold; 1993

[5] Fligor BJ. Risk for noise-induced hearing loss from use of portable media players: a summary of evidence through 2008. Persp ect Audiol 2009; 5: 10–20

[6] Hu BH, Henderson D, Nicotera TM. Involvement of apoptosis in progression of cochlear lesion following exposure to intense noise. Hear Res 2002; 166: 62–71

[7] Miller MH. Hearing conservation in industry. Curr Opin Otolaryngol Head Neck Surg 1998; 6: 352–357

[8] Musiek FE, Baran JA, Shinn J. Assessment and remediation of an auditory processing disorder associated with head trauma. J Am Acad Audiol 2004; 15: 117–132

[9] Sha SH, Schacht J. Antioxidants attenuate gentamicin-induced free radical formation in vitro and ototoxicity in vivo: D-methionine is a potential protectant. Hear Res 2000; 142: 34–40

[10] Tun C, Hogan A, Fitzharris K. Hearing and vestibular dysfunction caused by-blast injuries and traumatic brain injuries. Hear ing J 2009; 62; (11): 24–26

121 Sudden Idiopathic Sensorineural Hearing Loss

Christopher J. Linstrom

121.1 Introduction

Virtually every physician working in otolaryngology-head and neck surgery will at some time encounter a patient with sudden, unprovoked neurosensory hearing loss. This problem is sufficiently common that the general ear, nose, and throat physician should be able to recognize it, distinguish it from hearing loss with other likely causes, obtain a history and conduct a physical examination, order the appropriate initial diagnostic tests, and start the patient on proven forms of treatment in a timely fashion. The efficacy of treatment diminishes with the passage of time after the initial awareness of hearing loss. Thus, it is incumbent upon every otolaryngologist to have a sound awareness of this problem and to start treatment immediately, or to make a direct and timely referral to an otologist/neurotologist who will.

Sudden idiopathic sensorineural hearing loss (SNHL) was first described by DeKleyn in 1944. It is typically characterized by the new onset of *unilateral* hearing loss that develops within 72 hours. By convention, at least three midrange frequencies should be involved. There may be associated fullness and/or tinnitus in the affected ear. Imbalance or vertigo may also be present and is a negative prognosticator for the recovery of hearing, along with advanced age and lack of measurable hearing at the time of the first audiogram. Favorable prognostic factors are younger age and measurable hearing, especially word discrimination and an upward-sloping or "cookie bite" pattern on the first audiogram. Wide fluctuations of hearing are a negative prognosticator for the future recovery of hearing.

121.2 Incidence of Disease

Sudden idiopathic SNHL has an estimated incidence of 5 to 20 per 100,000 persons per year. This incidence is approximately the same as that for Meniere syndrome (15 per 100,000 per year). The true incidence may be underestimated because spontaneous recovery has been reported to occur in 32 to 65% of untreated or placebo-treated patients. A "window of opportunity" of several weeks to a few months exists, during which the oral or injected (transtympanic) administration of steroids may help the recovery of hearing. The likelihood of recovery diminishes as time passes. If the hearing loss is mild, many patients do not recognize it and therefore delay seeking medical attention. Aural fullness is often misdiagnosed as eustachian tube dysfunction, and the patient is treated for a cold or influenza before an audiogram establishes that a neurosensory loss of hearing has actually occurred. This further delays treatment. As more and more general practitioners become aware of this entity, the delays in diagnosis and treatment will inevitably lessen.

It is important for all physicians to realize that a tuning fork examination yields information only about the *physics* of audition (i.e., sounds heard by air conduction should be perceived as louder than sounds heard by bone conduction). A tuning fork examination yields very little reliable information about the actual level of audition. That must be determined in an audiometric booth by a properly trained and qualified audiologist, never by the patient himself or herself.

121.3 Applied Anatomy

The anatomy of the cochlear and vestibular apparatus has been described in other chapters of this book and will not be repeated here. Sudden idiopathic SNHL is purely neurosensory, not conductive, in nature. It is by definition not provoked by anything known to the patient and should not occur in the context of chronic suppurative otitis media with or without perforation or cholesteatoma. The antecedent history should in fact be "no history." Sudden idiopathic SNHL does not occur in the context of sudden changes in resting barometric pressure, as one would expect with a perilymphatic fistula. The patient ordinarily does not experience a warning sign that the ear is changing. The hearing loss is indeed sudden, not slow, in onset. The onset does not mimic the slow, gradual, and inevitable decline in hearing associated with an acoustic neuroma or another slowly growing tumor of the retrocochlear pathways of hearing.

121.4 The Disease Process

121.4.1 Etiology

There is no known "cause" for sudden idiopathic SNHL. This disease does not run in families, is not heritable, is not caused by a known infectious agent, and is not the end stage or tangential product of any known systemic illness, such as rheumatoid arthritis or other connective tissue disorders. If a cause of the hearing loss is known, then it is no longer "idiopathic."

121.4.2 Pathogenesis

Proposed causative theories suggest vascular etiology, a viral etiology, or both. Because this condition is not lethal, fresh autopsy specimens do not exist, and the pathophysiology of sudden idiopathic SNHL, although logically postulated, remains unproven. There is no animal in which sudden idiopathic SNHL is known to occur naturally. Although vascular occlusion of the cochlea in an animal model has been shown to produce SNHL, this is not idiopathic (i.e., the cause is known). In the absence of fresh histopathologic evidence, speculation is the best one can do. This, of course, is of little comfort to the patient, who is as mystified as the treating physician as to what precisely has occurred. Evidence to support a vascular theory of sudden idiopathic SNHL includes the following:

- Sudden onset, suggestive of infarction
- Case reports of sudden deafness occurring in association with known systemic vascular disease
- Histopathlogic demonstration of cochlear changes due to vascular occlusion in animal models

However, temporal bone studies of patients with sudden idiopathic SNHL who donated their temporal bones after natural death have not demonstrated labyrinthine ossification, the hallmark of labyrinthine ischemia. Evidence to support a viral theory includes the following:

- A temporal relationship between active viral upper respiratory illness and sudden idiopathic SNHL has been shown.
- Patients with sudden idiopathic SNHL have been shown to have antibody titers to several viruses.
- Postmortem histopathologic specimens of human temporal bones have shown atrophy of the organ of Corti, spiral ganglion, and tectorial membrane; unraveling of myelin; and relative preservation of the spiral ganglion cells. These findings are consistent with viral infection. However, no specimen exists for the acute period of this illness because it is not lethal. Thus, no comment can be made about the *causative* nature of these histologic findings.
- In animal laboratory experiments, inflammatory cytokines produced in response to viral disease may interrupt gap junction pathways in the cochlea, resulting in suddenly decreased function and the death of hair cells within the cochlea. Early treatment with corticosteroids has been seen to reverse this process.

121.4.3 Natural History and Progression

Most patient presenting with sudden idiopathic SNHL have reached a nadir of hearing loss at the time of presentation. Patients' hearing may infrequently fluctuate downward for 1 to 3 days before settling to its lowest point. What the ear should not do is fluctuate down, recover, then fluctuate down again in a repetitive cycle, which suggests cochlear hydrops. This is not the typical pattern of hearing loss associated with sudden idiopathic SNHL. Patients who present with measurable hearing have a better chance of recovery. Patients who present with little if any measurable hearing and either have vertigo or are older than approximately 60 years have a poorer prognosis for recovery.

121.4.4 Potential Disease Complications

The major potential complication of sudden idiopathic SNHL is that the disease entity is a "red herring"—the presentation of a retrocochlear lesion, such as an acoustic neuroma, another benign neoplasm, or metastatic disease to the temporal bone. Although sudden hearing loss due to benign retrocochlear disease is rare, it may occur. Thus, a thorough diagnostic evaluation of every patient with sudden idiopathic SNHL should include a retrocochlear radiographic study, preferably magnetic resonance (MR) imaging with or without contrast.

121.5 Disease Grading

There is no accepted staging system for patients presenting with sudden idiopathic SNHL. Prognostication of the response to treatment, as previously discussed, is predicated upon the amount of measured residual hearing at the time of the initial audiogram.

121.6 Medical Evaluation

Patients with sudden idiopathic SNHL are generally healthy, in midlife, with few if any underlying medical problems. If the patient is known to have hypertension, diabetes, or another medical problem, such as glaucoma, coronary artery disease, or systemic vascular disease, these should be carefully controlled by the internist because they will have a direct bearing on the form of treatment. It is important to know if women in the childbearing years are pregnant. Other than a careful medical history to elicit concomitant medical conditions that could be exacerbated by the administration of steroids, it is usually not necessary to perform any blood testing that the patient's primary care physician or internist would have on record. There is no serum marker for sudden idiopathic SNHL.

121.6.1 Presenting Complaints

The chief complaint of the patient is unilateral acute hearing loss. By accepted definition, it should have occurred over a time period of no more than 72 hours. It should never be bilateral hearing loss or sequentially bilateral loss; it is unilateral. Additional features, such as aural fullness, tinnitus, dizziness, and vertigo, may accompany the chief complaint, which is hearing loss.

121.6.2 Clinical Findings, Physical Examination

The patient should have a general head and neck examination that concentrates on the ear, and ordinarily there should be no physical findings that would *in themselves* explain the hearing loss.

121.6.3 Testing

A tuning fork test with at least one or two forks in the speech frequencies (e.g., 512 Hz, 1,024 Hz) should be done. The examiner should have a good idea that the hearing loss is neurosensory and not conductive in nature before sending the patient for an audiogram,

A standard *minimum* audiogram consists of pure tones presented *separately* by air and bone for each ear, a test of word recognition presented *separately* for each ear, and immittance testing including testing of the middle ear muscle response if possible, depending upon the anatomy. Audiograms that do not provide this minimal information should be immediately discarded and the hearing tested by a trained professional.

Regardless of the supposed diagnosis and treatment plan, if the hearing is indeed asymmetrically decreased, a radiographic evaluation of the retrocochlear pathways should be performed, ideally with well-done MR imaging of the temporal bones, base of the skull, and brain without and with gadolinium enhancement. Patients who are claustrophobic may be able to withstand open or "stand-up" MR imaging. The quality of these studies is ever improving. Patients who cannot undergo MR imaging for anatomical reasons (e.g., implanted ferromagnetic hardware) may undergo computed tomography (CT) of the temporal bones *with* contrast enhancement. The utility of auditory brainstem reflex (ABR) testing, compared with the cur-

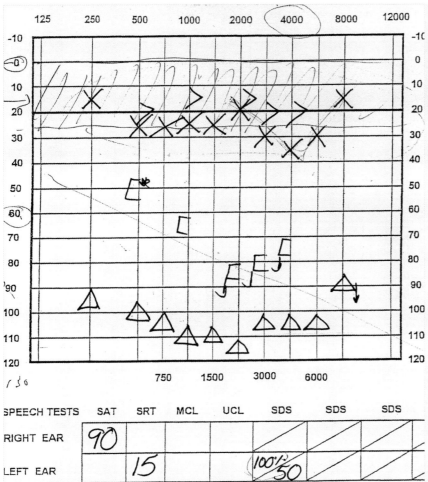

Fig. 121.1 Initial audiogram of 60-year-old man with sudden sensorineural hearing loss in the right ear.

rent level of diagnostic accuracy of MR imaging and CT with contrast, is simply too low for it to be recommended as a routine diagnostic tool. Well-done MR imaging with contrast is a definitive study in that its sensitivity for detecting and specificity for excluding retrocochlear disease are in the range of 98 to 99%.

121.6.4 Differential Diagnosis

Once retrocochlear pathology has been excluded, the main items in the differential diagnosis are Meniere syndrome, a perilymphatic fistula of the oval or round windows, autoimmune inner ear disease (which may present in a *sequential* fashion), otosyphilis, and structural abnormalities of the otic capsule that might predispose the patient to hearing loss.

Meniere Syndrome.

Endolymphatic hydrops may rarely present as sudden hearing loss without vertigo. The classic presentation is a collection of symptoms, usually unilateral: increasing fullness, pressure, and tinnitus in the affected ear, followed by a drop in hearing acuity and violent, unprovoked vertigo lasting one to several hours. The history is so characteristic that it usually yields the correct diagnosis by itself without additional testing. If vertigo is absent, one could postulate hydrops, but the characteristic

prodrome and collection of symptoms are absent in sudden idiopathic SNHL. In addition, unlike Meniere syndrome, sudden idiopathic SNHL is not episodic. Many patients with sudden idiopathic SNHL are in fact treated with steroids, a low-salt diet, and a salt-wasting diuretic early in the course of the illness. The lack of a second episode usually clears up any doubt as to what has actually occurred.

Perilymphatic Fistula

Perilymphatic fistula is almost always diagnosed after a sudden and violent change in the resting barometric environment of the ear, such as a violent sneeze, a rapid descent in an aircraft in which the ear pressure could not be equalized, or underwater scuba diving in which the pressure could not be equalized. The history is paramount to making a proper diagnosis. The history almost always includes a sudden loss of hearing accompanied by violent vertigo. It is ordinarily not something to guess about, but is readily apparent from the history.

Autoimmne Inner Ear Disease

Autoimmne inner ear disease is usually bilateral and presents as inexorable, downwardly fluctuating neurosensory hearing loss. The hearing loss is usually symmetric, although one ear may be farther down than the other. In rare cases, one ear loses hearing first, and then after a few months or even years, the

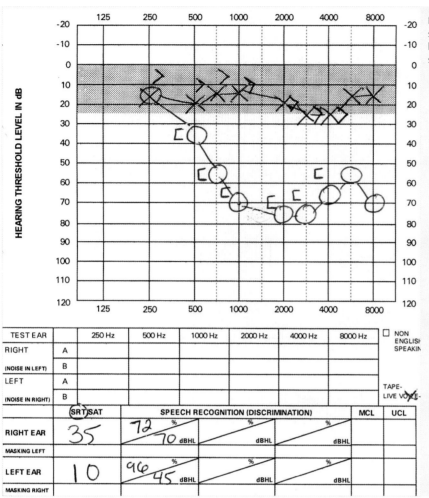

Fig. 121.2 One-year follow-up audiogram of the same patient shows some modest recovery of hearing in the right ear after treatment with oral steroids.

TEST EAR		250 Hz	500 Hz	1000 Hz	2000 Hz	4000 Hz	8000 Hz	☐ NON ENGLISH SPEAKIN
RIGHT	A							
(NOISE IN LEFT)	B							
LEFT	A							TAPE-
(NOISE IN RIGHT)	B							LIVE VOICE-

	SRT SAT	SPEECH RECOGNITION (DISCRIMINATION)			MCL	UCL
RIGHT EAR	35	72 % 70 dBHL	% dBHL	% dBHL		
MASKING LEFT						
LEFT EAR	10	96 % 45 dBHL	% dBHL	% dBHL		
MASKING RIGHT						

other ear begins to lose hearing. The main features of this condition are the pattern of fluctuation and the time course over a period exceeding 72 hours. The onset is ordinarily not sudden; rather, the inevitable downward pattern of loss occurs over a period of weeks and months.

Syphilis

Syphilis is the "great masquerader," and indeed late or latent syphilis may infrequently cause sudden acute hearing loss. One feature suggestive of otosyphilis is that the hearing in both ears may fluctuate in an alternating fashion; an ear will hear poorly on day, better the next day, and so on. Up and down, fluctuating, *bilateral* hearing loss is *not* seen with sudden idiopathic SNHL. Any patient with sudden idiopathic SNHL should be tested for historical exposure to *Treponema pallidum* with a fluorescent treponemal antibody absorption (FTA-ABS) test, or its equivalent.

Structural Abnormalities of the Otic Capsule

Structural abnormalities of the otic capsule, especially patent vestibular aqueduct, may predispose a person to sudden hearing loss. A history of head trauma or any head injury should be elicited. This is almost never found in an adult. In addition, if profound hearing loss of any nature is noted in a child, edge-

enhanced CT of the temporal bone without contrast should be performed to look for a structural abnormality of the temporal bone on both the affected side and the side with better hearing. The most common finding will be a patent vestibular aqueduct, usually with a greatest width of more than 1.8 to 2.0 mm. If this is discovered, the child must avoid all sports in which the head could be struck.

121.7 Treatment

121.7.1 Medical Treatment

Steroids

The mainstay of the treatment for sudden idiopathic SNHL is steroid administration, either orally or via transtympanic injection, or both. Most patients can be treated by at least one method. The 1980 landmark paper of Wilson et al, and those of many authors thereafter, have clearly demonstrated the benefits of exogenous steroid administration in the treatment of sudden idiopathic SNHL. Although there is no "recipe" for treatment, most patients will be able to withstand a treatment protocol of oral steroid, usually prednisone, taken as a single dose or in divided doses equaling 1 mg/kg of body weight per day. This will usually equal 60 to 80 mg per day for most adult patients. It is important for patients to be counseled that the treatment pro-

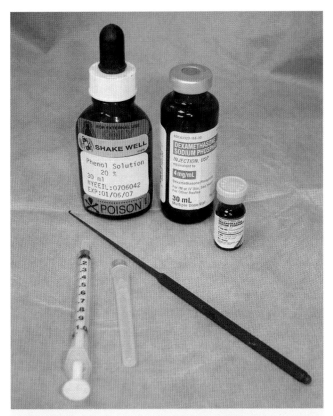

Fig. 121.3 Setup for an intratympanic injection of dexamethasone. A 1.0-mL tuberculin syringe is filled to approximately 0.5 mL with a 27-gauge long needle. The topical anesthetic, 20% phenol, is applied with a drop applicator (*long, black instrument*). The injection site is usually the near the round window. For multiple injections, one should choose different sites to decrease the chance of causing a tympanic membrane perforation.

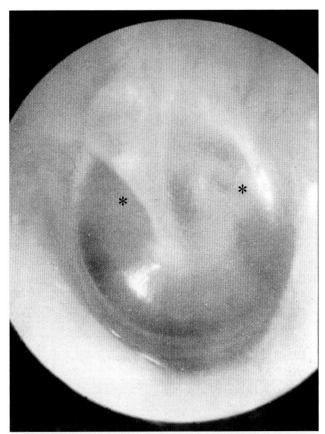

Fig. 121.4 Typical injection sites (*asterisks*) for a left eardrum.

gram is for a brief period only, that the potential side effects, although significant, are transient, and that there are no other medications whose efficacy has been proved to equal that of steroids. The exact anti-inflammatory mechanism of steroids remains unknown. They intimately affect the biochemical pathways of carbohydrates, inhibit multiple inflammatory cytokines, and produce multiple glucocorticoid and mineralocorticoid effects. Steroids stabilize cell membranes and make them more structurally intact and less leaky, thereby acting as anti-inflammatory agents. Even though their exact mechanism of action is unknown, steroids are known to be of benefit in sudden idiopathic SNHL, a form of nerve hearing loss in which hearing is potentially *restorable* (▶ Fig. 121.1 and ▶ Fig. 121.2).

Oral steroids are give in a "burst then taper" pattern, in which a high "shoulder" of medication is given for a period of 10 to 14 days, followed by a period of tapering of approximately 5 to 7 days. As the amount of exogenous steroid is decreased, the adrenal glands will again supply endogenous cortisol. Steroids have several potential side effects, and the patient should be made aware of them:

Weight Gain

A transient gain of 3 to 5 lb is common with the use of oral steroids because of both the retention of water and appetite stimulation. Ordinarily, the weight gain is transient, and compensatory weight loss will occur as the steroid is tapered.

Increased Serum Glucose

This is ordinarily not a problem for the patient who does not have diabetes. However, patients who have borderline diabetes or are known to have diabetes that is controlled with either oral hypoglycemic agents or insulin may have to alter their daily regimen while on exogenous steroids. Any physician who prescribes oral steroids must inquire about this, and the patient must either know how to regulate the serum glucose by himself or herself or seek the help of another treating physician. Patients with brittle, insulin-dependent diabetes may not be candidates for oral steroids.

Hypertension

Exogenous steroids cause water retention, and thus the patient's resting blood pressure may increase. For the normotensive patient, steroids ordinarily will be very well tolerated. Patients with labile hypertension must be managed carefully by an internist or cardiologist during the period of oral steroid use. These patients may require an increase in the dose of their regular antihypertensive agent or an additional medication to regulate the blood pressure.

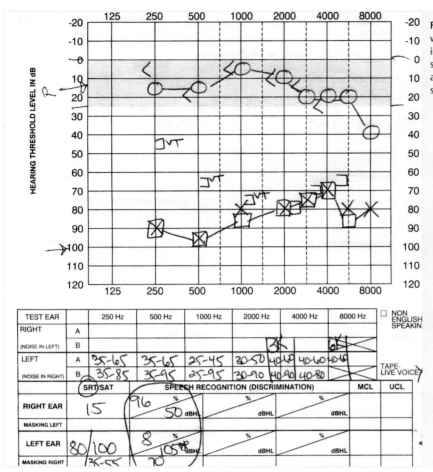

Fig. 121.5 Initial audiogram of a 65-year-old man with sudden idiopathic sensorineural hearing loss in the left ear. After treatment with oral corticosteroids, the patient showed some improvement and subsequently was treated with intratympanic steroid injections.

Gastritis

Oral steroids may cause rather pronounced gastritis and should be taken with food or with an over-the-counter or prescribed antacid or hydrogen ion blocker such as omeprazole, esomeprazole, or dexlansoprazole. These agents will ordinarily significantly reduce acid reflux while the patient is taking oral steroids.

Insomnia

Almost all adults report that exogenous steroids affect their normal patterns of sleep, usually the transition between a state of tiredness and sleep. Therefore, it is practical to attempt to take the full daily dose by about 2 PM, so that blood levels of the steroid are decreasing when the patient ordinarily tries to fall asleep in the evening. The tendency to insomnia ordinarily decreases as the daily dose is tapered.

Avascular Necrosis

Avascular necrosis of the weight-bearing joints is an idiopathic reaction to any exogenous steroid in any form that may occur in approximately 1 per 200,000 individuals. This may lead to a precipitous osteoarthritis causing necrosis of the articular surfaces of the weight-bearing joints, most especially the femoral heads. It is not dose-related. Any patient contemplating the use of oral steroids must be informed of the risk for this rare but significant potential complication.

Other Conditions

Patients who have poorly controlled glaucoma or who are pregnant will ordinarily not be allowed to take exogenous steroids. It is of great importance that the patient's overall care be coordinated with his or her primary care physician. In certain instances, the underlying medical problem(s) preclude the use of oral steroids, and the only other available method of treatment would be intratympanic administration.

Antiviral Medication

One of the two main putative pathophysiologic mechanisms of sudden idiopathic SNHL is viral infection of the cochlea. Antivirals agents such as acyclovir, valacyclovir, famciclovir, and ganciclovir may be used along with steroids in the treatment of sudden idiopathic SNHL when a viral etiology is strongly suspected. However, their benefit at this time is unproven, and they are no longer the mainstay of treatment for this condition.

Intratympanic (or Transtympanic) Steroids

It is known that exogenous steroid is of benefit to patients with sudden idiopathic SNHL. What is unknown at present is the preferred means of delivering the steroid, either per os or via the round or oval window, although this is the subject of active and intense inquiry. Patients who cannot or will not take oral steroids or who have failed a course of oral steroids may benefit from intratympanic steroids. The administration of steroid in

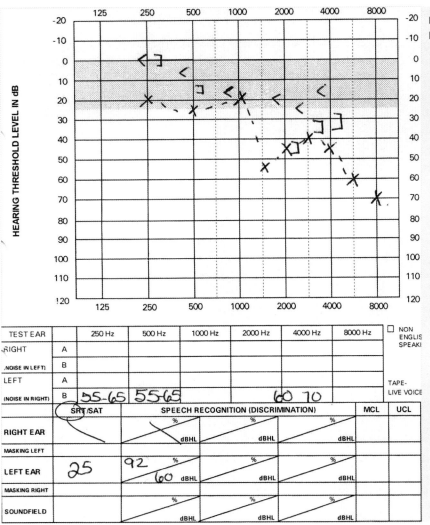

Fig. 121.6 Audiogram after oral and intratympanic corticosteroid treatment.

TEST EAR		250 Hz	500 Hz	1000 Hz	2000 Hz	4000 Hz	8000 Hz	☐ NON ENGLIS SPEAKI
RIGHT	A							
(NOISE IN LEFT)	B							
LEFT	A							TAPE-
(NOISE IN RIGHT)	B	55-65	5565			60 10		LIVE VOICE

	SRT/SAT	SPEECH RECOGNITION (DISCRIMINATION)						MCL	UCL
		%		%		%			
RIGHT EAR			dBHL		dBHL		dBHL		
MASKING LEFT									
LEFT EAR	25	92 % 60	dBHL	%	dBHL	%	dBHL		
MASKING RIGHT									
SOUNDFIELD		%	dBHL	%	dBHL	%	dBHL		

this fashion for this indication has been studied rigorously and has been shown to be of benefit for sudden idiopathic SNHL. The choice of steroid depends upon several factors; the pharmokinetics (the mineralocorticoids are more highly absorbed than the glucocorticoids), the relative discomfort to the patient depending upon the resting pH of the solvated steroid, and the availability of the steroid all affect the choice of steroid to be used.

Most treating physicians will choose dexamethasone (4 or 10 mg/mL) and administer about 0.5 mL through the topically anesthetized (20% phenol or trichloroacetic acid) tympanic membrane (▶ Fig. 121.3 and ▶ Fig. 121.4). The patient is placed in the Trendelenburg position for about 25 to 30 minutes and asked not to swallow in order to keep the steroid within the middle ear cleft. The patient is the brought to the supine position thereafter, the excess steroid is suctioned from the middle ear, and a few otic antibiotic drops are instilled into the external canal of the treated ear.

Other choices for steroid injection include hydrocortisone sodium succinate and methylprednisolone sodium succinate. These have been shown in a rodent model to achieve higher concentrations in the inner ear when given intravenously. However, injections of these agents into the middle ear cleft are quite painful, may induce an acute inflammation not unlike acute otitis media, and in general are less likely to be well tolerated. Patients may experience transient vertigo and discomfort after the first dexamethasone injection into the middle ear cleft, but most tolerate the medication very well. The same cannot be said for methylprednisolone and hydrocortisone, which are quite noxious to the middle ear.

A hearing test of the treated ear (pure tone, bone, discrimination, no immittance) is repeated 1 week after the second injection (given 3 to 7 days after the first injection). If the ear shows signs of improvement in either the speech recognition threshold (SRT) or the word discrimination score (WDS), the intratympanic injections continue until a "ceiling effect" of improvement in the SRT or, more likely, the WDS is achieved. Further injections will be unlikely to be of any additional benefit. If, on the other hand, there is no improvement in either the SRT or WDS after two injections, no further injections are performed (▶ Fig. 121.5, ▶ Fig. 121.6, ▶ Fig. 121.7, ▶ Fig. 121.8).

The main risk of intratympanic injection of steroid is perforation of the tympanic membrane. The use of a small-bore needle with the minimum amount of topical anesthetic will usually decrease this risk. For patients undergoing repeated injections, alternating the injection site will also decrease the risk. Treatment during pregnancy should be discussed and coordinated

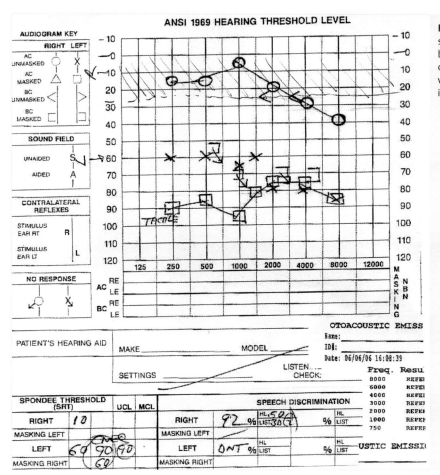

Fig. 121.7 A 61-year-old woman with sudden sensorineural hearing loss in the left ear 5 days before audiogram, with a brief (24-hour) period of vertigo but constant tinnitus. She was treated with dexamethasone orally followed by four intratympanic injections.

with the patient's obstetrician. Although the amount of injected steroid is small, at least some of it is likely to be ingested via the eustachian tube and gut and thus will be absorbed systemically.

121.7.2 Surgical Treatment

There is no known surgical treatment to restore neurosensory hearing loss that is idiopathic and sudden. Any other entity is not strictly sudden idiopathic SNHL. Middle ear exploration and the packing of suspected fistulas of the oval and round windows are of no value in sudden idiopathic SNHL.

121.8 Prognosis and Response to Treatment

The response of a patient to either oral or injected steroid depends upon several factors. The three most salient are the following:
1. The amount of measurable hearing (pure tone and speech recognition) at the time of the first audiogram.
2. The pattern of the first audiogram. An upward-sloping hearing loss and a "cookie bite" hearing loss with only the mid frequencies affected are good prognosticators, whereas both a severely downward-sloping pattern of loss and a "flat out" pattern of immeasurable hearing loss are poor prognosticators.

3. The time course between the occurrence of sudden hearing loss and the administration of steroids. A time delay of more than 2 weeks is certainly unfavorable. The sooner steroids are administered, the more likely a beneficial response.

The numbers vary widely depending upon the reported series of patients, the type of medical treatment given, and the criteria used to define "beneficial response" versus "little response" or "no response."

Patients with sudden idiopathic SNHL can be divided basically into three groups, as can patients with many other disease processes.

121.8.1 Good Responders

Patients with mild or moderate levels of hearing loss, good discrimination scores, and the absence of vertigo are likely to be the best responders. The patient with an upward-sloping or "cookie bite" audiogram and measurable residual hearing will show the most favorable response. Many will recover nearly normal or normal hearing, and routine audiometric follow-up is performed within 6 months.

121.8.2 Midlevel Responders

These patients present with worse levels of hearing and poorer initial discrimination scores, and they may have imbalance or vertigo along with hearing loss. They are likely to recover some

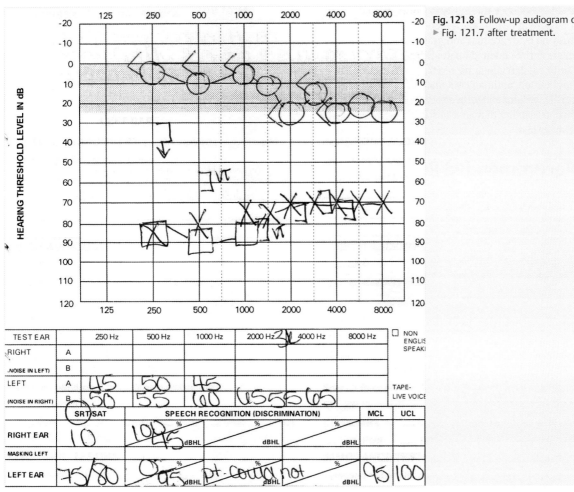

Fig. 121.8 Follow-up audiogram of the patient in ► Fig. 121.7 after treatment.

TEST EAR		250 Hz	500 Hz	1000 Hz	2000 Hz	4000 Hz	8000 Hz	☐ NON ENGLISH SPEAKI
RIGHT	A							
(NOISE IN LEFT)	B							
LEFT	A	45	50	45				
(NOISE IN RIGHT)	B	50	55	60	65 55 65			TAPE- LIVE VOICE

	SRT/SAT	SPEECH RECOGNITION (DISCRIMINATION)			MCL	UCL
RIGHT EAR	10	10 45 % dBHL	% dBHL	% dBHL		
MASKING LEFT						
LEFT EAR	75/80	95 % dBHL	Pt could not % dBHL	% dBHL	95	100

of their hearing, but it is almost never completely normal, and they may or may not become candidates for amplification in the affected ear. Follow-up audiograms should be obtained within 6 months and the status of the hearing assessed.

121.8.3 Poor Responders

These patients present with flat, "all gone" audiograms after therapy, tend to be older (past 60 years of age), and usually have violent vertigo along with their sudden hearing loss. In fact, these patients may have labyrinthitis. They should be counseled that it is highly unlikely that they will regain any hearing regardless of treatment and that they should use a sound-shunting device, such as a contralateral routing of signals (CROS) device or a bone-anchored hearing aid (BAHA). Many if not most of these patients have seen numerous physicians and otologists, have tried both oral and injected steroids, and are looking for a miracle. With empathy, the physician must be a realist, offer these patients a careful and thorough diagnosis, and help them to accept the loss of hearing on the affected side. One important step along the way is to emphasize that it is highly unlikely that the patient will lose hearing in the opposite (good) ear and that, were this to happen, the patient would never truly become deaf because he or she would be a candidate for cochlear implantation. It is important to reassure the patient that the sudden loss of hearing on one side does not in any way mean that the

second ear is condemned to the same fate. This is the (usually) unspoken fear of every patient, and it should be dispelled. With the physician's kindness and empathy, the patient with unrecoverable, profound sudden idiopathic SNHL may be helped to accept the loss of hearing and to take positive measures to improve his or her overall ability to communicate. Without a doubt, these are most difficult patients to treat.

121.9 Roundsmanship

- Sudden idiopathic SNHL occurs in approximately 1 to 2 per 100,000 persons per year. It is not precipitated by any known cause.
- Sudden idiopathic SNHL is almost always unilateral. If a patient should suffer sudden hearing loss in the contralateral ear, another cause, such as autoimmune hearing loss, should be investigated.
- Steroids are the treatment for sudden idiopathic SNHL. They may be given by mouth or injected through the tympanic membrane. They are the mainstay of treatment for recovery and should be offered unless there are medical contraindications to their use.
- There is a "window of opportunity" for the treatment of sudden idiopathic SNHL of about 4 to 6 weeks, after which time the likelihood of hearing recovery is greatly diminished. It is

of great importance that once this entity is suspected or diagnosed, proper treatment be initiated as soon as possible.

- There is currently no evidence that antiviral medication is of benefit to patients with Sudden idiopathic SNHL.
- Every patient with sudden idiopathic SNHL should undergo a retrocochlear evaluation, optimally MR imaging of the internal auditory canals without and with edge enhancement, to exclude the small possibility that an acoustic neuroma is the cause of the hearing loss.

121.10 Recommended Reading

[1] Adams JC. Clinical implications of inflammatory cytokines in the cochlea: a technical note. Otol Neurotol 2002; 23: 316–322

[2] Byl FM. Sudden hearing loss: eight years' experience and suggested prognostic table. Laryngoscope 1984; 94: 647–661

[3] Chen CY, Halpin C, Rauch SD. Oral steroid treatment of sudden sensorineural hearing loss: a ten year retrospective analysis. Otol Neurotol 2003; 24: 728–733

[4] De , K , leyn A. Sudden complete or partial loss of function of the octavus system in apparently normal persons. Acta Otolaryngol 1944; 32: 407–429

[5] Mattox DE, Simmons FB. Natural history of sudden sensorineural hearing loss. Ann Otol Rhinol Laryngol 1977; 86: 463–480

[6] Stachler RJ, Chandrasekhar SS, Archer SM et alAmerican Academy of Otolaryngology-Head and Neck Surgery. Clinical practice guideline: sudden hearing loss. Otolaryngol Head Neck Surg 2012; 146 Suppl :: S1–S35

[7] Tucci DL. Sudden sensorineural hearing loss: a viral etiology? Arch Otolaryngol Head Neck Surg 2000; 126: 1164–1165

[8] Tucci DL, Farmer JC, Kitch RD, Witsell DL. Treatment of sudden sensorineural hearing loss with systemic steroids and valacyclovir. Otol Neurotol 2002; 23: 301–308

[9] Wilson WR, Byl FM, Laird N. The efficacy of steroids in the treatment of idiopathic sudden hearing loss. A double-blind clinical study. Arch Otolaryngol 1980; 106: 772–776

122 Ototoxicity

Katrina R. Stidham

122.1 Introduction

The term *ototoxicity* is used to describe damage to the function of the inner ear, specifically the cochlea, balance canals, and/or auditory–vestibular nerves, due to an external exposure or toxin. The term is most often used to describe dysfunction caused by medical drugs, but ototoxicity can also be caused by the abuse of medical drugs or the use of street drugs. In addition, radiation damage to the inner ear may be referred to as ototoxicity. Finally, chemical exposures, as may be experienced in the workplace, can cause ototoxicity. Any agent that can cause temporary or permanent dysfunction of the inner ear is considered ototoxic.

122.2 Incidence of Disease

The incidence of ototoxicity depends on the individual ototoxin and dose administered. Individual incidence rates for specific agents are listed below.

122.3 Terminology

122.3.1 Cochleotoxicity

Cochleotoxicity is damage to the hearing organ (cochlea, cochlear nerve). Symptoms include hearing loss and tinnitus. Hearing loss is usually bilateral and symmetric (unless there has been a direct insult to one ear, as would occur in directed radiation therapy). Hearing loss typically begins at high frequencies and progresses to low frequencies.

122.3.2 Vestibulotoxicity

Vestibulotoxicity is damage to the balance organ (semicircular canals, utricle, saccule, vestibular nerves). Symptoms can vary from mild imbalance to more severe dizziness and vertigo with nausea and vomiting. Individuals with severe vestibulotoxicity may suffer from ataxia, head tilt, and oscillopsia.

122.4 Applied Anatomy

The cochlea is a tonotopic, snail-shaped organ. High-frequency sensitivity is located in the basal (outer) turn of the cochlea, and low-frequency sensitivity is situated in the apical (inner) turn. The nerve endings, known as hair cells, consist of three rows of outer hair cells and one row of inner hair cells. The outer hair cells act as an amplifier of the acoustic signal, while the inner hair cells convert the acoustic signal to an electrochemical signal. This signal is passed on to the spiral ganglion cells located in the central portion of the cochlea and ultimately transmitted to the brain.

The vestibular organ consists of the semicircular (balance) canals, utricle, and saccule. The vestibular epithelium is composed of two types of sensory hair cells, referred to as type I and type II cells. Increased and decreased discharges of the hair cells from each inner ear send signals to the brain regarding spatial orientation, acceleration, and angular rotation.

122.5 The Disease Process

122.5.1 Etiology

More than 130 drugs have been identified as potentially ototoxic. However, many cases of drug-induced ototoxicity have been anecdotally reported, often in patients without pretreatment audiograms. Some agents with known ototoxicity, such as nitrogen mustard and dihydrostreptomycin, are no longer clinically available. In addition to ototoxic drugs, there are multiple chemical exposures and radiation therapies with documented ototoxicity. The following are currently available agents with definite or probable ototoxic potential.

Chemotherapy Agents

Platinum Analogues: Cisplatin, Carboplatin

Both of these chemotherapeutic agents are known to be ototoxic, with a significant cochleotoxic effect. Cisplatin has a high incidence of documented ototoxicity, with an incidence of cochleotoxicity of up to 100% documented when ultra-high-frequency audiometric thresholds are included. Carboplatin, although less toxic than cisplatin, is still a risk, particularly in higher doses. Both agents are radiosensitizers and have a synergistic ototoxic effect with radiation therapy. Platins can cause early hearing loss but also can have progressive ototoxic effects for several months after the completion of treatment.

Antibiotics

Aminoglycosides: Gentamicin, Streptomycin, Tobramycin, Amikacin, Neomycin, Kanamycin

Aminoglycosides have been estimated to cause ototoxicity in anywhere from 2 to 45% of adults and 0 to 2% of infants. Amikacin, kanamycin, and neomycin are more cochleotoxic, whereas gentamicin and streptomycin tend to cause more vestibulotoxic damage. Tobramycin, although less toxic overall, has both cochleotoxic and vestibulotoxic effects. Long-term use with a higher cumulative dose increases the risk for ototoxicity, as can high peak and trough levels of individual doses. Concurrent use of diuretics can also increase the risk for ototoxicity. In addition, a subset of patients has been identified with a genetic susceptibility to aminoglycoside ototoxicity, due to a mutation in mitochondrial ribosomal RNA. These individuals are highly susceptible to aminoglycoside ototoxicity, with even one dose leading to severe hearing loss.

Aminoglycosides have historically been used in topical medications for the ear, including in Cortisporin Otic (neomycin) and tobramycin ophthalmic solutions. Neither of these drugs is actually FDA-approved for use in ears with perforated tympanic membranes or tympanotomy tubes. Although no convincing human data exist to prove that these drugs definitely cause ototoxicity when administered topically, care should be taken when these medications are prescribed, and if at all possible, an alternative ototopical agent should be used.

In recent years, a specific therapeutic benefit of aminoglycoside ototoxicity has been used to advantage in otology. Gentamicin is frequently used in the management of Meniere disease. The antibiotic is injected into the middle ear and allowed to perfuse the inner ear to create a controlled vestibulotoxic effect. This therapy has been more than 90% successful in controlling symptoms of Meniere disease in patients who fail to respond to conservative medical management.

Vancomycin

Vancomycin has been associated with several reports of increased tinnitus and anecdotal reports of decreased hearing. No definitive data exist on the true ototoxic effects of this antibiotic when it is administered alone. There is, however, evidence of increased risk for ototoxicity when it is administered concurrently with aminoglycosides.

Macrolides: Erythromycin, Clarithromycin, Azithromycin

Reports of macrolide ototoxicity are relatively infrequent. The effects are often reversible, although there have been a few reported cases of irreversible hearing loss. No systematic review of these antibiotics in regard to ototoxic effects has yet been completed.

Loop Diuretics: Furosemide, Bumetanide, Ethacrynic Acid

It is estimated that approximately 7% of patients taking loop diuretics may experience ototoxic symptoms in the form of tinnitus or hearing loss. The symptoms are usually self-limited and reversible in adults with no other comorbidities. Irreversible hearing loss has been reported in neonates and in patients with renal failure. Loop diuretics have also been shown to have a synergistic effect with other ototoxic medications, particularly aminoglycosides, leading to an increased risk for irreversible hearing loss.

Quinine Derivatives: Quinine, Hydroxychloroquine, Mefloquine

Quinine derivatives have been documented to cause both cochleotoxic and vestibulotoxic symptoms, with hearing loss, tinnitus, vertigo, and nausea. Hearing loss is usually reversible, but permanent hearing loss has been reported.

Aspirin and Nonsteroidal Anti-inflammatory Drugs

Tinnitus is a commonly recognized side effect of aspirin. The incidence of ototoxicity with aspirin is estimated to be 1% and is probably higher in elderly patients and those with dehydration. Symptoms of tinnitus and a mild to moderate flat hearing loss occur and are usually reversible within 24 to 72 hours after the medication has been discontinued. Nonsteroidal anti-inflam-matory drugs have a much lower rate of ototoxicity, but cases of irreversible loss have been documented.

Narcotics: Hydrocodone/Acetaminophen, Codeine/Acetaminophen, Propoxyphene

Each of these narcotics has been associated with ototoxicity, specifically with cochleotoxicity and hearing loss. Hearing loss has been documented primarily in patients with long-term and abusive use of these medications. Effects can be severe, with some patients progressing to profound hearing loss, necessitating cochlear implantation.

Radiation

Any patient who receives whole-brain irradiation or radiation involving the temporal bone is at risk for radiation ototoxicity. The groups most commonly affected include patients with primary or metastatic brain cancer and patients with head and neck cancer. The effects of radiation are dose-dependent, and there is also a documented synergistic effect of radiation and platins. Hearing loss can be acute or delayed. Patients are at long-term risk for the progression of hearing loss, which often becomes noticeable years after the completion of therapy.

Occupational Chemicals

Multiple chemical agents to which an individual may be exposed in an industrial environment can also lead to ototoxicity. Some documented ototoxins include the following: toluene, xylene, styrene, carbon disulfide, ethyl benzene, trichloroethylene, carbon monoxide, benzene, ethyl benzene, n-butanol, n-hexane, and solvent mixtures. In addition, chemical ototoxins have been proved to have a potentiating or synergistic effect with exposure to noise in worsening ototoxic damage. Thus, several professions that involve exposure to both chemical ototoxins and noise, including painting, printing, boat building, construction, furniture making, the manufacture of metal, leather, and petroleum, fueling vehicles, firefighting, and weapons firing, may be associated with a heightened risk for hearing loss or vestibular damage.

122.5.2 Pathogenesis

The pathogenesis of ototoxicity is not entirely understood and probably varies from agent to agent. In permanent cochleotoxicity, there appears to be damage to the stria vascularis, which leads to secondary damage to the hair cells. The outer hair cells are more commonly affected first, proceeding from basal to apical turn. The inner hair cells are affected secondarily, again proceeding from basal to apical turn. Thus, ototoxicity typically causes high-frequency hearing loss first. Damage to the spiral ganglion cells can be secondary to, or in some cases independent of, hair cell damage. Vestibular ototoxicity typically causes selective damage to type I hair cells, although type II cells can also be affected.

With many of the agents causing permanent ototoxic effects, an increase in the formation of oxygen free radicals and depletion of the antioxidant enzyme system lead to permanent cell death. Platin agents accumulate in the cochlea and are integrated into the DNA, leading to an overload of oxygen free radicals while the production of important antioxidant enzymes is downregulated, including superoxide dismutase, catalase, and glutathione peroxidase. Aminoglycosides have been found to bond with iron to form iron–aminoglycoside complexes. The complexes disrupt mitochondrial protein synthesis and lead to the formation of free oxygen radicals, which cause cell death. The iron–aminoglycoside complexes can persist in the inner ear for up to 6 months after administration, causing ototoxic effects long after the medication has been stopped.

In contrast, loop diuretics, which usually have temporary ototoxic effects, create a change in the ionic gradient between the fluid spaces (perilymphatic space and endolymphatic space) in the inner ear. This change can cause swelling of important supporting cells in the stria vascularis, which is usually reversible once the medication is cleared from the cochlea.

Other clinical and external factors may increase the likelihood that an agent will cause ototoxicity in an individual patient. Some of the factors that may increase the risk for ototoxicity are listed in the Box Risk Factors for Ototoxicity (p.977).

Risk Factors for Ototoxicity

- Renal disease/dysfunction
- Extremes of age: children younger than 5 years of age and the elderly
- Prior or concurrent cranial irradiation plus ototoxic medication
- Simultaneous administration of two ototoxic medications
- Genetic predisposition
- Poor hydration
- Prolonged medical therapy
- Noise exposure
- Preexisting hearing loss
- Immunocompromise

122.5.3 Natural History and Progression

The natural history and progression of ototoxicity are entirely dependent on the ototoxic agent to which the patient is exposed. Platin agents may cause hearing loss acutely as well as several months after treatment has been completed. Aminoglycosides can also stay in the inner ear for up to 6 months after treatment and cause hearing loss or balance dysfunction long after the completion of treatment. The effects of radiation therapy can be progressive for decades after the initial treatment. Finally, although many ototoxic medications have permanent effects, the effects of a few, including loop diuretics and aspirin, may be reversible with cessation of the medication.

122.6 Medical Evaluation

Patients with potential ototoxicity should always be medically evaluated to rule out other causes of their symptoms. Often, patients receiving ototoxic therapies are very ill and at risk for other problems that can affect hearing or balance function. All patients should have a careful examination of the ear to evaluate for possible cerumen impaction, middle ear effusion, and acute otitis media. Patients with asymmetric hearing loss and vestibular symptoms should have imaging, usually magnetic resonance imaging of the brain with contrast, to rule out other pathology that may be causing symptoms.

122.6.1 Presenting Complaints

The presenting complaints of a patient with ototoxicity depend on the associated ototoxic effects of the specific ototoxin administered. Patients with cochleotoxic effects will have tinnitus and hearing loss. The hearing loss can vary in severity from mild, high-frequency loss to profound hearing loss across all frequencies. Hearing loss is usually symmetric except in cases of direct radiation therapy to one ear. Patients with vestibulotoxicity may have mild dizziness, disequilibrium, and nausea, and those with more severe dysfunction may experience severe vertigo and vomiting. Those with total or nearly total vestibulotoxic effects can experience severe ataxia and oscillopsia.

122.6.2 Clinical Findings, Physical Examination

The ear examination for patients with both cochleotoxicity and vestibulotoxicity is usually normal. Subjective hearing loss may be appreciated on interview of the patient. Patients with vestibulotoxicity may have abnormalities on completion of their neurotologic examination. These can include nystagmus, inability to perform Romberg and tandem Romberg maneuvers, and unsteady gait or ataxia. Oscillopsia may be noted with ambulation.

Other bedside tests that can be performed include the dynamic visual acuity test and the horizontal head thrust test. In the dynamic visual acuity test, the patient is asked to look at an eye chart. The examiner then rotates the patient's head back and forth and asks the patient to read the smallest line again. Someone with an intact vestibulo-ocular reflex should be able to focus on the same line, whereas the patient with oscillopsia will be able to read only a much larger print. In the horizontal head thrust test, the examiner turns the patient's head quickly to one side and then the other and then asks the patient to fix the eyes on a specified point straight ahead. The examiner looks for catch-up saccades, which can be a sign of vestibular damage.

Bedside evaluations can be helpful in determining if a patient may have possible ototoxic effects, particularly when the consideration is to urgently stop a potentially ototoxic medication. However, for a complete and accurate evaluation, patients require formal testing.

122.6.3 Testing

The primary problem in evaluating ototoxicity is that damage is often done before measurable changes can be appreciated on standard testing and before subjective symptoms appear. In addition, patients may not be able to fully recognize or communicate the symptoms of ototoxicity. This is particularly a concern in very young patients and those who are very ill.

Cochleotoxicity Testing

The following tests are recommended for patients at risk for cochleotoxicity:

- High-frequency audiography: This tests frequencies up to 20,000 Hz to detect hearing loss before it reaches the lower frequencies of speech and language range.
- Distortion product otoacoustic emissions (DPOAEs): These measure outer hair cell function and have been shown to change before changes are documented on the audiogram.
- Auditory brainstem response (ABR) and auditory steady state response (ASSR): Both of these are objective parameters of electrical signals from the brain. They can be used to test or screen patients at risk who cannot complete standard audiometric testing.

Vestibulotoxicity Testing

- Videonystagmography (VNG): This assesses the integrity of the peripheral vestibular system through stimulation of the horizontal semicircular canals. The system is stimulated at a relatively low frequency of 0.002 to 0.004 Hz, lower than that typically experienced by the vestibulo-ocular reflex (VOR).
- Rotational chair testing: This stimulates the VOR at a more physiologic rate of 0.01 to 1.28 Hz. It can also provide information about possible dysfunction of the inner ear balance canals.
- Computerized dynamic posturography (CDP): This is a test of postural stability and assesses quantitatively how much balance dysfunction a vestibulotoxic insult may have caused.

122.7 Monitoring for Ototoxicity

Patients receiving ototoxic agents should be monitored throughout the course of their treatment for signs of ototoxicity. Practically, it is much easier to monitor for cochleotoxicity than for vestibulotoxicity because the testing is easier for the patient to undergo and can be completed in an inpatient setting. There are several sources for suggested guidelines, but no uniformly endorsed screening protocols, and most centers formulate a version of their own guidelines. Unfortunately, outside research and university hospitals, monitoring for ototoxicity is often not consistently completed. In addition, at least three different guidelines are used for defining ototoxicity, including the American Speech-Language-Hearing Association (ASHA) criteria, the Brock hearing loss criteria, and the Common Terminology Criteria for Adverse Events (CTCAE). The latter two break down hearing loss into grade levels. Unfortunately, these have been recognized in recent years as insufficiently sensitive to assess early ototoxicity accurately. To define the presence or absence of ototoxicity, the ASHA criteria should be used. All three of these ototoxic grading systems are outlined in the Box Ototoxicity Grading Systems (p. 978).

The following are suggested guidelines for ototoxicity monitoring.

122.7.1 Baseline Evaluation

A baseline evaluation should be completed for all patients before, or as close as possible to, the first ototoxic treatment. This should include (1) otoscopy/tympanometry; (2) pure-tone air conduction/bone conduction audiometry, including ultra-high-frequency audiometry; (3) DPOAE testing; and (4) ABR/ASSR testing, as indicated.

Ototoxicity Grading Systems

American Speech-Language-Hearing Association criteria for hearing loss
- Pure-tone threshold change of ≥ 20 dB at one frequency
- Pure-tone threshold change of ≥ 10 dB at two adjacent frequencies
- Loss of responses at three consecutive test frequencies at which responses were previously obtained when otoacoustic emissions or auditory brainstem response was used

Brock hearing loss grades
- Grade 0: hearing thresholds < 40 dB HL at all frequencies
- Grade 1: hearing thresholds ≥ 40 dB HL at 8,000 Hz
- Grade 2: hearing thresholds ≥ 40 dB HL at 4,000 to 8,000 Hz
- Grade 3: hearing thresholds ≥ 40 dB HL at 2,000 to 8,000 Hz
- Grade 4: hearing thresholds ≥ 40 dB HL at 1,000 to 8,000 Hz

Common Terminology Criteria for Adverse Events (CTCAE) hearing loss grades
- Grade 1: threshold shift of 15 to 25 dB relative to baseline, averaged at two or more contiguous frequencies in at least one ear
- Grade 2: threshold shift of 25 to 90 dB, averaged at two contiguous frequencies in at least one ear
- Grade 3: hearing loss sufficient to indicate therapeutic intervention, including a hearing aid (e.g., > 20 dB bilateral HL in speech frequencies, > 30 dB unilateral HL, and requiring additional speech– language services)
- Grade 4: indication for cochlear implant and requiring additional speech–language services

---

122.7.2 Monitoring during Treatment

Monitoring should continue during treatment, with the above protocol repeated at each level of monitoring. The frequency of monitoring may depend on the individual agent given and the frequency of treatment but in general should be as follows: (1) For patients undergoing cisplatin/carboplatin treatment, monitoring should be completed just before the next dose. (2) For patients receiving aminoglycosides or other ototoxic antibiotics, testing should be completed once or twice per week throughout treatment. (3) For patients receiving cranial radiation, testing should be completed before and after treatment.

Throughout the course of treatment, patients should be clinically monitored for any signs or symptoms of ototoxicity. Testing should be repeated urgently if any symptoms of ototoxicity arise. Patients who present with possible vestibulotoxic symptoms should undergo urgent vestibular testing when feasible. The treating physician should be notified immediately of any ototoxic symptoms and objective findings. At that time, the following should be considered when clinically an option: (1) reduction of dose; (2) change in dosing administration; (3) change to a less toxic or non-ototoxic treatment option (this option should be initiated immediately if vestibulotoxic symptoms from aminoglycoside treatment are noted).

122.7.3 Monitoring after Treatment

For all patients undergoing ototoxic therapies, monitoring should be completed for at least 1 year following treatment at the recommended intervals of 4 weeks, 3 months, 6 months, and 1 year. Patients with a documented shift in hearing will require evaluations at least yearly on a long-term basis to follow hearing loss. In addition, patients undergoing cranial irradiation should have testing every 6 months for the first few years and then yearly follow-up thereafter, even if no hearing loss is detected in the first few years.

122.8 Treatment

As previously noted, the initial and urgent intervention for ototoxicity is immediate suspension of the ototoxic agent if at all possible. Subsequent treatment is directed at the damage caused by ototoxicity.

For patients with cochleotoxicity, the long-term effects may include hearing loss and tinnitus. When hearing loss affects the speech and language spectrum, patients should be fitted with appropriate amplification, usually in the form of a hearing aid. For the rare patient with severe–profound hearing loss, cochlear implantation is very successful. Tinnitus can be managed with amplification, biofeedback, background noise, and, when needed, anxiolytics and antidepressants.

Patients with vestibulotoxicity should be initiated into a vestibular rehabilitation therapy program as soon as possible. Vestibular rehabilitation therapy can benefit many patients by improving their overall balance function and providing coping strategies for managing their loss of balance. Unfortunately, in patients with severely damaged vestibular function, long-term balance problems persist and may lead to permanent disability.

Research is ongoing to evaluate possible otoprotective measures that can be taken for patients receiving ototoxins without compromising the efficacy of the treatment for its intended purpose. Much of this research is focusing on the role of antioxidants in preventing ototoxicity. Promising data have been obtained from both animal and human studies, but currently otoprotective treatments are used only in research protocols and are not clinically available.

122.9 Roundsmanship

- Ototoxic agents can cause permanent damage to hearing and balance function both during and following the completion of treatment, with progressive effects often lasting for several months to years after the completion of therapy.
- Patients receiving an ototoxic treatment should be screened before treatment, then monitored closely throughout the course of therapy and after the completion of treatment.
- When possible, cessation or adjustment of the ototoxic medication should be considered to limit damage to the inner ear.
- Intervention with amplification and balance therapy is necessary to rehabilitate patients with ototoxic effects.

122.10 Recommended Reading

[1] Bhandare N, Jackson A, Eisbruch A et al. Radiation therapy and hearing loss. Int J Radiat Oncol Biol Phys 2010; 76 Suppl: S50–S57

[2] Friedman RA, House JW, Luxford WM, Gherini S, Mills D. Profound hearing loss associated with hydrocodone/acetaminophen abuse. Am J Otol 2000; 21: 188–191

[3] NoiseChem. Noise and Industrial Chemicals: Interaction Effects on Hearing and Balance. Key Action 4: Environment and Health 2001–2004. Final Report. . Accessed November 28, 2013

[4] Guthrie OW. Aminoglycoside induced ototoxicity. Toxicology 2008; 249: 91–96

[5] Jung TT, Rhee CK, Lee CS, Park YS, Choi DC. Ototoxicity of salicylate, nonsteroidal antiinflammatory drugs, and quinine. Otolaryngol Clin North Am 1993; 26: 791–810

[6] Mudd PA, Edmunds AL, Glatz FR, Campbell KCM, Rybak LP. Ototoxicity. http://emedicine.medscape.com/article/857679-overview. Accessed November 28, 2013

[7] Rybak LP, Mukherjea D, Jajoo S, Ramkumar V. Cisplatin ototoxicity and protection: clinical and experimental studies. Tohoku J Exp Med 2009; 219: 177–186

123 Auditory Neuropathy

Helen R. Salus

123.1 Introduction

The diagnostic term *auditory neuropathy* is used to describe a condition affecting a variety of individuals (mainly children) who meet the following criteria: (1) Their understanding of speech (speech recognition ability) is disproportionately poorer than what would be predicted from the pure-tone thresholds on the behavioral audiogram; (2) delays in speech and language development in children often occur in association with auditory neuropathy; (3) otoacoustic emissions (OAEs) are present, at least in the initial stages of the condition; (4) auditory brainstem responses (ABRs) are often abnormal and may be absent.

123.2 Terminology

From the point of view of neurology, the term *neuropathy* refers to pathology that is confined to the peripheral nerve fibers without involving the neuronal cell bodies. However, the term *auditory neuropathy* (AN) was proposed by Rapin and Gravel to be used when the pathologic changes encompass the spiral ganglion cells, or their axons, or cranial nerve (CN) VIII as a whole. Thus, AN is neither a sensory nor a central auditory disorder. Nonetheless, because of diagnostic limitations, the precise site of the lesion cannot be established in many patients who present with auditory neuropathy-like symptoms, causing some controversy regarding the appropriate use of the term *auditory neuropathy.*

Cases exist in which damage initially may be confined to sites peripheral to CN VIII (e.g., the inner hair cells [IHCs]), with later progression of disease from transsynaptic degeneration then affecting the spiral ganglia cells and their axons; these later pathologic changes meet the definition of *neuropathy.* The degeneration may further advance rostrally through the brainstem cochlear nuclei and central auditory pathway into the cortex. Neuropathies are categorized as demyelinating, axonal, or mixed. Demyelination impairs the conduction of signals in affected nerves. Axonal neuropathy (axonopathy) is characterized by axonal loss, with dropout of the fastest-conducting fibers. Typically, muscle abnormality is greater with axonal peripheral neuropathies than with demyelinating neuropathies. However, the boundary between demyelinating neuropathy and axonal neuropathy is not always clear because histologic evidence suggests focal secondary demyelination and remyelination in some cases.

The term *auditory dyssynchrony* is used more liberally than the term *auditory neuropathy.* Auditory dyssynchrony encompasses a broader spectrum of pathologies than auditory neuropathy; it includes conditions, such as IHC loss, that represent sensory rather than neural pathology. The more recently employed term *auditory neuropathy spectrum disorder* (ANSD) is preferred to the term *auditory dyssynchrony* by some clinicians and researchers. Related terms include *auditory neural synchrony disorder* and *auditory synaptopathy.*

123.3 Incidence

AN/ANSD is a relatively rare condition with onset at any age from birth to the seventh decade of life. In the majority of cases, the reported onset is before the age of 10 years. No estimates of gender prevalence have been reported. Approximately 25% of persons with AN/ANSD have no known associated developmental or medical risks. The majority of patients who have AN, however, present with risk factors such as prematurity, hyperbilirubinemia, genetic hearing disorders, or sensory motor neuropathies.

Estimates of the incidence of AN/ANSD vary from 1 to about 10% in schools for the deaf. Estimates of the incidence range from 0.5 to 15% in persons with sensorineural hearing loss. In one hospital study, AN (based on permanent hearing loss, present cochlear microphonic [CM], abnormal or absent ABR waveforms, and present transient evoked OAEs [TEOAEs] or distortion product OAEs [DPOAEs]) was noted in 5% of 428 children in whom hearing loss was diagnosed. In another study, of 5,199 children at risk for hearing loss (based on neonatal factors or family history) who received hearing screening, 0.23% were identified with AN based on absent ABR waveforms and present CM. In another study, of 17 patients with AN, the authors estimated a high prevalence of AN in China, although they did not state any specific prevalence.

123.4 Disease Characteristics

Persons with AN/ANSD exhibit specific diagnostic and behavioral characteristics consistent with absent neural function in the presence of normal cochlear or outer hair cell (OHC) function. They may have normal hearing sensitivity or hearing loss ranging from mild to profound in magnitude. Nonetheless, persons with AN/ANSD, even those with normal hearing sensitivity, exhibit speech recognition scores that are disproportionately poor relative to the magnitude of the hearing impairment. The difficulty in the identification/recognition of speech is further exacerbated in the presence of noise.

The diagnostic hallmarks of AN/ANSD are present (at least initially) OAEs and present CM (an electrical response occurring just before the ABR), together with an abnormal or absent ABR. Thus, normal OHC function (at least initially) and faulty or dyssynchronous neural responses are the characteristics of the disorder. The findings on neuroimaging evaluations typically are normal. Although AN/ANSD can affect persons of all ages, from infancy through adulthood, in the majority of cases, AN/ANSD is diagnosed in early childhood.

The condition was first reported in the 1970s as the seemingly paradoxical finding of a discrepancy between an absent ABR and recordable hearing thresholds (albeit with some elevation in thresholds). Initially, the disorder had been inappropriately termed a *central auditory dysfunction.* Later, it was labeled an *auditory neural synchrony disorder.* The term *auditory neuropathy* was introduced by Starr et al. The disorder (AN/ANSD) also can be associated with vestibular pathology.

123.5 Etiology and Pathophysiology

Much remains to be understood regarding the pathophysiology and etiology of AN/ANSD. These disorders are associated with several possible sites of lesion. In some cases, the disorder may involve isolated IHC dysfunction or a synaptic dysfunction between CN VIII and the hair cells; with the latter site of lesion, the disorder category would fall under the broader umbrella of ANSD rather than AN. Damage to the nerve itself can result in AN/ANSD. A combination of these problems may occur in some cases. Although the OHCs generally are more prone to damage than the IHCs, the OHCs often seem to function normally in persons with AN/ANSD. Loss of OAEs and progressive hearing loss are more likely to be a result of axonal loss in the efferent system—axonopathy or mixed neuropathy—than a result solely of a demyelinating neuropathy.

Although AN/ANSD often is diagnosed in persons with unremarkable medical histories, certain medical conditions can be associated with the disorder. There are reports of AN/ANSD diagnosed in patients with hyperbilirubinemia, hypoxia, mumps, Guillain-Barré syndrome, Friedreich ataxia, hereditary sensory and motor neuropathy (HSMN), Charcot-Marie-Tooth disease, Refsum disease, Mohr-Tranebjaerg syndrome, or olivopontocerebellar degeneration, and in patients with HIV/AIDS.

In the majority of patients with AN/ANSD, the condition is bilateral rather than unilateral. For example, Berlin et al identified bilateral AN/ANSD in 241 (93%) of 260 pediatric and adult patients. Of the 19 unilateral cases, 13 affected the left ear and 6 affected the left ear; 10 patients were male and 9 were female.

In one study, a review of the histories of 153 pediatric patients (from birth to 18 years of age) with a diagnosis of AN/ANSD revealed unremarkable history and pregnancy only in 38%. Multiple risk factors were identified in many of the patients: history of premature birth (48%), history of bilirubinemia (48%), history of exchange transfusion (20%), anoxia (17%), history of ototoxicity (29%), and history of artificial ventilation (23%). The findings of a review of the histories of 197 patients across all ages in the same study revealed that 32 (16%) of the patients had family members with ANSD, suggesting a genetic mutation(s) as the underlying cause. A mutation in the gene for otoferlin (a protein that may have a role in neurotransmitter release at the hair cell synapse) was documented in some of these participants; 6 of the 32 patients had mitochondrial disease, 3 had a diagnosis of HSMN (possibly encompassing Charcot-Marie-Tooth disease), 3 had optic nerve atrophy, 13 had cerebral palsy, and 3 had a history of kernicterus.

Many patients in whom AN/ANSD is identified in infancy and early childhood present with a history of serious neonatal illness and have a greatly increased risk for neurodevelopmental delays. Among the symptoms reported by the parents of young patients with AN/ANSD are apraxia, ataxia, cerebral palsy, hypotonicity, seizures, feeding problems, gross and fine motor skills delays, nystagmus, strabismus, sensory integration issues, tactile defensiveness, and autistic tendencies.

123.5.1 Inner Hair Cell/Primary Afferent Damage

Possible etiologies of IHC/primary afferent damage have been hypothesized to be ototoxicity from carboplatin or deferoxamine (Desferal; Novartis, East Hanover, NJ) treatment, excessive release of glutamate from the IHCs as a result of acoustic trauma or presbycusis, chronic cochlear hypoxia secondary to in utero hypoxia, perinatal anoxia, vascular accident and hematologic hemoglobin disorder, and genetic mutations (otoferlin). Selective IHC loss was documented in the cochleas of premature infants studied in neonatal intensive care unit autopsies. The findings of normal OAEs in conjunction with a corner audiogram (showing behavioral responses only for intense low-frequency sounds) and negative magnetic resonance (MR) imaging findings with regard to CN VIII status are consistent with IHC hypofunction with anterograde loss of afferents and other synaptic connections.

123.5.2 Interruption in the Afferent-to-Efferent Loop

Interruption in the afferent-to-efferent loop is supported by the findings of absent contralateral efferent OAE suppression in persons with AN/ANSD. The afferent part of the loop refers to the myelinated afferent fibers (type I) from the IHCs to the cochlear nuclei with fiber transmission to the superior olivary complex, whereas the efferent part of the loop refers to the olivocochlear bundle, which has contralateral medial synaptic connections to the cochlear OHCs.

123.5.3 Cranial Nerve Neuropathy

The most typical example of CN. VIII involvement representing AN sensu stricto would be HSMNs, including Charcot-Marie-Tooth disease, Friedreich ataxia, Refsum disease, and Mohr-Tranebjaerg syndrome (X-linked recessive disorder of mitochondrial metabolism).

123.6 Newborn Hearing Screening and Differential Diagnosis

123.6.1 Newborn Hearing Screening

Universal newborn hearing screening programs are now implemented in the majority of states in United States. The limitation of newborn hearing screening programs with regard to AN/ANSD lies in the fact that many of them employ OAE but not ABR screening procedures. The Joint Committee on Infant Hearing 2007 position statement includes auditory neuropathy/dyssynchrony in infants admitted to the neonatal intensive care unit within the definition of disorders targeted for identification via newborn hearing screening programs. Additionally, the 2007 position statement, in order to identify auditory neuropathy/dyssynchrony, mandates ABR testing for babies who spend more than 5 days in the neonatal intensive care unit. Nevertheless, a significant proportion of patients with AN/ANSD with onset

Table 123.1 Auditory pathway sites of lesion and physiologic test responses

Site of lesion	Pathology	Test										
		OAEs	CM	Compound AP	Acoustic	Tactile	Vestibular	OAE	ABR waves	ABR waves	MLD	Cortical
OHCs	Cochlear/sensory loss	−	+	+	+	+	+	−	+	+	+	+
OHCs and IHCs	Cochlear/sensory loss	−	−	−	−	+	+	−	−	−	−	−
IHCs[b] (OHCs OK)[a]	Cochlear/sensory loss	+	+	−	−	+	+	−	−	−	−	−
SGCs[b] (HCs OK)[a]	Neuronopathy/ganglion-opathy	+	+	−	−	+	+	−	−	−	−	−
CN VIII axons	CN VIII axonal neuropathy	+	+	−	−	+	+	−	−	−	−	−
CN VIII myelin (Schwann cells)	CN VIII demyelinating neuropathy	+	+	+	−	+	−	−	−	−	−	−
CN VIII axons and myelin	Mixed CN VIII neuropathy	+	+	+	−	+	−	−	−	−	−	−
Brainstem	Brainstem	+	+	+	−	−	−	−	+	−	−	−
Thalamus/cortex	Thalamocortical	+	+	+	+	+	+	+	+	+	−	−

Source: Adapted from Rapin I, Gravel J. "Auditory neuropathy": physiologic and pathologic evidence calls for more diagnostic specificity. Int J Pediatr Otorhinolaryngol 2003;67(7):707–728.
Abbreviations: ABR, auditory brainstem response; acoustic MEMR, ipsilateral and contralateral acoustic reflex tests; AP, action potential; CM, cochlear microphonic; CN, cranial nerve; HCs, hair cells; IHCs, inner hair cells; MEMR, middle ear muscle reflex; MLD, masking level difference; OAEs, otoacoustic emissions; OHCs, outer hair cells; SGCs, spiral ganglion cells; +, recordable response; −, nonrecordable response.
Note: Table applies only to cases of severe pathology.
[a]There were no reported cases of pathology limited to the synapses between the IHC axons and the dendrites of the SGCs.
[b]There were no reported cases selectively limited to the pathology of IHCs or SGCs.

before 2 years of age have no known risks. Thus, the chances of the condition going undetected in early infancy remain high.

123.6.2 Differential Diagnosis

The diagnostic protocol for AN/ANSD involves a multidisciplinary approach with an emphasis on audiologic and medical assessment. The audiologic battery to rule out AN/ANSD should include audiometric testing, suprathreshold speech recognition assessment, acoustic immittance testing (tympanometry and acoustic reflex testing), and OAE and ABR testing. In addition, masking level difference (MLD), electrocochleography (ECochG) for measurement of the compound action potential and CM, efferent suppression of OAEs (olivocochlear reflex) testing, and vestibular testing may be performed. Although vestibular pathology may exist in conjunction with AN/ANSD, confirmed peripheral vestibular nerve and/or vestibular nerve end-organ pathology in the absence of AN/ANSD signs cannot be accepted as indication of AN/ANSD.

The appropriateness of specific tests must be considered with reference to the maturation of the auditory mechanism and the behavioral test abilities of the specific patient. A categorization of the auditory pathway sites of lesion and expected electrophysiologic test responses (recordable versus nonrecordable) are presented in ► Table 123.1.

The OAE and ABR findings cannot differentiate between selective damage to IHCs and CN VIII damage. If a CN VIII site of lesion cannot be confirmed, then ANSD should be used as a diagnostic term; the diagnosis of AN is acceptable if the patient is diagnosed with other peripheral neuropathies.

123.7 Audiometry and Speech Recognition Testing

Pure-tone air and bone conduction testing of individuals with AN/ANSD produces diverse audiometric configurations. The results may vary from normal hearing sensitivity to hearing impairment ranging from mild to profound. Some patients may present with rising or unusual audiometric configurations. Most cases of AN/ANSD are bilateral, although asymmetric hearing loss was reported by Berlin et al in about 23% (24 of 103) of patients with bilateral AN/ANSD. In another study, of 16 children with AN/ANSD, mild to moderate hearing loss was observed in 5, moderate to severe hearing loss in 2, severe to profound hearing loss in 7, and fluctuating hearing loss in 2. The majority of these children (63%) presented with multiple associated risk factors: hyperbilirubinemia (24%), prematurity (19%.), genetic syndrome (10%), low birth weight (5%), and hydrocephalus (5%). The mean pure-tone average (based on 1,000, 2,000, and 4,000 Hz) for a group of 66 ears with AN/ANSD was 57 dB HL in another study.

The type of hearing impairment associated with AN/ANSD is sensorineural, or it is mixed if a problem (unrelated to AN/ANSD) affecting the outer and/or middle ear is superimposed on the sensorineural hearing impairment. Otitis media and other middle ear conditions may easily obscure the presence of

AN, particularly in infants and young children, who are more prone to otitis media than adults.

Discrepancies between measured behavioral thresholds and ABR results are reported in the literature.

A high proportion of individuals with AN/ANSD present with poor agreement between the pure-tone average suprathreshold speech recognition score for speech materials presented in a quiet background and the score for speech materials presented in background noise, which increases the difficulty of recognizing and identifying speech.

123.7.1 Acoustic Immittance

Because AN/ANSD is a neural pathology, the tympanometry results should be unremarkable. The high incidence of middle ear pathologies unrelated to AN/ANSD (e.g., otitis media) can make the diagnosis of AN/ANSD problematic.

The ipsilateral and contralateral acoustic reflexes were reported to be absent in persons with AN/ANSD when a low-frequency probe tone (typically 226 Hz) was used. However, inasmuch as a multitude of studies have shown absent acoustic reflexes in neonates and infants when low-frequency probe tones are used, future research needs to examine the acoustic reflex responses when middle- and high-frequency probe tones are used. Tactile middle ear muscle responses were shown to be present in patients with AN/ANSD.

123.7.2 Otoacoustic Emissions

Patients with AN/ANSD usually exhibit robust OHC activity on TEOAE tests and DPOAE tests. TEOAEs are present in ears with mild cochlear loss of up to about 30 dB HL, and DPOAEs can be present in ears with up to moderate hearing impairment. OAEs may be absent or diminish over time because of a deterioration in hearing sensitivity or as a result of a middle ear problem. However, no correlation exists between hair cell function and the magnitude of hearing loss, as the latter in AN/ANSD appears to be related to the degree of neural disease or disruption in the transmission of neural potentials in response to acoustic stimuli. Starr et al reported absent TEOAEs in 30% of 63 ears of patients with AN/ANSD; TEOAEs were absent bilaterally in 25% and were absent unilaterally in 5%. Of the 11 patients with AN/ANSD who had absent TEOAEs, 9 had previously had present TEOAEs.

In patients with absent OAEs due to middle ear pathology, the response of the cochlear hair cells can be assessed from the CM recorded by using surface electrodes with ABR instrumentation, particularly with insert earphones. In patients with AN/ANSD, as in individuals without hearing problems, the waveform is inverted, with changes in stimulus polarity (rarefaction phase vs condensation phase). The results of some studies reveal decreases in OAEs over time despite the absence of changes in the CM. Both OAEs and CMs are dominated by OHC activity. However, the tests may be differentially sensitive to various degrees of the OHC damage, or reflect different hair cell functions.

Efferent Suppression of Otoacoustic Emissions

In the phenomenon of efferent suppression of OAEs (olivocochlear reflex), amplitude reduction or phase change results from the inclusion of an additional stimulus. Efferent suppression is observed in healthy ears but is absent in patients with AN/ANSD. Berlin et al reported that the phenomenon of efferent suppression of TEOAEs when continuous contralateral broadband noise is used represents a small reduction of 2 to 3 dB over a 20-millisecond study interval but a larger reduction of 6 to 8 dB in normal individuals under microstructural analysis after stimulus cessation. The phenomenon was entirely absent in patients with probable AN/ANSD, as evidenced by hearing sensitivity close to normal limits and absent ABRs, and in patients with Charcot-Marie-Tooth disease, who had normal OAEs, substantial hearing impairment as evidenced by audiometric thresholds, absent acoustic reflexes, and absent ABRs.

123.7.3 Auditory Brainstem Response and Cochlear Microphonic

In an evaluation of patients suspected to have AN/ANSD, Teagle et al performed ABR testing by presenting high-intensity click stimuli via insert earphones, with separate recordings for condensation and rarefaction phase stimuli. The use of single-polarity stimulation facilitates identification of the CM. The CM can be differentiated from the neural response of the ABR because the CM waveform reverses with change in stimulus polarity from condensation to rarefaction phase (and vice versa), whereas the CM latency remains essentially unchanged despite increases or decreases in stimulus intensity. For each single-polarity stimulation, recordings should be obtained at two stimulus intensities that differ by 10 dB to determine whether latency changes are occurring with changes in stimulus level. To rule out stimulus artifact during recordings with single-polarity stimulation, the sound tubing of the insert phone can be disconnected or clamped and the recording repeated; disappearance of the waveform component assumed to be the CM establishes the component as being biological in nature rather than a recording artifact.

Some investigators have reported larger-amplitude and longer-duration CMs in some patients with AN/ANSD. For example, Starr et al observed significantly larger CM amplitudes in patients with AN than in normal individuals, and longer-duration CM responses (e.g., the phase-inverted CM responses peaked at about 0.4 millisecond in a normal subject and in a patient with AN but persisted to 3 milliseconds in the latter patient but to 0.7 millisecond in the former subject. The CM amplitude exceeded the age-adjusted limits, reflecting 2 standard errors of estimates for the control group in 40% of the patients with AN/ANSD.

Absent or abnormal ABR waveforms are typical in patients with AN/ANSD. Starr et al observed a present click-elicited ABR in 21% of a group of 33 patients (66 ears) with AN/ANSD; the ABRs were characterized by a low-amplitude wave V and an absent wave I. The absolute wave V latency was prolonged in 62.5% of the 16 recordings. No significant differences were observed between CM amplitude or pure-tone average (based on 1,000, 2,000 and 4,000 Hz) in patients with AN/ANSD and present ABRs versus CM amplitude or pure-tone average in patients with AN/ANSD and absent ABRs.

123.7.4 Summating Potential Recorded on Electrocochleography

The summating potential (SP) measured during ECochG (extratympanic recordings) with click stimuli was preserved in a study of three adult patients with AN/ANSD. Findings on the SP were inconclusive in a study of 57 ears with AN/ANSD; the SP was absent 50% of the ears with AN and in 50% of the 27 normal, control ears.

123.7.5 Masking Level Difference

The MLD is defined as the improvement in masked threshold between dichotic and diotic (or monotic) signal presentation. MLD is absent in patients with AN/ANSD. For example, the lack of any improvement in monaural masked thresholds (monotic condition) for low-frequency tones after the addition of correlated contralateral noise (dichotic condition), as observed in six patients by Starr et al, was consistent with AN/ANSD. Absent MLD in AN/ANSD differentiates the pathology from a cochlear or conductive hearing loss, in which the MLD is present, albeit reduced in magnitude when compared with that in normal subjects. The differential diagnosis value of MLD may, however, be obscured in patients with severe or asymmetric pure-tone configurations.

123.7.6 Vestibular Tests

The presence of a disorder of the vestibular branch of CN VIII and its end organs in patients with AN/ANSD was demonstrated in three patients with symptoms of vestibular disorder whose vestibular evaluations produced abnormal caloric and damped rotation measurements. Saccades, smooth pursuit eye movements, and optokinetic nystagmus were normal.

A comprehensive medical assessment should include a thorough history, physical examination, and laboratory testing. MR imaging is recommended as part of a pediatric evaluation to visualize labyrinthine and internal auditory canal morphology, CN VIII integrity, and brain structure. In cases of stenosis of the internal auditory canals, temporal bone pathology, inner ear malformation, or cochlear luminal obstruction, high-resolution computed tomography may be recommended, as well.

123.8 Management

The management of a patient, especially a pediatric patient, with variable audiometric results and an uncertain audiologic prognosis, combined with a history of major neonatal illness and a high risk for neurologic developmental problems, may require the involvement of multiple specialties. The team may include therapeutic and educational specialists (e.g., speech–language pathologist, educational audiologist, physical therapist, educational therapist).

Systematic monitoring of the auditory status is of the utmost importance in infants and young children, especially those with findings suggestive of AN/ANSD and no other neuropathologic manifestations. The perceptual consequences of the condition may jeopardize speech and language acquisition in affected children.

The case management of patients with AN/ANSD often includes a trial of conventional types of amplification and the use of assistive listening devices, particularly to determine cochlear implant candidacy. One recent study found that of 85 patients with AN/ANSD, 61% received no benefit from hearing aid amplification, 25% received benefit restricted to hearing environmen-

tal sounds, 11% received benefit sufficient to facilitate language acquisition, and 3% received good benefit. Of the 49 patients with AN/ANSD (47 of whom were younger than 12 years of age) who received a cochlear implant, outcomes were judged to be successful in 86%, reflective of slow progress in 2%, and uncertain in 4%; outcomes could not be assessed (implantation too recent) in 8%. Of the 260 patients with AN/ANSD, 13 (5%) had mild forms of pathology that did not necessitate intervention with hearing aids or cochlear implants, although all of these patients reported difficulty communicating in noisy situations. Many of these children require enrollment in communication rehabilitation programs.

Research studies report improvements after implantation in neural responses that were absent or abnormal preoperatively. A longitudinal investigation of 39 children with AN/ANSD (78 ears) and cochlear implants (60 implanted cochleas) revealed that the children with implants who had abnormal electrical ABRs achieved substantially poorer speech recognition scores than the children with implants who had normal electrical ABRs at 1 and 2 years after implantation.

123.9 Roundsmanship

- In patients with AN, the understanding of speech (speech recognition ability) is disproportionately poorer than what would be predicted from the pure-tone thresholds on behavioral audiogram.
- Delays in speech and language development in children often are seen in association with AN.
- OAEs are present, at least in early AN/ANSD (OHC function is usually intact or minimally impaired).
  - OAEs frequently are more robust than would be predicted from the behavioral audiogram.
  - Poor OAEs in AN/ANSD are suggestive of efferent involvement (axonal neuropathy).
  - Efferent suppression of OAEs is absent.
- Hearing sensitivity is normal or sensorineural hearing loss is present, ranging from mild to profound. It may be bilateral (asymmetric or symmetric) or unilateral.
- A severely abnormal (beginning at wave I) or absent ABR and evidence of a large CM suggest that the disorder arises from a cochlear and/or CN VIII pathology (rather than a more central process).
  - The ABR deteriorates with increasing degrees of IHC and primary cochlear afferent neuronal degeneration (consistent with progressive demyelination).
- The medical history is unremarkable, or the condition is comorbid with anoxia, hypoxia, hyperbilirubinemia, a genetic disorder (HSMN, Charcot-Marie-Tooth syndrome, mitochondrial enzymatic deficit, Friedreich ataxia, olivopontocerebellar degeneration), an immune disorder (e.g., Guillain-Barré syndrome), an infection (e.g., mumps), or another condition.
- The identification of newborns at risk for AN/ANSD requires OAE and ABR screening.
- The approach to management should be multidisciplinary (otorhinolaryngology, audiology, pediatrics, neurology, speech–language pathology, physical therapy, educational therapy, and other specialties, depending on the comorbidity).

○ Management should involve hearing aids and assistive listening devices, cochlear implants (some limited research findings suggest that a normal preoperative or perioperative electrical ABR is a predictor of improvement after implantation), and speech–language therapy.

123.10 Recommended Reading

[1] Amatuzzi MG, Northrop C, Liberman MC et al. Selective inner hair cell loss in premature infants and cochlea pathological patterns from neonatal intensive care unit autopsies. Arch Otolaryngol Head Neck Surg 2001; 127: 629–636

[2] Berlin CI, Hood LJ, Hurley A, Wen H. The First Jerger Lecture. Contralateral suppression of otoacoustic emissions: an index of the function of the medial olivocochlear system. Otolaryngol Head Neck Surg 1994; 110: 3–21

[3] Berlin CI, Hood LJ, Morlet T et al. Multi-site diagnosis and management of 260 patients with auditory neuropathy/dys-synchrony (auditory neuropathy spectrum disorder). Int J Audiol 2010; 49: 30–43

[4] Deltenre P, Mansbach AL, Bozet C et al. Auditory neuropathy with preserved cochlear microphonics and secondary loss of otoacoustic emissions. Audiology 1999; 38: 187–195

[5] Franck KH, Rainey DM, Montoya LA, Gerdes M. Developing a multidisciplinary clinical protocol to manage pediatric patients with auditory neuropathy. Semin Hear 2002; 23: 225–237

[6] Gibson W. Auditory neuropathy and persistent outer hair cells. Paper presented at: 7th International Cochlear Implant Conference; September 4–6, 2002; Manchester, England

[7] Gibson WPR, Sanli H. Auditory neuropathy: an update. Ear Hear 2007; 28 Suppl: 102S–106S

[8] Hood LJ, Berlin CI, Morlet T, Brashears S, Rose K, Tedesco S. Considerations in the clinical evaluation of auditory neuropathy/auditory dysynchrony. Semin Hear 2002; 23: 201–208

[9] Joint Committee on Infant Hearing. Year 2000 Position Statement: Principles & Guidelines for Early Hearing Detection & Prevention Programs. Audiology Today, Special Issue, August 2000

[10] American Academy of Pediatrics, Joint Committee on Infant Hearing. Year 2007 position statement: principles and guidelines for early hearing detection and intervention programs. Pediatrics 2007; 120: 898–921

[11] Kraus N, Ozdamar O, Stein L, Reed N. Absent auditory brain stem response: peripheral hearing loss or brain stem dysfunction? Laryngoscope 1984; 94: 400–406

[12] Madden C, Rutter M, Hilbert L, Greinwald JH, Choo DI. Clinical and audiological features in auditory neuropathy. Arch Otolaryngol Head Neck Surg 2002; 128: 1026–1030

[13] Rance G, Beer DE, Cone-Wesson B et al. Clinical findings for a group of infants and young children with auditory neuropathy. Ear Hear 1999; 20: 238–252

[14] Rapin I, Gravel J. "Auditory neuropathy": physiologic and pathologic evidence calls for more diagnostic specificity. Int J Pediatr Otorhinolaryngol 2003; 67: 707–728

[15] Sheykholeslami K, Kaga K, Murofushi T, Hughes DW. Vestibular function in auditory neuropathy. Acta Otolaryngol 2000; 120: 849–854

[16] Sininger YS, Oba S. Patients with auditory neuropathy: who are they and what can they hear? In: Sininger YS, Starr A, eds. Auditory Neuropathy: A New Perspective on Hearing Disorders. Albany, NY: Thompson Learning; 2001:15–35

[17] Sininger YS. Identification of auditory neuropathy in infants and children. Semin Hear 2002; 23: 193–200

[18] Starr A, Picton TW, Sininger Y, Hood LJ, Berlin CI. Auditory neuropathy. Brain 1996; 119: 741–753

[19] Starr A, Sininger Y, Nguyen T, Michalewski HJ, Oba S, Abdala C. Cochlear receptor (microphonic and summating potentials, otoacoustic emissions) and auditory pathway (auditory brain stem potentials) activity in auditory neuropathy. Ear Hear 2001; 22: 91–99

[20] Teagle HFB, Roush PA, Woodard JS et al. Cochlear implantation in children with auditory neuropathy spectrum disorder. Ear Hear 2010; 31: 325–335

[21] Trautwein P. Auditory neuropathy: diagnosis and case management. Paper presented at: 4th ACFOS International Conference: The Impact of Scientific Advances on the Education of Deaf Children; November 8–10, 2002; Paris, France

[22] Wang Q, Gu R, Han D, Yang W. Familial auditory neuropathy. Laryngoscope 2003; 113: 1623–1629

124 Tinnitus

Christopher J. Linstrom

124.1 Introduction

Tinnitus, which is an unpleasant sound coming from one or both ears or from the head, is an annoying problem for both the patient and the treating physician. It is usually accompanied by neurosensory hearing loss, but not always, and is rarely found in individuals with completely normal hearing in both ears. Tinnitus is usually bothersome when the sound environment is otherwise quiet (e.g., in the early morning and late evening hours). If tinnitus interferes with sleep, sleep deprivation may be significant. There is no medical or surgical "cure" for tinnitus. Many medicines have been tried; none are universally successful. There is no uniform antidote for tinnitus.

A proper evaluation for tinnitus includes a carefully taken history to exclude likely treatable causes of hearing loss (e.g., otosclerosis), an otologic examination, a well-done audiogram, and additional diagnostic tests as indicated by the complaint and the audiogram. Unilateral hearing loss or tinnitus should be investigated in an age-appropriate fashion, such as with enhanced magnetic resonance (MR) imaging with gadolinium contrast.

The treatment for tinnitus consists of positive and negative measures, as will be described below.

124.2 Incidence of Disease

Many individuals who have been exposed to an extremely loud noise of a sudden nature (e.g., a gun blast, an explosion near the ear, a train or fire engine horn close by) or to excessively loud noise for a prolonged period (in a nightclub, at a rock concert) will experience at least a transient change in their threshold of hearing and/or a temporary noise emanating from the ear or head. This may lead to tinnitus, which is usually short-lived. As the temporary threshold shift improves, so generally does the tinnitus. Although most patients with tinnitus have no antecedent history, the most common history is one of exposure to noise, especially in industry, military service, etc. The rare patient will have a known cause of tinnitus (e.g., otosclerosis) or may have had antecedent otologic disease treated medically or surgically that can be identified as the cause of tinnitus. Medical intervention (e.g., the use of an ototoxic aminoglycoside such as streptomycin, amikacin, or gentamicin) may be the cause of tinnitus.

124.3 Terminology

Tinnitus may be classified as continuous or pulsatile, erratic, and high-, medium-, or low-pitched. Other than whether the tinnitus is pulsatile (a vascular cause until proved otherwise) or nonpulsatile, the words used to describe the tinnitus ("No, doctor, I have chirping, not ringing") are irrelevant. What is relevant is that the sound is coming from *within* the ear or head, not from *without*.

124.4 Applied Anatomy

Most ears with tinnitus are normal in appearance and have no abnormal features. Very rarely, a wax impaction or even hair touching the tympanic membrane may cause tinnitus. Patients with otosclerosis at any stage may have tinnitus. Although retrocochlear imaging is often performed for unilateral or pulsatile tinnitus, the initial screen often images soft tissue (magnetic resonance [MR] imaging), not bone, because it is more likely that a soft-tissue abnormality will be found than a defect in bone.

124.5 The Disease Process

124.5.1 Etiology

The putative causes of tinnitus depend upon the anatomical part of the ear that is capable of causing tinnitus. The cause of tinnitus may also predict its treatment and outcome. If the patient has tinnitus accompanied by a pathologic process in the external auditory canal (e.g., wax impaction, acute otitis externa) or in the middle ear cleft (e.g., serous otitis media, acute otitis media, traumatic perforation of the tympanic membrane, glomus tympanicum), or a potentially reversible condition of the inner ear (e.g., otosclerosis, sudden idiopathic sensorineural hearing loss, Meniere syndrome), treatment of the underlying cause may relieve the tinnitus. All of these rarely cause only tinnitus. The vast majority of patients who complain of head and/or ear noise have neurosensory or mixed hearing loss in varying degrees. This is by far the most common cause of tinnitus, and any investigation should begin with an evaluation for this problem.

124.5.2 Pathogenesis

Depending upon whether the offending cause is reversible or nonreversible, and on whether exposure to the cause (loud industrial noise or music) continues, tinnitus may be unchanged, made worse, or in most cases tolerated by the brain. Indeed, once the patient has been assured that nothing serious has been discovered, such as a skull base tumor, the anxiety caused by the complaint is often markedly diminished to the point at which the patient can "live with it." This is true of the vast majority of patients. The rare patient, often one multitasking many very stressful life events (e.g., a sick child or parent, a difficult work situation, impending possible negative outcomes, future surgery), may be at an emotional crossroad in trying to deal with the problem and may require the assistance of a psychotherapist or another professional who can aid in stress management. For the average patient, a thorough investigation and reassurance with the use of common techniques such as masking (sound substitution) will go a long way toward managing the nuisance of tinnitus.

124.5.3 Natural History and Progression

The bother of tinnitus usually remains unchanged or may actually decrease as time passes. Rarely does it worsen, and if it does, this is often the result of progression of an underlying cause (e.g., a neoplasm) or continued noise exposure.

124.5.4 Potential Disease Complications

Tinnitus per se cannot cause a serious complication, such as death. As part of an underlying problem, it is not only annoying but also may be one of several complaints that warrant further investigation. Asymmetric hearing loss with unilateral tinnitus or pulsatile tinnitus of any nature requires appropriate investigations until serious disease has been excluded. Pulsatile tinnitus should be assumed to be of a vascular nature until proven otherwise.

124.6 Disease Grading

There is no accepted grading system for tinnitus. Tinnitus is a subjective complaint, and each patient is his or her own "metric." As previously discussed, tinnitus is classified as "pulsatile" or "nonpulsatile," as continuous or intermittent, and by the patient's description. One clinical quantifier is the sleep deficit. A patient who is sleep-deprived because of tinnitus is in a rather urgent state because sleep deprivation affects many aspects of a patient's life, especially work productivity. Every effort should be made to investigate the likely causes of tinnitus in a timely fashion and to offer some type of relief that will restore refreshing sleep. Such a patient may also have sleep apnea, and the history should include questions about anything that would be depriving the patient of sleep. The patient may need to be referred to an appropriate medical professional, who will likely obtain a sleep study and may prescribe a trial of nocturnal continuous positive airway pressure (CPAP).

The judicious and conservative use of soporifics, either over-the counter medications such as various antihistamines (diphenhydramine, chlorpheniramine maleate) or prescription medications such as zolpidem (Ambien; Sanofi-Aventis, Bridgewater, NJ) and diazepam (Valium; Genentech, South San Francisco, CA) may at least temporarily aid sleep. They are more psychologically than physically addicting and should be used with caution.

124.7 Medical Evaluation

The medical history in the patient with tinnitus is straightforward: time of onset; unilateral or bilateral; continuous, irregular, or pulsatile (always significant), etc. It is important to elicit the "sentinel event," if any, such as significant noise exposure. This may aid in directing the patient to obtain earplugs or muffs if continued noise exposure is likely.

124.7.1 Presenting Complaints

Patients will describe what they are hearing. The important features have been mentioned. Other than pulsatile tinnitus, the adjectival description of the sound has very little import, if any, for either diagnosis or treatment.

124.7.2 Clinical Findings, Physical Examination

After the head and neck, the ears are carefully examined, preferably under the microscope. Wax and debris should be cleaned because they may themselves rarely cause tinnitus. Most patients have a normal otoscopic examination. Tests of audition with tuning forks should be done.

The rare patient with objective tinnitus should be examined in a very quiet space, preferably an audiometric booth. All likely sources of a bruit or sound (neck, ears, mastoid areas, orbits) should be examined with a stethoscope in a quiet space.

124.7.3 Testing

The very first and key test to obtain for any patient with tinnitus is a well-done audiogram consisting of pure tones, masked bone, word discrimination, and immittance, performed separately for each ear. Self-administered audiograms may be widely erroneous and are to be condemned. A professionally performed audiogram is an absolute necessity for several reasons: (1) It establishes the level of audition separately for each ear. (2) It will graphically demonstrate any asymmetry of hearing. (3) It gives an idea of the likely frequency of the offending noise. (4) The presence or absence of the acoustic reflex and reflex decay may guide the examiner toward a more thorough retrocochlear evaluation.

The typical patient with tinnitus will have symmetric, downward-sloping hearing loss at frequencies between 1 and 6 kHz. High-tone loss is more commonly found on an audiogram than low-frequency loss. Patients with noise exposure will typically have a nadir around 4 kHz, consistent with noise exposure. Unless the patient has unilateral tinnitus, the investigation may stop at this point. Patients who have unilateral symptoms or asymmetry on the audiogram should undergo a retrocochlear investigation that is age-appropriate. If the patient is 85 years old and a retro-cochlear lesion is found, it is observed, not treated; one may choose auditory brainstem response (ABR) or stacked ABR testing, or surveillance with the audiogram repeated in 1 to 2 years. If, however, the patient is young enough that any discovered retrocochlear lesion will be treated, not just observed, then a more sensitive and specific test with greater predictive value should be obtained, ideally contrast-enhanced MR imaging or, if this is contraindicated, computed tomography (CT) of the brain with contrast focused on the cerebellopontine angles and internal auditory canals. These are more accurate by geometric proportions than ABR testing and have in large measure supplanted all other retrocochlear tests. Each method yields photographic proof of the anatomy of the retrocochlear system. However, the minimum size for identification is still in the range of 2 mm with contrast-enhanced MR imaging and larger with contrast-enhanced CT. If the patient is young enough that either stereotactic radiotherapy or surgery would be a consideration, then definitive imaging should be done and all other retrocochlear tests bypassed.

124.8 Treatment

124.8.1 Medical Treatment

1. The mainstay of medical treatment for virtually all forms of tinnitus is "masking," better described as "sound substitution." A sound of any nature from any source (e.g., fan, air purifier, radio, television, device that generates "white" or "pink" noise) that is less noxious to the ear than the sound emanating from the ear may be chosen to cover the offending sound. Every patient with tinnitus should understand the concept of masking and judiciously employ it. It is a technique for everyone with the problem. Many patients use masking techniques without being aware that they do so. Certainly, head or ear noise is in general less bothersome in a noisy, crowded environment than in a perfectly quiet room, such as a library. Patients intuitively understand this concept, and it should be explained and stressed. It is the cornerstone of all therapy.

2. Noise avoidance must be stressed. The ear with tinnitus will respond in a most bothersome fashion to continued noise exposure. The patient must be educated that acoustic instruments such as an unamplified orchestra or singer can rarely produce enough volume to cause noise-induced hearing loss. As long as the listener is in the body or nave of the auditorium, the cumulative volume will dissipate the intensity of the sound. (Of course, if one is sitting directly in front of the brass section of an orchestra, the effect is a bit more dangerous to hearing.) The same is *not* true of electrically amplified music. Many amplified bands, including bands with vocalists, will play at a decibel level almost equal to that of a jet aircraft taking off (130 to 140 dB). This level of sound is inhumanly loud; the ear is not designed to sustain such sound levels for any length of time, and significant noise-induced hearing loss can occur after even short intervals of exposure.

3. Avoiding central nervous system stimulants such as coffee, tea, and other methylxanthines may help to ameliorate tinnitus.

4. Acetylsalicylic acid (ASA), or aspirin, provokes tinnitus in a dose-related manner. For the rare patient who requires large doses of ASA to relieve joint or spine pain, reducing the dose or choosing a non-ASA medication may help tinnitus.

5. Many so-called "smart phones" such as the iPhone have associated free or modestly priced masking applications ("apps") that can be downloaded onto the phone and transmitted through an earpiece or headphone for masking purposes.

124.8.2 Surgical Treatment

Other than the eradication of vascular tumors or the correction of an arteriovenous malformation or a venous malformation such as a venous diverticulum, there is no specific surgical treatment to eradicate tinnitus. Patients with otosclerosis *and* tinnitus often state that the subjective annoyance of tinnitus is relieved after successful stapedotomy or stapedectomy. However, tinnitus is never the reason for this surgery because of the inherent risk to neurosensory hearing. Restoring the conductive component of the hearing loss toward the nerve line is the only reason to perform stapedectomy and accept its potential risks, chiefly the 0.3 to 0.5% incidence of complete deafness after primary surgery and the 1% incidence after revision surgery.

In the past, elective labyrinthectomy with the insertion of an electrical stimulating device near the round window membrane, and even cochlear implantation via the round window or cochleostomy, were attempted, all without success in eradicating tinnitus. Recently, attempts to diminish or ablate tinnitus have been made by inserting an electrode into the Heschl gyrus. However, one must weigh the risk of placing a foreign body into the brain against the potential benefit; success rates have been questionable. This technique is mentioned for the sake of completeness but is not to be recommended. There is no substitute for a thorough diagnostic plan and traditional therapy that must include masking.

124.9 Prognosis

Most patients with tinnitus are significantly relieved after a thoroughly performed series of diagnostic tests, as previously described, has been discussed with them and they are told that nothing untoward or life-threatening has been found. Normal test results are of great therapeutic benefit in cases of tinnitus. The patient will learn over time that head or ear noise is not an indication of something seriously wrong and will come to ignore it. This is the very best course of treatment—to ignore the problem. In most cases, the bother of tinnitus tends to subside with time.

Other patients cannot attend to mental tasks and need to employ some form of masking during waking hours. There are many forms which the patient may use, such as commonly found items around the home or office (e.g., fan, air freshener, radio, television, generator of "white" or "pink" noise).

124.10 Roundsmanship

- Tinnitus, an unpleasant sound emanating from the ear or the head, is a symptom, not a disease.
- The investigation of tinnitus requires an audiogram and occasionally, if the tinnitus is unilateral, a retrocochlear study (e.g., MR imaging).
- Masking is the mainstay of therapy for all patients with tinnitus.
- There is no medical or surgical antidote for tinnitus. Many over-the-counter and prescription medications exist touting relief from tinnitus. None have been proved statistically successful in carefully performed studies.
- The elimination of known offending agents, such as methylxanthines (e.g., caffeine, nicotine) and noise, may significantly help patients with tinnitus.
- Diagnostic thoroughness, masking, the rare use of medicines, and patience are the best methods of treating tinnitus.
- Most forms of nonpulsatile tinnitus improve with time. Noise exposure is extremely noxious to an ear with tinnitus.
- Truly pulsatile tinnitus is the symptom of a vascular lesion until proved otherwise.
- A rare patient may have objective pulsatile tinnitus, heard by the examiner as well as the patient. An appropriately designed vascular study (CT with contrast, MR angiography, MR venography, four-vessel angiography) must be done to obtain

a definitive diagnosis in these rare cases. Treatment of the underlying lesion may ameliorate the pulsatile tinnitus.

124.11 Recommended Reading

[1] Belli H, Belli S, Oktay MF, Ural C. Psychopathological dimensions of tinnitus and psychopharmacologic approaches in its treatment. Gen Hosp Psychiatry 2012; 34: 282–289

[2] Cianfrone G, Pentangelo D, Cianfrone E et al. Pharmacological drugs inducing ototoxicity, vestibular symptoms and tinnitus: a reasoned and updated guide. Eur Rev Med Pharmacol Sci 2011; 15: 601–636

[3] De Ridder D, De Mulder G, Verstraeten E et al. Auditory cortex stimulation for tinnitus. Acta Neurochir Suppl (Wien) 2007; 97: 451–462

[4] Savage J, Waddell A. Tinnitus. Clin Evid (Online) 2012–0506

[5] Seidman MD, Standring RT, Dornhoffer JL. Tinnitus: current understanding and contemporary management. Curr Opin Otolaryngol Head Neck Surg 2010; 18: 363–368

[6] Shulman A, Goldstein B. Principles of tinnitology: tinnitus diagnosis and treatment a tinnitus-targeted therapy. Int Tinnitus J 2010; 16: 73–85

[7] Soleymani T, Pieton D, Pezeshkian P, et al. Surgical approaches to tinnitus treatment: A review and novel approaches. Surg Neurol Int 2011; 2: 154

125 Retrocochlear Hearing Disorders

Robert Hong and Seilesh C. Babu

125.1 Introduction

An estimated 10% of individuals worldwide are afflicted with hearing loss. In the vast majority of cases, sensorineural hearing loss is cochlear in origin, often secondary to exposure to loud noise, aging, and/or genetics. However, in an important minority of cases, the lesions responsible for sensorineural hearing loss are retrocochlear—located medial to the cochlea in the auditory pathway. Retrocochlear lesions are considered to involve the auditory nerve. A lesion more central to the auditory nerve that involves the central nervous system, although technically also located medial to the cochlea, is for categorization purposes considered to be a central as opposed to a retrocochlear cause of hearing loss.

In considering the types of lesions that can lead to retrocochlear hearing loss, it is helpful to understand the anatomy of the auditory nerve. The auditory nerve is the part of the vestibulocochlear nerve (eighth cranial nerve) that is responsible for hearing. It exits the cochlea to run within the internal auditory canal (IAC), leaving the IAC at the porus acusticus to enter the cerebellopontine angle (CPA) before entering the brainstem to project to the cochlear nuclei of the medulla. Lesions of the auditory nerve can occur via compression of the nerve by tumors (or less commonly, adjacent blood vessels) within the IAC or CPA. The nerve can also be compressed via growth of the surrounding bone of the IAC, as is seen in proliferative bony disorders. Alternatively, retrocochlear hearing loss can be due to lesions that originate within the auditory nerve. Physiologic dysfunction of the nerve may occur, as in auditory dyssynchrony. The nerve may degenerate with age, as in neural presbycusis. The nerve may be missing, as in agenesis of the auditory nerve. Finally, the integrity of the nerve may be affected by a neurologic disorder that similarly affects other parts of the central nervous system, such as multiple sclerosis.

125.2 The Disease Process

125.2.1 Tumors of the Internal Auditory Canal and Cerebellopontine Angle

One of the most important reasons why otolaryngologists are asked to assess a patient with newly diagnosed sensorineural hearing loss is to evaluate the likelihood that a tumor may be causing the hearing deficit. The most common tumor found in the IAC/CPA is a vestibular schwannoma (acoustic neuroma), which is a benign tumor that may originate from either the superior or inferior branch of the vestibular nerve. This is typically a slow-growing tumor, with an average growth rate of 1 to 2 mm per year. As the tumor grows, it compresses and/or stretches the adjacent cochlear nerve, causing a retrocochlear hearing loss. Alternatively, a growing tumor may occlude the blood supply to the cochlear nerve, such as by compressing the internal auditory artery within the IAC, also leading to hearing loss. As the tumor grows further, it expands within the CPA,

compressing other, nearby cranial nerves and causing potentially life-threatening brainstem compression.

Other, less common tumors involving the IAC/CPA may also lead to retrocochlear hearing loss via similar mechanisms. The second most common tumor of the IAC/CPA is a meningioma, which is a benign tumor arising from the arachnoid villi. Neuromas originating from the other nerves within the IAC can also lead to hearing loss, including facial neuromas (facial nerve) and cochlear schwannomas (cochlear nerve). Other rare tumors that can arise in this region include lipomas, hemangiomas, and metastatic tumors (such as from breast, prostate, or lung cancer).

125.2.2 Neural Presbycusis

The progressive loss of sensorineural hearing associated with old age is termed *presbycusis*. Patients older than 55 years of age can be expected to lose hearing at an average rate of 9 dB per decade as a result of age-related degeneration of different structures within the auditory pathway. These structures include those found within the cochlea, such as the hair cells (sensory presbycusis), basilar membrane (mechanical presbycusis), and stria vascularis (metabolic presbycusis), as well as those found behind the cochlea, such as the first-order neurons of the auditory nerve (neural presbycusis). In neural presbycusis, which is the only type of presbycusis that leads to a *retrocochlear* hearing loss, the classic audiometric pattern is speech recognition scores that are lower than expected based on pure-tone audiometry in combination with a slowly down-sloping high-frequency sensorineural hearing loss.

125.2.3 Auditory Dyssynchrony

Auditory dyssynchrony (also known as auditory neuropathy) has become better known since the use of objective measures to assess hearing, particularly otoacoustic emissions (OAEs) and auditory brainstem response (ABR) testing, has become widespread as part of newborn hearing screening programs. Auditory dyssynchrony is defined by an abnormal ABR (reflecting auditory nerve dysfunction) in the context of normal OAEs (reflecting normal outer hair cell function within the cochlea) in a patient without other retrocochlear pathology (such as a tumor of the IAC/CPA). The exact site of the lesion responsible for auditory dyssynchrony is unknown and may vary from patient to patient; lesions of the inner hair cells of the cochlea, auditory nerve, or intervening neural synapse between the cochlea and auditory nerve may all fit this definition. Two groups of patients with auditory dyssynchrony have been described. The predominant group includes infants in whom the condition is found during the course of neonatal hearing screening. It has been estimated that auditory neuropathy is responsible for approximately 7% of cases of permanent hearing loss in children. Although the cause is often unknown, correlations between neonatal insults (especially hyperbilirubinemia and hypoxia) and auditory dyssynchrony have been found. The second group includes young adults, typically patients with multiple neuropathies. For example, neurologic disorders such as Charcot-Marie-Tooth syndrome and Friedreich ataxia may lead to degeneration of the auditory nerve with auditory dyssynchrony.

125.2.4 Temporal Bone Osseous Dysplasias

Rare disorders of the temporal bone involving abnormal bone remodeling may be associated with retrocochlear hearing loss. The mechanism by which hearing loss occurs is abnormal osseous growth around the internal auditory canal, causing stenosis of the IAC and compression of the auditory nerve. Osseous dysplasias do not exclusively cause retrocochlear hearing loss—for example, bony proliferation can also narrow the external auditory canal, resulting in a conductive hearing loss. Of these disorders, the ones most likely to lead to IAC stenosis are the osteopetroses (marble bone disease), a group of hereditary diseases characterized by immature, dense bone secondary to abnormal remodeling, in which a characteristic "chalky" sclerosis of bone is evident on computed tomography (CT). Two other bony dysplasias may also on rare occasions cause IAC stenosis and retrocochlear hearing loss. The first is fibrous dysplasia, in which normal bone is replaced by weak, immature fibro-osseous tissue that has a classic "ground glass" appearance on CT. The second is Paget disease, in which haphazard osteoclastic and osteoblastic activity leads to abnormal bone deposition and the appearance of multiple translucencies on CT, reflective of demineralized bone.

125.2.5 Other Disorders

A number of other etiologies of retrocochlear hearing loss have been described. Congenital absence of the auditory nerve is an important cause to consider in infants born with profound sensorineural hearing loss because it is a contraindication to cochlear implantation. Radiographic imaging demonstrating a narrow IAC (<3 mm in diameter) or magnetic resonance (MR) imaging demonstrating the absence of signal corresponding to the auditory nerve is consistent with this diagnosis. However, such radiographic findings do not guarantee the absence of functional auditory nerve fibers because children with apparent cochlear nerve aplasia on imaging have undergone implantation and demonstrated responses to auditory stimuli.

Disorders of the central nervous system can affect the auditory nerve and result in retrocochlear hearing loss. In patients with multiple sclerosis, demyelination of the auditory nerve can lead to hearing loss. Neurosyphilis is another disorder that can result in lesions of the auditory nerve and hearing loss. However, hearing loss as the sole presenting symptom is unusual in these disorders; patients often have lesions that affect multiple parts of the central nervous system and are not specific to the auditory nerve.

Another potential cause of retrocochlear hearing loss is compression of the auditory nerve by adjacent blood vessels. Vascular loops from nearby branches of the posterior or anterior inferior cerebellar artery have been implicated. However, such a diagnosis is controversial because many patients without hearing loss may also have blood vessels that appear on MR images to be touching the auditory nerve.

125.3 Medical Evaluation

125.3.1 History and Physical Examination

It is important to take a thorough history in the evaluation of a patient with hearing loss. The character of the hearing loss should be probed. A sudden or asymmetric sensorineural hearing loss, or the presence of unilateral nonpulsatile tinnitus, often prompts additional work-up for a retrocochlear etiology. All patients should be questioned about the presence of associated ear symptoms, including tinnitus, otorrhea, otalgia, and vertigo. Patients should also be asked about any history of exposure to loud noise, ear surgery, hearing aid use, and hearing loss in the family. When children are evaluated, it is important to ask the parents if the child passed a newborn hearing screen, to help determine if the hearing loss is congenital or acquired. The child's birth history and development should also be assessed for clues about the etiology and severity of the hearing loss.

The physical examination of the head and neck will often be normal in a patient with retrocochlear hearing loss. Otoscopic examination is useful in evaluating for other (nonretrocochlear) causes of hearing loss, such as a middle ear effusion or tympanic membrane perforation. The results of the Weber and Rinne tuning fork tests will be consistent with a sensorineural hearing loss. Occasionally, patients with a retrocochlear hearing loss may have other cranial nerve deficits, such as those associated with a large cerebellopontine angle tumor.

125.3.2 Audiometric Evaluation

All patients who have hearing loss should be evaluated with an audiogram at their initial visit. The audiometric evaluation is helpful in determining if additional work-up for a retrocochlear hearing loss is indicated. The finding of sensorineural hearing loss on pure-tone audiometry is consistent with both cochlear and retrocochlear etiologies. The following additional audiometric findings increase the clinician's suspicion of a retrocochlear loss, often prompting further testing.

Asymmetry of Hearing Loss.

Concern for a retrocochlear lesion (in particular a tumor of the IAC/CPA on the affected side) occurs when a patient demonstrates a significant asymmetry in sensorineural hearing loss. The exact criteria for *significant* asymmetry are controversial. Obholzer et al suggested the criteria of asymmetry of more than 15 dB at two adjacent pure-tone frequencies for unilateral hearing loss, and asymmetry of more than 20 dB at two adjacent frequencies for bilateral hearing loss. This yielded a sensitivity of 97% and a specificity of 49% when further testing with MR imaging was ordered to evaluate for an IAC/CPA tumor.

Poor Speech Discrimination Out of Proportion to Degree of Hearing Loss

Individuals with cochlear sensorineural hearing loss typically do not experience a significant degradation of their ability to understand speech until they have a hearing loss of at least

60 dB HL. In contrast, a patient with a retrocochlear loss may exhibit poor speech discrimination despite relatively good pure-tone thresholds. It has been shown that 75% of the auditory nerve fibers can be damaged before a decrease in pure-tone thresholds is seen, whereas good speech discrimination requires the preservation of the majority of such fibers. Thus, an IAC/CPA tumor that compresses the auditory nerve will result in an earlier deterioration of speech discrimination than of pure-tone thresholds.

Rollover

Rollover is a classic finding consistent with retrocochlear pathology, in which as the intensity of speech is increased, it becomes more difficult for patients to understand the speech. The theory is that in patients with a retrocochlear lesion, fatigue of the auditory nerve increases as sound intensity increases, making speech perception more difficult.

Decruitment

Decruitment is another classic finding in patients with retrocochlear pathology, in which as the intensity of a sound is increased, its perceived loudness increases at an abnormally slow rate. Some patients may even perceive a decrease in loudness as sound intensity increases. This is again related to an increased susceptibility to auditory nerve fatigue with a retrocochlear lesion. Decruitment, however, is not routinely assessed in an audiometric evaluation.

Abnormal Acoustic Reflexes

Acoustic reflex testing has also traditionally been used to determine the likelihood of a retrocochlear lesion by assessing contraction of the stapedius muscle in response to loud sounds. This reflex is thought to be important in protecting the ear from acoustic trauma. Two measurements have been correlated with retrocochlear lesions. The first is an abnormally elevated (if not absent) acoustic reflex threshold, in which a sound stimulus needs to be presented at an abnormally high intensity to trigger the reflex. The second is an abnormally fast acoustic reflex decay, in which the stapedius muscle is unable to sustain contraction during the presentation of a continuous loud sound. In both cases, these findings reflect increased fatigue of the auditory nerve, induced by a retrocochlear lesion, in response to high-intensity sound stimuli. However, although more than 75% of patients with a vestibular schwannoma will demonstrate abnormal acoustic reflexes, this test is no longer routinely used to rule out a retrocochlear lesion because of its high false-negative rate.

125.3.3 Further Work-up

If a patient is suspected of having a retrocochlear hearing loss, additional work-up is warranted. Some have suggested using ABR testing as the most cost-effective next step in the screening process, though this is controversial. ABR testing involves the measurement of auditory evoked potentials. Electrodes are placed on the patient's head to measure changes of electrical activity in response to the presentation of a sound stimulus.

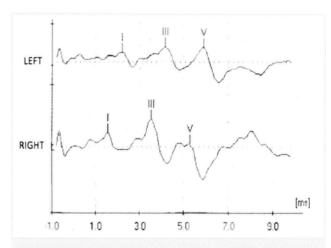

Fig. 125.1 Standard auditory brainstem response (ABR) of a patient with a left acoustic neuroma. The right ear demonstrates normal ABR waveforms. The left ear demonstrates prolonged absolute latencies for waves I, III, and V, consistent with the patient's diagnosis of an acoustic neuroma.

The measured activity occurs in a wavelike pattern, as the stimulus is transmitted in a peripheral to central direction through the auditory system: from the auditory nerve (waves I and II) to the cochlear nucleus (wave III) to the superior olivary complex (wave IV) to the lateral lemniscus (wave V) to the inferior colliculus (waves VI and VII). The presence of a retrocochlear lesion is suspected when the appearance of the expected waves of the ABR is delayed, either in a relative sense (the affected ear is compared with the opposite normal ear, or early waves are compared with later waves in the same ear) or in an absolute sense (▶ Fig. 125.1). A poor ABR waveform on the affected side is also consistent with a retrocochlear lesion. However, the use of ABR testing is limited for a number of reasons. First, it is not useful in patients with a severe (> 70 dB HL) hearing loss because the ABR waveform will be abnormal strictly because of the severity of hearing loss. Second, ABR testing is good for detecting larger tumors but may miss smaller ones (< 1 cm), with a reported sensitivity above 95% for tumors larger than 1 cm and a sensitivity of 79% for those smaller 1 cm. Thus, patients with a normal ABR can be relatively but not absolutely confident that they do not have an acoustic neuroma.

Recently, the use of stacked ABR testing to screen for acoustic neuromas has become more popular. In stacked ABR testing, masking noise of different frequencies is used in conjunction with the traditional auditory click stimulus to derive measured waveforms reflecting neural activity across the entire auditory spectrum. This is in contrast to the standard click-evoked ABR, in which the measured waveform is dominated by the response of high-frequency auditory nerve fibers. As a result, the stacked ABR test is more sensitive for detecting small acoustic tumors because a tumor affecting only low-frequency auditory nerve fibers would result in a normal standard ABR but an abnormal stacked ABR. Stacked ABR testing has been reported to have a sensitivity of 95% and a specificity of 88% for detecting small (≤ 1 cm) acoustic tumors. Patients with an abnormal ABR require additional MR imaging to evaluate for a retrocochlear lesion.

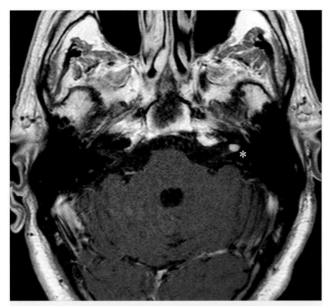

Fig. 125.2 Magnetic resonance image (T1 with gadolinium) demonstrating a small (0.5 cm) acoustic neuroma located in the left internal auditory canal. The neuroma enhances with contrast (*asterisk*).

The gold standard to evaluate for a retrocochlear lesion is MR imaging with gadolinium contrast, and many clinicians will bypass ABR testing in favor of MR imaging to obtain a definitive diagnosis more quickly. MR imaging can detect IAC/CPA tumors as small as a few millimeters in diameter, with these tumors demonstrating characteristic enhancement after the administration of contrast (▶ Fig. 125.2). However, some patients cannot undergo MR imaging—for example, because of the presence of metal in the body (e.g., cardiac pacemakers, shrapnel, hemostatic clips in the brain). If these patients need to be evaluated for a retrocochlear lesion, CT with intravenous contrast and/or ABR testing should be used. If CT is used, patients should be aware that it may miss tumors smaller than 1.5 cm.

125.3.4 Auditory Dyssynchrony versus Neural Presbycusis versus Central Auditory Processing Disorder

Some adults may complain of difficulty hearing, particularly in noisy environments, but have relatively normal pure-tone thresholds and speech discrimination scores (in quiet) on audiometric evaluation. The need for additional work-up from this point is controversial. Some clinicians will attribute these patients' complaints to neural presbycusis, particularly if they are older. Others will obtain OAE and ABR testing to evaluate for auditory dyssynchrony. (It should be noted, however, that the absence of OAEs does not rule out auditory dyssynchrony in adults, as many adults with normal hearing lose their OAEs with age.) Yet others will obtain testing to evaluate for a central auditory processing disorder (CAPD). CAPD is a controversial diagnosis in which difficulty hearing in the context of normal peripheral auditory function is attributed to problems with auditory processing by the central nervous system. No consensus criteria exist for the diagnosis of CAPD, although most

testing involves an evaluation with sensitized speech (in which speech is distorted in some manner to reduce intelligibility, such as with the addition of background noise). If CAPD is diagnosed, auditory rehabilitation is prescribed, although the effectiveness of such therapy is inconclusive.

125.4 Treatment

125.4.1 Retrocochlear Hearing Loss

Treatments with respect to hearing are similar for retrocochlear and cochlear hearing loss. Hearing amplification is useful for mild to moderate hearing loss, with a decrease in utility noted as the severity of hearing loss increases. Patients who have retrocochlear loss may find hearing aids relatively less helpful than those who have cochlear loss because amplification often makes speech sounds louder but not more understandable. Patients with bilateral severe to profound sensorineural hearing loss may be candidates for cochlear implantation, as long as the integrity of the cochlear nerve has not been compromised (e.g., by a tumor of the IAC).

125.4.2 Tumors of the Internal Auditory Canal and Cerebellopontine Angle

The treatment of tumors of the IAC and CPA is discussed in detail elsewhere in this book. Briefly, the options fall into three categories: observation, surgery, and stereotactic radiosurgery. Observation is typically reserved for older individuals with small tumors. If surgery is selected, the decision must be made either to sacrifice hearing (via a translabyrinthine approach) or to attempt to preserve hearing (via a middle cranial fossa or retrosigmoid approach). Stereotactic radiosurgery is another option for preserving hearing, although long-term outcomes have yet to be determined.

125.4.3 Auditory Dyssynchrony

Infants who are evaluated for hearing loss often have failed objective testing, typically OAE and/or ABR testing. The combination of normal OAE and abnormal ABR test results is consistent with auditory dyssynchrony. Infants with auditory dyssynchrony are typically followed until behavioral audiometric thresholds can be obtained, so that the degree of hearing loss can be determined. Patients with auditory dyssynchrony may have anywhere from a mild to profound sensorineural hearing loss. The initial treatment for auditory dyssynchrony is hearing amplification. Some children may derive a significant benefit from hearing aids. (In contrast, few adults with auditory dyssynchrony benefit; they report that hearing aids make speech louder but not more understandable.) Additional measures, such as preferential seating in classrooms and the use of FM systems, may be useful. Speech and language therapy should also be considered for all children with auditory dyssynchrony because both are often impaired as a consequence of the hearing impediment. Finally, cochlear implantation should be considered for children who continue to struggle with hearing despite amplification. Such a decision should be undertaken carefully because cases of spontaneous resolution of auditory dyssynchrony before 1 year of age have been reported. Additionally, although cochlear implantation is widely accepted for treating auditory dyssynchrony when it is associated with a severe to profound sensorineural hearing loss, its role in treating milder degrees of associated hearing loss requires further study.

125.5 Roundsmanship

- A retrocochlear etiology should be considered for all patients with sensorineural hearing loss. Initial clinical suspicion is heightened when patients demonstrate asymmetric sensorineural hearing loss, asymmetric nonpulsatile tinnitus, speech perception worse than expected based on pure-tone audiometry, or auditory fatigue.
- The gold standard for the evaluation of retrocochlear hearing loss is MR imaging of the internal auditory canal with gadolinium. Other tests that may have clinical value in selected cases include ABR testing and CT.
- Auditory neuropathy is a retrocochlear disorder most commonly diagnosed in young children with normal OAEs and abnormal ABRs. The mainstays of therapy include hearing amplification and speech–language therapy. Cochlear implanta-

tion is reserved for those who do not demonstrate significant improvement with these measures.

125.6 Recommended Reading

[1] Davis AC, Ostri B, Parving A. Longitudinal study of hearing. Acta Otolaryngol Suppl 1990; 476: 12–22

[2] Don M, Kwong B, Tanaka C, Brackmann D, Nelson R. The stacked ABR: a sensitive and specific screening tool for detecting small acoustic tumors. Audiol Neurootol 2005; 10: 274–290

[3] Fortnum H, O'Neill C, Taylor R et al. The role of magnetic resonance imaging in the identification of suspected acoustic neuroma: a systematic review of clinical and cost effectiveness and natural history. Health Technol Assess 2009; 13: iii–iv, ix–xi, 1–154

[4] Obholzer RJ, Rea PA, Harcourt JP. Magnetic resonance imaging screening for vestibular schwannoma: analysis of published protocols. J Laryngol Otol 2004; 118: 329–332

[5] Rance G. Auditory neuropathy/dys-synchrony and its perceptual consequences. Trends Amplif 2005; 9: 1–43

[6] Raveh E, Buller N, Badrana O, Attias J. Auditory neuropathy: clinical characteristics and therapeutic approach. Am J Otolaryngol 2007; 28: 302–308

[7] Schuknecht HF, Woellner RC. An experimental and clinical study of deafness from lesions of the cochlear nerve. J Laryngol Otol 1955; 69: 75–97

[8] Warren FM, Wiggins RH, Pitt C, Harnsberger HR, Shelton C. Apparent cochlear nerve aplasia: to implant or not to implant? Otol Neurotol 2010; 31: 1088–1094

126 Middle Ear Implants

George Alexiades

126.1 Introduction

Conductive hearing loss is one of the most common indications for middle ear surgery. A conductive hearing loss results when sound is not effectively transmitted through the ossicular chain to the inner ear. It may occur in many situations, such as cerumen impaction, otitis externa, tympanic membrane perforation, middle ear effusion, and ossicular erosion and/or fixation. Conductive hearing loss is commonly found in patients with cholesteatoma, chronic otitis media, and otosclerosis and is a frequent result of otologic surgery. This chapter will concentrate on the prostheses used when continuity of the ossicular chain is disrupted. Numerous techniques and materials are used for ossiculoplasty. Many of the materials that were in vogue years ago have been replaced by lighter, more biocompatible materials.

126.2 Incidence of Disease

It is unclear what the incidence of conductive hearing loss is because it is associated with many causative disease processes. Chronic suppurative otitis media, with or without cholesteatoma, and otosclerosis are the most common situations that result in ossicular problems. Other causes of conductive hearing loss include temporal bone trauma, osteogenesis imperfecta, and various genetic syndromes.

126.3 Terminology

Traditional ossicular chain reconstructions are classified according to the Wullstein classification on a scale of I through V. A type I tympanoplasty consists of a primary tympanic membrane repair (myringoplasty) with an intact ossicular chain. In a type II tympanoplasty, the tympanic membrane is grafted to the incus. The tympanic membrane is grafted directly to the stapes suprastructure in a type III tympanoplasty. In a type IV tympanoplasty, the tympanic membrane is grafted onto a mobile stapes footplate. A type V tympanoplasty has also been described and consists of grafting the tympanic membrane to the oval window or a lateral semicircular canal fenestration.

Middle ear implants are classified according to the point of origin from which the prosthesis spans the ossicular gap. The two major classes are partial ossicular reconstruction prosthesis (PORP) and total ossicular reconstruction prosthesis (TORP). A PORP is used when the incus is eroded but the stapes suprastructure is intact. A TORP is required when the incus and the stapes suprastructure are eroded but an intact, mobile stapes footplate remains. In situations in which there is a fixed stapes footplate, stapes prostheses, in a variety of shapes and materials, may be used. The two most common stapes prosthesis shapes are the wire–piston and the bucket handle. These typically span from the long process of the incus to a stapedotomy in the footplate or, in the case of a stapedectomy, to a vein or perichondrial graft placed over the oval window. In patients with erosion of the long process of the incus, a longer prosthe-

sis can be used to span the gap from the manubrium of the malleus to the stapedotomy/stapedectomy site.

126.4 Materials

Before the 1970s, autologous ossicular remnants, cartilage, or bone, as well as homografts, were used for ossicular chain reconstructions. The most common ossicular reconstruction in which the patient's own tissue is used is the incus interposition. In this instance, the long process of the incus is usually eroded by disease, resulting in ossicular discontinuity. The incus is removed and remodeled to fit on top of the stapes suprastructure and underneath the manubrium of the malleus, thus restoring continuity of the ossicular chain. In situations in which the incus is unavailable, multiple materials have been used over the years, ranging from gold, stainless steel, polytetrafluoroethylene (Teflon; DuPont, Wilmington, DE), fluoroplastic, and bioglass to hydroxyapatite, ionomeric cement, and titanium. Titanium has become the material of choice for PORPs and TORPs because it biocompatible, lightweight, and strong. ▶ Fig. 126.1 shows a typical titanium PORP in use today. The head of the prosthesis is wide and sits underneath the tympanic membrane, while the bottom of the prosthesis attaches to the stapes suprastructure. The shaft is usually adjustable in length. ▶ Fig. 126.2 shows a typical TORP, which has a similar head, but the shaft is longer and lies on the stapes footplate. In addition to being used as a material for prostheses, ionomeric cement has been used to fuse the incus remnant to the stapes suprastructure in cases of erosion of the long or lenticular process of the incus. Stapes prostheses are still made from a variety of materials: stainless steel, platinum, titanium, and fluoroplastic, or from combinations thereof (▶ Fig. 126.3).

126.5 Results

The rates of successful hearing depend on the type of prosthesis used. Stapedectomies have the highest success rate; closure of the air–bone gap to within 10 dB is achieved in approximately 90% of cases. When PORPs are used, closure to within 20 dB

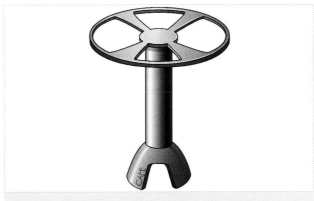

Fig. 126.1 Partial ossicular reconstruction prosthesis (PORP).

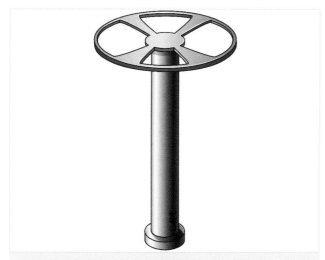

Fig. 126.2 Total ossicular reconstruction prosthesis (TORP).

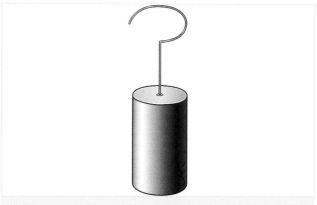

Fig. 126.3 Wire–piston stapes prosthesis.

occurs about 70 to 80% of the time, which is considered acceptable. TORPs fare even worse, with closure of the air–bone gap to within 20 dB achieved in only 50 to 60% of cases. The results of incus interposition grafts are comparable to those of PORPs. Comparisons of the various materials in use for ossiculoplasty yield varying results; however, the trend suggests that titanium is the material of choice today.

Hearing results after ossicular chain reconstruction ultimately depend upon the status of the mucosa and aeration of the middle ear cleft. Hearing results in situations of eustachian tube dysfunction will be poorer than those in cases of good middle ear aeration. In addition to the formation of a serous effusion, retraction of the tympanic membrane negatively impacts surgical success. Continued negative middle ear pressure is believed to be a significant risk factor for prosthesis extrusion and/or displacement.

126.6 Complications

The most common complication of ossicular reconstruction is persistent conductive hearing loss. The variables described earlier all affect the success of ossiculoplasty and do not depend merely upon choice of prosthesis material or proper sizing. Prosthesis migration and/or extrusion is another frequent complication of ossiculoplasty. It is currently recommended that a cartilage graft be laid between the head of the prosthesis and the tympanic membrane to act as a thin biological barrier and reduce extrusion rates. Rates of extrusion for currently available prostheses are in the range of 5 to 10% for PORPs and TORPs. As would be expected, the rates of extrusion increase over time. Stapes prostheses are generally more stable, and prosthesis displacement and/or erosion of the long process of the incus

resulting in ossicular discontinuity is uncommon (3 to 5%). Chorda tympani nerve stretch injury or transection occurs in approximately 15% of patients undergoing tympanoplasty and results in either temporarily or permanently altered taste; stretch injuries are more symptomatic than nerve transactions in these cases. Facial nerve injury is also exceedingly rare in ossiculoplasty without concomitant mastoidectomy and occurs in fewer than 1% of cases. Permanent sensorineural hearing loss is quite rare with the use of PORPs and TORPs; however, the incidence of sensorineural hearing loss is 0.5% in primary stapedectomy and 1% in revision stapedectomy.

126.7 Roundsmanship

- Although currently available ossicular reconstruction prostheses are made of a number of materials, titanium has become the material of choice because of its light weight and strength, and the ease with which the length of the prosthesis can be adjusted.
- Ossiculoplasty results in successful hearing in about 90% of patients with stapedectomies, 60 to 70% of those with PORPs, and 50 to 60% of those with TORPs.
- The status of the middle ear is critical in successful ossiculoplasty.

126.8 Recommended Reading

[1] Coffey CS, Lee FS, Lambert PR. Titanium versus nontitanium prostheses in ossiculoplasty. Laryngoscope 2008; 118: 1650–1658
[2] Truy E, Naiman AN, Pavillon C, Abedipour D, Lina-Granade G, Rabilloud M. Hydroxyapatite versus titanium ossiculoplasty. Otol Neurotol 2007; 28: 492–498
[3] Wullstein H. Techniques of tympanoplasty I, II, and III. AMA Arch Otolaryngol 1960; 71: 424–427
[4] Wullstein H. Techniques of tympanoplasty IV and V. AMA Arch Otolaryngol 1960; 71: 451–453

127 Otosclerosis and Stapedectomy

Seilesh C. Babu

127.1 Introduction

Otosclerosis is a disease that affects the otic capsule of the temporal bone, resulting in conductive, mixed, or rarely a sensorineural hearing loss. Causes of otosclerosis can remain elusive and have been known to include endocrine, metabolic, traumatic, and autoimmune disorders. Otosclerosis may also be hereditary.

127.2 History

Hearing restoration for otosclerosis via a fenestration procedure was described in 1938 by Lempert. Rosen and Shea furthered the work of their mentor by performing stapes mobilizations and stapedectomies. In 1956, Shea first performed a stapedectomy for otosclerosis. In 1969, Schuknecht and Applebaum introduced the technique of stapedotomy, in which the stapes superstructure is resected but the footplate is preserved. The adaptation of the laser to microsurgery has been a more recent innovation that has made stapes surgery more accurate and less risky.

127.3 Clinical Findings

The hearing loss associated with otosclerosis is typically conductive and presents in middle adult life. Occasionally, it may present earlier or may represent congenital stapes fixation. The treatment is similar for both presentations, but the risk for complete hearing loss needs to be discussed with family members when hearing loss presents early in a child and surgery is contemplated. A positive family history is found in approximately 50% of patients. In some patients, a mixed hearing loss and a gradual worsening of the sensorineural component develop as a result of cochlear involvement with otosclerosis. The degree of eventual sensorineural involvement is unpredictable. Otosclerosis is estimated to be unilateral in approximately 15% of cases. Tinnitus may be associated with otosclerosis and varies in intensity and character.

Audiometry reveals a low-frequency conductive hearing loss initially, which usually progresses to a larger air–bone gap as the degree of fixation increases at the footplate of the stapes. In other audiometric testing, impedance plethysmography often is normal or can show reduced tympanic membrane compliance. The stapedial reflexes classically are abnormal; however, they may be within normal limits depending on the degree of stapes fixation.

127.3.1 Carhart Notch

An apparent loss in bone conduction, first described by Carhart in 1950, occurs at around 2,000 Hz on audiometry in patients with otosclerosis. This is secondary to loss of the contribution of the middle ear to bone conduction. Upon vibration of the mastoid bone, the ossicular chain vibrates slightly out of phase, causing a movement of the stapes footplate relative to the coch-

lea. In otosclerosis, this does not occur. Carhart found that otosclerosis reduces bone conduction thresholds by 5 dB at 500 Hz, 10 dB at 1,000 Hz, 25 dB at 2,000 Hz, and 15 dB at 4,000 Hz.

127.4 Differential Diagnosis

The diagnosis of otosclerosis is based on the clinical and audiometric findings. Progressive conductive hearing loss, a normal otoscopic examination with an intact and mobile tympanic membrane, no evidence of eustachian tube dysfunction, a negative Rinne test result, and an absent stapedial reflex are typical findings in otosclerosis. Other processes should be considered in patients with conductive hearing loss. Ossicular discontinuity, middle ear effusion or disease, tympanosclerosis, Paget disease, osteogenesis imperfecta, and degenerative arthritis may all cause conductive deafness. In addition, causes of ossicular fixation should be considered, including lateral ossicular fixation and incus–anulus fusion. Another consideration is superior semicircular canal dehiscence. The stapedial reflex can help differentiate this condition from otosclerosis because the reflex should be intact in superior semicircular canal dehiscence; however, variable presentations of the reflex can occur depending on the degree of stapes fixation present. VEMP (vestibular evoked myogenic potential) testing and computed tomography (CT) of the temporal bone may be used to rule out superior semicircular canal dehiscence.

127.5 Management of Otosclerosis

127.5.1 Amplification

Patients may use hearing aids as an alternative to surgery. These carry little risk but will obviously not prevent further progression of the otosclerotic process. The disadvantage of the use of hearing aids for a long period is that it may reduce the success rate and may increase the complication rate of surgery years later as the otosclerosis progresses. If the patient has a significant mixed hearing loss before surgery, he or she may require a hearing aid after stapes surgery. However, the patient may require a less powerful, more effective hearing aid with better sound quality.

127.5.2 Medical Management

The value of medical therapy for otosclerosis is controversial. Medical therapy may be considered for patients with a predominantly sensorineural hearing loss.

Shambaugh first predicted that otosclerotic lesions could be stabilized with the use of sodium fluoride. This agent is thought to slow or halt the progression of otosclerotic hearing loss by neutralizing and inactivating the hydrolytic and proteolytic enzymes of otospongiotic lesions. Sodium fluoride promotes the maturation of active otospongiosis by reducing its vascularity and bone resorption activity and by increasing new bone formation, eventually inactivating otosclerosis.

Over-the-counter preparations of sodium fluoride include Monocal and Florical (Mericon Industries, Peoria, IL). Monocal is is absorbed in the intestine rather than in the stomach and may cause fewer side effects. Recommended doses vary, typically two tablets per day to minimize side effects, which include stomach upset, allergic itching, and increased joint pain. Fluorosis, the most severe side effect in the treatment of osteoporosis, has not been noted with lower doses of fluoride therapy. Women of childbearing age should be informed that fluoride medication can be teratogenic during the first 6 weeks of fetal development.

127.5.3 Surgical Management

Stapedectomy is typically considered for patients with an air–bone gap of at least 15 dB, reversal of Rinne testing with a 512-Hz tuning fork, speech discrimination scores of 60% or better, and no contraindication to surgery. The ear with the worse hearing should be addressed first. Early procedures entailed removal of the entire stapes footplate and the placement of grafted tissue over the oval window, followed by the piston. With newer technology, such as the microdrill and laser, stapedotomy (opening into the vestibule) has become a more common technique because it results in less trauma and better hearing.

Stapedectomy Prostheses

Many different prostheses of various materials have been developed for stapedectomy. Some of the designs that have proved most effective and are still in use today include the McGee piston and the Robinson bucket handle prostheses. The implantation of metallic prostheses must be carefully considered because of potential issues with magnetic resonance imaging compatibility. Appropriate nonferromagnetic metals, such as platinum, titanium, and stainless steel, may be used safely. Numerous types of prostheses are available and have been successfully used in stapes surgery. Surgeon preference usually leads to the selection of a safe and effective prosthesis.

Lasers in Stapedotomy

Several different types of lasers have been adapted for stapedotomy. Lasers allow vaporization of the stapes footplate with minimal vibratory effect. This technology also causes minimal thermal injury to the perilymph. Complex revision stapes surgery that traditionally was associated with high risk and low success rates is now performed much more effectively with laser.

Several types of lasers are available for otologic surgery, including argon, potassium titanyl phosphate (KTP), and carbon dioxide (CO_2) lasers. Argon and KTP lasers have similar wavelengths and properties. The wavelength of an argon laser is 488 nm, whereas the KTP laser wavelength is 532 nm. The visible wavelengths of these two lasers provide excellent target accuracy because the aiming beam and the surgical beam are the same. Both fiber-optic handheld probes and micromanipulators can be used with these lasers. Argon and KTP laser radiation is poorly absorbed in bone and perilymph, so that potential risk to the saccule and utricle is increased during use.

The wavelength of the invisible CO_2 laser is 10,600 nm. CO_2 lasers are absorbed in bone and perilymph, an ideal characteristic that allows stapedotomy to be performed safely. Studies have shown that use of the CO_2 laser in the open vestibule causes a rise in the perilymph temperature of only 0.3°C. One of the advantages of the CO_2 laser for stapedotomy, the high rate of absorption in the perilymph, results in a low penetration depth of only 0.01 mm.

Because the CO_2 laser beam is invisible, a second aiming beam (helium–neon [HeNe], 612 nm) is required, and the calibration of these two lasers must be ensured. Until recently, CO_2 laser was available for use only with a micromanipulator. Fiber-optic delivery of the CO_2 laser has now been introduced, allowing the benefit of handheld manipulation.

Stapedotomy Procedure

The procedure may be performed with intravenous sedation or general anesthesia. Antibiotics and often steroids are given preoperatively.

After sterile preparation and draping, local anesthetic is infiltrated into the ear canal and postauricular region. This should be done slowly and deliberately, and blanching of the ear canal skin should be observed to ensure adequate anesthesia and hemostasis.

A small piece of subcutaneous fascia or fat is harvested from a postauricular incision and saved for later use.

The speculum should then be secured in the speculum holder. The largest speculum that can comfortably fit into the ear canal should be used for the greatest exposure.

A 6- to 8-mm tympanomeatal flap is created. The chorda tympani nerve is preserved and the middle ear entered. Adequate exposure is attained by using a microdrill and/or curet on the osseous anulus (► Fig. 127.1) until the stapedial tendon and inferior portion of the tympanic facial nerve are well seen. Malleus and incus mobility are ensured, and stapes fixation is confirmed by manual palpation.

The incudostapedial joint is lasered before it is separated with a joint knife (► Fig. 127.2). To allow better stability of the stapes superstructure, the stapes tendon is lasered *after* the joint has been separated (► Fig. 127.3). The posterior crus of the stapes is then lasered (► Fig. 127.4) as close to the footplate as possible to prevent the stump of the crus from later interfering with placement of the piston. If the anterior crus is visible, it can also be lasered. The superstructure is then briskly down-fractured away from the facial nerve and removed (► Fig. 127.5).

Small fenestra laser stapedotomy can be performed via a rosette technique wherein multiple laser applications (► Fig. 127.6) with the 0.2-mm spot size are used to gradually create a 0.7-mm fenestra (► Fig. 127.7). Although the CO_2 wavelength will minimize the risk to the inner ear, care must still be taken not to allow the laser to pass through adjacent, previously created holes in order to prevent injury to the inner ear, especially if perilymph has leaked out to cause a dry fenestra. Absence of the perilymph takes away the natural protection of the vestibular end-organs. Those surgeons who choose to use visible spectrum lasers (KTP or argon) instead of the invisible

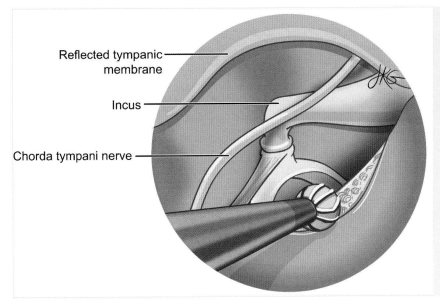

Fig. 127.1 Adequate exposure of the stapes footplate often necessitates removal of some of the osseous anulus.

Reflected tympanic membrane

Incus

Chorda tympani nerve

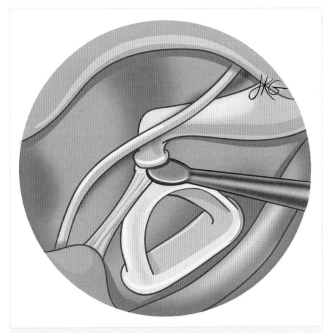

Fig. 127.2 Separation of the incudostapedial joint with a joint knife.

wavelength CO_2 laser must take even greater care because visible lasers can pass through perilymph, potentially causing injury to the inner ear.

Measurements may be taken from the incus to the stapes footplate opening. Typically, the stapes prosthesis measures 4.25 mm in length and 0.5 mm in diameter. These dimensions seem to be appropriate for 90 to 95% of patients undergoing surgery. The stapes piston is then inserted into the fenestra with a small alligator forceps.

Once its position is confirmed, the piston is crimped onto the incus (▶ Fig. 127.8), and then its position at both the incus and the footplate is confirmed under high-power magnification. The previously harvested fascia is cut into 3 mm pieces, which are moistened and packed around the piston at the fenestra. A

critical maneuver before closure is to move the malleus and look for movement of both the incus and piston. The tympano-meatal flap is then replaced. A whisper test confirms improved hearing, and several pieces of saline-soaked Gelfoam (Pfizer, New York, NY) are placed over the tympanomeatal flap and tympanic membrane. An antibiotic ointment that is not oto-toxic, such as bacitracin, is then instilled in the external auditory canal. Most patients may be discharged the same day if they live within an hour or two of the hospital.

Intraoperative Issues

Anatomical variants may be found at the time of middle ear exploration done for possible stapes surgery. When these are encountered, erring on the side of patient safety is of critical importance. If a low-hanging facial nerve contacting the stapes or a persistent stapedial artery is identified, the surgeon will not be faulted for aborting the procedure.

Narrow Oval Window Fenestra

A difficult scenario in stapes surgery is dealing with a narrow oval window niche. This limits the surgeon's ability to create an appropriately sized fenestra and makes it difficult to know if the fenestra created may in fact be too narrow, which will restrict movement of the piston. A narrow niche can often be markedly improved by using the laser to vaporize approximately 1 mm of promontory bone just below the stapes. This improves visibility and allows accurate placement of the piston.

Incus Erosion/Subluxation

Erosion of the incus is a common finding at revision stapedectomy. In dealing with incus erosion, the surgeon must assess whether reconstruction is possible with the remaining incus or whether reconstruction to the malleus or drum is necessary. In certain modification techniques, bone cement may be used to rebuild the incus and anchor the prosthesis. Alternative prostheses, such as the Big Easy offset piston and the Lippy-

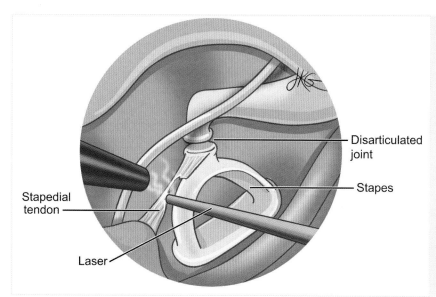

Fig. 127.3 The stapedial tendon is lysed with laser.

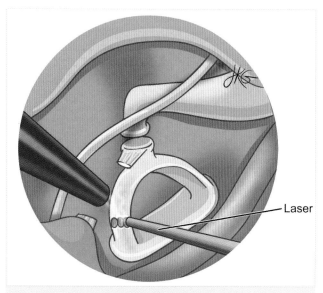

Fig. 127.4 The posterior crus of the stapes is lasered.

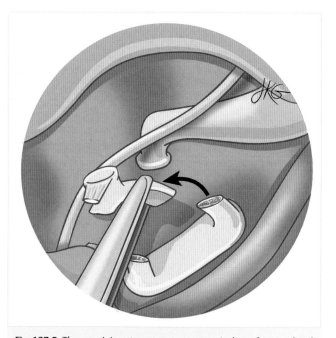

Fig. 127.5 The remaining stapes superstructure is down-fractured and removed.

modified Robinson prostheses, may also be effective if the incus erosion is mild to moderate. If incus erosion is severe, a malleus–to–oval window prosthesis may be used and the procedure performed by an experienced surgeon.

Postoperative Complications

In the postoperative patient with significant dizziness, tinnitus, and/or hearing loss, one must consider the most likely differential diagnosis. Etiologies include serous labyrinthitis, perilymphatic fistula, a deep piston, and reparative granuloma. Patients should be monitored closely; the timing and severity of symptoms as well as the physical examination findings are key factors in determining the likely cause and treatment.

Serous Labyrinthitis

The most common cause of postoperative inner ear symptoms after routine stapedotomy is thought to be "serous labyrinthitis," which occurs during routine "successful" stapes surgery. This complication may be associated with individual variations in inner ear sensitivity. Most patients appear to benefit from a short course of oral steroids. If rapid improvement is not noted, the packing should be removed (even at an early stage postoperatively), the ear examined, and the hearing assessed. Reparative granuloma, perilymph fistula, and a deep or long piston should be excluded.

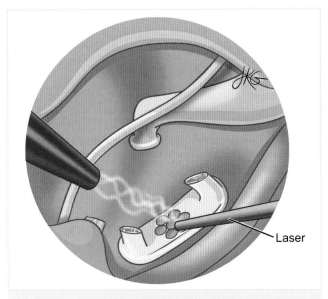

Fig. 127.6 A rosette pattern is lasered on the stapes footplate.

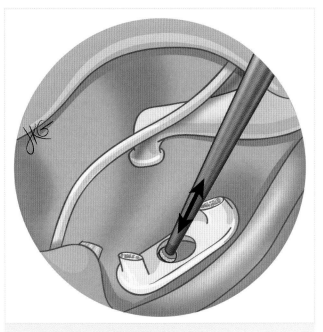

Fig. 127.7 Creating a small stapedotomy.

Oval Window Fistula

Oval window fistula was relatively common in the past when Gelfoam and blood were used in the fenestra instead of tissue seals. Oval window fistula after stapedectomy may occur in the early postoperative period or years later. Fluctuating or progressive hearing loss is noted, as well as tinnitus with or without vertigo. Trauma or a change in barometric pressure may precede the symptoms. The clinical examination may include fistula testing, typically performed simply with digital pressure or pneumotoscopy to elicit dizziness. Audiometric findings include sensorineural hearing loss, although hearing loss is not always present on the audiogram. The diagnosis is rarely seen when a tissue seal of fascia or vein has been used. Middle ear exploration and grafting of the oval window with tissue is indicated if a fistula is thought to be present.

Deep Piston/Prosthesis

The incidence of deep insertion of the piston within the vestibule is low in experienced hands. Most commonly, this complication occurs when the length of the chosen piston is more than the standard length of 4.25 mm. The diagnosis is strongly considered when either a longer prosthesis was used or the patient experienced dizziness intraoperatively during placement of the piston through the fenestra. As in patients with perilymph fistula, digital pressure or pneumotoscopy often elicits dizziness; however, the onset of symptoms is usually immediately after surgery, whereas fistulas may occur quite late. CT after stapedectomy has not been shown to be reliable in determining the depth of piston insertion within the vestibule. Thus, imaging after stapedectomy has limited value in identifying a piston that is too deep within the vestibule.

Other etiologies of vertigo should be considered, including benign paroxysmal positional vertigo (BPPV), a depressed footplate fragment, or reparative granuloma. BPPV in the postoperative period may be secondary to surgical injury to the utricle or due to the free flow of particles from the fenestra. This

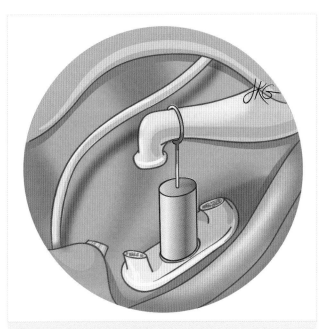

Fig. 127.8 Stapes prosthesis in place in stapedotomy and crimped on the long process of the incus.

condition is typically self-limiting, and patients often benefit from canalith repositioning maneuvers.

Reparative Granuloma

The hallmark of reparative granuloma is progressive sensorineural hearing loss after earlier postoperative hearing improvement. This may be associated with vertigo, aural fullness, or tinnitus. Often, the audiogram reveals a mixed hearing loss that is most severe in the high frequencies. If this diagnosis is considered, the packing in the external auditory canal should be removed and the ear examined. The tympanic membrane typically appears thickened, and bright red tissue is visualized along the tympanomeatal flap and lenticular process of the incus.

The cause of this rare complication is currently unknown. Surgical exploration should be considered if it is suspected. Significant granulation tissue around the oval window and prosthesis is noted on exploration. Multinucleated giant cells are noted histologically, signifying foreign body reaction. The granuloma should be lasered away, the prosthesis removed, and a tissue seal placed over the oval window. Another prosthesis is usually not placed, and depending on the hearing level, revision surgery in 6 months may be considered. Alternatively, a hearing aid or bone-anchored hearing aid may be considered.

Persistent Postoperative Conductive Hearing Loss

In the case that the postoperative audiogram shows no improvement in hearing, one must consider malleus fixation, a fenestra that is too tight, piston displacement, or superior canal dehiscence. After superior canal dehiscence is ruled out, the patient may be reexplored. If malleus head fixation is found, mobilization may be considered, which is ideally done after the incudostapedial joint (or piston) has been separated to minimize labyrinthine trauma. Refixation of the malleus after mobilization, though, is not uncommon. Thus, alternatively, an atticotomy may be performed to remove the malleus head and incus, with subsequent ossicular reconstruction performed between the malleus and oval window.

Postoperative Otitis Media

Acute otitis media in the postoperative period is a rare complication. This is an especially concerning condition because bacteria may enter the labyrinth and can rarely lead to meningitis. Antibiotic therapy should be instituted, myringotomy considered, and the patient's condition monitored closely.

Results of Stapes Surgery

Approximately 90% of patients undergoing primary stapes surgery have a conductive deficit of 10 dB or less when measured 6 to 12 months after stapedectomy. In these studies, about 5% of patients have an unsatisfactory result, with an estimated average air–bone gap of 15 dB or higher. The air–bone gap closure typically remains stable through time. A long-term sensorineural hearing loss affecting the high frequencies may occur with time and may be a consequence of presbycusis or cochlear otosclerosis.

The experience of the surgeon is clearly a predictor of stapes surgery outcomes. Experienced surgeons in one study more accurately placed the stapes prosthesis and caused less cochlear trauma than novice surgeons. The number of resident stapedectomies performed in training programs over the past several decades has declined significantly, and more recent graduates have become increasingly reluctant to perform stapes surgery. Consequently, although an otologic fellowship is not a prerequisite for performing stapes surgery, otolaryngologists should honestly evaluate their training, experience, and microsurgical skills before opting to perform stapes surgery.

127.6 Summary

Otosclerosis is a common cause of conductive hearing loss for which surgical treatment is highly successful, with a low incidence of complications in experienced hands. The nonsurgical treatment of otosclerosis includes fluoride therapy and amplification. Laser stapedotomy is the definitive treatment for hearing restoration.

Generous exposure of the middle ear, the use of laser technology, and compulsive attention to detail before, during, and after stapedectomy are critical elements to achieve optimal results and minimize complications.

127.7 Roundsmanship

- Otosclerosis typically presents with conductive or mixed (rarely sensorineural) hearing loss.
- A Carhart notch occurs because stapedial vibration at the round window at around 2,000 Hz on bone conduction testing is diminished in a patient with stapes fixation, resulting in a factitious finding of sensorineural hearing loss.
- Sodium fluoride reduces vascularity and bone-resorptive activity, thereby inactivating foci of otospongiosis.
- Although all patients should be measured to determine the appropriate length of a stapes prosthesis, most are treated appropriately with a length of 4.25 mm.
- Palpation of the malleus to observe piston motion should always be performed to ensure an intact sound-conducting mechanism.
- Common causes of postoperative vertigo include a long prosthesis, benign paroxysmal positional vertigo, a depressed footplate fragment, and reparative granuloma.

127.8 Recommended Reading

[1] Carhart R. The clinical application of bone conduction audiometry. Trans Am Acad Ophthalmol Otolaryngol 1950; 54: 699–707
[2] Caughey RJ, Pitzer GB, Kesser BW. Stapedectomy: demographics in 2006. Otol Neurotol 2006; 27: 769–775
[3] Cawthorne T. Otosclerosis. J Laryngol Otol 1955; 69: 437–456
[4] Lempert J. Improvement of hearing in cases of otosclerosis: a new, one stage surgical technic. Arch Otolaryngol 1938; 28; (1): 42–97
[5] Levin G, Fabian P, Stahle J. Incidence of otosclerosis. Am J Otol 1988; 9: 299–301
[6] McGee TM. The argon laser in surgery for chronic ear disease and otosclerosis. Laryngoscope 1983; 93: 1177–1182
[7] Perkins RC. Laser stepedotomy for otosclerosis. Laryngoscope 1980; 90: 228–240
[8] Rosen S. Restoration of hearing in otosclerosis by mobilization of the fixed stapedial footplate; an analysis of results. Laryngoscope 1955; 65: 224–269
[9] Schuknecht HF, Applebaum EL. Surgery for hearing loss. N Engl J Med 1969; 280: 1154–1160
[10] Shambaugh GE. Clinical diagnosis of cochlear (labyrinthine) otosclerosis. Laryngoscope 1965; 75: 1558–1562
[11] Shea JJ. Thirty years of stapes surgery. J Laryngol Otol 1988; 102: 14–19
[12] Sheehy JL, Nelson RA, House HP. Stapes surgery at the Otologic Medical Group. Am J Otol 1979; 1: 22–26
[13] Soifer N, Weaver K, Endahl GL, Holdsworth CE. Otosclerosis: a review. Acta Otolaryngol Suppl 1970; 269: 1–25

128 Baha and Other Osseointegrated Temporal Bone Implants

Katrina R. Stidham

128.1 Introduction

The bone-anchored hearing aid or Baha is an osseointegrated temporal bone implant that conducts sound through the skull and directly into the inner ear. It has been shown to be effective in treating patients with conductive hearing loss, mixed hearing loss, or unilateral profound hearing loss.

128.2 Terminology

128.2.1 Baha

Baha is a patented technology owned by Cochlear (Cochlear Baha Products and Services, Mölnlycke, Sweden). In the past, BAHA was an acronym for *bone-anchored hearing aid*, but the company has dropped use of the acronym and instead prefers to describe the technology as an osseointegrated temporal bone implant under the product line of Baha.

128.2.2 Osseointegration

Osseointegration is the active process of bone growing into or assimilating an implanted material. Osseointegration provides very strong fixation for a prosthesis, which essentially becomes an integrated part of the bone.

128.2.3 Osseointegrated Hearing Aid

The term *osseointegrated hearing aid* is is used to describe the Baha and any other hearing aids that are fixed by osseointegration.

128.2.4 Single-Sided Deafness

The term *single-sided deafness* (SSD) is used to describe a situation in which an individual has profound hearing loss in one ear with very poor discrimination that cannot be improved with conventional hearing aid technology.

128.3 Applied Anatomy

Sound normally passes in waveforms into the ear canal and to the eardrum. The sound waves cause the eardrum to vibrate, and the vibration drives movement of the ossicular chain. The ossicular chain, in turn, transmits the vibratory nature of the sound waves to the cochlea, where the acoustic signal is translated into an electrical signal, and the cochlear nerve transmits the information to the brain.

The cochlea is encased in bone that is contiguous with the skull. It has long been known that when a sound wave is applied directly to the skull, the skull can conduct the wave effectively to the inner ear. In this way, the normal passage of sound through air, which requires a functioning eardrum and ossicular

chain, is effectively bypassed. This phenomenon is known as bone conduction. It can be demonstrated by pressing a vibrating tuning fork to the skull. Bone conduction of sound is regularly used in audiometric testing to distinguish between conductive and sensorineural hearing loss. In situations of conductive hearing loss, in which there is a problem with sound conduction from the environment to the inner ear, bone conduction thresholds are normal, whereas air conduction thresholds are elevated.

128.4 Function and Components of Osseointegrated Hearing Aids

128.4.1 History of the Baha and Other Osseointegrated Hearing Aids

The concept of osseointegrated hearing aids began with research in the 1950s related to dental implants. At that time, Per Ingvar Brånemark discovered that titanium could be accepted as part of living bone. He described this process as osseointegration and began research on creating titanium dental implants. In 1977, Professor Brånemark and a colleague in otolaryngology, Anders Tjellström, suggested that bone-anchored implants could be used to help patients with conductive hearing loss who could not benefit from traditional amplification.

Before that time, patients with conductive hearing loss were treated with transcutaneous bone conduction hearing aids. Traditional bone conduction devices consist of a hearing aid that is placed on a metal headband on one side of the head and a transducer that presses against the skull on the opposite side of the head. The hearing aid picks up the sound and transfers it via a cable to the transducer, which in turn conducts sound through the skull to the inner ear. Unfortunately, bone conduction aids have several inherent problems. First, the soft tissue between the transducer and the skin attenuates the sound, reducing sensitivity and causing distortion. Second, because of the pressure needed to transmit the sound, the devices are very uncomfortable and have to be repositioned frequently. Third, with the need to wear a metal band across the head, cosmesis is a significant concern. Because of these combined problems, the overall compliance rate with traditional bone conduction hearing aids is low. However, for patients with atresia and severe stenosis, this type of hearing aid was previously the only option available for sound amplification.

The first Baha was placed in Sweden in 1977, and over the next several years, many technologic advances were implemented to improve the functionality of the device. The obstacle of combining the transducer and hearing aid in the same unit was overcome by elastically suspending the hearing aid below the transducer. The second problem was to create a coupling system that would allow the hearing aid to easily be coupled to and decoupled from the abutment while a high level of mechanical impedance was maintained. The coupling system also had to have a low profile and withstand debris from hair, sweat, and hair products. A unique flexing male-to-female coupling system was designed that, with a few modifications, is still in use today.

The Baha was first approved by the FDA in 1996 for use in adults with mixed and conductive hearing loss. It was subsequently approved for implantation in children 5 years of age and older in 1999, and was approved for bilateral fittings in 2002.

In the early 2000s, research was carried out to evaluate the functionality and benefit of the Baha in patients with unilateral profound hearing loss, also known as Single-Sided Deafness or SSD. These were patients, usually with a sudden severe shift in hearing, experiencing significant functional difficulties. Before the Baha, the only option for a patient with SSD was either no intervention or a CROS hearing aid. The CROS (contralateral routing of sound) hearing aid consists of a device with a microphone worn in the ear with poor hearing and an amplifier worn in the ear with good hearing. Sound is picked up on the side of the deficit and transmitted to the good ear. Because the Baha transmits sound through the entire skull, it essentially functions in the same way as the CROS device, and the patient does not have to wear an amplifier in the opposite ear. Initial research was positive, and the FDA approved the Baha for use in patients with SSD in 2002.

Recent developments have focused on improving the internal technology of the hearing aid. The initial devices were based on analogue technology. Recent generations of Baha devices are based on digital technology and have improved qualities, including automatic directional microphone, microphone position compensation, automatic noise reduction, and active feedback cancellation. All of these advances are designed to improve the functionality of the devices.

The Baha has also been modified for use in young children. An elastic headband, referred to as the softband, was approved by the FDA in 2002. It allows the device to be worn much more comfortably than it can with the conventional metal headband. The softband is indicated for children too young to undergo surgical placement of a titanium implant.

In 2009, Oticon Medical (Somerset, NJ) released a competing osseointegrated hearing aid that mimics Baha technology. It is marketed under the name Ponto and has many of the same features as the Baha. In June 2011, Sophono (Boulder, CO) released an implant with a magnetic attachment that does not have a percutaneous abutment. Cochlear has also recently developed a magnetic attachment for the Baha as well.

128.4.2 Components of the Baha

The Baha basically consists of three parts: the titanium implant, the abutment, and the external processor (▶ Fig. 128.1). The titanium implant and abutment are usually packaged and placed at surgery as a combined unit, but they can be separated if there is a need to change to a longer abutment. The external processor is coupled to the abutment via a unique flexing male component on the external processor that attaches to a fixed female component on the abutment. The external processor houses the transducer and the digital hearing aid.

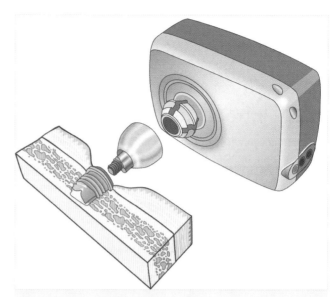

Fig. 128.1 Baha components include the titanium implant inset into bone; the abutment, which serves to link the external processor to the implant; and the external processor.

128.4.3 How the Baha Works

The external processor, through its coupling to the abutment (and ultimately the titanium implant), transmits sound directly through the skull.

In patients with a conductive hearing loss, the device bypasses the problematic natural amplifiers of the eardrum and middle ear bones and conducts sound waves directly to the inner ear. The device can be programmed to provide hearing thresholds within a normal range when the device is worn.

In patients with SSD, the device transmits sound through the skull to the opposite inner ear. The microphone picks up sounds on the side with poor hearing that would otherwise be missed. For persons with SSD, the Baha is particularly useful in environments with background noise or competing noise.

128.4.4 Indications and Testing for Use of the Baha

There are basically two categories of patients who are potential Baha candidates: those with conductive or mixed hearing loss and those with SSD.

Common diagnoses in patients with conductive hearing loss who are potential Baha candidates include aural atresia, congenital syndromic hearing loss (e.g., Treacher Collins syndrome, CHARGE [coloboma, heart disease, atresia of the nasal choanae, retarded growth and/or development, ear abnormalities or deafness] syndrome), chronic draining ear, and otosclerosis. The current FDA criteria for fitting the Baha system require a pure-tone average bone conduction threshold equal to or better than 45 dB HL, a speech discrimination score of 60% or better, and an air conduction threshold equal to or poorer than the bone conduction threshold.

Common diagnoses in patients with SSD include sudden sensorineural hearing loss, acoustic neuroma, trauma, Meniere disease, labyrinthitis, and congenital unilateral hearing loss. The

FDA criteria for fitting a Baha in a patient with SSD include profound hearing loss in the affected ear and essentially normal hearing in the opposite ear.

An individual patient in either group can evaluate the potential benefit of the device by listening with a demo device on a metal headband or test rod. The demo device is not as good as the implanted device because of the presence of soft tissue between the device and the skull, but it gives the patient a reasonable approximation of the benefit that may be anticipated.

128.5 Surgery for the Baha

128.5.1 Surgical Procedure for Placement

Surgery for placement of the Baha is a relatively simple procedure that takes approximately 30 minutes to complete. For adults, the procedure can be done with intravenous sedation and local anesthetic. For children, the procedure is completed with general anesthesia. Surgery requires a dedicated drill unit, drill tips, and implants, all produced by the implant manufacturer. Modifications to the technique have been developed over the years, and individual surgeons have different methods for incision and soft-tissue reduction. The following technique is the vertical incision method.

Before anesthesia is administered, a mark is made on the surgical side, approximately 5 cm behind the ear canal. It is important to ask the patient about specific preferences regarding hats or glasses, and to have the patient to bring these to the surgery center. Usually, the device can be positioned away from such hindrances. For patients with prior surgical defects, such as from a previous suboccipital approach to tumor, the incision will need to be modified to take in account present bony defects.

In the operating room, the area is shaved and prepared for surgery. Depth of soft tissue is measured using a needle prior to anesthetic injection nd appropriate abutment length is selected accordingly. A generous amount of local anesthetic with epinephrine is infiltrated into the area of the incision and surrounding soft tissue down to the skull. A 3-cm vertical incision is made.

The bone is then prepared for placement of the implant. A 10-mm area of periosteum in the center of the incision is opened to expose the bone beneath. With a guide drill, an opening is first created to a depth of 3 mm (▶ Fig. 128.2). The bone is carefully examined, and if it is adequate, the guide drill length is increased to 4 mm. If the bone is inadequate for drilling to a depth of 4 mm, the surgeon proceeds to the next step, using a 3-mm countersink and a 3-mm implant.

Following the determination of bone adequacy, the countersink drill bit is placed, and drilling is carried out with copious irrigation just to the depth that the countersink recess is created in the bone (▶ Fig. 128.3). The combined titanium implant and abutment is then opened, and without touching the implant, the surgeon uses the rotating hand piece to pick it up. A very slow rotation is used to place the implant, initially without irrigation until the first threads of the screw are in the bone and subsequently with copious irrigation until the implant is

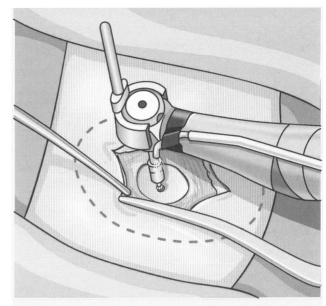

Fig. 128.2 A guide drill is used to gauge the depth of bone.

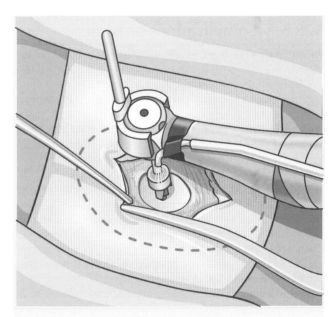

Fig. 128.3 Countersink drilling.

seated flush with the bone (▶ Fig. 128.4). The wound is closed around the implant, with the abutment left exposed. A healing cap is placed on the abutment, and a pressure dressing is applied (▶ Fig. 128.5).

Alternatively, a two-stage procedure can be completed, with placement of only the osseointegrated titanium implant; the skin is closed directly over it after soft-tissue reduction. After osseointegration is complete, the surgeon returns and makes a punch incision over the implant and attaches the abutment. Some surgeons choose the two-stage procedure for children in whom there is a concern about hitting or disrupting the abutment before full osseointegration.

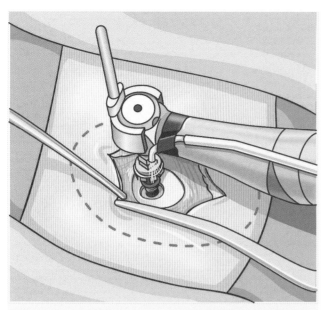

Fig. 128.4 Placement of the combined titanium implant and abutment.

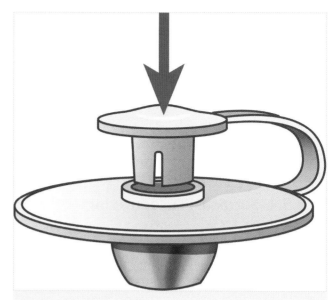

Fig. 128.5 The healing cap is positioned over the abutment.

128.5.2 Complications of Surgery

As with any surgical procedure involving placement of an implant, there can be intraoperative, immediate postoperative, and late postoperative complications.

Intraoperative complications are few and consist primarily of bleeding from soft tissue and bone. There is, however, a potential risk for dural exposure and cerebrospinal fluid leak. Many surgeons have not found dural exposure itself to be a problem, and the implant can be safely placed with exposed dura.

Postoperative and long-term complications have been reported in 8 to 59% of Baha patients. The most common long-term complications are soft-tissue overgrowth and skin infection at the abutment site. Other problems include abutment and fixture dislodgement, exposed bone at the abutment site, scalp paresthesia, persistent pain, failure of osseointegration, granulation tissue and bleeding at the abutment site, feedback problems, neuroma, keloid, and hematoma.

Skin irritation, infection, and overgrowth are thought to be due in part to the percutaneous nature of the implant and in part to the surgical approach and abutment design. Most of the skin irritation problems can be managed locally with topical steroids and antibiotic ointment. Cauterization and oral antibiotics are employed in more severe cases. When complete skin overgrowth occurs, surgery is necessary to reexpose the abutment and thin the skin. Some patients can be managed by placing a longer abutment, which usually resolves the problem. Recent modifications in surgical technique and abutment design have been associated with lower complication rates.

128.6 Hearing Benefits of the Baha

The Baha has been shown to provide objective and subjective benefit in patients with bilateral conductive and mixed hearing loss, unilateral conductive and mixed hearing loss, and SSD.

For patients who have bilateral conductive hearing loss, the benefits are the most obvious because their only other means to amplify hearing is often a bone conduction device worn on a headband. Patients who have bilateral conductive loss experience significant improvement in speech thresholds with a unilateral Baha fitting. However, the greatest benefit is achieved in patients who receive bilateral implants. Initially, this benefit was questioned because one device can obviously conduct sound to both cochleas. However, improvements in directional hearing and speech recognition in quiet and in noise with bilateral fittings compared with unilateral fitting have been documented. Patients who have bilateral implants also report a significant increase in quality of life on standardized questionnaires compared with those who have unilateral Baha placement.

Patients with unilateral conductive hearing loss have been noted to have better hearing in quiet and in background noise, with significant improvement on speech-in-noise tests. Sound localization is not changed for the majority of patients using the Baha, although a subset of patients have had definitive improvement in localization, as well. In general, greater benefits are seen in patients who have acquired conductive hearing loss compared with those who have congenital conductive hearing loss, due in part to overall better unaided scores for directional hearing and understanding in noise for the group with congenital hearing loss.

For patients with SSD, Baha has been documented to improve performance on speech-in-noise tasks. No improvement in localization has been documented. This lack of localization is attributed to the fact that all sound is directed into one functional cochlea, and normal cues of interaural timing and intensity are not restored with the amplification. Patients report significant subjective benefit in multiple hearing situations, including listening in quiet, listening in a group, listening at a dinner table, and listening to TV or radio. In addition, an increase in quality of life and a decrease in hearing handicap scores have been documented.

128.7 Roundsmanship

- Osseointegrated conductive hearing aids are beneficial for patients with conductive and mixed hearing loss, and for those with unilateral profound hearing loss.
- Osseointegration of the Baha allows it to conduct sound effectively through the skull to the inner ear.
- The most common complications of soft-tissue overgrowth and skin infection can usually be managed with topical medications. Revision of the abutment site may occasionally be required.
- The Baha improves sound localization in patients with bilateral conductive hearing loss when two devices are fitted.
- For patients with unilateral conductive hearing loss and single-sided deafness, the Baha improves hearing in noise but in general does not improve sound localization.

128.8 Recommended Reading

[1] Badran K, Arya AK, Bunstone D, Mackinnon N. Long-term complications of bone-anchored hearing aids: a 14-year experience. J Laryngol Otol 2009; 123: 170–176

[2] Bosman AJ, Snik AF, van der Pouw CT, Mylanus EA, Cremers CW. Audiometric evaluation of bilaterally fitted bone-anchored hearing aids. Audiology 2001; 40: 158–167

[3] Håkansson B. Birth of Baha. Baha Users Support Web site. http://www.baha-users-support.com/birth_of_baha.php

[4] Ho EC, Monksfield P, Egan E, Reid A, Proops D. Bilateral Bone-anchored Hearing Aid: impact on quality of life measured with the Glasgow Benefit Inventory. Otol Neurotol 2009; 30: 891–896

[5] Hobson JC, Roper AJ, Andrew R, Rothera MP, Hill P, Green KM. Complications of bone-anchored hearing aid implantation. J Laryngol Otol 2010; 124: 132–136

[6] Kunst SJ, Leijendeckers JM, Mylanus EAM, Hol MKS, Snik AFM, Cremers CW. Bone-anchored hearing aid system application for unilateral congenital conductive hearing impairment: audiometric results. Otol Neurotol 2008; 29: 2–7

[7] Newman CW, Sandridge SA, Wodzisz LM. Longitudinal benefit from and satisfaction with the Baha system for patients with acquired unilateral sensorineural hearing loss. Otol Neurotol 2008; 29: 1123–1131

129 Cochlear Implantation

Christopher J. Linstrom

129.1 Introduction

Hearing loss in any degree for any reason handicaps the ability of a person to communicate. Background noise worsens this handicap. For a patient with bilateral hearing loss so severe that medical care (amplification) or surgical care (e.g., eradication of chronic ear disease or a cholesteatoma, or correction of the conductive component of hearing loss in otosclerosis) has not brought the hearing up to an amplifiable level, a cochlear implant may be the next best alternative.

It is important to keep a few basic facts in mind. Firstly, a patient whose hearing can be amplified will generally communicate globally better than a patient with a cochlear implant. Secondly, a cochlear implant is *not* a hearing aid. It is an electrical representation of sound. It works in a very different way from any analog or digital hearing aid. Thirdly, unilateral hearing loss is *not* an indication for cochlear implantation; a normal or nearly normal ear will always function better than an ear with a cochlear implant. Furthermore, a cochlear implant is not a substitute for normal hearing. Finally, the cochlea and, most importantly the spiral ganglion cells from the eighth cranial nerve are housed in the hardest bone in the body, the petrous temporal bone. Although they are themselves soft-tissue structures, they are protected from many disease processes affecting the temporal bone, so that cochlear implantation is possible.

This chapter will focus on the evaluation of the patient with severe to profound hearing loss, on various means used to habilitate hearing, and on the steps taken before and during cochlear implantation with the goal of rehabilitating the patient who has a hearing handicap and restoring a better means of communication.

129.2 Incidence of Disease

It is estimated that 21 million Americans are sufficiently hearing-impaired to require some form of treatment, whether through amplification or surgery, including cochlear implantation. Of those with significant hearing loss, it is difficult to estimate how many would qualify for cochlear implantation. The minimum age for cochlear implantation in the United States is 12 months, although this number is being pushed downward. There is no upper age limit for cochlear implantation. The audiometric and general health status of the patient alone determines the upper age limit.

When a person is discovered to have hearing loss and seeks medical attention for this problem, the medical professional who encounters the patient should investigate several basic features. Is the hearing loss unilateral or bilateral? Was it of sudden or gradual onset? Does it fluctuate? Has there been a return of any hearing? What medical or surgical means has the patient used to habilitate his or her hearing? Is the hearing loss associated with any other ear-related problem, such as chronic ear disease? Is there any other complaint, such as dizziness/vertigo or facial nerve weakness? Is there a family history of hearing loss? Does the patient remember previously hearing well in the affected ear? What medical and/or surgical problems does the patient have, if any, that might cause hearing loss?

129.3 Terminology

Hearing is measured in decibels (dB) of hearing level. For standard audiometric measurement, the worse the hearing, the higher the decibel level of the hearing threshold, commonly measured as the speech reception threshold (SRT). The SRT is the level at which the subject is aware of 50% of the words in a list of equally weighted two-syllable words, although the number of syllables per word in the word list will vary depending upon the language tested. A second, complementary parameter to test hearing is the word recognition score (WRS), expressed as the percentage of correctly heard words from a list of single-syllable words presented *without* context. In English, the single-syllable word will be chosen from a list of "consonant–nucleus–consonant" (CNC) words presented by convention at 35 dB above the SRT. The WRS is a difficult test because every part of the word must be heard and recognized independently and divorced from any context. The SRT and WRS are separate but complementary tests and should be done independently for each ear. Of all test parameters, these two items will yield the greatest amount of information about the subject's level of audition.

Hearing loss may be classified as mild, moderate, severe, or profound. Each category implies approximately a 20-dB worsening of hearing. The term *deaf* to any hearing professional is associated with immeasurable hearing at or below 110 to 120 dB. Very few patients who claim to be "deaf" have this extremely poor level of hearing (▶ Fig. 129.1).

129.4 Applied Anatomy

The basic anatomy of the outer, middle, and inner ear has been presented in this book. For a consideration of cochlear

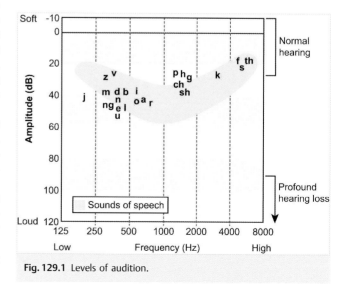

Fig. 129.1 Levels of audition.

implantation, the ear should have normal anatomy and eustachian tube function. In rare cases, the patient may have had severe chronic ear disease and already undergone otologic surgery. The patient and surgeon must bear in mind that a cochlear implant is a large foreign body, roughly the size of a silver dollar, with an electrode array (or two arrays in one FDA-approved model) at one end. Any preexisting otologic disease must be eradicated *before* a cochlear implant can be placed into the mastoid and inner ear. In some cases, cochlear implantation must be staged; first, the external and middle ear are exenterated of any disease and surgically overclosed. After a suitable period of about 4 to 6 months, if the ear is free of active disease, an implantation may be done. In patients who have had bacterial meningitis, the otic capsule may be filled in with scar tissue (labyrinthitis ossificans), or in rare cases of advanced otosclerosis, the otic capsule is distorted to such a degree that only a few electrodes of the array can be implanted. In other cases, a split electrode array is made, and the cochlea is fenestrated in two places to allow both an orthograde and a retrograde insertion of the electrodes. In general, the greater the number of active electrodes that are implanted, the better the patient's word recognition will be.

129.5 The Disease Process

Deafness has hundreds of causes, and the likely causes based upon the patient's history and physical examination must be investigated, as would be done in any medical or surgical process. Hearing loss in general may be classified as congenital or acquired. The most common causes of congenital hearing loss are heritable, and most of these are subclassified as nonsyndromic forms of hearing loss.

The most common cause of acquired hearing loss in children is bacterial meningitis, especially meningococcal meningitis. This gram-positive infection leads to a severe immune reaction that causes labyrinthitis ossificans, with severe scarring of the basal and higher turns of the cochlea. Many of these children will have a precipitous loss of hearing, and cochlear implantation should not be delayed because the window of opportunity between the onset of meningitis and the development of labyrinthitis ossificans is a matter of weeks to a few months. If a child has little measurable hearing, implantation should be done as soon as the severe hearing loss has been established and the child is well enough to undergo the procedure.

A more complete list of the causes of hearing loss is given in ▶ Table 129.1. All of these items will be factored into the differential diagnosis of hearing loss. The patient's history of hearing loss will usually determine which factors merit investigation.

129.6 Medical Evaluation

The history of the hearing impairment is the single most important step guiding the investigation and rehabilitation of the patient. The diagnostic steps will vary depending upon the patient's age and prior audition, if any.

129.6.1 Children

Most parents give hearing the benefit of the doubt for no more than 12 months. If the child is not reliably responding or starting to babble by the first birthday, the parents usually seek medical intervention. The child with suspected speech delay or suspected hearing loss eventually requires a professional evaluation of hearing. It is important to investigate this problem

Table 129.1 Common causes of hearing loss

Congenital hearing loss	Acquired hearing loss

• Familial/genetic
 ○ Syndromic versus nonsyndromic
• Gestational, delivery-related, perinatal
 ○ Prematurity, hypoxia, anoxia, hyperbilirubinemia
• Infectious
 ○ Rubella, toxoplasmosis, syphilis, cytomegalovirus infection, herpes
• Teratogens
 ○ Thalidomide
• Congenital malformations of the otic capsule
 ○ Michel aplasia
  – Agenesis of the otic capsule, both bony and membranous; middle and external auditory canal may be normal
 ○ Mondini-Alexander dysplasia
  – Partitioning defect of the bony and membranous labyrinth; subclassification termed by degree and location of partitioning defect
 ○ Scheibe dysplasia
  – Bony labyrinth normal; membranous dysplasia of the cochlea and saccule (pars inferior); membranous utricle and semicircular canals normal (pars superior)
 ○ Alexander dysplasia
  – High-frequency neurosensory hearing loss caused by partial aplasia of cochlear aqueduct
 ○ Bing-Siebenmann dysplasia
  – Vestibular labyrinth abnormal; cochlear labyrinth may be abnormal
	• Familial/genetic
	 ○ Syndromic versus nonsyndromic
	• Infectious
	 ○ Meningitis
	 ○ Chronic otitis media
	 ○ Cholesteatoma
	 ○ Labyrinthitis
	  – Serous (sterile)
	  – Bacterial
	  – Viral: mumps, measles, influenza
	• Trauma
	 ○ Head trauma (temporal bone, base of skull fracture)
	 ○ Iatrogenic trauma (otologic surgery)
	• Aminoglycosides
	 ○ Kanamycin, amikacin: primarily cochleotoxic
	 ○ Streptomycin, gentamicin: primarily vestibulotoxic, may affect cochlea if doses high enough
	• Metabolic
	 ○ Paget disease
	 ○ Cochlear otosclerosis
	• Autoimmune
	 ○ Autoimmune neurosensory hearing loss
	• Idiopathic
	 ○ Endolymphatic hydrops (Meniere syndrome)

Table 129.2 Important questions for cochlear implant candidates

For younger children (0 to 2 years)	For older children (older than 2 years)	For adults
Normal gestation?	Do the parents remember the child hearing well?	When did the patient become aware of the hearing loss?
Infections during pregnancy (e.g., genital herpes)?	History of frequent ear infections?	Was it sudden or progressive? Is there progression of loss?
Mother immunized for rubella and toxoplasmosis?	Over what period of time was hearing loss noted?	Is the hearing loss in one or both ears?
Delivered by cesarian section? If so, why?	Does the child remember hearing in each ear?	Does the hearing fluctuate?
Apgar scores (at 1 minute and at 5 minutes)?	Has the child ever had a serious head injury?	Does the patient have a history of chronic ear disease?
Neonatal jaundice?	Has the child ever been hospitalized for a serious ear infection?	Is there a history of significant noise (especially military or industrial) exposure?
Did the neonate have any phototherapy or exchange transfusion for jaundice?	Has the child ever had meningitis?	Familial history of hearing loss?
History of sepsis?	Has the hearing ever been measured?	Is the hearing loss related to puberty or to pregnancy?
Intravenous antibiotics, especially an aminoglycoside?	Has the child ever been treated for hearing loss?	Has the hearing loss previously been documented?
Neonatal hearing screening done?		
Familial history of hearing loss?		
Parental consanguinity?		
Parental hearing normal?		

with care and to be aware of the familial and social issues involved.

A single test does not yield all of the information about the child's hearing. If there is reasonable doubt about the level of audition, it is wise to state so at each point of the investigation, to be empathetic, but above all to be truthful based upon the current knowledge.

A number of specific questions are helpful when a patient with suspected speech delay or hearing loss is evaluated, and these differ for pediatric and adult patients (▶ Table 129.2). The adult patient will usually have a very good idea about the onset and progression of hearing loss in one or both ears, can generally give a thorough medical history, and may even be wearing a hearing aid.

129.6.2 Presenting Complaints

In addition to hearing loss, the parents of young patients and older patients themselves may describe related problems of tinnitus, imbalance, or very rarely facial nerve involvement. It is very rare for young children themselves to complain of dizziness. Young children do not have this mental concept or the vocabulary to describe it. The parent will usually notice that the child cannot sit upright alone or is very clumsy in walking, etc. These complaints must be investigated, and the collaboration of a pediatric neurologist is crucial for such cases.

Older patients will usually have a very good way of describing concomitant otologic complaints. As indicated, these should be investigated with the appropriate means and treated.

129.6.3 Physical Examination

For most patients presenting with hearing loss, the physical examination is usually noncontributory, but it is important to rule out chronic ear disease (especially cholesteatoma) in all patients.

With children, the parents will usually know if there is anything abnormal about the shape or size of a child's ear (e.g., in a case of congenital auricular atresia). This is noticed at birth in almost all cases. The parents usually know about other "syndromic" causes of hearing loss, such as Pierre Robin malformation, Alport disease, Goldenhar syndrome, and other first arch abnormalities, unless the otologist is the first medical professional to evaluate the child.

129.6.4 Testing

Audiometry

It is difficult to fully express how important each and every test of audition is; fundamental and profound recommendations with far-reaching effects are made based upon tests of audition. Each test must be designed in an age-appropriate manner for the subject with the knowledge that not every subject may be able to inform the examiner of the exact level of audition. For very young subjects, objective tests of audition are employed. For older subjects, the standard audiogram assumes that the patient understands the test and is willing to comply with the examiner to ascertain the true level of audition.

Objective Tests of Audition

Otoacoustic Emissions

The cochlea is not solely a passive conduit of sound from the footplate of the stapes, through the conversion of shearing forces of the perilymph to electrical impulses transmitted thence to the eighth cranial nerve. The cochlea interacts with the auditory environment in a very active way, producing a weak sound, called the cochlear microphonic, in response to sound stimulation. The otoacoustic emission (OAE) measures this sound of the cochlea produced in response to received sound. It occurs in the outer hair cells of the cochlea in response to sound stimuli. A probe with both a sound source and a highly sensitive microphone is placed into the external auditory canal. A weak sound stimulus is presented to the ear. The ear responds by producing a very weak sound (about 3 to 4 dB in amplitude) virtually immediately. Several different responses may be obtained, depending on the function used. If there is hearing loss from any etiology of approximately 40 dB or greater, the OAE will not occur. Thus, the OAE is of great value as an audiometric screening tool, especially in the neonatal period. It is a "pass or fail"–type of audition test. Patients who pass the screen are assumed to have at least cochlear hearing; those who do not are scheduled for retesting and for additional tests of audition.

Auditory Brainstem Reflex

The auditory brainstem reflex (ABR) is an evoked response of the cochlea, eighth cranial nerve, cochlear nerve nucleus, midbrain, and higher centers of hearing to a sound stimulus. It is obtained by an "averaging" computer that is calibrated to exclude competing bioelectrical signals, such as those from the electroencephalogram and electrocardiogram, and to allow only signals of predetermined latency and amplitude to pass. The ABR is used to test both cochlear and retrocochlear pathways of hearing. In neonates and babies who fail the OAE screen, the ABR is of great value both to determine the presence of audition and also to give some idea of the level at which audition can be expected to occur. Sound may be presented by air or to the mastoid bone. The ABR can establish the presence of audition or predict its level, or it can be used as a retrocochlear screen after an abnormal result of sound field, conditioned orientation response (COR), ABR, or standard audiometry testing.

Radiography

Structural abnormalities of the otic capsule, such as patent vestibular aqueduct, partitioning defects (e.g., Mondini deformity, single-sac abnormality), and dysplasia/aplasia (e.g., Michel aplasia), are best demonstrated by edge-enhanced computed tomography (CT) of the petrous temporal bone without contrast, which yields important information about the bone–air interface. Soft tissue is less well delineated on CT. For purposes of preoperative planning, CT is usually the only radiographic test required because it will provide important information about the structure of the inner ear, structure of the middle ear cleft, amount of mastoid pneumatization and aeration, and course of the facial nerve.

Magnetic resonance (MR) imaging with and without gadolinium contrast gives important information about soft tissue. Bone and air are both seen as a black silhouette on MR images.

If vascular abnormalities are suspected, MR angiography or MR venography may be designed *along with* MR imaging. It is important to note that MR angiography and MR venography cannot be added to the MR imaging data once the latter have been obtained. They are a different data set and must be requested "up front."

It is also important to remember that both CT and MR imaging are tests of anatomy, not of function. They will yield information about space requirements for an implant within the otic capsule but give no predictive information about the function of any cochlear implant.

Serology

For otherwise healthy children, the yield of routine blood testing for causes of neurosensory hearing loss is very poor. Nonsyndromic causes of hearing loss, such as a connexin deficiency, may be diagnosed by the appropriate special genetic tests. Most adult patients have very little in their medical history to suggest the utility of specific serologic testing. A "shotgun" approach to serologic screening should not be used because it is cumbersome to both patient and medical provider, rarely yields clinically important information, and represents an unnecessary expense. The physician should know what he or she is specifically looking for before ordering any test. For most patients, age-specific blood work will be required before implantation, and no other serologic testing.

129.6.5 Differential Diagnosis

See ▶ Table 129.1.

129.7 Treatment

129.7.1 Medical Treatment

Patients with downwardly fluctuating sensorineural hearing loss will have been or should be treated with an oral corticosteroid, with or without an antimetabolite such as methotrexate. Continuation of medical treatment depends on clinical success; patients who fail medical treatment and progress inexorably to severe or profound hearing loss will require implantation.

Some forms of neurosensory and mixed hearing loss may respond to medical treatment. The most common examples are sensorineural haring loss resulting from syphilis and autoimmune sensorineural haring loss. Both are treated with corticosteroids. If a patient tests positive for syphilis and has never been treated, intramuscular followed by oral penicillin (with probenecid) may be added to the treatment plan. The anti-inflammatory effect of steroids may help restore some hearing. For patients who have hypertension, diabetes, glaucoma, or osteoporosis, coordinated care with the appropriate medical specialists is necessary.

The medical treatment of hearing loss in almost all cases will include a trial of amplification. This is common sense, except in cases in which the audition is so poor that it is obvious from the audiogram that no hearing aid could possibly benefit the patient. For patients with measurable hearing, a trial of amplification of at least 6 weeks should be offered. The procedure of cochlear implantation includes some form of cochleostomy, which may be expected to remove any residual cochlear hearing. In rare cases, the residual cochlear hearing may be preserved, but the patient must be made aware that in every case it is likely that any residual measurable hearing will be gone.

The only exception to the trial of hearing amplification is in cases of bacterial meningitis, especially culture-proven meningococcal meningitis. The risk for the development of labyrinthitis ossificans is so great that the patient should undergo implantation as soon as profound hearing loss can be established and he or she is medically cleared for the procedure.

129.7.2 Surgical Treatment

Patient Selection

Patients who have been completely evaluated and have been given, when appropriate, a trial of amplification, and have failed, may then progress to a cochlear implant. Because of the irreversibility of cochlear implantation, a thorough and routine evaluation is required.

It is intuitive that the patient most likely to benefit from a cochlear implant would be one who has already developed a system of oral communication (i.e., can hear, speak, read, and write a language and has a good idea of how his or her own speaking voice should sound). Such a patient is a postlingually deafened adult.

A somewhat less favorable candidate would be a postlingually or perilingually deafened child, still less favorable a prelingually deafened child.

A prelingually deafened adult (born deaf, with little speech and communication via sign language) would be expected to have very little sound perception and prognostically would be expected be the poorest performer, as a consequence of the lack of the trophic effect of sound upon the spiral ganglion cell population, cochlear nerve, cochlear ganglion cell bodies, and cells of the midbrain and auditory cortex.

Because the cochlea is minimally functional or nonfunctional, an electrical stimulating device is placed that will depolarize the residual (and expectedly healthy) spiral ganglion cells with an envelope of electromagnetic information, regulated by time (pulses per millisecond) and place (frequency-specific stimulation). The electrical engineering specifics of the workings of a cochlear implant are too complex for a brief discussion. However, there are common themes in every cochlear implant that should be understood. All cochlear implants are designed with the the following basic features:

1. External receiver (directional microphone). This is usually worn at ear level and is positioned to pick up the sound source, the naturally occurring or analog signal. These signals include the human voice, music, noise, and other sounds. The received analog signal is transmitted to the external speech processor. This part of the cochlear implant resembles a behind-the-ear (BTE) hearing aid.
2. External speech processor. This is usually built into the BTE external receiver complex. It may also be designed to be clipped to a belt or placed in a back pack for very young children. The analog signal received by the directional microphone is filtered and digitized, converted into a digital representation of sound, and presented to the external transmitting coil as a digitized electronic signal. For reasons of efficiency and size, not all of the sound envelope can be represented. Enough of it is represented to eventually give the spiral ganglion cells and eighth cranial nerve information about *place* (pitch), *time* (rhythm), *amplitude* (loudness), and *timbre* (the quality of a sound). It is here that the analog signal is processed (external speech processor), converted into a digital envelope of sound information through various coding strategies, and then sent on its way to the external transmitting coil.
3. External transmitting coil. This part of the cochlear implant consists of a centrally placed, coated magnet surrounded by the transmitting antenna. The external transmitting coil is held by its magnet over a magnet of opposite polarity implanted within the internal receiver/stimulator. The transmitting antenna of the external transmitting coil passes the digitized electric signal via electromagnetic induction across the scalp to the internal receiver/stimulator. The external transmitting coil is connected to the external receiver and external speech processor by a wire and appears to be an added part to the BTE device. Thus, all ear-level cochlear implants have the same basic features, but the design and style of each manufacturer will vary.
4. Internal receiver/stimulator. This is the only part of a cochlear implant that is surgically implanted. It consists of an internal magnet, the polar opposite of the magnet of the external transmitting coil, and the receiver/stimulator apparatus.

A bony well in the outer table of the parieto-occipital cortex of the skull is usually drilled to accommodate the body (also called the "can") of the internal receiver/stimulator. Each manufacturer has a slightly different design of the "can" and will supply a sterile metallic pattern to help in planning the bony well (the sterile "dummy). The device will be anchored with permanent sutures after placement through soft tissue, through a suture hole drilled into the outer table and diploë, or over a small titanium post. The internal receiver/stimulator should be stabilized as it heals. The internal receiver/stimulator contains the multichannel electrode, which is composed of several proximal stiffening (inactive) electrodes and distal stimulating (active) electrodes.

The multichannel electrode has been demonstrated to definitively transmit an electronic representation of sound better than the single-channel electrode. As would be expected, each manufacturer will have a slightly different design for the electrode array; all are multichannel electrodes. The electrode array is placed into the cochlea through a cochleostomy drilled near the round window or through a cochleostomy that incorporates the round window. Recently, some implant surgeons have returned to placing the electrode array through the round window. Recent evidence indicates that placement of the electrode array into the scala tympani rather than into the scala vestibuli is associated with better performance. Infrequently, especially in "drill out" cases of labyrinthitis ossificans, the electrode array must be placed into the scala vestibuli. These patients will definitely be expected to have sound perception, but their overall performance may not be as good as with a scala tympani insertion. The spiral ganglion cell population and thereafter the cochlear nerve are stimulated via electromagnetic induction, which produces the perception of sound.

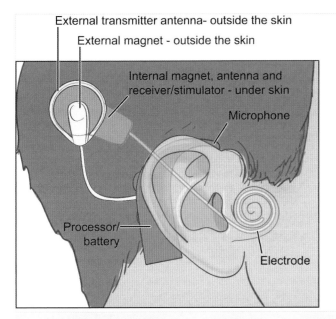

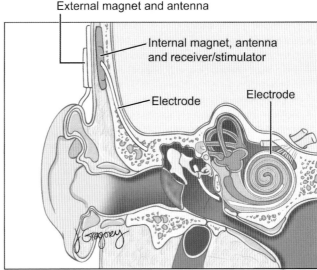

Fig. 129.2 Schematic representation of a cochlear implant.

A schematic representation of a cochlear implant is shown in ▶ Fig. 129.2. There are other designs available worldwide that have not yet obtained FDA approval for use within the United States. All have the same basic features, but they differ significantly not only in design but in coding strategy for conversion of the analog to digital envelope of sound and how this is represented and passed to the cochlea. Each of the three FDA-approved manufacturers has made extensive information available on the Internet, and the reader is referred to the Web site address provided at the end of this chapter.

Unusual Cases

Infrequently, underlying disease will lead to structural abnormalities that will either prevent complete insertion of the electrode array or necessitate placement of a split electrode array.

The most common causes of these structural abnormalities are labyrinthitis ossificans after meningitis, leading to incomplete insertion, and cochlear otosclerosis, causing severe distortion of the otic capsule. Other cases of dysgenesis of the otic capsule may require a straight electrode array, a shortened electrode array, or a non–modiolar-hugging array. In all cases, edge-enhanced, thin-section CT of the temporal bone performed before implantation will help the surgeon decide which array to use.

In rare cases, such as patients with hearing loss after surgical removal of or stereotactic irradiation for a neurofibroma of the eighth cranial nerve (neurofibromatosis type II), there will no longer be a useful cochlear nerve. In these patients, an auditory brainstem implant may be used, but its efficacy would not be expected to approach that of a standard cochlear implant because the tonotopic representation of sound structurally mirrored in the multichannel electrode array is not reproduced with the same precision and nuances as in the auditory brainstem

implant. In general, its utility would be for the awareness of environmental sounds and to aid in lip reading, but little else. It is of some benefit to these very difficult patients, but it lacks the robust reproduction of sound expected of a cochlear implant.

129.8 Prognosis

Many metrics are used to measure the efficacy of a cochlear implant. Almost all of them show a preoperative histogram worse than its postoperative counterpart, no matter what metric is used to measure the outcome. If the patient can be brought up to the level of soft speech, into an area called the "speech banana" (see ▶ Fig. 129.1), he or she can be expected a benefit of audition significantly above the preimplant level. Not all patients will derive the same benefit, especially if the lack of cochlear hearing has been long-standing over many years. Such a patient may obtain information about directionality but would not be expected to enjoy the same benefit as would a recently deafened, timely implanted patient. The latter patient would be expected to have a very robust spiral ganglion cell population and an otherwise healthy eighth cranial nerve, and to benefit much more than a patient who has been deaf for longer than 5 to 10 years. The more recently hearing ear is the ear that is usually implanted for this very reason.

129.9 Complications

- Flap failure and extrusion
- Soft failure
- Device failure/obsolescence
- Trauma
- External component breakage and loss

129.10 Roundsmanship

- A cochlear implant is *not* a hearing aid. It is an electrical (analog to digital) representation of sound. It works in a very different way from any analog or digital hearing aid.
- Unilateral hearing loss is *not* an indication for cochlear implantation. A normal or nearly normal ear will always function better than an ear with a cochlear implant.
- A cochlear implant is not a substitute for normal hearing.
- A cochlear implant converts analog sound energy to a digital representation, then transmits this via electromagnetic induction through the scalp to the internal receiver/stimulator and then to the cochlea.
- The indications for cochlear implantation are strict. Every effort should be made to rehabilitate the patient by medical and other surgical means before an implant is chosen.

129.11 Recommended Reading

[1] Linstrom CJ. Cochlear implantation. Practical information for the generalist. Prim Care 1998; 25: 583–617

[2] Dorman MF, Spahr T, Gifford R et al. An electric frequency-to-place map for a cochlear implant patient with hearing in the nonimplanted ear. J Assoc Res Otolaryngol 2007; 8: 234–240

[3] Finley CC, Holden TA, Holden LK et al. Role of electrode placement as a contributor to variability in cochlear implant outcomes. Otol Neurotol 2008; 29: 920–928

130 Vestibular Pathology: Evaluation and Clinical Syndromes

Ana H. Kim, Clare Dean, and Ronald A. Hoffman

130.1 Introduction

The proper diagnosis and management of balance disorders result from a thorough history and physical examination with subsequent appropriate laboratory evaluation. The basic anatomy and physiology of the vestibular system are covered in Chapter 113 of this book. However, the reader is reminded that vestibular pathology may arise from a dysfunction in any of the major vestibular pathways and centers (▶ Fig. 130.1).

130.2 History

130.2.1 The Chief Complaint

Balance symptoms that arise from disorders of the inner ear (semicircular canals, utricle, and saccule) can range from a vague sense of imbalance to a sense of being "off," or feeling "drunk," or that the body or the world is turning or moving. This last symptom, the sense of bodily motion, particularly that the body or the environment rotating, defines the word *vertigo*. It is important to remember that vertigo is a symptom, not a disease entity. It is critical to take all balance complaints seriously and not be of the opinion that only vertigo constitutes real pathology.

130.2.2 History of the Present Illness

The features documented in the history of the present illness must be focused on identifying the source of the balance problem. Is the dizziness constant or intermittent? Was the onset associated with any systemic illness? Is the dizziness positional? Are there any precipitating or relieving factors? Is there hearing loss? If so, is the hearing loss unilateral or bilateral, progressive or sudden, and does it fluctuate with episodes of dizziness? Tinnitus may be defined as "a noise in the ear or head." If present, it should be ascertained whether the tinnitus is unilateral or bilateral, constant or intermittent, pulsatile or nonpulsatile, and whether it occurs in concert with episodes of dizziness. Is there

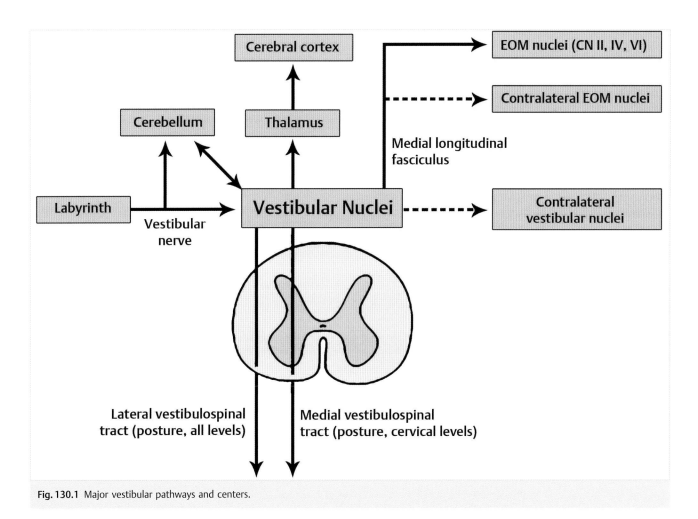

Fig. 130.1 Major vestibular pathways and centers.

a sense of ear fullness? If so, is it unilateral or bilateral, and is it associated with the episodes of dizziness? Has there been any recent head trauma or barotrauma? Does loud sound make the dizziness worse? Does lifting heavy objects or blowing the nose make the dizziness worse? Is there any history of ear pain or drainage? Is there any past medical history of ear infection or surgery? Are there any associated neurologic symptoms? In particular, are there any symptoms of migraine headache, cranial nerve symptoms, or cerebellar symptoms?

130.2.3 Review of Systems

A thorough review of systems is necessary to identify any new systemic diseases that might be associated with dizziness or hearing loss.

130.2.4 Past Medical History

A full past medical history is important, with emphasis upon general medical conditions that might cause dizziness, medications that might be associated with dizziness, and prior hospitalizations and the possible administration of ototoxic medications.

130.2.5 Family History

It is obviously important to assess for any familial history of hearing loss, dizziness, migraine headache, or other neurologic disorders.

130.2.6 Physical Examination

The neurotologic physical examination focuses on the ear and central nervous system. The core elements include the following:

- A thorough examination of the external and middle ear, including a fistula test if indicated
- Tuning fork testing as a hearing screen
- Assessment of cranial nerves III through XII, with an emphasis on eye movements and nystagmus (▶ Table 130.1)
  - Smooth pursuits: The patient follows the examiner's finger from one extreme of the visual field to the other in smooth pursuit. Some patients must be encouraged to concentrate when they do this. Poor pursuits suggest cerebellar pathology.
  - Saccades: The examiner holds up one finger to the left and one to the right of the patient's visual field. The patient is instructed to look from finger to finger. "Overshoot" of the target suggests cerebellar pathology.
  - Saccadic catch: The patient's gaze is fixed on the examiner's nose. The patient lowers the head 15 degrees to bring the horizontal semicircular canal into the horizontal plane. The head is moved from side to side slowly and then gently thrust to the left; this maneuver is then repeated to the right. The patient should be able to maintain a fixed gaze on the examiner's nose. If there is a saccadic catch, it suggests peripheral hypofunction on the side of the direction of head thrust associated with the catch.
  - Frenzel goggles: These are a valuable adjunct during an evaluation for induced nystagmus. The lenses prevent visual fixation, which powerfully inhibits nystagmus. The magnification of the lenses (20 diopters) and the lights enhance the clinician's observations.
    - Spontaneous nystagmus: The patient is instructed to gaze forward, to the left, and to the right. Nystagmus (the fast phase) beats away from a hypoactive ear or toward a hyperactive ear. First-degree nystagmus occurs only with the eyes in the direction of the slow phase. Second-degree nystagmus occurs with the eyes in the direction of the slow phase and in the center. Third-degree nystagmus occurs in all three stations of gaze. Upbeating or down-beating nystagmus strongly suggests central pathology.
    - Headshake-induced nystagmus: The head is lowered 15 degrees to bring the horizontal semicircular canal into the horizontal plane. The head is moved from side to side gently for 15 seconds. This is stopped, and the patient opens the eyes and looks forward. If there is a unilateral vestibular weakness of 60% or greater, there will usually be a headshake-induced nystagmus with the fast phase away from the hypoactive ear. Headshake-induced nystagmus in the presence of a normal caloric irrigation result on videonystagmography suggests a central velocity storage abnormality.
    - Dix-Hallpike maneuver–induced nystagmus: The patient sits on a flat table, the examiner turns the patient's head toward himself or herself, and then lays the patient back, head hanging over the edge of the table, as quickly as possible. The patient is observed in this position for induced nystagmus for 60 seconds.

Table 130.1 Eye movements

Class of eye movement	Main function
Fixation	Holds image of a stationary object on the fovea
Vergence	Moves eyes medially so image of single object is placed simultaneously on both foveas
Vestibular	Holds images steady on retina during brief head rotations
Optokinetic	Holds images steady on retina during sustained head movements
Smooth pursuit	Holds image of a moving target on fovea
Nystagmus	Resets eyes during prolonged rotation and direct gaze toward the oncoming visual scene
Saccades	Rapid eye movement that brings image of interest onto fovea

Table 130.2 Physical findings that differentiate peripheral from central vertigo

Characteristic	Peripheral vertigo	Central vertigo
Intensity	Severe	Mild
Fatigability	Fatigues, adaption	Does not fatigue
Eye closure	Symptoms worse with eye closure	Symptoms better with eye closure
Nystagmus	Horizontal, may be unilateral, rotary	No effect or enhances nystagmus
Ocular fixation	Suppresses nystagmus (may not suppress in acute phase)	No effect or enhances nystagmus
Associated symptoms	Nausea, hearing loss, sweating	Weakness, numbness, falls more likely

- Assessment of cerebellar function
  - Rapid finger to nose exercise
- Romberg and sharpened (tandem) Romberg testing

The physical findings that differentiate peripheral from central vertigo are summarized in ▸ Table 130.2.

130.2.7 Laboratory Testing

Laboratory testing will depend upon the history and physical examination findings. The most commonly performed tests include the following:
- Pure-tone and speech audiometry establishes the presence, degree, and type of hearing loss.
- Auditory evoked brainstem response (ABR) measures auditory potentials from the ear to the brainstem. ABR is not performed routinely in the evaluation of patients with a vestibular disorder. Historically, it has been used to screen for vestibular schwannoma.
- Electrocochleography (ECochG) measures cochlear potentials that reflect abnormalities in fluid dynamics. An elevated SP (summating potential)/AP (action potential) ratio may be encountered in endolymphatic hydrops or perilymph fistula and can be helpful in identifying the offending ear.
- Vestibular evoked myogenic potential (VEMP) testing has been well documented to be helpful in identifying patients with superior canal dehiscence syndrome.
- Videonystagmography assesses the function of the vestibular end-organs, the central vestibulo-ocular pathways, and oculomotor processes. A subtest of videonystagmography is warm and cold water caloric irrigation, in which the eye movements clinically observed with Frenzel goggles in response to caloric stimulation of the horizontal semicircular canal and superior vestibular nerve are objectively recorded. Caloric testing allows a selective determination of unilateral vestibular responsiveness.
- Rotational chair testing quantifies the vestibulo-ocular reflex and helps differentiate peripheral from central pathology.
- Dynamic posturography involves a battery of tests that help to assess the functional capacity of a patient with a balance disorder.
- Imaging studies
  - Magnetic resonance (MR) imaging
  - Computed tomography (CT) of the temporal bones
- Selected serologic studies
  - Syphilis (fluorescent treponemal antibody [FTA]), Lyme titer, autoimmune (antinuclear antibody [ANA], rheumatoid factor [RF], erythrocyte sedimentation rate [ESR])

130.3 Differential Diagnosis of Vertigo

The diagnostic paradigm for common causes of dizziness is described in this chapter. An overview of the algorithm for evaluation of the dizzy patient is shown in ▸ Fig. 130.2.

130.3.1 Peripheral Causes of Vertigo

Benign Paroxysmal Positional Vertigo

Benign paroxysmal positional vertigo (BPPV) is the most common type of vertigo in otherwise healthy adults. BPPV occurs when free-floating otoconia cause movement of the vestibular sensory epithelia. The most common cause of BPPV is head trauma, but it can be of viral or of unknown cause. Patients will describe the sudden onset of rotatory vertigo, lasting seconds to minutes, in specific positions. The vertigo is usually noticed in bed, when they roll over or look up or down. There may be a prior history of similar episodes in the past that resolved spontaneously. There should be no history of hearing loss or tinnitus and no associated neurologic symptoms. The physical examination will be normal with the exception of Dix-Hallpike testing, in which the patient will experience vertigo and nystagmus will be observed when the offending ear is down. The most typical form of BPPV involves the posterior semicircular canal; the nystagmus is rotatory and down-beating toward the lower ear. The minimum laboratory work-up is a pure-tone and speech audiogram, which should be normal or show a symmetric hearing loss. The treatment of BPPV consists of a head maneuver that moves and relocates the offending otoconia, known as the Epley maneuver.

Meniere Disease

Meniere disease results from an abnormal buildup of endolymph and presents as a classic symptom complex of ear fullness, drop in hearing, tinnitus, and vertigo. The symptoms may last minutes to days, resolve spontaneously, and recur at unpredictable and irregular intervals. Not all of the symptoms in the complex must be present to make the diagnosis. Meniere disease is of unknown etiology. It should be viewed as a common set of symptoms reflective of several possible underlying pathologies: too much endolymph production; too little endolymph absorption; or viral, genetic, toxic, or metabolic disorders. Unfortunately, we do not have the diagnostic tools to reliably elucidate these possibilities. Diseases that can mimic Meniere

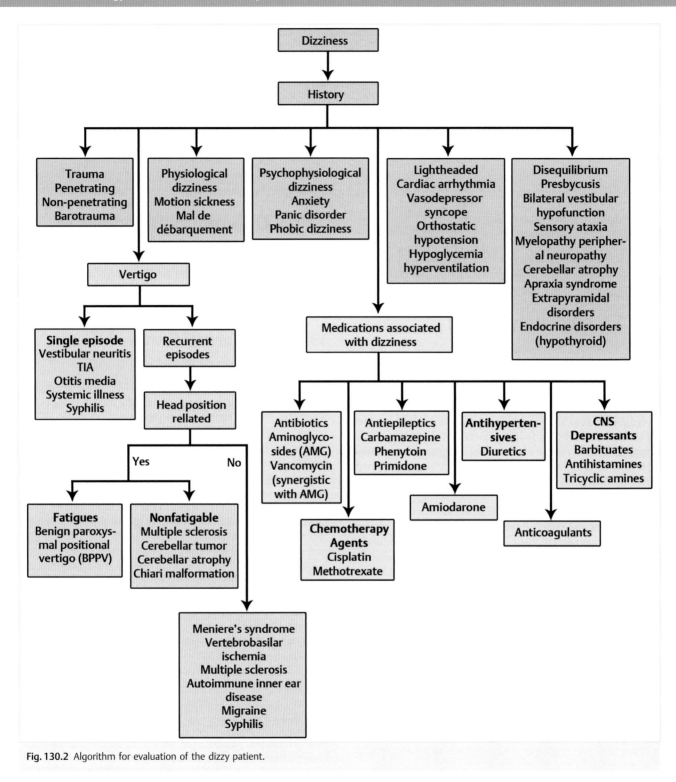

Fig. 130.2 Algorithm for evaluation of the dizzy patient.

disease include acoustic neuroma, perilymphatic fistula, Lyme disease, syphilis, autoimmune inner ear disease, and multiple sclerosis. If a specific etiology can be identified, Meniere syndrome is diagnosed as opposed to idiopathic disease. Meniere disease is bilateral in about 25% of patients. Over time, the hearing loss ceases to fluctuate and becomes more severe, and the acute attacks of vertigo "burn out" and give way to a constant sense of imbalance.

Physical findings are few. During an acute attack, nystagmus can be observed. Between attacks, abnormal tuning fork testing may be the only finding. Audiometry documents a sensorineural hearing loss, often more noticeable in the low frequencies, that fluctuates on repeated testing. ECochG may confirm hydrops. Vestibular testing is not usually necessary to make the diagnosis, which relies heavily on the patient's history. MR imaging with gadolinium enhancement is mandatory to rule out an acoustic neuroma, multiple sclerosis, and other central nervous system pathology.

Initial treatment is with salt restriction to 2 g a day, an oral diuretic, and vestibular suppressants as necessary. If medical therapy is not adequate, vestibular ablation can be performed. This is done most often with intratympanic gentamicin therapy. Surgical alternatives include endolymphatic sac decompression, labyrinthectomy, and vestibular neurectomy.

Delayed Endolymphatic Hydrops

This diagnosis is made when episodic vestibular symptoms, similar to those in Meniere disease, develop months or years after a sensorineural hearing loss of any cause. For example, this condition may develop after a congenital hearing loss, after an idiopathic sudden or progressive hearing loss, or following a "dead ear" after stapedectomy surgery. Some authors feel that the syndrome is a variant of Meniere disease, with endolymphatic hydrops developing as a sequela of prior otologic pathology, so that it is referred to as delayed endolymphatic hydrops. The diagnosis is confirmed by documented hearing loss and the absence of other ear pathology.

Viral Neuronitis

Viral neuronitis is due to inflammation of the vestibular portion of the eighth cranial nerve. The history is critical in establishing the presence of a systemic viral infection close to the time of the onset of vertigo. The presence of hearing loss or tinnitus excludes this diagnosis. Physical examination may reveal nystagmus, but the findings are otherwise normal. Pure-tone and speech audiometry should be normal. Treatment is with vestibular suppressants. The symptoms usually resolve within several days to weeks.

Labyrinthitis

This condition produces an acute vestibular crisis with a history similar to that of vestibular neuritis. However, the vertigo is accompanied by a sudden hearing loss, usually within a few hours before or after the onset of vertigo. The recovery period should be similar to that seen in vestibular neuritis. Hearing may be recovered, or the hearing loss may persist.

Perilymphatic Fistula

Perilymphatic fistula is an abnormal leakage of perilymph via the oval or round window. It is almost always the result of implosive or explosive pressure changes due to head trauma, barotrauma, or Valsalva maneuver. The history is the key to the diagnosis. Symptoms may be isolated dizziness or vertigo, with or without hearing loss or tinnitus. Perilymphatic fistula can mimic Meniere disease. On physical examination, pneumatic otoscopy can precipitate or exacerbate symptoms, a so-called positive "fistula test." There is no diagnostic laboratory test. The presence of a fistula can be confirmed only by surgical exploration of the middle ear. The treatment is surgical repair of the leak.

Dehiscent Superior Semicircular Canal Syndrome

Dehiscent superior semicircular canal syndrome is a loss of bone over the dome of the superior semicircular canal that exposes its endosteum to the dura. The cause is unknown. The most common symptom is episodic dizziness or vertigo, precipitated by loud noise or Valsalva maneuver. Hearing loss is common and may be a low-frequency conductive loss with preservation of the acoustic reflexes. Based on the history and audiometric findings, the patient undergoes CT of the temporal bones, which is the diagnostic study. The treatment is surgical resurfacing of the dehiscence.

130.3.2 Central Causes of Vertigo

Migraine Headache (Vestibular Migraine)

Migraine headache can be associated with dizziness or vertigo as an aura. The diagnosis in these cases is obvious. However, other patients present with episodic vertigo without headaches, so that the diagnosis is obscured. In these cases, the spells of vertigo are similar to those of Meniere disease, but without the associated hearing loss, tinnitus, or aural fullness. A personal or family history of classic migraine is key because all diagnostic tests of inner ear function and radiographic findings are normal.

Vertebrobasilar Vascular Insufficiency

The vertebrobasilar artery supplies the essential structures of the vestibular system, including the inner ear, cranial nerve VIII, and the cerebellum. As a result, transient symptoms may occur as a consequence of reduced blood flow resulting from hypotension (including orthostatic hypotension) or cardiac arrhythmias. Some patients with diabetes mellitus or atherosclerosis have balance complaints and may have multiple small ischemic areas in the brainstem. Others may have intermittent vertebrobasilar artery insufficiency associated with postural changes, certain head positions, or exercise.

Acoustic Neuroma

Acoustic neuroma is a misnomer because this entity is a schwannoma that usually arises on the vestibular portion of the eighth cranial nerve and so is more properly called a vestibular schwannoma. The usual presenting symptoms are hearing loss and/or tinnitus. When an acoustic neuroma is associated with dizziness, the dizziness is usually vague and nonspecific, not frank vertigo. On occasion, an acoustic neuroma can mimic Meniere disease. The physical examination is usually normal, except for tuning fork testing. When an acoustic neuroma is large, cranial nerve V and VII findings may be noted. Pure-tone and speech audiology reveals a unilateral or asymmetric sensorineural hearing loss. MR imaging with gadolinium enhancement is 100% sensitive and highly specific. Treatment options include continued observation, radiation, and surgery.

Multiple Sclerosis

Vertigo or dizziness is an initial symptom in 5 to 15% of patients with multiple sclerosis. Up to 50% of patients with multiple sclerosis become vertiginous at some time during the course of the illness. The vertigo may be transient or permanent and is usually accompanied by nystagmus. Cerebrospinal fluid and MR imaging studies are helpful in confirming the diagnosis.

Psychiatric Disorders

Patients with panic disorder and related anxiety disorders, such as agoraphobia, tend to have vestibular complaints. The pathophysiology is unclear. Patients may have difficulty distinguishing dizziness from anxiety attacks because they occur together. In addition, the dizziness may be nonspecific and possibly mask an underlying clinical depression.

130.4 Using the Clinical History to Guide Treatment Decisions

Most patients with acute vertigo will improve with supportive, expectant management. When this is not the case, and the symptoms have been present for months to years, it is important to determine whether the vestibular pathology is stable or unstable. If the symptoms are predictable and provoked by motion, then the patient has a stable vestibular lesion not yet completely compensated by the central nervous system. These patients are appropriate candidates for vestibular rehabilitation. On the other hand, if the symptoms occur spontaneously and without warning, the patient has an unstable peripheral dysfunction. Meniere disease is the prototype of an unstable vestibular dysfunction. These "unstable" patients are not suitable candidates for vestibular rehabilitation. They are managed with medical therapy, and if this fails, surgical interventions should be considered, depending on the etiology of the vestibulopathy.

130.5 Roundsmanship

- Frenzel goggles are a valuable adjunct during an evaluation for induced nystagmus. The lenses prevent visual fixation, which powerfully inhibits nystagmus.
- Up-beating or down-beating spontaneous nystagmus strongly suggests central pathology.
- Videonystagmography assesses the function of the vestibular end-organs, central vestibulo-ocular pathways, and oculomotor processes.
- Rotational chair testing quantifies the vestibulo-ocular reflex and helps differentiate peripheral from central pathology.
- Dynamic posturography involves a battery of tests that help to assess the functional capacity of the patient with a balance disorder.

130.6 Recommended Reading

[1] Epley JM. The canalith repositioning procedure: for treatment of benign paroxysmal positional vertigo. Otolaryngol Head Neck Surg 1992; 107: 399–404

[2] Fasunla AJ, Ibekwe TS, Nwaorgu OG. Migraine-associated vertigo: a review of the pathophysiology and differential diagnosis. Int J Neurosci 2012; 122: 107–113

[3] Herrera WG. Vestibular and other balance disorders in multiple sclerosis. Differential diagnosis of disequilibrium and topognostic localization. Neurol Clin 1990; 8: 407–420

[4] Hillier SL, McDonnell M. Vestibular rehabilitation for unilateral peripheral vestibular dysfunction. Cochrane Database Syst Rev 2011: CD005397

[5] House JW, Doherty JK, Fisher LM, Derebery MJ, Berliner KI. Meniere's disease: prevalence of contralateral ear involvement. Otol Neurotol 2006; 27: 355–361

[6] Kamei T. Delayed endolymphatic hydrops as a clinical entity. Int Tinnitus J 2004; 10: 137–143

[7] Maitland CG. Perilymphatic fistula. Curr Neurol Neurosci Rep 2001; 1: 486–491

[8] Merchant SN, Adams JC, Nadol JB. Pathophysiology of Meniere's syndrome: are symptoms caused by endolymphatic hydrops? Otol Neurotol 2005; 26: 74–81

[9] Minor LB. Superior canal dehiscence syndrome. Am J Otol 2000; 21: 9–19

[10] Moubayed SP, Saliba I. Vertebrobasilar insufficiency presenting as isolated positional vertigo or dizziness: a double-blind retrospective cohort study. Laryngoscope 2009; 119: 2071–2076

[11] Teggi R, Caldirola D, Colombo B et al. Dizziness, migrainous vertigo and psychiatric disorders. J Laryngol Otol 2010; 124: 285–290

[12] Theodosopoulos PV, Pensak ML. Contemporary management of acoustic neuromas. Laryngoscope 2011; 121: 1133–1137

131 Management of the Patient with Chronic Dizziness

Bryan D. Hujsak and Laura Lei-Rivera

131.1 Introduction

Dizziness ranks as one of the most frequent complaints in primary care medicine. Dizziness can arise from a number of causes, including but not limited to side effects of medications, cardiac conditions, psychological disorders, neurologic disorders, and dysfunction of the vestibular system. Dizziness arising from a vestibular disorder can be quite disabling. It may reduce not only quality of the life and well-being but also interpersonal relationships. The treatment of individuals with chronic dizziness can be quite challenging. It requires patience and confidence on the part of the practitioner to guide the patient through the murky waters of conflicting opinions and the multitude of medical tests used to rule out more life-threatening pathology. Many people with chronic dizziness do not show any outward signs of their disorder. As a result, they sometimes are unable to obtain the kind of empathy from friends, family, and health care practitioners that someone with a more visible disability receives. Sometimes, the symptoms they are experiencing may be attributed to the anxiety and depression that commonly accompany any disabling condition, limiting the care that might return them to their previous level of function. It is our hope that this summary of the management of patients with chronic dizziness will provide the reader with a deeper appreciation of the complexities involved in caring for this unique population of patients.

131.2 Classification of Vestibular Disorders

Vestibular disorders can be broadly defined as either stable or unstable lesions. Stable lesions are typically the result of a one-time insult to the system, such as vestibular neuritis or labyrinthitis. Episodic disorders that have been ameliorated through medical or surgical management can also be classified as stable. An example would be Meniere disease that has responded to a low-sodium diet and diuresis, ablative therapy with an intratympanic injection of gentamicin, vestibular nerve sectioning, or labyrinthectomy. Unstable lesions are those that continue to cause episodic bouts of vertigo, dizziness, and disequilibrium, potentially resulting in further degradation of the vestibular system. Examples include unmanaged Meniere disease, vestibular migraine, endolymphatic hydrops, and vestibular autoimmune disorders. Before any rehabilitation intervention is undertaken, it is critical that any episodic degenerative process be halted through medication or surgery, or the outcome will most certainly be less than optimal.

Vestibular disorders can be further classified as unilateral or bilateral, incomplete or complete, symmetric or asymmetric, and peripheral, central, or mixed. Peripheral disorders include any pathology that affects the vestibular end-organs or the vestibular portion of the eighth cranial nerve (e.g., vestibular neuritis). Bilateral peripheral dysfunction can be seen in patients with ototoxicity from the intravenous administration of an aminoglycoside or with Meniere disease. Any of these disorders can cause partial or complete loss of function. Central disorders include any pathology that affects the vestibular nuclei, the cerebellum, or any of the connecting pathways in between (e.g., cerebellar degeneration, hydrocephalus, vascular insult, brainstem traction injuries, and basilar migraine). Demyelination at the nerve root entry zone of cranial nerve VIII occurs with multiple sclerosis and can be classified as a mixed peripheral–central disorder. Other mixed disorders include vestibular schwannomas compromising the cerebellopontine angle and acquired brain injury with labyrinthine concussion as a sequela. Classification in these categories can assist in the prognosis and may determine the most appropriate approach to rehabilitation. A combination of vestibular function testing, the clinical examination, and the patient's report will aid the clinician in determining the type of vestibular dysfunction that is present.

131.3 Disablement Model

For most patients with vestibular dysfunction, once they have been stabilized medically, the symptoms of dizziness and imbalance resolve over time. As they begin to engage in their prior activities, gradually increasing the level of intensity, the system naturally recovers and adapts. However, in some individuals, barriers to this adaptive process prevent spontaneous recovery. Typically, it is these patients who require skilled rehabilitation to facilitate a more favorable outcome. Although the main objective of treatment is to eliminate the symptoms of dizziness and disequilibrium, this cannot always be achieved. In lieu of a complete recovery, management of the patient with chronic dizziness should emphasize a return to the patient's prior level of function with a minimum of symptoms.

Traditionally, treatment has focused on addressing the underlying pathology. According to the medical model, if the pathology is eliminated, the impact on the patient's life will also be diminished. Over time, this philosophy has fallen short, especially in disorders in which a complete cure is not available. In order to understand how pathology impacts an individual's ability to function, many disablement models have been developed. The currently accepted model in rehabilitation is the International Classification of Function, Disability, and Health (ICF), developed by the World Health Organization (WHO). This multidirectional interaction model takes into account how a health condition impairs body structure and function. It also takes into account how this impairment affects an individual's activity level and participation in activities of daily living. The ICF model is the first to formally acknowledge the influence of personal and environmental factors. Earlier models by WHO and Nagi considered pathology, impairments, functional disability, and handicap only in a bidirectional fashion. The significance of the ICF model lies in its broadened view of how the disease process impacts a person's ability to function in society (▸ Fig. 131.1).

In providing comprehensive management for patients with chronic dizziness, it is important for the practitioner to consider all levels of the ICF model. It is imperative that the patient

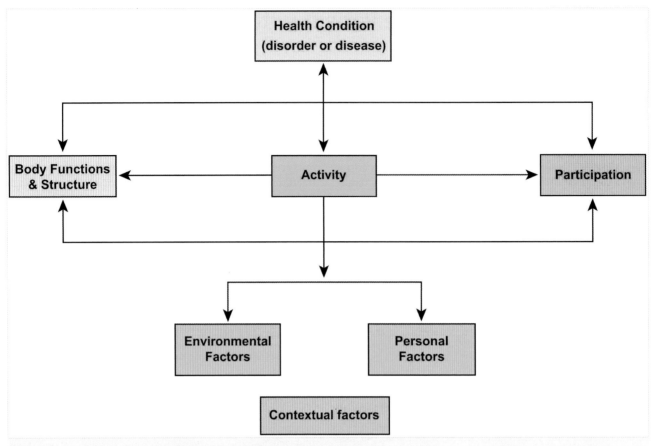

Fig. 131.1 International Classification of Function, Disability, and Health.

receive all possible medical and surgical care to minimize the impact of the health condition on body structure and function. Physical therapists, occupational therapists, and audiologists may provide skilled rehabilitation in order to facilitate adaptation of the system to any residual deficits. This helps to return the patient to premorbid levels of activity and participation. During the course of rehabilitation, these practitioners can also provide strategies that allow the patient to participate in activities of daily living with a minimum of symptoms. All practitioners participating in the care of these patients need to be mindful of the personal and environmental factors that either help or hinder the patient's recovery. If these barriers prove to be too large to overcome, consultation with psychiatry, psychology, and social work may be appropriate.

131.4 Principles of Treatment

The ultimate goal of rehabilitation is to return the individual to a premorbid level of function. Complete recovery can be defined as the patient's ability to tolerate all motions and activities without any remaining symptoms of vertigo, dizziness, or disequilibrium. Recent texts have delineated separate approaches for differing theoretical models of recovery. These have been described in a hierarchical fashion:

1. Adaptation/compensation
2. Habituation
3. Substitution

Separate modalities for each category are implemented in the hope of facilitating functional recovery. In terms of planning treatment strategies, the preferred result is one in which the central nervous system has adapted to the altered vestibular input caused by the pathology. Specific movements are prescribed that attempt to recalibrate the responses of the associated vestibular reflexes and their subsequent sensory integration. This is described as adaptation or compensation. A second treatment approach takes advantage of the neurologic phenomenon of habituation. A symptom-provoking stimulus, usually a head motion or position change, is presented to the patient in small increments followed by a specified recovery time. With repeated stimulation, the symptom response diminishes until the individual is no longer symptomatic with the particular movement. A third treatment approach is to substitute an alternative sensation for the missing vestibular information. In this approach, commonly used for patients with complete bilateral vestibular loss, vision and somatosensory information are optimized during the activity.

131.5 Treatment Modalities

The primary form of rehabilitative treatment is exercise. Early forms of exercise developed by Cawthorne and Cooksey recognized the need to move the eyes, head, and body in a repeated fashion. These maneuvers helped facilitate recovery by requiring the patient to move in directions that had been avoided

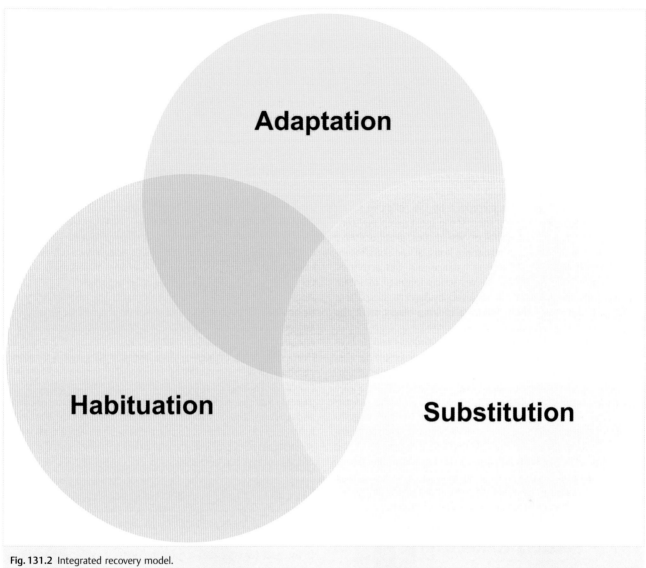

Adaptation

Habituation

Substitution

Fig. 131.2 Integrated recovery model.

because of a fear of dizziness. Although less sophisticated and specific than modern approaches, the continued use of these exercises may be effective with some patients, especially during the interim between consultation with the medical practitioner and the initiation of formal rehabilitation.

Although we can make clear theoretical distinctions among adaptation, habituation, and substitution, the movements used in treatment usually take advantage of all three effects. Initially, the dizziness provoked by the therapeutic motion may be too great for adaptation to be achieved, and tolerance of the motion through habituation may be required first. To a large degree, many patients spontaneously learn to substitute alternate senses to maintain their orientation. During visual fixation on stationary objects, visual cues override the erroneous signals generated by the vestibular system, improving equilibrium and minimizing dizziness. Also, many patients will maximize their proprioceptive input by increasing their double support time during gait, resulting in shorter, more deliberate steps. These substitution strategies become ineffective in conditions of absent visual stimuli (i.e., dark and dimly lit environments),

complex visual movements (i.e., crowds, stores), and uneven terrain (sand, grass, sidewalks; ▶ Fig. 131.2).

Modern approaches to treatment target three areas: gaze stability, postural reflexes, and sensory organization. Exercises are introduced at a level that challenges the patient's abilities but does not overwhelm his or her ability to complete the task. Each exercise is performed two to three times per day. Symptom provocation is not the primary objective in adaptation exercises, but it can be present as a minor side effect. If symptoms are provoked, the recovery time should be minimal because patients are instructed to recover from any symptoms before proceeding to the next exercise or activity.

Gaze stability exercises primarily address deficits in the vestibulo-ocular reflex. Patients are asked to fix their gaze on a simple, asymmetric target while oscillating the head through 30 degrees of yaw or pitch. This head motion is continued for a minimum of 90 seconds in both directions. If any degradation of the image is observed, patients are asked to slow down to maintain clarity and stability. Over time, they will be able move their head at a faster rate. More complex targets are progressively substituted for simple targets. Target motion adds another dimension to the exercise, approximating in vivo demands on the vestibular system.

Postural reflexes are challenged with both static and dynamic balance activities designed to improve the responsiveness of the vestibulospinal reflex. The vestibulospinal reflex is responsible for maintaining balance during changes in head or body position relative to the gravity axis (i.e., walking on an inclined surface) or displacement of the head outside the base of support (i.e., a head turn). These activities may include static standing with a progressively narrowed base of support, postural sway activities, gait with a progressively narrowed base of support, and gait with head turns.

Sensory organization is characterized by the reflexive selection of the appropriate orientation sense for a given environment. The brain selectively relies on visual cues, proprioceptive information, or vestibular information. If visual and somatosensory cues are manipulated during balance and gait activities, the system can be forced to use vestibular input to maintain balance. This manipulation is achieved by having the patient stand with the eyes closed, follow a moving object with the eyes, or stand on a compliant surface.

In addition to exercises, there are many products and devices that purport to be effective in managing chronic vestibular disorders. Some of these devices are based on the principle of sensory substitution, providing head and body position sensation via tactile stimulation of the body, feet, and even the tongue. Other devices provide controlled, measurable, sensory organization testing and training. Like the vestibular exercises previously described, they have their strengths and weaknesses and may not be effective with all patients. It is not our objective to promote or diminish the efficacy of these devices, but to urge clinicians to evaluate the evidence surrounding each device before incurring large expenses to their capital budget.

131.6 Barriers to Recovery

Most people respond favorably to therapy as long as the lesion is stable and the therapy provided is skilled and customized to the needs of the patient. Because therapeutic exercise is a very conservative form of management for vestibular disorders, it is important to recognize that not all patients are helped by vestibular rehabilitation. As with any disorder, failure via conservative management should compel the clinician to investigate the underlying cause. There are many reasons why a patient may not recover from lesions of the vestibular system. These barriers may also prevent progress with rehabilitation. Although not exhaustive, the following is a list of the more common causes.

One of the primary reasons for failure to adapt is that the patient has a misdiagnosed unstable lesion. Many times, patients are referred for therapy for what appears to be an unresolving vestibular neuritis. Unfortunately, the initial bout of vertigo assumed to be the result of neuritis is only the first of many episodes to follow. This is commonly seen in patients with Meniere disease or vestibular migraine. Once the pattern of episodic vertigo has been identified, the medical approach needs to be revised in order to stabilize the disorder.

Visual–perceptual forms of dysfunction are another major barrier to recovery. Of all sensory information processed by the brain, 90% is related to vision, and therefore distortions in this system can be very disorienting. It is a common misconception that the vestibular system is the "balance organ." The reality is that our visual system, not our vestibular system, is the primary orientation sense. Symptoms of dizziness can be compounded by or arise purely from visual–perceptual forms of dysfunction. These include, but are not limited to, cataracts, glaucoma, macular degeneration, visual field loss, refractive errors, and multifocal lenses. It is important to recognize that patients are usually the last to know that they cannot see as well as they should. This is because most pathology in the visual system occurs over time, and the brain is able to adapt to this slow deterioration. Therefore, a visual screen for acuity, dominance, vergence, confrontation visual fields, and extraocular eye movements should be a component of every clinician's examination.

Emotional disorders are another common cause of failed recovery. It is expected that any patient with a vestibular disorder will have some degree of anxiety and depression related to the condition. This is a normal emotional response that can be considered pathologic only when it prevents the patient from participating at a level that would promote adaptation. This type of anxiety and depression is different from primary clinical anxiety and depression and is classified as an adjustment disorder. Other emotional disorders, such as premorbid mood disorders, personality disorders, and psychoses, will also have a negative effect on treatment outcome. It is important to educate the patient that management of both the psychological disorder and the vestibular disorder is needed in order to maximize functional improvement. In these cases, close work with a psychiatrist, psychologist, or social worker versed in vestibular disorders can be quite effective.

131.7 Alternatives to Traditional Treatment

In the past two decades, a growing body of evidence supporting tai chi as a valuable complementary treatment for vestibular disorders has emerged in the Western scientific literature. Tai chi, a traditional Chinese method of exercise derived from a martial arts form, has gained popularity as a treatment paradigm for a variety of human ailments, including balance impairment.

Tai chi is an appropriate form of exercise for individuals of all ages with a wide range of abilities and conditions, including the medically complex. It has applications for balance dysfunctions, orthopedic and neurologic rehabilitation, pain management, cardiovascular and respiratory disorders, mood and mental disorders, fitness, and general well-being. The beneficial effects of tai chi for which the evidence is most compelling appear to be related to functional balance and fall prevention.

Vestibular rehabilitation is a well-accepted exercise program intended for the treatment of persons with balance impairment caused by damage to the peripheral vestibular system. However, individuals with balance deficits resulting from central nervous system pathology or the involvement of multiple components of the sensory system do not generally have the same outcomes. Although patients with central pathology can achieve clinical and functional gains, implementing tai chi training as an adjunctive therapy in the first group of patients may maximize treatment outcomes. In addition, the implementation of a tai chi program may help transition patients from supervised medical care to a longer-term community-based program. It is this lifestyle change that may have the most enduring effect of improving balance and wellness.

131.8 Conclusion

The management of patients with chronic dizziness arising from vestibular dysfunction can be very challenging, but also extremely rewarding. In order to achieve successful outcomes in this patient population, it is critical to properly classify the underlying disorder, involve the appropriate professionals in each patient's care, recognize influences beyond the pathology, and explore comorbidities in the face of slow or absent progress. Communication between the patient, physician, audiologist, and therapist is critical because the successful management of vestibular dysfunction is not an event, but a process.

131.9 Roundsmanship

- Vestibular rehabilitation is an effective form of conservative management for patients with *stable* peripheral and central vestibular dysfunctions.
- The management of patients with chronic dizziness requires considerations beyond pathology. Understanding the effects of physical impairment on social and environmental factors will result in optimal patient outcomes.

- Patients who do not respond to rehabilitation should be evaluated for comorbidities that may be preventing adaptation, habituation, and substitution. These may include visual–perceptual dysfunction, emotional disorders, or a previously unidentified unstable lesion.
- Adjunctive and alternative therapies like tai chi have been shown to be effective in promoting recovery and may also help in transitioning patients from medical care to participation in community-based activities.
- The effective management of patients with chronic dizziness may require additional support from psychology and social work to complement the medical and therapeutic care provided by the physician and physical therapist.

131.10 Recommended Reading

[1] Baloh RW. Clinical practice. Vestibular neuritis. N Engl J Med 2003; 348: 1027–1032
[2] Brown KE, Whitney SL, Marchetti GF, Wrisley DM, Furman JM. Physical therapy for central vestibular dysfunction. Arch Phys Med Rehabil 2006; 87: 76–81
[3] Herdman SJ, Whitney SL. Interventions for the patient with vestibular hypofunction. In: Herdman SJ, ed. Vestibular Rehabilitation. 3rd ed. Philadelphia, PA: F. A. Davis Company; 2007:310–312
[4] Hillier SL, Hollohan V. Vestibular rehabilitation for unilateral peripheral vestibular dysfunction. Cochrane Database Syst Rev 2007: CD005397
[5] Jette AM. Toward a common language for function, disability, and health. Phys Ther 2006; 86: 726–734
[6] Li F, Harmer P, Fisher KJ et al. Tai Chi and fall reductions in older adults: a randomized controlled trial. J Gerontol A Biol Sci Med Sci 2005; 60: 187–194
[7] Neuhauser HK, Radtke A, von Brevern M, Lezius F, Feldmann M, Lempert T. Burden of dizziness and vertigo in the community. Arch Intern Med 2008; 168: 2118–2124

132 Diagnostic Assessment and Management of Acute Facial Palsy

Christopher J. Linstrom

132.1 Introduction

The management of a patient presenting with facial paresis or paralysis may at first seem like a daunting task to the clinician, and it should be remembered that "all that palsies is not Bell's." A thorough history and physical examination, with the reasoned development of a differential diagnosis, understanding, and the judicious use of clinical testing, will enable the physician to arrive at a specific diagnosis and formulate an appropriate treatment plan in cases of acute facial paralysis. This chapter will review the pertinent anatomy and physiology of the facial nerve and facial movement, with an emphasis upon the accurate evaluation and supportive and definitive care of the patient with facial paralysis. A review of the common etiologies of acute facial dysfunction and a plan for the treatment of acute facial paralysis will be given, along with several clinical case examples. A separate section will review electrodiagnostic testing of the facial nerve.

132.2 Relevant Anatomy and Physiology

Like many other structures in the head and neck, the facial nerve, cranial nerve (CN) VII, respects the rule of "economy of

means." It is a composite nerve, primarily subserving motor function to the muscles of facial expression (branchial motor) but also, through the nervus intermedius of Wrisberg, carrying general sensory and special sensory fibers (taste) and preganglionic parasympathetic fibers (visceral motor) for lacrimation and salivation (to the submandibular and sublingual glands).

The facial nerve may be detected in embryonic life as early as the third week of gestation, when the embryo is 3 mm long. This collection of neural crest cells also gives rise to CN VIII and thus is called the facioacoustic primordium or crest.

The facial nerve becomes housed within the petrous temporal bone, taking the longest intraosseous course of any cranial nerve (▶ Fig. 132.1). It has two major points of flexion, the first (superior) and second (inferior) genus, before taking a somewhat vertical course to leave the temporal bone at the stylomastoid foramen, where it branches at the pes anserinus ("goose's foot") into two main divisions, the temporofacial (superior) and cervicofacial (inferior) branches. These then travel between the superficial and deep lobes of the parotid to innervate the muscles of facial expression via five named branches: the temporal, zygomatic, buccal, marginal mandibular, and cervical rami. Proximal to the point of ramification, the facial nerve gives off three and sometimes four small branches: (1) the nerve to the stapedius muscle (within the facial canal); (2) the posterior auricular nerve to the occipitalis muscle;

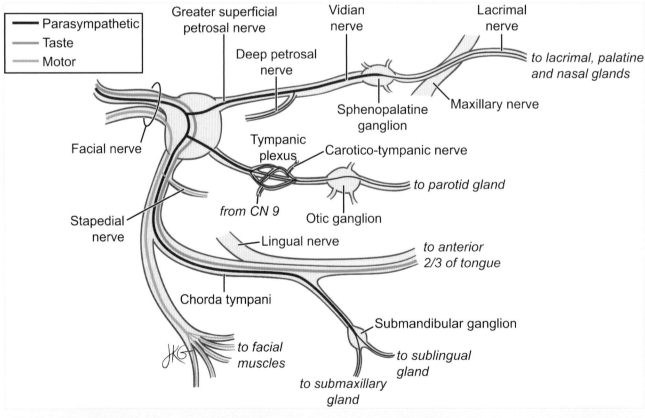

Fig. 132.1 Schematic of the facial nerve.

(3) the nerve to the posterior belly of the digastric muscle; and (4) the lingual branch, which the corda tympani joins to carry afferent special sensation (taste) for the anterior two-thirds of the tongue.

The nervus intermedius exits the brainstem near the motor nucleus of the facial nerve. Cell bodies for lacrimation and salivation, as well as vasomotor fibers destined for the nasal mucosa, arise in the superior salivatory nucleus and join the facial nerve after it has passed the abducens nucleus (CN VI); these structures travel together until the nerve reaches the geniculate ganglion. The greater superficial petrosal nerve takes off at this point, carrying preganglionic parasympathetic fibers for the pterygopalatine ganglion and eventually innervating the lacrimal, minor salivary, and mucosal glands of the palate and nose.

A small named contribution to the facial nerve, the corda tympani, carries special sensory fibers for taste from the anterior two-thirds of the tongue. Its cell bodies are located in the geniculate ganglion. These special sensory afferent fibers will eventually synapse in the medulla in the nucleus solitarius of the tractus solitarius. General sensation for the tongue, however, is mediated by the lingual nerve (CN V_3).

The principal motor functions of the facial nerve are indicated by its anatomical distribution. Teleologically, there are few branches to the extremes of the face because these areas do not serve either to protect the eye or to aid in alimentation. The muscles of facial expression, although of great importance, are of a secondary order because they are not required for life-sustaining functions. The facial nerve branches extensively and densely in the midface to innervate the orbicularis oculi, orbicularis oris, and buccinator, all necessary for life-sustaining functions. The orbicularis oculi and orbicularis oris serve both protective and expressive functions—hence the large amount of anatomy devoted to them.

The cornea, as will be described in greater detail below, is protected by an elaborate system. The afferent fibers of CN V_1 sense when the cornea becomes dry, and a reflex arc to efferent fibers of CN VII in the pons both stimulates lacrimation and initiates blinking. In health, it is an elegant and efficient system. With either an afferent sensory deficit or weakness of CN VII, this system may fail and place the cornea at risk for dryness and exposure.

132.3 Facial Paralysis: History

It is of the utmost importance to concentrate on the *time course* of facial paralysis. Paresis or paralysis of the face occurring over a matter of minutes (e.g., trauma) or hours (Bell palsy) is usually quite different from that occurring over a period of years (cholesteatoma involving the otic capsule, other inflammatory conditions of the temporal bone and facial nerve, facial nerve neuroma, or rarely acoustic neuroma). What was the overall general health of the patient at the time of the onset of facial dysfunction? Does the patient have any other metabolic disorders, such as diabetes? Did the paralysis occur during pregnancy? What was at first thought to be Bell palsy may in fact turn out to be something completely different after a careful history has been obtained.

Has the patient ever had an episode of paresis or paralysis similar to the current one on the same or opposite side of the face? Are there any additional findings that the patient has noticed, has been told about, or remembers from a prior episode (e.g., fissuring of the tongue [lingua plicata], as in Melkersson-Rosenthal syndrome)? Was facial paralysis accompanied by vesicular lesions around the ear or soft palate (herpes zoster oticus)? Was any other otologic complaint, such as pain, aural discharge, tinnitus, or vertigo, associated with the loss of facial nerve function? Did facial paralysis occur in the context of otologic surgery? If so, it is important to hear from the referring surgeon or to determine from the operative report the exact nature of the disease being treated, the surgical procedure, and the suspected site of injury to the facial nerve.

Trauma to the temporal bone resulting in facial paralysis requires special consideration. If the patient or an observer remembers the nature of the trauma or it is well documented, this may aid in estimating the likely nature and extent of a facial nerve injury. So often, a patient with severe multisystem trauma is taken to the emergency department of a hospital, stabilized, operated upon for general, orthopedic, or neurologic injury, placed in a surgical intensive care unit (ICU), and thereafter sent to a non-ICU bed on a surgical floor for a few days before a nurse or house officer notices facial weakness or paralysis. Other body systems may have taken precedence and required urgent medical or surgical intervention before any thought was given to facial nerve injury. In other cases, facial nerve function is observed and documented immediately upon arrival in the emergency department. In this latter case, the decision to treat or observe may be more straightforward, much as in the possible surgical management of Bell palsy.

If the patient with traumatic facial paralysis was observed early on to move the face, one can safely bet that at least part of the facial nerve was intact and functioning. If the patient subsequently lost facial function completely, one would treat much as one would with Bell palsy: anti-inflammatory agents (steroids) first, with surgical decompression of the nerve to be considered if the patient lost all clinical and electrical function and was otherwise a surgical candidate.

If, however, the trauma patient has been observed to have *no* active facial movement upon arrival or was not observed at all early on and now has been found to have facial paralysis and is stable enough for the facial nerve to be evaluated, the temporal bone should be imaged with edge-enhanced computed tomography (CT), which will yield the greatest amount of anatomical information for the bone, air, and soft-tissue interfaces. Further management will be based on this result and the overall health of the patient. A comatose patient is obviously not a candidate for a facial nerve decompression. However, the same patient may be much more functional 2 to 3 months later and still have a facial nerve paralysis. In this case, he or she may be able to endure a facial nerve decompression to definitively manage the nerve, as indicated.

Facial paralysis is much more than a cosmetic deficit. Because eyelid closure depends upon an actively functioning orbicularis oculi, facial nerve dysfunction for any reason places the cornea at risk. With every eye blink, two very important actions happen to the tear film. (1) It is wicked from a superolateral point of production in the lacrimal gland in an inferomedial direction toward the superior and inferior lacrimal puncta. (2) It is then everted, much as a sheet is turned upside down in a dryer.

These two active functions ensure that the tear film is kept fresh and actively moving across the globe to lubricate the cornea. With facial paralysis, this active function is severely impeded or ceases, placing the cornea at risk for exposure. If there is a concomitant corneal afferent sensory deficit (CN V_1), especially in patients who have undergone resection of a large posterior fossa tumor involving CN V, the cornea is now at severe risk for exposure keratitis, abrasion, ulceration, and eventually endophthalmitis. If the condition is left untreated, the patient may ultimately lose sight in the affected eye. Because of the grave potential risk to the globe, it is important that the clinician focus carefully on the eye, especially the health of the cornea. Clinical tests of tearing, such as the Schirmer test, yield information about the quantity but not about the nature of the tear film produced. This information may be obtained by sampling and analyzing the tear film, looking at the hormonal content of the tear film, especially estrogen. In actual practice, this is rarely done by an otolaryngologist. The estrogen concentration in the tear film of postmenopausal women, for example, is decreased in comparison with that in the tear film of premenopausal women, and this decrease is thought to contribute in large measure to the complaint of "dry eye" in patients with otherwise normal facial nerve function. Awareness of the grave consequences of exposure keratitis will ordinarily suffice for both the doctor and patient to keep the eye moist. It is wise to enlist the collaboration of an ophthalmologist experienced in the care of the anterior chamber to help in the care of these patients.

132.4 Physical Examination: Evaluation of Facial Nerve Function

In cases of facial nerve paralysis, detection is generally simple. However, a mild paresis of only one part of the face may be noticeable to the patient alone, especially when the patient is fatigued, and to no other observer.

It is wise to complete the general head and neck examination before focusing on the face. In this way, the likelihood of overlooking potential contributory pathologies, such as a lesion in the parotid, base of the tongue, retromolar trigone, or nasopharynx, will be diminished. Not all pathology involving the facial nerve occurs within the temporal bone. Once the general ear, nose, and throat examination has been performed and is negative, a careful examination of the facial nerve should be performed.

A quick examination will reveal which part of the face has impaired movement. The patient must be instructed not to bite, but simply to try to move the face. Can the patient raise the eyebrow (while the examiner holds down the opposite, "normal" side)? Is there active eyelid closure? Or is there simply passive relaxation of the upper lid with or without a Bell reflex (upward rotation of the globe, protecting the cornea.) Is there an active closed-lipped smile? Do the extremes of the face (frontalis, depressor anguli oris) move? Where is the greatest deficit—upper face versus lower face versus the whole face? Is there synkinesis?

Active movement *alone* counts. It is a common fault of physicians who should understand the subtleties of facial function to mistake relaxation of the levator (CN III) with active eyelid

closure. This is *not* active eyelid closure. Even a newborn baby will demonstrate "crow's-feet" formation at the lateral margins of the orbit while crying, and this pattern alone indicates active contraction of the orbicularis oculi and not relaxation of an adynamic upper lid. The examiner must elicit active motion as opposed to passive relaxation.

It is also important for the physician interested in treating patients with facial paresis/paralysis to study the normal face, to have a good idea of what is "normal."

132.5 Facial Nerve Grading Systems

Most facial nerve grading systems are based upon the clinical observation of facial nerve function and not upon objective measures of linear displacement, velocity, or acceleration from repose. Although numbers have been assigned in these systems, the numbers should be thought of as "bins," or levels of function. The various grades of function are not integers, and the assigned number cannot undergo mathematical subtraction or addition.

Two of the more commonly used systems will be described here: the House-Brackmann (H-B) grading system and the Fisch classification. Many other systems have been promulgated. The House-Brackmann system has been approved by the American Academy of Otolaryngology—Head and Neck Surgery (AAO-HNS) for general use in describing facial nerve function. Although it is commonly used to describe facial function at any time along the course of facial dysfunction, it was actually devised to describe a state of function after medical or surgical intervention (i.e., later on in the course of disease). The House-Brackmann system is easy to learn and apply to the patient (▶ Table 132.1). The face may be divided into an upper face (containing the eyes) and a lower face. The dividing line in this system is an actively closing eye (H-B III) and an eye that cannot close on its own (H-B IV). Patients with normal facial function in all divisions of the nerve are H-B I; patients with flaccid/adynamic hemifacial function are H-B VI. Mimimal paresis of the nerve but *with* active eyelid closure and no synkinesis is H-B II. Tone only of the face *without* active facial movement is H-B V. Any amount of synkinesis downgrades the patient to H-B III.

The ease of application of this system is also its greatest disadvantage. Not all H-B III patients are the same, as is true for patients in each H-B grade. There may be marked differences in the appearance of two hemifaces within the exact same classification, especially when the deficit is predominantly in the upper face. Nonetheless, the H-B system has proved to be of great utility in the evaluation and management of facial paralysis.

The second most commonly used system was developed by Fisch. He recognized the problem of sorting out facial function in rigid categories and tried to achieve a point-based grading system that might yield greater predictability for recovery from acute facial dysfunction. In his system, the hemiface is divided into five regions: frontal, eyelid, midface (buccal), mouth, and lower face, corresponding roughly to those regions innervated by the respective branches of the facial nerve: temporal, zygomatic, buccal, mandibular, and cervical rami.

Table 132.1 House-Brackmann classification of facial nerve function

Grade	Clinical description	Resting	Volitional
I	Normal	*Normal* facial function in all divisions	*Normal* facial function in all divisions
II	Mild dysfunction	Normal symmetry and tone; slight weakness noted	Mild dysfunction, usually at the extremes of the face; active eyelid closure
III	Moderate dysfunction	Obvious difference between the two sides	Greater dysfunction; active eyelid closure with forced movement
IV	Moderately severe dysfunction	Obvious, disfiguring asymmetry	Greater dysfunction; passive eye closure *only*
V	Severe dysfunction	Asymmetry at rest; tone only	Barely perceptible motion; passive eye closure *only*
VI	Total paralysis	Flaccid, adynamic face	Flaccid, adynamic face

Twenty points are awarded for each of the five facial regions, for a total of 100 points. Synkinesis subtracts points from the final score. A higher overall score is better than a lower score and is thought to predict greater return of function. Although this grading system takes a bit longer to calculate, it is intuitive and does attempt to use a clinical metric (i.e. regional observation) to predict outcome. However, it is not truly arithmetic in that the final grading system is ultimately subjective in design and cannot undergo strict mathematic functional analysis.

132.6 Testing

132.6.1 Objective Measurement of Facial Nerve Function

Many attempts have been made to measure facial nerve function in an objective way and thereby to remove observer bias from the calculation. Various methods have been quite ingenious in their ways of measuring facial nerve function.

Facial displacement may be measured linearly with surface electrodes and an electromyographic recording and measuring system. Neely et al and Holman et al used a subtracted-image, computer-assisted technique that measures the degree of facial surface deformation (per expression, per time segment) expressed as a summation of all pixels in the subtracted area. Light reflectance is taken as a two-dimensional marker of the three-dimensional surface deformation occurring during facial expression. Another system uses normal shadows of the various regions of the face and variations of luminance produced by changes of facial expression to calculate linear regional displacement. Landmark-based systems apply some type of fixed marker to the face, with facial movement from repose measured either by hand or via a video/computer digital interface.

These systems are advanced, eloquent, and supremely "believable" in that the data they generate are not subject to observer bias. Unfortunately, almost all of them have the built-in burden of advanced computation and are never real-time. Some require more than an hour of computer time to compute the data analysis for one requested movement (e.g., closed-lip smile). The clinical utility of objective facial nerve function systems is limited, but as a research tool they are superb. With faster "super computers" an objective, real-time metric of facial function may one day be possible.

132.6.2 Topognostic (Site-of-Lesion) Testing

Testing the various branches of the facial nerve for the presence or absence of function has been performed in an effort to locate the site of the lesion. The supposition for these tests is that decreased function at a given site identifies the approximate site of pathology and that the nerve proximal to this site is functioning. These suppositions are not always true. Topognostic testing has been shown to correlate poorly with the chronologic return of function. The accuracy of defining the absolute site of a lesion is also quite low. For these reasons, topognostic testing has largely been replaced by electrical testing of the facial nerve and radiographic imaging of the temporal bone. Perhaps the test of greatest utility is the Schirmer test because it may help identify an eye at risk for exposure keratitis. These tests are reviewed for historical interest (▶ Table 132.2).

1. The Schirmer test measures the capillary flow of tears onto a filter paper placed into the inferior fornix of the eye, indirectly measuring the function of the greater superficial petrosal nerve, which is the first branch of CN VII. Tear production is usually markedly reduced in Bell palsy.
2. The stapedius reflex measures the contraction of the stapedius muscle, innervated by the facial nerve. It is usually absent in facial paralysis due to Bell palsy.
3. The blink reflex measures an involuntary reflex arc of the afferent CN V_1 (corneal sensation) to the trigeminal nerve and thence to the brainstem, with connections in the pons and out through the efferent CN VII to the orbicularis oculi. The arc is intact only if some active function of VII remains.
4. The rate and amount of salivary gland production from the submandibular gland may be measured by direct microcatheterization of the Warthin duct. A quantitative decrease in salivary production from the affected side has been thought to help locate the site of facial nerve involvement but is nonspecific.
5. Taste (via the chorda tympani) has been used as a qualitative test of facial dysfunction but has proved to be of little clinical use as a predictor of return of function.

The greatest potential use of topognostic testing remains in cases of temporal bone trauma in which the patient retains a slight amount of facial movement and in which there is a discrete area of injury to the nerve, identified on a CT scan. In these cases, topognostic testing may give clinical clues to the

Table 132.2 Topognostic testing of the facial nerve

Clinical test	Branch of facial nerve
Tearing (Schirmer test)	Greater superficial petrosal nerve
Immittance (stapedial reflex) testing	Stapedial branch
Salivary secretion (cannulation of Warthin duct)	Lingual branch (preganglionic parasympathetic fibers from chorda tympani to lingual nerve)
Blink test	Reflex arc of cranial nerve V_1 (afferent) and cranial nerve VII (efferent)
Taste test	Chorda tympani nerve

precise area of injury. In the majority of cases, however, the face is flaccid and adynamic.

Because the point of greatest narrowing of the intratympanic facial nerve is at the meatal foramen and because supramaximal stimulation of the facial nerve with electroneuronography (compound muscle action potential) has been shown to be a better predictor of facial nerve outcome, topognostic testing is now of secondary utility and is indeed of historical interest in the diagnostic evaluation of idiopathic facial paralysis. The Schirmer test, along with slit-lamp fluorescein testing for punctate keratopathy, is still performed as part of a global assessment of corneal health. Other than this, topognostic testing is rarely done today because its utility is low compared with that of other tests.

132.6.3 Audiogram

All patients with facial paralysis, regardless of the suspected cause, should have an audiogram with a minimum battery of tests, performed separately for each ear, of pure tones, bone conduction (masked appropriately), word discrimination, and immittance with reflex decay, if the level of hearing permits. Otologic and neurotologic medical and surgical advice must be based upon a reliable audiogram performed by a trained and licensed audiologist.

Otoacoustic emission (OAE) testing and auditory brainstem response (ABR) testing may be considered if the patient is unresponsive or cannot otherwise cooperate with a behavioral audiogram. The OAE test is a "pass or fail" examination and will not detect the presence of audition below about 40 dB. Therefore, its utility is somewhat limited. If facial nerve neuroma is suspected as a part of retrocochlear pathology, the ABR test may be helpful as part of the test battery to determine if hearing can be preserved in the management of a neoplasm affecting the facial nerve.

As has already been described, the middle ear muscle reflexes (immittance) would be expected to be affected in facial paralysis, depending upon the site of the paralysis.

132.6.4 Electrical Testing of the Facial Nerve

The ordinarily possible test battery of the facial nerve is large and includes the following types of tests.

Minimal Excitability Test

This test employs a portable, battery-powered, transcutaneous stimulator of the facial nerve. A Hilger stimulator (WR Medical

Electronics, Stillwater, MN) or similar device is placed on the face near the stylomastoid foramen of both the normal (reference) and affected sides. The lowest stimulus intensity that excites all branches of the nerve on the unaffected side is considered the electrical baseline. A 2.0- to 3.5-mA difference between the normal and affected sides indicates impending denervation of the affected side. Advantages of this technique are its portability, relatively low electric current requirements, and relatively low level of discomfort for the test subject. The disadvantage is that the metric is subjective; the tester must judge that all branches are either moving or not. In addition, the test may excite larger branches more easily than smaller branches and give a false picture of the overall function of the nerve.

Maximal Excitability Test

A transcutaneous electrical device is employed to maximally saturate and stimulate both the unaffected and affected sides of the face. A subjective determination is made that the affected side is (1) the same as the normal side,(2) 50% diminished (minimally affected) when compared with the normal side,(3) 75% diminished (markedly affected) when compared with the normal side, or (4) 100% diminished (completely affected), with an absence of electrical stimulation. The advantage of this test is its ease of application. The obvious disadvantage is that it is a subjective test and lacks a metric to quantify the degree of facial dysfunction.

Supramaximal Tests (Electroneuronography/ Evoked Electromyography)

In electroneuronography (ENOG), a supramaximal stimulation of the facial nerve is applied at its junction with the face at the stylomastoid foramen, and the amplitude of the compound muscle action potential (cMAP) is recorded at the site of greatest amplitude. This technique allows a comparison of the response of the affected side with the unaffected side to be displayed and recorded and may be used to measure the relative integrity of working axons within the nerve. ENOG is very helpful for identifying nerve degeneration and for prognosticating the likelihood of return of function, as well as possible adverse sequelae of the affected nerve. ENOG is of clinical value when a nerve injury is "in evolution"—that is, after wallerian degeneration should have occurred (48 to 72 hours after the onset of paralysis) but within 2 to 3 weeks after the onset of facial paralysis. It is of little value after this time because of the dyssynchrony of fibers within an affected nerve. ENOG is also of secondary importance if any part of the affected side is actively moving, and the clinical examination *always* takes precedence over ENOG.

When used during this window, however, ENOG has been shown to reliably predict good versus poor prognosis for recovery. A 90% threshold is used; patients who retain at least 10% of electrical function on ENOG testing are thought to have a better clinical outcome than those with 10% or less of electrical function.

Because of its ability to offer an objective metric and its relative ease of application, this test now supersedes almost all others in clinical use. It has become the mainstay of clinical practice. Its chief drawback is its learning curve; an inexperienced technician may erroneously stimulate the masseter (V) and obtain falsely encouraging results. These false-positive results occur mainly in children and in patients with very thin necks.

The term *electroneuronography* is synonymous with the term *compound muscle action potential*, which is used more commonly by neurologists.

Electromyography of the Facial Muscles

The response of an individual muscle or its fibers to either the voluntary initiation of movement or electrical stimulation may be recorded at the neuromuscular junction with monopolar (bare-tip) or coaxial (concentric) needle electrodes. Voluntary and spontaneously generated facial motor responses are measured and compared with those in neighboring groups on the affected side and in equivalent groups on the unaffected side.

Quantification in units of electric potential, current flow, or resistance may be used to indicate relative function versus lack of the same in a given muscle group. The greatest utility of electromyography (EMG) is in the measurement of facial nerve integrity and the prognostication of expected return of function in patients with significant neurapraxia, such as after acoustic neuroma dissection, or possible neurotmesis after temporal bone fracture.

EMG recordings made 10 to 14 days after the onset of clinical paralysis reflect the dynamic resting membrane potentials of postsynaptic elements. In this phase, the muscle membrane, deprived of "trophic" substances that are normally transported through the axon, undergoes changes that destabilize the resting potential. These changes produce spontaneous depolarizations reflected in the EMG as fibrillation potentials and are interpreted as indicators of persistent denervation.

Successful reinnervation generates high-frequency polyphasic potentials that increase in amplitude and duration and replace fibrillation potentials. These polyphasic potentials may be used to measure the course of reinnervation.

Magnetic Stimulation

Transcranial electrical stimulation has been performed in an effort to stimulate the facial nerve proximal to a suspected intratemporal lesion, and continuous orthograde stimulation has been used during the dissection of skull base lesions in which the facial nerve is adjacent to the pathologic process. Although less selective than other means of facial nerve stimulation, it has been demonstrated that the stimulation of cortical representations of the facial nerve is possible. This method of facial nerve stimulation has not yet gained widespread use.

Of these tests, ENOG and needle EMG are by far the most frequently utilized clinically. They provide real-time information about the status of the nerve, so that the course of facial paralysis in electrical evolution can be followed and the likelihood of recovery can be predicted.

In practice, in a patient with acute *complete* facial paralysis, most otologists will rely upon ENOG (cMAP) to guide the decision between medical treatment (steroids, antivirals, and lubrication) and surgical decompression of the facial nerve.

132.6.5 Radiographic Evaluation

For patients who have idiopathic facial paralysis *without* accompanying hearing loss, early radiographic imaging is usually not indicated because it will not affect either the clinical decision-making process or the eventual outcome. Because idiopathic facial paralysis (Bell palsy) results in inflammation of the nerve, especially at the meatal foramen, it is expected that magnetic resonance (MR) imaging of the temporal bone and brain will demonstrate enhancement of the nerve. This is usually found and in no way indicates a retrocochlear neoplasm. However, the finding of nerve enhancement does not exclude a retrocochlear neoplasm. It does commit the patient and the third-party payer to a second, follow-up MR imaging session after inflammation would be expected to have subsided, about 6 months later. If hearing in the two ears is equal, it is a waste of time, money, and effort to obtain MR imaging in the *acute* phase because inflammation will cause a positive result. All patients with idiopathic facial paralysis would be expected to recover at least some function. In now famous demographic studies, Peitersen described the natural history of *untreated* (but observed) idiopathic facial paralysis. No one who had truly idiopathic (Bell) palsy was left with a flaccid, adynamic face. Approximately 71% had nearly perfect recovery; 29% had imperfect recovery of either a facial region or synkinesis. One of the important findings of this study was that all patients had some recovery of facial function. Those who had no recovery did not strictly have Bell palsy and were further studied to exclude retrocochlear neoplasia, including facial nerve neuroma and other lesions. For these rare patients, a retrocochlear imaging study would be appropriate at this time, not during the acute inflammatory phase.

If there is asymmetric neurosensory hearing loss, unilateral tinnitus, involvement of another cranial nerve, or any concomitant neurologic deficit, these must be investigated as they would be if facial paralysis were not part of the clinical picture. It is the unilateral hearing loss, tinnitus, or other conditions that drive the retrocochlear investigation, not acute facial weakness.

Facial paralysis occurring in the context of acute or chronic inflammatory or infectious disease should be investigated as the underlying disease would be—that is, ordinarily with computed tomography (CT) of the temporal bone. The expected course of the intratympanic facial nerve is easy to follow in the normal temporal bone. Its expected location may be lost in inflammatory or infectious disease, thus pinpointing the likely site of facial nerve involvement.

Temporal bone trauma is best investigated with CT of the temporal bone. With edge-enhanced studies, the temporal bone may be imaged in any plane, including planes at a right angle to and coaxial to the suspected direction of the injury. Any angle may be imaged with modern scanning equipment. In facial nerve trauma, one wants to best detail the bony architecture as it affects the normal and expected pathway of the intratympanic facial nerve. Ultimately, the decision must be made to observe or to operate, and the CT will better guide this decision than MR imaging. If there is complete loss of hearing along with facial paralysis, one would expect to find a transverse or mixed fracture of the temporal bone involving the otic capsule. If the otic capsule has been spared and if the patient has a conductive pattern of hearing loss, one would expect a longitudinal fracture of the temporal bone. Rarely, a discrete fracture line may be seen pointing to the geniculate ganglion with no other findings. Because the geniculate is "tethered" by the greater superficial petrosal branch, it is a likely site of injury and should be carefully inspected.

132.7 Differential Diagnosis

A complete listing of all the conditions that cause facial paralysis would be enormous, and it is impractical to investigate them in day-to-day clinical practice. It is important for the clinician to think broadly as he or she takes the patient's history and let the patient's story point toward the most likely cause of facial weakness. The time course of facial weakness is probably the most important part of the history. Also of great importance in the history is recurrence: has the patient ever had a similar episode on the same or opposite side? Does the patient have any known metabolic or neurologic problems, such as neurofibroma formation or a family history of these? The common causes of acute facial paralysis are presented in ▶ Table 132.3. For the general otolaryngologist practicing in a community setting, cases of acute facial paralysis will most frequently be Bell palsy (idiopathic) or associated with herpes zoster oticus, infectious/inflammatory conditions including Lyme disease, and temporal bone trauma. Other conditions are included for the sake of completeness but are rarely seen in a community-based practice.

132.8 Treatment

132.8.1 Medical Treatment

The mainstay of medical care for acute facial paralysis is lubrication and passive protection of the cornea, and the administration of corticosteroids. Any oral form of steroid may be chosen, with the dose equivalent of approximately 1 mg of prednisone per kilogram. Regardless of the cosmetic deficit, the patient must be instructed that the real problem at hand is ongoing exposure of the eye, and every effort must be taken to ensure that the cornea is kept moist.

There is controversial and inconclusive but nonetheless suggestive evidence from acute and convalescent serologic studies that idiopathic facial paralysis may be linked to a herpetic infection, especially herpes simplex type 1. Because of this, there is currently little objection to the addition of antiviral medications such as acyclovir and famciclovir to the medical treatment of acute idiopathic facial paralysis. For patients with known herpetic infections, such as Ramsey Hunt syndrome (herpes zoster oticus), antiviral medications would be indicated along with steroids, usually for 5 to 7 days. The patient's hepatic function may need to be monitored for higher or longer dosing regimens.

Rarely, acute facial paralysis may be part of a polyneuropathy involving both the seventh and eighth cranial nerves, as is occasionally seen in Ramsey Hunt syndrome. These patients may require acute hospitalization and sedation to control vertigo.

In addition to artificial tears and salves, many other nonsurgical techniques are readily available to help in acute facial paralysis. The affected eye may be taped shut or may be covered with a clear plastic moisture chamber. This is somewhat bulky but changes the local milieu of the cornea from dry to moist and may be required acutely in exposure keratitis. Patching the eye is less desirable because the levator palpebrae superioris (CN III) remains functional and unopposed and may keep the eyelid open underneath the patch, especially during sleep. The lower lid may be suspended with a thin adhesive tape if tone is absent and ectropion develops. A small fusiform piece of adhesive tape placed above the tarsal crease may help to keep the upper lid in a somewhat ptotic position, thus improving passive closure of the eyelid. Patients are instructed in these local measures, and it is important to enlist the aid of an ophthalmologist to prevent any ocular injuries in the setting of incomplete eye closure.

Parenteral steroid medications are rarely indicated in the treatment of acute facial paralysis. However, they may be indicated in a patient who is hospitalized following traumatic multisystem injury and whose face is not actively moving. Depending upon concomitant injuries and the general state of the patient, it may be desirable to treat with intravenous or intramuscular steroid medication. Similarly, in patients with multiple cranial nerve involvement and vertigo, intravenous treatment with steroids and sedation may be of benefit if nausea and vomiting are severe and persistent.

132.8.2 Surgical Treatment

Eyelid

The oculoplastic literature is replete with various techniques used to protect the cornea in acute paralysis. One need not formally train in oculoplastic surgery to readily and adequately treat acute paralytic corneal exposure. A few simple surgical techniques are easy to master and should be in the armamentarium of any surgeon treating patients with facial paralysis. Most patients will do very well with a temporary tarsorrhaphy or a gold or platinum weight properly placed to counterbalance the levator. The technique of lid loading is straightforward and easy to learn, and it may be performed under straight local anesthesia in an office-based procedure room. However, it is important for the nonophthalmologist to know his or her limits. The Asian paralytic eyelid or an eyelid with in-turning lashes for any reason is a very difficult eyelid to manage. These paralytic eyelids often do poorly with standard, simple surgical techniques, and patients should be referred immediately to the oculoplastic surgeon.

Tarsorrhaphy

Tarsorrhaphy is a static technique of corneal protection. It does not aid in wicking the tear film across the globe. Although it has been the mainstay of treatment of the acutely paretic eyelid, it has largely fallen into disfavor because other, dynamic techniques are readily available. Nonetheless, it is occasionally

Table 132.3 Differential diagnosis of facial paralysis

Etiology	Conditions	
Birth	Forceps delivery Myotonic dystrophy Möbius syndrome (facial diplegia associated with other cranial nerve deficits)	
Trauma	Cerebrocortical injuries Penetrating injury to the middle ear Brainstem injuries	Basilar skull fractures Barotrauma (altitude paralysis, scuba diving)
Neurologic	Opercular syndrome (cortical lesion in facial motor area)	Millard-Gubler syndrome (abducens palsy with contralateral hemiplegia due to lesion in base of the pons involving corticospinal tract)
Infectious	Necrotizing otitis externa Otitis media (acute or chronic)/mastoiditis Meningitis Parotitis Cholesteatoma (acquired or congenital) Chickenpox Herpes zoster oticus (Ramsay Hunt syndrome) HIV/AIDS Syphilis Lyme disease	Influenza Coxsackievirus infection Tuberculosis Mucormycosis Botulism Leprosy Malaria Scleroma
Metabolic	Diabetes mellitus Hyperthyroidism Hypertension	Pregnancy Acute porphyria
Vascular	Embolization for epistaxis (external carotid branches) Anomalous sigmoid sinus Intratemporal aneurysm of internal carotid artery Benign intracranial hypertension	
Neoplastic	Acoustic neuroma Meningioma Parotid tumors (benign or malignant) Sarcoma Facial nerve neuroma Metastatic carcinoma (breast, kidney, lung, prostate, thyroid); malignant melanoma	Fibrous dysplasia Hemangioblastoma Glomus jugulare Neurofibromatosis (von Recklinghausen disease) Hand-Schüller-Christian disease Leukemia
Toxic	Thalidomide (Miehlke syndrome: cranial nerves VI and VII with congenital malformed external ears and deafness) Lead intoxication	Carbon monoxide poisoning
Iatrogenic	Otologic, neurotologic, skull base, head and neck surgery Antitetanus serum Local anesthesia infiltration	Rabies vaccine Dental surgery, mandibular block anesthesia Embolization
Autoimmune/idiopathic	Bell palsy Temporal arteritis Guillan-Barré syndrome (ascending paralysis) Paget disease of bone Melkersson-Rosenthal syndrome (recurrent facial palsy, furrowed tongue [lingua plicata], faciolabial edema) Sarcoidosis (Heerfordt syndrome, uveoparotid fever, periarteritis nodosa, myasthenia gravis)	Multiple sclerosis Amyloidosis Hereditary hypertrophic neuropathy (Charcot-Marie-Tooth disease, Dejerine Sottas disease) Idiopathic thrombocytopenia purpura Osteopetrosis (marble bone disease) Kawasaki disease (infantile acute febrile mucocutaneous lymph node syndrome)

indicated, and the surgeon caring for patients with acute or chronic facial paralysis should understand the technique and be able to perform it.

The rare patient, especially one with a CN V_1 afferent deficit, may suffer from exposure keratitis despite common means of corneal protection. In certain instances, a lateral and/or medial tarsorrhaphy must be performed in order to narrow the area of corneal exposure and still allow frontal vision. The typical patient is elderly with a large, partially resected acoustic neuroma or meningioma extending anteriorly toward the petrous apex and involving the trigeminal nerve. The patient may already have been treated with irradiation or for whatever reason is no longer a candidate for skull base resection. These rare patients must be managed in concert with an ophthalmologist experienced in the care of the cornea.

Temporary

Under local anesthesia and with corneal protection, one or two sutures (e.g., 4–0 silk) are placed in the lateral and/or medial canthal areas between the upper and lower lids. If the need is expected to be temporary, the surgeon need not expose mucosa in order to create a controlled, apposed scar. A lateral tarsorrhaphy will limit lateral gaze; a medial tarsorrhaphy will limit medial gaze. The occasional patient may require both medial and lateral tarsorrhaphies. In this case, the field of vision will be severely limited.

Permanent

The technique is the same as that for temporary tarsorrhaphy with a few modifications. A small (2 × 3 or 4 mm) strip of skin and mucosa is removed from the upper and lower lids in the area of the intended tarsorrhaphy (lateral and/or medial). One or two mattress sutures are placed (with or without silicon bolsters) to appose the raw surfaces. These are left in place for 7 to 10 days, then removed in the office. The result should be a controlled and healed apposition of the upper and lower lids. Permanent tarsorrhaphy is indicated when an insensate cornea and paretic eyelid place the cornea at extreme risk.

Palpebral Spring

A palpebral spring may be thought of as an open safety pin under the upper eyelid. Because the levator muscle (CN III) is almost always normal and unopposed, the eyelid will have normal opening forces. These opening forces are opposed by a spring, made from biocompatible material (usually gold) and inserted under the upper lid to force it into the closed position This technique, although straightforward and relatively simple, in most cases requires revision because of slippage of the spring or because of the changing needs of opposing force as the eyelid recovers motor function. In large measure, it has been replaced by lid-loading techniques.

Lid Loading

The paralytic eyelid over time will be more and more at risk for exposure because the levator palpebrae superioris is unopposed and usually normal. Over time, the cornea will become progressively exposed and dry. In normal function, the tear film is actively pumped and wicked across the globe, as has been previously described. This process is diminished or absent in facial paralysis. Various techniques of loading the upper lid with various materials or implanting springs have been developed in an effort to counteract the tonic retraction of the unopposed levator. Although none of these methods is perfect when compared with normal, active eyelid closure or blink, some very simple techniques offer the patient with an affected cornea immediate benefit.

The most important technique is lid loading with a bar of pure (24-kt) gold or platinum weighing 0.6 to 1.6 g; weights are in increments of 0.2 g. The bar to be implanted is either taped or affixed to the paralytic eyelid with a temporary fixative, usually tincture of benzoin or double-sided adhesive tape. The patient is placed in a sitting position and is asked to relax the eyelid. The patient makes a decision about the most comfortable weight; the surgeon chooses the weight providing the best closure. Topical corneal anesthesia is provided with drops (0.5% tetracaine), and the lid is injected with 1% lidocaine with epinephrine 1:100,000. This outpatient procedure may be done under straight local anesthesia, with or without intravenous

sedation. Most patients will require a 1.0- to 1.2-g weight. The gold or platinum bar is implanted in a small pocket made at or above the level of the tarsal crease and is suture-fixed to the pretarsal soft tissue. A layered closure of the orbicularis oculi and skin must be performed because the foreign body (gold or platinum bar) crosses an incision line. When the eyelid is relaxed, gravity will allow the upper lid to close. It is important for the patient to be told that this technique provides better passive closure in the sitting or standing position, less so in the supine position. When facial function returns, the eyelid may feel excessively heavy because the now-functioning orbicularis oculi is reinforced with the weight. At this time, after consultation with the ophthalmologist, the weight may be removed.

Canthoplasty for Ectropion Repair

The paralytic lower eyelid may become ptotic over time and lead to further exposure of the cornea. Epiphora may become an additional problem due to sagging of the paralytic lower lid. This is especially so in patients age 55 and older in whom the normal supportive and elastic properties of the face have already weakened. For patients with facial paralysis who are older than 50 years of age, ectropion formation should be anticipated and the lower lid supported with a small lateral canthoplasty. This technique is easy to understand and master. The arch of the upper lid is drawn downward for about 6 mm. A line 4 to 5 mm medial to the lateral canthus is also drawn. The lower lid is injected with local anesthetic. The incisions to be made are grasped with straight hemostats placed in the inferior fornix, and the small triangle so clamped is removed. The inferior tarsal plate/lateral canthal tendon is supported with a suture of 5–0 clear nylon or other permanent suture placed at the lateral canthal tubercle. The skin is closed with interrupted sutures of 5–0 fast-absorbing gut.

Facial Nerve Decompression

Decompression of the facial nerve in the acute time period remains controversial. The main questions to be answered are the following: (1) In the acute situation, does facial nerve decompression *significantly* improve the outcome of facial paralysis over standard medical management? (2) Which patient should be selected for facial nerve decompression?

Very few well-designed, prospective, randomized clinical studies with large numbers of patients have attempted to answer these questions. The important work of Peitersen in studying the natural history of untreated idiopathic facial paralysis should loom large in the mind of any surgeon contemplating decompression of the facial nerve for a patient with Bell palsy. A further confounding factor is that the metric for the most part is *subjective* (i.e., the House-Brackmann or Fisch classification system). There is no universal, easy-to-apply objective system for measuring facial movement or expression, and electrical testing of the facial nerve is of value only within the first 10 to 14 days after the onset of facial paralysis.

For surgeons interested in this field, the seminal work of Professor Fisch must be carefully studied and mastered, with the acknowledgment that the numbers of patients both observed and treated are not large. In addition, to be recalled is that the outcome grading of facial movement was better by the surgeon and worse by the patient, the person with the problem. In general, based upon his work in patients with *idiopathic* facial paralysis, a window of opportunity of approximately 2 weeks exists between the onset of clinical paralysis (not paresis) and electrical degeneration of 90% or more by ENOG testing in which decompression of the facial nerve (and especially the meatal segment of the facial nerve) will beneficially affect the clinical outcome of the nerve. Both the time window and indication for decompression remain controversial in cases of acute idiopathic facial paralysis.

Of less controversy are cases of traumatic facial paralysis and, for many surgeons, herpes zoster oticus.

Patients with temporal bone trauma may be treated in the same way as those with Bell palsy, depending upon the timing of observation of the face, as has been previously described.

The natural history of facial function after herpes zoster oticus is bleak for patients with both clinical and electric paralysis. Approximately 50 to 60% of patients with facial paralysis due to herpes zoster oticus will have adverse sequelae: lack of reinnervation and/or synkinesis. Because of the poor natural history of herpes zoster oticus, the case for surgical decompression may be more compelling in patients with this condition than in those with idiopathic facial paralysis.

Delayed Surgery for the Eye

The various techniques previously described may be used for patients with chronic facial paralysis. What may not be delayed is adequate lubrication and protection of the cornea. For patients with facial paralysis for 3 weeks or longer, it is wise to consult with an ophthalmologist experienced in corneal care to offer guidance about corneal health and the risk for exposure keratitis.

Patients with chronic facial paralysis and brow ptosis may have severely limited field vision on the affected side. The paretic eyelid may retract under the ptotic brow (lateral hooding) and cause poor natural toilet of the cornea. All of these factors may predispose the eye to blepharitis, chronic conjunctivitis, and further infection. In the chronic state, the needs and level of activity of the patient, such as driving and reading, must be taken into account. The vision in both the affected and unaffected eyes should be carefully evaluated. The elderly patient may have cataract formation that will require treatment. Glaucoma may be found in one or both eyes. The overall health of the eye must be evaluated along with the requirements of facial movement.

When indicated, the ptotic brow may be lifted with a variety of straightforward techniques (endoscopically, directly above the brow line, or through a re-created forehead crease; see Chapter 56). The lifted brow will now be in a more neutral position just above the level of the superior orbital rim and allow the upper lid to be seen. The upper lid may require lid loading at this time to counterbalance the chronic retraction of the levator oculi. The lower lid may have undergone ectropion formation that may require correction. An experienced ophthalmologist must be consulted to help thoroughly evaluate the vision in both eyes, as well as the overall needs and goals of the patient.

Face

Many techniques exist for facial reanimation. The surgical catalogue is far too great to describe in detail for the purposes of this summary. The interested reader is referred Chapter 51 for further discussion.

Synkinesis after return of facial function may be relieved with the selective use of botulinum toxin (Botox; Allergan, Irvine, CA) to chemically denervate unwanted facial movement temporarily. If desired, a more permanent selective denervation may be achieved either chemically (with phenol or absolute alcohol) or surgically.

There is no surgical technique of facial reanimation that will *equal* a working, normal facial nerve. Reconstructive procedures are in essence attempts to restore facial symmetry (static procedures) or isolated and/or regional facial movement (dynamic procedures), but the patient will never possess the subtlety of mimetic facial expression provided by a normal, functioning facial nerve. This fact must be clearly understood by the patient (and physician) so that reasonable goals and expectations may be achieved. It is always better to underplay intended surgical results and have a delighted patient than to overstate them and have a disappointed one. Neither physician nor patient should yield to magical, unrealistic thinking.

The physician must carefully attend to the history and time course of the paralysis and the functional needs and goals of the patient. Consultation with other physicians and surgeons in related disciplines, especially ophthalmology, may be required to achieve the best overall plan for the patient. With all of these techniques, the best plan for restoring facial function to the individual who has facial paralysis may be reached.

132.9 Case Examples

132.9.1 Case 1: Recurrent Bell Palsy

A 13-year-old girl presented with a 7-day history of left facial paralysis. A prior episode of facial paralysis on the same side had occurred about 2 years prior. There were no other contributing findings: no fissuring of the tongue and no vesicles around the ear or in the nasopharynx. The hearing was within normal limits by tuning fork and audiometric examination. The left ipsilateral and right contralateral acoustic reflexes were absent, as expected. She had no facial movement on the left side (H-B VI/VI), but an intact Bell reflex (► Fig. 132.2). ENOG was obtained and showed complete degeneration of the left facial nerve (► Fig. 132.3). Nonenhanced CT of the petrous temporal bones was normal. Because by history she had recurrent facial paralysis, her parents were instructed that a surgical decompression of the left facial nerve would be advisable in order to increase the chances of a good outcome and help prevent recurrent episodes of left facial paralysis. They agreed to this and gave consent for the procedure. The patient underwent surgical decompression of the complete facial nerve (► Fig. 132.4). She healed well and has a very slight weakness of the left ramus mandibularis as her only sequela (► Fig. 132.5). She has been followed for longer than 10 years and has had no subsequent episodes of facial paralysis.

132.9.2 Case 2: Herpes Zoster Oticus

A 32-year-old man presented with right facial paralysis of 2 weeks' duration. He had no active eyelid closure and severe right facial dysfunction (H-B VI/VI). The facial paralysis had

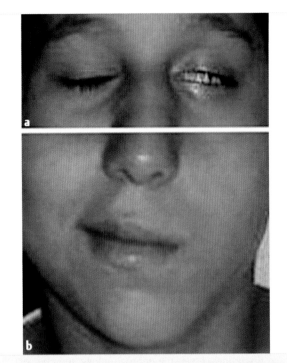

Fig. 132.2 Case 1. (a,b) Left facial paralysis with an intact Bell reflex.

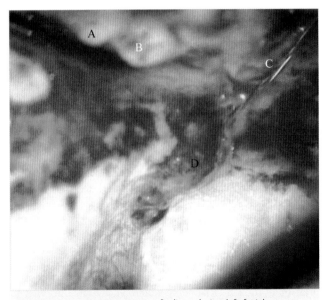

Fig. 132.4 Case 1: Intraoperative findings during left facial nerve decompression. *A*, head of malleus; *B*, short process of incus; *C*, left geniculate ganglion; *D*, labyrinthine segment of left facial nerve.

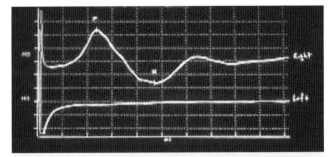

Fig. 132.3 Case 1: Electroneuronogram shows 100% degeneration of left facial nerve function.

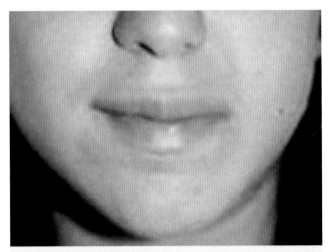

Fig. 132.5 Case 1: Postoperative result.

was normal, as was his level of audition. ENOG was obtained, which showed 64% degeneration of the seventh cranial nerve on the right (▶ Fig. 132.7).

The patient had previously been started on very low doses of corticosteroids, which were changed to prednisone 60 mg/d for 10 days with tapering thereafter. He had already been treated with famciclovir 2 g/d for 7 days, which was not continued. The patient was using artificial tears during the day and lubrication at night, but he still had excessive dryness of the right eye during the day. A gold weight was inserted in the right upper lid under local anesthesia approximately 1 week after presentation. Serial ENOG never revealed degeneration of the right facial nerve of more than 62%. At the second week after presentation, a slight twitch of motion was detected in the right frontalis region. The right side of the face returned to normal function without synkinesis. Patient has now been followed for at least 3 years and is normal with an H-B I classification.

132.9.3 Case 3: Temporal Bone Trauma (Gunshot Wound)

A 27-year-old man was brought to a New York City emergency room after sustaining a gunshot wound to the right side of his face at close range (▶ Fig. 132.8). He was unconscious on arrival

been preceded by an eruption of blisters around his right ear and lower face in the distribution of right CN V₁, and the patient presented to the office 8 days after the onset of facial paralysis.

The otoscopic examination was normal. The patient had a few healing blisters (▶ Fig. 132.6) around the right ear, none in the oropharynx or nasopharynx. The tuning fork test at 512 Hz

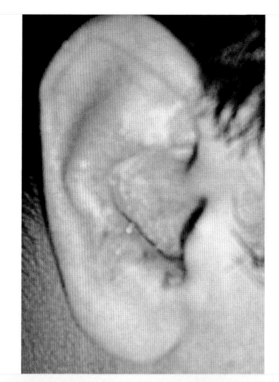

Fig. 132.6 Case 2: Vesicular eruption in the inferior right concha.

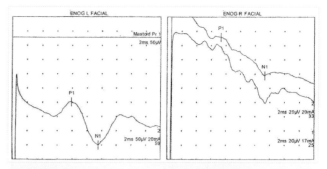

Fig. 132.7 Case 2: Electroneuronogram 3 days after the onset of right facial paralysis, showing partial degeneration of the right facial nerve. *ENOG*, electroneuronogram.

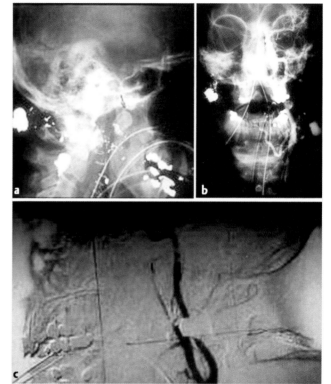

Fig. 132.9 Case 3: (a) Lateral and (b) frontal plain X-rays of the face and neck, with shrapnel in the right mastoid and left neck. (c) Angiogram of the left carotid artery, with shrapnel at the site of a pseudoaneurysm.

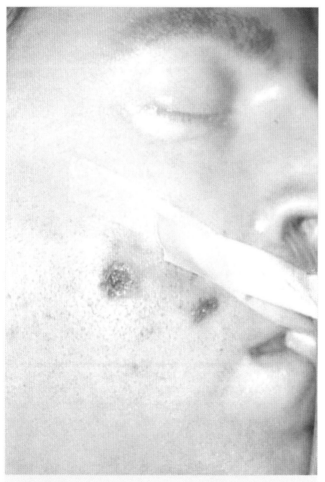

Fig. 132.8 Case 3: Gunshot wound to the right side of the face.

and was intubated and treated by the trauma team for vascular injuries to the right and left carotid arteries. The entry site of the bullet was seen on the right cheek. Plain films of the head and neck showed bullet fragments in the right mastoid, as well as around the bifurcation of the left common carotid artery (▶ Fig. 132.9). After he regained consciousness, a complete right facial paralysis was noted. The patient subsequently underwent a right tympanoplasty with mastoidectomy, evacuation of shrapnel in the mastoid and right and left neck, and a modified right neck dissection. The right facial nerve had been injured by the bullet, and a reparative neuroma in formation was noted and excised. The proximal and distal ends of the facial nerve were found and freshened; a gap of about 2.5 cm was left. A

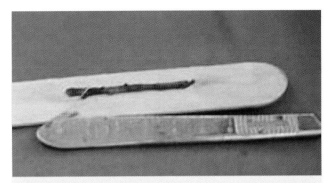

Fig. 132.10 Case 3: Segment of the great auricular nerve for grafting.

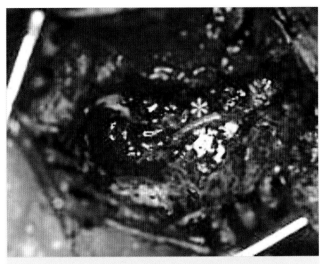

Fig. 132.11 Case 3: Interposition graft in place (*asterisk*).

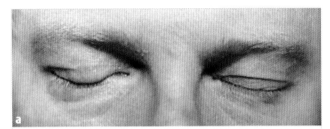

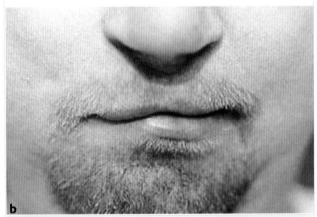

Fig. 132.12 Case 3: Postoperative views of (**a**) eye closure (right gold weight in place) and (**b**) closed-lip smile. Note the relative flattening of the right nasolabial fold, droopy right upper lip, and inward curl of the right lower lip.

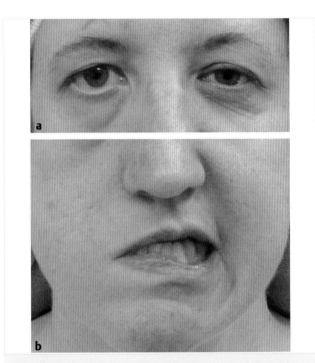

Fig. 132.13 Case 4: Preoperative view of right facial paralysis. (**a**) Close-up view of eyes shows ptosis of the right upper lid with rounding and malposition of the right lower lid. (**b**) Paralysis of the lower right face.

right great auricular nerve interposition graft was harvested (▸ Fig. 132.10) and was sutured in place in an end-to-end fashion (▸ Fig. 132.11). This patient also underwent placement of a gold weight in the right upper lid and a right lower lid shortening procedure at the same sitting.

The patient had additionally sustained significant injuries to his right external auditory canal and right temporomandibular joint and had to have subsequent surgery to repair these sites. He regained function to an H-B III/VI level with significant synkinesis (▸ Fig. 132.12). After removal of the injured tympanic ring and a wide meatoplasty, there was closure of the conductive deficit in the right ear to within 10 dB.

132.9.4 Case 4: Cholesteatoma

A 39-year-old woman presented with a 6-week history of worsening facial nerve function and hearing loss on the right. By the time she was seen, she had no active facial movement in any part of the right side of her face (▸ Fig. 132.13) and no hearing in the right ear by tuning fork examination.

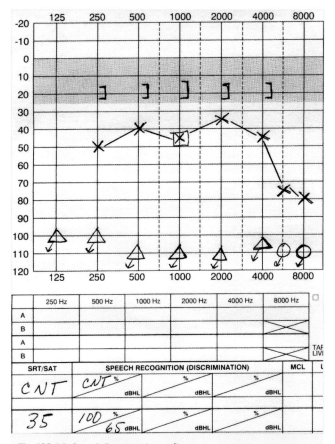

Fig. 132.14 Case 4: Preoperative audiogram.

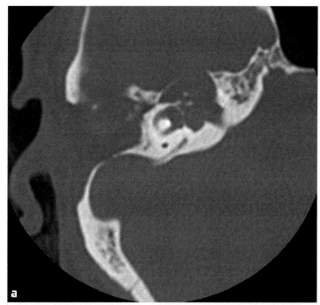

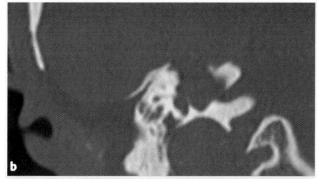

Fig. 132.15 Case 4: (a) Axial and (b) coronal computed tomographic scans demonstrating a large petrous apex lesion.

Two years before being seen, she had undergone two separate surgeries in Denmark to control "ear disease," the first on the left and the second on the right. The left ear became dry, and she was wearing a behind-the-ear hearing aid on this side. During the surgery on the right side, a cerebrospinal fluid (CSF) leak had occurred, and she subsequently underwent repair of the CSF leak and overclosure of the right ear with abdominal fat. She reported a right facial weakness at the time of these two surgeries that subsequently recovered.

An audiogram showed no measurable hearing on the right (▶ Fig. 132.14) and a mixed hearing loss on the left at 35 dB/ 100% word recognition score. The left canal-wall-down ear was safe and dry.

CT of the petrous temporal bones without contrast revealed an overclosed right ear with postoperative changes and a large tegmen defect of approximately 2 x 2 cm. The temporal lobe retained its normal contour. Soft tissue was seen immediately inferior to the temporal lobe, likely representing a fat graft. The right petrous apex was scalloped, and the normal appearance of the cochlea and intratympanic facial nerve was distorted. The normal bony appearance of the internal auditory canal was lost, with scalloping (▶ Fig. 132.15).

Images of the left temporal bone showed postsurgical changes consistent with a canal-wall-down technique. The otic

capsule was intact, and there were no erosive changes of the petrous apex, as seen on the right.

MR imaging of the brain without and with gadolinium enhancement showed findings similar to those on CT, including an intact right temporal dura and a low-lying temporal lobe. Soft tissue immediately under the temporal lobe had the signal characteristics of fat; the signal within the right petrous apex was of low intensity on T1-weighted images and brighter on T2-weighted images, supporting the diagnosis of cholesteatoma of the petrous apex (▶ Fig. 132.16).

Within a week of being seen, the patient underwent placement of a right upper lid gold weight and lateral canthoplasty, and she subsequently underwent a combined neurotologic/ neurosurgical procedure. After placement of a lumbar drain, a middle fossa craniectomy was performed. The tegmen defect was exposed from below and above. A small dural dehiscence was suture-repaired, and the tegmen defect, which was larger than anticipated, was repaired with a 5 x 3-cm calvarial bone and tensor fasciae latae graft in an extradural fashion (▶ Fig. 132.17).

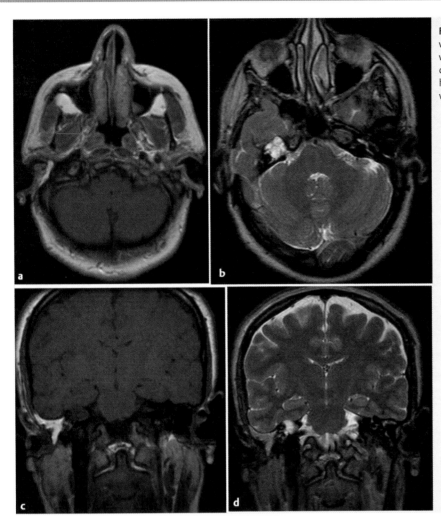

Fig. 132.16 Case 4: (a) T1-weighted and (b) T2-weighted axial and (c) T1-weighted and (d) T2-weighted coronal magnetic resonance images demonstrating low-intensity signals on T1 and high-intensity signals on T2 images, consistent with cholesteatoma of the right petrous apex.

After the temporal lobe had been reduced, a cholesteatoma within the right petrous apex was immediately seen. Because the right ear had no measurable hearing, a right translabyrinthine approach was used to exteriorize the cholesteatoma. The usual landmarks of the otic capsule and tympanic facial nerve were gone. All visible cholesteatoma and its accompanying matrix were carefully removed. The bone surrounding the internal auditory canal was weak and decalcified. At the level of the internal auditory canal, a CSF leak was again encountered, and this was stopped with a single piece of tensor fasciae latae, a fat graft, and fibrin glue. Facial nerve function is not expected, and the patient will likely require a microneurovascular muscle graft (see Chapter 51).

132.10 Conclusion

More than any other patient, the patient presenting with acute, subacute, or chronic facial paresis/paralysis may challenge the treating physician with the complexity of the required fact finding, investigations, and diagnostic and therapeutic planning. Because of the complex nature of the facial nerve (a combined nerve) and its long course through the temporal bone, the etiologies of facial nerve compression and paralysis are numerous and varied.

132.11 Roundsmanship

- A thorough and careful history will almost always point toward the correct pathway for an investigation of facial paralysis.
- The facial nerve must be viewed in light of the whole patient, and especially the function of the inner ear.
- Regardless of the patient's cosmetic concerns, the affected eye and specifically the cornea are of primary concern. Attention should be focused upon eye care. In many cases, ophthalmologic intervention will be required, most especially in the patient with a concomitant afferent sensory deficit.
- Once a facial nerve completely loses function, it is highly unlikely that recovery will be perfect. Sequelae such as synkinesis and regional paresis may occur, and the patient must be so informed.
- Timely surgical decompression of the facial nerve in the appropriate patient who has both clinical and electrical degeneration of the nerve remains a viable option and should be offered. Time is of the essence, with surgical intervention undetaken no more than approximately 2 to 3 weeks after the onset of paralysis.
- Traumatic injury to the facial nerve is the most compelling reason for surgical decompression.

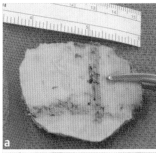
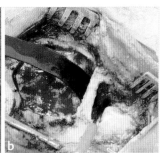
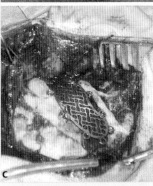

Fig. 132.17 Case 4: Repair of a right tegmen defect with calvarial bone graft (full thickness). (**a**) Bone graft design. (**b**) Right middle fossa and transmastoid view of tegmen defect. Retractor is protecting the temporal lobe, and the Freer elevator instrument points to the petrous apex. (**c**) Following repair of the right tegmen defect with bone, tensor fasciae latae, and titanium mesh.

132.12 Recommended Reading

[1] Donaldson JA, Duckert LG, Lambert PM, Rubel EW. Surgical Anatomy of the Temporal Bone. New York, NY: Raven Press; 1992

[2] Fisch U, Esslen E. Total intratemporal exposure of the facial nerve. Pathologic findings in Bell's palsy. Arch Otolaryngol 1972; 95: 335–341

[3] Fisch U. Surgery for Bell's palsy. Arch Otolaryngol 1981; 107: 1–11

[4] Fisch U. Prognostic value of electrical tests in acute facial paralysis. Am J Otol 1984; 5: 494–498

[5] Gantz BJ, Rubinstein JT, Gidley P, Woodworth GG. Surgical management of Bell's palsy. Laryngoscope 1999; 109: 1177–1188

[6] House JW, Brackmann DE. Facial nerve grading system. Otolaryngol Head Neck Surg 1985; 93: 146–147

[7] Linder TE, Pike VE, Linstrom CJ. Early eyelid rehabilitation in facial nerve paralysis. Laryngoscope 1996; 106: 1115–1118

[8] May M. The Facial Nerve. New York, NY: Thieme Medical Publishers; 1986

[9] Meier-Gallati V, Scriba H, Fisch U. Objective scaling of facial nerve function based on area analysis (OSCAR). Otolaryngol Head Neck Surg 1998; 118: 545–550

[10] Peitersen E. The natural history of Bell's palsy. Am J Otol 1982; 4: 107–111

[11] Sillman JS, Niparko JK, Lee SS, Kileny PR. Prognostic value of evoked and standard electromyography in acute facial paralysis. Otolaryngol Head Neck Surg 1992; 107: 377–381

133 Anatomy of the Skull Base and Infratemporal Fossa

Maura K. Cosetti and Christopher J. Linstrom

133.1 Introduction

The skull base, or floor of the intracranial cavity, is a complex anatomical region that forms the border between the brain and the structures of the face and upper neck. A basic understanding of skull base anatomy is critical for the accurate diagnosis and effective management of lesions in this area. For otolaryngologists and neurosurgeons alike, treatment planning and surgical decision making depend on the relationship between the disease process or lesion and the adjacent intracranial and neurovascular structures.

The skull base is composed of five bones: the frontal, ethmoid, temporal, sphenoid, and occipital; of these, the frontal and temporal bones are paired. Each bone houses multiple foramina (▶ Table 133.1) traversed by cranial nerves (CNs) I through XII (▶ Table 133.2) and by arteries and veins (described in detail in the following sections). A knowledge of the contents, locations, and relationships of these neurovascular foramina is crucial in both diagnosing and treating skull base disease, as well as in understanding routes of spread of intracranial and extracranial disease.

Clinically and anatomically, bony landmarks divide the cranial base into three general regions—the anterior, middle, and posterior fossae (▶ Fig. 133.1). The anterior fossa and middle fossa are separated by the lesser wings of the sphenoid bone and the planum sphenoidale, while the dorsum sellae, posterior

clinoid processes, and petrous temporal ridges separate the middle fossa from the posterior fossa. The skull base is longest in the anterior–posterior diameter and thinnest in the craniocaudal direction, measuring only 3 to 5 mm in all areas except the petrous temporal bone. This chapter will describe the anatomical boundaries, contents, and pertinent extracranial relationships of the anterior, middle, and posterior fossae. Important anatomical–clinical correlations will be highlighted. The anatomical borders, contents, and pertinent intracranial relationships of the infratemporal fossae will also be discussed.

133.2 Anterior Skull Base

133.2.1 Borders and Foramina

The anterior cranial fossa is bordered anteriorly by the orbital portion of the frontal bone, posteriorly by the lesser wing and body of the sphenoid bone, and centrally by the cribriform plate of the ethmoid bone. Bilaterally, the frontal bone forms the lateral boundary of the anterior cranial fossa and houses the supraorbital foramen. The central cribriform plate is the deepest and thinnest portion of the anterior cranial fossa and contains 15 to 20 small foramina that transmit the olfactory nerves (CN I) from the olfactory bulb intracranially to the superior nasal mucosa. In the anteromedial portion of the cribriform pate is the crista galli, a superiorly directed bony projection between

Table 133.1 Foramina of the skull base

Intracranial foramen	Bone(s) involved	Structure(s) transmitted
Anterior cranial fossa		
Cribriform plate	Ethmoid	CN I
Middle cranial fossa		
Optic canal	Sphenoid	CN II, ophthalmic artery
Superior orbital fissure	Sphenoid	CNs III, IV, V$_1$, VI; superior ophthalmic vein
Foramen rotundum	Sphenoid	CN V$_2$
Foramen ovale	Sphenoid	CN V$_3$, accessory meningeal artery, lesser petrosal nerve, emissary vein
Foramen spinosum	Sphenoid	Middle meningeal artery and vein
Foramen lacerum[a]		
Posterior cranial fossa		
Internal auditory meatus (porus acusticus)	Temporal	CNs VII, VIII; internal auditory artery and vein
Jugular foramen	Occipital, temporal	CNs IX, X, XI; internal jugular vein; inferior petrosal sinus
Foramen magnum	Occipital	Medulla oblongata, spinal root of CN XI, vertebral artery and vein, anterior and posterior spinal arteries and veins
Hypoglossal canal	Occipital	CN XII

Abbreviation: CN, cranial nerve.
[a]The foramen lacerum is not a true foramen. It is located at the junction of the sphenoid, temporal, and occipital bones and is covered by cartilage. The greater and deep petrosal nerves and the internal carotid artery pass over its intracranial surface.

Table 133.2 Cranial nerves and their function

Cranial nerve	Type of nerve	Function
Olfactory (I)	Sensory	Special visceral afferent for smell
Optic (II)	Sensory	Special visceral afferent for vision
Oculomotor (III)	Motor	All extraocular muscles except superior oblique and lateral rectus; striated muscle of the eyelid; pupillary constrictors
Trochlear (IV)	Motor	Superior oblique muscle; moves globe down and outward
Trigeminal (V)	Mixed	V_1: sensory to the upper face, nasal cavity, ethmoid and sphenoid sinuses V_2: sensory to the midface, hard and soft palate, maxillary sinus, maxillary dentition and gums V_3: motor to muscles of mastication, anterior belly of the digastric, mylohyoid, tensor tympani, tensor palatini; sensory to lower face and jaw, mandibular dentition and gums; taste to anterior two-thirds of the tongue (from CN VII) Autonomic[a]
Abducens (VI)	Motor	Lateral rectus muscle; moves globe laterally
Facial (VII)	Mixed	Motor: muscles of facial expression, stapedius, stylohyoid, posterior belly of digastric Sensory: taste sensation from anterior two-thirds of tongue carried via CN V_3 and chorda tympani Autonomic: parasympathetic fibers originate in nervus intermedius and travel via chorda tympani and greater superficial petrosal nerve to tongue; lacrimal gland; submandibular, sublingual, and lingual salivary glands
Vestibulocochlear (VIII)	Sensory	Cochlear nerve: hearing Superior and inferior vestibular nerves: balance
Glossopharyngeal (IX)	Mixed	Motor: pharyngeal musculature, parotid gland Sensory: taste sensation from posterior one-third of tongue; sensation from pharynx and tympanic cavity; visceral afferent from carotid sinus and body Autonomic: parasympathetic to parotid gland
Vagus (X)	Mixed	Motor: striated muscles in larynx, pharynx, and soft palate; palatoglossus muscle of tongue; smooth muscles in heart, blood vessels, trachea, bronchi, esophagus, stomach, small and large intestine Sensory: taste sensation from epiglottis; sensory from external ear canal, tympanic membrane, pharynx, larynx, thoracic and abdominal viscera Autonomic: parasympathetic to abdominal and thoracic viscera
Spinal accessory (XI)	Motor	Trapezius and sternocleidomastoid muscles
Hypoglossal (XII)	Motor	All muscles of tongue except palatoglossus (CN X)

Abbreviation: CN, cranial nerve.

[a]Parasympathetic neurons do not originate in CN V; however, branches of CN V are used as carriers for the peripheral distribution of parasympathetic input from CNs VII and IX.

the cerebral hemispheres onto which the falx cerebri attaches. Anterior to the crista galli is the foramen caecum, a variable opening in the frontoethmoidal suture line through which a nasal emissary vein may communicate with the intracranial superior sagittal sinus. Immediately lateral to the cribriform plate is the fovea ethmoidalis, or roof of the ethmoid cavity. The fovea is thicker and frequently more superior than the adjacent cribriform plate, although anatomical variance in this area is common. Knowledge of these relationships and individual patient anatomy is an essential component of presurgical planning in both intranasal sinus surgery and the extirpation of anterior skull base lesions. At the anterolateral and posterolateral aspects of the cribriform plate, the anterior and posterior ethmoidal branches of the ophthalmic artery, respectively, exit the intracranial cavity to enter the nasal cavity. Posteriorly, the cribriform plate of the ethmoid bone articulates with the central portion, or body, of the sphenoid bone, forming the planum sphenoidale. The optic chiasm or chiasmatic sits in the midline, while posterolaterally, the lesser wings of the sphenoid form the anterior clinoid processes and the roof of the optic canals.

133.2.2 Contents

The contents of the anterior cranial fossa include the frontal lobes of the brain, olfactory bulbs and tracts, and inferior and superior sagittal sinuses. The olfactory nerve (CN I) is a primary afferent sensory nerve consisting of bipolar neurons with short peripheral and long central projections. The peripheral olfactory receptor cells are located in the superior 2-cm^2 aspect of each nasal cavity, adjacent to the cribriform plate, superior nasal septum, and superior–lateral nasal wall. Hundreds of central processes traverse the cribriform plate as unmyelinated fascicles, or fila olfactoria, with approximately 20 fila or olfactory nerves on each side of the crista galli. These nerves culminate centrally in the ipsilateral olfactory bulb, an extension of the brain on the ventral surface of the frontal lobe closely apposed to the cribriform plate. Disruption of this region by trauma, planned anterior skull base surgery, or unintentional iatrogenic injury during endoscopic sinus surgery can lead to cerebrospinal fluid (CSF) leak as well as disorders of smell, such as anosmia or hyposmia (inability or decreased ability, respectively, to

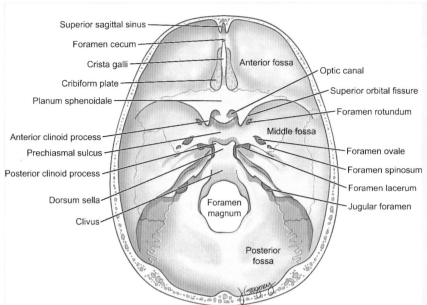

Fig. 133.1 Internal aspect of the skull base, with division into three distinct fossae.

Labels on figure:
Superior sagittal sinus
Foramen cecum
Crista galli
Cribiform plate
Planum sphenoidale
Anterior fossa
Optic canal
Superior orbital fissure
Foramen rotundum
Anterior clinoid process
Middle fossa
Prechiasmal sulcus
Foramen ovale
Posterior clinoid process
Foramen spinosum
Foramen lacerum
Dorsum sella
Jugular foramen
Clivus
Foramen magnum
Posterior fossa

detect odors). Following synapse in the olfactory bulb, secondary sensory neurons course posteriorly along the ventral frontal lobe as the olfactory tract. The venous contents of the anterior cranial fossa have implications for the intracranial spread of infection. The dural attachments to the frontal crest and the crista galli form the falx cerebri, which transmits the inferior and superior sagittal sinuses. These valveless venous channels drain the brain, meninges, and diploic spaces within the cranial bones, ultimately forming the internal jugular vein. In the anterior cranial fossa, the veins of Brechet, which are valveless, diploic veins of the posterior frontal bone, provide a venous route for the intracranial spread of frontal sinus infections. Patency of the foramen caecum, anterior to the crista galli, is the anatomical basis for developmental nasal anomalies such as nasal gliomas, encephaloceles, and meningoencephaloceles.

133.2.3 Extracranial Relationships

The major extracranial relationships of the anterior cranial fossa are with the orbits and paranasal sinuses. As previously described, the floor of the anterior cranial fossa serves as the roof of the orbits and the ethmoid and sphenoid sinuses and abuts the posterior wall of the frontal sinuses. Neoplastic lesions in these regions, such as esthesioneuroblastoma (a rare neoplasm originating from olfactory neuroepithelium), may extend into the anterior cranial fossa from below, whereas primarily intracranial processes may progress in the reverse direction. These relationships can also be exploited for surgical planning and used as routes of access to the anterior intracranial cavity.

The close proximity of the bony orbit to the anterior cranial and infratemporal fossae provides multiple routes for the transmission of intracranial or extracranial disease, including the posterior orbital foramina, such as the superior and inferior orbital fissures and the optic canals. Technically situated in the middle cranial fossa, the contents of the superior orbital fissure include the oculomotor nerve (CN III), trochlear nerve (CN IV), abducens nerve (CN VI), ophthalmic branch of the trigeminal nerve (CN V_1), and ophthalmic veins. The inferior orbital (in-

fraorbital) fissure transmits the maxillary branch of the trigeminal nerve (CN V_2) and infraorbital vessels, and unlike the superior orbital fissure, it communicates directly with the infratemporal and pterygomaxillary fossae. The optic canal contains the optic nerve (CN II) and ophthalmic artery.

133.3 Middle Skull Base

133.3.1 Borders

The middle cranial fossa is separated from the anterior skull base by the posterior aspect of the planum sphenoidale medially and by the lesser wings of the sphenoid bone laterally. The anterior wall and floor are formed by the greater wings and body of the sphenoid bone, while the posterior floor is composed of the anterior aspect of the petrous temporal bone. Laterally, the middle fossa is bounded by the squamous portion of the temporal bone and the anterior–inferior portion of the parietal bone. Posteriorly, the middle and posterior fossae are demarcated by the posterior clinoid processes medially and the petrous ridge of the temporal bone laterally. The petro-occipital fissure, a gap between the medial border of the petrous bone and the lateral border of the clivus, subdivides the middle cranial fossa into a central and two lateral compartments. Easily seen on radiologic imaging, this is an important landmark in preoperative surgical planning because of its close relationship with various middle fossa foramina.

Centrally located between the anterior and posterior clinoid processes, the sella turcica (Latin for "Turkish saddle") occupies the central compartment of the middle fossa and has three distinct regions (▶ Fig. 133.2). Anteriorly to posteriorly, these include the tuberculum sellae, which is an olive-shaped bony protuberance between the optic canals; the hypophyseal or pituitary fossa, which is a deep central depression that houses the pituitary gland; and the dorsum sellae. The dorsum sellae contains the sigmoid groove for the internal carotid artery as it navigates the middle fossa floor through the petrous apex into the cavernous sinus.

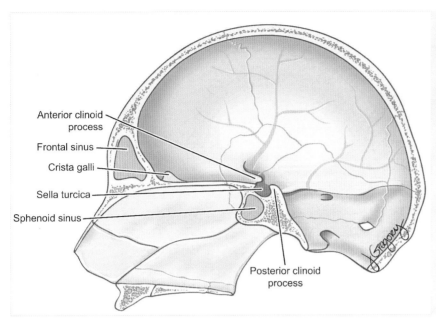

Fig. 133.2 Anatomical relationships near the sella turcica.

Anterior clinoid process

Frontal sinus

Crista galli

Sella turcica

Sphenoid sinus

Posterior clinoid process

Along the floor and lateral walls of the middle fossa, a groove for the middle meningeal artery is typically visible where it courses superoposteriorly and traverses the intracranial side of the pterion (an area of very thin bone where the parietal, squamous temporal, and frontal bones and the greater sphenoid wings meet). The pterion is easily fractured by head trauma, and resulting disruption of the middle meningeal artery is a common cause of epidural hematoma. The petrous ridge, or crest, along the superior aspect of the temporal bone demarcates the posterior boundary of the middle cranial fossa. In a depression on the superomedial aspect of the petrous temporal bone, the trigeminal (CN V) or gasserian ganglion lies within a dural envelope called the Meckel cave. This arachnoid-lined, CSF-filled cavity houses the ganglion and neural fascicles of CN V in the middle fossa. The three divisions of CN V then exit the middle fossa through individual foramina (discussed in the following section.)

Along the midpetrous ridge, the arcuate eminence is a bony protuberance representing the superior extent of the superior semicircular canal. An important landmark in the middle fossa approach to the internal auditory canal, the arcuate eminence can be used to localize the geniculate ganglion of the facial nerve (CN VII) and the internal auditory canal. Bony dehiscence over the geniculate ganglion is not uncommon, and careful elevation of the dura during middle fossa surgery is required to avoid facial nerve injury in this area. Laterally, the thin tegmen tympani and tegmen mastoideum form the roof of the middle ear and mastoid, respectively; trauma or iatrogenic injury to these regions during otologic or mastoid surgery may lead to dural disruption and CSF leak requiring repair.

133.3.2 Foramina

As previously discussed, the superior orbital fissure and optic canal are bony apertures in the anterior aspect of the middle cranial fossa. Posteroinferior to the superior orbital fissure and lateral to the sella turcica, the foramen rotundum transmits the second division of the trigeminal nerve (CN V_2) from the middle fossa through the lateral wall of the cavernous sinus to the pterygopalatine fossa. After exiting the skull, CN V_2 continues as the infraorbital nerve and provides sensory innervation to the cheek and maxillary dentition. Inferomedial to the foramen rotundum is the vidian canal, which transmits the vidian artery and nerve. The vidian nerve is composed of the greater superficial petrosal nerve and the deep petrosal nerve.

Unlike the first two divisions of CN V, the third division (CN V_3) does not pass through the cavernous sinus; instead, it exits directly from the Meckel cave through the foramen ovale. Also unlike the ophthalmic (CN V_1) and maxillary (CN V_2) divisions, the mandibular branch (CN V_3) carries both sensory and motor fibers providing innervation to the muscles of mastication (masseter, temporalis, and medial and lateral pterygoid muscles), the mylohyoid muscle, the tensor tympani and tensor veli palatini muscles, and the anterior belly of the digastric muscle. It also supplies sensation to the buccal mucosa, skin of the lower face, and mandibular dentition. In addition to CN V_3, the foramen ovale transmits the lesser superficial petrosal nerve, accessory meningeal branch of the maxillary artery, and emissary veins to the pterygoid plexus into the infratemporal fossa. Farther posterolaterally, the foramen spinosum contains the middle meningeal artery (described above). Formed by the greater wing of the sphenoid and the petrous apex of the temporal bone, the carotid canal transmits the internal carotid artery (also called at this level the petrous carotid artery) and its sympathetic plexus. Medial to the foramen ovale, the misnamed foramen lacerum is not a true foramen but rather the cartilaginous floor of the horizontal portion of the petrous internal carotid artery canal (▶ Fig. 133.3).

133.3.3 Contents

The middle cranial fossa houses a number of vital structures, including the temporal lobes, pituitary gland, cavernous sinuses, intracranial portion of the internal carotid arteries, trigeminal ganglia, and CNs I through VI. In the central compartment of the middle fossa, strong dural attachments form the

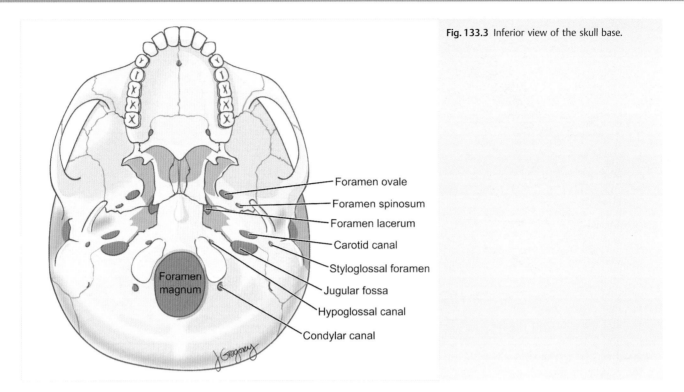

Fig. 133.3 Inferior view of the skull base.

- Foramen ovale
- Foramen spinosum
- Foramen lacerum
- Carotid canal
- Styloglossal foramen
- Jugular fossa
- Hypoglossal canal
- Condylar canal
- Foramen magnum

diaphragmatic sella, a circular band of dural reflections that envelope the pituitary gland. Superiorly, the infundibulum (pituitary stalk) and the hypophyseal veins perforate this structure.

The cavernous sinuses are paired, septate venous sinuses, lined with dura, that drain inferiorly to the two pterygoid plexus and internal jugular veins. Bounded laterally by the anterior and posterior petroclinoid dural folds and extending posteriorly from the superior orbital fissure to the petrous apex, this complex region of venous sinusoids is traversed by various critical neurovascular structures. Centrally, the horizontal portion of the intracranial internal carotid artery runs in the through the cavernous sinus close to the lateral wall of the sphenoid sinus. The following CNs traverse the lateral wall of the cavernous sinus (listed in a superior to inferior direction): oculomotor (CN III), trochlear (CN IV), ophthalmic (CN V_1), and maxillary (CN V_2). Only the abducens nerve (CN VI) actually courses through the venous sinusoids in the center of the sinus. With its complex neurovascular components, the cavernous sinus plays an important clinical role in the intracranial transmission of infection. Tributaries of the cavernous sinus include the valveless veins of the face, sinuses, and dentition, so that a rapid spread of infection from these anterior, extracranial sites into the cavernous sinus is possible.

133.3.4 Extracranial Relationships

Surgical approaches to the middle fossa exploit the close proximity of the pituitary and clivus to the sphenoid sinus and nasopharynx inferiorly. Sellar pneumatization allows the endoscopic or microscopic trans-sphenoidal excision of pituitary disease because the middle cranial fossa can be entered through the roof of the sphenoid sinus. During procedures in the sphenoid sinus, care must be taken to avoid injury or disruption of the lateral wall because the course of the internal carotid artery

and optic nerve is immediately lateral to the thin sinus wall. Occasionally, bony dehiscence results in exposure of the internal carotid artery, CN II, or vidian nerve within the sphenoid sinus. In the middle fossa approach to the internal carotid artery, a transtemporal route through the squamous portion of the temporal bone is used to access internal carotid artery disease superiorly.

The nasopharynx is located posterior and inferior to the sphenoid sinus and anterior to the clivus. The foramen lacerum and horizontal intracranial internal carotid artery, as previously described, lie immediately superior to the superior border of the nasopharynx. In the superior–lateral nasopharyngeal wall, the sinus of Morgagni is a clinically significant region of muscular dehiscence. Here, the levator veli palatini and cartilaginous eustachian tube penetrate the superior constrictor muscle; through this weak area, nasopharyngeal infections and neoplastic processes may gain access to and invade the skull base.

133.4 Posterior Skull Base

133.4.1 Borders

The posterior cranial fossa is separated from the middle fossa by the dorsum sellae medially and by the petrous ridges of the temporal bones laterally. In the midline, the basal part of the occipital bone (called the basiocciput) and the basisphenoid bone form the clivus and the anteromedial wall of the posterior fossa. Anterolaterally, this boundary is formed by the posterior face of the temporal bone. The remaining posterior, lateral, and inferior borders are formed by the occipital bone. The occipitomastoid suture, the junction of the occipital bone with the mastoid portion of the temporal bone, courses in an anteromedial to posterolateral direction along the posterior fossa floor. Superiorly, the tentorium cerebelli attaches to the petrous ridge of the temporal bone, creating a dural roof of the posterior fossa and a separation between the cerebellum below and the cerebral hemispheres above.

Centrally, the foramen magnum, the largest foramen of the skull base, is an opening in the floor of the posterior cranial fossa. The internal occipital crest courses in an anterior–posterior direction from the midline of the foramen magnum to the internal occipital protuberance and is the site of attachment for the falx cerebelli. This area is rich with venous sinuses; the dural folds of the falx cerebelli form the midline occipital venous sinus, which drains into the internal jugular vein. Superior to the internal occipital protuberance is a vertical groove for the superior sagittal sinus, while the horizontal grooves of the transverse sinuses are situated lateral to the bony protuberance. Laterally, the superior petrosal sinus is located at the junction of the transverse and sigmoid sinuses. Along the mastoid portion of the temporal bone, a sulcus for the sigmoid sinus can be identified coursing inferiorly toward the internal jugular foramen and vein. In the anterior midline, the paired inferior petrosal sinuses lie posterior to the clivus and anterior to the petrous apex.

133.4.2 Foramina

Like the floor of the middle cranial fossa, the floor of the posterior cranial fossa contains many important neurovascular structures and foramina, including CNs VII through XII, the medulla oblongata, and the jugular veins. The internal acoustic meatus, or porus acusticus, is located on the posterior face of the petrous temporal bone superior to the jugular foramen. This foramen transmits the facial (CN VII) and vestibulocochlear (CN VIII) nerves, the nervus intermedius, and the labyrinthine vessels (branches of the anterior inferior cerebellar artery) from the brainstem to the internal auditory canal of the temporal bone. Within the internal auditory canal, the facial nerve (CN VII) occupies the anterosuperior quadrant, separated from the superior vestibular nerve in the posterosuperior quadrant by a bony vertical crest ("Bill's bar," named for Dr. William House). Anteriorly, the bony transverse or falciform crest separates the facial nerve (CN VII) superiorly from the cochlear nerve inferiorly. At the lateral end of the internal auditory canal, or fundus, CN VIII innervates the inner ear; the superior and inferior vestibular nerves terminate in the vestibule and semicircular canals of the labyrinth, whereas the cochlear nerve traverses a multiply perforated osseous plate to enter the cochlear modiolus. The facial nerve, on the other hand, begins a complicated intratemporal course consisting of a short, narrow labyrinthine segment; a genu or bend, marking the location of the geniculate ganglion; and a horizontal, intratympanic segment that traverses the middle ear and ends in the descending or mastoid portion. The labyrinthine segment is the shortest and narrowest portion and thus the most susceptible to compression and injury from edema. After exiting the temporal bone through the stylomastoid foramen, located between the mastoid tip and styloid process, the nerve begins its extracranial course, ultimately innervating the muscles of facial expression. Also on the posterior face of the petrous bone, posterior and lateral to the porus acusticus, is the operculum or opening of the vestibular aqueduct (or endolymphatic duct) into the subarachnoid space of the posterior fossa. Enlargement of the duct is associated with congenital sensorineural hearing loss or a predisposition to the later development of hearing loss and can be associated with other anatomical abnormalities of the inner ear, such as Mondini deformity of the cochlea. The jugular foramen is formed by the processus jugularis of the petrous temporal bone anteriorly and the occipital bone posteriorly and can be found at the most posterior aspect of the petro-occipital fissure. The jugular foramen was previously divided into two portions, the anteromedial pars nervosa and the posterolateral pars vascularis, but a new division into three compartments has been suggested. Anteriorly to posteriorly, these include the following: (1) the petrous compartment, containing the inferior petrosal sinus; (2) the neural intrajugular compartment, containing CNs IX, X, and XI and their respective ganglia, the Jacobsen nerve (from CN IX), the Arnold nerve (from CN X), and the posterior meningeal artery (a branch of the ascending pharyngeal artery); and (3) the sigmoid compartment receiving the sigmoid sinus and beginning of the jugular bulb. In the neural compartment, the glossopharyngeal nerve (CN IX) is located anteriorly and is separated from the inferiorly located vagus nerve (CN X) and spinal accessory nerve (CN XI) by a dural septum. Inferomedial to the jugular foramen, inferior to the bony protuberance called the jugular tubercle, is the hypoglossal canal. Located in the condylar portion of the occipital bone, this foramen transmits the hypoglossal nerve (CN XII) and its venous plexus. Also formed completely of occipital bone, the large, central foramen magnum serves as the primary connection between the brainstem and spinal cord. It contains the cephalic component of CN XI, the vertebral and posterior spinal arteries, and the medulla oblongata.

133.4.3 Contents

An understanding of the anatomy of the posterior fossa, which houses the midbrain, pons, medulla, and cerebellar hemispheres, as well as CNs VI through XII and many critical vascular structures, is crucial for any surgeon working in this area. The posterior fossa arterial contents include the paired vertebral arteries, which enter the posterior skull base through the foramen magnum, then ascend vertically ventral to CNs IX, X, and XI. After giving off the posterior inferior cerebellar arteries, the vertebral arteries join to form the basilar artery at the base of the pons. The basilar artery ascends on the intracranial aspect of the clivus against the midline pons and gives rise to multiple branches. Inferiorly to superiorly, these are the anterior inferior cerebellar arteries, the multiple short and long pontine arteries, and the superior cerebellar arteries, which form the posterior aspect of the circle of Willis (▶ Fig. 133.4). Within the posterior fossa, the cerebellopontine angle is of unique importance to the otolaryngologist because of the location of the facial and vestibulocochlear nerves. The cerebellopontine angle extends from the abducens nerve (CN VI) and lateral aspect of the clivus anteriorly to the cerebellar flocculus posteromedially. Medially, it is bounded by the middle cerebellar peduncle, pons, and ventral cerebellum; it is bounded laterally by the posterior petrous temporal bone and inferiorly by CNs IX, X, and XI. The choroid plexus, a collection of CSF-producing ependymal cells, may pass through the foramen of Lushka into the cerebellopontine angle. Well-known surgical approaches to the internal auditory canal and cerebellopontine angle include the translabyrinthine

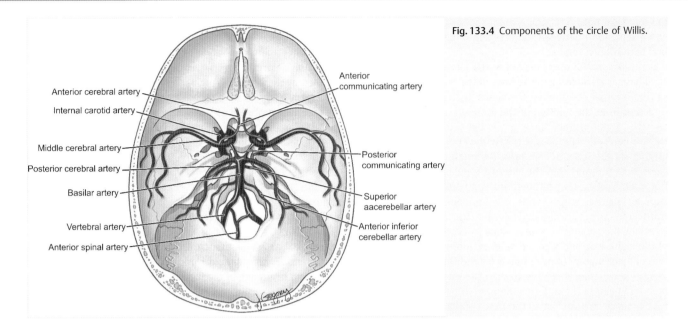

Fig. 133.4 Components of the circle of Willis.

Anterior cerebral artery

Internal carotid artery

Middle cerebral artery

Posterior cerebral artery

Basilar artery

Vertebral artery

Anterior spinal artery

Anterior communicating artery

Posterior communicating artery

Superior aacerebellar artery

Anterior inferior cerebellar artery

approach through the mastoid portion of the temporal bone, the retrosigmoid approach through an occipital craniotomy, and the middle fossa approach through the squamous temporal bone (previously described). Although further description is beyond the scope of this chapter, knowledge of the anatomy in this region is fundamental to understanding the presentation, diagnosis, and treatment of cerebellopontine angle pathology.

133.4.4 Extracranial Relationships

Extracranial structures inferior to the posterior fossa include the musculature of the suboccipital region, specifically the sternocleidomastoid muscle, which originates on the mastoid tip of the temporal bone, and the posterior belly of the digastric muscle. The posterior musculature includes, from superficial to deep, the trapezius, splenius capitis, splenius colli, and semispinalis capitis muscles. Beneath these muscles, inferior to the superior nuchal line and superficial to the ligaments connecting the atlas to the axis, lies the suboccipital triangle. The contents of this region include the occipital and vertebral arteries, a complex of veins, the greater occipital nerve, and the C1 nerve. Suboccipital surgical approaches can be used for access to the vertebral arteries and foramen magnum. Additional inferior extracranial relationships of the posterior skull base include the deep neck spaces, such as the retropharyngeal, danger, and prevertebral spaces, as well as the cervical spine. The fascia of these spaces begins at the skull base and extends to the level of the tracheal bifurcation, diaphragm, and coccyx, respectively.

133.5 Infratemporal Fossa

133.5.1 Borders and Foramina

The infratemporal fossae are irregular, complex anatomical spaces that lie medial to the zygomatic arches and mandibular rami bilaterally. Anteriorly, the infratemporal fossa is limited by the posterior surface of the mandible and the inferior orbital fissure. The roof, or superior boundary, includes the inferior surface of the greater wing of the sphenoid and the squamous temporal bone. Posteriorly, limits include the mastoid and tympanic temporal bone, while the inferior border comprises the superior aspect of the posterior belly of the digastric and the angle of the mandible. The infratemporal fossa communicates with the middle cranial fossa via various skull base foramina, notably the foramen spinosum and foramen ovale. Connection with the orbit is mediated by the inferior orbital fissure through the pterygopalatine fossa and pterygomaxillary fissure.

133.5.2 Contents

Muscular contents of the infratemporal fossa include the medial and lateral pterygoid muscles, the latter of which is divided into two muscular heads. The medial pterygoid runs from its origin on the medial side of the lateral pterygoid process and inserts on the medial surface of the mandible at the angle and ramus. Although both insert on the temporomandibular joint, the inferior belly of the lateral pterygoid arises from the lateral part of the lateral pterygoid process, and the superior belly attaches to the roof of the infratemporal fossa. Multiple braches of the mandibular nerve (CN V_3) traverse the infratemporal fossa, including the inferior alveolar, lingual, and buccal branches, the chorda tympani, and the otic ganglion. Exiting through the foramen ovale, CN V_3 carries motor fibers to the muscles of mastication and sensory fibers via the auriculotemporal, alveolar, lingual, and buccal branches. The chorda tympani branches from the facial nerve (CN VII) in the mastoid portion, courses through the middle ear and through the tympanic canaliculus in the petrotympanic suture, and enters the infratemporal fossa medial to the lateral pterygoid muscle, where it ultimately joins the lingual nerve. The primary arterial structure in the infratemporal fossa is the maxillary artery and its many branches. A branch of the external carotid artery, the maxillary artery enters the infratemporal fossa lateral to the lateral pterygoid muscle and proceeds anteriorly toward the pterygomaxillary fissure and pterygopalatine fossa. Venous drainage of the infratemporal fossa proceeds from the pterygoid venous plexus to the facial vein anteriorly and the maxillary vein posteriorly. An extensive venous anastomotic plexus connects the pterygoid plexus with the cavernous sinus, ophthalmic veins, and pharyngeal venous plexus.

133.6 Conclusion

A fundamental knowledge of the borders, foramina, and extracranial relationships is necessary for the otolaryngologist, neurosurgeon, or skull base subspecialist. Familiarity with the anatomical features of each particular region plays a key role in understanding the presentation, pathophysiology, and treatment of skull base lesions. Clearly, a knowledge of the complex anatomy of the cranial base is also the foundation for safe extirpation of lesions in this region.

133.7 Roundsmanship

- A thorough understanding of the anatomy of the posterior cranial fossa is an absolute prerequisite for performing safe otologic and neurotologic surgery.

- Although many of the structures described herein appear at first reading to be complex, they follow a logical order based upon regional embryogenesis and development.
- Safe skull base surgery requires not only a thorough grounding in the local anatomy but also a lifelong dedication to the acquisition and perfection of surgical skill based upon laboratory microdissection. There is no substitute for hands-on microsurgical training.

133.8 Recommended Reading

[1] Cruz OL. Anatomy of the skull base, temporal bone, external ear and middle ear. In: Cummings CW, Flint PW, Harker LA, et al, eds. Cummings Otolaryngology: Head and Neck Surgery. 4th ed. Philadelphia, PA: Elsevier Mosby; 2005: 2801–2814

[2] Harnsberger HR, Osborn AG, Ross J, Macdonald AJ, eds. Diagnostic and Surgical Imaging Anatomy: Brain, Head and Neck, Spine. Salt Lake City, UT: Amirsys; 2006:186–190

[3] Mark AS. Imaging of the labyrinth. In: Jackler RK, Brackmann DE, eds. Neurotology. Philadelphia, PA: Elsevier Mosby; 2005:332–348

[4] Stamm AC, Pignatari SS. Transnasasal endoscopic-assisted surgery of the skull base. In: Cummings CW, Flint PW, Harker LA, et al, eds. Cummings Otolaryngology: Head and Neck Surgery. 4th ed. Philadelphia, PA: Elsevier Mosby; 2005:3855–3876

134 Posterior Skull Base Diseases and Surgery

Seilesh C. Babu and Ryan G. Porter

134.1 Introduction

Although there are numerous diseases of the posterior fossa, the general otolaryngologist does not encounter most of them. This chapter will focus on the most common neoplasms that affect the seventh and eighth cranial nerve complex at the internal auditory canal and cerebellopontine angle (see Box Differential Diagnosis of Cerebellopontine Angle Tumors (p.1050)). Patients with these tumors often present first to the general otolaryngologist or primary care physician, and it is important that the diseases be identified and patients treated appropriately, or that they be referred to a subspecialist for further management. The two most common surgical approaches to the posterior fossa, the retrosigmoid (suboccipital) and the translabyrinthine approaches, will also be discussed.

Differential Diagnosis of Cerebellopontine Angle Tumors

- Vestibular schwannoma ("acoustic neuroma")
- Meningioma
- Epidermoid (cholesteatoma)
- Arachnoid cyst
- Facial schwannoma ("facial neuroma")
- Cochlear schwannoma (cochlear neuroma)
- Vascular lesions (e.g., hemangioma)
- Lipoma
- Metastatic carcinoma (e.g., breast carcinoma)

134.2 Applied Anatomy

Cranial nerves (CNs) VII (facial) and VIII (vestibulocochlear) exit the brainstem from their root entry zones at the pons and cross through the cerebellopontine angle (CPA) before entering the medial aspect of the internal auditory canal (IAC) at the porus acusticus. The nerves then travel in the IAC toward the fundus (lateral aspect of the IAC). The facial nerve travels anteriorly in the canal superior to the cochlear division of CN VIII. The superior vestibular and inferior vestibular branches of CN VIII travel posteriorly in the IAC. The facial and superior vestibular nerves are separated from the cochlear and inferior vestibular nerves at the fundus by the transverse crest. The facial nerve is separated anteriorly from the superior vestibular nerve by a vertical crest of bone ("Bill's bar," named for Dr. William House). After traveling through the fundus of the IAC, the nerves enter the inner ear, mastoid, or middle ear and ultimately innervate the cochlea, vestibular system, and facial and middle ear musculature.

The anterior inferior cerebellar artery, a branch of the basilar artery, is also located in the CPA. The anterior inferior cerebellar artery typically sends off an arterial branch to the inner ear through the IAC (the labyrinthine or internal auditory artery).

134.3 Epidemiology

The most common neoplasm affecting the CPA is the vestibular schwannoma (VS), also known as an acoustic neuroma. The incidence of VS is approximately 1 per 100,000 people. The second most common tumor affecting the CPA is the meningioma. In general, meningiomas are twice as common in females as in males and are most frequent after the fifth decade of life. Other tumors and lesions are much less common than VSs and meningiomas, but they must still be considered because their treatment may be markedly different.

134.4 Pathogenesis

VSs are benign neoplasms arising from Schwann cells on the vestibular portion of CN VIII. The inferior division of the vestibular nerve is affected by schwannomas almost twice as often as the superior division. VSs have two classic histologic patterns, Antoni A and Antoni B. The Antoni A pattern is characterized by compact cells and Verocay bodies, in which palisading nuclei line up beside anuclear, clear areas. A looser stroma, myxoid changes, and fewer cells characterize the Antoni B pattern (▶ Fig. 134.1). Tumors are typically mixtures of both Antoni A and Antoni B types, with the Antoni A pattern predominating.

The growth rate of VSs is variable. In an analysis by Sughrue et al of 982 patients in 34 published studies who had decent hearing and tumors 2.5 cm or smaller in size, the mean tumor growth rate was 2.9 ± 1.2 mm/y with a minimum 26-month follow-up. Additionally, patients with slower-growing tumors (≤ 2.5 mm/y) had higher rates of hearing preservation than did patients with faster-growing tumors (75% vs 32%, $p < 0.0001$).

Meningiomas are slow-growing and arise from arachnoidal cap cells. Although most meningiomas are sporadic, cranial irradiation (classically scalp irradiation for tinea capitis) and neurofibromatosis type II (NF2) are risk factors for development of the disease.

NF2 is an autosomal-dominant genetic disease due to a mutation of a gene on chromosome 22 (22q12) that causes a defect

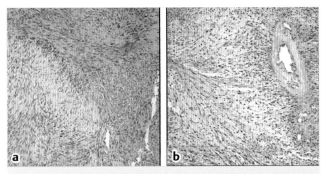

Fig. 134.1 (a) Antoni A and (b) Antoni B areas from a schwannoma. The cells are spindle-shaped, and the nuclei can be seen lining up or "palisading" in areas that represent characteristic Verocay bodies (H&E, x100).

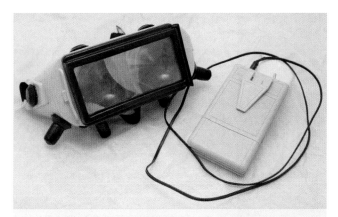

Fig. 134.2 Frenzel glasses are useful for magnifying a patient's eyes during an evaluation for nystagmus. They also obscure the patient's vision so that visual fixation is not possible.

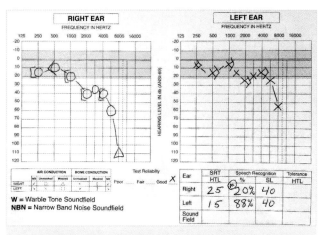

Fig. 134.3 An audiogram typical of a patient with a right-sided vestibular schwannoma shows an asymmetric sensorineural hearing loss with impairment of speech discrimination on the affected side.

in a tumor suppressor protein, merlin (also called schwannomin). Patients with NF2 are at increased risk for bilateral VSs as well as other central nervous system tumors, including meningiomas, other schwannomas, and ependymomas.

134.5 History and Physical Examination

Tumors of the CPA and IAC often present with unilateral hearing loss and tinnitus. A patient presenting with asymmetric hearing loss or asymmetric subjective tinnitus should prompt the clinician to investigate for retrocochlear pathology. Although some have been suggested, there are no universal guidelines on the degree of hearing asymmetry that should prompt further evaluation. A hearing loss of 10 db HL or more in multiple frequencies, especially in combination with impairment in auditory discrimination scores or other cranial nerve palsies, should raise suspicion for a neoplasm.

The work-up of any patient with a suspected lateral skull base lesion should include a detailed history and a head and neck examination, including otoscopy. A pertinent history includes the timing of the onset of hearing loss and tinnitus; history of otologic infections, previous head and neck surgery, imbalance, vertigo, falls, loss of coordination, or headaches; family history of brain tumors, including acoustic neuromas and meningiomas; past history of other neurologic tumors or any malignancies; and symptoms of cranial nerve dysfunction (e.g., facial hypesthesia, diplopia, dysphagia, aspiration, dysphonia, shoulder or tongue weakness). Symptoms of facial spasm or facial pain should lead the examiner to consider advanced disease or one of the rarer CPA pathologies.

Clinical vestibular testing should also be performed in all patients with suspected retrocochlear lesions because it can give clues about the status of the inner ears. Standard clinical vestibular testing should include observation for spontaneous nystagmus and post–head shake nystagmus, preferably with Frenzel goggles (▶ Fig. 134.2), which eliminate fixation; a head thrust test; a Dix-Hallpike test to rule out benign paroxysmal positional vertigo; Romberg testing; cerebellar testing; and a Fukuda stepping test. Common findings in a patient with VS include a

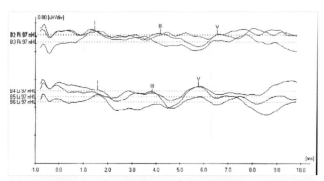

Fig. 134.4 Auditory brainstem response tracing from a patient with right-sided retrocochlear disease (vestibular schwannoma). The absolute latencies for waves III and V, as well as the interwave latency (I through V), are prolonged on the right side (*above*). The left side (*below*) is normal.

correction saccade after head thrust toward the lesion, post–head shake nystagmus with a fast phase away from the lesion, and a tendency to turn toward the lesion on Fukuda testing. Patients with large tumors can show signs of cerebellar dysfunction, loss of corneal reflex or facial hypesthesia resulting from CN V compression, or signs of lower cranial nerve dysfunction.

134.6 Testing

An audiogram, including speech reception testing, should be performed for every patient with suspected retrocochlear disease. Classic findings on standard audiometric testing include asymmetric sensorineural hearing loss and impaired speech discrimination on the side of the lesion (▶ Fig. 134.3). Additionally, "rollover" is sometimes noted, in which an increase in the loudness of the presented speech sounds actually leads to a decrease in speech recognition ability at the louder level.

Auditory brainstem response (ABR) testing has been used in the past to screen for retrocochlear lesions (▶ Fig. 134.4), but it lacks sensitivity for small lesions. The stacked ABR has been reported to increase sensitivity for smaller tumors, but it still has some problems, especially related to intersubject variability.

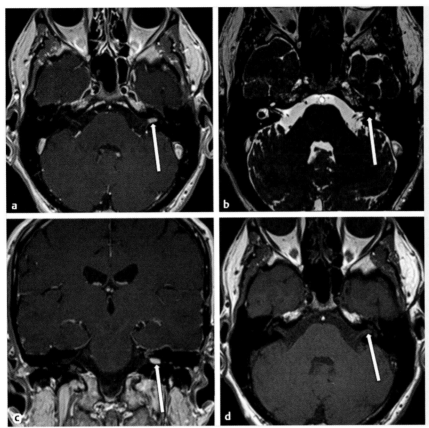

Fig. 134.5 T1-weighted magnetic resonance (MR) image after contrast shows enhancement of a left intracanalicular vestibular schwannoma (VS; *arrow*) on (**a**) axial and (**c**) coronal views. The VS is located where the cerebrospinal fluid signal is absent (*arrow*) in the left internal auditory canal on a (**b**) high-resolution, T2-weighted CISS (constructive interference steady state) sequence. The VS is not visible on noncontrast T1-weighted MR imaging. (**d**) The arrow points to the location of the tumor that is not visible.

The gold standard for the diagnosis of CPA tumors is gadolinium-enhanced magnetic resonance (MR) imaging of the brain, including thin-cut (≤ 3 mm) images through the IAC region. It is important to view T1 and T2 sequences, including contrast-enhanced images, in both coronal and axial sections. VSs, meningiomas, and malignancies typically enhance on contrasted T1 sequences. VSs and meningiomas are difficult to differentiate on MR imaging only. Meningiomas may exhibit a dural "tail sign" and/or hyperostosis of bone adjacent to the tumor. A dural "tail sign" refers to enhancement of a portion of the dura at the edges of the meningioma, giving the appearance of a "tail." T1 sequences without contrast may reveal CPA lipomas, and T2 images are useful for locating epidermoids and arachnoid cysts. High-resolution T2-weighted images are also useful for confirming the presence of a space-occupying lesion, such as a VS, in the IAC. The VS will prevent cerebrospinal fluid (CSF) signal at the site of the lesion, which will show up as a hypointense area on T2 imaging (▶ Fig. 134.5). Although relatively insensitive, this technique may be used as a screening tool in a low-risk patient if gadolinium was not administered. Standard MR imaging of the brain without dedicated, thin IAC cuts or without contrast may miss small lesions, and imaging should repeated if the level of suspicion is significant.

For patients who are not candidates for MR imaging (e.g., metallic implants, problems with access), thin-cut computed tomography (CT) of the brain and temporal bones with contrast is the next best option, but it is not as sensitive as MR imaging and will not likely show small lesions. CT with contrast or ABR screening may be a reasonable option if the patient is elderly or

in poor health because it is unlikely that a subcentimeter benign tumor would be treated even if identified.

If the patient has a known CPA tumor or abnormalities on the clinical vestibular tests previously described for the physical examination, videonystagmography (VNG) should be performed. VNG will often show a weak caloric response on the side with the lesion (▶ Fig. 134.6). VNG results can be used to counsel patients regarding their expected recovery following treatment; patients with preexisting large caloric deficits tend to recover faster because vestibular compensation in the contralateral inner ear and central nervous system (CNS) has already occurred before treatment. Some practitioners order facial nerve electroneurography before treatment to determine the subclinical insult to the facial nerve, which can help with patient counseling and treatment planning. Current studies have shown that electroneurography is not a good prognostic indicator of facial nerve function following tumor resection, although the studies have been done in limited patient populations. Further studies are needed to assess the prognostic role of electroneurography when the results are abnormal.

After a tumor has been identified on MR imaging, ABR testing is often performed as a baseline assessment before a hearing preservation approach is considered. If sufficient waveforms are present preoperatively, there will be a greater utility of intraoperative ABR testing to monitor the integrity of the cochlear division of the eighth nerve. Sedation is not typically needed to perform an ABR test in an adult, and many centers can obtain a baseline test in the office setting.

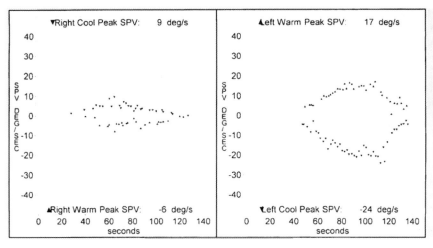

Fig. 134.6 Caloric testing (videonystagmography) from a patient with a right vestibular schwannoma. The test shows a 46% right-sided vestibular weakness. Both sides would be relatively symmetric in a patient with no vestibular dysfunction.

Table 134.1 American Academy of Otolaryngology—Head and Neck Surgery (AAO-HNS) hearing classification system

Class	Pure-tone threshold (dB)	Speech discrimination (%)
A	≤ 30 and	≥ 70
B	> 30 and ≤ 50 and	≥ 50
C	> 50 and	≥ 50
D	Any level	< 50

Source: Adapted from Committee on Hearing and Equilibrium guidelines for the evaluation of hearing preservation in acoustic neuroma (vestibular schwannoma). American Academy of Otolaryngology-Head and Neck Surgery Foundation, INC. Otolaryngol Head Neck Surg 1995;113 (3):179–80.

Table 134.2 Gardner-Robertson classification for hearing preservation

Class	Pure-tone average or speech reception threshold (dB)[a]	Speech discrimination (%)
1	0–30 and	70–100
2	31–50 and	69–50
3	51–90 and	49–5
4	91–maximum loss and	4–1
5	No response and	No response

Source: Adapted from Gardner G, Robertson JH. Hearing preservation in unilateral acoustic neuroma surgery. Ann Otol Rhinol Laryngol 1988;97 (1):55–66.
[a]Use the better score. If the pure-tone average or speech reception threshold score and the speech discrimination score do not qualify the patient for same class, use the class appropriate for the poorer of two scores.

Conventional audiometric results in patients with VSs and other tumors of the CPA are typically reported with one of two scales. The American Academy of Otolaryngology—Head and Neck Surgery (AAO-HNS) scale (▶ Table 134.1) uses the pure-tone average (PTA) of the air conduction thresholds at 0.5, 1, 2, and 3 kHz and the speech discrimination score (SDS). The Gardner-Robertson classification system (▶ Table 134.2) uses the poorer of the PTA or speech reception threshold (SRT) and the SDS to classify hearing in a range from class 1 (normal) to class 5 (no hearing).

134.7 Grading

VSs are often classified according to size: small (≤ 10 mm), medium (10 to 30 mm), large (30 to 40 mm), and giant (> 40 mm). By convention, only the extrameatal portion of the tumor is measured. Intracanalicular tumors are simply referred to as "intracanalicular." The extrameatal portion is measured with the axial MR imaging or CT scan that shows the largest portion of the tumor. Two linear measurements are taken, one of the maximal diameter in a plane parallel to the petrous ridge and one of the maximal diameter perpendicular to the first measurement. The square root of the product of the two measurements rounded to the nearest 0.5 cm is the tumor size (▶ Fig. 134.7).

Meningiomas can be classified according to the World Health Organization (WHO) grading system. WHO grade I meningio-

mas are the most common and typically have the most benign clinical course. The most common variants are the meningothelial, fibroblastic, and transitional patterns. WHO grade II (atypical) and WHO grade III (anaplastic) tumors are less common.

134.8 Treatment

There are four major treatment options for tumors of the CPA and IAC: (1) observation, (2) microsurgical resection, (3) stereotactic radiosurgery, and (4) multimodality therapy. Observation is an option for smaller asymptomatic tumors or for tumors that do not appear to be growing at a significant rate. In a study of the natural history of 552 patients followed with observation and serial MR imaging for VSs over a mean of 3.6 years, significant growth occurred in 17% of tumors that were confined to the IAC and in 28.9% of tumors that extended beyond the IAC. The tumors that grew typically did so within 5 years of diagnosis. However, not all tumors have an indolent course. Some tumors grow rapidly, and patients require treatment to avoid complications of tumor growth, including hearing loss, dizziness, brainstem compression, hydrocephalus, and eventual coma or death. It is reasonable to observe small tumors with serial audiograms and MR imaging. Typically, MR imaging and audiography will be repeated 6 months after the initial diagnosis of a tumor. If there is no significant change, testing may be repeated yearly. In a meta-analysis of patients with good hearing and small tumors, patients who had tumors with slower growth rates (≤ 2.5 mm/y) had higher rates of hearing preservation than did patients with faster-growing tumors (75% vs 32%, $p < 0.0001$).

Microsurgical resection can be categorized into hearing preservation and non–hearing preservation approaches. There are various criteria for deciding which approach to use, but the status of the patient's hearing and the tumor size are foremost in the decision-making process. "Serviceable hearing" is hearing that is realistically useful to the patient for understanding speech. Serviceable hearing includes hearing that is normal or nearly normal, as well as hearing thresholds that can realistically be rehabilitated with a hearing aid. A gross rule of thumb regarding serviceable hearing is the "50/50" rule. If a patient has a PTA (or an SRT) worse than 50 dB HL and an SDS worse than 50% (AAO-HNS class D or E, or Gardner-Robertson class 3, 4, or 5), the patient's hearing is considered to be generally not serviceable. Overall, the preservation of serviceable hearing (AAO-HNS class A or B) is possible in only about 40 to 50% of patients with tumors smaller than 2 cm.

Hearing preservation approaches include the middle cranial fossa approach and the retrosigmoid (RS) approach. A translabyrinthine (TL) approach is a non–hearing preservation procedure that gives the best overall view of the CPA with least amount of cerebellar retraction, at the expense of hearing. Factors affecting the decision-making process other than hearing status and tumor size include tumor location, patient age, vestibular function, and patient and surgeon preference (▸ Table 134.3). The TL and RS approaches will be described below. Intraoperative facial nerve monitoring is standard during all approaches to the CPA.

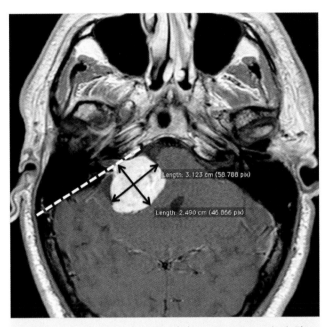

Fig. 134.7 Measurement of a right-sided acoustic neuroma (AN). The petrous ridge is marked with a white dashed line. The largest diameter in a plane parallel to the petrous ridge (3.12 cm) times the largest diameter perpendicular to the first measurement (2.49 cm) equals 7.77 cm². The square root of 7.77 equals 2.78. The final AN measurement equals 2.5 cm (2.78 rounded to the nearest 0.5 cm).

134.8.1 Translabyrinthine Approach

Although it does not allow hearing preservation, the TL approach is a versatile option that is useful for any tumor size or location. The TL approach offers the surgeon the best view of the entire IAC and CPA whereby even the fundus (the most lateral portion of the IAC near the meatal foramen) can be visualized. Additionally, the TL approach allows the surgeon to view the vestibular nerves with relative ease because the facial nerve lies medially in this plane of dissection (▸ Fig. 134.8).

The TL approach begins with an incision placed slightly posterior to a standard postauricular mastoidectomy incision, but in the same C-shape configuration. A generous mastoidectomy is accomplished first. Next, bone is removed from the sigmoid sinus, posterior fossa dura, and middle fossa dura. Some surgeons prefer to leave a small island of bone on the sigmoid sinus ("Bill's island") to protect the sinus from instrumentation and the rotating drill shaft during further tumor exposure and

Table 134.3 Advantages and disadvantages of the three major approaches to the cerebellopontine angle and internal auditory canal

	Middle cranial fossa	Translabyrinthine	Retrosigmoid
Advantages	Hearing preservation possible No intradural drilling Low rate of headache	Consistent identification of facial nerve Not limited by tumor size No intradural drilling Wide exposure to posterior fossa Low recurrence rates Auditory brainstem implant placement possible Low rate of headache Minimal or no cerebellar retraction	Not limited by extrameatal tumor size Hearing preservation possible Wide exposure at brainstem Auditory brainstem implant placement possible Consistent identification of facial nerve Neurosurgeons most familiar with this approach
Disadvantages	Limited to small tumors Temporal lobe retraction Limited posterior fossa exposure Increased recurrence risk if tumor is unfavorably positioned	Definite complete hearing loss Neurosurgeons less familiar with this approach Requires abdominal fat graft	Limited exposure for lateral internal auditory canal Possible intradural drilling Higher rate of postoperative headache Possible need for cerebellar retraction

Source: Adapted from Bennett M, Haynes DS. Surgical approaches and complications in the removal of vestibular schwannomas. 2007. Neurosurg Clin N Am 2008;19(2):331–343, vii.

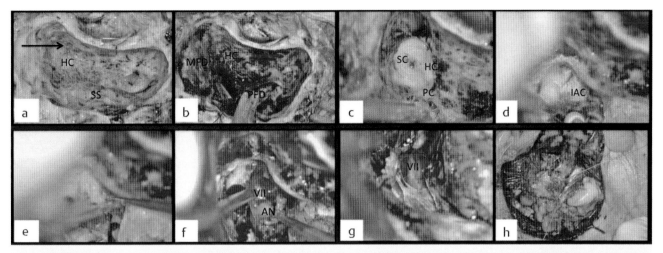

Fig. 134.8 Steps in the translabyrinthine resection of an acoustic neuroma. (**a**) Complete mastoidectomy. (**b**) Decompression of middle fossa, sigmoid sinus, and posterior fossa dura. (**c**) Labyrinthectomy. (**d**) Skeletonization of the internal auditory canal. (**e**) Removal of bone from the internal auditory canal. (**f**) Separation of tumor from the facial nerve. (**g**) Internal auditory canal after tumor removal. (**h**) Packing adipose tissue graft into the surgical defect. *AN*, acoustic neuroma; *IAC*, internal auditory canal; *HC*, horizontal semicircular canal; *IAC*, internal auditory canal; *MFD*, middle fossa dura; *PC*, posterior semicircular canal; *PFD*, posterior fossa dura; *SC*, superior semicircular canal; *SS*, sigmoid sinus; *solid arrow*, incus; *VII*, facial nerve.

resection. A labyrinthectomy is performed, and the IAC from the fundus to the porus acusticus is skeletonized. The goal is to remove bone approximately 270 degrees around the circumference of the IAC. Often, the cochlear aqueduct is opened while a trough is drilled inferior to the IAC and superior to the jugular bulb. When the cochlear aqueduct is opened, CSF flows from the opening, slightly decompressing the posterior fossa.

The dura of the posterior fossa inferior to the superior petrosal sinus and superior to the jugular bulb region is carefully opened. The seventh and eighth cranial nerves can be seen arising from the pons before they travel to the IAC through the CPA. Laterally, at the fundus of the IAC, "Bill's bar" can be palpated where it divides the facial nerve anteriorly from the superior vestibular nerve posteriorly. The transverse crest is seen separating the superior and inferior compartments of the IAC.

After tumor removal, the TL defect is usually closed with an abdominal fat graft because it is not possible to achieve a watertight dural closure following this approach. To prevent CSF rhinorrhea, the middle ear and eustachian tube are packed with periosteal or muscle tissue, and the mastoid antrum and air cells are covered with temporalis fascia and/or bone wax. The fat graft is gently packed into the craniotomy defect, and the wound is closed in layers over the fat.

134.8.2 Retrosigmoid Approach

The RS approach has the advantage of being familiar to most neurosurgeons, who may refer to it as the suboccipital approach. In reality, the two names are often used interchangeably, although the RS approach tends to be positioned slightly closer to the sigmoid and transverse sinuses. The RS approach has the ability to preserve hearing in selected cases, but hearing preservation with this approach is unlikely if exposure is needed in the lateral third of the IAC.

Intraoperative ABR monitoring is performed during an RS approach if hearing preservation is attempted. It is important to prevent antiseptic solution from accumulating in the external auditory canal because this will obscure ABR readings.

The RS approach begins with an incision similar to that of the TL approach. It is important to expose adequately the posterior portion of the mastoid tip and skull base. To minimize postoperative neck pain, care should be taken to incise the sternocleidomastoid muscle as close as possible to where it attaches to the skin near the mastoid rather than to cut through the belly of the muscle more inferiorly. A craniectomy is performed with cutting and diamond burs behind the sigmoid sinus and below the transverse sinus. A mastoid emissary vein is often encountered in the area posterior to the sigmoid sinus. Hemostasis is achieved with a combination of bipolar cautery and bone wax. Bone dust should be collected if an autologous cranioplasty is planned. Ultimately, an approximately 3-cm-diameter opening is made in the bone.

The posterior fossa dura is opened sharply along the posterior aspect of the sigmoid sinus and tacked open with braided nylon suture. Tumor may often be removed without drilling of the IAC, depending on how laterally the tumor extends past the porus acusticus. If the IAC must be drilled, Gelfoam (Pfizer, New York, NY) or other barrier materials are used to prevent the intradural accumulation of bone dust, which has been associated with postoperative headache and aseptic chemical meningitis.

The edges of the posterior fossa dura incision almost always become desiccated during tumor removal, but they can universally be rehydrated with irrigation so that they can be closed primarily for a watertight dural closure. The closure can be reinforced with a piece of muscle or synthetic dural repair matrix if necessary. It is important to separate the dural closure from the muscular closure to minimize the incidence of chronic postoperative headache. This can be accomplished by placing a mixture of bone dust and blood (bone pâté) over the dural closure, followed by an abdominal fat graft. Alternatively, hydroxyapatite bone cement has been used to reconstruct the cranial defect with promising results. The wound is then irrigated and closed in layers over the cranioplasty site.

134.8.3 Staged Surgery and Multimodality Therapy

Occasionally, an intraoperative change in the patient's general health condition or a particularly difficult tumor removal may require cessation of a tumor resection before complete removal. Other times, a poor surgical candidate or an elderly patient with a large tumor may require subtotal resection for brainstem decompression without being kept under general anesthesia for the length of time necessary for total tumor removal. In any of these cases, the patient with a subtotal or nearly total tumor resection will be left with three options: (1) serial observation of residual tumor, (2) second-stage surgery for complete resection, and (3) postoperative stereotactic radiosurgery ("multimodality therapy"). Tailoring the treatment algorithm based on all of the available information has been shown to give patients the best chance for a favorable facial nerve outcome, especially patients with large VSs.

134.9 Complications

The primary goal of surgery for CPA tumors is the preservation of life. Mortality and stroke are extremely rare in this modern era of skull base microsurgery, and efforts are now aimed at decreasing the morbidity of treatment. The early removal of unnecessary indwelling catheters (arterial lines, Foley catheters), early ambulation, pneumatic compression devices, perioperative antibiotics, and incentive spirometry help to minimize complications common to all surgical patients. Additionally, there are unique complications that may occur after skull base surgery.

The risk for CSF leak following the surgical resection of VS has been reported to be as high as 10.6% in one meta-analysis of 5,964 procedures and was not related to patient age or tumor size. CSF leak can manifest as CSF rhinorrhea, otorrhea, or drainage of fluid through the skin incision. CSF leaks are treated with stool softeners, bed rest, lumbar drain, and/or surgical revision. Bacterial meningitis, another complication, is more common in the presence of CSF leak and is treated with intravenous antibiotics. Aseptic meningitis can be caused by intradural bone dust or other meningeal irritants and is typically treated with corticosteroids. Postoperative patients with fevers and signs of meningeal irritation should be evaluated promptly with a lumbar puncture and CSF analysis.

Immediate or delayed facial palsy can also occur following surgical resection. Immediate facial palsy is typically due to a neurapraxia resulting from stretching the nerve during tumor removal. Neurapraxic injury is more common with larger tumors. Rarely, a complete ipsilateral facial paralysis is due to nerve transection or other iatrogenic trauma. Delayed facial palsy may be due to a reactivation of latent viruses or delayed surgical edema of the facial nerve. It can occur in up to 15% of patients, and some advocate the perioperative use of antiviral medication to minimize the incidence of this complication. Preoperative corticosteroids also help to control the rates of both immediate and delayed facial nerve weakness. The majority of patients with a delayed facial palsy recover most of their preoperative function, and 90% recover fully.

Headache is a common postoperative complaint following both the TL and RS approaches, but it is more common following RS surgery. As noted earlier, efforts to separate the dural closure from the nuchal musculature may help to control the rates of long-term post-craniotomy headaches.

Tinnitus is often present preoperatively. Although some patients notice improvement or resolution of their tinnitus after treatment, some patients actually develop a new onset of tinnitus. There have not been any accepted methods to improve or predict the outcomes of tinnitus.

Although not a complication, disequilibrium or vertigo is an expected postoperative symptom, especially after the TL approach. Patients usually have symptoms that are inversely proportional to their amount of weakness on preoperative caloric testing. Those with poorer preoperative inner ear function on the side of the tumor have begun central and contralateral compensation and are less affected by the acute loss of unilateral inner ear function. Early ambulation with assistance and focused vestibular rehabilitation beginning on postoperative day 1 are invaluable. Most patients do not need formal vestibular therapy after discharge.

134.10 Roundsmanship

- The two most common neoplasms of the CPA are vestibular schwannomas and meningiomas.
- The two non–hearing preservation approaches for the treatment of VS are the TL and the RS approaches.
- The four options for a patient with a diagnosis of VS are (1) observation, (2) microsurgical resection, (3) stereotactic radiosurgery, and (4) multimodality therapy (i.e., surgical resection + postoperative stereotactic radiosurgery).
- The gold standard for the diagnosis of VS is MR imaging of the brain and IAC with gadolinium contrast.
- NF2 is associated with an autosomal-dominant mutation in a gene located on chromosome 22 (22q12) that codes for a tumor suppressor protein, merlin.
- The most common grade of meningioma is WHO grade I.
- "Rollover" is seen when a patient with retrocochlear pathology has a decreasing SDS as speech is presented at louder levels.

134.11 Recommended Reading

[1] Bennett M, Haynes DS. Surgical approaches and complications in the removal of vestibular schwannomas. 2007. Neurosurg Clin N Am 2008; 19: 331–343

[2] Blevins NH, Jackler RK. Exposure of the lateral extremity of the internal auditory canal through the retrosigmoid approach: a radioanatomic study. Otolaryngol Head Neck Surg 1994; 111: 81–90

[3] Committee on Hearing and Equilibrium guidelines for the evaluation of hearing preservation in acoustic neuroma (vestibular schwannoma). American

Academy of Otolaryngology-Head and Neck Surgery Foundation, INC. Otolaryngol Head Neck Surg 1995; 113: 179–180

[4] Don M, Kwong B, Tanaka C. Interaural stacked auditory brainstem response measures for detecting small unilateral acoustic tumors. Audiol Neurootol 2012; 17: 54–68

[5] Gardner G, Robertson JH. Hearing preservation in unilateral acoustic neuroma surgery. Ann Otol Rhinol Laryngol 1988; 97: 55–66

[6] Jacob A, Robinson LL, Bortman JS, Yu L, Dodson EE, Welling DB. Nerve of origin, tumor size, hearing preservation, and facial nerve outcomes in 359 vestibular schwannoma resections at a tertiary care academic center. Laryngoscope 2007; 117: 2087–2092

[7] Kartush JM, Niparko JK, Graham MD, Kemink JL. Electroneurography: preoperative facial nerve assessment for tumors of the temporal bone. Otolaryngol Head Neck Surg 1987; 97: 257–261

[8] Louis DN, International Agency for Research on Cancer, World Health Organization. WHO Classification of Tumours of the Central Nervous System. Lyon, France: International Agency for Research on Cancer; 2000

[9] Porter RG, Leonetti JP, Ksiazek J, Anderson D. Association between adipose graft usage and postoperative headache after retrosigmoid craniotomy. Otol Neurotol 2009; 30: 635–639

[10] Selesnick SH, Liu JC, Jen A, Newman J. The incidence of cerebrospinal fluid leak after vestibular schwannoma surgery. Otol Neurotol 2004; 25: 387–393

[11] Stangerup SE, Caye-Thomasen P, Tos M, Thomsen J. The natural history of vestibular schwannoma. Otol Neurotol 2006; 27: 547–552

[12] Sughrue ME, Yang I, Aranda D et al. The natural history of untreated sporadic vestibular schwannomas: a comprehensive review of hearing outcomes. J Neurosurg 2010; 112: 163–167

135 Middle Cranial Fossa Anatomy and Surgery

Seilesh C. Babu and Matthew L. Kircher

135.1 Introduction

The middle cranial fossa (MCF), comprising the greater sphenoid wing and the temporal bone, forms the base of the skull upon which the temporal lobe rests. The anatomy, including the neurovascular structures that traverse the MCF and the cochleovestibular apparatus that lies within the petrous temporal bone, will be reviewed. Common disease processes and the basic surgical approaches relevant to the MCF will be the focus of this chapter.

The MCF approach was popularized by Dr. William House in the 1960s. The approach had been described previously, but it was the work of House that established this approach as a reliable surgical technique. Initially, its utility was in addressing vestibular schwannoma in patients with serviceable hearing and tumors that were relatively small and localized to the internal auditory canal. The indications for the MCF approach have since expanded to address multiple skull base pathologies, with the advantage that the labyrinth and its related structures can be approached from above, allowing the labyrinth to remain intact.

135.2 Common Indications for Middle Cranial Fossa Surgery

1. Middle and posterior cranial fossa neoplasms, including vestibular schwannomas, meningiomas, epidermoids, and arachnoid cysts
2. Petrous apex lesions, such as cholesterol granulomas, primary cholesteatomas, chondrosarcomas, and metastases
3. Superior semicircular canal dehiscence syndrome
4. Middle fossa encephalocele and cerebrospinal fluid (CSF) leak
5. Facial nerve decompression for facial nerve paralysis

135.3 Incidence of Disease

1. Vestibular schwannomas: Vestibular schwannomas account for more than 90% of neoplasms of the cerebellopontine angle (CPA) and internal auditory canal (IAC). Less common lesions include meningioma, epidermoid, and facial nerve schwannoma.
2. Petrous apex lesions: Petrous apex lesions are relatively rare and typically reported as small case series, even at large skull base surgical centers. However, incidental petrous apex findings are becoming more common because of the routine use of computed tomography (CT) and magnetic resonance (MR) imaging. Cholesterol granuloma is the most common lesion of the petrous apex.
3. Superior semicircular canal dehiscence (SSCD) syndrome: This entity was first described by Lloyd Minor in 1998. The incidence of anatomical canal dehiscence is 0.5%, with only a small subset of patients actually experiencing symptoms.

4. Middle fossa encephalocele: The incidence of tegmen defects in this region ranges from 6% to 22%; once again, only a small subset of patients with tegmen defects will develop an encephalocele and/or CSF.
5. Facial nerve paralysis: Bell palsy is the most common cause of facial paralysis, with most patients recovering full facial function. Trauma to the facial nerve may also occur after a temporal bone fracture or during surgical procedures. Studies have identified poor prognostic factors for facial recovery that include progression to full paralysis and paralysis that does not recover within 3 weeks. Electrodiagnostic techniques can quantify neural degeneration and predict the likelihood of recovery. Patients at risk for poor recovery are rare but may benefit from facial nerve decompression to improve function.

135.4 Applied Anatomy

When the middle fossa floor is viewed from above, the gasserian ganglion is located at the anterior aspect of the petrous apex and gives off the three subdivisions of the trigeminal nerve. The mandibular division, V_1, passes anteriorly through the superior orbital fissure. The maxillary and ophthalmic divisions, V_2 and V_3, pass through the foramen rotundum and foramen ovale, respectively. Posterior to the foramen ovale lies the foramen spinosum, through which the middle meningeal artery enters the MCF. The greater superficial petrosal nerve exits from the geniculate ganglion at the lateral aspect of the internal auditory canal (IAC) and runs in an anteromedial direction across the floor of the MCF in parallel alignment with the deeper and more lateral tensor tympani muscle and Eustachian tube. The horizontal portion of the carotid artery lies medial to the eustachian tube and inferior to the greater superficial petrosal nerve as it courses toward the cavernous sinus (▶ Fig. 135.1).

Posteriorly, the arcuate eminence approximates the position of the superior semicircular canal, which tends to be perpendicular to the petrous ridge, although the orientation may be variable in some patients. Medially, the superior petrosal sinus runs along the petrous ridge. The IAC lies in approximately the same plane as the external auditory canal and is found medially at the bisected angle of the superior semicircular canal and greater superficial petrosal nerve. The cochlea lies medial and inferior to the geniculate ganglion at the junction of the greater superficial petrosal nerve and IAC. The vestibule is situated anterolateral to the superior semicircular canal between the lateral end of the IAC and the middle ear space.

After the superior wall of the IAC is removed, the facial nerve can be seen in the anterosuperior portion of the IAC and the superior vestibular nerve in the posterosuperior portion, separated by "Bill's bar" in the lateral aspect of the IAC. The tegmen tympani and tegmen mastoideum are situated lateral to the labyrinth. This bone can be removed to reveal the epitympanum, the tympanic segment of the facial nerve, the ossicular chain, and the mastoid antrum.

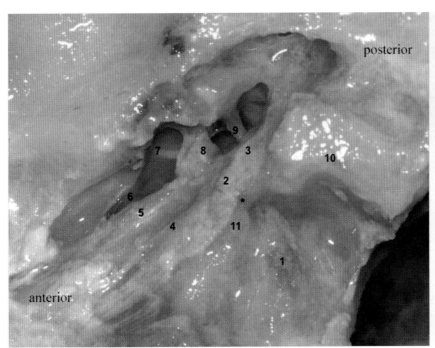

Fig. 135.1 View of the right side in the middle cranial fossa surgical approach. *1*, Internal auditory canal; *2*, geniculate ganglion; *3*, tympanic segment of facial nerve; *4*, greater superficial petrosal nerve; *5*, carotid artery; *6*, eustachian tube; *7*, tympanic membrane anulus; *8*, cochleariform process; *9*, long process of incus; *10*, superior semicircular canal; *11*, cochlea; *asterisk*, labyrinthine segment of facial nerve.

135.5 Etiology/Pathogenesis

1. Vestibular schwannoma: The most common lesion of the cerebellopontine (CPA) and IAC is vestibular schwannoma. A slow-growing benign tumor of the eighth cranial nerve sheath, it accounts for 8 to 10% of all intracranial tumors. These lesions exert pressure on surrounding neurovascular structures, thereby leading to auditory and vestibular symptomatology. The vast majority occur sporadically. Tumors with a genetic origin are typically manifestations of the neurofibromatoses types I and II.

2. Petrous apex lesion: The most common lesion of the petrous apex is cholesterol granuloma. Histologically, these lesions consist of a granulomatous response to cholesterol degradation components in blood. They develop in aerated portions of the temporal bone, including the petrous apex, distant to a lesion that prevents normal air cell aeration. Trauma or infection with hemorrhage is a major factor theorized to predispose to the formation of these lesions.

3. SSCD syndrome: SSCD syndrome is the result of bony dehiscence over the superior canal. There appears to be a developmental or congenital predisposition to these bony defects because the bone overlying the intact portions of the superior canal is significantly thinner in patients with unilateral dehiscence than in patients without SSCD. The onset of the signs and symptoms associated with SSCD syndrome typically occurs in adulthood, suggesting that patients with an already thin tegmen bone may be predisposed to the development of a dehiscence caused by overlying temporal lobe pulsations. The dehiscence effectively creates a third mobile window of the inner ear. Whereas sound pressure normally enters through the oval window and dissipates through the round window, the superior canal defect allows pressure to dissipate at this site. As a result, the superior canal is responsive to sound and pressure stimuli.

4. Middle fossa encephalocele: Congenital predisposition to middle fossa encephalocele is thought to result from a disturbance in the normal ossification and pneumatization of the temporal bone. This disturbance in turn creates a bony defect. However, encephalocele develops in only a small subset of patients with tegmen defects. Encephalocele formation and/or CSF leak is oftentimes associated with a locally destructive inflammatory process such as cholesteatoma or chronic otitis media, although surgical and nonsurgical trauma is also implicated. In addition, factors such as benign intracranial hypertension and obesity have been suggested.

5. Facial paralysis: Facial paralysis is most commonly due to Bell palsy, but herpes zoster oticus, temporal bone fracture, facial neoplasm, Melkersson-Rosenthal syndrome, Lyme disease, otitis media, and congenital causes must also be considered in the differential. Most commonly, facial nerve paralysis amenable to MCF decompression or repair is secondary to Bell palsy or to accidental or iatrogenic trauma.

135.6 Clinical Presentation
135.6.1 Vestibular Schwannoma

The typical clinical presentation of a vestibular schwannoma includes unilateral tinnitus and slowly progressive sensorineural hearing loss. Symptoms may be present for years before they are brought to the attention of a practitioner because these lesions tend to be slow-growing, averaging 2 mm of growth per year. Initially, a tumor confined to the IAC may be asymptomatic, but with growth, the cochleovestibular nerve, facial nerve, and labyrinthine vasculature become compressed. Many patients will describe a mild, nondebilitating imbalance because the contralateral labyrinth generally compensates well for single-sided vestibular loss. Also, the facial nerve tends to be relatively resistant to tumor compression and is affected only by very large tumors. Those tumors that continue to grow may expand the IAC and protrude into the CPA. Rarely, much larger lesions will compress the brainstem, leading to hydrocephalus and even death from tonsillar herniation.

135.6.2 Petrous Apex Lesion

Patients with petrous apex lesions may present with a variety of symptoms and clinical findings. Classically, Gradenigo syndrome describes retro-orbital pain, otorrhea, and ipsilateral sixth cranial nerve paresis secondary to petrous apicitis. Cholesterol granuloma and other petrous apex lesions may also be diagnosed incidentally on imaging studies. However, larger lesions may present with hearing loss and vestibular weakness due to IAC compression. In addition, patients may experience headache and/or retro-orbital, facial, or neck pain, depending on the portion of the temporal bone affected.

135.6.3 Superior Semicircular Canal Dehiscence Syndrome

Patients with SCCD syndrome are variably affected by vertigo brought on by loud sounds (Tullio phenomenon), tragal compression, Valsalva maneuver, or nose blowing. In addition, autophony and sometimes bizarre complaints such as "hearing" one's eye movements may be present. The Weber tuning fork test typically lateralizes to the affected ear, and patients also may hear a tuning fork placed on the lateral malleolus of the ankle. The clinical manifestations of SSCD syndrome are variable; some patients are affected solely by vestibular or auditory symptoms, whereas others will be affected by a combination. The application of positive pressure to the external auditory canal ultimately causes endolymph displacement, leading to an excitatory ampullofugal deflection of the superior canal. This excitation causes slow-component nystagmus directed upward and away from the affected ear with fast component nystagmus in the opposite direction. These evoked eye movements are in the plane of the superior canal.

135.6.4 Middle Fossa Encephalocele

This entity may present with a unilateral middle ear effusion, conductive hearing loss, a middle ear or mastoid mass, otorhinorrhea, or meningitis or another intracranial infectious process. A common scenario is an adult patient presenting with a unilateral middle ear effusion and conductive hearing loss. After a benign nasopharyngeal examination, myringotomy and tube placement are performed, and the patient notes a persistent clear otorrhea. Leakage may be intermittent and occur spontaneously or with increased intracranial pressure (i.e., Valsalva maneuver).

135.6.5 Facial Paralysis

Facial function should be documented with an established system, such as the House-Brackmann grading scale, to quantify the dysfunction and track outcomes. The clinical presentation in facial paralysis is of the utmost importance in determining the etiology, with special attention to the onset, duration, and

severity of paralysis. A complete history and physical examination, including otoscopy, should be performed in all patients. Middle ear and parotid lesions responsible for facial paralysis may be evident on examination.

The acute onset of paralysis or paresis with full recovery within 3 weeks is seen in the majority of patients with Bell palsy. Those patients with a gradual onset of weakness over 3 weeks, failure to resolve incomplete paresis, failure to regain function after 3 to 6 months, recurrent facial palsy, facial pain, or associated cranial neuropathy should be considered for further work-up.

Immediate facial paralysis after trauma indicates significant nerve impingement or transection. Delayed weakness indicates the gradual development of nerve edema and blockage of axoplasmic flow.

135.7 Testing
135.7.1 Vestibular Schwannoma

Auditory and vestibular studies assess the functional integrity of the audiovestibular system and are the preferred initial screening studies. Based on this information, the decision to perform imaging studies for a definitive anatomical diagnosis is made.

Audiometry

Asymmetric sensorineural hearing loss or impairment of speech discrimination disproportionate to pure-tone loss on a routine audiogram is suggestive of a retrocochlear lesion.

Auditory Brainstem Response Testing

The brainstem response to a broadband click is recorded, and the latencies of wave V for the two ears are compared. An adjusted interaural latency for wave V greater than 0.2 milliseconds is considered abnormal and suggestive of retrocochlear pathology.

Vestibular Testing

Electronystagmography and caloric testing may reveal unilateral vestibular weakness when retrocochlear pathology is present.

Imaging

CT can provide useful information regarding temporal bone pathology, but MR imaging with gadolinium is the imaging choice of study for the evaluation of vestibular scwhannoma. Schwannomas enhance with gadolinium and tend to be isointense or hypointense to brain on T1-weighted images and hyperintense on T2-weighted images.

135.7.2 Petrous Apex Lesion
Audiometry

Audiometry is a sine qua non before any intervention of the temporal bone.

Imaging

Characteristic CT and MR imaging findings are paramount in evaluating lesions of the petrous apex. The combination of CT and MR imaging provides the most complete radiologic assessment of petrous apex lesions, allowing the differentiation between benign and malignant lesions and normal anatomical variants.

135.7.3 Superior Semicircular Canal Dehiscence Syndrome

Audiometry

Routine audiogram may reveal a mild conductive hearing loss at lower frequencies and bone conduction thresholds below 0 dB nHL.

Vestibular Testing

Vestibular evoked myogenic potential (VEMP) responses have been used to assess for the presence of SSCD syndrome. In this test, nerve potentials evoked by clicks or tone bursts are recorded from surface electromyographic (EMG) electrodes placed over the ipsilateral sternocleidomastoid muscle while that muscle is tonically contracted. The reflex is thought to be activated by sound transmitted through the stapes footplate to the saccule and inferior vestibular nerve. The threshold for eliciting the VEMP response is lower in an ear affected with SSCD than in a normal ear.

Imaging

High-resolution CT scans reconstructed in the plane of and perpendicular to the plane of the superior semicircular canal can confirm the dehiscence of overlying bone. Of note, SSCD may be noted incidentally on imaging in patients without signs or symptoms of SCCD syndrome.

135.7.4 Middle Fossa Encephalocele

Laboratory

Collected fluid suspected to be CSF can be evaluated for a number of factors that are consistent with CSF composition. A glucose value that is 60% of serum levels, a protein concentration of less than 200 mg/dL, and a chloride level greater than normal serum levels are all consistent with CSF. However, it may be difficult to collect enough fluid to accurately assess these parameters. The identification of β_2-transferrin, a protein found in CSF and perilymph, is the most sensitive and specific laboratory test to confirm the presence of CSF, with only small trace amounts of fluid required for testing.

Imaging

High-resolution CT scans are needed to define bony defects in the tegmen tympani or mastoideum, and MR imaging is superior for defining soft-tissue and dural characteristics and confirming encephalocele communication with the intracranial cavity. CT with the intrathecal injection of metrizamide can show CSF leak fistulas for diagnosis and localization. The use of other radiopaque intrathecal agents, such as fluorescein and indigo carmine, has been reported. The main limitation is that small or intermittent leaks can lead to false-negative test results.

135.7.5 Facial Paralysis

Laboratory

Laboratory panels including blood glucose, erythrocyte sedimentation rate, angiotensin-converting enzyme, Lyme titers, and VDRL (Veneral Disease Research Laboratory) testing, may be sent to evaluate for systemic causes of facial paralysis.

Electrophysiology

Most physicians use electroneuronography (ENOG) and EMG to determine the level of nerve injury. In cases of incomplete paralysis, ENOG may give prognostic information, although in general these patients have a good prognosis for full facial nerve recovery. In patients with complete paralysis, ENOG can estimate the amount of nerve fiber degeneration. It is used between 4 and 21 days after paralysis to allow time for the onset of wallerian degeneration. Voluntary EMG potentials are measured as well because these may be present in a regenerating nerve and would indicate a greater chance of facial nerve recovery. Degeneration of more than 90% on EMOG without voluntary EMG potentials indicates a greater likelihood of poor facial nerve recovery, and facial nerve decompression may therefore be considered.

Imaging

Facial paralysis after temporal bone trauma should be evaluated with high-resolution CT of the temporal bone. Infectious or inflammatory processes may show evidence of enhancement along the fallopian canal with gadolinium-enhanced MR imaging. In this situation, edema at the meatal foramen is posited to be the common epicenter of neural injury. In addition, CT and MR imaging are complementary in evaluating neoplastic processes involving the facial nerve.

135.8 Treatment

135.8.1 Middle Cranial Fossa Surgery: Basic Technique

A preauricular incision is extended along the temporal region. Temporalis fascia is harvested as necessary. The temporalis muscle is divided, and a 5 x 5-cm craniotomy is performed centered over the zygomatic root. The floor of the middle fossa is exposed by elevating the dura in a posterior to anterior direction to avoid injury to the geniculate ganglion. Dural elevation continues medially to the level of the superior petrosal sinus. The principal landmarks for orientation to the IAC are the greater superficial petrosal nerve and the arcuate eminence, a marker for the superior semicircular canal. With the surgeon working at the bisected angle of these landmarks, wide skeletonization of the IAC begins medially. With progressively smaller diamond burs, the IAC is unroofed superiorly. Care must be taken in the lateral portion of the canal because of the proximity of the cochlea and vestibule. For tumor removal in the IAC, the dura of the IAC is opened and the facial nerve is freed from the tumor, with care taken to preserve the vascular structures as well. Once tumor removal is complete, the canal is sealed with autologous fat, fascia, or muscle, and the bone flap is replaced.

135.8.2 Potential Complications

CSF leak may occur if the dura is violated. This should be a consideration in older patients because the dura may be less resistant to injury and tear easily with elevation. Intracranial hematoma is a rare postoperative complication in which the patient may present with mental status change or severe headache. If this complication occurs, the patient must be returned to the operating room quickly for hematoma evacuation to prevent more serious sequelae. Language impairment caused by damage of the dominant temporal lobe must also be considered.

135.8.3 Disease-Specific Treatment Considerations

Vestibular Schwannoma

Treatement options include observation, stereotactic radiotherapy, and microsurgical resection. Vestibular schwannomas are typically slow-growing tumors. In fact, approximately one-third of tumors followed over a period of 5 years showed no growth on imaging. Nonetheless, serial MR imaging is indicated to track tumor progress because some tumors have been shown to display rapid growth. Poor operative candidates with tumors that display growth may be offered stereotactic radiotherapy as a primary treatment modality. In addition, patients who have undergone a subtotal resection because attempts at total resection might have caused undue facial nerve morbidity may receive adjuvant radiotherapy. Very large tumors causing brainstem compression are an absolute indication for surgery, with a higher risk for facial nerve dysfunction. Patients who have large tumors with significant CPA involvement may not be ideal candidates for primary radiation therapy because postradiation tumor swelling with hydrocephalus is a recognized complication. Ultimately, except for those with large tumors causing brainstem compression, patients may choose the treatment option that best suits them.

The primary surgical approaches used in the resection of a vestibular schwannoma are the translabyrinthine, retrosigmoid, and MCF approaches. The retrosigmoid and MCF approaches can potentially save hearing in selected patients. The translabyrinthine approach sacrifices hearing but is a more direct approach to the CPA and IAC, with the resultant advantage of requiring minimal brain retraction. The retrosigmoid approach is best suited for patients who have CPA-based lesions with limited IAC extension and serviceable hearing. Cerebellar retraction may be required for optimal exposure. The middle fossa approach is ideally suited for the resection of intracanalicular tumors in patients with serviceable hearing. The MCF approach requires temporal lobe retraction and thus provides limited medial exposure for lesions involving more than 1 cm of the CPA.

The success of hearing preservation depends in large part on maintenance of the cochlear blood supply. Disruption of the labyrinthine artery after IAC dissection despite cochlear nerve preservation can result in significant postoperative hearing loss. In addition, care must be taken to preserve the anterior inferior cerebellar artery, which may loop into the IAC.

Petrous Apex Lesion

The imaging characteristics of petrous apex lesions are paramount in establishing a diagnosis and determining the need for surgical intervention. Benign-appearing cystic lesions may be managed conservatively with observation. Solid tumors of the temporal bone and cholesteatoma are removed when first identified to prevent the further involvement of nearby vital structures. Drainage procedures are inadequate treatment for these lesions, and all reasonable efforts should be made to remove them entirely, while minimizing morbidity. Fortunately, the most common petrous apex lesion, cholesterol granuloma, is a benign cystic lesion that can be managed with drainage to an aerated portion of the temporal bone.

Drainage of a petrous apex cystic lesion is commonly performed via a transcanal infracochlear technique; however, anatomical constraints may sometimes limit this approach. The MCF craniotomy allows drainage of the cyst from above via the previously mentioned MCF surgical steps. Of note, the IAC is identified only as necessary to orient surgical landmarks. The cyst is opened, and a catheter is placed within the cyst and routed to an opening in the tegmen mastoideum to allow continued drainage.

Superior Semicircular Canal Dehiscence Syndrome

The severity of symptoms must be weighed against the risks and benefits of surgery. Some patients may choose lifestyle changes instead of surgery, simply avoiding stimuli that evoke symptoms (i.e., loud sounds, ambient pressure changes). Placement of a tympanostomy tube may be beneficial in some patients with principally pressure-induced symptoms. Autophony or a mild conductive hearing loss may be tolerable to some and intolerable to others. For those patients debilitated by symptoms, plugging or resurfacing of the superior canal may be offered.

This procedure may be done via a transmastoid or an MCF approach, each with inherent advantages and disadvantages. In general, the MCF approach requires temporal lobe retraction but offers a more direct examination of the superior semicircular canal for identification and manipulation. For canal occlusion, an MCF craniotomy is performed, and after exposure of the superior semicircular canal, harvested fascia is gently slid into the lumen of the bony superior canal, with care taken to preserve the underlying membranous superior canal. Overlying bone chips are then used to secure the fascia in place.

Besides the general risks inherent to MCF craniotomy, potential complications of superior semicircular canal occlusion include sensorineural hearing loss and initial worsening of imbalance symptoms postoperatively. Imbalance tends to improve with ambulation and physical therapy; however, recovery can be a longer and more difficult process in older patients.

Middle Fossa Encephalocele

Traumatic CSF leak tends to respond to conservative management with or without a lumbar drain. Middle fossa encephalocele with CSF leak requires surgical intervention to reconstitute the bony defect and prevent further encephalocele herniation. The current standard for encephalocele repair involves a multi-layered closure including a soft-tissue repair of the dura combined with a repair of the bone defect. The encephalocele is resected or reduced with bipolar cautery because it is inactive glial tissue. Temporalis fascia is typically used for soft tissue, with cortical bone grafts or hydroxyapatite synthetic bone cement used to reconstruct the bony defect. Transmastoid and middle fossa craniotomy approaches are routinely used to expose these leaks, often in combination. The transmastoid approach is best suited for isolated posterior tegmen defects. Anterior or medial sites are addressed via MCF craniotomy. In addition, multiple areas of tegmen dehiscence may be present and are best visualized from the MCF viewpoint. The potential for meningitis must be considered whenever a CSF leak is present.

Facial Nerve Paralysis

If a facial nerve has more than 90% degeneration on ENOG with absent EMG potentials, then patients may be offered MCF facial nerve decompression. Facial nerve decompression via MCF has been shown to have benefit only within 2 weeks after injury and is intended to reduce perineural edema and reestablish neural integrity along the labyrinthine, meatal foramen, and geniculate ganglion segments of the facial nerve in Bell palsy. Traumatic facial nerve injuries may also be explored through an MCF approach for decompression or repair via primary nerve anastomosis or grafting.

135.9 Roundsmanship

- The middle cranial fossa approach may be used to address small vestibular schwannomas in the internal auditory canal or with moderate extension into the cerebellopontine angle in patients who have good preoperative hearing.
- Cholesterol granuloma and other petrous apex lesions may be addressed with a middle cranial fossa approach.
- Superior semicircular canal dehiscence may be treated with canal occlusion via middle cranial fossa exposure of the canal dehiscence.
- Middle fossa encephalocele and CSF leak are commonly repaired via a middle cranial fossa craniotomy.
- Facial nerve decompression or repair via middle cranial fossa craniotomy may be used in patients with complete facial paralysis and electrophysiologic testing indicating a poor chance of facial nerve recovery.

135.10 Recommended Reading

[1] Arriaga MA, Haid RT, Masel DA. Antidromic stimulation of the greater superficial petrosal nerve in middle fossa surgery. Laryngoscope 1995; 105: 102–105

[2] Brackman DE, Arriaga MA. Neoplasms of the posterior fossa. In: Flint PW, Haughey BH, Lund VJ, et al, eds. Cummings Otolaryngology: Head and Neck Surgery. 5th ed. Philadelphia, PA: Mosby Elsevier; 2010

[3] Chen DA. Dural herniation and cerebrospinal fluid leaks. In: Brackman DE, Shelton C, Arriaga MA, eds. Otologic Surgery. 3rd ed. Philadelphia, PA: W. B. Saunders; 2010

[4] Crane BT, Carey JP, Minor LB. Superior semicircular canal dehiscence syndrome. In: Brackman DE, Shelton C, Arriaga MA, eds. Otologic Surgery. 3rd ed. Philadelphia, PA: W. B. Saunders; 2010

[5] Cruz OLM. Surgical anatomy of the lateral skull base. In: Flint PW, Haughey BH, Lund VJ, et al, eds. Cummings Otolaryngology: Head and Neck Surgery. 5th ed. Philadelphia, PA: Mosby Elsevier; 2010

[6] Gadre AK, Kwartler JA, Brackmann DE, House WF, Hitselberger WE. Middle fossa decompression of the internal auditory canal in acoustic neuroma surgery: a therapeutic alternative. Laryngoscope 1990; 100: 948–952

[7] Gantz BJ, Rubinstein JT, Gidley P, Woodworth GG. Surgical management of Bell's palsy. Laryngoscope 1999;109(8):1177–1188

[8] Massick DD, Welling DB, Dodson EE et al. Tumor growth and audiometric change in vestibular schwannomas managed conservatively. Laryngoscope 2000; 110: 1843–1849

[9] Shelton C, Hitselberger WE, House WF, Brackmann DE. Hearing preservation after acoustic tumor removal: long-term results. Laryngoscope 1990; 100: 115–119

136 Vascular Tumors of the Skull Base and Petrous Apex Lesions

Raj Murali, Dhruve S. Jeevan, Jayson A. Neil, and Christopher J. Linstrom

136.1 Jugular Foramen Lesions

Tumors of the skull base pose a significant management challenge as a consequence of the proximity of complex neurovascular structures. Advances in anesthesia, imaging modalities, and microsurgical techniques have enabled the surgical removal of these lesions. Because of their rarity and the complexity of their management, these tumors are best managed by a multidisciplinary team that often includes a neurosurgeon as well as an otolaryngologist.

A variety of vascular tumors can affect the skull base, including hemangiomas, hemangiopericytomas, lymphangiomas, juvenile nasopharyngeal angiofibromas, angiomatous meningiomas, and paragangliomas (glomus tumors). As a whole, they are uncommon entities, and thus accurate information about their incidence is unavailable. Many of these lesions are beyond the scope of this chapter, and we will focus our attention on tumors of the jugular foramen and paragangliomas.

The jugular foramen is a complex structure in the skull base at the junction of the temporal and occipital bones. The most common vascular tumors of this region are glomus jugulare tumors. These benign tumors arise from the neuroendocrine autonomic chemoreceptor cells (glomus bodies) of the jugular bulb and surrounding region and are included in a group of tumors referred to as paragangliomas. Paragangliomas occur at various sites and include carotid body, glomus vagale (inferior vagal ganglion), and glomus tympanicum (middle ear) tumors. Although the tumors are usually slow-growing and hypervascular, they occasionally can be more aggressive or even malignant.

136.1.1 Incidence of Disease

Glomus jugulare tumors are very rare, with an estimated annual incidence of 1 per 1.3 million persons. Nonetheless, glomus jugulare tumors remain the most common tumors of the middle ear and are second only to vestibular schwannomas as the most common tumors of the temporal bone. The mean age of patients at presentation is between 40 and 70 years, and the tumors are more common in females than in males by a 6:1 ratio. There is a left-sided predominance, with a multicentric incidence of 3 to 10% in sporadic cases and of 25 to 50% in familial cases.

136.1.2 Applied Anatomy

The jugular foramen is perhaps the most complex of all the skull base foramina (▶ Fig. 136.1, ▶ Fig. 136.2, ▶ Fig. 136.3, ▶ Fig. 136.4, ▶ Fig. 136.5, ▶ Fig. 136.6). It is an irregular gap in the skull base of the posterior cranial fossa between the temporal and occipital bones. Both neural and venous structures are transmitted through it. Sometimes, the terms *jugular foramen* and *jugular fossa* are used interchangeably to describe the jugular foramen. However, strictly speaking, the term *jugular fossa* should be limited to the deep, thumb-shaped depression that is seen on the external aspect of the skull base. Anatomically, this depression is just below the jugular foramen and houses the jugular bulb.

The foramen is separated by a fibrous band (jugular spine) into a larger posterolateral compartment (pars venosa) transmit-

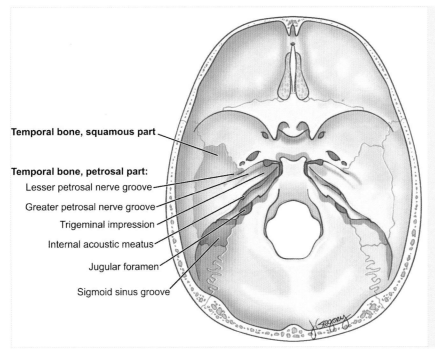

Fig. 136.1 Cranial base anatomy: superior view.

Temporal bone, squamous part

Temporal bone, petrosal part:
Lesser petrosal nerve groove
Greater petrosal nerve groove
Trigeminal impression
Internal acoustic meatus
Jugular foramen
Sigmoid sinus groove

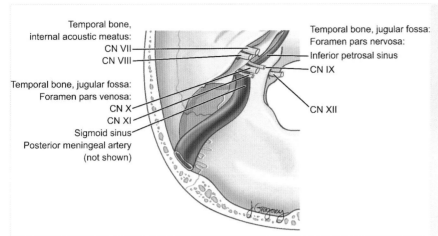

Fig. 136.2 Cranial base anatomy: superior view including selected vascular and nerve structures. *CN*, cranial nerve.

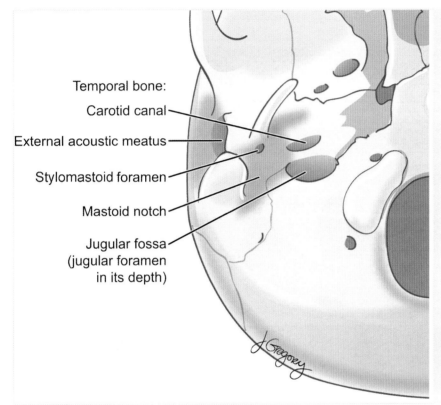

Fig. 136.3 Cranial base anatomy: inferior view. Source:

ting the jugular bulb, posterior meningeal artery, and cranial nerves (CNs) X and XI. The smaller anteromedial compartment (pars nervosa) receives the inferior petrosal sinus and CN IX (see ▸ Fig. 136.2, ▸ Fig. 136.4, ▸ Fig. 136.5, ▸ Fig. 136.6).

The inferior petrosal sinus and the sigmoid sinus join to form the internal jugular vein in the posterior compartment of the jugular foramen. At its origin, the internal jugular vein is somewhat dilated, and this dilatation is called the superior bulb. The lower cranial nerves are situated medial to the superior jugular bulb and posterior to the entry of the inferior petrosal sinus. The jugular canal then courses in an anterior, inferior, and lateral direction to exit the skull. The internal jugular vein runs down the side of the neck in a vertical direction, maintaining a lateral position first to the internal carotid artery and then to the common carotid. At the root of the neck, the jugular vein

unites with the subclavian vein to form the brachiocephalic vein (innominate vein); just before its termination is a second dilatation, the inferior bulb.

Many important structures lie in close proximity to the jugular foramen at the base of the skull, including the internal auditory canal, the middle ear, the medial external auditory canal (superiorly), the facial nerve (posterolaterally), and the internal carotid artery (anteriorly) within the carotid canal (see ▸ Fig. 136.1 and ▸ Fig. 136.2). At the exiting end of the jugular foramen, the internal carotid artery, internal jugular vein, and CNs VII, X, XI, and XII are all within a 2-cm area (see ▸ Fig. 136.3 and ▸ Fig. 136.4).

Both the glossopharyngeal nerve and the vagus nerve have parasympathetic branches arising from ganglia within the jugular foramen. The tympanic branch of the glossopharyngeal

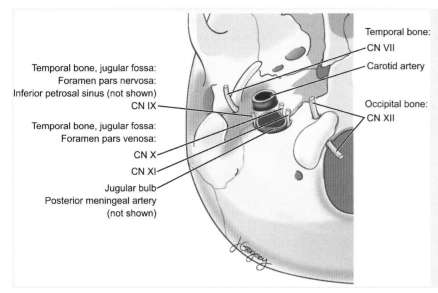

Fig. 136.4 Cranial base anatomy: inferior view including selected vascular and nerve structures. *CN*, cranial nerve.

Temporal bone:
CN VII
Carotid artery

Temporal bone, jugular fossa:
Foramen pars nervosa:
Inferior petrosal sinus (not shown)
CN IX

Occipital bone:
CN XII

Temporal bone, jugular fossa:
Foramen pars venosa:
CN X
CN XI
Jugular bulb
Posterior meningeal artery
(not shown)

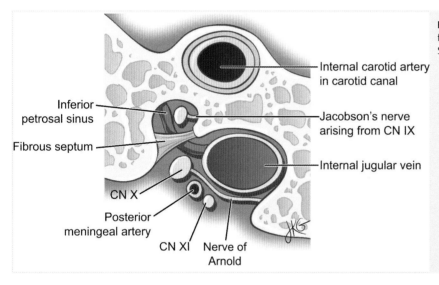

Fig. 136.5 Schematic diagram of the left jugular foramen and its contents. *CN*, cranial nerve. Source:

Internal carotid artery in carotid canal

Inferior petrosal sinus

Jacobson's nerve arising from CN IX

Fibrous septum

Internal jugular vein

CN X

Posterior meningeal artery

CN XI   Nerve of Arnold

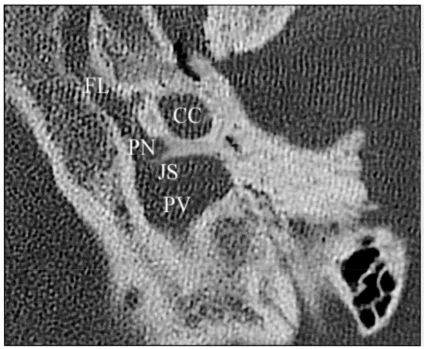

Fig. 136.6 Computed tomographic scan of the jugular foramen. CC, carotid canal; FL, foramen lacerum; JS, jugular spine; PN, pars nervosa; PV, pars vascularis.

FL
CC
PN
JS
PV

nerve and the auricular branch of the vagus nerve are the largest of these, and they form a complex plexus within the jugular foramen and the adjoining tympanic cavity. Glomus tumors are thought to originate in these autonomic ganglia.

Because a great deal of anatomical variation occurs in this area, careful study with computed tomography (CT) and magnetic resonance (MR) imaging is essential for calculating the precise locations of these structures in the skull base of an individual patient. For example, the jugular bulb in some patients may be very high-riding, almost as high as the internal auditory meatus itself. In such a case, the jugular bulb can be accidentally entered while the internal auditory meatus is being drilled, resulting in troublesome bleeding. Thin-cut CT studies of the temporal bone with axial, coronal, and sagittal reconstructions will delineate the anatomy of this region in detail. It is also essential for students to perform cadaver dissections of the temporal bone under the microscope to understand the three-dimensional anatomy of these structures.

136.1.3 The Disease Process: Etiology and Pathogenesis

Glomus jugulare tumors are examples of chemodectomas, or nonchromaffin paragangliomas. They originate from chromaffin-negative glomus cells derived from the embryonic neural crest, functioning as part of the sympathetic nervous system. Accordingly, they are categorized as originating from a neural cell line in the World Health Organization classification of neuroendocrine tumors. Chemodectomas also occur at other sites in the body, such as the carotid sheath, where they are referred to as carotid body tumors.

Glomus jugulare tumors are thought to originate from chemoreceptor cells located within the adventitia of the jugular bulb. They can be associated with either the tympanic branch of the glossopharyngeal nerve (Jacobson nerve) or the auricular branch of the vagus nerve (Arnold nerve), both of which are in close proximity to the jugular bulb. Many of these tumors secrete neuropeptides and catecholamines, occasionally in clinically symptomatic amounts that cause hypertension, excessive perspiring, tachycardia, and headaches.

The tumors are often well encapsulated and appear purplish to the naked eye. They tend to grow slowly, expanding into and destroying the surrounding bone of the jugular foramen. Within the temporal bone, they expand through the pathways of least resistance, such as air cells, vascular lumina, skull base foramina, and the eustachian tube. They invade and erode bone in a lobular fashion, often sparing the ossicular chain. As the tumor grows, it can compress the surrounding nerves in the jugular foramen and occlude the jugular bulb itself.

Glomus jugulare tumors are hypervascular, with a great tendency to recruit numerous blood vessels from the surrounding areas, and are often supplied by branches of the external carotid artery, especially the ascending pharyngeal and occipital arteries. Vascular growth factors may play an important role in this excessive vascularity. Large tumors may also invade the carotid artery wall and directly derive their blood supply from this vessel, or they may grow within the lumen of the jugular bulb.

Histologically, glomus tumors are made up of round to polygonal cells that congregate in small nests, known as zellballen.

These cells are dispersed between vascular channels. The principal cell, also known as the chief cell, is positive for chromogranin and neuron-specific enolase. The surrounding cellular matrix of the zellballen, made up of sustentacular cells, stains positive for S-100 protein and sometimes also for gliofibrillary acidic protein (GFAP).

Metastases from glomus tumors occur in approximately 4% of cases. A reduction in the proportion of chief cells and a poorer staining of sustentacular cells for S-100 and GFAP are reported to be correlated with a higher tumor grade. Metastatic lesions are distinguished from multicentric lesions on the basis of location and have been found in the lungs, lymph nodes, liver, vertebrae, ribs, and spleen. Malignancy of the tumor is likely related to *TP53* and *p16INK4A* mutations but is also characterized by the immunohistologic presence of MIB-1, Bcl-2, and CD3.

136.1.4 Medical Evaluation

Presenting Complaints

Symptoms due to glomus tumors often have an insidious onset and as a result go unnoticed, often with a delay in diagnosis. The signs and symptoms can be classified as those related to the ear, to the cranial nerves, or to other structures, and they can often be correlated with the anatomical compressive/erosive characteristics of the lesion.

The most common symptoms are hearing loss and pulsatile tinnitus. The hearing loss is usually conductive in nature, resulting from a secondary effusion or mass effect in the middle ear. Often, a characteristically pulsatile, reddish blue tumor can be seen behind the tympanic membrane on otoscopic examination. Other aural signs include dizziness, vertigo, a sensation of fullness in the ear, ear pain, and discharge from the ear.

Symptoms of cranial nerve compression can include hearing loss due to involvement of cranial nerve VIII and/or hoarseness of voice or difficulty swallowing due to involvement of CNs IX and X. The presence of jugular foramen (Vernet) syndrome, characterized by the simultaneous paresis of cranial nerves IX through XI (referred to as Collet-Sicard syndrome when CN XII is concomitantly involved), is pathognomonic for this tumor. The onset of the syndrome is usually delayed by almost a year after the initial symptoms of hearing loss and pulsatile tinnitus. The affected patient may exhibit dysphonia/hoarseness, soft palate dropping, deviation of the uvula toward the normal side, dysphagia, loss of sensory function in the posterior one-third of the tongue, decreased parotid gland secretion, loss of the gag reflex, and sternocleidomastoid and trapezius muscles paresis. In larger tumors, the facial nerve may be involved, and patients can present with a peripheral facial palsy. Very large tumors and recurrent tumors with a large intracranial extension can compress the brainstem, resulting in contralateral hemiparesis, ataxia, hydrocephalus, and increased intracranial pressure. Dural sinus involvement can lead to presentations similar to that of sinus thrombosis. Petrous carotid extension may herald Horner syndrome.

A few glomus tumors are hormonally active (2 to 4%) to the extent of causing symptoms and resulting in systemic hypertension and tachycardia (pheochromocytoma-like). Other related symptoms may include headache, perspiration, pallor, and nausea.

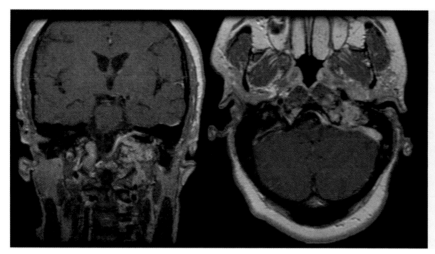

Fig. 136.7 MR images demonstrating a large, lobulated, intensely enhancing heterogeneous destructive tumor centered at the left jugular foramen and extending intracranially to the cerebellopontine angle and inferiorly below the base to the C2 level.

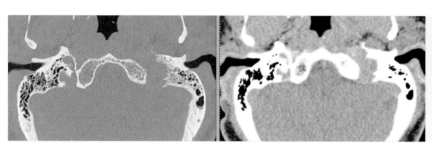

Fig. 136.8 Computed tomographic scans of the temporal bone and soft tissue demonstrating an invasive destructive tumor, consistent with glomus jugulare, at the left skull base. The tumor is destroying the left jugular foramen and left hypoglossal canal and is invading the medial left temporal bone, as well as the left occipital condyle.

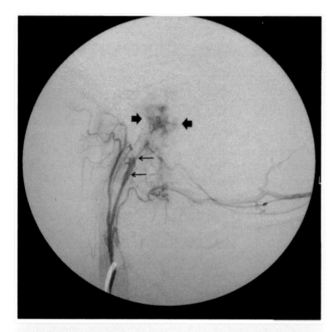

Fig. 136.9 Internal carotid arteriogram, lateral view, demonstrating the vascular blush of a glomus tumor (*short arrows*). The main feeding artery is the ascending pharyngeal artery (*long arrows*).

Testing

Glomus jugulare tumors are diagnosed through clinical examination and imaging rather than biopsy. Diagnostic biopsy is generally contraindicated because of the vascular nature of the tumors and poor accessibility. Identification and operative

planning can be aided by thin-cut CT of the temporal bone with bone and soft-tissue windows, with and without contrast. MR imaging with and without contrast is also useful, especially for larger tumors with intracranial extension (▶ Fig. 136.7). Cranial nerve and audiometric examinations are important for baseline investigation, along with urinary assay for catecholamines or their breakdown products.

Imaging studies are particularly helpful in identifying patients in whom the bone between the jugular foramen and the carotid canal is destroyed (▶ Fig. 136.8). This finding indicates that the tumor is encroaching upon the carotid artery and is important to recognize before surgery.

Almost all patients with glomus jugulare tumor should undergo vascular studies before surgery. Although CT angiography, MR angiography, and MR venography are useful, the gold standard remains cerebral angiography. Both the internal carotid and external carotid circulation and the vertebral circulation should be studied, with the venous phases included to show the sigmoid sinus and jugular vein on both sides. The classic finding on cerebral angiography is a tumor with a blush in the region of the jugular foramen, with arterial supply from the ascending pharyngeal and occipital arteries (▶ Fig. 136.9). The jugular bulb may be completely occluded by the tumor. In these cases, the venous drainage may be entirely contralateral. Cerebral angiography will also reveal the extent of collateral venous drainage, especially from the inferior petrosal sinus. Sometimes, the tumor may be seen as a filling defect within the jugular bulb.

Although formal cerebral angiography is not necessary, its advantage is that it allows the external carotid branches supplying the tumor to be embolized. Such embolization is extremely useful in limiting blood loss during surgical removal of this

Table 136.1 Glasscock-Jackson classification of glomus tumors

Tumor type	Description
I	Small tumor involving jugular bulb, middle ear, and mastoid
II	Tumor extending under internal auditory canal; may have intracranial extension
III	Tumor extending into petrous apex; may have intracranial extension
IV	Tumor extending beyond petrous apex into clivus or infratemporal fossa; may have intracranial extension

Table 136.2 Fisch classification of glomus tumors

Tumor type	Description
A	Tumor limited to middle ear
B	Tumor limited to middle ear or mastoid without involvement of infralabyrinthine space of temporal bone
C	Tumor involving infralabyrinthine and apical spaces of temporal bone, with extension into apex
C1	Tumor with limited involvement of vertical portion of carotid canal
C2	Tumor invading vertical portion of carotid canal
C3	Tumor invading horizontal portion of carotid canal
D1	Tumor with intracranial extension < 2 cm in diameter
D2	Tumor with intracranial extension > 2 cm in diameter

tumor and is usually performed as a preoperative maneuver 1 or 2 days before surgery. Cross-compression or trial balloon occlusion allows circle of Willis completeness to be evaluated in cases in which the carotid may be heavily involved in the tumor.

Classification of Glomus Jugulare Tumors

Many classification systems exist for these tumors. For example, they can be classified as functional or nonfunctional depending on whether they produce clinically symptomatic levels of catecholamines. They also can be classified on the basis of their location; tumors located primarily in the middle ear are referred to as glomus tympanicum tumors, and those whose main bulk is in the jugular foramen or middle ear are referred to as jugulotympanic tumors. Most commonly, the Glasscock-Jackson and Fisch-Mattox methods are used, which relate to morbidity and mortality. These classifications are based on extension of the tumor to surrounding anatomical structures (▶ Table 136.1 and ▶ Table 136.2).

136.1.5 Treatment

Medical Treatment

Because these tumors commonly present in the sixth and seventh decades of life, many are followed with imaging only and may not require surgical intervention. Patients who have symptomatic catecholamine-secreting tumors may be treated medically with α-blockers and β-blockers. These therapies are also instituted before any interventional procedures to prevent lethal hypertensive crises and arrhythmias. Octreotide has reportedly been used with success to control the growth of somatostatin receptor–positive tumors.

Gross total resection of some extensive tumors may be extremely difficult and carry unwarranted risk. In such cases, radiation therapy is often used for tumor control. It is certainly an option for patients with small tumors, residual tumors, or recurrent tumors, as well as for patients who refuse surgical treatment. Because of its long-term effects on bone and brain, radiation that is not stereotactically targeted is outdated.

Occasionally, glomus jugulare tumors are associated with metastatic disease. Radiation therapy is an option in these circumstances, and the successful treatment of pulmonary metastases with etoposide and cisplatin has been described.

Surgical Treatment

Complete surgical resection is the treatment modality of choice whenever possible but depends on the localization and extent of the tumor. Intraoperative monitoring with electroencephalography and somatosensory evoked potentials is routinely used. Type A and type B glomus tumors are best removed through standard middle ear or mastoid approaches. Type C and type D tumors require skull base techniques, and management is usually shared by a neurotologist and a neurosurgeon. These tumors are typically approached infratemporally. During surgery, the sigmoid sinus, jugular bulb, and presigmoid dura are completely exposed. The jugular vein, internal carotid artery, and lower cranial nerves are all isolated in the neck and traced up to the jugular foramen. The sigmoid sinus is occluded, and the jugular vein is tied off in the neck. The isolated jugular bulb is then excised with the tumor. Tumor may be present within the lumen of the jugular bulb itself. Many of the branches of the inferior petrosal sinus entering the jugular bulb will have to be coagulated and divided. The exact location of the internal carotid artery in large tumors can be detected with intraoperative ultrasound. The tumor can usually be removed from the adventitia of the internal carotid artery without damaging it.

The integrity of the lower cranial nerves can be preserved, but they have to be manipulated during surgery, which can cause temporary lower cranial nerve palsies. Postoperative cranial nerve deficits must be carefully diagnosed, and when they are present, early rehabilitation must be instituted. The facial nerve may require rerouting, especially in patients with larger tumors. Such rerouting is avoided if possible because it invariably causes at least a temporary facial palsy.

The surgical procedure is long and tedious, and a thorough knowledge of the regional anatomy gained by cadaver dissections is required. Complications include cranial nerve palsies, hearing loss, cerebrospinal fluid leakage, and blood loss. For patients who have very large tumors with significant intradural extension, it is often necessary to use a staged surgical approach.

136.1.6 Outcome and Prognosis

Glomus jugulare tumors are relatively slow-growing tumors that produce cranial nerve palsies, and many of these palsies are benign and cosmetically acceptable. However, long-term quality of life is reduced in patients with glomus tumors. Mortality ranges from 6.2% in those treated with radiation to 2.5% among those treated surgically. The overall mortality rate is 8.7%. Surgical treatment offers the best prognosis, with a 94% survival rate at 20 years and a 77% rate of symptom-free progression.

136.2 Other Vascular Tumors of the Skull Base

Although outside the scope of this chapter, it is necessary to mention some other important vascular tumors of the skull base. These tumors on the whole are relatively rare, and surgical resection remains the mainstay of treatment. Like all skull base lesions, they commonly present with symptoms of compression of important skull base structures.

Juvenile angiofibromas are found exclusively in adolescent boys and originate in the mucosa around the sphenopalatine foramen. The tumor consists of a dense fibrous mass interlaced with variable amounts of thinly walled, endothelium-lined vascular spaces. These tumors of the anterior skull base enlarge to present as nasopharyngeal masses with extension into the paranasal sinuses, orbit, pterygomaxillary space, and cavernous sinus. Epistaxis is a common presentation, along with other sinonasal symptoms. As for most skull base lesions, the treatment is

primarily surgical resection, although anti-androgenic hormonal treatment and radiation therapy have been described for selected patients.

Hemangiomas are true neoplasms; they can be capillary, cavernous, or mixed, depending on the type of blood vessels present in the lesion. Skull hemangiomas vary from small to very large and may be solitary or multiple. They proliferate rapidly after birth, then gradually shrink during childhood. Involvement of bone is uncommon. Hemangiomas of the skull base most commonly involve the orbital apex, where they affect vision by compressing the optic nerve or structures that pass through the superior fissure.

The term *angioblastic meningioma* was used in the early literature for a broad group of highly vascularized tumors of the meninges comprising both angiomatous meningiomas and hemangiopericytomas. These extremely rare vascular tumors of the skull base arise from the meningeal lining of the skull base. There is a high rate of recurrence after surgical resection.

136.3 Petrous Apex Lesions

The petrous apex forms part of the middle cranial fossa and lies at the anterior–superior border of the temporal bone (see ▸ Fig. 136.1). Petrous apex lesions are diagnosed primarily as complications of chronic otitis media. Improved imaging has made it possible to diagnose these lesions accurately and plan surgery in an area with complex anatomy. Lesions of the petrous apex are classified as infectious, inflammatory, neoplastic, or vascular abnormalities (▸ Table 136.3), with neoplastic and inflammatory lesions the most common pathologic processes. Generally, the presentation results from compression or other effects of these lesions on surrounding structures.

136.3.1 Incidence

Lesions of the petrous apex remain relatively rare. Once, infectious lesions resulting from middle ear complications were common, but their incidence is decreasing because of improved antibiotic therapy, improved techniques in surgery for chronic ear disease, and the earlier and more frequent placement of tympanostomy tubes. However, incidental lesions are becoming more common because of the routine use of imaging modalities.

136.3.2 Applied Anatomy

The temporal bone is made up of four portions: petrous, squamous, tympanic, and mastoid. The petrous portion is a pyramid with its apex directed anteromedially and its base directed

Table 136.3 Common lesions of the petrous apex

Type	Lesions
Inflammatory or congenital	Cholesterol granuloma, cholesteatoma, mucocele, epidermoid cysts
Infectious	Petrous apicitis, skull base osteomyelitis
Neoplastic	Meningioma; schwannoma (trigeminal, acoustic, jugular foramen); chordoma; chondroma; chondrosarcoma; glomus tumors; metastatic tumors
Vascular	Intrapetrous carotid artery aneurysm, dural arteriovenous fistula, hemangioma, hemangiopericytoma

posterolaterally (see ▶ Fig. 136.1). The base of the pyramid is the inner ear, the internal carotid artery, and the eustachian tube. The medial, pointed end of the petrous apex connects with the clivus. The anterosuperior or cerebral portion of the petrous apex forms the floor of the middle cranial fossa. The posterosuperior surface or cerebellar aspect of the petrous bone is vertical and marks the anterior limit of the posterior cranial fossa. The junction of the anterior and posterior surfaces is known as the petrous ridge. The inferior surface faces outward as the floor of the lateral skull base.

A number of neural and vascular structures are intimately related to the petrous apex. The trigeminal nerve and ganglion occupy the Meckel cave on the sloping anterosuperior surface of the petrous apex. CN VI traverses the Dorello canal in the petroclinoid ligament before entering the cavernous sinus. CNs VII and VIII enter the petrous bone through the internal auditory canal. The jugular foramen at the posterior and inferior surfaces is traversed by the jugular bulb and the lower cranial nerves. The internal carotid artery courses through the carotid canal in the anterolateral part of the petrous apex. The superior petrosal sinus is located along the petrous ridge. The tentorium is also attached in this location. The petrous apex is variably pneumatized.

136.3.3 Presenting Complaints

It is clear that lesions of the petrous apex can cause signs and symptoms referable to any of the structures mentioned in the preceding anatomical description. Hearing loss may be secondary to an effusion resulting from eustachian tube dysfunction or ossicular erosion resulting from chronic otitis media; sensorineural hearing loss may be secondary to invasion of the otic capsule or the cochleovestibular nerve. Tinnitus and vertigo can occur along with or independently of hearing loss. Facial paralysis occurs as a result of pressure on the facial nerve anywhere throughout its course in the temporal bone, especially near the geniculate ganglion. Headaches result from distortion of the dura near the lesion and are primarily retro-orbital or located at the vertex. Syncope, stroke, or amaurosis fugax can occur as a consequence of carotid artery occlusion. Other cranial neuropathies are associated with posterior lesions that affect CNs VIII through XII or with anterior lesions that affect CNs II through VI.

136.3.4 Inflammatory Lesions of the Petrous Apex

Cholesterol granuloma is the most common cystic lesion involving the petrous apex. The exact mechanism responsible for the formation of cholesterol granulomas in the petrous apex is not known. One theory is that they result from poor ventilation with a relative vacuum, resorption of air, mucosal hemorrhage, and hemoglobin breakdown leading to cholesterol formation. Hemorrhage seems to be a very important predisposing factor for the formation of cholesterol granulomas. Cholesterol crystals are produced during the anaerobic metabolism of free hemoglobin, and this process incites a giant cell foreign body reaction. The cycle of events is repeated and ultimately results in the formation of an expanding cholesterol granuloma. The

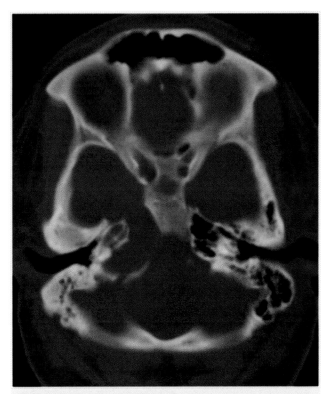

Fig. 136.10 Computed tomographic scan of the temporal bone demonstrating an expansile right petrous apex mass with thinned-out bony walls.

lesions contain a dark brown fluid with shining cholesterol crystals. The cysts occur either with or without an accompanying ear infection. Most of the cysts are unilateral and occur in adults. Symptoms include headache, diplopia from CN VI palsy, ear pain, dizziness, hearing loss, vertigo, and headaches. Sometimes, the cysts are an incidental finding on routine imaging studies. CT of the temporal bone (▶ Fig. 136.10) and MR imaging reveal the presence of an expansile petrous apex mass with thinned-out bony walls. On T1-weighted MR imaging, the lesion appears homogeneously hyperintense, whereas on T2-weighted MR imaging, a markedly hyperintense mass is revealed with a peripheral ring of low signal due to hemosiderin-laden macrophages (▶ Fig. 136.11). These MR imaging characteristics permit the differentiation of a cholesterol granuloma from an epidermoid cyst or arachnoid cyst. Small asymptomatic or incidental cholesterol granulomas can be managed with observation and periodic imaging studies alone. Large cholesterol granulomas can be drained through a transmastoid infralabyrinthine approach, and once the cystic cavity is ventilated, the lesion is unlikely to recur.

Infection of the petrous apex is also known as petrous apicitis. The triad of diplopia due to cranial nerve VI palsy, retro-orbital pain due to involvement of CN V, and otorrhea due to ear infection is known as Gradenigo syndrome. The infection is usually bacterial and is caused by pyogenic organisms.

Petrous apex infections can also be due to skull base osteomyelitis. Malignant otitis externa is a type of skull base osteomyelitis usually seen in diabetic or otherwise immunocompromised patients. The most common organism is *Pseudomonas*. In this

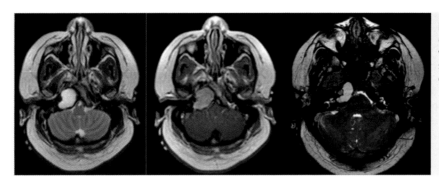

Fig. 136.11 T1-weighted (*left*) and T2-weighted (*middle*) magnetic resonance images and T1-weighted FIESTA (fast imaging employing steady-state acquisition) image (*right*) demonstrating a cholesteatoma of the right petrous apex.

setting, a relentless type of progressive osteomyelitis of the petrous bone occurs. The symptoms include chronic ear infection, drainage, ear pain, and cranial neuropathies as the disease advances. Treatment consists of prolonged and appropriate intravenous antibiotics accompanied by surgical drainage as indicated.

136.3.5 Neoplasms of the Petrous Apex

Benign tumors in the region of the petrous apex include meningiomas and schwannomas, usually of the trigeminal nerve. They often present as a cranial neuropathy, and the symptoms include dysfunction of CNs V, VI, VII, and VIII in this region. The tumors can also present with generalized headaches. Trigeminal schwannomas typically present with numbness in one or more distributions of the trigeminal nerve. The management of these tumors is surgical through a skull base approach. Petrous apex meningiomas, also known as petroclival meningiomas, require a lateral temporal approach with exposure both above and below the tentorium. The superior petrosal sinus and the tentorium are then divided to provide a wide access to the meningioma. These procedures are carried out with a team including both a neurotologist and a neurosurgeon.

Chordomas occur rarely and arise from notochord cells, primarily in the sphenoid and clivus. Tumors originating within the apex are rare, and spread is usually from the clivus. Surgery with postoperative radiation is the treatment plan of choice. Chordomas are difficult to excise completely and are only moderately radiosensitive. Average survival with aggressive treatment is only 4 years. Chondrosarcomas account for 0.15% of all intracranial neoplasms. Hearing loss, pulsatile tinnitus, vertigo/unsteadiness, CN VI palsy, and headaches are the presenting symptoms.

Breast and prostate carcinomas metastasize to the temporal bone, especially to the petrous apex and clivus. Kidney, lung, gastric, and thyroid carcinomas metastasize to the apex less commonly. When these lesions are discovered in the temporal bone, studies suggest that the lesion has already metastasized elsewhere. CT and MR imaging findings are specific to the primary tumor and depend on whether the tumor causes an osteogenic or osteoblastic reaction. The prognosis in patients with distant metastases remains poor.

An extensive three-dimensional understanding of the anatomy of the temporal bone is absolutely necessary to address disorders of the petrous apex surgically. This region is filled with critical structures that are unforgiving of subtle mistakes in surgical technique and of surgeons not intimately acquainted with the anatomy.

136.4 Roundsmanship

- A variety of vascular tumors can affect the skull base. These lesions include hemangiomas, hemangiopericytomas, lymphangiomas, juvenile nasopharyngeal angiofibromas, angiomatous meningiomas, and paragangliomas (glomus tumors).
- Although glomus jugulare tumors are rare, they remain the most common tumor of the middle ear and the second most common tumor of the temporal bone.
- Tumors of the skull base commonly affect multiple cranial nerves, particularly CNs VII through XII, which accounts for the significant morbidity associated with these lesions.
- Close proximity to vital cranial structures, including the carotid artery and jugular vein, makes the management of these tumors surgically challenging, and multidisciplinary teams are required.

136.5 Recommended Reading

[1] Borba LA, Araújo JC, de Oliveira JG et al. Surgical management of glomus jugulare tumors: a proposal for approach selection based on tumor relationships with the facial nerve. J Neurosurg 2010; 112: 88–98

[2] Fisch U, Mattox D. Microsurgery of the Skull Base. New York, NY: Thieme Medical Publishers; 1988:136–220

[3] Shah GV. Cholesterol granuloma of the petrous apex. In: Hoeffner EG, Mukherji SK, Gandhi D, Gomez-Hassan D, eds. Temporal Bone Imaging. New York, NY: Thieme Medical Publishers; 2008:136–139

[4] Horn KL, Hankinson HL. Tumors of the jugular foramen. In: Jackler RK, Brackmann DE, eds. Neurotology. 2nd ed. Philadelphia, PA: Mosby Elsevier; 2005:1037–1046

[5] Rhoton AL, Buza R. Microsurgical anatomy of the jugular foramen. J Neurosurg 1975; 42: 541–550

137 Stereotactic Radiation Treatment for Benign Tumors of the Posterior Cranial Fossa

Seilesh C. Babu and Sean R. Wise

137.1 Introduction

Over the past decade, stereotactic radiation has become an increasingly used treatment option for patients with acoustic neuromas, as well as those with other benign intracranial and skull base neoplasms. Advancements in imaging techniques, radiation delivery systems, and dose-planning software have contributed to improved patient outcomes.

The term *stereotactic radiation therapy* is used to define treatment modalities that deliver high-dose radiation in a highly conformal manner to a three-dimensional intracranial target through the use of multiple, precisely collimated beams of ionizing radiation. The goal of stereotactic radiation is tumor control with minimal toxicity to adjacent normal tissues. Such techniques have found particular application in the treatment of tumors within the posterior cranial fossa, where critical neurovascular structures, such as the brainstem, cerebellum, cochlea, vestibule, and multiple cranial nerves, lie in close anatomical proximity.

Stereotactic radiation techniques involve one of several types of ionizing radiation, and treatment may be delivered in a single dose (most commonly referred to as stereotactic radiosurgery) or in multiple fractions (generally referred to as fractionated stereotactic radiotherapy).

Advantages of radiation treatment include its ability to provide high rates of tumor control with minimal side effects. Additionally, such therapy is noninvasive and can be delivered as an outpatient procedure. The primary disadvantage of radiation therapy for such lesions is that the tumor generally persists following treatment. As a consequence, the potential for future tumor growth remains. The long-term outcomes and potential complications of various stereotactic radiation techniques remain a subject of continued investigation.

137.2 Types of Radiation

The most commonly used ionizing radiation sources for stereotactic radiosurgery or stereotactic radiotherapy are gamma photons and X-ray photons. Gamma photons are emitted through the decay of radioactive nuclei, typically cobalt 60. X-ray photons are generated from a linear accelerator (LINAC) through the collision of accelerated electrons and a target metal. Beams of heavier charged particles (e.g., protons) are also occasionally used consequent to their unique physical properties. The availability of particle beam therapy is generally limited, however, and it is found in only a few specialized facilities. The biological effectiveness of each of these sources is roughly equivalent.

137.3 Radiation Biology

Radiation delivered in the therapeutic range results in the production of free radicals within target cells through Compton scattering. The primary effect of radiosurgery is vascular fibrosis resulting in a diminished blood supply to the tumor. Evidence of more direct cellular injury has been demonstrated centrally where the radiation dose is greatest.

137.4 Stereotactic Radiation Delivery Systems

137.4.1 Gamma Knife

The gamma knife unit, developed by Leksell in 1968, contains a hemispheric array of 201 intersecting beams of cobalt 60 gamma radiation. Variously sized helmet collimators are used to further focus the individual sources of radiation to the unit's isocenter. The isocenter is the point in space where the radiation beams intersect, and essentially where the targeted tissue is positioned.

Before treatment, a stereotactic titanium frame with fiducial markers is rigidly fixed to the patient's skull. Magnetic resonance (MR) imaging or computed tomography (CT) is then acquired, with or without additional image merging. The frame ensures precise immobilization and provides the reference for defining the target in space relative to a Cartesian coordinate system. The treatment team then stereotactically localizes the tumor, and dosing software is employed to assist in developing a plan for treating the tumor effectively with high-dose radiation while sparing surrounding structures from the effects of radiation.

Treatment planning consists of placing one or more isocenters, or "shots," to fill the target of interest. Conformity to tumor is further refined through adjustments made in the collimators to vary the size and relative weight of each isocenter.

The amount of radiation delivered is the prescribed isodose, measured in units called grays (Gy). A steep falloff of radiation occurs at the periphery of the targeted volume. During treatment planning, this gradient is represented by isodose lines, which are the boundaries at which the radiation dose has fallen to a percentage of the prescribed dose. Gamma knife treatment plans commonly prescribe the 50% isodose line to the margin of the tumor (▶ Fig. 137.1).

When treatment planning is complete, the patient is positioned with the head frame fixed to the treatment couch and prescribed collimator helmet, and then advanced into the unit in a manner ensuring that the target volume resides at the unit's isocenter (▶ Fig. 137.2).

137.4.2 Linear Accelerator (LINAC)

An alternative radiosurgery technique involves the use of a LINAC. These systems employ accelerated photons and rely on a particle accelerator mounted on a gantry that rotates around the patient's head. Multiple beam positions or arcs are used to create a conformal radiation dose to the target. Tumor margin

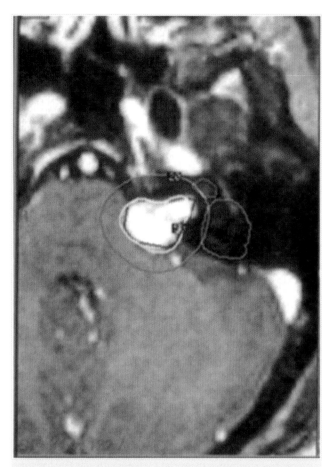

Fig. 137.1 Treatment plan for a left-sided acoustic neuroma depicting the tumor volume as well as the 50% and 20% isodose lines. Also note the contour lines of the cochlea and labyrinth; the dose distribution is tailored to minimize irradiation to these critical structures.

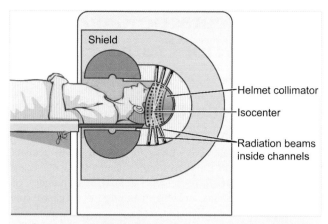

Fig. 137.2 Cross-sectional schematic of gamma knife unit.

systems in that image guidance technology is used that depends on real-time acquisition of the patient's bony anatomy to maintain orientation. The arm rotates the LINAC through a series of predetermined locations. This system also employs a non-isocentric treatment planning technique that improves the conformality and homogeneity of the delivered radiation. Additional advantages include greater patient comfort relative to rigid fixation systems, as well as the ability to provide stereotactic fractionated treatments (▶ Table 137.1).

137.5 Outcomes and Indications

Stereotactic radiation therapy is commonly used for a variety of intracranial neoplasms, both benign and malignant. Of primary interest to the otolaryngologist is the application of these techniques to several commonly encountered benign neoplasms involving the posterior cranial fossa, including acoustic neuromas, meningiomas, and glomus tumors. The indications for and outcomes of the treatment of such tumors are briefly reviewed.

137.5.1 Acoustic Neuroma

Acoustic neuromas are benign, slow-growing neoplasms originating from Schwann cells of the eighth cranial nerve. They account for approximately 15% of newly diagnosed intracranial neoplasms. Historically, the management of these tumors primarily involved observation or microsurgical resection. Stereotactic radiosurgery was reserved for patients deemed to be poor microsurgical candidates, and for those requiring adjuvant therapy for recurrent or residual disease following surgery. Over the last 20 years, the safety and efficacy of this treatment modality have been firmly established, and acoustic neuroma remains one of the most frequent targets for stereotactic radiosurgery.

Before 1992, treatment protocols for stereotactic radiosurgery involved relatively high doses of radiation, with prescribed isodoses typically of 16 Gy or more. Excellent rates of tumor control were achieved, but such protocols also resulted in significant morbidity in the form of facial weakness (21%) and facial numbness (27%). Since that time, reductions in doses to 12 to 13 Gy, as well as advancements in imaging technology and dose-planning software, have significantly improved treatment outcomes.

doses are similar to those employed with gamma knife, and traditional single-fraction stereotactic treatment still requires the use of a fixed head frame for patient immobilization.

Some LINAC systems have been modified so that stereotactic frames can be more readily removed and replaced. The primary advantage of such devices is that fractionated radiotherapy can be delivered while the targeting accuracy that is enabled through immobilization is preserved. Fractionated therapy enables efficient tumor control by making it possible to administer a higher total dose to the tumor while the surrounding normal tissues are spared from long-term radiation-induced injury because the total radiation dose is delivered over multiple sessions. This becomes particularly relevant in the treatment of larger tumors and those immediately adjacent to critical structures such as the brainstem, cranial nerves, and cochlea. A relative disadvantage of these systems is the potential for small tumor volume frameshifts between radiation fractions as the stereotactic frame is repeatedly removed and replaced.

137.4.3 Cyberknife

Cyberknife is an innovative, frameless, LINAC-based, stereotactic radiotherapy system in which a lightweight linear accelerator is mounted on a mobile robotic arm. It differs from other

Table 137.1 Comparison of stereotactic radiation delivery systems

	Gamma knife	LINAC	Cyberknife
Type of radiation	Gamma photons	X-ray photons	X-ray photons
Radiation source	Cobalt 60	Linear accelerator	Linear accelerator on mobile robotic arm
Radiation delivery	Hemispheric array of 201 intersecting radiation beams	Multiple converging radiation arcs from rotating gantry	Fixed beam delivered through multiple points to converge on target
Means to ensure localization accuracy	Fixed stereotactic head frame	Fixed frame or removable frame	Frameless, image-based guidance system
Treatment	Single session	Single or multiple sessions	Single or multiple sessions

Abbreviation: LINAC, linear accelerator.

Recent studies evaluating gamma knife stereotactic radiosurgery have reported tumor control rates ranging from 91 to 98%. Tumor control is generally defined as tumor stability or regression. Hearing preservation rates in these series vary widely (50 to 78%), and some data suggest that rates of preserved hearing may continue to decline with longer-term follow-up. When the current marginal doses of less than 13 Gy are used, the new onset of facial paralysis following treatment is rare. However, temporary facial paralysis is seen in approximately 1%. Similarly, the new onset of facial numbness or pain is uncommon but is occasionally encountered in 1 to 4% of cases. Less common complications after treatment that are rarely encountered include hydrocephalus (with the possible need for ventriculoperitoneal shunt placement), seizure, and rarely radiation-induced malignant transformation. The risks for such complications appear to be increased when larger tumors (> 2.5 cm) are treated.

In attempts to preserve hearing and decrease the rate of cranial neuropathies, a broad range of fractionated stereotactic radiotherapy protocols have been developed in the treatment of acoustic neuroma, ranging from hypofractionated regimens involving only three to six sessions to conventional regimens involving up to 30 fractions. Despite the theoretical advantages of stereotactic radiotherapy, rates for tumor control, hearing preservation, and cranial neuropathy appear similar whether patients are treated with conventionally fractionated, hypofractionated, or nonfractionated stereotactic techniques.

Despite initial data supporting the safety and efficacy of stereotactic radiation therapies, follow-up times in most studies to date have been relatively short. Late tumor growth, continued hearing decline, and delayed-onset cranial neuropathies have been encountered many years following initial treatment. Long-term follow-up will remain critical as we continue to evaluate outcomes.

The optimal strategy for the management of growing, small to medium-size acoustic neuromas remains controversial. For tumors 3 cm or smaller, similar outcomes are reported when microsurgery is compared with radiation. The ideal treatment plan for such patients depends on surgeon experience and institutional resources, as well individual medical factors and patient preferences. Stereotactic radiation is not generally recommended as primary treatment for tumors that are larger than 3.0 cm or that compress the brainstem because of the increased risks for associated brainstem injury. Radiation remains a safe and effective treatment option for the elderly, for patients medically unable or unwilling to undergo surgery, and for those with recurrent or residual disease following microsurgical resection.

137.5.2 Meningioma

Meningiomas account for approximately 25% of all intracranial tumors, and approximately 7 to 12% of them occur in the posterior cranial fossa. Meningiomas are usually benign, slow-growing neoplasms that arise from arachnoid cap cells. They can often reach substantial size before becoming symptomatic. Complete microsurgical resection remains the treatment of choice. However, when meningiomas occur within the regions of the posterior cranial fossa, total excision has been notoriously limited because of their intimate relationships with critical neural and vascular structures. Reported rates of gross total resection vary widely in different series (40 to 96%), and resection is frequently associated with significant morbidity (13 to 40%), mortality (0 to 13%), and recurrence (9 to 40%).

Over the last decade, stereotactic radiosurgery and stereotactic radiotherapy have become increasingly important in the treatment of meningiomas of the posterior fossa and skull base, not just as adjunctive therapy following incomplete resection or recurrent disease, but also as a viable treatment alternative to open surgery. In reviews of published studies, reported tumor control rates range from 82 to 100%. Adverse neurologic outcomes after treatment are generally encountered in fewer than 10% of cases. The overall results compare favorably with those after complete microsurgical resection. However, the follow-up intervals in most studies to date have been relatively short. Given the indolent nature of benign meningiomas, prolonged follow-up of these patients will be necessary to fully assess long-term outcomes.

When treatment for meningiomas within the posterior fossa becomes necessary, surgery is preferred if the tumor appears completely resectable with minimal risk, or if neurologic decompression is required because of progressive neurologic symptoms or significant mass effect. Radiation plays a limited role in the treatment of tumors larger than 3.0 cm, although staged radiosurgical treatment following initial surgical debulking may be considered for such patients. Radiation is most frequently indicated for patients with posterior fossa meningiomas who are of advanced age or have high operative risks, and for patients who refuse surgery or have residual or recurrent tumors.

137.5.3 Glomus Jugulare Tumor

Paragangliomas (glomus tumors) are slow-growing, usually benign, hypervascular tumors of neuroendocrine origin. Glomus jugulare tumors arise from rests of paraganglionic tissue in the adventitia of the jugular bulb. As such, they are intimately associated with cranial nerves IX, X, and XI. Spreading along pathways of least resistance, glomus tumors will commonly extend through the hypotympanic air cell tracts surrounding the jugular bulb and carotid artery to involve the jugular foramen and posterior cranial fossa. The standard treatment is microsurgical resection or radiation therapy. Because of the challenging location of glomus tumors at the skull base, their hypervascular nature, and their tendency to present at advanced stages, the optimal management is controversial. Microsurgical resection for these neoplasms is highly effective, with rates of tumor control of approximately 90%. However, surgery in this region risks significant morbidity and mortality.

Conventional fractionated radiation therapy has historically provided successful tumor control in those patients deemed unsuitable for surgery. When typical doses of 45 to 55 Gy are given in 20 to 25 fractions, tumor control rates of approximately 86 to 100% are reported. However, such results do not come without a risk for significant morbidity, including osteoradionecrosis, cranial neuropathy, and brain parenchymal necrosis.

In recent years, stereotactic radiosurgery techniques based on the gamma knife, modified LINAC, and cyberknife have been used in the treatment of glomus jugulare tumors in attempts to achieve satisfactory tumor control while minimizing treatment-related toxicity. In pooled analyses of published studies, gamma knife stereotactic radiosurgery with a mean marginal dose of 15.3 Gy yielded a tumor control rate of approximately 91% with minimal morbidity. The mean duration of follow-up in these various series was approximately 40 months. Recent short-term data have revealed excellent results when a combined, staged approach to radiosurgery was used following planned subtotal resection. With all of these approaches, longer-term follow-up will be required to better delineate overall risks and benefits.

The optimal management for glomus jugulare tumors remains a matter of controversy. However, in patients at an advanced age or with poor medical status, and in those with bilateral disease, radiosurgery offers a viable alternative to surgery as primary or adjunctive therapy. Microsurgical resection is generally indicated for patients who present with progressive neurologic deterioration, including those with hydrocephalus or increased intracranial pressure consequent to mass effect. Uncertainty regarding the radiologic diagnosis, a tumor diameter larger than 3 cm, and tumor extension below the skull base are additional relative contraindications to radiosurgery as primary therapy.

137.6 Roundsmanship

- The term *stereotactic radiosurgery* is applied when stereotactic radiation is delivered as a single dose, whereas the term *stereotactic radiotherapy* is used when multiple fractions are administered.

- The risk for complications following stereotactic radiosurgery for acoustic neuromas is significantly diminished by using a marginal dose of 12 to 13 Gy.
- Current evidence supports stereotactic radiation treatment for both primary and recurrent small to medium-size acoustic neuromas.
- Radiation treatment for posterior fossa tumors is limited to lesions smaller than 3 cm but may be used in combination with microsurgery.
- The long-term effects of stereotactic radiation therapy with respect to tumor control, hearing preservation, risks for cranial nerve dysfunction, malignant degeneration, and other potential complications warrant continued investigation in large studies.

137.7 Recommended Reading

[1] Anker CJ, Shrieve DC. Basic principles of radiobiology applied to radiosurgery and radiotherapy of benign skull base tumors. Otolaryngol Clin North Am 2009; 42: 601–621

[2] Battista RA. Gamma knife radiosurgery for vestibular schwannoma. Otolaryngol Clin North Am 2009; 42: 635–654

[3] Chen PG, Nguyen JH, Payne SC, Sheehan JP, Hashisaki GT. Treatment of glomus jugulare tumors with gamma knife radiosurgery. Laryngoscope 2010; 120: 1856–1862

[4] Chopra R, Kondziolka D, Niranjan A, Lunsford LD, Flickinger JC. Long-term follow-up of acoustic schwannoma radiosurgery with marginal tumor doses of 12 to 13 Gy. Int J Radiat Oncol Biol Phys 2007; 68: 845–851

[5] Di Maio S, Akagami R. Prospective comparison of quality of life before and after observation, radiation, or surgery for vestibular schwannomas. J Neurosurg 2009; 111: 855–862

[6] Friedman WA, Bradshaw P, Myers A, Bova FJ. Linear accelerator radiosurgery for vestibular schwannomas. J Neurosurg 2006; 105: 657–661

[7] Hasegawa T, Fujitani S, Katsumata S, Kida Y, Yoshimoto M, Koike J. Stereotactic radiosurgery for vestibular schwannomas: analysis of 317 patients followed more than 5 years. Neurosurgery 2005; 57: 257–265, discussion 257–265

[8] Kreil W, Luggin J, Fuchs I, Weigl V, Eustacchio S, Papaefthymiou G. Long term experience of gamma knife radiosurgery for benign skull base meningiomas. J Neurol Neurosurg Psychiatry 2005; 76: 1425–1430

[9] Lunsford LD, Niranjan A, Flickinger JC, Maitz A, Kondziolka D. Radiosurgery of vestibular schwannomas: summary of experience in 829 cases. J Neurosurg 2005; 102 Suppl: 195–199

[10] Mendenhall WM, Morris CG, Amdur RJ, Foote KD, Friedman WA. Radiotherapy alone or after subtotal resection for benign skull base meningiomas. Cancer 2003; 98: 1473–1482

[11] Pollock BE. Vestibular schwannoma management: an evidence-based comparison of stereotactic radiosurgery and microsurgical resection. Prog Neurol Surg 2008; 21: 222–227

[12] Starke RM, Nguyen JH, Rainey J et al. Gamma Knife surgery of meningiomas located in the posterior fossa: factors predictive of outcome and remission. J Neurosurg 2011; 114: 1399–1409

[13] Zachenhofer I, Wolfsberger S, Aichholzer M et al. Gamma-knife radiosurgery for cranial base meningiomas: experience of tumor control, clinical course, and morbidity in a follow-up of more than 8 years. Neurosurgery 2006; 58: 28–36, discussion 28–36

138 Lesions of the Petrous Apex

Christopher J. Linstrom

138.1 Introduction

Lesions of the petrous apex are uncommon in general otolaryngologic practice but will most likely be encountered in a practice limited to otology and neurotology. Certainly a lesion of the petrous apex must be considered as part of the differential diagnosis in a patient presenting with hearing loss, tinnitus, vertigo, disequilibrium, otalgia, or headache. The combination of any unilateral otologic complaint with weakness or paralysis of the sixth cranial nerve points to a lesion of the petrous apex. This chapter will focus on the clinical presentation, investigation, and treatment of the common lesions of the petrous apex.

138.2 Anatomy

The petrous (from the Greek πετρα, "stone") apex has the shape of a pyramid, with the point about 45 degrees medial and the base lateral, along the axis of the temporal bone. The medial surface of the pyramid corresponds to the medial surface of the temporal bone, with the other surfaces named in turn. The term *apex* is used to refer to that portion of the temporal bone medial to the otic labyrinth, the carotid artery, and the eustachian tube. These structures form the base of the petrous apex. The petrous apex abuts the internal auditory canal (IAC) and the canal for the petrous portion of the internal carotid artery. A small notch in the most superior and medial edge of the petrous pyramid identifies the Dorello canal. A small dural reflection creates the canal itself, through which passes cranial nerve VI. A small depression of the anterosuperior surface of the petrous apex identifies the position of the Meckel cave and the trigeminal ganglion; the arcuate eminence, seen more laterally, gives an approximation, but not a precise location, of the superior semicircular canal. The petrous apex is normally pneumatized by air cells that invaginate the apex from the middle ear along named tracts that may pass above or below the cochlea, although the degree and extent of pneumatization from left to right in an individual may vary considerably. The apex is dense in nonpneumatized bone. Variable amounts of fatty marrow may be present within the cancellous bone of the petrous apex.

138.3 Pathophysiology

The pathophysiology of a lesion in the petrous apex is determined by the lesion itself: arising from *within* the apex (e.g., cholesterol granuloma or epidermoid) or a vascular abnormality within the apex (e.g., aneurysm); coming from *above* (e.g., cerebrospinal [CSF] fluid cyst or cephalocele); growing into the area of the petrous apex from a *nearby* structure (e.g., meningioma arising from the dural lining adjacent to the petrous apex); or from *metastatic spread* of cancer to the petrous apex (e.g., metastatic breast, renal cell, lung, or prostate carcinoma and malignant melanoma). Several of these lesions will be considered in greater detail in the section on the differential diagnosis of lesions of the petrous apex.

138.4 Clinical Presentation and Physical Examination

The clinical history of lesions found within the petrous apex is often disproportionately mild compared with the actual findings on radiologic investigation. It is remarkable that until a lesion within the petrous apex reaches a size large enough to impinge upon the otic capsule, the IAC, or the euastachian tube, the patient may have only vague otologic complaints, such aural fullness without definite hearing loss or tinnitus, often accompanied by facial pressure or pain, a lack of sensation in an area of the face, or headache.

It is vital that the examining physician attend to the nature, duration, and location of the complaints. Knowledge of the anatomy of the petrous apex and its surrounding structures will point to the petrous apex if the history suggests pathology in this location. The history is probably the most important step in the investigative process, often outweighing the physical findings, which may be absent or mild.

Attention should be paid to those complaints that could stem from a lesion in the petrous apex: hearing loss, aural fullness, tinnitus, dizziness, facial hypesthesia or pain, weakness of the facial nerve, or headache. A complete otologic and head and neck examination should be done, with a focus on cranial nerves II through XII. A microscopic examination of the tympanic membrane is usually included, with care taken to examine each and every part of the drum. Crusting on the drum, especially near the pars flaccida, may hide disease. If at all possible, this should be softened and removed.

A minimal clinical examination of hearing includes a tuning fork examination at 512 Hz and possibly more frequencies, as necessary. The tuning fork examination must agree with the audiometric findings. If the patient describes pulsatile tinnitus, it is helpful to listen to the neck, ear, retromastoid area, and orbit in a quiet room, preferably in an audiometric booth. Clinical tests of balance should be performed if indicated. These may include tests of postural control, such as the Romberg, Quix, and Fukuda tests, as well as tests of the otolith system, such as the Dix-Hallpike maneuver. The test for head shake–induced nystagmus may help to point to the side and/or site of the putative problem.

138.5 Testing

138.5.1 Audiometry

All patients who have otologic complaints, regardless of the suspected lesion, should have an audiogram with a minimum battery of tests of pure tones, bone conduction (masked appropriately), word discrimination, and immittance with reflex decay, if obtainable. Each ear should be tested separately.

In rare cases, an auditory brainstem response test may demonstrate either a lack of wave I or, more commonly, increased I through III interwave latency on the side with hearing loss or known pathology. The abnormality on the auditory brainstem response test may revert toward normal after the lesion has been treated.

138.5.2 Radiology

Patients who have unilateral otologic complaints such as hearing loss, tinnitus, and fullness/pressure should be evaluated for a retrocochlear lesion with an appropriate study.

Although not every single dizzy patient will need a retrocochlear radiologic evaluation, many treating physicians feel that the patient is better served by testing more rather than less frequently. The decision pathway is relatively easy if the hearing is asymmetric. For most patients, the study of choice will be magnetic resonance (MR) imaging without and with gadolinium enhancement. MR imaging is highly sensitive and specific for the detection of soft-tissue lesions in the skull base, cerebellopontine angle, IAC, and brain. It is the test of choice for the detection of retrocochlear pathology, and many lesions of the petrous apex will be incidentally discovered by screening MR imaging.

A word of caution is indicated at this point. The degree of pneumatization of each petrous apex in an individual may normally vary from left to right. The petrous apex is pneumatized in approximately 30% of temporal bones. Signal from bone marrow in a nonpneumatized bone will be distinctly different from signal from a pneumatized petrous apex. If there are no corresponding clinical complaints (e.g., facial pain, hypesthesia, hearing loss, tinnitus, dizziness) and no objective signs of disease (e.g., unilateral sensorineural hearing loss, cranial nerve VI involvement), it is a safe bet that the increased signal on the T1-weighted image is from bone marrow. A quick look at the other petrous apex or a review of other marrow-containing areas of the skull may yield the answer. A T1-weighted image with fat suppression may already be part of the study and will demonstrate that the suspected lesion is marrow fat.

Once a lesion in or near the petrous apex has been discovered, additional imaging studies will most likely be planned. In an excellent review of radiographic imaging of the petrous apex, Curtin and Som postulated five questions that should be asked and answered with an appropriate study to properly identify a lesion of the petrous apex:

1. Is the abnormality arising in the petrous apex or from contiguous areas? (Is the lesion expansile from within the petrous apex itself, or infiltrative and destructive, either from within or without?)
2. Are the bony walls of the apex and the septa in the air cells smoothly remodeled? (Are the bony air cell walls of the petrous apex expanded (e.g., cholesterol granuloma, cholesteatoma, mucocele, aneurysm, meningocele, histiocytosis, giant petrous air cell) or destroyed (metastases to the petrous apex)?
3. What are the MR imaging signal characteristics of the lesion?
4. Is there enhancement of the internal "matrix" of the lesion? (Does the central part of the lesion have a blood supply?)
5. What is the relationship of the lesion to the carotid artery? (Is it bowed to the side, is the canal effaced, is it an aneurysm of the petrous carotid artery?)

These questions may usually be answered by complementary studies of the petrous apex. If the patient has undergone MR imaging, computed tomography (CT) would be the next test of choice. CT with a bone algorithm yields excellent information about bone and the interface of soft tissue, bone, and air, but it is far less sensitive and specific than MR imaging in detecting soft-tissue neoplasia. In patients who cannot otherwise undergo MR imaging with enhancement, CT with contrast may allow definition of the great vessels within the skull and neck and may give information about infectious or inflammatory processes and neoplasia. MR imaging, as previously discussed, will yield the most precise information about soft-tissue structures.

If additional sequences, such as MR angiography (MRA) and MR venography (MRV) are desired, it is important for the ordering physician to speak to the radiologist before planning the study. These sequences cannot be imported or added to MR data after they have been obtained and must be set up in advance. MRA and MRV yield information about first- and second-order named vessels. If one is concerned about a vascular lesion (e.g., aneurysm, arteriovenous malformation) or about the interface between a solid or cystic structure within the petrous apex and a named vessel, such as the petrous carotid artery, it may save the patient additional testing to obtain MRA and/or MRV at the same time as MR imaging. If the lesion is known to be vascular in nature (e.g., paraganglioma) and will need to be embolized, MRA and MRV yield little information that four-vessel angiography will not and for these lesions should not be ordered. Above all, it is vital that the otologist/neurotologist establish a comfortable working relationship with an experienced neuroradiologist and/or interventionalist who will take the time and effort to listen to the patient's history and attend to the radiologic requirements of the proposed imaging study.

138.6 Differential Diagnosis

The differential diagnosis of lesions of the petrous apex is large. They may be classified as benign or malignant, as expansile or erosive, or as arising from *within*, from *above*, from a *nearby* structure, or from *metastatic spread*.

Although a wide differential diagnosis should be kept in mind, the lesions most commonly encountered in an otologic/neurotologic practice will be cholesterol granuloma, cholesteatoma, and mucocele, with encephalocele/menigocele and aneurysm less commonly seen. It is important always to keep the patient's history in mind when developing the differential diagnosis.

Many sources differ in the classification and nomenclature of lesions of the petrous apex. A distillation of lesions described by many authors will be presented, as well as a brief description of the more common lesions.

138.6.1 Inflammatory/Infectious/Cystic Lesions

Cholesterol Granuloma

Manasse reported a case of "granulation tumor with foreign body cells" of the petrous apex in 1894. The term "cholesterin or cholesterol granuloma" has been used since this report.

The most common clinical entity an otologist will encounter within the petrous apex is cholesterol granuloma. There are several proposed mechanisms of formation. The second most common lesion will be cholesteatoma. The pathophysiology of these two lesions will be considered here.

Cholesterol granulomas have been produced in animal studies by two mechanisms: by introducing irritants into the middle ear cleft and by isolating a bony air-filled cavity that normally communicates with the atmosphere.

Beaumont produced cholesterol granuloma in a chick humerus by obstructing the foramen pneumaticum (the connection with the respiratory system) with a muscle pedicle. Histologic examination revealed no associated loss of blood or infection. Surgical trauma as a causative factor was excluded because an identical procedure performed on the contralateral humerus without complete occlusion of the foramen pneumaticum did not result in cholesterol granuloma formation. These findings support the "obstruction–vacuum" hypothesis of cholesterol granuloma formation.

Friedman was able to develop cholesterol granuloma by injecting sterile suspensions of cholesterol into the middle ear of a guinea pig. He proposed that the blood breakdown product cholesterol incited a foreign body reaction, thus leading to cholesterol granuloma formation. Sadé and Teitz disputed the necessity for hemorrhage as a predisposing factor for cholesterol granuloma formation.

A second major theory of the pathogenesis of cholesterol granuloma is that of "exposed marrow." The marrow-filled cavities of the petrous apex are eroded as air cells develop. This erosion may cause hemorrhage into the air cells; subsequent degradation into blood products such as cholesterin results in an inflammatory reaction and cyst development. The expansion of the cyst results from continued bleeding within the marrow cavities. These authors reported a small retrospective series of four patients with aggressive cholesterol granulomas in the mastoid. In all cases, there was a nearby blood source. The authors noted that an "obstruction–vacuum" postulate alone would not have explained the source of the hemorrhage, and that a blood source must have supplied these aggressive lesions.

A cholesterol granuloma may appear as granulation tissue or as a brown, green, or glistening yellow cystic mass; it is not a precursor of cholesteatoma.

It would appear that major factors predisposing to the formation of cholesterol granuloma are the following: (1) obstruction of the ventilation of an air-filled bony cavity that normally equilibrates with the atmosphere; (2) obstruction of drainage; (3) reaction to a foreign body, such as cholesterol; (4) the presence of bone marrow products, including blood, which lead to the development of cholesterol cysts; and (5) hemorrhage, although there is not unanimous agreement that this is a causative factor.

Epidermoid/Cholesteatoma

Cholesteatoma (more properly, keratoma) is not a true neoplasm but rather the accumulation of a living matrix of keratinizing squamous epithelium and its cellular debris in an enclosed space. It may be classified as congenital (arising de novo within the anatomical location) or acquired. Acquired cholesteatomas may be primary (arising from a retraction of a squamous epithelium–lined surface into the target) or secondary (arising from a break in the integrity of the target location, caused by either perforation or seeding from trauma). In patients with cholesteatoma of the petrous apex, the clinical and radiologic examination must look for a source outside the petrous apex, such as the pars flaccida (e.g., an attic retraction cholesteatoma). This is uncommonly found. If a "source" lesion is found, it is usually disproportionately small relative to the disease within the petrous apex. Cholesteatomas of the petrous apex are most commonly congenital.

Congenital cholesteatomas of the petrous apex may arise from epithelial cells trapped during embryogenesis by overclosure of the neural tube. Epithelial migration in the absence of other clinically obvious foci of cholesteatoma is another, although unlikely, possibility. Congenital cholesteatomas of the petrous apex may be clinically silent. If they expand to a volume sufficient to impinge upon structures within or adjacent to the petrous apex, the clinical manifestation will depend upon the size and location of the mass and may include hearing loss, aural fullness, facial pain or hypesthesia, headache, or blurred vision/diplopia. The clinical examination per se does not yield a pathologic diagnosis but rather points to the likely site of the lesion (e.g., in pathologies involving the fifth or sixth cranial nerve).

Effusion

Effusion of the middle ear and mastoid may cause a blocked feeling in the ear and a conductive hearing loss. This process may extend to the petrous apex. In some cases, the effusion is due to chronic mastoiditis in which the respiratory mucosa of the middle ear and mastoid has become hypertrophic. In these cases, the mucosa of the middle ear and mastoid will often remain hypertrophic and not revert to normal, thus becoming the source of an effusion rather than the result of an active infection. CT will usually reveal a nearly complete middle ear and mastoid but without erosion of bony septa or expansion of the apex. T1-weighted MR images will often be hypointense and T2 weighted images hyperintense. In rare cases, all of the hypertrophic mucosa must be removed during a mastoidectomy and/or a middle ear exploration to allow a new mucosa to develop for these spaces. Because the air cell system is contiguous, the mastoidectomy will usually provide drainage for the petrous apex.

Mucocele

Simple obstruction of the regular draining pathways of the petrous apex may rarely cause a mucocele. The apex expands as mucus continues to collect within it. The CT and MR imaging characteristics of a mucocele are similar to those of a cholesteatoma: a smooth, expansile appearance on CT that is isointense to CSF. On MR imaging, mucoceles are hypointense on T1- and hyperintense on T2-weighted images. However, the signal can vary depending upon the protein content of the fluid. Fluid with a low protein content is dark on T1-weighted images and bright on T2-weighted images. As the mucocele becomes chronic, the water fraction decreases and the protein content increases. This may alter the enhancing characteristics so that both T1- and T2-weighted images become bright.

Cerebrospinal Fluid Cysts and Cephaloceles

CSF cephaloceles are meningeal diverticula that may include only CSF (meningocele) or both CSF and brain (encephaloceles). If they arise from the dura of the Meckel cave, they are called petrous apex cephaloceles and typically contain only CSF. Encephaloceles typically arise from the middle fossa near the mastoid and tegmen tympani, and they are often associated with chronic ear disease or surgical trauma. CSF cephaloceles may be an incidental finding or may present with a variety of findings, including CSF otorhinorrhea, vertigo, hearing loss, diplopia, facial numbness, and meningitis.

Petrous Apicitis/Abscess

Gradenigo in 1904 described an infection of the ear with concomitant paralysis of the abducens nerve (cranial nerve VI). Profant first used the term *petrositis* to describe infection of the petrous apex combined with mastoiditis. Inflammation of the leptomeninges around the Dorello canal produces palsy of the sixth cranial nerve. Involvement of the adjacent trigeminal ganglion (cranial nerve V) may lead to periorbital and facial pain. The combination of otorrhea, lateral rectus palsy, and pain in the trigeminal distribution represents classic Gradenigo syndrome.

Cases of petrous apicitis are almost always found in a setting of acute or subacute otitis media. On both CT and MR imaging, the air cells are opacified, with enhancement of the dura over the petrous apex. Complications may arise in neighboring structures, such as intracranial abscess and venous thrombosis. The cavernous sinus, sigmoid sinus, and jugular vein are at risk because of their proximity to the apex. A variety of organisms may cause petrous apicitis, including *Mycobacterium tuberculosis*.

Skull Base Osteomyelitis/Necrotizing (Malignant) Otitis Externa

Malignant otitis externa, more properly called osteomyelitis of the skull base or necrotizing otitis externa, is a skull base osteomyelitis. *Pseudomonas* species are generally the predominant organisms. Toulmouche described a case of progressive osteomyelitis of the temporal bone in 1838 that was most likely the first reported case of necrotizing otitis externa. Risk factors for this disease include old age, diabetes, and immunosuppression for any reason. The typical complaint is deep-seated, boring pain in the ear that radiates toward the middle of the head. Granulations in the inferior margin of the external canal near the tympanic bone may be seen, but aural discharge is rare. A conductive hearing loss due to fluid or granulations within the middle ear may be diagnosed. Involvement of the facial nerve indicates more advanced disease. The treatment is medical, with dual antibiotic therapy and control of underlying medical conditions, such as diabetes. In extremely rare cases, surgical decompression of a phlegmon or abscess of the skull base may be necessary, as well. For further discussion, see Chapter 116.

Petrous Carotid Aneurysm

A smooth-bordered mass seen within the petrous apex may in fact be an aneurysmal dilatation of the petrous carotid and must always be included in the differential diagnosis. Violation of an aneurysm in this location would lead to catastrophic sequelae. An easy way to distinguish the lesion from the artery is to include MRA sequences along with the MR imaging to detail the soft tissues of the mass. MRA delineates first- and second-order vessels, will be formatted in many different planes, and will clearly show the mass to be separate from the lesion within the petrous apex. This is demonstrated in Case 3. If doubt remains after MRA, four-vessel angiography, with its attendant risks, can be performed.

Paget Disease and Fibrous Dysplasia

Paget disease of bone affects the skull base in sclerotic, lytic, and mixed forms. The skull base is rarely involved without simultaneous calvarial disease. In the base of the skull and petrous apex, the lesions are primarily lytic and may have an appearance similar to that of metastatic disease. Paget disease may cause demineralization or erosion of the otic capsule. It often involves the petrous temporal bones symmetrically.

Fibrous dysplasia has a typical appearance on CT of areas of bony thickening with a "ground glass" appearance. In the medullary region of the lesion, areas of dense ossification may be mixed with areas of fibrous tissue. Both T1- and T2-weighted MR images are of low signal intensity unless there are cystic areas, which are bright on both sequences. It is rare to find fibrous dysplasia isolated to the petrous apex.

138.6.2 Primary Neoplasms

Primary neoplasms of the petrous apex are rare, but a variety have been reported. These include giant cell tumor, xanthoma, endolymphatic sac tumor, hemangioma, hemangiopericytoma, chondroma/chondrosarcoma, aneurysmal bone cyst, plasmacytoma, undifferentiated carcinoma, various sarcomas, and by extension nasopharyngeal carcinoma. With the exception of aneurysmal bone cyst, these tumors tend to be cellular. The origin of aneurysmal bone cyst is controversial. Various pathologists believe that this expansile lesion is more properly classified as a giant cell tumor or that it may develop from a benign bone lesion. The appearance on CT and MR imaging is characteristic, with expanded bone and multiple cysts, most of which have air–fluid levels.

The endolymphatic sac tumor is a papillary adenoma arising from the endolymphatic sac or its adnexa. It tends to be more aggressive than similar lesions arising elsewhere in the temporal bone.

Chondroma/chondrosarcoma is thought to arise from embryonic rests of cartilage in the region of the foramen lacerum. Malignant chondrosarcoma is more common than its benign counterpart, chondroma. Chondrosarcomas appear as bulky, enhancing, irregular, destructive lesions with "popcorn" calcifications that arise from the midline. They are homogeneous on T1-weighted imaging and heterogeneous on T2-weighted imaging, with intense contrast enhancement.

Nager described sarcomas affecting the temporal bone under general categories of rhabdomyosarcoma, extraskeletal Ewing sarcoma, myxoma and fibromyxoma, and osteosarcoma. These malignancies have in common at least one primordial element from mesenchymal tissue. Although all of these cancers are uncommonly seen *solely* in the petrous apex, they may secondarily spread to this site as a consequence of their aggressive behavior.

Rhabdomyosarcoma is a highly malignant tumor of rhabdomyoblasts in varying stages of differentiation, with or without intracellular myofibrils or cross-striations. Three subtypes are distinguished: embryonal (including the botryoid type), alveolar, and pleomorphic. The first two are more common in children; the third is an adult neoplasm.

Extraskeletal Ewing sarcoma is a malignant tumor believed to arise from primitive mesenchymal tissue without obvious differentiation. It is often mistaken clinically and histologically for juvenile rhabdomyosarcoma. Approximately 70% of these tumors have been reported in patients younger than 20 years of age. It is rare in the temporal bone and is included for completeness.

Other sarcomatous lesions to be considered in the differential include myxoma, fibromyxoma, and osteosarcoma.

Eosinophilic Granuloma: Langerhans Cell Histiocytosis X

Langerhans cell histiocytosis may involve the skull base. Any bone can be involved, but the temporal bone is a common site. The clinical history often is that of an ear infection that will not heal despite appropriate aural toilet and antibiotic therapy. The temporal bone may be expanded or destroyed. The bone–lesion interface may be sharp on CT. The internal density of the lesion and the imaging characteristics on MR imaging may be variable. The patient tends to be young, further raising the index of suspicion. Other entities to be considered are teratoma, neuroma, and giant cell tumor.

Chordoma

Chordomas, derived from primitive notochord remnants, are midline masses arising from the clivus that may secondarily spread to the petrous apex. It is possible for notochord remnants to extend laterally toward the petrous apex, causing a primary tumor. Chordomas are bulky, lobulated, midline lesions on CT that enhance with contrast, are destructive of bone, and contain calcifications. They appear similar to chondrosarcomas on MR imaging, but they tend to arise more in the midline and are less brightly enhancing with gadolinium.

Meningioma

This benign tumor, arising from the meninges, comprises approximately 14% of all intracranial tumors and is the most common solid tumor involving the petrous apex. It appears rarely as a primary tumor, more commonly invading the apex secondarily. Meningiomas commonly present as broad-based tumors along the posterior petrous wall. They may exhibit calcification within and enhance with contrast, and they often have a characteristic dural "tail." Meningiomas tend to follow sites of dural penetration by cranial nerves VII through XII.

Paraganglioma

Paragangliomas (glomus tumors) usually do not arise from within but may grow into the petrous apex. It would extremely rare to find a glomus tumor primarily within the petrous apex in the absence of this lesion elsewhere.

138.6.3 Metastatic Neoplasms

Extratemporal primary cancers may metastasize via hematogenous routes to the temporal bone, specifically to the rich marrow spaces of the petrous apex. These include breast, prostate, lung, and renal cell carcinoma and malignant melanoma. The appearance is variable, depending upon the site of the primary. Metastatic cancer to the temporal bone may erode and remodel bone or be less invasive in appearance. A history of known cancer at any of these sites or the presence of additional metastatic disease anywhere raises the index of suspicion.

138.7 Treatment Paradigms

Few lesions of the petrous apex will be solely observed in otherwise healthy patients. Some, such as necrotizing otitis externa and petrous apicitis, will be treated medically, with very rare surgical intervention. However, the majority of lesions of the petrous apex will eventually require surgery for either drainage or resection. Many surgical approaches to the petrous apex exist, each tailored to the lesion and the extent of disease. The surgeon must carefully review the nature and extent of the lesion and its relationship to the important adjacent structures, such as the otic capsule, the petrous carotid artery, the jugular bulb, the facial nerve, and the eustachian tube. The surgeon must have several surgical approaches to lesions of the petrous apex available in the event that the selected approach fails to reach the pathology or adequately address the surgical requirements of treatment. If the lesion involves highly critical areas either adjacent to or within the petrous apex, such as the petrous carotid artery, the middle fossa dura, or the clivus, the patient's care is facilitated by a combined neurotologic and neurosurgical team approach.

Surgical approaches to the petrous apex may be classified according to the neighboring anatomy, the ability to preserve hearing, or the direction of the approach. Because the temporal bone is pneumatized by named air cell tracts invaginating the mastoid complex around the vestibular and cochlear labyrinths and the facial nerve, an easily understood classification scheme is based upon hearing conservation/hearing ablation and the named pathways of pneumatization around the otic capsule. It is understood that all approaches attempt to preserve and protect the facial nerve.

Flood and Kemink listed six requirements that must be fulfilled in approaching tumors of the petrous apex: (1) provide adequate exposure for complete excision or allow easy access to an exteriorized cavity; (2) preserve useful residual hearing if possible; (3) preserve facial nerve and other cranial nerve function when possible; (4) preserve the internal carotid artery; (5) avoid hazard to the brainstem; and (6) provide wound closure without CSF leak.

138.7.1 Hearing Conservation Approaches

These surgical approaches aim to reach the petrous apex while preserving the otic capsule in an attempt to preserve hearing.

The approaches follow established air cell tracts *above, below,* or *anterior* to the otic capsule. Many were first described in the preantibiotic era and were used to exteriorize abscesses of the petrous apex. None involves transposition of the facial nerve or of the petrous carotid artery. The jugular bulb is the third anatomical boundary.

Above the Labyrinth

Middle cranial fossa approach: This is an extension of the standard middle cranial fossa approach for decompression of the labyrinthine facial nerve and resection of lesions within the IAC, as described by William House in 1959 and thereafter. It may be a preferred approach for lesions, such as cholesteatomas, in which surgical removal and subsequent exenteration are the goals. It is difficult to drain lesions to other dependent areas of the temporal bone, although this has been described. The major landmarks to be preserved are the petrous carotid artery, the cochlea, and the facial nerve. This approach affords a "keyhole" window from above, through which a lesion may be more thoroughly exenterated. The middle fossa approach is further discussed in Chapter 135 .

Through the superior semicircular canal, along the path of the subarcuate artery: In patients with a well-developed perilabyrinthine air cell tract and a more posterior lesion, this approach may be contemplated. However, the diameter of the superior semicircular canal is no more than a few millimeters, and thus the vestibular and cochlear labyrinths are both placed at risk with this approach, which was developed to drain abscesses of the petrous apex and is mentioned here for historical interest.

Through the attic: This approach is rarely indicated for lesions of the petrous apex with extension above and posterior to the vestibular labyrinth. It may be of value for obtaining a biopsy but today would not in itself be considered a definitive approach. It is often combined with other approaches to the petrous apex, especially when the goal is to provide drainage or exteriorization and not definitive resection.

Through the root of the zygomatic arch: This is mentioned for historical completeness only and today would most likely be replaced by or combined with another technique, such as a middle cranial fossa approach.

Below the Labyrinth

Infracochlear (subcochlear) approach: This approach uses the triangular space bordered by the basal turn of the cochlea, the ascending petrous carotid artery, and the jugular bulb. In an anatomical study of 20 preserved temporal bones, Haberkamp found the average window created via this approach to be 9.41 x 7.33 mm; in none of his specimens was this approach impossible. In the living, well-defined axial and coronal CT scans with a bone algorithm are needed to estimate the space between the basal turn of the cochlea and the petrous carotid. If the space is more than approximately 3 to 4 mm, surgical drainage of the petrous apex will likely be possible. This approach is limited by a short distance between these two structures or by a high-riding jugular bulb. It is the most common otologic approach in current use and has been described by many authors.

Infralabyrinthine (retrofacial) approach: This approach is bordered by the posterior semicircular canal, the vertical (descending) facial nerve, and the jugular bulb. It is a straightforward approach, an anterior extension of a complete mastoidectomy. Preoperative axial CT with edge enhancement will help in the surgical planning. Haberkamp found the average window created via this approach to be 4.99 x 7.23 mm. The major limitation to this approach is a high-riding jugular bulb. In rare cases, the posterior semicircular canal may be blue-lined to allow a few extra millimeters of the operculum of the superior semicircular canal to be dissected. As in other approaches, the petrous apex is drained to a well-ventilated area, in this case the mastoid and subsequently to the eustachian tube. In the literature reviewed for this chapter, it is the second most commonly used approach.

Retrosigmoid (suboccipital) approach: This is the standard approach toward the posterior cranial fossa for the excision of lesions of the cerebellopontine angle and IAC. It is rarely used alone to approach the petrous apex, but it may be combined with another approach when intracranial extension of a petrous apex tumor produces signs of brainstem compression. The surgeon works at a great distance from the petrous apex, and the morbidity associated with this technique limits its usefulness as a primary approach to the petrous apex.

Infratemporal approach: The infratemporal approach to the skull base, with anterior transposition of the facial nerve, as is typically used in the resection of paragangliomas, allows the combined infracochlear and infralabyrinthine drainage of lesions of the petrous apex with preservation of hearing. Transposition of the facial nerve with attendant facial weakness is the major limiting factor with this approach.

Anterior to the Labyrinth

These approaches use the triangle formed by the cochlea, the petrous carotid artery, and the middle fossa dura. They were developed in the preantibiotic era and are rarely if ever indicated today.

Transsphenoidal approach: The history of this approach to the pituitary is a veritable history of modern advances in neuro-otology and neurosurgery. It was first popularized in North America by Harvey Cushing, although he claimed no credit for its discovery. It fell into disfavor because of poor anesthesia and limited visibility in an era devoid of the operating microscope. It was revived by Guiot and Jules Hardy after the advent of intraoperative radiofluoroscopy in 1958. Although this approach is aimed precisely at lesions of the sella turcica, it may be modified for lesions of the petrous apex. Gray et al have described the transnasal, transsphenoidal marsupialization of a cholesterol granuloma of the petrous apex and sphenoid sinus. This approach may be favored in patients who have lesions that expand the far anterior aspect of the petrous apex and in whom the petrous carotid artery has been laterally displaced. Preoperative planning may include edge-enhanced CT of the temporal bone and MR imaging with MRA to detail both the nature of the lesion and the exact location of the horizontal portion of the petrous carotid artery. An intraoperative navigational system or intraoperative fluoroscopic system is often used to confirm anatomical landmarks. The sphenoid sinus is approached in a transnasal fashion. The posterior wall of the sphenoid sinus is thinned with a diamond bur, and the anterior face of the petrous apex is opened. Removal of the intrasphenoid septum may facilitate exposure. A drain may be left in place, or a posteriorly based flap of septal mucosa may be rotated into the neo-osteum of the petrous apex, as described by Montgomery.

138.7.2 Hearing Ablation Approaches

These approaches are intended to reach the petrous apex via the cochlear and/or the vestibular labyrinth, the most direct pathway, at the expense of the vestibular or cochlear labyrinth. None of these approaches intentionally involves transposition of the facial nerve or of the petrous carotid artery. The jugular bulb is the third major boundary of these approaches.

Translabyrinthine Approach

In lesions of the petrous apex in which useful hearing is no longer present, the approach is through the labyrinth but *not* through the IAC. Combined with a canal wall down mastoidectomy and a sufficient meatoplasty, it yields a cavity that can be easily visualized and cleaned. The posterior and middle fossa dura may have been thinned by expansion of the lesion. It is important that toilet of the cavity be performed under microscopic vision, in an extremely gentle fashion and without the use of sharp instruments, in order to avoid a CSF leak. This is described later in Case 2.

Transcochlear Approach

This approach has been described by William House and is indicated in the patient with a lesion of the petrous apex in whom useful hearing is no longer present. It is important to follow the usual landmarks of the basal turn of the cochlea, the tympanic facial nerve, the eustachian tube orifice, and the petrous carotid artery carefully in order to prevent injury to vital structures. This approach, combined with a canal wall down mastoidectomy and a sufficient meatoplasty, will yield a cavity that is open and that can be cleaned.

Subtotal Petrosectomy

This is a "workhorse" approach, familiar to all skull base surgeons who have studied the work of Professor Ugo Fisch.

This technique leaves the otic capsule, the facial nerve, the carotid artery, and the jugular bulb as the only remaining anatomical landmarks within the temporal bone. The surgical goal is to exenterate all remaining disease from the external and middle ear clefts and all air cells of the mastoid. All squamous epithelium from the external auditory canal up to and including the tympanic membrane is removed, and the canal is overclosed. The ossicular chain, except for the mobile stapes footplate, is removed. Depending upon the pathology, the facial nerve may be decompressed, transposed, or grafted. The petrous carotid may be decompressed, according to need. There are many variations of this approach, including leaving the canal open for surveillance.

138.8 Clinical and Radiographic Follow-up

The lesion itself and the ability to preserve the function of the otic capsule in large measure determine the mode of surveillance for patients with lesions involving the petrous apex. If the lesion is being *observed*, clinical examination and serial audiograms at 6-month intervals or whenever the patient may experience a decrease in hearing are indicated. If the hearing remains unchanged, CT or MR imaging initially at 6 months and thereafter at longer intervals is commonly performed. The patient is instructed to attend to his or her symptoms. If these worsen at any time, new investigations will be ordered.

If the lesion has been *medically treated* (e.g., 6 to 12 weeks of intravenous antibiotics for necrotizing otitis externa involving the petrous apex), the patient should be examined and the hearing tested at shorter and then longer intervals. Many patients will require a full course of treatment only once. A gallium scan at 3 to 4 months after treatment should show significant improvement. However, it may never become completely clear and must be interpreted according to the clinical state of the patient. In an elderly patient or a patient of any age immunocompromised for any reason, the index of suspicion must be raised, especially if deep-seated otitic pain or pain at the base of the skull returns. In this case, in addition to the clinical examination and the audiometric and radiographic studies, radionuclide studies may need to be repeated.

If the patient has been treated *surgically*, the nature of the disease and the surgical approach will dictate the follow-up. If the disease has been exteriorized and can be visualized under the microscope, surveillance radiography may rarely be indicated. If, however, the disease has been drained to an area that is ordinarily not clinically accessible, such as to the mastoid in a canal wall up technique or to the hypotympanum, serial CT at the 6- and then the 12-month mark is indicated. Patients who have had subtotal excision of disease processes within the petrous apex with *overclosure* of the ear must know that lifelong surveillance at appropriate intervals is mandatory. Because there will always be a chance that a residuum of disease may continue to grow, appropriate imaging (CT, MR imaging, or other) at appropriate intervals must be organized along with the clinical examination. As long as the patient remains clinically and radiologically stable, the disease may be observed. Radiographic progression of disease, with or without progression of clinical symptoms, must be carefully assessed and a treatment plan outlined. The overall clinical state of the patient with any comorbidities will help determine what is to be done.

138.9 Case Illustrations

138.9.1 Case 1

A 56-year-old man with a 4-month history of tinnitus and decreased hearing in the right ear was referred for evaluation. He had no complaints of otitic pain or dizziness/vertigo and did not have facial pain. His ear, nose, and throat examination, which included cranial nerves II through XII, was unremarkable. His clinical tests of balance were normal. With a 512-Hz tuning

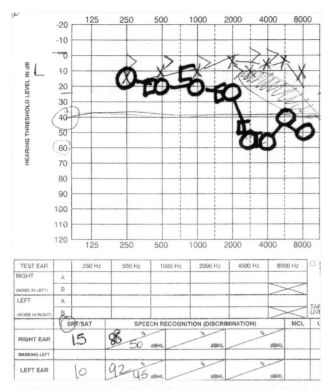

TEST EAR		250 Hz	500 Hz	1000 Hz	2000 Hz	4000 Hz	8000 Hz	
RIGHT	A							
(NOISE IN LEFT)	B							
LEFT	A							
(NOISE IN RIGHT)	B							

	SRT/SAT	SPEECH RECOGNITION (DISCRIMINATION)			MCL	U
RIGHT EAR	15	88 % 50 dBHL	% dBHL	% dBHL		
MASKING LEFT						
LEFT EAR	10	92 % 45 dBHL	% dBHL	% dBHL		

Fig. 138.1 Case 1. Preoperative audiogram, demonstrating asymmetric sensorineural hearing loss in the right ear.

fork, the Rinne tests were both positive, and the Weber test was midline.

A pretreatment audiogram demonstrated a significant asymmetry of hearing in the right ear at and above 2,000 Hz (▶ Fig. 138.1).

MR imaging of the brain demonstrated a 1.7 x 3.1 x 2.5-cm expansile lesion within the right petrous apex, high in signal on both T1- and T2-weighted images, with remodeling of bone and expansion into the cerebellopontine angle, consistent with cholesterol granuloma (▶ Fig. 138.2).

CT of the petrous temporal bone further detailed the bony architecture of this lesion. The scan demonstrated thinning and displacement of the posterior horizontal portions of the petrous carotid artery, as well as medial bowing and thinning of the petrous apex. Erosive changes were noted along the lateral margin of the porus acusticus, the clivus, and the basisphenoid. A careful review of the coronal images did not favor an infracochlear approach to the petrous apex but did show that a retrofacial (retrolabyrinthine) approach would be possible (▶ Fig. 138.3).

The patient elected to have the lesion surgically treated. He underwent a right retrofacial (infralabyrinthine) approach to the petrous apex, in which the standard landmarks of the posterior semicircular canal, the descending facial nerve, and the jugular bulb were used. The bone over the cystic space was thinned, and a 25-guage needle was used to aspirate dark brown fluid, confirming the cholesterol granuloma. The posterior face of the

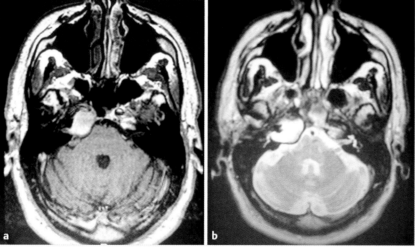

Fig. 138.2 Case 1. Preoperative (a) T1-weighted and (b) T2-weighted axial magnetic resonance images, both showing a high-intensity lesion of the right petrous apex.

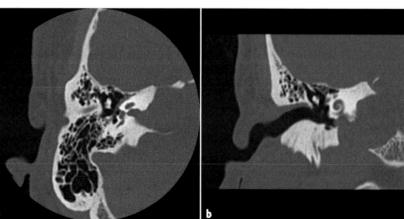

Fig. 138.3 Case 1. Preoperative (a) axial and (b) coronal computed tomographic scans, showing the ascending carotid artery abutting the cochlea.

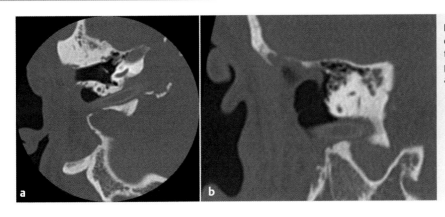

Fig. 138.4 Case 1. Postoperative (a) axial and (b) coronal computed tomographic scans, showing the Silastic (Dow Corning, Midland, MI) drain passing beneath the posterior semicircular canal and into the petrous apex.

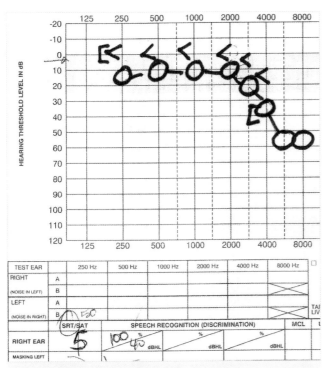

Fig. 138.5 Case 1. Postoperative audiogram, demonstrating modest improvement in hearing.

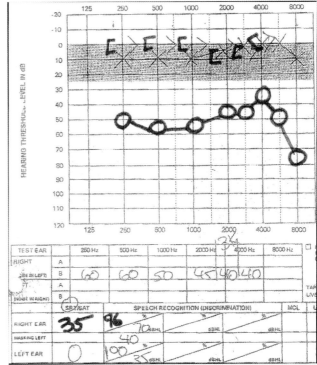

Fig. 138.6 Case 2. Preoperative audiogram, demonstrating right conductive hearing loss.

petrous apex was then opened with graduated diamond burs to a diameter of about 7 mm. This allowed gentle curettage with ringed forceps. Because of the known effacement and displacement of the petrous carotid artery, no attempt was made to strip the lining of the cystic space. A No. 5 Jackson-Pratt drain was placed within the petrous apex and brought out to the mastoid (▶ Fig. 138.4). An audiogram performed 1 month after surgery revealed a slight improvement in hearing at 2,000, 3,000, and 4,000 Hz, with 100% speech discrimination (▶ Fig. 138.5).

138.9.2 Case 2

A 19-year-old woman presented with right facial weakness, hearing loss and fullness in the right ear, dizziness, and right facial pressure/pain of approximately 6 months' duration. Examination revealed a right III/VI facial paresis and bulging in the right epitympanum. No discrete mass was seen. The 512-Hz fork lateralized to the right ear with bone conduction better

than with air conduction on the right side. The remainder of the examination was unremarkable.

An audiogram revealed a conductive hearing loss of 50 dB in the right ear with good word discrimination. The nerve line on the right ear was well preserved. Hearing in the left ear was normal (▶ Fig. 138.6).

CT of the temporal bone revealed an expansile lesion in the right petrous apex with extension toward the IAC and labyrinthine portion of the seventh cranial nerve, with significant bony erosion (▶ Fig. 138.7). MR imaging showed a lesion of the right petrous apex less bright on T1-weighted images and brighter on T2-weighted sequences, supporting the diagnosis of cholesteatoma of the petrous apex (▶ Fig. 138.8).

The patient subsequently moved to South America, and when she returned to New York a year later, she complained of worse hearing and worse facial function. On examination, she had complete (VI/VI) right facial paralysis. A repeat audiogram showed a conductive hearing loss of 60 dB on the right with

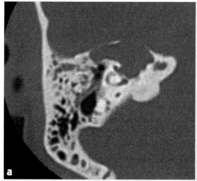
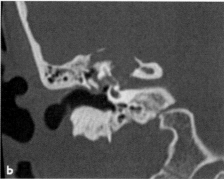

Fig. 138.7 Case 2. Preoperative (a) axial and (b) coronal computed tomographic scans of the right temporal bone, showing an expansile lesion of the right petrous apex.

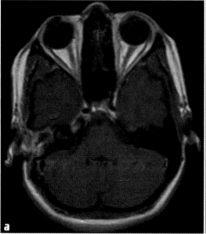
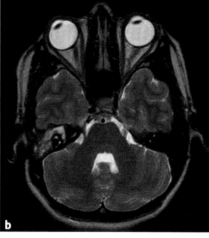

Fig. 138.8 Case 2. Preoperative (a) T1-weighted and (b) T2-weighted axial magnetic resonance images, showing a lesion of the petrous apex brighter on T2 than on T1 sequences, consistent with cholesteatoma.

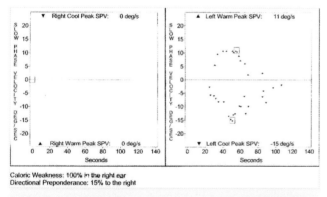

Caloric Weakness: 100% in the right ear
Directional Preponderance: 15% to the right

Fig. 138.9 Case 2. Preoperative bithermal calorics, showing absent responses in the right ear. *SPV*, slow-phase velocity.

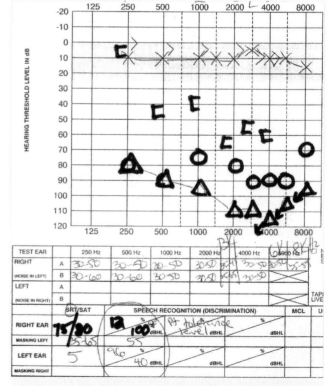

Fig. 138.10 Case 2. Postoperative audiogram, with no serviceable hearing in the right ear.

92% speech discrimination. Electroneurography showed 100% right-sided weakness to bithermal caloric irrigation (▶ Fig. 138.9). Preoperative electroneuronography showed 100% degeneration of the right facial nerve. The patient underwent a right infratemporal fossa and transmastoid dissection of the mass, as well as placement of gold weight in the right upper lid. In an effort to preserve hearing, the labyrinth was kept intact. The cholesteatoma was unroofed above the superior semicircular canal and removed with suction and curettage. The postoperative audiogram showed that little useful hearing remained on the right (▶ Fig. 138.10). The patient was followed conservatively with serial débridement, and the facial nerve slowly improved over a 1-year period, but follow-up MR imaging revealed little change in the overall size of the lesion. Because the hearing was no longer useful, the patient underwent a right labyrinthectomy, dissection of the cholesteatoma, and meatoplasty. Postoperatively, the patient's right facial nerve function recovered to a House-Brackmann grade III/VI.

138.9.3 Case 3

A 46-year-old woman was referred for evaluation of a "suspicious finding" on her CT scan by a general otolaryngologist. This patient had a lifelong history of left ear infections and had undergone two otologic procedures on the left ear in 2005 and 2006, resulting in a canal wall down mastoidectomy defect. She described tinnitus in the left ear as well as infrequent episodes of dizziness, but not vertigo. There were no other significant otologic complaints.

Microscopic examination revealed mild retraction of the right pars flaccida. There was a canal wall down mastoid cavity

on the left with a grafted, blunted drum. No ossicles were visualized on the left, but there was no obvious residual cholesteatoma either. Tuning fork testing at 512 Hz lateralized toward the left, with air conduction greater than bone conduction on the right side but reversed on the left. The facial nerve was normal bilaterally, as were clinical tests of balance.

An audiogram performed on June 5, 2008, revealed a mixed hearing loss in the left ear with good bone reserve and a conductive component of 45 dB, 96% word recognition score (WRS). The hearing on the right was normal at 5 dB, 96% WRS (▶ Fig. 138.11).

Noncontrast CT of the petrous temporal bone done on June 16, 2008 revealed postoperative changes consistent with a canal wall down tympanoplasty and mastoidectomy on the left, as well as an expansile mass in the inferior left petrous apex with osseous remodeling that measured 13 mm in greatest dimension (▶ Fig. 138.12), suggestive of an aneurysm of the petrous carotid artery.

MR imaging and MRA without and with gadolinium enhancement was performed and interpreted with the findings of the previous CT scan. The lesion in the left petrous apex was seen to be distinct from the petrous carotid artery (▶ Fig. 138.13). It

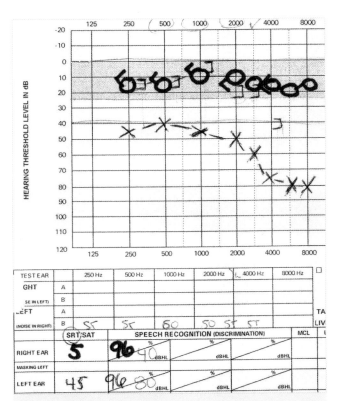

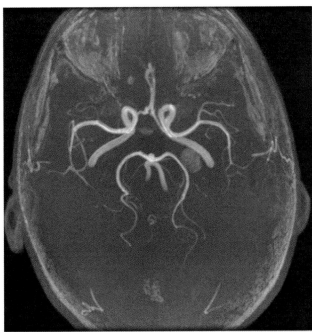

Fig. 138.13 Case 3. Magnetic resonance angiography of the brain. The lesion in the left petrous apex is distinct from the internal carotid artery.

Fig. 138.11 Case 3. Postoperative audiogram (following left canal wall down mastoidectomy).

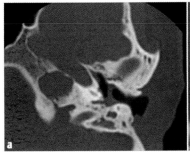
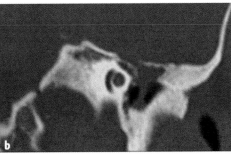

Fig. 138.12 Case 3. (a) Axial and (b) coronal computed tomographic scans of the left temporal bone, illustrating an expansile lesion in the petrous apex.

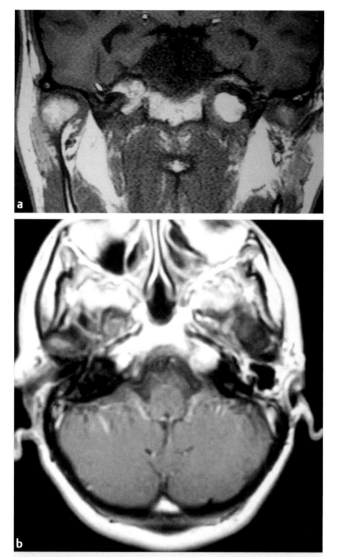

Fig. 138.14 Case 3. T1-weighted (a) coronal and (b) axial magnetic resonance images, showing a hyperintense mass in the inferior aspect of the left petrous apex.

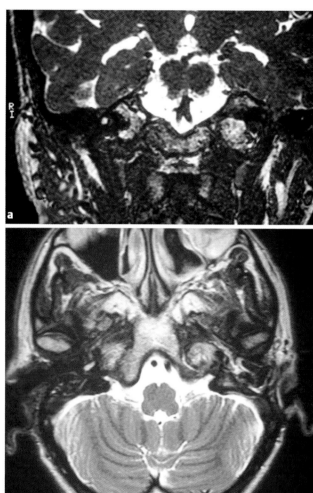

Fig. 138.15 Case 3. T2-weighted (a) coronal and (b) axial magnetic resonance images, showing a heterogeneous mass in the left petrous apex.

was hyperintense on T1-weighted images (▶ Fig. 138.14) and heterogeneous on T2-weighted images (▶ Fig. 138.15), suggesting a cholesterol granuloma. Given the lack of symptoms, the patient is being observed.

138.9.4 Case 4

A 14-year-old girl was evaluated for hearing loss in both ears. The child had a history of recurrent otitis media and prior myringotomy and tube placement at the time of a tonsillectomy and adenoidectomy. The otoscopic examination revealed retracted tympanic membranes, with a whitish mass seen in the posterior–superior quadrants bilaterally. Tuning fork testing at 512 Hz was heard midline, with bone conduction greater than air conduction bilaterally. An audiogram showed bilateral conductive hearing loss, worse on the left side. The speech recognition threshold (SRT) and WRS were 30 dB, 92% on the right and 40 dB, 88% on the left (▶ Fig. 138.16). The child's mother was advised that investigation of the problem was urgently required

with CT of the temporal bones and most likely otologic surgery. Despite frequent phone calls and a telegram, the patient was lost to follow-up for approximately 8 months. At that time, CT of the petrous temporal bones was obtained that demonstrated significant scalloping of the petrous apex and otic capsule, worse on the left. Despite thorough discussion with the child's parent regarding the need for treatment, the patient did not return for care for almost 2 years; at that time, repeat CT revealed worsening of the erosion of both petrous apices with significant scalloping of the otic capsule (▶ Fig. 138.17). The mother finally consented to surgery, and a left tympanoplasty with a canal wall down mastoidectomy approach was performed. Cholesteatoma was found underneath osteitic bone and was exteriorized as much as possible, with no attempt made to remove the matrix. Facial nerve monitoring demonstrated an intact facial nerve, and facial nerve function was normal postoperatively. A follow-up audiogram demonstrated an intact left bone line (▶ Fig. 138.18). Although the patient's mother was advised of the need for right ear surgery, the child has again been lost to follow-up.

138.10 Summary

Although rare in general otolaryngologic practice, lesions of the petrous apex will likely be encountered by the otologist/neurotologist. Most cases are referred, the patient having been seen by one or several other physicians before lesion imaging. Of the large body of possible lesions presented in the preceding text, several are by far more common than all of the others combined, especially cholesterol granuloma and cholesteatoma. Other lesions include mucocele and discrete metastatic disease from several primary tumors.

The history, physical examination, and audiometric and radiologic evaluation of the patient presenting with a lesion of the petrous apex have been reviewed. Above all, the cooperation of a skilled neuroradiologist is essential to help clinch the diagnosis before surgery.

The rare medical and more commonly performed surgical treatments of lesions of the petrous apex have been described. The surgical approach to lesions of the petrous apex is determined by the nature of the complaint, the age and underlying health of the patient, the amount of residual hearing, and the

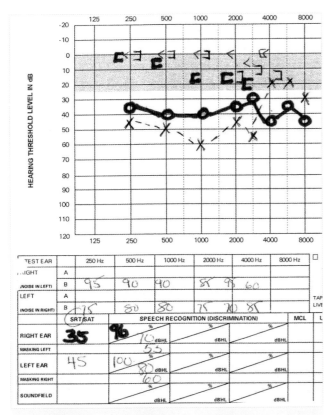

Fig. 138.16 Case 4. Preoperative audiogram, demonstrating bilateral conductive hearing loss.

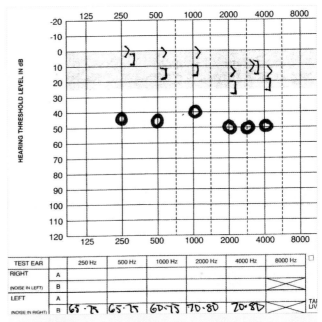

Fig. 138.18 Case 4. Postoperative audiogram, showing intact sensorineural hearing in the left ear.

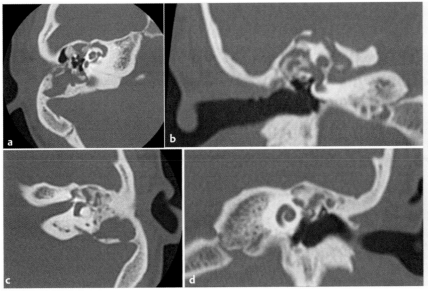

Fig. 138.17 Case 4. Preoperative (a) axial and (b) coronal computed tomographic scans of the right temporal bone, and (c) axial and (d) coronal computed tomographic scans of the left temporal bone, showing erosion of both petrous apices and scalloping of both otic capsules.

anatomical extent of the lesion. Cystic lesions should be drained to a nearby aerated structure. Solid lesions may be excised or rarely treated with stereotactic radiation. The common surgical approaches to lesions of the petrous apex have been reviewed.

Surveillance for lesions of the petrous apex must be planned according to the age of the patient and the nature of the lesion. It is the rare patient who will be "cured" and in whom follow-up will eventually cease. For the majority of patients, the disease process will be rendered less potentially aggressive, whether by medical care, excision, or drainage, so that clinical and radiographic follow-up at regular intervals will determine the future course of treatment.

138.11 Roundsmanship

- Lesions of the petrous apex may be classified as primary or secondary.
- Describe the anatomical boundaries of the petrous apex.
- Cholesterol granuloma is the most common primary lesion of the petrous apex.
- Breast, prostate, lung, and renal cell carcinoma and malignant melanoma are the most common metastatic lesions of the petrous apex.

138.12 Recommended Reading

[1] Chole RA. Petrous apicitis: surgical anatomy. Ann Otol Rhinol Laryngol 1985; 94: 251–257

[2] Curtin HD, Som PM. The petrous apex. Otolaryngol Clin North Am 1995; 28: 473–496

[3] Fisch U. Infratemporal fossa approach to tumours of the temporal bone and base of the skull. J Laryngol Otol 1978; 92: 949–967

[4] Friedman I. Epidermoid granuloma and cholesterol granuloma. Ann Otol Rhinol Laryngol 1959; 58: 57–79

[5] Gradenigo G. Sulla leptomeningite circoscritta e sulla paralisi dell' abducente diodigine otica. G Accad Med Torino 1904; 10: 59

[6] Haberkamp TJ. Surgical anatomy of the transtemporal approaches to the petrous apex. Am J Otol 1997; 18: 501–506

[7] House WF, De la Cruz A, Hitselberger WE. Surgery of the skull base: transcochlear approach to the petrous apex and clivus. Otolaryngol ogy 1978; 86: 770–779

[8] Isaacson B, Kutz JW, Roland PS. Lesions of the petrous apex: diagnosis and management. Otolaryngol Clin North Am 2007; 40: 479–519, viii

[9] Jackler RK, Cho M. A new theory to explain the genesis of petrous apex cholesterol granuloma. Otol Neurotol 2003; 24: 96–106, discussion 106

[10] Linstrom CJ, McLure TC, Gamache FW, Saint-Louis LA. Bilateral cholesterol granulomas of the petrous apices: case report and review. Am J Otol 1989; 10: 393–401

[11] Nager GT. Mesenchymal neoplastic processes. In: Nager GT, Hyams VJ, eds. Pathology of the Ear and Temporal Bone. Baltimore, MD: Williams & Wilkins; 1993:448–482

[12] Sadé J, Teitz A. Cholesterol and cholesteatoma. Acta Otolaryngol 1983; 95: 547–553

Index